ADULT AND PEDIATRIC UROLOGY

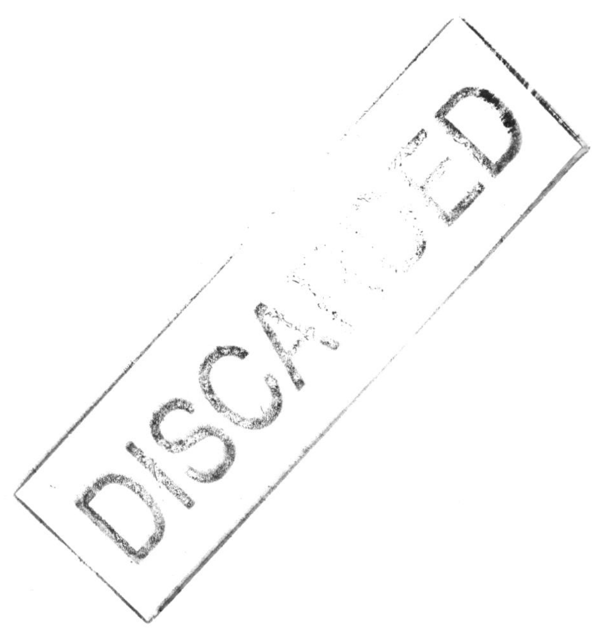

Volume 1

ADULT AND PEDIATRIC UROLOGY

FOURTH EDITION

Editors

Jay Y. Gillenwater, MD

Hovey S. Dabney Professor
Department of Urology
University of Virginia Medical School;
Professor of Urology
University of Virginia Hospital
Charlottesville, Virginia

John T. Grayhack, MD

Professor
Department of Urology
Northwestern University Medical School;
Attending
Department of Urology
Northwestern Memorial Hospital
Chicago, Illinois

Stuart S. Howards, MD

Professor
Departments of Urology and Physiology
University of Virginia
Charlottesville, Virginia

Michael E. Mitchell, MD

Professor
Department of Urology
University of Washington;
Chief
Division of Pediatric Urology
Children's Hospital and Regional Medical Center
Seattle, Washington

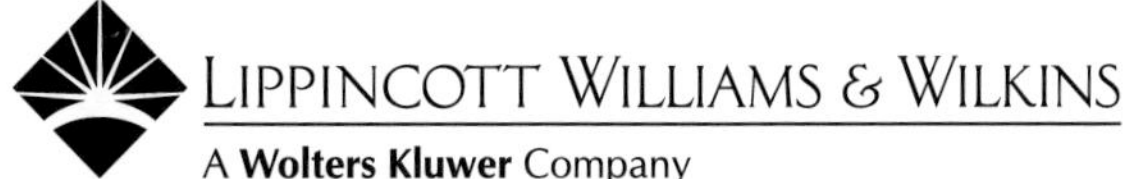
LIPPINCOTT WILLIAMS & WILKINS
A **Wolters Kluwer** Company
Philadelphia • Baltimore • New York • London
Buenos Aires • Hong Kong • Sydney • Tokyo

Acquisitions Editor: Anne M. Sydor
Developmental Editor: Brian Brown and Jenny Kim
Supervising Editor: Mary Ann McLaughlin
Production Editor: Suzanne Kastner
Manufacturing Manager: Colin Warnock
Cover Designer: Mark Lerner
Compositor: Graphic World Inc.
Printer: Courier Westford

530 Walnut Street
Philadelphia, PA 19106 USA
LWW.com

Printed in the USA

Library of Congress Cataloging-in-Publication Data

Adult and pediatric urology / [edited by] Jay Y. Gillenwater . . . [et al.].—4th ed.
p. ; cm.
Includes bibliographical references and index.
ISBN 0-7817-3220-4
1. Genitourinary organs–Diseases. 2. Urology. 3. Pediatric urology. I. Gillenwater, Jay Y. (Jay Young), 1933-
[DNLM: 1. Urologic Diseases. 2. Urologic Diseases—Child. 3. Urologic Diseases—Infant. WJ 100 A2437 2002]
RC871 .A26 2002
616.6—dc21

2001033883

Care has been taken to confirm the accuracy of the information presented and to describe generally accepted practices. However, the authors, editors, and publisher are not responsible for errors or omissions or for any consequences from application of the information in this book and make no warranty, expressed or implied, with respect to the currency, completeness, or accuracy of the contents of the publication. Application of this information in a particular situation remains the professional responsibility of the practitioner.

The authors, editors, and publisher have exerted every effort to ensure that drug selection and dosage set forth in this text are in accordance with current recommendations and practice at the time of publication. However, in view of ongoing research, changes in government regulations, and the constant flow of information relating to drug therapy and drug reactions, the reader is urged to check the package insert for each drug for any change in indications and dosage and for added warnings and precautions. This is particularly important when the recommended agent is a new or infrequently employed drug.

Some drugs and medical devices presented in this publication have Food and Drug Administration (FDA) clearance for limited use in restricted research settings. It is the responsibility of health care providers to ascertain the FDA status of each drug or device planned for use in their clinical practice.

10 9 8 7 6 5 4 3 2 1

CONTENTS

CONTRIBUTING AUTHORS

Mark C. Adams, MD Associate Professor, Department of Urologic Surgery, Department of Pediatrics, Vanderbilt University Medical Center; Division of Pediatric Urology, Vanderbilt Children's Hospital, Nashville, Tennessee

Vaseem Ali, MD, MRCOG Associate Professor, Department of Obstetrics and Gynecology, University of Texas Medical School at Houston, Herman Hospital, Houston, Texas

Beth Andersen, MD Children's Hospital and Regional Medical Center, University of Washington, Seattle, Washington

Jeffrey C. Applewhite, MD Department of Urology, Wake Forest University School of Medicine, Wake Forest University Baptist Medical Center, Winston-Salem, North Carolina

Anthony Atala, MD Associate Professor, Department of Surgery, Harvard Medical School; Associate in Surgery, Department of Urology, Children's Hospital, Boston, Massachusetts

David M. Barrett, MD Clinical Professor, Department of Urology, Tufts University School of Medicine, Boston, Massachusetts; Chief Executive Officer, Lahey Clinic, Burlington, Massachusetts

Georg Bartsch, MD Chief and Professor of Urology, Department of Urology, University of Innsbruck, Innsbruck, Austria

Laurence S. Baskin, MD Chief, Pediatric Urology, Department of Urology, University of California–San Francisco, San Francisco, California

Mark F. Bellinger, MD Clinical Professor, Department of Surgery/Urology, University of Pittsburgh; Attending Physician, Department of Pediatric Urology, Children's Hospital of Pittsburgh, Pittsburgh, Pennsylvania

George S. Benson, MD Medical Officer, Food and Drug Administration, Rockville, Maryland

David A. Bloom, MD Professor of Surgery; Chief of Pediatric Urology, Department of Urology, University of Michigan, Ann Arbor, Michigan

Bernard Bochner, MD Attending Physician, Department of Urology, Memorial Sloan-Kettering Cancer Center, New York, New York

Michel A. Boileau, MD Bend Urology Associates, Bend, Oregon

John W. Brock III, MD Professor, Departments of Urologic Surgery and Pediatrics; Director, Pediatric Urology, Vanderbilt University Medical Center, Nashville, Tennessee

Wade Bushman, MD, PhD Assistant Professor, Department of Urology, Northwestern University Medical School; Consultant, Rehabilitation Institute of Chicago, Chicago, Illinois

Douglas A. Canning, MD Associate Professor, Department of Urology, Hospital of the University of Pennsylvania; Chief, Division of Urology, Children's Hospital of Philadelphia, Philadelphia, Pennsylvania

Michael C. Carr, MD, PhD Assistant Professor, Department of Urology, University of Pennsylvania; Attending Surgeon, Department of Urology, Children's Hospital of Philadelphia, Philadelphia, Pennsylvania

Patrick C. Cartwright, MD Associate Professor, Departments of Surgery and Pediatrics, University of Utah; Attending Surgeon, Division of Pediatric Urology, Primary Children's Medical Center, Salt Lake City, Utah

Marc Cendron, MD, FAAP Associate Professor, Departments of Surgery (Urology) and Pediatrics, Dartmouth Medical School, Hanover, New Hampshire; Director, Pediatric Urology Services, Section of Urology, Dartmouth Hitchcock Medical Center, Lebanon, New Hampshire

Samuel Chacko, DVM, PhD Professor of Pathobiology, Director of Basic Urologic Research, Department of Pathobiology, University of Pennsylvania, University of Pennsylvania Medical Center, Philadelphia, Pennsylvania

Queena Chou, MD, FRCSC Assistant Professor, Department of Obstetrics and Gynecology, University of Western Ontario; Staff Physician, Department of Obstetrics and Gynecology, St. Joseph's Health Care London, London, Ontario, Canada

Peter L. Choyke, MD Professor of Radiology, Department of Radiology, Uniformed Services University of the Health Sciences; Chief of MRI, Department of Radiology, National Institutes of Health, Bethesda, Maryland

Ralph V. Clayman, MD Professor of Urology and Radiology, Co-director, Division of Minimally Invasive Surgery, Department of Surgery and Radiology, Washington University, Barnes-Jewish Hospital, St. Louis, Missouri

J. Quentin Clemens, MD Assistant Professor, Department of Urology, Northwestern University Medical School, Northwestern Memorial Hospital, Chicago, Illinois

Clare E. Close, MD Assistant Professor, Department of Surgery and Pediatrics, University of Nevada School of Medicine, Las Vegas, Nevada

Christopher S. Cooper, MD Assistant Professor, Department of Urology, University of Iowa College of Medicine; Assistant Professor, Department of Urology, Children's Hospital of Iowa, Iowa City, Iowa

Douglas E. Coplen, MD Assistant Professor, Department of Surgery, Division of Urology, Washington University-St. Louis; Director of Pediatric Urology, Division of Pediatric Urology, St. Louis Children's Hospital, St. Louis, Missouri

John M. Corman, MD Assistant Clinical Professor, Department of Urology, University of Washington; Staff Urologist, Section of Urology, Virginia Mason Medical Center, Seattle, Washington

Joseph N. Corriere, Jr., MD Professor of Surgery, Department of Surgery, Division of Urology, The University of Texas, Houston, Texas

Barbara Y. Croft, PhD Program Director, Biomedical Imaging Program, National Cancer Institute, Bethesda, Maryland

Jean B. deKernion, MD Chairman, Department of Urology, UCLA School of Medicine; Attending Urologist, UCLA Medical Center, Los Angeles, California

Michael E. DiSanto, PhD Research Assistant Professor, Division of Urology, University of Pennsylvania School of Medicine, Philadelphia, Pennsylvania

Jack S. Elder, MD Professor of Urology and Pediatrics, Case Western Reserve University; Director of Pediatric Urology, Rainbow Babies & Children's Hospital, Cleveland, Ohio

R. Sherburne Figenshau, MD Assistant Professor, Department of Urologic Surgery, Washington University, St. Louis, Missouri

Stuart M. Flechner, MD Section, Renal Transplantation, Urological Institute and Cleveland Clinic Foundation; Transplant Center, Cleveland Clinic Hospital, Cleveland, Ohio

Indiber S. Gill, MD, MCh Head, Section of Laparoscopic and Minimally Invasive Surgery, Cleveland Clinic Urological Institute, Cleveland Clinic Foundation, Cleveland, Ohio

Jay Y. Gillenwater, MD Hovey S. Dabney Professor, Department of Urology, University of Virginia Medical School; Professor of Urology, University of Virginia Hospital, Charlottesville, Virginia

Meidee Goh, MD, MPH Lecturer, Section of Urology, Department of General Surgery, University of Michigan, Ann Arbor, Michigan

Richard W. Grady, MD Assistant Professor, Department of Urology, The University of Washington Medical Center; Attending, Section of Pediatric Urology, Children's Hospital and Regional Medical Center, Seattle, Washington

John T. Grayhack, MD Professor, Department of Urology, Northwestern University Medical School; Attending, Department of Urology, Northwestern Memorial Hospital, Chicago, Illinois

Kenneth E. Greer, MD Chair and Professor, Department of Dermatology, University of Virginia, Charlottesville, Virginia

Marko Gudziak, MD Department of Urology, Royal Melbourne Hospital, Melbourne, Victoria, Australia

Faruk Hadziselimovic, MD Professor, Department of Pediatrics, University Basel, Basel, Switzerland; Chief, Department of Pediatrics, Kindertagesklinik, Liestal, Switzerland

M. Craig Hall, MD Associate Professor, Director, Urologic Oncology, Department of Urology, Wake Forest University School of Medicine; Staff, Department of Urology, Wake Forest University Baptist Medical Center, Winston-Salem, North Carolina

Terry W. Hensle, MD Professor of Urology, Department of Urology, Columbia University College of Physicians and Surgeons; Director, Pediatric Urology, Children's Hospital of New York, New York, New York

James R. Herman, MD, PhD Assistant Professor, Department of Surgery/Urology, University of Kentucky Chandler Medical Center, Lexington, Kentucky

Stuart S. Howards, MD Professor, Departments of Urology and Physiology, University of Virginia, Charlottesville, Virginia

Robert Huben, MD Associate Professor, Department of Urology, State University of New York at Buffalo; Chief, Urologic Oncology, Roswell Park Cancer Institute, Buffalo, New York

Dale Huff, MD Senior Pathologist, Department of Pathology, The Children's Hospital of Philadelphia, Philadelphia, Pennsylvania

Douglas A. Husmann, MD Professor, Department of Urology, Mayo Clinic, Rochester, Minnesota

Alan D. Jenkins, MD Associate Professor of Urology, Department of Urology, University of Virginia, Charlottesville, Virginia

Judith M. Joyce, MD Associate Chief, Nuclear Medicine, Western Pennsylvania Hospital, Pittsburgh, Pennsylvania

Edward D. Kim, MD Associate Professor, Departments of Urology and Urologic Surgery, The University of Tennessee Graduate School of Medicine, Knoxville, Tennessee

Stephen A. Koff, MD Professor of Surgery, Department of Surgery, The Ohio State University College of Medicine and Public Health; Chief, Section of Pediatric Urology, Children's Hospital, Columbus, Ohio

Stanley J. Kogan, MD Clinical Professor of Urology, Department of Urology, Weil Medical College, New York Medical College, Cornell University; Attending Pediatric Urologist, Department of Urology, New York Hospital, Cornell Medical Center, Westchester Medical Center, New York, New York

Harry P. Koo, MD Associate Professor, Department of Surgery, Virginia Commonwealth University; Director of Pediatric Urology, Department of Surgery, Medical College of Virginia, Richmond, Virginia

James M. Kozlowski, MD, FACS Associate Professor of Urology, Surgery, and Tumor Cell Biology, Chief, Section of Urologic Oncology, Vice Chair, Department of Urology, Northwestern University Medical School, Chicago, Illinois

John N. Krieger, MD Professor, Department of Urology, University of Washington; Chief of Urology, VA Puget Sound Health Care System, Seattle, Washington

Jaime Landman, MD Endourology Fellow, Department of Surgery, Division of Urology, Washington University Medical Center, Barnes-Jewish Hospital, St. Louis, Missouri

Fredrick Leach, MD, PhD Principal Investigator and Senior Staff Urologist, Urologic Oncology Branch, National Cancer Institute, Bethesda, Maryland

Richard A. Leder, MD Associate Clinical Professor of Radiology, Division of Abdominal Imaging, Department of Radiology, Duke University Medical Center, Durham, North Carolina

W. Marston Linehan, MD Chief, Urologic Oncology Branch, National Cancer Institute, Bethesda, Maryland

Marguerite C. Lippert, MD Associate Professor, Department of Urology, University of Virginia Health Science Center, Charlottesville, Virginia

Larry I. Lipshultz, MD Professor, Scott Department of Urology, Chief, Division of Male Reproductive Medicine & Surgery, Baylor College of Medicine, Houston, Texas

Fray F. Marshall, MD Professor and Chairman, Department of Urology, Emory University, Atlanta, Georgia

Jack W. McAninch, MD, MS Professor of Urology, Department of Urology, University of California-San Francisco; Chief of Urology, Department of Urology, San Francisco General Hospital, San Francisco, California

David L. McCullough, MD Professor and Chairman, Department of Urology, Wake Forest University School of Medicine; Chief, Department of Urology, Wake Forest University Baptist Medical Center, Winston-Salem, North Carolina

W. Scott McDougal, MD Walter Kerr, Jr., Professor of Urology, Harvard Medical School; Chief of Urology, Department of Urology, Massachusetts General Hospital, Boston, Massachusetts

Elspeth M. McDougall, MD, FRCSC Professor, Department of Urologic Surgery, Vanderbilt University Medical Center, Nashville, Tennessee

Edward J. McGuire, MD Professor, Department of Urology, The University of Michigan, Ann Arbor, Michigan

Kevin T. McVary, MD, FACS Associate Professor, Department of Urology, Northwestern University Medical School, Chicago, Illinois

Kiarash Michel, MD Clinical Attending, Department of Surgery, Division of Urology, Harbor–UCLA; Attending, Department of Surgery, Division of Urology, Cedars–Sinai Medical Center, Los Angeles, California

Douglas F. Milam, MD Assistant Professor, Department of Urologic Surgery, Vanderbilt University Medical Center, Nashville, Tennessee

Michael E. Mitchell, MD Professor, Department of Urology, University of Washington; Chief, Division of Pediatric Urology, Children's Hospital and Regional Medical Center, Seattle, Washington

James E. Montie, MD Professor of Surgery, Department of Urology; Chairman, Department of Urology, University of Michigan Medical Center, Ann Arbor, Michigan

Khaled H. Mutabagani, MD, PhD Assistant Professor, Department of Physiology, King Abdul Aziz University College; Pediatric Surgeon, Department of Surgery, New Jeddah Clinic Hospital, Jeddah, Saudi Arabia

Charles E. Myers, Jr., MD Professor of Medicine and Urology, University of Virginia School of Medicine, Charlottesville, Virginia

Robert B. Nadler, MD Assistant Professor, Head, Section of Endourology, Laparoscopy, and Stone Disease, Department of Urology, Northwestern University Medical School; Department of Urology, Northwestern Memorial Hospital, Chicago, Illinois

Peter Nichols, MD Professor, Department of Pathology, University of Southern California School of Medicine; Director, Department of Pathology, University of Southern California/Norris Cancer Hospital, Los Angeles, California

Brian E. Nicholson, MD Instructor, Department of Urology, University of Virginia, Charlottesville, Virginia

J. Curtis Nickel, MD, FRCSC Professor, Department of Urology, Queen's University; Staff Urologist, Department of Urology, Kingston General Hospital, Kingston, Ontario, Canada

H. Norman Noe, MD Professor of Urology, Chief Pediatric Urology, University of Tennessee; Professor, Department of Urology, LeBonheur Children's Hospital, St. Jude Children's Hospital, Memphis, Tennessee

Robert O. Northway, MD Chief Resident, Department of Urology, Emory University, Atlanta, Georgia

Andrew C. Novick, MD Chairman, Urological Institute, The Cleveland Clinic Foundation, Cleveland, Ohio

Helen O'Connell, MD, FRACS Senior Academic Associate, Department of Surgery, University of Melbourne; Urologist, Department of Urology, Royal Melbourne Hospital, Melbourne, Victoria, Australia

Robert A. Older, MD Professor of Radiology and Urology, Department of Radiology, University of Virginia Health System, Charlottesville, Virginia

David K. Ornstein, MD Assistant Professor, Department of Surgery/Urology, University of North Carolina, Chapel Hill, North Carolina

Joseph Ortenberg, MD Professor, Departments of Urology and Pediatrics, Louisiana State University; Director of Urologic Education, Department of Surgery, Children's Hospital, New Orleans, Louisiana

Jayashree Parekh, MD Assistant Professor, Department of Radiology, University of Virginia Health System, Charlottesville, Virginia

J. Chadwick Plaire, MD Children's Urology Associates, Las Vegas, Nevada

Sepp Poisel, MD Associate Professor, Senior Physician, Department of Anatomy & Histology, Müllerstrasse, Innsbruck, Austria

Glenn M. Preminger, MD Professor of Urologic Surgery, Department of Surgery; Director, Comprehensive Kidney Stone Center, Department of Surgery, Duke University Medical Center, Durham, North Carolina

Derek Raghavan, MD, PhD Professor of Medicine and Urology, Department of Medical Oncology, University of Southern California, Keck School of Medicine; Chief, Division of Oncology, University of Southern California, Norris Comprehensive Cancer Center, Los Angeles, California

Parvati Ramchandani, MD Professor, Department of Radiology, Division of Genito-Urinary Radiology, University of Pennsylvania Medical Center, Philadelphia, Pennsylvania

Martin I. Resnick, MD Lester Persky Professor and Chairman, Department of Urology, Case Western Reserve University School of Medicine; Director, Department of Urology, University Hospitals of Cleveland, Cleveland, Ohio

Michael L. Ritchey, MD C.R. Bard, Inc., Edward J. McGuire Distinguished Chair in Urology, Professor of Surgery and Pediatrics, Director, Division of Urology, University of Texas–Houston Medical School, Houston, Texas

Chad W.M. Ritenour, MD Assistant Professor, Department of Urology, Emory University, Atlanta, Georgia

Ronald Ross, MD Professor, Department of Preventive Medicine, University of Southern California, Keck School of Medicine; Deputy Director, University of Southern California/Norris Comprehensive Cancer Center, Los Angeles, California

Randall G. Rowland, MD, PhD Professor and Glenn Chair of Urology, Department of Surgery/Urology, University of Kentucky; Chief, Division of Surgery/Urology, University of Kentucky Medical Center, Lexington, Kentucky

Susan E. Rowling, MD Assistant Professor, Department of Radiology, University of Pennsylvania, Presbyterian Medical Center, University of Pennsylvania Health System, Philadelphia, Pennsylvania

Grannum R. Sant, MD C.M. Whitney Professor and Chairman, Department of Urology, Tufts University School of Medicine; Urologist-in-Chief, New England Medical Center, Boston, Massachusetts

Richard A. Santucci, MD Assistant Professor, Department of Urology, Wayne State University School of Medicine; Chief, Department of Urology, Detroit Receiving Hospital, Detroit, Michigan

Anthony J. Schaeffer, MD Professor and Chair, Department of Urology, Northwestern University Medical School; Northwestern Memorial Hospital, Chicago, Illinois

Hal C. Scherz, MD Assistant Clinical Professor, Department of Urology, Emory University; Chief Pediatric Urology, Georgia Urology, Children's Healthcare of Atlanta, Atlanta, Georgia

Francis X. Schneck, MD Clinical Assistant Professor, Department of Urology, University of Pittsburgh; Children's Hospital, Pittsburgh, Pennsylvania

J. Bayne Selby, Jr., MD Professor of Radiology, Department of Radiology, Medical University of South Carolina; Co-Director, Vascular/International Radiology, Medical University Hospital, Charleston, South Carolina

Donald G. Skinner, MD Professor and Chairman, Department of Urology, University of Southern California, Norris Comprehensive Cancer Center, Los Angeles, California

Steven J. Skoog, MD Professor, Department of Surgery and Pediatrics, Oregon Health Sciences University; Director, Pediatric Urology, Doernbecher Children's Hospital, Portland, Oregon

Joseph A. Smith, Jr., MD Professor and Chairman, Department of Urologic Surgery, Vanderbilt University, Nashville, Tennessee

Warren Snodgrass, MD Associate Professor, Department of Urology, Pediatric Section, University of Texas Southwestern Medical Center at Dallas; Physician, Department of Urology, Pediatric Section, Children's Medical Center, Dallas, Texas

Brent W. Snow, MD Professor of Surgery and Pediatrics (Pediatric Urology), Division of Urology (Pediatric Urology), University of Utah Hospital/ Primary Children's Medical Center, Salt Lake City, Utah

Howard M. Snyder III, MD Professor of Surgery in Urology, Department of Surgery, University of Pennsylvania School of Medicine; Associate Director, Pediatric Urology, Children's Hospital of Philadelphia, Philadelphia, Pennsylvania

R. Ernest Sosa, MD Associate Professor of Urology, Weill Medical College; Associate Attending Physician, Department of Urology, New York–Presbyterian Hospital, New York, New York

J. Patrick Spirnak, MD Professor, Department of Urology, Case Western Reserve University; Director, Department of Urology, Metrohealth Medical Center, Cleveland, Ohio

William D. Steers, MD Jay Y. Gillenwater Professor and Chair, Department of Urology, University of Virginia, Charlottesville, Virginia

John P. Stein, MD Assistant Professor, Department of Urology, University of Southern California; Assistant Professor, Department of Urology, Norris Comprehensive Cancer Center, Los Angeles, California

William R. Strand, MD Associate Professor, Department of Urology, University of Texas Southwestern Medical Center at Dallas; Associate Professor, Department of Pediatric Urology, Children's Medical Center, Dallas, Texas

H. Strasser, MD Associate Professor, Department of Urology, University of Innsbruck, Innsbruck, Austria

Stevan B. Streem, MD Head, Section of Stone Disease and Endourology, Urological Institute, The Cleveland Clinic Foundation, Cleveland, Ohio

Gerald Sufrin, MD Professor and Chair, Department of Urology, University at Buffalo; Director, Department of Urology, Kaleida Health, Buffalo, New York

Charles D. Teates, MD Professor, Department of Radiology, University of Virginia Health System, Charlottesville, Virginia

Dan Theodorescu, MD Paul Mellon Chair in Urologic Oncology, Professor of Urology, Associate Professor of Molecular Physiology, University of Virginia, Charlottesville, Virginia

E. Darracott Vaughan, Jr., MD Professor of Urology, Department of Urology, Weill-Cornell University Medical Center; Chairman, Urologist-in-Chief, Department of Urology, New York-Presbyterian Hospital, New York, New York

Suzie N. Venn, MS, FRCS Senior Lecturer and Consultant, Institute of Urology, UCLH, London and St. Richard's Hospital, Chichester, United Kingdom

R. Dixon Walker, MD Professor, Department of Surgery and Pediatrics, University of Florida College of Medicine; Chief, Pediatric Urology, Shands Children's Hospital, Gainesville, Florida

McClellan M. Walther, MD Senior Investigator, National Institutes of Health, National Cancer Institute, Urologic Oncology Branch, Bethesda, Maryland

George D. Webster, MB, FRCS Professor of Urologic Surgery, Department of Surgery, Division of Urologic Surgery, Duke University Medical Center, Durham, North Carolina

Alan J. Wein, MD Professor and Chair, Division of Urology, University of Pennsylvania School of Medicine; Chief of Urology, University of Pennsylvania Health System, Philadelphia, Pennsylvania

Jeffrey P. Weiss, MD Clinical Adjunct Assistant Professor of Urology, Weill/ Cornell University Medical College, New York, New York

Robert M. Weiss, MD Professor and Chief, Section of Urology, Department of Surgery, Yale University School of Medicine; Attending and Head of Urology, Department of Surgery, Yale–New Haven Hospital, New Haven, Connecticut

B. Dale Wilson, MD Department of Dermatology, Roswell Park Cancer Institute, Buffalo, New York

J. Stuart Wolf, Jr., MD Assistant Professor, Department of Urology, University of Michigan, Ann Arbor, Michigan

Arthur W. Wyker, Jr., MD Clinical Professor of Urology, University of Virginia Health Sciences Center, Charlottesville, Virginia

Norman Zambrano, MD Instructor, Department of Urology, Catholic University of Chile, Santiago, Chile; Chief, Urology Service, Sotero Del Rio Hospital, Puente Alto, Santiago, Chile

Stephen A. Zderic, MD Associate Professor of Urology, Department of Surgery, University of Pennsylvania School of Medicine; Associate Professor, Pediatric Urology, Division of Pediatric Urology, Children's Hospital of Philadelphia, Philadelphia, Pennsylvania

PREFACE

Adult and Pediatric Urology has been revised after only five years because of the rapid introduction of new information about urologic disease. The text, as in previous editions, has been written to serve as a practical reference for residents and practicing urologists. We have attempted to make the text readable and user-friendly and to provide a comprehensive description of the subject, rather than an encyclopedic dissertation. The authors have tried to assimilate all the important information about each subject and to evaluate it in order to reach the best conclusion or consensus. Practicing urologists and residents alike have commented favorably on the content and presentation of the material in the previous editions. We believe the new edition continues to present excellent coverage of the topics in a clear and concise manner.

The fourth edition consists of three volumes. The first two volumes cover adult urology. Most chapters have been completely rewritten. The coverage on prostatic diseases has been expanded; completely new chapters on anatomy, diagnostic imaging, surgical management of calculus disease, bladder cancer, diseases of the retroperitoneum, alternative therapies, office urology, AIDS, and spinal cord injury have been included. The third volume, under the very capable leadership of Michael Mitchell, covers pediatric urology. We have arranged the pediatric volume by pathophysiology and treatment modality to facilitate easy clinical referencing. The sections on hypospadias, exstrophy, laparoscopic surgery, and reconstruction techniques have been radically changed to include current techniques in state-of-the-art technologies.

With this new edition, we are pleased to present a companion CD-ROM that contains all of the text, figures, and tables found within the three volumes. In addition, we have used the power of electronic publishing to provide material that cannot be presented in print by including video clips of surgical procedures. These video clips concentrate on aspects of the procedures that cannot be conveyed adequately in still images. We hope the adage that a picture is worth a thousand words will be proven true and that these videos will provide a valuable resource for our readers. We also hope that the portable and searchable nature of the CD-ROM will further enhance the user-friendly nature of the fourth edition of *Adult and Pediatric Urology.*

No text is any better than its authors, editors, and publishers. Working with Jack Grayhack, Stuart Howards, and Michael Mitchell has been both pleasant and intellectually stimulating. Each of the editors has worked closely with his authors to ensure the best coverage possible for a wide array of subjects. The authors enthusiastically responded and produced scholarly, critical, and informative chapters that are easy to read. Anne Sydor, Brian Brown, and Jenny Kim of Lippincott Williams & Wilkins have been invaluable partners in this endeavor. I know of no other group who could have transformed so much manuscript into a completed textbook in such a compressed time frame. We believe the result to be an up-to-date, thorough, and eminently readable textbook of general urology.

For the editors
Jay Y. Gillenwater, MD

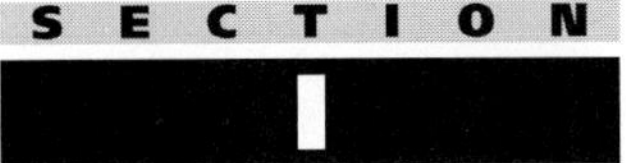

ADULT UROLOGY

1

SURGICAL ANATOMY OF THE GENITOURINARY SYSTEM

GEORG BARTSCH
H. STRASSER
SEPP POISEL

ABDOMINAL WALL

Superficial Abdominal Muscles

Figure 1.1 shows an external view of the anterior abdominal wall.

Lateral Group

External oblique muscle
Internal oblique muscle
Transversus abdominis

External Oblique Muscle

The external oblique muscle arises by eight slips from the external surfaces of the fifth through twelfth ribs. Its five upper slips interdigitate with the origins of serratus anterior, its three lower slips with the origins of latissimus dorsi. Its posterior fibers descend almost vertically to the iliac crest, and the adjacent anterior fibers pass obliquely forward and medially in their downward course.

About a fingerwidth from the lateral border of the rectus abdominis muscle, the external oblique fibers terminate in an aponeurosis. The aponeuroses of both external oblique muscles unite at the *linea alba,* where they attach to the pubic symphysis and the adjacent anterior surfaces of the superior pubic ramus.

The portion of the aponeurosis between the anterosuperior iliac spine and the pubic tubercle is thickened to form a tendinous band, the *inguinal ligament.* Just above and medial to the inguinal ligament is the *superficial inguinal ring,* bounded by the medial crus, lateral crus, and intercrural fibers. The latter are reinforcing fibers of the external oblique aponeurosis.

Internal Oblique Muscle

The internal oblique muscle originates from the deep layer of the lumbodorsal fascia, from the intermediate line of the iliac crest, from the anterorsuperior iliac spine, and from the lateral portion of the inguinal ligament. Its muscular fibers fan out broadly to their sites of insertion. The uppermost posterior fibers are inserted into the inferior borders of the

G. Bartsch and H. Strasser: Department of Urology, University of Innsbruck, Innsbruck, Austria.
S. Poisel: Department of Anatomy & Histology, Müllerstrasse, Innsbruck, Austria.

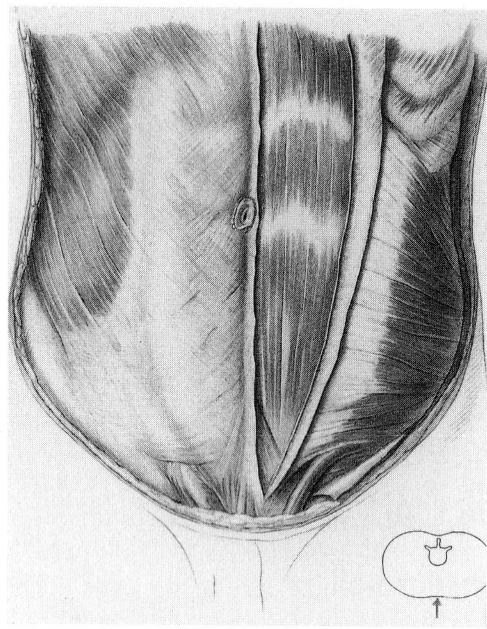

FIGURE 1.1. External view of the anterior abdominal wall. The anterior rectus sheath and external oblique muscle on the left side have been removed.

last three ribs. The intermediate fibers form an aponeurosis at the lateral border of the rectus abdominis muscle. This aponeurosis splits into an anterior and a posterior layer that pass around the rectus abdominis to form the rectus sheath before uniting with the contralateral aponeurotic fibers at the linea alba. The posterior rectus sheath terminates about three fingerwidths below the umbilicus at the *arcuate line.* The lower fibers of the internal oblique are continued onto the spermatic cord in males to form the *cremaster muscle.* In females, a few muscle fibers accompany the round ligament of the uterus within the inguinal canal.

Transversus Abdominis

The deepest of the three lateral abdominal muscles, the transversus abdominis, arises by six slips from the internal aspects of the seventh through twelfth costal cartilages, interdigitating with the slips of the costal part of the diaphragm.

Fibers also arise from the deep layer of the lumbodorsal fascia, the inner lip of the iliac crest, and the lateral part of the inguinal ligament. The transversus abdominis fibers pass in a horizontal direction and terminate in an aponeurosis along the laterally convex *semilunar line.* Above the arcuate line, this aponeurosis forms the posterior layer of the rectus sheath. Below the arcuate line, it unites with the anterior lamina of the internal oblique aponeurosis and helps form the anterior layer of the rectus sheath. Each transversus aponeurosis fuses with its counterpart at the linea alba.

Medial Group

Rectus abdominis
Pyramidalis

Rectus Abdominis

The rectus abdominis muscle arises by three slips from the external surfaces of the fifth through seventh costal cartilages, from the xiphoid process, and from ligaments in this region. The muscle tapers in its straight, descending course, especially in its lower one-fourth, and inserts by a short, strong tendon into the pubic crest. The fiber mass of the rectus abdominis is interrupted by three or more transverse tendinous bands, the *tendinous intersections,* which are intimately attached to the anterior rectus sheath.

Rectus Sheath. The rectus sheath that envelops the rectus abdominis muscle is formed by the aponeuroses of the three lateral abdominal muscles. It is divided into an *anterior layer* (anterior rectus sheath) and a *posterior layer* (posterior rectus sheath). As noted, the aponeurosis of the internal oblique muscle splits into two parts that pass behind and in front of the rectus abdominis to reach the linea alba. Above the umbilicus, or more precisely above the arcuate line, the anterior wall of the sheath consists of the external oblique aponeurosis and, deep to it, the anterior layer of the internal oblique aponeurosis. Below the level of the arcuate line, the aponeuroses of all three abdominal muscles pass in front of the rectus abdominis muscle.

The posterior layer of the internal oblique aponeurosis is reinforced above the arcuate line by the aponeurosis of the transversus abdominis. Below the arcuate line, the posterior wall of the rectus sheath is formed entirely by the transversalis fascia.

Pyramidalis

The pyramidalis muscle arises broadly from the superior pubic ramus, anterior to the insertion of the rectus abdominis. It passes upward, gradually narrowing as it ascends, to insert on the linea alba. The pyramidalis is absent in approximately 20% of the population.

Lumbar Trigone and Variations

The lumbar trigone is a triangular interval bounded by the iliac crest, the posterior border of the external oblique muscle, and the anterior (lateral) border of the latissimus dorsi. The shape and size of the triangle are highly variable depending on the degree of overlap of its bordering muscles and their tendons of origin. If the musculotendinous plates overlap sufficiently, a lumbar trigone is not formed (Fig. 1.2A).

If the muscles are less prominently developed, a lumbar triangle is present. The floor of the lumbar trigone may be

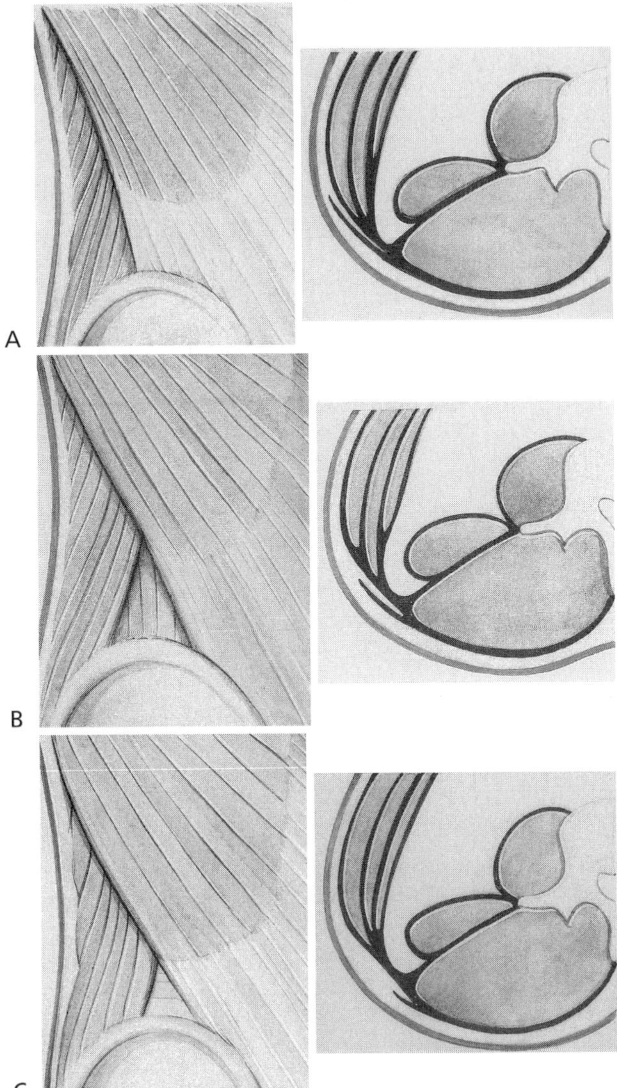

FIGURE 1.2. Variations of the lumbar trigone. **A:** Lumbodorsal fascia (superficial layer) overlies the external oblique muscle. **B:** Lumbodorsal fascia overlaps the internal oblique muscle. **C:** Lumbodorsal fascia forms a triangle (lumbar trigone) with the external oblique muscle.

formed by the internal oblique, if this muscle is well developed (Fig. 1.2B), or by the deep layer of the lumbodorsal fascia (Fig. 1.2C). In the latter case, the lumbodorsal fascia is the only solid structural component of the posterior abdominal wall in the lumbar trigone.

Latissimus Dorsi

The *vertebral part* of the latissimus dorsi muscle arises from the spinous processes of the fifth through twelfth thoracic vertebrae and its *iliac part* from the lumbodorsal fascia and the posterior iliac crest. The *costal part* of the latissimus dorsi muscle arises from the external surfaces of the tenth through twelfth ribs, and a variable *scapular part* originates from the inferior angle of the scapula. The fibers of the latissimus dorsi pass laterally upward with varying degrees of obliquity to the humerus, where they insert into the crest of the lesser tubercle (Figs. 1.3 and 1.4).

Serratus Anterior

The serratus anterior muscle overlies the lateral chest wall and arises by nine and sometimes ten slips from the outer surfaces of the upper nine (or eight) ribs. It is inserted along the entire medial border of the scapula. Its tripartite insertion consists of a *superior part* to the superior angle of the scapula, an *intermediate part* to the medial scapular margin, and an *inferior part* to the inferior angle of the scapula.

Intercostal Muscles

The intercostal muscles partially occupy the intercostal spaces and are composed of an internal and an external layer.

The *external intercostal muscles* run forward from the costal tubercle to the margin of the rib cartilage. The external intercostals become membranous between the costal cartilages, each continuing forward to the septum as the *external intercostal membrane.* The external intercostal fibers run obliquely downward, passing laterally downward in

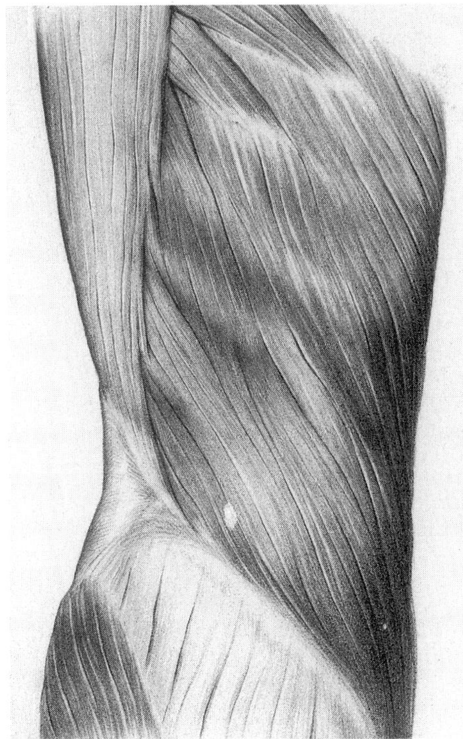

FIGURE 1.3. External view of the lateral abdominal wall.

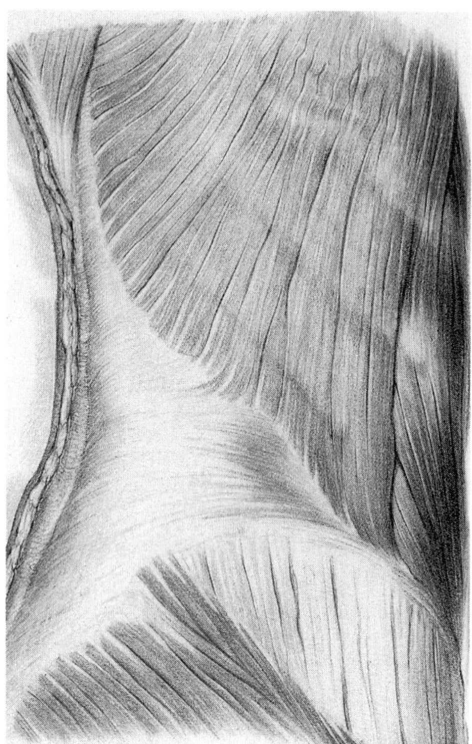

FIGURE 1.4. External view of the posterolateral abdominal wall, inferior portion.

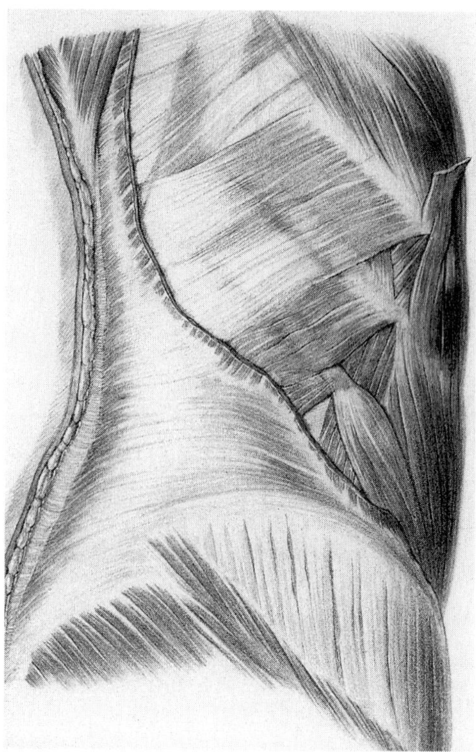

FIGURE 1.5. External view of the posterolateral abdominal wall, inferior portion. The latissimus dorsi has been removed to show the origins of the external oblique muscle.

their posterior portion and medially downward in their anterior portion.

The *internal intercostal muscles* extend obliquely forward and upward from the costal angle to the sternum. The last two internal intercostal muscles are often fused with the internal oblique muscle, showing no apparent boundary. In the intercostal space between the costal angle and vertebral column, each internal intercostal muscle is replaced by an *internal intercostal membrane.*

Serratus Posterior Inferior

The serratus posterior inferior muscle arises from the superficial layer of the lumbodorsal fascia at the level of the lower two thoracic vertebrae and the upper two lumbar vertebrae (Fig. 1.5). It runs obliquely upward and laterally to attach by four slips to the inferior margins of the lower four ribs, somewhat lateral to their costal angles.

Diaphragm

The diaphragm forms a musculotendinous partition between the abdominal and thoracic cavities (Fig. 1.6). Its central tendinous portion is termed the *central tendon,* and its muscular portion is divisible into a *sternal part,* a *costal part,* and a *lumbar part.*

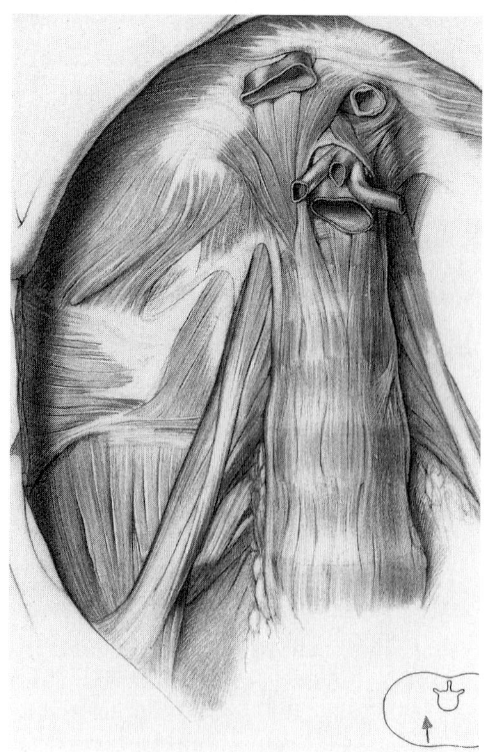

FIGURE 1.6. Internal view of the posterosuperior abdominal wall.

Lumbar Part

The lumbar part of the diaphragm arises by a *medial crus* and a *lateral crus.* A portion of the medial crus is sometimes split off to form an intermediate crus. The *right medial crus* arises from the anterior surfaces of the bodies of the first through fourth lumbar vertebrae; the *left medial crus* arises from the bodies of the first through third lumbar vertebrae. Both medial crura form the *aortic aperture* (aortic hiatus), which is bordered by the median arcuate ligament.

The *right medial crus* consists of three muscular bundles, the first arising from the lumbar vertebrae and merging directly with the central tendon. The second arises from the median arcuate ligament and forms the right border of the *esophageal aperture* (esophageal hiatus) of the diaphragm. The third muscular bundle, located posterior to the second, also originates from the median arcuate ligament and forms the left border of the esophageal aperture.

The *lateral crus* arises from the two tendinous arches of the medial and lateral arcuate ligaments. The medial arcuate ligament (medial lumbocostal arch or psoas arcade) extends from the lateral surface of the first (second) lumbar vertebral body to the first (second) costal process, passing over the origins of the psoas major muscle. The lateral arcuate ligament (lateral lumbocostal arch or quadratus arcade) extends from the costal process to the tip of the twelfth rib, passing over the quadratus lumborum muscle. The muscle fibers run steeply upward from both tendinous arches to the central tendon.

Costal Part

The costal part of the diaphragm arises from the inner surfaces of the cartilages of the lower six ribs, interdigitating with the transversus abdominis. The muscle fibers arch to their insertion at the anterolateral border of the central tendon.

Sternal Part

The sternal part, the smallest part, of the diaphragm arises by one or more small slips from the internal surface of the xiphoid process and from the posterior layer of the rectus sheath. The muscle fibers pass almost transversely to the anterior border of the central tendon.

Deep Abdominal Muscles

Psoas major
Quadratus lumborum

Psoas Major

The superficial part of the psoas major arises from the lateral surfaces of the twelfth thoracic vertebra and the first four lumbar vertebrae, and its deep part from the first through fifth costal processes. It unites with the fibers of the iliacus muscle and, enveloped by the iliac fascia, inserts into the lesser trochanter of the femur as the *iliopsoas muscle.*

The *psoas minor* is a variant present in fewer than 50% of individuals. It arises from the twelfth thoracic and first lumbar vertebrae and is attached to the iliac fascia and, via the fascia, to the iliopubic eminence.

Iliacus

The iliacus muscle arises from the iliac fossa and inserts conjointly with psoas major into the lesser trochanter of the femur. Their composite, the iliopsoas, passes through the *lacuna musculorum* (muscular compartment) beneath the inguinal ligament to reach the thigh.

Quadratus Lumborum

The quadratus lumborum is a flat muscle that lies adjacent to the vertebral column and stretches between the twelfth rib and iliac crest. It consists of two parts that cannot be completely separated from each other: a posterior part arising from the iliac crest and iliolumbar ligament and inserting into the costal processes of the first through third (or fourth) lumbar vertebrae and twelfth rib, and an anterior part passing from the costal processes of the lower three or four lumbar vertebrae to the last rib.

Pelvic Floor

The pelvic floor constitutes the posterior inferior boundary of the abdominal cavity (Fig. 1.7). It consists of the *pelvic diaphragm* and the *urogenital diaphragm.*

Pelvic Diaphragm

The pelvic diaphragm is composed of the *levator ani* and *coccygeus* muscles.

The *levator ani* muscle group consists of the puborectalis prerectal fibers, pubococcygeus, and iliococcygeus, which in some individuals are bounded superiorly by the sacrococcygeus and rectococcygeus muscles. The levator ani arises from the pubic bone lateral to the symphysis, from the tendinous arch of the levator ani (part of the obturator fascia), and from the ischial spine.

The most medial fibers of the puborectalis muscles form the *levator crura,* which bound the *levator hiatus* (genital hiatus). The prerectal fibers are attached to the perineum and separate the urogenital hiatus from the anal hiatus. The levator hiatus is traversed by the urethra in males and by the urethra and vagina in females. The rectum leaves the true pelvis behind the prerectal fibers. The pubococcygeus and iliococcygeus muscles are attached to the coccyx and anococcygeal ligament.

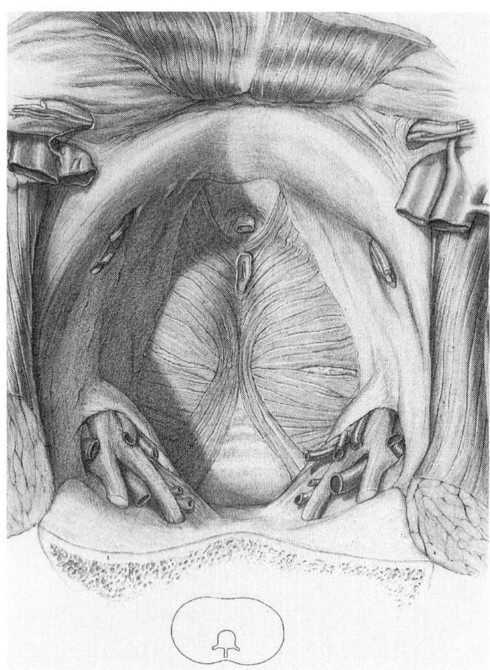

FIGURE 1.7. Internal view of the inferior abdominal wall (pelvic floor).

The *coccygeus* muscle passes from the ischial spine to the coccyx and completes the pelvic diaphragm posteriorly.

Striated Urethral Sphincter (Rhabdosphincter)

The rhabdosphincter and the transverse perineal ligament close the levator hiatus inferiorly. Contrary to standard descriptions, the muscle fibers of the rhabdosphincter are arranged in a loop-shaped fashion on the ventral and lateral aspects of the membranous urethra of the male and the caudal two-thirds of the female urethra. On gross anatomic and histologic examination, comparatively strong smooth muscular and connective tissue can be found dorsal to the membranous urethra (i.e., in the region of the perineal body). Both ends of the omega-shaped sphincter insert at the perineal body. The sphincter loop is continuous with muscle bundles that run along the anterior and lateral aspects of the prostate in the male and extend cranially to the bladder neck. Thus the rhabdosphincter of the urethra does not form a complete collar around the urethra. It should rather be described as a muscular coat ventral and lateral to the membranous urethra and the prostate of the male and the caudal two-thirds of the female urethra, the core of which is the omega-shaped loop around the urethra. Furthermore, the rhabdosphincter is separated from the ventral portions of the levator ani muscle by a sheet of connective tissue. Neither in anatomic dissections nor in serial histologic sections can any evidence of the classic muscular "urogenital diaphragm" be found. The transverse perineal ligament is traversed by the urethra and the rhabdosphincter.

RETROPERITONEAL SPACE

Anatomy

Definition, Boundaries, and Contents

The *retroperitoneal space* is the space between the posterior parietal peritoneum and the posterior abdominal wall. It is bounded superiorly by the diaphragm, and it blends inferiorly with the connective-tissue stratum of the subperitoneal space.

The lateral boundaries of the retroperitoneal space are imprecisely defined. They are essentially formed by the close apposition of the posterior parietal peritoneum to the transversalis fascia on the inner aspect of the lateral abdominal muscles, the thin subserous connective-tissue layer forming a virtual boundary in that region.

The contents of the retroperitoneal space can be described as having either a primary or a secondary retroperitoneal location. Portions of the duodenum, pancreas, and ascending and descending colon reach the retroperitoneum secondarily. Primary retroperitoneal structures are the kidneys and renal pelves, ureters, adrenal glands, and large nerves and vessels (Fig. 1.8).

Kidneys

Position. The kidneys are paired viscera that flank the vertebral column in the retroperitoneal space. Externally, the kidney presents a *medial border,* a *lateral border,* an *anterior surface,* a *posterior surface,* an *upper pole,* and a *lower pole.* The medial border presents a deep fissure, the *renal hilum,* which leads into the *renal sinus.* The upper pole of the kidney is more rounded than the lower pole because of its relation to the adrenal gland.

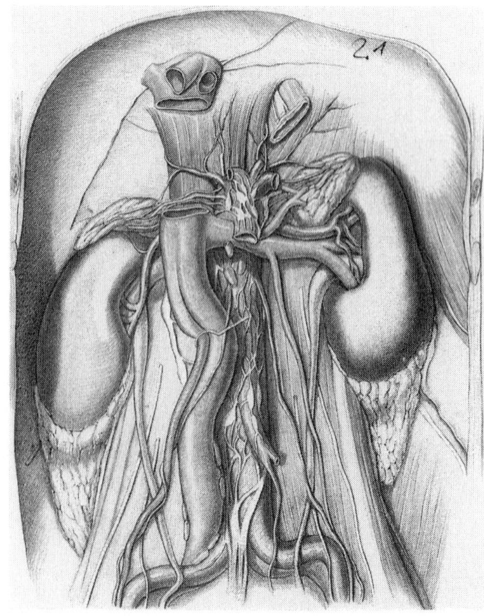

FIGURE 1.8. Topography of the organs, vessels, and nerves of the retroperitoneal space and posterior abdominal wall.

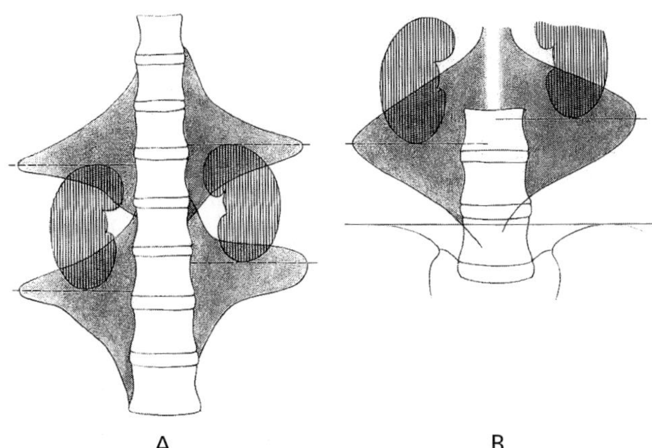

FIGURE 1.9. Range of variation in the levels of the renal poles. **A:** Position of the renal poles in relation to the lumbar spine. **B:** Position of the lower renal pole in relation to the iliac crest. The shaded areas indicate the range of variation.

The terms of orientation for the kidney are somewhat imprecise because the organ is oriented at an angle to the cardinal planes. The anterior surface of the kidney is angled posterolaterally from the frontal plane, so the renal hilum normally is directed anteromedially. The long axes of both kidneys are convergent superiorly, so the upper poles of the kidneys are separated by a smaller distance (7 to 8 cm) than the lower poles (11 to 15 cm).

The level of the kidneys in relation to the vertebral column is subject to marked individual variations. Renal position also depends on individual body posture and the phases of respiration. Changes in renal position are more common and pronounced in children than in adults.

The right kidney in adults usually lies somewhat lower than the left kidney. The upper pole of the right kidney typically occupies a level between the body of the twelfth thoracic vertebra and the upper third of the first lumbar vertebra. The upper pole of the left kidney generally is higher than the right upper pole by half the height of a vertebral body. The lower pole of the right kidney usually is at the level of the third lumbar vertebra, and the lower pole of the left kidney occupies a correspondingly higher position (Fig. 1.9).

The relation of the lower pole of the kidney to the highest point of the iliac crest is subject to the same individual variations. The right lower pole is approximately 3 cm above the iliac crest, on average, and the left lower pole is approximately 1 cm higher (Fig. 1.9).

Relations. The kidneys are embedded in the perirenal fat capsule, which is separated from the outer, pararenal fat by Gerota's fascia. The relations of the anterior surface of the kidney are shown in Figs. 1.10 and 1.11.

The posterior relations of the kidney are virtually identical on the right and left sides (Fig. 1.12). The cranial half of the posterior renal surface is in contact with the diaphragm. Their area of contact depends on the renal level and therefore is usually greater on the left side than on the right. The kidney apposes to the lateral crus of the lumbar part of the diaphragm. Between the lumbar and costal parts of the diaphragm is a variable amuscular interval, the lumbocostal trigone, which constitutes a site of least resistance. In this area, only the thin diaphragmatic fasciae separate the kidney and its fat capsule from the pleural cavity.

The caudal half of the posterior surface of the kidney is related to the quadratus lumborum muscle and the deep

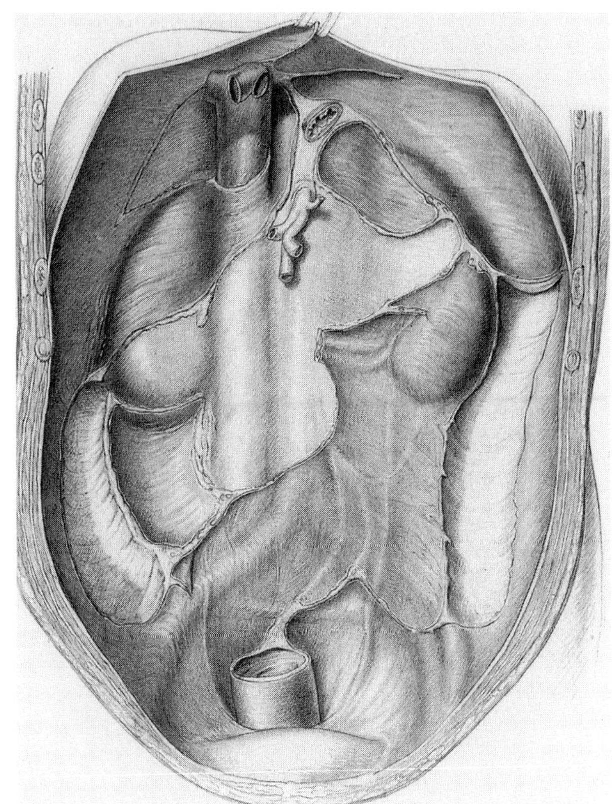

FIGURE 1.10. Relation of the kidneys to the parietal peritoneum and mesenteric roots.

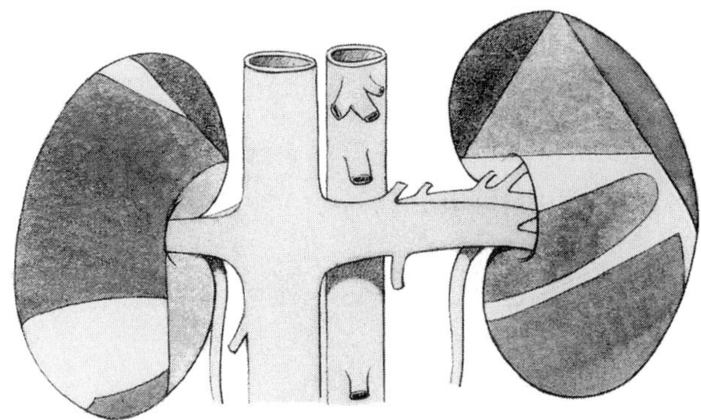

FIGURE 1.11. Contact areas of the kidneys, anterior aspect.

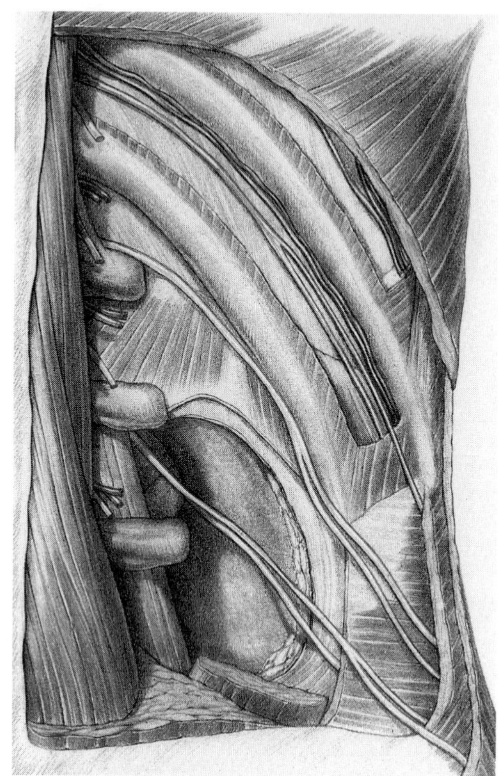

FIGURE 1.12. Posterior relations of the right kidney.

lumbodorsal fascia. The subcostal, iliohypogastric, and ilioinguinal nerves descend obliquely in a medial-to-lateral direction between the kidney and posterior abdominal wall.

The posterior part of the medial border of the kidney lies on the psoas major muscle. With a normal renal position, the twelfth rib passes obliquely downward and laterally to cross the upper third of the posterior renal surface. Between the twelfth rib and kidney are the diaphragm and the costodiaphragmatic recess of the pleural cavity. Attention must be given to the inferior reflection of the pleura in retroperitoneal approaches to the kidney that include a rib resection.

Capsules. Each kidney is enveloped by three capsules (Fig. 1.13): the fibrous capsule (capsule proper), the perirenal fat capsule, and Gerota's fascia (renal fascia, Gerota's capsule). The innermost *fibrous capsule* closely invests the renal parenchyma and is easily separated from the healthy kidney.

Surrounding the fibrous capsule is the *perirenal fat capsule,* which develops postnatally and is fully developed by puberty. The perirenal fat is connected to the inner fibrous capsule and the outer Gerota's fascia by loose connective tissue, which creates a mobile plane. The fat capsule is less well developed on the anterior surface of the kidney than posteriorly, and it envelops the kidney and adrenal gland. Composed of structural fat, the perirenal fat capsule has the primary function of keeping the kidney in place.

The outermost renal covering is *Gerota's fascia,* which forms a "sac" enclosing the kidney, adrenal gland, and perirenal fat capsule. Gerota's fascia is functionally and structurally distinct from the fascia that envelops the muscles and is more like the connective-tissue fascia that invests the organs in the true pelvis.

Gerota's fascia consists of two layers commonly termed the *prerenal (anterior)* and *retrorenal (posterior) fascia.* The fascial layers are fused approximately two fingerwidths lateral to the lateral renal border and above the adrenal gland. Gerota's fascia is also attached superiorly to the fascia of the diaphragm. The two layers of Gerota's fascia are separated below the kidney to allow passage of the ureter and blood

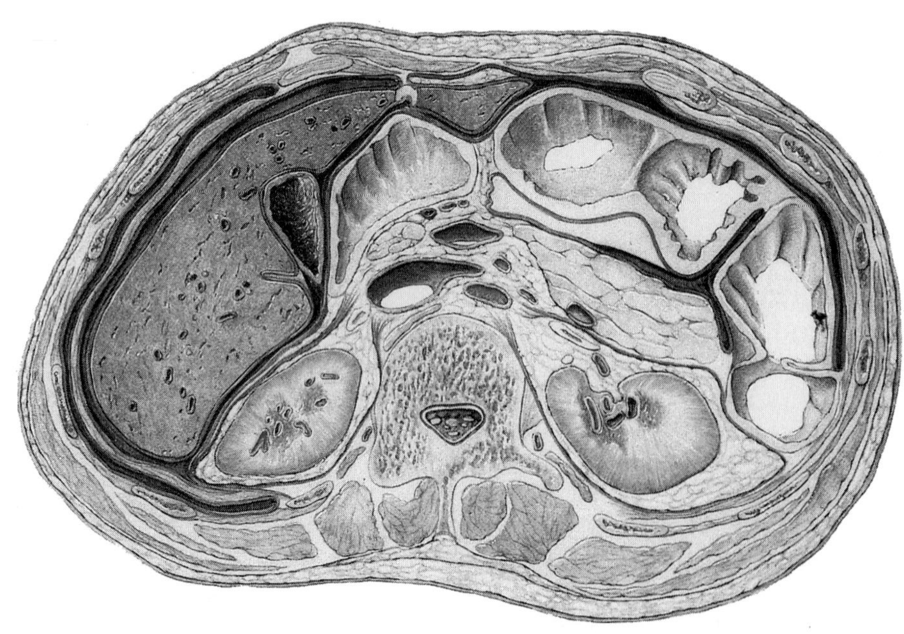

FIGURE 1.13. The transverse section through the abdomen at the level of the first lumbar vertebra (L1).

vessels. The prerenal and retrorenal layers fuse medially with the connective tissue surrounding the major blood vessels and nerves of the retroperitoneal space. The retrorenal fascia is firmly adherent to the muscular fascia of the posterior abdominal wall.

Lateral to the saclike Gerota's fascia is the *pararenal fat,* which differs from the perirenal fat capsule in that it is not composed of structural fat, so its volume is subject to marked individual and nutrition-dependent variations.

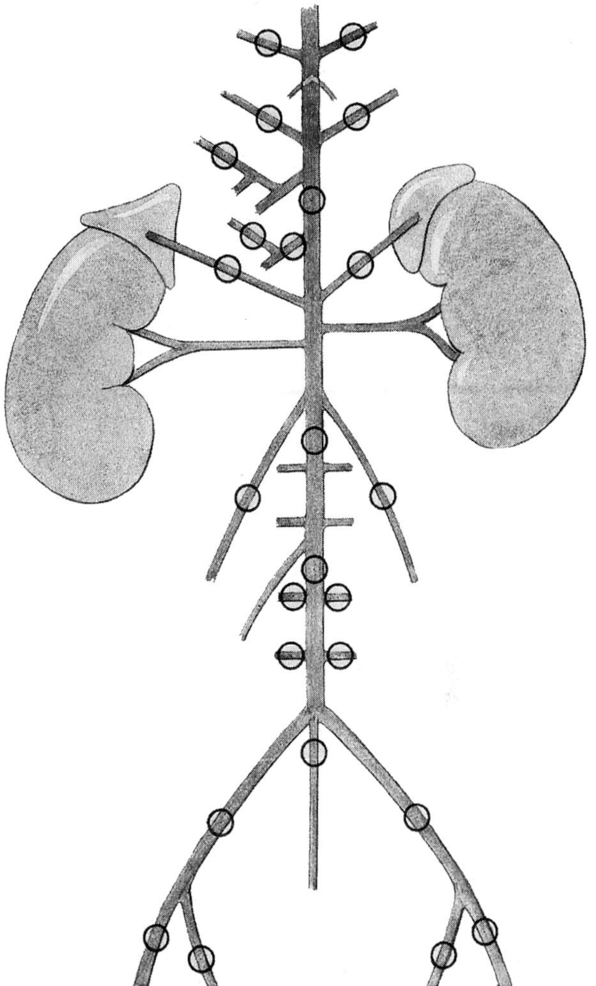

FIGURE 1.14. Schematic diagram of the abdominal aorta and kidneys. *Circles* indicate the potential origins of accessory (or aberrant) renal arteries.

Renal Vessels

Arteries. Normally, each kidney receives its blood supply from a single renal artery. Both renal arteries spring from the lateral aspect of the abdominal aorta, the right artery usually arising at a slightly lower level than the left. The origin of the renal arteries is usually situated below that of the superior mesenteric artery, between the inferior third of the first lumbar vertebra and the middle third of the second lumbar vertebra.

The right renal artery runs obliquely downward and laterally to the hilum of the kidney, passing behind the inferior vena cava. The accompanying renal vein is usually anterior to and above the artery, but in approximately 30% of cases, the artery is in front of the vein (Fig. 1.15). Anterior to the right renal hilum and vessels is the descending portion of the duodenum.

The left renal artery is shorter than the right and usually passes to the renal hilum above and partially behind the left renal vein. The hilum and renal vessels are covered anteriorly by the body of the pancreas and the splenic vessels.

The renal arteries divide at a variable distance from the hilum into two (57%) or three (43%) main branches (anterior, posterior, and inferior) that supply corresponding portions of the renal parenchyma. The branching of the renal arteries does not follow any consistent pattern in terms of right–left or gender distribution.

Variations in the number, course, and origin of the renal artery are common. In approximately 40% of cases, the kidney is found to have an atypical arterial supply. The presence of accessory or aberrant renal arteries is especially common. An "accessory" artery is a supernumerary artery that supplies the kidney as a separate vessel; "aberrant" arteries enter the renal parenchyma outside the hilum, generally at the upper or lower pole. Thus an accessory artery may or may not be aberrant. An aberrant artery may arise from the renal artery itself. Possible variations of the renal arteries are illustrated in Figs. 1.14 through 1.17.

Veins. The renal veins are interconnected by numerous anastomoses in the renal parenchyma and renal sinus, a pattern consistent with the general tendency for the venous system to form plexuses. The trunk of the renal vein is usually formed in the hilum by the convergence of two (53%) or three (34%) main tributaries that pass in front of the renal pelvis. A small tributary passing behind the renal pelvis occurs in approximately one-third of patients.

Outside the renal sinus, the veins usually are anterior to the renal arteries. The left renal vein commonly opens into the inferior vena cava at a higher level than the right renal vein. With a normally positioned inferior vena cava, the left renal vein is substantially longer (6 to 11 cm) than the right (2 to 4 cm). The right renal vein runs a straight, direct course from the hilum to the inferior vena cava; the left vein runs medially forward and passes in front of the aorta, just below the origin of the superior mesenteric artery, before entering the inferior vena cava. Phylogenetically, the left renal vein originates as part of the cardinal venous system and consequently receives the left suprarenal and testicular (or ovarian) veins.

Lymphatics

The intrarenal lymph vessels of the kidney accompany the arteries to the renal sinus and present in the hilum as

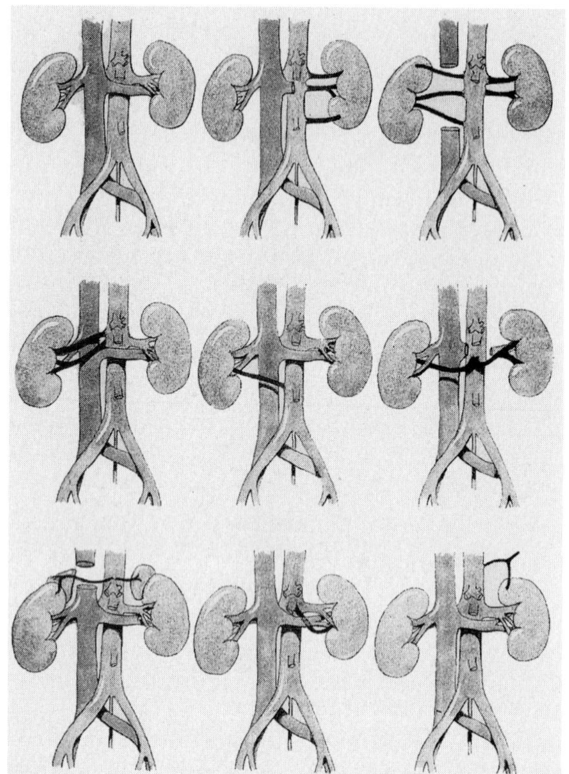

FIGURE 1.15. Typical patterns of aberrant and accessory renal arteries.

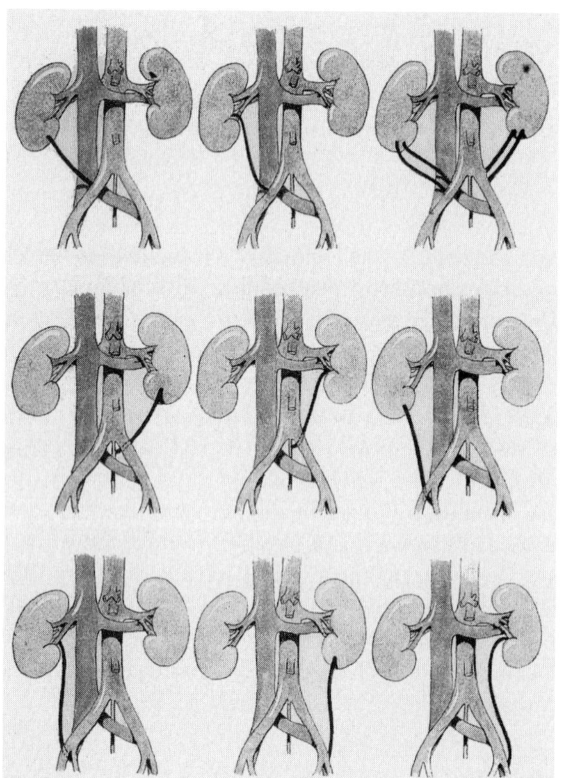

FIGURE 1.16. Typical patterns of aberrant and accessory renal arteries.

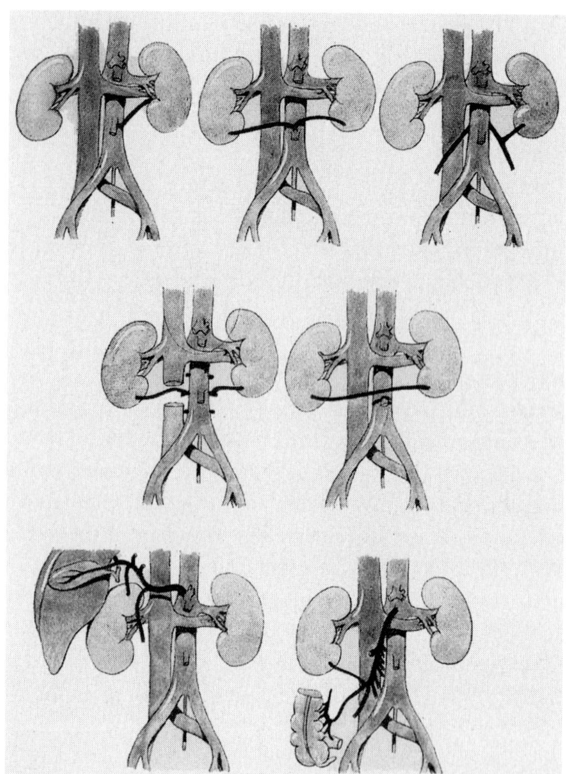

FIGURE 1.17. Typical patterns of aberrant and accessory renal arteries.

prevascular, retrovascular, and intervascular bundles. Regional lymph nodes encountered on the right side are the right lumbar (postcaval) lymph nodes and the intermediate nodes and rarely the preaortic nodes. The renal lymphatics on the left side drain into the left lumbar lymph nodes (lateral aortic and preaortic nodes) (Fig. 1.18).

The lymph vessels draining the renal capsules pass to the lumbar lymph nodes separately from the lymph vessels of the renal parenchyma. A few lymph vessels from the renal capsule pass through the diaphragm and end in the intercostal nodes. Anastomoses have been described between the lymph vessels of the renal capsules and those of the liver, colon, cecum, and uterine tube.

Renal Nerve Supply

The kidneys derive their nerve supply from the renal plexus, which is formed by sympathetic and parasympathetic fibers from the celiac plexus and abdominal aortic plexus, as well as direct fibers from the sympathetic trunk (lumbar part). The renal plexus accompanies the renal arteries to the hilum. Autonomic nerve fibers can be identified along the arteries as far as the efferent vessels of the renal glomeruli.

Renal Pelvis

The *renal pelvis* is a hollow muscular organ that forms the initial segment of the excretory portion of the urinary tract. The tension of the muscular wall of the renal pelvis varies

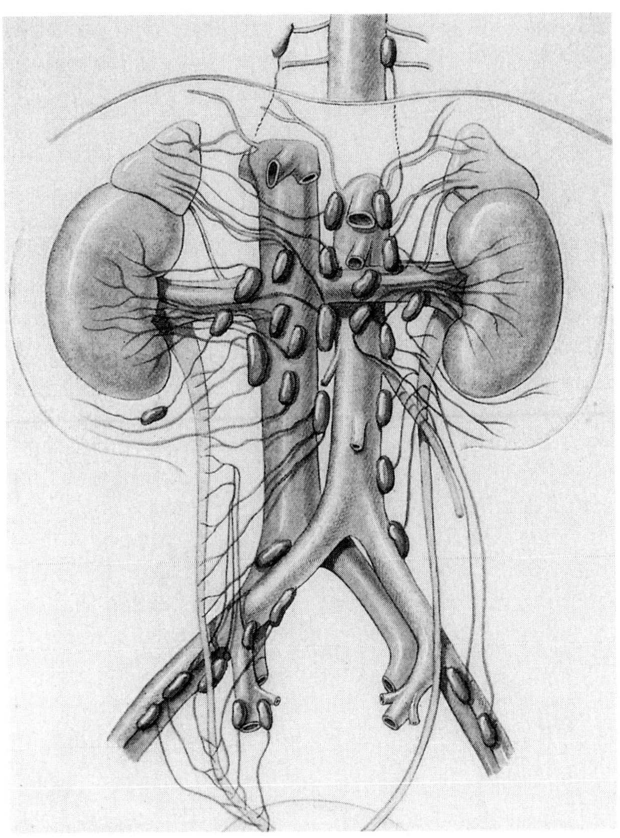

FIGURE 1.18. Lymph nodes and lymphatic vessels of the retroperitoneal space.

with its momentary functional state, so the shape of the renal pelvis also varies.

The renal pelvis begins with 7 to 13 *minor calices* at the renal papillae. The minor calices generally unite to form two or three *major calices* that make up the true renal pelvis (dendritic type). In some cases, all of the minor calices may open directly into the renal pelvis, which then exhibits an ampulelike dilation (ampullary type of pelvis). Forms intermediate between these extremes are common. At the time of operation, the renal pelvis is easily accessible at the hilum through a posterior approach, except for the rare cases in which all of the pelvis is contained within the renal sinus. The only structures that cross the posterior aspect of the renal pelvis are the main posterior branch of the renal artery and the variable posterior branch of the renal vein.

The renal pelvis derives its arterial supply (Fig. 1.8) from one or more branches of the renal artery and is drained by the renal vein. Lymphatic drainage (Fig. 1.18) is to the lumbar lymph nodes. The nerves of the renal pelvis are derived from the renal plexus.

Ureter

The renal pelvis becomes continuous with the ureter below the hilum, with no distinct ureteropelvic boundary. Their junction is at the level of the second or third lumbar vertebra.

The ureter is considered to consist of an *abdominal (proximal) part* and a *pelvic distal part* whose junction occurs at the point where the ureter is crossed by the iliac vessels.

The *abdominal (proximal) part* of the ureter passes downward and slightly medially from the renal pelvis on the fascia of the psoas major, encased within a sheath of fibrofatty tissue. The lateral distance of the ureter from the costal processes of the lumbar vertebrae is variable. In infancy, the proximal part of the ureter is tortuous and may even exhibit proximal kinks that disappear by approximately 1 year of age.

The topographic relations of the ureters to anterior structures are different on the right and left sides because of the asymmetric development of the abdominal viscera. At its origin, the *right ureter* is overlapped by the descending part of the duodenum. In its descent, it is crossed anteriorly by the right colic artery and ileocolic artery, which pass below the secondary parietal peritoneum (originally the ascending mesocolon) to the cecum and ascending colon. The right ureter passes below the testicular or ovarian vessels in its retroperitoneal course. Just before entering the true pelvis, the right ureter is crossed by the root of the mesentery, giving it an indirect relation to the terminal segment of the ileum. A mobile cecum and a transversely oriented appendix also may relate anteriorly to the right ureter.

The initial part of the *left ureter* descends lateral and posterior to the superior duodenal fold, which conveys the inferior mesenteric vein to the splenic vein. As it descends further, the left ureter is crossed by the branches of the inferior mesenteric artery (left colic artery and sigmoid arteries), which lie below the secondary parietal peritoneum (originally the descending mesocolon). The left ureter, like the right, is crossed at varying levels by the testicular or ovarian vessels. Just before entering the true pelvis, the left ureter is crossed by the attachment of the sigmoid mesocolon and can be found at this level within the *intersigmoid recess.*

The right ureter is usually adherent to the peritoneum and must be separated from it during surgery. The left ureter has no firm attachments to the secondary parietal peritoneum, and only the portion in the intersigmoid recess is directly apposed to the peritoneum.

Vessels and Nerves of the Ureter. The connective tissue surrounding the ureter (the adventitia) is permeated by an *arterial anastomotic network* (Fig. 1.8) composed basically of longitudinal vessels interconnected by transverse anastomoses. This periureteral arterial plexus is supplied by all arteries that have a close topographic relation to the ureter. The proximal part of the ureter is consistently supplied by one or two ureteral branches from the renal artery, from the testicular or ovarian artery, and occasionally by direct branches from the abdominal aorta. At the junction of the abdominal and pelvic parts of the ureter, the plexus is supplied by branches of the iliac vessels (common iliac, external or internal iliac).

In surgical procedures on the kidney or renal pelvis, care must be taken not to injure the ureteral branches of the renal artery. These branches provide the essential blood supply to the proximal part of the ureter, and their caliber and connections with the periureteral plexus give them the capacity to supply the entire proximal part of the ureter.

Vascular plexuses in the muscular and submucous coats of the ureter receive blood from the adventitial plexus and contribute to the ureteral blood supply.

The *veins* draining the proximal part of the ureter essentially follow the course of the arteries. The venous drainage is directed toward the renal veins and the testicular or ovarian veins.

The *lymph vessels* draining the proximal part of the ureter (Fig. 1.18) start at networks of lymph capillaries in the muscular wall and adventitia. They pass from the proximal ureter to the lumbar lymph nodes, on the right side draining into the lateral caval and precaval nodes and on the left into the lateral aortic and preaortic nodes. Lymphatics draining the lower portion of the proximal ureter are distributed to the common iliac nodes. Connections generally are present between these two drainage pathways.

The abdominal part of the ureter derives its *nerve supply* from the renal plexus superiorly and from the abdominal aortic plexus inferiorly. The adventitia of the ureter contains a dense network of nerve fibers that receive branches from the plexus surrounding the testicular or ovarian artery.

Adrenal Gland

The paired adrenal glands (Fig. 1.8) are set on the upper pole and anteromedial surface of the corresponding kidney. They are surrounded by the perirenal fat capsule and Gerota's fascia. Because of the close relation of the adrenal gland to the kidney and the confining renal fascial sac, adrenal tumors can produce a distortion of the renal outline.

The right adrenal gland has the approximate shape of a pyramid whose base rests on the upper pole of the right kidney. The left adrenal gland is semilunar in shape and apposes to the upper part of the medial border of the left kidney. It usually extends to the renal hilum and is in contact with the renal vessels.

The posterior surface of the *right adrenal gland* is in contact with the diaphragm, and its inferior surface is related to the kidney. The anterosuperior surface of the gland is related to the bare area of the liver. Its anterior surface is behind the inferior vena cava medially, and the inferior part of its anterior surface is covered by parietal peritoneum.

The *left adrenal gland,* like the right, is only partially covered by peritoneum, which invests the upper half of its anterior surface. Thus part of the gland projects into the omental bursa and may relate topographically to the abdominal part of the esophagus. The anteroinferior surface of the left adrenal gland is in contact with the body of the pancreas and the splenic vessels. The lateral part of the posterior surface of the gland apposes to the kidney, and the medial part is in contact with the left crus of the diaphragm.

Vessels and Nerves of the Adrenal Gland. Normally, at least three arteries contribute to the *arterial blood supply* of the adrenal gland (Fig. 1.8). These arteries are the superior, middle, and inferior suprarenal arteries, which arise from the inferior phrenic artery, abdominal aorta, and renal artery, respectively.

The superior suprarenal artery normally does not supply the gland as a single vessel (Fig. 1.8) but divides into 3 to 30 branches before entering the gland. Multiple superior suprarenal arteries also may occur. The middle suprarenal artery arises from the abdominal aorta at a variable level but always above the renal artery. The vessel may be absent or multiple (Fig. 1.8). The inferior suprarenal artery enters the undersurface of the adrenal gland by several branches that may arise separately from the renal artery or from accessory or aberrant vessels.

The *venous drainage* of the adrenal gland is generally handled by a single vessel, the suprarenal vein, which leaves the glandular tissue at the anterior surface of the adrenal gland. The right suprarenal vein takes a short, direct, transverse course to the inferior vena cava. The left suprarenal vein passes over the inferior part of the anterior surface of the gland and terminates at the left renal vein.

The *lymph vessels* (Fig. 1.18) from the adrenal cortex accompany the inferior phrenic and middle suprarenal arteries, and those from the adrenal medulla accompany the suprarenal vein. They terminate at the lumbar lymph nodes.

The *nerves* enter the posterior and medial aspects of the adrenal gland. The parasympathetic and sympathetic nerve fibers that form the *adrenal plexus* originate from the celiac plexus and the splanchnic nerves. Direct fibers from the sympathetic trunk can contribute to the formation of the adrenal plexus.

Major Vessels and Nerves of the Retroperitoneal Space

Abdominal Aorta. The descending aorta enters the retroperitoneal space through the aortic aperture in the diaphragm (Fig. 1.8). The thoracic duct traverses the aperture behind the aorta, and the aorta is occasionally accompanied by a splanchnic nerve.

The aorta usually enters the abdominal cavity on the median plane but deviates toward the left side as it descends further, apposed to the upper four lumbar vertebrae and intervertebral discs. It ends at the level of the fourth lumbar vertebra by dividing into its terminal branches—the common iliac arteries and the median sacral artery.

The inferior vena cava ascends to the right and slightly in front of the aorta. The left lumbar veins course between the vertebral column and aorta in a space that also contains the postaortic lymph nodes. The abdominal aorta is covered anteriorly by the autonomic aortic plexus (celiac, superior and inferior mesenteric) with corresponding ganglia and by the preaortic lymph nodes. Directly lateral to the aorta are the lateral aortic lymph nodes.

As the abdominal aorta descends, it passes behind the body of the pancreas, the left renal vein, and the horizontal (inferior) portion of the duodenum. Below the mesenteric root, the abdominal aorta is easily accessible to a transperitoneal surgical approach.

The branches of the abdominal aorta may be paired or unpaired, and the branches in both groups can be classified as visceral or parietal.

The unpaired visceral branches are as follows:

1. The celiac trunk, arising within the aortic aperture at the level of the twelfth thoracic vertebra
2. The superior mesenteric artery, arising at the level of the first lumbar vertebra
3. The inferior mesenteric artery, arising at the level of the third lumbar vertebra

The paired visceral branches are as follows:

1. The middle suprarenal arteries, arising at the level of the first lumbar vertebra
2. The renal arteries, usually arising at the same level from the aorta just below the suprarenal arteries
3. The testicular or ovarian arteries, arising at a variable level from the anterolateral aspect of the abdominal aorta and usually at different levels on the right and left sides

The unpaired parietal branch of the abdominal aorta is one of its terminal branches, the median sacral artery.

The paired parietal branches are as follows:

1. The inferior phrenic arteries, arising in the aortic aperture as the first branch of the abdominal aorta
2. Four pairs of lumbar arteries, arising from the back of the aorta at the levels of the first through fourth lumbar vertebral bodies

Inferior Vena Cava. The inferior vena cava (Fig. 1.8) is formed by the union of the two common iliac veins approximately one fingerwidth below and to the right of the aortic bifurcation. The lower part of the inferior vena cava is overlapped anteriorly by the right common iliac artery and relates posteriorly to the body of the fifth lumbar vertebra.

The inferior vena cava ascends on the right side of the aorta and parallel to it until reaching the level of the lower pole of the right kidney, where it diverges slightly to the right from the abdominal aorta and travels in a groove on the posterior surface of the liver. The inferior vena cava enters the thoracic cavity through the vena cava foramen in the diaphragm (at the level of Th 10) and immediately opens into the right atrium of the heart. It is accompanied through the diaphragm by the right phrenicoabdominal branch of the phrenic nerve.

The anterior surface of the inferior vena cava is covered in its lower portion by peritoneum (primary parietal peritoneum) up to the level of the mesenteric root. As it ascends, the inferior vena cava loses its peritoneal covering (secondary retroperitoneal structure) and is apposed to the duodenum and pancreas (Fig. 1.10). Ascending further in the posterior wall of the epiploic foramen, the vena cava is again covered with peritoneum and is adherent to the bare area of the liver in the groove for the inferior vena cava.

The inferior vena cava has both parietal and visceral tributaries. The parietal tributaries are as follows:

1. The common iliac veins
2. The median sacral vein, which follows the course of the homonymous artery and may empty into the left common iliac vein
3. The lumbar veins, whose arrangement corresponds to that of the homonymous arteries
4. The inferior phrenic veins, which enter the inferior vena cava just before it pierces the diaphragm

The visceral tributaries are as follows:

1. The right testicular or ovarian vein, which opens into the inferior vena cava just below the termination of the right renal vein
2. The renal veins (discussed in connection with the kidney)
3. The right suprarenal vein
4. The hepatic veins, usually three in number, which generally enter the inferior vena cava in their course through the hepatic groove for the inferior vena cava

Variations of the inferior vena cava are common and usually result from developmental anomalies (Fig. 1.19). The retroperitoneal venous system develops from three paired, longitudinally oriented parallel channels: the caudal cardinal vein, supracardinal vein, and subcardinal vein, which are continuous caudally with the sacrocardinal vein. Further differentiation of the venous system is characterized by a progressive asymmetry in favor of the right side, with anastomoses between the right and left cardinal veins assuming key importance.

The development of the vena caval system is shown in Fig. 1.19. It can be seen that the caudal cardinal veins largely disappear, whereas the supracardinal veins persist in part as the azygos and hemiazygos veins. Simply stated, the subcardinal veins develop into the inferior vena cava on the right side and into the suprarenal and testicular or ovarian veins on the left side.

Embryonic development of the inferior vena cava may be disrupted, arrested, or misdirected at any stage by extrinsic or intrinsic factors that are not yet fully understood. Each primarily formed cardinal vein (except for the lower portion of the caudal cardinal vein) may persist wholly or in part during definitive development, giving rise to such variants as

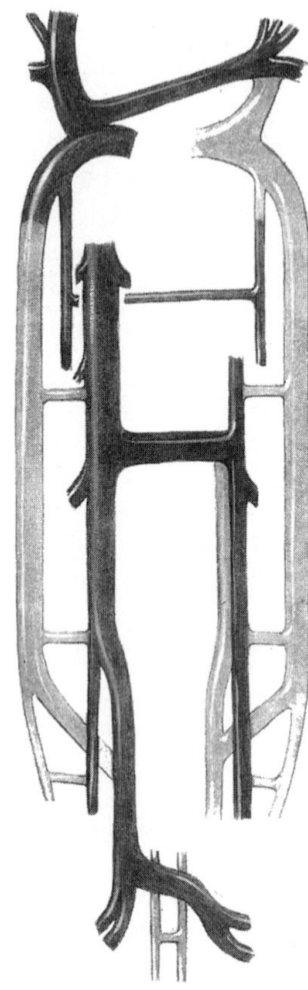

FIGURE 1.19. Development of the vena caval system. Vessels that do not persist are colored light gray.

a *double inferior vena cava* (2.2%) or *left inferior vena cava* (0.2%). All abnormal configurations of the inferior vena caval system are based on the persistence or anomalous involution of embryonic vascular channels.

Lymph Vessels. The *lymph vessels* and regional lymph nodes of the retroperitoneal space are discussed earlier in this chapter in connection with specific organs. The *thoracic duct* and its tributaries are discussed here.

The thoracic duct begins at the upper end of the cisterna chyli in the retroperitoneal space. The cisterna receives the lumbar and intestinal lymphatic trunks and is situated in front of the first and second lumbar vertebral bodies, behind and to the right of the abdominal aorta. The normally positioned cisterna chyli is found between the aorta and inferior vena cava, just below the left renal vein. After a short intraabdominal course, the thoracic duct enters the thorax through the aortic aperture, passing behind the aorta, and ascends through the posterior mediastinum.

Nerves. The large *nerve trunks* in the retroperitoneal space are derived mainly from the abdominal portion of the autonomic nervous system.

The anterior and posterior vagal nerve trunks enter the abdominal cavity through the esophageal aperture of the diaphragm. Only the posterior vagal trunk reaches the retroperitoneal space primarily, the bulk of its fibers passing between the left adrenal gland and the left medial crus of the diaphragm to the celiac ganglion.

Two nerves belonging to the sympathetic nervous system, the greater and lesser splanchnic, enter the retroperitoneal space through an aperture in the medial crus of the diaphragm. The greater splanchnic nerve runs between the medial crus of the diaphragm and the adrenal gland to the celiac ganglion. The fibers of the lesser splanchnic nerve terminate partly in the ganglion and may have direct connections with the renal plexus.

The two sympathetic trunks enter the retroperitoneal space after passing between the medial and lateral crura of the diaphragm. Both trunks lie on the psoas major muscles near their origin from the vertebral bodies. The left sympathetic trunk lies slightly behind and to the left of the abdominal aorta, and the right sympathetic trunk is posterior to the inferior vena cava. Connections between the right and left sympathetic trunks are generally present and course between the lumbar vertebral bodies and the aorta or inferior vena cava (Fig. 1.20).

The sympathetic trunks and their ganglia send branches (the lumbar splanchnic nerves) to the preaortic plexuses and their ganglia. The lumbar portion of the sympathetic trunk blends smoothly with the sacral portion at the arcuate line.

Application of Surgical Approaches

Supracostal Approach

The supracostal approach affords broad exposure of the retroperitoneal space (kidney, adrenal gland, proximal ureter) while avoiding the need for rib resection. Several anatomic circumstances make this approach possible: The eleventh and twelfth ribs terminate freely in abdominal muscle, both ribs articulate only with the corresponding vertebral body, and the twelfth rib is easily displaced downward following release of the muscles that insert on the twelfth rib or arise from it.

Exposure of the Lumbodorsal Fascia

After division of the subcutaneous fat, the thoracic fascia is divided, exposing the latissimus dorsi and external oblique muscles (Fig. 1.21).

Incision of the Lumbodorsal Fascia

The lumbodorsal fascia is incised at the tip of the twelfth rib, exposing the pararenal fat between the lumbodorsal fascia and Gerota's fascia. The lumbodorsal fascia can be opened over the fat by bluntly dissecting forward (Fig. 1.22).

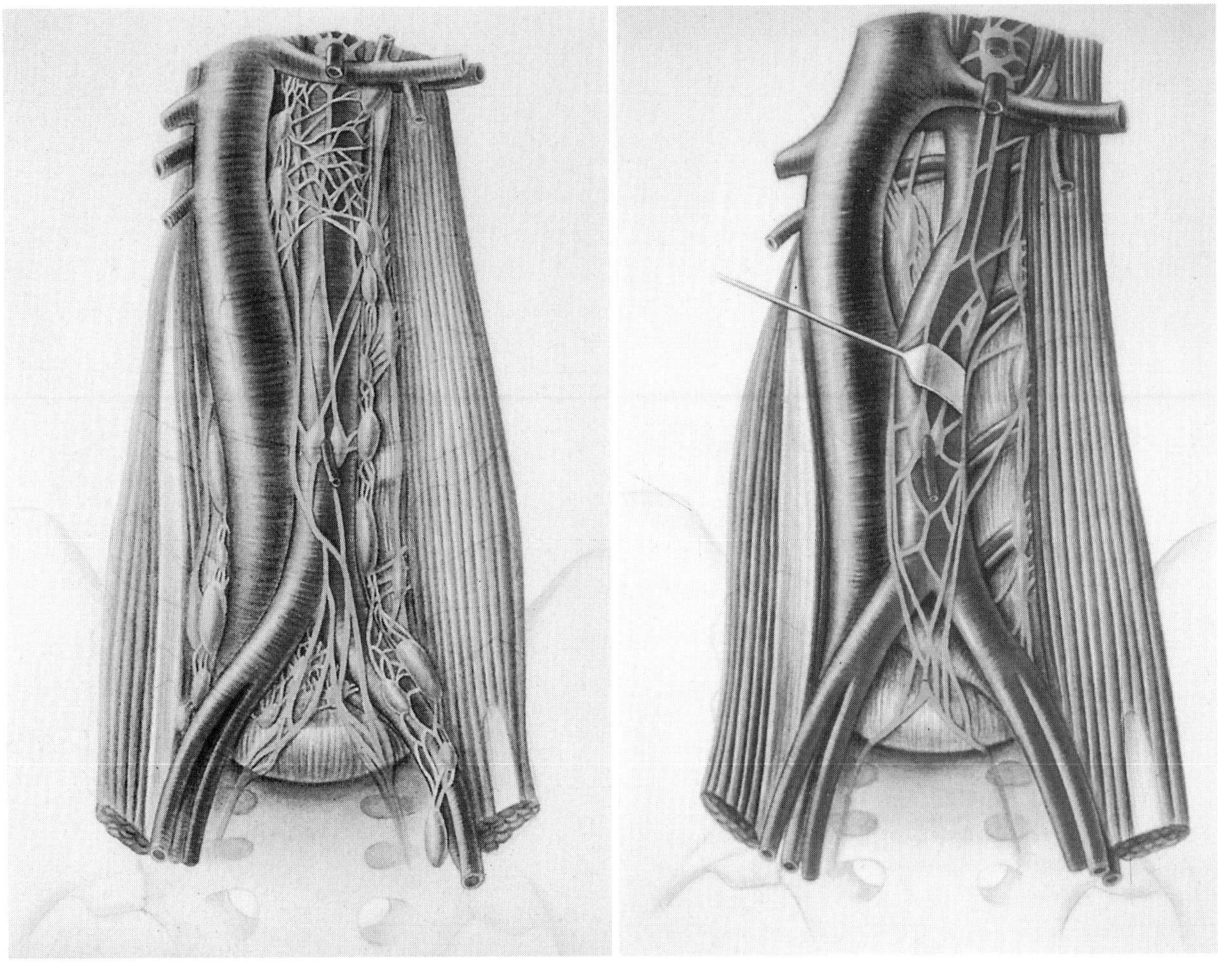

A

B

FIGURE 1.20. **A:** Right sympathetic trunk is situated dorsal to inferior vena caval vein, while left trunk is dorsal and lateral to abdominal aorta. **B:** L-3 ganglion is seen clearly on the left side because abdominal aorta is retracted medially.

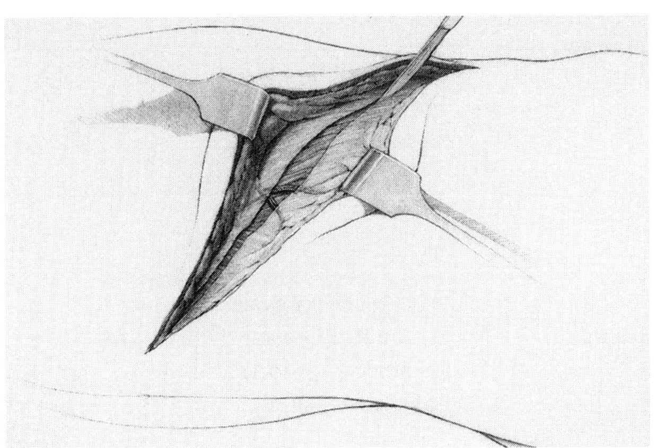

FIGURE 1.21. Exposure of the latissimus dorsi and external oblique muscles.

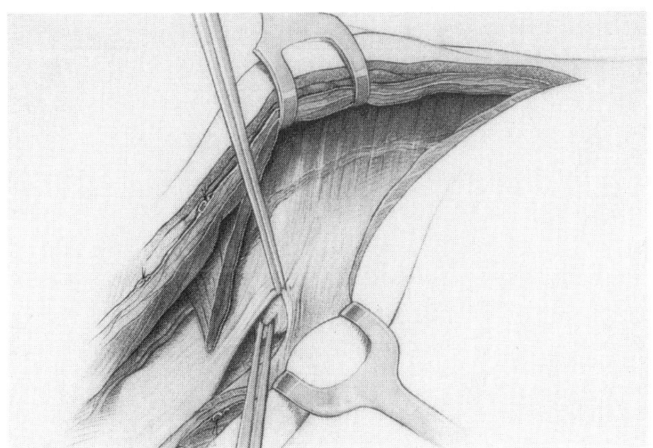

FIGURE 1.22. Incision of the lumbodorsal fascia.

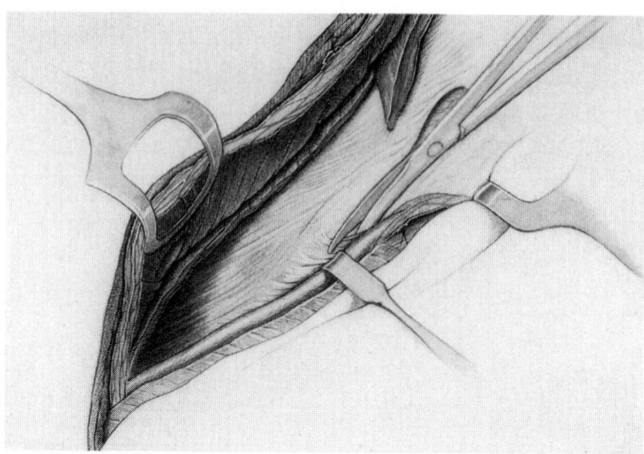

FIGURE 1.23. The thoracic cavity is opened extrapleurally, preserving the intercostal vessels and nerves.

As the twelfth rib is displaced downward and forward with a retractor, the lumbodorsal fascia is dissected from the inner periosteum of the rib (Fig. 1.23). This affords extrapleural entry to the thoracic cavity while sparing the intercostal nerves and vessels. The route of this approach is shown schematically in Fig. 1.24.

Dissection of the Lumbodorsal Fascia and Diaphragm from the Twelfth Rib

The lumbodorsal fascia and then the diaphragm are separated from the twelfth rib under vision, using the finger or a small sponge stick to guide the dissection. The incision at the twelfth rib can be carried over the quadratus lumborum muscle to the lateral arcuate ligament as part of the dissection, with the pleural cavity and lung remaining outside the operative field (Fig. 1.25).

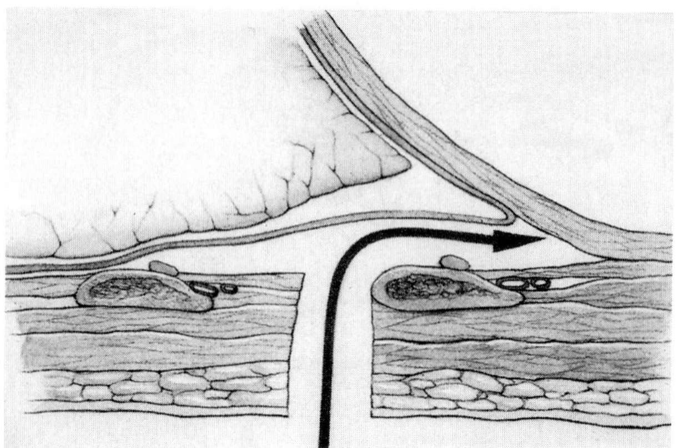

FIGURE 1.24. Schematic view of the dissection of the lumbodorsal fascia from the deep periosteum of the rib.

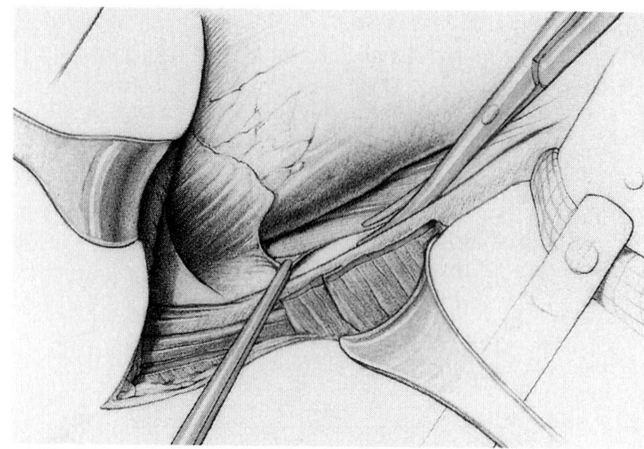

FIGURE 1.25. The pleural space and lung are outside the operative field. The quadratus lumborum muscle is visible below the lateral arcuate ligament.

Foley Muscle-splitting Approach

The Foley muscle-splitting approach gives access to the ureteropelvic junction and proximal ureter through a transfascial route.

Exposure of the Transversus Abdominis and Its Tendon of Origin

The latissimus dorsi and external oblique muscles are retracted, and a retractor is placed in the proximal part of the incision to expose the tendon of origin of the transversus abdominis and, anteriorly, the fibers of the internal oblique muscle (Fig. 1.26). The internal oblique is separated from the transversus abdominis along the line indicated and is

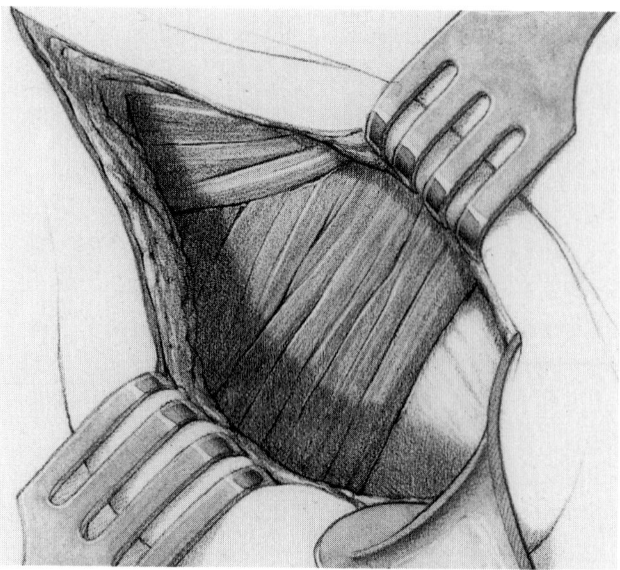

FIGURE 1.26. The internal oblique is separated from the transversus abdominis and its tendon of origin.

retracted forward with a second retractor. The tendon of origin of the transversus abdominis is incised in the direction of its fibers (Fig. 1.27).

Posterior Approach to the Adrenal Gland

The thoracic fascia is exposed. The latissimus dorsi and serratus anterior muscles are identified. Exposure is maintained with two retractors. The latissimus dorsi and serratus anterior are transected with a scalpel. The erector spinae muscle can be seen in the medial portion of the wound (Fig. 1.28).

The periosteum of the eleventh rib is divided with diathermy, and the rib is progressively isolated with a straight periosteal elevator and a curved stripper. The eleventh rib is resected as far medially as possible (Fig. 1.29).

Incision of the Rib Bed

The posterior rib bed is opened with a scissors, exposing the diaphragm. Care is taken to preserve the intercostal neurovascular bundle during incision of the rib bed.

With the aid of a wooden tissue protector or small sponge stick, the diaphragm is carefully divided with diathermy. The plane between the diaphragm and Gerota's fascia is carefully developed, and the diaphragm is incised anteriorly and posteriorly to establish entry into the retroperitoneal space. Gerota's fascia is identified (Fig. 1.30).

Thoracoabdominal Approach

The thoracoabdominal approach provides excellent exposure of the entire abdominal and retroperitoneal space. Because the intrathoracic portion of the inferior vena cava can also be exposed, this approach is useful for the removal of stage II and stage III tumor thrombi involving the vena

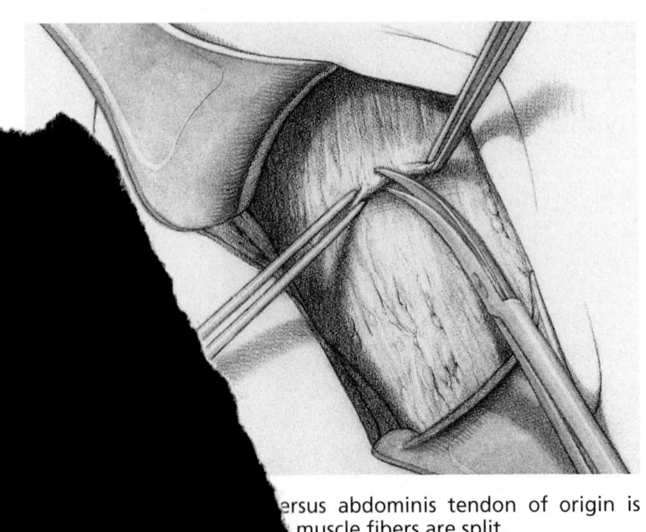

ersus abdominis tendon of origin is muscle fibers are split.

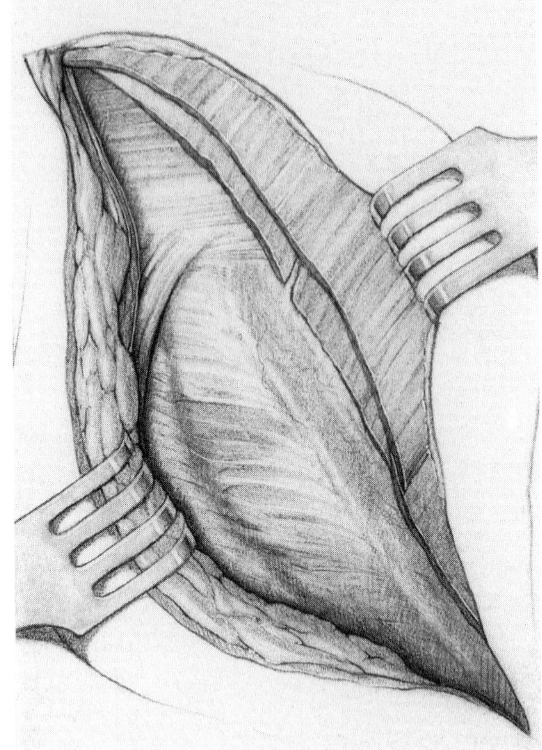

FIGURE 1.28. Exposure of the eleventh rib. The transected muscles are retracted.

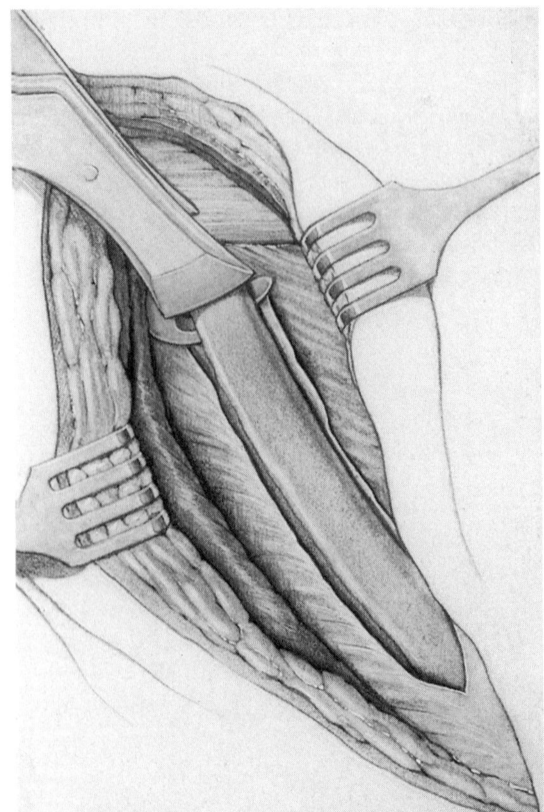

FIGURE 1.29. The eleventh rib is transected with rib shears.

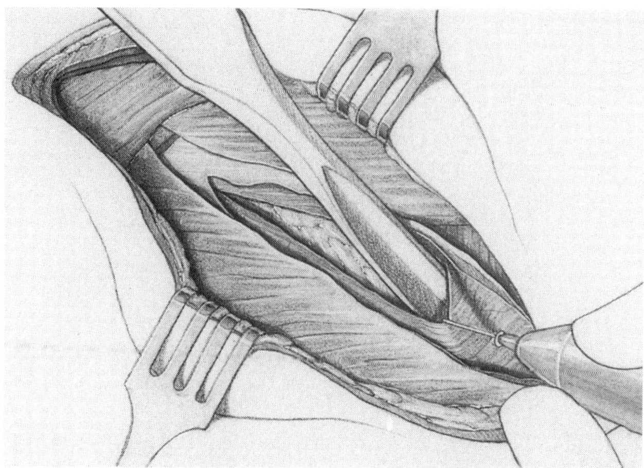

FIGURE 1.30. The diaphragm is divided with diathermy over a wooden tissue protector. Gerota's fascia is identified.

cava. A modification, the primary thoracoretroperitoneal approach, is useful for lymph node dissection in patients with testicular tumors.

Laparotomy and Thoracotomy

Starting at the anterior axillary line, the latissimus dorsi, serratus anterior, and external oblique muscles are transected with diathermy in line with the skin incision. The external and intercostal muscles are visible on the chest wall. Starting at the costal arch, the incision is first extended inferomedially, dividing the fibers of the rectus muscle in the epigastrium. The rectus abdominis is then bluntly freed laterally while sparing the nerves and vessels; this technique prevents denervation of the rectus musculature. The superior epigastric vessels are ligated. The rectus muscle is retracted laterally to expose the posterior layer of the rectus sheath. Small retractors maintain exposure in both the abdominal and thoracic portions of the field (Fig. 1.31).

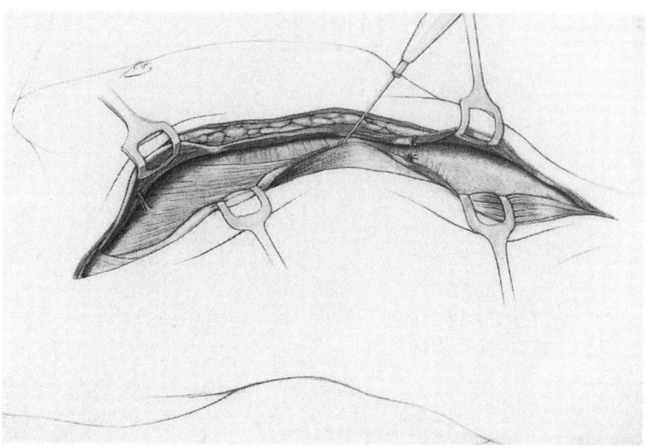

FIGURE 1.31. The serratus anterior and external oblique are transected, exposing the posterior rectus sheath.

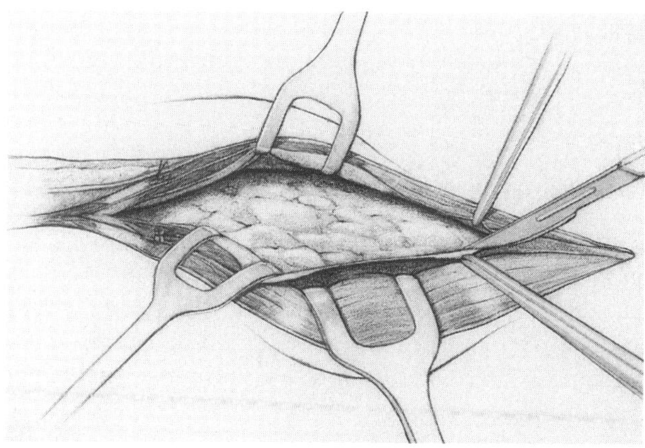

FIGURE 1.32. Entry into the abdominal cavity.

In the abdominal part of the incision, the posterior rectus sheath is picked up with forceps on both sides along with the transversus abdominis fibers and peritoneum, and all three layers are transected to establish entry into the peritoneal cavity. The greater omentum can be identified. The abdominal cavity is opened to the level of the umbilicus (Fig. 1.32).

Division of the Costal Arch. Before the costal arch is divided, the plane defined by the transversus abdominis and diaphragm is exposed. Once this plane has been identified, the costal arch is undermined at the osteochondral junction and divided. With this maneuver, the underlying intercostal arteries and veins can be dealt with under direct vision.

This dissection of the transversus abdominis and diaphragm is important in the primary thoracoretroperitoneal approach. In this modification, which avoids primary entry into the abdominal cavity, the approach is begun inferomedial to the costal arch and the peritoneum is retracted medially (Fig. 1.33).

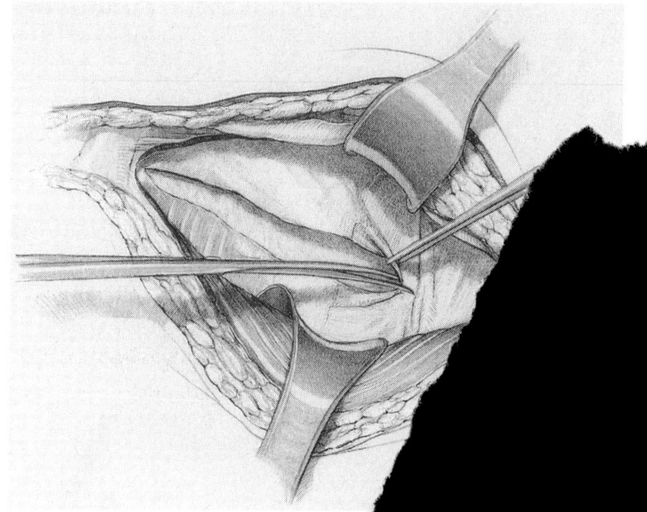

FIGURE 1.33. Primary thoracore

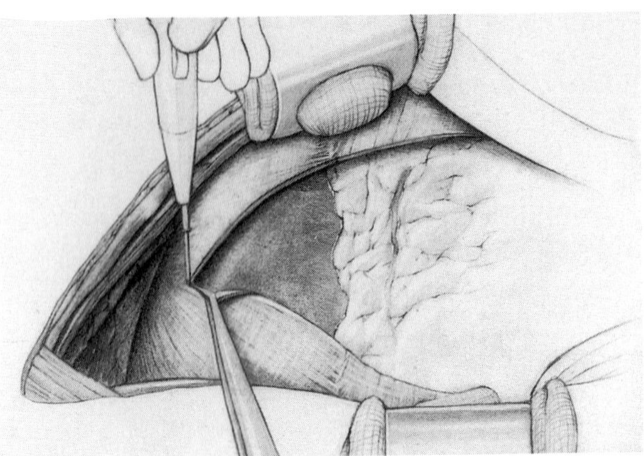

FIGURE 1.34. Division of the diaphragm.

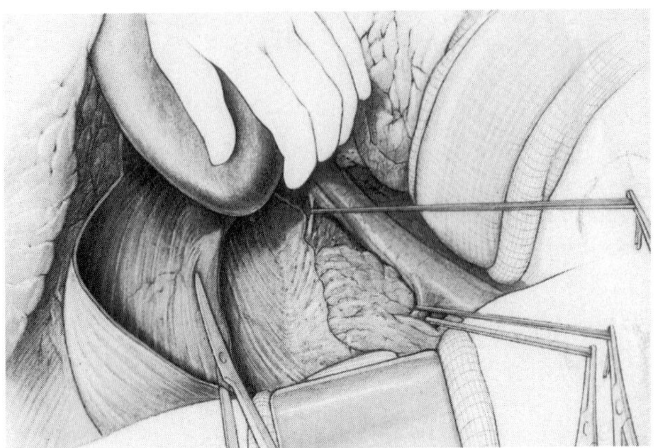

FIGURE 1.35. The right triangular ligament is sharply released from the diaphragm. The right adrenal gland and suprarenal vein are seen.

Division of the Diaphragm. The transversus abdominis fibers are divided close to the costal arch, followed by incision of the diaphragm. The diaphragm is incised as far laterally as possible to preserve the phrenic nerve branches (Fig. 1.34).

Modification of the Thoracoabdominal Approach for a Stage II or III Tumor Thrombus in the Vena Cava. After the abdominal cavity and chest have been opened, the incision in the mesocolon is carried along the colon and is continued along the mesentery to the duodenojejunal flexure. This line of incision permits a general mobilization of the large and small bowels, establishing access to a broad area of the retroperitoneal space. The left renal vein can be identified over the aorta and elevated to expose the superior mesenteric artery. The right renal artery is identified in the aortocaval space.

The peritoneum is dissected off the diaphragm. The right triangular ligament is incised at its attachment to the diaphragm so that the right lobe of the liver can be mobilized and deflected medially upward, exposing the hepatic veins. In this way, the entire retroperitoneal course of the vena cava can be visualized (Fig. 1.35) together with the right adrenal gland and suprarenal vein.

Use of the fifth interspace approach also permits exposure of the intrathoracic portion of the inferior vena cava. The parietal layer of the pericardium is incised above the diaphragm. After stay sutures are preplaced on both sides, the intrathoracic part of the vena cava can be freed and encircled with a tourniquet snare (Fig. 1.36).

Approach to the Retrocrural Lymph Nodes

Most positive suprahilar nodes are found in the retrocrural zone. The usual path of lymph flow from the retroperitoneum into the chest is periaortic and posterior (Figs. 1.37 and 1.38). The lymphatic pathways traverse the diaphragm via the aortic hiatus. They first drain into the cisterna chyli and then into the posterior mediastinal nodes.

The thoracic duct begins at the upper end of the cisterna chyli in the retroperitoneal space. The cisterna receives the lumbar and intestinal lymphatic trunks and is situated in front of the first and second lumbar vertebral bodies, behind and to the right of the abdominal aorta.

Dissection of the Lateral Crus, Exposure of the Inferior Phrenic Artery

The descending colon is retracted medially with the isolated left colic flexure. The left inferior phrenic artery and vein are

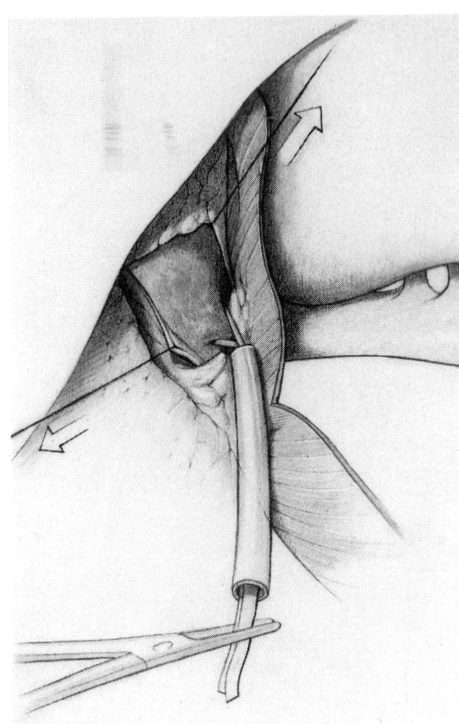

FIGURE 1.36. Exposure of the intrathoracic portion of the inferior vena cava.

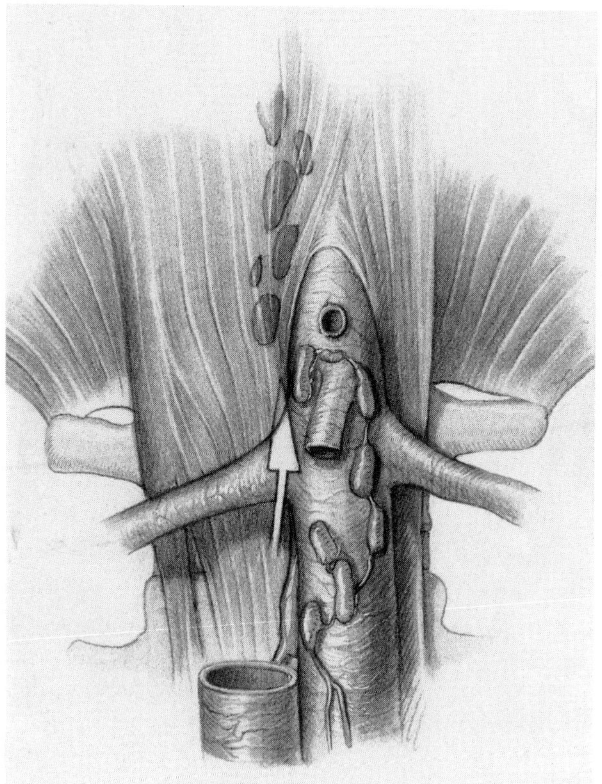

FIGURE 1.37. Path of lymph flow to the suprahilar region and the chest.

identified at the lateral crus, dissected, and ligated (Fig. 1.39). A middle suprarenal artery from the aorta is also ligated, and the adrenal gland is then freed from the lumbar part of the diaphragm and lateral crus and displaced inferolaterally (Fig. 1.40).

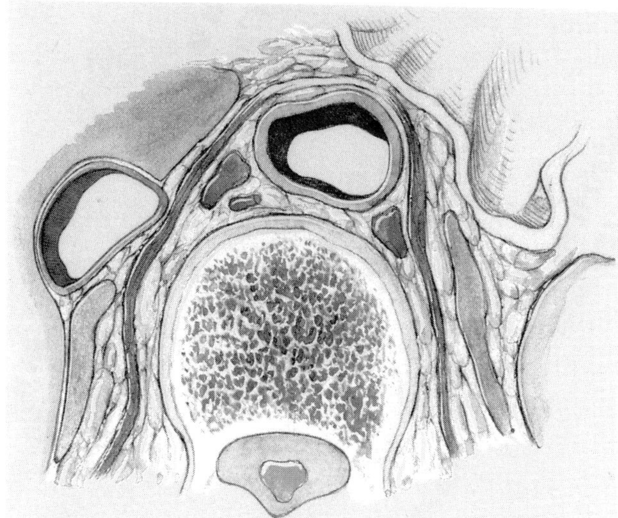

FIGURE 1.38. Transverse section. Location of retrocrural nodes in relation to the diaphragm and the aorta (schema).

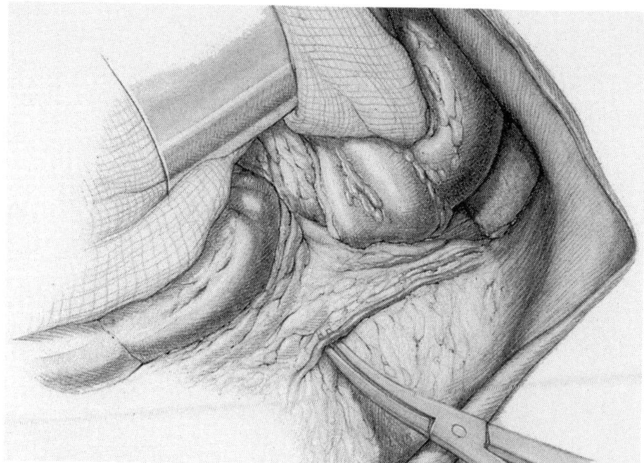

FIGURE 1.39. Exposure of the left inferior phrenic artery and vein.

Incision of the Aortic Aperture

After exposure of the abdominal aorta, the left renal artery is identified and dissected free. After ligation of the inferior phrenic artery, the aortic aperture is incised over the abdominal aorta, starting at the median arcuate ligament. If enlarged lymph nodes are found at the celiac trunk and superior mesenteric artery, both vessels must be dissected free (Fig. 1.41). The incision in the aortic aperture is carried to the esophageal hiatus. The inferior phrenic artery is again ligated close to the aorta (Fig. 1.42).

This approach provides exposure of the retroaortic space (Fig. 1.43). When the aorta is mobilized, attention must be given to the last two posterior intercostal arteries and first lumbar arteries at the lateral or posterior aspect of the vessel. These arteries may give origin to the great radicular artery (of Adamkiewicz), which contributes significantly to the blood supply of the spinal cord. Therefore segmental arteries must be preserved, especially on the left side of the body.

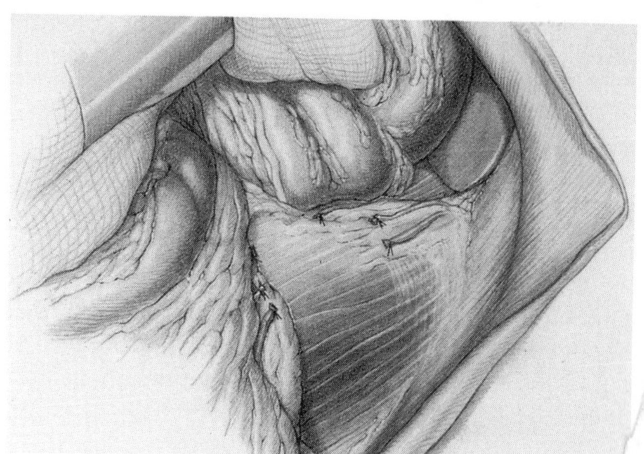

FIGURE 1.40. The left inferior phrenic artery and vein are gated, and the lumbar part of the diaphragm is exposed.

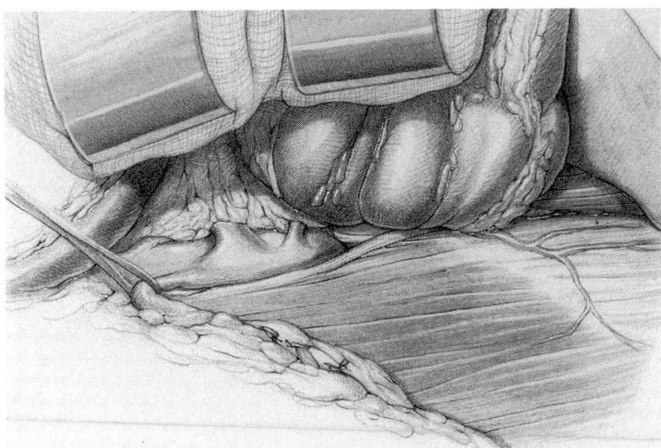

FIGURE 1.41. Dissection of the aorta and renal artery. The line of incision from the aortic hiatus to the esophagus is shown.

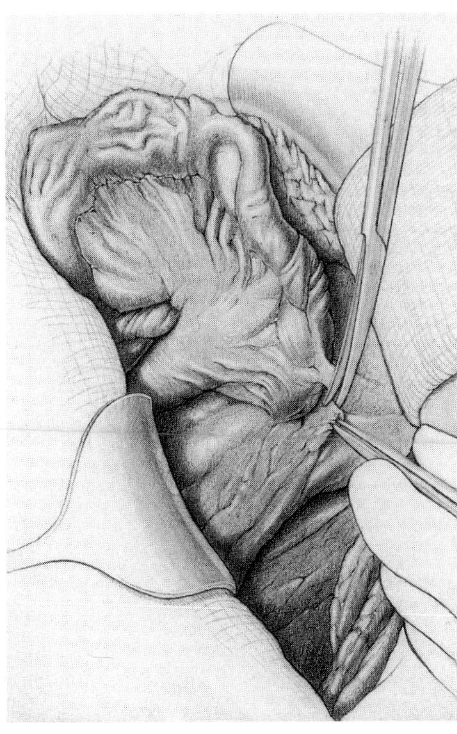

FIGURE 1.44. Incision of the inferior duodenal fold. The vascular pedicle of the kidney is approached between the aorta and inferior mesenteric vein.

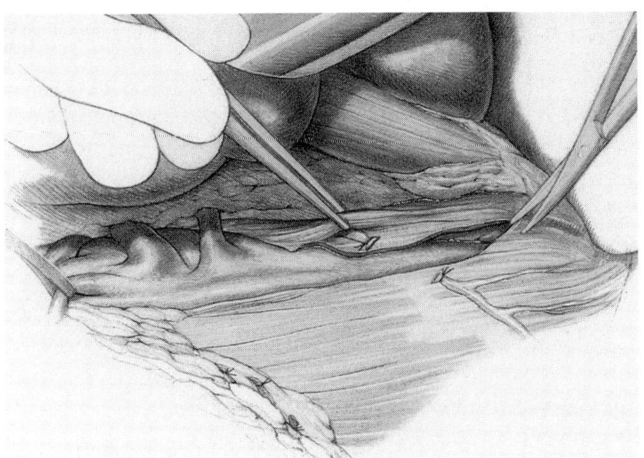

FIGURE 1.42. Incision over the abdominal aorta.

Anterior Subcostal Approach

Dissection of the Renal Vessels

For dissection of the renal vessels on the left side, the peritoneum is incised longitudinally between the aorta and inferior mesenteric vein, starting at the inferior duodenal fold (ligament of Treitz) (Fig. 1.44). This incision gives direct access to the vascular pedicle of the left kidney between the aorta and inferior mesenteric vein. The renal artery and vein can be dissected and snared (Fig. 1.45).

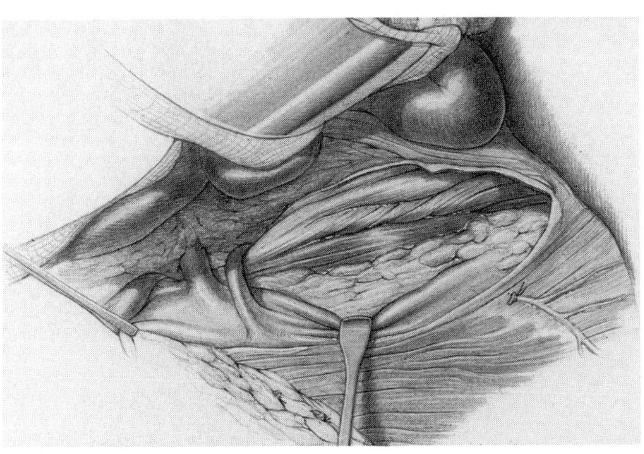

FIGURE 1.43. Exposure of the retroaortic and retrocrural spaces.

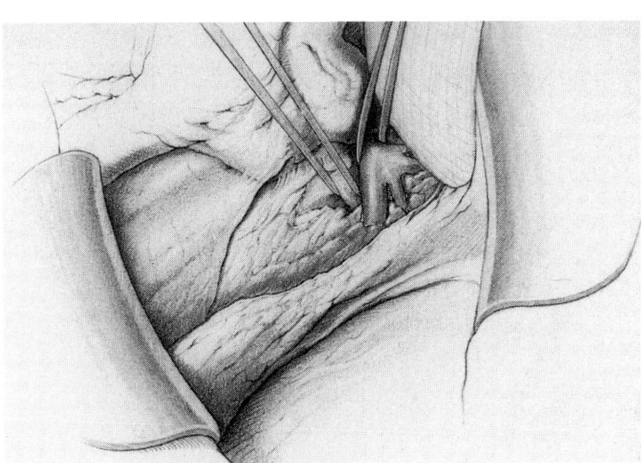

FIGURE 1.45. Exposure and isolation of the renal artery and vein.

Midline Transperitoneal Approach

Exposure of the Retroperitoneal Space

Starting at the inferior duodenojejunal fold, the retroperitoneal space is opened by incising distally along the root of the mesentery while the small bowel is packed away to the right side and the descending colon and left colic flexure are retracted to the left side (Fig. 1.46).

Next, the ascending part of the duodenum is dissected free along the line of the incision. For a suprahilar approach on the left side, the incision in the parietal peritoneum is extended farther upward and to the left so that the inferior mesenteric vein can be dissected and ligated (Fig. 1.47). This establishes broad access for the suprahilar lymph node dissection.

The line of incision is now extended farther toward the right common iliac artery from the abdominal aorta so that the cecum can be dissected from the underlying retroperitoneal connective tissue (Fig. 1.48).

The incision is extended along the right paracolic sulcus and ended at the inferior border of the epiploic foramen (of Winslow) (Fig. 1.49). This provides access for dissecting the ascending colon and right colic flexure from Gerota's fascia.

This extended incision (from the inferior duodenojejunal fold to the epiploic foramen) permits the entire small bowel, cecum, ascending colon, and right colic flexure to be mobilized (and if necessary exteriorized from the abdominal cavity). The abdominal aorta and inferior vena cava are visible below fibrous and fatty tissues, respectively, at the center of the retroperitoneal space (Fig. 1.50).

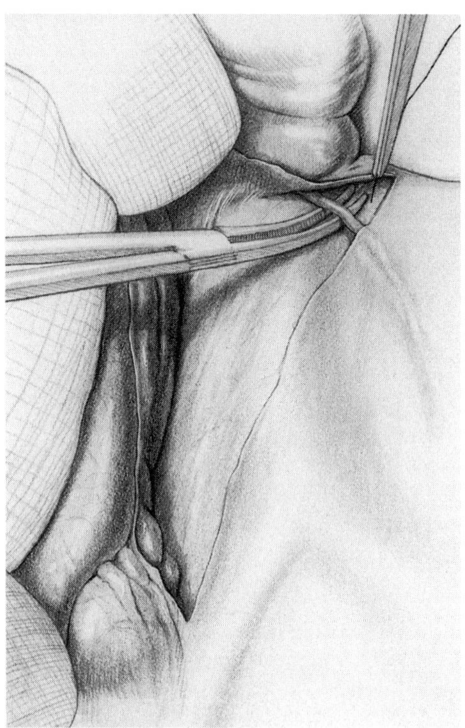

FIGURE 1.47. Left suprahilar approach. The inferior mesenteric vein is exposed and ligated.

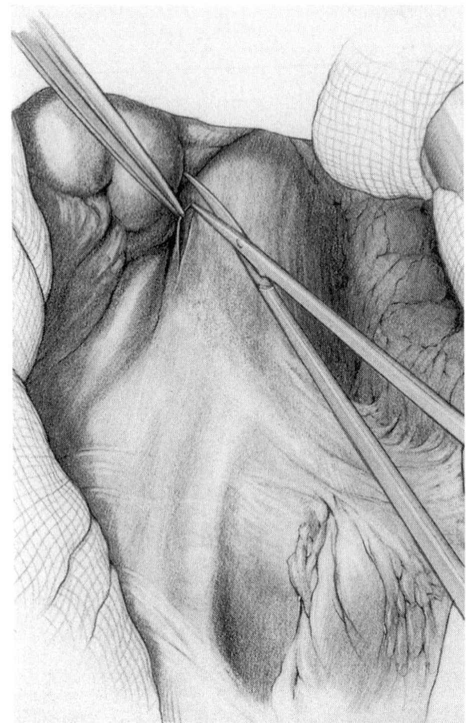

FIGURE 1.46. The retroperitoneal space is opened along the root of the mesentery, starting at the inferior duodenojejunal fold.

Incision of the Retroperitoneal Fascia

The fibrous and fatty tissue overlying the center of the vena cava and abdominal aorta is now opened, and the lymph node dissection is carried out using a split-and-roll technique (Fig. 1.51).

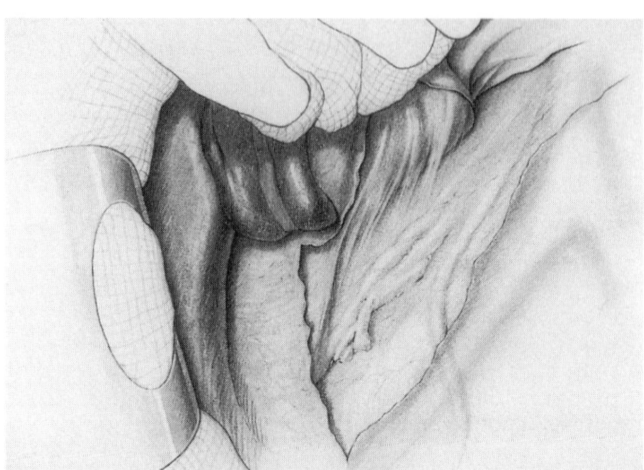

FIGURE 1.48. The incision is extended from the abdominal aorta over the right common iliac artery.

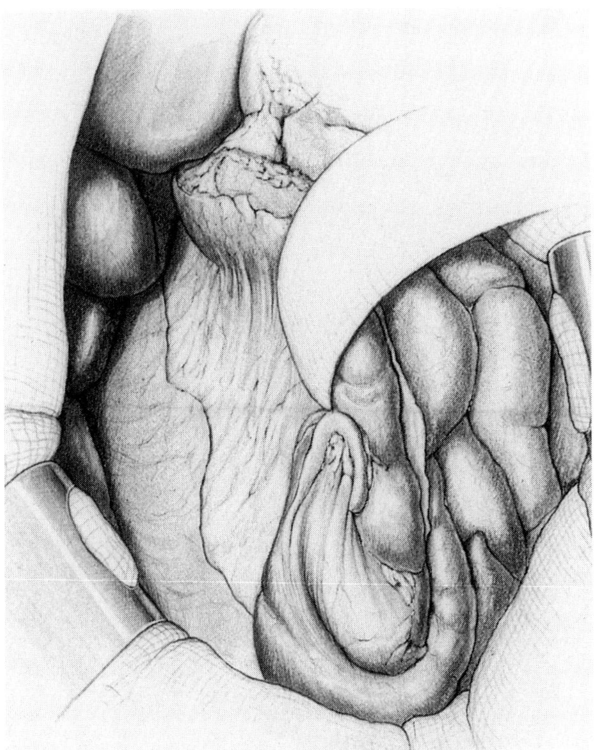

FIGURE 1.49. The incision in the right paracolic sulcus is extended to the inferior border of the epiploic foramen.

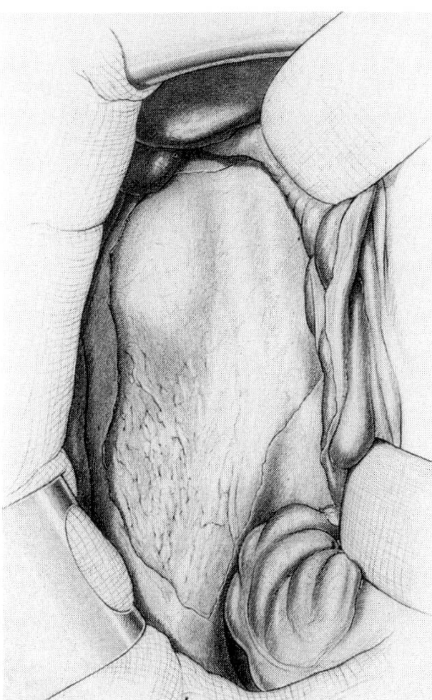

FIGURE 1.50. View of the incision from the ligament of Treitz to the inferior border of the epiploic foramen. The entire retroperitoneal space is visible.

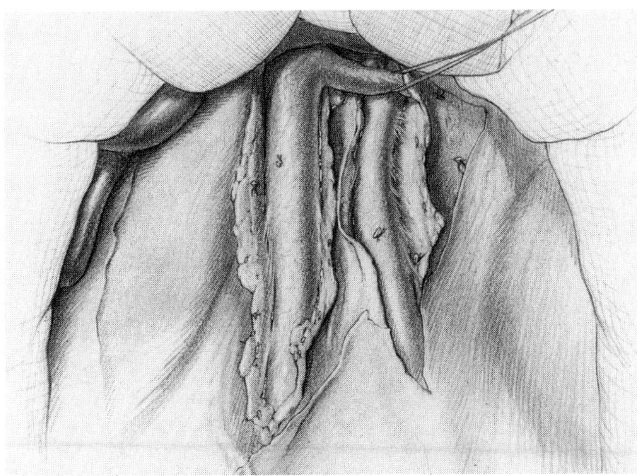

FIGURE 1.51. Split-and-roll technique of retroperitoneal lymph node dissection.

Nerve-sparing Retroperitoneal Lymph Node Dissection

Seminal emission and ejaculation are primarily under sympathetic control. The efferent fibers originating from T-12 to L-3 travel to the superior and on to the inferior hypogastric plexus (or pelvic plexus). The pelvic plexus also includes parasympathetic fibers originating from the pelvic nerves.

The sympathetic trunk consists of a series of spindle-shaped ganglia interconnected by short interganglionic rami to form a continuous chain of ganglia (Fig. 1.20). This trunk extends along the spinal column on either side from the base of the skull to the tip of the coccyx. It is connected to the spinal cord via the rami communicantes, which may behave in a number of different manners. Often, there are branches that course not only to the corresponding ganglia of the sympathetic trunk but also to the adjoining ganglia. In the lumbar region, where the rami communicantes are relatively long, their course is particularly variable. They pass beyond the tendinous origins of the psoas major, and a variable number of ganglia can be found at different levels at the anterolateral aspects of the vertebral bodies medial to the psoas major. The right sympathetic trunk is situated dorsal to the inferior vena cava, and the left trunk is located dorsal and lateral to the abdominal aorta. The transverse rami connect the two sympathetic trunks. Only rarely are the two trunks arranged symmetrically in the lumbar region. Furthermore, fusions of ganglia occasionally are encountered. The lumbar splanchnic nerves are the continuation of postganglionic fibers of the lumbar ganglia. They travel to the paraaortic nervous plexus and eventually reach the superior hypogastric plexus, a continuation of the abdominal aortic plexus, located on either side of the abdominal aorta between the origins of the superior and inferior mesenteric arteries.

The superior hypogastric plexus is situated ventral to the aortic bifurcation and extends across the common iliac vein in the direction of the promontory (Fig. 1.20). The right and left hypogastric nerves connect the superior hypogastric plexus with the inferior hypogastric plexus, which is on either side of the rectum in the lesser pelvis.

The afferent impulses triggering emission and ejaculation are conveyed via the pudendal nerve, whereas the efferent impulses inducing emission are transported to the target organs via the thoracolumbar sympathetic fibers (T-12 to L-3), the paravertebral ganglia, and the superior hypogastric plexus. The efferent impulses inducing ejaculation are conveyed via the parasympathetic fibers of the pelvic nerves (S-2 to S-3) and cause the bulbocavernous and ischiocavernous muscles to contract, which results in antegrade ejaculation.

The L-2 and L-3 ganglia are located close to each other; they may even fuse so that there is no interganglionic ramus. The lower margin of the L-3 ganglion is situated approximately one fingerwidth above the origin of the inferior mesenteric artery. If the abdominal aorta is displaced toward the median, the left L-3 ganglion is exposed medial to the psoas major on the lateral aspect of the L-3 vertebra. The right L-3 ganglion can be exposed by displacing the inferior vena cava toward the median (Fig. 1.20). The ganglion is located slightly ventral to the ventrolateral junction of the L-3 vertebral body. As mentioned, the two trunks are interconnected by the lumbar splanchnic nerves that arise from these ganglia.

Nerve-sparing Surgery

The aim of nerve-sparing surgery is to protect the sympathetic ganglia lying in the groove between the psoas muscle and the vertebral column. The sympathetic nerve fibers crossing over the distal aorta and its bifurcation must also be preserved (Fig. 1.52).

The sympathetic fibers can be identified with the help of magnifying lenses; the efferent fibers can be seen distally where they cross the common iliac artery. By reflecting the lymphatic tissue off the psoas muscle, the surgeon can identify the sympathetic trunk and trace the fibers distally from their origin at the sympathetic trunk. The sympathetic fibers are placed in vessel loops (Fig. 1.53). Subsequently, the lymphatic tissue is split over the aorta and rolled off.

The nerve-sparing technique can also be used in postchemotherapy surgery; however, in this type of elective surgery, patient selection is extremely important.

Suprahilar Node Dissection for High-stage Disease (Testicular Tumors)

Direct extension from an infrahilar tumor may project into the suprahilar zone; in this case, it is usually precrural and can be rolled down and away from the great vessels in the same way as tumors in the infrahilar region. Suprahilar disease can be managed by an anterior midline approach; the thoracoabdominal (thoracoretroperitoneal) approach should be used for tumors in the retrocrural zone.

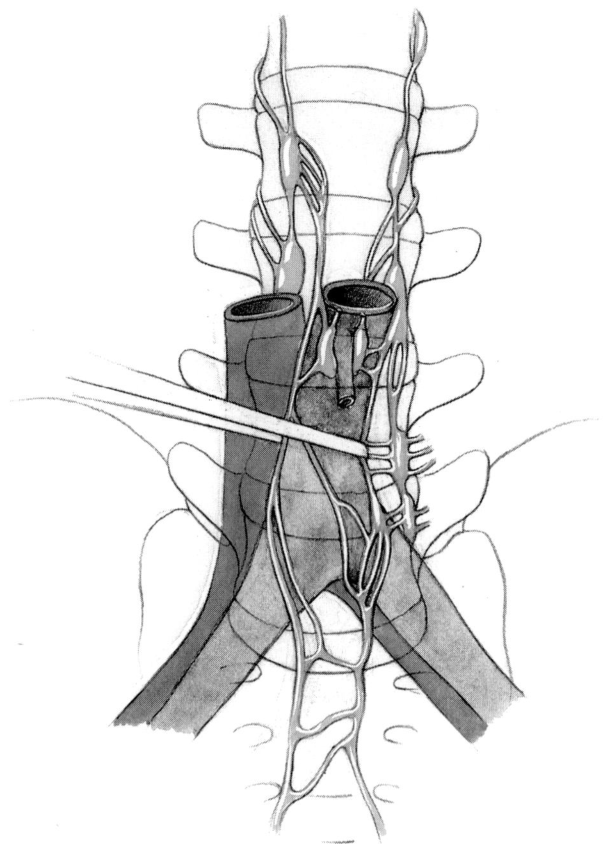

FIGURE 1.52. Nerve-sparing retroperitoneal dissection. Schematic drawing showing the sympathetic trunk, ganglia, and nerve fibers.

In the anterior midline approach, the root of the small bowel mesentery is incised. The posterior attachments to the cecum and the mesocolon are dissected free using the plane of Toldt as an avascular field of dissection. After dissection of the duodenum and the head of the pancreas, the Kocher maneuver is performed.

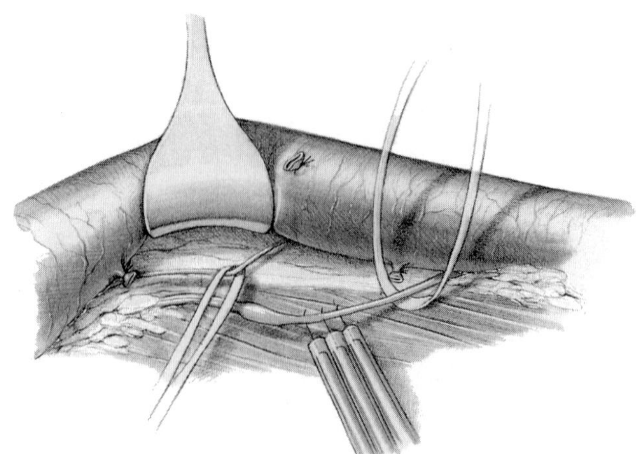

FIGURE 1.53. The nerve fibers to be spared are placed in vessel loops. Using an electric stimulator, ejaculation can be elicited intraoperatively.

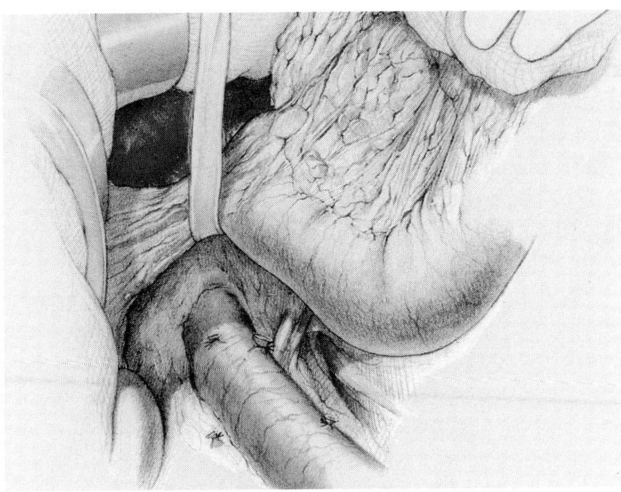

FIGURE 1.54. Exposure of the right suprahilar region; the hepatoduodenal ligament is placed in a vessel loop.

On the right side, access to the suprahilar nodes is gained by an incision below the hepatoduodenal ligament, which is dissected free and placed in a vessel loop to expose the suprahilar portion of the vena cava (Fig. 1.54).

To gain access to the left suprahilar region, the left inferior mesenteric vein is ligated and divided, and the left colonic mesentery is incised and mobilized. The incision in the left mesocolon is made in an oblique manner, parallel to the inferior margin of the pancreas. After this maneuver, the lower vein of the pancreas can be fully mobilized and retracted from the anterior surface of Gerota's fascia (Fig. 1.55).

The superior mesenteric artery is identified at the point where it crosses over the left renal vein (Fig. 1.55). Care must be taken to prevent excessive tension on this artery and to preclude injury to it by a retractor because it serves as a vascular pedicle for the small and large bowels. Therefore pads are placed on the pancreas and the pedicle of the superior mesenteric artery.

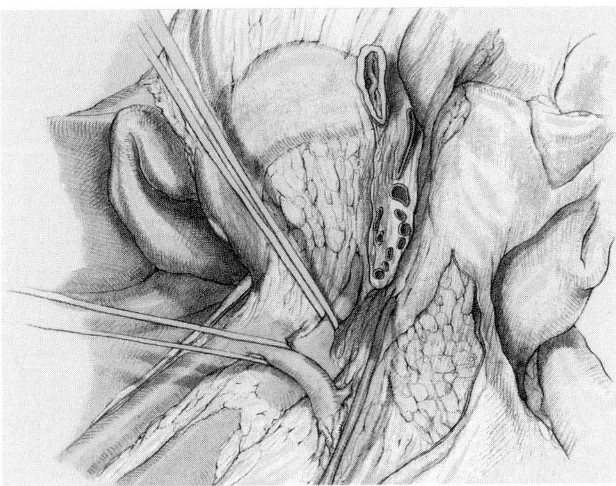

FIGURE 1.55. Anatomic approach to the suprahilar lymph node dissection, view from the right side.

Dissection of the crura is started at the base of this pedicle and, on completion of the infrahilar node dissection, should be continued to the suprahilar region. The lymphatic connections between the infrahilar and suprahilar regions can be identified by elevating the renal vessels with malleable vein retractors.

PELVIS

Anatomy

Pelvic Part of the Ureter

The pelvic (distal) part of the ureter makes up approximately half of its total length. It follows basically the same course in males and females, but its relations are gender specific (Figs. 1.56 and 1.57). The entrance of the ureter into the true pelvis is located anterior or slightly medial to the sacroiliac joint. There the ureter is related to the iliac vessels, crossing either the common iliac vessels or the external and internal iliac vessels, depending on the position of these vessels and the level of their bifurcation. Because of the left-sided position of the abdominal aorta, the right ureter typically crosses the iliac vessels below their point of bifurcation; the left ureter generally crosses the common iliac vessels (Figs. 1.56 and 1.57).

The first part of the pelvic portion of the ureter describes an anteriorly convex arch. It lies medial to the internal iliac artery and its branches, and it crosses the obturator nerve on the lateral pelvic wall just below the parietal peritoneum (Fig. 1.56). In the female, the ureter usually passes behind the ovary on the floor of the ovarian fossa (Fig. 1.57).

After crossing the pelvic vessels, the ureter diverges from the parietal peritoneum to enter the pararectal connective tissue (paraproctium). Just before or after this point, a sheet of connective tissue leaves the ureteral adventitia to establish a direct connection between the ureter and the rectal retinaculum.

After the ureter enters the pararectal connective tissue, its topographic relations display gender-specific differences.

In the male, the ureter passes through the pararectal connective tissue from behind forward, then turns slightly medially and closely approaches the tip of the seminal vesicle. There it crosses below the vas deferens. Surrounded by the veins of the vesical plexus, the ureter reaches and passes medially and obliquely through the bladder wall.

In the female, the ureter describes an inferiorly convex bend as it passes from the rectal retinaculum into the cardinal ligament (lateral cervical ligament). There it passes behind the uterine artery, which consistently gives off branches to the ureteral adventitia in this area. These branches travel in a thin sheet of connective tissue that is incorrectly termed the *vental mesoureter* (Fig. 1.57).

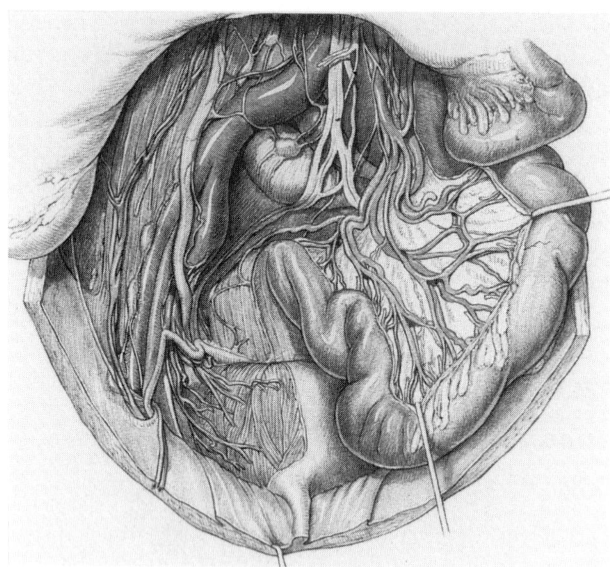

FIGURE 1.56. Pelvic dissection in a male. The peritoneum has been partially removed.

Generally, the ureter runs approximately 1.5 to 2 cm lateral to the uterine cervix, although this distance can vary from 1 to 4 cm if the uterus occupies a paramedian position.

In its further course to the bladder, the female ureter is related to the fornix and anterior wall of the vagina. The left ureter generally is more extensively apposed to the front of the vagina than the right ureter, so it is more vulnerable to trauma in vaginal operations. In all discussions of ureteral relations, it should be kept in mind that a distended bladder or rectum can cause displacement and even tortuosity of the ureters.

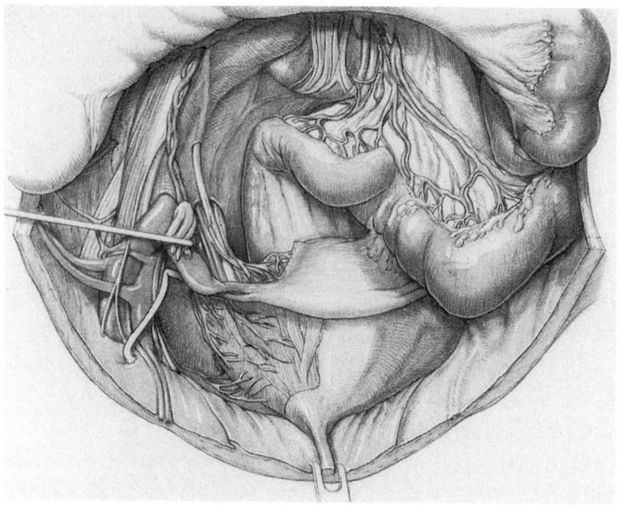

FIGURE 1.57. Pelvic dissection in a female. The peritoneum has been partially removed.

Vessels and Nerves of the Pelvic Ureter

The *arteries* of the pelvic part of the ureter form a plexus in the ureteral adventitia that, in the initial part of the pelvic ureter, is supplied by ureteral branches of the iliac vessels. These may arise from the common iliac artery or from the internal or external iliac artery. Ureteral branches from the iliolumbar and superior gluteal arteries are less commonly observed.

As the ureter descends further, its adventitial arterial plexus receives blood from the superior vesical artery, the artery of the vas deferens or uterine artery, the vaginal artery, and the inferior vesical artery. Branches from the middle rectal artery also may reach the connective-tissue sheath of the ureter (Figs. 1.56 and 1.57).

The *veins* of the pelvic part of the ureter reach the veins accompanying the arteries either directly or by way of the venous plexuses of the pelvis (vesical, prostatic, uterine, and vaginal plexuses).

The *lymph vessels* of the pelvic ureter drain into the regional lymph nodes on the pelvic wall: the external iliac, internal iliac, interiliac, and common iliac nodes.

The *nerves* of the pelvic ureter form dense networks in the adventitia, muscular wall, and mucosal layer of the ureter. They originate from the pelvic plexus, which in turn receives sympathetic fibers via the lumbar and sacral splanchnic nerves and the hypogastric plexus. Parasympathetic fibers reach the pelvic plexus via the pelvic splanchnic nerves from the sacral cord (Fig. 1.58).

Relations of the Male Bladder to Adjacent Organs

The relations of the bladder to adjacent organs correlate closely with its relations to the pelvic connective tissue and peritoneum.

Peritoneal Covering of the Bladder

The bladder is attached to the peritoneum by loose connective tissue. This enables it to function as an expansile urinary reservoir that is mobile with respect to the peritoneum. Only a greatly distended bladder is fixed by its peritoneal covering (Fig. 1.59).

The parietal peritoneum is continued from the anterior abdominal wall onto the bladder apex and covers the posterior surface of the bladder to the level of the tips of the seminal vesicles, sometimes extending to the level of the ureteral orifices. There the peritoneum is reflected onto the anterior wall of the rectum to form the rectovesical pouch, which is the lowest point of the peritoneal cavity. The entrance to the rectovesical pouch is bounded by the two sagittally oriented rectovesical folds. These peritoneal folds are backed with connective tissue that provides posterior support for the bladder base.

The peritoneum is recessed between the bladder and anterior abdominal wall to form the supravesical fossae

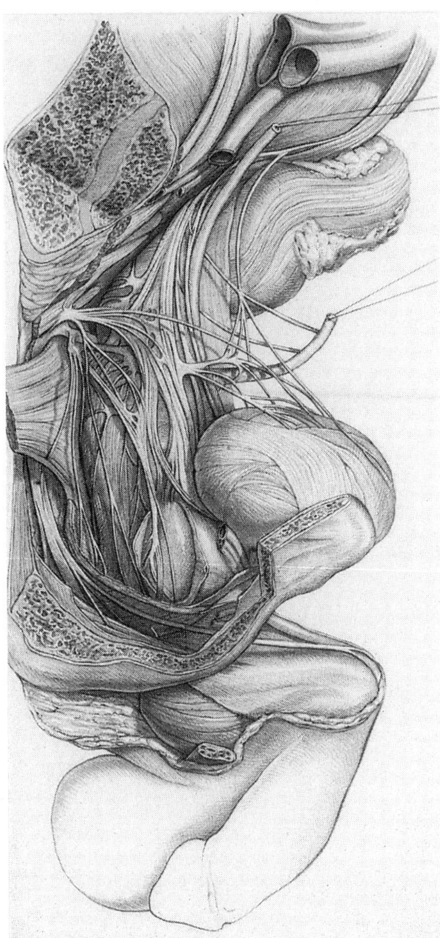

FIGURE 1.58. Nerves in a male pelvis, viewed from the right side: Portions of the coxa have been removed.

(Fig. 1.59). The right and left supravesical fossae are separated by the median umbilical fold. The supravesical fossa is bounded laterally by the medial umbilical fold. The peritoneal covering of the posterior bladder wall contains a reserve fold of peritoneum, the transverse vesical fold, which is progressively obliterated as the bladder distends.

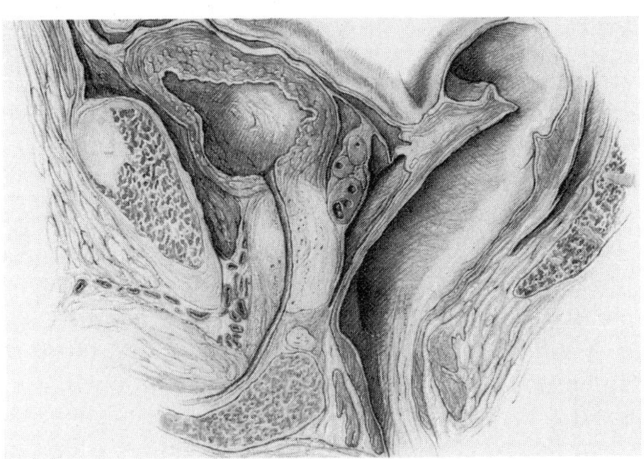

FIGURE 1.59. Midsagittal section through the pelvis.

Bladder and Pelvic Connective Tissue

The pelvic connective tissue consists of three main parts: the pelvic fascia (parietal and visceral), the neurovascular sheaths, and the loose connective tissue occupying the spaces of the pelvic viscera.

The *visceral pelvic fascia* is derived from the parietal pelvic fascia above the urogenital diaphragm at the site where the urethra pierces the diaphragm. The visceral fascia is reflected onto the prostate, and it invests the bladder as the vesical fascia.

The *neurovascular sheaths* are sheetlike condensations of intrapelvic connective tissue that invest and transmit nerves and blood vessels and that also perform retinacular functions. Portions distributed to the bladder and prostate assist in the fixation of the bladder base. The *puboprostatic ligament* (pubovesical ligament) extends from the symphysis and adjacent portions of the pubic bone to the prostate and continues onto the bladder neck. It binds the prostate and bladder to the anterior pelvic wall. The *paracystic connective tissue* (bladder retinaculum) passes to the bladder from the lateral pelvic wall. Between the paracystic connective tissue and *pararectal connective tissue* (rectal retinaculum) is the *rectovesical septum,* which represents the central portion of the lateral neurovascular sheath.

Loose connective tissue occupies the *spaces* between the condensations of the neurovascular sheaths and visceral fasciae. The *prevesical space* located between the anterior abdominal wall and bladder is bounded anteriorly by the transversalis fascia and posteriorly by the vesical fascia. The prevesical space is continuous inferiorly with the *retropubic space.* This space is bounded anteriorly by the posterior surface of the pubic symphysis, posteriorly by the prostatic fascia, and inferiorly by the urogenital diaphragm.

The rectovesical and retropubic spaces communicate laterally with the *paravesical space.* This mobile tissue plane is bounded posteriorly by the paracystic connective tissue, medially by the vesical fascia, and laterally and inferiorly by the parietal pelvic fascia.

Between the rectum and bladder is the *rectovesical space.* The rectovesical septum and the seminal vesicles subdivide this space into two separate compartments termed the *vesicogenital space* and the *rectogenital space* (Figs. 1.59 through 1.62).

Vessels and Nerves of the Bladder

The *arteries* of the bladder may arise directly from the internal iliac artery or from one of its visceral branches (Figs. 1.56 and 1.58).

The superior vesical artery is almost always multiple. Usually, there are two superior vesical arteries, their number ranging from one to four. The superior vesical arteries generally arise from the patent, unobliterated portion of the umbilical artery but occasionally are derived from the obturator artery (4.5%). They supply the base and body of the bladder and generally anastomose with the inferior vesical artery.

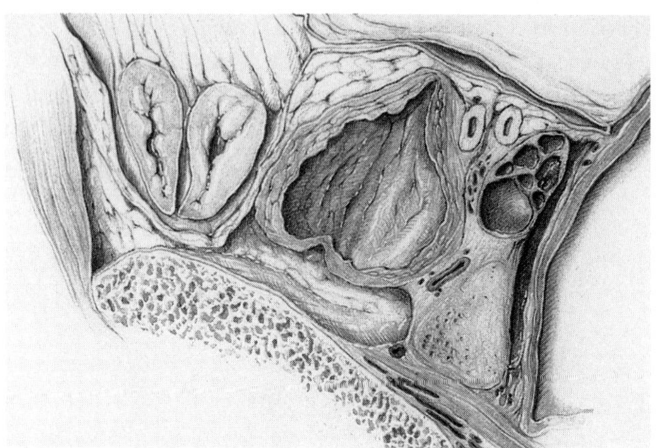

FIGURE 1.60. Paramedian section through the pelvis.

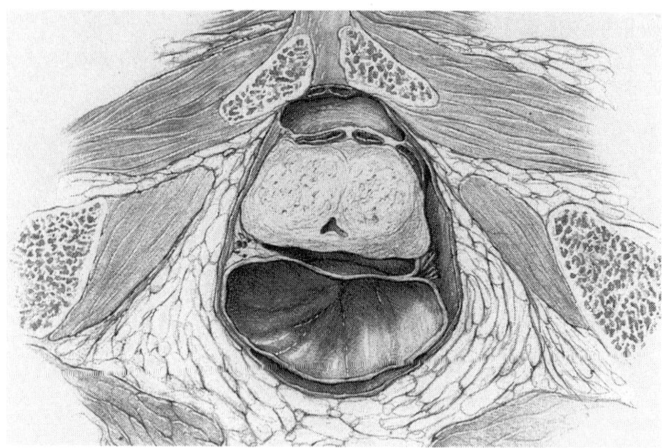

FIGURE 1.62. Transverse section through the pelvis at the level of the prostate.

The inferior vesical artery is usually a direct branch of the internal iliac but may arise from a nearby vessel such as the internal pudendal artery (25%) or inferior gluteal artery (4%). It supplies the bladder base in addition to the prostate and seminal vesicles.

The *veins* of the bladder commence as intramural plexuses. The larger vessels emerging from the bladder wall form the vesical plexus, which communicates with the venous plexus of the prostate. Both plexuses drain into the internal iliac vein.

The *lymph vessels* of the bladder communicate with one another in the paravesical space and may end directly at the external iliac and interiliac lymph nodes or may reach them by way of smaller nodes (anterior, lateral, and posterior vesical nodes). Connections with the internal iliac lymph nodes are occasionally observed.

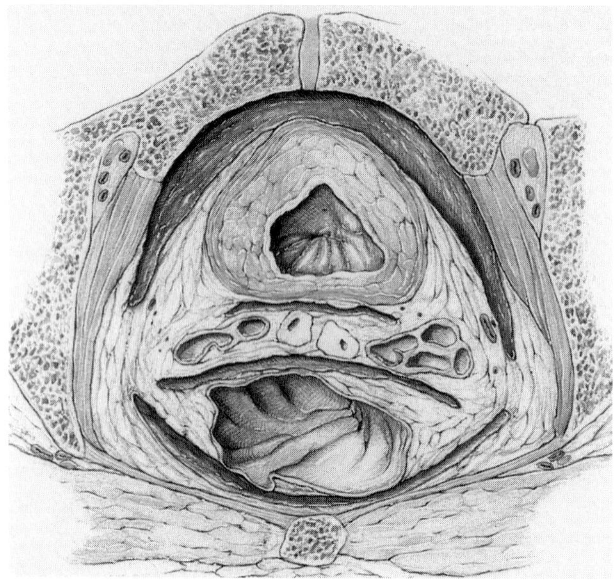

FIGURE 1.61. Transverse section through the pelvis at the level of the seminal vesicles.

The *nerves* supplying the bladder are derived from the pelvic plexuses (Fig. 1.59). The parasympathetic fibers (pelvic splanchnic nerves) of these plexuses originate from the second to fourth sacral segments and supply the detrusor muscle. The sympathetic fibers reach the vesical plexus from the first two lumbar segments by way of the hypogastric plexus.

Prostate

The prostate is enveloped by an external connective-tissue layer, the *prostatic capsule*, and by its visceral fascia, the *prostatic fascia.* The lateral portion of the prostatic fascia, the paraprostatic connective tissue, is well developed posteriorly to form Denonvilliers' fascia. Between the prostate and rectum is the *rectoprostatic space* (Figs. 1.59 and 1.60).

The rectoprostatic space communicates superiorly with the *rectovesical space,* which is subdivided by the seminal vesicles and spermatic ducts into a *rectogenital space* and a *vesicogenital space* (Figs. 1.61 and 1.62). The prostate is fixed to the symphysis anteriorly by the *puboprostatic ligaments,* and it is supported posteriorly by connective-tissue slips from the rectal retinaculum.

Relations of the Female Bladder to Adjacent Organs

The relations of the female bladder to the pelvic connective tissue are obviously gender specific. The parietal fascia of the pelvic floor is reflected onto the bladder at the bladder neck to form the vesical fascia.

The pubovesical ligaments in the female pelvis, derived from the intrapelvic neurovascular-retinacular sheaths, bind the bladder to the pubic symphysis.

The paracystic connective tissue passes from the lateral pelvic wall to the bladder. Tough connective-tissue fibers are distributed to this tissue from the cardinal ligament of the uterus.

The relation of the loose connective tissue to the female

bladder is the same anteriorly (prevesical space) and laterally (paravesical space) as in the male. Posteriorly, between the body of the bladder and the cervix, loose connective tissue occupies the *vesicouterine space.* The *vesicovaginal space* is located more caudally between the bladder base and the front of the vagina.

The relation of the female bladder to the pelvic connective tissue accounts in large part for its relations to adjacent organs.

The female urethra has two clinical subdivisions: a superior part and an inferior part. The superior part, comprising the cranial one-fourth of the urethra, can move relative to the vagina because of the loose connective tissue in the *urethrovaginal space.* The inferior part lacks a true space, and in that area, the vagina and urethra are fused together by their visceral fasciae. The anterosuperior portion of the female urethra is fixed by the lowermost fibers of the pubovesical ligaments, known also as the *pubourethral ligaments.*

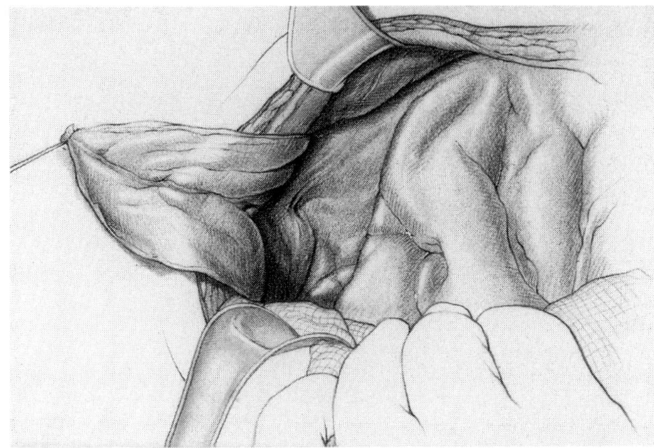

FIGURE 1.64. The freed vesicoumbilical plate is retracted inferiorly.

Application of Surgical Approaches

Anterior Pelvic Exenteration in the Male: Approach to the Nerve-vessel–guiding Plates

Dissection of the Vesicoumbilical Plate

The urachus is isolated near the umbilicus and divided (Fig. 1.63). Entry into the peritoneal cavity at a more inferior level is established by dissecting the *vesicoumbilical plate* (medial umbilical fold, median umbilical fold, transversalis fascia, peritoneal fat, and peritoneum) downward *en bloc* to the lateral umbilical ligaments (Fig. 1.64).

Dissection of the Lateral Bladder Pedicle (Lateral Bladder Retinaculum)

The right-handed surgeon places the fourth and fifth fingers of the left hand on the bladder and medial border of the lateral paracystic connective tissue with the third finger on the internal iliac artery. The index finger is swept medially behind the internal iliac artery into the depths of the pelvis. With this maneuver, the surgeon can displace the lateral retinaculum (lateral bladder pedicle) toward the bladder and the rectovesical septum (posterior bladder pedicle) toward the rectum. With the left index finger behind the lateral pedicle, the internal iliac artery is identified, followed by the anterior branches of the internal iliac artery, the lateral umbilical fold, the superior vesical artery, the inferior vesical artery, and the obturator artery. These vessels are individually isolated, identified, and ligated (Figs. 1.65 and 1.66).

Variants of the Internal Iliac Artery

The branching pattern of the internal iliac artery is extremely variable. The most common variants of the parietal branches of the internal iliac artery are shown in Fig. 1.67. The internal iliac artery usually divides at a variable level into an anterior and a posterior trunk. The origin of the obturator artery is largely independent of the primary bifurcation of the internal iliac artery.

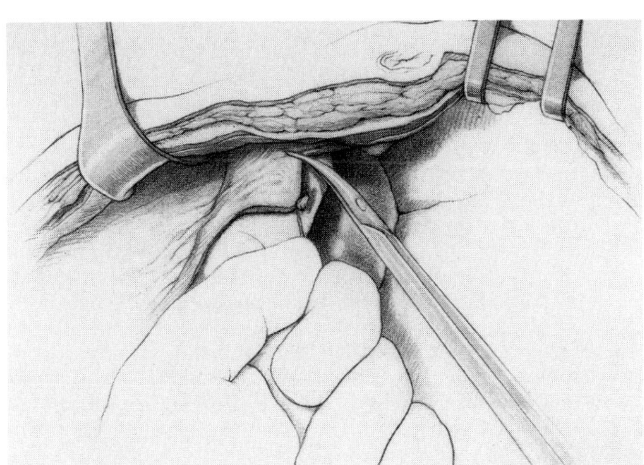

FIGURE 1.63. Dissection of the vesicoumbilical plate.

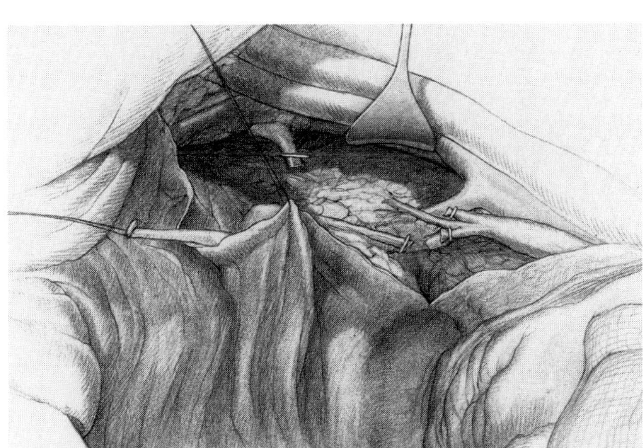

FIGURE 1.65. Dissection of the lateral bladder pedicle.

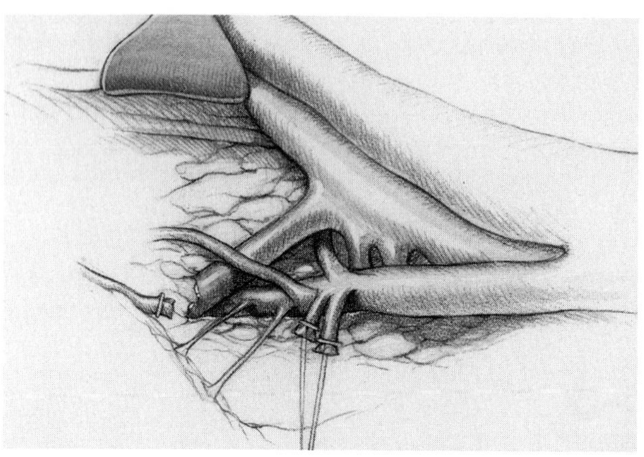

FIGURE 1.66. Close-up view of the dissection of the lateral bladder pedicle. The obturator artery, superior vesical artery, and inferior vesical artery are identified and clipped.

The *obturator artery* may arise from the anterior trunk of the internal iliac artery (Fig. 1.67A, B, and H; 41.5%) or from the posterior trunk (Fig. 1.67C and F). It also may arise from a common trunk for the internal pudendal and inferior gluteal arteries (Fig. 1.67E and I). The obturator artery springs from the internal pudendal artery in approximately 4% of cases (Fig. 1.67G and J) and from the inferior gluteal artery in 5% (Fig. 1.67).

In 19% of cases, the obturator artery arises from the inferior epigastric artery and in 1% from the external iliac. The obturator artery is duplicated in approximately 5% of cases, one vessel arising from the external iliac artery and the other from the internal iliac artery or its branches.

The visceral branches of the internal iliac artery are also subject to considerable variation:

The *umbilical artery (patent section)* consistently gives rise to the superior vesical arteries and the artery of the vas deferens. Rarely, it gives off a middle rectal artery, the vaginal artery, or both.

The *inferior vesical artery* may arise directly from the internal iliac artery or one of its anterior branches. It generally anastomoses with the uterine artery (86%).

The *artery of the vas deferens* may be a direct branch of the internal iliac artery (rare) but usually arises from the umbilical artery. It is absent in 23% of cases and may give origin to a superior vesical artery.

The *middle rectal artery* is rarely absent and normally springs directly from the internal iliac. It also may arise from the vaginal artery or, very rarely, from the sacral arteries.

The *superior vesical arteries,* numbering from one to four, usually arise from the patent section of the umbilical artery but may branch from the uterine artery (9%), the artery of the vas deferens (9%), or the obturator artery (4.5%).

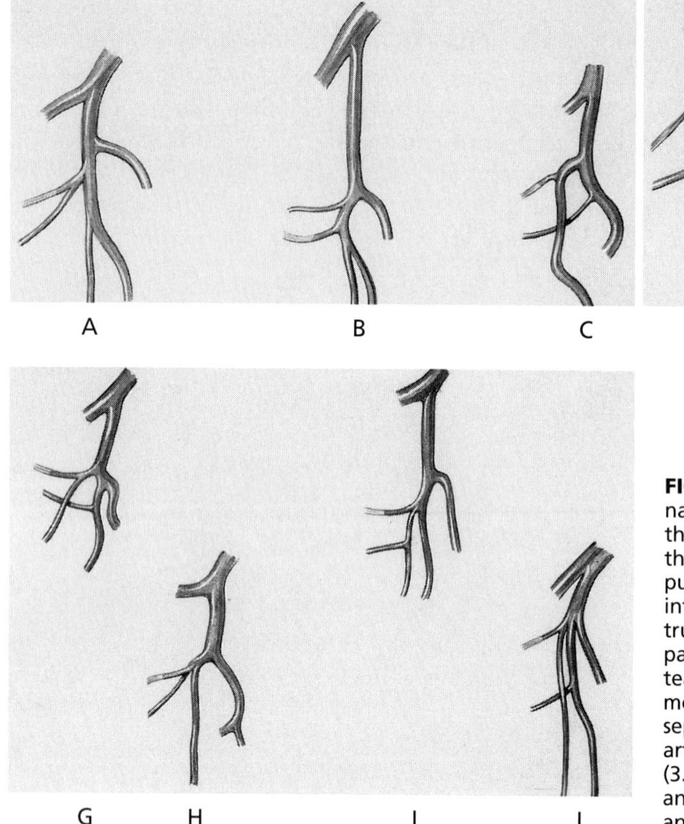

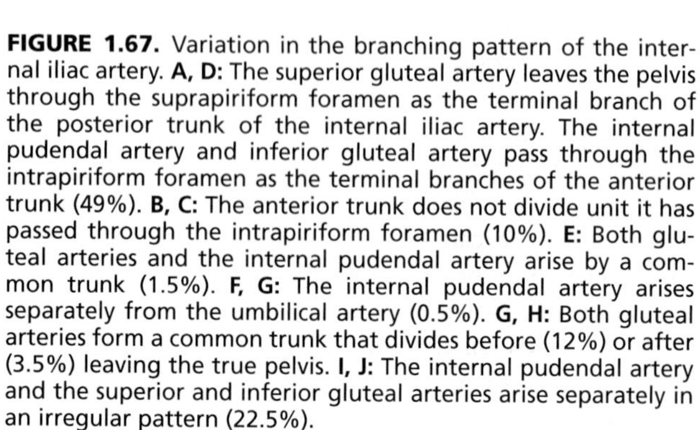

FIGURE 1.67. Variation in the branching pattern of the internal iliac artery. **A, D:** The superior gluteal artery leaves the pelvis through the suprapiriform foramen as the terminal branch of the posterior trunk of the internal iliac artery. The internal pudendal artery and inferior gluteal artery pass through the intrapiriform foramen as the terminal branches of the anterior trunk (49%). **B, C:** The anterior trunk does not divide unit it has passed through the intrapiriform foramen (10%). **E:** Both gluteal arteries and the internal pudendal artery arise by a common trunk (1.5%). **F, G:** The internal pudendal artery arises separately from the umbilical artery (0.5%). **G, H:** Both gluteal arteries form a common trunk that divides before (12%) or after (3.5%) leaving the true pelvis. **I, J:** The internal pudendal artery and the superior and inferior gluteal arteries arise separately in an irregular pattern (22.5%).

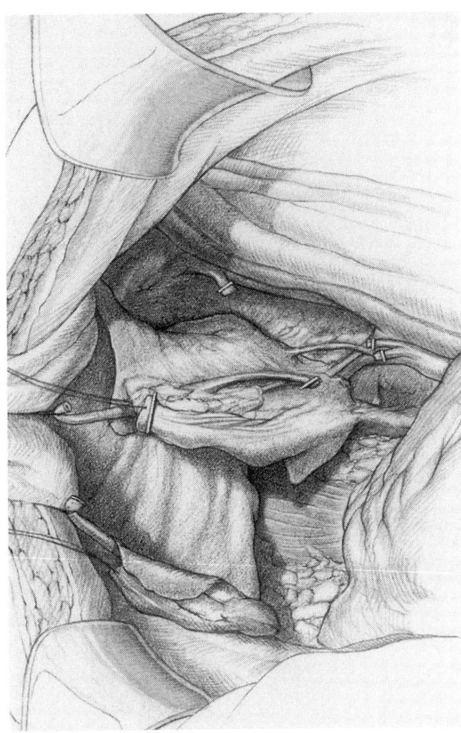

FIGURE 1.68. Exposure of the rectovesical septum (posterior bladder pedicle). The anterior branches of the internal iliac artery have been ligated, and the incision in the cul de sac has been completed. The right vas deferens and clipped ureter are retracted forward along with the freed lymph node package.

Anastomoses between the superior and inferior vesical arteries are generally present.

The *uterine artery* is usually a direct branch of the internal iliac but may arise conjointly with the vaginal or middle rectal artery. Duplication can occur. When necessary, the uterine artery can adequately assume the supply function of the vesical arteries.

Exposure of the Rectovesical Septum (Posterior Bladder Pedicle)

The neurovascular sheath transmits the arteries and veins of the seminal vesicles and prostate in addition to the pelvic splanchnic nerves. The space between the rectal fascia and Denonvilliers' fascia is developed. The posterior bladder pedicle is held between the second and third fingers as the second finger presses downward on the rectum, and the posterior pedicle is progressively ligated as far as the endopelvic parietal fascia. As traction is placed on the vas deferens and ureter to enlarge the space between the rectal fascia and Denonvilliers' fascia, individual portions of the posterior pedicle can be clipped or ligated under direct vision. The posterior pedicle is then progressively divided to the endopelvic parietal fascia (Fig. 1.68). The pelvic wall comes into view on the lateral side of these neurovascular bundles as they are progressively isolated and clipped or tied (Fig. 1.69).

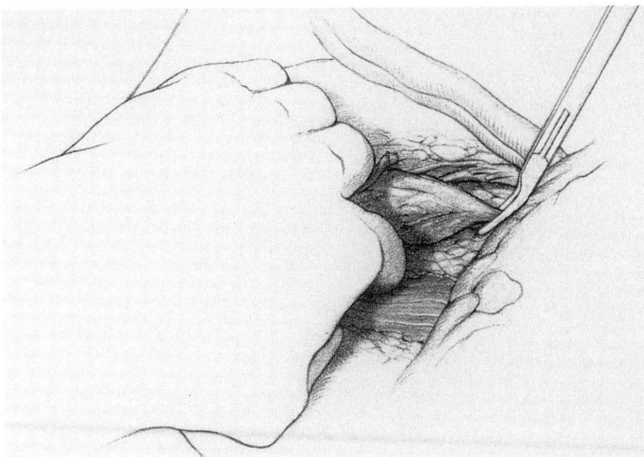

FIGURE 1.69. The posterior bladder pedicle is held between the second and third fingers while the second finger presses the rectum downward. The posterior pedicle is then progressively ligated.

Anterior Pelvic Exenteration in the Female

Exposure of the Posterior Bladder Pedicle

The peritoneum of the rectouterine pouch is incised from the pelvic wall aspect, and the specimen is retracted inferiorly by the vesicoumbilical plate and a uterine traction suture (Fig. 1.70). After division of the peritoneum over the rectum in the area of the rectouterine pouch, the posterior bladder pedicle, which includes the cardinal ligament in the female, is progressively ligated or clipped as far as the parietal pelvic fascia.

Opening the Posterior Vaginal Wall

The posterior bladder pedicle is clipped or ligated approximately 3 to 4 cm past the cervix, and the posterior vaginal wall is opened (Fig. 1.71). Much as in an anterior exenteration in the male, the remaining posterior pedicle is encircled

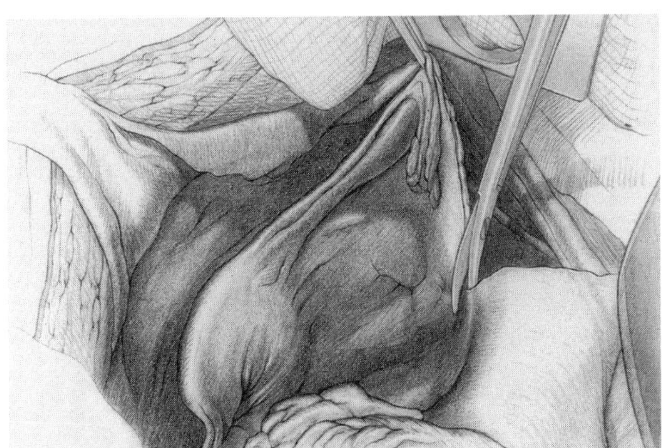

FIGURE 1.70. Line of incision in the peritoneum. Starting at the pelvic wall, the peritoneum is divided just over the rectum in the area of the rectouterine pouch.

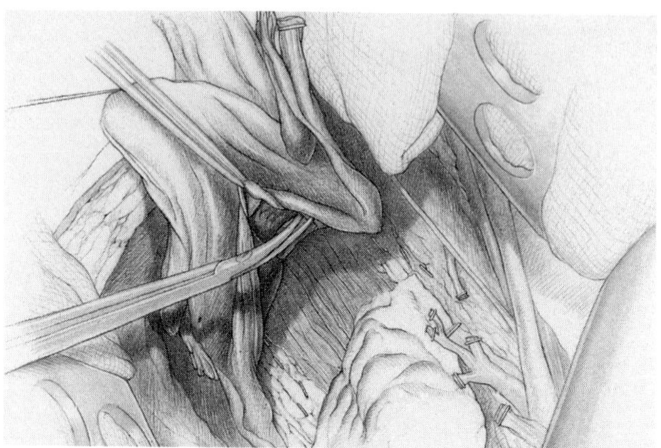

FIGURE 1.71. Exposure and division of the posterior bladder pedicle, which in the female includes the cardinal ligament. The posterior vaginal wall is opened 3 to 4 cm caudal to the cervix.

(the second finger is in the vagina) and progressively ligated forward to the parietal pelvic fascia.

Continence Following Radical Prostatectomy and Orthotopic Reconstruction Following Female and Male Anterior Exenteration

Anatomy and Innervation of the Rhabdosphincter: Male

Macroscopic Anatomy. The muscle fibers of the rhabdosphincter are arranged in a loop-shaped fashion on the ventral and lateral aspects of the membranous urethra (Fig. 1.72). On gross anatomic examination, comparatively strong smooth muscular and connective tissue can be noted dorsal to the membranous urethra (i.e., in the region of the perineal body). Both ends of the omega-shaped sphincter insert at the perineal body. The sphincter loop is continuous with muscle bundles that run along the anterior and lateral aspects of the prostate and extend cranially to the bladder neck. Thus, in the adult male, the rhabdosphincter of the urethra does not form a complete collar around the membranous urethra. It should rather be described as a muscular coat ventral and lateral to the membranous urethra and prostate, the core of which is the omega-shaped loop around the urethra. Furthermore, the rhabdosphincter is separated from the ventral portion of the levator ani muscle by a sheet of connective tissue.

Histology. The histologic findings in adult men confirm the data gained by gross anatomic examination (Fig. 1.73). The rhabdosphincter is a vertical muscular coat ventral and lateral to the prostate and membranous urethra extending from the bulb of the penis toward the region of the bladder neck. In all investigated specimens, striated muscle fibers corresponding to the deep transverse perineal muscle cannot be identified.

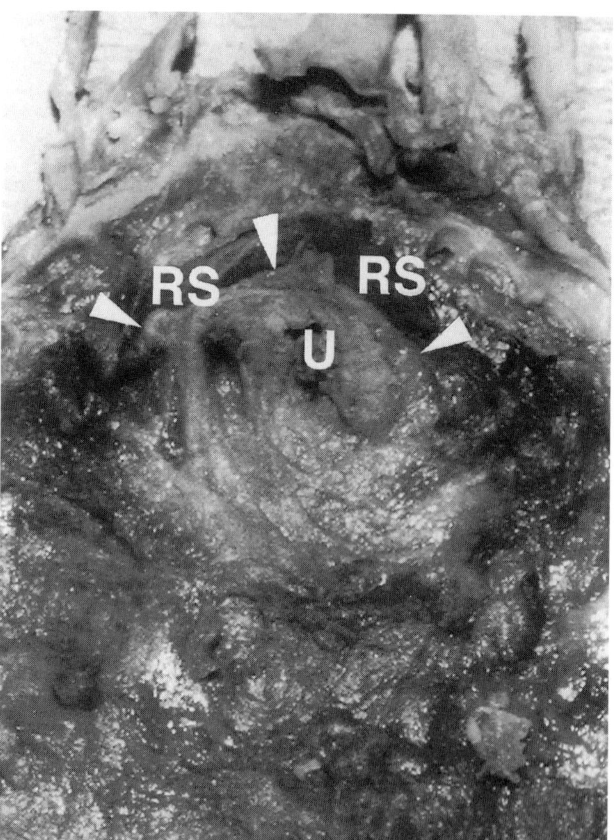

FIGURE 1.72. Anatomic specimen (adult rhabdosphincter, cranial view). RS, rhabdosphincter; U, urethra.

Nerve Supply. The pudendal nerve derives from the second, third, and fourth sacral spinal nerves. It takes a completely different course than the autonomic fibers of the pelvic plexus. The rhabdosphincter of the male urethra is supplied by fine branches of the pudendal nerve. These branches are given off lateral to the rhabdosphincter and

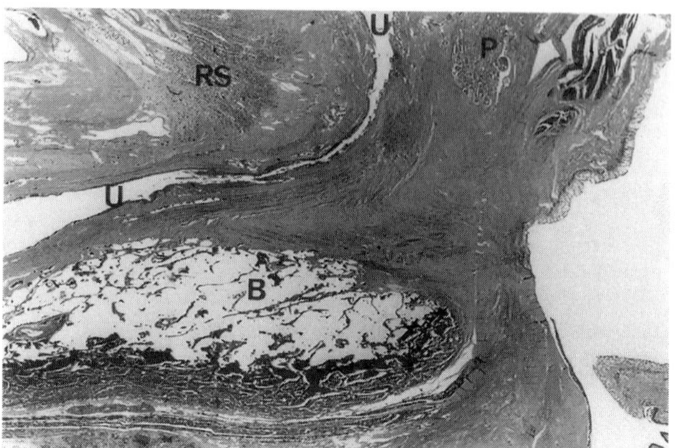

FIGURE 1.73. Histologic specimen (adult, sagittal section). B, bulb of penis; P, prostate; RS, rhabdosphincter; U, urethra.

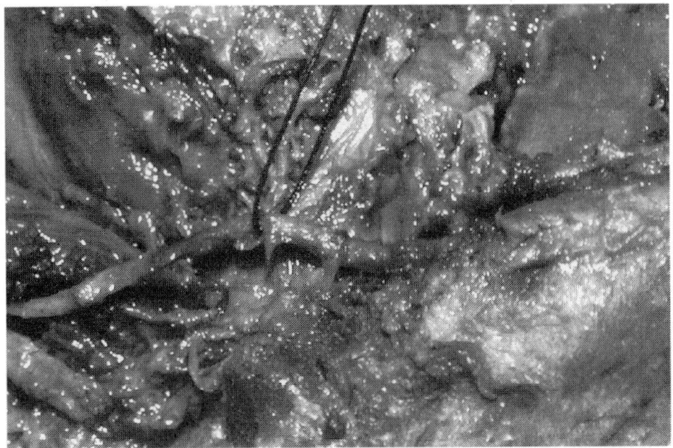

FIGURE 1.74. Anatomic specimen (adult, lateral view; the right hip bone has been completely removed).

reach the muscle at its dorsolateral aspects; the mean distance from the membranous urethra to the point of entry of these fibers into the rhabdosphincter is 0.7 to 1.3 cm (Figs. 1.74 and 1.75).

Anatomy and Innervation of the Rhabdosphincter: Female

On macroscopic examination, the sphincteric muscle is encountered on the ventral and lateral aspects of the urethra. Microscopically, this muscle corresponds to the omega-shaped rhabdosphincter in the male.

On histologic examination, in the cranial two-thirds of the urethra, three smooth muscle layers can be identified forming an outer and an inner longitudinal and a middle transverse layer. The inner longitudinal layer is delicate, thinning out toward the external meatus. The middle transverse layer is considerably thicker than the longitudinal layers (Fig. 1.76A–C). In serial transverse sections of the caudal urethra, there are abundant aspects, whereas dorsally there are mainly fibrous structures with only a few striated fibers. In transverse sections, the rhabdosphincter has an omega-like shape (Fig. 1.77).

The autonomic fibers that supply the pelvic visceral organs emerge from the pelvic plexuses. They then course in a sagittal layer of connective tissue containing vessels and nerves (the vessel nerve plate) lateral to the rectum, in which they course to the ventral pelvic organs. The hypogastric and pelvic splanchnic nerves have been identified in this vessel nerve plate between the rectum and the pelvic wall. The cranial portion of the pelvic plexus is located close to the lateral margin of the rectouterine pouch; its ventral and caudal portions extend to the lateral aspect of the cervix (Fig. 1.78).

The pudendal nerve courses alongside the internal pudendal vessels on the lateral aspects of the ischiorectal fossa inside the pudendal canal. The inferior rectal nerves, perineal nerves, and dorsal nerve of the clitoris branch off in the region of the pelvic floor. Arising from the terminal branch of the pudendal nerve, several thin branches run to the rhabdosphincter, which they enter on its lateral aspect (Fig. 1.79).

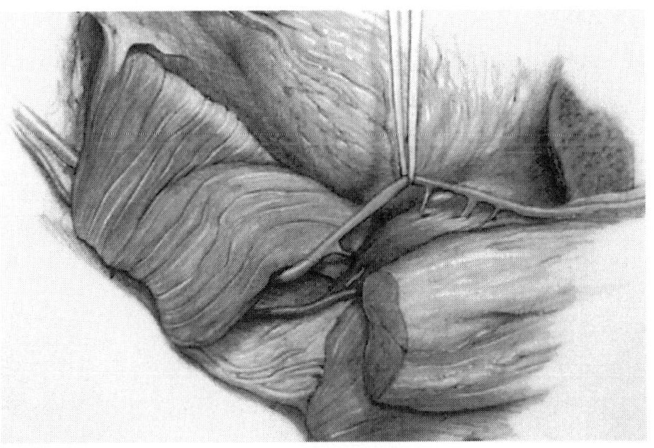

FIGURE 1.75. Corresponding drawing to Fig. 1.74.

Radical Prostatectomy

Retropubic Versus Perineal Approach

The perineal approach, by preserving the paraprostatic tissue (lateral pelvic fascia), avoids injury to the dorsal vein complex. In a perineal prostatectomy, the prostate is removed within the paraprostatic tissue, whereas the retropubic prostatectomy removes the prostate together with all paraprostatic tissue. The retropubic approach involves incision of the paraprostatic tissue (lateral pelvic fascia) and division of the dorsal vein complex (arrow). Thus, in contrast to the perineal approach, the retropubic approach includes removal not just of Denonvilliers' fascia but also of the paraprostatic tissue (lateral pelvic fascia) (Fig. 1.80).

Retropubic Radical Prostatectomy

Exposure and Division of the Striated Urethral Sphincter (Rhabdosphincter) and Membranous Urethra. After division of the dorsal venous complex, the anterolateral aspects of the striated urethral sphincter (rhabdosphincter) can be identified. It forms an omega-shaped loop anterior and lateral to the membranous urethra, its two crura inserting into the central tendon of the perineum (Fig. 1.81). In anatomic dissections, after the prostate has been removed, the membranous urethra, the omega-shaped rhabdosphincter, and the central tendon can be seen on the inner aspect of the transverse perineal ligament. The deep dorsal penile vein, the dorsal penile artery, and the dorsal penile nerve course between the inner and outer fasciae of the transverse perineal ligament. The deep dorsal penile vein runs between the arcuate ligament and transverse

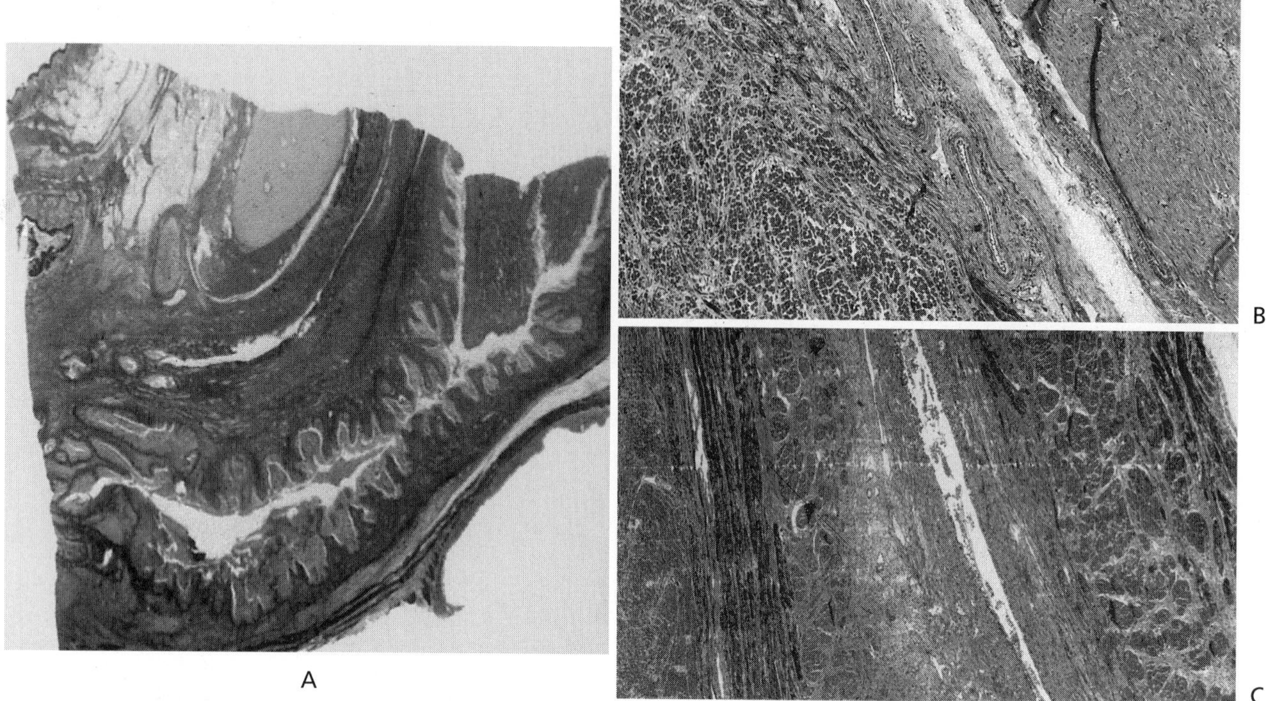

FIGURE 1.76. **A:** Median sagittal section of pelvic floor in fetal specimen. **B:** View of cranial two-thirds of female urethra: three layers of smooth muscle forming outer and inner longitudinal and middle transverse layers. **C:** In caudal third of the urethra, the rhabdosphincter is visible, with major portion in ventral and ventrolateral aspects of the urethra.

perineal ligament, and the dorsal penile artery and nerve run directly through the tissue of the transverse perineal ligament (Fig. 1.81).

Exposure of the Rectogenital Space. The membranous urethra is divided on the line shown. The posterior prostatic fascia is divided at its attachment, the rectourethral septum (the apex of the wedge-shaped perineal body), and the rectogenital space is opened. The rectal fascia is identified at the posterior aspect of the rectogenital space.

Exposure of the Vesicogenital Space. The prostate is now resected with the paraprostatic tissue between the rectogenital space and levator ani muscle. The seminal vesicles and the ampullae of the spermatic ducts are dissected from the bladder detrusor, following the course of the rectogenital space. The prostate is transected at the bladder neck and dissected out of the rectogenital space.

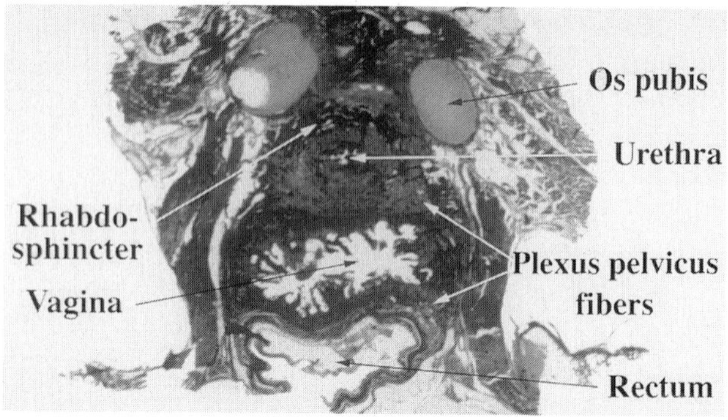

FIGURE 1.77. Transverse histologic section shows omega-shaped rhabdosphincter in caudal third of the urethra.

Modification: Nerve-sparing Radical Prostatectomy

In the modification of the nerve-sparing radical prostatectomy, the neurovascular bundle (base of the paraprostatic tissue) of the prostate is preserved. This bundle contains the cavernous nerves, fibers from the pelvic plexus to the membranous urethra, arterial branches to the prostate, the venous prostatic plexus, and prostatic lymph vessels (Fig. 1.82); to approach the neurovascular bundle, the paraprostatic tissue on the lateral surface of the prostate is incised and released. Located on the posterolateral aspect of the prostate, the neurovascular bundle is deeply embedded in the parietal layer of the fascia (paraprostatic tissue).

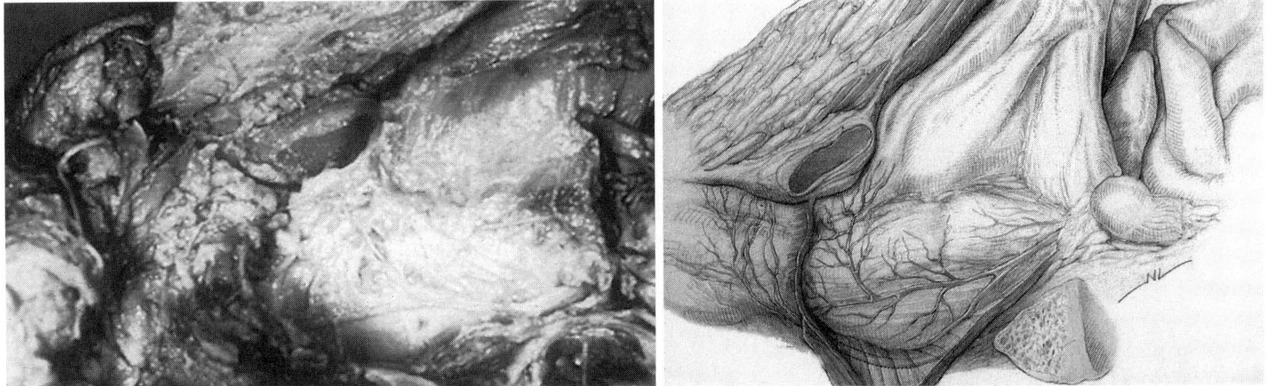

FIGURE 1.78. **A:** Lateral view of fetal specimen shows autonomic nerve supply to urethra relative to pelvic organs. **B:** Corresponding drawing to **A.**

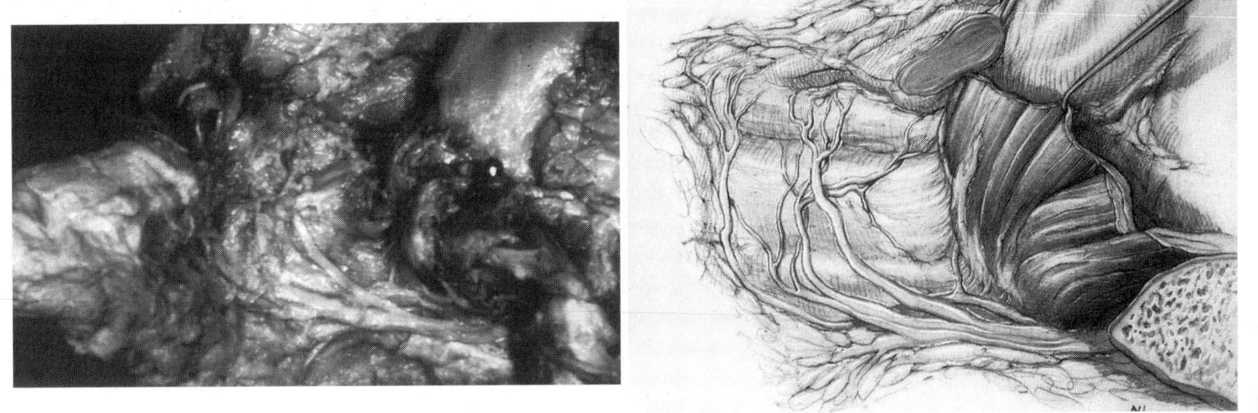

FIGURE 1.79. **A:** Several thin branches emerging from the pudendal nerve course to caudal third of urethra entering the rhabdosphincter at the lateral aspects. **B:** Corresponding drawing to **A.**

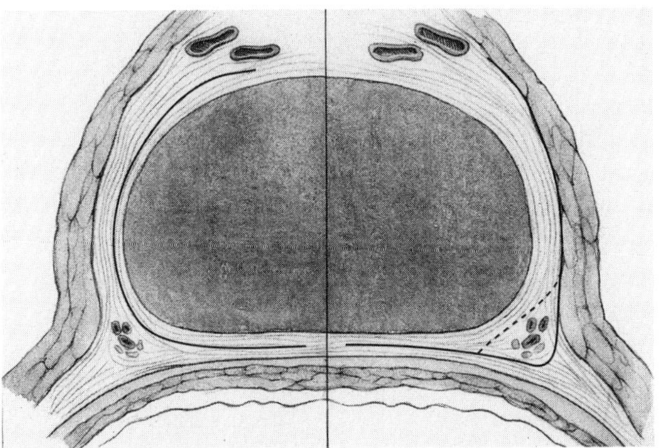

FIGURE 1.80. Approaches for perineal **(left)** and retropubic **(right)** prostatectomy. The significance of the paraprostatic tissue (lateral pelvic fascia) in each approach is shown (... = nerve-sparing approach for a retropubic radical prostatectomy).

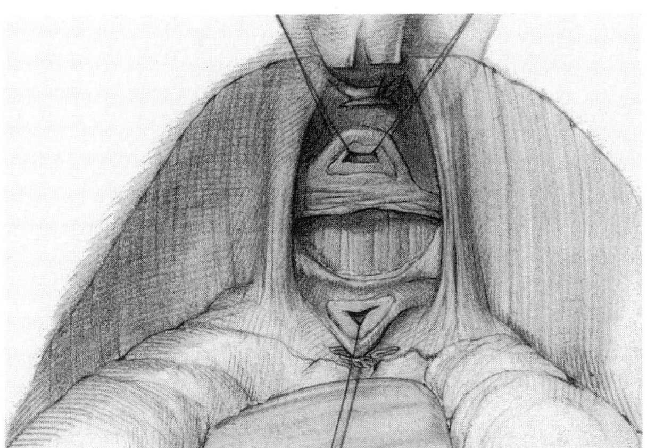

FIGURE 1.81. The rectourethral septum is incised, Denonvilliers' fascia is exposed, and the rectogenital space is entered. The rectal fascia is visible in the depths of the field.

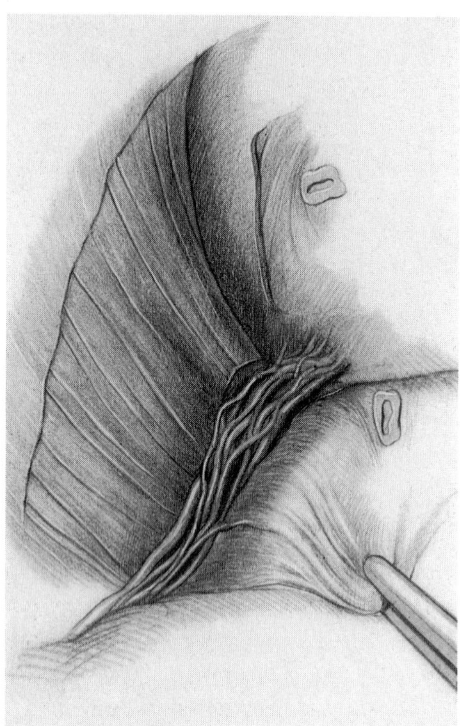

FIGURE 1.82. In this anatomic specimen, the left neurovascular bundle has been dissected out of the posterolateral portion of the paraprostatic tissue.

INGUINAL REGION

Anatomy

The inguinal canal obliquely traverses the abdominal wall in the medial portion of the inguinal region. The canal has a lateral-to-medial orientation, its lateral part being situated more deeply than its medial part. It has an average length of 4 to 5 cm in men and is about 5 mm longer in women.

The external (superficial) inguinal ring forms the external opening of the inguinal canal. Located in the external oblique aponeurosis, the ring is bounded by two thickenings in the aponeurosis termed the *medial* and *lateral crura* (Fig. 1.83). Both crura join at the superolateral aspect of the external ring and are sometimes reinforced in that area by transverse intercrural fibers. The development and location of these fibers are subject to marked individual variations, and the fibers can be dissected at the external inguinal ring in only 27% of the population.

The external inguinal ring is exposed by incision of the external spermatic fascia. The ring is elliptical in shape and highly variable in size and length. In 80% of cases, the superolateral border of the external ring is located above the medial half of the inguinal ligament. In the remaining 20%, its boundary is more superolateral and, in extreme cases, may extend to the anterosuperior iliac spine.

The slitlike internal opening of the inguinal canal, the internal (deep) inguinal ring, represents an evagination of the transversalis fascia. It is covered internally by parietal peritoneum, so surgical exposure of the internal ring requires incision of the peritoneum.

The layers of the lateral abdominal wall contribute in varying degrees to the substance of the inguinal canal walls. The anterior wall is formed by the external oblique aponeurosis, which is continued onto the spermatic cord as the thin external spermatic fascia. The floor of the canal is formed by the inguinal ligament.

The caudal fibers of the transversus abdominis muscle form the roof of the inguinal canal. The internal oblique muscle does not contribute to formation of the canal roof. Its caudal fibers are continued onto the spermatic cord as the cremaster muscle. The cremaster, which forms the middle coat of the spermatic cord, varies greatly in development among different individuals, and the middle covering is considered to consist of both the spermatic fascia and the cremaster muscle. Normally, a definite plane of cleavage can be developed between the internal oblique and transversus abdominis muscles in the region of the inguinal canal.

The posterior wall of the inguinal canal is formed by the transversalis fascia. Medial to the internal ring this fascia is strengthened by the variable interfoveolar ligament (Hessel-

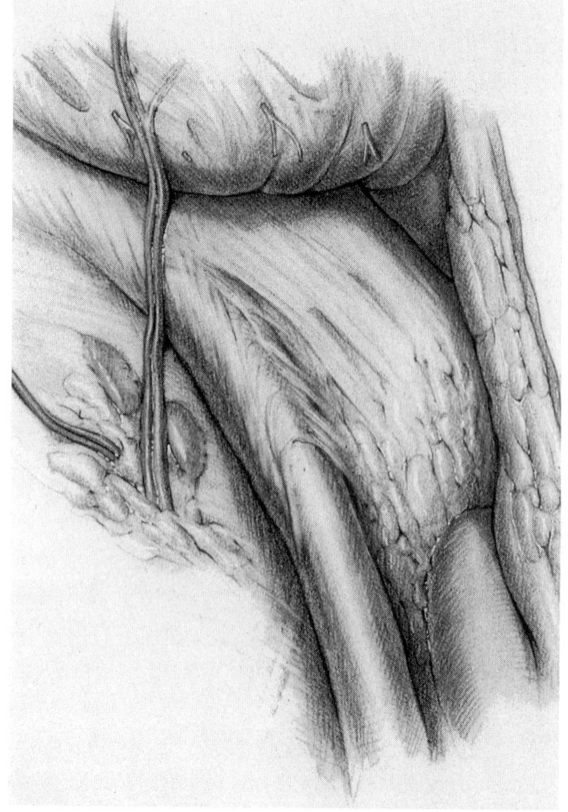

FIGURE 1.83. Inguinal region. Subcutaneous plane.

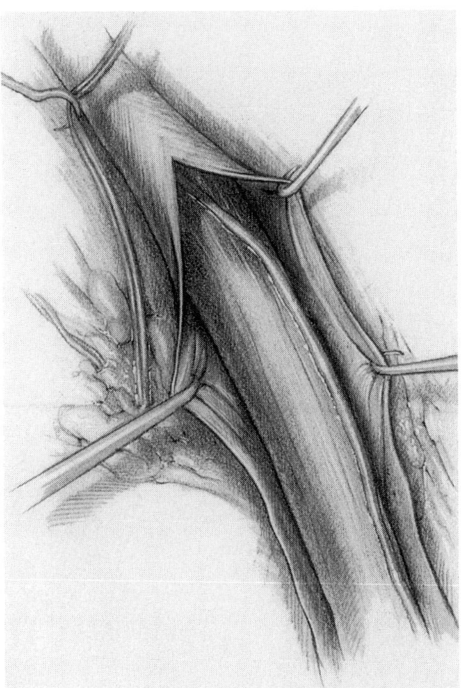

FIGURE 1.84. Spermatic cord after incision of the external spermatic fascia.

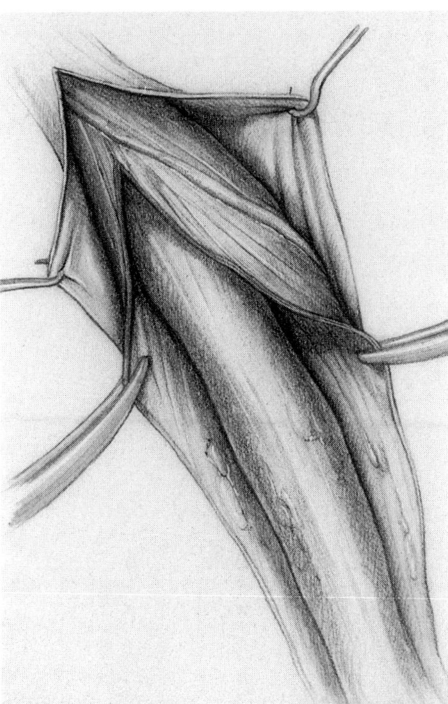

FIGURE 1.85. Spermatic cord after incision of the cremasteric fascia.

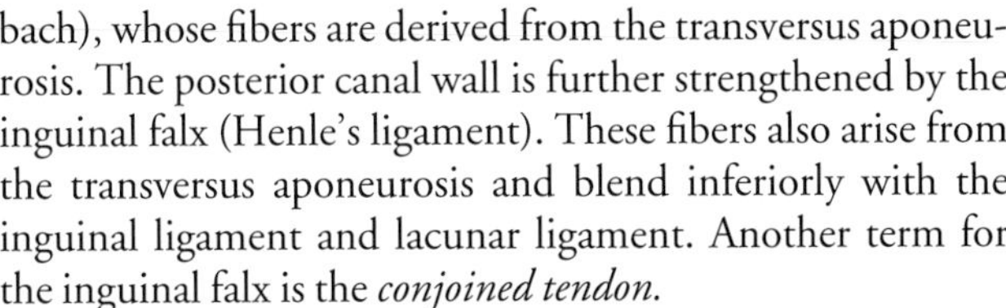

bach), whose fibers are derived from the transversus aponeurosis. The posterior canal wall is further strengthened by the inguinal falx (Henle's ligament). These fibers also arise from the transversus aponeurosis and blend inferiorly with the inguinal ligament and lacunar ligament. Another term for the inguinal falx is the *conjoined tendon.*

The layered dissections in Figs. 1.83 through 1.87 serve to clarify the arrangement of the individual abdominal tissue planes in the inguinal canal. The firm subcutaneous fatty layer in the inguinal region, permeated by fibrous strands and known also as *Camper's fascia,* is removed to expose the external oblique aponeurosis. This aponeurosis is continued onto the spermatic cord as the external spermatic fascia (Fig. 1.83). Incision of the outer coat of the spermatic cord exposes the middle layer, composed of the cremasteric fascia and the cremaster muscle, which is a continuation of the internal oblique muscle. The genital branch of the genitofemoral nerve can also be identified in this plane (Fig. 1.84). The external oblique aponeurosis can now be split further laterally and superiorly to expose the anterior terminal branch of the iliohypogastric nerve. The middle coat of the spermatic cord is divided to expose the internal spermatic fascia, which intimately invests the cord structures (Fig. 1.85). Division of the caudal fibers of the internal oblique muscle uncovers the portion of the transversus abdominis that forms the roof of the inguinal canal (Fig. 1.86). As the last step in the dissection, the internal coat of the spermatic cord is incised to expose the cord structures

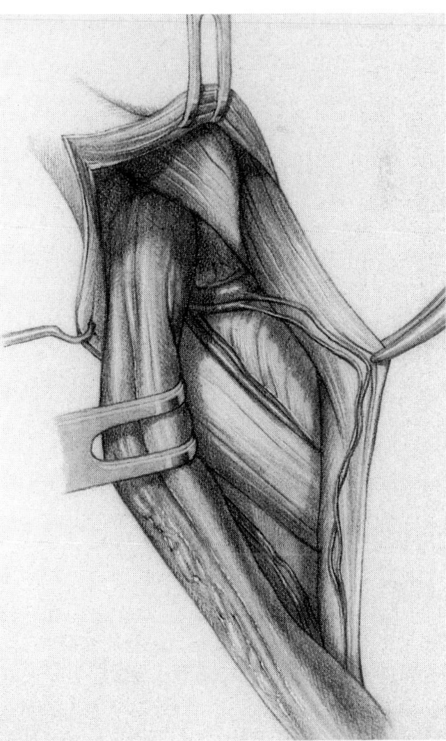

FIGURE 1.86. Spermatic cord after splitting of the internal oblique.

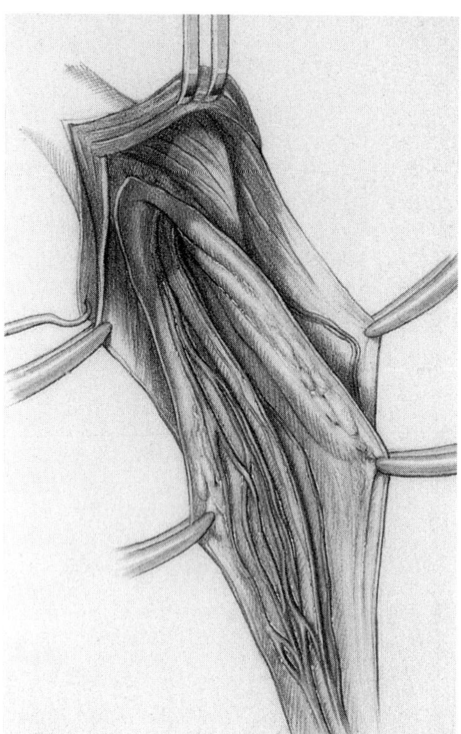

FIGURE 1.87. Spermatic cord after incision of the internal spermatic fascia.

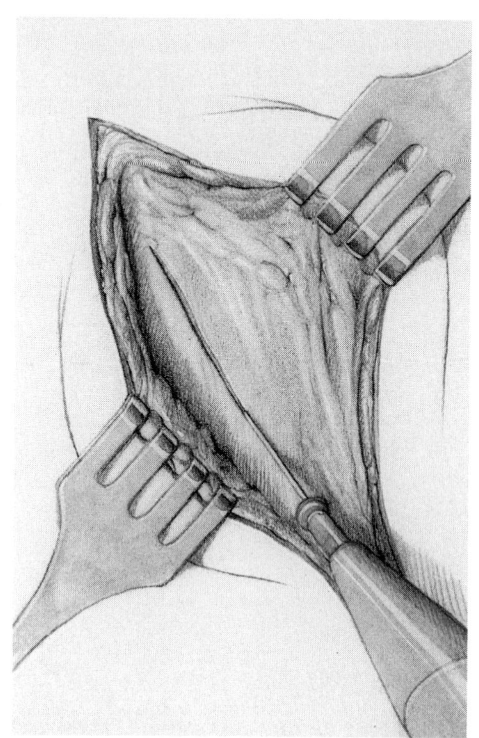

FIGURE 1.88. Exposure of the external inguinal ring.

themselves: the vas deferens, testicular artery, and pampiniform plexus (Fig. 1.87).

Inguinal Approach

Exposure of the External Inguinal Ring

The subcutaneous fat and Camper's fascia are divided along with branches of the superficial epigastric vessels and the superficial circumflex iliac vessels. The external oblique aponeurosis is identified (Fig. 1.88).

Exposure of the Internal Inguinal Ring

The external oblique aponeurosis and the most anterior portion of the external spermatic fascia are divided, sparing the genital branch of the genitofemoral nerve on the cremaster muscle medially. The internal oblique muscle and cremasteric fascia are exposed (Fig. 1.89).

Further exposure of the inguinal canal is accomplished by incision of the cremasteric fascia and internal oblique muscle (Fig. 1.90). The iliohypogastric nerve and genitofemoral nerve are visible on the medial side.

The internal oblique muscle is divided, exposing the transversus abdominis (Fig. 1.91). Following release of the cremaster muscle (whose fibers arise from the internal oblique), the spermatic cord with the surrounding internal spermatic fascia (derived from the transversalis fascia) is undermined and snared (Fig. 1.91). The internal fascia of the spermatic cord is dissected from the transversalis fascia to increase the length of the cord (Fig. 1.92). The external oblique aponeurosis and the incised internal oblique and transversus abdominis muscles are retracted upward in the proximal wound angle, allowing for further dissection of the spermatic cord, which is freed up into the internal inguinal ring (Figs. 1.93 and 1.94). The inferior epigastric vessels can be seen medial to the inguinal ring.

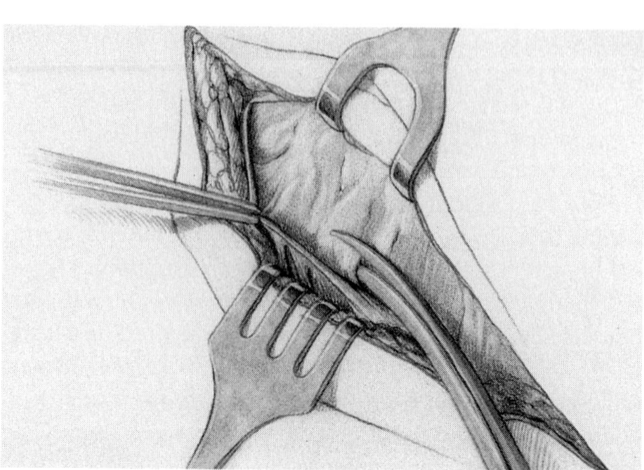

FIGURE 1.89. Division of the external oblique aponeurosis.

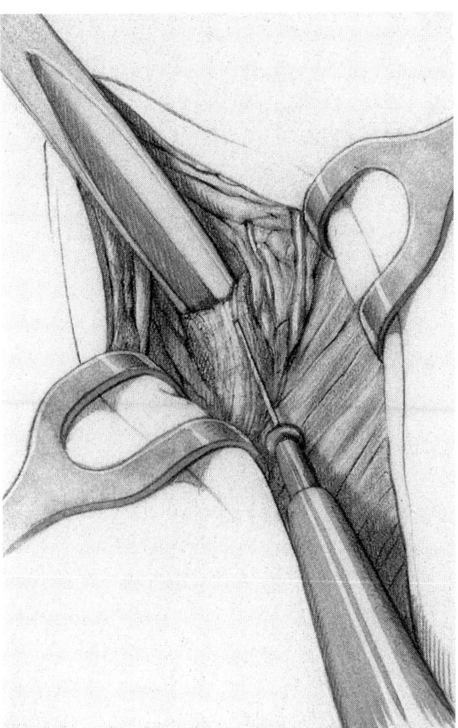

FIGURE 1.90. The cremasteric fascia and internal oblique are divided.

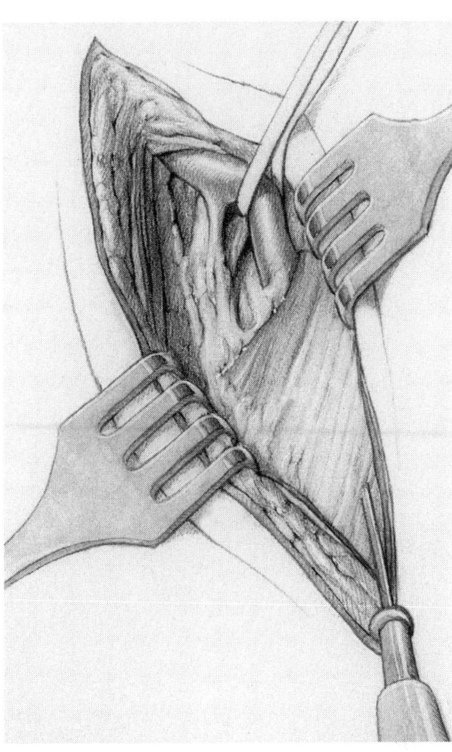

FIGURE 1.91. Mobilization of the spermatic cord and division of the transversus abdominis.

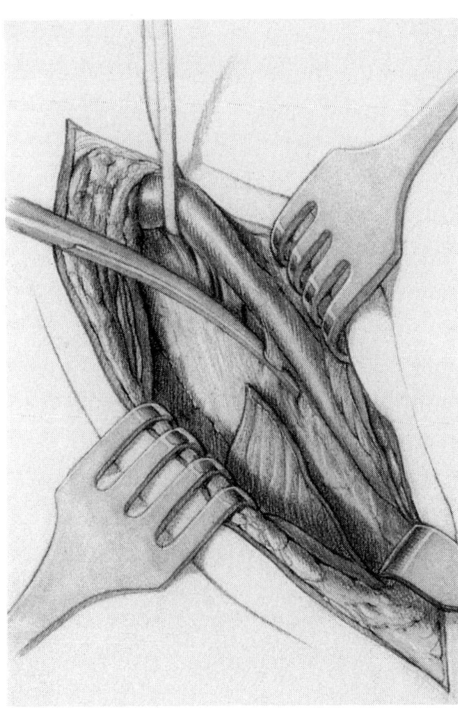

FIGURE 1.92. The spermatic cord is dissected from the transversalis fascia, and the internal ring is exposed.

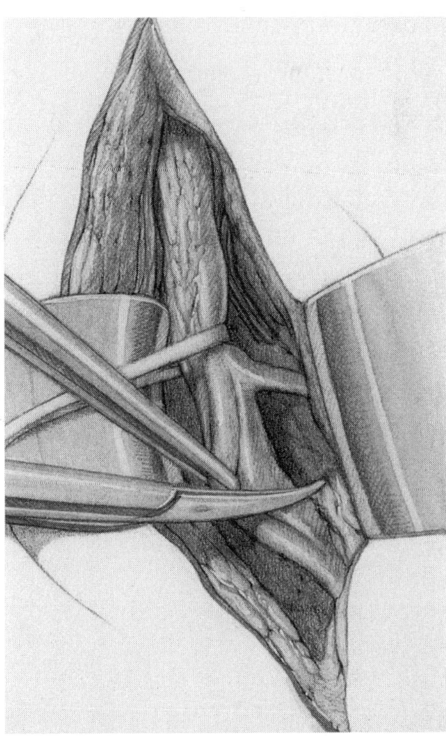

FIGURE 1.93. After incision of the internal spermatic fascia, the vas deferens and its artery are separated from the pampiniform plexus and testicular artery.

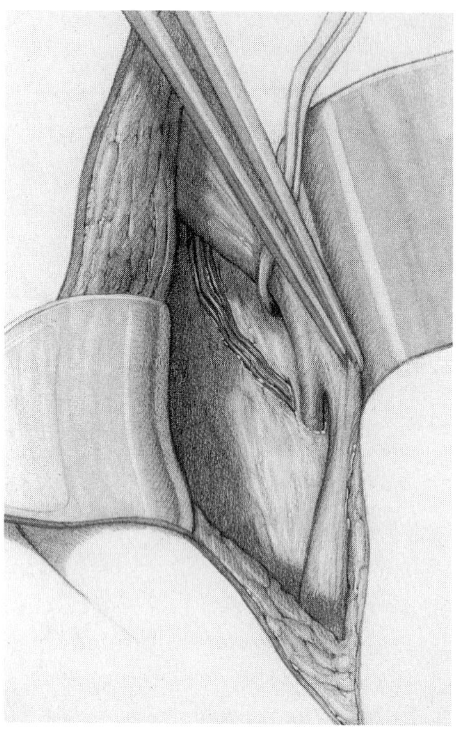

FIGURE 1.94. The inferior epigastric artery and the accompanying inferior epigastric veins are dissected free on the medial aspect of the spermatic cord.

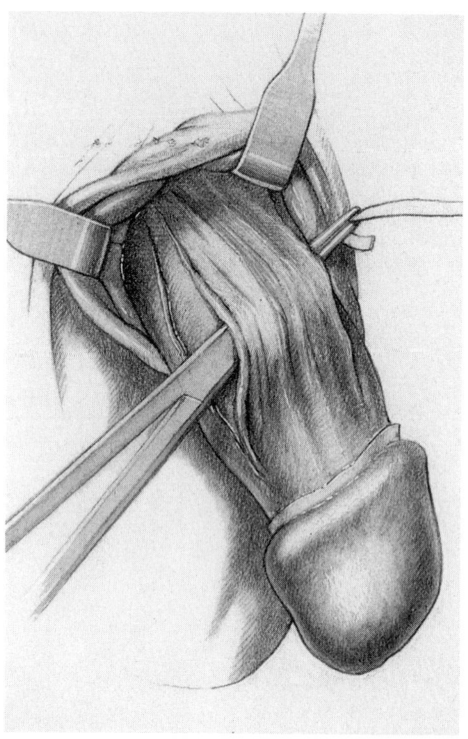

FIGURE 1.96. The neurovascular bundle is undermined and snared with a vascular tape.

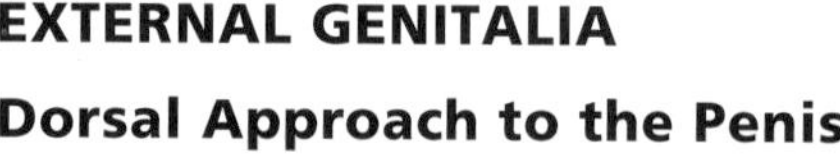

EXTERNAL GENITALIA

Dorsal Approach to the Penis

Exposure of the Dorsal Neurovascular Bundle

The superficial and deep penile fasciae are dissected and incised to the tunica albuginea along the lateral side of the penis (Fig. 1.95). A counterincision is made on the opposite side, and the neurovascular bundle (deep dorsal vein, artery, and nerve) is underrun and snared with a tape (Fig. 1.96).

The anatomic dissection in Fig. 1.97 shows the structures of the dorsal neurovascular bundle: the deep dorsal penile vein, the dorsal penile artery, and the dorsal nerve of the penis, located between the deep penile fascia and the tunica albuginea.

The fascial planes of the penis are shown in schematic cross section in Fig. 1.98.

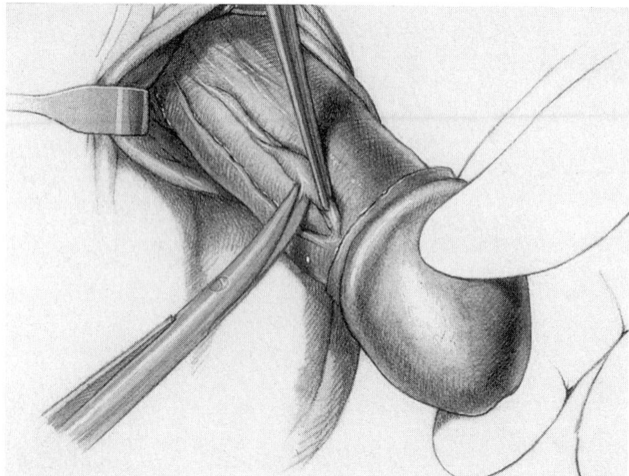

FIGURE 1.95. The superficial and deep fasciae of the penis are divided down to the tunica albuginea.

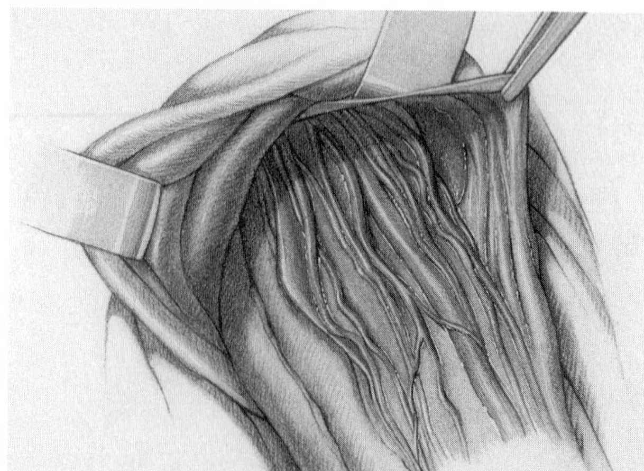

FIGURE 1.97. Anatomic dissection showing the structures of the neurovascular bundle: the deep dorsal penile vein, dorsal penile artery, and dorsal penile nerve.

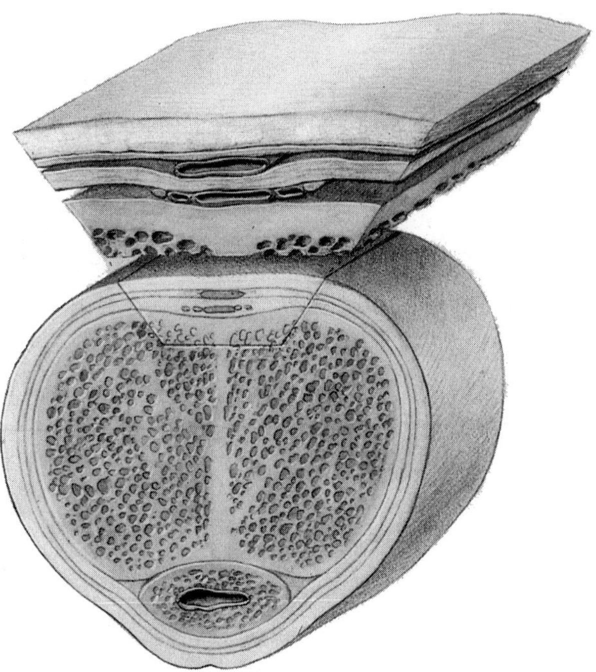

FIGURE 1.98. Schematic cross section of the penis.

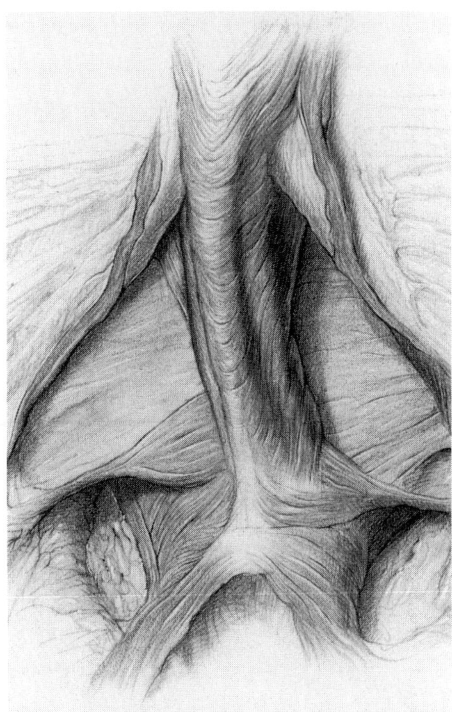

FIGURE 1.99. Anatomic dissection showing the pelvic floor structures from the inferior aspect.

PERINEUM

Anatomy of the Male Urethra and Pelvic Floor

The dissection shown in Fig. 1.99 demonstrates the relations of the corpus spongiosum to the pelvic floor. The corpus spongiosum is covered by the bulbospongiosus muscle and relates to the inferior aspect of the transverse perineal ligament, to which it is attached by loose connective tissue. The so-called "urogenital diaphragm" consists essentially of tough, transversely oriented connective-tissue fibers—the transverse perineal ligament. All pelvic muscles, as well as the levator ani of the pelvic diaphragm and the external anal sphincter, converge at the central tendon of the perineum. These structures are demonstrated more clearly by removal of the corpus spongiosum at the bulb of the penis along with the bulbospongiosus muscle (Fig. 1.100).

In another dissection (Fig. 1.101), the pubic bone has been partially removed to demonstrate the neurovascular supply of the penis (dorsal penile artery and nerve, deep dorsal penile vein). Removal of the pubic symphysis and corpora cavernosa renders a view of the transverse perineal ligament (Fig. 1.102).

Figure 1.103 shows the individual structures of the urogenital diaphragm in greater detail. Visible features include the pubic arcuate ligament, the transverse perineal ligament, and the external urethral sphincter, which forms a

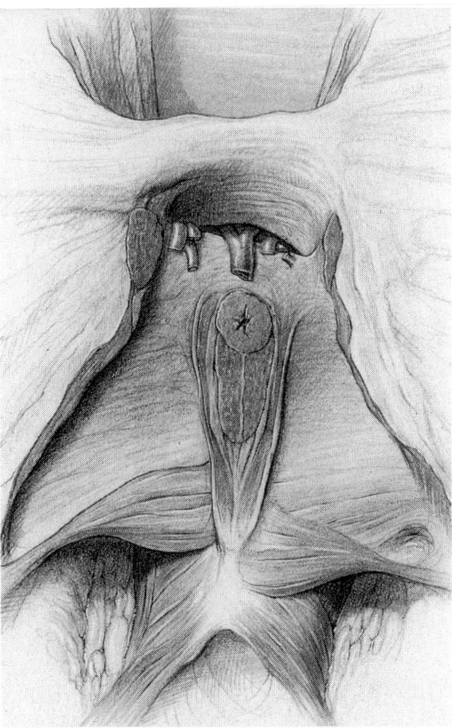

FIGURE 1.100. Transverse perineal ligament after removal of the corpus spongiosum (anatomic dissection).

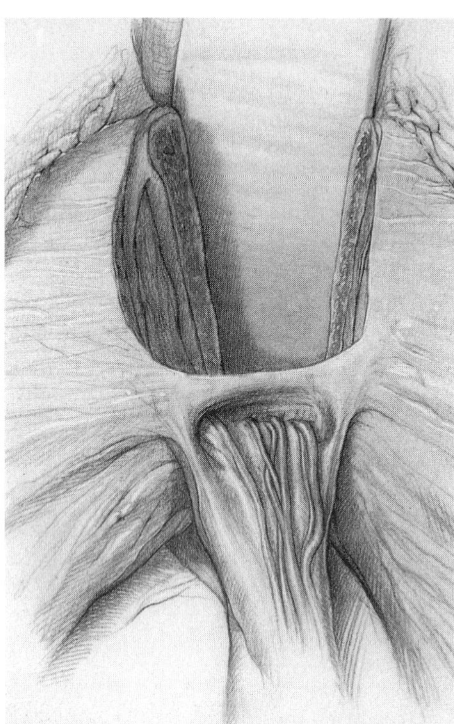

FIGURE 1.101. Dorsal neurovascular supply of the penis (anatomic dissection).

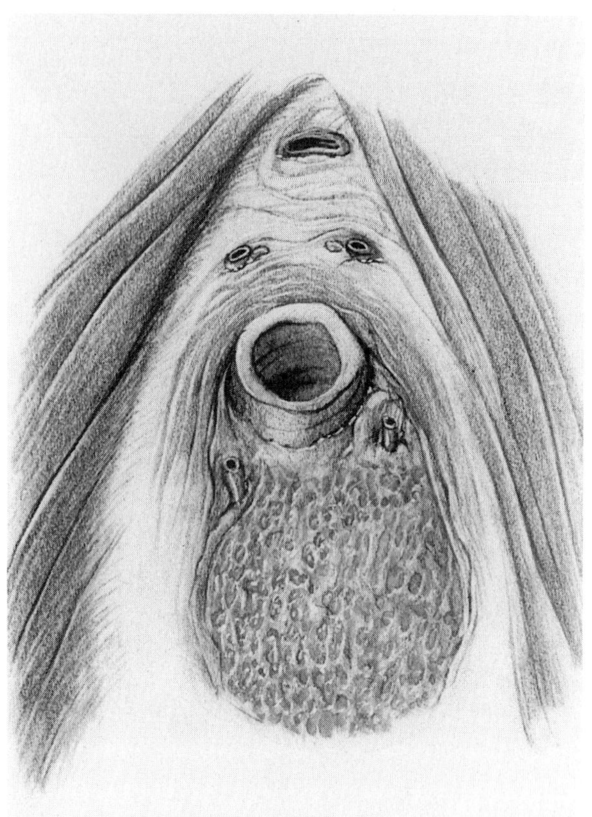

FIGURE 1.103. Close-up view of the transverse perineal ligament and rhabdosphincter (caudal view).

"horseshoe" about the anterior and lateral aspects of the membranous urethra. The structures that pierce the transverse perineal ligament are also seen: the deep dorsal penile vein, the dorsal penile artery and nerve, and the membranous urethra. The bulb of the penis has been divided, leaving a remnant on the diaphragm.

In Fig. 1.104, the anterior circumference of the membranous, urethra (from 9 to 3 o'clock) has been removed to demonstrate the lateral muscular portions of the striated

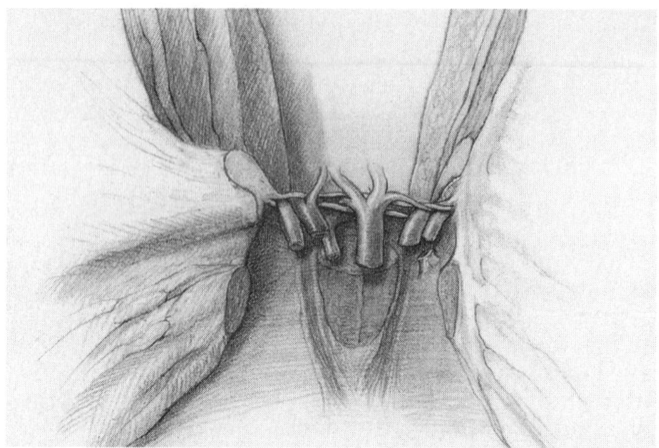

FIGURE 1.102. Appearance after resection of the corpora spongiosa and cavernosa (anatomic dissection).

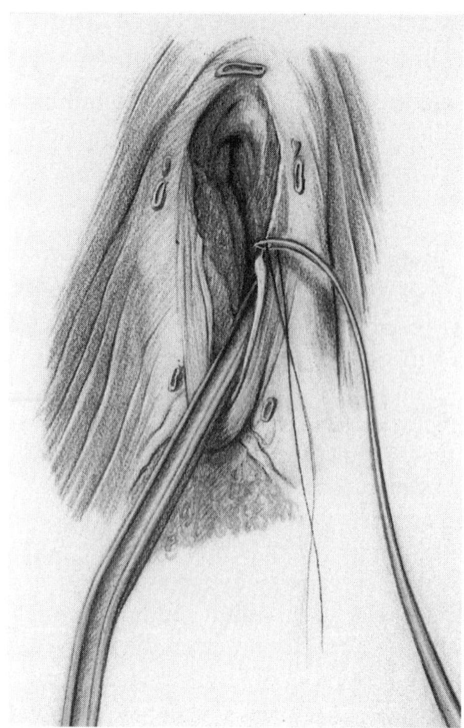

FIGURE 1.104. The urethral lumen is held open with a grooved probe. The lateral muscular portion of the rhabdosphincter can be seen.

urethral sphincter (rhabdosphincter). The artery of the bulb of the penis (bulbar artery) runs lateral to the membranous urethra. The dorsal penile artery and nerve perforate the transverse perineal ligament. The deep dorsal penile vein lies between the public arcuate ligament and transverse perineal ligament.

Perineal Approach to the Posterior Urethra

Dorsal Approach Through the Perineal Body

The dorsal approach is made through the wedge-shaped perineal body, which extends from the central tendon to the rectourethral septum (Fig. 1.105). The dissected bulb of the penis is held upward by its posterior surface, and individual bulbospongiosus muscle fibers are severed. The dorsal aspect of the bulb is sharply separated from the inferior urogenital fascia and the transverse perineal ligament (Fig. 1.106).

Figure 1.107 illustrates the details of this approach. The corpus spongiosum is dissected free from the bulbospongiosus muscle, and the bulb is then dissected from the pelvic floor (transverse perineal ligament). The origins of the

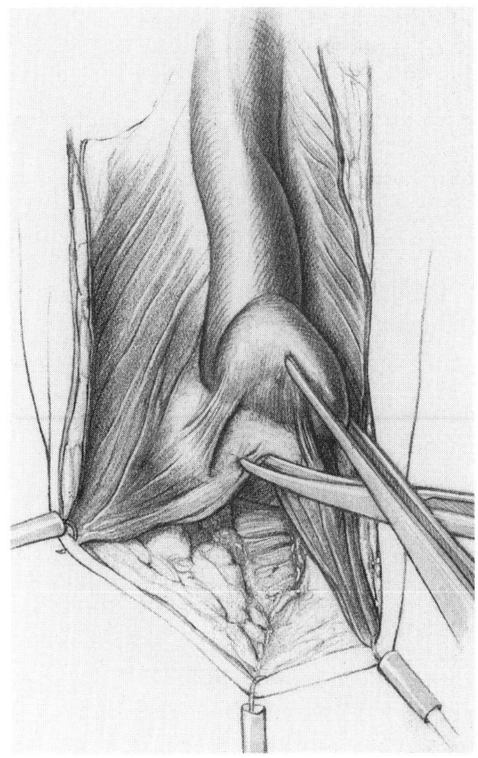

FIGURE 1.106. The bulbospongiosus muscle is removed. The tendinous origin of the bulbospongiosus is incised from front to back at the central tendon of the perineum.

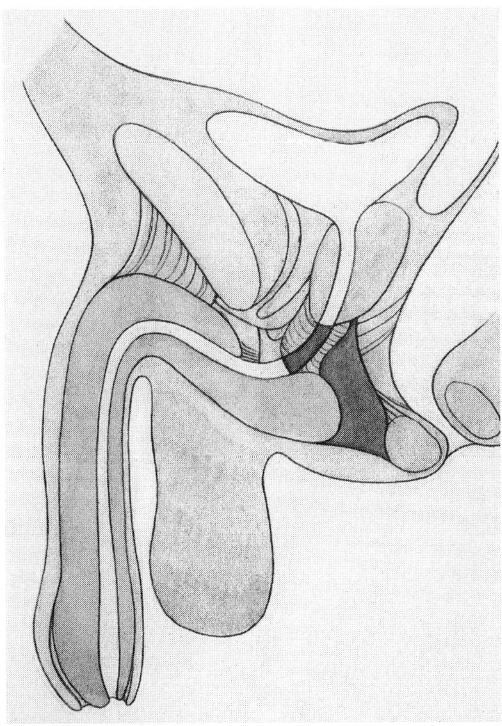

FIGURE 1.105. Schematic of the dorsal approach through the perineal body.

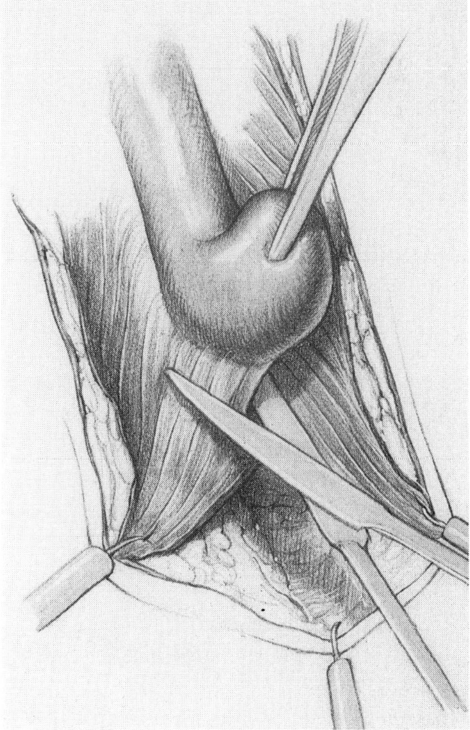

FIGURE 1.107. The bulbospongiosus fibers are detached from the dorsal aspect of the bulb.

bulbospongiosus at the central tendon are divided. The bulbar artery and vein also are divided at this stage.

Dissection of the Rectourethral Septum

Dissection of the rectourethral septum is used for the treatment of rectoprostatic fistulae or a very markedly displaced proximal prostatic urethral stump. The thick connective tissue at the apex of the perineal body is incised transversely.

Division of the rectourethral septum provides access for the dissection of Denonvilliers' fascia. The rectogenital septum is opened, and the posterior surface of the prostate is dissected free. A rectoprostatic fistula can be exposed by this perineal route.

Adult and Pediatric Urology, 4/e, edited by Jay Y. Gillenwater, John T. Grayhack, Stuart S. Howards, and Michael E. Mitchell.
Lippincott Williams & Wilkins, Philadelphia © 2002

2

STANDARD DIAGNOSTIC CONSIDERATIONS

ROBERT B. NADLER
WADE BUSHMAN
ARTHUR W. WYKER, JR.

In evaluating a patient, the urologist relies primarily on a skillfully taken history supplemented by a careful physical examination and appropriate laboratory studies. More often than not, a careful and detailed history of the patient's chief complaints indicates the probable diagnosis even before a physical examination is made or any laboratory test is performed. Because a thorough understanding of urologic signs and symptoms is critical to proper evaluation, they are analyzed here in some detail. A special effort has been made to explain the mechanism of each sign or symptom and to discuss the differential diagnosis.

SIGNS AND SYMPTOMS

Frequency

Frequency is the most common urologic symptom. When it occurs at night, it is termed *nocturia;* it is particularly bothersome and often is the reason for medical consultation. To properly evaluate these symptoms, the urologist should appreciate the wide range of frequency and nocturia in the general population. Study of a normal adult population revealed an average diurnal frequency of four to five times for men and five to six times for women. Ninety percent voided between three and nine times per day, and nocturia was common one to two times in both sexes (6). *Significant urinary frequency* is generally defined as voiding at least every 2 hours and *significant nocturia* as more than two times; however, normalcy varies with each patient. Usually, it is a significant increase in an individual's urinary frequency or nocturia that precipitates medical attention.

Etiology and Mechanism

A change in urinary frequency may result either from a decrease in functional capacity of the bladder or from an increase in urine production. An excellent screening test is the determination of *urine output per voiding.* The voided volume will be low when the bladder capacity is reduced and normal or high with polyuria. This information should

R.B. Nadler: Assistant Professor of Neurology, Head Section of Endourology, Laparoscopy, and Stone Disease, Northwestern University Medical School, Chicago, IL 60611.

W. Bushman: Assistant Professor of Urology, Northwestern University Medical School, Chicago, IL 60611.

A.W. Wyker, Jr.: Clinical Professor of Urology, University of Virginia Health Sciences Center, Charlottesville, VA 22908.

be obtained as part of a 24-hour diary of fluid intake and voiding (Fig. 2.1).

A reduced functional bladder capacity may occur secondary to inflammation of the bladder, pressure on the bladder from extravesical lesions, infravesical obstruction, radiation damage, or neurologic disease. Normal bladder mucosa is pain and pressure sensitive, and when inflamed, its threshold is greatly decreased, so it takes fewer stimuli to initiate the desire to void. Acute bacterial cystitis is by far the most common cause of bladder inflammation. Other causes include cancer, stones, foreign bodies, drugs (e.g., cyclophosphamide), nonbacterial cystitis (viral, fungal, parasitic, interstitial), and inflammatory processes in the adjacent bowel or vagina. Extravesical lesions pressing on the bladder may cause frequency by mechanically interfering with normal bladder expansion or by causing an irritable focus in the

VOIDING DIARY

INTAKE: All fluids and liquid based foods such as ice cream, jello, soup, etc.
OUTPUT: Amount of each urination
ACTIVITY: Note activity (working, relaxing at home, sleeping, etc.)

	DAY ONE			DAY TWO			DAY THREE		
TIME	**INTAKE**	**OUTPUT**	**ACTIVITY**	**INTAKE**	**OUTPUT**	**ACTIVITY**	**INTAKE**	**OUTPUT**	**ACTIVITY**
6AM									
7AM									
8AM									
9AM									
10AM									
11AM									
12N									
1PM									
2PM									
3PM									
4PM									
5PM									
6PM									
7PM									
8PM									
9PM									
10PM									
11PM									
12M									
1AM									
2AM									
3AM									
4AM									
5AM									

FIGURE 2.1. Sample of a 24-hour form for a diary of fluid intake and voiding.

bladder wall. Common causes include pregnant uterus, fibroids, ovarian masses, and pelvic malignancies.

Infravesical obstruction provokes frequency by several mechanisms. Detrusor hypertrophy occurs along with changes in the neural regulation of bladder function such that the urge to void occurs at smaller than normal volumes. The result is an increase in urinary frequency. These patients typically note a decrease in the size and force of their urinary stream. With chronic obstruction, the bladder detrusor muscle may decompensate. Failure to empty the bladder, with elevated postvoid residual urine volumes, further diminishes the functional capacity of the bladder. Benign prostatic hyperplasia is the most common cause of infravesical obstruction. Other causes include carcinoma of the prostate, bladder neck obstruction, urethral stricture, and posterior urethral valves (in boys).

Neurologic disease causes urinary frequency by allowing uninhibited detrusor contractile activity during bladder filling. This may occur with disease affecting either the cerebral cortex (e.g., after a stroke) or spinal cord (e.g., spinal cord injury), as well as diseases affecting the central nervous system diffusely (e.g., multiple sclerosis). Urinary symptoms may be the presenting symptoms of an occult neurologic disease process, and a possible neurogenic cause should always be considered in the differential diagnosis of urinary frequency.

An increase in frequency, typically without any other urinary symptoms, will accompany increased urinary production. Causes of polyuria include ingestion of excess fluid, diabetes mellitus, chronic renal failure, and diabetes insipidus. In diabetes mellitus, the unreabsorbed glucose is an osmotic diuretic causing the polyuria. In chronic renal failure, there is impaired ability to concentrate the urine that causes *polyuria,* defined as a daily urine output in excess of 2,500 mL. Diabetes insipidus occurs with inadequate production or release of antidiuretic hormone (ADH) from the pituitary gland (central diabetes insipidus) or with inadequate fluid reabsorption by the kidneys despite normal ADH levels (nephrogenic diabetes insipidus) (36). The acquired concentrating defect in nephrogenic diabetes insipidus may occur with electrolyte disorders (hypokalemia and hypercalcemia), kidney disorders (pyelonephritis and obstructive nephropathy), drugs (e.g., lithium), and sickle cell disease and trait.

Emotional stress can cause urinary frequency. Characteristically, the patient experiences episodic frequency during stressful periods punctuated by periods of normalcy. Stress has been shown to induce a significant rise in intravesical pressure. Straub and associates (35) performed cystometrograms while interviewing normal subjects. Stressful topics evoked a significant rise in the intravesical pressure, usually accompanied by a desire to void. After reassurance and relaxation, the intravesical pressure returned to normal. Interestingly, discussion of emotion-laden material produced a bladder response only when it *disturbed the subject.* Some subjects seemed to enjoy venting their feelings, and they experienced no rise in their intravesical pressure.

Urgency

Urgency of urination is a sudden, strong desire to void. This symptom is usually attributed to an involuntary contraction of the detrusor muscle. Associated symptoms of urinary frequency are often attributable to lower-amplitude detrusor contractions occurring during bladder filling. When uninhibited detrusor activity occurs as a consequence of neurologic disease or injury, it is termed *detrusor hyperreflexia.* In the absence of neurologic disease, it is termed *detrusor instability.* It is a common feature of infravesical obstruction or inflammatory conditions of the bladder, but it is also commonly idiopathic in origin. Patients may prevent leakage and temporarily delay voiding by maintaining voluntary contraction of the external sphincter until the detrusor contraction has abated; however, urge incontinence is a regularly accompanying feature.

In patients with urgency, the urologist should look for evidence of irritative lesions of the lower urinary tract, intravesical obstruction, and neurologic disorders. Urinalysis is critical to look for pyuria and bacteriuria, which may indicate an infection, or hematuria, which might indicate a malignancy or stone. Similarly, an ultrasound or catheterized postvoid residual can rule out outflow incontinence and urgency in these patients.

Diminished Urine Flow

The determinants of urine flow during voiding are detrusor contraction strength, any contribution of abdominal straining, and infravesical resistance to urine flow. Although commonly referred to as *obstructive symptoms,* hesitancy, diminished or interrupted stream, need to strain, postvoid dribbling, and a sensation of incomplete emptying may occur with either impaired detrusor function or infravesical obstruction. There are many causes of detrusor hypocontractility. It may be idiopathic. It can also occur as a result of central nervous system disease (e.g., Parkinson's), peripheral neuropathy (e.g., diabetes mellitus), chronic overdistention, or longstanding infravesical obstruction. Infravesical obstruction, although uncommon in women, may occur with a large cystocele or tight urethral stricture. These are usually evident on physical examination. Among the causes of infravesical obstruction in men, bladder neck obstruction from benign prostatic hyperplasia is the most common. Although the constellation of irritative and obstructive voiding symptoms in men has generally been attributed to benign prostatic hyperplasia (BPH), a common diagnostic challenge is posed by men with obstructive symptoms in whom detrusor hypocontractility or infravesical obstruction may coexist. Measures used to assess the relative contribution of each factor include endoscopic evaluation of the

INTERNATIONAL PROSTATE SYMPTOM SCORE (I-PSS)

Patient's Name

Date of Birth   Date Completed

	Not at all	Less than 1 time in 5	Less than half the time	About half the time	More than half the time	Almost always	Your score
1. Incomplete emptying Over the past month, how often have you had a sensation of not emptying your bladder completely after you finished urinating?	0	1	2	3	4	5	
2. Frequency Over the past month, how often have you had to urinate again less than two hours after you finished urinating?	0	1	2	3	4	5	
3. Intermittency Over the past month, how often have you found you stopped and started again several times when you urinated?	0	1	2	3	4	5	
4. Urgency Over the past month, how often have you found it difficult to postpone urination?	0	1	2	3	4	5	
5. Weak stream Over the past month, how often have you had a weak urinary stream?	0	1	2	3	4	5	
6. Straining Over the past month, how often have you had to push or strain to begin urination?	0	1	2	3	4	5	
	None	**1 time**	**2 times**	**3 times**	**4 times**	**5 times or more**	
7. Nocturia Over the past month, how many times did you most typically get up to urinate from the time you went to bed at night until the time you got up in the morning?	1	2	3	4	5	6	
Total I-PSS Score							

FIGURE 2.2. The AUA symptom index.

urethra and bladder neck for visual evidence of obstruction and urodynamic pressure-flow studies to measure detrusor pressure and urine flow during voiding.

The American Urological Association (AUA) symptom index (Fig. 2.2) is a widely used measure to quantify irritative and obstructive symptoms in men. This measure is not specific for obstruction, and because a number of studies have shown that BPH or bladder obstruction is often not the cause of bladder symptoms (3,8,29,37), obstructive and irritative voiding symptoms are now commonly described by the nonbiased term *lower urinary tract symptoms* (LUTS) (1).

Urinary Retention

The patient with *acute* urinary retention typically experiences distress with an uncomfortably distended bladder and the inability to void more than small volumes of urine. Catheter drainage brings prompt symptomatic relief. Symptoms of patients with *chronic* retention usually include frequency, weak urine flow, and a sensation of incomplete emptying. Patients may experience the frequent leakage typical of overflow incontinence. The serum creatinine may be increased as a result of obstructive nephropathy. Generally, these patients experience little discomfort from their distended bladder, even though the residual urine volumes obtained by catheterization can be larger than those found in patients with acute urinary retention. Urinary retention, whether acute or chronic, can occur as a product of intravesical obstruction, impaired detrusor function, neurologic disease, or in rare cases, psychogenic causes. The role of the urologist is to provide bladder decompression and to identify the underlying condition or precipitating events that contribute to retention. Particular attention should be paid in cases of young men and women of all ages to rule out an occult neurogenic cause.

Urinary Incontinence

Urinary incontinence is the *involuntary* loss of urine. Blandy (4) described it as follows: "There is almost no symptom more degrading or miserable than incontinence of urine: it inevitably brings, at any stage after early childhood, shame, stink, soreness, and ostracism."

Mechanism

The diagnostic approach to the incontinent patient emphasizes a careful history that notes the frequency and pattern of leakage, recognizes significant associated voiding symptoms, and identifies pertinent associated medical conditions. A careful physical examination and postvoid residual urine volume determination are essential.

Normal bladder function embraces two distinct activities: urine storage and urine evacuation. Incontinence may result from a problem with the urine storage phase because of an abnormal increase in bladder pressure during filling or because of a defective urinary sphincter mechanism. Alternatively, incontinence may result from a problem with the evacuation phase that prevents adequate emptying of the bladder. The classic forms of urge, stress, and overflow incontinence correspond neatly to this classification of incontinence mechanisms. Because most incontinent patients have one of these typical forms and a diagnosis usually can be made on the basis of history and physical examination alone, these types of incontinence are described in some detail. On evaluation, some patients are found to have atypical patterns of incontinence. These patients often have complex underlying mechanisms of voiding dysfunction and incontinence and may require more comprehensive urodynamic evaluation for accurate diagnosis.

Classification of Urinary Incontinence

Stress Incontinence

Women with stress incontinence have a characteristic history. They leak with coughing, sneezing, jogging, laughing, getting up from a chair, or engaging in other activities that cause a sudden rise in intraabdominal pressure. The normal mechanism to prevent leakage with straining depends on equal transmission of the increased pressure to the bladder and urethra. In women with the most common type of stress incontinence, a deficiency of pelvic support allows the urethra to herniate into the vagina (urethrocele). Less pressure is transmitted to the urethra than to the bladder, and the uncompensated rise in intraabdominal pressure results in leakage. The degree of leakage is proportional to the degree of straining. Characterized by leaking with minimal activities such as standing or walking, extremely severe stress incontinence is more likely the result of a deficiency in the intrinsic urethral sphincter mechanism rather than urethral hypermobility. Loss of the urethral sphincter function may occur with aging, from radiation therapy, from pelvic trauma, or from prior pelvic or antiincontinence surgery (5). The result is significant leakage with very small rises in intravesical pressure. Stress incontinence in the neurologically intact male without previous pelvic surgery is rare. Variable degrees of stress incontinence may be observed in men following prostatectomy; this incontinence is most often caused by deficient function of the intrinsic or extrinsic component of the distal urethral sphincter (30).

Overflow Incontinence

Overflow incontinence is distinguished by chronic failure of bladder emptying. This may occur with either intravesical obstruction or impaired detrusor function. Patients often have overt bladder decompensation with chronically high residual urine, often greater than 1,000 mL. The distended bladder is usually easily palpable and percussible in the lower abdomen. The intravesical pressure is consistently elevated, so slight increases in intraabdominal pressure may raise the intravesical pressure enough in women to overcome urethral resistance. Intermittent leakage may also occur because of uninhibited contractile activity in the stretched detrusor muscle. This is the mechanism of leakage in men with this form of urinary incontinence, most commonly seen with severe obstruction from BPH.

Urge Incontinence

Urge incontinence is an episodic form of urine leakage that occurs with involuntary contractions of the bladder detrusor muscle. The patient typically complains of a precipitous, unsuppressible urge to void. Patients may be able to forestall or minimize leakage for a brief period by contracting the external sphincter, but the typical patient experiences small- to large-volume leakage from what is essentially an involuntary voiding reflex. The most common cause is idiopathic detrusor instability. Specific causes also include inflammation adjacent to or in the bladder, longstanding intravesical obstruction, and varying forms of neurogenic bladder (detrusor hyperreflexia). Urge incontinence is particularly common in patients with a history of stroke and often occurs 3 to 6 months after the neurologic event. A careful history and 24-hour voiding diary usually reveal that episodes of leakage are most apt to occur with a full bladder, as a result of generous fluid intake, during periods of diuresis, or when regular toileting has been delayed. A cystometrogram may demonstrate uninhibited detrusor activity during filling. This can be useful in the cognitively impaired patient who cannot provide a useful history; however, the characteristic history provided by most patients makes this test superfluous.

Nocturnal Enuresis

Nocturnal enuresis is the repeated, involuntary loss of urine during sleep (17). If present since birth, it is termed *primary enuresis*. Bed-wetting spontaneously ceases with increasing age, being present in 15% of 5-year-old children, 5% of

10-year-old children, and 1% of 15-year-old children. If nocturnal enuresis follows a significant "dry" interval, it is termed *secondary enuresis.*

Etiology

Primary enuresis is caused by maturational lag of the central nervous system with delayed development of inhibitory control of the bladder. This delayed maturation theory is supported by the following findings in enuretics: (a) the high incidence of a spontaneous cure with time; (b) the presence of a bladder capacity smaller than that in normal children, with resultant increased frequency of voiding (Tables 2.1 and 2.2); and (c) the documented hereditary aspect of enuresis. The evaluation of the child with uncomplicated primary nocturnal enuresis includes a physical examination, screening neurologic examination, urinalysis, and urine culture. If these are normal, reassurance and observation are indicated. In patients with a history of urinary infection or primary *diurnal* enuresis, evaluation should include an ultrasound of the bladder and kidneys to rule out obstruction.

Secondary enuresis often occurs in association with emotional stress in the child's life, and a diligent search should be made for contributing emotional factors. Examples are a disruption of the family by divorce or the birth of a sibling. Other causes for secondary enuresis include neurologic disease and obstruction. Therefore the evaluation of the child with secondary enuresis should include a careful physical examination, screening neurologic examination, radiographs of the lumbosacral spine to detect vertebral abnormalities, urinalysis and culture, and an ultrasound of the bladder and kidneys.

Hematuria

Hematuria is a dramatic indicator of disease in the urinary tract, yet it is often ignored by patients and physicians alike. The passage of blood-stained urine may be the first sign of serious disease in the urinary tract, and a single episode of hematuria warrants a thorough urologic investigation.

TABLE 2.1. PHYSIOLOGIC MAXIMUM BLADDER CAPACITY

Age (yr)	Normal Children	Enuretic Children
4	296	180
5	301	238
6	359	279
7	394	217
8	428	272
9	457	281
10	473	353

Reprinted with permission from Esperanca M, Gerrard JW. Nocturnal enuresis: studies in bladder function in normal children and enuretics. *Can Med Assoc J* 1969;101:324.

TABLE 2.2. FREQUENCY OF VOIDING IN 24 HOURS

Age (yr)	Normal Children	Enuretic Children
4	5.3	11.9
5	5.7	11.0
6	6.4	10.0
7	5.5	8.4
8	5.3	9.7
10	4.6	10.7

Reprinted with permission from Esperanca M, Gerrard JW. Nocturnal enuresis: studies in bladder function in normal children and enuretics. *Can Med Assoc J* 1969;101:324.

Classification

It is helpful clinically to classify hematuria in two ways: first by quantity and second by the time of its appearance during voiding. Quantitatively, it is called *microscopic hematuria* if demonstrable only under the microscope and *gross hematuria* if it is evident to the naked eye. Microscopic hematuria is more commonly nephrologic in origin, whereas gross hematuria is more commonly urologic in origin. Blood noted chiefly at the beginning of urination is called *initial hematuria,* and it indicates disease in the urethra. Similarly, blood noted only between voidings or as stains on underclothing or pajamas, while the voided urine is clear, indicates disease at the urethral meatus or in the anterior urethra. Blood noted chiefly at the end of urination is called *terminal hematuria,* and it indicates disease near the bladder neck or in the prostatic urethra. Uniformly bloody urine, *total hematuria,* occurs with disease in the bladder, ureters, or kidneys.

Significance

The significance of hematuria varies with the age of the patient (Table 2.3). Gross painless hematuria is often the first manifestation of a urinary tract tumor. The episodic nature of the bleeding and the absence of other symptoms should not lull either the patient or physician into a false sense of security. In one review of 1,000 patients with gross hematuria (19), tumors were found in 21.5%. Two-thirds of these were bladder tumors.

Microscopic hematuria may also signal the presence of a tumor. Although evaluation of 500 patients with asymptomatic microscopic hematuria revealed tumors in only 2.2% (15), a more recent study from the same institution evaluating 200 consecutive patients with asymptomatic microscopic hematuria found tumors in 12.5% (7). This figure reflects the newer diagnostic modalities available today, particularly urine cytology.

TABLE 2.3. THE MOST COMMON CAUSES OF HEMATURIA BY AGE AND SEX

0–20 yr
Acute glomerulonephritis
Acute urinary tract infection
Congenital urinary tract anomalies with obstruction
20–40 yr
Acute urinary tract infection
Stones
Bladder tumor
40–60 yr (men)
Bladder tumor
Stones
Acute urinary tract infection
40–60 yr (women)
Acute urinary tract infection
Stones
Bladder tumor
60 yr (men)
Benign prostatic hyperplasia
Bladder tumor
Acute urinary tract infection
60 yr (women)
Bladder tumor
Acute urinary tract infection

The other common urologic causes of hematuria are infection and stones. Less common causes include BPH, trauma, sickle cell disease or trait, tuberculosis, renal infarction, renal vein thrombosis, coagulation and platelet deficiencies, exercise-related causes (e.g., jogging), hypercalciuria, and vasculitis.

Diagnostic Approach

After a careful history and physical examination, the fundamental means of diagnosis are urinalysis, cytologic examination of the urine, intravenous urography, and cystoscopy. For gross hematuria, cystoscopy at the time of bleeding can be helpful in localizing the bleeding to the left or right upper urinary tract. After these fundamental studies have been completed, the diagnosis is apparent in approximately 75% of cases. For the remaining 25% with unexplained hematuria, further investigation can then be carried out with retrograde pyelography, ureteroscopy, and computed tomography (CT). Although hematuria cannot occur without a cause, in 5% to 10% of cases, no definite cause can be found (10).

Pain

Mechanism

The chief cause of pain in the urinary tract is distention from increased intraluminal pressure. The severity of the pain is not primarily related to the degree of distention but to the rapidity with which it develops. Gradual distention of the ureter, renal pelvis, or calyces may cause little or no pain. When intrapelvic pressures have been measured in patients with an acutely obstructing ureteral calculus, the higher the pressure, the more severe the pain. With longstanding obstruction, distention may be marked, but the pressure in the renal pelvis is normal or only minimally elevated and the patient experiences little or no pain. The concept that pain from obstruction is related to increased intraluminal pressure and distention is extremely useful clinically. Urologists are often asked to evaluate patients with pain in the back, flank, or abdomen. When an intravenous urogram at the time of a pain episode is normal with no dilation of the ureter, pelvis, or calyces and no delay of the nephrogram or excretory phase, one can state with confidence that pain is not caused by obstruction. Two other causes of renal pain are distention of the renal capsule and acute renal ischemia. Both produce steady, usually mild pain in the costovertebral angle region.

Type and Location

Pain caused by distention may be steady or intermittent. Intermittent pain, particularly when it is severe, is often termed *renal colic* and is most commonly caused by an obstructing stone in the lower ureter. With each peristaltic wave, more urine is pumped into the obstructed portion of the ureter, with a resultant increase in the hydrostatic intraluminal pressure and pain intensity.

Steady pain, most typical of distention of the renal capsule and acute renal ischemia, also occurs in up to 50% of patients with distention of the ureter, renal pelvis, or calyces. The constant level of pain with obstruction and distention is thought to reflect an absence of ureteral pressure waves.

The distribution of urinary tract pain has been carefully mapped out by distending the renal pelvis and various portions of the ureter with small balloon catheters (24). The location of renal and ureteral pain is shown in Fig. 2.3.

Urinary tract pain does not occur in the central portion of the abdomen but is lateralized to the outer abdomen, flank, and costovertebral angle region. Ureteral pain follows a line along the lateral edge of the rectus muscle (Table 2.4).

Pain Pathways and Referred Pain

Kidney and ureter pain impulses are carried in afferent fibers that accompany the sympathetic nerves and enter the spinal cord by means of the posterior spinal roots. Renal and ureteral pain can be abolished by sympathectomy of T-7 to L-3 or by sectioning posterior spinal roots T-11 and T-12 and L-1 and L-2.

Referred pain is pain projected to an area distant from the point of stimulation. It may occur in addition to or in the absence of true visceral pain. The exact mechanism of

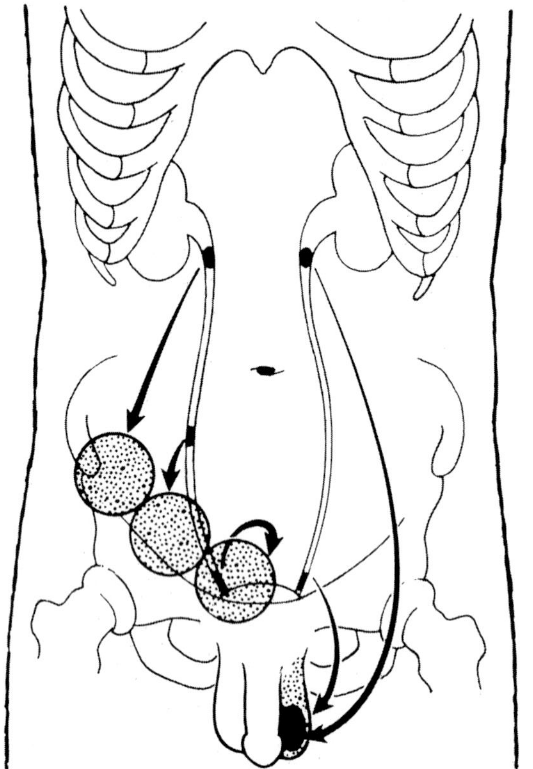

FIGURE 2.3. Sites of urologic pain. (Reprinted with permission from Wyker A, Gillenwater JY. *Method of urology.* Baltimore: Williams & Wilkins, 1975.)

referred pain is unknown, but the site of painful stimulus and the site of referred painful sensation usually share a common segmental innervation. Spinal cord segments T-11 and T-12 receive sensory fibers from both the upper ureter and testis, so distention of the upper ureter may cause referred pain to the ipsilateral testis. In similar manner, distention of the lower ureter may cause referred pain to the ipsilateral scrotum.

Pain in the Lower Urinary Tract

Bladder distention initially causes fullness and then pain in the suprapubic region and end of the penis associated with an intense desire to void (urgency). Normal bladder mucosa is sensitive to stimuli, and this sensitivity is greatly increased by inflammation. Suprapubic discomfort is typical. Stimulation of the trigone, ureteral orifices, or anterior urethra causes referred pain to the end of the penis. Pain from prostatic inflammation is usually described as perineal discomfort, which may radiate to the inguinal regions and lower back. Acute testicular pain such as that with trauma, torsion, or epididymo-orchitis often radiates to the groin.

TABLE 2.4. SITES OF URINARY TRACT PAIN

Site of Balloon Distention	Site of Uretral Pain
Renal pelvis	Costovertebral angle
Upper ureter	Flank
Middle ureter	Middle inguinal canal
Lower ureter	Suprapubic area

Pain on Urination

Pain on urination is usually caused by inflammation of the lower urinary tract. Patients may localize their discomfort to the suprapubic area or to the end of the penis or urethra. Milder degrees of pain are often described as a burning sensation. The most common cause is bacterial infection. Other causes include nonbacterial cystitis, cancer, stone or foreign body in the bladder or urethra, and excess phosphates in the urine (phosphaturia).

It is important to determine when pain or burning is noted during urination. If it begins with the onset and stops abruptly at the end, the primary pathology is probably in the urethra. When the bladder is primarily involved, as in acute bacterial cystitis, patients experience some discomfort during urination, but often the most severe pain occurs after voiding has ceased.

Chronic Pelvic Pain

Chronic pelvic pain syndrome (CPPS) is a more accurate subclassification of prostatitis and prostatodynia developed in 1995. The National Institutes of Health (NIH) prostatitis classification system is based on the presence of acute and chronic bacterial prostatitis and the presence of white blood cells (WBCs) in the expressed prostatic secretions (EPS) (28). Patients typically have any combination of perineal, penile, testicular, or low back pain. The classification is based on the following culture and EPS data. *Type I* refers to patients with acute bacterial prostatitis, as documented by culture. *Type II* refers to patients with chronic bacterial prostatitis as documented by culture of the EPS. *Type IIIa* refers to patients with CPPS, more than 10 WBCs per high-power field (HPF) (400×) in their EPS, and negative cultures. *Type IIIb* refers to patients with CPPS, no inflammation in their EPS (fewer than 10 WBCs), and negative cultures. *Type IV* refers to patients with asymptomatic inflammatory prostatitis (patients without CPPS who are found incidentally to have more than 10 WBCs per HPF in their EPS). The cause of CPPS, especially type IIIa, remains elusive, although oxidative stress (32) and cytokines (2,16,26) may play an important role. Treatment at this time is most successful with biofeedback (9) and nonsteroidal antiinflammatory medications. The NIH Chronic Prostatitis Symptom Index (NIH-CPSI) is a nine-part questionnaire developed and validated to quantitate the pain of urinary symptoms and effect that CPPS has on the quality of life in these patients (21). This questionnaire, similar to the AUA symptom index, is an important step for the practicing clinician to initially evaluate the patient and record the efficacy of the aforementioned treatments.

Sexual Dysfunction

Normal sexual function is difficult to define because of significant individual variation and the prevalence of age-related changes. However, most of these patients complain of diminished libido, erectile dysfunction, or both. Diminished libido may occur with acute and chronic illness or with psychologic or emotional stresses, and the existence of possible causative factors should be sought in the patient's history. The most common organic basis for diminished libido, a disturbance of the pituitary-gonadal hormonal axis, is evaluated by examining for evidence of hyperestrinism or hypogonadism (gynecomastia, decreased testicular volume) and obtaining a morning sample of serum testosterone. If the testosterone value is below the normal range, a free and total testosterone is repeated, along with measurements of follicle-stimulating hormone, luteinizing hormone, and prolactin. Hypergonadotropic hypogonadism (low testosterone, increased luteinizing hormone) is usually idiopathic, and pharmacologic testosterone supplement may yield a beneficial effect. Patients with hypogonadotropic hypogonadism (low testosterone, low luteinizing hormone) or with other evidence of pituitary endocrinopathy (elevated prolactin) merit a complete endocrine evaluation to rule out a hypothalamic or pituitary defect.

Erectile dysfunction, generally defined as failure to achieve and maintain an erection satisfactory for intercourse, is the most common complaint. The incidence increases with age, such that nearly 25% of men at age 65 are affected. There are many potential causes, and a careful history provides essential clues to the diagnosis. The manner of onset of erectile dysfunction, the degree of difficulty in attaining erection during masturbation versus with a sexual partner, a progression in the degree of dysfunction over time, and the presence or absence of nocturnal erections often distinguish an organic versus a psychogenic etiology. Typically, an organic etiology shows a gradual onset with progressive dysfunction over time, equal difficulty with a partner or during masturbation, and a loss of nocturnal erection. Psychogenic impotence more typically shows an abrupt or stuttering pattern of erectile dysfunction without a gradually progressive pattern, a situational pattern of erectile dysfunction, or maintenance of nocturnal erections.

Medical conditions contributing to erectile dysfunction include diabetes mellitus, neurologic disease, hypertension, hypercholesterolemia, peripheral vascular disease, a heavy smoking history, and some medications (e.g., antihypertensives). Psychologic factors that can contribute to erectile dysfunction include strained emotional relationships, performance anxiety, and unresolved inner conflicts associated with sexual behavior.

An occasional patient will report absence of emission. This may occur with autonomic denervation of the accessory sex organs as a complication of retroperitoneal surgery or longstanding diabetes mellitus, incompetency of the bladder neck following surgery, or diminished ejaculate volume from hypogonadism. The complaint of penile curvature and pain with erection (Peyronie's disease) is typically due to the presence of a fibrous plaque between the tunica albuginea and corpus cavernosum. It is usually palpable at the site of curvature reported by the patient.

Fever

To the urologist, as to most physicians, fever suggests the presence of infection. The most common cause is an acute urinary tract infection where significant temperature elevation is usually taken to indicate upper tract involvement. High spiking temperatures with shaking chills and systemic signs of sepsis should prompt radiographic imaging, usually with CT or ultrasound, to rule out upper tract obstruction. Infection with obstruction is a urologic emergency. Prompt drainage with a ureteral stent or percutaneous nephrostomy tube is essential to avert sepsis and allow effective antimicrobial treatment.

Occasionally, a patient will have an obstructing stone and a low-grade fever. A small amount of urinary extravasation from the renal pelvis, which can occur with acute ureteral obstruction, may produce a low-grade fever. In men lacking bacteriuria on urinalysis, high spiking fevers, and other signs of infection, empiric antibiotic coverage with close observation is reasonable. In women, the incidence of asymptomatic bacteriuria is more common and the possibility of infection above the point of obstruction considerably greater. The risks and benefits of prompt intervention to relieve obstruction versus antimicrobial coverage and observation must be considered on a case-by-case basis.

Acute bacterial prostatitis usually manifests as an acute febrile illness characterized by perineal discomfort, urinary frequency, hesitancy, diminished force of stream, and dysuria. Urinalysis usually reveals pyuria, and examination reveals a markedly tender, boggy prostate. Acute bacterial prostatitis or prostatic abscess may also occur in hospitalized patients with indwelling Foley catheters and should be considered as an occult source of fever and bacteremia. Physical examination is usually sufficient for diagnosis but may be aided by the use of transrectal ultrasound or CT to document a prostatic abscess. Prostate-specific antigen (PSA) determination often reveals significant elevation as a result of the acute or chronic inflammatory prostatic process (26).

Epididymitis with scrotal pain and swelling may be accompanied by fever. In men younger than 35 years of age, epididymitis can be caused by sexually transmitted diseases such as gonorrhea or *Chlamydia.* In older patients and in patients with recent instrumentation, it is more likely due to urinary pathogens.

Renal Insufficiency

The urologist is often asked to evaluate patients with renal insufficiency for potentially reversible causes of renal dysfunction. Renal ultrasound is the best screening test for obstruction because it is neither nephrotoxic nor invasive and is very sensitive for detecting hydronephrosis associated with obstruction. When obstruction is the *sole* cause of renal insufficiency in a patient with two kidneys, it must be bilateral. Supravesical causes include conditions such as pelvic malignancy and retroperitoneal fibrosis causing bilateral ureteral obstruction, as well as obstructive processes (e.g., stone disease) affecting each unit independently. More commonly, bilateral hydronephrosis is seen with conditions affecting bladder function. These conditions include increased intravesical filling pressures from uninhibited detrusor contractions or diminished compliance, neurogenic bladder dysfunction, or severe outlet obstruction with failure to empty and elevated postvoid residual urine volumes. Therefore the screening evaluation for obstruction in the patient with renal insufficiency includes a postvoid residual determination by ultrasound or catheterization. Unilateral obstruction may contribute to renal insufficiency when only one kidney is present or when the normal compensatory response of the contralateral kidney is prevented by preexisting impairment of renal function. Clues to this possibility may be provided by a renal ultrasound showing a small (atrophic) contralateral kidney or one with echotexture changes consistent with chronic intrinsic renal disease.

A renovascular cause of diminished renal function is another potentially reversible condition that the urologist may identify. It should be considered when there is no evidence of obstruction, no history or findings on urinalysis to support either acute or chronic intrinsic renal disease, or a history of conditions predisposing to vascular disease, such as hypertension, hypercholesterolemia, or diabetes mellitus, is present.

Medical History

Any urologic complaint must be framed in the context of the patient's medical history. In addition to inquiring about all previous genitourinary conditions or surgeries, the urologist must identify past or current disorders with potential effects on the genitourinary system (e.g., tuberculosis, diabetes mellitus). Each specific finding (e.g., microscopic hematuria) also prompts a search for pertinent conditions (e.g., sickle cell trait). The family history may be significant for genetic syndromes associated with urologic manifestations (autosomal-dominant polycystic kidney disease, Alport's syndrome, von Hippel–Lindau disease, tuberous sclerosis), as well as for diseases with known familial associations (stone disease, prostate cancer).

PHYSICAL EXAMINATION

Kidney

A kidney must be grossly enlarged or displaced to cause a perceptible bulge in the upper abdomen or flank. If a perinephric abscess is suspected, the patient should be in the knee–elbow position for an examination. The normal shallow depression below the lowermost rib may be obliterated by fullness and edema secondary to an underlying abscess.

Because of their location in the uppermost portion of the abdominal cavity, normal kidneys are usually not palpable. An exception is the newborn in whom both kidneys may be palpable during the first 48 hours of life because of the hypotonicity of all muscles. In approximately 10% of adults, usually thin women, the lower pole of the right kidney can be felt. Two maneuvers aid palpation: deep breathing and bimanual examination. The posterior hand lifts the soft tissue in the costovertebral angle, and the anterior hand presses deeply into the abdomen. The normal kidney is movable because it is fixed only by its vascular pedicle, and with deep inspiration, the descending diaphragm pushes the kidney down toward the examining fingers. The kidney is most easily felt between the fingers of both hands as a firm, smooth mass slipping upward as expiration starts. A renal mass is characteristically ballottable, unlike the liver and spleen, which usually can only be palpated with the anterior hand. Tenderness caused by inflammation in or around the kidney is best detected by exerting firm pressure in the costovertebral angle region.

In patients with hypertension, it is important to listen over the renal artery areas for the presence of a bruit. These murmurs are best heard anteriorly after complete exhalation.

Transillumination is occasionally helpful in newborns or small children with large, easily palpable abdominal masses. With the room as dark as possible, the mass should be manipulated against the abdominal wall with one hand while a high-intensity light (e.g., fiberoptic light cord) is firmly applied to the mass with the other hand. If the mass is cystic rather than solid, it will transilluminate, creating a reddish glow.

Ureter

In males, the ureter is not palpable by either abdominal or rectal examination, but in females, the lower ureter can be felt on vaginal examination. One or two fingers are gently pushed upward and outward, and at the limit of the fingertips, the ureter lies close to the bony pelvic wall and lateral to the ovary. From this point, the ureter can be followed to its junction with the bladder by carrying the fingers downward and inward. If the ureter is normal, it is usually not identifiable because it is soft and nontender. If a stone is present, both the stone and ureter are usually palpable. The ureter can be felt as a tender tubular mass proximal to the stone.

Urinary Bladder

The normal empty or nearly empty bladder is neither palpable nor percussible because of its anatomic location in the pelvis. When it contains approximately 125 mL of urine, it rises out of the pelvis into the lower abdomen, projecting one fingerbreadth above the pubis. It rises progressively toward the umbilicus with further filling. If the bladder contains more than 500 mL of urine, it may be identifiable as a bulge in the middle lower abdomen. This swelling rising out of the pelvis is best appreciated by observing from the side, with the eyes more or less level with the lower abdomen. The distended bladder may be palpated as a firm, round, movable mass rising out of the pelvis into the lower abdomen. Whether or not a mass is palpable, the lower abdomen should be percussed from the umbilicus to the pubis. If the patient has a distended bladder, the normally resonant note is replaced by dullness. Percussion over a distended bladder may also cause the patient to experience a desire to void because of the sudden induced rise in intravesical pressure. An accurate measurement of bladder volume is obtained by catheter drainage or by bladder ultrasound.

To assess the extent of a bladder tumor, bimanual examination is performed when the patient is anesthetized and the bladder is empty. Intravesical masses are usually ballottable; fixation usually signifies gross perivesical extension.

Prostate and Seminal Vesicles

The prostate and seminal vesicles are palpated through the anterior rectal wall (Fig. 2.4). Rectal examination is best performed with the patient standing on the floor, knees slightly bent and elbows resting on the edge of the examining table. Bedridden patients are best examined in the lateral decubitus position, with their knees pulled up into their chest. The typical prostate is 4 cm wide, 2.5 to 3 cm high, and 4.5 cm long with a volume of 20 mL. Volume can be measured with the index finger, which is approximately 1.5 cm wide, or estimated based on the examiner's experience. Transrectal ultrasound with its accurate volume measurement allows the examiner a means to constantly evaluate his or her volume estimates. The normal gland is smooth, slightly movable, and nontender, and it has a rubbery consistency. Two distinct lobes can be felt separated by a median furrow with distinct lateral sulci. Indurated areas and nodules should be noted and a biopsy performed if appropriate. If the physician's finger is long enough, he or she may be able to feel the soft, tubular seminal vesicles above the prostate. Coming off the base of the prostate somewhat obliquely, they are most easily felt when they are distended or tender. EPS for microscopic examination can be obtained from most patients by deliberately massaging each prostate lobe in a lateral to medial direction.

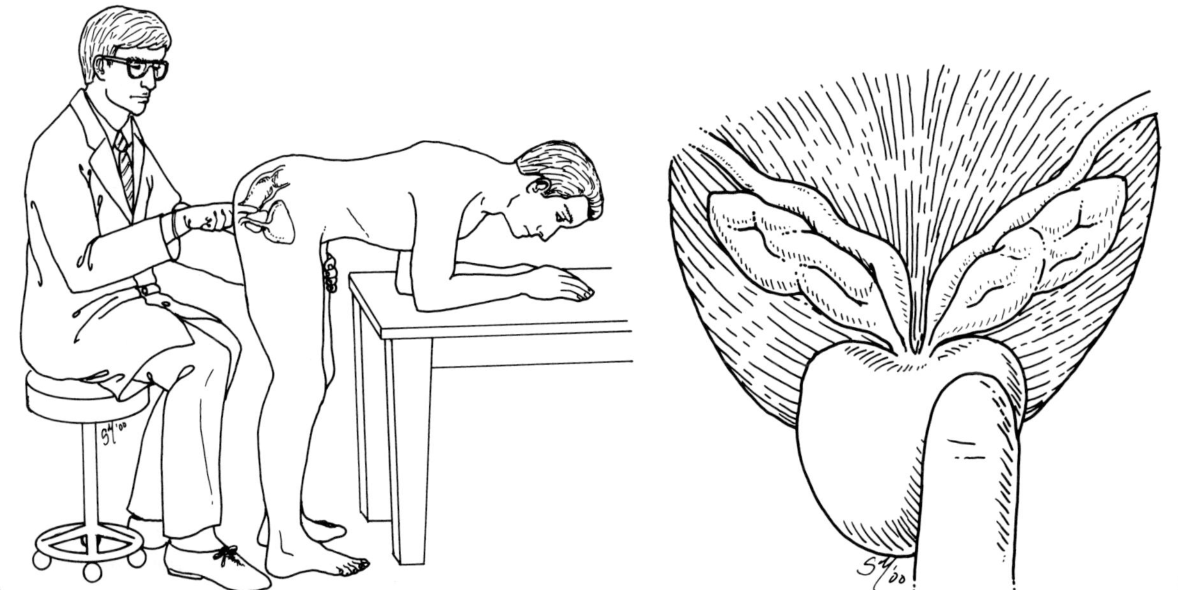

FIGURE 2.4. Palpation of the prostate and seminal vesicles. **A:** The prostate is best examined with the patient standing, knees slightly bent and elbows resting on the edge of the examining table. **B:** The examiner's index finger can be used to estimate the size of the prostate. (Reprinted with permission from Wyker A, Gillenwater JY. *Method of urology.* Baltimore: Williams & Wilkins, 1975.)

Scrotum and Testes

After the scrotal skin and perineum are inspected, the testes and epididymides should be palpated between the thumb and finger. The comma-shaped epididymis is closely attached to the posterolateral side of the testis. The physician can get his or her fingers into the groove between the epididymis and testis everywhere except superiorly, where the two structures are anatomically joined. In many men, a small ovoid lump, the rudimentary appendix testis, can be felt in or near the groove between the upper pole of the testis and the epididymis. The cord structures at the neck of the scrotum should be sifted through the physician's fingers. The solid cordlike vas is easily identified and followed to its junction with the tail of the epididymis. The other soft, stringy structures in the cord cannot be defined. To rule out the presence of the gravity-dependent varicocele, the cord must also be examined with the patient standing. If a varicocele is present, the intrascrotal varicosities secondary to valvular incompetence of the internal spermatic vein become distended in the upright position and feel like a bag of worms. Varicoceles tend to be left sided or bilateral due to the longer left gonadal vein attaching to the left renal vein. A solitary right-sided varicocele should alert the examiner to the risk of a retroperitoneal process.

Penis

If the patient is uncircumcised, the foreskin should be retracted to rule out phimosis with an obstructing, small aperture. To inspect the urethral meatus, the examiner must pinch the glans between the thumb and finger placed at the 6 and 12 o'clock positions. If the urethral meatus is not in the normal location, it can be found by following the midline raphe to its end on the undersurface of the penis. The shaft of the penis is palpated, looking particularly for the firm, fibrous plaques of Peyronie's disease. The floor of the urethra from the corona to the bulb should be palpated, looking for induration secondary to a stricture.

Pelvic Examination

Complete urologic examination of a woman includes a pelvic examination performed with the patient in lithotomy position. The vestibule and introitus are examined for evidence of mucosal atrophy, inflammation, or discharge. Any abnormal discharge is sampled for microscopic examination. The urethral meatus is examined and the urethra palpated for a mass or tenderness. Caruncle, a common benign finding in older women, is often seen as a purplish mass on the inferior aspect of the meatus. Calibration of the urethra is sometimes done to rule out urethral stenosis but is not a routine practice. Examination of the vaginal vault for cystocele, enterocele, or rectocele is performed in the course of a speculum examination of the cervix. Bimanual examination is carried out to identify any pelvic mass or tenderness.

URINALYSIS

A standard urinalysis consists of the following: determination of the physical characteristics of the urine, dipstick chemical tests, and microscopic examination of the urinary sediment. This key examination should not be delegated to uninterested laboratory personnel but should be performed by the physician. For reliable urinalyses, the urine must be collected properly and examined promptly.

Collection of the Urine Specimens

Of necessity, most urinalyses are performed on a random specimen freshly voided by the patient. However, the most information can be obtained if a first-morning specimen is examined. It is the best one for detecting formed elements in the urine and for determining whether urinary infection is present. The formed elements—red blood cells (RBCs), WBCs, and casts—are preserved in this characteristically acid and concentrated urine, whereas they may be lysed and disappear in dilute or alkaline urine. Bacterial colony counts are usually highest in this specimen because the bacteria have had more time to multiply during overnight incubation in the bladder.

For women, a voided sample is obtained by a clean-catch collection. The adequacy of the specimen for bacteriologic study depends on adequate cleansing with water of the periurethral areas to remove colonizing bacteria; avoiding bactericidal soap, which could produce a false-negative culture; and separation of the labia during collection. Only the midportion of the voided specimen should be collected. Urethral catheterization is performed when the patient is unable to perform the midstream collection properly because of handicap or body habitus, when microscopic examination of the voided specimen shows evidence of contamination by abundant squamous cells or mixed bacterial flora, or when previous culture of a voided specimen was positive for multiple organisms. The relatively minor drawbacks to urethral catheterization are the discomfort of the catheterization procedure itself and the potential for iatrogenic infection in up to 2% of patients from bacteria introduced into the bladder during the catheterization procedure.

For men, examination of the midstream urine (voided bladder 2) is the minimum urine examination, but the four-glass urine collection technique allows for the most thorough examination of the urine and prostate fluid. Stamey, Govan, and Palmer (33) originally described the four-glass urine collection technique as a method to distinguish urethral, bladder, and prostate infection in men. This technique was later modified by Meares and Stamey to include the EPS and is regarded as the gold standard for the evaluation of the lower urinary tract in males (25). The technique provides samples for both microscopic analysis and bacterial culture, allowing for a quantitative assessment of the urine for leukocytes, erythrocytes, macrophages, and bacteria (27). General practice is for circumcised men to void into sterile containers, being careful not to touch their glans penis or hands to the inside of the container, which could introduce bacteria that typically colonize the skin. There is some debate among urologists whether cleansing the glans penis with an alcohol pad or bactericidal soap is necessary in circumcised men, but it is the authors' practice not to do so. However, uncircumcised men should retract the foreskin and clean the glans penis with an alcohol pad or bactericidal soap before providing a four-glass urine sample (27).

Voided Bladder 1

The voided bladder 1 (VB1) specimen should include the first 10 mL of urine. The VB1 represents the urethral cells and bacteria, which are washed out with the first 10 mL of urine. This specimen is important in the diagnosis of urethritis (27).

Voided Bladder 2

The voided bladder 2 (VB2) specimen represents the bladder urine. It should be collected from a midstream urine specimen by placing the sterile specimen container into the urine stream after voiding 100 to 200 mL (27).

Expressed Prostatic Secretions

The EPS should be collected into a sterile container while the examiner digitally massages the prostate. The uncircumcised patient should hold back his foreskin, and the examiner should be careful not to contaminate the sterile container by touching the patient's penis to it. Even with vigorous massage, the EPS may be unobtainable owing to anxiety and guarding on the part of the patient. Often, if the patient is left alone in a quiet room, he can relax his external sphincter and consequently "milk" his urethra manually and collect a drop or two of EPS for examination. The EPS should be examined at high power (400×) for leukocytes, erythrocytes, macrophages, RBCs, fat bodies, and bacteria (27).

Voided Bladder 3

The voided bladder 3 (VB3) specimen is another method to examine the EPS. It represents the first 10 mL of urine voided after massaging the prostate and includes any EPS that may be trapped in the prostatic urethra. It allows for the examination of the EPS when a drop of fluid is unobtainable by digital massage. No longer than 30 minutes should elapse after a prostatic massage to collect this specimen. The VB1, VB2, and VB3 specimens should be centrifuged for 5 minutes and the sediment examined at high power (400×) for leukocytes, macrophages, erythrocytes, bacteria, and fungal hyphae, with their numbers recorded. The VB1, VB2, EPS, and VB3 specimens should then be immediately plated and cultured or temporarily stored in a refrigerator at 4°C, until they can be cultured later that day (27).

For infants and small children, strap-on collection devices are used to collect specimens for routine analysis. However, these specimens are often unsatisfactory for culture, and specimens for culture are most often obtained by catheterization with a well-lubricated 5-Fr feeding tube. Suprapubic aspiration may be performed in small infants. Although this has the best reliability in terms of specimens for bacteriologic study, it is not practical for routine use.

Urine should be examined within 30 minutes of collection. If it is allowed to stand, bacterial growth may alkalize the urine with resultant destruction of RBCs, WBCs, and casts. If the urine cannot be examined promptly, it should be refrigerated.

Physical Characteristics of Urine

Color

The color of normal urine is determined by the concentration of urochrome, an endogenously formed yellow-brown pigment excreted at a uniform rate. Because the amount of pigment excreted each hour is the same, the color of the urine varies directly with the urine output. With high urine flow rates, the urine is pale, almost water colored, whereas with low urine flow rates it is a deep yellow color. The appearance of an abnormal urine color may occur from a number of causes. Certain urinary pigments may impart a pink-to-red color to the urine, mimicking hematuria. These include anthocyanins in beets and berries (beeturia), phenolphthalein (present in some laxatives), vegetable dyes (used for food coloring), heavy concentration of urates, phenazopyridine (Pyridium), and *Serratia marcescens* infection in infants (red diaper syndrome). Myoglobinuria occurring as a result of muscle breakdown is also a cause of nonhematuric tea-colored urine. Characteristically, the urinary sediment shows no RBCs, but the dipstick test is positive.

Pneumaturia

Pneumaturia is the passage of gas in the urine and generally is caused by a fistula between the intestinal tract and the urinary tract. Because gas is lighter than water, it always rises to the top of the bladder and consequently is passed at the end of urination (terminal pneumaturia). This fistula may occur at any level, from the stomach to the rectum of the intestinal tract and from the kidney to the urethra of the urinary tract, but the large majority involve the bladder and the sigmoid colon or terminal ileum. The most common causes are diverticulitis of the sigmoid colon, carcinoma of the colon, and Crohn's disease.

Urinary tract infections caused by gas-forming bacteria and prior introduction of air into the bladder by means of insertion of a catheter or cystoscopy are occasional causes of pneumaturia.

Chyluria (Milky Urine)

Chyluria is the passage of lymph or chyle in the urine caused by the presence of an intrarenal, lymphatic-urinary fistula (11). The cause of this fistula is obstruction of the lymphatics superior to the kidney, usually the thoracic duct. With obstruction, there is increased back-pressure in the retroperitoneal and renal lymphatics, and eventually they rupture into a calyceal fornix. The most common cause of chyluria is filariasis resulting from *Wuchereria bancrofti.* The adult filarial worms invade the suprarenal lymphatics, causing obstruction and severe inflammation. Less common causes include posterior mediastinal and retroperitoneal tumors, tuberculosis, and trauma.

The passage of milky urine occurs intermittently, varying with the amount of fat ingested and sometimes with the patient's posture. Chylous urine contains fibrinogen, and fibrin clots may cause renal colic or urinary retention. The milky-colored appearance of the urine is usually diagnostic but may be confirmed by tests that confirm the presence of fat in the urine.

Clarity

Freshly voided urine is usually clear. Cloudiness of the urine is fairly common, however, and is usually caused by excessive amounts of crystals—amorphous phosphate in alkaline urine or amorphous urates in acid urine. This crystalluria is usually not clinically significant. The crystals can be dissolved, rendering the urine clear, by adding acid to dissolve the amorphous phosphates or by heating to dissolve the amorphous urates. Heavy pyuria, usually secondary to a bacterial infection, is a less common cause of cloudy urine.

Specific Gravity

The specific gravity of a solution is the measure of its density, an approximate measure of total solute concentration. The specific gravity of water is 1.000, plasma 1.010, and urine 1.003 to 1.040. Normally functioning kidneys conserve and excrete water as needed, accounting for the wide range of 1.003 to 1.040. Poorly functioning kidneys lose this ability, so urine specific gravity remains fixed at around plasma level (1.010).

Determination of the specific gravity of a random urine specimen is useful not only in assessing a patient's hydration status but also in interpreting the significance of dipstick chemical tests and urinary sediment findings. Substances such as WBCs, RBCs, and protein are generally excreted into the urine at a fairly constant rate. When the urine specific gravity is less than 1.007 as a result of a high urinary flow rate, the urine concentration of these elements may be significantly reduced. Also, in this hypotonic environment, RBCs are lysed, so patients with microhematuria may lack RBCs in the urinary sediment.

Chemical Tests

The standard urinalysis includes a dipstick assessment of nine different parameters. The pH, glucose, protein, ketone, bilirubin, and urobilinogen semiquantitative chemical tests provide the urologist with a powerful screening tool for metabolic abnormalities. The nitrite test serves as a screening for bacterial infection. Dipstick tests for blood and leukocyte esterase are commonly used in many settings as screens to determine the need for microscopic examination, but in the urologist's office, they are always used to complement the microscopic examination of the urinary sediment.

Urine pH varies between 5.0 and 8.0. It is usually more acidic in the early morning because of the excretion of a fixed acid load in the smaller volume of urine produced at night, and it is typically more alkaline after meals (alkaline tide). Specific medical conditions may be associated with characteristic changes in the range of urinary pH. Patients who form uric acid stones usually have a consistently acidic urine with a pH below 5.5. Patients with renal tubular acidosis type I (distal) are unable to acidify the urine below pH 5.5, even in the face of acid loading. This is in contrast to patients with type II renal tubular acidosis (proximal), who display the normal range of urinary pH (31). Alkaline urine above pH 8.0 is often associated with infection by urea-splitting organisms such as *Proteus.* Because leukocytes are lysed in very alkaline urine (above pH 8), it may sometimes be difficult to identify WBCs in the urinary sediment of patients with *Proteus* infection.

Detection of glucosuria by dipstick test indicates that the renal threshold for glucose reabsorption in the renal tubules (approximately 180 mg/dL) has been exceeded. This can occasionally be seen in normal patients, but most commonly, it is the result of hyperglycemia caused by diabetes mellitus. Although the semiquantitative dipstick test provides an approximate measure of the concentration of glucose in the urine, the clinician should realize that the degree of glucosuria is not necessarily an accurate indicator of the degree of hyperglycemia. Further medical evaluation and serum glucose determination are required. Elevated serum ketones, which may occur in diabetic ketoacidosis and in catabolic situations such as starvation, result in ketonuria detectable by the dipstick test.

The test for bilirubin will be positive when there are significant amounts of conjugated bilirubin filtered by the kidney and excreted in the urine. This is most commonly seen in liver disease and biliary obstruction. Urobilinogen, absorbed via the enterohepatic circulation, is normally present in small amounts in the urine. Increased levels are seen with hemolysis, gastrointestinal hemorrhage, and hepatocellular disease. Diminished levels may result from antibiotic suppression of the gut bacterial flora, and urobilinogen may disappear with complete biliary obstruction.

The dipstick test is the most commonly used screening test for urinary protein, detecting protein concentrations as low as 10 mg/dL. Normal supernatant urine usually gives a negative test for protein because the daily protein excretion of normal individuals is usually less than 50 mg.

Proteinuria is defined as the excretion of more than 150 mg of protein in 24 hours. The dipstick has a pH-sensitive indicator dye that changes color with various concentrations of protein. Although more sensitive to negatively charged protein (albumin) than to positively charged protein (Bence Jones), it does give a positive test when the concentration of Bence Jones protein is greater than 50 mg/dL. When the dipstick is positive, the 24-hour protein excretion in the urine should be determined by analysis of a timed 24-hour collection.

There are four types of proteinuria: glomerular, tubular, overflow, and functional. Glomerular is the most common form of proteinuria, found in patients with significant glomerular damage. A defect in the glomerular filter permits increased filtration of normal plasma proteins, and because albumin has the highest concentration in the plasma, glomerular proteinuria is predominantly an albuminuria. Massive proteinuria with excretion of 4 g/day or more is characteristic of the nephrotic syndrome.

Proteinuria secondary to tubular or interstitial disorders of the kidney occurs when the proximal tubules are unable to reabsorb the normally filtered proteins. In tubular proteinuria, one usually finds increased amounts of low-molecular-weight proteins smaller than albumin in the urine, and the total protein excretion is usually 1 to 2 g/day.

Overflow proteinuria is caused by the presence in plasma of abnormal quantities of low-molecular-weight proteins that are filtered across the normal glomerular capillary wall and saturate the proximal tubular resorptive mechanism. Examples include Bence Jones proteinuria, myoglobinuria, and hemoglobinuria. This is the least common type of proteinuria.

When proteinuria occurs in the absence of any clear-cut renal or systemic disease, it is termed *functional* or *physiologic proteinuria.* The mechanisms responsible for this type of proteinuria are unknown but are probably hemodynamic. Functional proteinurias are characteristically intermittent and mild, with protein excretion rarely exceeding 1 g/day. Clinical states that may cause this type of proteinuria include fever, exercise, emotional stress, and renal venous hypertension (congestive heart failure). Orthostatic (postural) proteinuria is a special form of functional proteinuria seen in healthy young adults. These individuals excrete protein in their urine in the upright position but excrete little or none on recumbency.

Urinary Sediment

Examination of the urinary sediment is performed on a centrifuged sample of urine. All specimens should be mixed thoroughly before a sample is taken because formed elements fall to the bottom during storage. Approximately 15 mL is centrifuged for 3 to 5 minutes, the supernatant removed, the pellet resuspended in the residual fluid, and a drop placed under a cover slip for examination. Before the specimen is examined, the pH and specific gravity of the urine should be noted because of their potential to influence stability of the formed elements such as WBCs and RBCs in the specimen.

White Blood Cells

Pyuria is increased WBC excretion in the urine (20,22) and may be detected by a dipstick test for leukocyte esterase or by counting the number of WBCs in the centrifuged, unstained urinary sediment. A WBC excretion rate of 400,000 WBCs per hour may be considered the upper limit of normal. If this excretion rate of 400,000 WBCs per hour is divided by the average urine output per hour of 50 mL, the upper limit of WBC concentration in the urine would be 8,000 WBCs/mL. This translates to urinary sediment findings of 4 to 5 WBCs per HPF, and for clinical purposes, pyuria may be defined as more than 5 WBCs per HPF. This method of quantitating pyuria is imprecise. Factors that may alter the microscopic findings significantly include presence or absence of contamination of the urine specimen, urine production rate at the time the urine specimen was obtained, and the specifics of preparing and examining the urinary sediment.

Leukocyte esterase, an isoenzyme specific for leukocytes, is the basis for the leukocyte esterase test strip. Both false-positive and false-negative results may occur, and the dipstick test is best combined with microscopic examination of the urinary sediment. When leukocytes are not seen despite a positive dipstick test in the setting of alkaline urine (pH greater than 8.0), such as might occur with *Proteus* infection, alkaline lysis of the leukocytes should be suspected.

Pyuria is the body's response to the inflammation of the urinary tract, but it is not a particularly sensitive sign of infection. Although most patients with acute bacterial infection such as cystitis have pyuria, significant bacteriuria may be present without pyuria. A urine culture is the only reliable means to diagnose infection. Pyuria is also not a specific sign of infection. Although many physicians equate the two (pyuria and urinary infection), this is a dangerous concept that can lead to patients being inappropriately treated for long periods with antibiotics for presumed infection. Pyuria has numerous causes, including tumors, stones, glomerulonephritis, foreign bodies, drugs (e.g., cyclophosphamide), fungal infection, and tuberculosis. When pyuria exists with a negative culture, a diligent search must be initiated to discover and treat the underlying cause.

Red Blood Cells

The average individual usually excretes approximately 30,000 RBCs per hour but may excrete up to 100,000 RBCs per hour. If the urine output is 50 mL/hour (1,200 mL/day), up to 2,000 RBCs/mL may be excreted, and this concentration of RBCs gives urine findings of 1 or fewer RBC per HPF. Greater than 1 RBC per HPF may be considered microscopic hematuria, but a commonly accepted benchmark for clinically significant hematuria is greater than 3 RBCs per HPF (23).

Osmotic Rupture of Red Blood Cells by Hypotonic Urine

The dipstick test for hematuria complements microscopic examination of the urinary sediment. RBCs are relatively resistant to alkaline lysis but are readily lysed in hypotonic urine. When the urine specific gravity is 1.007 or lower, the dipstick test will be positive even though no RBCs can be seen in the urinary sediment.

Urine containing 100,000 RBCs/mL with a urinary sediment finding of 30 RBCs per HPF was used as the standard in Table 2.5.

It is clinically important to know whether the RBCs present in the urinary sediment are glomerular or nonglomerular in origin because glomerular RBCs are diagnostic of glomerulonephritis. Two findings identify the glomeruli as the source of the RBCs: dysmorphic RBCs and RBC casts. Fairley and Birch (13) and Fassett and associates (14) used a phase microscope to study RBC morphology and reported that these dysmorphic RBCs were characteristic of glomerular bleeding. The marked RBC membrane distortions are thought to be caused by osmotic and physical changes during the passage of RBCs through the nephron. These findings have been confirmed by others. Stamey and Kindrachuk (34), in their excellent manual, showed many fine photographs contrasting dysmorphic RBCs of glomerular origin with RBCs of nonglomerular origin (Fig. 2.5). They also demonstrated that these dysmorphic RBCs could be identified under standard light microscopy, as well as phase-contrast microscopy.

Casts

The basic foundation of all renal casts is a special protein, Tamm-Horsfall globulin, secreted by the tubular epithelial cells. A small number of these basic hyaline casts are excreted normally, so their presence in the urinary sediment is not clinically significant. If RBCs, WBCs, or sloughed tubular epithelial cells are present in the renal tubular lumina, they may become incorporated within the cast. If these casts are detected in the urinary sediment, the presence of renal disease should be suspected. Because Tamm-Horsfall protein is soluble at a pH of 7.1 or higher, *all* casts disappear in alkaline urine.

TABLE 2.5. OSMOTIC RUPTURE OF RED BLOOD CELLS BY HYPOTONIC URINE

Urine Specific Gravity	RBCs/HPF	Dipstick	% Lysis
1.001	0	++++	100
1.005	0	++++	100
1.007	0	++++	100
1.010	30	+	0
1.015	30	+	0
1.020	30	+	0
1.025	30	+	0
1.028	30	+	0

RBCs/HPF, red blood cells per high-power field.

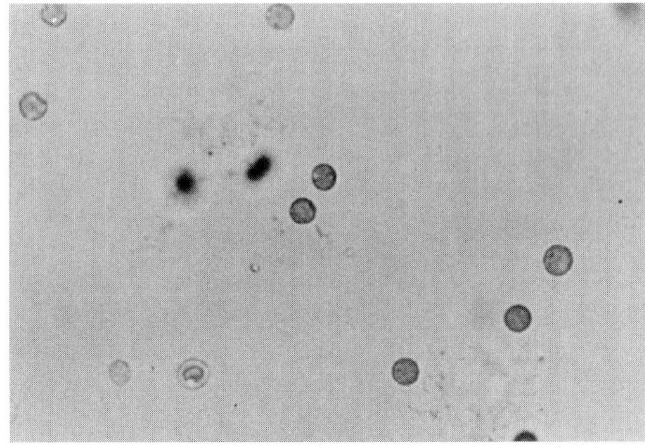

Normal Red Blood Cells

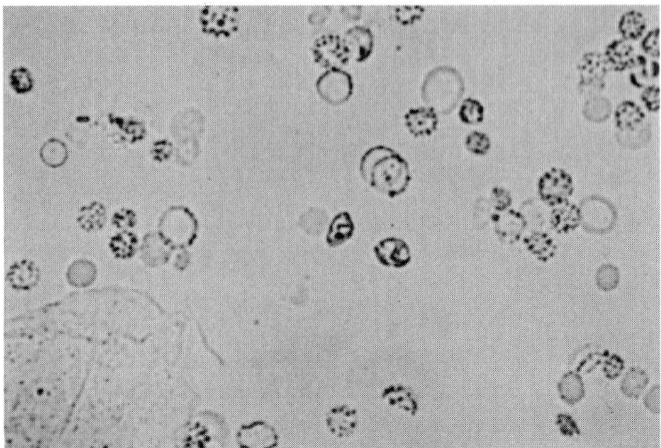

Dysmorphic Blood Cells

FIGURE 2.5. Normal and dysmorphic red blood cells. (Reprinted with permission from Stamey TA, Kindrachuk RW. *Urinary sediment and urinalysis: a practical guide for the health science professional.* Philadelphia: WB Saunders, 1985.)

Bacteria

Nitrite is a product of bacterial metabolism in many species of Gram-negative bacteria, and its presence in the urine is a strong indicator of significant bacteriuria. The false-positive rate for the dipstick test is low, and it may reliably be used as the basis for empiric antibiotic therapy pending results of culture and sensitivity. The more significant false-negative rate of the dipstick test, even in the presence of bacteriuria, can be due to a number of factors, including the presence of non–nitrite-producing organisms or very dilute urine. Urine culture is the only reliable means to exclude bacteriuria.

On microscopic examination, an effort should be made to detect bacteria because more than ten bacteria per HPF usually signifies greater than 10^5 colony-forming units (cfu) per milliliter (18). The morphology of any observed bacteria should be noted. A polymicrobial appearance or the presence of filamentous bacilli characteristic of lactobacillus in a woman's voided specimen strongly suggests contamination by vaginal or periurethral flora. In patients to be treated for suspected urinary tract infection, the identification of rods, streptococci (enterococci), or cocci (staphylococci) in the urine may guide the selection of antibiotic therapy. The presence of fungal elements or trichomonads should likewise be noted.

Because the most common uropathogens are aerobic species (Gram-negative rods, enterococci, and staphylococci), the standard urine culture is a test for aerobic organisms. A positive culture result is generally considered to be greater than 10^5 cfu/mL on a voided specimen, but as few as 10^3 cfu/mL may represent significant bacteriuria if the specimen is obtained in sterile fashion (e.g., catheterization). Similarly, localizing quantitative cultures on split-voiding fractions may reveal low-level bacteriuria in one fraction (e.g., VB3) that is nonetheless significantly greater than the other fractions, thereby showing bacterial infestation in the source of that fraction (e.g., prostate). Less commonly, fungi or microbacteria may be the cause of urinary tract infection. Fungi may grow on routine culture media with prolonged incubation; however, if fungal infection is suspected, the fungal culture should be specifically requested. Sterile pyuria with or without microscopic hematuria is a cardinal feature of genitourinary tuberculosis. Diagnosis is made by submitting at least three morning urine specimens to be examined for acid-fast bacteria and cultured for acid-fast bacteria for up to 8 weeks.

REFERENCES

1. Abrams P, Blaivas J, Griffiths D, et al. The objective evaluation of bladder outlet obstruction (urodynamics). In: Cockett A, Houry S, Aso Y, et al., eds. *The second international consultation on benign prostatic hyperplasia (BPH).* Channel Islands: Scientific Communications International, 1993.
2. Alexander RB, Ponniah S, Hasday J, et al. Elevated levels of proinflammatory cytokines in the semen of patients with chronic prostatitis/chronic pelvic pain syndrome. *Urology* 1998; 52:744.
3. Ameda K, Koyanagi T, Nantani M, et al. The relevance of preoperative cystometrography in patients with benign prostatic hyperplasia: correlating the findings with clinical features and outcome after prostatectomy. *J Urol* 1994;152:443.
4. Blandy J. *Operative urology.* Oxford, England: Blackwell Scientific Publications, 1978.
5. Blaivis JG, Olsson CA. Stress incontinence: classification and surgical approach. *J Urol* 1988;139:727.
6. Burgio KL, Engel BT, Locher JL. Normative patterns of diurnal variation across 6 age decades. *J Urol* 1991;145:728.
7. Carson CC III, Segura JW, Greene LF. Clinical importance of microhematuria. *JAMA* 1979;241:149.
8. Chancellor MB, Rivas DA. American Urological Association symptom index for women with voiding symptoms: lack of index specificity for benign prostatic hyperplasia. *J Urol* 1993; 150:1706.
9. Clemens JQ, Nadler RB, Schaeffer AJ, et al. Biofeedback, pelvic floor re-education and bladder training for male chronic pelvic pain syndrome. *Urology* 2000;56:951.
10. Copley JB, Hasbargen JA. Idiopathic hematuria: a prospective evaluation. *Arch Intern Med* 1987;147:434.
11. Diamond E, Schapira HE. Chyluria—review of the literature. *Urology* 1985;26:427.
12. Esperanca M, Gerrard JW. Nocturnal enuresis: studies in bladder function in normal children and enuretics. *Can Med Assoc J* 1969;101:324.
13. Fairley KF, Birch DF. Hematuria: a simple method of identifying glomerular bleeding. *Kidney Int* 1982;21:105.
14. Fassett RG, Horgan BA, Mathew TH. Detection of glomerular bleeding by phase-contrast microscopy. *Lancet* 1982;1: 1432.
15. Greene LF, O'Shaughnessy EJ Jr, Hendricks ED. Study of five hundred patients with asymptomatic microhematuria. *JAMA* 1956;161:610.
16. Hochreiter WW, Nadler RB, Koch AE, et al. Evaluation of the cytokines interleukin 8 and epithelial neutrophil activating peptide 78 as indicators of inflammation in prostatic secretions. *Urology* 2000;56:1025.
17. Kaplan WE. Office management of nocturnal enuresis. *AUA Update Series* 1989;19:146.
18. Kunin CM. The quantitative significance of bacteria visualized in the unstained urinary sediment. *N Engl J Med* 1961; 265:589.
19. Lee LW, Davis E Jr. Gross urinary hemorrhage: a symptom, not a disease. *JAMA* 1953;153:782.
20. Little PJ. Urinary white-cell excretion. *Lancet* 1962;1:1149.
21. Litwin M, McNaughton Collins M, Fowler F Jr, et al. The National Institutes of Health Chronic Prostatitis Symptom Index (NIH-CPSI): development and validation of a new outcome measure. *J Urol* 1999;162:369.
22. Mabeck CE. Studies in urinary tract infections: IV. Urinary leucocyte excretion in bacteriuria. *Acta Med Scand* 1969; 186:193.
23. Mariani AJ. The evaluation of adult hematuria. *AUA Update Series* 1989;23:178.
24. McLellan AM, Goodell H. Pain from the bladder, ureter and kidney pelvis. *Res Publ Assoc Nerv Ment Dis* 1942;23:252.
25. Meares EM, Stamey TA. Bacteriologic localization patterns in bacterial prostatis and urethritis. *Invest Urol* 1968;5:492.

26. Nadler RB, Koch AE, Calhoun EA, et al. IL-beta and TNF-alpha in prostate secretions are key indicators in the evaluation of men with chronic prostatitis. *J Urol* 2000;164:214.
27. Nadler RB, Schaeffer AJ. Lower urinary tract cultures. In: Nickel JC, ed. *Textbook of prostatitis.* Oxford, England: Isis Medical Media Ltd, 1999:205.
28. National Institutes of Health. Summary statement. National Institutes of Health/National Institute of Diabetes and Digestive and Kidney Disease's Workshop on Chronic Prostatitis. Bethesda, Md, 1995.
29. Nitti VW, Kim Y, Combs AJ. Correlation to the AUA symptom index with urodynamics in patients with suspected benign prostatic hyperplasia. *Neurol Urol* 1994;13:521.
30. Presti JC, Schmidt RA, Narayan PA, et al. Pathophysiology of urinary incontinence after radical prostatectomy. *J Urol* 1990; 143:975.
31. Rothstein M, Obialo C, Hruska KA. Renal tubular acidosis. *Endocrinol Metab Clin North Am* 1990;19:869.
32. Shahed A, Shoskes DA. Oxidative stress in prostatic fluid of men with chronic pelvic pain syndrome: correlation with bacterial growth and treatment response [Abstract]. *J Urol* 2000;163 (4 Suppl):24.
33. Stamey TA, Govan DE, Palmer JM. The localization and treatment of urinary tract infection: the role of bactericidal urine levels as opposed to serum levels. *Medicine* 1965;44:1.
34. Stamey TA, Kindrachuk RW. *Urinary sediment and urinalysis: a practical guide for the health science professional.* Philadelphia: WB Saunders, 1985.
35. Straub LR, Ripley HS, Wolf S. Disturbances of bladder function associated with emotional status. *JAMA* 1949;141:1139.
36. Verney EB. The antidiuretic hormone and the factors which determine its release. *Proc R Soc Lond (Biol)* 1947;135:25.
37. Yalla SV, Sullivan MP, Lecamwasam HS, et al. Correlation of the American Urological Association symptom index with obstructive and obstructive prostatism. *J Urol* 1995; 153:674.

3

IMAGING

3A

EXCRETORY UROGRAPHY

ROBERT A. OLDER

Excretory urography remains a basic radiologic examination of the urinary tract and is the foundation for the evaluation of suspected urologic disease. Despite development of the newer diagnostic modalities, such as isotope scanning, ultrasonography, computed tomography (CT), and magnetic resonance imaging (MRI), excretory urography has maintained a prominent role in uroradiology. Some indications have been altered and will continue to change with the newer imaging modalities. Noncontrast spiral CT has become the study of choice for suspected ureteral stones (88). The initial evaluation of suspected urinary tract structural abnormalities, hematuria, pyuria, and renal calculus disease is performed with excretory urography. The examination is relatively inexpensive and simple to perform, with few contraindications.

R.A. Older: Department of Radiology, University of Virginia Health System, Charlottesville, VA 22908.

When properly performed, excretory urography can provide valuable information about the renal parenchyma, pelvicalyceal system, ureters, and urinary bladder. Diagnostic results depend largely on the method by which excretory urography is performed. A closely monitored examination with specific radiographs determined by the needs of a patient provides the optimal examination. A study using only predetermined radiographs that are reviewed at a later time often provides inadequate diagnostic information. During urography, each radiograph should be evaluated immediately after it is obtained to determine which questions have been answered and which have not. Any necessary additional radiographs can then be obtained.

It is reasonable to have certain standard radiographs obtained in the immediate postinjection phase of a urogram. Further radiographs, however, should be determined on the basis of initial findings and not limited to a preset series.

TABLE 3A.1. COMMONLY USED IONIC CONTRAST MEDIA FOR EXCRETORY UROGRAPHY

Trade Name	Generic Name	Concentration (%)	Osmolality (mOsm/kg)	Iodine Content (mg/mL)
Renografin-60	Meglumine and sodium diatrizoate	60	1,420	288
Reno-M-60	Meglumine diatrizoate	60	1,500	282
Hypaque-50	Sodium diatrizoate	50	1,550	300
Hypaque-M-60	Meglumine diatrizoate	60	1,415	282
Conray-60	Meglumine iothalamate	60	1,400	282

CONTRAST MEDIA

Chemical Properties and Excretion

The first compounds introduced for clinical use in excretory urography during the early 1930s were diiodinated compounds that were hampered by low radiopacity and moderate toxicity. More often than not, retrograde pyelography was necessary to evaluate the urinary tract properly. The ability to achieve adequate opacification of the pelvicalyceal system and the renal parenchyma resulted from the introduction of the triiodinated benzoic acid derivatives in the early 1950s. Since then, several salts of triiodinated benzoic acid compound have been marketed for excretory urography with slight structural differences but similar physiologic and radiographic properties (Table 3A.1 and Fig. 3A.1).

The ionic compounds are water-soluble salt solutions that are hypertonic with an osmolality 2.5 to 6.0 times that of plasma. The cations are either sodium or meglumine (methylglucamine). The large number of different ionic contrast media merely represents variations of concentration and cations for the anions diatrizoate or iothalamate. The name often denotes a specific iodine concentration along with the cation and anion used. For urography, only the 50% or 60% agents are routinely used.

Researchers have described objective differences in the pyelogram when comparing sodium and meglumine as the cation (9,21,75). In the laboratory, the sodium salt has produced higher urinary iodine concentrations, whereas meglumine has given better distention of the pelvicalyceal system because of a greater diuresis. Neither of the two cations produces any significant difference in the nephrogram (21,24,36). With the doses used in present-day excretory urography, the advantages and disadvantages are minimal. Good-quality urography can be achieved using either of the salts.

For urography, low-osmolar contrast and nonionic contrast are essentially the same. Ioxaglate, a low-osmolar, but ionic, dimer is used predominantly in angiography. Low-osmolar contrast media are now used in more than 60% of

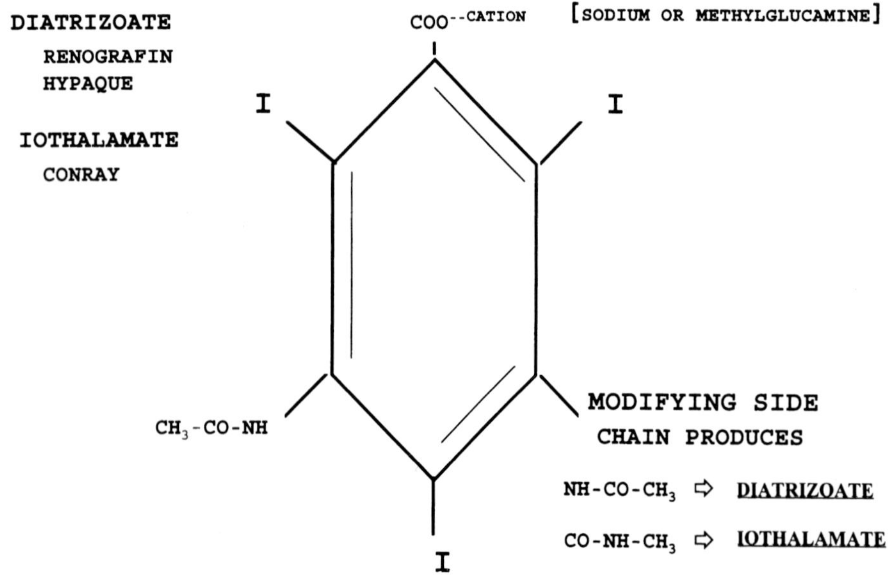

FIGURE 3A.1. Molecular structure of currently used ionic urographic contrast media. (From Older RA, Resnick MI, eds. *Basic radiologic techniques in diagnosis of genitourinary disease,* ed 2. New York: Thieme Medical Publishers, 1994, with permission.)

all radiographic procedures. They contain the same iodine concentration as the conventional agents but are much less hypertonic (Table 3A.2). These new compounds have approximately half the osmolality of the conventional compounds. To reduce the osmolality of the contrast media, two basic approaches are used. Three of these compounds (iohexol, iopamidol, and ioversol) are nonionic formulations that consist of three iodine atoms attached to a fully substituted, uncharged benzene ring (Fig. 3A.2). Because no balancing cation is needed, osmolality is reduced to half that of the conventional agents at the same iodine content. The fourth agent (ioxaglate) is an ionic dimer that consists of two linked benzene rings, each with three iodine molecules, and a single negative charge balanced by a cation. Thus there are two particles to six iodine atoms, also halving the osmolality at an equal iodine concentration. This feature is a definite benefit in angiography, where ioxaglate is used primarily because the lower osmolality of ioxaglate causes less pain in intraarterial injections. The lower-osmolality compounds also cause fewer physiologic responses. The newer media produce less peripheral vasodilation and less effect on myocardial contractility and cardiac electrophysiology. These decreased effects may be caused by the lower osmolality or due to a lower chemotoxicity (10).

Clinical studies have demonstrated that the nonionic agents can produce a urogram equal to or better than ionic media (3,89). The lower osmolality and solute load allow the nonionic agents to produce a denser pyelogram with higher urinary iodine concentration (23,89). There is a potential for decreased distention of the collecting system because of reduced diuretic effect, but this has not been a significant problem. No significant difference in the nephrogram has been noted (23,89). Therefore using nonionic contrast does not decrease the diagnostic efficacy of urography.

Contrast material is almost entirely excreted by glomerular filtration with little or no tubular excretion. Approximately 0.5% to 2.0% is excreted by the liver and bowel. Most of this is excreted by the biliary system, although the small intestine, stomach, and salivary glands can excrete small amounts. *Vicarious excretion* is the term used when extrarenal excretion is apparent on the radiograph (8). Contrast medium may be seen in the gallbladder and colon 24 hours after injection in patients with decreased renal function, in whom extrarenal routes of excretion take on greater importance. Occasionally, this phenomenon is also seen in patients with normal renal function after they have received large doses of contrast medium (Fig. 3A.3) (70). The amount of contrast excretion by the kidney and collecting system with resultant radiopacity is related to plasma concentration and glomerular filtration rate (GFR) (17). Because GFR is fixed in the individual, only the plasma concentration can be manipulated. Increasing the amount of contrast material will increase the radiopacity of the urinary tract to a certain extent. At doses greater than 2 mL/kg, the radiopacity will not continue to increase significantly, but the risk of toxicity is increased. The method of injection will also alter the quality of the urogram. When a drip infusion is used, the plasma concentration plateau is slowly reached and falls off over a longer period. The drip infusion technique never achieves a plasma level as high as the bolus injection (Fig. 3A.4) (17) and is of no benefit, save convenience. The intensity of the nephrogram is related to the plasma concentration. Studies have shown that immediately after bolus injection, a peak plasma concentration is achieved, which then declines rapidly. The nephrogram will be maximal during this period of peak plasma concentration (32).

Following glomerular filtration, approximately 85% of the water resorption that concentrates the urine and increases radiopacity occurs in the proximal convoluted tubules. Additional resorption occurs in the distal convoluted tubules and collecting ducts, being regulated by antidiuretic hormone (ADH) and depending on the state of hydration. Because of this small contribution, the effectiveness of dehydration in increasing radiopacity is minimal, especially in light of the larger contrast doses used today. A comparison of patients with and without fluid restriction favored the fluid-restricted group in terms of radiographic scoring, but the difference was not statistically significant (22).

TABLE 3A.2. LOW-OSMOLALITY CONTRAST MEDIA

Trade Name	Generic Name	Concentration (%)	Osmolality (mOsm/kg)	Iodine Content (mg/mL)
Omnipaque 300	Iohexol	64.7	709	300
Omnipaque 350	Iohexol	75.5	862	350
Isovue 300	Iopamidol	61	616	300
Isovue 370	Iopamidol	76	796	370
Optiray 320	Ioversol	68	702	320
Hexabrix	Ioxaglate (sodium 19.6%, meglumine 39.3%)	58.9	600	320

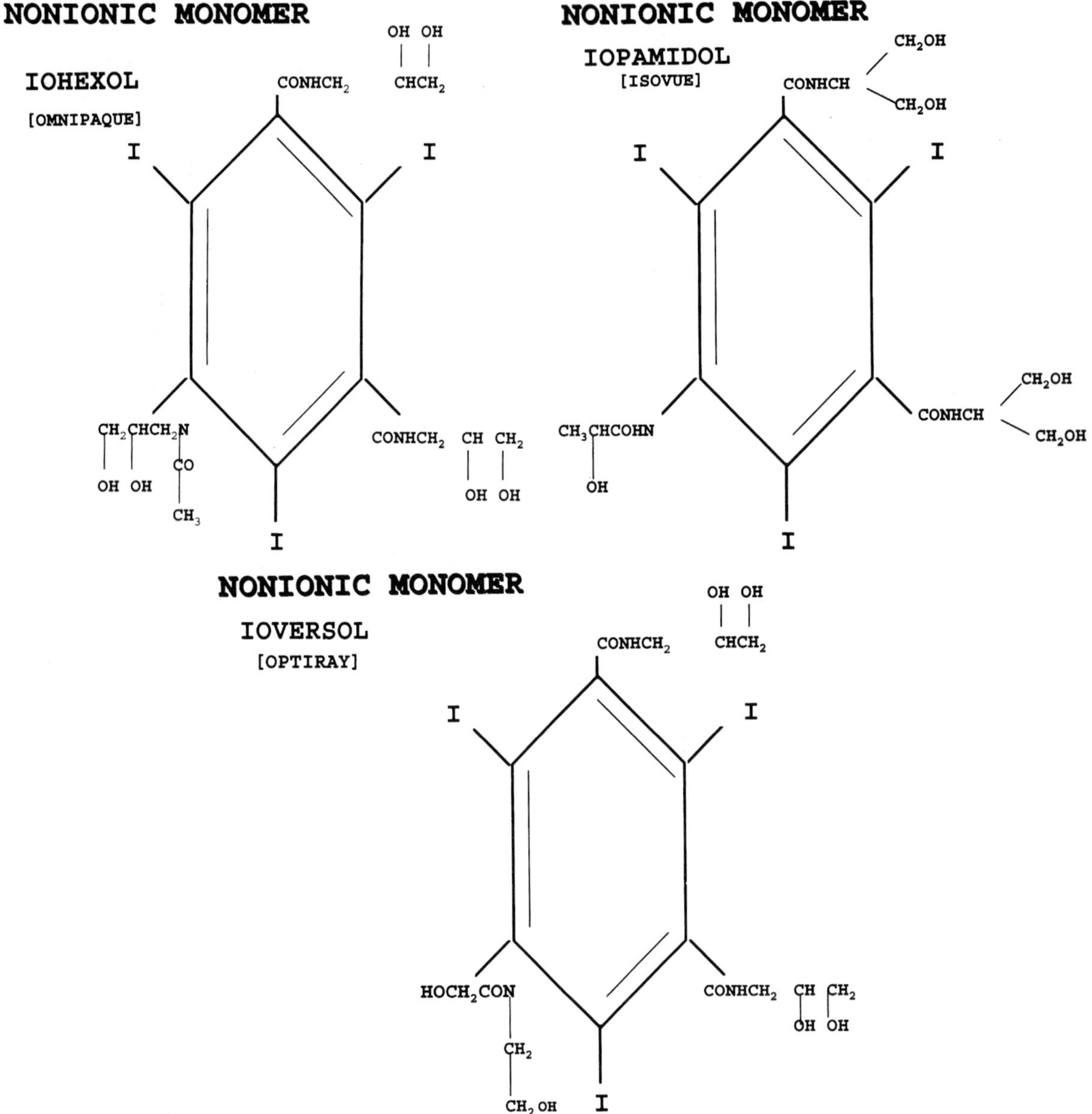

FIGURE 3A.2. Molecular structures of currently used nonionic urographic contrast. (From Older RA, Resnick MI, eds. *Basic radiologic techniques in diagnosis of genitourinary disease*, ed 2. New York: Thieme Medical Publishers, 1994, with permission.)

In most clinical situations, significant dehydration is not actually achieved. However, fluid restriction will limit fluid intake and the use of diuretic substances such as coffee, and it can avoid a state of excessive hydration with increased flow rate (43,64). We have found these urograms generally of better quality than those with no fluid restriction. Nephrotoxicity is the primary concern in fluid restricting a patient, and this should not be done in any patient with preexisting renal disease. Therefore, if it cannot be determined whether a patient has preexisting renal disease, fluid restriction should be avoided. In patients with normal renal function, overnight fluid restriction will probably improve the quality of the examination.

Physiologic Considerations

Following intravenous (IV) injection of ionic contrast material, there are several subjective effects, the intensity of which vary with the rate of injection and the individual. A sense of warmth and a "flushing" sensation are almost universal and may be misinterpreted as a reaction. A metallic taste and circumoral tingling are commonly observed. Sensations of pelvic and perineal warmth are not unusual and may be distressing to some patients. These uncomfortable side effects are virtually eliminated with nonionic contrast media.

Several physiologic responses have been noted with intravascular injection of contrast media. There is usually a mild and transient decrease in the systemic blood pressure along with a transient decrease in the heart rate (90). Pulmonary arterial pressure has been found to be transiently increased by contrast medium (76). Renal blood flow is initially increased but is followed by a decrease in renal blood flow proportional to the dose administered (31). A depressant effect on the myocardium has been shown with decreased myocardial contractility that is thought to be secondary to calcium binding and a depressant effect on the sinoatrial (SA) and atrioventricular (AV) nodes (46,79). It has been suggested that subclinical bronchospasm occurs in most patients (80). These effects are all transient and seem inconsequential but may play a part in the untoward reactions seen in a small percentage of patients.

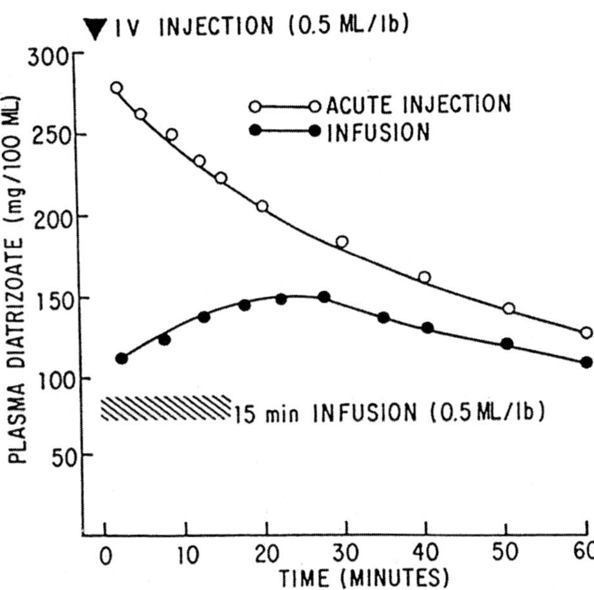

FIGURE 3A.4. Plasma diatrizoate concentration as a function of time and type of injection. IV, intravenous. (From Cattell WR. Excretory pathways for contrast media. *Invest Radiol* 1970;5:473, with permission.)

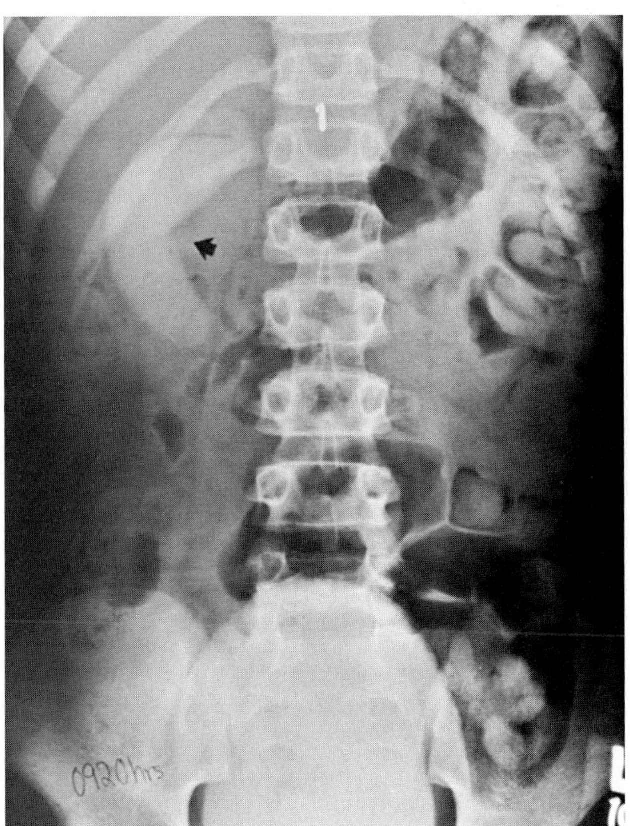

FIGURE 3A.3. Vicarious excretion of contrast material with opacification of the gallbladder *(arrowhead)*. X-ray film taken supine 24 hours after large dose of intravenous contrast material.

CONTRAST MEDIA REACTIONS

Incidence and Classification

Adverse reactions to intravascular contrast media are well known and are a source of concern, but fortunately, most cases are mild and insignificant. Several large series of patients have demonstrated an overall incidence of contrast reactions of all types ranging from 5% to 8% (85,86,97). However, major respiratory or cardiovascular reactions are reported to occur in fewer than 1% of patients. The reported frequency of fatal reactions ranges between 1 in 14,000 and 1 in 75,000 (4,42,84).

Contrast reactions are usually classified as mild, moderate, or severe. In most series, 95% or more of all reactions are classified as mild to moderate. A sense of heat and flushing, along with most cases of nausea and vomiting, should not be considered adverse reactions but rather common side effects of the contrast material. Mild reactions include mild urticaria and minimal respiratory symptoms. Moderate reactions include extensive urticaria, angioneurotic edema, and bronchospasm. Severe reactions include intense bronchospasm with laryngeal edema along with potentially lethal cardiovascular responses such as marked hypotension, pulmonary edema, and ventricular arrhythmias that can lead to cardiovascular collapse.

Etiology

Although adverse reactions to contrast media have been studied extensively over the years, their pathogenesis remains somewhat obscure. Most evidence points toward a multifactorial concept in which several poorly understood responses to contrast media may lead to an adverse reaction.

Certain reactions such as urticaria, erythema, and bronchospasm appear to be allergic. They resemble an allergic reaction and respond as an allergic reaction to antihistamines and epinephrine. However, the allergy concept is controversial, with many researchers disputing its validity. Failure to find the classic immunoglobulin E (IgE)-type antibodies to contrast media in humans and the fact that individuals may react without prior exposure to contrast media do not support the allergy model (35,55,59). However, work by Brasch (11) supports the theory that contrast material may act as haptens and induce specific antihapten antibodies. Anticontrast media antibodies of both the immunoglobulin G (IgG) and IgE classes have been produced in rabbits. Contrast reactions in individuals without prior exposure are explained on the basis of antibody cross-reactivity, where the contrast media are similar to other antigens to which the individual has had prior exposure, such as other halogenated benzene rings found in food additives, pesticides, and other substances.

Some of the most severe reactions, however, do not resemble allergic reactions. Sudden major cardiovascular responses such as profound hypotension, pulmonary edema, ventricular arrhythmias, and myocardial infarction involve responses that are poorly understood. Hypertonicity and direct chemotoxicity of the contrast material have been suggested as etiologies (30,77). Enhanced vagal tone as the result of stimulation of the vasomotor center of the medulla and accentuation of contrast medium–induced myocardial toxicity has been suggested as the etiology in the sudden deaths of fluid-depleted dogs following IV injection of contrast material (47).

Lalli (52,53) has developed an interesting hypothesis based on the effect of contrast medium on the central nervous system (CNS) after crossing the blood–brain barrier. He believes that all reactions are ultimately neurogenic, centered on the hypothalamus and medulla. The combination of anxiety and contrast materials stimulating the hypothalamus can lead to a variety of neurogenic responses, such as hypotension, ventricular arrhythmias, and pulmonary edema. He thinks that anxiety plays a large role in contrast reactions and that examinations performed in a quiet, nonthreatening manner will reduce the number of adverse reactions.

A significant decrease in mild, moderate, and severe reactions has been demonstrated with nonionic contrast materials. The decrease is approximately a factor of 5 (45,73,98). Initially, there was controversy regarding the methodology of the comparative contrast studies, but the data have continued to indicate much greater safety for nonionic contrast materials (16), and safety is no longer a controversial issue.

Relationship to Previous Reactions and Hypersensitivity States

Studies have shown that individuals with known hypersensitivity states have contrast reactions on the order of twice those of the normal population, 10% to 12% versus 5%. Individuals who have had a previous contrast material reaction have a threefold increase; 15% to 16% of these individuals have a recurrent contrast reaction (85,97). The nature of the recurrent reaction is variable, with minor reactions being repeated more often than life-threatening reactions.

Value of Pretesting and Premedication

IV injection of a test dose of contrast medium has not been proved useful as a screen for potential contrast reactions. Yocum, Heller, and Abels (99) demonstrated some value in high-risk patients with pretesting, but it involved a sophisticated protocol using multiple serial dilutions of the contrast material. A standard 0.5- to 1.0-mL IV test injection is of little use and may precipitate life-threatening reactions (85).

Investigators have shown that the incidence of recurrent reactions can be reduced by half or greater of the expected incidence with prophylactic antihistamines and corticosteroids (38,48,99). Steroid premedication can reduce the risk of an adverse reaction for ionic contrast to a level close to that of nonionic contrast. However, steroid premedications are not effective unless given for at least 12 hours before the administration of contrast (56,58), and this has limited the feasibility of routine premedication in all patients (25). The combination of a steroid preparation with a nonionic agent further reduces the risk of an adverse reaction (57); this is our approach to patients with previous adverse reactions to contrast or those with a significant allergy history in general. For convenience, we use Decadron 4 mg orally every 6 hours for 24 hours before the examination. Although steroid preparations and nonionic contrast can reduce the risk of an adverse reaction, they do not completely eliminate the possibility, and the need for a contrast examination should be examined closely in this group of patients.

Treatment of Contrast Material Reactions

Contrast reactions usually occur immediately or within minutes following the injection. However, severe reactions can occur after 15 minutes or even later. All physicians, nurses, and technologists involved in urography should be well trained in the recognition of the early signs of a contrast reaction and in resuscitation. Prompt recognition of a reaction and immediate treatment can be lifesaving. In all excretory urograms, the IV needle or catheter used for delivering the contrast should be left in place for the duration of the examination in case a reaction develops and

IV access is needed. Blood pressure and electrocardiographic (ECG) monitoring equipment, as well as oxygen, should always be close at hand. In each room, there should be ready access to epinephrine, atropine, and diphenhydramine. In cases of cardiovascular collapse, a "crash cart" containing a defibrillator, an endotracheal set, and drugs useful during cardiac arrest should be nearby. Table 3A.3 summarizes therapeutic measures for contrast reactions with drug doses.

Mild reactions usually do not require treatment except for reassurance and comforting. One must cast a suspicious eye on all reactions, however, because they may progress to a more serious nature. If the urticaria is symptomatic, 25 to 50 mg of diphenhydramine given intramuscularly or intravenously is effective.

Progressive urticaria should be treated with diphenhydramine 0.25 to 50 mg intravenously or intramuscularly in adults. If urticaria is profound, one should consider cimetidine, ranitidine, or epinephrine (12,93). Bronchospasm alone can be treated with a β_2-agonist administered via metered-dose inhaler (13,14,93) or subcutaneous epinephrine (1:1,000) (20). Severe bronchospasm and evidence of laryngeal edema should be treated immediately with IV epinephrine because such a reaction may suddenly worsen and subcutaneous epinephrine at this point would be useless because of poor absorption. A dose of 1 mL of 1:10,000 epinephrine should be given intravenously (slowly, 2 to 5 minutes) (93). Epinephrine is short lived, and repeated doses may be necessary at 5- to 15-minute intervals.

Isolated hypotension may be treated initially with leg evaluation, oxygen, and fluids. If not responsive, IV epinephrine can be used (93). In hypotensive patients, it is extremely important to check the pulse rate. Bradycardia in a hypotensive patient indicates a vasovagal type of response, and treatment with 0.6 to 1 mg of IV atropine is usually extremely effective; 2 to 3 mg of atropine can be given over 10 to 20 minutes.

Severe cardiovascular reactions that involve hypotension, loss of consciousness, and airway obstruction require immediate therapy. In total cardiovascular collapse, additional IV lines and establishment of an adequate airway are mandatory when embarking on cardiopulmonary resuscitation. IV epinephrine is the treatment of choice for anaphylactoid reactions and should be given as soon as such a reaction is diagnosed. Prompt therapy can reverse an anaphylactoid reaction within minutes, whereas epinephrine given after full development of the reaction may not reverse it for hours. IV epinephrine is a potent medication, however, and is usually not needed for mild reactions. Rapid assessment of the patient as to the severity of a reaction is therefore essential.

Corticosteroids are of no value during the immediate reaction but may be helpful if the reaction takes a prolonged course. Methylprednisolone can be given (100 to 1,000 mg intravenously) (2).

TABLE 3A.3. ACUTE REACTIONS TO CONTRAST MEDIA: TREATMENT

Urticaria

Mild: Observation.

Moderate: Diphenhydramine 25–50 mg PO/IM/IV (pediatric: 1–2 mg/kg IV/IM up to 50 mg).

Severe: Add cimetidine 300 mg, diluted to 20 mL, slow IV (pediatric: 5–10 mg/kg diluted to 20 mL, slow IV); *or* ranitidine 50 mg, diluted to 20 mL, slow IV (pediatric: use not established); *or* epinephrine IV, 1:10,000, 1.0 mL (0.1 mg) slowly over 2–5 min.

Bronchospasm (Isolated)

Oxygen: 6–10 L/min.

β_2-Agonist metered-dose inhaler (2–3 deep inhalations): Metaproterenol (Alupent), terbutaline (Brethaire), albuterol (Proventil).

Epinephrine: SC, 1:1,000, 0.1–0.2 mL (0.1–0.2 mg) (pediatric: 0.01 mg/kg up to maximum of 0.3 mg) (SC can be used if blood pressure normal); IV, 1:10,000, 1 mL (0.1 mg), slowly (e.g., over 3–5 min) (pediatric: 0.1 mL/kg IV up to 0.1 mg, may repeat every 5–15 min as needed).

Anaphylaxis-like Reaction (Generalized)

Oxygen: 6–10 L/min.

Suction, as needed.

Elevate patient's legs if hypotensive.

Intravenous fluids: Normal saline; Ringer's solution.

Epinephrine: IV, 1:10,000, 1 mL (0.1 mg), slowly (e.g., incrementally over 3–5 min), may repeat (pediatric: 0.1 mL/kg IV up to 0.1 mg, may repeat every 5–15 min as needed)
(*avoid* epinephrine in patients taking noncardioselective β-adrenergic blocking drugs); alternative drug therapy: isoproterenol 1:5,000 solution (0.2 mg/mL), 1 mL (diluted to 10 mL), titrate to effect at 1 mL/min (20 mg/min).

Antihistamines: H_1 blocker—diphenhydramine 50 mg, IV (*caution:* may exacerbate or cause hypotension); H_2 blocker—cimetidine 300 mg, diluted to 20 mL, slowly IV (pediatric: 5–10 mg/kg, diluted slowly); ranitidine 50 mg, diluted to 20 mL, slowly IV (pediatric: use not established).

β_2-Agonist metered-dose inhaler (2–3 inhalations): Metaproterenol (Alupent), terbutaline (Brethaire), albuterol (Proventil).

Corticosteroids: Methylprednisolone 100–1,000 mg IV, can be repeated.

Hypotension (Isolated)

Elevate patient's legs.

Oxygen: 6–10 L/min.

Intravenous fluids (primary therapy): Rapidly, 0.9% sodium chloride for injection (normal saline) or Ringer's solution.

If not responsive, consider vasopressor such as epinephrine 1:10,000 dilution 1 mL (0.1 mg) slowly over 2–5 min (93).

Vagal Reaction (Hypotension and Bradycardia)

Elevate patient's legs.

Oxygen: 6–10 L/min.

Intravenous fluids: Rapidly, 0.9% sodium chloride for injection (normal saline) or Ringer's solution.

Atropine: Adults 0.6–1.0 mg IV, repeat q3–5min to 2–3 mg total (pediatric: 0.02 mg/kg IV; maximum dose 0.6 mg; may repeat to maximum of 1 mg for infants and 2 mg for adolescents).

Nephrotoxicity

Acute renal insufficiency following the use of intravascular contrast medium is a well-known potential complication that is fortunately uncommon in excretory urography. Acute renal insufficiency may be manifested by a transient rise in the serum creatinine or by acute oliguric renal failure. Some cases can be diagnosed during the urogram by development of an abnormally persisting, dense nephrographic pattern (Fig. 3A.5) (69,71). The true incidence of nephrotoxicity in excretory urography is not clear but is probably lower than 5% (66,94).

Although renal toxicity is unlikely to occur from an IV injection of iodinated contrast material in a patient with normal renal function, patients with preexisting renal disease have consistently been shown to be at greater risk for contrast-induced nephropathy (7,37,60,94). VanZee and associates (94) found renal failure following urography to occur in only 0.6% of patients with normal renal function, but this increased to between 3.2% and 31% depending on the severity of preexisting renal disease. Minimal elevations of serum creatinine do not necessarily prohibit the use of iodinated contrast media when necessary for diagnosis, but preexisting renal disease does increase the risk of the examination, and this should be balanced against potential gain.

Studies have compared the nephrotoxicity of ionic and nonionic contrast media and have shown a decrease in nephrotoxicity with the low-osmolar contrast (41,60). A meta-analysis demonstrated significant benefit when low-osmolar contrast media are used in patients with prior renal impairment (7).

Acute renal insufficiency associated with contrast medium is generally self-limited. The serum creatinine usually peaks in 2 to 3 days and returns to the preexisting level within 1 to 3 weeks. Most patients completely recover, with few requiring dialysis.

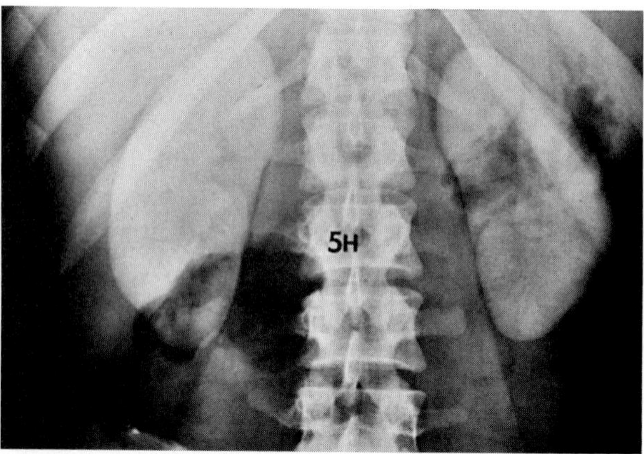

FIGURE 3A.5. Persistent dense nephrogram at 5 hours related to contrast-induced renal failure. (From Older RA, Resnick MI, eds. *Basic radiologic techniques in diagnosis of genitourinary disease,* ed 2. New York: Thieme Medical Publishers, 1994, with permission.)

The theories on the pathogenesis of contrast-induced renal failure include direct toxic effects of the contrast medium on the proximal tubular cells and ischemia resulting from damage to the renal microcirculation. Nephrotoxicity has been attributed to the hypertonicity of the contrast medium, resulting in a unique vacuolization of the cytoplasm of the proximal tubular epithelium termed *osmotic nephrosis* (67). Others think that acute tubular necrosis may result from ischemia due to vasoconstriction or sludging of the red blood cells in the renal microcirculation. Katzberg and associates (47) suggested that the hypertonicity of the contrast medium reduces the GFR by increasing the hydrostatic pressure in Bowman's capsule and the proximal tubules. In certain cases, precipitation of uric acid within the proximal tubules may lead to acute renal failure. Contrast material has a known uricosuric effect and may result in acute urate nephropathy in individuals with hyperuricemia.

A few cases of acute oliguric renal failure resulting in the death of patients with multiple myeloma have been reported following excretory urography. Because of these reports, some authorities considered multiple myeloma an absolute contraindication to excretory urography. However, excretory urography in patients with multiple myeloma is probably no different from that in patients with other forms of renal impairment (68,95). When necessary, excretory urography must be performed with caution, and dehydration should be avoided.

In high-risk patients who require a contrast examination, both dehydration and large contrast medium loads should be avoided. IV hydration performed overnight, as well as after the examination, may be helpful in preventing renal problems. Nonionic contrast media should be used in these patients. Sequential diagnostic studies that use intravascular contrast material should not be scheduled without allowing adequate intervals for observation and recovery (70).

Concurrent Use of Metformin (Glucophage) and Contrast Media

The concurrent use of metformin, an oral antihyperglycemic agent, and iodinated contrast media is of concern. A decrease in renal function could potentially decrease metformin excretion, which could subsequently lead to development of lactic acidosis. To prevent this potential complication, it is currently recommended that metformin be discontinued either before or at the time of a radiographic procedure in which iodinated contrast is to be used. The metformin should be withheld for 48 hours after the procedure and reinstated only after renal function has been reevaluated and shown to be normal (2).

Low-osmolality Contrast Media

Early experience with low-osmolar contrast demonstrated a decreased incidence of mild reactions and suggested a lower

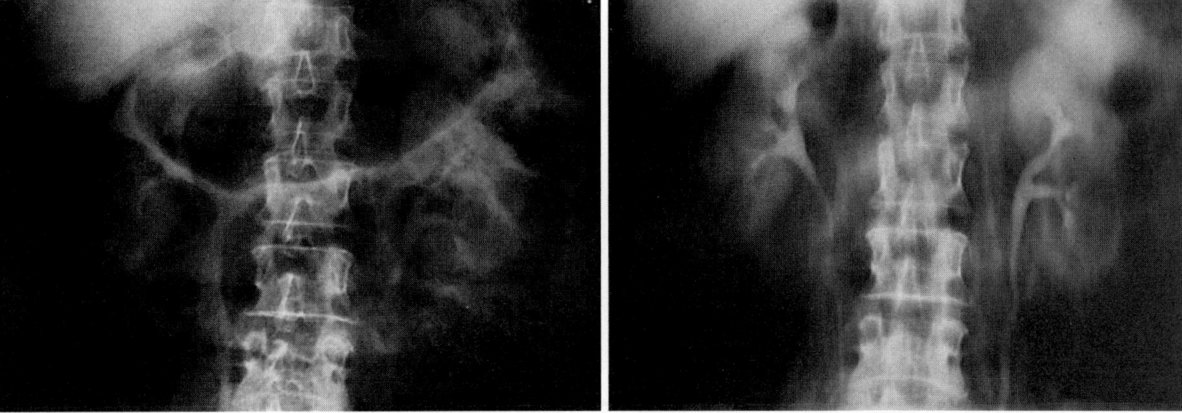

FIGURE 3A.6. **A:** Limited visualization due to overlying bowel content. **B:** Tomography dramatically improved visualization. (From Older RA, Resnick MI, eds. *Basic radiologic techniques in diagnosis of genitourinary disease,* ed 2. New York: Thieme Medical Publishers, 1994, with permission.)

incidence of moderate and severe contrast reactions. However, the early studies contained relatively small numbers of patients, making it difficult to arrive at a consensus on significant contrast reactions. Two studies involving large patient populations found a significantly decreased incidence of serious contrast reactions. In a Japanese study involving more than 300,000 patients, the incidence of all contrast reactions was four times less with the new agents. Even more striking, the incidence of severe reactions was six times less with the low-osmolality agents (45). This was corroborated by an Australian study involving more than 100,000 patients (73). Significantly increased safety of the low-osmolar agents is now accepted worldwide.

The disadvantage of the newer compounds is their higher cost compared with the conventional agents. This cost difference, which has been as high as 20:1, has decreased to approximately 4:1. (74). In European countries, there is almost universal use of nonionic media (92). In the United States, there is still controversy (27,87) regarding universal use of low-osmolar contrast media, but the significant cost reductions have made this a more feasible alternative.

TECHNIQUE

Several parameters must be considered to properly perform excretory urography. An adequate number of well-trained personnel should be employed to obtain good-quality radiographs, as well as to closely monitor the patient during the entire procedure. Emergency drug boxes and monitoring equipment should be available in every room where urography is performed. A physician should supervise all contrast administration and should remain close by in case complications arise. Regularly scheduled x-ray machine maintenance with established quality control guidelines for the technologists is essential.

Before the examination, the physician should have a completed x-ray request outlining the current problem and pertinent medical history (e.g., diabetes, nephrolithiasis, allergies). Laboratory values to assess renal function, blood urea nitrogen (BUN), and creatinine are important baselines, especially in debilitated or elderly individuals. Old films should be requested and reviewed.

For many years, bowel preparation was used to improve image quality of the urogram. Although helpful in some patients, these preparations often were not successful, and at the University of Virginia, we no longer use routine bowel preparation. A randomized prospective study found no difference in terms of overall quality between a prepared and an unprepared group of patients (34). Other studies have shown not only a lack of significant improvement of quality but also significant unpleasant side effects to these preparations (6). The need for bowel preparation has been reduced by the routine availability of tomography, which allows visualization of the kidneys despite considerable overlying bowel content (Fig. 3A.6).

Contrast Media: Dosage and Administration

An average dose of 0.5 to 1.0 mL of 60% contrast material per pound of patient's weight, with a maximum dose of 100 mL, is a generally accepted rule of thumb. Twenty grams of iodine was the dose recommended in the categorical genitourinary course at the 1978 Radiologic Society of North America (RSNA) Annual Meeting (63), and this dose has not changed significantly (64). This would be the equivalent of approximately 75 mL of contrast agent for a 150-pound patient. Dosage schedules for the newer nonionic contrast media were initially similar to the ionic agents because the concentrations were similar. However, cost considerations have necessitated that there be no waste when the very expensive nonionic contrast is used, and many institutions have gone to a dose of 50 mL because most of the available nonionic media come in standard vials of 50 mL. A dose of 50 mL of iohexol was compared with a larger, weight-based dose and showed no significant diagnostic difference (33). Kennan, List, and Kengsakul (49) also evaluated lower dosages for nonionic contrast and found that with a 42% reduction in the amount of contrast, diagnostic images were still obtained. Currently, packaging of the nonionic media is more flexible, and a dose equivalent of 75 mL of a 60% solution could be used with no wasted contrast agent.

IV contrast is rapidly administered through a 19- or 21-gauge butterfly scalp vein needle or catheter-type needle, which is taped and left in place until the procedure is finished. Thus venous access is established throughout the examination in case of a reaction. The contrast medium should be administered as quickly as possible to demonstrate a good nephrogram phase. The antecubital fossa and dorsum of the hand are preferred sites for contrast injection, but central lines may be used as well. If venous access is unavailable, a foot vein may be cannulated. However, after the contrast material is given, the leg should be elevated and 100 mL of saline solution flushed through the line to decrease the possibility of thrombophlebitis. Ionic contrast medium is very irritating, and care should be taken to avoid extravasation into the subcutaneous tissues because skin slough can occur.

Radiographs: Technical Factors

Both the preliminary radiograph and the routine tomographic radiographs should be obtained using kilovolt peaks (KVPs) in the range of 60 to 70. The visibility of contrast media decreases with higher KVPs.

Many types of film–screen combinations are available; use depends on personal preference, as well as what is available at a particular institution. Radiation dose can be reduced by using a high-speed system, and high-quality urograms can be obtained with such a system. At the University of Virginia, we use high-speed film in combination with intensifying screens, which gives a speed of 600. This type of high-contrast film is well suited for stone detection.

Collimation to the area of interest is crucial to eliminate image degradation produced by scattered radiation. One of the most common errors in urography is failure to collimate properly, and technologists should be encouraged to collimate as close to the area of interest as possible.

Various radiographic views and maneuvers allow the physician the flexibility to tailor each examination to a patient's particular problem (54). The one mandatory film is "the scout," or *kidney, ureter, and bladder preliminary* (KUB). This view is a supine abdominal radiograph (14 inches by 17 inches) taken before contrast injection that includes the kidneys to the pubic symphysis (Fig. 3A.7). Two exposures may be necessary in large patients to cover the entire anatomy. A careful review of the film for technique and underlying abnormalities is required. The size, shape, and position of both renal outlines should be observed. Abnormal calcifications (e.g., renal and ureteral calculi, gallstones, aneurysm, fibroids) should be identified. Oblique views before contrast administration may be needed to prove that a calcification is indeed renal in origin (Figs. 3A.8 and 3A.9). Bony architecture should be scrutinized for pathology, such as metastasis (Fig. 3A.10). The bowel gas pattern should be evaluated for possible obstruction and abnormal gas collections (Figs. 3A.11 and 3A.12). The lung bases are often included on the film and may reveal occult pulmonary disease. Radiopaque substances, such as tablets, foreign bodies, and recently administered barium, will be demonstrated and may even preclude the examination.

The nephrogram phase is evaluated with a collimated film (11 inches by 14 inches) immediately after injection. The nephrogram phase demonstrates the densest opacification of the renal parenchyma and should be obtained within 1 minute after injection (Fig. 3A.13). The kidneys are compared and evaluated for size, shape, and position. In lieu of a 1-minute film, however, nephrotomography is often preferred. Three tomograms at 1-cm intervals in the supine position are taken at 30, 60, and 90 seconds after injection, providing excellent visualization of the renal contours (Fig. 3A.14). The nephrogram can be delayed (obstruction) (Fig. 3A.15), misplaced (pelvic, thoracic/kidney), irregular (mass) (Fig 3A.16), or prolonged (hypotension).

A 5-minute collimated film (11 inches by 14 inches) is obtained to demonstrate the pyelogram phase with opacification of both collecting systems and proximal ureters (Fig. 3A.17). Calyceal distortion, irregularity, or filling defect may signal underlying disease. Tomography can be used to better delineate the calyces, as can oblique views. Oblique views are also helpful in further evaluating filling defects and in clarifying pseudofilling defects such as might be related to overlapping calyces or crossing vessels. Posteriorly and anteriorly positioned masses may also be more apparent on oblique views because these present a different surface of the kidneys.

Relative obstruction of the ureters with an inflatable compression device placed across the lower abdomen after the nephrogram phase achieves optimal distention of the collecting systems and proximal ureters (Fig. 3A.18). Contraindications include suspected ureteral obstruction, abdominal aortic aneurysm, and recent abdominal or renal surgery. Another alternative is to place the patient in the Trendelenburg position after the 1-minute film to enable better filling of the collecting system. Both the compression device and Trendelenburg position are maintained until a 10-minute collimated kidney film is taken (14 inches by 11 inches). The patient is brought up into the reverse Trendelenburg position, or the compression device is released, and an immediate full (14 inches by 17 inches) film is taken in

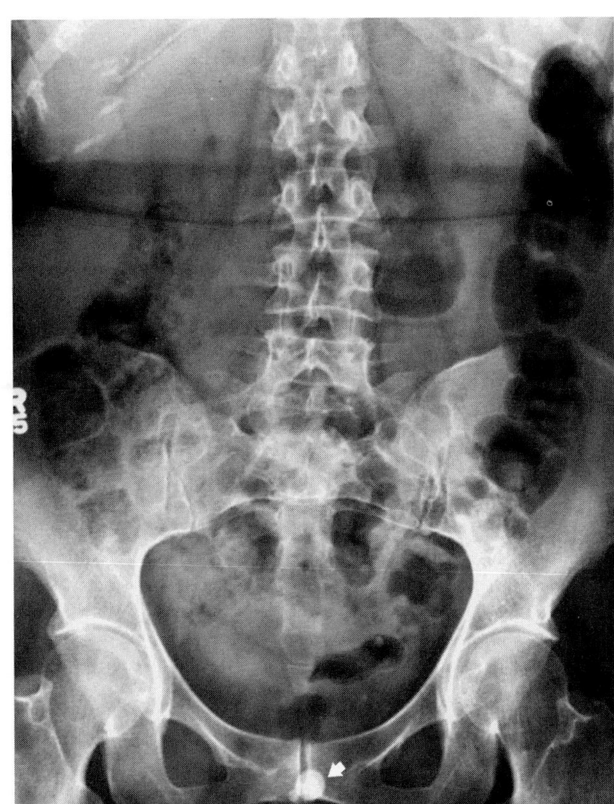

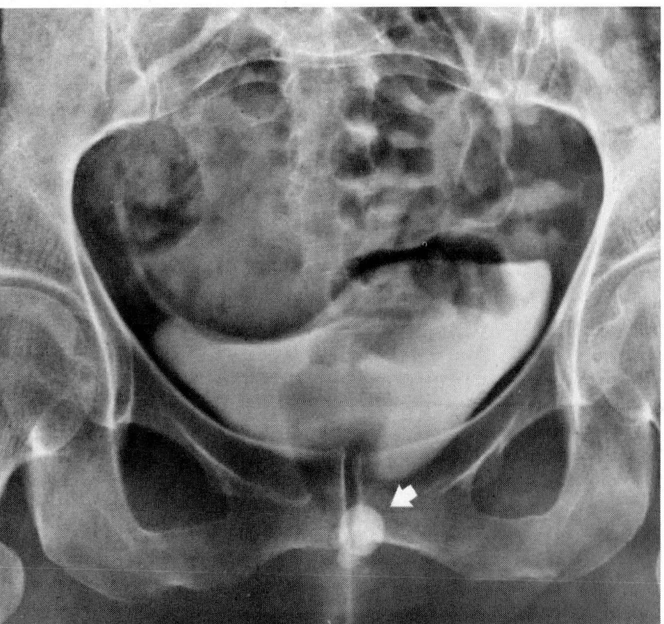

A B

FIGURE 3A.7. A: The preliminary radiograph should include area from kidneys to pubic symphysis. Calcification overlying pubic symphysis *(arrow)* is a calculus within a urethral diverticulum. **B:** Coned-down bladder radiograph following contrast media injection demonstrating urethral diverticulum. The urethral calculus would have been missed if the radiograph before contrast injection did not include the pubic symphysis.

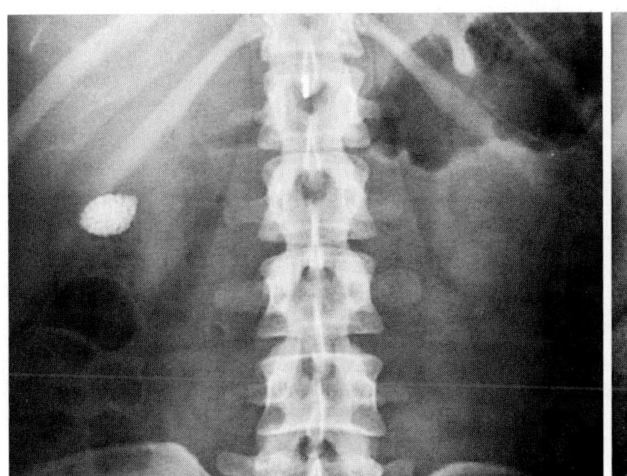

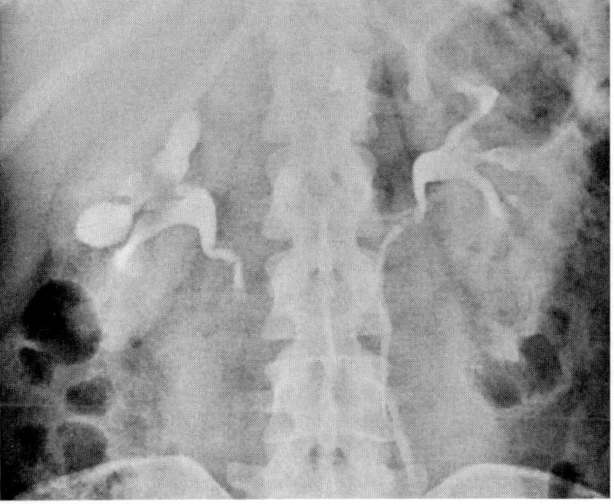

A B

FIGURE 3A.8. Faceted stones **(A)** with a typical appearance for gallstones, but **(B)** shown to be within a calyceal diverticulum with excretory urography.

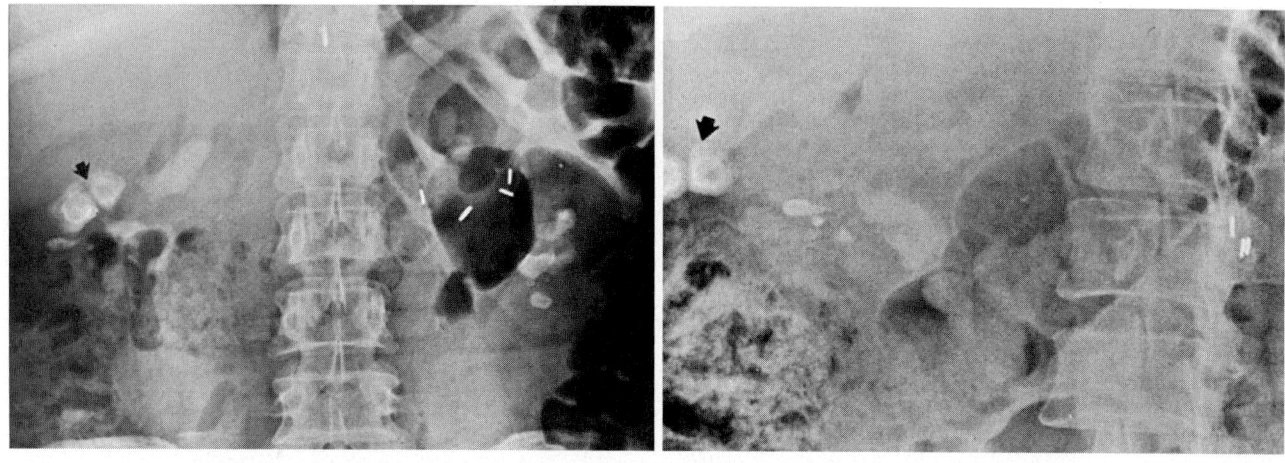

FIGURE 3A.9. **A:** Preliminary radiograph demonstrates calcific densities overlying both renal shadows. Two laminated calcific densities *(arrow)* overlying the right renal shadow are probably gallstones. **B:** Radiograph in the right posterior oblique projection confirms the presence of gallstones *(arrow)* in addition to renal calculi.

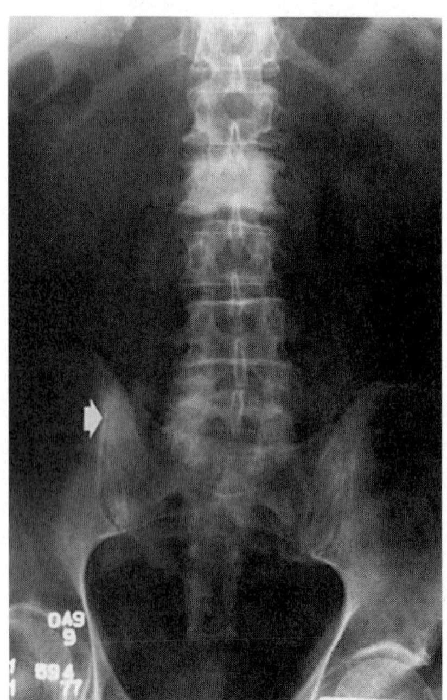

FIGURE 3A.10. Blastic metastases to pelvis *(arrow)* and spine (L-2).

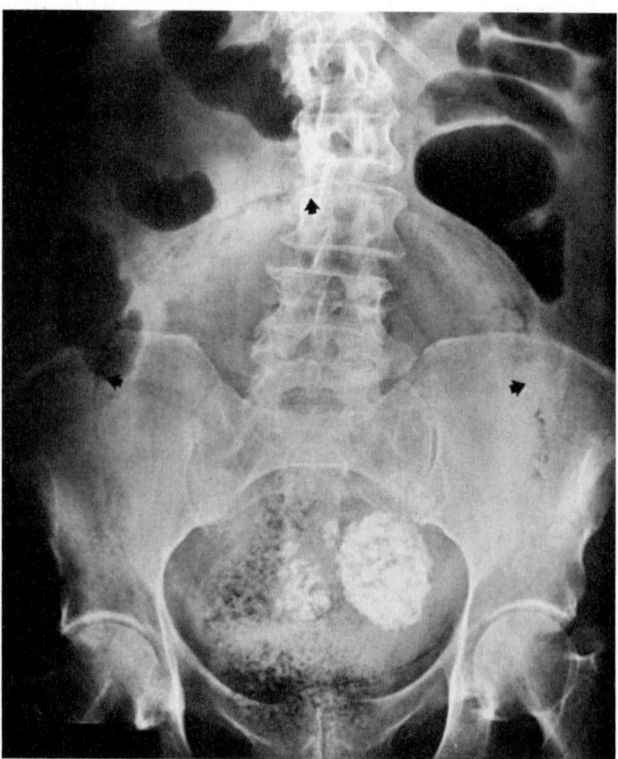

FIGURE 3A.11. Preliminary radiograph demonstrates significant distention of the bladder with air within the wall *(arrows)* in a patient with emphysematous cystitis. Large calcified uterine fibroids are noted within the pelvis.

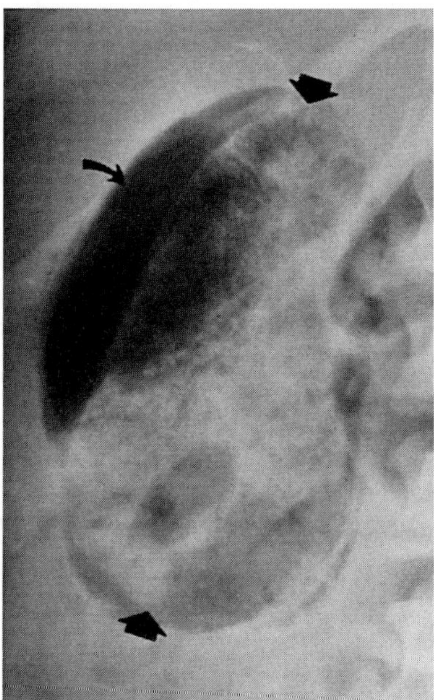

FIGURE 3A.12. Emphysematous pyelonephritis. Gas extends throughout the right kidney parenchyma *(black arrows)* and also to subcapsular space *(curved arrow)*. (From Older RA, Resnick MI, eds. *Basic radiologic techniques in diagnosis of genitourinary disease,* ed 2. New York: Thieme Medical Publishers, 1994, with permission.)

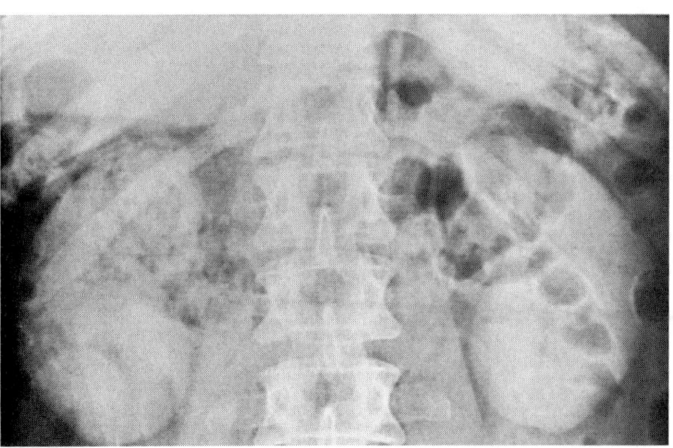

FIGURE 3A.13. The nephrogram phase demonstrates parenchymal opacification of both kidneys. Kidney size and contour abnormalities are best evaluated during the nephrogram phase.

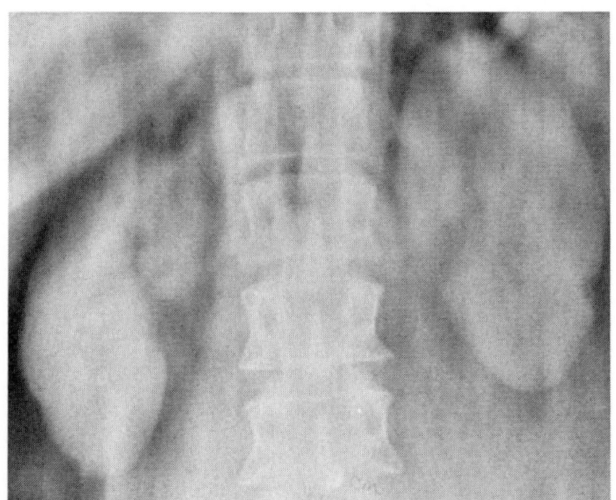

FIGURE 3A.14. Immediate postinjection tomogram clearly demonstrates the renal parenchyma bilaterally.

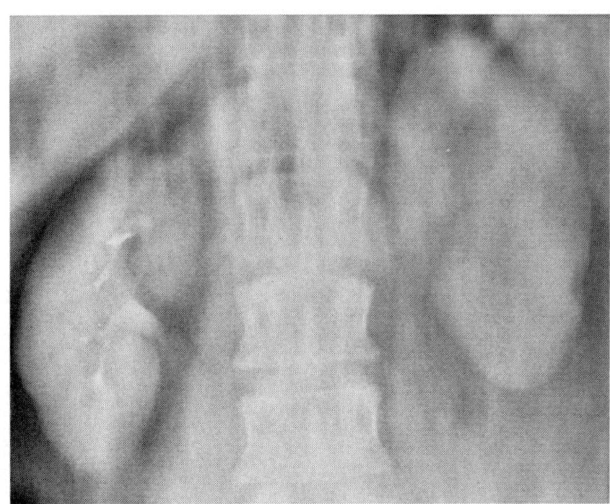

FIGURE 3A.15. Left-sided obstruction with delayed visualization of calyces. Same patient as Fig. 3A.14.

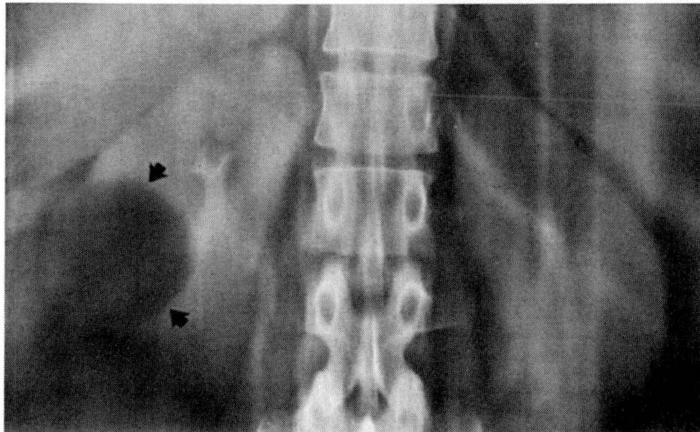

FIGURE 3A.16. Nephrotomography demonstrates a large, well-circumscribed mass in the lower pole of the right kidney *(arrows)* consistent with a renal cyst. Nephrotomograms provide excellent detail of renal contour abnormalities.

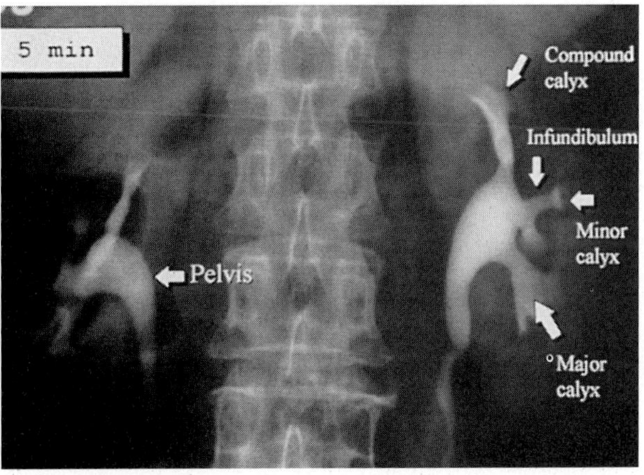

FIGURE 3A.17. Coned, 5-minute film of kidneys.

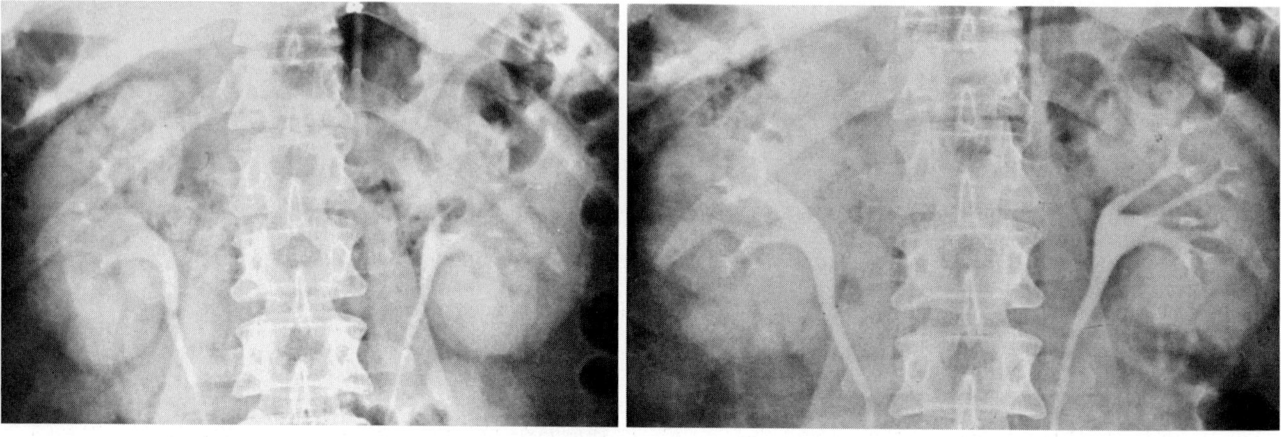

FIGURE 3A.18. A: Radiograph taken 5 minutes after contrast injection demonstrates the pyelogram phase with opacification of the collecting system and proximal ureters. **B:** Radiograph following the use of a compression device in the same patient. Note distention of collecting systems with improved visualization of the calyces and infundibula.

hopes of catching the contrast medium flowing down both ureters to the bladder. The ureters and bladder are usually well demonstrated (Fig. 3A.19).

If necessary, the bladder can be evaluated with a collimated view (11 inches by 14 inches) for better anatomic detail (Fig. 3A.20). The lower ureteral segment and ureterovesical junction can be better delineated with oblique views either before or after voiding (Figs. 3A.21 and 3A.22). If there is inadequate definition or a suspicious finding in the distal ureters or bladder, a prone film (11 inches by 14 or 14 inches by 17 inches) will distend the anterior portions of the collecting system as they become dependent, that is, the middle and distal portions of the ureters. This is often helpful in localizing an obstruction (Fig. 3A.23). Lesions involving the anterior wall of the bladder are better visualized as well.

Postvoid radiographs most often are used to assess bladder outlet obstruction resulting from prostatic hypertrophy in older adults. In the presence of a possible obstructive process involving the upper urinary tract, the postvoid radiograph can also be of benefit by demonstrating drainage. The combination of the patient's walking to the bathroom and emptying his or her bladder often aids significantly in evaluating the drainage of the upper tracts.

Fluoroscopy often provides additional information about urinary tract physiology. In combination with spot filming, fluoroscopy can reveal renal dynamics and relationships not seen with standard static radiographs.

TOMOGRAPHY

Tomography provides better visualization of the urinary tract by blurring out the surrounding structures. It is one of the most important refinements of the excretory urogram. Simple linear tomography is generally sufficient. We at Virginia use a short arc of 20 degrees, which will produce a tomographic cut of approximately 0.5 cm. Three such tomographic cuts are generally sufficient to visualize the kidneys.

The major contribution of tomography is in evaluating the renal parenchyma; therefore tomograms should be obtained immediately after the bolus injection of contrast when the nephrogram is most intense (Fig. 3A.14). This has been shown to increase detection of renal masses (39,72). Later in the urogram, during filling of the collecting structures, tomography can be used on a selective basis. It is most helpful when there is considerable overlying bowel content or poor concentration of the contrast

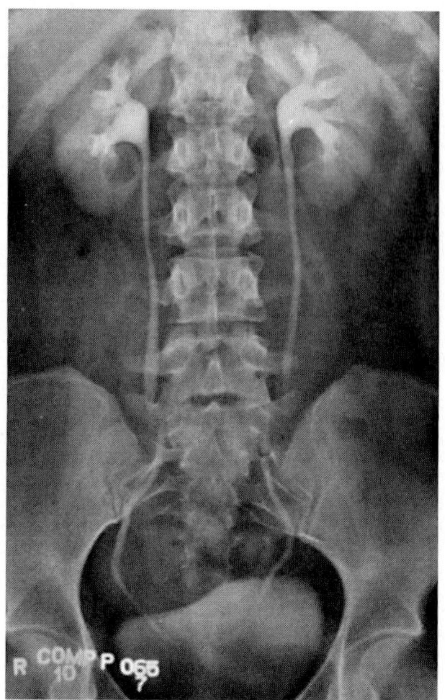

FIGURE 3A.19. Postcompression abdominal film demonstrating the ureters and bladder.

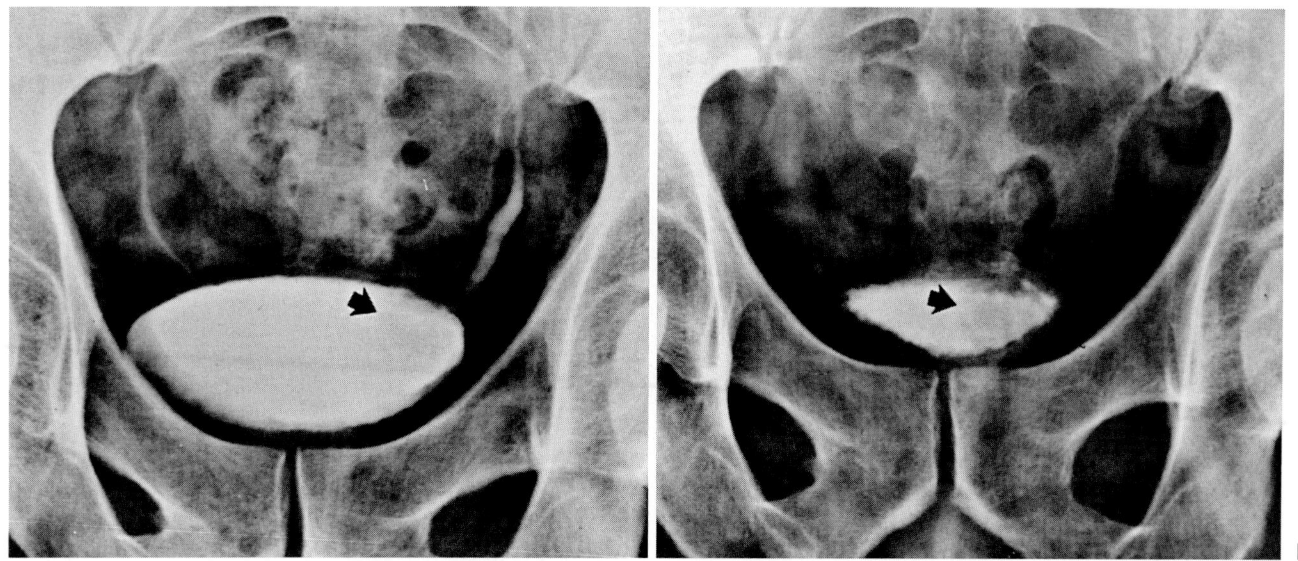

FIGURE 3A.20. A: The filled bladder suggests a filling defect near the left bladder wall *(arrow).* **B:** The postvoid radiograph confirms the defect *(arrow)* proved to be bladder carcinoma.

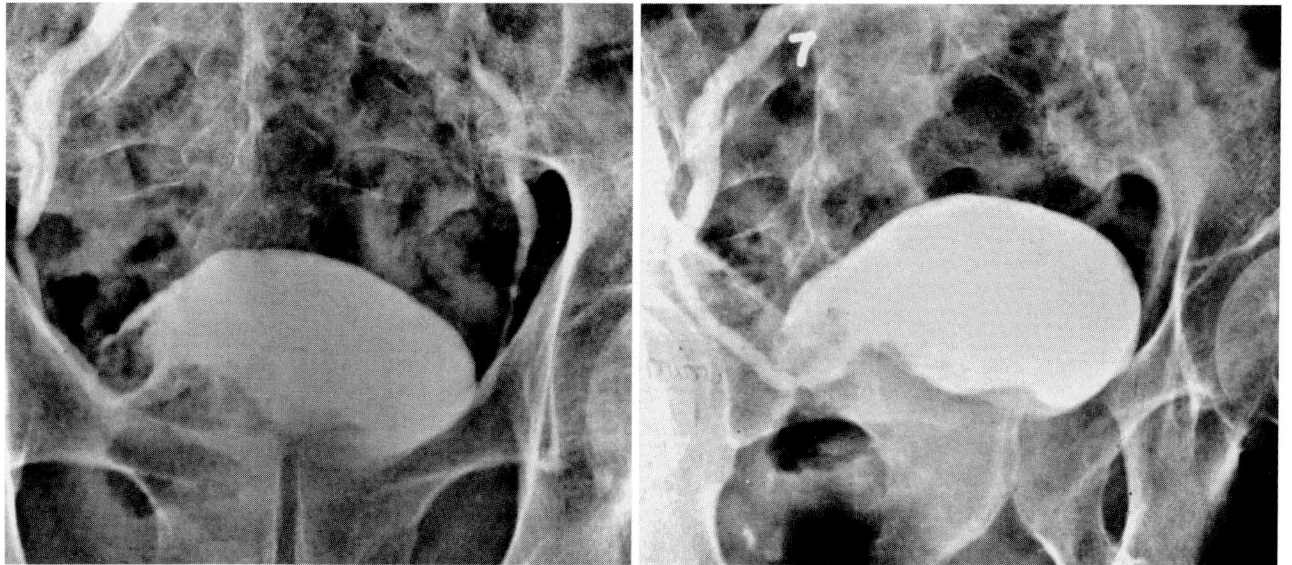

FIGURE 3A.21. A: Coned-down radiographs of the bladder suggest a mass involving the inferior aspect of the right wall of the bladder. **B:** Radiograph taken in the left posterior oblique projection confirms irregular mass near the insertion of the right ureter consistent with carcinoma.

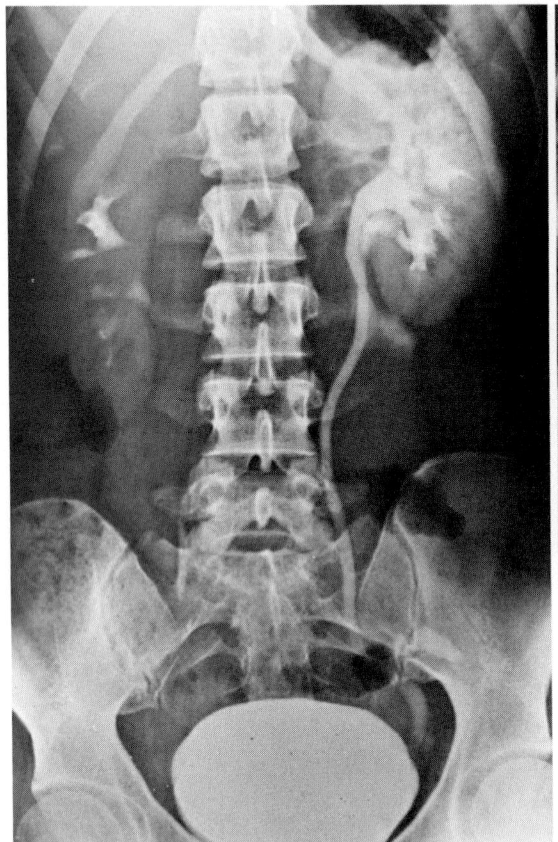

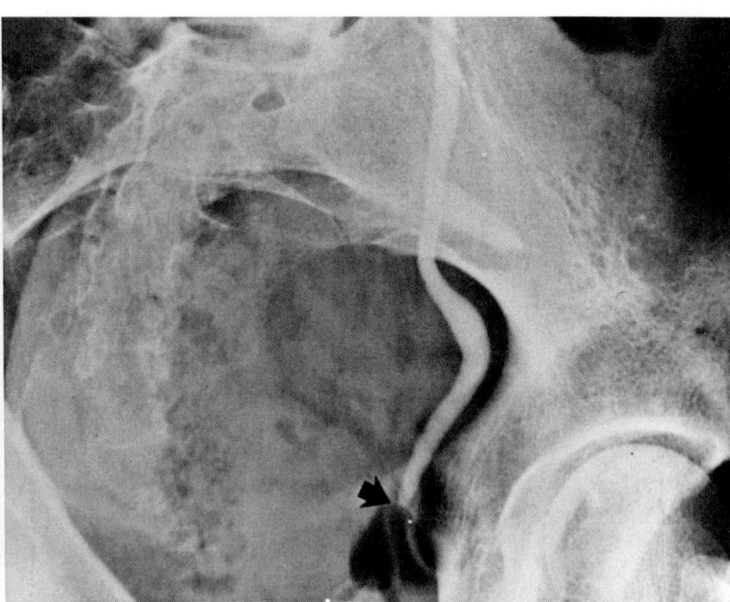

FIGURE 3A.22. A: Two-hour radiograph in a patient with left-sided renal colic. There is dilation of the left ureter down to the level of the bladder. The point of obstruction is not demonstrated. Note the peripelvic extravasation of contrast resulting from forniceal rupture. B: Postvoid radiograph in the left posterior oblique projection demonstrates the level of obstruction *(arrow)* due to a uric acid stone.

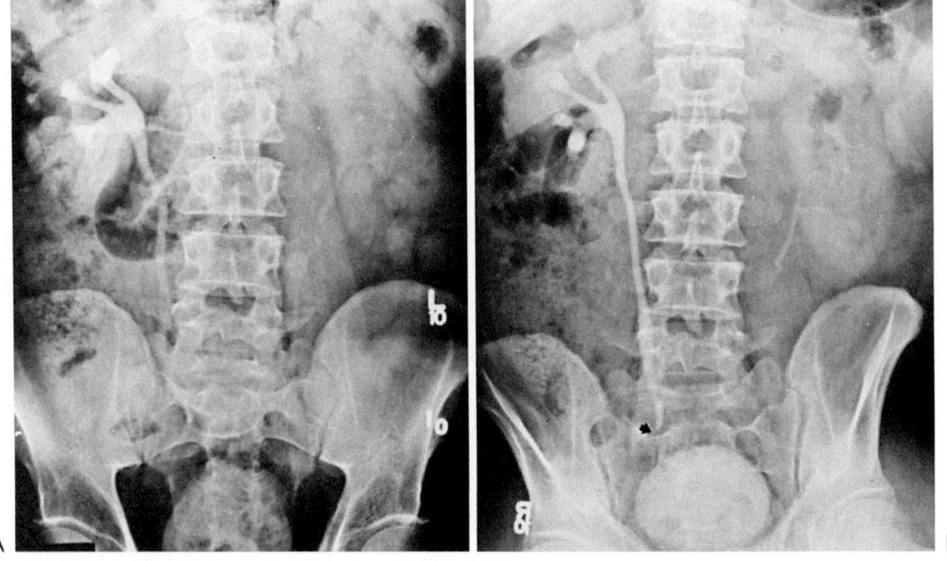

FIGURE 3A.23. A: Ten-minute radiograph in a patient with right renal colic. There is hydronephrosis and dilation of the ureter with poor definition of the level of the obstruction. B: Prone radiograph demonstrates excellent opacification of the ureter with identification of the level of the obstruction *(arrow)*.

medium. This will often salvage an otherwise nondiagnostic examination.

DIGITAL RADIOGRAPHY

Two types of digital radiography are available for use in urologic diagnosis. At present, digital radiography is not used extensively in the diagnosis of urologic disease, but with the potential for dose reduction and more efficient storage, its use will probably increase.

Digital luminescent radiography (Fig. 3A.24) does not use standard film but rather uses photo-stimulable plates with substances such as phosphorous and barium-fluorohalide europium-doped crystals. This system has the advantage of significant dose reduction. Because the imaging plates used have a much wider linear dynamic range than conventional screen–film combinations, imaging can be performed at decreased radiation doses (29,65,100). Dose reductions up to 50% for urography (65) and as great as 90% in urethrocystography (100) have been achieved. In addition, repeat examinations are significantly reduced, if not eliminated, by this system. Studies that have compared the diagnostic capabilities of digital systems with standard radiographic systems have shown no significant decrease in image quality or diagnostic accuracy with the digital systems (28,29).

The second type of digital system, digital fluororadiography, converts the fluoroscopic image to a digital image as shown in Figure 3A.25. The optical image of the TV tube is converted by an analog–digital converter into a series of electrical signals, which are then converted into the digital image. The digital image is converted back to an analog image and can either be sent to the monitor for viewing or printed out as a hard copy. The images can be manipulated later by changing window settings, brightness, or edge enhancement as needed. In contrast to standard radiography, the image is immediately available for review, allowing more rapid decision making as to further films.

THE PEDIATRIC PATIENT

Excretory urography in children requires special attention to several technical factors. First, establishment of rapport between the physician and the child and parents is crucial before obtaining radiographs. Explaining the procedure in a step-by-step fashion helps alleviate some of the anxiety regarding the examination. In the older age group, the clinician should direct the explanation primarily to the child.

Anesthesia or sedation is rarely indicated in excretory urography. In infants and preschool children, a "cradle" device is placed directly on the x-ray table for immobilization of the patient. Heat lamps, pediatric drug boxes, and resuscitative equipment should be available in each x-ray room.

Bowel preparation is not indicated in children. An adequate state of hydration is essential, especially in infants and younger children, to avoid dehydration from the diuresis caused by the excess solute load of the contrast medium. Abstinence from food for about 5 hours is sensible in most children to keep the stomach empty in case of emesis after contrast administration (19).

The contrast dosage in children is basically the same as for adults on a weight basis. Between 0.5 and 1.0 mL/lb (between 1 and 2 mL/kg) of patient's weight is a safe and effective amount of contrast medium to give a satisfactory

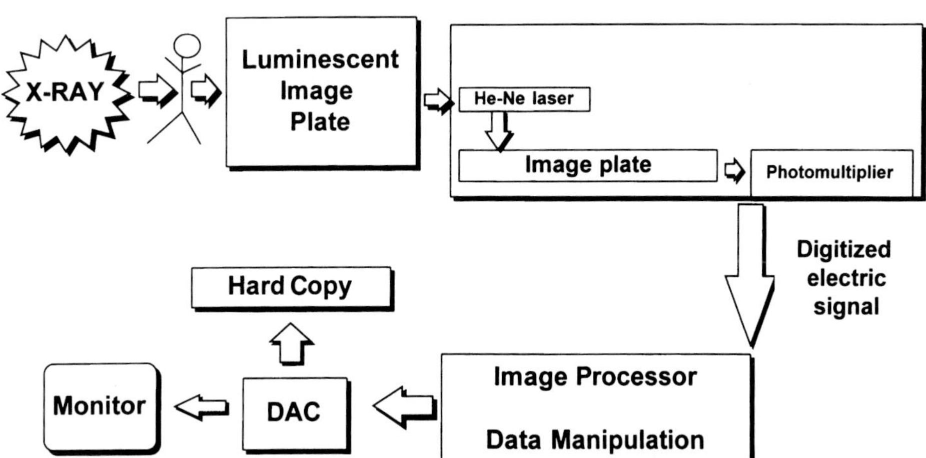

FIGURE 3A.24. Digital luminescent radiography. The luminescent plate is exposed and its energy state raised. Laser scanning releases radiation, which is converted to an electric signal and digitized. The digital image is processed and converted through a digital–analog converter to an analog image for the monitor or hard copy. (From Older RA, Resnick MI, eds. *Basic radiologic techniques in diagnosis of genitourinary disease,* ed 2. New York: Thieme Medical Publishers, 1994, with permission.)

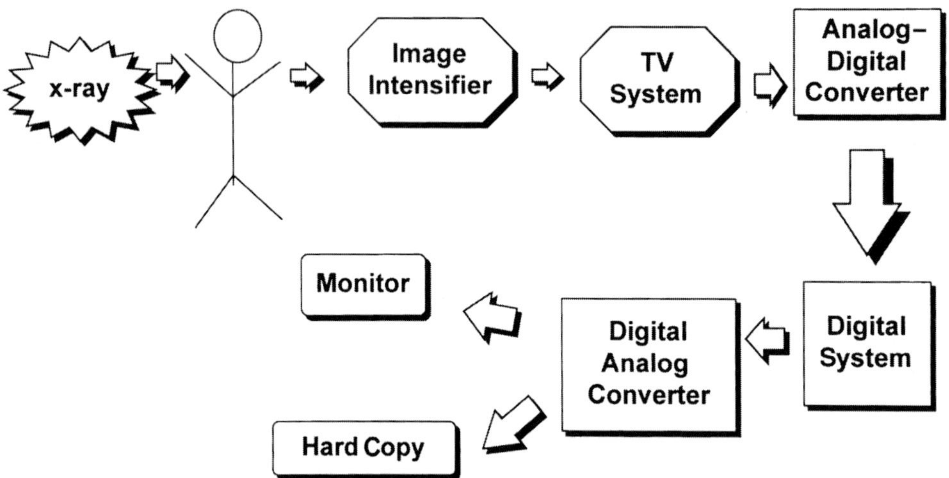

FIGURE 3A.25. Digital fluororadiography. (From Older RA, Resnick MI, eds. *Basic radiologic techniques in diagnosis of genitourinary disease,* ed 2. New York: Thieme Medical Publishers, 1994, with permission.)

urogram. Nonionic contrast is indicated for infants and also recommended for young children. Venous access in young children may be difficult to obtain. The veins on the dorsum of the hand or foot are usually the most accessible for cannulation with a 25-, 23-, or 21-gauge butterfly needle. Other sites include the antecubital fossa and scalp veins in infants. Pneumothorax is a complication of external jugular vein injections, and the femoral vein should be avoided because of the reported risk of septic arthritis of the hip (19). Bolus injection technique is recommended, and the needle should remain in place until the study is terminated. Immediately after giving the bolus, a carbonated beverage or juice may be given to the patient. This allows distention of the gastric bubble for optimal visualization of the kidneys, as well as providing calories and fluid intake for the child.

The filming sequence in the pediatric age group is aimed at obtaining the most information from a minimum number of radiographic exposures. Collimation should be used when possible.

A preliminary film, which includes the kidneys to the pubic symphysis, should be scrutinized carefully for underlying skeletal anomalies such as sacral agenesis and spinal dysraphism. A search for abdominal masses, an abnormal bowel gas pattern, and any calcifications should also be conducted.

In most cases, the entire pediatric excretory urogram can be completed with two postcontrast films. The nephrogram phase is demonstrated with a 1-minute collimated view of the kidneys. A large 10-minute film usually demonstrates both collecting systems, ureters, and the bladder. A postvoid bladder film is usually not obtained in children. However, additional views may be indicated for a particular clinical history or to clarify further abnormalities seen while performing the urogram.

Tomography is not used routinely for children but, if available, can often resolve a diagnostic problem, especially in a child with considerable overlying bowel content. There is a reluctance to use tomography in children because of radiation concerns. One or two tomograms actually may decrease the number of radiographs needed in a difficult diagnostic case and could possibly obviate the need for a follow-up imaging study, such as CT, which might involve even greater radiation.

INDICATIONS FOR EXCRETORY UROGRAPHY

The following list includes current indications for excretory urography. Some of these, such as obstruction, also use other technology; others, such as trauma, are controversial.

Stone disease
Preoperative extracorporeal shock wave lithotripsy (ESWL)
Acute abdominal pain or colic
Suspected obstruction
Blunt trauma thought to involve only the urinary tract
Hematuria, especially if abnormality of the collecting structures is suspected
Complicated or unusual infection, including tuberculosis
Postoperative evaluation of urologic procedures
Preoperative evaluation for endourologic procedures
Suspected transitional cell carcinoma
Questionable abnormality on isotope or ultrasound studies

These indications represent a combination of those indications that have persisted for many years, as well as relatively new indications, such as preoperative ESWL. Many previously accepted indications for urography are no longer considered justified. The evaluation of hypertension is one of these (51,78). Uncomplicated urinary tract infections, preoperative studies for various types of surgery (91), and enuresis are no longer studied routinely (51,78). Trauma has become a somewhat controversial indication with differing opinions regarding the value of urography.

Indications for urography have also been reduced by increasing availability of alternative methods of diagnostic imaging. A broad knowledge of the other imaging modalities is necessary to determine the proper examination. Urography is still widely used for obstruction, but ultrasound has become the primary screening study for this entity, and improvements in the diuretic renogram also erode the territory of urography. However, urography has the advantage of providing a unique combination of anatomy and function and for this reason continues to be used in suspected obstruction.

Urography and ultrasound are complementary examinations; this is particularly true in stone disease. There are those who have advocated replacement of the urogram by a combination of ultrasound and an abdominal film (40). However, a determination in each case as to which study would be most helpful is what should be done. Ureterovesical junction stones are detectable by a skilled ultrasonographer, but stones more proximal in the ureter are often difficult to find and can be demonstrated more easily by urography. Urography is generally more available, and interpretive experience also favors urography (18). To detect small ureteral stones, a sonographer with considerable experience and patience is needed.

Renal calculi can be evaluated by either technique. Some stones are more apparent with an abdominal radiograph or tomography, whereas others are better seen with ultrasound. Stone dimensions and degree of fragmentation following ESWL are better demonstrated with radiographs, but small stones, nonopaque stones, and small amounts of fragmented stone debris are often better demonstrated with ultrasound.

Noncontrast spiral CT has gained wide acceptance as the initial evaluation of renal colic and suspected ureteral stones. This has further reduced the use of intravenous pyelography (IVP), especially as an emergency procedure (88).

CT or ultrasound is used to study abdominal masses and retroperitoneal disease, which are no longer studied with urography. Similarly, urography is no longer used for evaluation of adrenal disease, but CT, MRI, or isotope techniques are used. Urography is still used as a primary study for hematuria. The urogram provides not only parenchymal information but also visualization of the collecting structures. Although sensitivity of excretory urography for detection of mass lesion is significantly less than CT (96), urography is excellent for lesions, such as transitional cell carcinoma, papillary necrosis, and other abnormalities of the collecting structures that might produce hematuria.

Patients in whom excretory urography may no longer be the study of choice are those with an above-average risk of complication. This may be an allergic reaction, abnormal cardiovascular response, or nephrotoxicity related to the contrast medium.

Urography can be performed in patients with a history of allergies to contrast media; however, if the reaction was severe, other modalities, such as ultrasound, CT without contrast, or radioisotope scanning, would probably be a better choice. Patients with significant heart disease have been shown to have a higher incidence of arrhythmias during bolus injection for urography; in these patients, other modalities should be considered. Urography is no longer used for evaluation of renal failure. Diagnostic ultrasound has improved to the extent that it can accurately determine whether obstruction is present, often the question being asked in a patient with renal failure (26,40,81,82). In addition, the potential toxicity of iodinated contrast media is now well established. Patients with mild renal failure are at significant risk for contrast-induced renal toxicity (1,5,7,15,50,60,69–71,83,94). Contrast-induced renal failure is a major cause of renal failure in the hospital population (44).

The indications for excretory urography in children have undergone changes in the past few years and are very limited. Ultrasonography and CT have virtually replaced the excretory urogram in the evaluation of abdominal and renal masses, hydronephrosis, and abdominal pain and as a screen for associated renal anomalies in children with other congenital anomalies (61). Ultrasonography is evolving into the initial screening procedure for pediatric urologic disease because of excellent detail in children and lack of radiation exposure.

Excretory urography is sometimes used in evaluating urinary tract infection in children in whom reflux has been demonstrated on voiding cystourethrography. The excretory urogram provides better definition of cortical scarring associated with vesicoureteral reflux (62), but ultrasound is often sufficient for this purpose. Excretory urography is also indicated in calculus disease, in nonmedical hematuria, and in children who have recently undergone urologic surgery.

REFERENCES

1. Alexander RD, Berkes SL, Abuelo JG. Contrast media–induced oliguric renal failure. *Arch Intern Med* 1978;138:381.
2. American College of Radiology Committee on Drugs and Contrast Media. *Manual on contrast media,* 4th ed. Reston, VA: ACR, 1998.
3. Amin MM, Cohan RH, Dunnick NR. Ionic and nonionic contrast media: current status and controversies. *Applied Radiology* 1993;Nov:41.
4. Ansell G. Adverse reactions to contrast agents: the scope of the problem. *Invest Radiol* 1970;5:374.
5. Ansari Z, Baldwin D. Acute renal failure due to radio-contrast agents. *Nephron* 1976;17:28.
6. Bailey SR, Tyrell PNM, Hale M. A trial to assess the effectiveness of bowel preparation prior to intravenous urography. *Clin Radiol* 1991;44:335.

7. Barrett BJ, Carlisle EJ. Metaanalysis of the relative nephrotoxicity of high- and low-osmolality iodinated contrast media. *Radiology* 1993;188:171.
8. Becker JA. Vicarious excretion of urographic media. *Radiology* 1968;90:243.
9. Benness GT. Urographic contrast agents. A comparison of sodium and methylglucamine salts. *Clin Radiol* 1970;21:150.
10. Bettman MA, Morris TW. Recent advances in contrast agents. *Radiol Clin North Am* 1986;24:347.
11. Brasch RC. Allergic reactions to contrast media: accumulated evidence. *AJR Am J Roentgenol* 1980;134:797.
12. Bush WH Jr, Muller RN, Mattrey RF. *Treatment of adverse reactions in trends in contrast media.* Berlin: Springer-Verlag, 1998.
13. Bush WH Jr. Treatment of systemic contrast medium reactions. *Society of Uroradiology Syllabus* 1994, Jan 11.
14. Bush WH, Swanson DP. Acute reactions to intravascular contrast media: types, risk factors, recognition, and specific treatment. *AJR Am J Roentgenol* 1991;157:1153.
15. Byrd L, Sherman RL. Radiocontrast-induced acute renal failure: a clinical and pathophysiologic review. *Medicine* 1979; 58:270.
16. Caro JJ, Trindade E, McGregor M. The risks of death and of severe nonfatal reactions with high vs low osmolality contrast media: a meta-analysis. *AJR Am J Roentgenol* 1991;156:825.
17. Cattell WR. Excretory pathways for contrast media. *Invest Radiol* 1970;5:473.
18. Choyke PL. The urogram: are rumors of its death premature? *Radiology* 1992;184:33.
19. Chrispin AR, Godon I, Hall C, et al. *Diagnostic imaging of the kidney and urinary tract in children.* Berlin: Springer-Verlag, 1980.
20. Cohan RH, Leder RA, Ellis JH. Treatment of adverse reactions to radiographic contrast media in adults. *Radiol Clin North Am* 1996;34:1055.
21. Dacie JE, Fry IK. A comparison of sodium and methylglucamine diatrizoate in clinical urography. *Br J Radiol* 1971;44:51.
22. Dawson P. Intravenous urography revisited. *Br J Urol* 1990; 66:561.
23. Dawson P, Heron C, Marshall J. Intravenous urography with low-osmolality contrast agents: theoretical considerations and clinical findings. *Clin Radiol* 1984;35:173.
24. Dray RJ, Winfield AC, Muhletale CA, et al. Advantages of nonionic contrast agents in adult urography. *Urology* 1984; 24:297.
25. Dunnick NR, Cohan RH. Cost, corticosteroids, and contrast media. *AJR Am J Roentgenol* 1994;162:527.
26. Ellenbogen PH, Scheible FW, Talner LB, et al. Sensitivity of gray scale ultrasound in detecting urinary tract obstruction. *AJR Am J Roentgenol* 1978;130:731.
27. Ellis JH, Cohan RH, Sonnad SS, et al. Selective use of radiographic low-osmolality contrast media in the 1990s. *Radiology* 1996;200:297.
28. Fajardo LL, Hillman BJ. Image quality, diagnostic certainty, and accuracy: comparison of conventional and digital urograms. *Urol Radiol* 1988;10:72.
29. Fajardo LL, Hillman BJ, Hunter TB, et al. Excretory urography using computed radiography. *Radiology* 1987;162:345.
30. Fischer HW, Cornell SH. The toxicity of the sodium and methylglucamine, salts of diatrizoate, iothalamate, and metrizoate: an experimental study of their circulatory effects following intracarotid injection. *Radiology* 1965;85:1013.
31. Forrest JB, Howards SS, Gillenwater JY. Osmotic effects of intravenous contrast agents on renal function. *J Urol* 1981; 125:147.
32. Fry IK, Cattel WR. The nephrographic pattern during excretion urography. *Br Med Bull* 1972;28:227.
33. Gavant ML, Ellis JV, Klesges ML. Diagnostic efficacy of excretory urography with low-dose, nonionic contrast media. *Radiology* 1992;182:657.
34. George CD, Vinnicombe SJ, Balkissoon ARA, et al. Bowel preparation before intravenous urography: is it necessary? *Br J Radiol* 1993;66:17.
35. Gillenwater JY. Reactions associated with excretory urography—current concepts. *J Urol* 1971;106:122.
36. Golman K. Urography: physiological considerations on the excretion of contrast media. *J Belge Radiol* 1977;60:229.
37. Gomes AS, Baker JD, Martin-Paredero V, et al. Acute renal dysfunction after major arteriography. *AJR Am J Roentgenol* 1985;145:1249.
38. Greenberger PA, Patterson R, Tapio CM. Prophylaxis against retested radiocontrast media reactions in 857 cases: adverse experience with cimetidine and safety of β-adrenergic antagonists. *Arch Intern Med* 1985;145:2197.
39. Greene LF, Segura JW, Hattery RR, et al. Routine use of tomography in excretory urography. *J Urol* 1973;110:714.
40. Haddad MC, Sharif HS, Shahed HS, et al. Renal colic: diagnosis and outcome. *Radiology* 1992;184:83.
41. Harris KG, Smith TP, Cragg AH, et al. Nephrotoxicity from contrast material in renal insufficiency: ionic versus nonionic agents. *Radiology* 1991;179:849.
42. Hartman GW, Hattery RR, Witten AM, et al. Mortality during excretory urography: Mayo Clinic experience. *AJR Am J Roentgenol* 1982;139:919.
43. Hattery RR, Williamson B, Hartman GW, et al. Intravenous urographic technique. *Radiology* 1988;167:593.
44. Hou SH, Bushinsky DA, Wish JB, et al. Hospital-acquired renal insufficiency: a prospective study. *Am J Med* 1983;74:243.
45. Katayama H, Yamaguchi K, Takshima T, et al. Adverse reactions to ionic and nonionic contrast media. *Radiology* 1990; 175:621.
46. Katzberg RW, Moris TW, Schulman G, et al. Reactions of intravenous contrast media: part I. Severe and fatal cardiovascular reactions in a canine dehydration model. *Radiology* 1983; 147:327.
47. Katzberg RW, Morris TW, Schulman G, et al. Reactions to intravenous contrast media: part II. Acute renal response in euvolemic and dehydrated dogs. *Radiology* 1983;147:331.
48. Kelly JF, Patterson R, Lieberman P, et al. Radiographic contrast media studies in high-risk patients. *J Allergy Clin Immunol* 1978;62:181.
49. Kennan RJ, List A, Kengsakul C. Low-dose intravenous urography: results and technique modifications. *Australas Radiol* 1990;34(2):137.
50. Krumlovsky FA, Simon N, Santhanam S, et al. Acute renal failure: association with administration of radiographic contrast material. *JAMA* 1978;239:125.
51. Kumar R, Schreiber MH. The changing indications for excretory urography. *JAMA* 1985;254:403.
52. Lalli AF. Urographic contrast media reactions and anxiety. *Radiology* 1974;112:267.
53. Lalli AF. Contrast media reactions: data analysis and hypothesis. *Radiology* 1980;134:1.
54. Lalli AF. *Tailored urologic imaging.* Chicago: Year Book Medical Publishers, 1980.
55. Lasser EC. Basic mechanisms of contrast media reactions: theoretical and experimental considerations. *Radiology* 1968;91:63.
56. Lasser EC. Pretreatment with corticosteroids to prevent reactions to IV contrast material: overview and implications. *AJR Am J Roentgenol* 1988;150:257.

57. Lasser EC, Berry CC, Mishkin MM, et al. Pretreatment with corticosteroids to prevent adverse reactions to nonionic contrast media. *AJR Am J Roentgenol* 1994;162:523.
58. Lasser EC, Berry CC, Talner LB, et al. Pretreatment with corticosteroids to alleviate reactions to intravenous contrast. *N Engl J Med* 1987;317:845.
59. Lasser EC, Walters AJ, Lang JH. An experimental basis for histamine release in contrast material reactions. *Radiology* 1974; 110:49.
60. Lautin ME, Freeman NJ, Schoenfeld AH, et al. Radiocontrast-associated renal dysfunction: a comparison of lower-osmolality and conventional high-osmolality contrast media. *AJR Am J Roentgenol* 1991;157:59.
61. Lebowitz RL, Ben-Ami T. Trends in pediatric uroradiology. *Urol Radiol* 1983;5:135.
62. Leonidas JC, McCauley RGK, Klauber GC, et al. Sonography as a substitute for excretory urography in children with urinary tract infection. *AJR Am J Roentgenol* 1985;144:815.
63. McClennan BL. The optimal urogram. In: Pfister RC, ed. *Syllabus categorical course in genitourinary tract radiology.* Chicago: Radiological Society of North America, Nov 26–Dec 1, 1978:1–21.
64. McClennan B. Urography—anatomy and technique. In: Putman CE, Ravin CE, eds. *Textbook of diagnostic imaging.* Philadelphia: Saunders, 1988:1161–1168.
65. Merritt CR, Tutton RH, Bell KA, et al. Clinical application of digital radiography: computed radiographic imaging. *Radiographics* 1985;5:397.
66. Moore RD, Steinberg EP, Powe NR, et al. Frequency and determinants of adverse reactions induced by high-osmolality contrast media. *Radiology* 1989;170:727.
67. Moreau J, Droz D, Sabto J, et al. Osmotic nephrosis induced by water-soluble triiodinated contrast media in man. *Radiology* 1975;115:329.
68. Myers GH, Witten DM. Acute renal failure after excretory urography in multiple myeloma. *AJR Am J Roentgenol* 1971; 113:583.
69. Older RA. Contrast-induced renal failure—a radiologic problem and a radiologic diagnosis. *Radiology* 1979;131:553.
70. Older RA, Miller JP, Jackson DC, et al. Angiographically induced renal failure and its radiographic detection. *AJR Am J Roentgenol* 1976;126:1039.
71. Older RA, Korobkin M, Cleeve DM, et al. Contrast-induced acute renal failure: persistent nephrogram as clue to early detection. *AJR Am J Roentgenol* 1980;134:339.
72. Older RA, McLelland R, Cleeve DM, et al. Importance of routine vascular nephrotomography in excretory urography. *Urology* 1980;15:312.
73. Palmer FJ. The RACR survey of intravenous contrast media reaction: final report. *Australas Radiol* 1988;32:426.
74. Palmisano SM. Low-osmolality contrast media in the 1990s: prices change. *Radiology* 1997;203:309.
75. Pearson MC, Gilkes R, Hall JH, et al. Sodium or methylglucamine? A comparison of iothalamate in urography. *Br J Radiol* 1974;44:55.
76. Peck WW, Slutsky RA, Hackney DB. Effects of contrast media on pulmonary hemodynamics: comparison of ionic and nonionic agents. *Radiology* 1983;149:371.
77. Pfister RC. Reactions to urographic contrast media. In: *Syllabus for the categorical course in genitourinary radiology.* Chicago: Radiological Society of North America, Nov 30–Dec 5, 1975.
78. Pollack HM, Banner MP. Current status of excretory urography—a premature epitaphy? *Urol Clin North Am* 1985; 12:585.
79. Popio KA, Ross AM, Oravec JM, et al. Identification and description of separate mechanisms for two components of Renografin cardiotoxicity. *Circulation* 1978;58:520.
80. Rosenfield AT, Littner NR, Ulreich S, et al. Respiratory effects of excretory urography: a preliminary report. *Invest Radiol* 1977;12:295.
81. Sanders RC, Conrad MR. The ultrasonic characteristics of the renal pelvicalyceal echo complex. *J Clin Ultrasound* 1977; 5:372.
82. Scheible W, Talner LB. Gray scale ultrasound and the genitourinary tract: a review of clinical application. *Radiol Clin North Am* 1979;17:281.
83. Shafi T, Chou S, Porous JG, et al. Infusion intravenous pyelography and renal function: effects in patients with chronic renal insufficiency. *Arch Intern Med* 1978;138:1218.
84. Shehadi WH. Adverse reactions to intravascularly administered contrast media: a comprehensive study based on a prospective survey. *AJR Am J Roentgenol* 1975;124:145.
85. Shehadi WH. Contrast media adverse reactions: occurrence, recurrence, and distribution patterns. *Radiology* 1982;143:11.
86. Shehadi WH, Toniolo G. Adverse reactions to contrast media. *Radiology* 1980;137:299.
87. Silverman PM. Universal versus selective use of low-osmolality contrast media in the 1990s: a radiologist's perspective. *Radiology* 1997;203:311.
88. Smith RC, Verga M, McCarthy S, et al. Diagnosis of acute flank pain: value of unenhanced helical CT. *AJR Am J Roentgenol* 1996;166:97.
89. Spataro RF. New and old contrast agents: pharmacology, tissue opacification, and excretory urography. *Urol Radiol* 1988;10:2.
90. Stanley RJ, Pfister RC. Bradycardia and hypotension following use of intravenous contrast media. *Radiology* 1976;121:5.
91. Talner LB. Routine urography in men with prostatism. *AJR Am J Roentgenol* 1986;147:960.
92. Thomsen HS, Dorph S. High-osmolar and low-osmolar contrast media. *Acta Radio* 1993;34:205.
93. Thomsen HS, Bush WH. Treatment of the adverse effects of contrast media. *Acta Radiol* 1998;39:212.
94. VanZee BE, Hoy WE, Talley TE, et al. Renal injury associated with intravenous pyelography in nondiabetic and diabetic patients. *Ann Intern Med* 1978;89:51.
95. Vix VA. Intravenous pyelography in multiple myeloma. *Radiology* 1966;87:896.
96. Warshauer DM, McCarthy SM, Street L, et al. Detection of renal masses: sensitivities and specificities of excretory urography/linear tomography, US, and CT. *Radiology* 1988;169:363.
97. Witten DM, Hirsh FD, Hartman GW. Acute reactions to urographic contrast medium: incidence, clinical characteristics and relationship to history of hypersensitivity states. *AJR Am J Roentgenol* 1973;119:832.
98. Wolf GL. Safer, more expensive iodinated contrast agents: how do we decide? *Radiology* 1986;159:557.
99. Yocum MW, Heller AM, Abels RI. Efficacy of intravenous pretesting and antihistamine prophylaxis in radiocontrast media–sensitive patients. *J Allergy Clin Immunol* 1978;62:309.
100. Zoeller G, May C, Vosshenrich R, et al. Digital radiography in urologic imaging: radiation dose reduction in urethrocystography. *Urol Radiol* 1992;14:56.

3B

CYSTOGRAPHY AND URETHROGRAPHY

RICHARD A. LEDER

INTRODUCTION

Cystography and urethrography are imaging studies performed of the bladder and/or urethra before, during, and after the administration of contrast material. The goal of cystography and/or urethrography is to detect abnormalities of the lower urinary tract. Abnormalities of the bony pelvis, or pelvic soft tissues that may affect the bladder or urethra, may also be detected. This should be accomplished using the minimum radiation necessary to provide sufficient anatomic detail for the diagnosis of normal or abnormal urinary findings.

These examinations are performed under the direct supervision of physicians who have received documented formal training in the performance, interpretation, and reporting of uroradiologic studies. The supervising physician must be familiar with multiple disease processes of the lower genitourinary tract and understand the cystographic and urethrographic manifestations of these diseases. Furthermore, the physician performing these studies must be knowledgeable of alternative imaging techniques that may be required, such as ancillary studies either after a cystogram or urethrogram or as a replacement for these techniques. In particular cases, the lower tract evaluation may be accomplished with ultrasonography, computed tomography, nuclear medicine, or magnetic resonance imaging (MRI).

The physicians and technologists performing these studies should have an understanding of and experience in proper film technique; film sequencing; and the volume, concentration, and method of administering contrast material. Cystography and/or urethrography should be performed after an appropriate history and preprocedure screening are performed. Risk factors must be assessed before these examinations are performed. Some patients may require a steroid premedication regimen. The signs and symptoms of an adverse reaction from the administration of contrast material must be well known to the physicians and support staff caring for patients undergoing these examinations. Understanding of and proficiency in the recognition and treatment of adverse contrast reactions are required. Medication and resuscitative equipment must be immediately available to treat adverse contrast reactions.

Imaging findings and interpretations should be reported in a timely fashion in compliance with the American College of Radiology standards on communications. Urgent or acute findings should be communicated promptly to the ordering physician (1).

CONTRAST MATERIAL

Contrast for urethrography must be sufficiently viscus and dense for proper visualization of the urethra. The meglumine salts of diatrizoate or iothalamate are most useful for this examination. Sixty percent (weight/volume) solutions are typically used in retrograde urethrography to provide maximal opacification of the urethra. Meglumine salts of diatrizoate and/or iothalamate are also the most widely used contrast agents for cystography. Solutions containing 15% (weight/volume) contrast media are optimal for cystography. Solutions that contain greater than 15% contrast media may result in very dense opacification of the bladder, and subtle abnormalities may not be detected. Higher

R.A. Leder: Division of Abdominal Imaging, Department of Radiology, Duke University Medical School, Durham, NC 27710.

concentrations of contrast media may be irritating to the bladder mucosa. Systemic reactions following retrograde urethrography are extremely rare. Although uncommon, systemic reactions to contrast media may occur during cystography (5). Patients who have had adverse reactions to intravenous contrast material may be studied using either nonionic low-osmolar contrast or potentially both a steroid premedication and nonionic contrast (25).

The initial interview of patients undergoing either cystography or urethrography must include an allergy history, particularly a history of allergic reactions to contrast material. If the patient is thought to be at sufficient risk for a allergic reaction, nonionic contrast can be used. For cystography, dilute Isovue-300 (iopamidol 61% Bracco Diagnostics Inc. Princeton, New Jersey) is used. For urethrography, nondilute Isovue 300 can be used for the injection of contrast into the urethra.

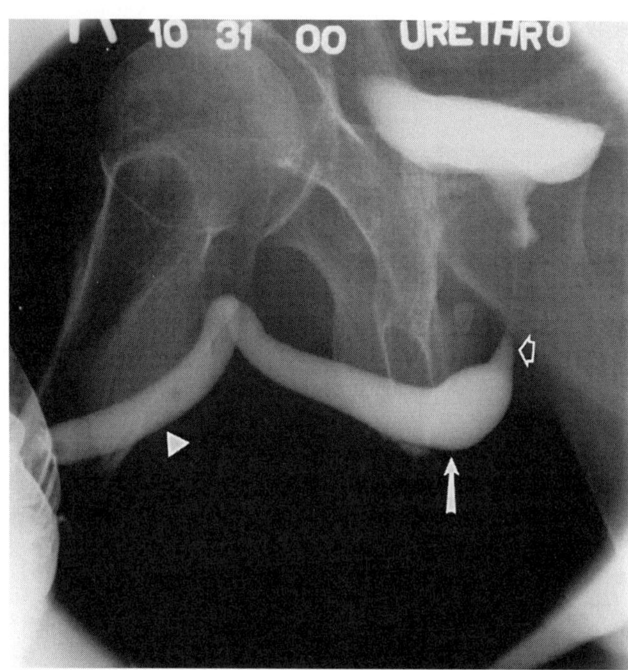

FIGURE 3B.1. Normal retrograde urethrogram, prior transurethral resection of the prostate (TURP). Contrast injected into the penile urethra shows excellent filling of the penile *(arrowhead)* and bulbar urethra *(arrow)*. The cone of the bulbous urethra is well depicted *(open arrow)*. The prostatic urethra is dilated in this patient status post TURP. A small air bubble is seen in the penile urethra.

URETHROGRAPHY

Normal Anatomy

The male urethra extends from the bladder neck to the external meatus, extending through the prostate gland and urogenital diaphragm. The urogenital diaphragm attaches anteriorly and laterally to the inferior rami of the public arch and the ischia. Posteriorly, the triangle is attached to the perineum and is continuous with the anal fascia. Near its apex, the diaphragm is perforated by the urethra approximately 1 cm below the symphysis pubis. This diaphragm divides the urethra into two portions: the anterior portion below the urogenital diaphragm and the posterior urethra above.

The anterior urethra extends from the inferior aspect of the urogenital diaphragm to the external meatus. The anterior urethra is divided into two parts by the penoscrotal junction inferiorly and the suspensory ligament superiorly. The penile urethra lies anterior to the penoscrotal junction. Distally, the penile urethra is dilated to form the fossa navicularis. Proximal to the penoscrotal junction lies the bulbous urethra. The bulbous urethra dilates slightly in its most inferior aspect and proximally terminates in a symmetric cone shape (Fig. 3B.1). The glands of Littre lie along the anterior urethra (Fig. 3B.2). Cowper's glands empty into the dilated portion of the bulbous urethra. The corpus spongiosum surrounds the anterior urethra.

The posterior urethra extends from the bladder neck to the urogenital diaphragm. The posterior urethra is composed of two parts: the membranous urethra and the prostatic urethra. The membranous urethra lies within the urogenital diaphragm and is 1 to 1.5 cm in length and 5 to 7 mm in caliber. The prostatic urethra extends through the prostate gland to the bladder neck. Anatomic features that may be noted when examining the posterior urethra include the verumontanum. This is a mound of smooth muscle on the posterior wall of the prostatic urethra. The superior aspect of the verumontanum lies above the middle of the prostatic urethra. The verumontanum extends inferiorly into the distal third of the prostatic urethra, tapering distal to form the urethral crest. There are three small orifices in the verumontanum. The superior opening is the prostatic utricle. Below and to the side of the prostatic utricle are the orifices of the ejaculatory ducts. On the side of the verumontanum is the prostatic sinus into which the prostatic ducts drain.

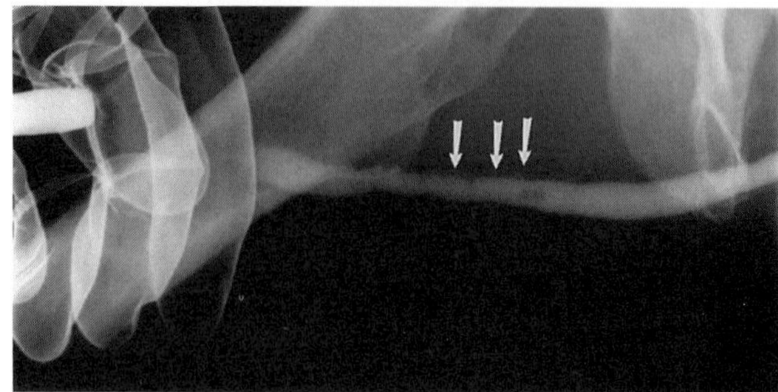

FIGURE 3B.2. Glands of Littre. Contrast has been injected into an Intracath placed in the penile meatus. Small contrast outpouchings are seen in the anterior urethra *(arrows)*. These are the glands of Littre. Air bubbles are incidentally noted in the penile urethra.

To understand urethrography, one must appreciate the presence of the urinary sphincters. The internal sphincter, which is composed of smooth muscle, surrounds the proximal portion of the prostatic urethra at the bladder neck. The intrinsic sphincter is also composed of smooth muscle and lies below the verumontanum. The external sphincter is composed of striated muscle and lies at the level of the membranous urethra. The internal sphincter of the bladder neck maintains passive continence. This internal sphincter is a circular band of smooth muscle, which is sympathetically controlled; it relaxes when bladder contraction occurs. Damage may occur in cases of traumatic pelvic injury or postsurgical obliteration, as can occur after a transurethral prostatic resection (TURP). The intrinsic sphincter consists of a 5-mm band of circular smooth muscle encircling the membranous urethra and extending proximally to surround the distal prostatic urethra. If damage occurs to the internal sphincter, passive continence may be maintained by the intrinsic sphincter. The intrinsic sphincter serves to empty the posterior urethra back into the bladder at the end of micturition. The external sphincter surrounds both the intrinsic sphincter and the membranous urethra. This sphincter is voluntarily controlled and is composed of striated muscle. Active continence is maintained by the external sphincter (22,23).

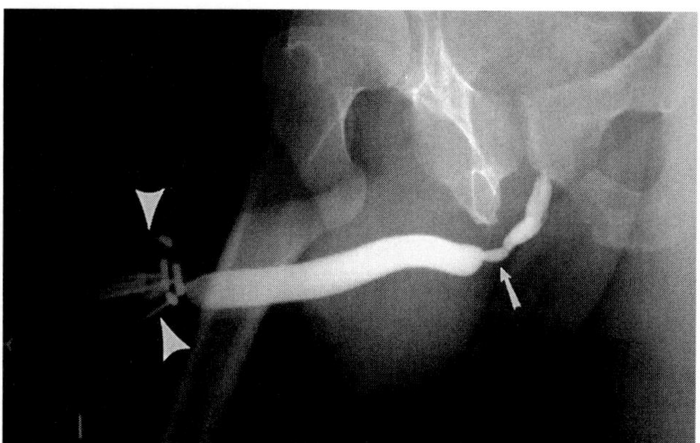

FIGURE 3B.3. Brodney clamp. A Brodney clamp *(arrowheads)* is seen positioned over the glans of the penis. Contrast has been injected in a retrograde fashion, and a bulbar urethral stricture *(arrow)* is demonstrated.

Technique

Although the technique of retrograde urethrography varies, the aim is to achieve consistent visualization of the urethra after the installation of contrast. Films must be exposed during the retrograde injection of contrast to adequately visualize the posterior urethra. The milking action of the intrinsic sphincter rarely allows opacification of the posterior urethra if contrast is not actively flowing through this portion of the urethra.

The initial film before a urethrogram is a coned film of the pelvis taken in a right posterior oblique position. The supervising physician reviews this film for abnormalities related to the pelvis, pelvic soft tissues, or bony structures. The patient is interviewed regarding possible heart murmurs, valve replacement, or the presence of a joint replacement. If any of these conditions exist, these patients are started on prophylactic antibiotics before the placement of a catheter and the injection of contrast. A 60-mL syringe is then filled with Reno-30 (diatrizoate meglumine 30%, Bracco Diagnostic Inc., Princeton, New Jersey). One standard technique requires the placement of a Foley catheter approximately 1 inch into the penis. A small amount of saline is injected into the balloon of a Foley catheter, with the dilated balloon fixed in the fossa navicularis. Films are obtained during the retrograde injection of contrast material. Typically, a 14- or 16-Fr Foley catheter is used for this study. Contrast material should be preinjected through the Foley catheter to purge air from the lumen. Patients are placed in a 45-degree right posterior oblique position so that the shaft of the penis is draped over the soft tissues of the thigh. After an initial volume is injected, resistance may be encountered due to spasm of the external sphincter. If there is spasm of the external sphincter, there will often be leakage of contrast from the meatus. In an attempt to overcome spasm of the external sphincter, patients are asked to attempt to void. Simultaneous to this action, contrast is injected in the hopes of filling the posterior urethra. Gentle pressure on the plunger of the syringe typically overcomes this resistance. There will be a noticeable decrease in effort when contrast begins to flow into the posterior urethra and bladder. This examination does not require fluoroscopic imaging (34).

Currently, we inject contrast into a syringe connected to a 19-by-⅞ butterfly needle apparatus from which the needle has been removed. This tubing is placed into the urethral meatus. Traction is placed on the penis, and manual compression is made close to the glans penis. Using this technique and appropriate penile traction, the hands of the individual injecting contrast will be outside the collimated beam. Alternatively, radiation-reduction gloves can be worn. The postinjection film is evaluated for adequate filling of all urethral segments. If necessary, additional images can be performed after repeat injection(s).

Other techniques are available for the performance of urethrography, including the use of a Brodney clamp (Fig. 3B.3) (11). This apparatus is no longer available at our institution. Nonetheless, practitioners have aimed to improve the diagnostic quality of retrograde urethrography using alternative techniques, including the use of an external compression "device." One such technique includes the placement of a 20-Fr Foley catheter with a 30-mL balloon placed under the penis. A bandage, 3 to 4 cm wide and approximately 60 cm long, is cut from the edge of a sterile disposable polythene drape; this is then wound around the penis and the catheter. The balloon of the external Foley catheter is inflated with air to produce firm pressure on the urethra. This technique aims to achieve external compression and serve as a penile clamp for retrograde urethrography (15).

Other imaging techniques include pericatheter retrograde urethrography. This can be accomplished by placing an Intra-Cath alongside an indwelling Foley catheter, permitting the injection of contrast adjacent to an indwelling Foley catheter. Compression distally should prevent spillage of contrast. The use of a pericatheter device can also serve the same purpose. A pericatheter device either 1 or 0.5 cm wide may be advanced along an indwelling catheter, through the meatus, and into the urethra until the injection arm of the device reaches the penile meatus. The standard device is 7 cm long; a smaller version is 4 cm long (18). The use of a disposable retrograde urethrogram catheter ("golf tee" catheter) made of soft blended plastic polymer has also been described. This catheter is 9 cm in overall length and has a 14-Fr outer diameter. The proximal end is flared and fits over a Toomey (standard catheter tip) syringe. The catheter is advanced to the level of the proximal flare, effectively occluding the penile meatus. Gentle pressure is applied around the base of the glans penis to prevent leakage of contrast. Mild traction is applied to stretch the urethra (24).

Although not our standard practice, a technique of double-contrast urethrography has also been described. Contrast coating of a urethral lesion has been described using 10 mL of iodized oil (Lipiodol) emulsion into the urethra, followed by 20 mL of air (43). A "choke" voiding urethrogram may be obtained by leaving a catheter in place and allowing the patient to void against pressure. This can be performed after the bladder is filled for a cystogram or after an intravenous urogram is performed. Meatal compression voiding urethrography (MCVU) using a Zipser clamp is described as a simple and accurate alternative to retrograde and noncompression voiding urethrography. Bladder filling with contrast either via a urethral catheter or as a result of an excretory urogram is first accomplished. The patient places the Zipser clamp behind the corona of his penis and signals the technologist when he begins to void. A radiograph is exposed, and the patient is told to stop voiding. If adequate urethral visualization is accomplished in full distention, the examination is concluded (8,13).

A recently described technique for retrograde urethrography includes the use of an appropriate-sized Bommelaer vacuum uterine cannula. This cannula is applied to the penile glans by increasing the negative pressure of the vacuum to a maximum of 25 mm Hg. After correct coupling of the cannula to the glans, contrast material is injected and spot films obtained. This technique permits better visualization of the distal tip of the anterior urethra, an area typically obscured by the presence of a Foley catheter. Patients experience less discomfort with this procedure compared with the Foley technique because the inflation of the balloon in the fossa navicularis is avoided. Opacification of the posterior urethra was reported to occur at a similar rate to that seen when using a Foley balloon method (3,27).

Urethrography of the Male Urethra

Radiographic landmarks seen during the performance of retrograde urethrography include the cone shape of the proximal bulbous urethra, the verumontanum within the prostatic urethra, and the bladder neck. Between the tip of the cone of the bulbous urethra and the inferior aspect of the verumontanum lies the membranous urethra. The penile urethra extends from the external meatus to the penoscrotal junction. The bulbous urethra lies between the inferior aspect of the urogenital diaphragm, where it exhibits a symmetric cone shape; it extends to the penoscrotal junction. The verumontanum is visualized as a smooth oblong-filling defect in the posterior wall of the prostatic urethra. Occasionally, a Cowper's duct or utricle may fill with contrast. Cowper's ducts are seen as faint lines of contrast adjacent of the proximal portion of the bulbous urethra. Cowper's ducts are posterior and lateral to the membranous urethra and extend from Cowper's glands to enter the cavernous portion of the bulbous urethra (41). The opaci-

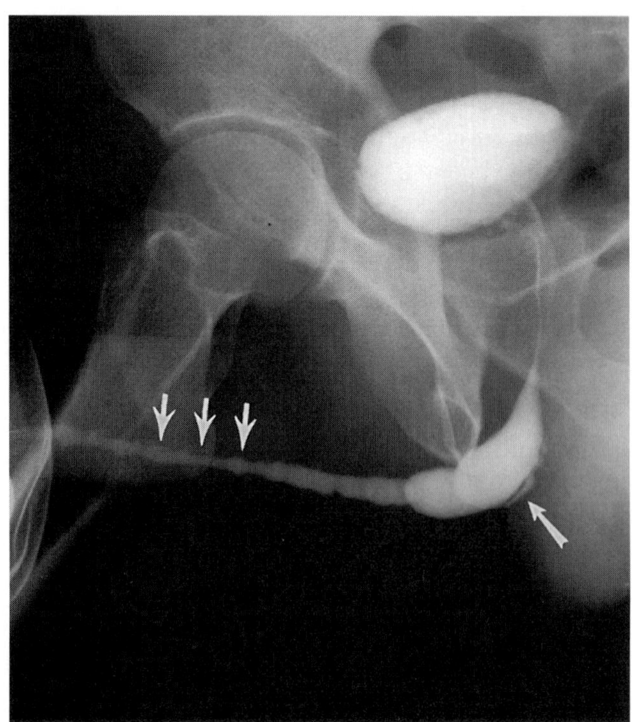

FIGURE 3B.4. Glands of Littre/Cowper's duct. There is a diffuse beaded appearance of the anterior urethra consistent with a long anterior urethral stricture. The bulbous urethra is dilated. A small amount of contrast is seen in Cowper's duct *(single arrow)*. Small contrast collections on the ventral surface of the urethra are consistent with the glands of Littre *(multiple arrows)*.

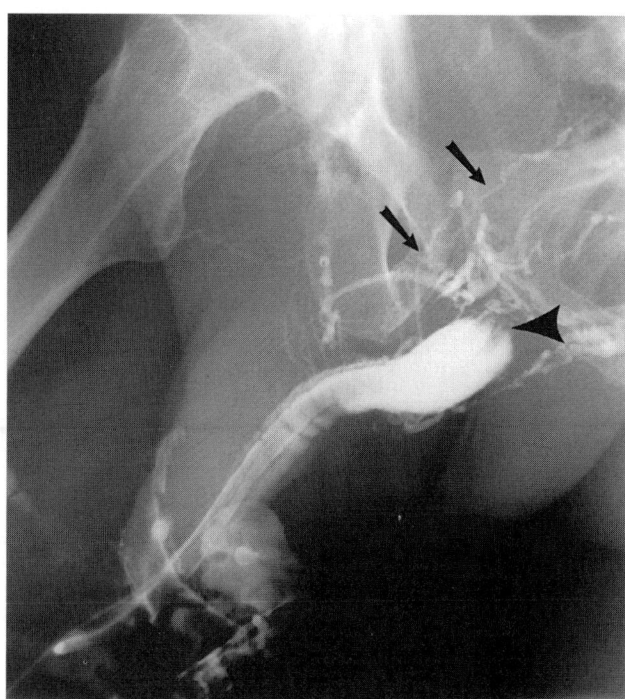

FIGURE 3B.5. Urethral extravasation. Contrast has been injected along side an indwelling Foley catheter. There is gross extravasation of contrast in the region of the membranous urethra *(arrowhead).* Filling is seen of the periurethral soft tissues, with widespread filling of pelvic veins *(arrows).*

fied utricle appears as a small tear drop–shaped cavity protruding posteriorly from region of the verumontanum. The glands of Littre appear as small linear collections of contrast material parallel to the superior margin of the anterior urethra. This is often associated with chronic infection or urethral stricture disease. Strictures may also account for opacification of Cowper's ducts and glands (Fig. 3B.4).

Rupture of the urethra during retrograde urethrography, although rare, can produce opacification of the corpus spongiosum, the paired corpora cavernosa, and the draining veins of the penis. Rupture may be secondary to a tight external sphincter or stricture, both processes causing increased intraurethral pressure during the injection of contrast material and an iatrogenic urethral tear. Corporal filling and venous filling may also be produced by trauma (whether caused by a Foley catheter or Brodney clap), previous urethral instrumentation, or external trauma (2) (Fig. 3B.5).

Urethrography of the Female Urethra

The female urethra is approximately 4 cm long and extends from the internal to the external urethral orifice. It courses in an oblique and downward fashion and is slightly curved. The urethral meatus is anterior to the vaginal opening; contrast material does not usually enter the vagina during voiding.

Standard voiding cystourethrography in females includes preliminary films of the pelvis to establish a baseline reference. The bladder is then partially filled, and supine views can be obtained to evaluate for potential reflux. After the bladder is completely filled, patients are placed in a standing position. Lateral, anteroposterior, and oblique fluoroscopic images can be obtained during the voiding and postvoid stages. These procedures can be videotaped. Films are scrutinized for the presence of a urethral diverticulum, evidence of urethral prolapse or hypermobility, and stress incontinence (29).

Double-balloon urethrography is described as a more sensitive diagnostic test for diagnosing a female urethral diverticulum (12). This technique requires the placement of a Bardex Davis model catheter (Bard Urological Division). The catheter is inserted into the bladder, and the balloon is inflated to 30 mL and pulled back until it is seated in the trigone. A sliding balloon is then pushed against the external meatus and inflated to 20 mL to produce a seal. Contrast is injected into the central lumen of the catheter. If leakage is seen into the bladder around the proximal balloon, the pressure and/or position of the balloon must be adjusted to reestablish the seal. In a recently reported study, double-balloon urethrography had a greater sensitivity (100%) than voiding cystourethrography (44%) relative to a confirmed surgical diagnosis (16) (Fig. 3B.6). Other authors have suggested that although the voiding cystourethrogram is not as sensitive as the double-balloon technique, it can still be used as a screening test. If the results of voiding cystourethrography are inconclusive and clinical suspicion persists, a double-balloon examination or MRI can be performed (28,33,40). Transrectal sonography has also been described in the diagnosis of urethral diverticula in women (39).

A variation in the double-balloon technique has been described. Dilute contrast may be used to inflate the intravesical and external balloons of the double-balloon catheter. The proximal balloon is inflated with 25% concentration contrast medium (Renografin 60, Conray 60, or Hypaque 50 diluted with saline) and then drawn snugly down to the internal urethral meatus. The external balloon is inflated with 50% contrast medium. Nondilute contrast medium is injected into the main lumen of the catheter. This is performed on the radiologic examination table, which facilitates fluoroscopic and spot films and provides suitable positioning of the patient during the injection of contrast material. The variation in concentration of contrast between the proximal and distal balloons and the full-strength contrast in the diverticulum permit more precise delineation of the relationship of the diverticulum to the bladder base, the internal sphincter, and the external urinary meatus (19).

An alternative examination in the investigation of potential female urethral diverticula simply requires obtaining a postvoid film after cystography. Comparison between a preliminary coned film of the pelvis and the postvoid film

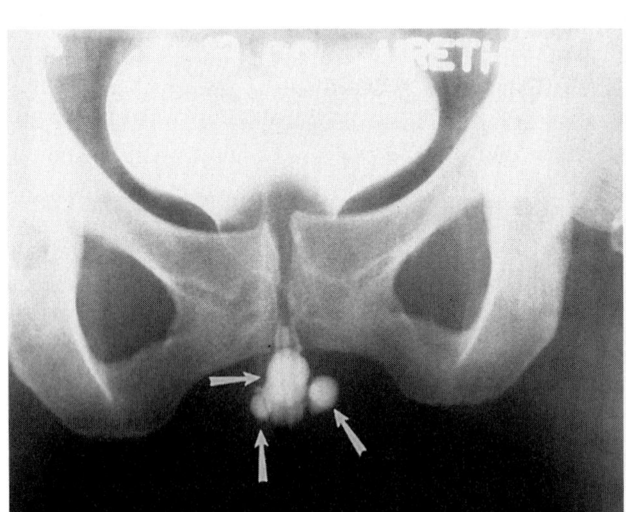

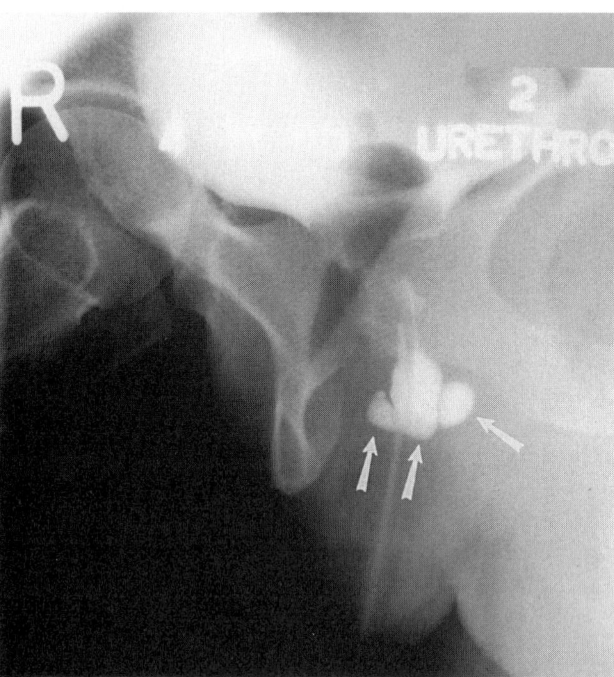

FIGURE 3B.6. A, B: Multiple urethral diverticula. Double-balloon retrograde urethrography reveals multiple diverticular outpouchings *(arrows)*. This patient previously had a normal voiding cystourethrogram.

may show accumulation of contrast in an expected periurethral location (Fig. 3B.7). This is an easy technique to use and does not require a double-balloon catheter.

Also described is the use of an Allis clamp to grasp the vaginal mucosa while a rubber olive-tip Brodney device is applied snugly to the urethral meatus. This maneuver is stated to result in elongation of the urethra, preventing compression and accordion-like shortening of the urethra (38). In our experience, patients who are suspected of having diverticular disease are best imaged with either a double-balloon technique or MRI.

Urethrography: Findings

Lesions that can be diagnosed on urethrography include traumatic injuries, congenital anomalies, obstructions, strictures, acquired diverticula, and neoplastic lesions. Congenital anomalies include hypospadias, posterior and anterior urethral valves, and urethral duplications. These anomalies, when severe, are usually treated surgically during childhood. Congenital duplication of the urethra is rare. Most duplications are incomplete and asymptomatic, requiring no treatment. A less common but clinically important entity is a complete patent duplication. These patients are symptomatic, with a double stream being the most common symptom. In all cases, the ventral channel proves to be the more normal urethral channel. These lesions have been classified into type I (blind and complete urethral duplication), type

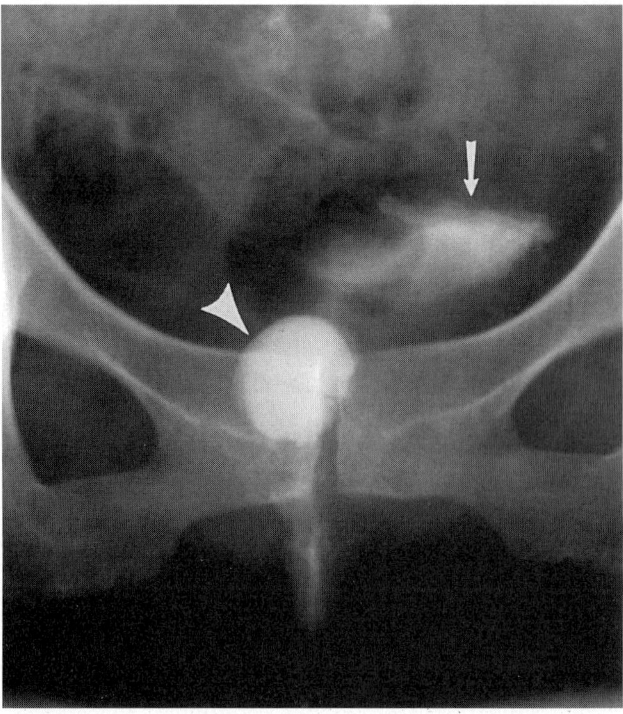

FIGURE 3B.7. Female urethral diverticulum. A rounded contrast collection is seen overlying the right public symphysis *(arrowhead)*. This is separate from the small residual contrast in the bladder *(arrow)*. Filling of this urethral diverticulum is demonstrated on the postvoid film from a cystogram.

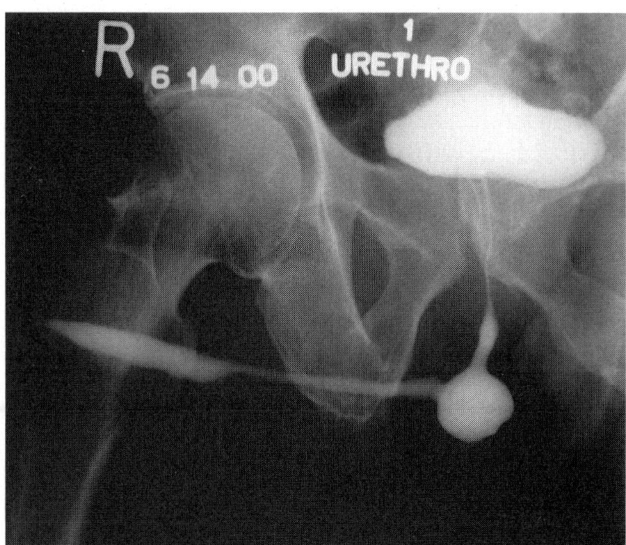

FIGURE 3B.8. Urethral diverticulum. Contrast is seen filling a bulbar urethral diverticulum. The distal bulbar urethra and proximal penile urethra are diffusely strictured.

IIA (complete patent duplication with two meatus), type IIA1 (two noncommunicating urethras arising independently from the bladder), type IIA2 (a second channel arising from the first and coursing independently to a second meatus), type IIB [complete patent urethral duplication with one meatus (two urethras arising from the bladder or posterior urethra reuniting to form a common distal channel)], and type III (urethral duplication as a component of partial or complete caudal duplication) (32). Cysts of Cowper's duct may be congenital in children but are typically acquired in adults secondary to urethral infection. A localized collection at the floor of the bulbous urethra is the typical appearance (9,35).

The presence of a double-density sign points to the diagnosis of a male urethral diverticulum. The double-density sign in the bulbous urethra is confirmed as a posterior urethral diverticulum after obtaining an oblique view accounting for the creation of this double density (31) (Fig. 3B.8).

Congenital saccular anterior urethral diverticula are uncommon. Congenital diverticula are termed *saccular* or *diffuse* on the basis of their anatomic configuration. A localized protrusion from the lumen into the ventral wall of the anterior urethra is a saccular-type diverticula. A generalized dilation of the entire anterior urethra, also termed *megalourethra* or *urethral ectasia,* is characterized as a diffuse type. Saccular-type diverticula may produce anterior urethral obstruction via a valvelike mechanism. The radiographic appearance of a saccular diverticulum is characteristic. Contrast will fill an oval outpouching on the ventral aspect of the anterior urethra. The diverticulum involves the midportion of the penile urethra but can involve the bulbous urethra as well. There is a broad communication between the urethral lumen and the diverticulum. Primary differential considerations when detecting this entity are anterior urethral valves and a dilated Cowper's gland duct (17). Female urethral congenital anomalies are extremely rare. An ectopic ureter may insert into the female urethra and fill during voiding. An ectopic ureter may masquerade as a urethral diverticulum (6).

Urethral stricture disease is common as a result of infection, instrumentation, or trauma. Gonorrheal infection may lead to fibrous scar formation. Inflammatory strictures are found most commonly in the bulbar urethra. The glands of Littre are more abundant in this portion of the urethra and presumably harbor infectious bacteria. Urethritis may also be secondary to conditions such as tuberculosis and schistosomiasis, causing abscesses in the periurethral tissues and perineal fistula formation. The "watering-can" perineum describes the presence of urethral cutaneous fistulae in patients with longstanding strictures (36). Often, these strictures are the result of postgonococcal disease.

Acquired female urethral diverticula occur posterior to the midurethra, although rarely they may occur anteriorly. These originate from infected periurethral glands, which may form an abscess that ultimately ruptures into the urethra. Filling defects within a urethral diverticulum may be secondary to debris, the presence of calculus disease, or rarely, a tumor (10).

Primary carcinomas of the urethra are uncommon but are seen more commonly in women than in men. Most tumors are squamous cell carcinomas; a smaller percentage are transitional cell carcinomas or adenocarcinomas. In men, carcinomas are often associated with an anterior urethral stricture (42).

A well-known artifact in urethrography is the pseudostricture of the urethra. This is caused by pressure on the under surface of the penis by a collecting vessel. This should not be mistaken for a stricture. A short proximal stricture can appear to be long on a voiding study if flow through the narrowed area is not forceful enough to distend the urethra. A smooth uniform narrowing of the entire anterior urethra distal to the penoscrotal junction causes this characteristic pseudostricture. If doubt remains, a retrograde examination or repeat voiding urethrography should be performed (20).

CYSTOGRAPHY

Technique

The first film exposed during the performance of a cystogram is a scout kidney, ureter, bladder (KUB). This is typically exposed using 65 kV and 900 mA at 60 ms. This plain film is evaluated for the presence of abnormal calcifications; abnormal gas collections; and any potential abnormalities related to the kidneys, ureters, or pelvis. Before a Foley catheter is placed, patients are interviewed regarding their history of cardiac valvular disease and the presence of

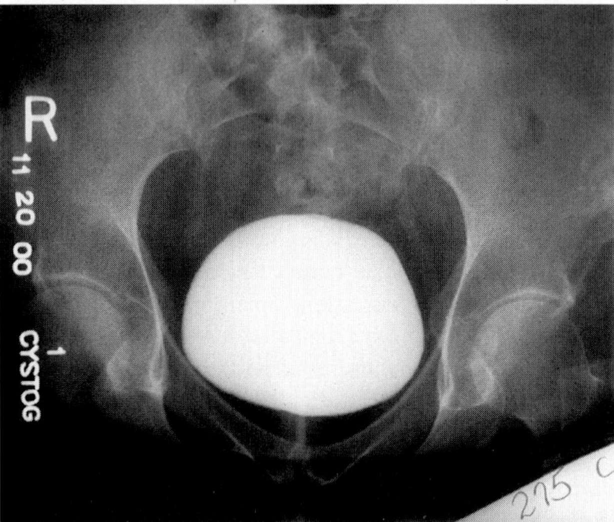

FIGURE 3B.9. Normal cystogram. Contrast (275 mL) fills this normal bladder as part of a pretransplant evaluation. There is no reflux. Calcification is seen in the iliac arteries bilaterally.

any joint replacement. Patients who have either a heart murmur (mitral or aortic prolapse/regurgitation), a prosthetic heart value, or an orthopedic joint replacement are placed on prophylactic antibiotics before the placement of the Foley catheter for the cystogram.

Typically, a 14-Fr, 16-inch Dover Rob-Nel catheter (Sherwood Medical, St. Louis, Missouri) is placed into the bladder. A bottle of Cystografin (diatrizoate meglumine 18%, Bracco Diagnostics Inc., Princeton, New Jersey) is infused into the Rob-Nel catheter. Contrast is infused until the patient complains of fullness. At this point, a supine KUB is exposed in addition to a left posterior oblique film. The supervising physician checks these films. The catheter is then removed, and a voiding film is obtained in a right posterior oblique. If the patient is unable to void for this film, an oblique film is exposed with the patient straining. The supervising physician reviews this film. Subsequent to this, the patient is allowed to void completely and a postvoid film is obtained in a frontal supine position. When cystography is performed, every effort should be made to administer as much contrast as the patient can comfortably retain. In the posttrauma setting, this is particularly important to avoid missing bladder extravasation. Ideally, 300 to 500 mL of contrast is administered.

Normal Anatomy

The bladder is oval shaped, with its greatest dimension in the vertical or horizontal position (especially in women). The bladder wall appears smooth when there is full distention and the bladder is normal (Fig. 3B.9). Continence is maintained at the level of the bladder neck. Filling of the posterior urethra may occur in patients who have had a prostatectomy or in patients who have an incompetent internal sphincter. A small amount of air may be seen within the bladder when air is introduced during instrumentation. The bladder base is flat in a supine position and cone shaped when the patient is erect. Voiding occurs when the smooth muscles of the bladder detrusor contract. There are three layers of muscle in the bladder: outer and inner longitudinal muscle and middle circular muscle. Pelvic floor musculature will relax during micturition, and the bladder will descend and change its appearance.

Films are evaluated for the presence of reflux, diverticula, possible mural lesions, and extravasation. If voiding films are desired, these are typically obtained with the patient in an upright position. A receptacle, which is radiolucent, is given to the patient. Filming is performed in an oblique position (Fig. 3B.10). As described previously, this technique can be modified by having the patient void against resistance. This can be accomplished by pinching the distal aspect of the penis or by using a penile clamp such as a Zipser clamp.

Indications

Cystoscopy remains the gold standard for the urologic evaluation of the bladder; radiographic investigation is performed in a number of settings, including the evaluation

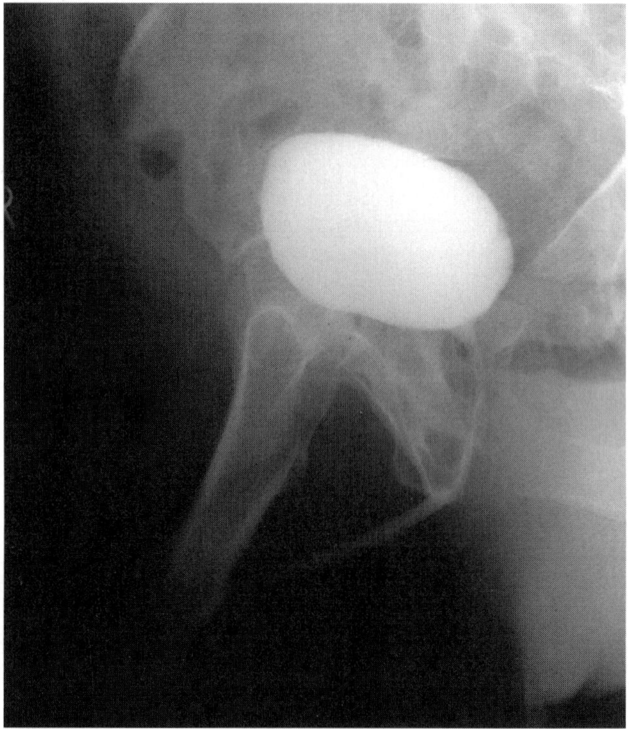

FIGURE 3B.10. Voiding film, normal voiding cystourethrogram. Contrast fills a normal-appearing bladder. There is no evidence of reflux. Filling is seen of a normal-appearing urethra.

of possible vesicoureteral reflux, evaluation of bladder diverticular disease, investigation of a potential bladder injury in a trauma patient, and common in our practice, documenting the bladder appearance in patients before a renal transplant.

The vast majority of cystograms are performed in the posttrauma setting; cystography may also be performed in postsurgical patients who have had radical retropubic prostatectomies. Reconstructive techniques of the vesicourethral anastomosis after radical retropubic prostatectomy involve placement of a urethral catheter for stenting the anastomosis and drainage of the bladder. Traditionally, this catheterization period is approximately 2 to 3 weeks. Cystographic evaluation in these postoperative patients permits evaluation of postoperative extravasation, allowing extension of the catheterization period. An abnormal appearance of the bladder contour in cystography suggests the presence of an intrapelvic fluid collection such as a hematoma or lymphocele. Ultrasound or computed tomography (CT) may be performed to diagnose these fluid collections as well as guide potential drainage (4,21).

Posttrauma cystograms should include standard frontal, oblique, and occasionally lateral views. In severely immobile patients, oblique views are often omitted. Postdrainage films in these patients assume added importance. Small amounts of extravasation should be readily identified on the postdrainage film (37). Recently, more attention has been paid to the diagnosis of bladder injury using CT because most posttrauma patients will have CT scans to exclude intraabdominal injuries. These studies should be evaluated closely for the presence of a bladder injury. CT cystography in the detection of bladder rupture has a reported overall sensitivity and specificity of 95% and 100%, respectively (7). Other authors have addressed the radiographic and clinical predictors of bladder rupture and compared CT cystography with conventional cystography in the evaluation of bladder injuries. These results show that CT cystography is clearly an accurate method for evaluating bladder injuries (14,26,30).

REFERENCES

1. American College of Radiology (ACR). ACR standard for adult cystography and urethrography. *Am Coll Radiol* 1992;13:1.
2. Amis ES, Newhouse JH, Cronan JJ. Radiology of male periurethral structures. *AJR Am J Roentgenol* 1988;151:321.
3. Barange XS, Schorlemmer WC, Vijande RA, et al. Barcelona retrograde urethrography: a new device and technique. *J Urol* 1999;161:1863.
4. Berlin JW, Ramchandani P, Banner MP, et al. Voiding cystourethrography after radical prostatectomy: normal findings and correlation between contrast extravasation and anastomotic. *AJR Am J Roentgenol* 1994;162:87.
5. Bettenay F, Campo J. Allergic reaction following micturating cystourethrography. *Urol Radiol* 1989;11:167.
6. Curry NS. Ectopic ureteral orifice masquerading as a urethral diverticulum. *AJR Am J Roentgenol* 1983;141:1325.
7. Deck AJ, Shaves S, Talner L, et al. Computerized tomography cystography for the diagnosis of traumatic bladder rupture. *J Urol* 2000;164:43.
8. Fitts FB, Mascatello VG, Mellins HZ. The value of compression during excretion voiding urethrography. *Radiology* 1977; 125:53.
9. Flanagan JL. Urethrography: recognition of Cowper's glands and ducts. *Clin Radiol* 1982;33:71.
10. Fortunato P, Schettini M, Gallucci M. Diverticula of the female urethra. *Br J Urol* 1997;80:628.
11. Golji H. New method of cystourethrography. *Urology* 1980; 135:554.
12. Greenberg M, Stone D, Cochran ST, et al. Female urethral diverticula: double-balloon catheter study. *AJR Am J Roentgenol* 1981;136:259.
13. Hillman BJ. Evaluation of postsurgical urethra and urethral strictures by meatal compression-voiding urethrography. *Urology* 1981;17:95.
14. Horstman WG, McClennan BL, Heiken JP. Comparison of computed tomography and conventional cystography for detection of traumatic bladder rupture. *Urol Radiol* 1991; 12:188.
15. Houghton-Allen B. A penile clamp for retrograde urethrography using external compression by a balloon catheter. *Aust Radiol* 1997;41:6.
16. Jacoby K, Rowbotham RK. Double balloon positive pressure urethrography is a more sensitive test than voiding cystourethrography for diagnosing urethral diverticulum in women. *J Urol* 1999;162:2066.
17. Kirks DR, Grossman H. Congenital saccular anterior urethral diverticulum. *Radiology* 1981;140:367.
18. Knoll LD, Furlow WL, Karsburg W. Pericatheter retrograde urethrography: introduction of a new device and technique. *J Urol* 1989;142:1533.
19. Kohorn EI, Glickman MG. Technical aids in investigation and management of urethral diverticula in the female. *Urology* 1992; 40:322.
20. Lebowitz RL. Pseudostricture of the urethra: urinal artefact on urethrography. *AJR Am J Roentgenol* 1978;130:570.
21. Leibovitch I, Rowland RG, Little JS, et al. Cystography after radical retropubic prostatectomy: clinical implication of abnormal findings. *Urology* 1995;46:78.
22. McCallum RW. The adult male urethra: normal anatomy, pathology, and method of urethrography. *Radiol Clin North Am* 1979;17:227.
23. McCallum RW, Colapinto V. The role of urethrography in urethral disease. Part I. Accurate radiological localization of the membranous urethra and distal sphincters in normal male subjects. *J Urol* 1979;122:607.
24. McLellan GL, Turetsky DB, Swartz DA. New catheter for retrograde urethrography. *Urology* 1991;37:582.
25. Miller KT, Moshyedi AC. Systemic reaction to contrast media during cystography. *AJR Am J Roentgenol* 1995;164:1551.
26. Morgan DE, Nallamala LK, Kenney PJ, et al. CT cystography: radiographic and clinical predictors of bladder rupture. *AJR Am J Roentgenol* 2000;174:89.
27. Muruka FJ. Ascending urethrography using the Leech-Wilkinson intra-uterine cannula in adult male patients. *East Afr Med J* 1989;66:603.
28. Neitlich JD, Foster HE, Glickman MG, et al. Detection of urethral diverticula in women: comparison of a high resolution fast spin echo technique with double balloon urethrography. *J Urol* 1998;159:408.
29. Pelsang RE, Bonney WW. Voiding cystourethrography in female stress incontinence. *AJR Am J Roentgenol* 1996;166: 561.

30. Peng MY, Parisky YR, Cornwell EE, et al. CT cystography versus conventional cystography in evaluation of bladder injury. *AJR Am J Roentgenol* 1999;173:1269.
31. Preminger GM, Steinhardt GF. Male urethral diverticulum: the double density sign. *Urology* 1985;26:417.
32. Psihramis KE, Colodny AH, Lebowitz RL, et al. Complete patent duplication of the urethra. *J Urol* 1986;136:63.
33. Romanzi LJ, Groutz A, Blaivas JG. Urethral diverticulum in women: diverse presentations resulting in diagnostic delay and mismanagement. *J Urol* 2000;164:428.
34. Sandler CM. Questions and answers. *AJR Am J Roentgenol* 1994;163:1263.
35. Selli C, Nesi G, Pellegrini G, et al. Cowper's gland duct cyst in an adult male. *Scand J Urol Nephrol* 1996;31:313.
36. Sharfi ARA, Elarabi YE. The "watering-can" perineum: presentation and management. *Br J Urol* 1997;80:933.
37. Spirnak JP. Pelvic fracture and injury to the lower urinary tract. *Surg Clin North Am* 1988;68:1057.
38. Steinhardt GF, Landes RR. Countertraction retrograde urethrography in women: an improved diagnostic technique. *J Urol* 1982;128:936.
39. Vargas-Serrano B, Cortina-Moreno B, Rodriguez-Romero R, et al. Transrectal ultrasonography in the diagnosis of urethral diverticula in women. *J Clin Ultrasound* 1997;25:21.
40. Wang AC, Wang CR. Radiologic diagnosis and surgical treatment of urethral diverticulum in women. *J Reprod Med* 2000; 45:377.
41. Yaffe D, Zissin R. Cowper's glands duct: Radiographic findings. *Urol Radiol* 1991;13:123.
42. Yoder IC, Papanicolaou N. Imaging the urethra in men and women. *Urol Radiol* 1992;14:24.
43. Yokoyama M, Watanabe K, Iwata H, et al. Case profile: double-contrast urethrography for visualizing small lesions in distal urethra. *Urology* 1982;19:440.

Adult and Pediatric Urology, 4/e, edited by Jay Y. Gillenwater, John T. Grayhack, Stuart S. Howards, and Michael E. Mitchell.
Lippincott Williams & Wilkins, Philadelphia © 2002

3C

COMPUTED TOMOGRAPHY

PARVATI RAMCHANDANI
SUSAN E. ROWLING

FUNDAMENTALS OF COMPUTED TOMOGRAPHY IMAGING

Computed tomography (CT) plays a crucial role in the diagnosis, management, and follow-up of many urologic disorders. A detailed discussion of the physical principles involved in the production of a CT image is beyond the scope of this chapter. However, a basic understanding of the physics of CT and its recent technologic advances is helpful to the ordering clinician to ensure appropriate patient referral and optimal scanning protocols.

CT is similar to conventional radiographic tomography in that a single slice or section of a patient is imaged. However, an important difference is that the x-ray beam passes only through the area of interest and not through adjacent structures, thus eliminating degradation of the image by superimposition of structures outside the slice. The entire urinary tract is directly shown in cross section, so overlying gas or bony structures do not obscure the areas of interest, as can occur with intravenous urography (IVU) or ultrasonography. Compared with magnetic resonance imaging (MRI), CT has better spatial resolution, is more widely available, usually has shorter scanning time, and is of lower cost. However, when an apparent renal mass is indeterminate in imaging features on CT, the greater contrast sensitivity of MRI may allow better detection of intratumoral enhancement. CT and MRI may therefore be complementary for such lesions. Anatomic regions such as the retroperitoneal structures, which are only indirectly imaged by conventional means, are directly visualized by cross-sectional techniques such as CT.

The creation of an image by CT relies on the inherently different attenuation characteristics of the various tissues in the body. CT has much higher contrast sensitivity than conventional radiographs and thus allows the differentiation of tissues with much smaller density differences than is possible with plain radiographs. Thus calculi that are nonopaque on abdominal films (e.g., uric acid stones) are seen as dense structures on CT scans.

Basically, a CT image is a two-dimensional representation of the distribution of different x-ray attenuation coefficients, or densities, of the various tissues within a narrow cross section of the subject's anatomy. The x-ray tube circles around the patient, emitting narrowly collimated x-ray beams from multiple different angular projections that pass through the subject and are sensed on the opposite side by a series of x-ray detectors. By reconstruction, an image is produced that is comprised of quantified grayscale values,

P. Ramchandani and S.E. Rowling: Department of Radiology, University of Pennsylvania Medical Center, Philadelphia, PA 19104.

known as *pixels,* that assign density values to individual points within the section. Each pixel value is directly related to the linear attenuation coefficient of the corresponding volume element of the slice, called a *voxel.* The density measurements are then standardized using the Hounsfield scale, named after Sir Godfrey Hounsfield, the inventor of the first clinically viable CT scanner (4,12,34). This scale assigns water a CT number, or Hounsfield Unit (HU), of zero and assigns all other tissue values ranging from −1,000 to approximately +2,000, depending on their attentions relative to water. Using this scale, air is −1,000 HU, fat is approximately −50 to −100 HU, fluid is 0 to +20 HU, soft tissue is between +40 and +60 HU, and cortical bone is between +1,000 and +2,000 HU. CT numbers may vary slightly between manufacturers and are a function of scanner kV (4,12).

The attenuation value of a specific tissue is measured by placing a cursor over the region of interest (ROI) on the workstation and instructing the computer to give the average CT number for that region. The number actually represents the average attenuation of the voxels within the cursor. Therefore measurements are most accurate if the ROI cursor is smaller than the structure being measured, if the cursor is placed well within its boundaries, and if the structure fills the entire slice width of the voxel. Measurements are subject to partial-volume artifact if the structure being measured is smaller than the slice width (4). For example, if the slice thickness is 10 mm and the ROI cursor is placed over a 5-mm renal cyst within the slice, the attenuation measurement will be erroneously high, representing the average of the cyst fluid and the adjacent 5 mm of renal parenchyma. Partial-volume artifact also occurs if an object extends only partially into a CT slice or if two different structures extend into the same slice; it is also exacerbated by patient motion and differences in respiration between slices, leading to respiratory misregistration. Partial-volume artifact is diminished when shorter scan times, thin-section collimation, and single breath-hold scanning techniques are used (4).

Following reconstruction, a CT image is processed to make certain anatomy or pathology more conspicuous by changing the window level and window width. The dynamic range of CT scanners is 4,096 different grayscale values. However, because a maximum of 256 gray levels can be displayed in a typical image, a small subset of the entire grayscale range must be chosen to optimize contrast within specific tissue types (12). The window level controls the image brightness. A midgray level in the center of the display range is selected. The window width defines the range of densities, from black to white, around the midgray level that will be displayed in the image. For example, the typical window level for soft tissue imaging within the abdomen and pelvis is 50 HU with a window width of 200 HU. Therefore only tissues with CT numbers of −50 to +150 HU will be displayed. Those with numbers less than −50 HU will be black, and those values greater than +150 will be white (12). Selecting a narrower window width will enhance contrast, as well as noise, but may be helpful in identifying subtle mass lesions, particularly those in the liver. In contrast, imaging the lung parenchyma requires a lower window level of approximately −700 HU and a wider width of 2,000 HU to enable display of a larger range of densities, including air-filled lung and soft tissue (12). A CT scan of the abdomen and pelvis is routinely reviewed in soft tissue, liver, bone, and lung windows. A liver window or similar narrow window is often helpful in improving lesion conspicuity within the kidneys, particularly when there is intense contrast enhancement of the renal parenchyma.

CT scanning geometry has evolved from first- to fourth-generation scanners. Rapid scan times and optimal spatial resolution require a large number of x-ray detectors, an integral feature of third- and fourth-generation scanners. First-generation scanners had a single x-ray tube and detector. Most modern scanners use third-generation geometry, in which the x-ray tube and a large number of detectors (referred to as a *detector array*) are rigidly fixed opposite one another and rotate together around the patient as the detector samples the fan of divergent rays. In fourth-generation scanners, the detector array forms a complete 360-degree outer ring that samples x-ray beams from the inner x-ray tube and generator as they rotate around the patient. The major advantage of the later-generation models is a faster scan time of 1 second or less and improved spatial resolution (4,12).

Helical computed tomography (HCT), or spiral CT imaging, became commercially available in the early 1990s (4,36,37). In conventional CT scanning, the x-ray tube focal spot lies within a single plane, the table and patient are stationary as data are collected from each slice of anatomy, and the table is moved incrementally between each slice acquisition until the entire area of interest is imaged. During HCT, the table and patient are not stationary during image acquisition, but rather move at a predetermined constant speed while the x-ray tube, and usually the detector array, rotate 360 degrees around the patient. Therefore the x-ray tube focal spot forms a continuous helix around the patient, rather than multiple contiguous circular planes, enabling rapid acquisition of a volumetric data set. Whereas conventional CT images are typically reconstructed from the entire 360-degree angular view set, HCT images are reconstructed from half (180 degrees) of the available view set (4). Because the acquired views do not lie in a plane, the view set is not comprised of actual projections of the slice, but rather is interpolated from the adjacent volumetric data to create the image slice. For this reason, HCT is subject to increased volume averaging artifact. However, the benefits of diminished motion and respiratory misregistration outweigh the mild increase in partial-volume averaging. One of the greatest advantages of HCT is the ability to improve z-axis resolution by retrospectively selecting a narrower collimation using overlapping reconstruction. This feature is important when attempting to characterize small lesions based on attenuation measurements (4,26).

The development of HCT has enabled imaging of large anatomic regions in a single breath hold, which helps eliminate problems of respiratory misregistration between adjacent slices and helps improve lesion characterization. HCT also enables imaging during the optimal phase, or multiple phases, of enhancement following bolus injection of iodinated intravenous contrast media. In addition, identical image levels are more consistently achieved before and after intravenous contrast media for assessment of lesion enhancement characteristics (26). The risk of imaging during suboptimal phases of contrast enhancement, common in conventional CT imaging, is much reduced with HCT. The three-dimensional data set acquired during HCT imaging has also been critical in the development of three-dimensional CT reconstruction and CT angiography (CTA) (66). The more recent development of multidetector-row HCT (MDCT), also known as *multislice HCT,* and subsecond gantry rotation times, has further revolutionized CT imaging. Much more rapid scan times, improved longitudinal resolution, greater longitudinal coverage, and diminished radiation doses and intravenous contrast load are now possible (66).

COMPUTED TOMOGRAPHY OF THE KIDNEYS

Technique

Complete evaluation of the kidneys requires precontrast and postcontrast imaging. Thus, in patients with a suspected or known renal mass, or those with hematuria, both precontrast and postcontrast scanning should be performed. However, for some indications, such as evaluation of a patient with suspected acute renal colic, unenhanced (noncontrast) scanning alone is generally sufficient to answer the clinical question. Although many renal abnormalities may be detectable on postcontrast images, definitive evaluation of renal masses requires assessment of enhancement in the mass, for which thin-section images through the kidneys both before and after the administration of intravenous contrast media are necessary. It is imperative to use identical scanning parameters before and after contrast administration to ensure that attenuation measurements are obtained from exactly the same location within a lesion and that any change in attenuation can be attributed to lesion enhancement.

The dose of intravenous contrast depends on patient size but generally is between 100 and 150 mL (20 to 50 g of iodine). Oral contrast is given to all patients except those being evaluated for acute renal colic.

The kidneys can be imaged in three distinct phases after contrast administration: the corticomedullary phase (CMP), the nephrographic phase (NP), and the excretory phase (EP) (Fig. 3C.1). The CMP occurs between 25 and 80 seconds after initiation of the contrast bolus, when much of the contrast remains in the renal cortical capillaries, proximal tubules, and peritubal spaces (8,41,86). Because the medullary pyramids are lower in attenuation compared with the cortex, there is an increased chance of either missing a central low-attenuation mass or mistaking a normal pyramid for a mass (Figs. 3C.2 and 3C.3). More rarely, the enhancing renal cortex may obscure an intensely enhancing vascular cortical neoplasm (86). The NP occurs between 85 and 130 seconds after the initiation of contrast administration as contrast filters through the glomeruli, loops of Henle, and collecting ducts, creating homogeneous parenchymal enhancement. EP images are obtained 3 to 5 minutes after intravenous contrast administration. At this point, the renal parenchyma remains homogeneous but is diminished in attenuation compared with the NP (86). EP images are typically recommended if a urothelial tumor is suspected because contrast in the collecting system increases the conspicuity of a low-attenuation mass. They are also often helpful in distinguishing central renal cell carcinomas (RCCs) from transitional cell tumors located within a calyx or renal pelvis (81). Delayed images obtained after 15 minutes may be helpful in characterizing incidentally identified renal masses when preliminary unenhanced images were not obtained. It has been shown that the attenuation of renal neoplasms diminishes with time as the contrast "washes-out," whereas the density of high-attenuation cysts does not change with time (54,86).

Recognition of these phases of normal renal enhancement and the effect on renal mass detection, conspicuity, and characterization is very important. Masses may be difficult to recognize and characterize if imaging is performed during the CMP alone (Figs. 3C.2 and 3C.3). Of all renal lesions detected in the NP, only 67% to 72% are also detected in the CMP of imaging (8,18,78). In one study (18), the addition of NP imaging to CMP imaging resulted in a 4.4-fold increase in detection of medullary lesions, and a 1.2-fold increase in the detection of cortical lesions. False-positive results are also more common in the CMP of imaging (5,18,78). However, renal venous involvement is best seen during the CMP of enhancement (45).

Current scanning protocols for renal mass characterization are performed as follows. During HCT, unenhanced (precontrast) images are obtained through the kidneys at 5-mm increments. Intravenous contrast is then administered using a mechanical power injector at a rate of 2 or 3 mL per second. Following initiation of the contrast bolus, contiguous 5-mm scans are obtained through the kidneys. CMP images are acquired after a delay of 30 to 40 seconds, and NP images acquired after a delay of 100 seconds. If indicated, EP images are acquired 3 to 5 minutes after

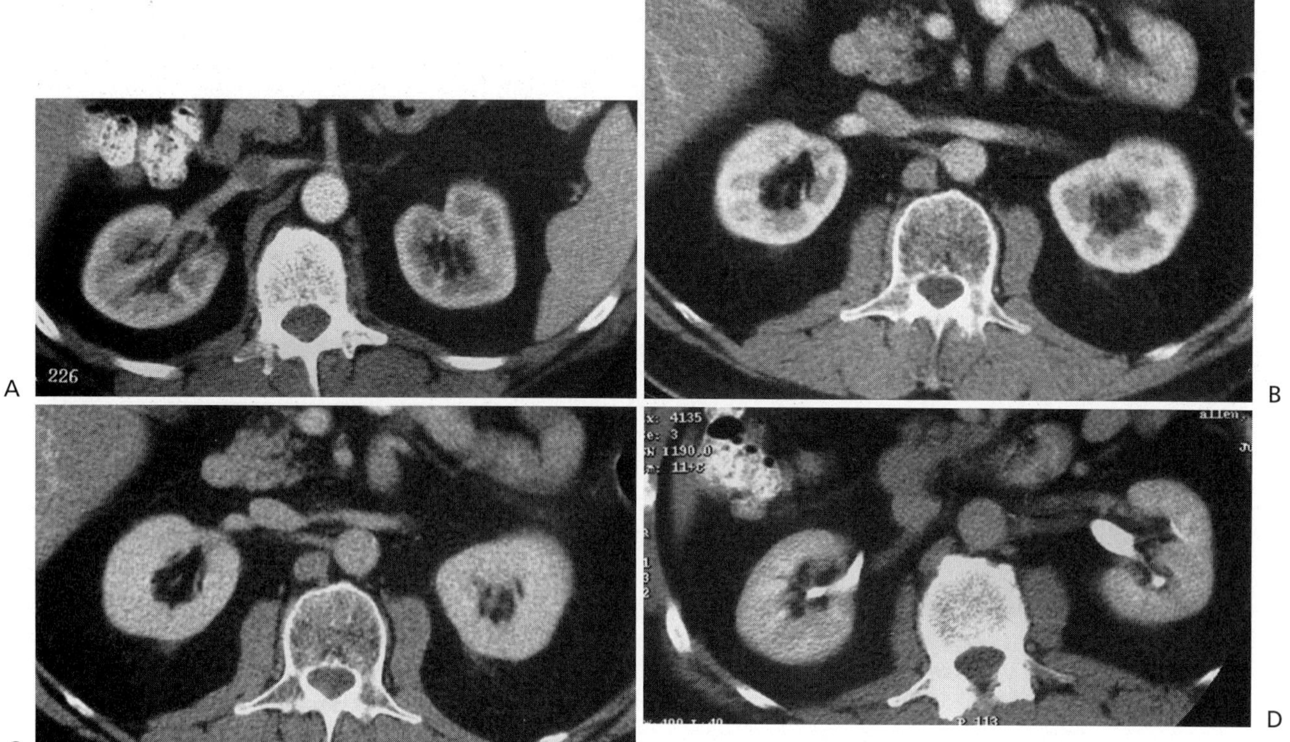

FIGURE 3C.1. Phases of renal contrast enhancement. In corticomedullary phase **(A, B)**, the renal cortex and medulla are very distinct. Note flow artifact in cava on **A** and course of renal vessels. In nephrographic and excretory phases **(C, D)**, the parenchymal enhancement is homogeneous, making it easier to detect renal masses.

contrast bolus (18,45,78,86,88). It has been shown that the timing of the NP is variable and depends on multiple factors, such as the patient's cardiac output and renal function and the dose and rate of injection of the contrast media. Therefore it may be helpful to use a bolus-tracking device such as Smart-Prep (GE Medical Systems, Milwaukee, Wisconsin), which triggers the onset of HCT at the completion of the CMP (7) and ensures true NP imaging. As stated, postcontrast series should use scanning parameters identical to those used during the initial unenhanced series. If the entire abdomen is to be imaged, it is possible to scan the remainder of the abdomen and pelvis between the CMP and NP images (86).

Vascular-phase imaging, or CTA, is recommended in patients who are undergoing preoperative planning for nephron-sparing surgery, repair of ureteropelvic junction obstruction, or donor nephrectomy (32). Specific techniques for CTA are considered in Chapter 3F. With the advent of MDCT, it is now possible to perform high-quality CTA of the renal arteries and aorta and high-resolution imaging of the kidneys for lesion detection in a single examination. In the past, renal lesions were often suboptimally evaluated during the CMP of enhancement obtained during CTA.

FIGURE 3C.2. Renal cyst obscured on corticomedullary phase (CMP) of enhancement. Image on right in nephrographic phase (NP) demonstrates a small cyst *(arrow)*, which is a much more subtle finding on the CMP image on the left.

Anatomic Considerations

The perinephric fat outlines the surface of the kidney; the renal capsule cannot be distinguished from the renal parenchyma. The fat in the renal sinus is of low attenuation and outlines the collecting system and the blood vessels, which course anteromedially. The perirenal fascia and the septa extending from the kidney to the anterior or posterior renal fascia are visible as linear soft tissue densities (48). The anterior renal fascia is usually seen on the left, less com-

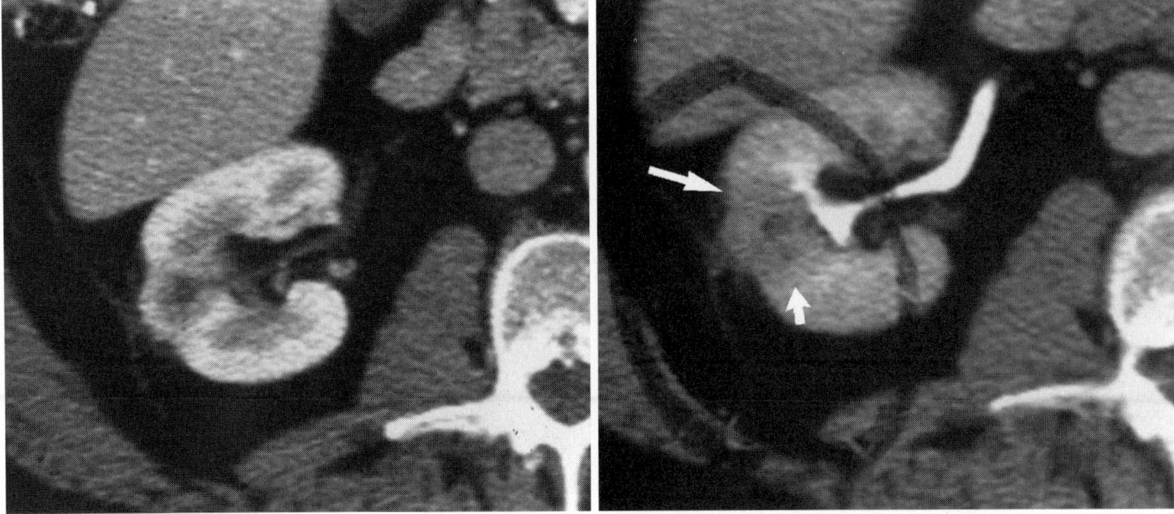

FIGURE 3C.3. Small renal cell carcinoma, poorly seen on corticomedullary phase (CMP) imaging. On CMP image **A,** there is an irregular bulge in the renal contour. The different enhancement of this lesion is much more obvious *(arrows)* on the excretory phase imaging **(B).** (Artifact on image circling area of interest).

monly on the right, and it separates the structures in the anterior pararenal space, such as the pancreas, retroperitoneal duodenum, and the ascending and descending colon, from the kidneys. The posterior renal fascia is commonly seen posterior to both kidneys.

The right adrenal gland is superior to the upper pole of the kidney, just dorsal to the inferior vena cava (IVC). The left adrenal gland is more anteriorly and medially located, with the splenic vein just anterior to it as a consistent landmark (30).

The renal parenchyma is of homogeneous soft tissue density on noncontrast images with attenuation values of 30 to 60 HU. The renal pelvis and proximal infundibula may be seen as water-density structures, particularly if the renal pelvis is extrarenal. The calyces are not identifiable without contrast excretion. After intravenous contrast administration, the renal vessels and cortex enhance brightly. In the first 60 seconds after contrast administration (the CMP), there is sharp distinction between the cortex and the medulla (Fig. 3C.1A and B), but the medulla also soon enhances brightly (the NP) (Fig. 3C.1C). On delayed images, dense urine is seen in the collecting system in patients with normal renal function (Fig. 3C.1D). The ureter courses anteroinferiorly over the psoas muscle.

The renal veins lie ventral to the arteries, with the longer left renal vein (Fig. 3C.1B) coursing between the aorta and the superior mesenteric artery to the IVC (which may be oval or slitlike at this level). The right renal vein is shorter and, with a more oblique course into the cava, and may not always be well imaged on CT scans. The right renal artery crosses behind the cava to enter the kidney (Fig. 3C.1B) while the left courses directly to the kidney (Fig. 3C.1C and D).

Normal Variants and Congenital Anomalies

Pseudotumors, named variously as the column of Bertin, dromedary hump, or hilar lip, may occur in the kidneys due to variations in the pattern of lobar fusion and may simulate renal masses on IVU and sonography. Compensatory hypertrophy due to focal scarring can also simulate a mass. All pseudotumors are isointense to the renal parenchyma on precontrast and postcontrast imaging and are readily distinguished from true renal masses.

Anomalies such as retroaortic renal vein; retrocaval ureter (Fig. 3C.5); circumaortic renal vein; and persistent, duplicated, or left-sided IVC can be recognized on CT, as can renal agenesis (Fig. 3C.6), malpositioned or ectopic kidneys,

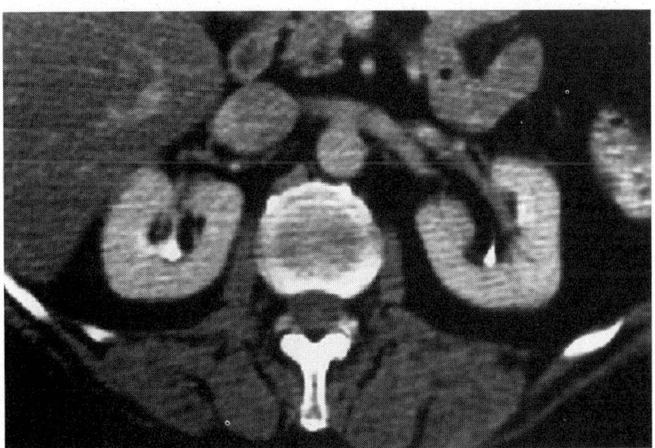

FIGURE 3C.4. Course of renal vessels. Note that the right renal artery courses behind the cava. The renal sinus fat surrounds the vessels.

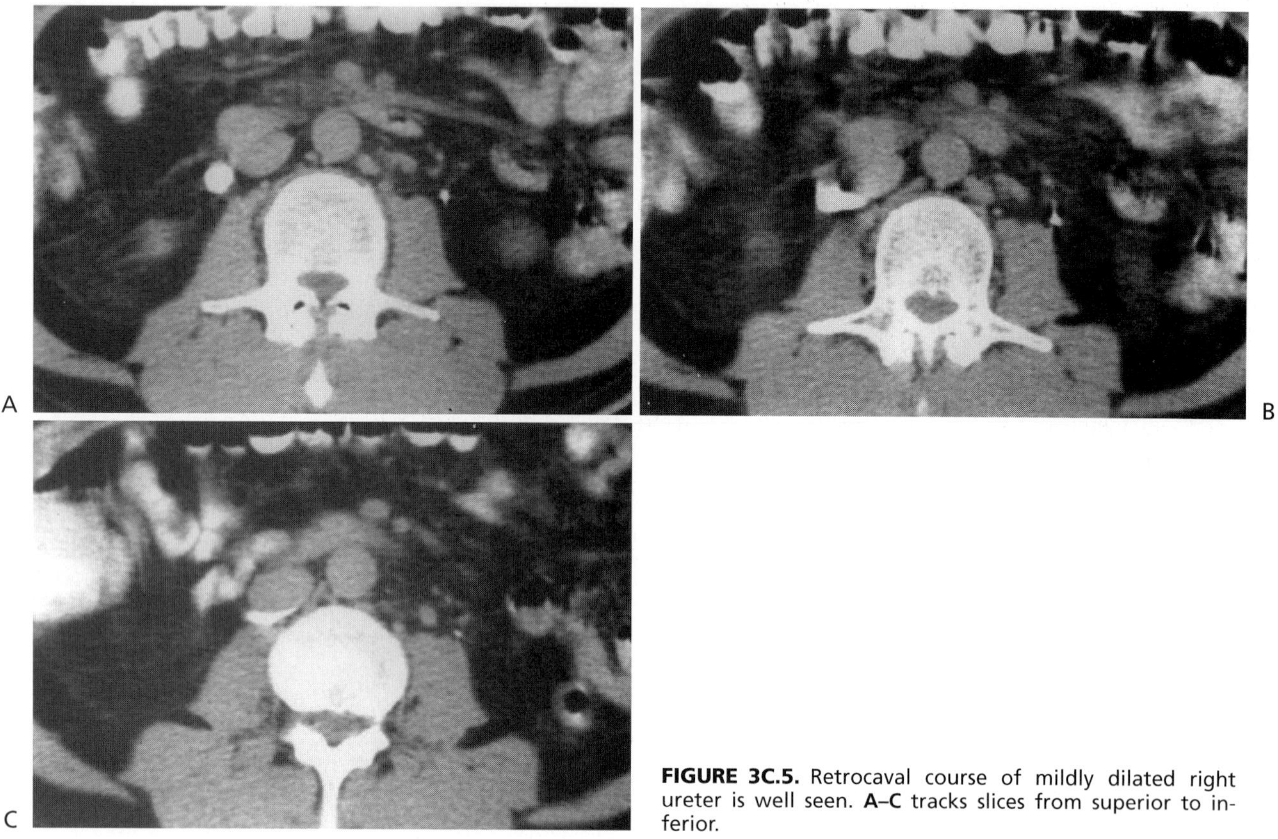

FIGURE 3C.5. Retrocaval course of mildly dilated right ureter is well seen. **A–C** tracks slices from superior to inferior.

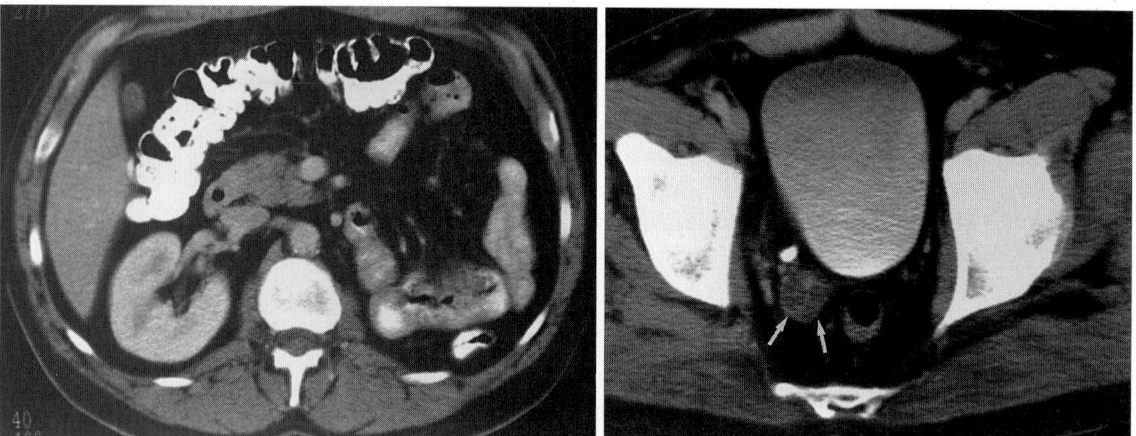

FIGURE 3C.6. A 30-year-old man with left renal agenesis and absent left seminal vesicle. There appears to be cystic change in the right seminal vesicle also *(arrows).*

and fusion anomalies such as horseshoe kidneys or cross-fused ectopy. With renal agenesis, it is imperative to look for genital anomalies as well (Fig. 3C.6). CT is very accurate at distinguishing true renal agenesis from atrophic, nonfunctioning kidneys. Ectopic ureteral insertions, whether associated with duplication anomalies or not, can also be demonstrated.

Renal Masses

Renal Cell Carcinoma

The burgeoning use of CT in modern-day clinical practice is making the incidental discovery of RCCs an increasingly familiar scenario. Such masses may be detected during a CT scan being performed for symptoms referable to organ systems other than the urinary tract or for the workup of vague signs and symptoms. In a Japanese survey (3), incidentally discovered renal cell cancers increased from 20 in 1980 to 338 in 1988. Increasingly, more RCCs are detected at a smaller size (less than 3 cm in diameter) (1,19); in one study, 25% of incidentally discovered cancers were found to be smaller than 3 cm as compared with only 5% in the pre-CT era (71) (Fig. 3C.7). Contrast-enhanced CT is more sensitive than either sonography or IVU in detecting renal masses smaller than 3 cm (94% versus 79% and 67%, respectively) (1,84).

CT is the recommended investigative modality when a renal mass is indeterminate in its characteristics on sonography, if a patient has a malignancy that metastasizes to the kidneys, or if there is a palpable flank mass. It is also the imaging modality of choice for evaluating a suspected renal mass and for staging a known neoplasm.

Imaging Features of Renal Cell Carcinoma

1. Distortion or bulge of the renal contour can occur. Because RCCs arise from the cortex, 95% of these lesions are exophytic (87) (Fig. 3C.8).

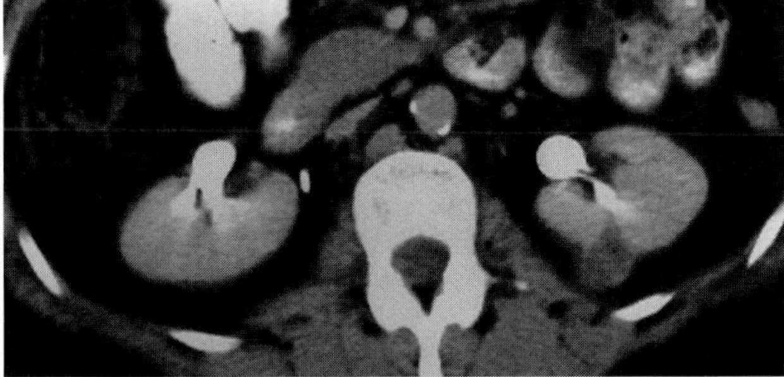

FIGURE 3C.7. Small left renal cell carcinoma discovered incidentally in a 42-year-old woman being evaluated for right abdominal pain. The mass is exophytic and enhances less than the normal renal parenchyma, expected findings with renal carcinoma.

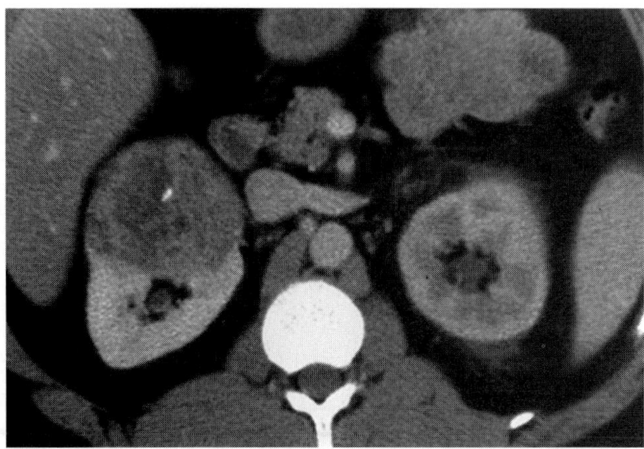

FIGURE 3C.8. Exophytic right renal cell carcinoma with a focus of calcification. On this contrast-enhanced scan, the mass is enhancing heterogeneously.

2. On unenhanced images, small lesions are homogeneous and isodense to the kidneys. Large masses vary from being nearly isodense to the kidneys (Fig. 3C.9) and slightly heterogeneous to being hypodense with necrotic areas (Fig. 3C.10A) or hyperdense due to hemorrhage (85). Calcification is seen in approximately 30% of cases when the tumors are larger than 3 cm (Figs. 3C.8, 3C.9, and 3C.10); smaller lesions are calcified about 3 % of the time (85,87).
3. After contrast administration, all RCCs enhance, but less so than the normal renal parenchyma. Most small tumors tend to have homogeneous enhancement, whereas larger tumors may show heterogeneity in enhancement (Figs. 3C.9 B and 3C.10B), particularly if there is central necrosis. Papillary RCCs tend to demonstrate central cystic or necrotic degeneration and calcification, and they enhance less than the non–papillary cell types.

Staging of Renal Cell Carcinoma

The classification schemes for staging RCC are not reiterated here.

Stage I disease (confined within renal capsule) is difficult to distinguish from stage II disease (extension into perinephric fat but contained within Gerota's fascia) by CT scanning. Thickening of the renal fascia and the bridging septa (Fig. 3C.9) is more often the result of vascular engorgement and enlargement and edema in the perinephric region than the result of tumor extension (35). This shortcoming of CT is not usually a clinically significant issue because both stage I and II tumors are surgically respectable.

CT has a sensitivity of greater than 95% for the detection of regional lymph node metastases to the renal hilum or retroperitoneum (stage III disease) (Fig. 3C.11). Nodes larger than 1 cm in short axis diameter are considered to be enlarged by CT criteria. Lymphadenopathy can be caused by metastatic disease or reactive hyperplasia; these condi-

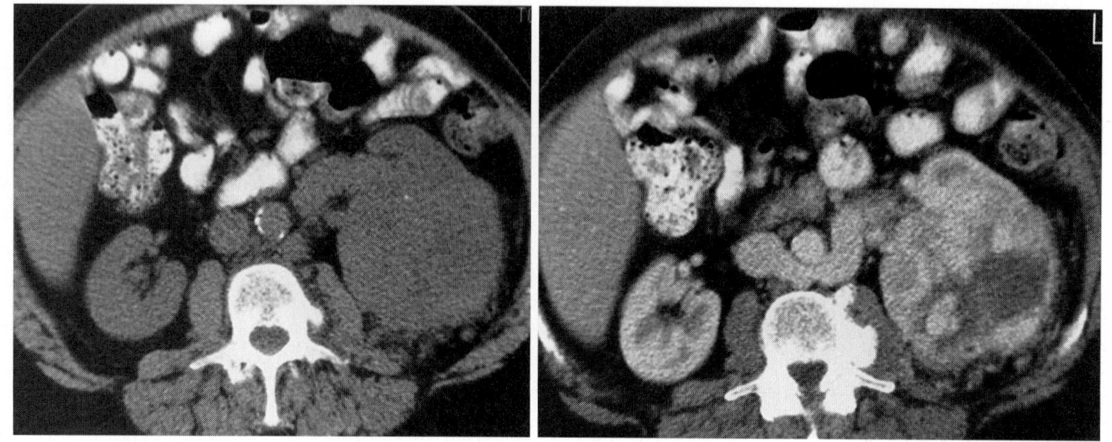

FIGURE 3C.9. Large left renal cell carcinoma. **A:** Unenhanced image demonstrates a small amount of calcification in the mass. **B:** Following contrast enhancement, there is irregular enhancement and a shaggy border to the mass, more likely due to perinephric collateral vessels than to perinephric extension. Note that the left renal vein is retroaortic.

tions are indistinguishable on CT imaging (76). Cystic necrosis may be seen in the nodes that are often hypervascular (Fig. 3C.11).

Tumor extension into the renal vein or IVC is well evaluated with contrast-enhanced CT (Fig. 3C.12), with reported sensitivity and specificity rates in the range of 80% and 96% (35,38). A good bolus of contrast within the vascular structures facilitates evaluation of the venous structures—the tumor thrombus is seen as a filling defect in the brightly enhanced blood within the vessel. It is important not to misdiagnose streaming artifact in the IVC (from unopacified blood returning from the lower extremities or the renal veins) as tumor thrombus (Fig. 3C.1A). Enlargement of the renal vein may suggest the presence of tumor thrombus but can also be related merely to increased flow from a hypervascular neoplasm. Tumor thrombus is easier to detect in the left renal vein than in the right renal vein.

Adrenal involvement, whether due to direct extension in large tumors or to contralateral hematogenous metastasis, is well evaluated with CT (29).

Direct tumor spread to contiguous organs is detectable on CT as loss of the expected tissue planes between the kidneys and the adjacent organs such as the liver, spleen, psoas muscle, or pancreas. However, imaging in the axial plane alone (as with routine CT scanning) has the disadvantage that volume averaging of oblique tissue interfaces makes it difficult to determine whether a renal lesion merely abuts an adjacent organ such as the liver or actually invades it (Fig. 3C.10B). In such cases, MRI is often useful for further evaluation because imaging can be performed in the appropriate plane to answer the question.

CT or MRI scanning of the abdomen combined with CT scanning of the chest is the current recommendation for assessment of distant metastatic disease in patients with RCC.

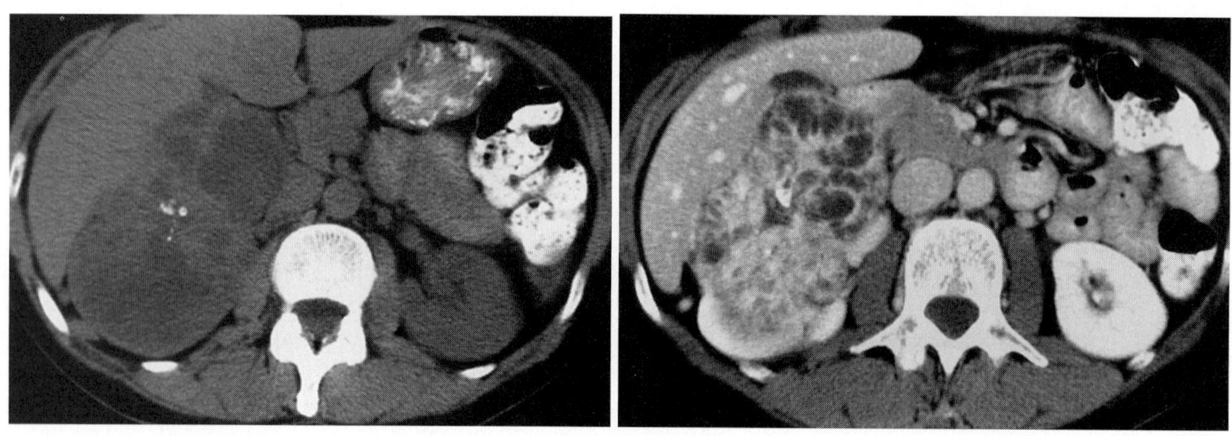

FIGURE 3C.10. Large, necrotic renal cell carcinoma. **A:** Unenhanced image shows calcification and low-attenuation areas in the mass, representing areas of cystic necrosis. **B:** There is avid, heterogeneous enhancement after contrast administration. The areas of cystic necrosis do not enhance.

Chest CT is highly sensitive for detecting metastatic disease, but its low specificity is a drawback because abnormalities related to granulomatous disease may be indistinguishable from metastatic disease (55). Radionuclide bone scanning is not recommended as a routine procedure and is indicated in patients with symptoms worrisome for metastatic disease.

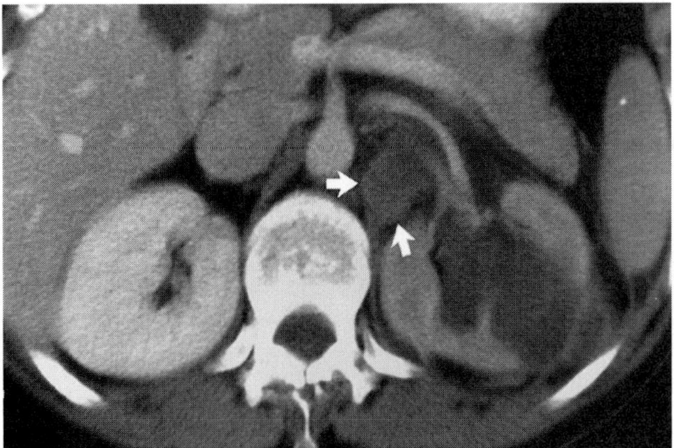

FIGURE 3C.11. Lymph node metastasis with left renal cell carcinoma. Contrast-enhanced scan shows nonenhancing areas of cystic necrosis with a large paraaortic node, which also appears to be necrotic *(arrows)*. There were multiple other enlarged nodes on other cuts (not shown). The renal vein is compressed by the nodal enlargement, which is likely the cause of the decreased nephrogram in the left kidney.

Because 5% of RCCs are bilateral, careful attention must be paid to the contralateral kidney in every case.

Accuracy of CT in Diagnosis of RCC

Contrast-enhanced CT scanning has an overall accuracy in the 95% range for the diagnosis of RCC, with the diagnosis of small renal masses proving the most difficult. False-positive diagnosis of RCC can be as high as 17% (67), even with contemporaneous imaging techniques. When a renal mass is indeterminate in nature on CT imaging, MRI can sometimes be helpful in demonstrating enhancement within the lesion, therefore better characterizing it. Alternatively, follow-up scans may demonstrate growth of the lesion. RCCs grow at a mean rate of 0.5 cm per year, a rate much faster than seen with benign lesions (6).

Postoperative Findings

Recurrence in the operative bed, liver, remaining kidney, adrenal glands, and the retroperitoneum can be assessed on follow-up CT examinations. The migration of normal structures into the operative bed, such as bowel, may simulate a recurrent tumor. Baseline scans are therefore of value in serial follow-up, particularly in patients who have undergone nephron-sparing surgery, so that the postoperative alterations in the appearance of the kidney are not misdiag-

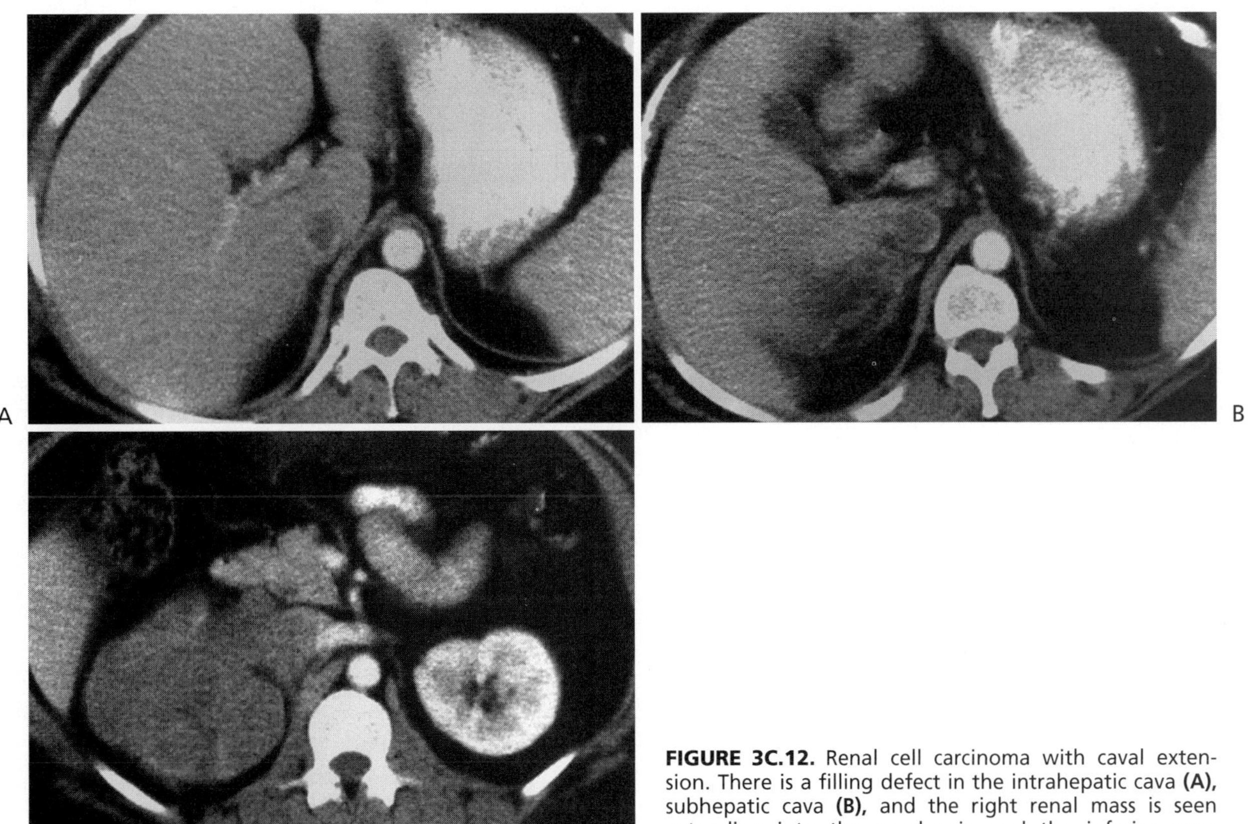

FIGURE 3C.12. Renal cell carcinoma with caval extension. There is a filling defect in the intrahepatic cava **(A)**, subhepatic cava **(B)**, and the right renal mass is seen extending into the renal vein and the inferior vena cava **(C)**.

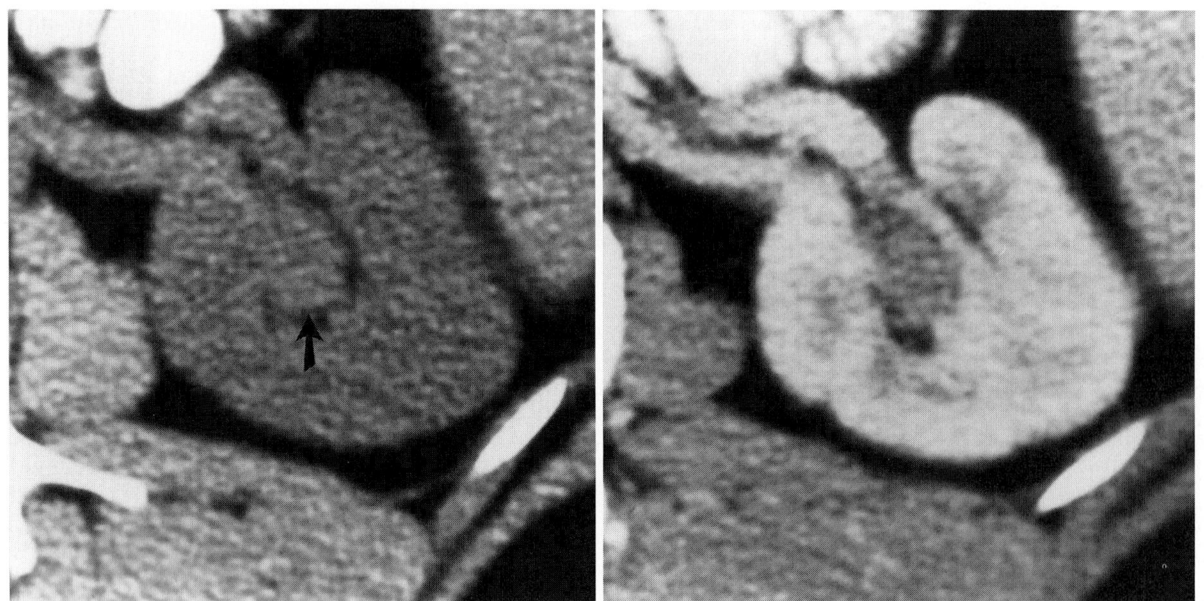

FIGURE 3C.13. Transitional cell carcinoma in the left renal pelvis. There is a soft tissue mass in the left renal sinus *(arrow)* on the unenhanced image **(A)**, which enhances slightly after contrast **(B)**. The sinus fat does not appear to be invaded.

nosed as tumor recurrence (39). Wedge-shaped or concave defects may be seen at the site of resection, and there may also be fat pads placed at the resection site.

Urothelial Tumors

Urothelial tumors are the second most common primary malignancies of the kidney, with transitional cell carcinoma (TCC) accounting for the vast majority (approximately 85% to 90%). Squamous cell carcinomas (SCCs) are the next most common, accounting for 6% to 7% of primary renal pelvic tumors. Other rarer urothelial tumors are not considered here.

CT Imaging Features of Urothelial Neoplasms (14,57,81,82)

Although most cases of TCC are diagnosed on IVU or retrograde pyelography, an occasional case may be picked up serendipitously on CT.

1. An intraluminal soft tissue mass in the pyelocalyceal system or ureter, which is isodense on precontrast images (31 to 48 HU), may be seen (57). TCC enhances less than the adjacent parenchyma after contrast administration (attenuation values of 43 to 82 HU) (Fig. 3C.13). In the EP, the mass may be outlined by the excreted contrast (Fig. 3C.14). With contemporaneous imaging techniques, TCC lesions larger than 1 cm can be visualized (81).
2. Stippled calcification may be seen on the surface of the mass.
3. Rather than a well-defined mass, there may be concentric or eccentric thickening of the wall of the renal pelvis or ureter. Early flat or plaquelike lesions that would not be identifiable on IVU can often be detected on CT.
4. There may be hydronephrosis proximal to the lesion in the collecting system. An obstructive lesion will cause alterations in the nephrogram, which may be delayed, dense, striated, or persistent (Fig. 3C.15).
5. The reniform shape of the kidney is maintained even with large TCCs that infiltrate the renal sinus and the renal parenchyma.
6. Venous involvement (renal vein or the IVC), lymph node involvement, or distant metastases may be seen with stage IV tumors.

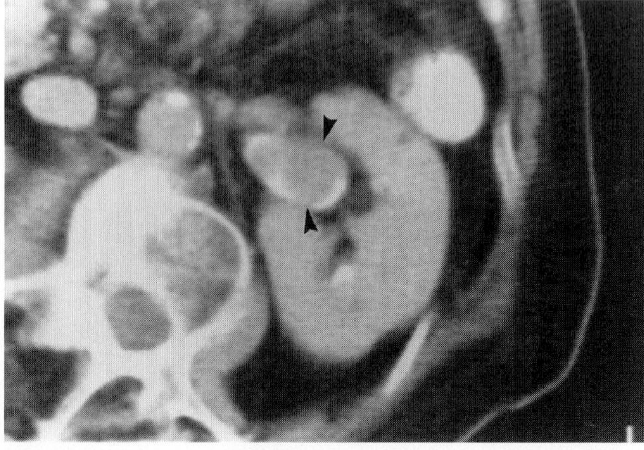

FIGURE 3C.14. Transitional cell carcinoma in the left renal pelvis is seen as a filling defect *(arrowheads)*.

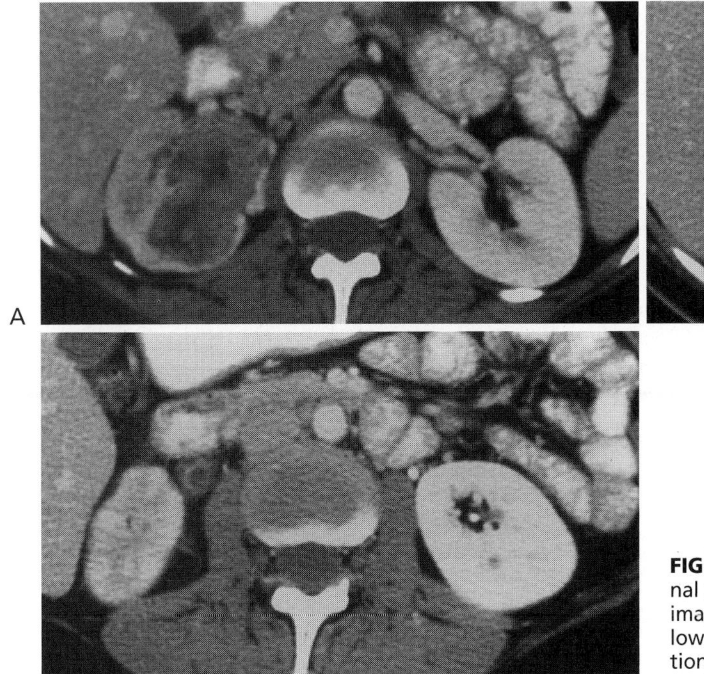

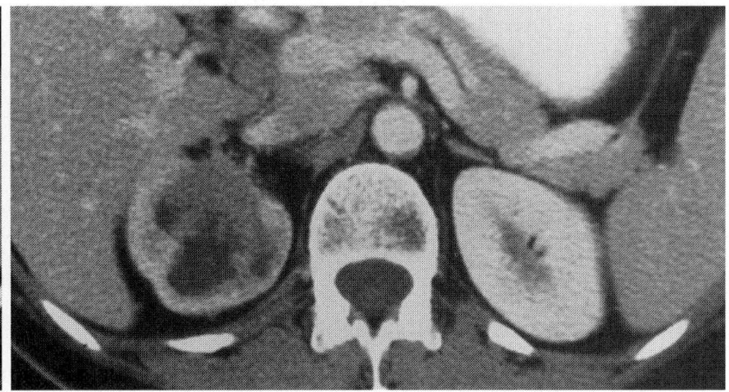

FIGURE 3C.15. Transitional cell carcinoma of the right renal pelvis, which is partially obstructing. Contrast-enhanced images demonstrate a mass in the right renal pelvis and lower pole collecting system **(A, B)**. Because of the obstruction, the right nephrogram is delayed compared with the left kidney **(C)**.

Utility of CT in Patient with TCC

CT is highly accurate in distinguishing stage III and IV disease from stage I and II disease because parenchymal invasion, tumor extension through the wall of the renal pelvis or ureter, lymphadenopathy, and other metastatic spread are well demonstrated. CT imaging can therefore be crucial in staging such patients if conservative management is being contemplated. Furthermore, in patients with high-grade obstruction in whom IVU is nondiagnostic, the level of obstruction can be demonstrated on CT and the obstructing ureteral lesion easily distinguished from obstruction due to a stone or other periureteral pathology (42).

The distinction between stage I disease (limited to mucosa) and stage II disease (invasion of muscle) is not possible with CT.

CT is extremely useful in the characterization of a radiolucent filling defect seen on urography and in distinguishing radiolucent calculus from a urothelial tumor or blood clots (57). On nonenhanced CT, all renal calculi have densities greater than 200 HU (as compared with mean density of 39 HU for TCC lesions), whereas blood clots are often denser than normal parenchyma (50 to 90 HU). Following administration of a bolus of contrast, TCC lesions show slight enhancement, but blood clots do not enhance.

Squamous Cell Carcinomas

SCCs are aggressive and tend to present late in their course, usually as an infiltrating renal mass rather than as an intraluminal or mucosal lesion. The kidney is usually enlarged and not functioning. Staghorn renal calculi are often associated, and in fact, calculi have been reported in 4 of 5 patients with renal SCC on CT. There may be infiltration of adjacent organs at presentation (56).

Angiomyolipoma

Angiomyolipomas (AMLs) are benign renal neoplasms that contain varying proportions of mature adipose tissue, smooth muscle, and blood vessels; one or two of these elements may predominate. The radiographic appearance can therefore range the spectrum from being nearly completely fatty to nearly all soft tissue (10,50,83). The detection of regions of fat within a lesion is confirmatory of the diagnosis of an AML; the density measurements in the fatty areas range from −10 to −50 HU. Calcification is usually not present, and if hemorrhage has occurred, it too will be evident (Figs. 3C.16, 3C.17, and 3C.18).

Most AMLs are asymptomatic and found incidentally on imaging. Lesions larger than 4 to 5 cm, being more prone to hemorrhage, may become clinically apparent because of hematuria or symptoms associated with perinephric or retroperitoneal hemorrhage. There may also be mass effect caused by displacement of adjacent organs. AMLs can increase in size over time, particularly lesions that are larger than 4 cm; thus follow-up is warranted for such lesions (74).

Typically, AML is a unilateral lesion in a middle-aged woman. Numerous bilateral AMLs should raise the suspi-

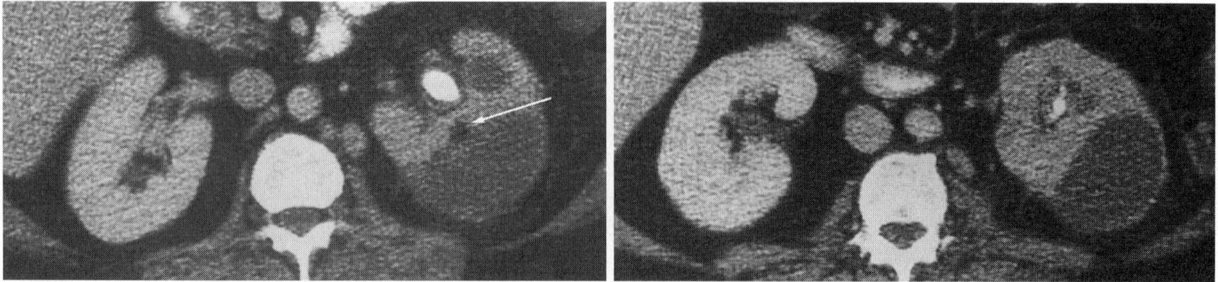

FIGURE 3C.16. Tiny angiomyolipoma *(arrow)* in the left kidney, which has caused a subcapsular hematoma. Note the compression of the renal contour. Patient also has a calculus in the renal pelvis.

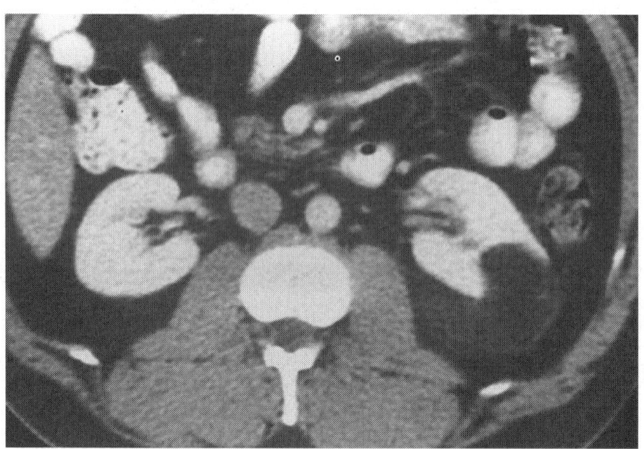

FIGURE 3C.17. Angiomyolipoma in the left kidney with a predominantly fatty composition. Note that the density of the lesion is similar to the retroperitoneal fat. Soft tissue strands are also seen within the mass, representing the other components.

cion of tuberous sclerosis (TS) because 80% of patients with TS have AMLs; 30% also have renal cysts. Sporadic occurrence of bilateral AMLs in patients without TS can also occur.

Fat within a renal mass is indicative of an AML. However, there are reports of RCCs that may appear to have fat within them because the tumor has engulfed renal sinus fat or undergone osteoid metaplasia with resultant fat and marrow deposition within the tumor (31).

Other Renal Tumors

Oncocytoma is an uncommon solid renal neoplasm with a distinctive histologic appearance. The CT features of this lesion are largely indistinguishable from those of an RCC (22).

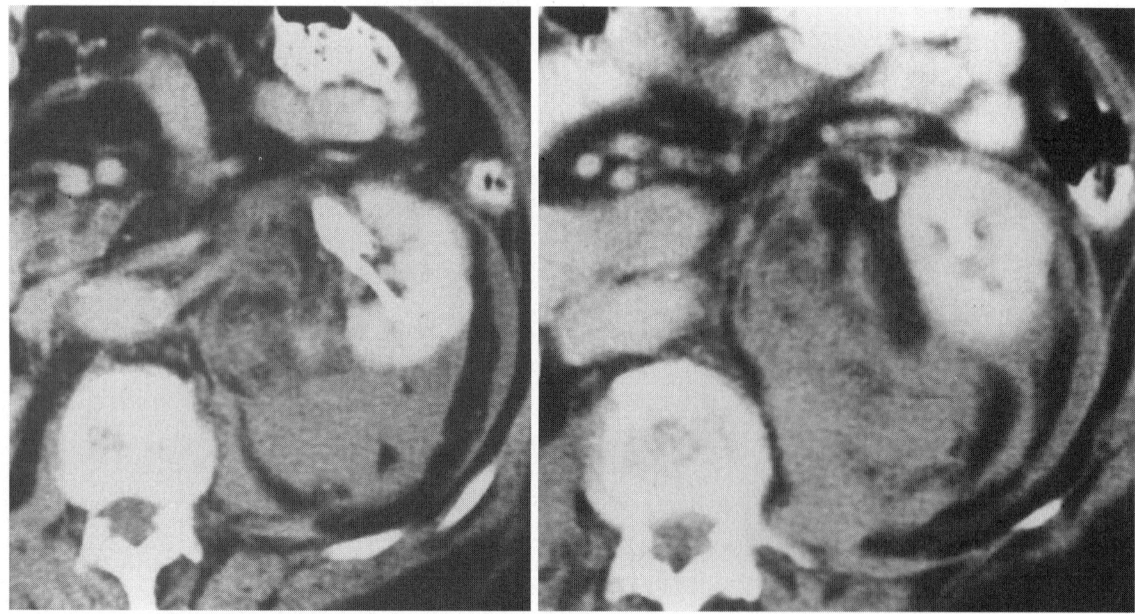

FIGURE 3C.18. Angiomyolipoma that has bled. Note the high-density blood that has accumulated in the perinephric space. Fat within the angiomyolipoma (AML) is also visible as dark patches. The kidney is displaced by the hemorrhage.

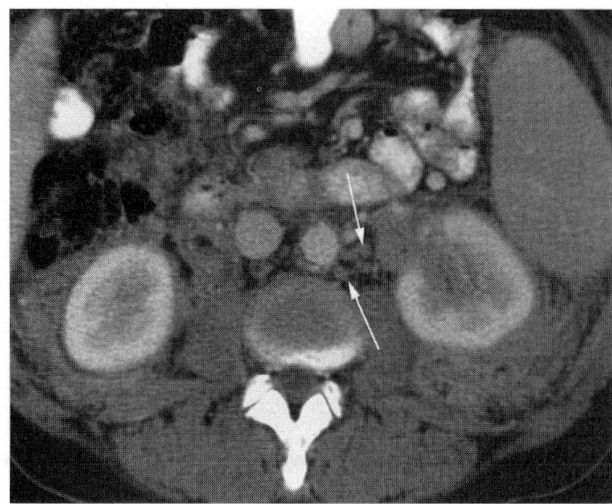

FIGURE 3C.19. Lymphoma presenting as a rind of soft tissue in the perinephric region bilaterally. There are also several small retroperitoneal lymph nodes *(arrows).*

Renal sarcomas are similar in radiographic appearance to RCCs. Leiomyosarcomas are the most common primary renal sarcoma, and they can arise from the renal capsule or the walls of renal veins or the IVC.

Lymphomatous involvement of the kidney is usually due to hematogenous or direct spread from an extrarenal source. Primary renal lymphoma is very rare because there is no lymphomatous tissue within the kidney. Non-Hodgkin's disease involves the kidneys far more frequently than Hodgkin's disease (92% versus 8%). The CT appearance is variable (65). There may be multiple discrete masses (31% cases), a solitary mass (23%), or tumor infiltration in the perirenal space (40%) (Fig. 3C.19).

Renal metastases are seen in association with metastatic disease elsewhere in a patient with a known primary malignancy. They are usually multiple and bilateral and are smaller than a 1 cm (33). An individual lesion may be indistinguishable from RCC, and percutaneous biopsy may be necessary to establish the diagnosis, if required.

Renal medullary carcinoma is a highly aggressive tumor that arises in the medulla near the renal papilla and then invades the parenchyma. It has been described in young patients, commonly but not exclusively African Americans, with sickle cell trait or hemoglobin SC disease. The central infiltrative pattern of tumor growth and extensive necrosis in a young patient should suggest the diagnosis. Mean survival from first symptoms to death is about 15 weeks (21).

Renal Cystic Masses

Simple Renal Cysts

Simple renal cysts are ubiquitous lesions that increase in number and size with age (20). Cysts should be of homogeneous water density (less than 20 HU) with thin or imperceptible walls, have a sharp interface with the renal parenchyma, and demonstrate no enhancement after contrast administration (Fig. 3C.20). No follow-up is necessary for lesions that meet these criteria.

Complicated Cysts

Cysts that are complicated by hemorrhage or infection will have an alteration in their imaging characteristics and may be confused with cystic renal neoplasms such as cystic RCCs or Wilms' tumor. The Bosniak classification system for renal cysts was devised to help categorize complicated renal cysts and predict the risk of malignancy (11). A *type I* lesion meets all of the aforementioned criteria for a simple cyst. A *type II* cyst (Figs. 3C.21, 3C.22, and 3C.23) is minimally complicated and demonstrates thin septations or minimal calcification on septa or the walls or is of high density (40 to 90 HU before contrast administration). These lesions have minimal risk for malignancy. *Type III* lesions may have one or more features suggestive of malignancy but no definite sign of malignancy. Such lesions exhibit thick or nodular walls or septations, thick or irregular calcification, and heterogeneous density but no enhancement of the walls or the septa in the lesion. Approximately 50% of these lesions will prove to be malignant, and surgical treatment or close follow-up is required for these lesions. *Type IV* lesions demonstrate unquestionable enhancement of a component of the lesion and are considered cystic tumors (Figs. 3C.24 and 3C.25).

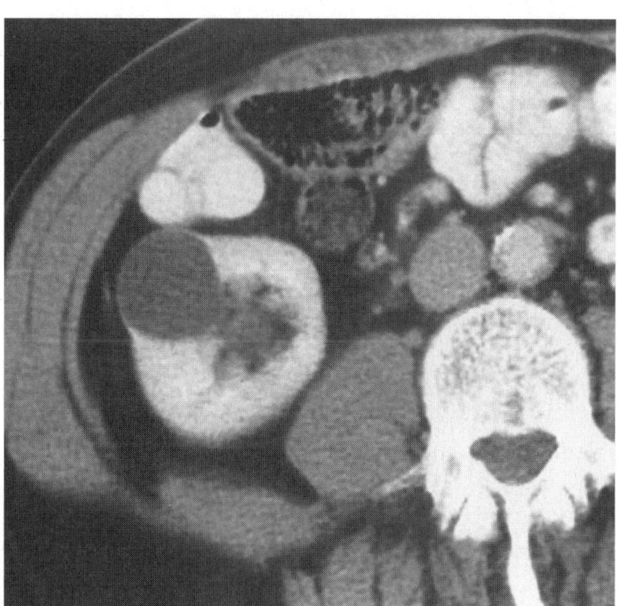

FIGURE 3C.20. Simple renal cyst. The walls are thin, and there is no enhancement within the lesion.

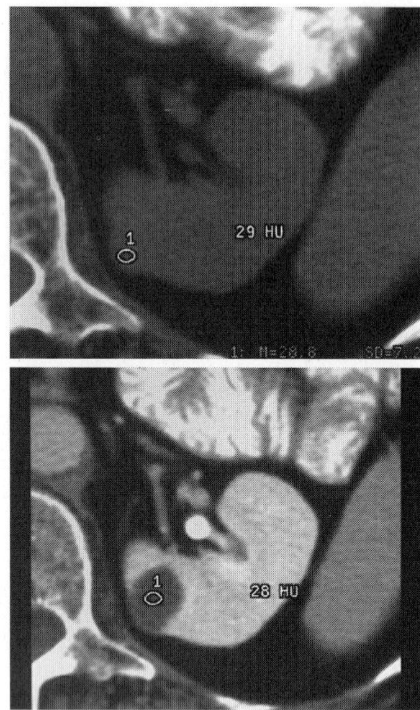

FIGURE 3C.21. High-density cyst. Bosniak II lesion. The lesion is of higher density (29 HU) than expected for a simple cyst (0 to 20 HU). However, there is no enhancement after contrast administration. The increased density is related to the presence of hemorrhage or proteinaceous material within the lesion.

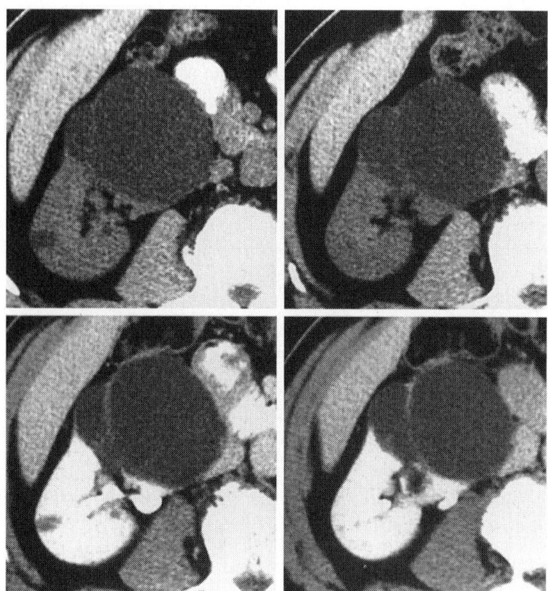

FIGURE 3C.22. Septated cyst. Bosniak II lesion. Nonenhaced images *(top row)* and enhanced images *(bottom row)* demonstrate thin septations within the cystic lesion.

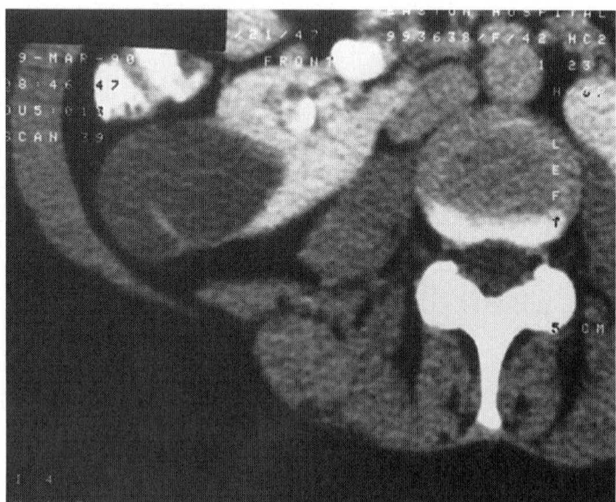

FIGURE 3C.23. Bosniak II cyst. Short thin septation in right renal cyst.

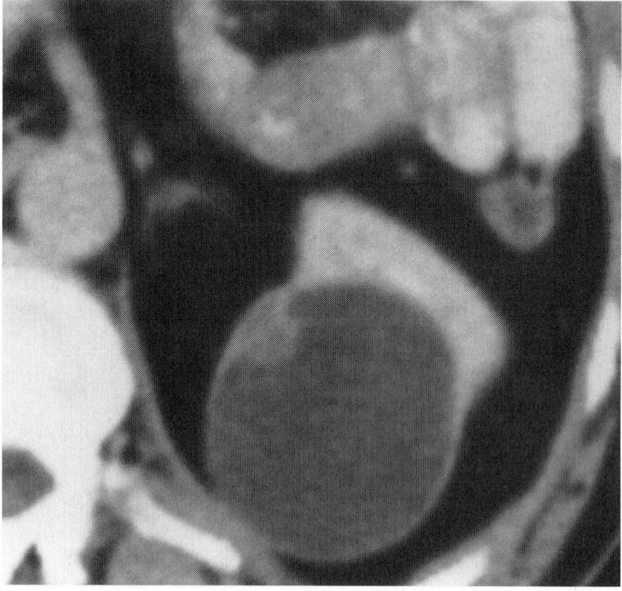

FIGURE 3C.24. Cystic renal cell carcinoma. Bosniak IV lesion. There is an enhancing nodule within the lesion that is predominantly cystic.

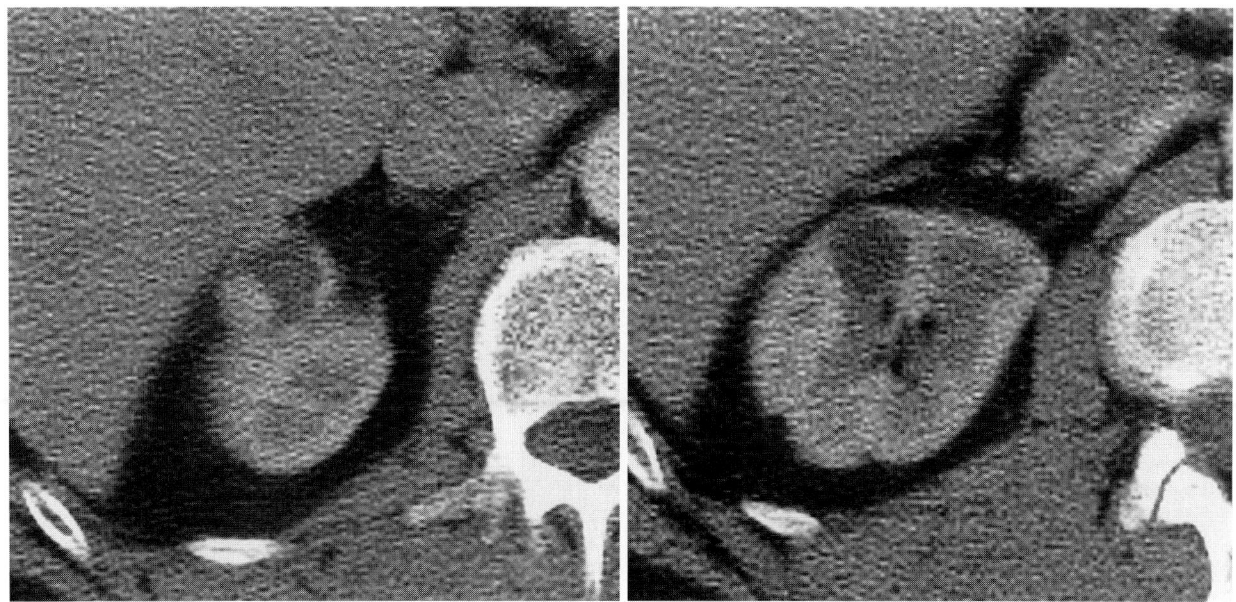

FIGURE 3C.25. Cystic renal cell carcinoma. Small right renal lesion has a thick irregular wall superiorly **(A)** and a relatively cystic appearance in its inferior aspect **(B).** However, nodular thickening in any portion of the lesion makes it a category IV lesion.

Multilocular Cystic Nephroma

A localized cystic disease of unknown etiology with no known hereditary pattern of inheritance, multilocular cystic nephroma (MCN) is a benign neoplasm. Multiple epithelial-lined cysts are separated by fibrous septa of varying thicknesses; a minority of lesions may have microscopic foci of nephroblastoma or sarcoma in the septa. The septations often enhance on contrast-enhanced CT, making it difficult to reliably exclude cystic RCC or Wilms' tumor, even when MCN is strongly suspected by imaging. Surgery is therefore indicated for these lesions (15).

Parapelvic Cysts

Parapelvic cysts occur in the renal sinus and may simulate hydronephrosis on noncontrast scans. Images in the EP of the CT scan will demonstrate mass effect on the collecting system.

Cystic Renal Diseases

Autosomal-dominant polycystic kidney disease (ADPKD) causes cyst formation in the kidneys, liver, pancreas, and spleen (Fig. 3C.26). The kidneys are often greatly enlarged, and multiple cysts of varying sizes are seen throughout the parenchyma. Cysts may show hemorrhage (and therefore be hyperdense) and calcification in the walls. Calculi are also common (51).

Multiple bilateral simple renal cysts in an individual patient may be difficult to differentiate from ADPKD. The absence of a family history, normal renal function, lack of cysts in other organs (e.g., the liver), and normal renal size favor the diagnosis of multiple simple cysts.

Acquired Cystic Kidney Disease

Patients with chronic renal failure, particularly those receiving chronic dialysis, can develop numerous cysts in the kidneys; 90% of patients may demonstrate renal cysts after 5 to 10 years of dialysis therapy (52). There is also an increased incidence of RCC, which is three to six times greater than the annual incidence of renal carcinoma in the general population (62). Early in the course, the kidneys are small in size but increase in volume with time. The appearance may be indistinguishable from ADPKD, but no cysts occur in organs other than the kidneys.

Syndromes Associated with Renal Cysts

Many syndromes are associated with renal cysts; such diseases are also referred to as *pluricystic kidney disease* (64) and are not discussed here.

Two syndromes in which renal cysts occur in association with neoplasms are of particular importance to urologists. *TS* is associated with AMLs in 40% to 80% of patients, and renal cysts are seen in approximately 15% of patients. There may also be a slight increased incidence of RCC (9,16).

von Hippel–Lindau disease is an autosomal-dominant hereditary disease associated with renal cysts and cancers, pancreatic cysts, pheochromocytomas, and retinal and cen-

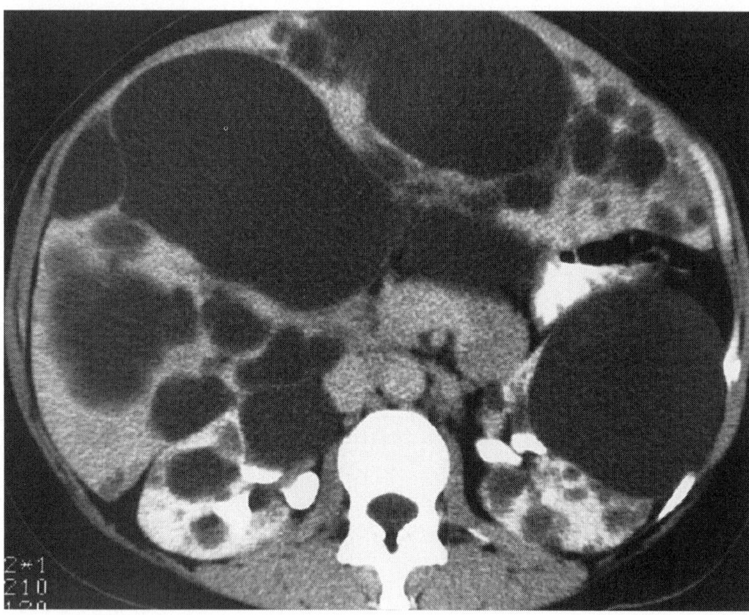

FIGURE 3C.26. Autosomal-dominant polycystic kidney disease. Innumerable large cysts in the kidneys and liver are pathognomonic of the disease.

tral nervous system hemangioblastomas (17). Approximately 60% of patients will have renal cysts, and 29% of patients develop clear cell renal carcinomas. As many as 600 microscopic tumorlets may be present in the parenchyma of each kidney.

Renal Inflammatory Processes

In patients with clinically suspected *acute pyelonephritis,* CT is used not for its diagnosis, but rather to detect complications when the clinical response to appropriate therapy is not satisfactory. CT is the best imaging method to delineate the extent of the renal inflammatory process and also evaluate for extrarenal extension of the disease (72,73).

The CT findings in acute pyelonephritis (40) are as follows: (a) The most common finding is the presence of one or more round or wedge-shaped areas of decreased attenuation, seen only on contrast-enhanced scans. These areas enhance less than the normal parenchyma (Fig. 3C.27). Delayed scans may show increased density in these same areas due to eventual filling of tubules that are obstructed by the surrounding edema (Figs. 3C.28 and 3C.29). This is likely the CT equivalent of a focal, delayed obstructive nephrogram. These zones of acute pyelonephritis have straight borders rather than rounded contours and extend from the renal collecting system to the capsule. (b) Striated bands of alternating low and high density may be seen within the wedge-shaped areas (striated nephrogram), representing slow flow of contrast-opacified urine through tubules that are obstructed by adjacent bands of interstitial edema. (c) Thickening of the renal fasciae and perinephric septa may occur as a result of edema. (d) Global or focal enlargement of the kidney may be seen. (e) Severe infections may lead to focal or global scarring and atrophy, detected on follow-up scans.

Emphysematous pyelonephritis (EPN) is a severe gas-forming infection in which gas is seen within the renal parenchyma itself. Identification of this entity requires aggressive treatment. Emphysematous pyelitis, on the other hand, is a gas-forming infection limited to the collecting system; it does not portend the same grave prognosis as does EPN.

The most common abnormality in *renal abscess* is an area of low attenuation on noncontrast images, which represents the liquefied center of the abscess cavity. Following contrast administration, a thick and irregular rind of enhancement

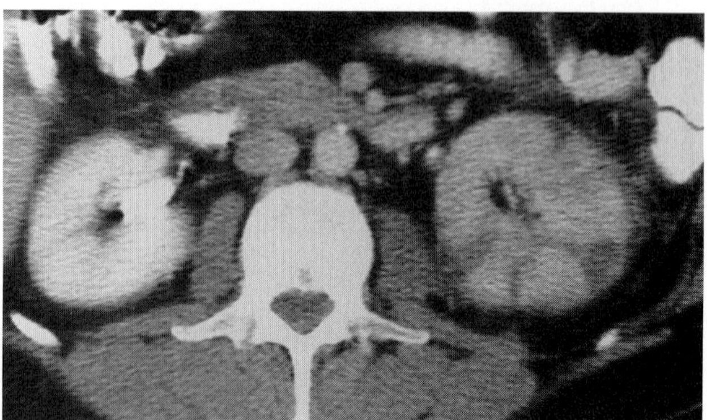

FIGURE 3C.27. Acute pyelonephritis of left kidney. Contrast-enhanced computed tomography scan. Note perinephric fascial thickening due to edema and wedge-shaped defects in the parenchyma that extend from the collecting system to the capsule. The nephrogram is delayed overall compared with the right kidney.

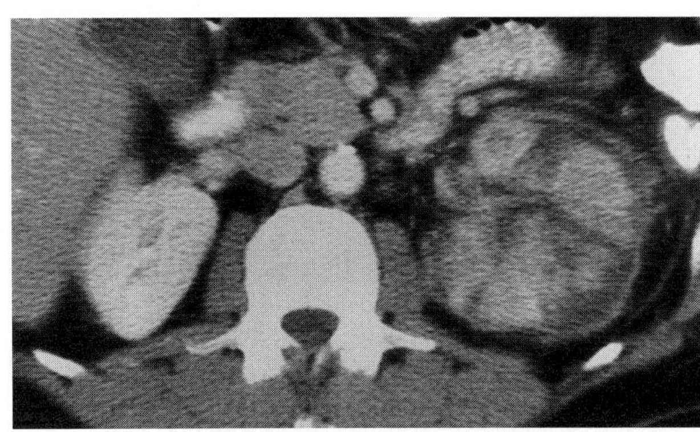

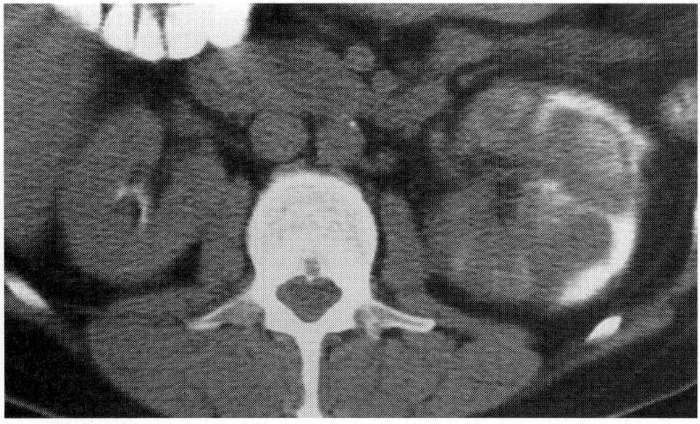

FIGURE 3C.28. Acute pyelonephritis. Contrast-enhanced scans. **A:** Early images demonstrate wedge-shaped filling defects in the parenchyma. **B:** Delayed images demonstrate a striated nephrogram with persistent opacification of some regions, likely obstructed tubules.

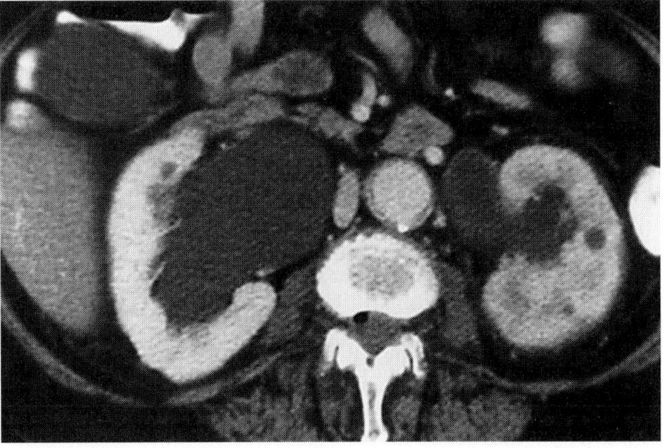

FIGURE 3C.29. Acute pyelonephritis of the left kidney in a patient with bilateral hydronephrosis due to bladder outlet obstruction. Note the patchy and irregular nephrogram in the left kidney. This appearance cannot be separated radiographically from changes due to acute obstruction. There is also a small cyst in the left kidney.

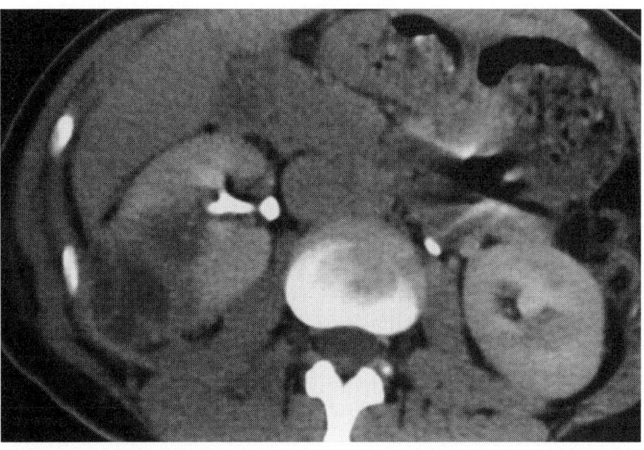

FIGURE 3C.30. Renal abscess. Irregular abscess cavities in the right kidney. Patient has right renal calculi (not shown). Note the asymmetric right perinephric fascial thickening.

is seen surrounding the abscess cavity (Fig. 3C.30). The remainder of the kidney may range from being normal in appearance to showing signs of acute pyelonephritis (72).

Xanthogranulomatous pyelonephritis is an uncommon chronic infection associated with calculi and obstruction. The kidney is enlarged, and calculi, often staghorn, are present. The kidney is usually nonfunctioning. Perinephric extension is seen in 14% of patients, and fistulae may also occur (77).

Renal Trauma

CT is very accurate in the categorization of renal injuries, and it is the imaging modality of choice when significant renal injuries are suspected (25,61). Both oral and intravenous contrast should be used in such patients; delayed imaging is often required to detect contrast extravasation (Fig. 3C.31), which indicates laceration of the collecting system.

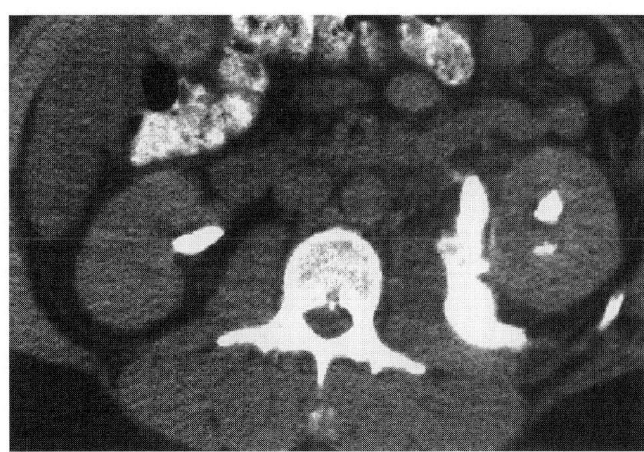

FIGURE 3C.31. Contrast extravasation in a patient who sustained blunt trauma. Delayed images demonstrate contrast tracking along the left perinephric space. The patient had extravasation from the collecting system in the left kidney (not shown).

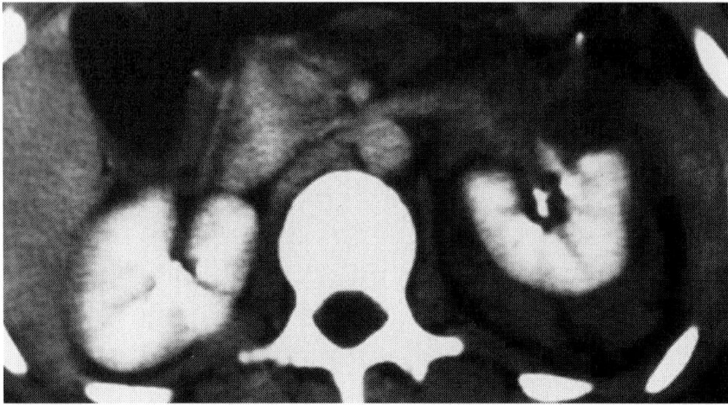

FIGURE 3C.32. Renal laceration. Note laceration in the right kidney. Both kidneys are functioning well. There is a perinephric hematoma on the left side (appears dark due to the contrast setting on the scan).

The grading system of renal injuries by the American Association for the Surgery of Trauma (AAST) cannot be addressed here. However, there is a close relationship between the grading system and CT abnormalities seen in this setting.

Renal contusion (grade I lesion) causes decreased enhancement of a focal area; it may be slightly hyperdense on nonenhanced scans because of hemorrhage. Grade II and III lesions are cortical lacerations that do not extend into the collecting system and are seen as defects in the parenchyma (Fig. 3C.32). Deep corticomedullary lacerations (grade IV injuries) extend into the collecting system and result in extravasation of contrast from the collecting system. Renal fractures, a shattered kidney (grade V injuries) (Fig. 3C.33), and renal vascular injury are also well depicted by CT.

Subcapsular hematomas are typically lenticular in shape and compress the adjacent kidney, whereas perinephric hematomas may displace the kidney. These may accompany any of the injuries described previously.

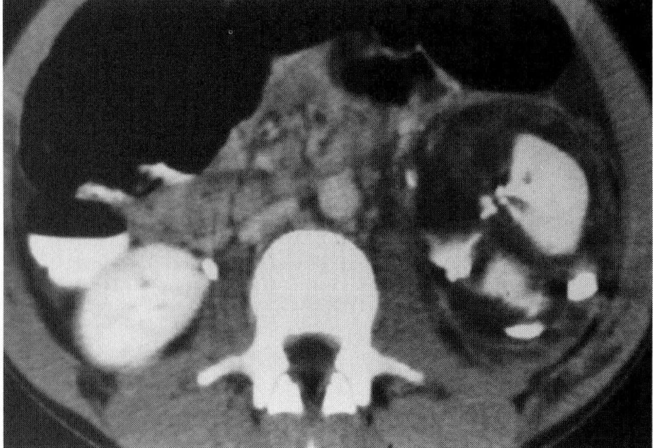

FIGURE 3C.33. Renal fractures and left perinephric hematoma. Delayed images also demonstrated contrast extravasation (not shown).

COMPUTED TOMOGRAPHY IN CALCULUS DISEASE OF THE URINARY TRACT

CT is more sensitive than abdominal radiography or nephrotomography in detecting calculi and calcifications (58,59). Spiral CT was more accurate than radiography and nephrotomography in both detecting and measuring renal calculi in a phantom *in vitro* (58). In another series (59), no residual stones were missed on noncontrast CT after percutaneous nephrostolithotomy, whereas plain film radiography detected only 46% of residual calculi.

Stones within the collecting system are obscured by excreted contrast within the collecting system; therefore, as with IVU, it is imperative that scans be obtained before the administration of contrast for accurate detection of calculi. All kidney stones are homogeneously dense on CT, except for the rare pure matrix stone and calculi that occur in patients infected with HIV who are being treated with protease inhibitors (13). Stones of different compositions have considerable overlap in their CT attenuation values, making prediction of the chemical type problematic by CT densitometry. Nonopaque/poorly opaque calculi such as uric acid and cystine stones have CT numbers in the range of 300 to 500 HU, whereas calcium stones are in the range of 500 to −1,000 HU.

When a filling defect is seen on an IVU or retrograde pyelogram, CT is valuable in differentiating nonopaque stones from blood clots or neoplasms because calculi are of so much higher density. CT is also useful in the preprocedural evaluation of patients with stones and congenital anomalies of the kidney or the bony structures, which make percutaneous procedure technically more complex.

HCT has proved to be particularly advantageous in the evaluation of the patient with acute renal colic and suspected ureteral calculi; it is replacing excretory urography for this indication (26,68,70). The advantages of CT are manifold: (a) No prescan preparation is necessary, unlike for an IVU; (b) the entire urinary tract from the kidney to the bladder can be imaged in a single breath hold, in less than a minute; (c) the location and size of a stone in the ureter can be accurately delineated; (d) no intravenous contrast material administration is necessary; (e) more anatomic information about the kidney and ureter can be obtained than from ultrasound; and (f) other intraabdominal processes that may be mistaken clinically for renal colic can be diagnosed (e.g., appendicitis, diverticulitis, bleeding aortic aneurysm, adnexal masses).

CT imaging for the evaluation of acute renal colic is performed without the administration of intravenous or oral contrast media because both may obscure a stone. However, this protocol should be altered and oral contrast media administered if there is any suspicion of bowel pathology. Intravenous contrast may become necessary if it is unclear whether a calcification lies within or adjacent to the ureter. Oral and intravenous contrast are also occasionally helpful in confirming that acute ureteral obstruction is the cause of flank pain and in excluding other causes of flank pain. In as many as one-third of patients evaluated by CT for acute flank pain, significant abnormalities outside the urinary tract may be detected (47,69).

Ureteral calculi causing acute renal colic demonstrate the following findings: (a) stone within the ureter and (b) hydroureteronephrosis and asymmetric perinephric stranding (Fig. 3C.34). These two signs together have a positive predictive value of 97%, and the absence of these signs has a negative predictive value of 93%. Overall, for the detection of ureteral calculi in the setting of acute flank pain, HCT has accuracy and positive and negative predictive values of 98% (69,70). The main difficulty in identifying ureteral calculi is the confusion created by phleboliths (Fig. 3C.35). Stones that are larger than 6 mm, located in the proximal third of the ureter, or not associated with perinephric stranding are less likely to pass spontaneously (27,80) (Fig. 3C.36).

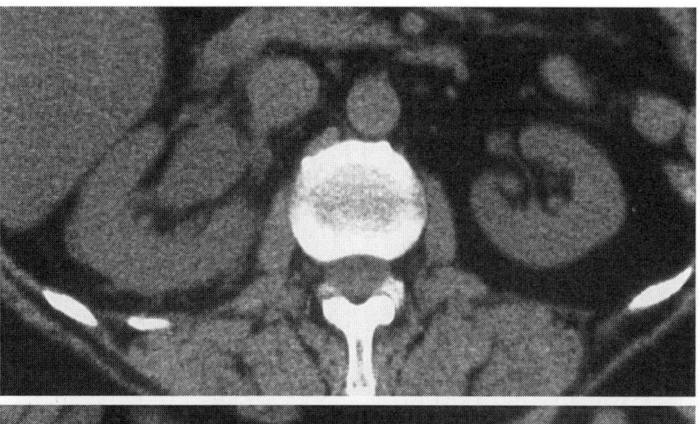

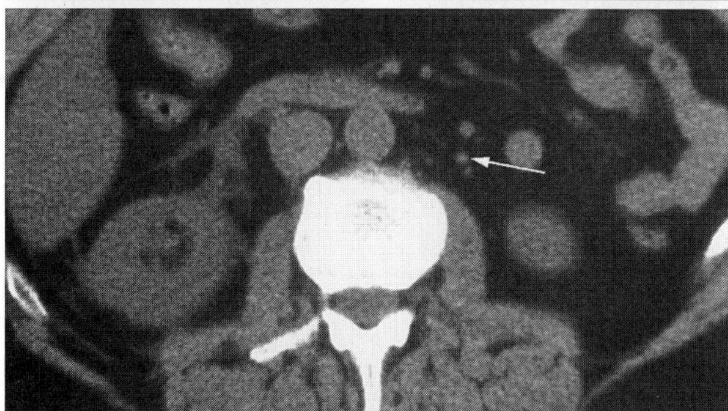

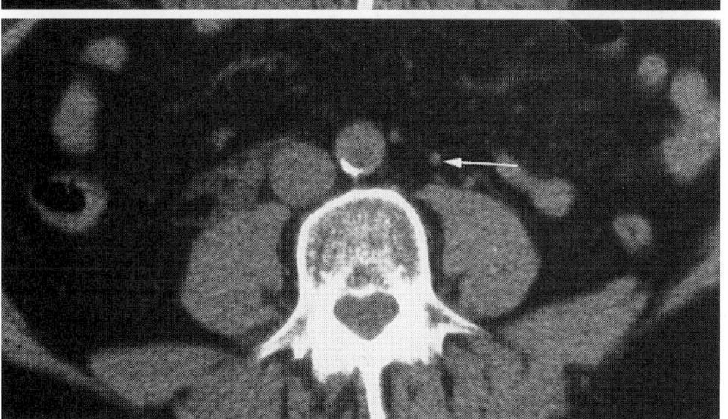

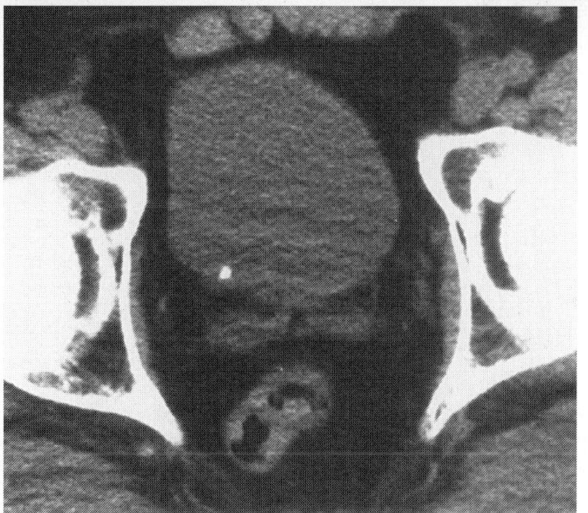

FIGURE 3C.34. Right renal colic due to a calculus at the right ureterovesical (U-V) junction. Note stranding in the perinephric **(A)** and periureteral **(B, C)** regions, right hydroureteronephrosis and stone at right U-V junction **(D)**. Left ureter, long arrow **(B, C)**.

COMPUTED TOMOGRAPHY OF THE ADRENALS

The normal adrenal glands and most masses can be identified on nonenhanced scans (Fig. 3C.37). Intravenous contrast administration is often helpful in characterizing adrenal masses, and the routine use of oral contrast prevents unopacified bowel loops from being mistaken for adrenal masses. Other structures that may be confused as being adrenal masses are vascular structures such as dilated or tortuous splenic arteries, splenic veins, or a dilated inferior phrenic vein.

Adenomas

Both nonhyperfunctioning (nonfunctional) and hyperfunctioning adenomas are morphologically similar in appearance (Fig. 3C.38). Therefore imaging findings have to be correlated with clinical findings and biochemical evidence. CT has approximately 85% sensitivity in detecting adrenal adenomas; tumors that are missed are usually smaller than 1 cm. A focal bulge or enlargement of the gland is indicative of the presence of a mass. Adenomas are rounded, homogeneous, soft tissue masses with well-defined margins, and they have densities that range from 0 to 20 HU on nonenhanced scans. If there is abundant fat within the lesion, the density measurements will be close to that of water (0 HU). On enhanced scans, adenomas have a density between 30 and 37 HU at 30 to 60 minutes after contrast injection (46,79), whereas nonadenomas measure greater than 41 HU.

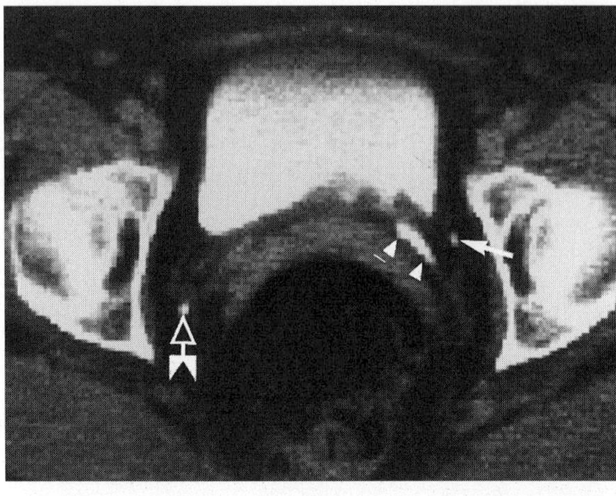

FIGURE 3C.35. Contrast-enhanced scan demonstrates the opacified left ureter *(arrowheads)* and an adjacent phlebolith *(long arrow)*. Broken arrow, right ureter.

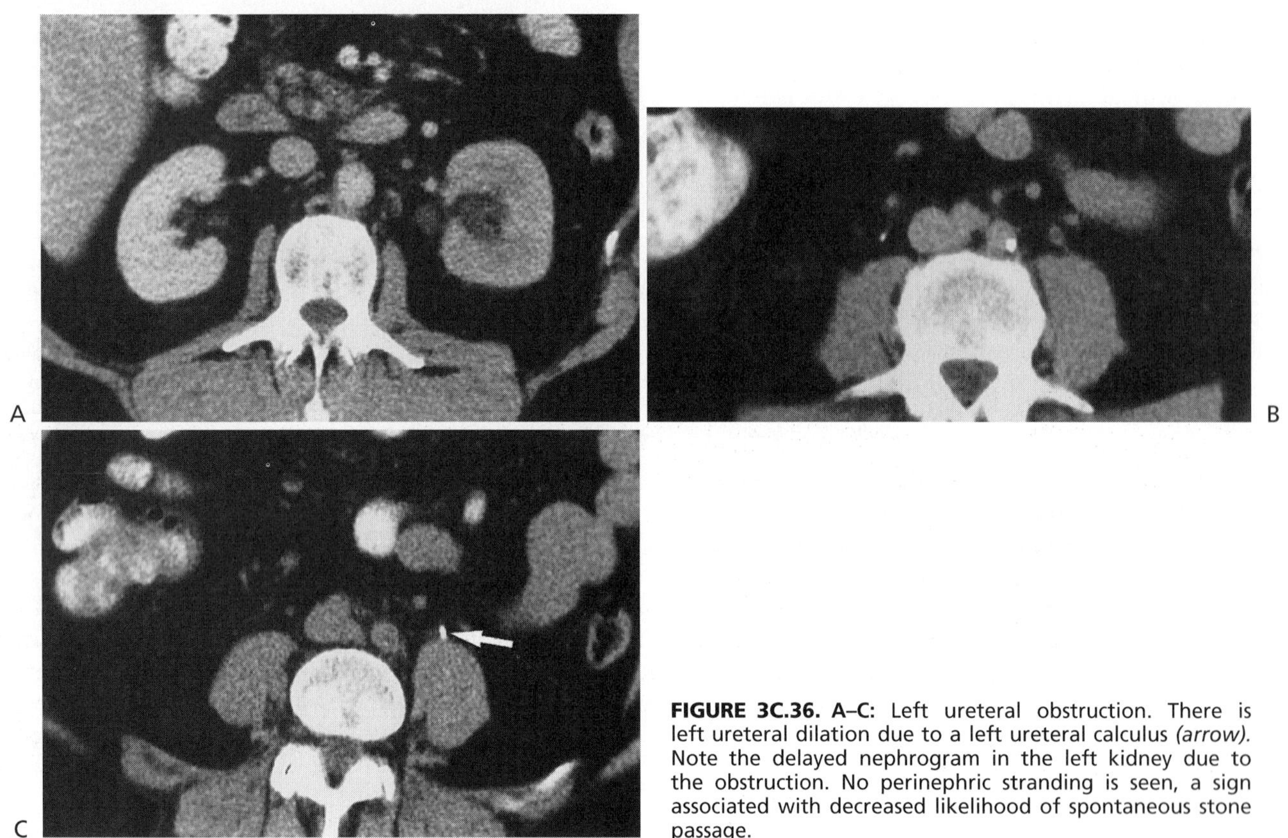

FIGURE 3C.36. **A–C:** Left ureteral obstruction. There is left ureteral dilation due to a left ureteral calculus *(arrow)*. Note the delayed nephrogram in the left kidney due to the obstruction. No perinephric stranding is seen, a sign associated with decreased likelihood of spontaneous stone passage.

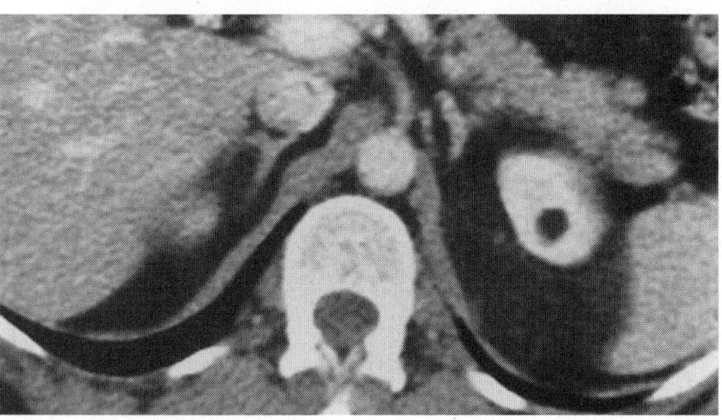

FIGURE 3C.37. Normal right and left adrenal glands. Upper pole of right kidney is immediately posterior to the right adrenal. There is a small cyst in the upper pole of the left kidney.

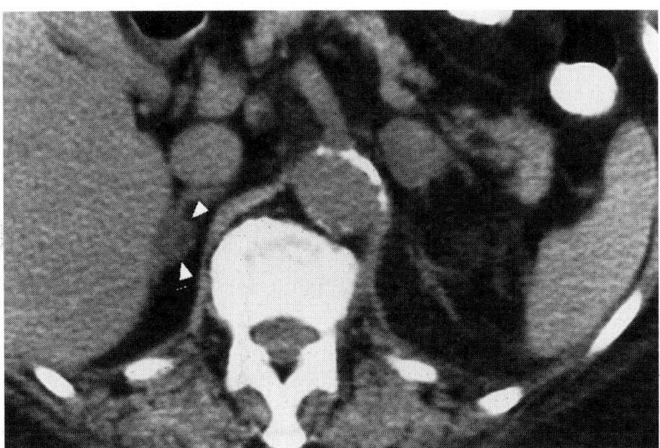

FIGURE 3C.38. Adenoma arising from the inferior aspect of the lateral limb of the right adrenal gland *(arrowheads)*.

Adrenal Hyperplasia

In adrenal hyperplasia, there is symmetric enlargement of the adrenal glands but retention of the normal shape. However, there is overlap in the CT appearance of normal and hyperplastic glands in that many patients with clinical evidence of hyperplasia may have normal-appearing adrenal glands. Bilateral enlargement is indicative of hyperplasia.

Adrenal Carcinomas

Adrenal carcinomas tend to be large, undergo central necrosis, and invade adjacent organs. If the mass is very large, the organ of origin may be difficult to determine, particularly if the adjacent organs are invaded and the normal adrenal gland is obliterated by the tumor. An adrenal carcinoma may be difficult to distinguish from a renal adenocarcinoma on CT. Calcification is seen in one-third of cases (28); venous extension, liver metastases, and lymphadenopathy may also be seen.

Incidental Adrenal Mass

Most incidentally discovered adrenal masses are benign. However, an adrenal mass in a patient with a known primary mass raises the question of adrenal metastases. If the mass is of low density, as described earlier, it is most likely is a benign adenoma. In one series, mean attenuation values were 2.2 HU for adenomas and 29.8 HU for metastases (49). If the threshold for nonenhanced CT density is set at 10 HU, the sensitivity-to-specificity ratio for diagnosis of an adenoma is 74%:96%. If the adenoma is lipid poor, the density will be higher and it may be difficult to distinguish it from a metastasis by CT. MRI may be warranted in such a case for further characterization.

Pheochromocytoma

Pheochromocytomas are hypervascular neoplasms with a tendency for hemorrhagic necrosis, even when benign. Heterogeneous enhancement of the mass is seen with contrast, an appearance that may be indistinguishable from that of an adrenal carcinoma. Thus correlation with biochemical tests is crucial for the diagnosis. Approximately 90% of pheochromocytomas arise from the adrenal glands, whereas 10% are extraadrenal.

If the patient has known hypertensive episodes, adequate pharmacologic adrenergic blockade should be in place before contrast administration so that a hypertensive crisis is not precipitated (intravenous injection of contrast can raise plasma catecholamine levels) (23,63).

Myelolipoma

Myelolipoma is a benign, nonfunctioning neoplasm of the adrenal gland containing variable amounts of fat and myeloid elements. Calcification may also be seen in the lesion (Fig. 3C.39). Large lesions may hemorrhage, although this is uncommon. The presence of foci of fat within an adrenal lesion is diagnostic of a myelolipoma (43).

Retroperitoneum

Lymphadenopathy

With CT, size alone is used to diagnose abnormalities in lymph nodes because intranodal architecture is not depicted on CT. Retroperitoneal and pelvic lymph nodes that are greater than 10 mm in short axis diameter are considered abnormal, although multiple smaller (6 to 8 mm) nodes are also cause for suspicion. Massively enlarged retrocaval and retroaortic nodes can displace these vascular structures.

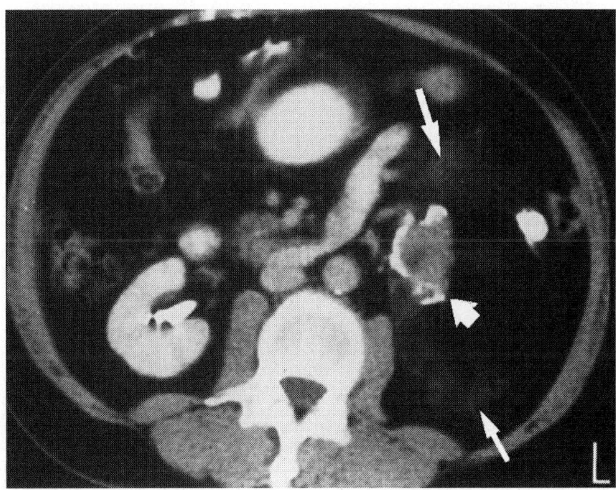

FIGURE 3C.39. Large left adrenal myelolipoma. The entire adrenal gland is replaced with low-density fatty tissue *(long arrows)*. Note the large calcification within the lesion *(short arrow)*.

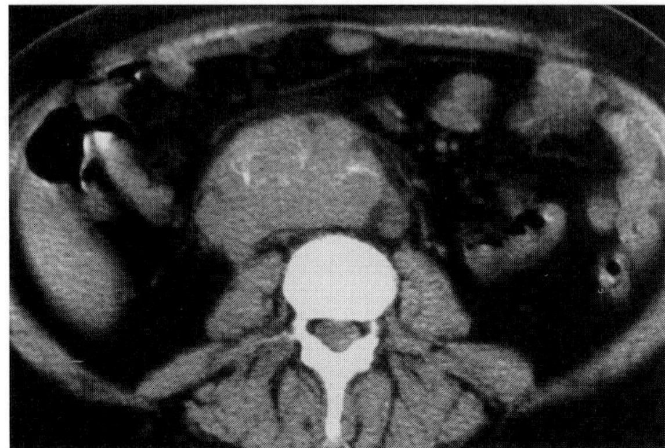

FIGURE 3C.40. Retroperitoneal lymphadenopathy in a patient with testicular cancer. There is a small amount of calcification in the nodes, likely the result of therapy. The vascular structures are not identifiable on this unenhanced scan.

CT is the preferred imaging method for staging patients with testicular neoplasms (Fig. 3C.40). Residual retroperitoneal masses that remain visible on CT scans after treatment can represent posttreatment fibrosis or teratoma, but they cannot be reliably differentiated from residual viable tumor (75).

Primary Retroperitoneal Tumors

Retroperitoneal tumors are well depicted on CT, and their effect on the urinary tract is also elegantly demonstrated. Most solid retroperitoneal tumors are of soft tissue attenuation and cannot be distinguished on CT.

Retroperitoneal Fibrosis

Fibrous tissue proliferation around the aorta and the IVC is the hallmark of retroperitoneal fibrosis (RPF). A soft tissue density that obscures the contours of the IVC and the aorta is seen (Fig. 3C.41). The process may extend into the pelvis, and there may be vascular or ureteral encasement. On noncontrast CT, the density of the soft tissue is similar to that of muscle. Following contrast administration, variable enhancement is seen. Malignant forms of RPF cannot be distinguished from the benign ones (2).

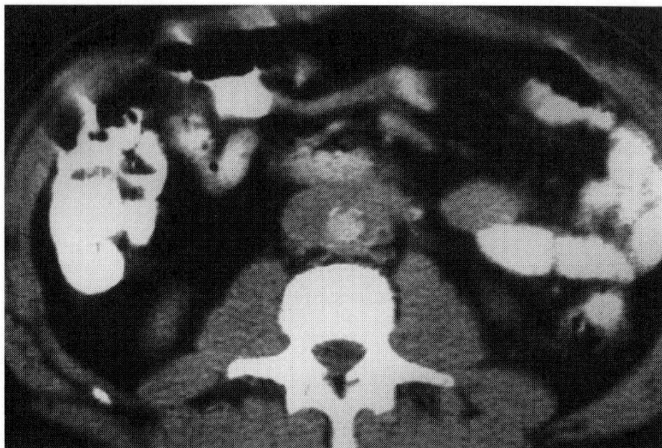

A

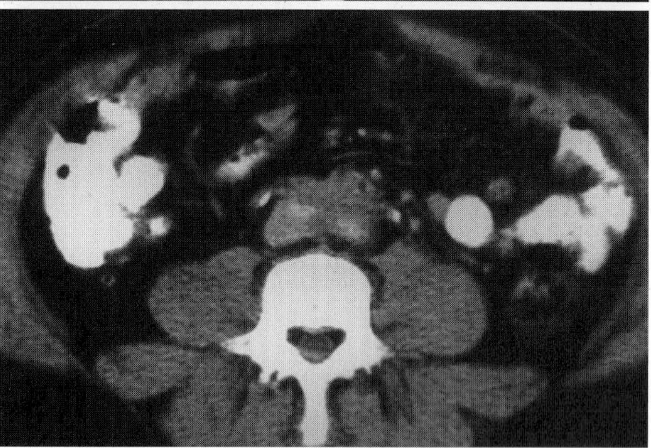

B

FIGURE 3C.41. Retroperitoneal fibrosis. **A:** There is soft tissue encasement of the aorta and the cava, obscuring the tissue planes that lie between them. **B:** The process extends caudally to encase the common iliac vessels also.

COMPUTED TOMOGRAPHY OF THE PELVIS

The entire abdomen and pelvis is imaged so rapidly with current scanners that on the initial scans through the pelvis, the urinary bladder is often not opacified with contrast excreted by the kidneys. Delayed images through the pelvis are required if assessment of the bladder wall is necessary, as in patients with bladder cancer. Pelvic lymph nodes larger than 1 cm in short axis diameter are considered abnormally enlarged. Normal-sized nodes may be difficult to differentiate from adjacent vessels and nerves without intravenous contrast.

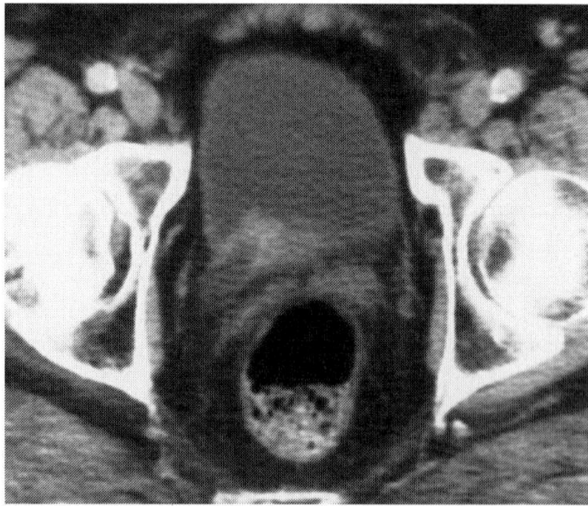

FIGURE 3C.42. Bladder cancer at the right ureteral orifice. There is ureteral dilation, which may be partially mechanical. No definite perivesical extension is seen.

Urinary Bladder

Tumors

CT scanning cannot reliably assess the presence or depth of muscle invasion of bladder tumors. However, gross invasion of perivesical structures can be ascertained, as can lymphadenopathy.

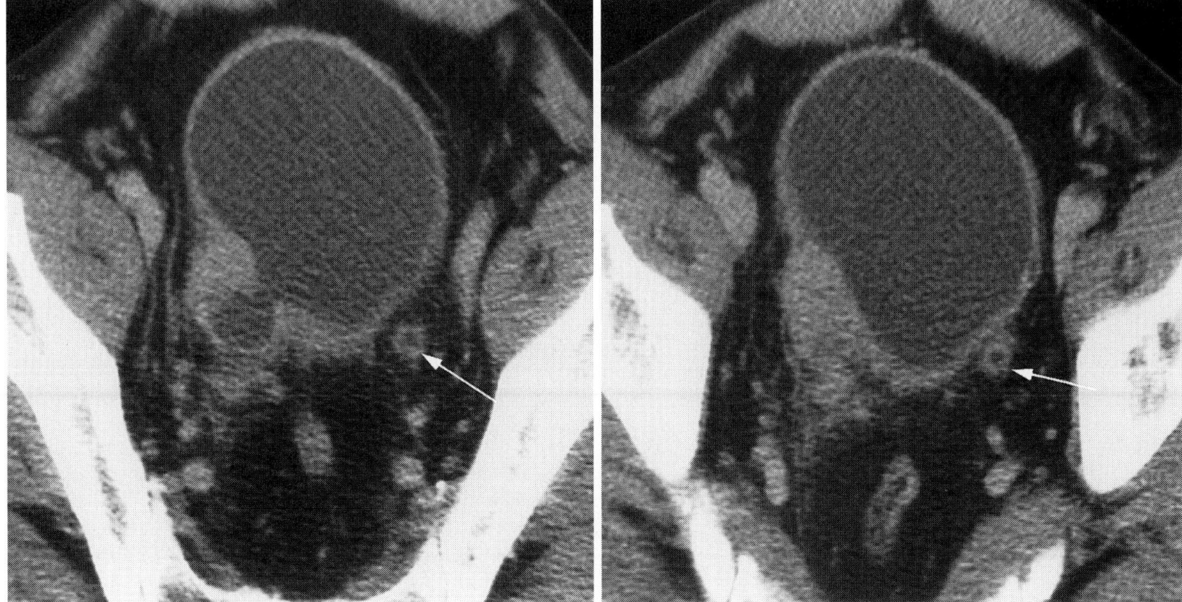

FIGURE 3C.43. Bladder cancer involving a right posterior bladder diverticulum. Note the soft tissue mass within the diverticulum **(A)** and perivesical extension of the mass **(B)**. The left distal ureter is thickened *(arrow)* **(A, B)**, raising the possibility of tumor involvement.

Bladder tumors are seen as sessile or pedunculated masses that project into the lumen or as focal or diffuse wall thickening (Fig. 3C.42). Perivesical extension causes blurring of the soft tissue planes; in more advanced cases, a soft tissue mass projecting into the adjacent tissues will be seen (Fig. 3C.43). The overall accuracy for detecting perivesical extension is 65% to 85%, and the accuracy for detecting lymph node involvement is 70% to 90% (44).

Trauma

Because CT is often the initial study performed in patients with blunt abdominal or pelvic trauma, CT cystography is a convenient way to assess for bladder injury. It is important to adequately distend the bladder actively and not rely on passive filling of the bladder with excreted contrast (Fig. 3C.44). With these caveats in mind, the sensitivity of CT cystography is comparable to that of conventional cystography for diagnosing bladder injuries (53).

Prostate

The main utility of CT in patients with prostate cancer is in the detection of lymphadenopathy (Fig. 3C.45). The sensitivity for the detection of intraprostatic tumor, transcapsular extension, and seminal vesicle involvement is low (24,60).

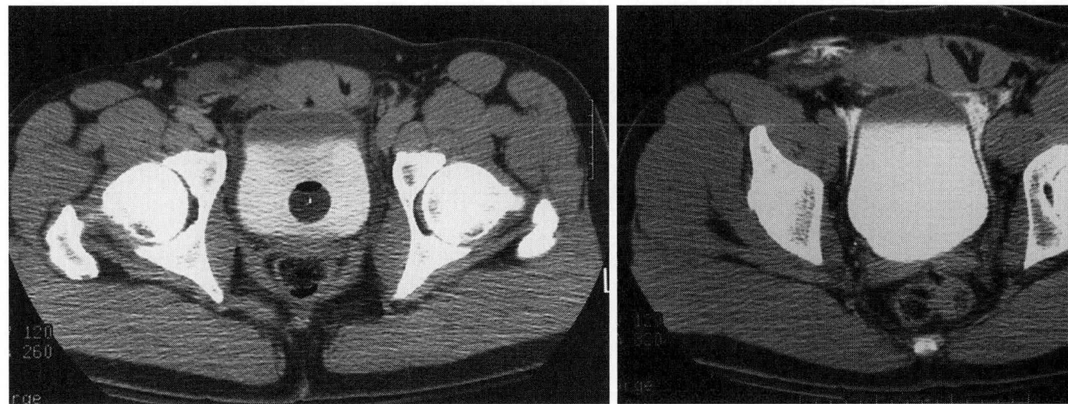

FIGURE 3C.44. Extraperitoneal bladder rupture. Patient in a motor vehicle accident. **A:** Images with passive bladder filling demonstrate no extravesical contrast. **B:** When bladder is filled till there is a detrusor contraction, contrast extravasation from urinary bladder becomes obvious.

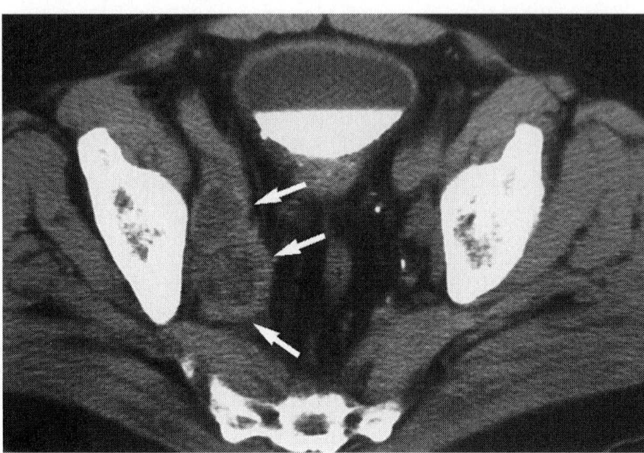

FIGURE 3C.45. Large, necrotic obturator lymph nodes *(arrows)* in a patient with prostate cancer.

In postoperative patients being evaluated for local recurrence, artifact emanating from metal clips can obscure the surgical bed.

REFERENCES

1. Amendola MA, Bree RL, Pollack HM, et al. Small renal cell carcinomas: resolving a diagnostic dilemma. *Radiology* 1988; 166:637.
2. Amis ES. Retroperitoneal fibrosis. *AJR Am J Roentgenol* 1991; 157:321.
3. Aso Y, Homma Y. A survey on incidental renal cell carcinoma in Japan. *J Urol* 1992;147:340.
4. Barnes GT, Lakshminarayanan AV. Conventional and spiral computed tomography: physical principles and image quality considerations. In: Lee JKT, Sagel SS, Stanley RJ, Heiken JP, eds. *Computed Body Tomography with MRI correlation,* vol II. Philadelphia: Lippincott-Raven, 1998:1.
5. Bennet HF, Werden SA, Brink JA, et al. Dual phase spiral CT of renal masses-comparison of cortical and nephrographic enhancement phases. *AJR Am J Roentgenol* 1998;170:S99.
6. Birnbaum BA, Bosniak MA, Megibow AJ, et al. Observations on the growth of renal neoplasms. *Radiology* 1990;176:695.
7. Birnbaum BA, Jacobs JE, Langlotz AP, Ramchandani P. Assessment of bolus-tracking technique in helical renal CT to optimize nephrographic phase imaging. *Radiology* 1999;211:87.
8. Birnbaum BA, Jacobs JE, Ramchandani P. Multiphasic renal CT: comparison of renal mass enhancement during the corticomedullary and nephrographic phases. *Radiology* 1996;200:753.
9. Bjornsson J, Short MP, Kwiatkowski DJ, et al. Tuberous sclerosis-associated renal cell carcinoma: clinical, pathological and genetic features. *Am J Pathol* 1996;149:1201.
10. Bosniak MA, Megibow AJ, Hulnick DH, et al. CT diagnosis of renal angiomyolipoma: the importance of detecting small amounts of fat. *AJR Am J Roentgenol* 1988;151:497.
11. Bosniak MA. The current radiological approach to renal cysts. *Radiology* 1986;158:1.
12. Boyd DP, Parker DL, Goodsitt MM. Principles of computed tomography. In: Moss MA, Gamsu G, Genant HK, eds. *Computed tomography of the body with magnetic resonance imaging,* vol III, 2nd ed. Philadelphia: WB Saunders, 1992:1355.
13. Bruce GR, Munch LC, Hoven AD, et al. Urolithiasis associated with the protease inhibitor indinavir. *Urology* 1997;50:513.
14. Buckley J, Urban BA, Soyer P, et al. Transitional cell carcinoma of the renal pelvis: a retrospective look at CT staging with pathologic correlation. *Radiology* 1996;201:194.
15. Castillo OA, Boyle ET Jr, Kramer SA. Multilocular cysts of kidney: a study of 29 patients and review of literature. *Urology* 1991;37:156.
16. Choyke PL. Inherited cystic diseases of the kidney. *Radiol Clin North Am* 1996;34:925.
17. Choyke PL. von Hippel-Lindau disease. In: Pollack HM, McClennan BL, eds. *Clinical urography,* 2nd ed. Philadelphia: WB Saunders, 2000:1333.
18. Cohan RH, Sherman LS, Korobkin M, et al. Renal masses: assessment of corticomedullary-phase and nephrographic-phase CT scans. *Radiology* 1995;196:445.
19. Curry NS. Small renal masses (lesions smaller than 3 cm): imaging evaluation and management. *AJR Am J Roentgenol* 1995; 164:355.
20. Dalton D, Neiman H, Grayhack JT. The natural history of simple renal cysts: a preliminary study. *J Urol* 1986;135:905.
21. Davidson AJ, Choyke PL, Hartman DS, et al. Renal medullary carcinoma associated with sickle cell trait: radiologic findings. *Radiology* 1995;195:83.
22. Davidson AJ, Hayes WS, Hartman Ds, et al. Renal oncocytoma and carcinoma: failure of differentiation with CT. *Radiology* 1993;186:693.
23. Disler DG, Chew FS. Adrenal pheochromocytoma. *AJR Am J Roentgenol* 1992;158:1056.
24. Engeler CE, Wasserman NF, Zhang G. Preoperative assessment of prostatic carcinoma by computed tomography: weaknesses and new perspectives. *Urology* 1990;40:346.
25. Federle M. Renal trauma. In: Pollack HM, McClennan BL, eds. *Clinical urography,* 2nd ed. Philadelphia: WB Saunders, 2000: 1772.
26. Fielding JR, Silverman SG, Rubin GD. Helical CT of the urinary tract. *AJR Am J Roentgenol* 1999;172:1199.
27. Fielding JR, Silverman SG, Samuel S. Spiral CT of ureteral stones: predicting need for intervention. *Radiology* 1997; 205:508.
28. Fishman EK, Deutch BM, Hartman DS, et al. Primary adrenocortical carcinoma: CT evaluation with clinical correlation. *AJR Am J Roentgenol* 1987;148:531.
29. Gill IS, McClennan BL, Kerbl K, et al. Adrenal involvement from renal cell carcinoma: predictive value of computerized tomography. *J Urol* 1994;152:1082.
30. Hattery RR, Sheedy PF, Stephens DH, et al. Computed tomography of the adrenal gland. *Semin Roentgenol* 1981;16:290.
31. Helenon O, Meran S, Paraf F, et al. Unusual fat-containing tumors of the kidney: a diagnostic dilemma. *Radiographics* 1997; 17:129.
32. Herts BR, Coll DM, Lieger ML, et al. Triphasic helical CT of the kidneys: contribution of vascular phase scanning in patients before urologic surgery. *AJR Am J Roentgenol* 1999;173:1273.
33. Honda H, Coffman CE, Berbaum KS, et al. CT analysis of metastatic neoplasms of the kidneys. *Acta Radiol* 1992;33:39.
34. Hounsfield GN. A method of an apparatus for examination of the body by radiation such as X or gamma radiation. British patent no. 1283915, 1972.
35. Johnson CD, Dunnick NR, Cohan RH, et al. CT staging of 100 tumors. *AJR Am J Roentgenol* 1987;148:59.
36. Kalender WA, Seissler W, Klotz E, et al. Spiral volumetric CT with single-breath-hold technique, continuous transport, and continuous scanner rotation. *Radiology* 1990;176:181.

37. Kalender WA, Seissler W, Vock P: Single breath-hold spiral volumetric CT by continuous patient translation and scanner rotation. *Radiology* 1989;73:414.
38. Kallman DA, King BF, Hattery RR, et al. Renal vein and inferior vena cava tumor thrombus in renal cell carcinoma: CT, US, MRI, and venacavography. *J Comput Asst Tomogr* 1992;16:240.
39. Kauczor H-U, Schadmand-Fischer S, Filipas D, et al. CT after enucleation of renal cell carcinoma. *Abdom Imaging* 1994; 19:361.
40. Kawashima A, Sandler CM, Goldman SG, et al. CT of renal inflammatory disease. *Radiographics* 1997;17:851.
41. Kenney PJ, McClennan. The kidney. In: Lee JKT, Sagel SS, Stanley RJ, Heiken JP, eds. *Computed body tomography with MRI correlation*, vol II. Philadelphia: Lippincott-Raven, 1998:1087.
42. Kenney PJ, Stanley RJ. Computed tomography of ureteral tumors. *J Comput Asst Tomogr* 1987;11:102.
43. Kenney PJ, Wagner BJ, Rao P, et al. Myelolipoma: CT and pathologic features. *Radiology* 1998;208:87.
44. Kim B, Semelka SC, Ascher SM, et al. Bladder tumor staging: comparison of contrast-enhanced CT, T1- and T2-weighted MR imaging, dynamic gadolinium enhanced imaging and late-gadolinium enhanced imaging. *Radiology* 1994;193:239.
45. Kopka L, Fischer U, Zoeller B, et al. Dual-phase helical CT of the kidney: value of the corticomedullary and nephrographic phase for evaluation of lesions and preoperative staging of renal cell carcinoma. *AJR Am J Roentgenol* 1997;169:1573.
46. Korobkin M, Brideur FJ, Francis IR, et al. Delayed enhanced CT for differentiation of benign from malignant adrenal masses. *Radiology* 1996;200:737.
47. Krinsky G. Unenhanced helical CT in patients with acute flank pain and renal infarction: the need for contrast material in selected cases. *AJR Am J Roentgenol* 1996;167:282.
48. Kunin M. Bridging septa of the perinephric space: anatomic, pathologic and diagnostic considerations. *Radiology* 1986; 158:361.
49. Lee MJ, Hahn PF, Papanicolaou N, et al. Benign and malignant adrenal masses: CT distinction with attenuation coefficients, size and observer analysis. *Radiology* 1991;179:415.
50. Lemaitre L, Claudon M, Dubvelle F, et al. Imaging of angiomyolipomas. *Semin US CT MRI* 1997;18:100.
51. Levine E, Grantham JJ. Calcified renal stones and cyst calcification in autosomal dominant polycystic kidney disease: clinical and CT study in 84 patients. *AJR Am J Roentgenol* 1992;159:77.
52. Levine E, Slusher SL, Grantham JJ, et al. Natural history of acquired renal cystic disease in dialysis patients: a prospective longitudinal study. *AJR Am J Roentgenol* 1991;156:501.
53. Lis LE, Cohen AJ. CT cystography in the evaluation of bladder trauma. *J Comput Asst Tomgr* 1990;14:386.
54. Marcari MJ, Bosniak MA. Delayed CT to evaluate renal masses incidentally discovered on contrast enhanced CT: demonstrating vascularity by de-enhancement [Abstract]. *Radiology* 1998: 209:301.
55. McClennan BL. Oncologic imaging: staging and follow up of renal and adrenal carcinoma. *Cancer* 1991;67:1199.
56. Narumi Y, Sato T, Hori S, et al. Squamous cell carcinoma of the uroepithelium: CT evaluation. *Radiology* 1989;173:853.
57. Nyman U, Oldbring J, Aspelin P. CT of carcinoma of the renal pelvis. *Acta Radiol* 1992;33:31.
58. Olcott EW, Sommer GF, Napel S. Accuracy of detection and measurement of renal calculi: in vitro comparison of three dimensional spiral CT, radiography and nephrotomography. *Radiology* 1997:204:19.
59. Pearle MS, Watamull LM, Mullican MA. Sensitivity of noncontrast helical computerized tomography and plain film radiography compared to flexible nephroscopy for detecting residual fragments after percutaneous nephrostolithotomy. *J Urol* 1999; 162:23.
60. Platt JF, Bree RL, Schwab RE. The accuracy of CT in the staging of carcinoma of the prostate. *AJR Am J Roentgenol* 1987;149(2):315.
61. Pollack HM, Wein AJ. Imaging of renal trauma. *Radiology* 1989;172:297.
62. Port FK, Ragheb NE, Schwartz AG, et al. Neoplasms in dialysis patients: a population-based study. *Am J Kidney Dis* 1989; 14:119.
63. Raisanen J, Shapiro B, Glazer GM, et al. Plasma catecholamines in pheochromocytoma: effect of urographic contrast media. *AJR Am J Roentgenol* 1984;143:43.
64. Ramchandani P, Pollack HM. Renal cystic disease. *Imaging* 1992;4;225.
65. Reznek RH, Mootoosamy I, Webb JAW, et al. CT in renal and perirenal lymphoma: a further look. *Clin Radiol* 1990;42:233.
66. Rubin GD, Shiau MC, Schmidt AJ, et al. Computed tomographic angiography: historical perspective and new state-of-the-art using multi detector-row helical computed tomography. *J Comput Assisted Tomogr* 1999;23S:S83.
67. Silverman PM, Cooper CJ, Weltman DI, et al. Helical CT: practical considerations and potential pitfalls. *Radiographics* 1995;15:25.
68. Smith RC, Dalrymple NC, Neitlich J. Noncontrast helical CT in the evaluation of acute flank pain. *Abdom Imaging* 1998; 23:10.
69. Smith RC, Verga M, Dalrymple NC, et al. Acute ureteral obstruction: value of secondary signs on helical unenhanced CT. *AJR Am J Roentgenol* 1996;167:1109.
70. Smith RC, Verga M, McCarthy S, et al. Diagnosis of acute flank pain: value of unenhanced helical CT. *AJR Am J Roentgenol* 1996;166:97.
71. Smith SJ, Bosniak MA, Megibow AJ, et al. Renal cell carcinoma: earlier discovery and increased detection. *Radiology* 1989; 170:699.
72. Soulen MC, Fishman EK, Goldman SM, et al. Bacterial renal infection: role of CT. *Radiology* 1989;171:703.
73. Soulen MC, Fishman EK, Goldman SM. Sequelae of acute renal infections: CT evaluation. *Radiology* 1989;173:423.
74. Steiner MS, Goldman SM, Fishman EK, et al. The natural history of renal angiomyolipoma. *J Urol* 1993;150:1782.
75. Stomper PC, Kalish LA, Garnick MB, et al. CT and pathologic predictive features of residual mass histologic findings after chemotherapy for nonseminomatous germ cell tumors: can residual malignancy or teratoma be excluded? *Radiology* 1991;180:711.
76. Studer UE, Scherz S, Scheidegger J, et al. Enlargement of regional lymph nodes in renal cell carcinoma is often not due to metastases. *J Urol* 1990;144:243.
77. Sussman SK, Gallmann WH, Cohan RH, et al. CT findings in xanthogranulomatous pyelonephritis with coexistent renocolic fistula. *J Comput Asst Tomogr* 1987;11:1088.
78. Szolar DH, Kammerhuber E, Altziebler S, et al: Multiphasic helical CT of the kidney: increased conspicuity for detection and characterization of small (<3-cm) renal masses. *Radiology* 1997; 202:211.
79. Szolar DH, Kammerhuber F. Quantitative CT evaluation of adrenal gland masses: a step forward in the differentiation between adenomas and nonadenomas. *Radiology* 1997;202:517.
80. Takahashi N, Kawashima A, Ernst RD, et al. Ureterolithiasis: can clinical outcome be predicted with unenhanced helical CT. *Radiology* 1998;208:97.

81. Urban BA, Buckley J, Soyer P, et al. CT appearance of transitional cell carcinoma of the renal pelvis, part 1: Early-stage disease. *AJR Am J Roentgenol* 1997;169:157.
82. Urban BA, Buckley J, Soyer P, et al. CT appearance of transitional cell carcinoma of the renal pelvis, part 2: advanced-stage disease. *AJR Am J Roentgenol* 1997;169:163.
83. Van Baal JG, Smits NJ, Keeman JN, et al. The evolution of renal angiomyolipomas in patients with tuberous sclerosis. *J Urol* 1994;152:35.
84. Warshauer DM, McCarthy SM, Street L, et al. Detection of renal masses; sensitivities and specificities of excretory urography/linear tomography, US and CT. *Radiology* 1988;169:363.
85. Yamashita Y, Takahashi M, Watanabe O, et al. Small renal cell carcinoma: pathologic and radiologic correlation. *Radiology* 1992;184:493.
86. Yuh BI, Cohan RH. Different phases of renal enhancement: role in detecting and characterizing renal masses during helical CT. *AJR Am J Roentgenol* 1999;173:747.
87. Zagoria RJ, Wolfman NT, Karstaedt N, et al. CT features of renal cell carcinoma with emphasis on relation to tumor size. *Invest Radiol* 1990;25:261.
88. Zeman RK, Zeiberg A, Hayes WS, et al. Helical CT of renal masses: the value of delayed scans. *AJR Am J Roentgenol* 167:771.

Adult and Pediatric Urology, 4/e, edited by Jay Y. Gillenwater, John T. Grayhack, Stuart S. Howards, and Michael E. Mitchell.
Lippincott Williams & Wilkins, Philadelphia © 2002

3D

ULTRASOUND

J. PATRICK SPIRNAK
MARTIN I. RESNICK

The development of ultrasound instrumentation effective in the evaluation and treatment of many medical conditions dates back to the 1940s, when Firestone first described a technique using ultrasonic waves to detect flaws in metal castings (71). During World War II, the principles of ultrasound were used to develop sonar (sound navigation ranging), a tracking technique useful in identifying submerged enemy submarines. The first medical use of ultrasound was reported by an Austrian psychiatrist, Karl Dussik (29), who attempted to locate brain tumors with the use of two opposing ultrasound transducers. In the early 1950s, Howry and Bliss (46) used discarded naval equipment and studied and recorded the echo patterns obtained from a variety of soft tissue structures. They initially used water immersion techniques, and it was not until the early 1960s that they began experimenting with handheld scanners applied directly to the body surface. Since the early 1970s, with the development of real-time capability, grayscale imaging, high-frequency transducers, color-flow Doppler, and power Doppler, ultrasound has gained an important role in the clinical evaluation of many urologic abnormalities. The emerging use of ultrasound contrast agents promises to enhance and expand many of these applications.

BASIC PRINCIPLES OF ULTRASOUND

Ultrasound consists of sound waves of frequencies beyond the audible range of the human ear [greater than 20,000 Hz (cycles per second)]. For medical purposes, diagnostic ultra-

J.P. Spirnak and M.I. Resnick: Department of Urology, Case Western Reserve University, Cleveland, OH 44106.

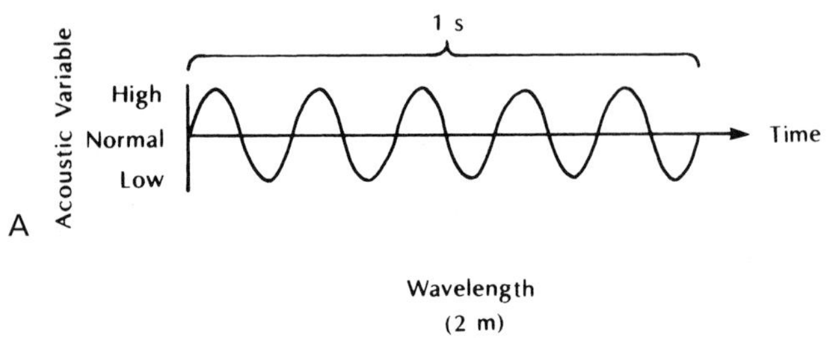

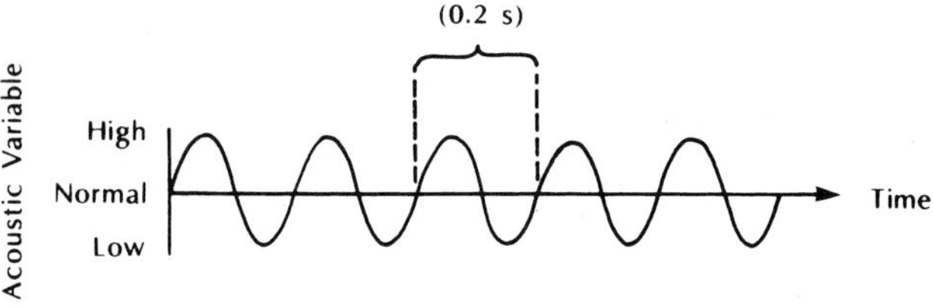

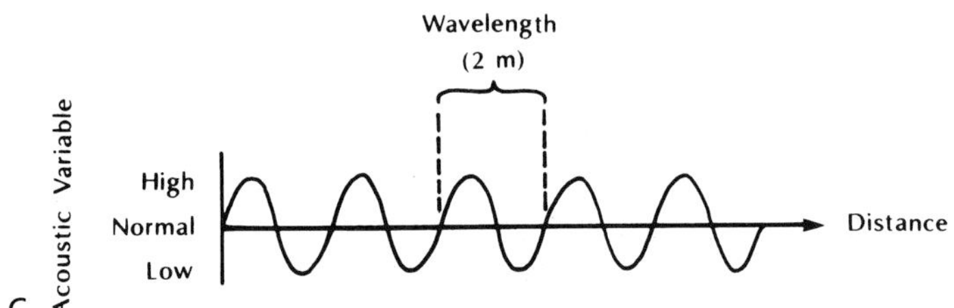

FIGURE 3D.1. **A:** Frequency. The number of complete variations (cycles) that an acoustic variable goes through in 1 second. In this diagram, five cycles occur in 1 second. One hertz is 1 cps. One megahertz is 1 million cps. **B:** Period. The time for one complete cycle. The period in this diagram is 0.2 seconds. **C:** Wavelength. The distance over which one cycle occurs. In this diagram each cycle is 2 m. (Adapted with permission from Kremkau FW. *Diagnostic ultrasound principles, instruments and exercises,* ed 3. Philadelphia: Saunders, 1989.)

sound equipment uses sound waves between 2 million and 10 million MHz. Sound travels in a wave form that is dependent on the medium in which it travels and has a multitude of variables, including density, pressure, temperature, and particle motion (54). Sound waves are described in terms of frequency, period, amplitude intensity (determined by the source), propagation speed (determined by the medium), and wavelength (determined by the source and medium) (Fig. 3D.1).

The source of the ultrasound beam is a transducer consisting of a piezoelectric transmitter and receiver (Fig. 3D.2A). The piezoelectric crystal generates a wave at a frequency that is dependent on the strength of the current applied to it and the size of the crystal. Sound waves are produced by the deformation of the crystal associated with electrical excitation. Short impulses, approximately 10 ms each, of alternating current are applied to the crystal, and the ultrasound beam thus generated is focused by the transducer into a beam several millimeters in width. The thickness of the crystal determines the frequency of the generated sound waves. The sound waves are focused with an acoustic lens that produces a narrow beam only a few millimeters in diameter with good lateral resolution.

The body and its contents are the molecular medium that propagates the generated sound waves. In the presence of a homogeneous fluid medium (e.g., renal cyst, full urinary bladder), the sound waves are propagated in an uninterrupted manner. No sound waves are reflected back to the transducer, and therefore this area appears without echoes *(anechoic).* If the sound waves encounter a different density of tissue, a portion is reflected back to the source and that area is imaged. If the area or structure has a greater number of reflected waves than surrounding regions, it is termed *hyperechoic,* and if the echoes are less, the region appears *hypoechoic* (Fig. 3D.2B). The reflecting boundary is called an acoustic interface, and it exists because of the differing acoustic impedances between the two media. *Acoustic impedance* is the product of a medium density and the speed of sound in the medium. The greater the difference in acoustic impedance between the two media, the greater the amount of sound reflected back from the interface. Typically less than 1% of incident energy is reflected.

Whether the sound waves are reflected also depends on the relative size of the interface and the frequency of the generated wavelength. Sound waves of higher frequencies are generally reflected by smaller surface interfaces but have less depth of penetration, thereby giving better spatial reso-

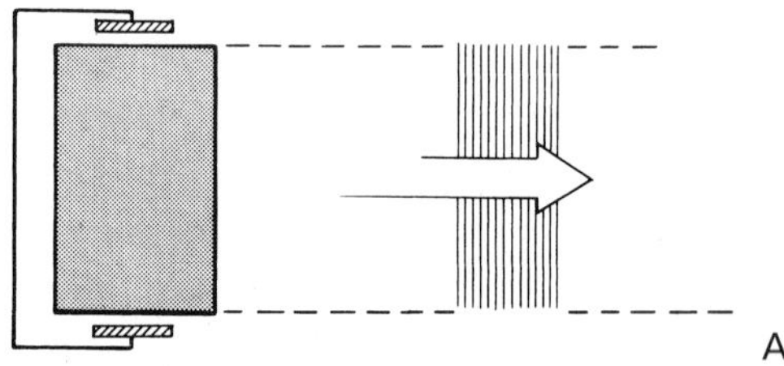

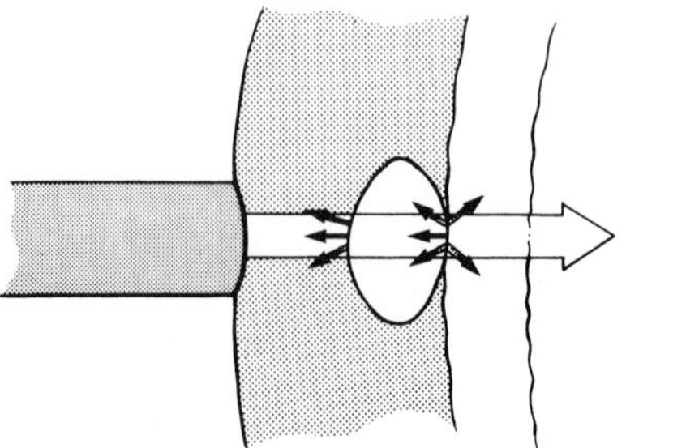

FIGURE 3D.2. **A:** High-frequency sound waves are transmitted after excitation of a piezoelectric crystal. **B:** Transmitter sound waves are reflected at tissue interfaces where there is a change in acoustic impedance. Reflected sound waves obey laws of optics—the angle of incidence is equal to the angle of reflection.

lution at the expense of decreased sound wave penetration. The use of lower-frequency sound waves sacrifices spatial resolution but makes it possible to image deeper structures. Appropriate transducer selection is critical for the success of the evaluation, and it is generally best to select the highest frequency that permits adequate tissue penetration and visualization of the desired structures. For example, higher-frequency transducers (7 MHz) are used for transrectal prostate imaging and lower-frequency ones (3.5 MHz) are used to view the kidneys.

During the course of the examination, the ultrasound transducer functions not only as a source of the sound waves but also as a receiver of the sound waves that have been reflected from the different tissue interfaces (Fig. 3D.3). The sound waves' energy is converted in the transducer by the piezoelectric crystal to electrical energy, which is then processed and displayed as a dot on a cathode ray tube (oscilloscope). The sound waves reflected back to the transducer are highly dependent on the angle of the reflector (Figs. 3D.4 and 3D.5). Amplitude, or A-mode, records reflect echoes as spikes arising from a horizontal baseline and represent one of the earliest displays used in medical ultrasound (Fig. 3D.6). The main application of this mode is to measure the distances from the margins of a mass to the skin surface or to determine the internal architecture of the mass, but with the development of two-dimensional and real-time imaging this mode is rarely used. The brightness modulated display, or B-mode, is a two-dimensional image obtained while the transducer is moved along a given arc; the resultant display is of a cross-sectional image of the examined area. With the development of scan converters and real-time imaging, images are now displayed in varying shades of gray (grayscale imaging). Gray-scale imaging offers a significant improvement in the quality of images compared with those obtained with early B scanners. Use of Doppler, in particular color-flow and power Doppler, has allowed measurement of flow and detection of flow in vascular structures.

The transducer and its mechanism of action (mechanical sector and radial; array-linear, curved, and phased) are other important components of the instrumentation. In both forms of imaging, the sound waves sweep repeatedly through the tissue and structures to be imaged. Mechanical scanners use a variety of principles and can be composed of rotating transducers or groups of transducers, oscillating

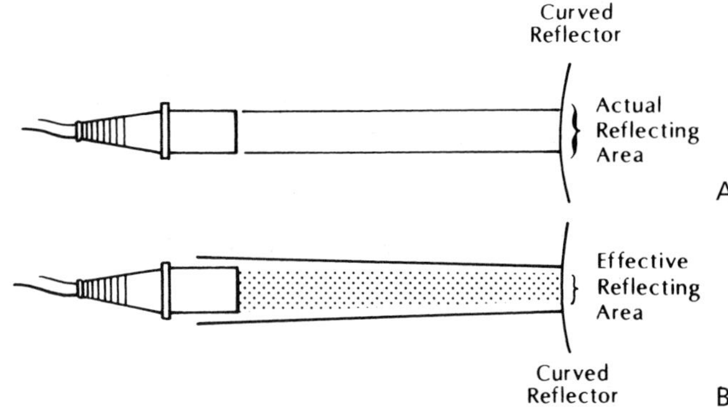

FIGURE 3D.4. Curved reflector. **A:** Propagated sound waves. **B:** Reflected sound waves received by transducer in shaded areas. (Adapted with permission from Kremkau FW. *Diagnostic ultrasound principles, instruments and exercise,* ed 3. Philadelphia: Saunders, 1989.)

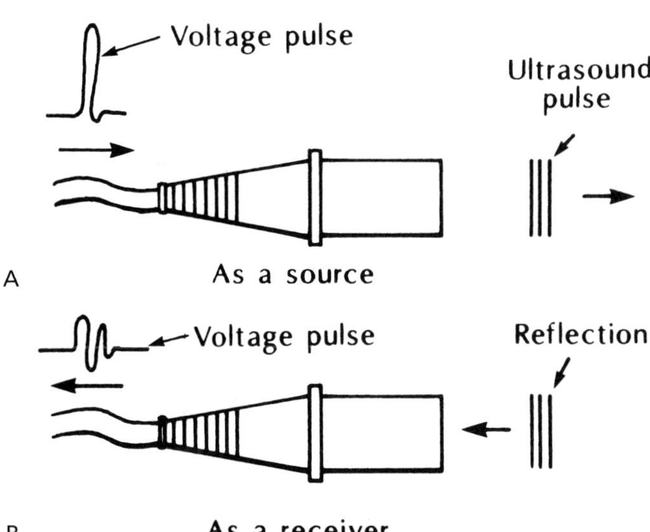

FIGURE 3D.3. Transducer operating in pulsed mode. **A:** Electrical pulses are converted to ultrasound pulses. **B:** Neural ultrasound pulses are converted to electrical pulses. (Adapted with permission from Kremkau FW. *Diagnostic ultrasound principles, instruments and exercise,* ed 3. Philadelphia: Saunders, 1989.)

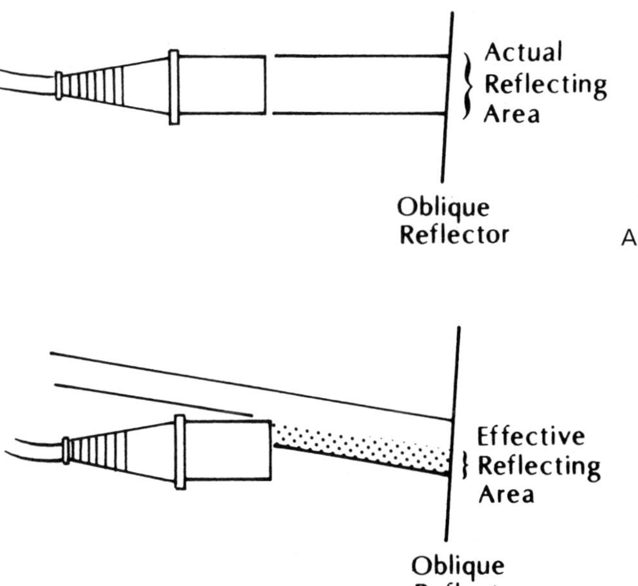

FIGURE 3D.5. Oblique reflector. **A:** Propagated sound waves. **B:** Reflected sound waves reached by transducer in shaded area. The remaining sound waves miss the transducer. (Adapted with permission from Kremkau FW. *Diagnostic ultrasound principles, instruments and exercise,* ed 3. Philadelphia: Saunders, 1989.)

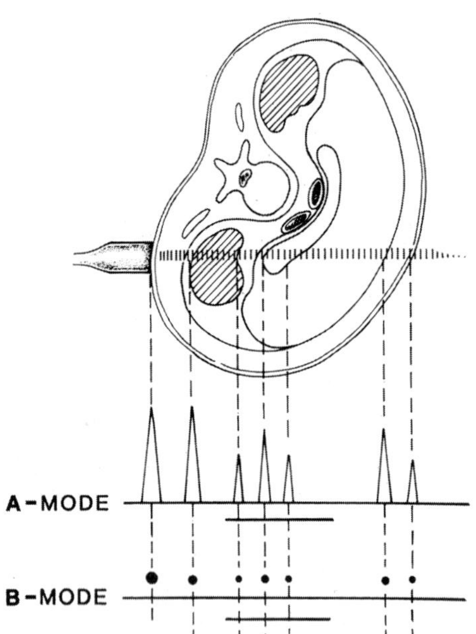

FIGURE 3D.6. Amplitude mode (A-mode) delineates reflected echoes as spikes arising from a horizontal baseline. The echo amplitude is plotted against distance between transducer and reflecting tissue interface. Brightness modulated display (B-mode) is a composite two-dimensional image obtained while transducer is moved along a given arc. Echoes are shown as multiple dots or points on the oscilloscope screen, the brightness of which is dependent on the intensity of the echo.

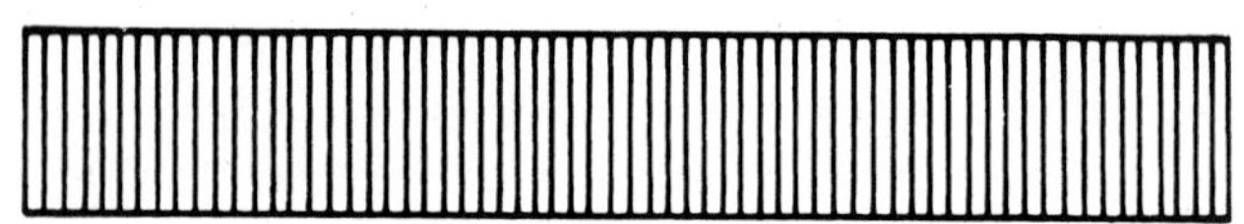

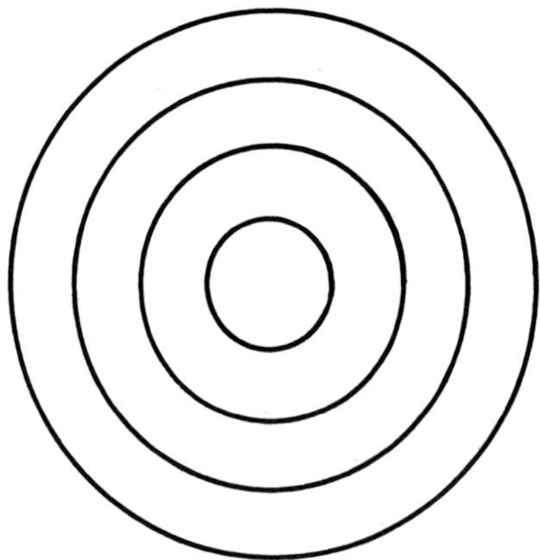

FIGURE 3D.8. Frontal view. **A:** Linear-array transducer with 64 elements. **B:** Annular array with four elements. (Adapted with permission from Kremkau FW. *Diagnostic principles, instruments and exercise,* ed 3. Philadelphia: Saunders, 1989.)

transducers, and the combination of oscillating transducers and reflectors (Fig 3D.7). In most instances, the oscillating or rotating component is surrounded by a cup of liquid that is incorporated within the transducer assembly. Various ingenious techniques have been devised (54). Array transducers operate by the application of voltage pulses to single elements or groups of elements in succession (Fig. 3D.8). In the linear-array scanner, many small elements are aligned side by side much like the teeth of a comb, and the plane of the structure to be imaged is determined by the orientation of the scanner. In most instances, the scanner provides a real-time image. Phased-array and curved-array systems operate by applying voltages to all elements in the assembly. By allowing small time differences that can be controlled electronically, the pulsed sound waves can be shaped and steered in an infinite number of directions (Fig. 3D.9).

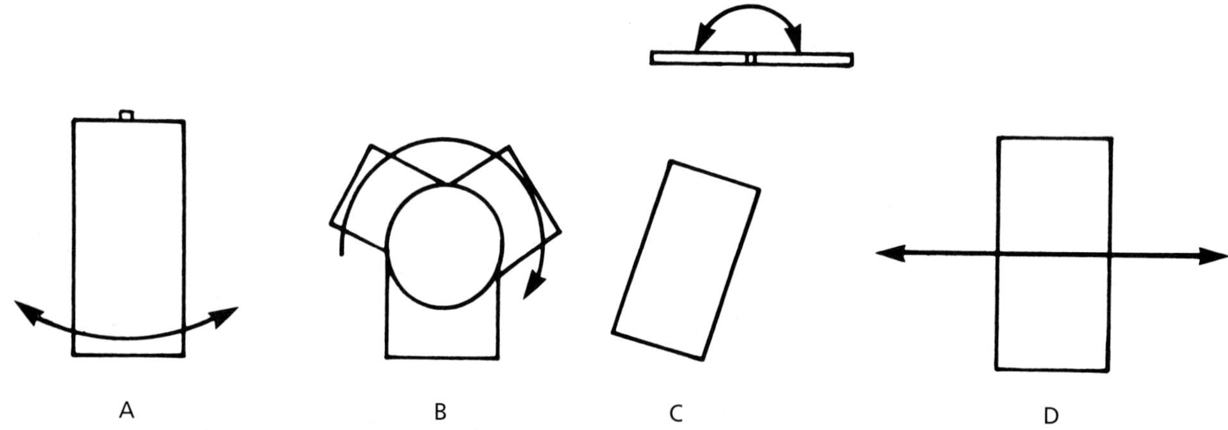

FIGURE 3D.7. Mechanical real-time transducers. **A:** Oscillating. **B:** Rotating. **C:** Oscillating. **D:** Linearly translating. (Adapted with permission from Kremkau FW. *Diagnostic ultrasound principles, instruments and exercise,* ed 3. Philadelphia: Saunders, 1989.)

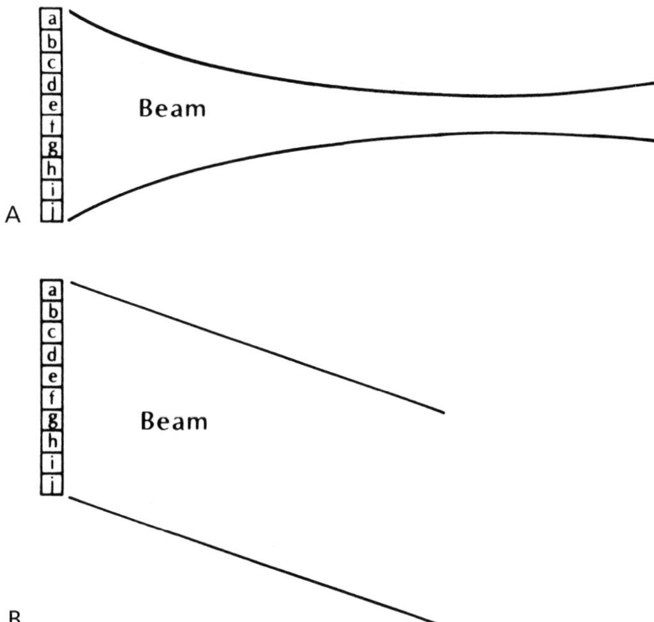

FIGURE 3D.9. Linear phased-array scanner. **A:** Beam focusing is accomplished by applying voltage pulse to the upper and lower elements earlier than the middle elements. **B:** Beam steering is accomplished by applying voltage pulses to the upper elements earlier than the lower elements. (Adapted with permission from Kremkau FW. *Diagnostic ultrasound principles, instruments and exercise,* ed 3. Philadelphia: Saunders, 1989.)

With the linear-array system, real-time images are obtained. By orienting the transducer differently, a variety of scanned planes can be realized. Much work will continue to enhance the quality and resolution of the image received.

Doppler instrumentation is based on the principle of a change in reflected frequency caused by reflector motion. Differences between incident and reflected frequencies are related to the speed of the reflector or media boundary—the greater the speed, the greater the difference. *Doppler shift* refers to the difference between the incident frequency and the reflected frequency, and the Doppler equation provides a quantitative relationship between the flow speed and frequency change. The development of color-flow techniques and power Doppler has permitted assessment of the direction of blood flow in arteries and veins, which has been useful in evaluation of a variety of benign and malignant urologic disorders.

Doppler instruments provide either continuous or pulsed voltages to the transducer. Continuous-wave instruments detect flow that occurs anywhere along the transmitted beam, but recently, pulsed-wave instruments have been introduced that provide information at a specific depth. Echoes can be received from different depths, depending on the receiver length and location, which can be controlled by the operator. Combination instruments are now available with the development of real-time cross-sectional ultrasound imaging in association with pulsed Doppler instrumentation (Fig. 3D.10). These instruments have allowed for the measurement of blood flow within specific blood vessels with the advent of color-flow technique and have been used in the assessment of blood flow within the kidney, testes, and penis. Power Doppler has greater sensitivity than conventional color Doppler, and it is particularly of value for assessing small vessels with low flow velocity (38). Echo-contrast development consisting of microbubble technology continues and offers much potential in clinical practice (15,107).

The images available for interpretation with most diagnostic ultrasound instruments are grayscale views; stop-action views can be obtained from a real-time examination. Real-time ultrasonography offers the advantage of dynamic imaging similar to that obtained with fluoroscopy. The obtained images are representations of a spectrum of echoes arising from the surface and substance of the given structure in two dimensions. With current scanners, a complete cross section of a structure is formed one line at a time. After one line is drawn, the transducer is moved slightly and pulsed again to draw another line. Typically 10,000 lines per second are drawn, enabling a complete image of the structure to be obtained. A permanent record of the scan can be recorded on Polaroid film, radiographic film, videotape, computer floppy disks, laser disks, and thermal paper.

Newer, less expensive equipment is making ultrasound examination of the urinary tract practical in the office setting. In addition, the equipment can be used for vascular flow studies, which is useful in the evaluation of men with erectile dysfunction and for assessing blood flow to a testicle when torsion of the spermatic cord is suspected. It can also be used in conjunction with urodynamic studies to image the bladder, bladder neck, and proximal urethra. Ultrasound examinations performed at the time of an office visit can speed diagnosis and treatment and reduce the cost of patient care.

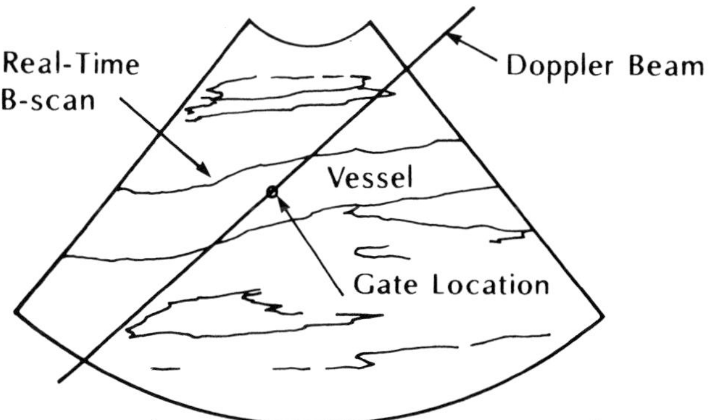

FIGURE 3D.10. Combination of real-time imaging and pulsed Doppler instrument. Blood flow measurement can be obtained within specific blood vessels. (Adapted with permission from Kremkau FW. *Diagnostic ultrasound principles, instruments and exercise,* ed 3. Philadelphia: Saunders, 1989.)

RENAL ULTRASOUND

When ultrasound images of the kidneys are obtained, patients can be scanned in the supine, decubitus, or prone positions and images are obtained in the transverse and longitudinal planes (Fig. 3D.11). In the past, the kidneys were usually examined with the patient in the prone position; however, the frequent location of the upper poles beneath the rib cage often led to incomplete or unsatisfactory studies. Currently, the right kidney is best examined with the patient in the supine position, using the liver as an acoustic window. The best images of the left kidney are usually obtained with the patient in the right lateral decubitus position, with the spleen as an acoustic window. When indicated, different views can also be obtained in the oblique plane by moving the transducer through different arcs relative to the longitudinal and transverse planes.

Renal Anatomy

The adult kidneys are paired, retroperitoneal structures lying between the twelfth thoracic and second lumbar vertebrae. Each kidney is approximately 10 cm long, 5 cm wide, and 2 to 5 cm thick. The right kidney is typically lower than the left. Ultrasonography continues to be an excellent modality to determine renal size. The upper pole of the right kidney is in contact with the adrenal superomedially and the duodenum anteromedially, and the posterior aspect of the right lobe of the liver overlies its anterior surface. Overlying the lower pole of the right kidney is the hepatic flexure of the colon and loops of small bowel. The anterior surface of the left kidney is in contact with the spleen, left adrenal, stomach, pancreas, descending colon, and small bowel. Posteriorly, the kidneys are in contact with the twelfth rib, diaphragm, transversus abdominis muscle, quadratus lumborum muscle, and psoas major muscle.

Each kidney is surrounded by a closely adherent, dense, fibrous capsule, which is surrounded by perinephric fat and enclosed in Gerota's fascia. On ultrasound examination, the renal outline is determined by the acoustic interface formed by the renal capsule and surrounding fat. Transverse scans show the kidney to be round or bean-shaped, whereas longitudinal images reveal an elliptic configuration (Fig. 3D.12). The renal parenchyma is relatively homogeneous, with the cortex appearing more echogenic than the medulla. Located in the center of the longitudinal renal scan is a dense echo complex consisting primarily of peripelvic fat, renal vessels, lymphatic vessels, and normal collecting system. The renal medullary pyramids appear somewhat less echogenic (more sonolucent) than the renal cortex and are often identified abutting on the dense sinus fat. The arcuate arteries separate the cortex from the renal medulla and, when visualized, allow for an accurate assessment of the renal cortical thickness. The renal vascular pedicle often can be identified with real-time scanning techniques. Doppler instrumentation has permitted assessment of blood flow in the main renal artery, and its branches have been used to evaluate patients with suspected renal vascular lesions and to assess for renal viability in the presence of severe hydronephrosis (13,65). Color-flow and power Doppler studies have provided detailed images of both the extrarenal and renal vasculature and are being increasingly used in patient evaluations (38,79,81).

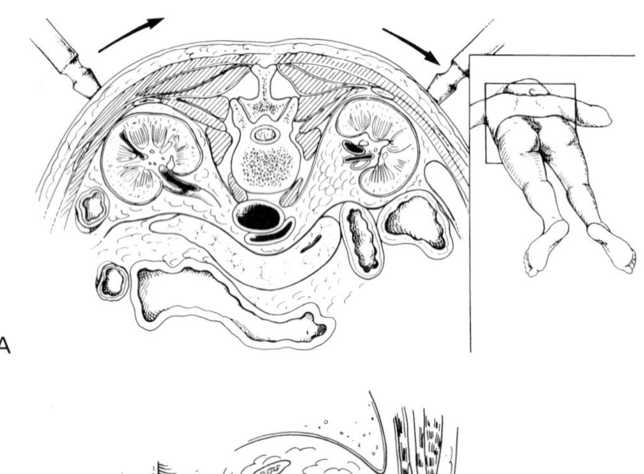

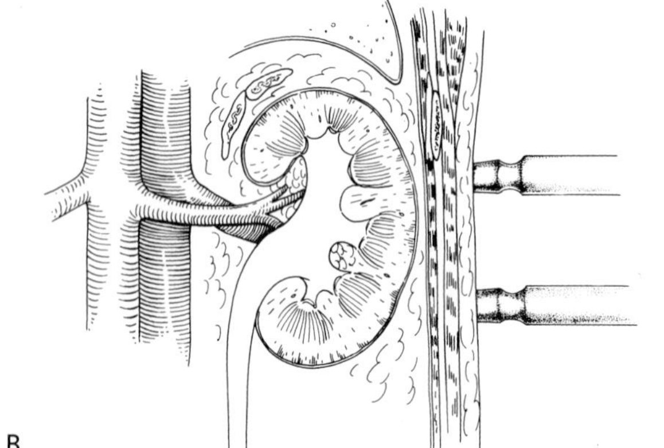

FIGURE 3D.11. Image planes of a transverse renal scan **(A)** and a longitudinal renal scan **(B)**.

Indications for Renal Ultrasound

Renal Mass

The question of a renal mass is usually raised by an abnormality found on excretory urography. In the adult, simple renal cysts are the most commonly diagnosed renal mass lesion. They are rarely seen in children. They occur with increasing frequency beyond age 30 years, and in an autopsy series, approximately 50% of all patients older than 50 years had at least one renal cyst (53). Ultrasound can identify cystic masses as small as a few millimeters in diameter. Solid mass lesions 1 to 2 cm wide also are routinely identified. The ability to identify a renal mass lesion depends on the depth of the lesion beneath the skin and the patient's body habitus.

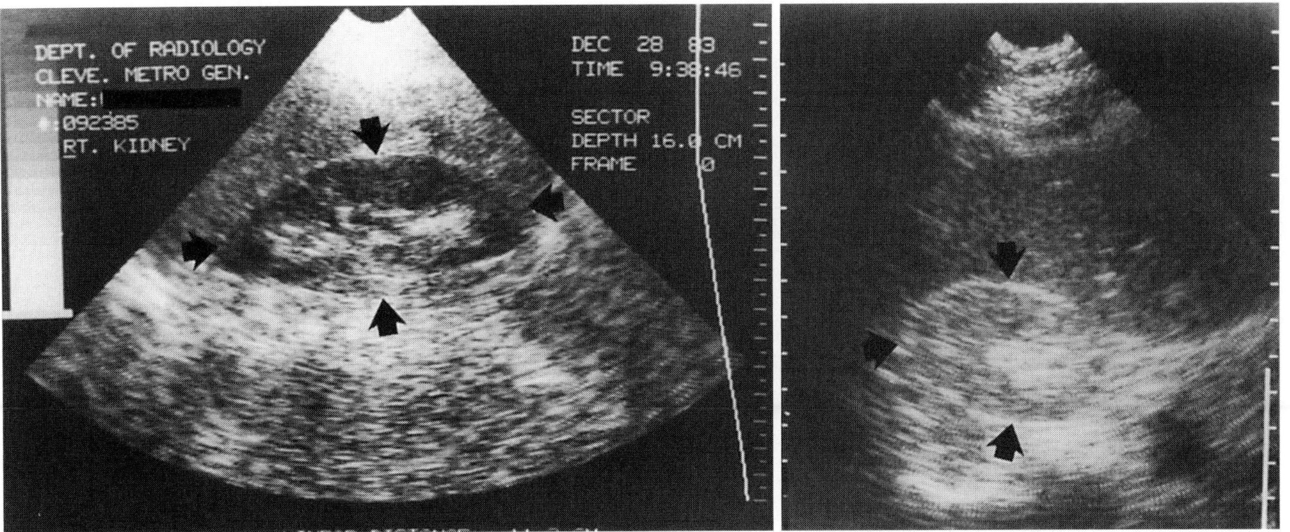

FIGURE 3D.12. Longitudinal **(A)** and transverse **(B)** scans of normal kidney. Note sharp demarcation of renal capsule *(arrows);* pelvic-calyceal system noted centrally as echogenic area.

Ultrasound has been extremely valuable in differentiating a simple renal cyst from other renal masses and is therefore the first study obtained in the evaluation of a suspected renal mass. On ultrasound, a renal cyst is typically spherical or slightly ovoid, demonstrates no internal echoes, has a clearly identifiable thin wall separate from the surrounding renal parenchyma, and allows enhancement of ultrasound transmission beyond the cyst (Fig. 3D.13). When these criteria are strictly adhered to, diagnostic accuracy rates approaching 100% have been reported (93). If a renal mass meets all of these criteria and the patient is asymptomatic, no further evaluation is required. If, however, the patient is symptomatic (pain or hematuria), cyst aspiration under ultrasound guidance can be performed to confirm the diagnosis. Aspirated fluid is routinely sent for cytologic study, lactate dehydrogenase, culture, and cholesterol determinations. While cyst puncture is performed, contrast material and air may be injected into the cyst to better define the cyst's margins and contours of the wall. Typically, computed tomography (CT) with and without injection of intravenous contrast agent is useful in assessing these symptomatic patients, thus avoiding the need for cyst aspirations. CT can also be used to help delineate a complex mass initially imaged with ultrasound, but occasionally, these studies are unable to exclude the presence of a renal malignancy, and often renal biopsy or surgical exploration is required to establish the correct diagnosis.

The finding on ultrasound of a solid or indeterminate (complex) renal mass raises the possibility of the presence of a renal malignancy and dictates that additional evaluation be performed. Ultrasound characteristics of a solid renal mass include the presence of internal echoes, poor delinea-

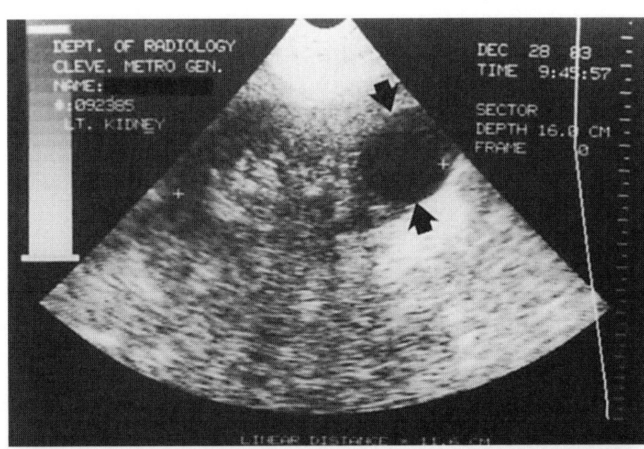

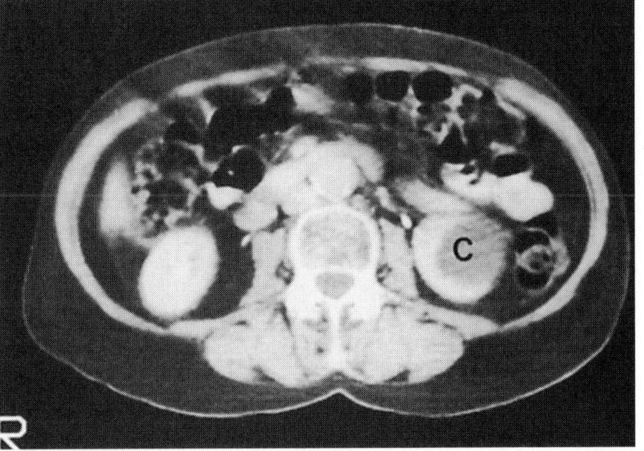

FIGURE 3D.13. A: Longitudinal renal scan showing characteristic findings of a simple renal cyst *(arrows).* **B:** Cyst *(C)* demonstrated on computed tomography scan.

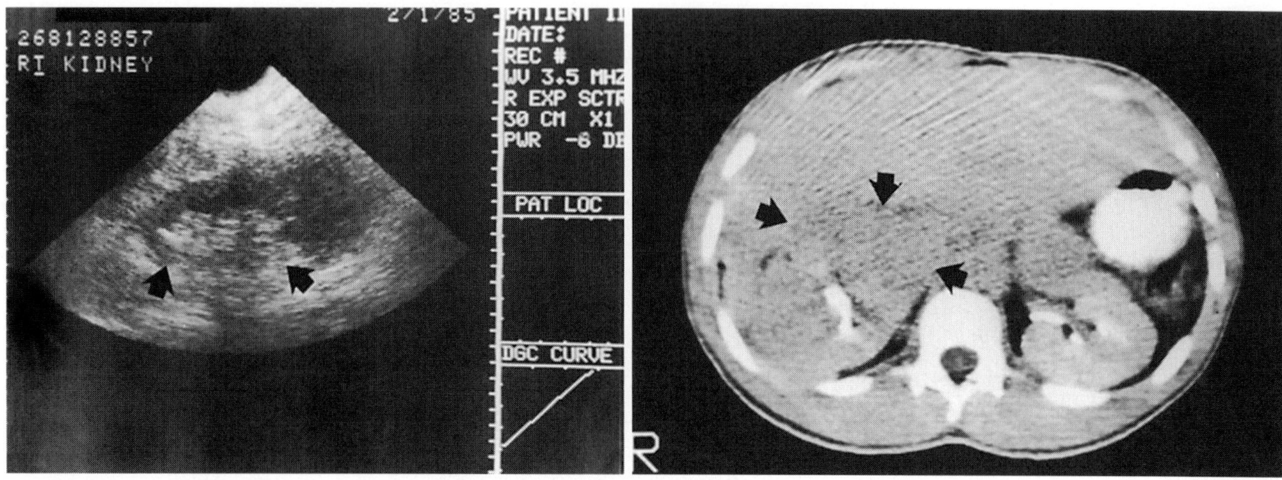

FIGURE 3D.14. Longitudinal renal ultrasound **(A)** and computed tomography scan **(B)** demonstrating findings of a hypernephroma *(arrows).*

tion of the posterior wall, and the lack of enhancement on through transmission (Fig. 3D.14).

The ultrasonic diagnosis of solid lesions is not as accurate as that of cystic lesions, and a false-negative rate has been reported to be as high as 14% (110). Therefore the diagnosis of a solid lesion requires further evaluation and possibly exploration. Color-flow and power Doppler studies have been used to differentiate solid renal masses (e.g., renal cell carcinoma versus renal lymphoma), and they have also been used to detect intravascular extension of invasive renal malignancies (37,55).

Angiomyolipoma, a benign tumor, seems to be the only solid renal mass with typical ultrasonographic features that allow presumptive diagnosis and safe differentiation from other solid mass lesions (62). If the lesion contains a high concentration of fat, it will be extremely echogenic, even more so than a solid renal mass. Hyperechogenicity coupled with the CT findings of fat lucency allows the diagnosis to be made with certainty (92) (Fig. 3D.15). Computer-aided tissue echo quantification has permitted the differentiation of small hyperechoic renal cell carcinomas from angiomyolipoma (111).

In the presence of a complex cystic lesion, the most likely diagnosis is necrotic tumor, hematoma, or abscess. The clinical course coupled with the findings on angiography or CT allows an accurate, certain diagnosis. When the diagnosis remains obscure, aspiration biopsy or exploration is often required.

A relatively new application is the use of ultrasound intraoperatively to monitor the cryoablation of small renal masses (126). Ultrasound has also been reported to be of value in the evaluation of the patient with acute renal trauma by determining the presence of urinary extravasation, perirenal hematoma, and renal fracture.

Collecting System Masses

Renal ultrasound has been extremely helpful in evaluating a noncalcified mass of the collecting system detected on excretory urography. A noncalcified or poorly calcified renal calculus (uric acid) demonstrates classic ultrasound findings. Typically, these calculi demonstrate increased echogenicity with acoustic shadowing (Fig. 3D.16). Other common soft tissue masses of the collecting system include tumors primarily of transitional cell origin, blood clots, and sloughed renal papilla (Fig. 3D.17). These abnormalities, although usually easily distinguishable from a nonopaque stone, often require urologic studies (e.g., ureteroscopy, biopsy) to arrive at the correct diagnosis. Intraluminal ultrasonography has

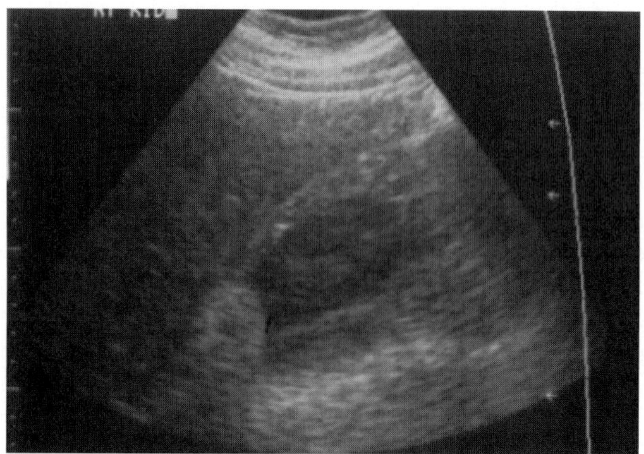

FIGURE 3D.15. Sagittal ultrasound of the right kidney shows a hyperechoic lesion at the superior aspect of the kidney. Computed tomography examination demonstrated fat within the tumor, indicative of an angiomyolipoma. (Permission granted by Urologic Multimedia, Inc.)

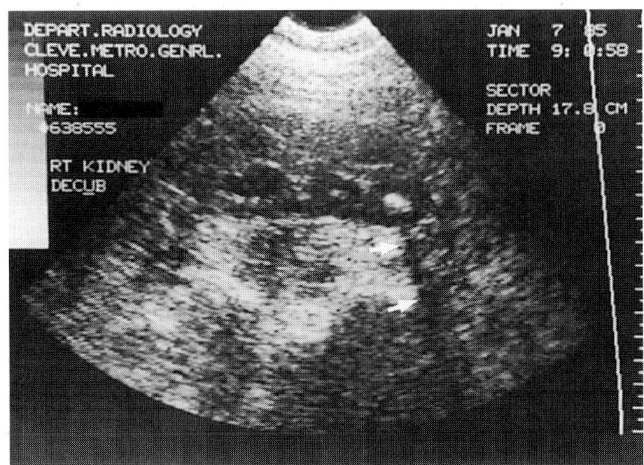

FIGURE 3D.16. Longitudinal scan demonstrating stone in the lower pole calyx. Stone is highly echogenic. Note area of acoustic shadowing *(arrows)*.

allowed assessment of the ureter and collecting system, which has been of value when other imaging studies have failed (118).

Renal Failure and Hydronephrosis

Although accounting for only 5% of all cases of renal failure, ureteral obstruction is potentially reversible and is usually accompanied by hydronephrosis. As a screening study to rule out obstruction as the cause of renal failure, ultrasound has a sensitivity approaching 100% (49,116). Patients with renal failure resulting from parenchymal disease characteristically have small kidneys with diffuse increases in echogenicity. Doppler studies also have been useful in monitoring the renal vasculature in both critically ill patients and those with renovascular disease (40,91). Color-flow studies with measurement of resistive index (RI) have been used to assess parenchymal viability in an attempt to differentiate those kidneys that are worth repairing from those with minimal chance of recovery that should be removed (13).

Studies also have indicated that minimum hydronephrosis can be substantial when there is a clinical question of the presence of renal obstruction (51). The renal sinus that normally appears as a region of intense echogenicity because of many dense interfaces becomes interspaced with hypoechoic regions with the development of hydronephrosis. These hypoechoic regions represent the dilated calyces and infundibula (Fig. 3D.18). As the dilation of the collecting system becomes more pronounced, this central echogenic region may be unidentifiable altogether (Fig. 3D.19). This finding aids in the diagnosis of longstanding hydronephrosis and parenchymal thinning. The dilated intrarenal collecting system can be imaged with longitudinal scans to reveal a dilated renal pelvis and, at times, upper ureter (Fig. 3D.20).

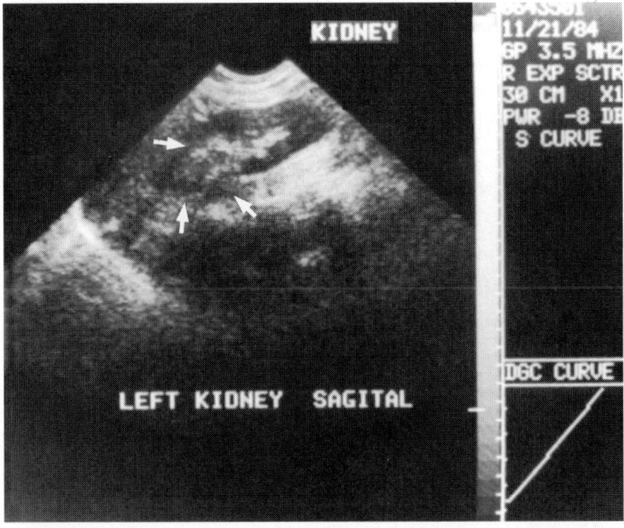

FIGURE 3D.17. Longitudinal renal scan demonstrating upper pole mass *(arrows)*. Surgical exploration revealed transitional cell carcinoma.

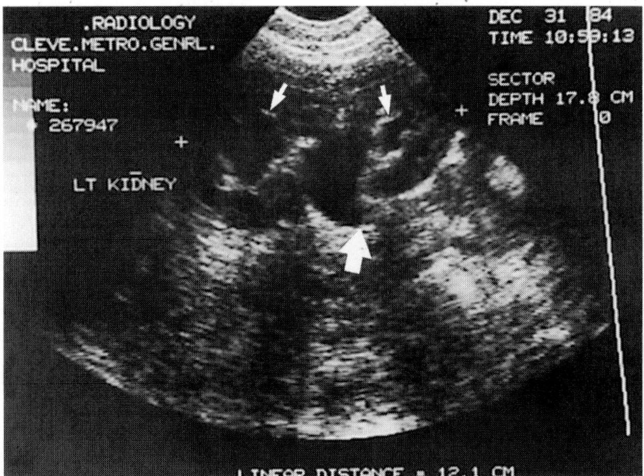

A

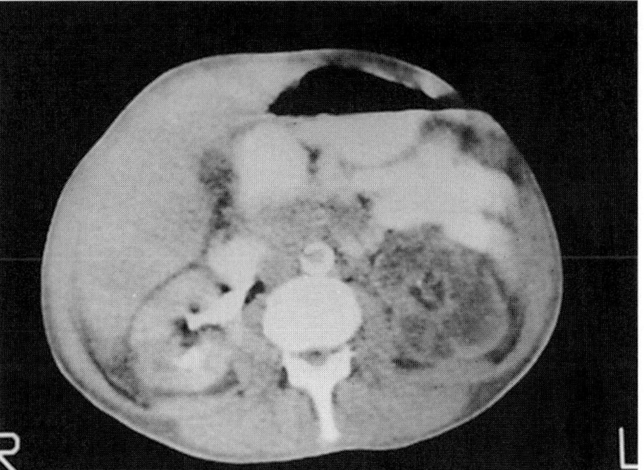

B

FIGURE 3D.18. A: Longitudinal scan demonstrating hydronephrosis secondary to ureteropelvic junction obstruction *(large arrow)*. Note dilated calyces *(small arrows)*. **B:** Computed tomography scan of same patient showing hydronephrotic kidney.

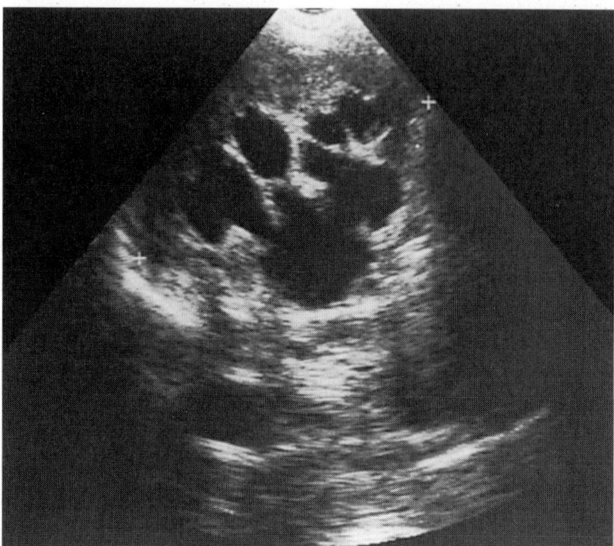

FIGURE 3D.19. Longitudinal scan demonstrating severe hydronephrosis with thinning of the renal parenchyma.

Lesions that may be misinterpreted as hydronephrosis include congenital megacalycosis, calyceal diverticulum, pelvic cysts, and a prominent extrarenal pelvis. False-positive studies can also be secondary to instances of high urinary output.

The assessment of the presence or absence of hydronephrosis has many implications in urologic practice. Although important in the evaluation of patients with impaired renal function, its assessment has application in evaluations made before and after treatment of many patients. Ultrasonography has been useful in the follow-up of patients after extracorporeal shock wave lithotripsy for the detection of hydronephrosis. Although abdominal radiographs are helpful in determining the presence of residual stone fragments, particularly in the ureter, ultrasound is a valuable adjunct in evaluating for the presence of hydronephrosis.

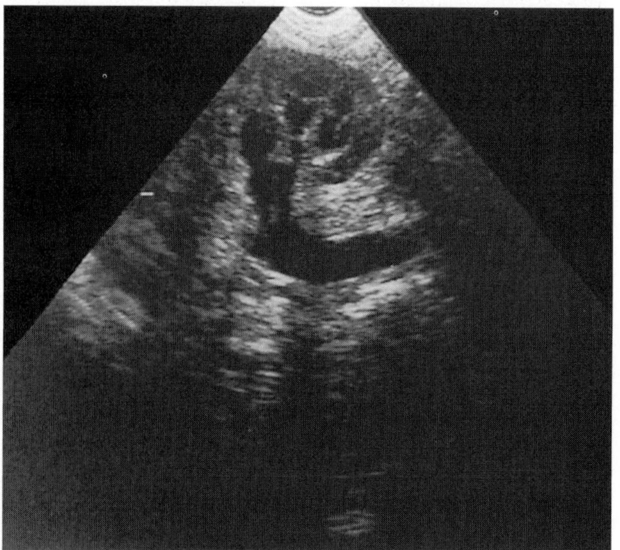

FIGURE 3D.20. Longitudinal scan demonstrating dilation of renal pelvis and upper ureter.

In addition, the technique is useful in follow-up of patients who have ureteral stones that are being observed and allowed to pass. The development or resolution of hydronephrosis can be easily assessed with this technique. False-negative studies can occur when urinary output is low or in instances when collecting system dilation is prevented by the presence of severe perineal and ureteral disease (e.g., inflammation, tumor).

Experience has indicated that Doppler studies are also useful in the evaluation of patients with acute renal obstruction. Changes in flow patterns and resistive indices are proving to be of increasing value to the clinician evaluating these patients (90,91,104). Other useful applications of ultrasonography relate to the postoperative follow-up of patients. Individuals undergoing urinary diversion or other surgical procedures on the urinary tract (e.g., pyeloplasty, ureteroneocystostomy) can be evaluated during the postoperative period to also assess for the development of resolution of preexisting hydronephrosis. Finally, the routine follow-up of patients with a variety of urologic disorders is improved with ultrasound assessment. Those with neurogenic bladders (e.g., spinal cord injury, myelomeningocele) can be assessed with this technique, as can those with malignancies (e.g., prostate carcinoma) and long-term postoperative patients (urinary diversion). Further evaluation and treatment can then be undertaken if hydronephrosis is detected.

RENAL TRANSPLANTATION

Because of its superficial position in the pelvis, the transplanted kidney is particularly well suited for ultrasound evaluation, which has also proved to be useful in evaluating posttransplant diminishing urine output. The short-term changes in renal volume associated with refection can usually be differentiated from an obstructive cause. It is also possible to detect the presence of perirenal hematomas, lymphoceles, and urinomas that may occur in the transplant patient.

Power Doppler and color-flow studies have been used to detect the presence of acute rejection. These studies have been helpful not only in the detection of acute rejection but also for the differentiation of acute rejection from the various other causes of renal failure (e.g., obstruction) (90,95,100,102,120).

PERIRENAL EVALUATION

Ultrasonography is useful in the evaluation of the perirenal space. Perirenal fluid collections may represent hematoma

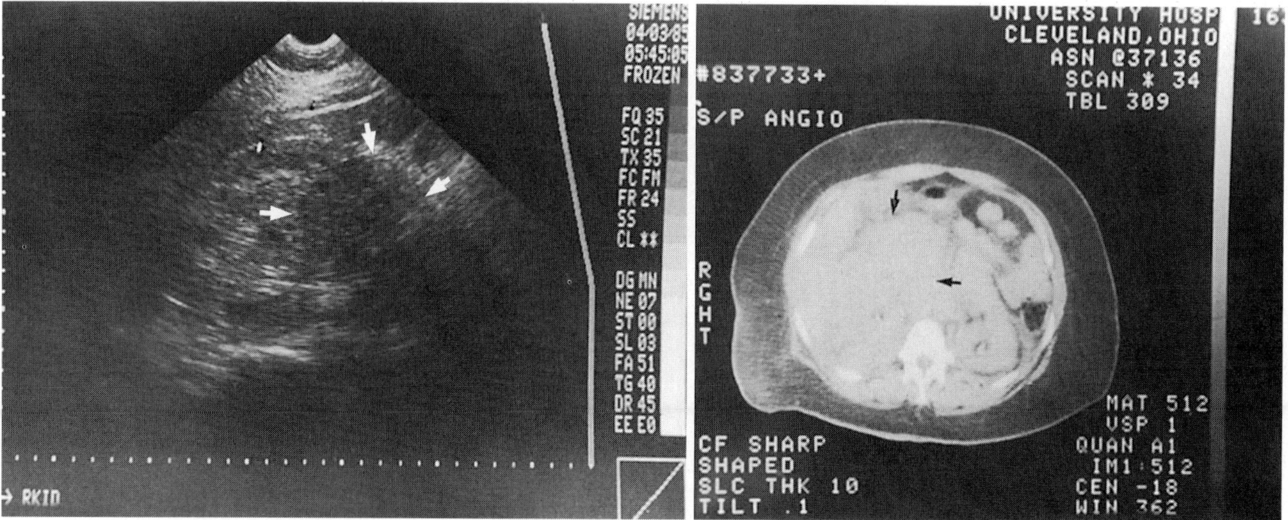

FIGURE 3D.21. **A:** Large perirenal hematoma after blunt abdominal trauma *(arrows).* **B:** Computed tomography scan of same patient.

or urinoma, which usually are associated with an antecedent history of trauma or prior renal surgery (Fig. 3D.21). Urinomas tend to be cystic, whereas hematomas may be solid, cystic, or a combination of both, depending on the stage of clot breakdown. Ultrasound offers an accurate, noninvasive, radiation-free means of following the presence and course of perinephric hematomas resulting from blunt trauma.

The presence of a perinephric abscess is usually suggested by a febrile course unresponsive to the usual antibiotic regimen. Sonographically, the perinephric collection appears as a complex mass with the internal architecture dependent on the amount and type of pus and the presence or absence of gas within the abscess (Fig. 3D.22). Ultrasound can be used to assist in percutaneous drainage of these collections, which in many instances has supplanted the need for open surgical procedures.

FIGURE 3D.22. Transverse scan showing complex perirenal mass, proved to be multiloculated perinephric abscess. Note multiple loculations *(arrows).*

SCREENING PROCEDURES

Renal ultrasonography has a role in the evaluation of suspected adult polycystic renal disease. The sonographic appearance is that of enlarged kidneys with randomly distributed cysts (Fig. 3D.23). Early cystic renal changes are ultrasonically visualized before any other signs or symptoms are apparent in affected individuals.

FETAL RENAL ULTRASOUND

Obstetric ultrasonography is often performed during the course of pregnancy and is useful in the evaluation of fetal size, gestational age, fetal lie, and placental position. Recent advances in ultrasound technology have improved the visualization of fetal anatomy and have led to increased identification of unsuspected congenital anomalies. Between 15 and 17 weeks of gestation, it is possible to identify the fetal kidneys by ultrasound approximately 50% of the time (58). By 20 weeks of gestation, it is unusual not to be able to identify the kidneys accurately. It is therefore currently possible to diagnose accurately the presence of in utero hydronephrosis; however, in most instances, it is impossible to differentiate its many etiologies: posterior urethral valves, primary megaureter (Fig. 3D.24), ureteropelvic junction obstruction, multicystic kidney (Fig. 3D.25), duplication anomalies with or without ureteroceles (Fig. 3D.26), vesicoureteral reflux, or prune-belly syndrome (22,28,50,127). The diagnosis of fetal hydronephrosis best serves to alert the

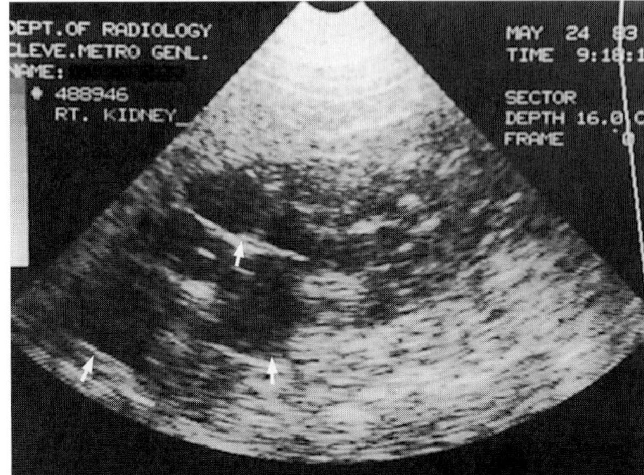

A

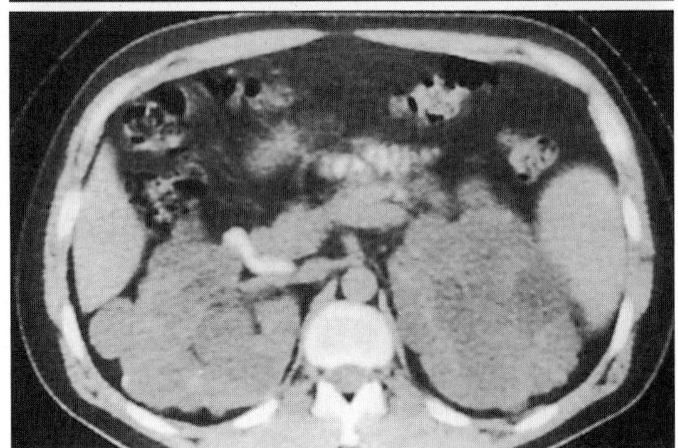

B

FIGURE 3D.23. **A:** Transverse scan showing multiple cysts *(arrows)* in an enlarged kidney. Changes typical of adult polycystic kidney disease. **B:** Computed tomography scan of same patient.

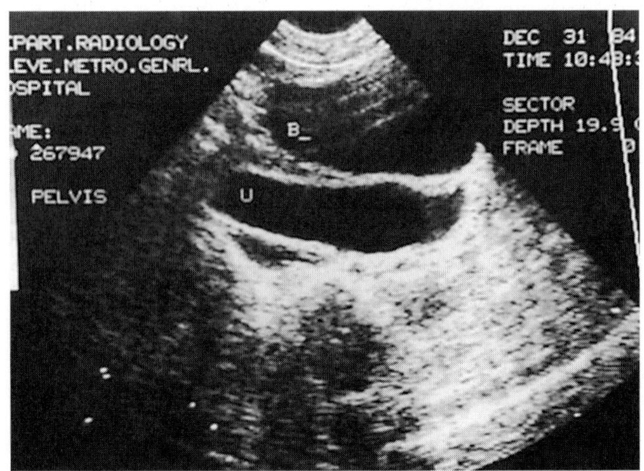

FIGURE 3D.24. Longitudinal pelvic scan showing dilated megaureter. B, bladder; U, ureter.

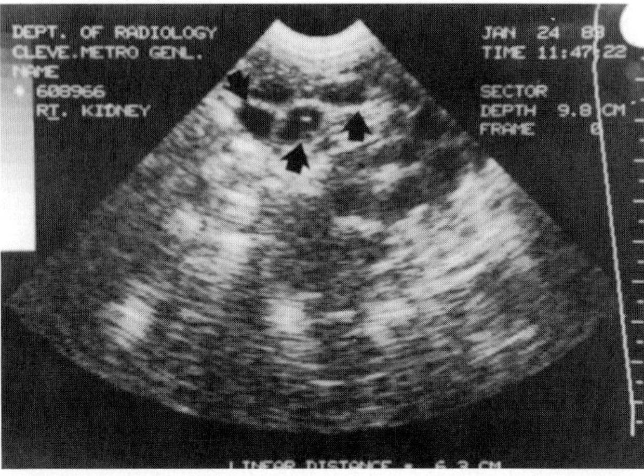

FIGURE 3D.25. Ultrasonic changes of multicystic kidney. Note multiple cysts *(arrows)*.

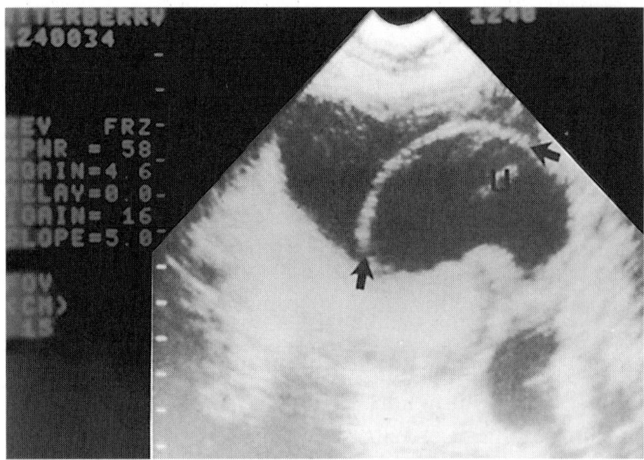

FIGURE 3D.26. Longitudinal scan of bladder demonstrating presence of ureterocele *(U)*. Note thin wall of ureterocele *(arrows)*.

primary physician to the need for additional urologic evaluation in the early neonatal period. When indicated, appropriate surgical intervention may be expeditiously performed.

RETROPERITONEAL SCANNING

The retroperitoneal space is a difficult area to examine with conventional radiographic methods, but it is well suited for sonographic studies. It is possible to identify lymph node enlargement, primary retroperitoneal tumors, and aortic aneurysms with a considerable degree of accuracy (Fig. 3D.27). Ultrasound may be helpful in determining the cause of ureteral deviation in patients with obstruction detected on excretory urography. In patients with retroperitoneal nodal metastases (e.g., testicular tumor), ultrasound

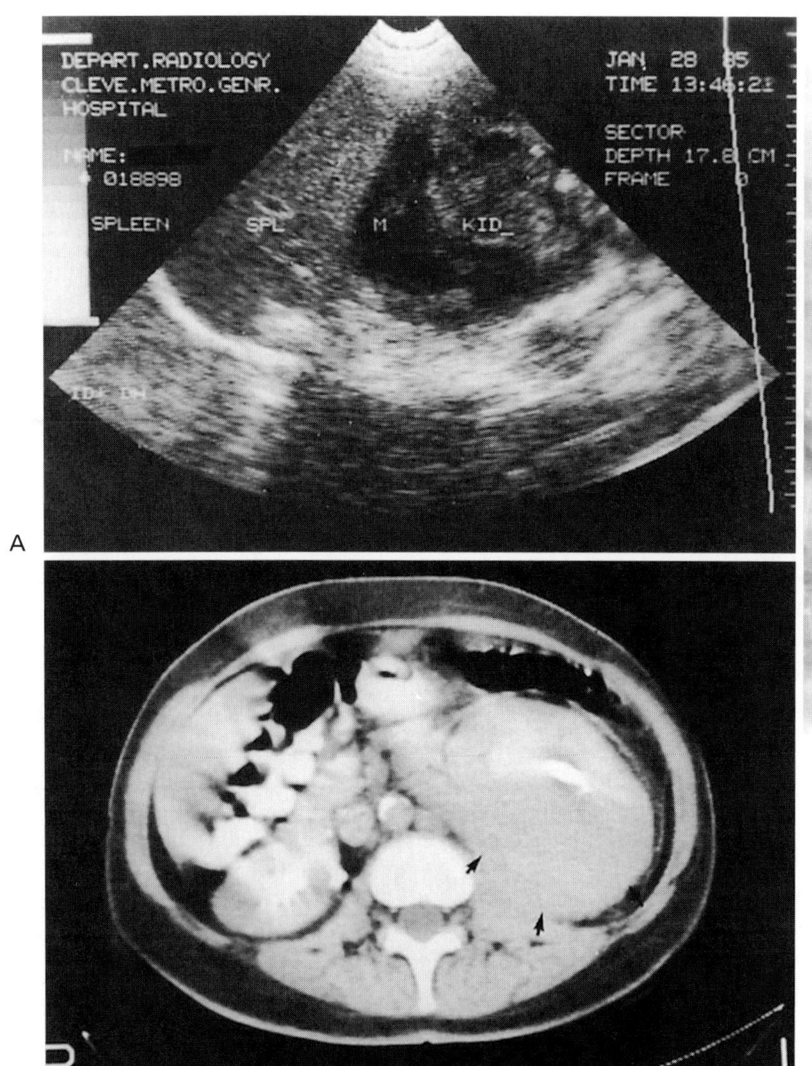

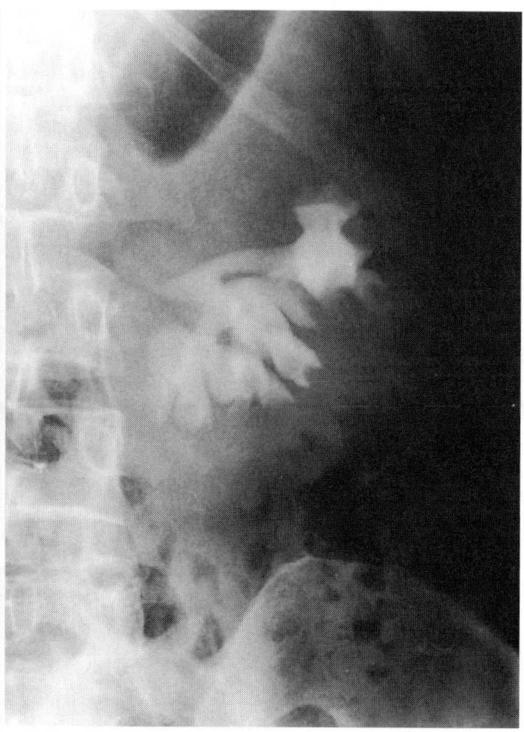

FIGURE 3D.27. A: Longitudinal scan of retroperitoneum demonstrating left perirenal mass. KID, kidney; M, mass; SPL, spleen. Surgical exploration revealed lymphoma. Intravenous urogram **(B)** and computed tomography **(C)** from same patient.

remains an excellent way to follow up the response to chemotherapeutic regimens without the risk of repeated radiation exposure. More commonly, CT studies are used to assess the retroperitoneum and in most instances are the primary studies used. When indicated, ultrasound-guided biopsies can be performed of suspicious structures. Ultrasound examination of the retroperitoneum also has been used to identify and locate accurately the undescended testicle. The study is helpful in identifying the inguinal testis, but it is less accurate in localizing the intraabdominal testis.

ULTRASONOGRAPHY OF THE ADRENAL GLAND

Because of their small size and protected location beneath the rib cage, it is often difficult to study the normal adrenal glands sonographically (9). Similarly, the evaluation of adrenal masses smaller than 3 cm is probably best performed with other radiographic techniques (e.g., CT, magnetic resonance imaging). Radionuclide and serum studies may also prove invaluable.

SCROTAL ULTRASONOGRAPHY

The superficial location and the maneuverability of the intrascrotal contents make the anatomic area well suited for sonographic evaluation. The primary use for scrotal ultrasound is in differentiating intratesticular lesions (tumors) from abnormalities arising from the paratesticular tissues. With the currently available high-frequency "small-parts" transducers, grayscale real-time techniques, and color-flow and power Doppler availability, a complete scrotal examination can be performed in minutes while providing excellent tissue resolution. The procedure is usually performed by first immobilizing the testicle with the free hand and then

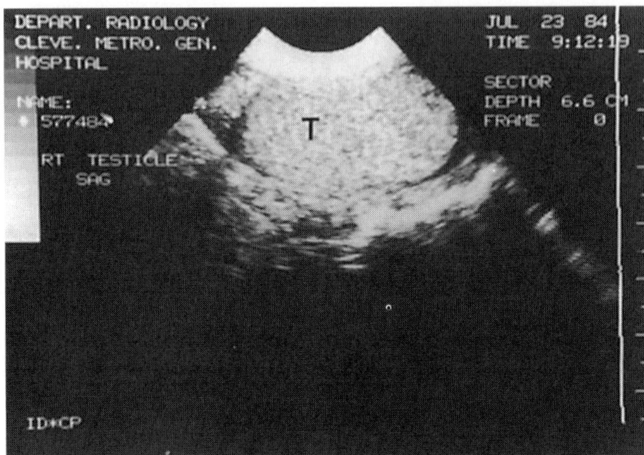

FIGURE 3D.28. Scrotal ultrasound showing sonographic appearance of normal testicle *(T).*

placing the transducer directly in contact with the scrotal skin. Mineral oil or acoustic gel is routinely used as a coupling agent to help reduce artifact (27).

Normal Ultrasonic Scrotal Anatomy

Sonographically, the scrotal wall appears as a hyperechoic strip 3 to 4 mm thick. Between the scrotal wall and the testicle is an anechoic area, usually no more than a few millimeters in width, which represents a small amount of fluid normally present between the visceral and parietal layers of the tunica vaginalis. The normal testicle measures about 4 by 3 by 3 cm and is characterized by a homogeneous, fine granular echo pattern (Fig. 3D.28). The tunica albuginea appears as a thin hyperechoic layer surrounding the testicle. Posteriorly, the tunica albuginea reflects into the testicle to form the mediastinum testis, a structure that usually is seen only with the newer small-parts transducers. The epididymis runs along the posterolateral aspect of the testicle. The head, or globus major, is seen above the superior pole of the testicle and, when normal, appears to be either hyperechoic or of the same echogenicity as the testicle. The body and tail of the epididymis sonographically appear as a coarser echo pattern than the testicle. The vas deferens, when visualized, appears as a circular hyperechoic area on transverse scans. Doppler and color-flow studies allow for assessing testicular perfusion, thus detecting vascular abnormalities associated with the spermatic cord. These studies have also been of value in the evaluation of patients with testicular trauma and intratesticular masses.

Applications of Scrotal Ultrasound

Patients with scrotal swelling and pain represent a diagnostic challenge and require prompt evaluation. Scrotal ultrasound has been helpful in differentiating the presence of inflammatory lesions (orchitis or epididymitis) from spermatic cord torsion, traumatic testicular disruption, and testicular or paratesticular tumors. Sonographically, epididymitis appears as a hypoechoic enlargement (inflammatory edema), usually involving the globus major. A reactive hydrocele may also be present (Fig. 3D.29). In the presence of epididymo-orchitis, the testicle adjacent to the involved epididymis may demonstrate areas. Individuals with presumed epididymo-orchitis who fail to respond to antibiotic therapy may demonstrate a testicular or scrotal abscess on ultrasound examination. When acute scrotal swelling occurs as a result of trauma, ultrasound has been helpful in differentiating testicular rupture from a normal testicle surrounded by hematoma (Fig. 3D.30). Acutely, the ischemic testicle is enlarged, with decreased echogenicity compared with the normal testicle. Color-flow studies can assess testicular perfusion and are invaluable in evaluating children with an acutely painful testicle (8,14,86,114). When properly

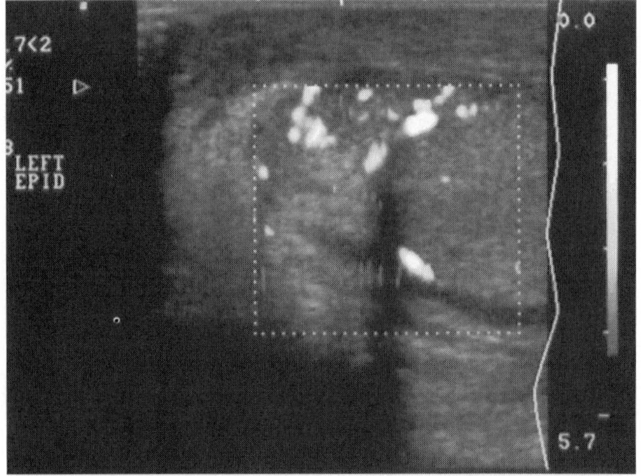

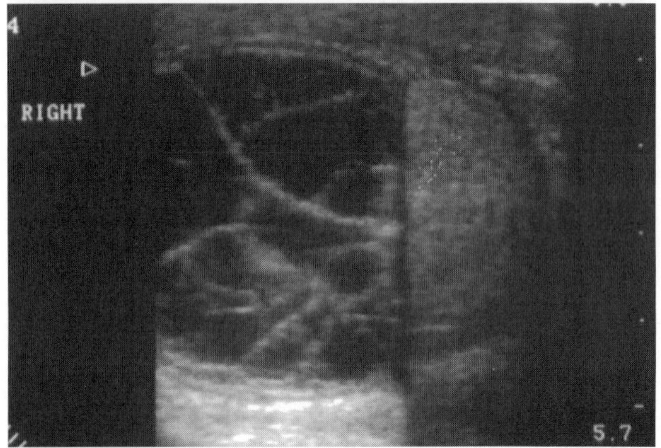

FIGURE 3D.29. A: Scrotal examination using power Doppler shows marked hyperemia involving a swollen left epididymis. These are typical features with acute epididymitis. **B:** Ultrasound of a different patient demonstrates a reactive hydrocele related to acute epididymitis. This shows a weblike pattern with multiple thick septations. (Permission granted by Urologic Multimedia, Inc.)

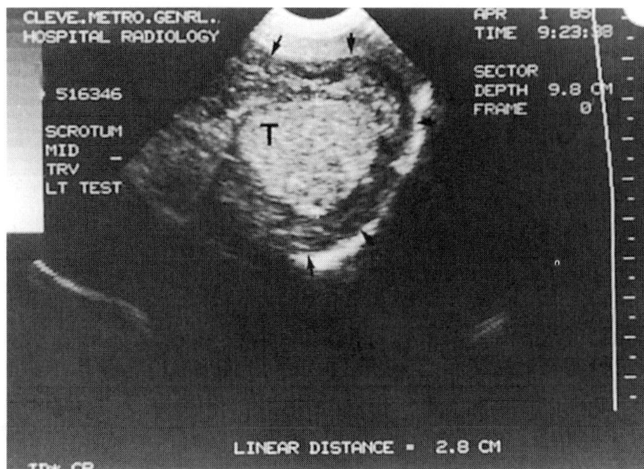

FIGURE 3D.30. Scrotal ultrasound demonstrating large hematoma *(arrows)* surrounding normal testicle *(T)*.

FIGURE 3D.32. Scrotal ultrasound demonstrating large inhomogeneous testicular mass *(arrows)*. Pathologic examination revealed embryonal cell carcinoma.

performed, these studies are as reliable as radionuclide imaging and approach an accuracy of 98%.

A *hydrocele* is a fluid collection that occurs between the visceral and parietal layers of the tunica vaginalis, making accurate testicular examination difficult to perform on physical examination. Scrotal ultrasound has been helpful in identifying hydroceles secondary to a malignant process. In the presence of a hydrocele, the quality of the testicular sonogram may be improved because of the fluid, which acts as a biologic water bath. Typically, a simple hydrocele appears as an anechoic area surrounding the testes anterolaterally (Fig. 3D.31). The presence of a hypoechoic inhomogeneous mass in the testicle is suggestive of a malignancy and warrants surgical exploration (Fig. 3D.32). Unlike embryonal cell carcinoma, seminoma sonographically has a more homogeneous pattern (Fig. 3D.33). Nonseminomatous testicular tumors often demonstrate increased flow on Doppler studies. Individuals with repeated bouts of epididymal infection may also have scrotal pain and swelling. Ultrasonically, a diagnosis of chronic epididymitis is suggested by an enlarged hyperechoic epididymis (Fig. 3D.34).

Scrotal ultrasound, particularly when combined with Doppler studies, has been helpful in identifying the subfertile male patient with a nonpalpable or subclinical varicocele (30,88). The clinical significance of the subclinical or nonpalpable varicocele continues to be debated. Testicular microlithiasis is usually bilateral and has been found to be associated with testicular malignancies and infertility (2,77). The disorder is usually identified incidentally and, when found without clinical evidence of malignancy, is followed with periodic ultrasound examinations. Ultrasound studies have also been used to assess postpubertal testicles having undergone prepubertal orchidopexy (121) and in following the remaining testes after unilateral orchiectomy for testicu-

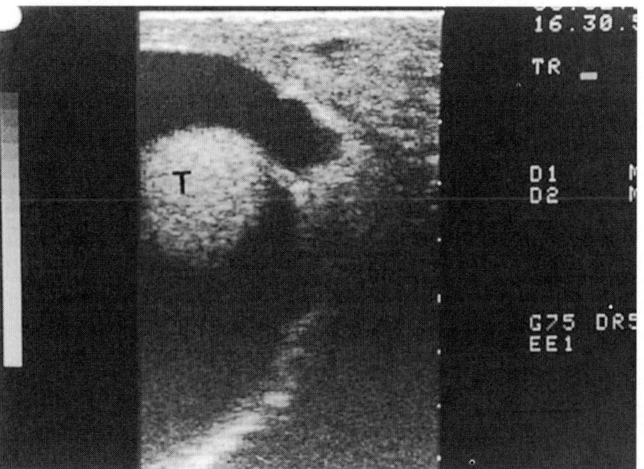

FIGURE 3D.31. Scrotal ultrasound demonstrating characteristic findings of normal testicle *(T)* surrounded by large hydrocele.

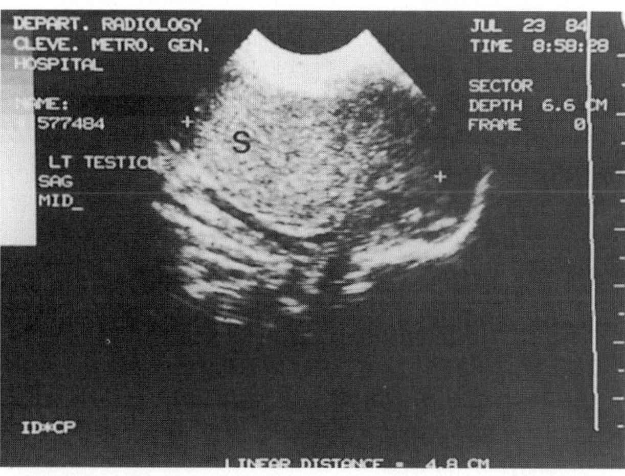

FIGURE 3D.33. Homogeneous testicular mass *(S)* pathologically proved seminoma.

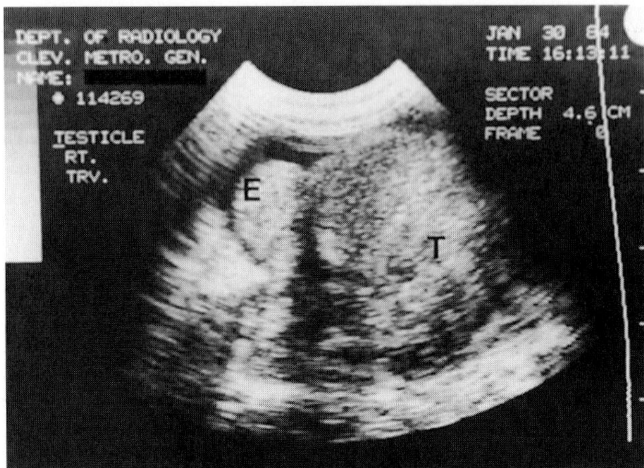

FIGURE 3D.34. Scrotal ultrasound demonstrating changes typical of chronic epididymitis. Note enlarged hyperechoic epididymis *(E)* and normal testicle *(T)*.

lar germ cell tumors (63). Ultrasonography has also been used to assess not only the location of undescended testes, but their histologic characteristics as well (6).

TRANSRECTAL ULTRASONOGRAPHY OF THE PROSTATE

Since its inception in the 1960s, abdominal and scrotal ultrasound has gained an important role in the evaluation of many urologic disorders. However, because of the relatively inaccessible pelvic location of the prostate, ultrasonic evaluation of this structure with conventional techniques has not been as widely accepted. In the late 1950s, Wild and Reid were the first to develop and test a transrectal ultrasonic probe (43). Although their initial experience with the transrectal approach resulted in visualizing only the rectal wall, the possible usefulness of this technique as a means to evaluate the lower urinary tract and particularly the prostate was clearly demonstrated. In 1964, Takahashi and Ouchi (115) used a transrectal probe equipped with a radial scanning device and obtained poor-quality tomographic pictures of the prostate, which had no clinical value. It was not until 1967 that Watanabe and associates (122,123) obtained the first clinically useful transrectal ultrasonic tomograms of the prostate. Since then, additional advances in instrumentation and technique have allowed for more reliable ultrasonic visualization of this pelvic organ. Today, the use of transrectal ultrasonography is helpful in the assessment of both benign and malignant disorders of the prostate and has been particularly valuable in biopsy and assessment of treatment of patients with carcinoma of the prostate.

Instrumentation

The transducer and its mechanism of action (mechanical sector and radial, array-linear, and phase) are important components of the current instrumentation used in this technology. Most transducers used for imaging the prostate vary in frequency from 6.0 to 7.5 MHz. This allows for excellent visualization of the posterior prostate, but because of the limited penetration of high-frequency sound, visualization of the anterior prostate is limited, especially when associated with significant enlargement. There is increasing interest in the role of color-flow Doppler studies; however, the utility of these studies continues to be debated (12,47,68,82,105). Different types of transducers are available, but most are typically biplanar and use radial or sector transducers. This allows imaging of the prostate in the transverse and sagittal planes. The transducer of the radial scanner rotates 360 degrees and propagates sound waves perpendicular to the long axis of the transrectal probe. Within the human body and with respect to the prostate gland, the sound waves are directed perpendicular to the long axis of the body and prostate. The direction is called *transaxial* or *axial,* and it is similar to the transverse plane of a CT image. Linear-array and mechanical sector scanners have eliminated the need for the rectal balloon, and the probe is placed in direct contact with the rectal wall. A decided advantage of these instruments is that transrectal prostate core biopsies and aspirations can be performed under ultrasonic guidance. In the phased-array scanner, many small transducers are aligned side by side, and when the scanner is oriented parallel to the long axis of the body, the sonographic images obtained are in the longitudinal or sagittal plane. Mechanical sector and phased-array scanners can provide images in either plane, and new biplanar probes incorporate both types of transducers in one unit.

Transverse images yield more information about the lateral margins and symmetry of the prostate, whereas longitudinal images delineate the apex and base of the gland more clearly. The longitudinal orientation appears to be more ideal for ultrasound guidance of prostate biopsy, even though the technique was first demonstrated with a radial scanner. Use of axial and longitudinal projections provides increased sensitivity in the examination of the prostate, and probes with both capabilities have been developed and will likely continue to be the standard.

Technique of Examination and Prostatic Biopsy

Technically, transrectal ultrasonography is minimally invasive and easy to perform. The entire examination takes 15 to 20 minutes and can be performed in the office on an outpatient basis without the need for anesthetics. Before beginning the examination, the clinician should perform a rectal examination to exclude the presence of anal or rectal abnormalities that may contraindicate transrectal probe insertion. In addition, a careful digital examination of the prostate should be undertaken. The examination may be performed with the patient in the lithotomy, lateral decubitus, knee-chest, or sitting position. Before performing the

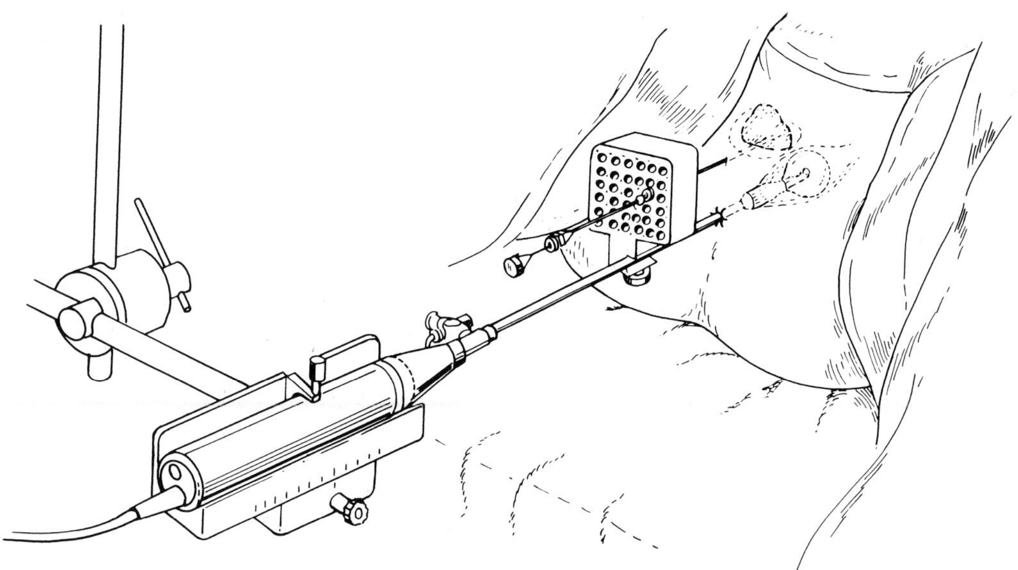

FIGURE 3D.35. Diagram demonstrating transperineal biopsy with radial transducer.

study a cleansing enema can be administered, but this is not necessarily done routinely. The transrectal probe is then inserted approximately 8 to 9 cm above the anal verge, and serial sonograms are obtained. It is important to perform the study systematically. When transverse images are obtained, sonograms are typically obtained at increments of 5 mm beginning at the bladder and seminal vesicles and progressing toward the apex. When a longitudinal scanner is used, images are obtained at increments of 5 degrees right and left of center. All images should be appropriately marked and hard copies obtained so that they may be referred to at a later date. Permanent records can be obtained with Polaroid film, multiple format cameras, thermal printers, videotape, laser disks, and computer floppy disks.

Applications

Over the past 10 years, significant advances have been made in the technology and methodology associated with transrectal ultrasonographically guided biopsies of the prostate. Although initial reports used the transperineal route (43), more recent experience has been with transrectal approaches (60). In addition, data are being obtained on the relative merits of both core and aspiration techniques (60). Spring-loaded devices also have been used in association with ultrasound-guided systematic or sextant core biopsies, and they have resulted in sampling of the prostate with a reduction in the pain associated with the procedure (117). Technologic improvements in ultrasound instrumentation have resulted in the development of transducers that permit viewing of the prostate in a variety of planes, which also has increased the accuracy of biopsy techniques (32,60).

Transperineal biopsies have generally been performed with the aid of radial or linear-array scanners (Figs. 3D.35 and 3D.36), but since the development of transrectal techniques, these procedures are performed rarely. The biopsy is performed under sterile conditions, and the perineum is cleansed and draped in the standard manner. Biopsies can be performed with the patient in either the lithotomy or lateral decubitus position, depending on the examiner's preference. When the radial scanner is used, often a grid with multiple holes is placed against the perineum and the site of needle entry corresponds to the grid that appears on the viewing screen (97). When an area of interest is imaged, the biopsy needle is inserted in the appropriate site on the

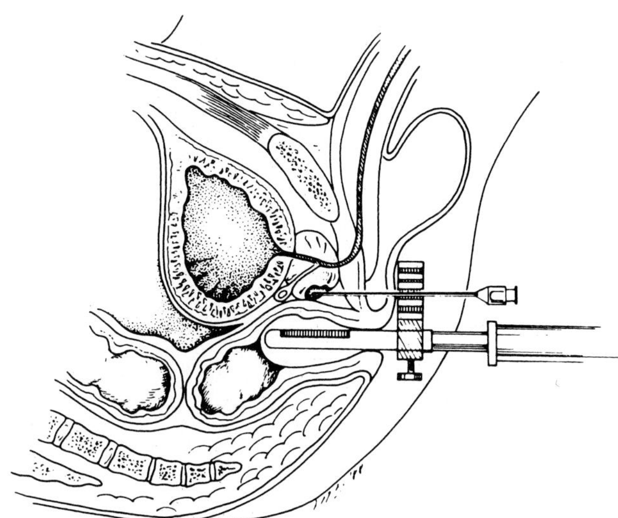

FIGURE 3D.36. Diagram demonstrating transperineal biopsy with linear-array transducer.

grid and the movement of the needle is monitored on the viewing screen. One of the disadvantages of this system is that the needle cannot be tracked or followed continuously during the entire biopsy. If care is not exercised, tissue may be obtained that is cephalad or caudad to the particular area to be sampled. This disadvantage can be overcome with the use of a linear-array transducer. It is of interest that the techniques developed for biopsy have recently been used for interstitial radiation of the prostate. The approach allows for accurate seed implantation, which is a treatment modality for carcinoma of the prostate that is being used with increasing frequency.

Transrectal biopsies are performed most commonly with a biplanar probe (Fig. 3D.37). Before performing the transrectal biopsy, many clinicians prefer to administer broad-spectrum oral antibiotics 1 hour before the procedure and to give the patient a cleansing enema. As with the transperineal biopsy, the procedure can be performed with the patient in either the lateral decubitus or the lithotomy position, based on the examiner's preference. Some clinicians use the knee-chest position because they believe the drainage of blood from the gland and associated collapse of prostatic and periprostatic veins improves the ultrasound image. Most of the newer instruments have markers that appear on the viewing screen when the transducer is in the biopsy mode, and these correspond to the path of the needle. Aligning the area from which a biopsy specimen is to be taken with these markers ensures that reliable biopsies can be obtained (Fig. 3D.38). Devices also have been developed for obtaining either aspiration or core biopsy. Although higher than with the perineal biopsy, the risk of sepsis remains low (less than 1%).

The normal prostate is viewed as a symmetric triangular ellipsoid structure that is delineated circumferentially by the continuous prostatic capsule (Fig. 3D.39). The capsule or margin is usually well defined, highly echogenic, continuous, and free of distortion. The anteroposterior diameter appears shorter than the transverse diameter because the posterior portion of the prostate becomes concave as a result of compression by the probe during the examination. The internal sonographic structure of the prostate is composed of multiple fine diffuse homogeneous echoes that probably represent acoustic interfaces created by numerous glands that are present. The posterior peripheral zone can usually be delineated from the more anterior, fibromuscular stroma and the central and transition zones.

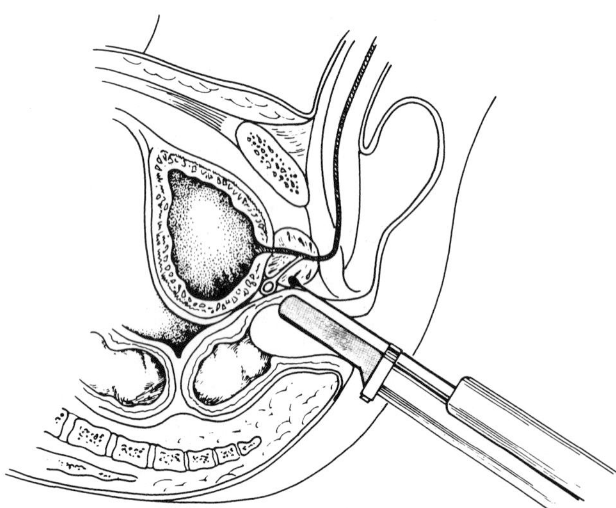

FIGURE 3D.37. Diagram demonstrating transrectal biopsy with end-fire multiplane probe.

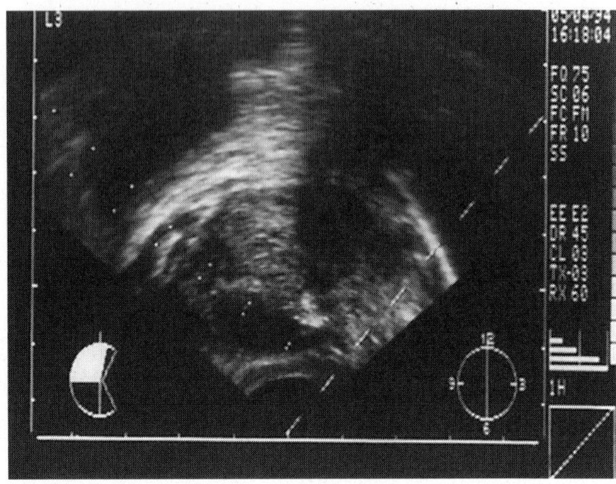

FIGURE 3D.38. Sagittal scan with markers indicating path of biopsy needle.

Benign prostatic hyperplasia is limited to the transition zone and appears as diffuse enlargement, with the greatest increase in size occurring in the anteroposterior diameter. The prostate margin remains well defined but thicker than is found in the normal gland. The hyperplastic portion of the gland consists of multiple fine homogeneous echoes believed to represent small adenomas located in fibrous tissue between glandular elements and multiple microcysts created by dilated prostatic ducts containing secretions, corpora amylacea, and microcalculi (Fig. 3D.40). Often, the transition zone that gives rise to benign prostatic hyperplasia can be differentiated from the more echogenic peripheral zone from which 70% of carcinomas arise. It is often difficult to distinguish the transition zone from the central zone in the presence of significant hyperplasia. Prostatic calculi, often present at the interface of the peripheral and transition zones, commonly can be identified by their marked echogenicity in association with typical "shadowing" (Fig. 3D.41).

Unlike the usual homogeneous sonographic appearance of the normal hyperplastic prostate, the ultrasonic characteristics of carcinoma of the prostate are varied. Early studies with B-mode and initial gray-scale imaging reported that prostate cancers appeared as echo-dense or hyperechoic areas (52). With improvement in instrumentation and the

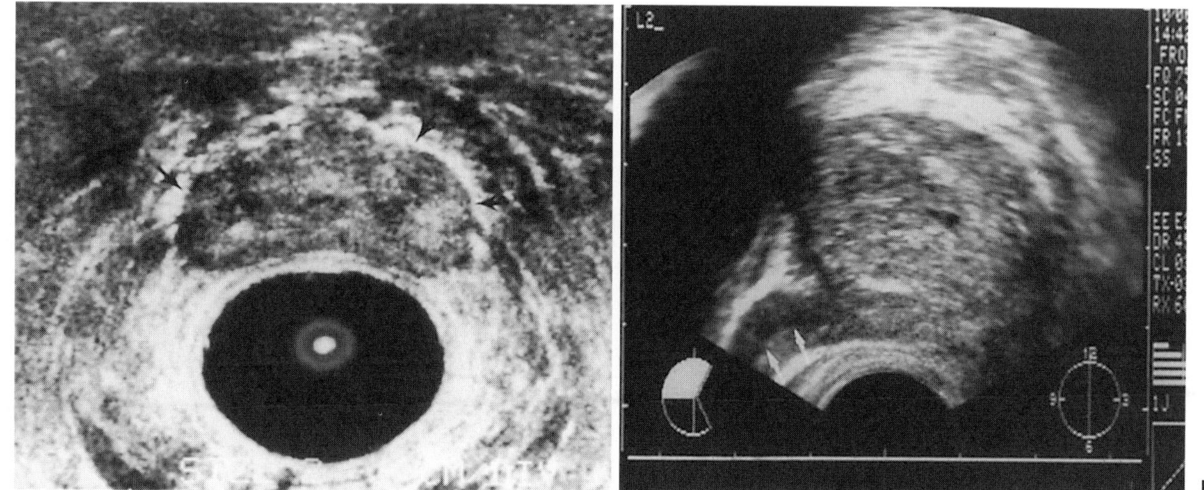

FIGURE 3D.39. **A:** Transverse image of normal prostate. **B:** Sagittal image of normal prostate. Note relationship of seminal vesicles *(arrows)* to prostate. Urinary bladder is to the left.

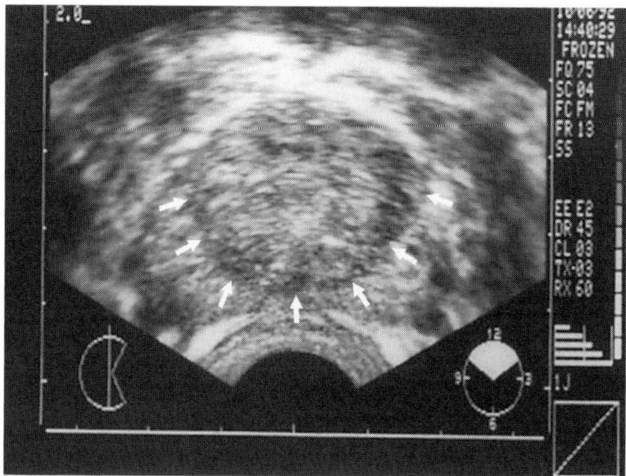

FIGURE 3D.40. Transverse image demonstrating typical appearance of benign prostatic hyperplasia. *Arrows* indicate transition zone border.

use of higher-frequency transducers, the appearance of tumors changed. Some investigators began to demonstrate that prostatic malignancies, particularly when they are small and localized, appear as hypoechoic areas located in the peripheral zone (Fig. 3D.42), but others demonstrated that tumors can be hyperechoic, hypoechoic, isoechoic, or of mixed echogenicity (24,59,98). There does not appear to be a reliable correlation between histologic grade and ultrasonic pattern other than the fact that small tumors that tend to be well differentiated often appear hypoechoic and larger, and high-grade tumors tend to have a mixed pattern. Isoechoic tumors tend to have a mixed pattern. Isoechoic tumors tend to be better differentiated. Newer, high-resolution equipment visualizes a prostate tumor as an echopenic focus before it obtains a more echogenic appearance. A desmoplastic reaction and associated calcification

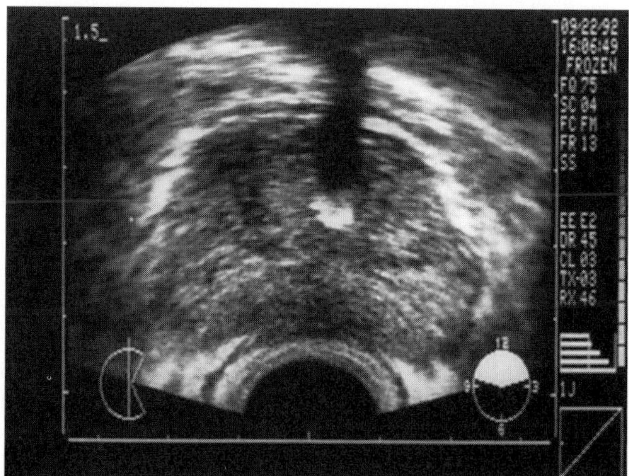

FIGURE 3D.41. Transverse image demonstrating hyperechogenicity and shadowing associated with prostatic calculi.

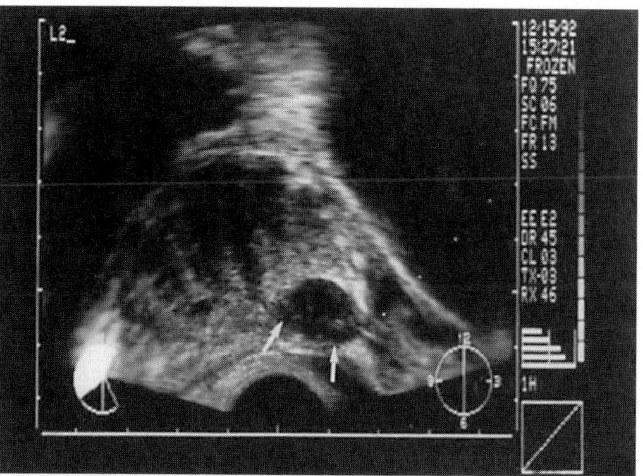

FIGURE 3D.42. Transverse image demonstrating appearance of peripheral zone hypoechoic carcinoma *(arrows)*.

are often associated with tumor growth and invasion. These changes may contribute to the mixed pattern observed with advanced tumors (99).

Unfortunately, many structures and benign processes within the prostate can have ultrasonic characteristics similar to the hypoechoic appearance of small prostate malignancies, including small nodules of hyperplasia, cysts, infarcts, inflammatory processes, cystic atrophy, blood vessels, and muscle tissue. Many carcinomas are isoechoic and cannot be imaged with this technique. In addition, anterior tumors often cannot be distinguished reliably from the normally hypoechogenic appearance of this region of the gland.

Improvements in technology have resulted in the development of newer devices that may improve the ability of ultrasonography to detect and stage prostate malignancies. Color Doppler, power Doppler, ultrasound contrast agents, and three-dimensional studies have all been used, but unfortunately, none has been able to locally determine the extent of disease once the diagnosis of carcinoma has been established (26,33,68,82,105).

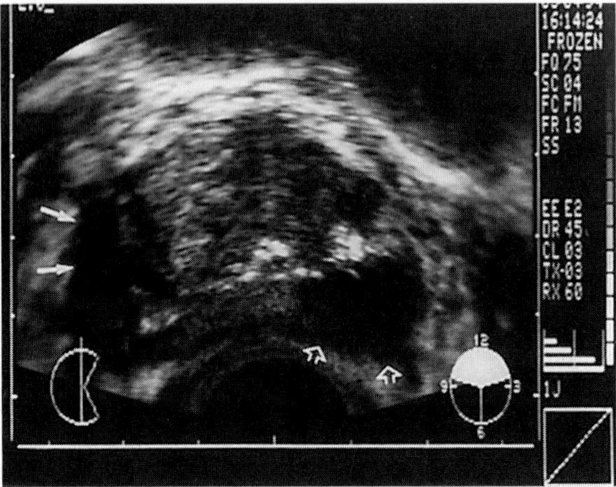

FIGURE 3D.43. Transverse image demonstrating distortion of border of prostate *(arrows)* associated with invasive carcinoma. Note hyperechogenicity of tumor.

Clinical Applications

Although transrectal prostatic ultrasonography has had its greatest use in the assessment of patients with carcinoma of the prostate, other applications include the evaluation of patients with both acute and chronic prostatitis and men with infertility (48). Experiences indicate that the technique is useful in the assessment and the detection of seminal vesicle abnormalities that may be associated with infertility, and ductal obstruction also has been confirmed with this technique.

Sekine and associates (108) have developed a transrectal electronic linear-array scanner that allows one to obtain longitudinal sonograms of the lower urinary tract. With real-time imaging, dynamic studies obtained while the patient is voiding may provide valuable diagnostic information on voiding dysfunction (87,109).

Staging

Transrectal ultrasonography has been useful in the evaluation of patients already diagnosed as having carcinoma of the prostate. The technique is valuable in assessing prostatic size and in detecting unrecognized invasive disease. Early reports show that the stage of prostatic carcinomas, as determined by transrectal ultrasonography, corresponded with the stage diagnosed pathologically on radical prostatectomy specimens (Fig. 3D.43). Pontes and associates (94) demonstrated a sensitivity of 89% and 100% for preoperative ultrasonic detection of capsular and seminal vesicle involvement, respectively. The specificity of detecting capsular penetration and seminal vesicle involvement was only 50% and 28%, respectively, because of the inability of the study to detect microscopic disease. Fujino and Scardino (34) reported the ability of ultrasound to detect invasive disease in 8 of 18 patients who had no extension of the disease by rectal examination. Lee and colleagues (61) introduced the concept of obtaining biopsy specimens from areas with a high probability of invasion, such as the apex and point at which the seminal vesicles enter the central zone. Areas of microscopic invasion that were not evident on digital rectal or routine ultrasound examination have been detected. More recent experience has indicated that ultrasound staging is limited, and its value in clinical decision making remains questionable (4,66,101,112). Others have attempted to characterize specific components of the tumor to assist in ultrasound staging, but the value of this methodology is limited (119).

Measurement of Prostate Gland Size

Transrectal ultrasonography is useful in documenting prostate gland volume, and it is accurate within 5% in determining true prostatic weight (39). This ability allows ultrasound to provide information regarding the response of the tumor to therapy. These determinations are based largely on total gland volume and not tumor volume. Prostate ultrasonography has documented reduction in prostate size after administration of endocrine therapy when used as treatment for patients with disseminated cancer. Within 3 to 6 months after either orchiectomy or estrogen therapy, a sonographically detectable 20% to 30% decrease in prostate volume occurs (17,96). Changes with estrogen therapy are slightly slower to occur than those with surgical castration.

Further usefulness of ultrasound has been demonstrated in the evaluation of prostate cancer patients treated with radiotherapy and chemotherapy. Studies have indicated that the maximum reduction in the size of the prostate occurs usually by 9 months after radiotherapy and 3 months after chemotherapy (34). As a response to therapy, in addition to decrease in size, the prostate resumed a more symmetric shape, the margin reformed and thickened, the degree of extracapsular extension diminished, and the seminal vesicles became normal in appearance. These techniques also have been used to measure prostatic size to document response to endocrine agents (e.g., 5α-reductase inhibitors) in the treatment of benign prostatic hyperplasia. A similar reduction in prostate size has been recognized.

Ultrasound-guided Biopsy, Interstitial Radiation Therapy, and Cryotherapy

As noted, transrectal prostatic ultrasonography is useful as an aid in the placement of the biopsy needle within a specific suspicious area of the prostate. Transrectal ultrasonically guided biopsies are widely used (Fig. 3D.44), and new aspiration and core biopsy needles with spring-load guns continue to be developed. Problems exist because not all tumors can be visualized ultrasonically, and more studies are required to correlate the area of the ultrasound biopsy with the physical findings. Hodge and colleagues (42) used ultrasound-guided biopsy to ensure accurate placement of the biopsy needle in the peripheral zone of the prostate. Multiple "systematic" biopsies are performed, and with this approach, more than 50% of patients with palpable abnormalities (e.g., firm areas, nodules) have been diagnosed as having carcinoma. It has also been recognized that the larger the prostate, the lower the yield in establishing a diagnosis of carcinoma (64). Ultrasound-guided biopsies have a role in the evaluation of patients with or suspected of having prostate cancer [e.g., abnormal digital rectal examination, elevated or change in prostate-specific antigen (PSA)].

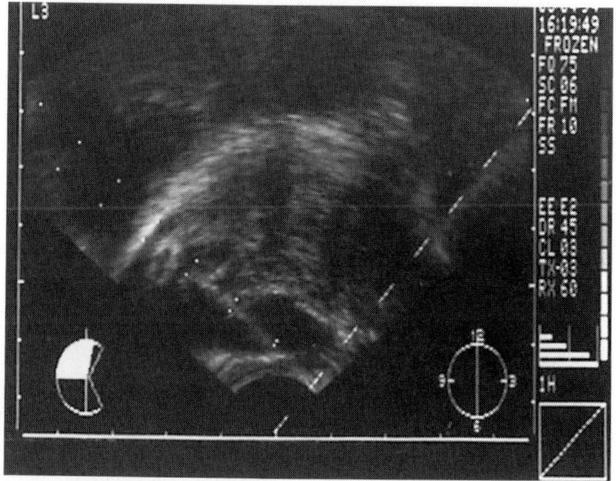

FIGURE 3D.44. Sagittal image with biopsy guide with visualization of hyperechoic needle demonstrating the use of ultrasound guidance to assist in a biopsy.

Repeat ultrasound-guided biopsies after a negative digitally directed biopsy are thought to be worthwhile in patients with suspicious palpable abnormalities. In patients with nonpalpable but suspected prostate malignancy (e.g., elevated PSA), ultrasound-directed biopsy of sonographically suspicious areas or when performed in a sextant manner has been shown to assist in establishing the diagnosis of prostate cancer. Experience indicates that the diagnosis of cancer can be increased by obtaining a greater number of cores (e.g., more than six) and by performing biopsies on more lateral aspects of the prostate to enhance sampling of the peripheral zone. In addition, the technique has a role in the evaluation of patients treated with definitive radiation therapy who have no palpable abnormalities, but suspicion of recurrence based on change in serum PSA.

As noted earlier, ultrasound can also be used to direct radioactive seed implantation into the prostate when using this treatment modality (44). Permanent implantation of radioactive seeds offers some advantages over external beam radiation, and the implantation technique is less time-consuming for the patient and staff than a full course of external beam therapy. In addition, a higher concentration of seeds can be placed in and around the area of malignancy. The disadvantage of this technique is that extracapsular tumors with ill-defined margins may not be irradiated adequately and that regional lymphatic vessels are not treated appropriately. These problems may be overcome by combining interstitial therapy with external beam or endocrine therapy. Studies are in progress to assess these alternatives. Ultrasound has also been used to monitor the "ice ball" during cryoablation for treating prostatic malignancies. The monitoring not only ensures adequate treatment of the malignancy but also helps protect the rectum from injury.

Its important to recognize that ultrasound is unable to visualize a significant number of tumors located within both the peripheral and transition zones. In addition, the presence of these tumors may only be suggested by the finding of an elevated PSA with a prostate that may be free of palpable abnormalities. Ultrasound may be useful in assisting in biopsy, but ultrasound should not be used as a discriminator as to who should or should not be biopsied. This decision should be made on the basis of clinical indications (i.e., abnormal digital rectal examination or elevated serum PSA).

ULTRASONOGRAPHY OF THE URINARY BLADDER

The urinary bladder is an extraperitoneal musculomembranous sac that functions primarily as a urinary storage reservoir. In children younger than 6 years of age, the bladder is predominantly an intraabdominal organ lying beneath the anterior abdominal wall. In adults, it is a pelvic organ lying, when empty, beneath the symphysis pubis. When dis-

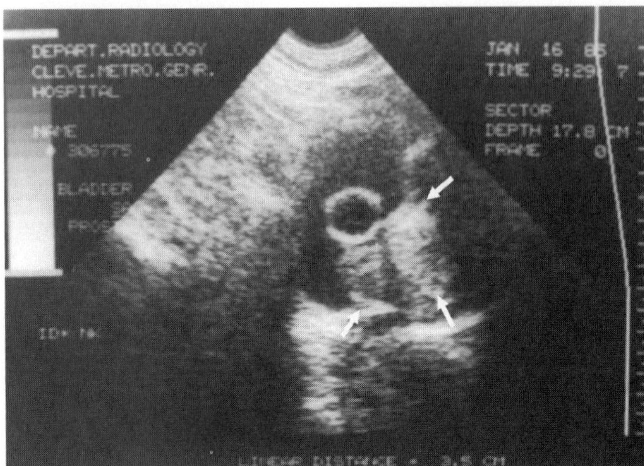

FIGURE 3D.45. Longitudinal abdominal scan showing urinary bladder and enlarged prostate *(arrows)*. Note Foley catheter balloon at the bladder neck.

tended, the bladder assumes a globular shape and is easily studied with the transabdominal approach. Recently, transrectal and transurethral approaches have been used to study and define subtle bladder abnormalities.

Transabdominal Scanning

Transabdominal ultrasound imaging of the bladder is usually performed with the patient in the supine position and the bladder distended. Although it is not necessary to have a Foley catheter in place, its presence is helpful in identifying the bladder neck (Fig. 3D.45). Usually, a 3.5-MHz transducer is used to obtain transverse and longitudinal images.

Transrectal Scanning

Transrectal ultrasonic imaging of the bladder is performed with the same equipment and technique as previously described (Fig. 3D.46).

Transurethral Scanning

Although both transabdominal and transrectal approaches have been helpful in evaluating bladder abnormalities, subtle changes in the bladder wall (e.g., muscular invasion by tumors) are often not discernible. Experience by Gammelgaard and Holm and others suggests that the bladder may be best studied with the transurethral approach (80).

The scanner for transurethral ultrasonography consists of a motor that rotates a long rod, which is connected at the opposite end to an interchangeable transducer. The scanner fits within a standard resectoscope sheath and is interchangeable with the usual optical system. Two 5.5-MHz transducers are available. One emits the ultrasonic beam at 90 degrees to the instrument, whereas the other emits the beams at 135 degrees to the probe in retrograde fashion and is useful in studying the bladder neck region. With these two transducers, complete visualization of the entire bladder is possible. Probes with multiple and variable angulations are also available. During routing cystoscopy, when further evaluation of a detected bladder lesion is desired, the telescope is removed from the sheath and is replaced with the sterilized scanner. Dynamic scans using the transducers are obtained. The entire bladder wall can be rapidly scanned in a matter of minutes.

Normal Bladder

Ultrasonically, the normal bladder appears as a globular structure, the shape of which varies depending on the patient's position and degree of distention. The bladder wall is hyperechoic and appears as a symmetric, smooth surface. When distended, the fluid-filled bladder is anechoic (Fig. 3D.47).

Clinical Application

Bladder tumors are a common urologic problem, the treatment of which depends on an accurate assessment of the grade of the primary tumor. With currently available staging modalities, errors may occur in nearly 50% of cases (10). Large, exophytic tumors appear ultrasonically as echogenic masses projecting into the lumen of the echo-free bladder (Fig. 3D.48). These areas are fixed to the wall; unlike blood clots or stones, they do not move as the patient changes position. Ureteroceles, although fixed to the bladder wall, are easily recognized by their thin echogenic wall surrounding a relatively anechoic center. Bladder stones readily move about with changes in intravesi-

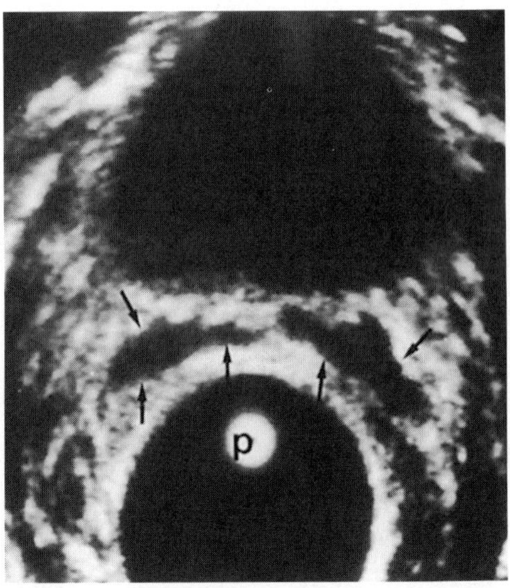

FIGURE 3D.46. Transrectal scan of normal bladder and seminal vesicles *(arrows)*. Rectal probe *(p)* is in place.

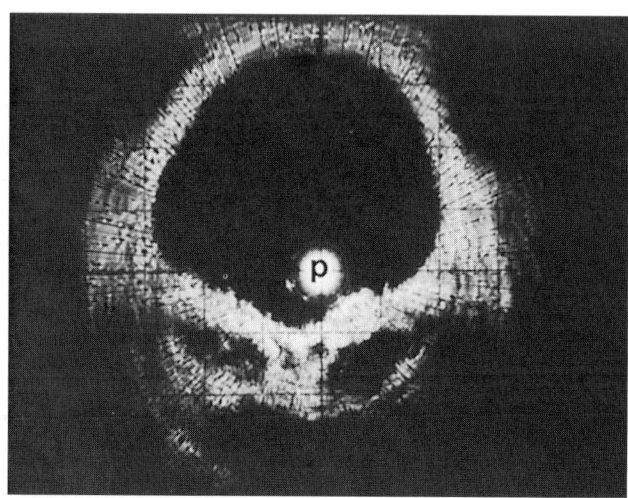

FIGURE 3D.47. Transurethral scan of normal urinary bladder. Note seminal vesicles posterior to the bladder. p, transurethral probe.

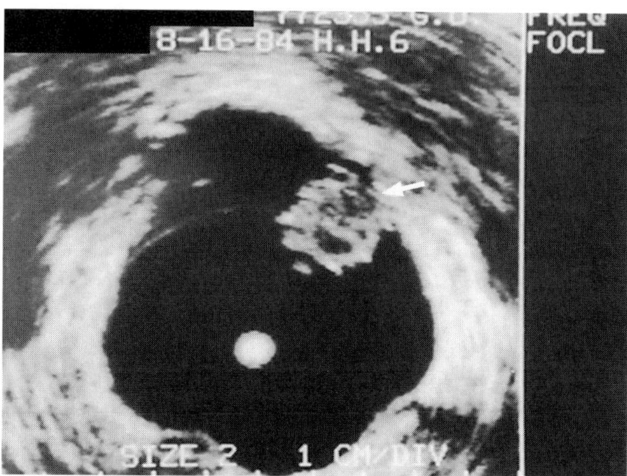

FIGURE 3D.49. Transurethral bladder scan demonstrating superficial bladder tumor. Note lack of bladder wall invasion *(arrow).*

cal volume and patient position, and like renal stones, they appear as dense hyperechoic areas associated with sonic shadowing.

Superficial bladder tumors or minimally infiltrative tumors (stage T_1 or T_2) do not cause distortion or fixation of the bladder wall, and they demonstrate a well-defined base (Figs. 3D.49 and 3D.50). Multiple scans obtained during bladder filling demonstrate free movement of the bladder wall.

Infiltrative tumors tend to be broad based, and the bladder wall may be fixed and distorted. Stage T_3 tumors that have completely extended through the bladder wall are visualized as an extravesical mass (Fig. 3D.51).

Probably the most common use of bladder ultrasonography has been in the estimation of residual urine in patients with voiding disorders. The study is helpful in estimating total bladder capacity and postvoid residual urine when urethral instrumentation is not desired or is contraindicated (16,79,103). The most commonly used formula is that of a prostate ellipse:

$$\text{Volume} = 0.5 \times \text{Diameter}_1 \times \text{Diameter}_2 \times \text{Diameter}_3$$

where $diameter_1$ is width, $diameter_2$ is height, and $diameter_3$ is length.

When these measurements are used, the correlation between catheterized and estimated residual volume has been

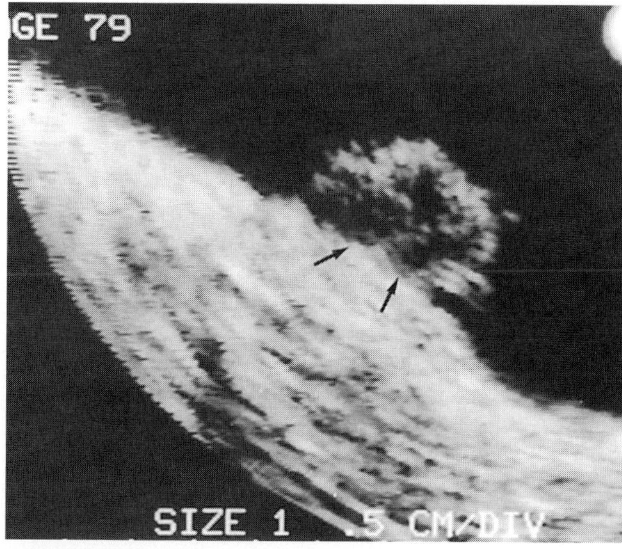

FIGURE 3D.48. Transurethral bladder scan demonstrating large, exophytic bladder.

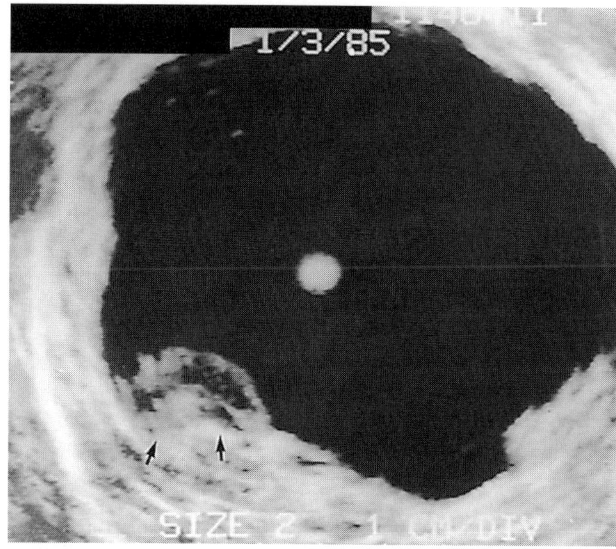

FIGURE 3D.50. Transurethral bladder scan demonstrating minimally invasive tumor *(arrows).*

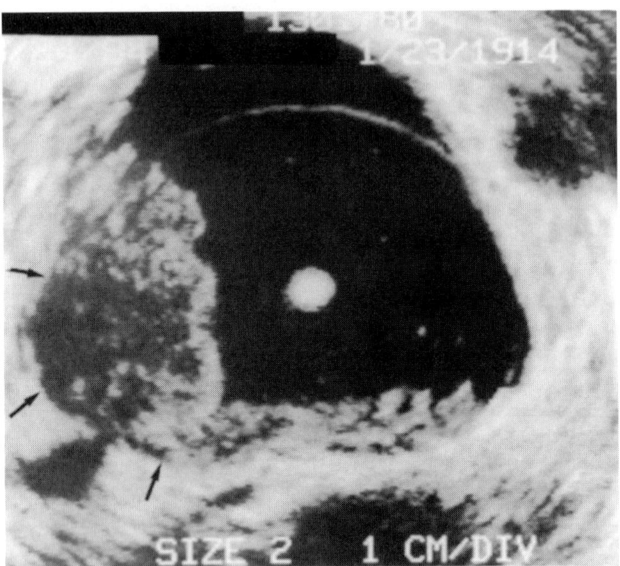

FIGURE 3D.51. Transurethral bladder scan demonstrating tumor invasion beyond bladder wall *(arrows).*

reported to be as high as 98%. A three-dimensional device was recently described for this purpose (70).

Other applications include assessment of patients for vesicoureteral reflux (23,36,124) and increasingly assessment of abnormalities in bladder structure and function. Although limited, perineal and transvaginal ultrasonography has been reported to be of assistance in identifying the presence of vesicovaginal fistula (1,125). The technique of "video urodynamics" has been used with Doppler sonography (84,85), and urethral abnormalities have also been identified in assessing patients with stress urinary incontinence and other urethral disorders (7,31,56,57). It is likely that with continued technologic improvements these studies will be expanded because of their availability and cost-to-benefit ratio.

PENILE ULTRASONOGRAPHY

Ultrasonography of the penis has been used primarily in three clinical areas: assessment of Peyronie's disease, evaluation of urethral strictures, and assessment of impotence. This latter category is discussed in detail in the chapter related to the assessment of men with erectile dysfunction.

Peyronie's disease is an uncommon problem that is related to the excessive deposition of collagen and associated calcium in the tunica albuginea of the corpus cavernosum. Patients usually have pain and deformity of the penis associated with erection, and on physical examination a palpable area of "plaque" is often evident. Ultrasound has been used to visualize the area of fibrosis, and shadowing often can be noted secondary to the areas of calcification. Correlation has also been noted with xeroradiography (3,21). The ultrasound studies may have a role in the diagnosis of the condition but possibly may have a more important one in documenting progression or regression of the areas of abnormality.

Another interesting application of penile ultrasonography relates to the assessment of the distal male urethra. Experience has indicated that this technology is useful in the assessment of patients for urethral strictures, and excellent correlative data have been obtained with standard radiographic urethrography. An advantage of this technique is that the periurethral tissue can be seen clearly, and it is believed that this method of imaging may allow for a more informative decision regarding the most appropriate treatment of urethral stricture (19,20,35,76). Other interesting applications relate to imaging of urethral calculi (113).

Doppler ultrasound studies are widely used in the assessment of men with erectile dysfunction. Both inflow and outflow abnormalities can be readily identified. The penile arteries can be readily identified with current technology and changes in flow identified following intracorporeal injection with vasoactive agent. Recent experience also indicates these studies may be of value in determining the role of oral agents in treating patients with erectile dysfunction (20,25,41,73,78,83,106).

INTRAOPERATIVE ULTRASONOGRAPHY

Intraoperative real-time renal scanning displays a cross section of renal tissue and, using multiple images, allows accurate, three-dimensional stone localization. Most intraoperatively used portable ultrasound units use a frequency of 7 to 10 MHz and are modifications of the small ophthalmic ultrasound probe. The study is of value when performing open stone surgery. After adequately mobilizing the kidney, it is scanned in multiple planes until the stone is identified by its characteristic dense echo pattern and the presence of acoustic shadowing (Fig. 3D.52). Fine-needle probes are then passed to the stone and a nephrotomy made directly over the stone. With this technique, an experienced ultrasonographer can identify stones 2 mm or more in diameter.

Ultrasound probably has greater application at time of partial nephrectomy when removing small renal malignancies. Assimos and associates (5) reported the role of intraoperative ultrasonography in assisting in partial nephrectomy in patients with small renal tumors. The study is helpful in delineating the location and extent of these lesions. An additional application used intraoperative ultrasound to assess tumor involvement of the renal vein in patients with adrenal malignancy (67). More recently, ultrasonography has been used in association with laparoscopic cryoablation of renal malignancies. Ultrasound can monitor the formation of the "ice ball," thus ensuring adequate treatment (126).

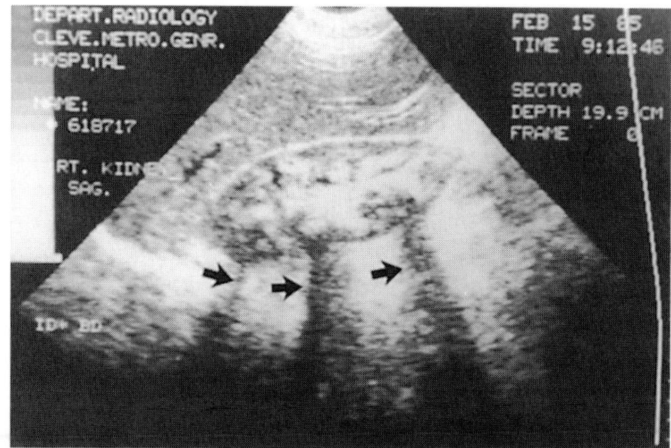

A

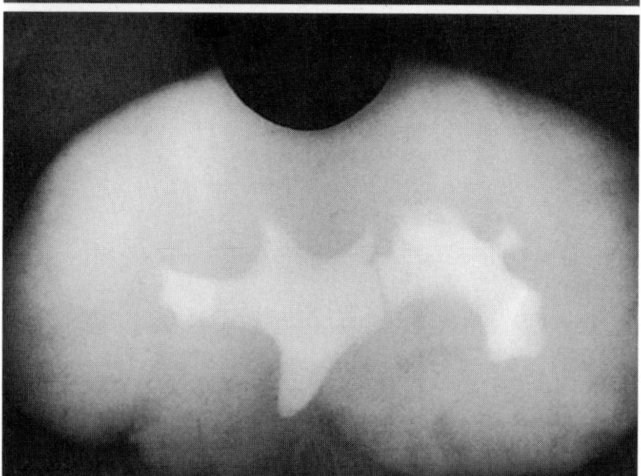
B

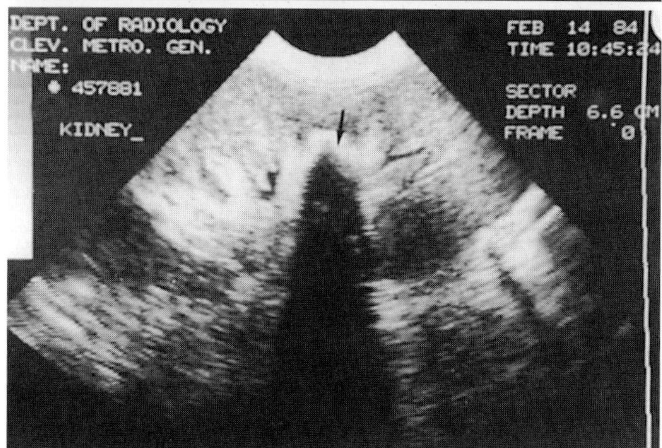

C

FIGURE 3D.52. A: Preoperative renal scan of large staghorn calculus. Note multiple areas of acoustic shadowing *(arrows).* **B:** Intraoperative radiograph before nephrotomy. **C:** Intraoperative ultrasound localizing small retained stone fragment *(arrow).*

REFERENCES

1. Abulafia O, Cohen HL, Zin DL, et al. Transperineal ultrasonographic diagnosis of vesico-vaginal fistula. *J Ultrasound Med* 1998;17:333.
2. Aizenstein RI, Didomenico D, Wilbur AC, et al. Testicular microlithiasis: association with male infertility. *J Clin Ultrasound* 1998;26:195.
3. Altaffer LF, Jordan GH. Sonographic demonstration of Peyronie's plaques. *Urology* 1981;17:292.
4. Andriole GL, Copten DE, Mikkelsen DJ, et al. Sonographic and pathological staging of patients with clinically localized prostatic cancer. *J Urol* 1989;142:1259.
5. Assimos DG, Boyce WH, Woodruff RD, et al. Intraoperative renal ultrasonography: a useful adjunct to partial nephrectomy. *J Urol* 1991;146:1218.
6. Atilla MK, Sargon H, Yilmaz O, et al. Undescended testes in adults: clinical significance of resistive index values of the testicular artery measured by Doppler ultrasound as a predictor of testicular histology. *J Urol* 1997;158:841.
7. Baldwin DD, Hadley HR. Epithelial inclusion cyst formation after free vaginal wall swing sling procedure for stress urinary incontinence. *J Urol* 1997;157:952.
8. Barth RA, Shortliffe LD. Normal pediatric testes: comparison of power Doppler and color Doppler ultrasound in the detection of blood flow. *Radiology* 1997;204:389.
9. Becker JA, Schneider M. Techniques and applications of sonography and computed tomography. In: Witten DM, Myers GH, Utz DC, eds. *Emmett's clinical urography,* ed 4. Philadelphia: Saunders, 1977.
10. Bodner D, Bryan PJ, Lipuma JP, et al. Ultrasonography of the urinary bladder. In: Resnick MI, Sanders RC, eds. *Ultrasound in urology,* ed 2. Baltimore: Williams & Wilkins, 1984.
11. Bodner D, Lipuma J, Resnick MI. Basic principles and utilization of ultrasound in urological malignancies. In: Javadpour N, ed. *Principles and management of urologic cancer,* ed 2. Baltimore: Williams & Wilkins, 1983.
12. Bree RL. The role of color Doppler and staging biopsies in prostate cancer detections. *Urology* 1997;49[Suppl 34]:31.
13. Brkljacic B, Drinkovic I, Sabljar-Matovinovic M, et al. Intrarenal duplex Doppler sonographic evaluation of unilateral native kidney obstruction. *Am Inst Ultrasound Med* 1994; 13:197.
14. Brown JM, Taylor KJW, Alderman JL, et al. Contrast enhanced ultrasonographic visualization of gonadal torsion. *J Ultrasound Med* 1997;16:309.
15. Calliada F, Campani R, Bottinelli O, et al. Ultrasound contrast agents: basic principles. *Eur J Radiol* 27[Suppl 2]:3157.
16. Cardenas DD, Kelly E, Krieger JN, et al. Residual urine volumes in patients with spinal cord injury: measurement with a portable ultrasound instrument. *Arch Phys Med Rehabil* 1988; 69:514.
17. Carpentier PJ, Schroeder FH, Schmitz PIM. Transrectal ultrasonometry of the prostate: prognostic relevance of volume changes under endocrine management. *World J Urol* 1986; 4:159.
18. Chio RK, Pomeroy BD, Chen WS, et al. Hemodynamic patterns of pharmacologically induced erection: evaluation by color Doppler sonography. *J Urol* 1998;159:109.
19. Chiou RK, Anderson JC, Tran T, et al. Evaluation of urethral strictures and associated abnormalities using high-resolution and color Doppler ultrasound. *Urology* 1996;47:102.
20. Chiou RK, Conovan JM, Anderson JC, et al. Color Doppler ultrasound assessment of urethral artery location: potential implication for technique of visual internal urethrotomy. *J Urol* 1998;159:796.
21. Chou YH, Tiu CM, Pan HB. High resolution real-time ultrasound in Peyronie's disease. *J Ultrasound Med* 1987;6:67.
22. Cohen HL, Zinn HL, Patel A, et al. Prenatal sonographic diagnosis of posterior urethral valves: identification of valve and thickening of the posterior urethral wall. *J Clin Ultrasound* 1998;26:366.
23. Contractor H, Darqe K, Wiesel M, et al. Diagnosis of vesicoureteral reflex by use of echo-enhanced voiding ultrasonography. *J Urol* 1999;161:197.

24. Dahnert WF, Hamper UM, Eggleston JC, et al. Prostatic evaluation by transrectal ultrasonography with histopathologic correlation: the echogenic appearance of early carcinoma. *Radiology* 1986;158:97.
25. DeMeyer JM, Thiho. The resistance index represents the corporeal pressure and not the cavernous wall resistance. *J Urol* 1997;157:830.
26. Downey DB, Fensten A. Three-dimensional power Doppler detection of prostate cancer. *Am J Radiol* 1995;165:741.
27. Dubinsky TJ, Chen P, Maklad N. Color-flow and power Doppler imaging of the testes. *World J Urol* 1998;16:35.
28. Duel BP, Mogbo K, Barthold JS, et al. Prognostic value of initial renal ultrasound in patients with posterior urethral valves. *J Urol* 1998;160:1198.
29. Dussik KT. Über die Möglichkeit hoch frequente mechanische Schwingungen als diagnostiches Hilfmittel zu vewenden. *Z Ges Neurol Psych* 1942;174:153.
30. Eskew LA, Watson NE, Wolfman N, et al. Ultrasonographic diagnosis of varioceles. *Fertil Steril* 1993;60:693.
31. Fontana D, Poriglia F, Morra I, et al. Transvaginal ultrasonography in the assessment of organic disease of female urethra. *J Ultrasound Med* 1999;18:237.
32. Fornage BD, Touche DH, Deglaire M, et al. Real-time ultrasound-guided prostatic biopsy using a new transrectal linear-array probe. *Radiology* 1983;146:547.
33. Forsberg F, Ismail MI, Hagen EK, et al. Ultrasound contrast imaging of prostate tumors. Personal communication, 1999.
34. Fujino A, Scardino PT. Transrectal ultrasonography for prostatic cancer: its value in staging and monitoring response to radiotherapy and chemotherapy. *J Urol* 1985;133:806.
35. Gluck CD, Bundy AL, Fine C, et al. Sonographic urethrogram: comparison to roentgenographic techniques in 22 patients. *J Urol* 1988;140:1404.
36. Gudinchet F, Oberson JC, Frey P. Color Doppler ultrasound for evaluation of collagen implants after endoscopic injection treatment of refluxing ureters in children. *J Clin Ultrasound* 1997;25:201.
37. Habboub HK, Abu-Yousef MM, Williams RD, et al. Accuracy of color Doppler sonography in assessing venous thrombus extension into renal cell carcinoma. *Am J Radiol* 1997;168:267.
38. Hamper UM, DeJong MR, Caskey CI, et al. Power Doppler imaging: clinical experience and correlation with color Doppler ultrasound and other imaging modalities. *Imaging Therapeutic Tech* 1997;17:499.
39. Hastak SM, Gannelgaard J, Holm HH. Transrectal ultrasonic volume determination of the prostate—a preoperative and postoperative study. *J Urol* 1982;127:1115.
40. Helenon O, Melko P, Correas JM. Renovascular diseases; Doppler ultrasound. *Semin Ultrasound CT MRI* 1997;18:136.
41. Ho LU, Sathyanarayana, Lewis RW. Two injection color duplex Doppler characterization of patients with successful Viagra use. *J Urol* 1999;161:270.
42. Hodge KK, McNeal JE, Terris MK, et al. Random systematic versus directed ultrasound-guided transrectal core biopsies of the prostate. *J Urol* 1989;142:66.
43. Holm HH, Gammelgaard J. Ultrasonically guided precise needle placement in the prostate and seminal vesicles. *J Urol* 1982;125:385.
44. Holm HH, Juul N, Pedersen JF, et al. Transperineal ^{125}iodine seed implantation in prostatic cancer guided by transrectal ultrasonography. *J Urol* 1983;130:282.
45. Holm HH, Northeved A. A transurethral ultrasonic scanner. *J Urol* 1974;111:238.
46. Howry DH, Bliss WR. Ultrasonic visualization on soft tissue structures of the body. *J Lab Clin Med* 1952;40:579.
47. Ismail MT, Pefersen RO, Alexander AA, et al. Color Doppler imaging in predicting the biological behavior of prostate cancer: correlation with disease free survival. *Urology* 1997;50:906.
48. Jarrow JP. Transrectal ultrasonography of infertile men. *Fertil Steril* 1993;60:1035.
49. Jeffrey R, Frederle M. CT and ultrasonography of acute renal abnormalities. *Radiol Clin North Am* 1983;21:515.
50. Kaefer M, Peter CA, Retik AB, et al. Increased renal echogenicity: a sonographic sign for differentiating between obstructive and nonobstructive etiologies of in utero bladder distension. *J Urol* 1997;158:1026.
51. Kamholtz RG, Cronan JJ, Dorfman GS. Obstruction and the minimally dilated renal collecting system: US evaluation. *Radiology* 1989;170:51.
52. King WW, Wilkiemeyer RM, Boyce WH, et al. Current status of prostatic echography. *JAMA* 1973;226:444.
53. Kissane JM. Congenital malformations. In: Heptinstall RH, ed. *Pathology of the kidney*, ed 2. Boston: Little, Brown, 1974.
54. Kremkau FW. *Diagnostic ultrasound principles, instruments and exercises*, ed 3. Philadelphia: Saunders, 1989.
55. Kuijpers D, Kruyt RH, Oudkerk M. Renal masses: value of duplex Doppler ultrasound in the differential diagnosis. *J Urol* 1994;151:326.
56. Kuo HC. Transrectal sonography of the female urethra in incontinence and frequency-urgency syndromes. *J Ultrasound Med* 1996;15:363.
57. Kuo HC. Transrectal sonographic investigation on urethral and paraurethral structures in women with stress urinary incontinence. *J Ultrasound Med* 1998;17:311.
58. Lawson TL, Foley WD, Berland LL, et al. Ultrasonic evaluation of fetal kidneys. *Radiology* 1981;138:153.
59. Lee F, Gray JM, McLeary RD, et al. Transrectal ultrasound in the diagnosis of prostate cancer: location, echogenicity, histopathology and staging. *Prostate* 1985;7:117.
60. Lee F, Littrup PJ, Kumasaka GH, et al. The use of transrectal ultrasound in the diagnosis: guidance in an automatic biopsy system. *Radiology* 1987;165:215 (abst).
61. Lee F, Littrup PJ, Torp-Pederson ST, et al. Prostate cancer: comparison of transrectal ultrasound and digital rectal examination for screening. *Radiology* 1988;168:389.
62. Lee TG, Henderson SC, Freeny PC, et al. Ultrasound findings of renal angiomyolipoma. *J Clin Ultrasound* 1978;6:150.
63. Leibovitch I, Ramon J, Hayman Z, et al. Annual ultrasonographic (US) screening of the remaining testis following unilateral radical orchiectomy for testicular germ cell tumor (GCT). A prospective multicenter study. *J Urol* 1999;181:183.
64. Letran JL, Meyer GE, Loberiza FR, et al. The effect of prostate volume in the yield of needle biopsy. *J Urol* 1998;160:1718.
65. Lewis BD, James EM. Current applications of duplex and color Doppler ultrasound imaging: abdomen. *Mayo Clin Proc* 1989; 64:1158.
66. Liebrass RH, Pollack A, Lankford SP, et al. Transrectal ultrasound for staging prostatic carcinoma prior to radiation therapy. An evaluation based on disease outcome. *Cancer* 1998;85: 1577.
67. Long LP, Choyke PL, Shawker TA, et al. Intraoperative ultrasound in the evaluation of tumor involvement of the inferior vena cava. *J Urol* 1993;150:13.
68. Louvar E, Littrup PJ, Goldstein A, et al. Correlation of color Doppler flow in the prostate with tissue microvascularity. *Cancer* 1998;83:135.
69. Lytton B. Intraoperative ultrasound for nephrolithotomy. *J Urol* 1983;130:213.

70. Marks LS, Dorey FJ, Macairan ML, et al. Three-dimensional ultrasound device for rapid determination of bladder volume. *Urology* 1997;50:341.
71. Martin JF. History of ultrasound. In: Resnick MI, Sanders RC, eds. *Ultrasound in urology,* ed 2. Baltimore: Williams & Wilkins, 1984.
72. Massagli TL, Cardenas DD, Kelly EW. Experience with portable ultrasound equipment and measurement of urine volumes: inter-user reliability and factors of patient position. *J Urol* 1989;142:969.
73. McGahan JP, Blake LC, White RD, et al. Color-flow sonographic mapping of intravascular extension of malignant renal tumors. *J Ultrasound Med* 1993;12:403.
74. McGahan JP, Richards JR, Jones D, et al. Use of ultrasonography in the patient with acute renal trauma. *J Ultrasound Med* 1999;18:207.
75. McMahon C, Touma K, Johnston H. Color-flow duplex ultrasonography of the proximal cavernosal arteries. *J Urol* 1999; 161:271.
76. Merkle W, Wagner W. Sonography of the distal male urethra—a new diagnostic procedure for urethral strictures: results of a retrospective study. *J Urol* 1988;140:1409.
77. Miller RL, Wissman R, White S, et al. Testicular microlithiasis: a benign condition with a malignant association. *J Clin Ultrasound* 1996;24:197.
78. Montorsi F, Guazzoni G, Barbieri L, et al. The effect of intercorporeal injection plus genital and audiovisual sexual stimulation versus second injection on penile color Doppler sonography parameters. *J Urol* 1996;155:536.
79. Murphy KJ, Rubin HM. Power Doppler: it's a good thing. *Semin Ultrasound CT MRI* 1997;18:13.
80. Nakamura S, Niijima T. Transurethral real-time scanner. *J Urol* 1981;125:781.
81. Nazzi MAS, Hoballah JJ, Miller EU, et al. Renal Hilar Doppler analysis is of value in the management of patients with renovascular disease. *Am J Surg* 1997;174:164.
82. Newman JS, Bree RL, Rubin JM. Prostate cancer: diagnosis with color Doppler sonography with histologic correlation of each biopsy site. *Radiology* 1995;195:86.
83. Oats CP, Pickard RS, Powell PH, et al. The use of duplex ultrasound in the assessment of arterial supply to the penis in vasculogenic impotence. *J Urol* 1995;153:354.
84. Ozawa H, Kumon H, Yokoyama T, et al. Development of non-invasive velocity flow video urodynamics using Doppler sonography. Part I. Experimental urethra. *J Urol* 1998;160: 1787.
85. Ozawa H, Kumon H, Yokoyama T, et al. Development of non-invasive velocity flow video urodynamics using doppler sonography. Part II. Clinical application in bladder outlet obstruction. *J Urol* 1998;160:1792.
86. Paltiel HJ, Connolly LP, Atala A, et al. Acute scrotal symptoms in boys with an indeterminate clinical presentation: comparison of color Doppler sonography and scintigraphy. *Radiology* 1998; 207:223.
87. Perkash I, Friedland GW. Transurethral ultrasonography of the lower urinary tract: evaluation of bladder neck problems. *Neurol Urodynamics* 1986;5:299.
88. Petros JA, Andriole GL, Middleton WD, et al. Correlation of testicular color Doppler ultrasonography, physical examination and venography in the detection of left varicoceles in men with infertility. *J Urol* 1991;145:785.
89. Platt JF. Doppler ultrasound of the kidney. *Semin Ultrasound CT MRI* 1997;18:22.
90. Platt JF. Duplex Doppler evaluation of acute renal obstruction. *Semin Ultrasound CT MRI* 1997;18:147.
91. Platt JF. Advances in ultrasonography of urinary tract obstruction. *Abdom Imaging* 1998;23:3.
92. Pode D, Meretik S, Shapiro A, et al. Diagnosis and management of renal angiomyolipoma. *Urology* 1985;25:461.
93. Pollack HM, Banner MP, Arger PH, et al. The accuracy of gray-scale renal ultrasonography in differentiating cystic neoplasms from benign cysts. *Radiology* 1982;143:741.
94. Pontes JE, Eisenkraft S, Wantanabe H, et al. Preoperative evaluation of localized prostatic carcinoma by transrectal ultrasonography. *J Urol* 1985;134:289.
95. Renowden SA, Griffiths DF, Nair S, et al. Renal transplant sonography: correlation of Doppler and biopsy results in cellular rejection. *Clin Radiol* 1992;46:265.
96. Resnick MI, Willard JW, Boyce WH. Transrectal ultrasonography in the evaluation of patients with prostatic carcinoma. *J Urol* 1980;124:482.
97. Resnick MI. Transrectal ultrasound-guided versus digitally directed prostatic biopsy: a comparative study. *J Urol* 1988; 139:754.
98. Rifkin MD, Friedland GW, Shortliffe L. Prostatic evaluation by transrectal endosonography: detection of carcinoma. *Radiology* 1986;158:85.
99. Rifkin MD, McGlynn ET, Choi H. Echogenicity of prostate cancer correlated with histologic grade and stromal fibrosis: endorectal US studies. *Radiology* 1989;170:549.
100. Rifkin MD, Needleman L, Pasto ME, et al. Evaluation of renal transplant rejection by duplex Doppler examination: value of the resistive index. *AJR Am J Roentgenol* 1987;148:759.
101. Rifkin MD, Zerhouni EA, Gatsonis CA, et al. Comparison of magnetic resonance imaging and ultrasonography in staging early prostate cancer. Results of multi-institutional cooperative studies. *N Engl J Med* 1990;323:621.
102. Rob PM, Jansen O, Richter V, et al. Diagnosis of renal transplant failure by real-time and duplex Doppler sonography. *Clin Invest* 1993;71:531.
103. Roehrborn CG, Peters PC. Can transabdominal ultrasound estimation of postvoiding residual (PVR) replace catheterization? *Urology* 1988;31:445.
104. Roy C, Tuchnann C, Pfleger D, et al. Potential role of duplex Doppler sonography in acute renal colic. *J Clin Ultrasound* 1998;26:427.
105. Sakarya ME, Arslan H, Unal O, et al. The role of power Doppler ultrasonography in the diagnosis of prostate cancer: a preliminary study. *Int J Urol* 1998;82:386.
106. Schwartz AN, Lowe M, Berger RE, et al. Assessment of normal and abnormal erectile function: color Doppler flow sonography versus conventional techniques. *Radiology* 1991;180:105.
107. Sehgal CM, Argen PH, Pugh CR, et al. Comparison of power Doppler and B-scan sonography in renal imaging using a sonographic contrast agent. *J Ultrasound Med* 1998;17:751.
108. Sekine H, Oka K, Takehara Y. Transrectal longitudinal ultrasonotomography of the prostate by electronic linear scanning. *J Urol* 1982;127:62.
109. Shapeero LG, Friedland GW, Perkash I. Transrectal sonographic voiding cystourethrography: studies in neuromuscular bladder dysfunction. *Am J Radiol* 1983;141:83.
110. Sherwood T. Renal masses and ultrasound. *BMJ* 1975;4:682.
111. Sim JS, Seo CS, Kim SH, et al. Differentiation of small hyperechoic renal cell carcinoma from angiomyolipoma: computer-aided tissue echo quantification. *J Ultrasound Med* 1999;18:261.
112. Smith JA, Scardino PT, Resnick MI, et al. Transrectal ultrasound versus digital rectal examination for the staging of carcinoma of the prostate: results of a prospective multi-institutional trial. *J Urol* 1997;157:902.

113. Solivetti FM, D'Ascenzo R, Orazi C, et al. Ultrasound diagnosis and management of urethral stones. *J Ultrasound Med* 1989;8:685.
114. Suzer O, Azcam H, Kupeli S, et al. Color Doppler imaging in the diagnosis of acute scrotum. *Eur Urol* 1997;32:457.
115. Takahashi H, Ouchi T. The ultrasonic diagnosis in the field of urology on the diagnosis of prostatic disease. In: *Proceedings of the 4th meeting of the Japanese Society Ultrasound Medicine.* Osaka, Japan, 1964.
116. Talner LB, Scheible W, Ellenbogen PH, et al. How accurate is ultrasonography in detecting hydronephrosis in azotemic patients? *Urol Radiol* 1981;3:1.
117. Terris MK, McNeal JE, Stamey TA. Detection of clinically significant prostatic cancer by transrectal ultrasound-guided systematic biopsies. *J Urol* 1992;148:829.
118. Uchidi K, Akaza H. Intraluminal ultrasonography in urology: development of endoscopic ultrasonography using flexible miniature probe. *J Urol* 1999;161:92.
119. Ukimura O, Troncosa P, Ramirez EI, et al. Prostate cancer staging: correlation between ultrasound determined tumor contact length and pathologically confirmed extraprostate extension. *J Urol* 1998;159:1251.
120. Vergesslich KA, Khoss AE, Balzar E, et al. Acute renal transplant rejection in children: assessment by duplex Doppler sonography. *Pediatr Radiol* 1988;18:474.
121. Ward JF, Stock J. Ultrasonic appearance of post pubertal testicles having undergone prepubertal orchidopexy. *J Urol* 1999;181:157.
122. Watanabe H, Date S, Ohe H. A survey of 3000 examinations by transrectal ultrasonotomography. In: *Proceedings of the 25th annual convention of the American Institute of Ultrasound in Medicine.* 1980.
123. Watanabe H, Igari D, Tanahashi Y, et al. Development and application of new equipment for transrectal ultrasonography. *J Clin Ultrasound* 1974;2:91.
124. Weinberg B, Yeung N. Sonographic sign of intermittent dilatation of renal collecting system in 10 patients with vesicoureteral reflux. *J Clin Ultrasound* 1998;26:65.
125. Yang JM, Su TH, Wang KA. Transvaginal sonographic findings in vesico-fistula. *J Clin Ultrasound* 1994;22:201.
126. Zegal HG, Holland GA, Jennings SB, et al. Intraoperative ultrasonographically guided cryoablation of renal masses. *J Ultrasound Med* 1998;17:571.
127. Zeiji C, Roefs B, Boer K, et al. Clinical outcome and follow-up of sonographically suspected in utero urinary tract anomalies. *J Clin Ultrasound* 1999;27:21.

Adult and Pediatric Urology, 4/e, edited by Jay Y. Gillenwater, John T. Grayhack, Stuart S. Howards, and Michael E. Mitchell.
Lippincott Williams & Wilkins, Philadelphia © 2002

3E

MAGNETIC RESONANCE IMAGING

PETER L. CHOYKE

Magnetic resonance imaging (MRI) is an important method of imaging the urinary tract. Not only has image quality and speed improved, but there are now many new applications for MRI in urology. With the advent of surface coils, contrast agents, and faster pulse sequences, the scope of information that can be derived from MRI has greatly expanded. This chapter reviews the basic principles underlying MRI, describes advances in magnetic resonance (MR) technology, and summarizes the current role of MRI in the genitourinary tract.

BASIC PRINCIPLES

More than half of the human body is composed of water, and each molecule of water contains two hydrogen protons. Hydrogen protons are ubiquitous and can be found not only in water but also attached to the aliphatic chains of fatty acids. Regardless of their chemical environment, each hydrogen proton, when it is placed in a magnetic field, will align either with or against the direction of the applied magnetic field. A slight preponderance of the protons will align in the same direction as the field because this is a lower-energy state. This small excess of protons aligned with the field as opposed to against the field is responsible for the MR signal.

Not only do the protons align with (or against) the externally applied magnetic field, but they also precess or rotate around the axis of the main magnetic field. This precession occurs at a precise frequency that is dependent on the strength of the externally applied magnetic field and is known as the *resonant,* or *Larmor, frequency.*

If a radio frequency (RF) pulse, tuned precisely to the resonant frequency, is applied to protons, they will absorb this energy and begin to deviate from alignment with the external magnetic field. Commonly, these RF pulses are left on long enough to deviate the protons 90 or 180 degrees with respect to the main magnetic axis, although any angle can be obtained. When the RF pulse is completed, however, the protons will quickly relax to their resting state; that is, they realign with the magnetic field. This relaxation process has two components. First, the axis of each proton returns to alignment with the main magnetic field. This process is termed *T_1 relaxation.* Also, protons dephase with respect to each other; that is, they start aligned, or "in phase," with each other but end up randomly distributed. An analogy has been drawn with runners who begin a race at the same starting line but later may be spread around the track depending on their speed and endurance. Similarly, protons are initially aligned during exposure to an RF pulse but will separate from each other with time. This process is termed *T_2 relaxation.* T_1 and T_2 relaxation occur simultaneously, and neither process can be isolated from the other. Thus a T_1-weighted scan means that most of the effects are due to T_1 relaxation but T_2 relaxation also influences the image. Similarly, T_2-weighted images are influenced by T_1 differences among tissues.

Each tissue has its own properties with regard to T_1 and T_2. These are summarized in Table 3E.1. Fat, for instance, has the most rapid T_1 (relaxes quickly to equilibrium), whereas urine has a very long T_1 (relaxes slowly to equilibrium). On T_1-weighted images, fat is bright and urine is dark. The T_2 of urine is longer than that of fat, so on

P.L. Choyke: Department of Radiology, Uniformed Services University of Health Sciences, National Institute of Health, Bethesda, MD 20892.

TABLE 3E.1. SIGNAL INTENSITIES IN T_1- AND T_2-WEIGHTED IMAGES

Tissue	T_1*	T_2
Fat	High	Less high
Muscle	Low	Low
Liver	Medium	Medium
Adrenal	Medium	Medium
Cyst	Low	High
Pheochromocytoma	Medium	Very high
Kidney		
Cortex	Medium	High
Medulla	Medium (less than cortex)	High
Cyst	Low	High
Hemorrhagic cyst	High	High
Tumor	Medium	Higher (variable)
Urine	Low	High
Bladder wall	Low	Low
Prostate		
Transition zone (TZ)	Medium	Low
Peripheral zone (PZ)	Medium (higher than TZ)	High
Tumor	Medium	Lower than PZ
Seminal vesicles	Low	High
Cortical bone	Low	Low
Marrow	Very high	High
Metastases	Medium	Low
Blood		
Fast flow	Low	Low
Slow flow	Medium to high	High
Tumor thrombus	Medium	Medium
Lymph nodes	Medium	Medium

*Low, black; medium, gray; high, white.

T_2-weighted images, urine is brighter than surrounding pelvic fat.

T_1 and T_2 weighting is achieved by varying the timing of the pulse sequences applied to the resting protons. In a typical T_1-weighted image, a 90-degree RF pulse (a pulse that deviates protons 90 degrees) is followed by a 180-degree RF pulse. This second pulse is used to refocus the dephased protons. This is analogous to interrupting the race described previously and having the runners turn around and run back to the starting line. The slower runners have a head start over the faster runners, so all the runners reach the starting line at approximately the same time. For protons, this signal, or "echo," can be measured at the time the protons become rephased (i.e., arrive at the "finish line"). The 90- and 180-degree sequence is repeated at short intervals until enough sequences have been acquired to form an image. By keeping the repetition time (TR) or time between repeated sequences to a minimum and also by minimizing the echo time between the 90- and 180-degree RF pulses (TE/2), T_1 weighting is achieved. Conversely, by lengthening the TR and TE, T_2 weighting is achieved. Typical values for a T_1-weighted spin echo scan are TR = 500 ms and TE = 15 ms, and typical values for a T_2-weighted spin echo scan are TR = 2000 ms and TE = 100 ms, although these numbers vary depending on manufacturer and model and the particular imaging requirements.

Other factors besides T_1 and T_2 influence an image. Flowing blood can cause an increased or decreased signal in vessels, depending on the imaging technique. Iron and other metals can induce strong local magnetic field gradients that degrade the image due to "susceptibility effects." The proton concentration and physical state can also affect the signal: cortical bone and calcifications in the urinary tract have few free protons and thus yield very low signal intensities on all pulse sequences.

Paramagnetic contrast agents can be also used to modify the T_1 relaxation process in tissues. Gadolinium ion is *paramagnetic;* that is, it becomes "magnetic" when placed in a magnetic field. Gadolinium shortens the T_1 value of protons that come nearby, thus leading to enhancement of blood and vascular tissues. Because unchelated gadolinium ion is highly toxic, it must be tightly chelated to a harmless carrier that speeds its removal from the body by glomerular filtration. Gadolinium chelate enhancement on MRI is analogous to iodinated contrast media enhancement on computed tomography (CT); tumors are enhanced but less so than renal parenchyma, and the collecting system and bladder become opacified while cystic ischemic or necrotic areas are not enhanced. Paradoxically, at very high concentrations of gadolinium, there is a darkening of signal as a result of shortening of T_2.

The magnet that supplies the external magnetic field in which the patient lies can be a permanent magnet, a resistive electromagnet, or a superconducting electromagnet. The advantages of the permanent magnet are that it does not require a large power source and it can have a more open architecture than other types of magnets. This is desirable for claustrophobic patients, pediatric patients, or interventional procedures requiring MR guidance. Resistive electromagnets are relatively energy inefficient, requiring large amounts of electric current. The advantage of the supercooled magnet is that it can generate a much higher magnetic field because the coil windings become superconducting at liquid helium temperatures. Higher field strength means higher signal for a given period of scanning, and this allows for faster imaging or higher-resolution images (or both). Field strength is measured in units of Tesla (T) (1 Tesla = 10,000 gauss). For reference, the earth's magnetic field varies from 0.5 to 2 gauss. Magnetic field strengths for MRI units currently on the market vary from 0.02 to 3 T.

There have been several recent technical improvements in MRI. One innovation is called *fast spin-echo* or *turbo spin-echo imaging.* This technique produces T_2-weighted scans in much less time than conventional T_2-weighted scans. This time reduction results in fewer artifacts resulting from motion. Fast spin-echo acquires groups of phase encodings during each excitation, greatly improving the efficiency of scanning.

Another innovation is the suppression of the fat signal in MRI. Fat is ubiquitous in the abdomen and pelvis. Because the protons in fat are in a different molecular milieu than the protons of water, they have a slightly different resonant frequency. With the application of an RF pulse that selectively suppresses the signal from fat but not water, the image is "fat suppressed." By removing the fat from an image, the dynamic range of the image (gray scale) is changed, and the scan becomes more sensitive to slight increases in signal intensity due to enhancement. Instead of fat representing the brightest signal, the contrast-enhancing structure becomes the brightest signal and is easier to see. Fat-suppressed scans show greater enhancement for a given dose of gadolinium chelate and thus are more sensitive for detecting disease.

Another type of fat suppression is known as *chemical shift imaging.* Because protons in fat and water resonate at different frequencies, there are times when the protons in fat and water are in phase and times when they are completely opposed to each other. It is possible to time the imaging to "catch" the protons when they are either in phase or out of phase with each other. If one compares fat–water in-phase and fat–water out-of-phase images and detects a loss of signal for the latter, one can infer that the tissue in question contains some lipid. This is particularly useful in detecting adrenal adenomas, angiomyolipomas, and dermoids, as is described later. Because in-phase and out-of-phase images must be obtained with different pulse sequences, it is often helpful to normalize the signal intensity of the adrenal adenoma to another organ, such as the liver, muscle, or the spleen.

One of the main criticisms of MRI has been that it is too slow and thus motion artifacts degrade the image. It is now possible to obtain MR images during a single breath hold by using a type of scan known as *gradient echo imaging.* Instead of applying a second 180-degree RF pulse after the initial 90-degree RF pulse, magnetic gradients are used to refocus the MR signal. It is now routinely possible to obtain MR images at a rate of 50 to 100 ms per image. This is useful for following a contrast bolus within a renal lesion or in assessing contrast enhancement within a bladder lesion. Even faster imaging may become routinely available with echo planar imaging, or "snapshot" MRI.

Another development in MRI technology is magnetic resonance angiography (MRA). MRA can be used to image the abdominal vasculature, including the aorta and renal arteries and veins. An intravenous bolus of gadolinium chelate is administered and a three-dimensional (3D) acquisition is obtained through the abdomen during a single breath hold (10 to 20 seconds). These images can be reconstructed as projection images much like a conventional angiogram.

Surface coils have enabled high-resolution images to be obtained from targeted areas. The advantage of surface coils is that the signal is unattenuated by distance. Meanwhile, because the signal is collected only from the area of interest and not from the rest of the body, which often acts as an antenna for extraneous RF, signal to noise is further improved. This enhances the signal-to-noise ratio, which in turn can be used to obtain higher-resolution or faster images. Surface coils can be thought of as magnifying lenses for MRI. Endorectal surface coils for prostate imaging are one example of surface coils, but other noncavitary types of surface coils are commonly used for pelvic and renal imaging. Phased-array surface coils are combinations of coils that take advantage of the gain in signal-to-noise ratio afforded by multiple surface coils but allow a wider field of view to be scanned.

It is important to be aware of contraindications to MRI. Patients with pacemakers, implanted infusion pumps, cochlear implants, or any other implanted electronic devices should not be scanned with the device in place because it may be ruined or cause aberrant function. Patients with cerebral aneurysm surgical clips should generally not undergo MRI because these clips can become magnetic and torque. Newer aneurysm clips are MR compatible. Most other surgical clips, heart valves (with the exception of early Starr-Edwards valves), and orthopedic pins and screws are made of nonmagnetic stainless steel and are not contraindications for MRI. Patients with shrapnel imbedded in their bodies may experience movement of the fragment or pain during MRI. A metal worker who has chips of metal lodged in the eye may develop intraocular hemorrhage and blindness and should be evaluated with orbital radiographs before MRI if there is any question of an ocular metallic foreign body. In general, consultation with a radiologist is recommended if there is any doubt about the safety of a device. Claustrophobia is a relative contraindication for MRI but usually can be ameliorated by mild, oral anxiolytics. Because young children (younger than 5 years) usually cannot hold still long enough for an MRI, they must be sedated if adequate studies are to be obtained. There are no contraindications to gadolinium chelate administration except for severe renal dysfunction (creatinine clearance less than 20 mL per minute), in which case dialysis is recommended after use of the contrast. Gadolinium chelates have been used as a substitute for iodinated contrast in conventional x-ray angiography in patients with poor renal function, but there are reports of nephrotoxicity using this direct intraarterial method.

Limitations of MRI include the inability to detect calcification, susceptibility to flow and other motion artifact, and lack of a good oral contrast agent with which to differentiate normal bowel from pathology.

The cost of MRI not only has made it less attractive but also has made it a high-profile target for regulators. With increasing competition in the medical marketplace, MRI has become less expensive. This is achieved by efficiencies in throughput and overhead. Manufacturers are also offering

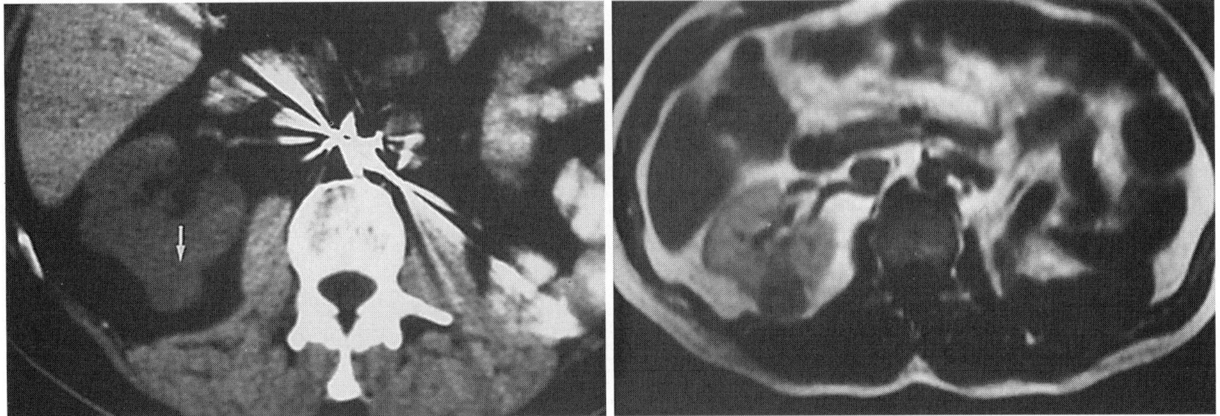

FIGURE 3E.1. A 47-year-old patient with prior nephrectomy for renal cell carcinoma and a severe contrast allergy. **A:** Noncontrast computed tomography (CT) scan 2 years after nephrectomy demonstrated a nonspecific bulge in the posterior kidney *(arrow)*. Because intravenous iodinated contrast media could not be given, a magnetic resonance imaging (MRI) scan was performed with gadolinium. **B:** An enhancing mass corresponding to the lesion seen on CT that proved to be a recurrent renal cell carcinoma.

smaller, less expensive MRI units. As a result, one of the barriers to the use of MRI, its cost, is becoming less of an issue.

ROLE OF MAGNETIC RESONANCE IMAGING IN THE GENITOURINARY TRACT

Kidney

When it was introduced, MRI was not generally considered helpful in the management of most renal masses compared with CT and ultrasound because of severe motion artifacts and nonspecificity (14). However, U.S. Food and Drug Administration (FDA) approval of contrast agents with gadolinium has made MRI more clinically applicable (16). MRI with gadolinium chelate enhancement is directly analogous to CT with iodinated contrast. However, because CT is less expensive and more available, it is still the preferred technique for evaluating parenchymal abnormalities of the kidney. MRI can be substituted for CT when there is a severe iodinated contrast allergy or renal dysfunction (39,91) (Figs. 3E.1, 3E.2, and 3E.3). The original gadolinium chelate introduced in 1988 was gadopentetate dimeglumine (GD-DTPA) (Magnevist, Berlex Laboratories); since

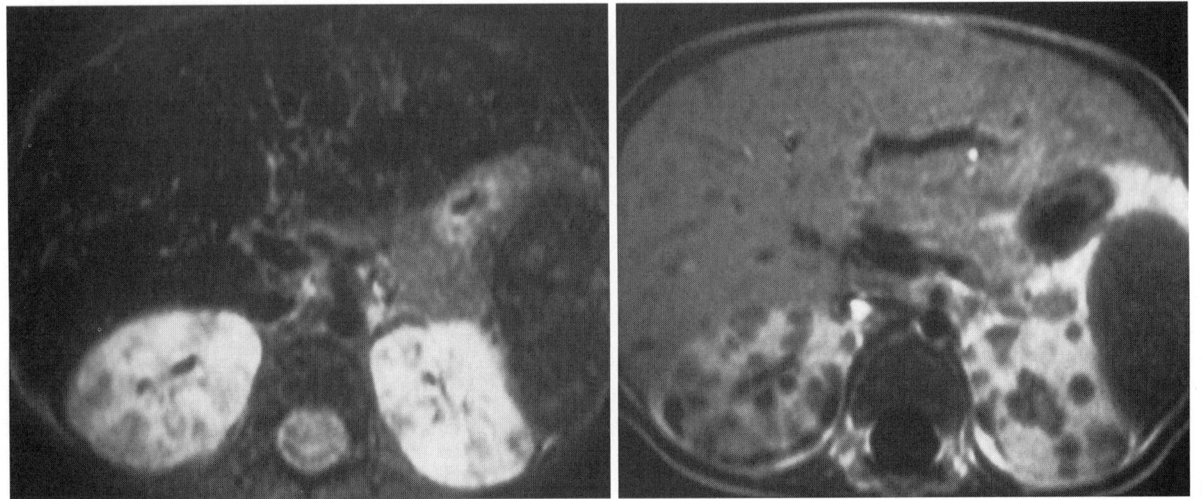

FIGURE 3E.2. Use of gadolinium-enhanced MRI in the presence of renal failure. This patient had been treated for acute myelogenous leukemia and developed fevers. Renal function was significantly diminished (serum creatinine = 2.9 mg/dL). **A:** Noncontrast T_2-weighted scan demonstrates nonspecific heterogeneous signal within the renal parenchyma. **B:** Postgadolinium-enhanced MRI demonstrates multiple distinct filling defects in the kidney and liver. These proved to be fungal *(Candida)* abscesses.

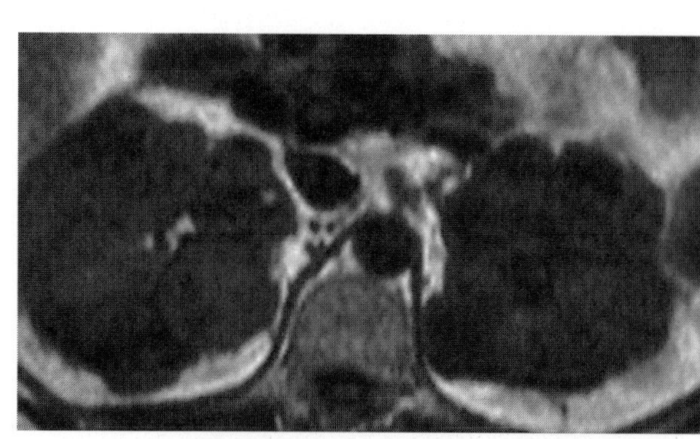
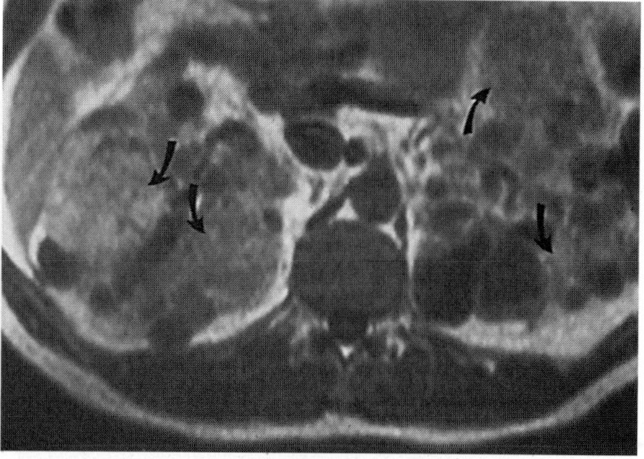

A B

FIGURE 3E.3. Use of gadolinium-enhanced magnetic resonance imaging (MRI) scan for detecting renal masses in renal failure. This 38-year-old patient was thought to have autosomal-dominant polycystic kidney disease. When a family member was discovered to have symptoms of von Hippel Lindau disease, he was reevaluated. Because of his renal failure, gadolinium-enhanced MRI was performed. **A:** Precontrast T_1-weighted image demonstrates enlarged kidneys with a typical appearance of autosomal dominant polycystic kidney disease. **B:** Contrast-enhanced MRI, however, demonstrates multiple areas of enhancement consistent with renal cell carcinomas *(arrows).* This was confirmed surgically by bilateral nephrectomy and subsequent transplant.

1993, two other compounds, gadoteridol (Gd-D03A) (ProHance, Squibb) and gadodiamide (Gd-DTPA-BMA) (Omniscan, Winthrop), have become available in the United States. All of these contrast agents are thought to have the same enhancement properties and offer a very high safety profile. Allergic reactions requiring treatment occur in less than 1% of the population. Gadolinium chelates do not cross-react with iodinated contrast agents, and they are not thought to have the same nephrotoxic potential as iodinated contrast agents, although allergies to both agents can be seen (32). Any patient with a strong history of multiple allergies should be considered at increased risk of reacting to a gadolinium chelate.

Gadolinium chelates have been proposed as alternatives to iodinated contrast or conventional angiograms in patients with renal dysfunction. Because gadolinium is a heavy metal, it attenuates x-rays sufficiently to be a potential substitute for iodinated contrast. However, this approach should be viewed with caution because renal failure may occur after intraarterial gadolinium chelate administration.

Occasionally, contrast-enhanced CT and ultrasound results are indeterminate or contradictory regarding the type of renal lesion present. A common example is the hemorrhagic cyst, which may be hyperdense on CT and thus difficult to evaluate for enhancement, whereas the ultrasound may demonstrate echogenic debris within the lesion (Fig. 3E.4). MR has better sensitivity for enhancement

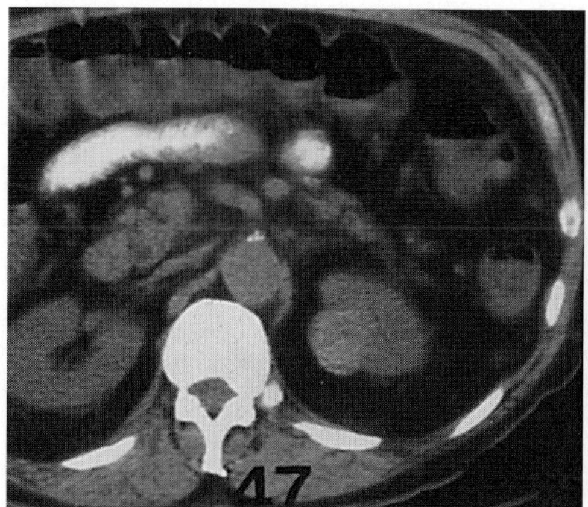

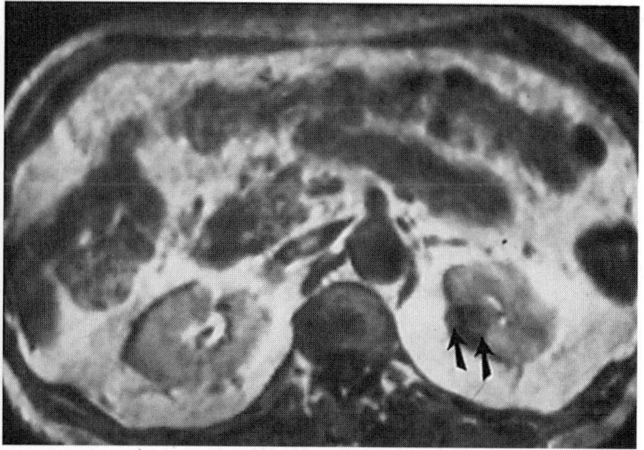

A B

FIGURE 3E.4. Magnetic resonance in the evaluation of indeterminate renal masses. **A:** This hemorrhagic cystic lesion in the left kidney measured 47 HU on computed tomography. Postcontrast scan showed no enhancement. **B:** Postcontrast gadolinium study demonstrates two small nodules of enhancement in the wall *(arrows)* of the lesion, which were foci of low-grade renal carcinoma.

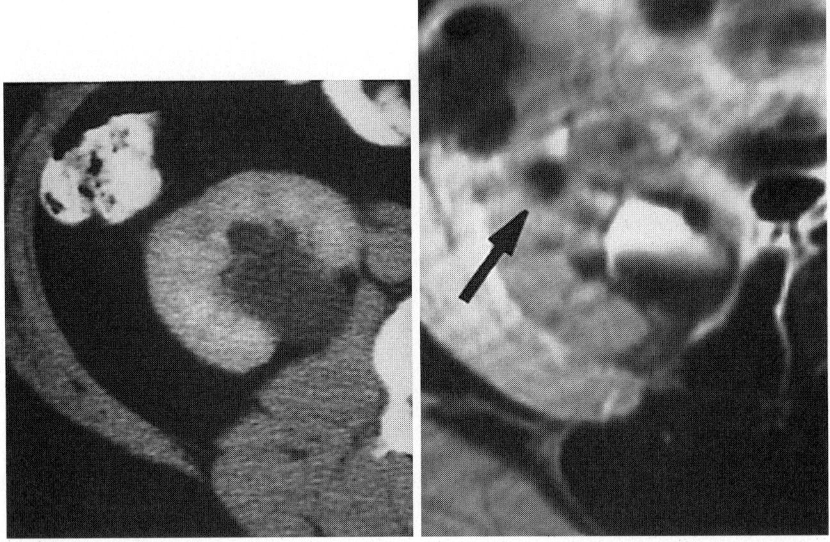

FIGURE 3E.5. The value of magnetic resonance imaging (MRI) in indeterminate renal masses. **A:** Contrast-enhanced computed tomography (CT) scan shows an inhomogeneous renal parenchyma but no definite focal masses. **B:** Postcontrast T_1-weighted image demonstrates a cystic mass in the right kidney with a small mural nodule *(arrow),* as well as several additional smaller lesions in the parenchyma. The patient had a ureteropelvic junction stenosis, accounting for the dilated renal pelvis. The fluid level in the renal pelvis on the MRI is due to the more concentrated gadolinium layering below the less concentrated (bright), more dilute urine.

within some masses than does CT and can detect small mural neoplasm (Fig. 3E.5). In such cases, contrast-enhanced MRI may be useful as a "tie breaker" study to help guide proper management. The multiplanar capabilities of MRI may also be useful in certain instances when CT and ultrasound may be limited by patient size (Fig. 3E.6).

When an MRI of the kidney is performed for renal masses, a torso-phased array coil should be used to boost signal. It is important that thin-section (5 to 7 mm) T_1-weighted MRI be performed before and after contrast media. This allows the direct measurement of lesion enhancement. The same parameters must be used before and after contrast to enable comparison of signal intensity. Unlike CT density measurements, MR signal intensity units are arbitrary and thus "rules" have not been generated regarding abnormal enhancement. If possible, fat-suppressed T_1-weighted images should be used because of the augmented sensitivity to contrast enhancement with this technique (72,79,80). However, conventional T_1 weighting should not be discarded because fat-saturated scans can hide vascular neoplasms (Fig. 3E.7). Cysts will not enhance and will remain very low in signal intensity, whereas solid lesions, such as renal cancers, will increase in signal intensity after contrast medium administration. Careful attention to the wall of the cyst may reveal a small mural cancer (Figs. 3E.7 and 3E.8). T_2-weighted MRI should also be performed to detect cysts, which will be very high in signal intensity, but tumors will also tend to be high in signal intensity except for rare cases of tumor or hemorrhage (Fig. 3E.9). MRI cannot differentiate benign oncocytomas and malignant renal cell carcinomas (23). Some authors advocate that serial scanning be performed during breath holding and contrast enhancement to demonstrate the enhancement pattern (22,49), but this is generally not necessary.

Another application of renal MRI is in staging renal cancers for venous invasion. Enhanced CT can be equivocal with respect to caval thrombus due to streaming of contrast media in the inferior vena cava (IVC) during a bolus of iodinated contrast media. MRI can be used to detect thrombi within the renal veins and IVC when the CT is equivocal (56). MRI has proven to have a 90% to 100% positive predictive value for tumor thrombus in the IVC (Figs. 3E.10, 3E.11, and 3E.12) (1,27,29,37,61,78). MRI often cannot differentiate stage I from stage II renal cancers, although this is not a clinical problem. Extrinsic compression of the IVC due to bulky adenopathy may make assessment of thrombus difficult (36). Depending on the imaging technique, either the normal-flowing blood can have a low signal intensity with the tumor thrombus intermediate in signal or the normal-flowing blood can be high in signal intensity with tumor thrombus appearing as a low-signal defect (Fig. 3E.10). Scans should be obtained in all three planes to ensure that the IVC is fully evaluated; flow artifacts can cause false-positive results if only one plane is used. MRI can be used for nonneoplastic causes of renal vein thrombosis, such as with glomerulonephritis or lupus nephritis. MRI is also useful in identifying potential adjacent organ invasion, including the liver, pancreas, and

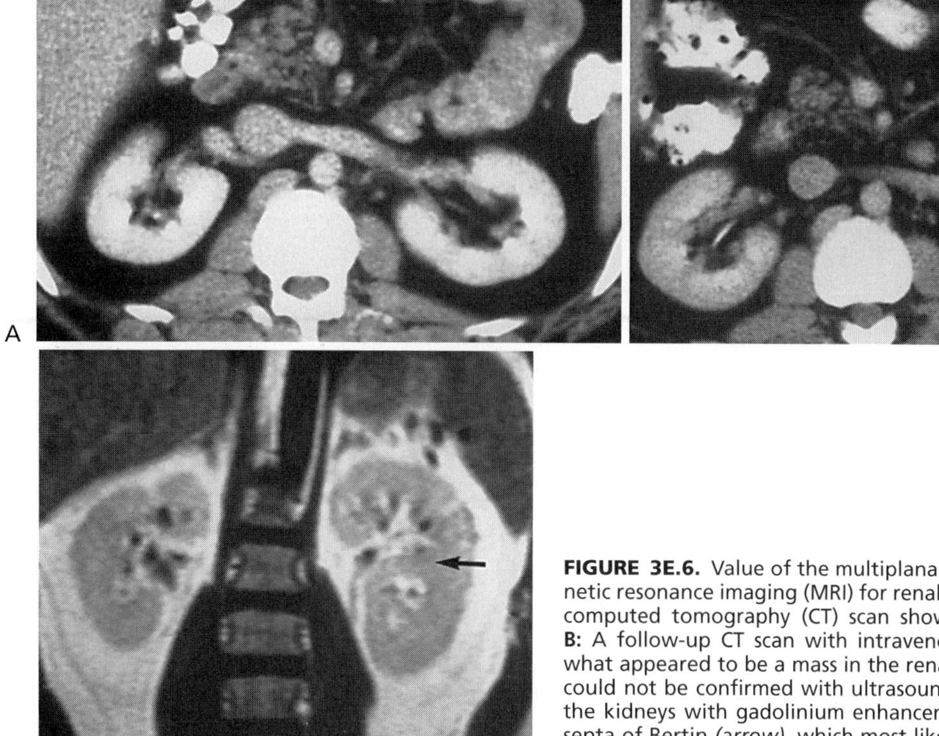

FIGURE 3E.6. Value of the multiplanar capabilities of magnetic resonance imaging (MRI) for renal imaging. **A:** Baseline computed tomography (CT) scan showed normal kidneys. **B:** A follow-up CT scan with intravenous contrast showed what appeared to be a mass in the renal pelvis *(arrow)*. This could not be confirmed with ultrasound. **C:** Coronal MRI of the kidneys with gadolinium enhancement demonstrates a septa of Bertin *(arrow)*, which most likely accounts for findings on this CT scan. No renal mass is identified with MRI.

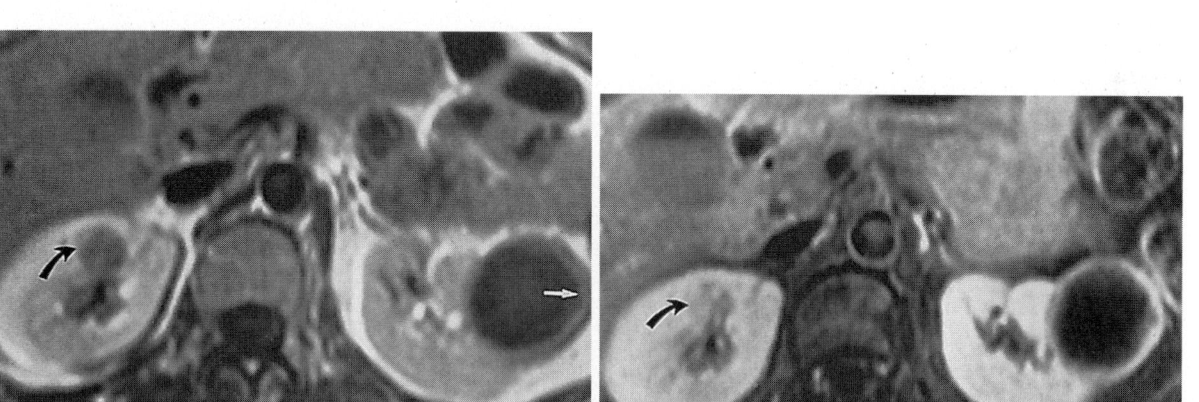

FIGURE 3E.7. The advantage of fat-suppressed T_1-weighted images for detecting enhancement in renal masses. **A:** Conventional contrast-enhanced T_1-weighted image demonstrates a thickened wall of a cystic left kidney *(white arrow)*, but definite enhancement is not seen. A right-sided mass *(curved arrow)* is readily seen in the right kidney. **B:** Fat-suppressed T_1-weighted image after intravenous contrast demonstrates markedly enhanced wall of the cystic mass, which proved to be a renal cell carcinoma. The contralateral solid mass *(curved arrow)* is harder to identify on the fat-suppressed image.

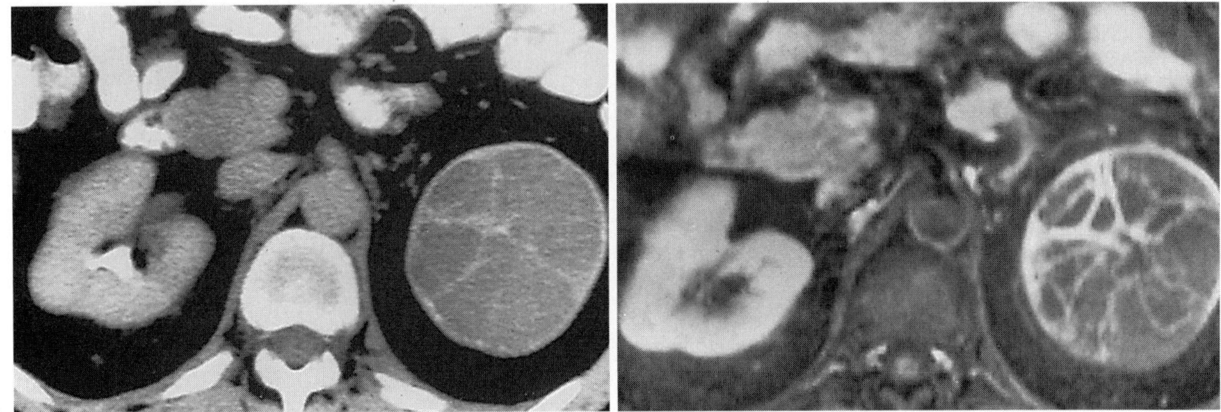

FIGURE 3E.8. The value of fat-suppressed T_1-weighted enhanced magnetic resonance imaging (MRI) for detecting mural enhancement. **A:** Contrast-enhanced computed tomography (CT) scan demonstrates a large cystic mass in the left kidney. It is not evident how much enhancement there is in the wall of the mass. **B:** Fat-suppressed T_1-weighted image after gadolinium enhancement demonstrates markedly enhanced irregular walls of the cystic mass, suggesting a malignancy. This lesion proved to be a cystic renal cell carcinoma.

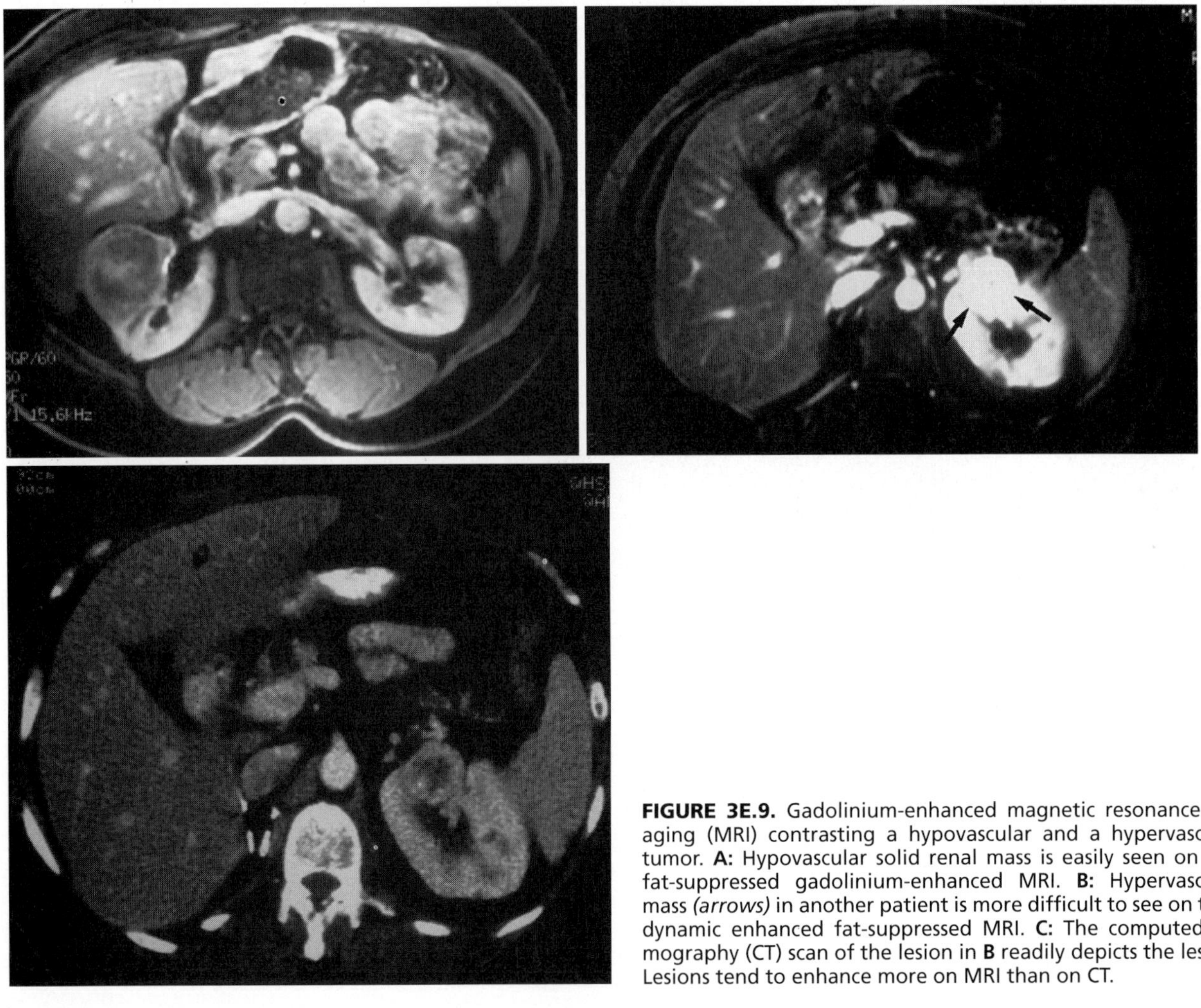

FIGURE 3E.9. Gadolinium-enhanced magnetic resonance imaging (MRI) contrasting a hypovascular and a hypervascular tumor. **A:** Hypovascular solid renal mass is easily seen on this fat-suppressed gadolinium-enhanced MRI. **B:** Hypervascular mass *(arrows)* in another patient is more difficult to see on this dynamic enhanced fat-suppressed MRI. **C:** The computed tomography (CT) scan of the lesion in **B** readily depicts the lesion. Lesions tend to enhance more on MRI than on CT.

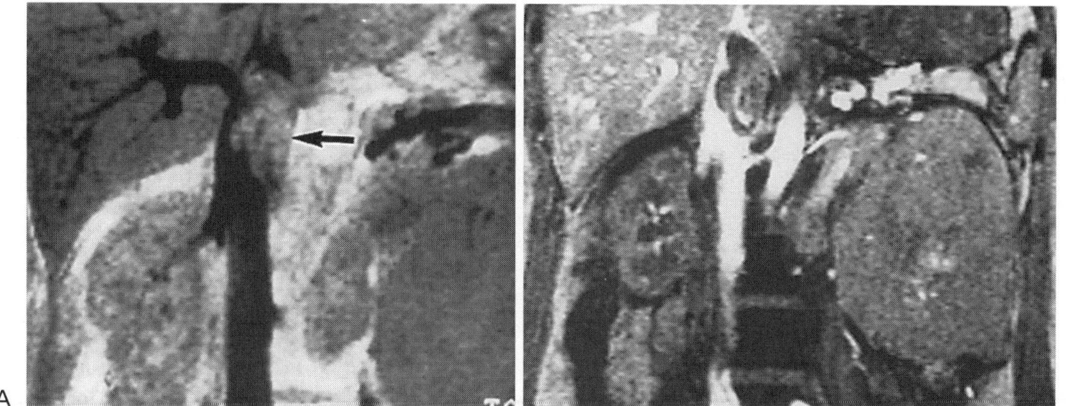

FIGURE 3E.10. Two techniques for identifying tumor thrombus within the inferior vena cava. **A:** There is a large left-sided renal mass. A tumor thrombus *(arrow)* is identified within the inferior vena cava. Because of the spin-echo technique used, the flowing blood appears dark and the tumor thrombus is relatively higher in signal intensity. **B:** When a gradient-echo technique is used, the flowing blood becomes bright in signal intensity, whereas the tumor thrombus is dark. Either technique can be used for detecting a thrombus within the inferior vena cava.

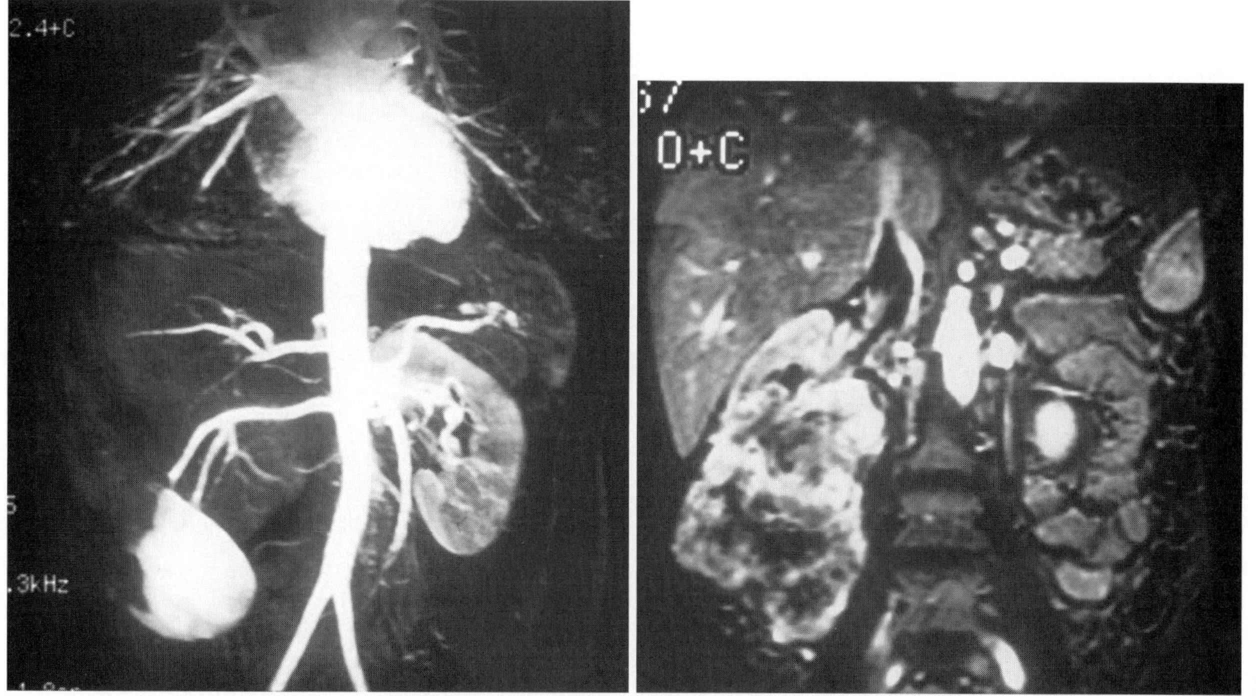

FIGURE 3E.11. New methods of staging renal cancers with magnetic resonance imaging (MRI). **A:** Magnetic resonance angiogram (MRA) of a patient with a large right renal cancer demonstrates the elongation of the right renal artery and extrarenal branching of this vessel. **B:** Delayed MRA from another case demonstrates filling defect in the inferior vena cava arising from the right renal cancer. The absence of enhancement within the thrombus distally (bland thrombus) contrasts with the more proximal portion of the thrombus that shows enhancement.

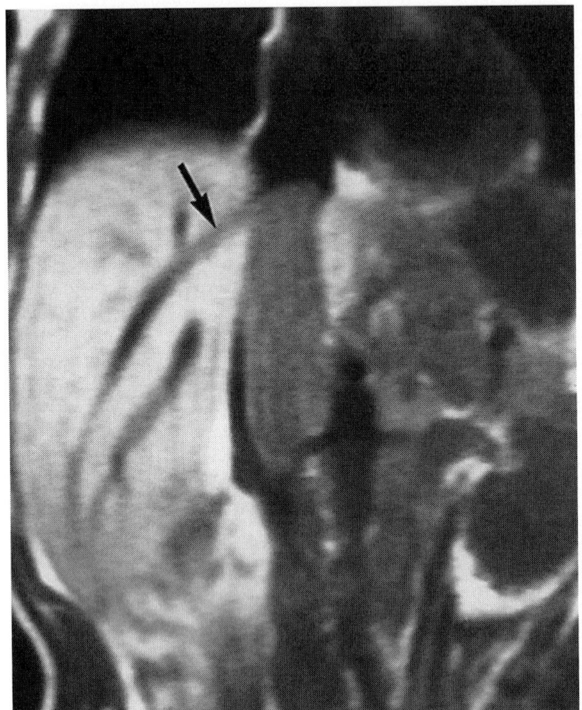

FIGURE 3E.12. Inferior vena caval thrombus caused by large left-sided renal cell carcinoma. T_1 coronal magnetic resonance imaging demonstrates a large thrombus within the inferior vena cava with extension of the thrombus into the right hepatic vein *(arrow).*

spleen. The bones should always be evaluated on the sagittal image because MRI may be more sensitive than bone scan for detecting early bone metastases in the spine (40).

MRI is useful in detecting fat within angiomyolipomas (AMLs). CT demonstrates fat within an AML, which is diagnostic, but occasionally the fat may be obscured by previous hemorrhage or may not be visible. T_1-weighted images obtained before and after fat suppression will confirm that the mass is an angiomyolipoma if it contains fat, but neither CT nor MRI can differentiate a nonfatty AML from a renal cancer.

Renal lymphoma is often a multifocal process and can result in renal insufficiency (39). Noncontrast CT and ultrasound can be insufficient to identify renal lymphoma; however, MRI with gadolinium chelate enhancement will readily demonstrate the multiple masses within the renal parenchyma typical of renal lymphoma (Fig. 3E.2). In fact, this technique is readily applied to any patient with a parenchymal defect caused by renal infection, hemorrhage, or infarct (44) (Fig. 3E.13).

The evaluation of renal arteries by MRA is an important application of MRI. Sensitivity for renal artery stenosis varies from 90% to 100% overall to 90% for proximal renal artery and 82% for branch renal artery stenosis. Several studies have shown MRA to be a highly accurate method of detecting main renal artery stenosis (6,25,28,59). Although this technique is sensitive, it may overestimate the degree of stenosis because of flow-related artifacts (Fig. 3E.14). Because renal MRA is noninvasive, it is the preferred method of diagnosing renal artery stenosis and is more reliable than Doppler ultrasound. It is now possible to measure renal arterial velocity directly from an MR angiogram using phase-contrast MRA (6,52,76).

One particularly useful application of MRA is in the renal transplant recipient, in whom renal arterial anastomotic stenosis is common (54,63). MRA is particularly well suited for these patients because surface coils can be used, which increase the available signal, thus permitting high-resolution images. Moreover, the use of iodinated contrast media is often contraindicated in patients with poorly functioning renal transplants. MRI can provide information about the integrity of the renal transplant parenchyma, obstruction of the ureter, and perinephric collections (31,33). Gadolinium chelate–enhanced imaging is useful in this setting to document renal infarctions and focal lesions such as tumors and infections. MRA can also be used to evaluate potential living related donors

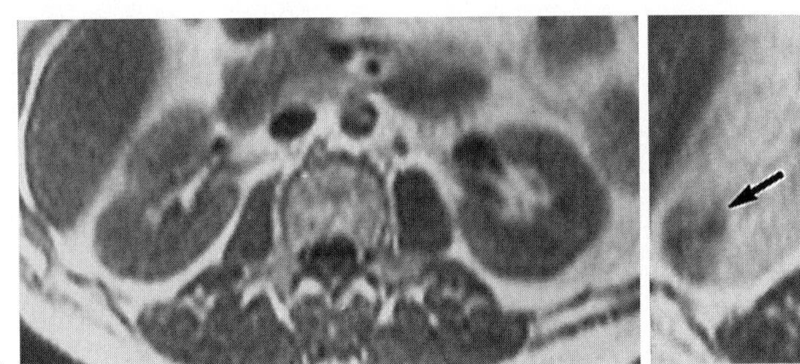

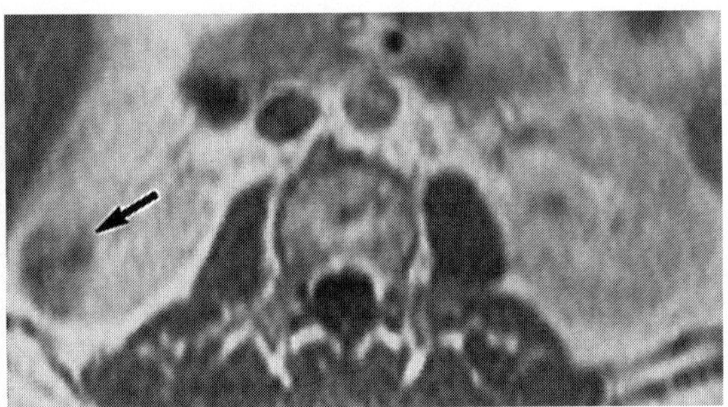

FIGURE 3E.13. Role of magnetic resonance imaging (MRI) in detecting renal infection in an immunocompromised patient. This patient was immunocompromised as a result of aplastic anemia. Previous exposure to nephrotoxic antibiotics had impaired his renal function. **A:** Precontrast T_1-weighted image shows no detectable abnormality. **B:** Postcontrast T_1-weighted image demonstrates a focal defect in the periphery of the right kidney *(arrow).* Subsequent percutaneous biopsy demonstrated cryptococcus.

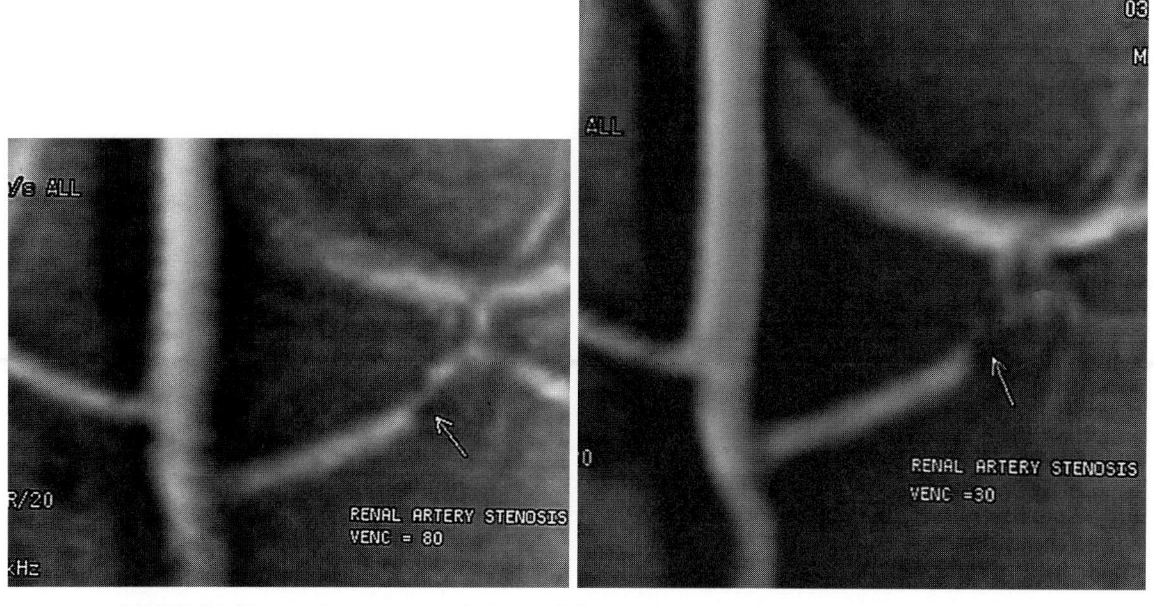

FIGURE 3E.14. Renal artery stenosis *(arrows)* detected with magnetic resonance angiography (MRA). **A:** This stenosis is demonstrated by MRA using appropriate parameters (VENC-80). **B:** Using other parameters (VENC-30), the stenosis appears more severe than it actually is.

for vascular or parenchymal abnormalities before transplantation (3,64).

Adrenal

CT is the best method of evaluating the adrenals based on its sensitivity and availability (49). Often, however, CT findings are nonspecific, and MRI can then be used to characterize the features of an adrenal mass to determine if it is malignant (26). MRI of the adrenal gland may be particularly useful in confirming the presence of pheochromocytomas and in differentiating adrenal adenomas from metastatic disease.

Pheochromocytomas are often cystic and contain large amounts of free water. This is easily recognized as a high-signal-intensity mass on T_2-weighted images (55,95) (Fig. 3E.15). Naturally, not all pheochromocytomas are very high in signal intensity; hemorrhage within the tumor can cause lower signal intensity on T_2-weighted images (51). Nevertheless, the high-signal appearance of most pheochromocytomas and paragangliomas makes MRI useful for quickly identifying adrenal and ectopic sites of pheochromocytoma. Metaiodobenzyl guanidine (MIBG) studies are often more difficult to obtain and interpret. Other sites of paragangliomas, such as the organ of Zuckerkandl, the retroperitoneum, the bladder, the carotid bulb, and the jugular foramen, are also well suited to the multiplanar capabilities of MRI. Thus most pheochromocytomas, regardless of location, can be identified by MRI. Many other pathologic processes can have high signal intensity on T_2-weighted MRI,

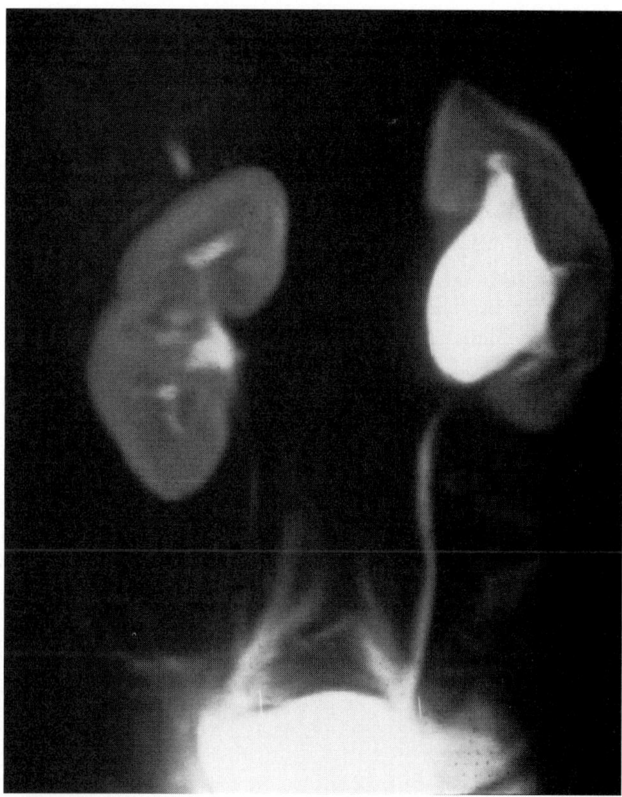

FIGURE 3E.15. A magnetic resonance urogram demonstrating a left ureteropelvic junction narrowing and hydronephrosis. This image was acquired using a fast T_2-weighted breath-hold scan.

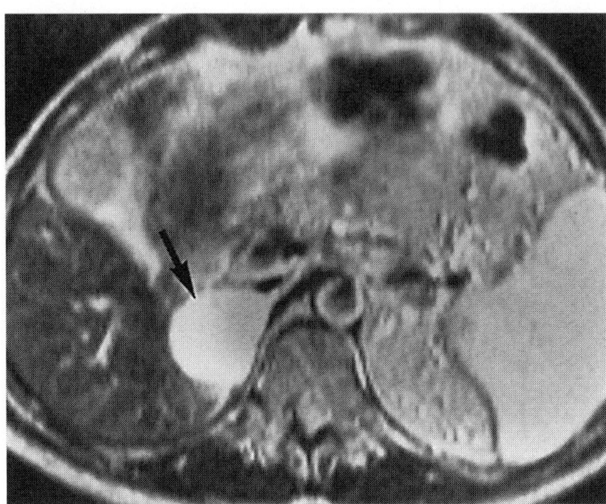

FIGURE 3E.16. High-signal-intensity adrenal mass not representing a pheochromocytoma. This T_2-weighted image demonstrates a very-high-signal-intensity lesion in the right adrenal gland. There is no clinical or chemical evidence of a pheochromocytoma. This patient had melanoma with metastases to the right adrenal gland.

including metastases and cysts; however, these can usually be distinguished by the clinical setting (Fig. 3E.16). If bilateral or ectopic pheochromocytomas are discovered, a hereditary cause such as multiple endocrine neoplasia (MEN) II, MEN III (MEN IIb), von Hippel Lindau, or neurofibromatosis must be considered (66) (Fig. 3E.17). Neumann and co-workers (66) have shown that hereditary forms of pheochromocytoma occur more frequently than previously thought among patients with apparently sporadic pheochromocytomas. MRI can be helpful when retroperitoneal surgical clips obscure evaluation on CT (Fig. 3E.18).

Adrenal adenomas and adrenal metastases are common findings on CT, yet it is difficult to separate one from the other on the basis of CT alone. One important parameter is lesion size. Lesions smaller than 2 cm are more likely to be benign, but size alone is not sufficient to predict behavior (57). The adrenal adenoma contains intracellular lipid because it is composed of cortical tissue, which produces and stores steroid-based hormones. Thus low-density (less than 10 Hounsfield units [HU]) measurements on CT within a small (less than 2 cm) mass are virtually diagnostic of an adenoma (49,50,94). Very-low-density measurements (less than −10 HU) suggest a myelolipoma. However, many adenomas are greater than 15 HU in density. Metastatic lesions to the adrenals usually do not contain lipid but are generally high in extracellular water due to the leakiness of neoplastic vessels. The differences in histology and physiology can be exploited with several different strategies, each of which focuses on signal intensity differences between the tightly packed lipid-containing cells of adenomas and the loosely packed cells with a relatively large amount of extracellular water of metastases. The original attempts to differentiate these two entities with MRI included the ratio of signal intensity of the mass to that of the liver or fat on T_2-weighted images (12,70). Adenomas tend to have a low adrenal mass-to-liver signal ratio, whereas metastases tend to have a higher ratio. However, considerable overlap exists using these techniques (9,94). Another technique is to use dynamic enhanced MRI during rapid contrast media infusion (48). Metastases enhance at a much faster rate and attain higher-signal-intensity changes than adenomas. Although this technique appeared to be successful in one study, dynamic enhancement has not been widely applied (48,85).

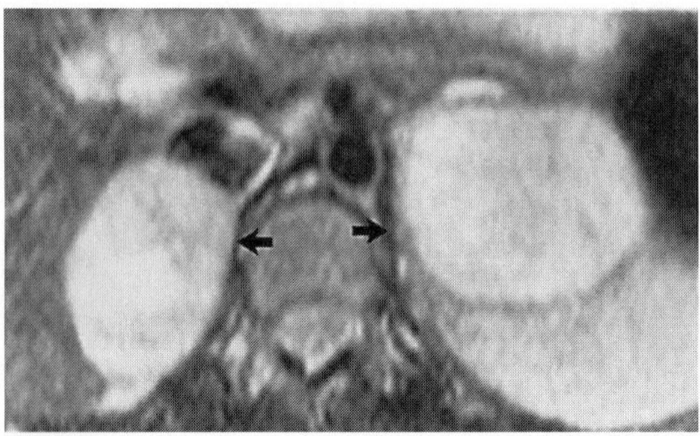

FIGURE 3E.17. Bilateral pheochromocytomas in a patient with MEN IIb syndrome. This young woman experienced hypertensive crisis during childbirth. Subsequent workup revealed bilateral pheochromocytomas *(arrows)* on T_2-weighted magnetic resonance imaging. Bilateral pheochromocytomas are usually associated with hereditary forms of pheochromocytoma.

Mitchell and associates (60) showed that reliable differentiation of adrenal adenomas and metastases could be achieved using chemical shift MRI. In this technique, fat- and water-bound protons are imaged with in-phase and out-of-phase scans. If the signal intensity of the adrenal mass decreases on the out-of-phase image relative to the in-phase image, the lesion contains lipid and therefore represents an adenoma (Fig. 3E.19). Lesions that show either no change or an increase in signal within the mass on the out-of-phase image do not contain lipid and therefore are more likely to be malignant. Initially, this technique was reportedly almost 100% accurate (60,93); however, subsequent data have shown some overlap between adenomas and metastases (15,47,70,85). Nevertheless, the chemical shift technique appears to be the most successful strategy for separating adenomas and metastases by MRI (82). Lesions deemed to be adenomas by MRI deserve follow-up until this technique is more established. Advocates of MRI argue that MRI is at least as effective as percutaneous adrenal biopsy and does not carry with it the 2% to 10% complication rate of adrenal biopsy (11,81,82,92). Of course, additional functional assessment for a chemically active adenoma is useful in identifying benign but functional lesions that should be removed (18).

Ureter and Bladder

MRI of the ureter is now possible, although it does not yet have the resolution of plain film radiography. In MR

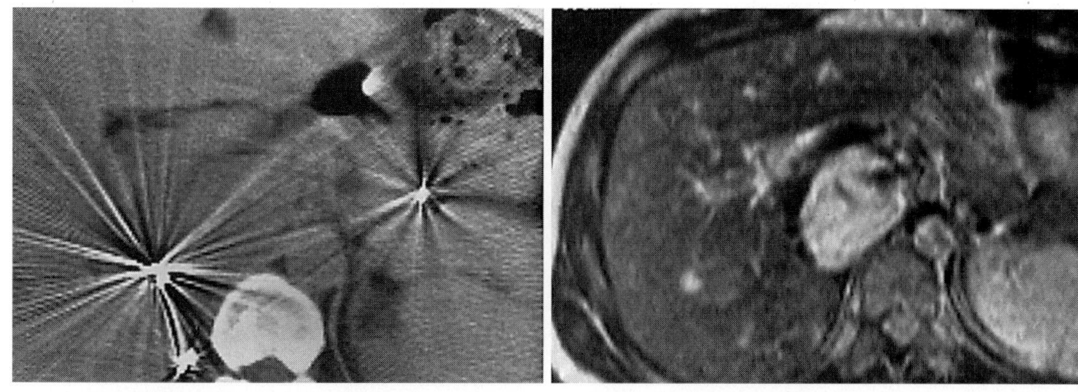

A B

FIGURE 3E.18. The advantage of magnetic resonance imaging (MRI) in detecting retroperitoneal lesions when multiple surgical clips are present. This patient had resection of adrenal carcinoma several years before. **A:** Multiple clips obscure the retroperitoneum on this precontrast computed tomography (CT) scan. **B:** T_2-weighted image demonstrates a recurrence adjacent to the inferior vena cava. The MRI is less influenced by surgical clip artifact than is the CT.

urography, strongly T_2-weighted scans are obtained through the ureters in the coronal plane (4). Alternatively, T_1-weighted scans are obtained after low-dose administration of gadolinium chelates with a small dose of furosemide (Lasix) to enlarge the ureter (67). Stenoses, obstructions, and filling defects caused by stones or tumors can be seen with these techniques. They are especially useful in pediatric and pregnant patients, in whom exposure to ionizing radiation is undesirable (7). MR urography provides a noninvasive method of surveying the ureters for causes of hematuria.

FIGURE 3E.19. Chemical shift magnetic resonance imaging to determine that an adrenal mass is benign. *Top image* is an out-of-phase T_1-weighted scan that demonstrates a low-signal left adrenal mass. *Bottom image* shows an increase in signal in the same lesion when scanned with an in-phase T_1-weighted scan. The decrease in signal within the left adrenal mass is highly suggestive of a benign process such as an adrenal adenoma or hyperplasia.

A routine role for MRI in bladder disease has not been established. MRI is clearly not as good as cystoscopy for diagnosing bladder tumors or evaluating hematuria. MRI has been used to document tumors within diverticula, to characterize suspected intravesical pheochromocytomas, and to aid in the identification of urachal tumors.

MRI has been suggested as a method for staging bladder cancer invasion of the bladder wall (10). Assessment of tumor invasion is currently limited by sampling error and accuracy, especially in the assessment of extravesical extension. It has only recently become pragmatic even to consider bladder cancer staging by MRI because the spherical nature of the bladder means that there are an infinite number of planes perpendicular to the bladder wall. To obtain truly perpendicular sections at all points in the bladder requires 3D imaging, which has now become feasible (5). One of the major improvements in bladder MRI was the use of pelvic phased-array coils, which boost the available signal significantly. With a 3D data set, the bladder wall can be "sectioned" in any plane perpendicular to the bladder wall at the tumor site (Fig. 3E.20). Thus the depth of muscle invasion becomes possible to measure. Fat-suppression techniques have also proven useful in identifying invasion of the perivesical fat.

Several different methods of assessing the bladder wall for tumor invasion have been suggested. Highly T_2-weighted images of the bladder wall demonstrate a trilayer appearance to the bladder wall corresponding to the mucosa, submucosa-lamina propria, and muscularis layers. The degree of disruption of these bands can be used to indicate the depth of tumor invasion and is accurate in 73% of patients (5). The other method of assessing bladder wall invasion is with dynamic enhanced MRI, which is performed after a bolus injection of a gadolinium chelate contrast agent. Normally, after contrast administration, an enhancing

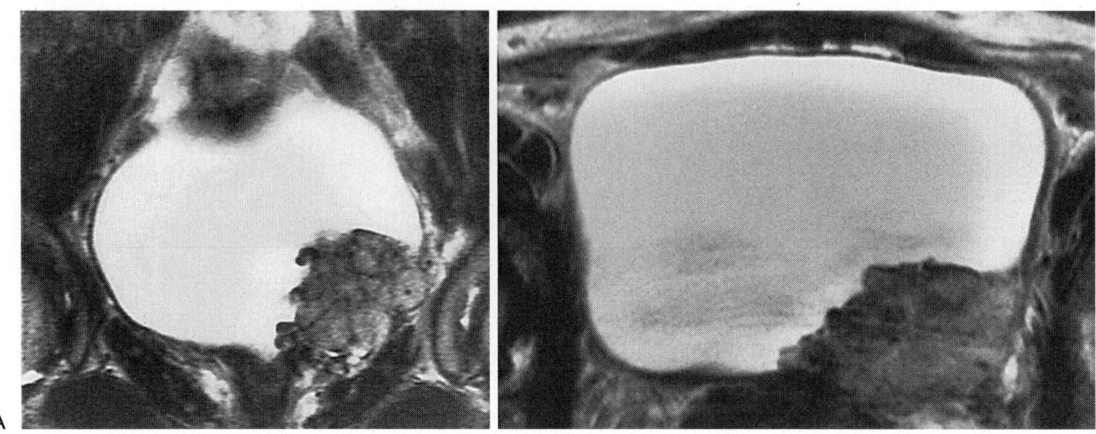

FIGURE 3E.20. Transmural invasion of bladder tumor using phased-array surface coils. **A:** A coronal T_1-weighted magnetic resonance imaging (MRI) demonstrates a papillary mass within the base of the bladder with extension outside the bladder wall. **B:** Axial T_1-weighted MRI demonstrates the extent of the mass through the wall in another plane.

trilayer appearance is seen corresponding to the three layers seen with T_2 weighting. The layers are disrupted to varying degrees by the invading tumor (5,62,83,86,89). This technique has achieved greater than 90% accuracy in some centers (5) (Fig. 3E.21).

The major limitation of MRI for local staging is that microscopic disease cannot be detected. The clinical importance of this is uncertain, but it lessens the accuracy of MRI staging. Also, tumors at the bladder outlet can be difficult to evaluate because the anatomy of the layers of the bladder wall is somewhat different at this site. Nevertheless, overall, extravesical extension is detected with a sensitivity of approximately 93% (65,86). Endorectal surface coils and phased-array surface coils placed on the low pelvis have been used to improve the signal-to-noise ratio and hence the resolution of the images. Conventional body coil MRI is used to detect lymphadenopathy; however, MRI is no more accurate than CT for assessing adenopathy because both modalities depend on changes in size as the criterion for positivity. As is well known from CT, nodes may be enlarged by hyperplastic changes, and small nodes may be infiltrated with tumor.

A recent development in MRI has been the dynamic assessment of pelvic floor relaxation. In this study, a rapid T_2-weighted image is obtained sagittally through the bladder base, uterus, and rectum at rest and then again during a straining maneuver (97). Cystoceles, uterine prolapse, rectal prolapse, and enteroceles are surprisingly well seen without having to resort to cystoproctolography, which is an uncomfortable and embarrassing procedure (53,96). The MR procedure is equally applied in men and in women, although it is usually a greater clinical issue in women because it is associated with incontinence (17,30,58).

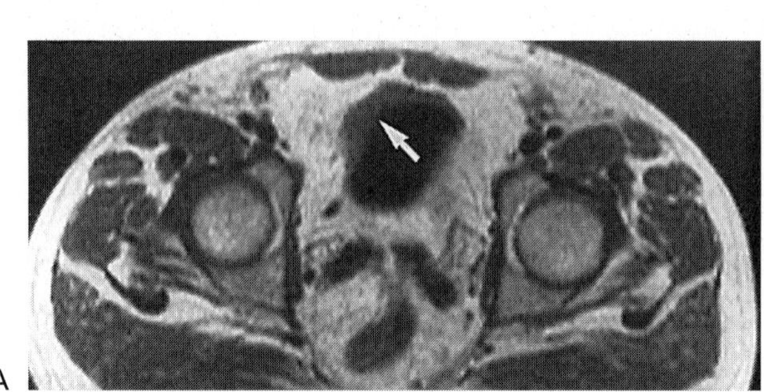

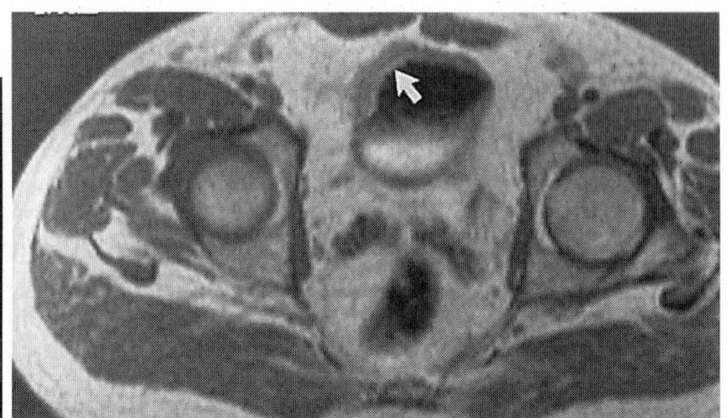

FIGURE 3E.21. The use of gadolinium enhancement to detect bladder wall tumors. **A:** Precontrast T_1-weighted magnetic resonance imaging scan demonstrates a thick rind of bladder tumor against the anterior lateral wall *(arrow)*. **B:** Postcontrast enhancement demonstrates enhancement of the tumor with small projections into the perivesical fat. The mucosal surface of the tumor is enhanced to a greater extent than the transmural component of the tumor.

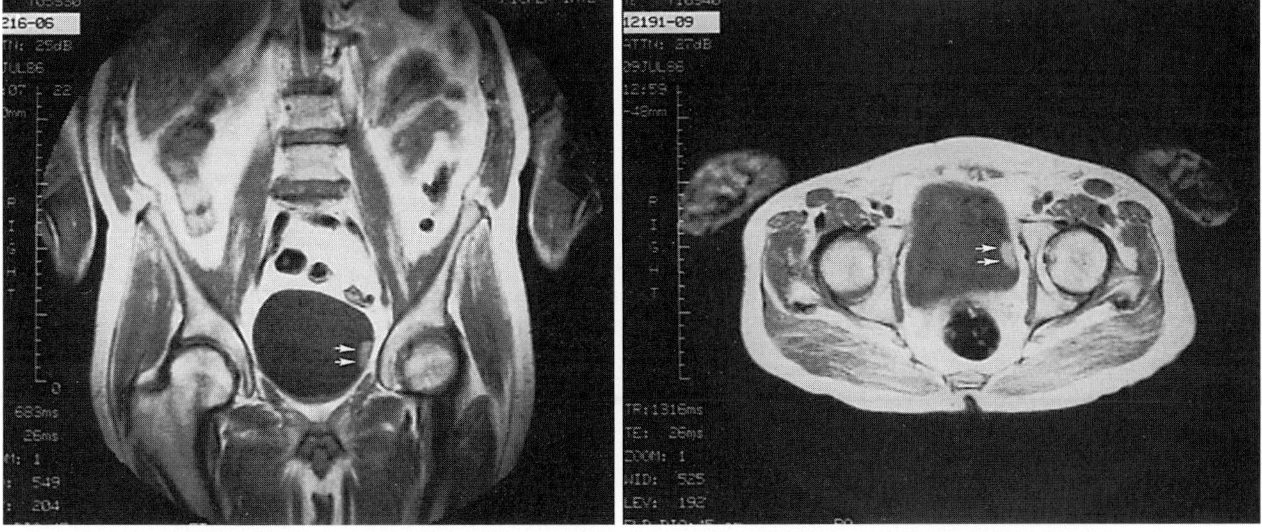

FIGURE 3E.22. Superficial bladder cancer on T_1-weighted magnetic resonance imaging. The small tumor *(double arrows)* is seen in the coronal **(A)** and axial **(B)** planes. Note that the bladder wall is undisturbed and there is no evidence of transmural invasion. No adenopathy is present. The natural contrast between the tumor and the urine in the bladder allows the tumor to be delineated.

Prostate

MRI of the prostate offers the possibility of accurate local staging of prostate cancers. With sufficient resolution, it is possible to visualize the neurovascular bundle and prostatic capsule with reliability. Results with whole body coil imaging, however, were disappointing, and it became clear that endorectal coils were needed for accurate staging (43,71). With the advent of endorectal surface coils, prostate MRI became a feasible method of staging local spread of prostate cancer. The endorectal coil allows a significant gain in signal-to-noise ratio, which permits high-resolution images. Thus fine detail of the prostatic surface and internal anatomy can be obtained (Figs. 3E.22, 3E.23, and 3E.24). Initial reports demonstrated a very high sensitivity for extracapsular disease versus localized disease (75); however, a subsequent multiinstitutional trial has had difficulty reproducing these results (69,90). As more experience has been gained it has become clear that MRI is useful in specific instances in which the risk of extracapsular disease is high based on prostate-specific antigen (PSA) and tumor grade (46).

To be successful, prostate MRI must be performed with an endorectal surface coil, which is inflated in the rectum with 60 to 100 mL of air and with a phased-array pelvic coil placed anteriorly on the pelvis (42). Glucagon (1 mg intramuscularly) is administered to reduce bowel motion. T_2-weighted images must be obtained with the highest resolution (3 to 4 mm thick with the smallest possible field of view). Field of view must be limited, and a large matrix size must be used. Axial and oblique coronal views through the prostate long axis should be obtained. Contrast enhancement, especially when applied dynamically, is useful in some instances (84,88).

T_2-weighted axial endorectal coil images and oblique coronal T_2-weighted images allow the apex to be evaluated more fully. Scanning should be extended through the seminal vesicles on both planes. T_1-weighted body coil images should be obtained through the pelvis to detect lymphadenopathy. As with bladder cancer, the criterion for lymph node involvement on MRI is increased size, which has well-known limitations.

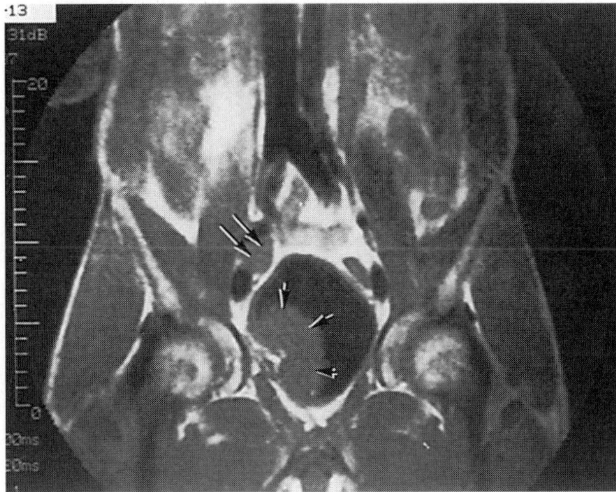

FIGURE 3E.23. Coronal T_1-weighted magnetic resonance imaging scan of large muscle invasive bladder cancer *(short arrows)* and tumorous pelvic lymph node *(long arrows)*.

The normal T_2-weighted image of the prostate demonstrates a high-signal peripheral zone with a central hypointense region corresponding to the central gland (central and transitional zones). The urethra is often high in signal intensity because of the presence of small amounts of urine and glandular tissue in the prostatic urethra. The central gland is surrounded by a hyperintense peripheral zone, which is the site of most prostate cancers. The posterior median raphe in the peripheral zone is often hypointense. Surrounding the peripheral zone on all but the posterior wall is the high-signal periprostatic venous plexus (Santorini's plexus), which serves as a marker for the margin of the prostate. The neurovascular bundles are seen at approximately the 5 and 7 o'clock positions on the axial views. Denonvilliers' fascia is seen as a thick low-signal band between the prostate and rectum (Fig. 3E.24). The seminal vesicles appear as multiple locules of high signal intensity above the prostate. The vas deferens are thick-walled structures medial to thin-walled seminal vesicles.

Prostate cancers appear as areas of relative hypointensity compared with the peripheral zone (68) (Fig. 3E.25). Of course, this appearance is not universal. Several hyperintense prostate cancers (mucinous adenocarcinoma) have been reported; moreover, hypointense lesions can represent biopsy artifact, hyperplasia, infarction, and other nonneoplastic disorders. To avoid a potentially misleading biopsy artifact, MRI should not be performed within 3 weeks of a biopsy.

The seminal vesicles, normally high in signal intensity, become focally hypointense when involved with tumor on T_2-weighted images. However, this can be mimicked by epithelial hyperplasia of the glandular lining of the seminal vesicle or by atrophy. Thus hypointense seminal vesicles are suspicious but not absolutely diagnostic of extracapsular extension. Contrast-enhanced MRI may show areas of tumor, which should enhance while benign entities remain low in signal intensity (84).

The reported accuracy of endorectal coil imaging varies from 51% to 82% depending on patient mix and experience (69,90). Overall, the staging accuracy is approximately 68% to 70% in most studies (13,69). Most staging errors with MRI occur from understaging, which will not deny patients potentially curative surgery. False-positive studies are unusual but are more problematic because they would deny potentially curative surgery. Another issue is that intraobserver disagreement occurs with some frequency using endorectal coil MRI, and proper training is essential before these studies begin to yield clinically useful data (35,73). However, with improvements in MRI technique it is expected that image interpretation will become more uniform and reliable. For instance, accuracy can be greatly improved by using a computer-based algorithm that considers both MR and clinical features of the patient. MR has also been proposed as a method of guiding placement of brachytherapy seeds (19). MR spectroscopy (MRS) has recently been proposed as a diagnostic technique. There is a growing recognition that extracapsular disease per se is not necessarily a contraindication to radical prostatectomy (46,74). Better methods of determining inherent biologic aggressiveness of tumors are being sought. One method, MRS, is based on the metabolic signature of cancers relative to the rest of the prostate. Using ^1H spectroscopy, the normal prostate is unusually rich in citrate and choline. Cancers are lower in citrate, resulting in abnormal choline-to-citrate ratios. Data indicate that the magnitude of substrate ratios such as choline to citrate reflects the biologic

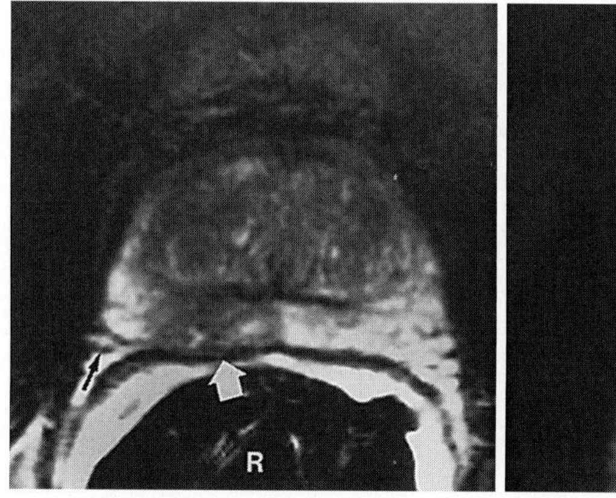

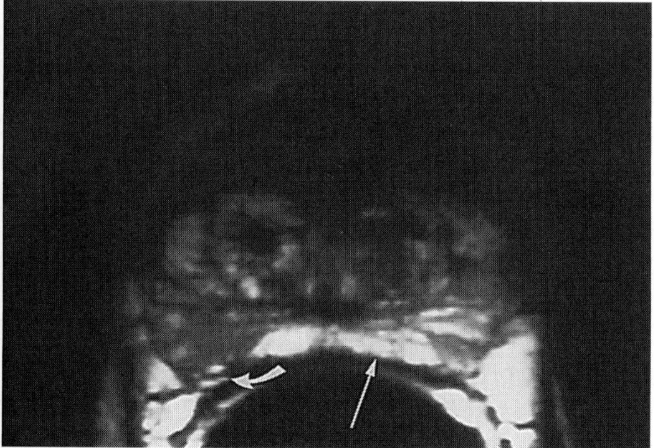

FIGURE 3E.24. Endorectal coil magnetic resonance imaging scan showing stage B prostate cancer. A transverse section demonstrates the thick Denonvilliers' fascia *(white arrows).* The tumor, which is low in signal intensity, can be seen in the background of the high-signal-intensity peripheral zone. The neurovascular bundle *(black arrow)* is spared. R, rectum. (Courtesy of Dr. Ronald M. Summers, NIH.)

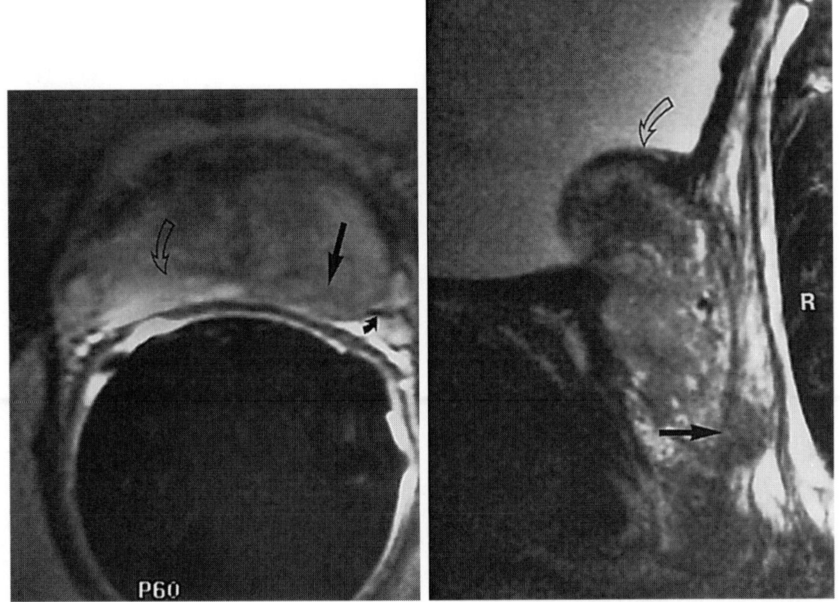

FIGURE 3E.25. Endorectal coil magnetic resonance imaging scan showing T_3 prostate cancer. **A:** The transverse image demonstrates the hypointense tumor *(black arrow)* involving the left prostatic hemisphere. The tumor abuts and involves the neurovascular bundle. *Curved arrow* demonstrates normal peripheral zone. **B:** Sagittal view demonstrates the bulging of the capsule *(straight arrow)* from the tumor. Prostatic hyperplastic nodules are seen within the bladder base *(curved arrow).*

aggressiveness independent of other factors such as PSA and Gleason score.

Testicle

MRI does not currently have a routine role in the evaluation of testicular disease. This is because of the combined success of physical examination and testicular sonography for diagnosing the most testicular diseases. There is experimental evidence that MRI may be useful in the evaluation of testicular torsion and neoplasia. However, it is unlikely that MRI will be a mainstream test for these indications.

The testicles are normally very bright on T_2-weighted images. Testicular MRI must be performed with surface coils to achieve high-resolution images. Tumors are even more hyperintense but often are heterogeneous in signal intensity. Cysts and dilated rete testis will be uniformly hyperintense on T_2-weighted images. Therefore MR is useful when the differential consideration of a testicular ultrasound is dilated rete testis versus a neoplasm. Testicular tumors enhance significantly with intravenous contrast media, but the appearance on MRI is nonspecific regarding histology (21). MRI may be valuable in local staging of the scrotum because small disruptions of the tunica albuginea may be missed on ultrasound and physical examination. However, MRI does not contribute sufficient information to be justified routinely.

Dynamic enhanced testicular MRI has been used to evaluate testicular ischemia in animals. Enhancement is very delayed or absent on the torqued side, and time activity curves analogous to the radionuclide scan can be obtained (20). Delayed washout of the contrast medium may be related to venous compression. Better anatomic detail is possible with MRI than with sonography, and the torqued spermatic cord can be directly visualized. Advantages of MRI are that it does not require radiation, it can provide a semiquantitative assessment of perfusion, and it may provide more information about the viability of the testicle than either nuclear medicine or color-flow Doppler studies. Disadvantages include its cost, limited availability on an emergency basis, and requirement for intravenous contrast.

Penis

The anatomy of the penis is readily depicted on MRI (38). On T_1-weighted images, the corpora are relatively low in signal. The corpora are high in signal intensity on T_2-weighted imaging. The urethra is not seen unless a Foley catheter is in place (Fig. 3E.26). Absence of a high signal within the corpora can be seen in thrombosis associated with priapism (45,77) (Fig. 3E.27). The plaques of Peyronie's disease can also be detected with MRI and can be used to guide and monitor treatment (34,87). Fractures of the penis, in the setting of pelvic crush injuries, can be evaluated for surgical repair using MRI (2,8,24).

Investigators have evaluated the potential of dynamic enhanced MRI for determining the cause of erectile dysfunction (41). They have found delayed enhancement of corpora in patients with arterial insufficiency. Valvular disease results in a rapid washinn and washout of contrast media (41). The future of penile MRI for erectile dysfunction will depend on the success of procedures to correct erectile dysfunction.

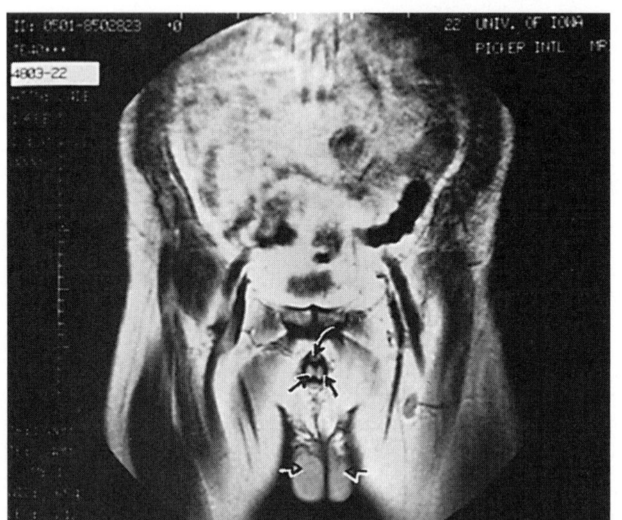

A

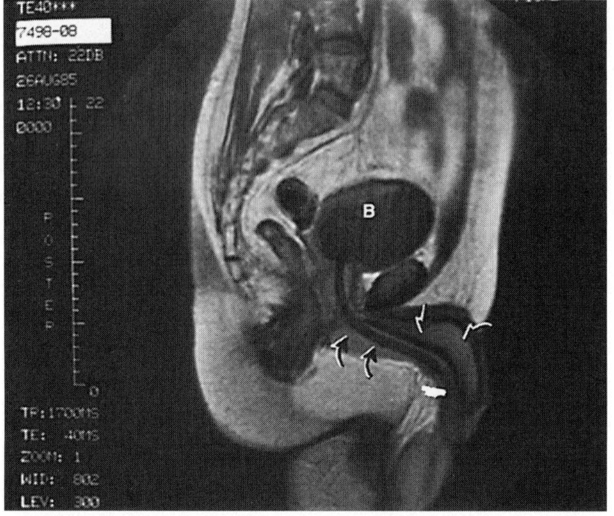

B

FIGURE 3E.26. A: Coronal T_1-weighted magnetic resonance imaging (MRI) scan of normal pelvis showing corpus spongiosum *(curved arrow),* corpora cavernosa *(straight arrows),* and testicles *(open arrows).* **B:** Sagittal T_1-weighted MRI of normal pelvis showing corpus cavernosum *(straight arrow)* and bulbocavernosus muscle *(curved arrows).* There is a catheter in the bladder **(B).**

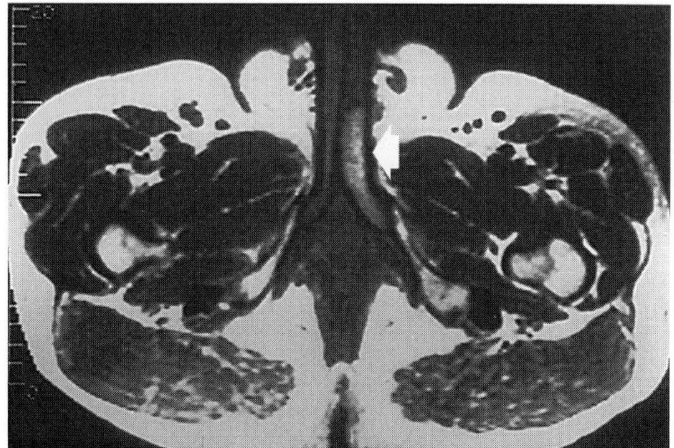

A

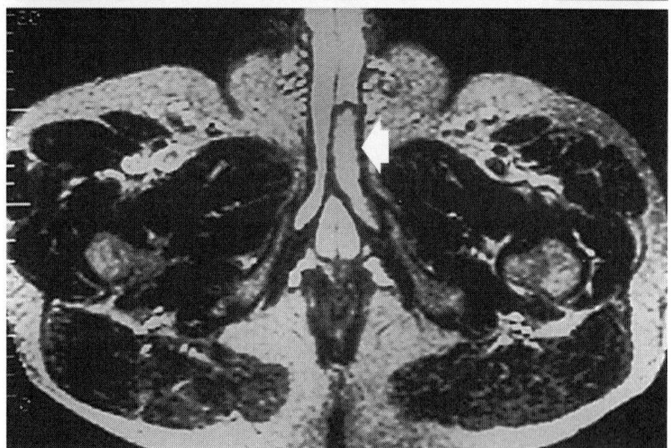

B

FIGURE 3E.27. Partial penile thrombus with priapism. **A:** T_1-weighted image demonstrates a high-signal-intensity thrombus *(arrow)* within the left corpora cavernosa. **B:** T_2-weighted image demonstrates a high-signal-intensity rim. (Reprinted with permission from Kimball DA, Yuh WTC, Farmer RM. MR diagnosis of penile thrombus. *J Comput Tomogr* 1988;12:604.)

MAGNETIC RESONANCE IMAGING IN THE FUTURE

There are several exciting trends in MRI. MR technology continues to improve in total imaging time, spatial resolution, and flexibility. Recently, determination of the functional status of organs has become possible with dynamic enhancement or changes in perfusion. Focus is now directed at the brain because it is the most straightforward organ to assess, but functional studies may soon be directed at other organs, including the kidneys and testicles. This may affect the assessment of renal function and primary testicular infertility. MRS may also prove to be a useful diagnostic tool.

Open-bore magnets that decrease patient anxiety but also allow for invasive procedures under MRI are widespread. These may permit biopsy or even operative procedures to be performed with real-time MR guidance. The quality of open-bore magnets has greatly improved, although the flexibility of such units remains limited.

New contrast agents are being developed to improve the tissue specificity of MRI. Such agents may be able to distinguish malignant and benign nodes noninvasively. Ultrasmall iron dextran particles already have shown promise in this area in animals. Tissue-specific antibody imaging may also be possible. The goal of this research is to improve the tissue specificity of MRI and allow noninvasive "MR biopsies" to be reliably performed, and this continues to be an active area of research.

Acknowledgments

The author wishes to thank Barbara McCoy for her secretarial assistance and Ronald M. Summers, MD, PhD, for valuable advice.

REFERENCES

1. Amendola MA, King LR, Pollack HM, et al. Staging of renal cancer using MRI at 1.5 Tesla. *Cancer* 1990;66:40.
2. Armenakas NA, McAninch JW, Lue TF, et al. Posttraumatic impotence: magnetic resonance imaging and duplex ultrasound in diagnosis and management. *J Urol* 1993;149:1272.
3. Bakker J, Ligtenberg G, Beek FJA, et al. Preoperative evaluation of living renal donors with gadolinium-enhanced magnetic resonance angiography. *Transplantation* 1999;67:1167.
4. Balci NC, Mueller-Lisse UG, Holzknecht N, et al. Breathhold MR urography: comparison between HASTE and RARE in healthy volunteers. *Eur Radiol* 1998;8:925.
5. Barentz JO, Ruijs SHJ, Strijk SP. The role of MR imaging in carcinoma of the urinary bladder. *AJR Am J Roentgenol* 1993; 160:937.
6. Binkert CA, Hoffman U, Leung DA, et al. Characterization of renal artery stenoses based on magnetic resonance renal flow and volume measurements. *Kidney Int* 1999;56:1846.
7. Borthne A, Nordshus T, Reiseter T, et al. MR urography: the future gold standard in pediatric urogenital imaging? *Pediatr Radiol* 1999;29:694.
8. Boudghene F, Chem R, Wallays C, et al. MR imaging in acute fracture of the penis. *Urol Radiol* 1992;14:202.
9. Burt M, Heelan RT, Coit D, et al. Prospective evaluation of unilateral adrenal masses in patients with operable non small cell lung cancer. Impact of magnetic resonance imaging. *J Thorac Cardiovasc Surg* 1994;107:584.
10. Buy JM, Moss AA, Guinet C, et al. MR staging of bladder carcinoma: correlation with pathologic findings. *Radiology* 1988; 169:695.
11. Candel AG, Gattuso P, Reyes CV, et al. Fine needle aspiration biopsy of adrenal masses in patients with extraadrenal malignancy. *Surgery* 1993;114:1132.
12. Chang A, Glazer HS, Lee JKT, et al. Adrenal gland: MR imaging. *Radiology* 1987;163:123.
13. Chelsky MJ, Schnall MD, Seidmon EJ, et al. Use of endorectal surface coil MRI in staging prostate cancer. *J Urol* 1993; 150:391.
14. Choyke P, Kressel H, Pollack H, et al. Focal renal masses: magnetic resonance imaging. *Radiology* 1984;152:471.
15. Choyke PC. From needles to numbers. *World J Urol* 1998; 16:29.
16. Choyke PL. Focal renal masses: magnetic resonance imaging. *Radiology* 1988;169:572.
17. Comiter CV, Vasavada SP, Barbaric AL, et al. Grading pelvic prolapse and pelvic floor relaxation using dynamic magnetic resonance imaging. *Urology* 1999;54:454.
18. Copeland PM. The incidentally discovered adrenal mass: an update. *Endocrinologist* 1999;9:415.
19. Cormack RA, Kooy H, Tempany CM, et al. A clinical method for real-time domestic guidance of transperineal I-125 prostate implants using interventional magnetic resonance imaging. *Int J Radiat Oncol Biol Phys* 2000;46:207.
20. Costabile R, Choyke PL, Frank JA, et al. Dynamic enhanced magnetic resonance imaging of testicular perfusion in the rat. *J Urol* 1993;149:1195.
21. Cramer BM, Schlegel EA, Thueroff JW. MR imaging in the differential diagnosis of scrotal and testicular disease. *Radiographics* 1991;11:9.
22. Dalla-Palma L, Panzetta G, Pozzi-Mucelli RS, et al. Dynamic magnetic resonance imaging in the assessment of chronic medical nephropathies with impaired renal function. *Eur Radiol* 2000;10:280-286.
23. Defossez SM, Yoder IC, Papinicolaou N, et al. Nonspecific magnetic resonance appearance of renal oncocytomas: report of 3 cases and review of the literature. *J Urol* 1991;145:552.
24. Dixon CM, Hricak H, McAninch JW. Magnetic resonance imaging of traumatic posterior urethral defects and pelvic crush injuries. *J Urol* 1992;148:1165.
25. Dong Q, Schoenberg SO, Carlos RC, et al. Diagnosis of renal vascular disease with MR angiography. *Radiographics* 1999;19: 1535.
26. Francis IR, Gross MD, Shapiro B, et al. Integrated imaging of adrenal disease. *Radiology* 1992;184:1.
27. Fritzsche PH, Millar C. Multimodality approach to staging renal cell carcinoma. *Urol Radiol* 1992;14:3.
28. Ghantous VE, Eisen TD, Sherman AH, et al. Evaluating patients with renal failure for renal artery stenosis with gadolinium-enhanced magnetic resonance angiography. *Am J Kidney Dis* 1999;33:36.
29. Goldfarb DA, Novick AC, Lorig R, et al. Magnetic resonance imaging for the assessment of vena caval tumor thrombi: a comparative study with venacavography and computerized tomography scanning. *J Urol* 1990;144:1100.
30. Gufler H, Laubenberger J, DeGregorio G, et al. Pelvic floor descent: dynamic MR imaging using a half-Fourier RARE sequence. *J Magn Reson Imaging* 1999;9:378.
31. Hanna S, Helenon O, Legendre C, et al. MR imaging of renal transplant rejection. *Acta Radiol* 1991;32:42.
32. Haustein J, Niendorf HP, Krestin G. Renal tolerance of gadolinium-DTPA/dimeglumine in patients with chronic renal failure. *Invest Radiol* 1992;27:153.
33. Helenon O, Attlan E, Legendre C, et al. Gd-DOTA enhanced MR imaging and color doppler US of renal allograft necrosis. *Radiographics* 1992;12:21.
34. Helweg G, Judmaier W, Buchberger W, et al. Peyronie's disease: MR findings in 28 patients. *AJR Am J Roentgenol* 1992;158: 1261.
35. Holtz P, Zerhouni EA. MR imaging in adenocarcinoma of the prostate. Interobserver variation and efficacy for determining stage C disease. *AJR Am J Roentgenol* 1992;158:559.
36. Horan JJ, Robertson CN, Choyke PL, et al. The detection of renal carcinoma extension into the renal vein and IVC: prospective comparison of venacavography and MRI. *J Urol* 1989; 142:943.
37. Hricak H, Demas BE, Williams RD, et al. Magnetic resonance imaging in the diagnosis and staging of renal and perirenal neoplasms. *Radiology* 1985;154:709.

38. Hricak H, Marotti M, Gilbert TJ, et al. Normal penile anatomy and abnormal penile conditions: evaluation with MR imaging. *Radiology* 1988;169:683.
39. Iselin CE, Leder RA, Lacey J, et al. Renal lymphoma in an azotemic patient: usefulness of magnetic resonance imaging. *Scand J Urol Nephrol* 1999;33:129.
40. Kabala JE, Gillatt DA, Persad RA, et al. MRI in the staging of renal cell carcinoma. *Br J Radiol* 1991;64:683.
41. Kaneko K, De Mouy EH, Lee BE. Sequential contrast enhanced MR imaging of the penis. *Radiology* 1994;191:75.
42. Kier R, Wain S, Troiano R. Fast spin-echo MR images of the pelvis obtained with a phased-array coil: value in localizing and staging prostatic carcinoma. *AJR Am J Roentgenol* 1993;161:601.
43. Kim D, Edelman RR, Kent KC, et al. Abdominal aorta and renal artery stenosis: evaluation with MRI angiography. *Radiology* 1990;174:727.
44. Kim SH, Han MC, Han JS. Exercise induced acute renal failure and patchy renal vasoconstriction: CT and MR findings. *J Comput Assist Tomogr* 1991;15:985.
45. Kimball DA, Yuh WTC, Farner RM. MR diagnosis of penile thrombosis. *J Comput Assist Tomogr* 1988;12:604.
46. Kindrick AV, Grossfeld GD, Stier DM, et al. Use of imaging rests for staging newly diagnosed prostate cancer: trends from the CaPSURE database. *J Urol* 1998;160:2102.
47. Korobkin M, Aisen AM, Francis IR, et al. Differentiation of adrenal adenomas from non-adenomas using chemical shift and gadolinium enhanced MRI imaging. Paper presented at the Annual Meeting of the Society of Uroradiology, Jan 1994.
48. Krestin GP, Freidmann G, Fishbach R, et al. Evaluation of adrenal masses in oncologic patients: dynamic contrast enhanced MR vs. CT. *J Comput Assist Tomogr* 1991;15:104.
49. Lee JKT. Recent advances in magnetic resonance imaging of renal masses. *Can Assoc Radiol J* 1991;42:158.
50. Lee MJ, Hahn PF, Papanicolau N, et al. Benign and malignant adrenal masses: CT distinction with attenuation coefficients, size and observer analysis. *Radiology* 1991;179:415.
51. Lee MJ, Mayo-Smith WW, Hahn PF, et al. State of the art imaging of the adrenal gland. *Radiographics* 1994;14:1015.
52. Lee VS, Rofsky NM, Krinsky GA, et al. Single-dose breath-hold gadolinium-enhanced three-dimensional MR angiography of the renal arteries. *Radiology* 1999;211:69.
53. Lienemann A, Anthuber C, Baron A, et al. Diagnosing enteroceles using dynamic magnetic resonance imaging. *Dis Colon Rectum* 2000;43:205.
54. Luk SH, Chan JHM, Kwan TH, et al. Breath-hold 3D gadolinium-enhanced subtraction MRA in the detection of transplant renal artery stenosis. *Clin Radiol* 1999;54:651.
55. Maurea S, Cuocolo A, Reynolds JC, et al. MIBG scintigraphy in preoperative and postoperative evaluation of paragangliomas: comparison with CT and MRI. *J Nucl Med* 1993;34:173.
56. McClennan BL, Deyoe LA. The imaging evaluation of renal cell carcinoma: diagnosis and staging. *Radiol Clin North Am* 1994; 32:55.
57. McGahan JP. Adrenal gland: MR imaging. *Radiology* 1988; 166:284.
58. Mikuma N, Tamegawa M, Morita K, et al. Magnetic resonance imaging of the male pelvic floor: the anatomical configuration and dynamic movement in healthy men. *Neurourol Urodyn* 1998;17:591.
59. Miller S, Schick F, Duda SH, et al. GD-enhanced eD phase-contrast MR angiography and dynamic perfusion imaging in the diagnosis of renal artery stenosis. *Magn Reson Imaging* 1998; 16:1005.
60. Mitchell DG, Crovello M, Matteucci T. Benign adrenocortical masses: diagnosis with chemical shift imaging. *Radiology* 1992; 185:339.
61. Myeni L, Hricak H, Carroll PR. MRI of renal carcinoma with extension into the vena cava: staging accuracy and recent advances. *Br J Urol* 1991;68:57.
62. Narumi Y, Kadota T, Inoue E, et al. Bladder tumors: staging with gadolinium enhanced oblique MRI imaging. *Radiology* 1993;187:145.
63. Neimatallah MA, Dong Q, Schoenberg SO, et al. Magnetic resonance imaging in renal transplantation. *J Magn Reson Imaging* 1999;10:357.
64. Nelson HA, Gilfeather M, Holman JM, et al. Gadolinium-enhanced breathhold three-dimensional time-of-flight renal MR angiography in the evaluation of potential renal donors. *J Vasc Interv Radiol* 1999;10:175.
65. Neuerburg JM, Bohndorf K, Sohn M, et al. Staging of urinary bladder neoplasms with MR imaging: is Gd-DTPA helpful? *J Comput Assist Tomogr* 1991;15:780.
66. Neumann HP, Berger DP, Sigmund G, et al. Pheochromocytomas, multiple endocrine neoplasia type 2, and von Hippel–Lindau disease [Comments]. *N Engl J Med* 1993;329:1531 [published erratum appears in *N Engl J Med* 1994;331:1535].
67. Nolte-Ernsting CCA, Bucker A, Adam GB, et al. Gadolinium-enhanced excretory MR urography after low-dose diuretic injection: comparison with conventional excretory urography. *Radiology* 1998;209:147.
68. Perrotti M, Han KR, Epstein RE, et al. Prospective evaluation of endorectal magnetic resonance imaging to detect tumor foci in men with prior negative prostatic biopsy: a pilot study. *J Urol* 1999;162:1314.
69. Quinn SF, Franzini DA, Demlow TA, et al. MR imaging of prostate cancer with an endorectal surface coil technique: correlation with whole-mount specimens. *Radiology* 1994;190:323.
70. Reinig KD, Rush CG, Pelster HL, et al. Real-time visually and haptically accurate surgical simulation. *Stud Health Technol Inform* 1996;29:542.
71. Rifkin MD, Zerhouni EA, Gatsonis CA, et al. Comparison of magnetic resonance imaging and ultrasonography in staging early prostate cancer. Results of a multi-institutional cooperative trial [Comments]. *N Engl J Med* 1990;323:621.
72. Rominger MB, Kenney PJ, Morgan DE, et al. Gadolinium-enhanced MR imaging of renal masses. *Radiographics* 1992;12: 1097.
73. Schiebler ML, Yankaskas BC, Tempany C, et al. MR imaging in adenocarcinoma of the prostate: interobserver variation and efficacy for determining stage C disease. *AJR Am J Roentgenol* 1992;158:559.
74. Schmid HP, Oerpenning F, Pummer K. Diagnosis and staging of prostatic carcinoma: what is really necessary? *Urol Int* 1999; 63:57.
75. Schnall MD, Connick T, Hayes CE, et al. MR imaging of the pelvis with an endorectal-external multicoil array. *J Magn Reson Imaging* 1992;2:229.
76. Schoenberg SO, Essig M, Bock M, et al. Comprehensive MR evaluation of renovascular disease in five breath holds. *J Magn Reson Imaging* 1999;10:347.
77. Schroeder-Printzen I, Schroeder-Printzen J, Weidner W, et al. Diagnosis and therapy of erectile dysfunction: a function of legal health insurance? *Urologe A* 1994;33:252.
78. Semelka RC, Hricak H, Stevens SK, et al. Combined gadolinium-enhanced and fat-saturation MR imaging of renal masses. *Radiology* 1991;178:803.

79. Semelka RC, Shoenut JP, Kroeker MA, et al. Renal lesions: controlled comparison between CT and 1.5-T MR imaging with nonenhanced and gadolinium-enhanced fat-suppressed spin-echo and breath-hold FLASH techniques [Comments]. *Radiology* 1992;182:425.
80. Semelka RC, Shoenut JP, Kroeker RM. T2-weighted MR imaging of focal hepatic lesions: comparison of various RARE and fat-suppressed spin-echo sequences. *J Magn Reson Imaging* 1993; 3:323.
81. Silverman SG, Mueller PR, Pinkney LP, et al. Predictive value of image-guided adrenal biopsy: analysis of results of 101 biopsies. *Radiology* 1993;187:715.
82. Slapa RZ, Jakubowski W, Januszewicz A, et al. Discriminatory power of MRI for differentiation of adrenal non-adenomas vs adenomas evaluated by means of ROC analysis: can biopsy be obviated? *Eur Radiol* 2000;10:95.
83. Sohn M, Neuerburg J, Teufl F, et al. Gadolinium-enhanced magnetic resonance imaging in the staging of urinary bladder neoplasms. *Urol Int* 1990;45:142.
84. Sommer FG, Nghiem HV, Herfkens R, et al. Gadolinium-enhanced MRI of the abnormal prostate. *Magn Reson Imaging* 1993;11:941.
85. Stutley JE, Reinig JW, Leonhardt CM, et al. Adrenal MR imaging: comparison of four methods for distinguishing benign adrenal masses from metastases and pheochromocytomas. Paper presented at the 79th Scientific Assembly of the Radiologic Society of North America, Nov 1993.
86. Tachibana M, Baba S, Deguchi N, et al. Efficacy of Gd-DTPA enhanced magnetic resonance imaging for differentiation between superficial and muscle invasive tumor of the bladder: a comparative study with computerized tomography and transurethral ultrasonography. *J Urol* 1991;145:1169.
87. Tamburrini O, Della Sala M, Sessa M, et al. Functional magnetic resonance of Peyronie's disease in the chronic stable phase. *Radiol Med (Torino)* 1993;86:851.
88. Tanaka N, Samma S, Joko M, et al. Diagnostic usefulness of endorectal magnetic resonance imaging with dynamic contrast-enhancement in patients with localized prostate cancer: mapping studies with biopsy specimens. *Int J Urol* 1999;6:593.
89. Tanimoto A, Yuasa Y, Imai Y, et al. Bladder tumor staging: comparison of conventional and gadolinium enhanced dynamic MR imaging and CT. *Radiology* 1992;185:741.
90. Tempany CM, Zhou X, Zerhouni EA, et al. Staging of prostate cancer: results of Radiology Diagnostic Oncology Group project comparison of three MR imaging techniques. *Radiology* 1994;1:47.
91. Terens WL, Gluck R, Golimbu M, et al. Use of gadolinium-DTPA-enhanced MRI to characterize renal mass in patient with renal insufficiency. *Urology* 1992;40:152.
92. Tikkakoski T, Taavitsainen M, Paivansalo M, et al. Accuracy of adrenal biopsy guided by ultrasound and CT. *Acta Radiol* 1991; 32:371.
93. Tsushima Y, Ishizaka H, Matsumoto M. Adrenal masses: differentiation with chemical shift fast low angle shot MR imaging. *Radiology* 1993;186:705.
94. Van Erkel AR, van Gils AP, Lequin M, et al. CT and MR distinction of adenomas and nonadenomas of the adrenal gland. *J Comput Assist Tomogr* 1994;18:432.
95. Van Gils AP, Falke TH, van Erkel AR, et al. MR imaging and MIBG scintigraphy of pheochromocytomas and extraadrenal functioning paragangliomas. *Radiographics* 1991;11:37.
96. Vanbeckevoort D, Van Hoe L, Oyen R, et al. Pelvic floor descent in females: comparative study of colpocystodefecography and dynamic fast MR imaging. *J Magn Reson Imaging* 1999;9:373.
97. Weidner AC, Low VHS. Imaging studies of the pelvic floor. *Obstet Gynecol Clin North Am* 1998;25:825.

3F

VASCULAR IMAGING

J. BAYNE SELBY, JR.

The dramatic advances that have occurred in radiologic imaging techniques over the last 20 years make it difficult for editors of textbooks to decide what is worthy of inclusion and what should be discarded. The solution in this chapter was to give different imaging modalities used for urologic investigations their own section. This works fine until one addresses imaging of urology conditions that have a predominantly vascular basis. The current state of imaging in regard to vascular disease can at times require the use of any or all of the different modalities. Angiography, still the gold standard for visualization of vascular issues, is being rapidly supplemented by computed tomographic angiography (CTA), magnetic resonance angiography (MRA), color Doppler ultrasound, and nuclear medicine. With the current emphasis on cost containment, efficient workups, and clinical pathways, trying to determine when and where to use each of these modalities can be perplexing. This chapter attempts to define the strengths and weaknesses of each imaging technique by approaching the subject from a clinical question standpoint. Technical descriptions of the different modalities, except for angiography, are covered in other chapters.

J.B. Selby, Jr.: Department of Radiology, Medical University of South Carolina; Vascular/International Radiology, Medical University Hospital, Charleston, SC 29425.

TECHNIQUE OF ANGIOGRAPHY

The basics of angiography have not changed since Seldinger (22) described his technique for percutaneous puncture of the common femoral artery in 1953. However, the tools have undergone significant improvements, with a resultant increase in success rates and decrease in complications. Although angiography is still an invasive procedure compared with ultrasound or computed tomography (CT), this fact alone should not prevent a patient from having an angiogram if indicated. Most series quote the incidence of serious complications from angiography in the range of 0.5% to 2.5% (14,23,24); however, these studies were all done before 1980, when catheters were larger and stiffer, fluoroscopic visualization was inferior to that available today, and digital subtraction angiography had not been developed. In addition, nonionic contrast was not available at that time. No large series of complications from angiography have been published recently, but it is reasonable to assume that the basic procedure is safer than it was 25 years ago.

The most important aspect of preprocedure evaluation of the patient is assessment of renal function. The amount of contrast material used for a study is usually not an issue in otherwise healthy individuals, but diabetic patients and patients with impaired renal function are more susceptible to acute renal failure (4,5,10,17). A baseline creatinine level should always be obtained and any recent trends noted. The risk of acute renal failure is greater in someone with a creatinine of 2.5 mg/dL that has been rising over the last week than in a patient who has been stable at that level. There is no clear consensus on whether bleeding parameters should be checked, although the majority still check prothrombin time, partial thromboplastin time, and platelets. Anyone with a history of bleeding tendencies should have appropriate laboratory studies. Most angiographers require an international normalized ratio of less than 1.5 before proceeding with angiography.

In the past, most patients were admitted to the hospital the night before a procedure. This is no longer true unless the patient happens to already be an inpatient. Therefore particular attention must be paid to adequate hydration before the study (7). Outpatient angiography is now common. Outpatients usually arrive early in the morning, are evaluated, receive an intravenous catheter and groin preparation, and are then taken to the angiography suite.

The procedure is usually performed using conscious sedation such as midazolam and fentanyl, as well as local anesthesia at the arterial puncture site. Sterile preparation and drape is observed. Access is obtained through either common femoral artery. If the femoral arteries are unavailable for any reason, angiography can be performed from an axillary artery approach. Translumbar aortography is no longer performed. Nonionic contrast material is nearly always used in angiography. The risk of contrast reaction is much less. There is currently debate over whether nonionic contrast carries a lower risk of nephrotoxicity. This is covered in more detail in other chapters. Carbon dioxide and gadolinium are sometimes used as contrast agents in patients with severely compromised renal function (2,12,26). Procedures are most often performed using a 5-Fr catheter. For many interventions, microcatheters, which can be placed through a 5-Fr catheter, are used.

After the procedure is completed, the catheter is removed from the groin and pressure is held for approximately 15 minutes. Historically, patients had to lie flat with their legs straight for 6 hours after the procedure, but many sites now allow patients to ambulate earlier. Also, a number of percutaneous closure devices have recently become available. These devices act by using either a suture or a collagen plug to obtain immediate hemostasis. As more experience is gained with these devices, the recovery period will continue to shorten.

As mentioned earlier, many imaging techniques can be used to aid in the diagnosis and treatment of vascular-related problems. The remainder of this chapter provides guidance on the appropriate use of various imaging modalities in a number of common clinical problems. This is not meant to be a thorough discussion of each entity because these are covered in later chapters.

RENOVASCULAR HYPERTENSION

It is fair to say that this is one area where the treatment of the disease has progressed more rapidly than the diagnosis. Angioplasty and metal stents have significantly simplified the treatment of renovascular hypertension over the last 15 years (Fig. 3F.1), but our ability to accurately detect the presence of the disease has changed little. It is also fair to say that there is more variability from institution to institution in the diagnostic techniques used than in any other of the clinical situations discussed here.

All the imaging techniques are aimed at identifying a renal artery stenosis. This must then be correlated with other clinical data to determine the likelihood that the stenosis is related to the hypertension. Venography with renal vein sampling for renin is the one exception. Lateralization of elevated renin to one kidney is presumptive evidence of renovascular hypertension. Angiography can be done at the same time to determine the presence or absence of a stenosis. Unfortunately, it takes a number of days to get the renin assay results back, so if this approach is taken, angioplasty/stent placement must be postponed until the results are available. In practice, renal vein sampling for renin is not usually performed at most institutions except in questionable cases or when it is unclear how to proceed. One example is the case in which no arterial stenosis is found but peripheral renins are clearly elevated. Renal vein sampling may indicate which kidney is the culprit. Another example is the case in which a stenosis is found but does not appear significant. Obtaining renal vein renins can then be used to determine whether to bring the patient back for treatment of the questionable stenosis.

As far as imaging of a stenosis is concerned, angiography is still the gold standard; however, CTA (18) and MRA (8) have both made dramatic improvements over the last 10 years. The success of these two modalities is highly dependent on the experience and interest of the radiologists at a given institution. At medical centers with little experience in either CTA or MRA, their reliability is variable. Many centers have begun using these as a standard screening examination, and in experienced hands, the accuracy exceeds 85%. More important, the negative predictive value can be greater than 95% (18). Angiography is still performed at the time of treatment, but using CTA or MRA can greatly reduce the number of negative angiograms. CTA and MRA have the advantage of being noninvasive, but they both require intravenous contrast material. Gadolinium is now used for almost all MRA, and CTA requires rapid intravenous contrast injection. Computerized three-dimensional (3D) reconstruction techniques show promise of replacing standard two-dimensional imaging in the near future. This allows examination of the artery in 360 degrees and increases the sensitivity of the examination.

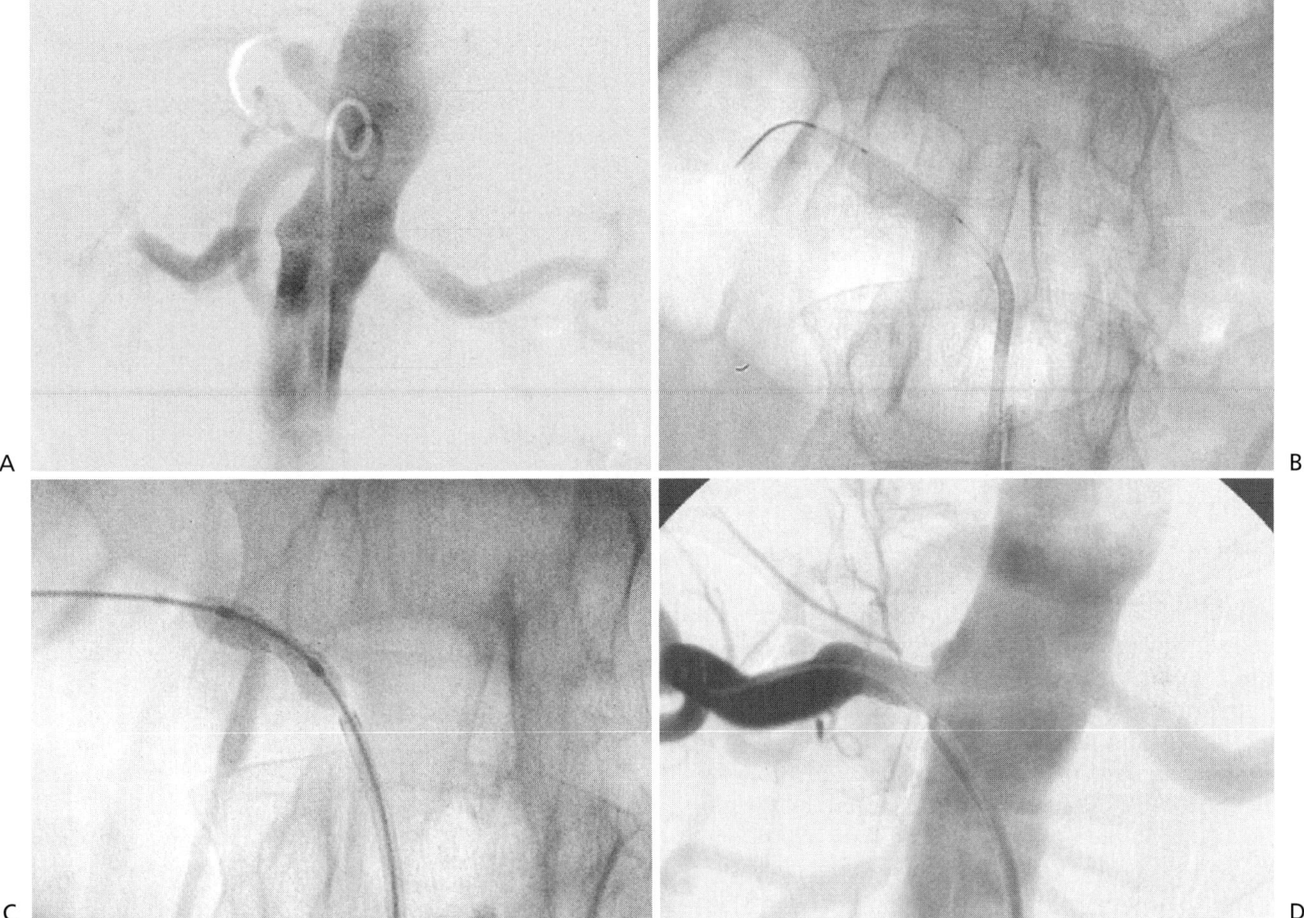

FIGURE 3F.1. Patient with difficult to control hypertension on four medications. Creatinine elevated at 1.7 mg/dL. **A:** Digital subtraction angiography demonstrates a 99% stenosis in the right renal artery and a less severe stenosis on the left. **B:** A balloon-on-a-wire low-profile system is used to dilate the lesion. **C:** Because of a residual 40% stenosis, a balloon-expandable stent is placed. **D:** Stent in place and no residual stenosis.

Nuclear medicine renal scans, with or without captopril, can be useful in cases of unilateral stenosis (6). Interpretation becomes more difficult if both sides show symmetric function. At institutions where CTA and MRA have not been pursued, renal scans remain the primary screening tool for renal artery stenosis.

The use of ultrasound in the evaluation of arterial stenoses has become common. In fact, many vascular surgeons perform carotid endarterectomy based on ultrasound findings alone in some cases. Unfortunately, the renal arteries lie deep within the body, making ultrasound examination difficult and, in some cases, impossible. Although there have been technologic improvements in ultrasound transducers, this method remains the most operator dependent of all imaging methods. Some operators have obtained a high success rate using this as a screening examination, but they are in the minority.

In summary, many options are now available for imaging renal artery stenoses, but only angiography maintains a high accuracy rate from institution to institution. The best approach is to discuss this issue with the radiologists at a given medical center and ask them which technique they prefer for screening. In cases with a strong clinical impression of renovascular hypertension, it may be quickest and most cost-effective to proceed directly to angiography.

RENAL TUMOR DIAGNOSIS

Imaging of tumors is covered in other sections, but there is a vascular-related topic worth mentioning: determination of renal vein and inferior vena cava (IVC) invasion by tumor.

Invasion of the IVC by renal cell carcinoma was a diagnosis made by venography up until the advent of ultrasound. Now CT and magnetic resonance imaging (MRI) also have that capability. Interestingly, this is one area where angiography (venography) may not represent the gold standard. CT and MR are both capable of detecting a thrombus in the IVC. Both modalities have pitfalls, as does venography, primarily related to flow phenomena (21). Ultrasound, on the other hand, is limited only if the IVC cannot be well visualized. Ultrasound also has the advantages of requiring no contrast and being the least expensive. Comparisons of the different modalities consistently show that ultrasound should be the first choice. Venography can be reserved for those cases in which the IVC is not well seen. Although ultrasound is the best examination, if a CT or MRI has already been obtained and the question of caval invasion is answered in an unequivocal manner, there is no need to pursue additional studies.

RENAL TUMOR EMBOLIZATION

There are usually no specific arterial questions that must be answered when working up renal tumors, and CT and MRI have done away with the old technique of intraarterial epinephrine in the diagnosis of small lesions. However, percutaneous arterial embolization should be kept in mind for very large tumors or when there are other reasons to make extra efforts to decrease blood loss, such as when operating on a patient who will not accept blood transfusions. In these instances, preoperative embolization can be helpful (Fig. 3F.2). Angiography is performed in the standard manner, and the number of renal arteries is defined. Transcatheter embolization is then performed with alcohol (13), Gelfoam, or another embolic material. Embolization of renal cell carcinomas is one of the older applications of this technique, and therefore much experience has been gained. The procedure should be straightforward for any fellowship-trained interventional radiologist. The patient should proceed to surgery within the next 48 hours because parasitization of vessels by the tumor occurs rapidly.

OCCULT HEMATURIA

Occasionally, a patient with hematuria undergoes the standard battery of tests and no cause can be found. In this context, if bleeding is seen coming out of a ureter during cystoscopy, angiography should be the next step. An arteriovenous malformation becomes a possibility, and the other imaging modalities will not reliably demonstrate these lesions. Angiography, on the other hand, will not only make the diagnosis, but embolization can be undertaken (3), often at the same sitting.

Modern angiographic catheters and embolic materials make this procedure very simple. A standard renal arteriogram is done in multiple projections. If an arteriovenous malformation or arteriovenous fistula is found, embolization can be undertaken at the same sitting. If a 5-Fr catheter can easily be advanced selectively into the branch vessel that is the culprit, embolization can be performed with no additional maneuvers. If not, microcatheters can be used that almost always allow catheterization of third-, fourth-, or even fifth-order branches (Fig. 3F.3). Coils are used for embolization with Gelfoam occasionally needed as an adjunct. This is clearly the best modality for making the diagnosis, and the fact that a minimally invasive treatment is available at the same time is a plus.

LIVING RENAL DONOR WORKUP

In recent years, CTA has become the procedure of choice (25). CT is less invasive than angiography, gives functional information not available on MRA, and is probably less expensive. In comparison with ultrasound and MRA, CT has been shown to be superior in depicting accessory renal arteries (9,19) (Fig. 3F.4). Standard CT examinations for this indication require three parts. An initial noncontrast scan should be obtained to exclude any calcifications in the kidneys. This is followed by a true CTA examination. Our protocol uses 3-mm-thick slices 1 mm apart from the celiac axis to the bifurcation. We inject 3.8 mL of 150 mL of Omnipaque 350 per second, with a 12-second delay. A delayed scan is then performed to evaluate the kidney and ureters.

The standard axial images are reviewed along with 3D reconstructions. The fact that 3D images can be rotated 360 degrees (Fig. 3F.5) can be a major advantage in determining the number and location of renal arteries. Using a posterior view can be helpful in visualizing the left renal artery where it lies behind the vein. When both sets of images are used, it is only in rare cases that angiography is still needed. An additional advantage to the 3D reconstructions at our institution is that the surgeons prefer those images to take to the operating room.

MRA with gadolinium has become a good method of visualizing the renal arteries at institutions with experience in this technique; however, it does not have the advantages of CT in picking up calcifications or in demonstrating function by contrast material in the collecting system.

URETEROPELVIC JUNCTION OBSTRUCTION

Preoperative assessment for treatment of ureteropelvic junction obstruction includes defining the location and number of crossing vessels. Until recently, this has been one of the few situations in which there has been no substitute for angiography. CTA is now proving to be of value for this condition (20). Adding 3D reconstructions has the potential to give minimally invasive surgeons even more informa-

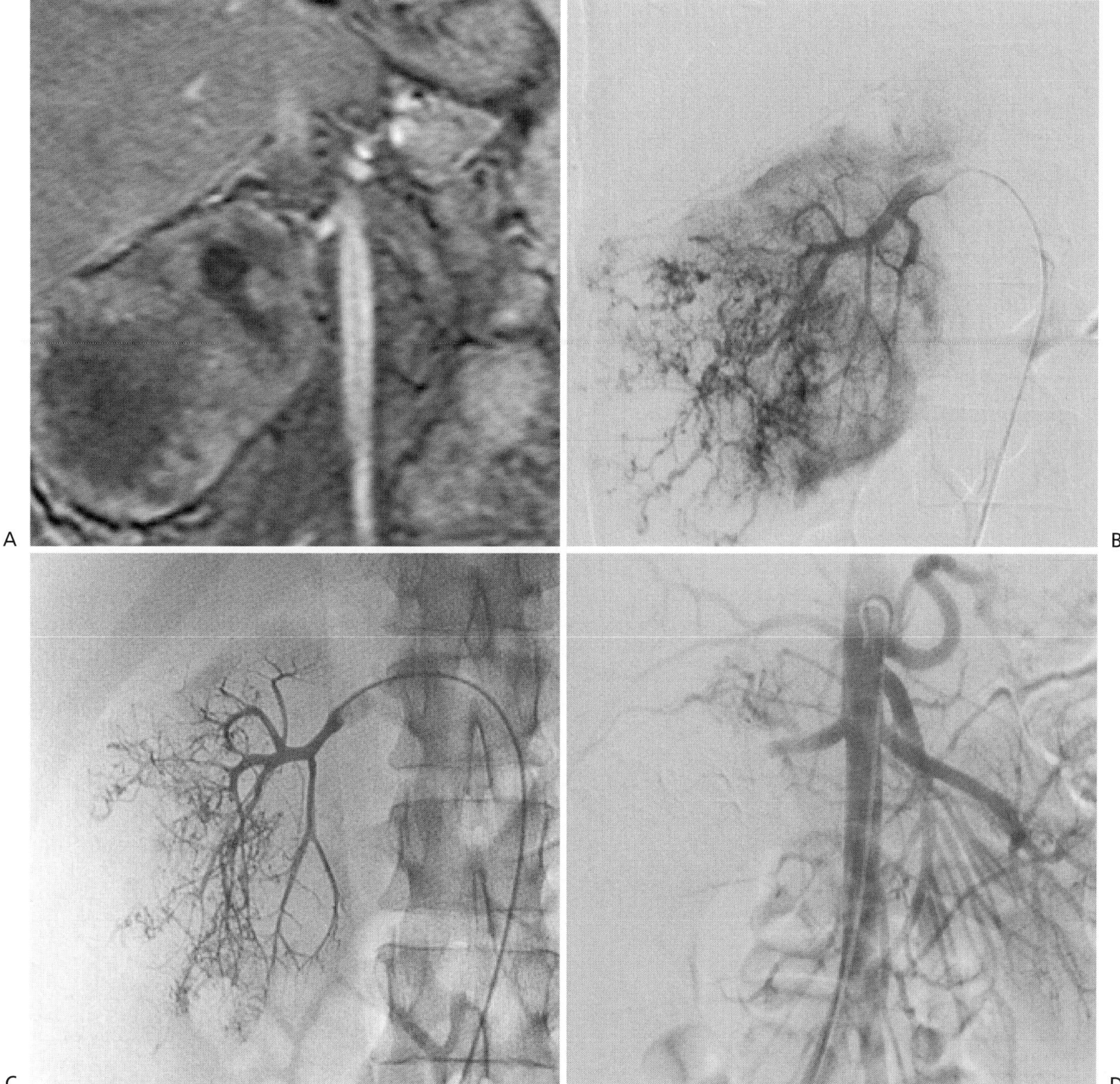

FIGURE 3F.2. This patient is a 56-year-old man with right flank mass and hematuria. **A:** Magnetic resonance imaging scan demonstrates renal cell carcinoma fed by enlarged renal artery. **B:** Digital subtraction angiography confirms single renal artery. **C:** Absolute alcohol is used to embolize tumor preoperatively. Occlusion balloon is in place to prevent reflux. **D:** Follow-up angiogram shows no flow through renal artery.

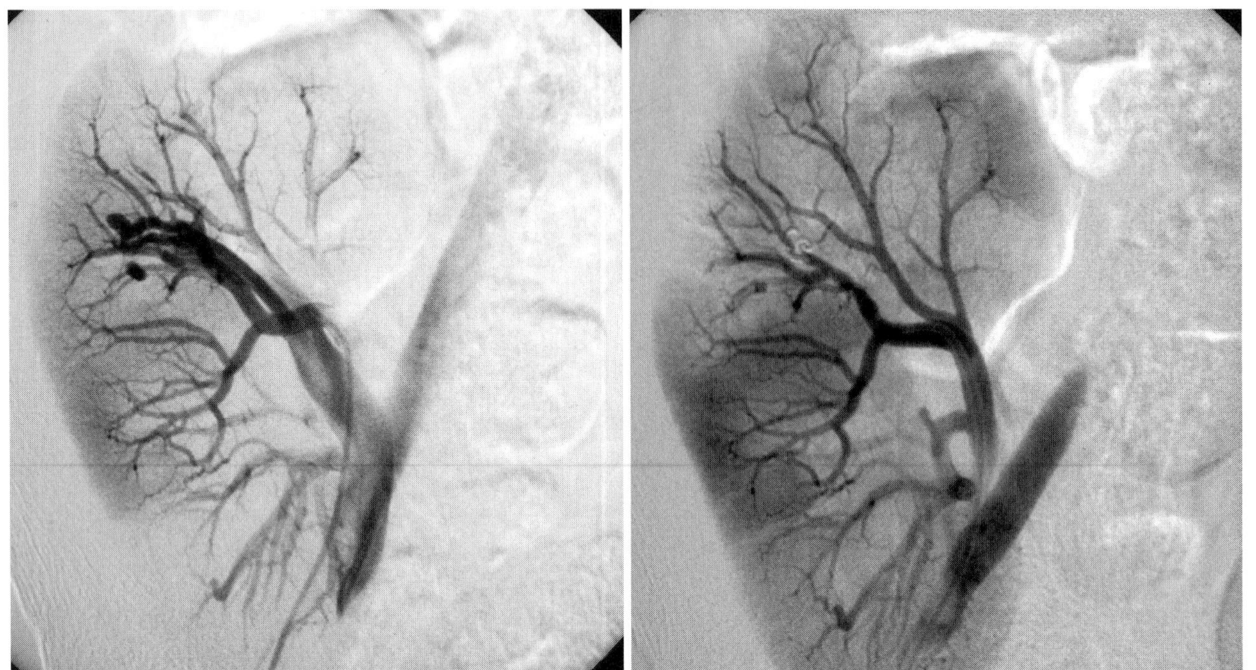

FIGURE 3F.3. Renal transplant patient with persistent hematuria following biopsy. **A:** Renal artery injection shows small pseudoaneurysm and early draining vein emptying into iliac vein. **B:** Following placement of two microcoils, fistula is occluded with minimal loss of parenchyma.

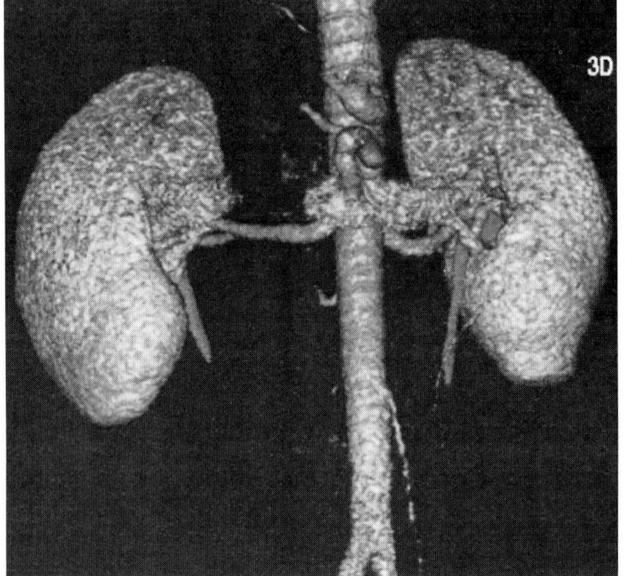

FIGURE 3F.4. Living renal donor computed tomography angiogram shows single arteries to each kidney and left renal vein passing anterior to the aorta. Different color schemes can be used depending on the preference of the viewing physicians. See also Color Figure 3F.4.

tion. Because this is a relatively new application of CT, it may be helpful to do a comparison with angiography until sufficient experience is gained to be sure the findings of CTA are reliable.

TRAUMA

Angiography remains the gold standard for trauma to the kidney where vascular injury is suspect. CT is the best overall screening tool, but doing a true CT angiogram in this situation is difficult and unreliable. If either occlusion of the renal artery is suspected or if the patient is actively bleeding from the kidney, emergency angiography should be undertaken immediately.

Occlusion of the renal artery or avulsion of the renal pedicle, once diagnosed by angiogram, should be taken immediately to the operating room. There is no minimally invasive technique at this time that can be used to treat this condition.

Bleeding from the kidney can be treated with transcatheter embolization. Angiography will demonstrate the bleeding site, and then a standard embolization technique, such as that mentioned in the occult hematuria section, can be used. This is one instance in which the embolization technique is not only less invasive but is probably easier to

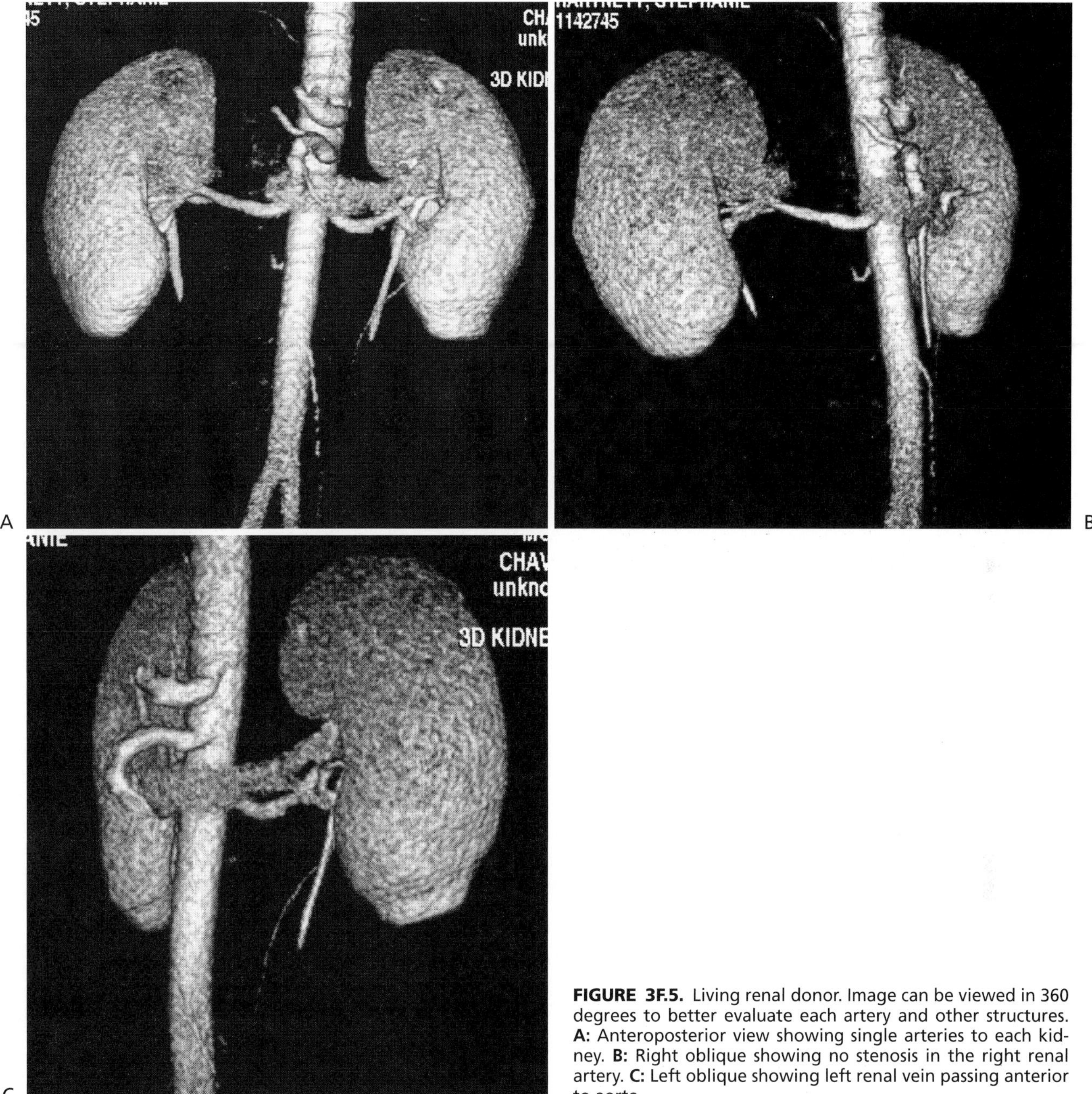

FIGURE 3F.5. Living renal donor. Image can be viewed in 360 degrees to better evaluate each artery and other structures. **A:** Anteroposterior view showing single arteries to each kidney. **B:** Right oblique showing no stenosis in the right renal artery. **C:** Left oblique showing left renal vein passing anterior to aorta.

perform than trying to control bleeding from a branch vessel surgically.

TRANSPLANT KIDNEYS

The fact that a transplanted kidney is in a different location has important ramifications for vascular imaging. Because of the superficial location, ultrasound is very accurate in determining the presence or absence of a stenosis. The main difficulty lies in separating the transplant artery from the internal iliac artery and its branches. If ultrasound finds high velocities suggestive of renal artery stenosis, angiography can be undertaken for confirmation and to treat with angioplasty or stent placement. Nuclear medicine studies can be undertaken to evaluate renal blood flow and excretion, but they are not as helpful in renal artery stenosis because there is no "other" kidney for comparison.

Ultrasound can also be useful in evaluating any other vascular abnormalities that might occur. Because these kidneys often undergo biopsy, there is the potential for pseudoaneurysm or arteriovenous fistula formation. Ultrasound can often detect either one of these conditions. Angiography again is reserved for confirmation and treatment. Three-dimensional CT has recently been suggested to be of value in the vascular evaluation of transplant kidneys (11). Although this work is relatively recent, with the current explosion in fast CT techniques, it can be expected that the application of CT in the transplant setting will increase.

There is an additional attribute of transplant kidneys that makes a difference in angiography. Because angiography is often undertaken in the setting of a rising creatinine, it is helpful to limit iodinated contrast material or even exclude it completely. Carbon dioxide can be used as a very good contrast material, particularly with latest-generation digital equipment. Transplant kidneys are particularly well suited to this because the kidney lies anterior to the feeding vessel. Carbon dioxide contrast, being lighter than blood, will tend to fill anterior structures better. Unfortunately, because of the same reasoning, native kidneys do not visualize as well with carbon dioxide contrast material. Special maneuvers such as turning the patient onto his or her side must be performed. Some institutions have also begun using gadolinium, a non–iodine-based contrast material, to evaluate the kidneys.

IMPOTENCE AND PRIAPISM

Impotence is increasingly being recognized as a more common problem than previously believed. With this recognition has come greater emphasis on diagnostic arterial studies. Ultrasound with Doppler (16) can be helpful, but angiography remains the most sophisticated study (1). Internal pudendal arteriography can be performed from a femoral artery puncture. Intraarterial vasodilators and pharmacologic erection are necessary for a complete evaluation. Although the techniques are straightforward, this is not a procedure routinely used at all medical centers. Therefore the experience of any individual should be considered before requesting these studies.

Priapism is a rare but exceptionally painful condition. Imaging studies are not usually required, but Doppler ultrasound is being increasingly used when necessary. When the veins do not appear to be the problem, investigation of the arterial system with angiography can be helpful. Catheterization of the hypogastric arteries is required. Microcatheters can then be used to selectively catheterize the internal pudendal arteries. If high-flow priapism is thought to exist and other treatment methods have failed, embolization has been successful (27).

MRA and CTA, although becoming increasingly used in place of angiography, have not yet been shown to be of benefit in either of these two conditions.

VARICOCELE

Varicocele is another condition that rarely needs any imaging technique; however, venography may be used to evaluate the venous drainage in cases in which there is a recurrent varicocele or where embolotherapy is requested. CTA and MRA with 3D reconstructions can both show enlarged gonadal veins, but because embolotherapy is undertaken at the same time as venography, there is usually no reason to obtain cross-sectional imaging studies. Venography is usually performed from a femoral vein approach with catheterization of the left renal vein. The gonadal vein is then catheterized, and contrast material is injected with the table tilted in reverse Trendelenburg position. The main vein and any collateral channels are identified, and embolization can be performed. This procedure is particularly helpful in patients with anatomic variants of venous drainage (15).

A wide variety of embolic materials have now been used for this indication. Initially, detachable balloons were most common, but sclerotherapy agents and injection of boiling contrast material have subsequently been used. The introduction of microcatheters with the resultant decrease in spasm of the veins has led to increased use of metal coils. In Europe, sclerotherapeutic agents are used more commonly (15).

REFERENCES

1. Bookstein JJ. Penile angiography: the last angiographic frontier. *AJR Am J Roentgenol* 1988;150:47.
2. Caridi JG, Stavropoulos SW, Hawkins IF. Carbon dioxide digital subtraction angiography for renal artery stent placement. *J Vasc Interv Radiol* 1999;10:635.
3. Clark RA, Gallant TE, Alexander ES. Angiographic management of traumatic arteriovenous fistulas: clinical results. *Radiology* 1983;147:9.
4. Cochran ST, Wong WS, Roe DJ. Predicting angiography-induced acute renal function impairment: clinical risk model. *AJR Am J Roentgenol* 1983;141:1027.
5. D'Elia JA, Gleason RE, Alday M, et al. Nephrotoxicity from angiographic contrast material. *Am J Med* 1982;72:719.
6. Eardley KS, Lipkin GW. Atherosclerotic renal stenosis: is it worth diagnosing? *J Hum Hypertens* 1999;13:217.
7. Eisenberg RL, Bank WO, Hedgock MW. Renal failure after major angiography can be avoided with hydration. *AJR Am J Roentgenol* 1981;136:859.
8. Gilfeather M, Yoon H, Siegelman ES, et al. Renal artery stenosis: evaluation with conventional angiography versus gadolinium-enhanced MR angiography. *Radiology* 1999;210:367.
9. Halpern EJ, Nazarian LN, Wechsler RJ, et al. US, CT, and MR evaluation of accessory renal arteries and proximal renal arterial branches. *Acad Radiol* 1999;6:299.
10. Harkonen S, Kjellstrand CM. Exacerbation of diabetic renal failure following intravenous pyelography. *Am J Med* 1977; 63:939.

11. Hofmann LV, Smith PA, Kuszyk BS, et al. Three-dimensional helical CT angiography in renal transplant recipients: a new problem-solving tool. *AJR Am J Roentgenol* 1999;173:1085.
12. Kaufman JA, Geller SC, Waltman AC. Renal insufficiency: gadopentetate dimeglumine as radiographic contrast agent during peripheral vascular interventional procedures. *Radiology* 1996;198:579.
13. Klimberg I, Hunter P, Hawkins IF, et al. Preoperative angioinfarction of localized renal cell carcinoma using absolute ethanol. *J Urol* 1985;133:21.
14. Lang EK. A survey of the complications of percutaneous retrograde arteriography. *Radiology* 1963;81:257.
15. Lenz M, Hof N, Kersting-Sommerhoff B, et al. Anatomic variants of the spermatic vein: importance for percutaneous sclerotherapy of idiopathic varicocele. *Radiology* 1996;198:425.
16. Lue TF, Hricak H, Marich KW, et al. Evaluation of arteriogenic impotence with intracorporeal injection of papaverine and the duplex ultrasound scanner. *Semin Urol* 1985;1:21.
17. Mason RA, Arbeit LA, Giron F. Renal dysfunction after arteriography. *JAMA* 1985;253:1001.
18. Prokop M. Protocols and future directions in imaging of renal artery stenosis: CT angiography. *J Comput Assist Tomogr* 1999; 23[Suppl 1]:101.
19. Qanadli SD, Mesurolle B, Coggia M, et al. Abdominal aortic aneurysm: pretherapy assessment with dual-slice helical CT angiography. *AJR Am J Roentgenol* 2000;174:181.
20. Rouviere O, Lyonnet D, Berger P, et al. Ureteropelvic junction obstruction: use of helical CT for preoperative assessment—comparison with intraarterial angiography. *Radiology* 1999; 213:668.
21. Selby JB, Pryor JL, Tegtmeyer CJ, et al. Inferior vena caval invasion by renal cell carcinoma: false positive diagnosis by venacavography. *J Urol* 1990;143:464.
22. Seldinger SI. Catheter replacement of the needle in percutaneous arteriography. A new technique. *Acta Radiol* 1953;39:368.
23. Sigstedt B, Lunderquist A. Complications of angiographic examinations. *AJR Am J Roentgenol* 1978;130:445.
24. Silverman JF, Wexler L. Complications of percutaneous transfemoral coronary arteriography. *Clin Radiol* 1976;27:317.
25. Slakey DP, Florman S, Lovretich J, et al. Utility of CT angiography for evaluation of living kidney donors. *Clin Transplant* 1999;13:104.
26. Spinosa DJ, Matsumoto AH, Angle JF, et al. Renal insufficiency: usefulness of gadodiamide-enhanced renal angiography to supplement CO_2-enhanced renal angiography for diagnosis and percutaneous treatment. *Radiology* 1999;210:663.
27. Steers WD, Selby JB. Use of methylene blue and selective embolization of the pudendal artery for high flow priapism refractory to medical and surgical treatments. *J Urol* 1991;146: 1361.

Adult and Pediatric Urology, 4/e, edited by Jay Y. Gillenwater, John T. Grayhack, Stuart S. Howards, and Michael E. Mitchell.
Lippincott Williams & Wilkins, Philadelphia © 2002

3G

NUCLIDE STUDIES

BARBARA Y. CROFT
JUDITH M. JOYCE
JAYASHREE PAREKH
CHARLES D. TEATES

Radioactive tracers have been used for more than 30 years to measure renal function and to image the urinary tract. Because of the kidneys' rich vascularity, unique function, and high metabolic rate, a number of radiopharmaceuticals have been used to study this organ system. The anatomic placement of the urinary tract is favorable for external counting and imaging, except that the bladder is anterior and the kidneys are posterior. Nuclear medicine has made unique and valuable contributions to the study of the genitourinary tract, but it cannot compete with other modalities such as radiography and sonography for high-resolution anatomic imaging. On the other hand, none of the other imaging modalities has the ability of nuclear medicine for functional imaging or quantitation.

This chapter outlines the pharmaceuticals used in genitourinary evaluation, radiation dose from nuclear procedures in relation to radiographic procedures, instrumentation, and clinical applications. Nuclear medicine procedures applicable to patients with genitourinary disease that are not specific to the genitourinary system are not discussed in any detail. Included among the latter techniques are procedures for imaging infection (gallium citrate Ga-67 scans and indium In-111 oxine-labeled or technetium-99m [^{99m}Tc] HMPAO-labeled white blood cell [WBC] scans), bone imaging (e.g., ^{99m}Tc methylene diphosphonate), lung scanning (^{99m}Tc macroaggregated albumin and xenon-127 gas or xenon-133 gas), and cardiovascular studies (thallium-201 images of myocardial perfusion or ^{99m}Tc-tagged red blood cells [RBCs] for evaluation of cardiac function). These and other nuclear procedures are beyond the scope and intent of this chapter.

B.Y. Croft: Biomedical Imaging Program, National Cancer Institute, Bethesda, MD 20852.
J.M. Joyce: Western Pennsylvania Hospital, Pittsburgh, PA 15224.
J. Parekh and C.D. Teates: Department of Radiology, University of Virginia, Charlottesville, VA 22908.

RENAL RADIOPHARMACY

Pharmaceuticals

Chemical Structures

The chemical structures for the various compounds in use in nuclear medicine renal work range from the simple to the

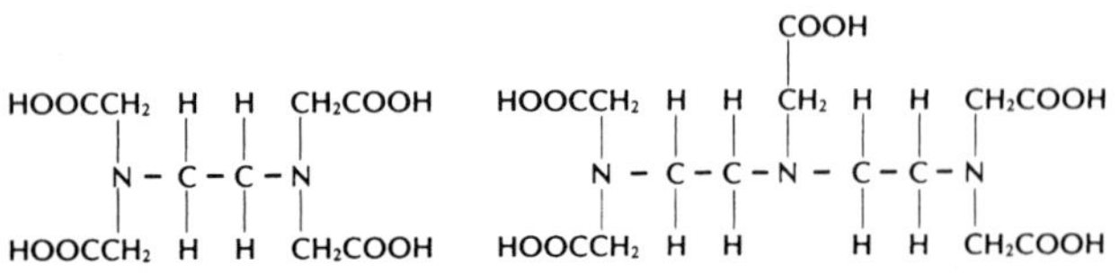

FIGURE 3G.1. Chemical structures of *(left)* ethylenediamine tetraacetic acid (EDTA) and *(right)* diethylene triamine pentaacetic acid (DTPA).

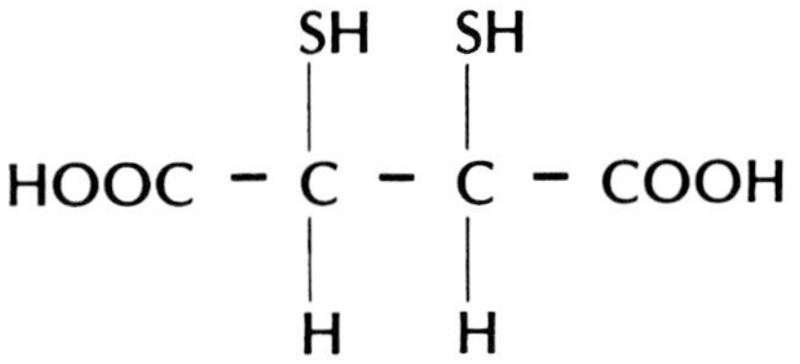

FIGURE 3G.3. Chemical structure of dimercaptosuccinic acid (DMSA).

complex. The compounds themselves vary in their pharmacology from the general to the specific.

Xenon-127 and xenon-133 are the simplest compounds in use; they are also nonspecific. Xenon is a monatomic gas, belonging to the noble, or "inert," gas group. It is sparingly soluble in water or isotonic saline and quite soluble in fat. Xenon-127 has the better half-life for storage, the better energy for imaging, and confers the smaller radiation dose, but xenon-133 has been the more available and cheaper isotope.

The radioactive nuclide most used in nuclear medicine is ^{99m}Tc, which has a 6-hour half-life and a 140-keV gamma ray energy. It is ideal for examinations taking less than 1 day using the Anger camera, the most common nuclear medical imaging instrument today. The radionuclide is obtained in the pertechnetate form, TcO_4^-, from a "generator." A new generator is delivered to most laboratories weekly. There is a supply of sterile, pyrogen-free ^{99m}Tc in most nuclear medicine laboratories at all times. The pertechnetate form may itself be used in studying renal blood flow and cystograms. Other technetium radiopharmaceuticals are compounded from purchased kits and available pertechnetate.

Most of the compounds in use have been chosen because of specific interaction with the kidneys. For example, ethylenediamine tetraacetic acid (EDTA) is a chelating compound with the ability to bond a positive metal ion; the nitrogens provide electrons for the covalent bonds, as do the oxygens of the acetic acids. The compound in routine use in nuclear medicine is diethylenetriamine pentaacetic acid (DTPA). It bonds its three nitrogens and five acidic oxygens to positively charged metal ions. EDTA and DTPA are shown schematically in Fig. 3G.1. The method for naming these compounds has been to assume that biomedical people could not remember the chemical names and that the

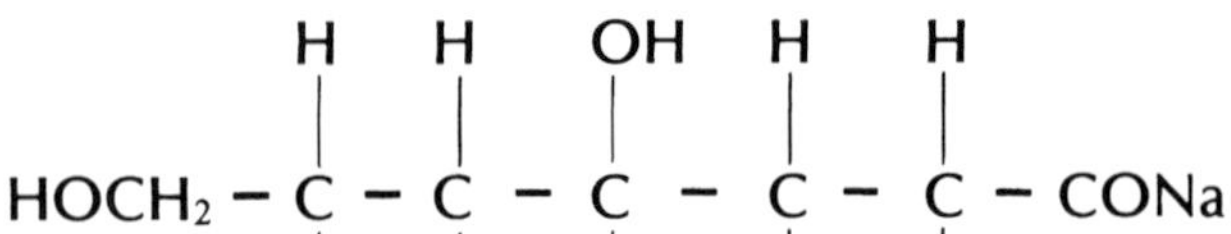

FIGURE 3G.2. Chemical structure of sodium glucoheptonate (GH).

initials were not sonorous enough, so parts of the chemical names or initials have been turned into the simpler names *edetate* and *pentetate.*

Commercial kits are available for compounding ^{99m}Tc DTPA, ^{99m}Tc glucoheptonate (GH) (Fig. 3G.2), and ^{99m}Tc meso-2,3-dimercaptosuccinic acid (DMSA) (Fig. 3G.3). All three kits contain stannous chloride as a reducing agent, so Tc^{4+} will be the positive ion species chelated by the organic compound. The package inserts should be consulted for special instructions in using the radiopharmaceuticals.

More recently, ^{99m}Tc mercaptoacetyltriglycine (MAG_3) (Fig. 3G.4) has been introduced for renal tubular function studies (51). It has the advantages of ^{99m}Tc and kit formulation using stannous ion. It has been approved by the U.S. Food and Drug Administration (FDA) for renal imaging and for studying renal function.

The chromium isotope, ^{51}Cr, has been chelated to EDTA for renal work. The half-life of ^{51}Cr is 27.8 days, and although the chemical characteristics of ^{51}Cr EDTA are favorable (5), the yield of radioactive decay products available for counting is low. Therefore ^{51}Cr EDTA is used for examinations requiring blood sampling but not those requiring imaging.

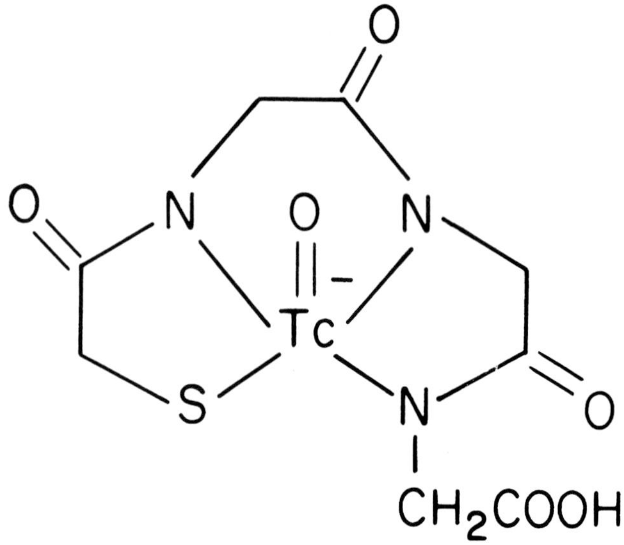

FIGURE 3G.4. Chemical structure of ^{99m}Tc MAG_3.

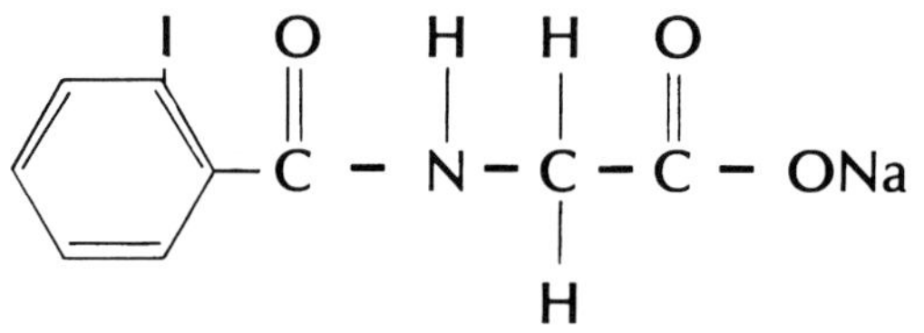

FIGURE 3G.5. Chemical structure of sodium o-iodohippurate (OIH).

The iodine isotopes, ^{123}I and ^{131}I, have been attached to the ortho position of hippuric acid to create compounds for renal tubular function studies. The structure is given in Fig. 3G.5. Because ^{123}I has a 13.2-hour half-life, ^{123}I hippurate (Hippuran) must be made on site with recently purchased ^{123}I or must be purchased for the studies for that day. The ^{131}I hippurate, with an 8-day half-life, may be kept on hand at all times if demand for its use is sufficient.

BIOLOGIC BEHAVIOR

Xenon is more soluble in fat than in blood. If the patient is caused to rebreathe from a closed system containing radioactive xenon mixed with air or oxygen, the patient becomes more and more radioactive, with fat accumulating the major part of the activity. If the patient is then caused to breathe air alone, the washout of the xenon from the tissues can be observed with nuclear medical instruments. The rate of washout correlates with the blood flow to the organ or area. This technique has been used in many organs in the body.

The specific behavior of ^{99m}Tc DTPA and ^{51}Cr EDTA is considered later in this chapter in the discussion of glomerular filtration rate (GFR). A variable amount (10% or less) of injected ^{99m}Tc DTPA is bound to protein.

^{99m}Tc GH is injected intravenously (IV). The material is found in the plasma, and blood clearance is rapid (1,4), similar to DTPA. The GH clears by both tubular secretion and glomerular filtration. Approximately 70% of the material is excreted in the urine of normal subjects. Approximately 6% of the dose is retained in each kidney, largely in the cortex, permitting imaging of the cortex 3 to 4 hours after injection. A normal variation is clearance by the liver into the gallbladder and intestines.

^{99m}Tc DMSA is slowly injected IV. It is distributed in the plasma, loosely bound to plasma proteins. The activity clears from the plasma with a half-time of 60 minutes and concentrates in the renal cortex. Approximately 16% of the activity is excreted within 2 hours, increasing to 25% by 6 hours. At 2 hours, 15% is concentrated in each kidney; this increases to 20% by 6 hours (1). Imaging is best performed 3 hours or more after injection.

Iodinated hippurate has been used extensively in the examination of renal function; there is a voluminous literature on the use of this compound. The biologic behavior of iodinated hippurate is discussed in the section on effective renal plasma flow. Most of the hippurate is actively secreted by renal tubules. In a normal person, 70% of the compound is excreted in the urine in 30 minutes.

^{99m}Tc MAG_3, also known as *mertiatide,* is another renal tubular agent; it is confined to the plasma, having less RBC binding than sodium iodohippurate (OIH) (35). The plasma protein binding of MAG_3 is approximately twice as great as that of OIH. MAG_3 has a plasma clearance of approximately half that of OIH, probably as a result of decreased glomerular filtration and lower tubular secretion.

Dosimetry

Both nuclear studies and radiographic procedures result in patient exposure to ionizing radiation. The major difference between the two procedures is that radioactive pharmaceuticals produce patient exposure from internal sources, whereas that from a radiographic diagnostic procedure results from external irradiation. Exposure from radiographic procedures can be accurately determined if the unit is accurately calibrated and the exposure factors are known. In nuclear procedures, the patient dosage is determined by the biologic handling of the pharmaceutical, the physical behavior of the radionuclide, and patient dosage. Alterations in patient physiology, as for example in renal failure, affect the absorbed dose of radiation markedly if the radiopharmaceutical behavior is altered by the disease process. In recent years, patient exposure has been reduced in both areas by improvements in radiopharmaceuticals, nuclear instrumentation, radiographic and fluoroscopic equipment, and film and screen sensitivity. The patient exposures listed in Tables 3G.1 and 3G.2 are considered average exposures and may not be accurate for a given patient or a particular institution. There are inaccuracies in published radiation dose calculations for a number of these materials (55). Personnel exposures should be low with both types of procedures if appropriate protective measures such as syringe shields and equipment shielding are used. The procedure potentially resulting in the highest exposure is fluoroscopy because a typical fluoroscope exposes the patient and personnel to as much as 10 rad per minute.

Certain terms must be defined to understand exposure to ionizing radiation. The patient dose of a radiopharmaceutical is measured by the number of atoms disintegrating per second. The term most commonly used in nuclear medicine is *millicurie (mCi),* defined as 3.7×10^7 disintegrations per second. A *microcurie (μCi)* is 3.7×10^4 disintegrations per second.

The Système Internationale (SI) units are coming into more common use; the SI unit for radioactive decay is the becquerel (Bq), which is 1 disintegration per second. Because many disintegrations occur per second, reference is often made to megabecquerels (MBq), 10^6 disintegrations

TABLE 3G.1. TYPICAL ABSORBED DOSES (RAD) FROM COMMON RADIONUCLIDE STUDIES

Agent	Usual Dosage (mCi)	Kidney	Bladder Wall	Gonads	Whole Body
^{99m}Tc DTPA					
Adult[a]	15.0	1.35	1.73[b]	0.16[b]	0.09
10-year-old	9.75	0.68	7.8[b]	—	0.29
^{99m}Tc glucoheptonate					
Adult[d]	15.0	2.55	4.2[b]	0.2[b]	0.15
10-year-old[c]	9.75	1.95	7.8[b]	0.2[b]	0.07
^{99m}Tc DMSA					
Adult[e]	5.0	3.8	1.4[b]	0.1[b]	0.08
10-year-old[c]	3.25	2.3	0.98[b]	0.07[b]	0.07
^{99m}Tc MAG_3					
Adult[f]	5.0	0.07	2.4[b]	0.08[b]	0.03
10-year-old	3.25	0.08	1.2[b]	0.06[b]	0.02
^{131}I hippurate					
Adult[g]	0.2	0.03	1.1[b]	0.02[b]	0.006[h]
10-year-old[c]	0.13	0.01	1.0[b]	0.003[b]	0.008
^{123}I hippurate[i] (p,5n)					
Adult[j]	1.0	0.03	1.0[b]	0.03[b]	0.02
10-year-old[i]	0.65	0.01	0.05[b]	0.003[b]	0.009
^{99m}Tc cystography[i]	1.0	—	0.07	0.002	

[a]Package insert, Cinitichem, Inc., Tuxedo, NY, 1988.
[b]Bladder and gonad doses determined by frequency of voiding.
[c]Koenigsberg and colleagues (30).
[d]Package insert, E.I. du Pont de Nemours & Co., Billerica, Md, 1987.
[e]Esser and colleagues (14).
[f]Stabin (47).
[g]Package insert, Squibb Diagnostics, Princeton, NJ, 1989.
[h]Unblocked thyroid dose as high as 8.7 rad.
[i]Dimitriou and colleagues (11).
[j]Croft calculation, based on ^{131}I hippurate values.

per second, and to gigabecquerels (GBq), 10^9 disintegrations per second. Therefore 1 mCi is equal to 37 MBq, 37×10^6 Bq. Obviously, a radionuclide with a long half-life in the patient will usually expose the patient to more ionizing radiation than another radiopharmaceutical with a shorter effective half-life. The effective half-life is influenced both by the physical decay rate of the nuclide and by the biologic turnover of the pharmaceutical.

TABLE 3G.2. ADULT DOSES FROM RADIOGRAPHIC PROCEDURES

Procedure	Dose
Intravenous urograms	
(No. of films/examinations)	(5.31)
Mean exposure/examination	3.133 R
Mean marrow dose/examination	0.103 rad
Mean male gonadal dose/examination	0.207 rad
Mean female gonadal dose/examination	0.588 rad
Mean dose to total body/examination	0.278 rad
Fluoroscopy	
Exposure/min	2–10 rad

Reprinted with permission from Gorson RO, Lassen M, Rosenstein M. Patient dosimetry in diagnostic radiology. In: Waggener RG, Kereiakes JG, Shalek RJ, eds. *CRC handbook of medical physics,* vol 2. Boca Raton, Fla: CRC Press, 1984:474, 487, 488.

Two terms are commonly used as measures of x-ray and patient exposure. The *roentgen* (R) is a measure of ionization of air by x-rays or gamma rays. There is no physical difference between an x-ray and a gamma ray. An x-ray originates from atomic electrons, and a gamma ray originates in the nucleus of an atom. One R results in 2.082×10^9 ion pairs in 1 mL of air at standard atmospheric pressure. The term *roentgen* is usually used to express the output of an x-ray machine. The amount of energy absorbed by a patient's tissue is expressed in rad. The *rad* is defined as 100 ergs absorbed per gram of tissue. In most tissues, exposure to 1 R results in approximately 1 rad of absorbed energy. The two terms are used somewhat interchangeably, but it should be remembered that the roentgen is a measure of exposure, whereas the rad is a measure of energy absorbed by tissue.

The SI unit for exposure to ionizing radiation is the coulomb per kilogram, and for absorbed radiation is the gray (Gy), with 100 rad equal to 1 Gy. Table 3G.3 gives the conversion factors to SI units.

Table 3G.1 lists typical absorbed doses in patients receiving the five most common radionuclide studies of the urinary tract. The bladder receives the highest exposure

TABLE 3G.3. CONVERSION FACTORS TO SI UNITS

	Customary Units	SI Units
Radioactive materials	1 curie (Ci)	3.7×10^{10} becquerels (Bq)
	2.7×10^{-11} Ci	1 Bq
Absorbed dose	1 rad	0.01 gray (Gy)
	100 rad	1 Gy

from most of these pharmaceuticals, but this dose can be reduced considerably by frequently emptying the bladder. Free iodine, present to some extent in ^{131}I hippurate, will result in exposure to the thyroid. The dose of the thyroid can be reduced by more than 90% by giving Lugol's solution, saturated solution of potassium iodide, or other blocking agents before the study.

The doses listed from radiographic procedures in Table 3G.2 are based on a survey performed by the Bureau of Radiologic Health between 1964 and 1970. The patient exposures can be reduced somewhat from the values listed by using better collimation of the x-ray beam, by using improved films and screens, and by reducing the number of films or fluoroscopic exposures.

INSTRUMENTATION

Two types of instruments are most often used to detect ionizing radiation in clinical applications. The oldest and simplest technique uses a gas detector. In this type of instrument, a charge is placed across electrodes in a chamber containing some type of gas. Gamma rays or x-rays cause the gas to ionize, thereby resulting in current flow across the electrodes. The amount of voltage between the electrodes determines the amount of current flow, the sensitivity of the detector, and the useful range of radiation that the instrument can accurately measure. The walls of the chambers can be altered to allow detection of very poorly penetrating radiation or highly penetrating radiation.

Two types of gas detectors are commonly used in nuclear medicine laboratories. A Geiger-Müller (GM) survey meter is usually used for detecting contamination in the nuclear medicine laboratory. This gas detector operates with a relatively high voltage, making the detector sensitive for small amounts of radiation. A typical range of usefulness is between 0 and 50 millirads per hour (1 rad = 1,000 mrad). The ionization chamber is usually attached to a rate meter and an electronic package by an electrical cord that allows survey of work areas. The probe is relatively nondirectional. The standard survey meter is intended for detection of x-rays and gamma rays and is not very suitable for low-energy beta ray detection.

The second type of gas detector usually found in the laboratory is a dose calibrator. At one time, most of the radiopharmaceuticals administered in nuclear medicine laboratories had relatively long half-lives and were purchased as needed from a pharmaceutical supplier in precalibrated doses. Patient doses were withdrawn from a precalibrated vial, and activity was calculated based on the known activity per cubic centimeter. As discussed previously, many of the radiopharmaceuticals carry the radioactive label ^{99m}Tc.

Technetium is eluted daily from a shielded ion exchange column containing molybdenum-99. The elution is unpredictable, and therefore the patient dose must be accurately measured in the laboratory. Highly accurate dose calibrators currently available allow the measurement of bulk quantities of individual patient doses of radiopharmaceuticals. The dose calibrators use a gas-filled ionization detector. Physically, the detector is a well chamber that allows the vial or syringe to be inserted for high-efficiency counting. These instruments are capable of accurately measuring over a wide range of activity, typically from approximately 1 μCi to more than 2,000 mCi. One millicurie equals 1,000 μCi. The dose calibrators are designed to give a digital readout of activity and are usually accurate to within 5%. The dose calibrators must be checked daily against known standard amounts of activity. These chambers operate with a relatively low voltage to allow measurements of high radiation intensities, and they are not accurate for measuring low-energy x-rays, low-energy gamma rays, or beta rays.

The other major category of detectors of ionizing radiation uses solid crystals. In most laboratories, the detector is sodium iodide, doped with an impurity such as thallium. Sodium iodide is hygroscopic, and therefore the crystal is completely enclosed in a barrier impervious to water, such as aluminum or glass. Ionizing radiation is absorbed by the crystal, converting the energy to visible light. Thus the sodium iodide crystal is called a scintillation crystal or scintillation detector. The light produced by each ionizing event is quite small and is detected by a nearby photomultiplier (PM) tube, which has a photocathode that converts light energy into a small electronic pulse. The electronic pulse is amplified more than 1 million times within the PM tube, making it large enough to be amplified and processed in standard electronic circuits. Thus an ionizing event in the crystal produces light that is converted into an electronic pulse. The magnitude of the pulse is related to the amount of energy contained in the ionizing event. The pulse can be analyzed to determine the energy of the x-ray or gamma ray that hit the crystal. Pulses can be integrated over a variable time to give counts per second or counts per minute. The count rate can be displayed on a meter or a digital printout, or it can be stored in a computer.

A single crystal detector is usually mounted in some type of lead or other heavy-metal shielding so that the crystal is sensitive to x-rays or gamma rays from a localized region (Fig. 3G.6). Typically, a single crystal–single PM tube system is used for measuring count rate from the thyroid for thyroid uptake determination or monitoring the count rate in the kidneys during a renogram. Under these circumstances, the probe and its collimator are positioned so that

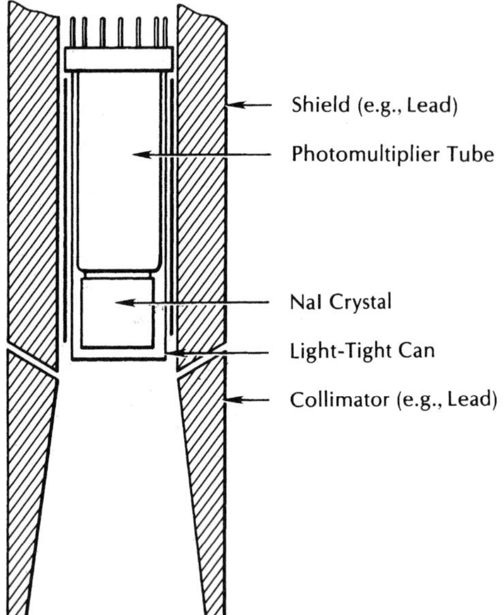

FIGURE 3G.6. Typical probe detector system. The sodium iodide (NaI) crystal and photomultiplier (PM) tube are shielded by lead to restrict the field of view to the desired anatomic region. The crystal is enclosed in a polished can to increase the reflection of light to the PM tube and protect the crystal from degradation by moisture.

the crystal monitors the count rate in the organ and nearby tissues being surveyed. The successful use of this detector assumes that the organ can be accurately localized from anatomic landmarks.

A sodium iodide scintillation detector can be manufactured in the form of a "well counter." This is used for counting in vitro samples. In effect, the sample is inserted into a hole in the protected crystal so that high counting efficiency is achieved. As with the scintillation probe, the activity can be counted over time to determine sample activity.

The imaging device used in most departments is the Anger camera. The camera contains a single crystal, measuring up to 50 cm in diameter, that is round, square, or rectangular in shape and 0.25 to 0.375 inches thick. Behind the crystal, there is a matrix of PM tubes, typically numbering anywhere from 37 to 91, which look at the intensity of light from each scintillation in the crystal (Fig. 3G.7). The light striking the multiple PM tubes is analyzed so that the location of the scintillation is determined, as well as the total energy from the x-ray or gamma ray. The front of the crystal is protected by a collimator. The multiple holes in the collimator determine the origin of the photons that hit the crystal. Ordinarily, most Anger cameras are used with a parallel-hole collimator that sees a field of view 25 to 50 cm in size depending on the size and shape of the system. The thickness of lead septa between holes is selected for the appropriate energy of the photons being imaged, that is, low energy (up to 160 keV) and medium energy (160 to 360 keV). The hole diameter and collimator thickness are selected for desired resolution and counting efficiency.

The camera electronics include an energy discriminator (spectrometer) to be sure that only the appropriate energy is accepted. The crystal detects stray cosmic rays, scattered x-rays, and so forth, as well as the desirable photons emitted by the nuclide being imaged. The image quality will suffer unless the unwanted radiation is excluded by energy discrimination.

The final image that is viewed depends on where the signal is sent once it leaves the PM tubes and analyzers. It may enter a cathode ray tube (CRT) that puts a series of dots on the screen. By using time-lapse photography of the CRT, an image is generated on Polaroid film or transparency film. The same signals may be sent to a computer for storage and later manipulation.

Computers have been used in nuclear medicine for years to digitize and store the information from the scintillation probe or Anger camera for later manipulation. Over the years, the storage capacity and sophistication of programs have improved greatly. When using a computer to store and manipulate data, it is essential that the information be stored in an adequate format. If images are integrated for 1 minute each, for instance, the data cannot be later analyzed at 1-second intervals. Therefore the appropriate prescription for the storage must be determined before initiating the study. Most commercial computers now have several software programs that allow histogram displays of activity versus time. These curves can be stripped or analyzed to allow washin and washout rate determinations, fractionation of individual renal function, and analysis of blood clearance rates to determine GFR and effective renal plasma flow. In addition, computer manipulation is essential to enhance images from an Anger camera and perform specialized procedures such as single photon emission com-

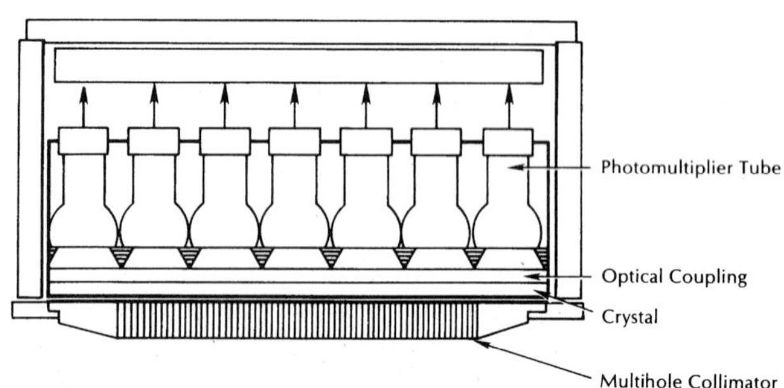

FIGURE 3G.7. Diagram of a cross section through a 37 photomultiplier (PM) tube gamma camera. The PM tubes are arranged in a hexagonal array, with three rings of tubes surrounding a central tube. Gamma rays or x-rays pass through the collimator and interact with the crystal, producing light. The location of the scintillation and the total energy absorbed are determined from the signal output by the PM tubes. The amplified signal is analyzed for energy levels and sent to the cathode ray tube or computer for recording.

puted tomography (SPECT). SPECT creates tomographic images in much the same way as computed tomography (CT) scanning, by combining images from multiple positions as the camera rotates about the patient.

PROCEDURES

The following sections describe the range of procedures available in nuclear medicine to assist the renal diagnostician. For easy reference, the examinations, radiopharmaceuticals, and typical doses of radioactivity are outlined in Table 3G.4.

Renal Imaging

Renal images are typically performed with Anger cameras. The arrival of activity can be recorded in the form of renal vascular studies. This information can also be analyzed by computer to compare the washin rates for the two kidneys. Most of the technetium pharmaceuticals can be used for the vascular sequence, provided adequate amounts of activity (15 to 20 mCi) are injected, but the later static views show varying features depending on the pharmaceutical used. The vascular sequence is typically recorded on film and by the computer at one frame per 2 seconds, but the framing rate can be tailored to the patient's age and the injected dose. In general, faster sequences are desired for children. The limiting factor on the renal vascular sequences is generally the low information density due to a small number of counts per image, so higher imaging rates may actually cause deterioration of the images. Because of its ability to add frames together, the computer is often a more satisfactory method than film for recording and displaying this information.

The static images of the kidneys are collected immediately after the vascular sequence and up to several hours later. Static images may contain as many as 1 million counts and require up to several minutes' accumulation time. ^{99m}Tc DTPA is filtered and concentrated in the tubules and is then excreted through the collecting system. Activity in the calyces, renal pelvis, and ureters decreases after 5 to 10 minutes, and delayed views beyond 30 minutes have little value unless the patient has obstruction.

The ^{99m}Tc MAG_3 imaging sequence is very similar to DTPA; it is best used in a dynamic fashion for vascular imaging and the renogram referred to later.

^{99m}Tc GH and DMSA show progressive accumulation in the kidneys over several hours; delayed views will show better images of the renal cortex after the background and collecting system activity have decreased. Patient hydration will influence the washout rates from the kidneys just as with a renogram. This effect is used in the "furosemide (Lasix) renogram," discussed under Hydronephrosis and Hydroureter later in this chapter.

TABLE 3G.4. RADIOPHARMACEUTICALS AND ACTIVITY DOSAGE FOR GENITOURINARY EXAMINATIONS

Examination	Agent	Dose of Activity
Renal blood flow imaging	^{99m}Tc compound	15 mCi
Effective renal plasma flow		
Imaging	^{131}I hippurate	200 μCi
Blood sampling only	^{131}I hippurate	30 μCi
Imaging	^{123}I hippurate	1.0 mCi
Imaging	^{99m}Tc MAG_3	10 mCi
Blood sampling only	^{99m}TC MAG_3	300 μCi
Glomerular filtration rate		
Imaging	^{99m}Tc DTPA	15 mCi
Blood sampling only	^{99m}Tc DTPA	300 μCi
Blood sampling only	^{125}I iothalamate	100 μCi
Blood sampling only	^{51}Cr EDTA	100 μCi
Renal cortical imaging	^{99m}Tc DMSA	5 mCi
Cystography	^{99m}Tc pertechnetate	1 mCi
Testicular imaging	^{99m}Tc pertechnetate	15 mCi

Renograms

Initially, renograms were performed using multiple, single-crystal probes positioned over the patient's back. The probes were positioned by external anatomic landmarks, but this often did not locate the kidneys in the field of view of the probes. Later, workers positioned the probes by injecting a small amount of renal tracer (e.g., ^{203}Hg chlormerodrin) and finding the maximum count rate before injection of ^{131}I hippurate. More recently, most renograms have been performed with Anger cameras, even though the sensitivity of a camera is somewhat less than that of a probe. The versatility of data recorded from a camera more than offsets the disadvantage of the higher pharmaceutical dose required. A renogram may be performed using external probes with as little as 30 μCi of ^{131}I hippurate. Renograms performed on Anger cameras typically use 200 μCi of the same agent. With the camera, the accumulated information is usually stored by a computer for later analysis of individual kidney count rates and generation of renogram curves. The camera-generated data are acquired by the computer at intervals of 10 to 15 seconds for as long as 30 minutes to 1 hour.

The term *renogram* simply indicates that an activity versus time graph is being generated from the kidney activity. Classically, the renogram study was performed with ^{131}I hippurate, but other agents such as ^{99m}Tc DTPA or MAG_3 may be used. The shape of the renal curve is obviously affected by the pharmaceutical used. The shape is also affected by patient preparation and positioning. For instance, the classic renogram is performed with the patient

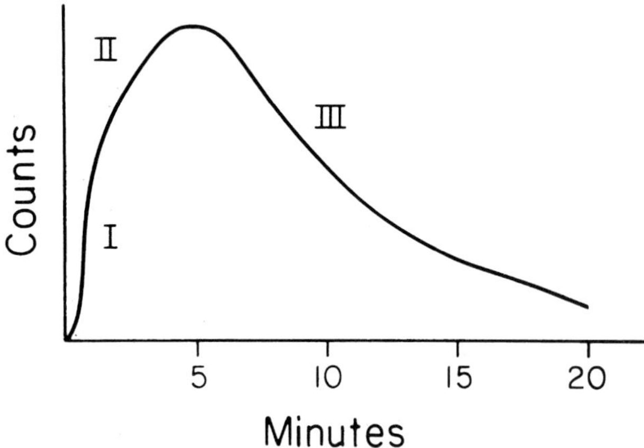

FIGURE 3G.8. Renogram curve showing count rate versus time. The shape is affected by the radiopharmaceutical injected intravenously. The idealized curve shown is typical of that following hippurate injection in a moderately hydrated patient, recording activity with a gamma camera and computer. Phase I is vascular content in kidney and background. As the kidney extracts the tracer, activity rises in phase II. When the collecting system starts emptying through the ureter, activity falls in phase III.

mildly dehydrated and seated in front of the Anger camera. Drainage from the upper collecting system is more consistent in the upright position, but unfortunately, there is more tendency for the patient to move. Patients who cannot maintain this position comfortably and consistently may be imaged in the supine position. Follow-up patient studies should always be performed in the same position, if possible.

Hydration state affects the timing and shape of the renogram curves. Phase I (Fig. 3G.8), lasting approximately 30 seconds, represents the arrival of the IV-injected pharmaceutical in the blood pool of the kidney and adjacent tissues. There will be a phase I increase in count rate regardless of the status of the kidney because there is blood pool activity in all tissues. The activity during this phase is poorly related to renal blood flow. Phase II typically lasts 4 to 6 minutes and terminates when activity in the kidney reaches a maximum. As the kidney extracts the radiopharmaceutical from blood, the count rate gradually rises. Because the blood levels fall rapidly during the first few minutes, activity in the urine is maximum initially and gradually falls with time. When this most active urine leaves the region of interest being analyzed, the count rate will start to fall. Thus the rate of increase in count rate during phase II is directly related to the renal blood flow and renal function. The rate of increase of activity is not affected by hydration, but the duration of phase II is inversely related to the urine formation rate.

Phase III starts at the peak of renal activity and illustrates a gradual fall in count rate as the most concentrated activity is washed from the collecting system. The time that is required for the count rate to fall to half of the peak value is called the half-time for washout, and this time is affected by urine formation rate. Numerous other aspects of the shape and timing of the renogram curve have been analyzed, but none is specific for disease process. However, if hydration state and positioning are consistent, changes in the slope of phase II, the time to peak, and the half-time for washout do reflect changes in renal status.

Mathematical Model: Two-Component Model

To be able to quantitate the results of functional studies, a model is developed to describe the organ function. A connection is made between the numbers that are available from the noninvasive examination and the properties that it is desired to measure. In the case of the kidneys, the quantities to be measured include renal plasma flow, GFR, and individual kidney function. Whether renal plasma flow or GFR is measured depends on the pharmaceutical used in the measurement.

The estimation of renal blood flow and function can be computed by the Fick principle, which when applied to the kidney gives the following formula:

$$\text{Clearance} = U_V/(A - V)$$

where U is the concentration of the test substance in the urine, V is the volume of urine, A is the concentration of the substance in the renal artery, and V is the concentration of the substance in the renal vein. If the substance is completely removed by the kidney, the renal vein concentration can be assumed to be zero; the arterial concentration may be assumed to be equal to the peripheral venous concentration. Thus the formula is simplified as follows:

$$\text{Clearance} = U_V/A$$

To perform a clearance measurement using Fick's principle, blood is sampled and a total urine collection is made during continuous IV infusion of the agent for three 20-minute periods. The assumption is made that the body reaches a steady state in which the input of the measured substance is the same as the output. One can further assume that measurements of the quantity of the substance in the infusion and the peripheral venous concentration are sufficient. If the separate function of each kidney is desired, catheters must be placed in each ureter.

It was discovered by Sapirstein and co-workers (42) that a single injection of the test substance could be substituted for continuous infusion with no compromise in the total functional information.

In a renal function examination using a radiopharmaceutical, the numbers that are available are the relative concentration in the kidneys as attenuated by tissue and the amount of activity per unit volume in the blood during the examination. The relative concentration in the urine in the bladder during the examination may be compared with the absolute concentration in voided urine at the end of the examination, especially in transplant patients whose kidney and bladder are close enough together for imaging at the same time. Note that unless complex techniques are resorted to, only samples removed from the patient can be quantitated in an absolute way.

It has been observed that the radioactivity per unit volume of plasma of radiopharmaceuticals injected for renal examination decreases according to a biexponential curve as a function of time. This means that the curve of plasma activity as a function of time shown in Fig. 3G.9 can be decomposed into two straight lines (on a semilogarithmic scale as shown in Fig. 3G.10). Each of these lines is described by its intercept with the activity axis, which is its concentration at time equals zero, and its half-time, or the amount that disappears per unit time. Thus one curve yields four numbers.

If, in turn, we consider a model of renal function (Fig. 3G.11), it is possible to write differential equations describing the loss of material from one compartment and the gain of an equal amount by another, following the arrows of the model and using the language and symbolism of reaction-rate chemistry. The model pictured is called an *open two-compartment mammillary model* (33). Such differential equations can be solved to yield mathematical functions that describe the concentration in each compartment as a function of time. For this model, the function that describes the concentration in the vascular compartment as a function of time is a biexponential curve. Thus the kinetic variables in the model can be related to the numbers generated from patient plasma sampling. The renal clearance is a function of all four numbers, which come from both parts of the curve:

$$\text{Clearance} = \ln(2)(A_1 \times t_1 + A_2 \times t_2)$$

where A_1 and A_2 are the fractions of the injected dose per milliliter for each of the two parts of the curve at time zero, and t_1 and t_2 are the half-times for the two parts of the curve.

The measurements of the plasma disappearance curve may be made in several different ways. One method is to

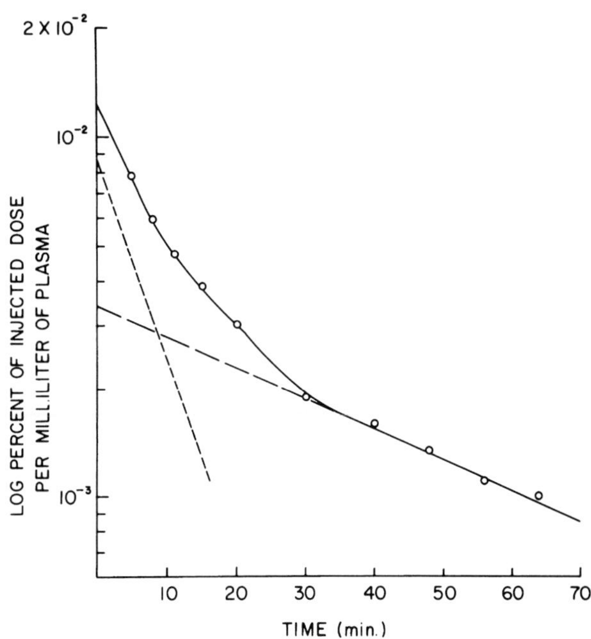

FIGURE 3G.10. The semilog graph of percent of injected dose per milliliter of plasma versus time shows a biexponential functionality. The two exponential parts are shown.

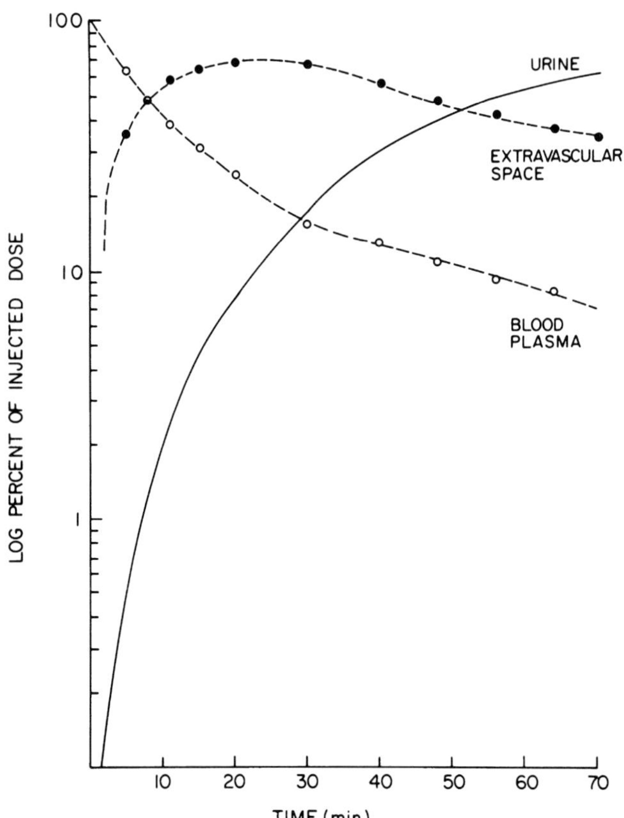

FIGURE 3G.9. The semilog graph of percent of injected dose versus time illustrates the amount of sodium o-iodohippurate in the blood, urine, and extravascular space.

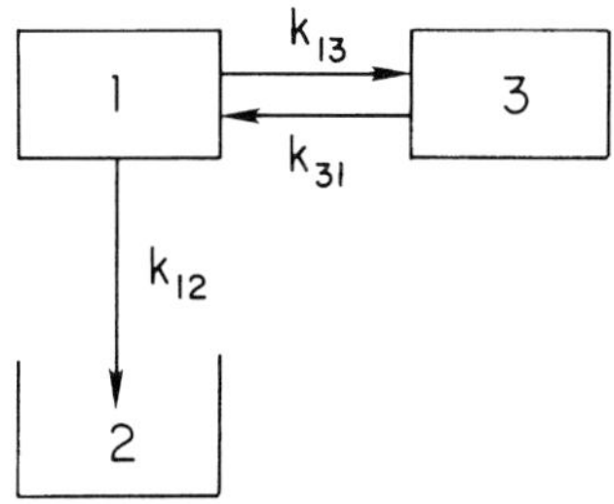

FIGURE 3G.11. The open two-compartment mammillary model. Compartment *1* is the plasma, compartment *3* is the extravascular space, and compartment *2* is the urine. There is kinetic equilibrium between compartments *1* and *3*, and there is no return from compartment *2*. *k* indicates the rate constant for transfer from compartment i to compartment j.

take plasma samples over a time suitable for defining the two parts of the curve; ten samples are sufficient to permit curve-fitting and the discrimination of poor samples. Some laboratories have simplified this method to taking one blood sample at a particular time with the subsequent calculation of renal clearance by a relationship connecting the clearance to the single-sample activity and several constants. A second method involves the measurement of a major blood pool in the body, such as the cranium or the heart, with a probe detector, combined with a blood sample that is compared with a standard to permit calibration of the plasma disappearance curve.

Clearly, using eight to ten blood samples to define the biexponential curve is the more accurate method, although simplification of the test procedure is necessary in some instances. In such a case, a method that accurately defines the longer half-life part of the curve should be sufficient to eliminate the difficulties of a single sample. In this case, the clearance equation becomes as follows:

$$\text{Clearance} = \ln(2)(A \times t)$$

where A is the fraction of the injected dose per milliliter of plasma at time zero, and t is the half-time of the line.

It should be pointed out that the simplified methods may not allow the accurate comparison of one patient to an absolute scale but may permit the progress of that patient's disease to be observed with changes in the renal function value because a particular patient's measurement is reproducible.

Constant Infusion Methods

Constant infusion methods, in which there is an IV infusion of saline containing the radioactive material, seem simple and appealing. Once a steady state is reached, measurements of urine and blood concentrations and interval urine volumes are all that is required to perform a clearance measurement.

The apparent simplicity is not real. The patient must be given a priming dose of the material to ensure that the blood and extravascular space will come to equilibrium during the constant infusion period, and the patient must be well hydrated to be able to urinate on command at given intervals. Urinary retention, normally up to 100 mL, is greater than this in certain diseases, and highly variable. Bladder retention can be estimated with external detectors, but this complicates the examination.

Computer Processing for Fractionation

The fractionation of renal clearance into values for the individual kidneys is accomplished by reference to the images acquired by the Anger camera at 15-second intervals after injection of the tracer dose. Regions of interest are drawn around the kidneys; background-corrected activity versus time curves are generated. From this point, two different methods can be used to complete the calculation.

In the slope method, the slopes of the curves for the two kidneys between 60 and 150 seconds after injection are calculated using least-square methods. The two slope values are added together, and the fractional contribution of each kidney's slope to the total is calculated. This is the fractional contribution that each kidney makes to the clearance.

In the integrated count method, the counts for each kidney between 60 and 150 seconds after injection are found, after background correction; this is a relative measure of the activity multiplied by time in each kidney. The two integrated counts are added, and the fractional contribution of each kidney to the total is calculated. Once again, this is the fractional contribution that the kidney makes to the clearance.

Both of these methods give similar results for kidneys that function well. The results for poorly functioning kidneys are open to more uncertainty for several reasons: The selection of the background region becomes more critical; the difference between kidneys and background is small and shows great variability; and the statistical uncertainties of radioactive detection are more serious for lower counts, so all the calculations have greater uncertainty.

When percentages are used for comparisons, they must always add up to 100%. This means that if one kidney remains the same after some elapsed time but the other improves in clearance, the one that remains the same will appear to have lost function on a percentage basis. It is thus incumbent on the observer to look at both the percentages and the absolute clearance values.

Glomerular Filtration Rate

The glomeruli produce an ultrafiltrate of the plasma by means of a physical process, which is nonselective for substances of low molecular weight. The volume of this ultrafiltrate, expressed in milliliters per minute, is defined as the GFR. The formation of the filtrate is regulated by the hydrostatic pressure gradient, osmotic pressure, the filtration surface, and membrane porosity.

To measure GFR, the agent must have the following characteristics (45):

1. Be nontoxic, physiologically inert, and chemically stable
2. Be easily and accurately measured in blood and urine
3. Be fully filterable through the glomerular membrane
4. Not combine with plasma proteins
5. Not be resorbed, synthesized, destroyed, or excreted by tubules
6. Have a constant clearance with high or low urinary flow, and greater or lesser concentrations of the agent in the plasma

7. Have a clearance equal to that of other tracers already proved adequate for GFR measurement, such as inulin
8. Be eliminated exclusively by the kidneys

The standard for comparison for GFR measurements is inulin clearance in a protocol that includes continuous IV infusion and three 20-minute complete urine collections and three blood samples drawn during the urine sampling periods. The protocol is not practical for clinical use.

The use of radioactively labeled compounds has simplified GFR measurement by simplifying the measurement of the agent. Of the radioactively labeled materials, ^{99m}Tc DTPA comes closest to fulfilling the criteria for GFR measurement. It can also be used in combination with an imaging examination to visualize renal and ureteral anatomy and to quantitate the fraction of the GFR attributable to each kidney (fractionation). Inulin, labeled with the beta-minus emitter carbon-14, can also be used with the standard continuous infusion method or in a plasma sampling mode, as can sodium iothalamate and other radiographic contrast agents, labeled with ^{125}I or ^{131}I. DTPA and EDTA have also been used. The ready availability of ^{99m}Tc DTPA makes its use simpler than any of the other materials mentioned here.

The measuring process is described earlier in this chapter. Ten plasma samples obtained during 1.5 to 2 hours of blood sampling after a single IV injection should be sufficient to define the two parts of the biexponential curve. The single-sample technique uses a function of the form where *A, B,* and *C* are constants, and *S* is the fraction of the injected dose per milliliter of plasma in the 3-hour sample (7).

The radionuclide technique described by Gates (18) is an alternative method of measuring the GFR. The calculation is based on the renal uptake on Anger camera images during the 2- to 3-minute interval following tracer (^{99m}Tc DTPA) arrival in the kidneys. The GFR is computed by using the following formula:

$$\mathrm{GFR} = \mathrm{A(L + R) - B}$$

where *L* and *R* represent the depth-corrected percentages of renal uptake for the left and right kidneys and *A* and *B* are constants. The formula was derived from linear regression analysis comparing the renal uptake of ^{99m}Tc DTPA with 24-hour creatinine clearance in 51 adult studies.

The advantage of this method is that it allows rapid determination of split renal function, as well as total GFR, without blood samples. The accuracy of this method, however, has been called into question. Ginjaume and co-workers (19) compared four methods of measuring GFR and found that the effective volume technique using one blood sample taken at 2 hours was the best compromise between accuracy and convenience and that the Gates method presented practical problems due to uncertainty in background subtraction and kidney-depth approximation.

The mean value of GFR in the normal adult is approximately 130 mL per minute in men and 120 mL per minute in women, with an uncertainty of 10%. The GFR of the newborn is between 20% and 40% of the adult value and increases progressively until, at age 1 year, it becomes equal to adult values in relation to the standard surface area.

Effective Renal Plasma Flow

If the renal tubules can be assumed to remove a substance totally from the blood during perfusion, a study of the concentration of that substance could yield values of renal blood flow. Most of the substances used in such a measurement are concentrated in the plasma, so the measurement is of renal plasma flow (RPF).

The ideal substance for estimating RPF should have the following characteristics:

1. Be nontoxic, physiologically inert, and chemically stable
2. Be easily and accurately measured in blood and urine
3. Be fully secreted by renal tubules
4. Be readily dissociated from any plasma protein complex in its transit through the kidney
5. Not be resorbed, synthesized, or destroyed by tubules
6. Have a saturable clearance so that high concentrations have lesser clearance values
7. Have nearly total renal extraction
8. Be eliminated exclusively by the kidneys

Both because only a portion of renal blood flow is presented to renal secretory tissue as opposed to the small fraction that normally perfuses the nonsecretory tissue (perirenal fat, pelvis, and capsule) and because no substance perfusing the kidney will be totally extracted, the calculated clearance will be less than the total renal plasma flow, so it is termed *effective renal plasma flow* (ERPF). Extraction efficiency of the tubules may be decreased in disease, as may renal blood flow.

Para-aminohippurate (PAH) was found to meet the aforementioned criteria best. Sodium iodohippurate (OIH) was found to be similar in behavior to PAH; in addition, it can be labeled with radioactive isotopes of iodine, such as ^{131}I, ^{123}I, and ^{125}I, making detection of the material simpler than in the previously used chemical methods. ^{131}I and ^{123}I have the added advantage of ready imaging with the Anger camera.

Because ^{131}I OIH disappears from the blood according to a biexponential function, the open two-compartment mammillary system is appropriate for analysis. Again, the examination protocol may be combined with imaging so that the images and fractional ERPF for each kidney are obtained along with the total ERPF value. The protocol may be based on serial blood sampling between 5 and 70 minutes after IV injection of ^{131}I OIH, to define the biexponential curve, or a less accurate single-sampling method can be used. Tauxe and co-workers (49) performed an elaborate analysis, which suggested that it was feasible to use a single blood sample, at 44 minutes after injection, and a polynomial to calculate the ERPF:

$$ERPF = A + B/S + C/S$$

where *A, B,* and *C* are constants, and *S* is the fraction of the injected dose per milliliter of plasma.

Normal ERPF values lie above 600 mL per minute, with a 10% uncertainty. Approximately 50% of the function should be attributable to each kidney. Filtration fraction is the comparison of GFR and ERPF measurements. The normal value is approximately 0.2. Tauxe (48) documents ERPF values in normal patients and patients with unilateral nephrectomy.

Renal plasma flow can also be measured with ^{99m}Tc MAG_3 (40,41). As the agent becomes widely available and more controlled studies are performed, the ERPF ratio between MAG_3 and OIH will be better known. From the University of Alabama research, the 44-minute MAG_3 concentration is 0.563 times the OIH value (41).

Nuclear Cystography

Although cystograms may be performed after the bladder has filled following an IV injection of a radiopharmaceutical, the study is more accurate in detecting ureteral reflux if the tracer is placed directly in the urinary bladder. From 3/10 to 1 mCi of ^{99m}Tc pertechnetate is mixed with 250 to 500 mL of sterile saline in an IV bottle. The IV bottle should not be more than 3 feet above the bladder. After the tubing is attached to the catheter, the bladder is slowly filled and the time and volume are recorded. At the same time, sequential images are recorded by the camera and computer. The patient is then instructed to void with the catheter in place; if voiding is impossible, the catheter is withdrawn.

The recording sequence varies somewhat among laboratories, but in general, frames are recorded on film and in the computer at 15- to 30-second intervals. Posterior projections are used. Images or computer curves may reveal reflux up the ureters. The severity of reflux is usually gauged by the volume of infused fluid required to produce significant reflux. Increasing volumes instilled before reflux occurs implies improvement.

Scrotal Imaging

Nuclear imaging to evaluate scrotal pathology has been used since 1973 with excellent accuracy reported. Its primary role is the differentiation of testicular torsion from epididymitis in patients with an "acute" scrotum. The standard radionuclide used is ^{99m}Tc pertechnetate.

In our procedure, the patient is given an oral dose of potassium perchlorate 30 minutes before radionuclide dose to block thyroid uptake. Potassium iodide can also be used. Positioning includes taping the penis to the abdominal wall and supporting the testicle on a tape sling to rest the testicle on a slightly higher plane than the thigh. A large-field-of-view camera is positioned anteriorly, and no shielding is used.

A bolus of 20 mCi of ^{99m}Tc pertechnetate is injected IV. A flow sequence of 3 seconds per frame at 70-mm image size is used, and then static images with a LEAP collimator are obtained immediately and at 5 and 10 minutes for 500,000 counts per view. The analysis is described in the following section.

CLINICAL APPLICATIONS

Acute Renal Failure

Acute renal failure may be caused by anatomic or physiologic abnormalities. Anatomic causes of renal failure include occlusion of renal arteries and veins and obstruction of the urinary tract at any level. Physiologic causes of acute renal failure include blood volume depletion ("prerenal") and acute tubular necrosis (ATN). The first step in evaluation of acute renal failure is sonography to evaluate the status of the collecting system (3). Contrast studies are not recommended because of their potential adverse effect on renal function. If the sonogram shows no evidence of dilation of the collecting system, the next step is dynamic renal scintigraphy.

We recommend ^{99m}Tc DTPA or ^{99m}Tc MAG_3. The technetium compounds provide better anatomic detail than either ^{123}I hippurate or ^{131}I hippurate. An important part of this examination is the visual evaluation of renal blood flow. The flow portion of dynamic imaging is the essential part in the evaluation of renal arterial blood flow. Analysis is based on observing the symmetry and the intensity of kidney visualization. The peak of activity in the kidney should be no more than 3 seconds after the peak of activity in the aorta. The intensity of activity in a normal-sized kidney should equal or exceed the early activity in the spleen (16).

Unilateral delay or decrease in kidney visualization on the flow study signifies a vascular abnormality. The possible vascular abnormalities include renal artery occlusion secondary to embolism, thrombosis, or dissection of an aortic aneurysm; renal artery laceration secondary to trauma; renal artery stenosis; and renal vein thrombosis. Unilateral delay can also be caused by severe unilateral ureteral obstruction or damage from infection or other disease. The sonographic findings are helpful in this differential.

Bilateral delay or decrease in renal perfusion is less specific. This pattern could be due to bilateral vascular compromise, severe prerenal circulatory failure, severe renal causes of failure (including ATN), and severe bilateral ureteral obstruction (Fig. 3G.12). Obstruction is again excluded by the sonographic findings.

The static images are analyzed for renal size and position along with symmetry, uniformity, and promptness of up-

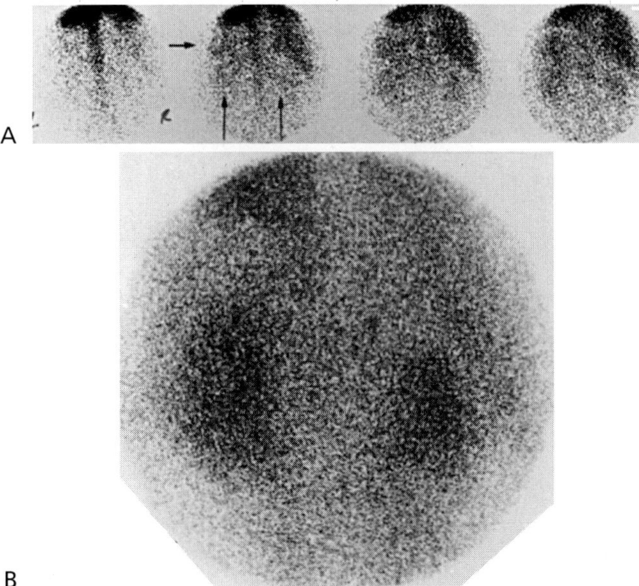

FIGURE 3G.12. Woman, 64 years old, with acute tubular necrosis following partial resection of her small bowel. **A:** ^{99m}Tc DTPA vascular sequence shows symmetrically poor renal blood flow. *Vertical arrows,* kidneys; *horizontal arrow,* spleen. **B:** Static image at 20 minutes demonstrates moderate bilateral uptake. No bladder activity was demonstrated.

take bilaterally. In normal kidneys, the immediate postdynamic images demonstrate symmetric, homogeneous activity in the renal cortices. Within 5 minutes, background activity lessens and the collecting systems are well visualized.

Renal size and position can suggest the cause, as well as prognosis, of the disease process. Bilaterally, normal-sized kidneys suggest recent onset and potential reversibility. Small kidneys indicate chronic disease, congenital or acquired, and irreversibility. Large kidneys can be seen in polycystic disease, an infiltrating disease such as amyloidosis, or renal vein thrombosis (44).

Evaluation of symmetry and uniformity of uptake on the static views compared with the flow study can also suggest underlying causes. Asymmetry of uptake with a corresponding flow abnormality correlates with a vascular problem. Lack of uniformity of uptake is caused by localized parenchymal disease. Wedges or segments of decreased activity that correlate with vascular distributions imply vascular abnormalities. Mass lesions may also cause nonuniformity and are discussed later in this chapter.

Promptness of uptake is also an important indicator. Delay in uptake in the kidneys suggests poor renal function secondary to parenchymal compromise. Causes include prerenal circulatory failure; renal disease, such as ATN; and postrenal obstruction. When severe enough, this compromise can decrease the flow as described previously.

In the severely oliguric or anuric patient, renal function may be so severely compromised that ^{99m}Tc DTPA or ^{99m}Tc GH scans are inadequate. In that case, ^{131}I hippurate is recommended because renal concentration can occur with as little as 3% of normal function (38). ^{99m}Tc MAG_3 provides results that are comparable to those with hippurate in patients with impaired renal function (50).

Chronic Renal Failure

In evaluating the azotemic patient, excretory urography becomes inadequate when the plasma creatinine level exceeds 5 mg per 100 mL. Large bolus doses of organic iodides may improve visualization radiographically but adversely affect already compromised renal function. ^{99m}Tc MAG_3 is the recommended agent for evaluation of chronic renal failure. Technetium compounds are chosen because flow studies can be performed. Additional experience with ^{99m}Tc MAG_3 shows that this compound is preferred to hippurate or DTPA. As in acute renal failure, the size, position, promptness, symmetry, and uniformity of renal uptake of the kidneys are important in guiding investigation and narrowing the diagnostic possibilities (46).

Masses and Pseudomasses

In evaluating a renal mass, the purpose of noninvasive tests is to narrow the diagnostic possibilities and avoid intervention if the mass is benign. The current resolution of scintigraphy is not as good as that of radiography. Lesions as small as 1 cm have been detected on phantoms, but a larger lesion centrally placed in the kidney may not be detected by scintigram. On the other hand, peripheral lesions or those obscured by fat or bowel gas may be better visualized. Therefore radiologic and radionuclide techniques are complementary in evaluation of renal masses.

Ultrasound is generally the recommended first procedure for initial characterization of a renal mass. If lobulation is noted, a normal variant, or "pseudomass," of the kidney may be present, such as a hypertrophied column of Bertin, splenic impression, dromedary hump, or fetal lobulation. The next step is nuclear imaging with ^{99m}Tc DMSA, used because of its concentration in the parenchyma. If the lobulation is secondary to a pseudomass, the static images will demonstrate normally functioning parenchyma. In some cases, the pseudomass may actually be more intense because of the increased thickness of the parenchyma (37).

If lobulation is not seen sonographically and the mass is atypically cystic, complex, or solid, CT or angiography is recommended. In determining whether a mass is vascular or nonvascular, radionuclide vascular flow studies are 80% to 85% accurate, a rate lower than the other two modalities.

Whether the mass is neoplasm, infarction, abscess, cyst, or localized pyelonephritis, the renal study will be abnormal due to replacement of normal parenchyma that concentrates radionuclide. A typical cyst or infarct will demonstrate no activity on blood flow or on early and delayed images. A

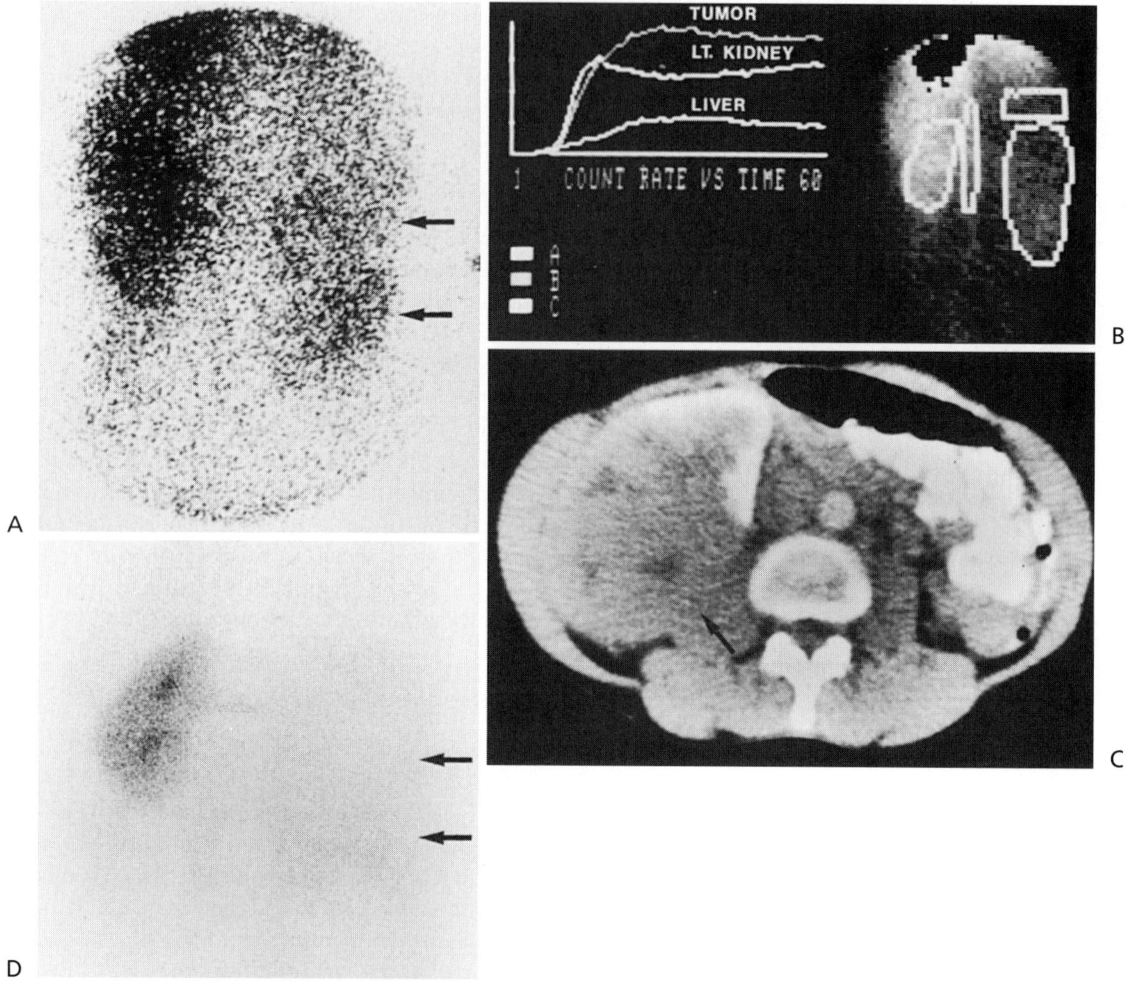

FIGURE 3G.13. Woman, 38 years old, with right hypernephroma. ^{99m}Tc glucoheptonate study showed initial delay of flow to right kidney (0 to 30 seconds). **A:** View at 40 seconds shows definite vascularity of tumor *(arrows).* **B:** Histogram of blood flow to abdominal organs demonstrates initial delay in blood flow to tumor, then increased activity compared with left kidney. Normal delay in flow to liver is seen, corresponding to portal venous supply. **C:** Static views at 5 minutes show minimal function of right kidney, particularly in the upper pole. **D:** Computed tomography scan shows large right renal mass *(arrows)* with crescentic area of functioning renal tissue present along anteromedial aspect. Bowel loops in the left abdomen are opacified with oral contrast agent.

typical renal carcinoma will demonstrate activity on blood flow and early images but a photon-deficient area on delayed images (Fig. 3G.13). An abscess or localized pyelonephritis may be similar to a cyst or tumor, depending on the size and amount of hyperemia.

Hydronephrosis and Hydroureter

One of the most important applications of renal scintigraphy is in the evaluation of urinary tract obstruction. Renal imaging can help in the diagnosis, determination of timing for surgical intervention, and evaluation of therapy. It is also valuable in assessing renal function, which cannot be evaluated reliably by intravenous pyelography (IVP). In the setting of acute obstruction, any renal function implies salvageability, whereas in chronic obstruction, poor function suggests permanent damage.

When the ultrasound examination shows urinary tract dilation, the next question is whether obstruction is present. Conventional urography and radionuclide scanning are unreliable in differentiating obstructive from nonobstructive hydronephrosis.

Perfusion studies introduced by Whitaker (54) obtaining pressure–flow relationships have provided a more functional approach. The procedure requires placing a catheter into the renal pelvis to obtain pressure readings. This is an invasive procedure that can involve a significant radiation dose when done fluoroscopically.

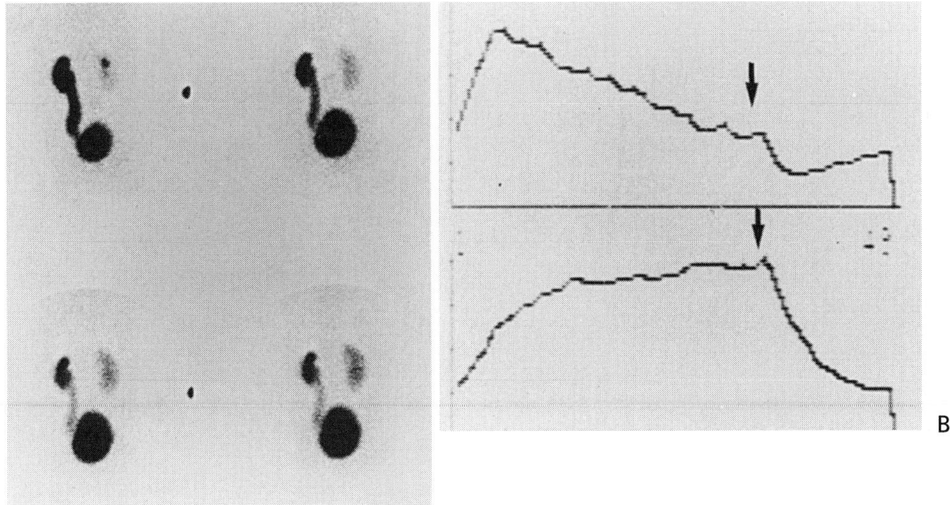

FIGURE 3G.14. Boy, 2 years old, following left ureteral reimplantation. ^{99m}Tc DTPA study. **A:** Posterior images demonstrate left hydronephrosis and hydroureter and a normal right kidney. The top left image was taken 30 minutes after radionuclide injection, at time of furosemide administration. Subsequent images were taken at 5-minute intervals showing radionuclide excretion. **B:** The right kidney *(top curve)* has excreted most of the radionuclide before furosemide administration. The *bottom curve* shows decreasing counts in the left kidney only after furosemide *(arrow)* signifying no evidence of obstruction.

Using parenteral diuretics allows radionuclide renography to be modified to obtain similar information by noninvasive methods. Published reports indicate a high degree of accuracy in distinguishing the dilated obstructed system from the nonobstructed (53).

The success of diuretic renography is directly dependent on strictly following the procedure. First, the patient must be well hydrated either by oral or IV methods. The patient needs to void just before injection or have a Foley catheter inserted for constant drainage. We prefer ^{99m}Tc DTPA because of its excellent visualization of the collecting system and inject 15 mCi (or the appropriate pediatric dose). MAG_3 is used in newborns or where renal function is poor. Images are taken every 5 minutes and continuously on computer until the *entire* collecting system is filled with radionuclide. (If this takes longer than 1 hour, the study decreases in reliability.) The patient then voids and is injected with furosemide, 1 mg/kg, up to 40 mg IV. Images are taken every 5 minutes for the next 30 minutes.

Computer analysis of the renal collecting system activity is performed, resulting in computer curves of the counts. Three curve patterns are possible. A definite decrease in counts with time after furosemide administration represents a nonobstructive pattern (Fig. 3G.14), whereas a definite increase is obstructive (Fig. 3G.15). A plateau signifies an indeterminate pattern, which could be secondary to poor renal function and poor response to furosemide, or a very large atonic hydronephrotic sac. Providing the renal function is good, $T_{1/2}$ (half-time for washout) of less than 10 minutes is normal; greater than 20 minutes indicates obstruction; and 10 to 20 minutes is indeterminate. These numbers are not absolute, and the volume of the affected collecting system is related to the half-time of washout. A distended bladder can also delay the washout, and catheterization of the bladder is often necessary. Efforts have been made to develop consistent methods for performing diuretic renograms for better consistency among institutions (9).

Vesicoureteral Reflux

Reflux nephropathy is a recognized problem in the pediatric population, and it is evaluated in the workup of urinary tract infection. It is also recognized in some adults as a cause of hypertension, proteinuria, and renal failure. The traditional study is a voiding cystourethrogram, which can deliver a radiation dose of several hundred millirads to several rads. The retrograde radionuclide cystogram gives a fraction of this radiation dose depending on several factors, including the amount of material instilled and the time the solution remains in the bladder before voiding (8).

The traditional voiding cystourethrogram can categorize reflux into grades of severity by visualizing the morphology of the urinary tracts. The radionuclide grading is determined by the volume in the bladder when reflux occurs and the amount of reflux. The anatomy of the collecting system, as well as the base of the bladder and urethra, cannot be assessed (Fig. 3G.16). However, the residual volume after voiding can be accurately determined.

The quantity of reflux that is significant in a single study

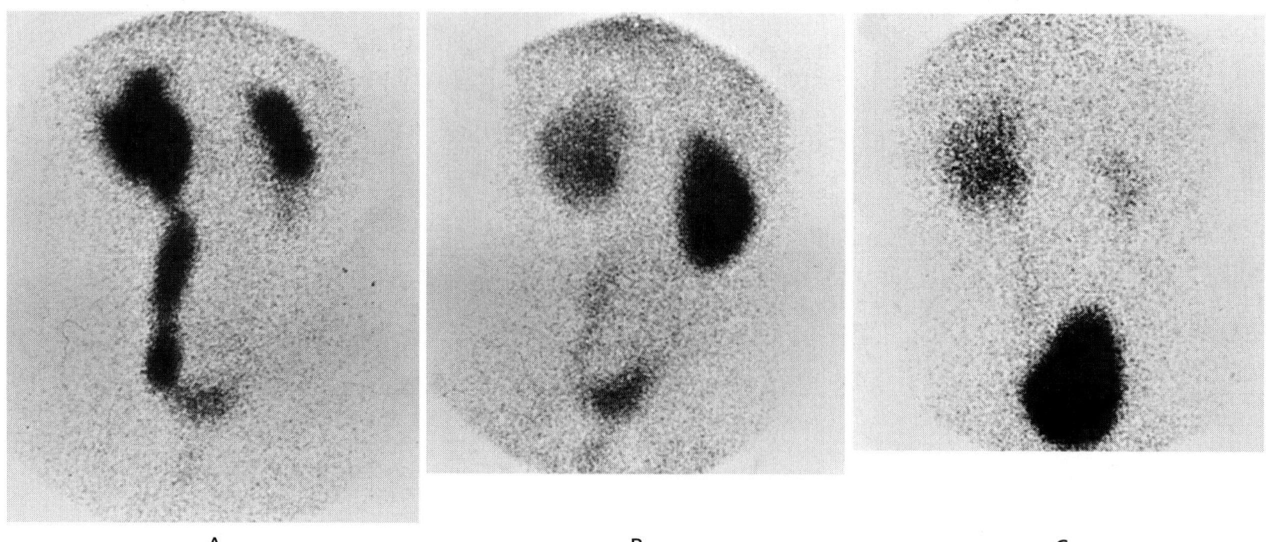

A B C

FIGURE 3G.15. Boy, 5 years old, with dilated, nonobstructed collecting system on the left and a dilated, obstructed collecting system on the right. Furosemide ^{99m}Tc DTPA study. **A:** Posterior image taken at 30 minutes after radionuclide injection, at time of furosemide administration. **B:** Twenty minutes after furosemide administration, the nonobstructed left system has emptied and the obstructed right side has accumulated more. **C:** Postoperative image at 25 minutes after furosemide administration shows resolution of obstructed right system.

is not yet defined. Serial studies can be of value for comparison to determine whether improvement has occurred. Accurate records of the volumes of solution instilled resulting in reflux are important, as is quantitation of reflux by visual and computer analysis. An increased volume instilled before reflux implies improvement (32). More recently, grading of reflux by radionuclide cystography has been correlated with the criteria for grading established by the International Reflux Study Committee (56). Despite the emphasis in the international study on calyceal detail (26), the correlation is stated to be 80% to 100%.

Studies have now shown that kidney infection, associated with reflux, often causes sufficient damage to result in scarring, proteinuria, or hypertension. Sonography and contrast urograms are relatively insensitive for detection of initial damage (13,43). Renal scans and SPECT with ^{99m}Tc DMSA significantly increase the detection rate and are the recommended screening procedures (Fig. 3G.17).

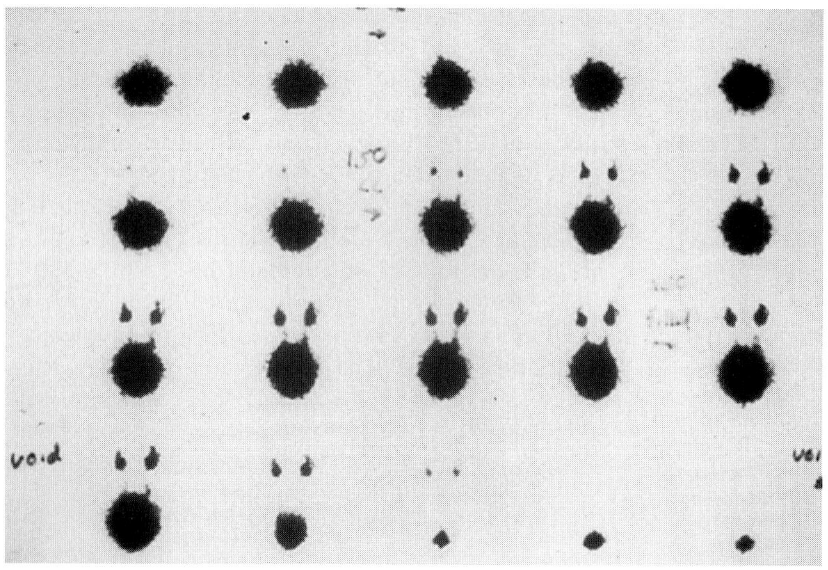

FIGURE 3G.16. Retrograde ^{99m}Tc pertechnetate voiding cystoureterogram demonstrates activity in both ureters and kidneys. The left side refluxes first as the bladder fills, indicating worse reflux. After voiding, activity cleared from the upper tracts.

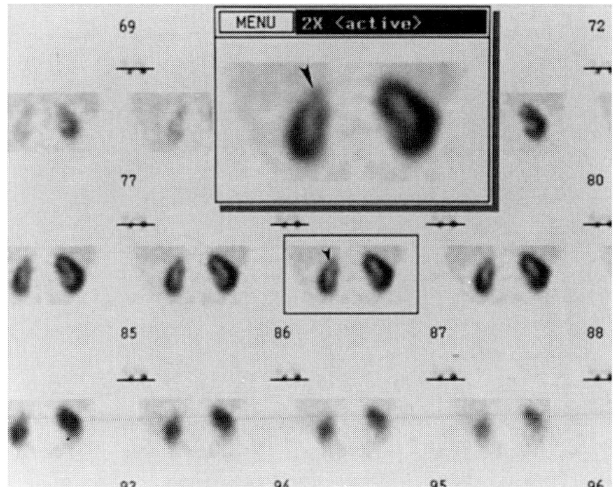

FIGURE 3G.17. Boy, 8 years old, with chronic renal insufficiency and recurrent urinary tract infections. ^{99m}Tc DMSA coronal SPECT images show the right kidney to be smaller than the left kidney with a significant scar in the upper pole *(arrowheads).* The selected image is magnified. This size defect is often difficult to demonstrate on planar views.

Renovascular Abnormalities

Renal artery stenosis not only plays a role in hypertension but also is a potentially treatable cause of renal failure. In most patients, renal damage has already occurred. Damage can cause abnormalities on the renal images that resemble other diseases, making the results nonspecific. However, this test can still be valuable in following patients with documented renal artery stenosis.

As with renal artery embolism, dynamic radioisotope scanning with technetium compounds is preferred (Fig. 3G.18). On the initial flow images, decreased perfusion of the affected kidney is noted along with reduced concentration followed by a prolonged parenchymal transit time. The sensitivity is 60% to 85%. Serial studies can guide in timing for intervention and evaluation of open surgical or angioplastic treatment.

Some centers prefer hippurate scanning to evaluate unilateral renovascular disease. Emphasis is on observing differences in the time interval between injection and peak activity (transit time) and on the symmetry of the downslope of the third phase on the renogram curve. The affected kidney will show a prolonged transit time and a slower decline in the excretory phase. A difference of 20% or more in these parameters is generally considered the criterion for positive diagnosis. Accuracy from 87% to 96% has been claimed (34). Analysis of ERPF and fractionation of renal function allow measurement of individual renal flow (Fig. 3G.19).

Recent studies have shown that the specific effects of angiotensin-converting enzyme inhibitors (captopril) on renal function add both sensitivity and specificity to the radiorenogram. Various authors have advocated using ^{99m}Tc DTPA, ^{99m}Tc MAG_3, or ^{131}I hippurate. Although success has been obtained with all three tracers, the theoretical reasons for using an enzyme inhibitor would seem to favor the use of DTPA. In part, the lack of optimal sensitivity of radiorenograms is due to the intrarenal compensation for a decrease in renal perfusion pressure distal to a stenotic renal artery. It has been demonstrated that the release of renin and subsequent formation of angiotensin II cause a

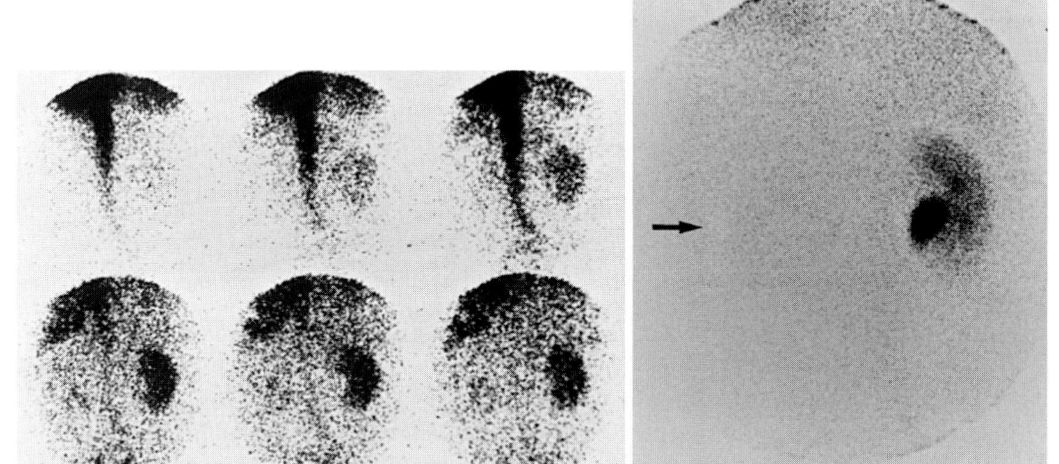

FIGURE 3G.18. Man, 65 years old, with sudden onset of left flank pain and hematuria. **A:** ^{99m}Tc glucoheptonate flow study shows good flow to the right kidney and minimal flow to the left. **B:** Delayed view demonstrates minimal left renal uptake *(arrow);* the right kidney appears normal. The combination of significantly decreased flow to the entire left kidney and delayed uptake is compatible with left renal artery embolus.

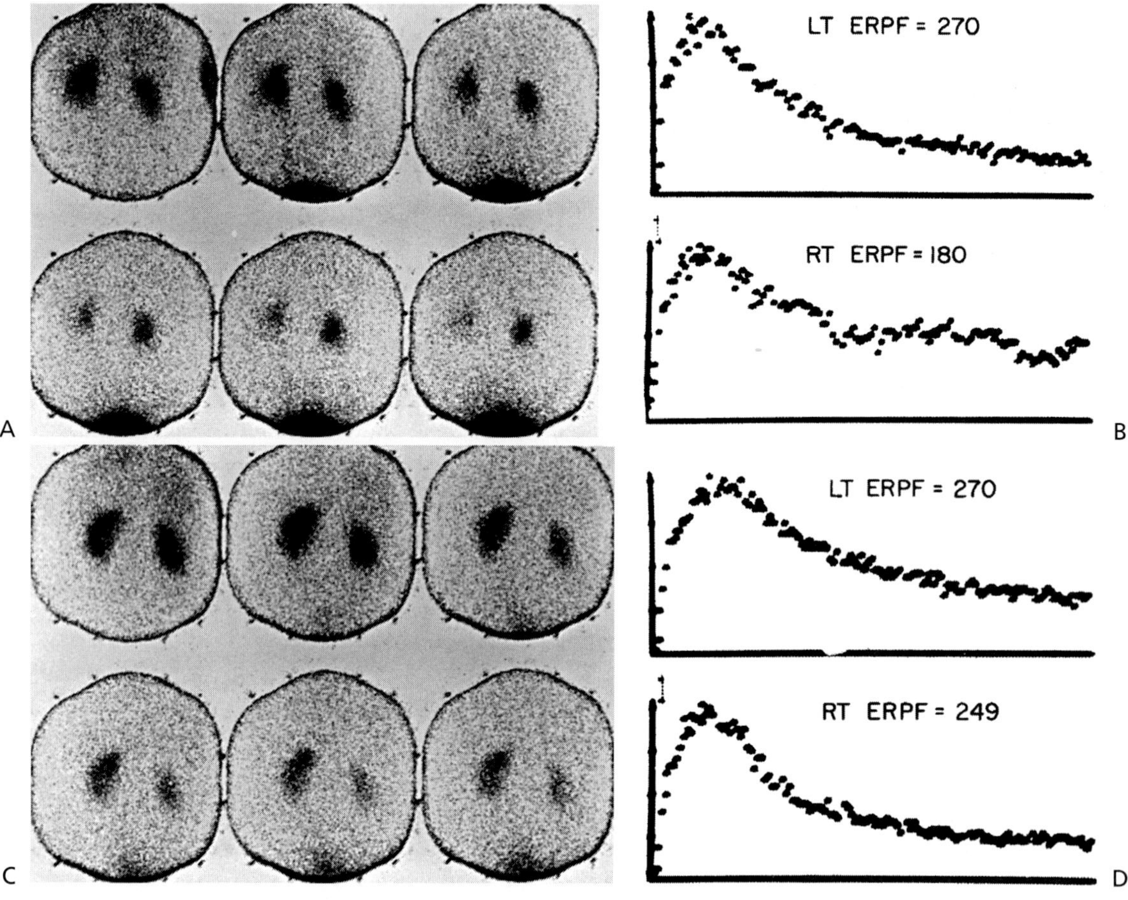

FIGURE 3G.19. Angioplasty of renal artery. **A, B:** Preangioplasty for right renal artery stenosis. ^{131}I hippurate scan shows delayed clearance of the right kidney on the static views and the renogram curve. The effective renal plasma flow (ERPF) was diminished on the right (180 mL per minute) compared with the left. **C, D:** Postangioplasty there was improvement in clearance of the right kidney and the ERPF on the right increased to 249 mL per minute.

selective vasoconstriction in the efferent renal arterioles, thus maintaining glomerular filtration pressure. Only when the renal artery stenosis becomes more severe is this compensation inadequate to maintain renal function. Recent studies have shown that comparing renal excretion of ^{99m}Tc DTPA, ^{99m}Tc MAG_3, or ^{131}I hippurate before and after oral administration of 25 to 50 mg of captopril improves the sensitivity of the renogram from 60% to more than 90% (Fig. 3G.20). In addition, there is increased specificity because a lack of response indicates that the compensation mechanism is inoperative (17). Although blockage of the converting enzyme affects the renograms performed with hippurate, MAG_3, and DTPA, the use of the latter agent would seem to be preferred because it is excreted by only glomerular filtration, the physiologic process most affected when compensatory efferent arteriolar vasoconstriction is blocked. However, studies have shown excellent results with MAG_3 (12,15,36).

Renal vein thrombosis is an uncommon entity that can be imaged with radionuclides. Technetium compounds are preferable because flow studies and detailed static views can be obtained. Typically, in renal vein thrombosis, the involved kidney is enlarged, with decreased flow and poor, delayed uptake (Fig. 3G.21).

Transplant Evaluation

Radionuclide imaging is a routine part of the assessment of renal function following renal transplant. Our technique involves injection of the patient with ^{99m}Tc MAG_3. Routine images are taken in the anterior position as previously described because of the kidney's position. Computer analysis produces the renogram curves. We look at the total transplant counts, shape of the renogram curve, bladder-to-kidney count ratio at 30 minutes, and static views. Total transplant counts are helpful to compare in serial studies; we have no absolute value for determination of function based on one individual scan. Estimation of renal function with the Gates technique is more quantitative (18).

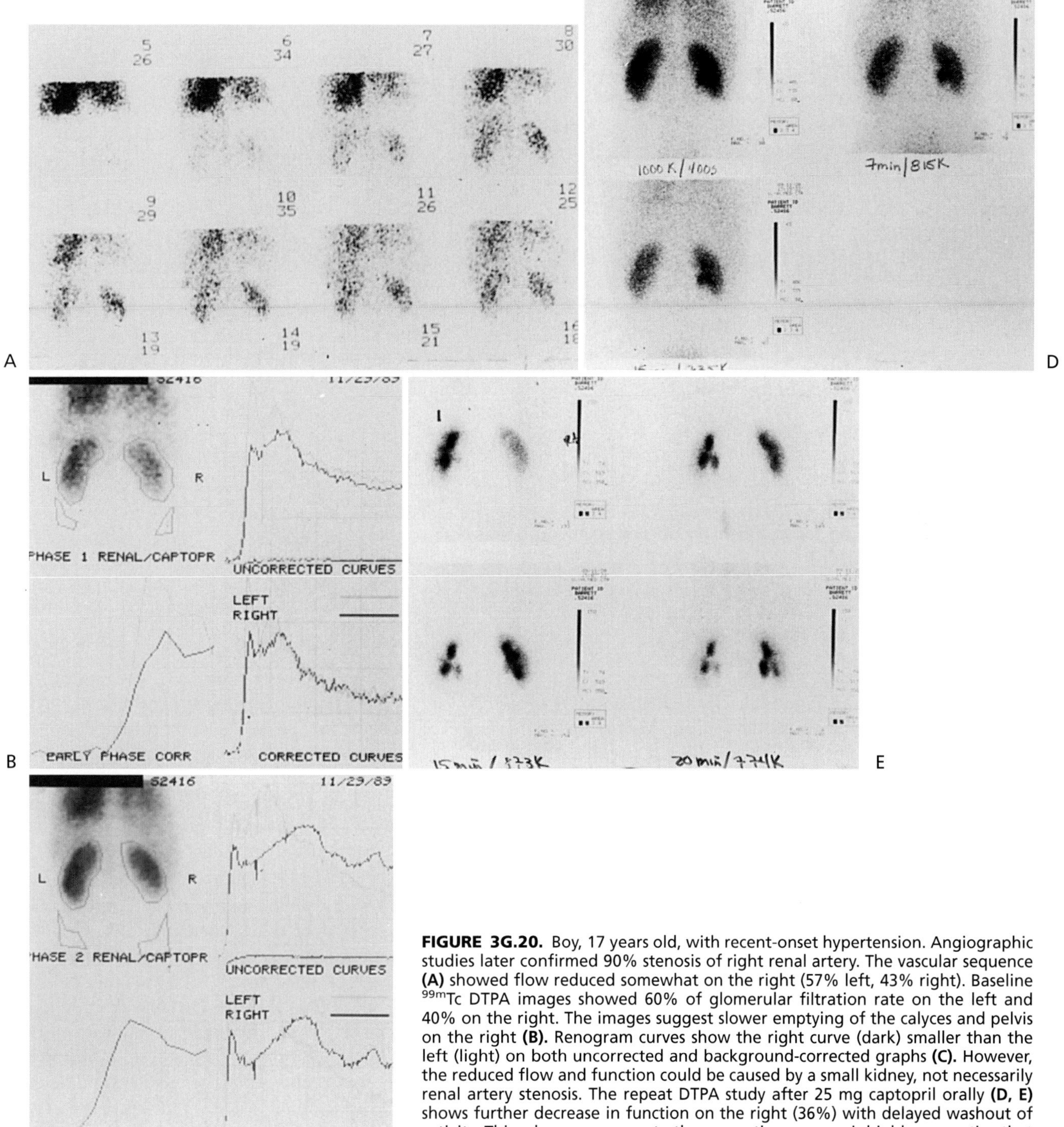

FIGURE 3G.20. Boy, 17 years old, with recent-onset hypertension. Angiographic studies later confirmed 90% stenosis of right renal artery. The vascular sequence **(A)** showed flow reduced somewhat on the right (57% left, 43% right). Baseline ^{99m}Tc DTPA images showed 60% of glomerular filtration rate on the left and 40% on the right. The images suggest slower emptying of the calyces and pelvis on the right **(B).** Renogram curves show the right curve (dark) smaller than the left (light) on both uncorrected and background-corrected graphs **(C).** However, the reduced flow and function could be caused by a small kidney, not necessarily renal artery stenosis. The repeat DTPA study after 25 mg captopril orally **(D, E)** shows further decrease in function on the right (36%) with delayed washout of activity. This adverse response to the converting enzyme is highly suggestive that arterial stenosis with renin release is a causative factor in the hypertension.

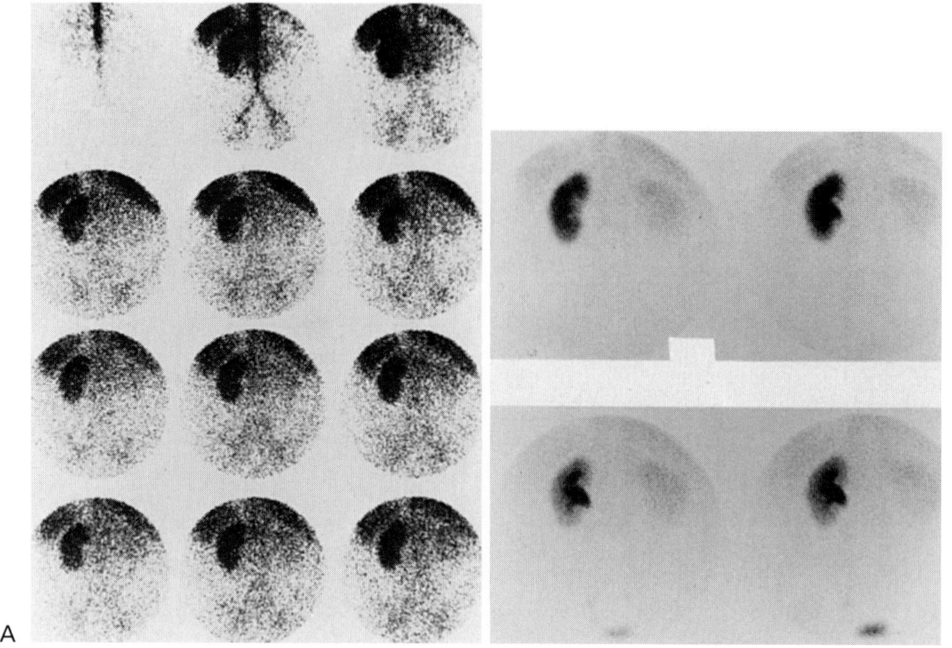

FIGURE 3G.21. Man, 27 years old, developed hematuria after retroperitoneal resection for testicular cancer. ^{99m} Tc glucoheptonate study. **A:** Renal flow study shows poor flow to right kidney. **B:** Static images at 5-minute intervals postinjection show poor right renal uptake. The combination of asymmetric poor flow along with poor function implies renal vein thrombosis. However, usually the involved kidney is also enlarged.

The bladder-to-kidney ratio is determined by drawing regions of interest around the kidney and the bladder and obtaining total counts at a specific time (23). The normal ratio at 30 minutes is 3:1 to 5:1 with hippurate, but it can be up to 10:1 or more with MAG_3. For this parameter to be useful, the Foley catheter must be clamped, which cannot usually be done until after the first week. Also, native kidneys may still have some function and falsely imply good transplant function.

In the early postoperative period (up to 4 weeks), serial radionuclide scanning and sonography are helpful in following renal function and determining the cause of oliguria or anuria. Total absence of flow and function, along with a photopenic area on the static images, can be caused by renal artery or vein thrombosis, hyperacute rejection, or severe urinary obstruction. Obstruction can usually be diagnosed by ultrasound; however, nonobstructed dilation of the collecting system can occasionally occur after transplantation. Diuretic renography may be helpful in differentiating obstruction from nonobstruction if adequate function is present.

Diminished early radionuclide uptake with progressively increasing activity in later views and poor excretion can be seen with ATN, acute rejection, and urinary obstruction. This pattern implies preserved blood flow but decreased concentrating and excreting capability. A kidney with ATN typically can extract hippurate or MAG_3 from the blood but has difficulty transporting it into the tubular lumen ("tubular block"). Cadaver transplants virtually always show an element of ATN in the early postoperative period. Postoperative ATN will resolve without therapy, after 1 day to several weeks.

As the kidney improves after ATN, the total excreted counts will increase and the bladder-to-kidney ratio will improve (Fig. 3G.22). The shape of the curve may not change initially but contains more counts; after further improvement, the curve will start peaking in the first 10 minutes. Any reversal of this sequence or failure of improvement implies rejection. However, other processes, such as infection or renal artery stenosis, also cause a deterioration in renal function. Considerable confusion has been added to this evaluation in recent years because of the toxicity of the immunosuppressive agent cyclosporine. Unfortunately, by usual techniques it is not possible to differentiate between cyclosporine toxicity and rejection. After 6 months, a renogram is of little value unless serial studies are maintained; serial laboratory values (creatinine and blood urea nitrogen [BUN]) are more pertinent and economical.

Leaks may develop at the ureterovesical anastomosis, at the cystotomy site, or from a renal biopsy site (Fig. 3G.23). These can be well demonstrated by collection of the radionuclide outside of the urinary tract. Hematomas or lymphoceles (Fig. 3G.24) appear as photon-deficient areas around the kidney or between the kidney and bladder.

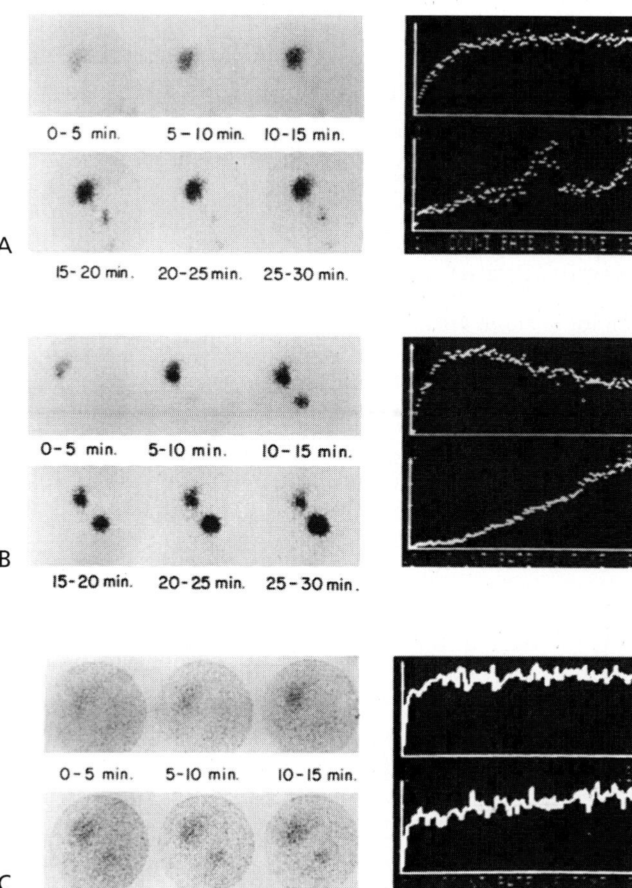

FIGURE 3G.22. Man, 54 years old, with end-stage renal disease who received a cadaver transplant kidney in the right iliac fossa. A series of renograms was performed using 200 μCi of ^{131}I hippurate. **A:** Baseline study 24 hours after transplantation. Sequential camera images *(left)* show progressive accumulation of activity in kidney with transport to urinary bladder. The renogram curves *(right)* reflect progressive kidney accumulation, the plateau occurring after approximately 10 minutes as the tracer emptied into the urinary bladder. The lower curve, from the urinary bladder, shows intermittent emptying because the Foley catheter was not clamped. **B:** The transplant function gradually improved as the acute tubular necrosis cleared. On this study performed 6 weeks after transplantation, the renogram curve *(above)* shows a peak at approximately 8 minutes with a gradual fall in count rate during phase III. Tracer gradually accumulated in the bladder, with a bladder-to-kidney ratio of 2.8:1 at 30 minutes. **C:** Repeat study at 3 months after transplantation. Serum creatinine levels were increased with significant deterioration in renal function. Note the very flat renogram curve *(above)* and minimal accumulation of activity in the urinary bladder. Not only has the bladder-to-kidney ratio deteriorated to 0.6:1, but the total excreted activity in the kidney and bladder fell to approximately 25% of prior values. The patient underwent therapy for rejection with a subsequent improvement in renal function.

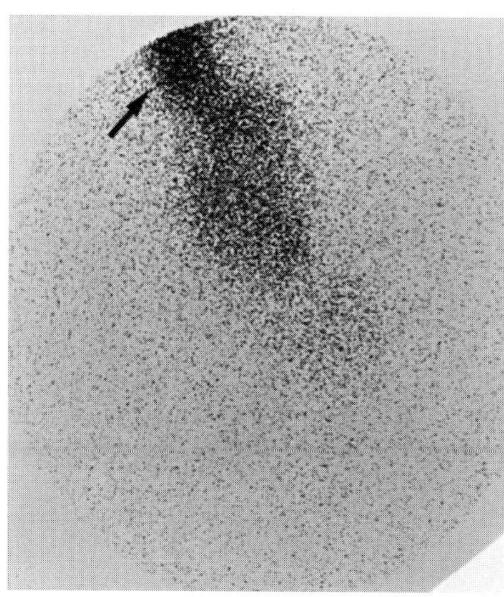

FIGURE 3G.23. Man, 24 years old, 3 weeks after a cadaver transplant. ^{131}I hippurate study shows extravasation of radionuclide at the superior margin of the transplant *(arrow)* representing a urinary anastomotic leak.

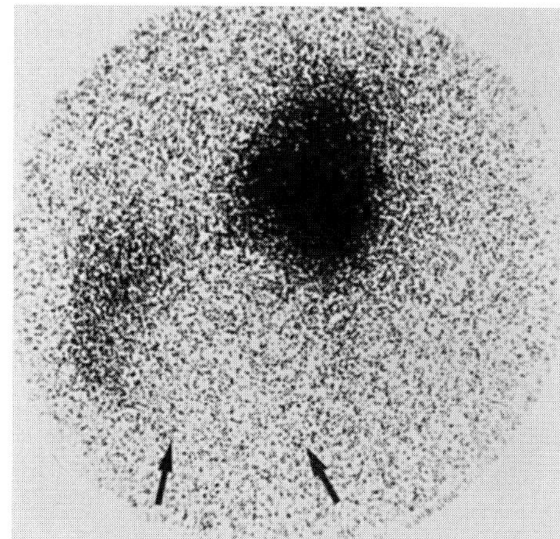

FIGURE 3G.24. Man, 42 years old, developed nephrotic syndrome after transplant. ^{131}I hippurate study shows large photopenic area *(arrows)* compressing the left lateral aspect of the bladder, which proved to be a lymphocele obstructing urinary excretion.

Some centers use technetium compounds to evaluate renal transplants, including evaluation of renal blood flow dynamically. In the normally perfused transplant, activity on the flow or dynamic images should do the following:

1. Appear in the graft within 6 seconds of its appearance in the adjacent iliac artery
2. Obtain maximum activity per unit area equal to or greater than that in the adjacent artery
3. Clearly fall after the peak

Renal blood flow is usually preserved in ATN but deteriorates in rejection. The evaluation of the static views is similar to that of the hippurate images. We have found the MAG_3 renogram to be better than that from hippurate or DTPA alone.

Other agents used include ^{99m}Tc sulfur colloid, gallium citrate Ga-67, and labeled platelets. Although such studies may be useful, they are not routine and are beyond the scope of this chapter.

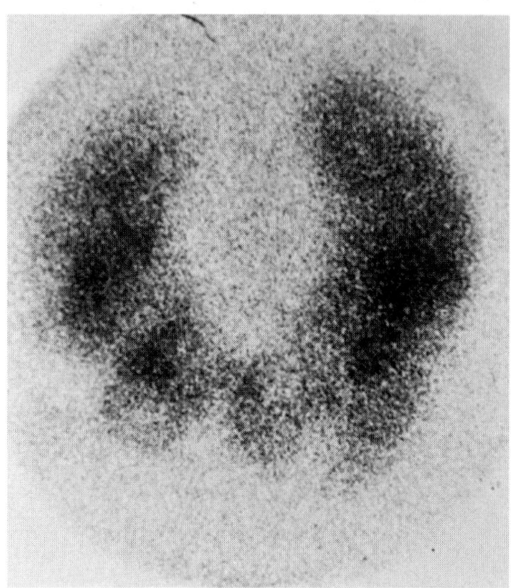

FIGURE 3G.25. Boy, 8 years old, with recurrent urinary tract infections. ^{99m}Tc iron hydroxide DTPA study demonstrates a horseshoe kidney. This anterior view shows the bridging tissue better than a posterior view.

Congenital Anomalies

Congenital anomalies such as horseshoe kidney (Fig. 3G.25), crossed fused ectopia, and ectopic kidneys are easily demonstrated by radionuclide scanning. ^{99m}Tc DTPA and MAG_3 are the agents of choice.

A renal mass in the infant or child should first be evaluated by ultrasound. A solid mass should then be studied by CT. A cystic mass can be either a multicystic dysplastic kidney or hydronephrosis, which can sometimes be difficult to differentiate sonographically. A MAG_3 scan is the next recommended study. Nonvisualization of the corresponding kidney on early and delayed views confirms dysplasia (Fig. 3G.26). However, delayed films may show some activity secondary to a small amount of residual functioning tissue, which is usually irregularly located in a photopenic mass. A more uniform cortical rim sign with gradual filling of the central collecting system is typical of hydronephrosis. The time of appearance of these features during the scanning period depends on the severity of obstruction.

TRAUMA

The excretory urogram and CT are the traditional modes of initial evaluation of the kidneys in the trauma setting. Many reports have shown the sensitivity of radionuclide image for detection of extent of damage and the evaluation of renal function. However, we advocate CT scanning for initial evaluation because other organs and the retroperitoneum can be evaluated simultaneously. Nuclear imaging can be valuable in following renal function after trauma.

The agent of choice is ^{99m}Tc MAG_3 or DTPA, because blood flow to the kidneys can be rapidly evaluated. If there is no immediate blood flow to either kidney on the flow study or initial static images, immediate angiography or surgical exploration may be necessary. Extravasation and obstruction can also be detected by scanning.

Scrotal Imaging

Scrotal imaging provides an accurate means of distinguishing between the most common causes of "acute" scrotum: epididymitis and testicular torsion. Less common causes include hydroceles and testicular tumors.

In classic acute epididymitis, hyperemia occurs in the head, body, and tail of the epididymis. The radionuclide angiogram shows significantly increased perfusion through the spermatic cord vessels. On the static views, increased tracer activity usually extends laterally, corresponding to the location of the epididymis (Fig. 3G.27).

If the inflammatory process spreads to the testis, it is termed *epididymo-orchitis.* The radionuclide activity then extends also medially to involve the testis. Extensive scrotal swelling or rotation of the scrotum in positioning may produce medial activity in the absence of testicular involvement.

If the inflammation is confined to a small area of the epididymis, focal hyperemia occurs only in the infected

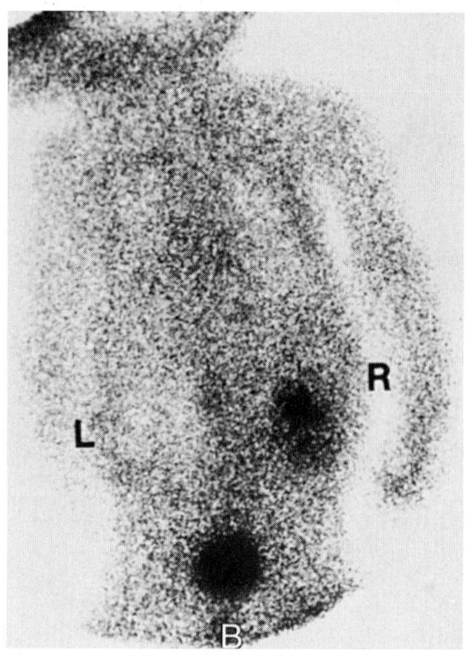

FIGURE 3G.26. Boy, 3 days old, with cystic left kidney on ultrasound. ^{99m}Tc glucoheptonate study demonstrates a normal right kidney and a photon-deficient area in the region of the left kidney that remained photopenic, compatible with a multicystic kidney. Bladder activity *(B)* was evident on this delayed static image.

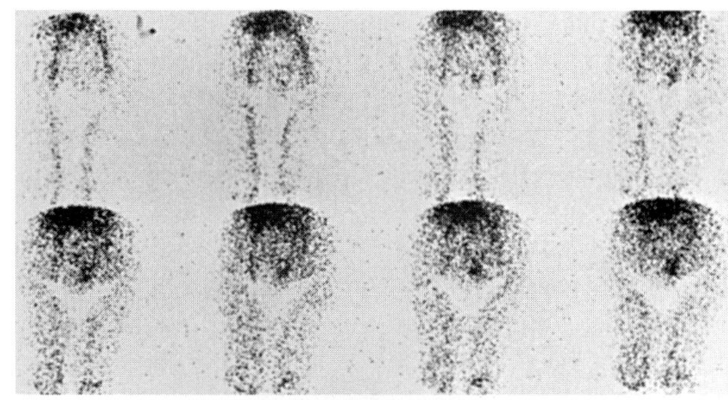

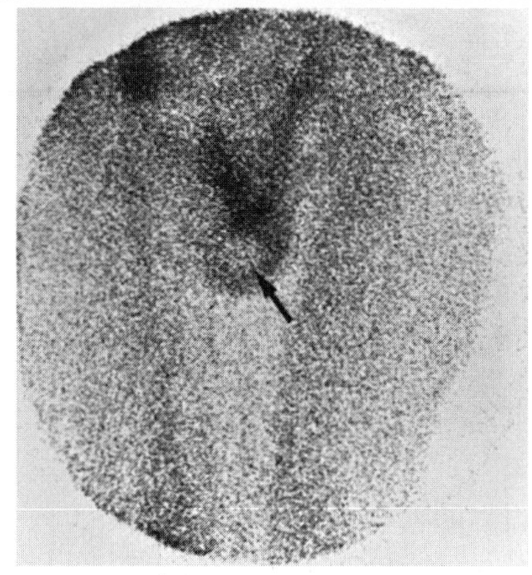

FIGURE 3G.27. Boy, 11 years old, with left testicular swelling. **A:** ^{99m}Tc pertechnetate flow study shows increased blood flow to the left epididymis. **B:** Increased activity along the lateral aspect of the left scrotum on the static views is present, compatible with epididymitis. The right scrotum *(arrow)* contained a hydrocele, causing the photopenic appearance. The differentiation between a photopenic and ischemic testicle and a hydrocele is easy after physical examination and transillumination.

part, and the radionuclide angiogram may often show "normal," barely perceptible activity. Later images may show a focal "spot" of increased activity.

Torsion of the spermatic cord has been described as displaying four radionuclide patterns (25). The first is seen if spontaneous detorsion occurs within 4 hours after torsion, which usually results in a normal scan. Occasionally, mild hyperemia is present throughout the entire hemiscrotum.

In early testicular torsion of less than 7 hours' duration, the testicle is often viable. The radionuclide angiogram shows no increase of perfusion through the vessels or to the scrotum. The scrotal scans demonstrate a cold area in the location of the testicle. In this second pattern, minimal, if any, activity is seen in the dartos, making the cold area often difficult to see.

Midphase testicular torsion occurs approximately 7 to 24 hours after torsion, when the testicle may still be viable. A reactive edema and erythema are present, resulting in increased activity in the scrotal region. This results in a halo of activity around the cold testicle (Fig. 3G.28), the third pattern.

The final pattern of "missed testicular torsion" occurs usually more than 24 hours after torsion. The testicle may still be viable if the twist is less than 360 degrees. The radionuclide angiogram will often show dartos perfusion. An intense halo of activity with a cold center is present and occasionally increased activity in the region of the spermatic cord. A testicular abscess can have a similar pattern. This symmetric halo should not be confused with the asymmetric curvilinear activity in epididymitis.

A hydrocele is a collection of fluid between the layers of the tunica vaginalis. It may be primary or secondary to epididymitis, testicular torsion, tumor, trauma, or posthernia repair. On the radionuclide angiogram, the perfusion is normal or a reflection of the underlying cause. The scrotal scan demonstrates a lucency around the central nidus of testicular tissue.

Radionuclide scanning of testicular tumors is usually performed to exclude other causes of the pain and swelling. The radionuclide angiogram may show normal or moder-

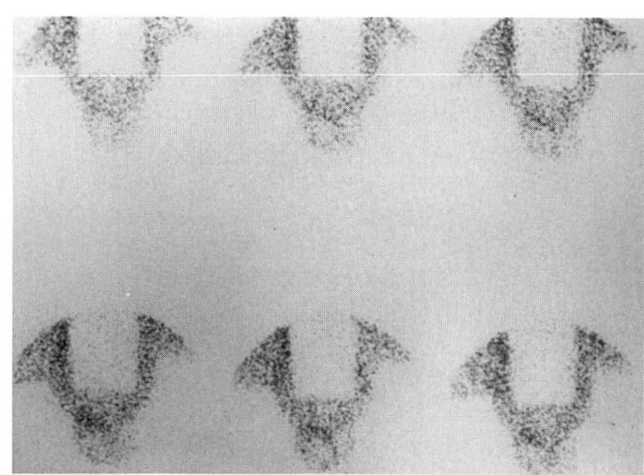

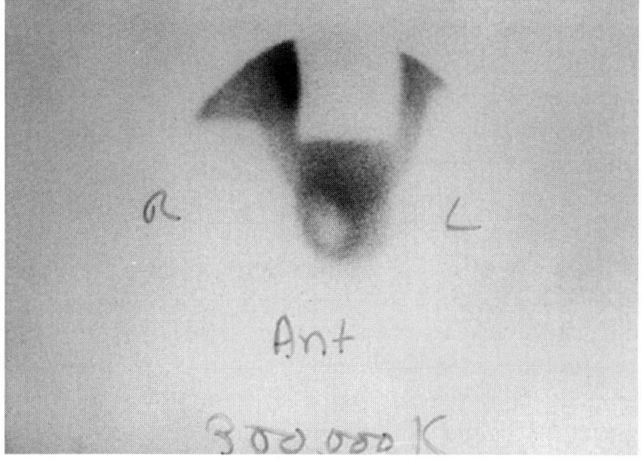

FIGURE 3G.28. Midphase testicular torsion. **A:** Flow study shows no hypervascularity but a developing focal area of increased uptake along the superior aspect of the right testis on later views. **B:** Delayed view shows photopenic area of right testis with surrounding increased uptake along all borders. Because the shield obscured the spermatic vessels, we no longer advocate its use.

ately increased perfusion. If increased, the scrotal perfusion is diffuse rather than linear or halolike. A cool area may represent a focal area of central necrosis or relative tissue avascularity (25).

EVALUATION OF PROSTATE CANCER

Adenocarcinoma of the prostate is the most commonly diagnosed malignancy in men. As in the case of all malignancies, appropriate therapeutic intervention requires accurate staging. Clinical examination, serum prostate-specific antigen (PSA) level, Gleason score, and imaging modalities such as bone scintigraphy, CT, and magnetic resonance imaging (MRI) are used for staging prostate carcinoma. However, the sensitivity of CT and MRI is poor in detecting lymph node metastases (52). A monoclonal antibody (Capromab pendetide) that reacts with prostate-specific membrane antigen (PSMA) has been commercially available for imaging prostate carcinoma for several years. PSMA is a glycoprotein produced by both the benign and malignant epithelial cells of the prostate gland. Capromab pendetide is a murine immunoglobulin (IgG_1) that is radiolabeled with indium-111 and reacts with more than 95% of prostate carcinomas (21). It is available for injection in a kit form (10). In-111 chloride is used for radiolabeling. After IV injection, Capromab pendetide is slowly cleared from the bloodstream. It is eliminated via the kidneys and by the gastrointestinal tract.

The incidence of adverse events following the antibody infusion is low (4%). The incidence of human antimurine antibody (HAMA) titers greater than 8 ng/mL after a single IV injection is reported to be 8%. The FDA has approved it for single injection. The incidence of HAMA levels greater than 8 ng/mL after repeated injections is reported to be 19%, but the incidence of adverse reactions is only 5%, with altered biodistribution present in 7% (21,31).

Anterior and posterior imaging of the chest, abdomen, and pelvis is performed at 72 to 96 hours. On a normal scintiscan, activity is seen in the liver, kidneys, bone marrow, urinary bladder, and bowel. Occasionally, significant bowel activity can cause interference with image interpretation, and a laxative 24 hours before imaging is routinely used. Sometimes, additional delayed imaging at 96 to 120 hours is necessary. Planar imaging is followed by SPECT imaging of the pelvis and abdomen (Fig 3G.29). We recommend simultaneous blood pool imaging with ^{99m}Tc-labeled RBCs at 72 to 96 hours to provide an outline of the blood vessels and improve the specificity (29). Image coregistration with pelvic CT using blood vessels as anatomic landmarks is technically feasible and improves specificity (20). Some authors use a subtraction analysis software that subtracts the ^{99m}Tc-RBC data set from the In-111 data set to allow easier identification of the metastatic sites (39).

Altered biodistribution manifested by intense liver, bone marrow, and urinary bladder uptake is sometimes seen. The etiology for this phenomenon is unknown, but it decreases the sensitivity of the test. Accumulation of the antibody is seen in areas of inflammation such as arthritis, fractures, surgical incision sites, and reactive lymph nodes. Accumulation in Paget's disease of the bone and necrotic tumors has also been reported (21).

Since the availability of this antibody, many clinical studies have been performed. It is useful in patients with new diagnosis of prostate carcinoma who are at high risk for metastatic disease and in patients with elevated PSA after radical prostatectomy.

Hinkle and colleagues (24), in a multicenter trial, studied 51 patients with prostate carcinoma at high risk for metastases with the antibody scan. All of the patients underwent prostatectomy and open pelvic lymphadenectomy. They reported the sensitivity and specificity for detecting extraprostatic disease as 75% and 86%, respectively. The accuracy and positive predictive value was 81% and 79%, respectively. A study by Burgers and co-workers (6) also compared the imaging findings on the antibody scan with CT or MRI and surgery. They reported an accuracy of 92% for detecting prostate cancer and 81% for extraprostatic lesions with the antibody imaging compared with an accuracy of 53% and 48% with other imaging modalities such as CT or MRI. They also reported "skip metastases" in two patients at the level of aortic bifurcation. These patients had negative pelvic lymph nodes at surgery (6). Although these statistics are better than CT or MRI, the results vary considerably. Babaian and colleagues (2) reported a sensitivity and specificity of 44% and 86%, respectively, in a study of 19 patients undergoing pelvic lymph node dissection. However, all of these studies were reported before the use of ^{99m}Tc-RBC blood pool imaging.

In 181 patients with recurrent prostate cancer after radical prostatectomy and rising PSA, antibody imaging was performed to evaluate local recurrence and distant metastases (27). All patients had prostatic fossa biopsied. Immunoscintigraphy showed disease in 60% of patients, with localization more frequently to the prostatic fossa (34%). Extraprostatic localization was seen in 42%. Abdominal lymph nodes showed localization in 23% and pelvic lymph nodes in 22% of the patients. Only 50% of the patients with positive scans in the prostatic fossa had the finding confirmed by biopsy. The overall sensitivity was 49%, specificity 71%, positive predictive value 50%, and negative predictive value 70%. The investigators concluded that single biopsy of the prostatic fossa is insensitive because of the sampling error involved. The accuracy for detecting distant metastases was not evaluated by this study because the extraprostatic sites of antibody localization were not confirmed by other conventional imaging modalities or biopsies in this study (27).

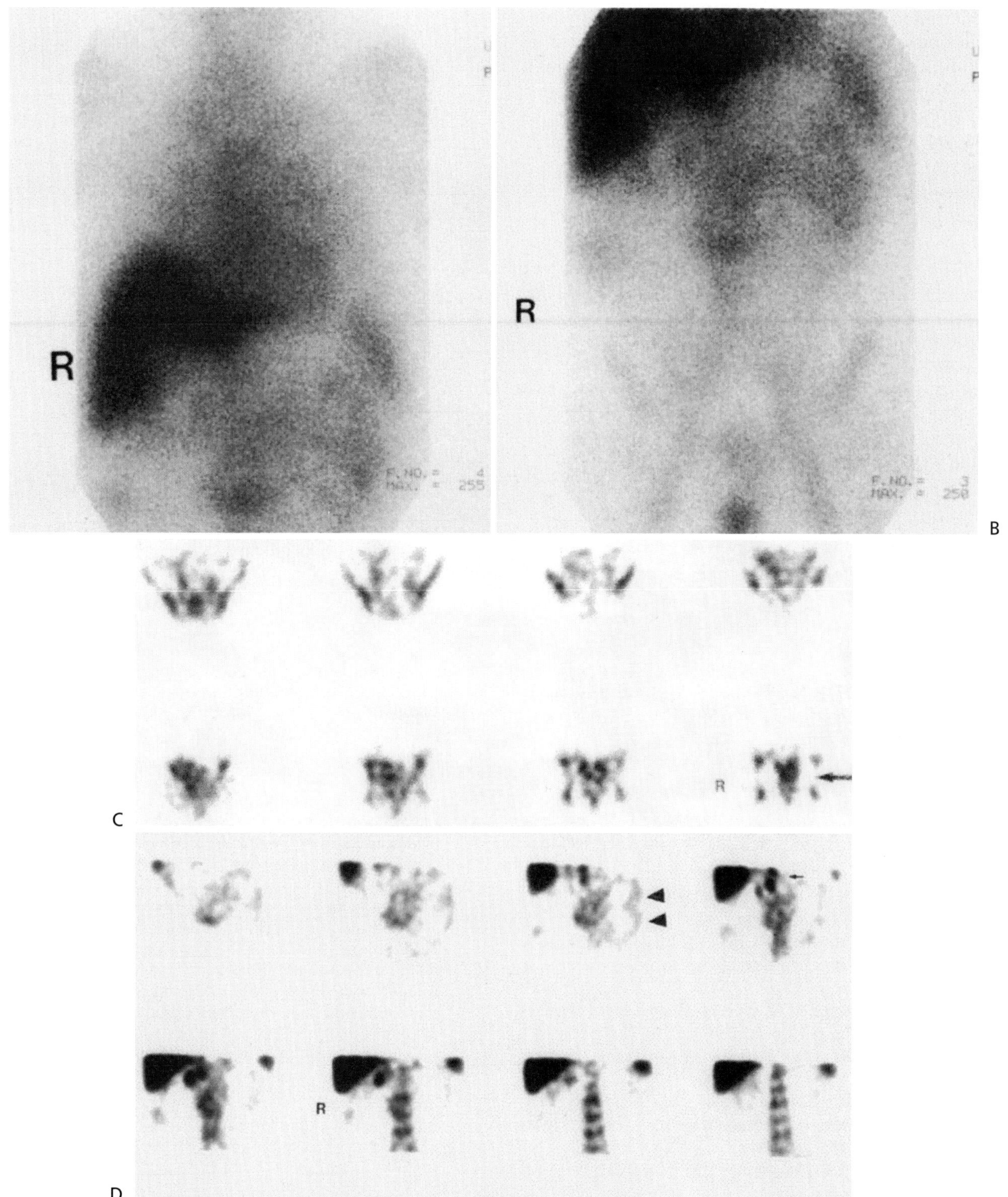

FIGURE 3G.29. Man, 65 years old, with newly diagnosed prostate cancer. **A:** Anterior planar image of the chest and abdomen was obtained 96 hours after the injection of In-111 Capromab pendetide. Uptake is seen in the blood pool of the heart, liver, and bowel. **B:** Anterior planar image of the abdomen and pelvis shows uptake in the iliac vessels, bowel, and bone marrow. **C:** Transverse SPECT images of the pelvis show uptake in the prostate *(arrow),* consistent with carcinoma. **D:** Coronal SPECT images of the abdomen (day 5) show uptake in the bowel *(arrowheads),* as well as focal uptake in the midline suggestive of periaortic lymph nodes.

Thirty-two patients with failed radical prostatectomy were evaluated with the antibody scan (28). After pelvic radiotherapy, these patients were followed for 13 months. Seventy percent of patients with antibody localization only to the prostate bed had a durable complete response; 22% had a positive extraprostatic and extrapelvic localization (28).

Haseman and colleagues (22) imaged 14 patients with elevated PSA with Capromab pendetide imaging and F-18 fluorodeoxyglucose (FDG) positron emission tomography (PET) imaging. All patients had biopsies of the prostatic fossa. In the limited number of patients studied, antibody scan was superior to PET imaging in the detection of both local recurrence and lymph node metastases (22). However, more studies are needed to confirm this finding.

Antibody imaging with Capromab pendetide is used for patients with a new diagnosis of prostate cancer and high risk of metastatic disease and in patients with failed radical prostatectomy. Capromab pendetide imaging is challenging, and experience, along with dual isotope imaging with ^{99m}Tc-RBC labeling, is of great help.

REFERENCES

1. Arnold RW, Subramanian G, McAfee JG, et al. Comparison of Tc-99m complexes for renal imaging. *J Nucl Med* 1975;16:357.
2. Babaian RJ, Sayer J, Podoloff DA, et al. Radioimmunoscintigraphy of pelvic lymph nodes with In-111 labeled monoclonal antibody CYT356. *J Urol* 1994;152:1952.
3. Bell EG, McAfee JG, Makhuli ZN. Medical imaging of renal diseases: suggested indications for different modalities. *Semin Nucl Med* 1981;11:105.
4. Boyd RE, Robson J, Hunt FC, et al. Tc-99m gluconate complexes for renal scintigraphy. *Br J Radiol* 1973;46:604.
5. Brien TG, O'Hagan R, Muldowney FP. Chromium-51-EDTA in the determination of glomerular filtration rate. *Acta Radiol Ther Phys Biol* 1969;6:523.
6. Burgers JK, Hinkle GH, Haseman M. Monoclonal antibody imaging of recurrent and metastatic prostate cancer. *Semin Urol* 1995;13:103.
7. Constable AR, Hussein MM, Albrecht MP, et al. Renal clearance determination from single plasma samples. In: Hollenberg NK, Lange S, eds. *Radionuclides in Nephrology.* New York: Thieme-Stratton, 1980.
8. Conway JJ, Lowell RK, Belman AB, et al. Detection of vesicoureteral reflux with radionuclide cystography. *AJR Am J Roentgenol* 1972;115:720.
9. Conway JJ, Maizels M. The "well tempered" diuretic renograms. *J Nucl Med* 1992;33:2047.
10. Prostascint Capromab Pendetide package insert. Cytogen Corporation, Princeton, NJ.
11. Dimitriou P, Fretzayas A, Nicolaidou P, et al. Estimates of dose to the bladder during direct radionuclide cystography: concise communication. *J Nucl Med* 1984;25:792.
12. Dondi M, Fanti S, DeFabritiis A, et al. Prognostic value of captopril renal scintigraphy in renovascular hypertension. *J Nucl Med* 1992;33:2040.
13. Elison BS, Taylor D, Vanderwall H, et al. Comparison of DMSA scintigraphy with intravenous urography for the detection of renal scarring and its correlation with vesicoureteric reflux. *Br J Urol* 1992;69:294.
14. Esser PJ, McAfee JG, Subramanian G. Appendix: radioactive tracers. In: Freeman LM, ed. *Freeman and Johnson's clinical radionuclide imaging,* ed 3. Orlando: Grune & Stratton, 1984.
15. Fommei E, Ghione S, Palla L, et al. Renal scintigraphic captopril test in the diagnosis of renovascular hypertension. *Hypertension* 1987;10:212.
16. Freeman LM. The kidneys. In: Freeman LM, ed. *Freeman and Johnson's clinical radionuclide imaging,* ed 3. Orlando: Grune & Stratton, 1984.
17. Fumio G, Jackson EK, Branch RA, et al. The effects of renal perfusion pressure on angiotensin II–induced changes in glomerular filtration rate. *Pharmacologist* 1983;25:344.
18. Gates GF. Split renal function testing using ^{99m}Tc DTPA. *Clin Nucl Med* 1983;8:400.
19. Ginjaume M, Casey M, Barker M, et al. A comparison between four simple methods for measuring glomerular filtration rate using technetium-99m DTPA. *Clin Nucl Med* 1986;11:647.
20. Hamilton RJ, Blend MJ, Pelizzari CA, et al. Using vascular structure for CT-SPECT registration in the pelvis. *J Nucl Med* 1999;40:347.
21. Haseman MK, Reed NL. Capromab pendetide imaging of prostate cancer. *Nucl Med Annual.* Lippincott-Raven, 1998:51–82.
22. Haseman HK, Reed NL, Rosenthal SA. Monoclonal antibody imaging of occult prostate cancer in patients with elevated prostate-specific antigen positron emission tomography and biopsy correlation. *Clin Nucl Med* 1996;21:704.
23. Hayes M, Moore TC, Taplin GV. Radionuclide procedures in predicting early renal transplant rejection. *Radiology* 1972; 103:627.
24. Hinkle GH, Burgers JK, Neal CE, et al. Multicenter radioimmunoscintigraphic evaluation of patients with prostate carcinoma using indium-11 Capromab pendetide. *Cancer* 1998;83:739.
25. Holder LE, Melloul M, Chen D. Current status of radionuclide scrotal imaging. *Semin Nucl Med* 1981;11:232.
26. International Reflux Study Committee. Medical versus surgical treatment of primary vesicoureteral reflux: a prospective international reflux study in children. *J Urol* 1981;125:277.
27. Kahn D, Williams RD, Manyak MJ, et al. In-111 Capromab pendetide in the evaluation of patients with residual or recurrent prostate cancer after radical prostatectomy. *J Urol* 1998;159: 2041.
28. Kahn D, Williams RD, Haseman HK, et al. Radioimmunoscintigraphy with In-111–labeled Capromab pendetide predicts prostate cancer response to salvage radiotherapy after failed radical prostatectomy. *J Clin Oncol* 1998;16:284.
29. Kelty NL, Holder LE, Khan SH. Dual-isotope protocol for indium-111 Capromab pendetide monoclonal antibody imaging. *J Nucl Med Technol* 1998;26:174.
30. Koenigsberg M, Freeman LM, Blaufox MD. Radionuclide and ultrasound evaluation of renal morphology and function. In: Edelman CM Jr, ed. *Pediatric kidney disease.* Boston: Little, Brown, 1978.
31. Lamb HM, Faulds D. Capromab pendetide: a review of its use as an imaging agent in prostate cancer. *Drugs Aging* 1998;12:293.
32. Majd M, Belman AB. Nuclear cystography in infants and children. *Urol Clin North Am* 1979;6:395.
33. Matthews CME. The theory of tracer experiments with ^{131}I-tagged sodium *o*-iodohippurate. *Phys Med Biol* 1957;2:36.
34. McAfee JG, Reba RC, Chodos RB. Radioisotopic methods in the diagnosis of renal vascular disease: a critical review. *Semin Roentgenol* 1967;2:198.

35. Müller-Suur R, Müller-Suur C. Glomerular filtration and tubular secretion of MAG_3 in the rat kidney. *J Nucl Med* 1989;30: 1986.
36. Nally JV Jr, Gupta BK, Clarke HS Jr, et al. Captopril renography for the detection of renovascular hypertension: a preliminary report. *Cleve Clin J Med* 1988;55:311.
37. Older RA, Korobkin M, Workman J, et al. Accuracy of radionuclide imaging in distinguishing renal masses from normal variants. *Radiology* 1980;136:443.
38. O'Reilly PH, Shields RA, Testa HJ. Renovascular hypertension and renal failure. In: O'Reilly PH, Shields RA, Testa HJ, eds. *Nuclear medicine in urology and nephrology.* London: Butterworths, 1979.
39. Quintana JC, Blend MJ. The dual isotope ProstaScint imaging procedure: clinical experience and staging in 145 patients. *Clin Nucl Med* 2000;25:33.
40. Russell CD, Thorstad B, Yester MV, et al. Comparison of technetium-99m MAG_3 with iodine-131 Hippuran by a simultaneous dual channel technique. *J Nucl Med* 1988;29:1189.
41. Russell CD, Thorstad BL, Yester MV, et al. Quantitation of renal function with technetium-99m MAG_3. *J Nucl Med* 1988; 29:1931.
42. Sapirstein LA, Vidt DG, Mandel MJ, et al. Volumes of distribution and clearance of intravenously injected creatinine in the dog. *Am J Physiol* 1955;181:330.
43. Shanon A, Feldman W, McDonald P, et al. Evaluation of renal scars by technetium labeled dimercaptosuccinic acid scan, intravenous urography and ultrasonography: a comparative study. *J Pediatr* 1992;120:399.
44. Sherman RA, Byan KJ. Nuclear medicine in acute and chronic renal failure. *Semin Nucl Med* 1982;12:265.
45. Smith HW. *The kidney: structure and function in health and disease.* New York: Oxford University Press, 1951:47.
46. Staab EV, Hopkins J, Patton DD, et al. The use of radionuclide studies in the prediction of function in renal failure. *Radiology* 1973;106:141.
47. Stabin M. Personal communication, 1990.
48. Tauxe WN. Prediction of residual renal function after unilateral nephrectomy. In: Tauxe WN, Dubovsky EV, eds. *Nuclear medicine in clinical urology and nephrology.* Norwalk, Conn: Appleton-Century-Crofts, 1985.
49. Tauxe WN, Maher FT, Taylor WF. Effective renal plasma flow: estimation from theoretical volumes of distribution of intravenously injected ^{131}I orthoiodohippurate. *Mayo Clin Proc* 1971; 46:524.
50. Taylor A Jr, Eshima D, Christian PE, et al. Evaluation of ^{99m}Tc mercaptoacetyltriglycine in patients with impaired renal function. *Radiology* 1987;162:365.
51. Taylor AT Jr, Eshima D, Christian PE, et al. Technetium-99m MAG_3 kit formulation: preliminary results in normal volunteers and patients with renal failure. *J Nucl Med* 1988;29:616.
52. Tempany CM, Zhou X, Zerhouni EA, et al. Staging of prostate cancer: results of Radiology Diagnostic Oncology Group project comparison of three MR imaging techniques. *Radiology* 1994; 193:47.
53. Thrall JH, Koff SA, Keyes JW Jr. Diuretic radionuclide renography and scintigraphy in the differential diagnosis of hydroureteronephrosis. *Semin Nucl Med* 1981;11:89.
54. Whitaker RH. Methods of assessing obstruction in dilated ureters. *Br J Urol* 1973;45:15.
55. Wooten WW, Eshima D, Taylor A Jr. Radiation exposure by technetium-99m MAG_3 [Letter]. *J Nucl Med* 1989;30:720.
56. Zhang G, Day DL, Loken M, et al. Grading of reflux by radionuclide cystography. *Clin Nucl Med* 1987;12:106.

Adult and Pediatric Urology, 4/e, edited by Jay Y. Gillenwater, John T. Grayhack, Stuart S. Howards, and Michael E. Mitchell.
Lippincott Williams & Wilkins, Philadelphia © 2002

4

URINARY TRACT INFECTIONS

ANTHONY J. SCHAEFFER

Urinary tract infections are common, affect men and women of all ages, and vary dramatically in their presentation and sequelae. Although the urinary tract is normally free of bacterial growth, bacteria that generally ascend from the rectal reservoir may cause urinary tract infections. When bacterial virulence increases or host defense mechanisms decrease, bacterial inoculation, colonization, and infection of the urinary tract occur. Clinical manifestations can vary from asymptomatic bacterial colonization of the bladder to irritative voiding symptoms associated with bacterial infection, upper tract infections associated with fever and chills, and bacteremia associated with severe morbidity, including

A.J. Schaeffer: Department of Urology, Northwestern University Medical School, Chicago, IL 60611.

sepsis and death. The clinical challenges are (a) to identify patients at risk; (b) to prevent or minimize infections by reducing factors that increase the risk of infection; (c) to accurately and efficiently diagnose infections; and (d) to provide prompt, effective, and safe therapy in a cost-effective manner. This chapter defines various types of infection and reviews the epidemiology and bacterial and host factors instrumental in urinary tract infections. The clinical manifestations and diagnostic techniques used to identify the site and severity of infection are then discussed. Pertinent antimicrobial agents and their use are reviewed. Common clinical scenarios are discussed, beginning with the clinical and laboratory findings, the differential diagnoses, and sequential management steps necessary to achieve satisfactory results.

DEFINITIONS

Urinary tract infection is an inflammatory response of the urothelium to bacterial invasion. *Bacteriuria* is a commonly used term that means bacteria in the urine. It has been assumed to be a valid indicator of either bacterial colonization or bacterial infection of the urinary tract. Although this is usually true, studies in animals (153,232) and humans (75) have indicated that bacteria may colonize the urothelium without causing bacteriuria. *Pyuria,* the presence of white blood cells (WBCs) in the urine, is generally indicative of infection and a significant inflammatory response of the urothelium to the bacterium. Bacteriuria in the absence of pyuria is generally indicative of bacterial colonization without infection of the urinary tract. Alternatively, bacteriuria may represent bacterial contamination of an abacteriuric specimen during collection. The possibility of contamination increases as the reliability of the collection technique decreases from suprapubic aspiration, to catheterization, to voided specimens. The term *significant bacteriuria* has a clinical connotation and is used to describe the number of bacteria in a suprapubically aspirated, catheterized, or voided specimen that exceeds the number usually caused by bacterial contamination from the skin, the urethra, or the prepuce or introitus, respectively. Hence, it represents a urinary tract infection.

Infections are often defined by their presumed site of origin. *Cystitis* describes a clinical syndrome associated with dysuria, frequency, urgency, and occasionally suprapubic pain. These symptoms, although generally indicative of cystitis, may also be associated with infection of the urethra or vagina or noninfectious conditions such as interstitial cystitis, bladder carcinoma, or calculi. Conversely, patients may be asymptomatic and have infection of the bladder and possibly the upper urinary tract.

The term *bacterial nephritis* should be reserved for interstitial renal inflammation primarily caused by the immediate or late effects of bacterial infection in the renal parenchyma. *Pyelonephritis* refers to bacterial nephritis involving the renal parenchyma and collecting system. *Acute pyelonephritis* refers to a clinical symptom complex or pathologic lesion characterized by fever, chills, and flank pain, or tenderness that is always associated with urinary tract infection. It may, however, have no morphologic or functional components detectable by routine clinical modalities. *Chronic pyelonephritis* describes a shrunken, scarred kidney that can only be diagnosed when there is postinfectious morphologic, radiologic, or functional evidence of renal disease. However, it need not be associated with urinary tract infection at the time of study.

Acute prostatitis is a febrile urinary tract infection associated with prostate tenderness and swelling and irritative voiding symptoms. *Chronic bacterial prostatitis* is a subtle condition characterized by recurrent relapsing urinary tract infections caused by persistence of the pathogen in the prostatic secretory system between courses of antimicrobial therapy. *Nonbacterial prostatitis* refers to an inflamed prostate without bacterial infection.

Urinary tract infections may also be described in terms of the anatomic or functional status of the urinary tract and the health of the host. Infections occurring in a functionally and anatomically normal urinary tract and a healthy host are considered *uncomplicated* infections. A *complicated* infection is associated with factors that increase the chance for acquiring bacteria and decrease the efficacy of therapy (Table 4.1). The urinary tract is functionally or anatomically abnormal, the host is compromised, or the bacteria have increased virulence. Renal diseases that reduce the concentrating ability of the kidney or neurologic conditions that alter bladder-emptying capabilities are commonly encountered functional abnormalities. Examples of common anatomic abnormalities include obstruction associated with calculi or enlargement of the prostate or congenital or acquired sites of residual urine, such as calyceal or bladder diverticula.

Infections may be defined by their relationship to other urinary tract infections. A *first* or *isolated infection* is one that occurs in an individual who has never had a urinary tract infection or has one remote from a previous urinary tract

TABLE 4.1. FACTORS THAT SUGGEST COMPLICATED URINARY TRACT INFECTION

- Functional or anatomic abnormality of urinary tract
- Male gender
- Pregnancy
- Elderly
- Diabetes
- Immunosuppression
- Childhood urinary tract infection
- Recent antimicrobial use
- Indwelling urinary catheter
- Urinary tract instrumentation
- Hospital-acquired infection
- Symptoms for greater than 7 days at presentation

infection. An *unresolved infection* is one that has not responded to antimicrobial therapy. A *recurrent infection* is one that occurs after documented, successful resolution of an antecedent infection. If the infection is a new event associated with reintroduction of bacteria into the urinary tract from outside, the term *reinfection* is appropriate. If the recurrent infection is due to bacteria reemerging from a focus within the urinary tract, the term *bacterial persistence* or *bacterial relapse* is used. These definitions require careful clinical and bacteriologic assessment and are important because they influence the type and extent of the patient's evaluation and therapy.

The presumed source of bacteria that causes the infection can be used to further define infections. *Domiciliary infections,* or *outpatient-acquired infections,* occur in individuals who are not institutionalized at the time they incur the infection. *Nosocomial infections,* or *health care–associated infections,* occur in individuals who are hospitalized or institutionalized and, often, in those who are catheterized (i.e., catheter-associated nosocomial urinary tract infections). Domiciliary infections are usually caused by common fecal bacteria (i.e., Enterobacteriaceae) and are generally susceptible to most antimicrobial therapy, whereas nosocomial infections are frequently caused by *Pseudomonas* and other more antimicrobial-resistant strains.

EPIDEMIOLOGY

Urinary tract infections are among the most common infectious diseases acquired by humans, affecting more than 7 million people annually in the United States and accounting for substantial morbidity (140). Urinary tract infections affect approximately 30% of women between the ages of 20 and 40, a prevalence 30 times more than in men, and at least half of all women will experience one or more infections during their lifetime (140,190). However, with increasing age, the ratio of women to men with bacteriuria progressively decreases. At least 20% of women and 10% of men older than 65 years of age have bacteriuria (23). Many adults previously had urinary tract infections as children (104). Once a patient has an infection, he or she is likely to develop subsequent infections. Longitudinal studies in young women with symptomatic recurrent infections have shown an overall attack rate of 0.2 infections per month (182). Infections tended to occur in clusters that were followed by remission-free intervals that averaged approximately 1 year. However, most remissions were followed by recurrent urinary tract infection, thus underscoring the importance of genetic factors in the pathogenesis of recurrent urinary tract infections in women.

Risk factors can be compounded. The prevalence of bacteriuria increases with institutionalization or hospitalization and concurrent disease. In a study of women and men older than 68 years of age, Boscia and Kaye (23) found that 24% of functionally impaired nursing home residents had bacteriuria compared with 12% of healthy domiciliary subjects (24). It is well established that in the presence of obstruction, infection stones, or diabetes mellitus, urinary tract infections in adults can lead to progressive renal damage (96). In the absence of these complicating factors, it is difficult to implicate infection in the pathogenesis of severe renal disease in adults.

PATHOGENESIS

Successful invasion of the urinary tract is determined in part by the virulence characteristics of the bacteria, the inoculum size, and the inadequacy of host defense mechanisms. These factors also play a role in determining the ultimate level of colonization and damage to the urinary tract.

Routes of Infection

Ascending Route

Most bacteria enter the urinary tract from the fecal reservoir via ascent through the urethra into the bladder. This route is enhanced in individuals with significant soilage of the perineum with feces, women using spermicidal agents (142), and patients with intermittent or indwelling catheters.

The weight of clinical and experimental evidence strongly suggests that most episodes of pyelonephritis are caused by retrograde ascent of bacteria from the bladder through the ureter to the renal pelvis and parenchyma. Although cystitis is often restricted to the bladder, in approximately 50% of instances, there is further extension of the infection into the upper urinary tract (32). Although reflux of urine is probably not required for ascending infections, edema associated with cystitis may cause sufficient changes in the ureterovesical junction to permit reflux. Once the bacteria are introduced into the ureter, they may ascend to the kidney unaided. However, this ascent would be greatly increased by any process that interferes with the normal ureteral peristaltic function. Gram-negative bacteria and their endotoxins, as well as pregnancy and ureteral obstruction, have a significant antiperistaltic effect.

Bacteria that reach the renal pelvis can enter the renal parenchyma by means of the collecting ducts at the papillary tips and then ascend upward within the collecting tubules. This process is hastened and exacerbated by increased intrapelvic pressure from ureteral obstruction or vesicoureteral reflux, particularly when it is associated with intrarenal reflux.

Hematogenous Route

Infection of the kidney by the hematogenous route is uncommon in normal individuals. However, the kidney is occasionally secondarily infected in patients with *Staphylococcus aureus* bacteremia from oral sites or with *Candida fungemia.* Experimental data indicate that infection is enhanced when the kidney is obstructed (322).

Lymphatic Route

Direct extension of bacteria from the adjacent organs via lymphatics may occur in unusual circumstances, such as a severe bowel infection or retroperitoneal abscesses. There is little evidence that lymphatic routes play a significant role in the vast majority of urinary tract infections.

Urinary Pathogens

Most urinary tract infections are caused by facultative anaerobes usually originating in the bowel flora. Uropathogens such as *Staphylococcus epidermidis* and *Candida albicans* originate in the flora of the vagina or perineal skin.

Escherichia coli is by far the most common cause of urinary tract infections, accounting for 85% of community-acquired and 50% of hospital-acquired infections. Other Gram-negative Enterobacteriaceae, including *Proteus* and *Klebsiella,* and Gram-positive *Enterococcus faecalis* and *Staphylococcus saprophyticus* are responsible for the remainder of most community-acquired infections. Nosocomial infections are caused by *E. coli, Klebsiella, Enterobacter, Citrobacter, Serratia, Pseudomonas aeruginosa, Providencia, Enterococcus faecalis,* and *S. epidermidis* (175). Less common organisms such as *Gardnerella vaginalis, Mycoplasma* species, and *Ureaplasma urealyticum* may infect patients with intermittent or indwelling catheters (81,167).

The prevalence of infecting organisms is influenced by the patient's age. For example, *S. saprophyticus* is now recognized as causing approximately 10% of symptomatic lower urinary tract infections in young, sexually active females (192), whereas it rarely causes infection in males and elderly individuals. A seasonal variation with a late summer to fall peak has been reported (148).

Virulence characteristics play a role in both selecting the organism that will invade the urinary tract and determining its level of infection within the urinary tract. It is generally believed that uropathogenic strains, such as *E. coli,* are selected from fecal flora not by chance but rather by the presence of virulence factors that enable them to adhere to and colonize the perineum and urethra and migrate to the urinary tract where they establish an inflammatory response in the urothelium (298,399). Subsequently, other virulence factors that play a role in the persistence and expansion of infection include resistance to serum bactericidal activity (21), hemolysin (150), and aerobactin (164). Half of all second urinary tract infections are caused by the same strain that causes the first and has identical virulence factors (94).

Bacterial Adherence in the Pathogenesis of Urinary Tract Infections

It is well established that bacterial adherence to epithelial cells is an essential early step in the initiation of urinary tract infections. This interaction is influenced by the adhesive characteristics of the bacteria, the receptive characteristics of the epithelial surface, and the fluid bathing both surfaces. Bacterial adherence is a specific interaction that plays a role in selecting the organism, the host, and the site of infection. Portions of this section on bacterial adherence have been published (298).

Bacterial Adhesins

The bacterial cell structures that seem to be most important in binding the bacteria to epithelial cells are long filamentous protein appendages called pili, or fimbriae (Fig. 4.1). Bacteria may produce a number of antigenically and functionally different pili on the same cell; others produce a single type; and in some, no pili are seen (179). A typical piliated cell may contain 100 to 400 pili. These supramolecular structures are usually 5 to 10 nm in diameter, up to 2 μm long, and appear to be composed primarily of subunits known as pilin, which have molecular weights of 17 to 27 kDa, depending on the type of pili (179). *Pili* are defined functionally by their ability to mediate hemagglutination (HA) of specific types of erythrocytes. The most well-described pili are type 1 and P pili. Type 1 pili are commonly expressed on both nonpathogenic and pathogenic *E. coli* and appear to facilitate bacterial colonization of the vaginal mucosa and bladder. These pili mediate HA of guinea pig erythrocytes (67). The reaction is inhibited by the addition of mannose; thus type 1 pili are termed *mannose-sensitive HA* (MSHA) (275,357). P pili have receptors that adhere to α-D-Galp-(1-4)β-D-Galp belonging to the globoseries of glycolipids (168,196), which are found on P blood group antigens and in uroepithelium (356). Adher-

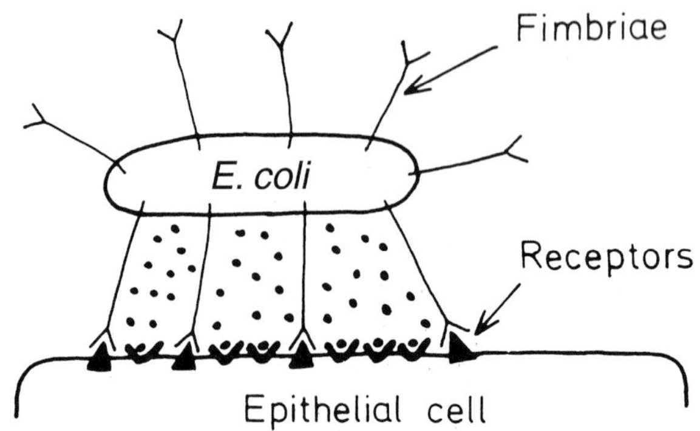

FIGURE 4.1. Bacterial adherence. Adhesins on pili mediate attachment to specific epithelial cell receptors. (Reprinted with permission from Schaeffer AJ. The role of bacterial adherence in urinary tract infection. *AUA Update Series* 1989;8:18.)

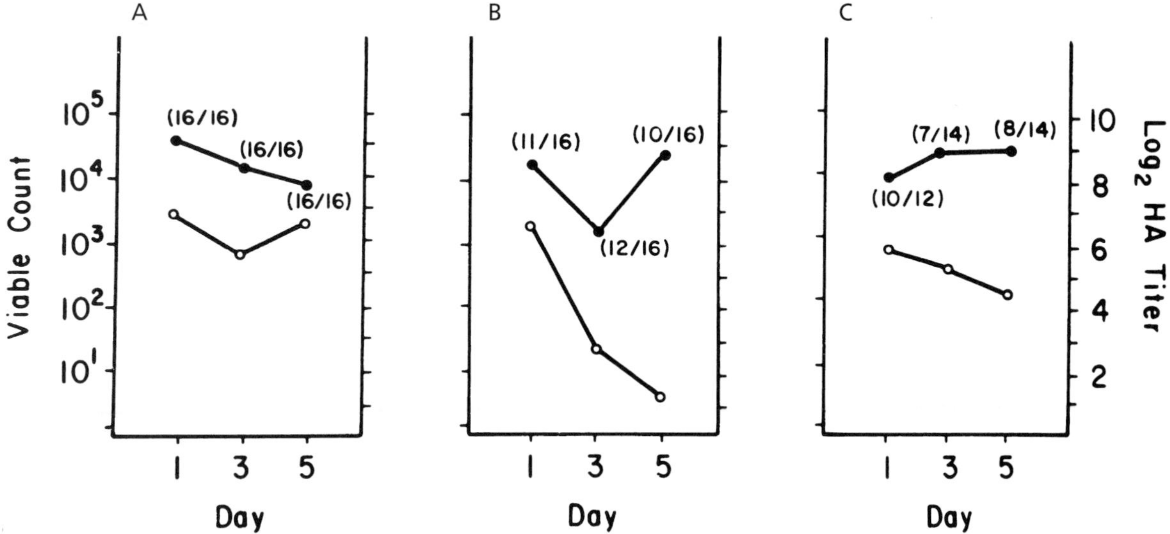

FIGURE 4.2. Time study after intravesical inoculation with strain I-149 that compared the mean viable-bacteria count *(open circle)* and HA titer *(closed circle)* for bladders **(A)**, kidneys **(B)**, and urine specimens **(C)** from the same animals. Each point is the mean of all the animals tested. The numbers in parentheses show the proportion of animals inoculated that gave positive cultures. The HA titers were tested after 18 hours of growth on agar. The HA titer of bacteria recovered from the kidney decreased significantly by day 5 (P <.001). (Reprinted with permission from Schaeffer AJ, Amundsen SK, Schmidt LN. Adherence of *E. coli* to human urinary tract epithelial cells. *Infect Immun* 1979;24:753.)

ence of P-piliated strains to human red blood cells is not inhibited by mannose; hence, P pili are termed *mannose-resistant HA* (MRHA) (169,275,357).

Bacterial pili are subject to rapid phase variation *in vitro* and *in vivo* wherein bacteria revert between states of expression and nonexpression of pili. For example, some bacteria grown in a broth medium express pili, whereas the same strain grown on the same medium in a solid state will cease production of pili. Occurrence of phase variation may contribute to the pathogenesis of infections (72,154).

Evidence for the role of type 1 and P pili in urinary tract infection has been established by *in vitro* and *in vivo* studies. Svanborg Eden and associates (355) were the first to report a correlation between bacterial adherence *in vitro* and severity of urinary tract infections. They showed that *E. coli* strains from girls with acute pyelonephritis had high adhesive ability, whereas strains from girls with asymptomatic bacteriuria or normal feces had low bacterial adherence. Between 70% and 80% of the pyelonephrogenic strains had adhesive capacity, but only 10% of the fecal isolates adhered. This association is not observed in individuals with abnormal urinary tracts. Lomberg and colleagues (200), for example, showed that in girls, recurrent pyelonephritis with gross reflux (in which most of the scarring historically occurs) was minimally associated with P-piliated *E. coli* strains.

Type 1 pili consist of a helical rod composed of repeating Fim A subunits joined to a 3-nm wide distal tip structure containing the adhesin Fim H (165). Binding of the Fim H adhesin to mannosylated host receptors present on the urothelium is critical to the ability of *E. coli* to colonize the bladder and cause cystitis (52,190,360). Animal studies showed that *E. coli* expressing type 1 pili, but not those not expressing pili, can cause urinary tract infections (159). Furthermore, anti–type 1 pili antibodies and competitive inhibitors protected animals from experimental urinary tract infections (7,153).

An animal model of ascending urinary tract infections and studies of isolates from different sites in patients with urinary tract infection provide evidence that phase variation can occur during *E. coli* urinary tract infection *in vivo.* Type 1 piliated *E. coli* that were capable of phase variation were introduced into the mouse bladder in the piliated phase, and the bacteria recovered from the bladder and urine 24 or more hours after inoculation were tested for piliation. All of the animals had bladder colonization, and 78% of the bacteria recovered showed type 1 piliation. The bacteriologic state of the urine often differed from that of the bladder. The urine was sterile in 59% of the animals with bladder colonization, and the bacteria recovered from the urine were often nonpiliated. Phase variation also occurred over time. When bladder and kidney cultures were examined 1, 3, and 5 days after intravesical inoculation of piliated bacteria, organisms recovered from the bladder remained piliated, whereas organisms recovered from the kidney and urine showed significantly less piliation (297a) (Fig. 4.2).

Studies in humans using indirect immunofluorescence of fresh urine bacteria have confirmed *in vivo* expression and phase variation of pili. Kisielius and associates (178) analyzed the urine of adults with lower urinary tract infection and detected type 1 pili in 31 of 41 specimens and P pili in 6 of 18 specimens. The piliation status of the bacterial population in the urine was heterogeneous, varying from predominantly piliated to a mixture of piliated and nonpiliated cells (Fig. 4.3). Strains isolated from different sites in the urogenital tract showed variation in the state of piliation. These results demonstrate that *E. coli* type 1 and P pili are expressed and subject to phase variation *in vivo* during acute urinary tract infections.

This process of phase variation has obvious biologic and clinical implications. For example, the presence of type 1 pili may be advantageous to the bacteria for initially adhering to and colonizing the bladder mucosa. Subsequently, type 1 pili may be unnecessary for strains in suspension in urine, and in fact detrimental because they enhance apoptosis, phagocytosis, and killing by neutrophils (232,318). In the kidney, P pili may then take over as the primary mediator of bacterial attachment via their binding to the glycolipid receptors (348).

Epithelial Cell Receptivity

The significance of epithelial cell receptivity in the pathogenesis of ascending urinary tract infection has been studied initially by examining adherence of *E. coli* to vaginal epithelial cells and uroepithelial cells collected from voided urine specimens. Fowler and Stamey (92) established that certain indigenous microorganisms (e.g., lactobacilli, *S. epidermidis*) avidly attached themselves to washed epithelial cells in large numbers. When vaginal epithelial cells were collected from patients susceptible to reinfection and compared with such cells obtained from controls resistant to urinary tract infection, the *E. coli* strains that cause cystitis adhered much more avidly to the epithelial cells from the susceptible women. These studies established increased adherence of pathogenic bacteria to vaginal epithelial cells as the first demonstrable biologic difference that could be shown in women susceptible to urinary tract infection.

Subsequently, Schaeffer and colleagues (298) confirmed these vaginal differences in women, but in addition, they observed that the increased adherence was also characteristic of buccal epithelial cells. As can be seen in Fig. 4.4, there is a striking similarity in the ability of both cell types to bind the same *E. coli* strain. In addition, there was a significant relationship between vaginal cell and buccal cell receptivity. Seventy-seven different *E. coli* strains were tested for their ability to bind to vaginal and buccal epithelial cells. A direct nonlinear relationship between buccal and vaginal adherence in controls and patients was confirmed for urinary, vaginal, and anal isolates. Thus high vaginal cell receptivity was associated with high buccal cell receptivity.

These observations emphasize that the increase in receptor sites for *E. coli* on epithelial cells from women with recurrent urinary tract infections is not limited to the vagina and thus suggest that a genotypic trait for epithelial cell receptivity may be a major susceptibility factor in urinary tract infections. This concept was extended by examining the human leukocyte antigens (HLAs), which are the major histocompatibility complex in humans and have been associated statistically with many diseases (299). The A3 antigen was identified in 12 (34%) of the patients, a frequency significantly higher than the 8% frequency observed in healthy controls. Thus HLA-A3 may be associated with increased risk of recurrent urinary tract infections.

A 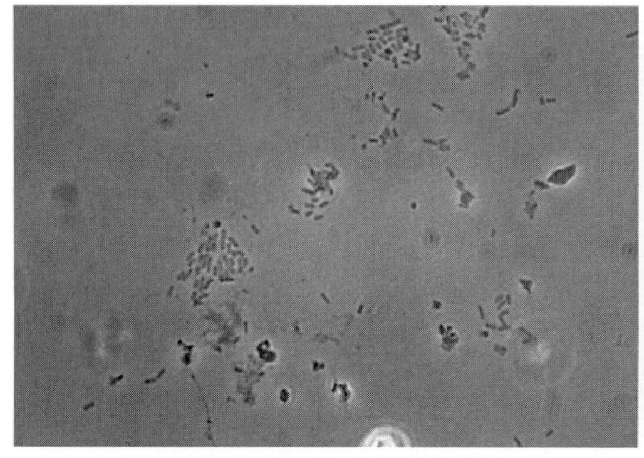

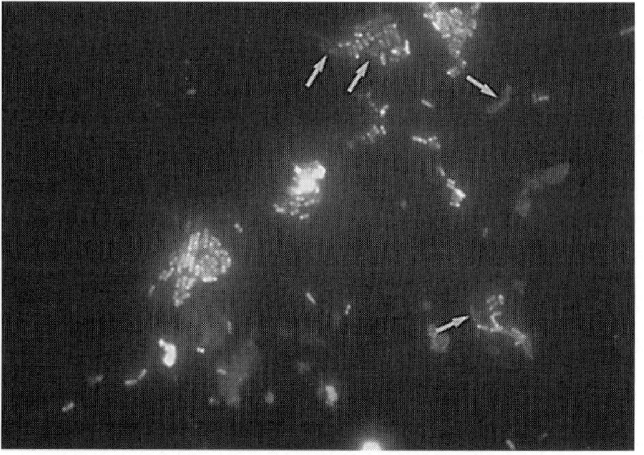 B

FIGURE 4.3. Phase-contrast micrograph **(A)** and immunofluorescence **(B)** stained with antiserum to type 1 pili of strain I-149 and with fluorescein-5-isothiocyanate (FITC)-conjugated second antibody of nonadherent *E. coli* in the urine of a patient with acute urinary tract infection showing a mixture of piliated and nonpiliated *(arrows)* cells. (Reprinted with permission from Kisielius PV, Schwan WR, Amundsen SK, et al. *In vivo* expression and phase variation of type-1 and P pili by *Escherichia coli* in the urine of adults with acute urinary tract infections. *Infect Immun* 1989;57:1656.)

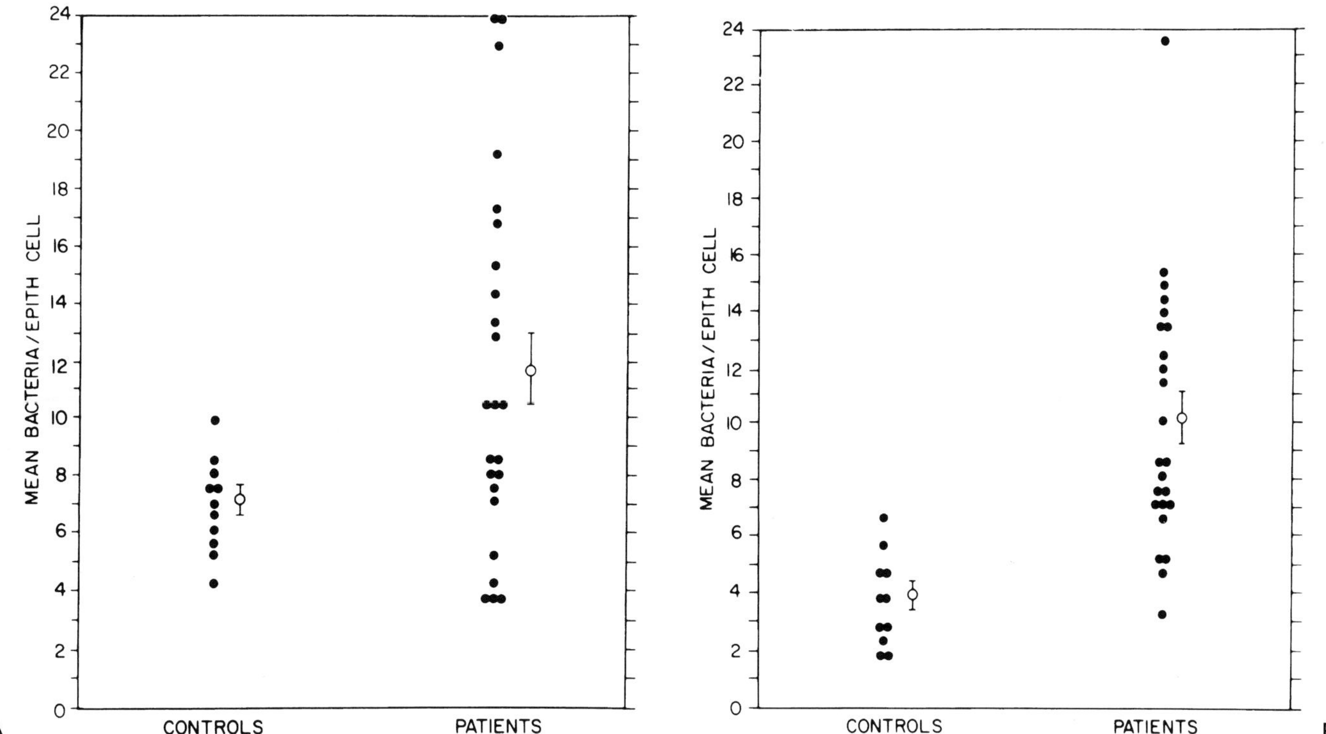

FIGURE 4.4. *In vitro* adherence of *E. coli* to vaginal **(A)** and buccal **(B)** cells from healthy controls and patients with recurrent urinary tract infections. Values represent an average of 14 **(A)** and 11 **(B)** determinations in each individual. The *open circles* and *bars* represent the means plus standard error. (Reprinted with permission from Schaeffer AJ et al. Association of *in vitro Escherichia coli* adherence to vaginal and buccal epithelial cells with susceptibility of women to recurrent urinary-tract infections. *N Engl J Med* 1981;304:1062.)

Bladder urothelial cells deposit on their apical surfaces a quasi-crystalline array of hexagonal complexes made up of four integral membrane glycoproteins known as *uroplakins* (132,353). *In vitro* binding assays have shown that two of the uroplakins, UPIa and UPIb, bind *E. coli* expressing type 1 pili (397). Blood group antigens, carbohydrate structures bound to membrane lipids or proteins, also constitute an important part of the uroepithelial cell membrane. The presence or absence of blood group determinants on the surface of uroepithelial cells may influence an individual's susceptibility to a urinary tract infection. Sheinfeld and associates (313) determined the blood group phenotypes in women with recurrent urinary tract infection and compared them to age-matched women controls. Women with Lewis Le(a-b-) and Le(a+b-) phenotypes had a significantly higher incidence of recurrent urinary tract infections than women with Le(a-b+) phenotypes. There was no significant difference in the distribution of ABO or P blood group phenotypes. The Lewis antigen controls fucosylation. The protective effect in women with the Le(a-b+) phenotype may be due to fucosylated structures at the vaginal cell surface or in the overlying mucus, which decreases availability of putative receptors for *E. coli* (238). In addition, Stapleton and co-workers (349) have shown that unique *E. coli*–binding glycerides are found in vaginal epithelial cells from nonsecretors but not from secretors. These studies individually and collectively support the concept that there is an increased epithelial receptivity for *E. coli* on the introital, urethral, and buccal mucosa that is characteristic of women susceptible to recurrent urinary tract infections and may be a genotypic trait.

Variation in Receptivity

A small variation in both vaginal cell and buccal cell receptivity may be observed from day to day in healthy controls. Adherence ranges from 1 to 17 bacteria per cell and appears to be both cyclic and repetitive. When adherence was correlated with the days of a woman's menstrual cycle, higher values were noted in the early phase, diminishing shortly after the time of expected ovulation (day 14) (Fig. 4.5). The number of bacteria per epithelial cell often correlated with the value obtained on the same day of the menstrual cycle 1 or 2 months previously. Premenopausal women are particularly susceptible to attachment of uropathogenic *E. coli* and nonpathogenic lactobacilli at certain times during the menstrual cycle and to *E. coli* during the early stages of pregnancy. The importance of such hormones

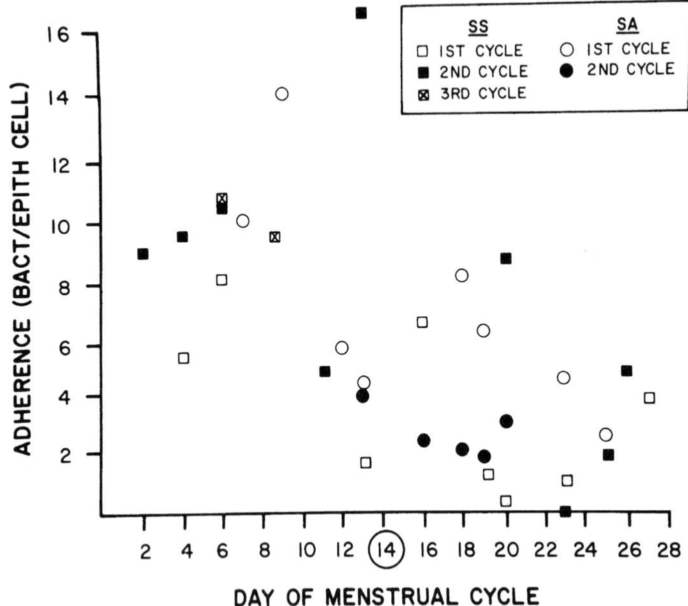

FIGURE 4.5. Relationship between the adherence of *E. coli* and the day of the menstrual cycle on which uroepithelial cells were obtained from two women with no history of urinary tract infections. Adherence was measured on the same day that the cells were collected. (Reprinted with permission from Schaeffer AJ, Amundsen SK, Schmidt LN. Adherence of *E. coli* to human urinary tract epithelial cells. *Infect Immun* 1979;24:753.)

as estrogens in the pathogenesis of urinary tract infection is therefore a matter of great interest, especially because the clinical urologist may see women who have recurrent cystitis at regular intervals, possibly in response to these hormonal changes.

Reid and Sobel (275) found that uropathogens attached in larger numbers to uroepithelial cells from women older than 65 years of age than to cells from premenopausal women 18 to 40 years of age. Raz and Stamm (274) noted that susceptibility to recurrent urinary tract infection was increased by the lowered estrogen levels found in the postmenopausal women and that estrogen replacement decreased uropathogenic bacterial colonization and the incidence of urinary tract infection.

The possibility that vaginal mucus might influence bacterial receptivity was investigated by Schaeffer and colleagues (302). Type 1 piliated *E. coli* bound to all of the vaginal fluid specimens (372). The binding capacity of vaginal fluid from women colonized with *E. coli in vivo* was greater than that from noncolonized women (293). The importance of vaginal fluid in bacteria–epithelial cell interactions was investigated in an *in vitro* model that measured the effect of vaginal fluid on the binding of bacteria to an epithelial cell line (100). Vaginal fluid from colonized women enhanced binding of bacteria to epithelial cells. Conversely, vaginal fluid from noncolonized women inhibited adherence. Thus the vaginal fluid appears to influence adherence to cells and presumably vaginal mucosal colonization. Subsequent studies demonstrated that secretory immunoglobulin A (IgA) is the primary glycoprotein responsible for vaginal fluid receptivity (272).

Natural Defenses of the Urinary Tract

Periurethral and Urethral Region

The normal flora of the vaginal introitus, the periurethral area, and the urethra usually contain microorganisms such as lactobacilli, coagulase-negative staphylococci, corynebacteria, and streptococci that form a barrier against uropathogenic colonization (79,211,263). Changes in the vaginal environment related to estrogen and pH may alter the ability of these bacteria to colonize. More commonly, however, acute changes in colonization have been associated with use of antimicrobial agents and spermicidal agents that alter the normal flora and increase the receptivity of the epithelium for uropathogens. The importance of vaginal colonization with uropathogens is supported by the classic longitudinal observations of Stamey and associates (337) on women who were prone to recurrent urinary tract infections. Episodes of bacteriuria were often preceded by uropathogenic colonization of the vaginal introitus and periurethral areas with bacteria from the fecal flora that subsequently infected the bladder. Between episodes of bacteriuria, women with recurrent urinary tract infections showed a higher prevalence and a greater density of perineal colonization with urinary pathogens than did healthy control subjects (300,330). Other studies have shown reduced titers of cervical IgA (339) and low vaginal pH (336) associated with increased susceptibility to urinary tract infections.

Little is known about the factors that predispose patients to urethral colonization with uropathogens. The proximity of the urethral meatus to the vulvar and perianal areas suggests that contamination occurs frequently. The nature of urethral defense mechanisms other than flow of urine is largely unknown. Bacterial multiplication in the normal urethra may be inhibited by the indigenous flora (42). Although colonization of the periurethral and urethral regions is prerequisite to most infections, the ability of the organisms to overcome the normal defense mechanisms of the urine and the bladder is clearly pivotal.

Urine

In general, fastidious organisms that normally colonize the urethra will not multiply in urine and rarely cause urinary tract infections (40). In contrast, urine will usually support the growth of nonfastidious bacteria (8). Urine from normal individuals may be inhibitory, especially when the inoculum is small (173). The most inhibitory factors are the osmolality, urea concentration, organic acid concentration, and pH. Bacterial growth is inhibited by either very dilute urine or a high osmolality when associated with a low pH. Much of the antibacterial activity of urine is related to a high urea and organic acid content (324). From a clinical perspective, however, these conditions do not appear to significantly distinguish between patients who are susceptible or resistant to infection.

The presence of glucose in the urine may increase infections. This is consistent with the increased frequency and severity of infection in diabetes (8). Urine obtained from pregnant women exhibits a more suitable pH for growth of *E. coli* in all stages of gestation (9). Uromodulin (Tamm-Horsfall protein), a kidney-derived mannosylated protein that is present in an extraordinarily high concentration in the urine (greater than 100 mg/mL), may play a defensive role by saturating all the mannose-binding sites of the type 1 pili, thus potentially blocking bacterial binding to the uroplakin receptors of the urothelium (68,188).

Bladder

Bacteria presumably make their way into the bladder fairly often. Whether small inocula of bacteria persist, multiply, and infect the host depends in part on the ability of the bladder to empty (58). Additional factors responsible for defense include antiadherence mechanisms and antibacterial properties of the bladder mucosa. Alterations in any or all of these defense mechanisms presumably enhance the ability of bacteria to colonize and infect. The mucopolysaccharides that coat the surface of the uroepithelial cells may modulate receptivity and prevent bacterial attachment. However, damage to the bladder mucus may allow bacteria to gain access to the urothelium.

One consequence of bacterial colonization of the bladder is the exfoliation and excretion of infected and damaged superficial cells. Mulvey and colleagues (232) demonstrated that this process is mediated by type 1 piliated bacteria that induce programmed cell death. However, some bacteria can resist this innate host defense mechanism by invading into deeper tissue. The possibility that these factors may be modified to reduce susceptibility to infection has been explored primarily through immunization in animal and human systems. For example, in a monkey model, vaccination with P fimbria has been shown to reduce adherence of P-fimbriated *E. coli* to uroepithelial cells and prevent acute pyelonephritis (280). Similarly, vaccination of mice with Fim H adhesin prevents cystitis in mice (191). Vaccination in women may reduce colonization of the vaginal introitus and subsequent ascending bacteria (369).

Kidney

The renal medulla and renal papilla have been identified as highly susceptible to infection because of high osmolality, low pH, low blood flow, and a high concentration of ammonia, which is thought to inactivate complement (17). Hyperosmolality of the renal medulla also favors the conversion of bacteria to a cell-wall–deficient state that is resistant to cell-wall–active antimicrobials and may lead to persistent infection despite therapy (118). The cortex, on the other hand, is much more resistant to infection. No natural barrier or defense mechanism against bacterial adherence has been identified in the kidney. Tamm-Horsfall protein may bind bacteria and prevent or diminish adherence and colonization, but its role requires further study.

During pyelonephritis and cystitis, an acute inflammatory response occurs. This response is aimed at limiting bacterial spread and persistence within the kidney. However, the infiltrating phagocytic cells drawn to the infection may also contribute to local tissue damage and result in renal scarring (281).

Immune Mechanisms

The urinary tract is part of the secretory immune system. Most of the human and experimental animal studies have focused on the immune response to bacterial infections of the upper tract and colonization of the vaginal introitus. Kidney infections are accompanied by both serum and local kidney immunoglobulin synthesis and the appearance of type-specific antibodies in the urine. Antibodies in serum against the O antigen and, to a lesser extent, the K antigen of the infecting *E. coli* strain have been found (289). Serum antibodies directed at type 1 and P pili have also been identified after acute pyelonephritis (65,277). In pyelonephritis, IgG and SIgA also appear in the urine and may become evident before antibodies are detected in the serum. These antibodies are synthesized locally within the kidney and may enhance bacterial opsonization and ingestion of the invading microorganisms by local phagocytic cells. These antibodies may have further protective function. Svanborg Eden and Svennerholm (354) showed that IgG and SIgA derived from the urine of patients with acute pyelonephritis reduced *in vitro* adherence of the same strain of *E. coli* to uroepithelial cells. Similarly, immunization with *E. coli* P pili resulted in immunoglobulin production in experimental animals that prevented ascending pyelonephritis by reducing the adhesive capacity of the invading autologous uropathogenic *E. coli* (249,280).

The role of urinary immunoglobulins in preventing infection of the bladder is less clear. IgA-producing lymphocytes have been demonstrated in the submucosa of infected rat bladders (133). Infection of the lower urinary tract is usually associated with a reduced or undetectable serologic response, reflecting the superficial nature of this type of cystitis. However, Uehling and Wolf (368) showed that bladder immunization of rats with bacterial antigens decreases *in vivo* adherence of *E. coli* to bladder mucosa and that bladder immunization with killed bacteria may also protect rats against pyelonephritis (367). The protective function of urinary immunoglobulins was also emphasized by the observations of Riedasch and associates (278) that lower urinary levels of SIgA were associated with an increased risk of urinary tract infection in humans.

Uehling and colleagues (369) have also demonstrated that vaginal immunization with mixtures of *E. coli* may prevent or reduce uropathogenic colonization of the introitus and reduce subsequent urinary tract infections. This line of research may lead to the development of vaccines to reduce the incidence of recurrent infection.

Evidence supports a protective role of cell-mediated immunity in urinary infections. Profound depression of or even absent T-cell function has not been associated with increased frequency of urinary tract infection or altered course of infection. The innate immune system response to an infection in the bladder or kidneys is primarily of local inflammation, which is followed by an adaptive response characterized in part by an antibody response to the infecting bacteria. Neutrophils from the urinary tract appear to be essential for bacterial clearance, and their recruitment plays a pivotal role in resistance to urinary tract infections (122). In mice, a urinary tract infection will spontaneously resolve in most cases; however, in mice with specific genetic backgrounds, a urinary tract infection can persist. This suggests that the presence or absence of specific host genes may determine how effectively a urinary tract infection will be resolved (145). The role of immune deficiencies in human susceptibility to urinary tract infections warrants investigation.

Alterations in Host Defense Mechanisms

Obstruction

Obstruction to urine flow at all anatomic levels is a key factor in increasing host susceptibility to urinary tract infection. Obstruction inhibits the normal flow of urine, and the resulting stasis compromises bladder and renal defense mechanisms. Stasis also contributes to the growth of bacteria in the urine and their ability to adhere to the urothelial cells. In the animal model of experimental hematogenous pyelonephritis, the kidney is relatively resistant to infection unless a ureter is ligated. Under these circumstances, only the obstructed kidney becomes infected (119). Clinical observations support the role of obstruction in pathogenesis of urinary tract infection and in increasing severity of infection. Mild episodes of cystitis or pyelonephritis can become life-threatening when obstruction to urine flow becomes present. Although obstruction clearly increases the severity of infection, it need not be a predisposing factor. For example, men with large residual urine may remain uninfected for years. However, if they are catheterized, even small inocula may lead to severe infections that are difficult to eradicate.

Vesicoureteral Reflux

Hodson and Edwards (136) first described the association of vesicoureteral reflux, urinary tract infection, and renal clubbing and scarring. Children with gross reflux and urinary tract infections usually develop progressive renal damage manifested by renal scarring, proteinuria, and renal failure. Those with a lesser degree of reflux usually improve or completely recover spontaneously or after treatment of the urinary tract infection. In adults, the presence of reflux does not appear to decrease renal function unless there is stasis and concurrent urinary tract infections.

Underlying Disease

There is a high incidence of renal scarring in patients with underlying conditions that cause chronic interstitial nephritis, virtually all of which produce primary renal papillary damage. These conditions include diabetes mellitus, sickle cell disorders, adult nephrocalcinosis, hyperphosphatemia, hypokalemia, analgesic abuse, sulfonamide nephropathy, gout, heavy-metal poisoning, and aging (97). An increased incidence of clinical overt urinary tract infections appears to occur in women with diabetes mellitus, but there is no substantial increase among diabetic men (90,250,371). Autopsy studies have shown the incidence of pyelonephritis to be fourfold to fivefold higher in diabetic than in nondiabetic individuals (279). However, such studies may be misleading because it is difficult to distinguish renal parenchymal changes resulting from pyelonephritis from the interstitial inflammatory changes of diabetic nephropathy.

Although most urinary tract infections in diabetic patients are asymptomatic, diabetes appears to predispose the patient to more severe infections. One study using antibody-coated bacteria techniques to localize the site of infection showed the upper urinary tract to be involved in nearly 80% of diabetic patients with urinary tract infections (90). This evidence of increasing immunologic response in diabetic patients who acquire bacteriuria suggests renal parenchymal involvement and a potential increase in morbidity. Once established, upper urinary tract infections are often complicated by emphysematous pyelonephritis, papillary necrosis, perinephric abscess, or metastatic infection (384).

Other conditions that may increase the susceptibility of the kidney to infection include hypertension and vascular obstruction (97). Association of renal infection with several other renal diseases, including glomerulonephritis, atherosclerosis, and tubular necrosis, which are not associated with papillary necrosis, does not lead to pyelonephritis and scarring.

Pregnancy

The prevalence of bacteriuria in pregnant women varies from 4% to 7%, and the incidence of acute clinical pyelonephritis ranges from 25% to 35% in untreated bacteriuric women (331). This is probably the result of dilation of the ureters and pelvis of the kidney secondary to pregnancy-related hormonal alterations. It is not surprising that untreated bacteriuria in the first trimester is accompanied by a substantial incidence of acute pyelonephritis, because Fairley and associates (82) documented that half of these women have upper tract bacteriuria. Untreated bacteriuria involving these dilated upper tracts would be expected to produce a significant number of abnormalities that should be radiologically apparent. Kincaid-Smith and Bullen (177) performed a culture on 4,000 women at their first antenatal visit. Of 240 bacteriuric women, 148 returned for intravenous urography 6 weeks after delivery. Approximately 40% of these patients had radiologic abnormalities consistent with pyelonephritis or analgesic nephritis. Brumfitt and colleagues (28) showed that the incidence of radiologic abnormalities in bacteriuria of pregnancy was proportional to the difficulty in clearing the infection. Patients who responded promptly to a single course of therapy had a 23% incidence of radiologic abnormalities, but those who remained bacteriuric despite repeated therapeutic efforts had a 65% incidence of radiologic changes. Thus prolonged bacteriuria and pyelonephritis of pregnancy appear to be associated with significant radiologic abnormalities. However, there is little evidence to suggest that bacteriuria of pregnancy or acute pyelonephritis of pregnancy causes these renal radiologic abnormalities.

CLINICAL MANIFESTATIONS

Symptoms and Signs

Pyelonephritis is classically associated with fever, chills, and flank pain. Nausea and vomiting are commonly present. Cystitis is usually associated with dysuria, frequency, urgency, suprapubic pain, and hematuria. Lower tract symptoms are commonly present and usually predate the appearance of upper tract symptoms by several days. Renal or perirenal abscess may cause indolent fever and flank mass and tenderness. In the elderly, the symptoms may be much more subtle (e.g., epigastric or abdominal discomfort), or the patient may be asymptomatic (282). Patients with indwelling catheters often have asymptomatic bacteriuria, but fever associated with bacteremia may occur rapidly and become life-threatening.

Diagnosis

Presumptive diagnosis of urinary tract infection is made by direct or indirect analysis of the urine and is confirmed by urine culture. Assessment of the urine provides clinical information about the status of the urinary tract. The urine and the urinary tract are normally free of bacteria and inflammation. False-negative urinalysis and culture can occur in the presence of urinary tract infection, particularly early in an infection when the numbers of bacteria and WBCs are low or diluted by increased fluid intake and subsequent diuresis. Occasionally, the urine may be free of bacteria and WBCs despite bacterial colonization and inflammation of the uroepithelium (75,153). False-positive urinalysis and culture are caused by contamination of the urine specimen with bacteria and WBCs during collection. This is most likely to occur in voided specimens but can also occur during urethral catheterization. Suprapubic aspiration of bladder urine is least likely to cause contamination of the specimen; therefore it provides the most accurate assessment of the status of bladder urine.

Urine Collection

In circumcised men, voided specimens require no preparation. For men who are not circumcised, the foreskin should be retracted and the glans penis washed with soap and then rinsed with water before specimen collection. The first 10 mL of urine (representative of the urethra) and a midstream specimen (representative of the bladder) should be obtained. Prostatic fluid is obtained by performing digital prostatic massage and collecting the expressed prostatic fluid on a glass slide. In addition, collection of the first 10 mL of voided urine after massage will reflect the prostatic fluid added to the urethral specimen. Catheterization of a male patient for urine culture is not indicated unless the patient cannot urinate.

In women, contamination of a midstream urine specimen with introital bacteria and WBCs is common, particularly when the woman has difficulty spreading and maintaining separation of the labia. Therefore the female should be instructed to spread the labia, wash and cleanse the periurethral area with a moist gauze, and then collect a midstream urine specimen. Cleansing with antiseptics is not recommended because they may contaminate the voided specimen and provide a false-negative urine culture. If the voided specimen shows evidence of contamination as indicated by vaginal epithelial cells and lactobacilli on urinalysis, catheterization should be performed and a midcatheterized specimen collected. Suprapubic aspiration is highly accurate, but because it carries some morbidity, there is limited clinical usefulness except for a patient who cannot urinate on command, such as patients with spinal cord injuries.

Urinalysis

Urinalysis provides rapid identification of bacteria and white cells and presumptive diagnosis of urinary tract infection. Usually, the sediment from an approximately 5- to 10-mL specimen obtained by centrifugation for 5 minutes at 2,000 rpm is analyzed. Microscopic bacteriuria is found in more than 90% of infections with counts of 10^5 colony-forming units (CFU) per milliliter of urine or greater and is a highly specific finding (161,340). However, bacteria are usually not detectable microscopically with lower colony count infections (10^2 to 10^4/mL). Significant pyuria can be determined simply and reliably with a microscope by accurately examining the centrifuged sediment or by using a hemocytometer to count the number of WBCs in the unspun urine. Approximately 1 to 2 WBCs per high-power field (HPF) in sediment from a centrifuged specimen represents about 10 WBCs/mm^3 in an unspun specimen. More than 2 WBCs per HPF in a centrifuged specimen or 10 WBCs/mm^3 of urine correlates well with the presence of bacteriuria and is rarely seen in nonbacteriuric patients (344). In clinical studies, determination of pyuria in voided urine specimens has a reported sensitivity of 80% to 95% and a specificity of 50% to 76% for urinary tract infection (depending on the definition of infection, the patient population, and the method used to evaluate for pyuria) (308,340,386,393).

Microscopic hematuria is found in 40% to 60% of cases of acute cystitis and is uncommon in other dysuric syndromes (343,386). Thus microscopic bacteriuria and hematuria lack sensitivity but are highly specific for urinary tract infections.

Urine Culture

Confirmation of urinary tract infection requires documentation of bacteria by culture. Urine should be cultured immediately or refrigerated at 40°C. Direct surface plating is the traditional quantitative culture technique used by most microbiology laboratories. A known amount of urine is streaked on split agar plates. Half of the plate contains a nonselective medium, such as blood agar, for growth of any bacteria, and the other half contains a selective medium, such as MacConkey, which is specific for Gram-negative bacteria. Each bacterial rod or cluster of cocci will form a single colony after overnight growth in an incubator. Dip-slide culture is a simpler, less expensive, and somewhat less accurate technique. An agar-coated slide is dipped in the urine and replaced into its sterile container. An approximate colony count is determined after overnight incubation at room temperature by comparing the appearance of the slide with a series of pictures provided by the manufacturer.

The definition of significant bacteriuria as greater than 10^5 CFU/mL was originally published by Kass and Finland (171) to differentiate infected from contaminated urine in voided specimens from women with asymptomatic bacteriuria. Most bacteria, when allowed to incubate for several hours, will reach colony counts to this level. However, this cutoff has limitations because about one-third of women with acute symptomatic cystitis caused by *E. coli, S. saprophyticus,* and *Proteus* have colony counts in midstream urine specimens between 10^2 and 10^4 CFU/mL (329,345). Thus, in dysuric women, the appropriate threshold value for defining significant bacteriuria is 100 CFU/mL or greater (345).

In a clinical setting, false-positive urine cultures are problematic. Women susceptible to infections often carry large numbers of pathogenic bacteria on the perineum that could contaminate a voided urine specimen. Contaminated cultures often show more than one organism and include indigenous bacteria such as lactobacilli. Diagnostic accuracy of voided specimens in women can be optimized by detailed history, proper collection techniques, and carefully performed urinalysis.

Midstream urine specimens in men or catheterized specimens in women are less likely to be contaminated, and hence counts of 10^2 CFU/mL are usually diagnostic of significant bacteriuria. Any uropathogen identified in a urine specimen obtained by suprapubic aspiration should be considered significant.

Rapid Screen Methods

Biochemical and enzymatic tests have been devised to detect bacteriuria and pyuria (261). The Griess test detects the presence of nitrite in urine that is formed when bacteria reduce the nitrate normally present in urine. Tests for detecting pyuria by determining leukocyte esterase activity have also been developed (46). In a study comparing traditional urine culture with these indirect tests, the combination of nitrite and leukocyte esterase tests (either test positive) had a sensitivity of 71% and a specificity of 83% when compared with 10^3 CFU/mL or greater of urine cultures (262). However, several investigators (155,258) noted substantial variability in the sensitivity and specificity results, which could be markedly influenced by the types of patients and infections chosen to evaluate the tests. This concept of spectrum bias was illustrated by a study that reported differences in the sensitivity of reagent strip testing, ranging from 56% to 92%, by changing only the groups of patients included in the analysis. Although false-positives are relatively uncommon, the borderline sensitivity of these tests, especially among patients with less characteristic symptoms of urinary tract infections, does not allow these inexpensive tests to replace careful microscopic urinalysis in symptomatic patients (311). Their main role is in screening asymptomatic patients (261).

IMAGING

Imaging studies are not required in most cases of urinary tract infections because clinical and laboratory findings alone are sufficient for correct diagnosis and adequate management of most patients. However, febrile infections, infection in an otherwise healthy male, signs or symptoms of urinary tract obstruction, failure to respond to appropriate therapy, and a pattern of recurrent infections suggesting bacterial persistence within the urinary tract warrant imaging for identification of underlying abnormalities that require modification of medical management or percutaneous or surgical intervention.

Excretory urography has traditionally provided excellent anatomic assessment of the urinary tract and remains the best examination for detection of lesions of the collecting system and ureter. Ultrasonography and computed tomography (CT) scans have gained considerable acceptance. Ultrasonography serves as a rapid, noninvasive means of evaluating the renal collecting system, parenchyma, and surrounding retroperitoneum for evidence of infection, and it is particularly useful for identifying hydronephrosis, calculi, and abscess. A single radiograph for calculi should accompany ultrasonography. Ultrasonography examination is also useful for diagnosing postvoid residual urine. CT clearly is the modality of choice for identifying inflammatory processes that involve the renal, perirenal, and pararenal spaces and radiolucent calculi. Magnetic resonance imaging may provide some advantages in delineating the extent of inflammation.

Although gallium-67 scanning has been reported to be useful in the diagnosis of pyelonephritis and renal abscess, it is uncommonly required and may be positive in noninfectious entities. Indium-111–labeled WBC studies have limited efficacy in establishing the presence of an inflammatory focus, particularly when the patient's clinical presentation does not suggest an infectious process.

ANTIMICROBIAL THERAPY

Therapy for urinary tract infections must ultimately eliminate bacterial growth in the urinary tract. This can occur within hours if the proper antimicrobial agent is used. Efficacy of the antimicrobial therapy is critically dependent on the antimicrobial levels in the urine and the duration that this level remains above the minimum inhibitory concentration of the infecting organism (141). Hence, resolution of infection is closely associated with the susceptibility of the bacteria to the concentration of the antimicrobial agent achieved in the urine (215,333,338). Inhibitory concentrations in urine are achieved after oral administration of all commonly used antimicrobial agents, except for the macrolides (erythromycin). The concentration of the antimicrobial agent achieved in blood is not important in treatment of uncomplicated urinary tract infections. Blood levels are critical in patients with bacteremia and febrile urinary infections consistent with parenchymal involvement of the kidney and prostate.

In patients with renal insufficiency, dosage modifications are necessary for agents that are cleared primarily by the kidneys and cannot be cleared by another mechanism. In renal failure, the kidneys may not be able to concentrate an antimicrobial agent in the urine; hence, difficulty in eradicating bacteria may occur. Urinary tract obstruction may also reduce concentration of antimicrobials within the urine.

The antimicrobial selection and the duration of therapy must consider the spectrum of activity of the drug against the known pathogen or the most probable pathogens based on the presumed source of acquisition of infection, whether the infection is judged to be uncomplicated or complicated, potential adverse effects, and cost. An often underemphasized but important characteristic is the drug's impact on the fecal and vaginal flora and the hospital bacterial environment. Bacterial susceptibility will vary dramatically in patients exposed to antimicrobials and in individuals in inpatient and outpatient settings. It is imperative that each clinician keep abreast of changes that affect antimicrobial use patterns.

Bacterial Resistance

In the last several years, the frequency and spectrum of antimicrobial-resistant urinary tract infections have increased in both the hospital and community. The increasing frequency of drug resistance has been attributed to combinations of microbial characteristics, bacterial selection pressure due to antimicrobial use, and societal and technologic changes that enhance the transmission of drug resistance (50). Bacterial resistance may occur because of natural (inherited) chromosomal-based resistance or by acquired chromosomal- or extrachromosomal (plasmid)-mediated resistance due to exposure of an organism to antimicrobials. Inherited resistance exists in a bacterial species because of the absence of the proper mechanism on which the antimicrobial agent can act. For example, *Proteus* and *Pseudomonas* species are always resistant to nitrofurantoin. Chromosomal-mediated resistance can be acquired by urinary bacteria during therapy for urinary tract infections. Before antimicrobial therapy, relatively resistant mutants of a bacterial strain may be present in the urine at very low concentrations. The remainder of the bacteria, which are susceptible to the administered antimicrobial agent, will be eradicated by therapy, but within 24 to 48 hours, a repeat urine culture will show high bacterial counts of the resistant mutant. In essence, the antimicrobial therapy has selected out the resistant mutant. This phenomenon is most likely to occur when the antimicrobial level in the urine is close to or below the minimum inhibitory concentration of the drug. Underdosing and noncompliance, as well as diuresis induced by increased fluid intake, can contribute to this process.

Resistance may also be acquired and transferable via extrachromosomal plasmids, which contain the genetic material for the resistance. This so-called R-factor resistance occurs in the fecal flora and is much more common than selection of preexisting mutants in the urinary tract. All antimicrobial classes are capable of causing plasmid-mediated resistance with the exception of the fluoroquinolones and nitrofurantoin. Hence, patients previously exposed to β-lactams, aminoglycoside, sulfonamide, trimethoprim (TMP), and tetracycline will often have R-factor resistance to both the antimicrobial to which the bacteria were exposed and also to other antimicrobials. In addition, the plasmids carrying the resistant genetic material are transferable both within species and across genuses. Thus, for example, a patient receiving tetracycline may harbor several fecal strains that are resistant to tetracycline, ampicillin, sulfonamides, and TMP. Because the fecal flora is the major reservoir for bacteria that ultimately colonize the urinary tract, infections that occur after antimicrobial therapy and that can cause plasmid-mediated resistance are commonly caused by organisms with multidrug resistance.

Antimicrobial resistance is also influenced by the duration and amount of antimicrobial used. For example, documented increased use of fluoroquinolones in the hospital setting has been directly associated with increased resistance of bacteria (particularly *Pseudomonas*) to the fluoroquinolones. Resistance tends to increase the longer the antimicrobial is used. Conversely, reduction in duration of therapy and in the amount of the drug use can lead to reemergence of more susceptible strains.

Most studies reporting antimicrobial resistance have been based on surveys of laboratory isolates, generally without correlation with clinical or epidemiologic factors (e.g., the presence and nature of symptoms, age, sex, and whether the infection was complicated). Gupta and colleagues (117) determined the prevalence of and trends in antimicrobial resistance among uropathogens isolated from a large, well-defined population of women with acute uncomplicated cystitis. Over a 5-year period, the prevalence of resistance to trimethoprim/sulfamethoxazole, ampicillin, and cephalothin increased significantly, whereas resistance to nitrofurantoin and ciprofloxacin remained uncommon. However, fluoroquinolone resistance of *E. coli* has increased from less than 1% to 7% in hospitalized patients. Previous use of fluoroquinolones and the presence of underlying urologic diseases were the strongest determinants for urinary tract infections caused by resistant strains (76).

Antimicrobial Formulary

Trimethoprim/sulfamethoxazole

The combination of trimethoprim/sulfamethoxazole (TMP-SMX) has been the most widely used antimicrobial for the treatment of acute urinary tract infections. TMP alone is as effective as the combination for most uncomplicated infections and may be associated with fewer side effects (163); however, the addition of SMX contributes to efficacy in the treatment of upper tract infection via a synergistic bactericidal effect and may diminish the emergence of resistance (31). TMP alone or in combination with SMX was effective against most common uropathogens, with the notable exception of *Enterococcus* and *Pseudomonas* species. TMP and TMP-SMX are inexpensive and have minimal adverse effects on the fecal flora. Disadvantages are relatively common adverse effects, consisting primarily of skin rashes and gastrointestinal complaints (49).

Nitrofurantoin

Nitrofurantoin is effective against common uropathogens, but it is not effective against *Pseudomonas* and *Proteus* species (157). It is rapidly excreted from the urine but does not obtain therapeutic levels in most body tissues, including the gastrointestinal tract. Therefore it is not useful for upper tract and complicated infections (387). It has minimal effects on the resident fecal and vaginal flora and has been used effectively in prophylactic regimens for more than 30 years. Acquired bacterial resistance to this drug is exceedingly low.

Cephalosporins

All three generations of cephalosporins have been used for the treatment of acute urinary tract infections (387). In general, as a group, activity is high against Enterobacteriaceae and poor against enterococci. First-generation cephalosporins have greater activity against Gram-positive organisms, whereas second-generation cephalosporins have activity against anaerobes. Third-generation cephalosporins are more reliably active against community-acquired and nosocomial Gram-negative organisms than other β-lactam antibiotics. Their cost should limit their use to complicated infections and situations where parenteral therapy is required and resistance to standard antibiotics is likely. Cephalosporins produce less resistance among fecal bacteria than the aminopenicillins, but the incidence of *Candida* vaginitis is nearly the same (157).

Aminopenicillins

Ampicillin and amoxicillin have been used often in the past for the treatment of urinary tract infections, but the emergence of resistance in up to 30% of common urinary isolates has lessened the usefulness of these drugs (141). The effects of these agents on the normal fecal and vaginal flora can predispose patients to reinfection with resistant strains and often lead to *Candida* vaginitis (157). The addition of the β-lactamase inhibitor clavulanate to amoxicillin greatly improves activity against β-lactamase–producing bacteria resistant to amoxicillin alone. However, its high cost and frequent gastrointestinal side effects limit its usefulness. The extended-spectrum penicillin derivatives (e.g., piperacillin, mezlocillin, azlocillin) retain ampicillin's activity against enterococci and offer activity against many ampicillin-resistant Gram-negative bacilli. This makes them attractive agents for use in patients with nosocomially acquired urinary tract infections and as the initial parenteral treatment of acute uncomplicated pyelonephritis acquired outside of the hospital, although less expensive agents are equally effective.

Aminoglycosides

When combined with TMP-SMX or ampicillin, aminoglycosides are the first drugs of choice for febrile urinary tract infections. Their nephrotoxicity and autotoxicity are well recognized; hence, careful monitoring of patients for renal and auditory impairment associated with infection is indicated. Once-daily aminoglycoside regimens have been instituted to maximize bacterial killing by optimizing the peak concentration-to-minimum inhibitory concentration ratio and reduce potential for toxicity (239). Administering an aminoglycoside as a single daily dose can take advantage not only of its concentration-dependent killing ability but also of two other important characteristics: time-dependent toxicity and a more prolonged postantibiotic effect (103,401). The regimen consists of a fixed 7-mg/kg dose of either gentamicin or tobramycin. Subsequent interval adjustments are made by using a single concentration in serum and a nomogram designed for monitoring of once-daily aminoglycoside therapy (Fig. 4.6). This regimen is clinically effective, reduces the incidence of nephrotoxicity, and provides a cost-effective method for administering aminoglycosides by reducing ancillary service times and serum aminoglycoside determinations.

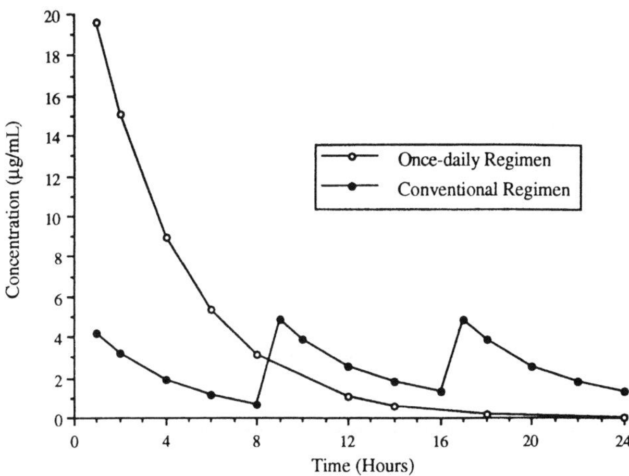

FIGURE 4.6. Simulated concentration-versus-time profile of once-daily (7 mg/kg every 24 hours) and conventional (1.5 mg/kg every 8 hours) regimens for patients with normal renal function.

Aztreonam

Aztreonam has a similar spectrum of activity as the aminoglycosides, and as with all β-lactams, it is not nephrotoxic. However, its spectrum of activity is less broad than the third-generation cephalosporins. It should be used primarily in patients who have penicillin allergies.

Fluoroquinolones

Fluoroquinolones share a common predecessor in nalidixic acid and inhibit DNA gyrase, a bacterial enzyme integral to replication. The fluoroquinolones have a broad spectrum of activity that makes them ideal for the empiric treatment of urinary tract infections. They are highly effective against Enterobacteriaceae, as well as *Pseudomonas aeruginosa.* Activity is also high against *S. aureus* and *S. saprophyticus,* but in general, antistreptococcal coverage is marginal. Most anaerobic bacteria are resistant to these drugs; therefore the normal vaginal and fecal flora are not altered (396). Bacterial resistance initially appeared to be uncommon, but it is being reported at an increasing rate because of indiscriminate use of these agents (374,396).

These drugs are not nephrotoxic, but renal insufficiency prolongs the serum half-life, requiring adjusted dosing in patients with creatinine clearances of less than 30 mL per minute. Adverse reactions are uncommon; gastrointestinal disturbances are more common. Hypersensitivity, skin reactions, mild central and peripheral nervous system reactions, and even acute renal failure have been reported (138). Administration of the fluoroquinolones to immature animals has caused damage to the developing cartilage; therefore they are currently contraindicated in children, adolescents, and pregnant or nursing women (47). There are important drug interactions associated with the fluoroquinolones. Antacids containing magnesium or aluminum interfere with absorption of fluoroquinolones (63). Certain fluoroquinolones (enoxacin and ciprofloxacin) elevate plasma levels of theophylline and prolong its half-life (396).

For most uncomplicated urinary tract infections, the fluoroquinolones have been only slightly more effective than TMP-SMX. However, as resistance to TMP-SMX increases, the fluoroquinolones have distinct advantages in empiric treatment of patients recently exposed to antimicrobials and in the outpatient treatment of complicated urinary tract infections (61,117). They may be considered as first-line agents in areas where a significant level of resistance (greater than 20%) exists (in common bacteria) to agents such as ampicillin and TMP-SMX.

BLADDER INFECTIONS

Uncomplicated Cystitis

Most cases of uncomplicated cystitis occur in women. Approximately 25% to 30% of women 20 to 40 years of age have a history of urinary tract infections (190). Although it is much less common, young men may also experience acute cystitis without underlying structural or functional abnormalities of the urinary tract (185). Risk factors include sexual intercourse and use of spermicides (93,139). Sexual transmission of uropathogens has been suggested by demonstrating identical *E. coli* in the fecal and urinary flora of sex partners.

The presenting symptoms of cystitis are variable but usually include dysuria, frequency or urgency, and suprapubic pain. Because acute cystitis, by definition, is a superficial infection of bladder mucosa, fever, chills, and other signs of dissemination are not present. Some patients may experience suprapubic tenderness, but most have no diagnostic physical findings. In women, physical examination should include the possibility of vaginitis, herpes, and urethral pathology, such as a diverticulum.

E. coli is the causative organism in approximately 75% to 80% of cases of acute cystitis in young women (192). *S. saprophyticus,* a commensal organism of the skin, is the second most common cause of acute cystitis in young women, accounting for 10% to 20% of these infections (166). Other organisms less commonly involved include *Klebsiella* and *Proteus* species and *Enterococcus.* In men, *E. coli* and other Enterobacteriaceae are the most commonly identified organisms.

Laboratory Diagnosis

The presumptive laboratory diagnosis of acute cystitis is based on microscopic urinalysis, which indicates microscopic bacteriuria, pyuria, and hematuria. Indirect dipstick tests for bacteria (nitrite) or pyuria (leukocyte esterase) may also be informative but are less sensitive than microscopic examination of the urine. Urine culture remains the definitive test, and in symptomatic patients, the presence of 10^2 CFU/mL or more of urine usually indicates infection (345).

Routine urine cultures are often not necessary. It is generally more cost-effective to manage many patients who have symptoms and urinalysis findings characteristic of uncomplicated cystitis without an initial urine culture because treatment decisions are usually made and therapy is often completed before culture results are known (181). This position was supported by a cost-effectiveness study (38) in which it was estimated that the routine use of pretherapy urine cultures for lower urinary tract infection increases costs by 40% but decreases the overall duration of symptoms by only 10%.

Thus, in patients with symptoms and signs suggesting acute cystitis and in whom no complicating factors are present, a urinalysis that is positive for pyuria, hematuria, or bacteriuria, or a combination, should provide sufficient documentation of urinary tract infection and a urine culture may be omitted. A urine culture should be obtained for patients in whom symptoms and urine examination findings leave the diagnosis of cystitis in doubt, however. Pretherapy cultures and susceptibility tests are also essential in the management of patients with recent antimicrobial therapy or urinary tract infection. In these situations, various pathogens may be present and antimicrobial therapy is less predictable and must be tailored to the individual organism (341).

Differential Diagnosis

Cystitis must be differentiated from other inflammatory infectious conditions in which dysuria may be the most prominent symptom, including vaginitis, urethral infections caused by sexually transmitted pathogens, and miscellaneous noninflammatory causes of urethral discomfort (180). Characteristic features of the history, physical examination, and voided urine or other specimens allow patients with dysuria to be assigned to one of these diagnostic categories. Vaginitis is characterized by irritative voiding associated with vaginal irritation and is subacute in onset. A history of vaginal discharge or odor and multiple or new sexual partners is common. Frequency, urgency, hematuria, and suprapubic pain are not present. Physical examination reveals a vaginal discharge, and examination of vaginal fluid demonstrates inflammatory cells. Differential diagnosis includes herpes simplex virus, gonorrhea, *Chlamydia,* trichomoniasis, yeast, and bacterial vaginosis. Urethritis causes dysuria that is usually subacute in onset and is associated with a history of discharge and new or multiple sexual partners. Frequency and urgency of urination may be present but are less pronounced than in patients with cystitis, and fever and chills are absent. Urethral discharge with inflammatory cells or initial pyuria in the male is characteristic. The common causes of urethritis include gonorrhea, *Chlamydia,* herpes simplex virus, and trichomoniasis. Appropriate cultures and immunologic tests are indicated. Urethral injury associated with sexual intercourse, chemical irritants, or allergy may also cause dysuria. A history of trauma or exposure to irritants and a lack of discharge or pyuria are characteristic.

Management

Antimicrobial Selection

Oral antimicrobial agents for treatment of acute uncomplicated cystitis are listed in Table 4.2. TMP and TMP-SMX are effective and inexpensive agents for empiric therapy. They are recommended in areas where the prevalence of resistance to these drugs among *E. coli* strains causing cystitis is less than 20% (377). When used alone, TMP is as efficacious as TMP-SMX and is associated with fewer side effects, presumably because of the absence of the sulfa component (123). Nitrofurantoin has maintained an excellent level of activity over three decades and is well tolerated, but it is more expensive than TMP-SMX. It is not associated with plasmid-mediated resistance, however, so it is an excellent choice for patients with recent exposure to most other antimicrobials. The high *in vitro* resistance to ampicillin and sulfonamide and the high cost of amoxicillin/clavulanate and the cephalosporins limit their usefulness. The fluoroquinolones offer excellent activity, and they are well tolerated. Their use for uncomplicated cystitis should be limited to patients with allergy to less costly drugs, to patients with previous exposure to antibiotics causing bacterial resistance, and to areas where the prevalence of resistance to TMP or TMP-SMX is 20% or greater (377).

Duration of Therapy

The traditional approach of 7 to 14 days of therapy for acute uncomplicated cystitis overtreats most patients, is more costly, and is associated with more side effects than shorter-term therapy (312). As an alternative, investigators initially proposed single-dose therapy wherein patients were given 1 to 2 days of conventional therapy in one dose. Although single-dose therapy was nearly as effective as 7-day therapy in healthy women with cystitis (85,266), resolution of symptoms was sometimes slower. Furthermore, it proved less effective in the presence of recent urinary tract infections, with the use of spermicides, and when more than 10^5 CFU/mL of urine was present (85).

Three-day therapy now appears to be the preferred regimen in uncomplicated cystitis in women (244,377). In an excellent review of more than 300 separate clinical trials of single-dose, 3-day or 7-day treatment with TMP, TMP-SMX, fluoroquinolones, and β-lactam antimicrobial therapies, it was concluded that, irrespective of the antimicrobial used, single-dose therapy is not as effective as 3-day therapy. Three-day therapy is as effective as a 7- to 10-day course of treatment (377). Three-day therapy with TMP-SMX, TMP, amoxicillin, or cloxacillin has been associated with cure rates similar to longer courses of therapy and an incidence of adverse effects as low as that seen with single-dose therapy and lower than seen with longer courses of therapy (3,44,189,218). Seven-day therapy often causes more adverse effects and therefore is recommended only for women with symptoms of 1 week or more, men, and individuals with possible complicating factors. Other options include nitrofurantoin, perhaps as 7-day therapy, and fosfomycin single-dose therapy; each of these requires further study. β-Lactams as a group are less effective in treatment of cystitis than TMP, TMP-SMX, and the fluoroquinolones.

Cost of Therapy

The cost of treating a urinary tract infection involves not only the initial evaluation and cost of the drug but what occurs subsequently. The most important prediction of high cost-effectiveness is high efficacy against the most common urinary pathogen—*E. coli*. The lower the effectiveness against this bacterium, the greater the number of revisits, cases of progression to pyelonephritis, and follow-up costs. Antimicrobial cost is a poor prediction of cost-effectiveness as illustrated by the finding that the most expensive and least

TABLE 4.2. ORAL ANTIMICROBIAL AGENTS FOR UNCOMPLICATED CYSTITIS

Drug	Dosage	Cost Per Day[a]
TMP-SMX	1 double-strength tablet b.i.d. (160/800 mg)	$0.28
Trimethoprim	100 mg b.i.d.	$0.38
Sulfasoxazole	1 g, followed by 500 mg q.i.d.	$0.32
Ciprofloxacin	500 mg b.i.d.	$8.30
Enoxacin	400 mg b.i.d.	$6.84
Levofloxacin	500 mg q.i.d	$8.58
Nitrofurantoin	100 mg q.i.d.	$3.24
Amoxicillin	250 mg t.i.d.	$0.68
Cephalexin	500 mg q.i.d.	$4.52

[a]Prices in dollars reflect the average wholesale price to the pharmacist as of February 2000. When products were available from multiple sources, the least expensive generic supply prices were used. The price to the patient is dependent on the pharmacist's professional fee structure.

expensive drugs, the fluoroquinolones and TMP-SMX, are approximately equally cost-effective (283). Both of these drugs are more cost-effective than nitrofurantoin and amoxicillin.

UNRESOLVED URINARY TRACT INFECTIONS

Unresolved infection indicates that initial therapy has been inadequate in eliminating bacterial growth in the urinary tract. If the symptoms of urinary tract infection do not resolve by the end of treatment or if symptoms recur shortly after therapy, urinalysis and urine culture with susceptibility testing should be obtained. If the patient's symptoms are significant, empiric therapy with a fluoroquinolone is appropriate pending results of the culture and susceptibility testing.

The causes of unresolved bacteriuria during antimicrobial therapy are shown in Table 4.3. Most commonly, the bacteria are resistant to the antimicrobial agent selected to treat the infection. Typically, the patient has received the antimicrobial therapy in the recent past and developed fecal colonization with resistant bacteria. β-Lactams, tetracycline, and sulfonamides are notorious for causing plasmid-mediated R factors that simultaneously carry resistance to multiple antimicrobial agents. The second most common cause is development of resistance in a previously susceptible population of bacteria during the course of treatment of urinary tract infections. This problem occurs in approximately 5% of the patients receiving antimicrobial therapy. It is easy to recognize clinically because culture on therapy shows that the previous susceptible population has been replaced by resistant bacteria of the same species. It can be shown that resistant organisms were actually present before contact with the initial antimicrobial agent, but they were present in such low numbers that it was impossible to detect by *in vitro* susceptibility studies before therapy. When the antimicrobial concentration in the urine is insufficient to kill all the bacteria present, the more resistant forms will emerge. This characteristically is seen in patients who are underdosed or who are poorly compliant and hence have inadequate dose regimens. The third cause is the presence of an unsuspected, second pathogen that was present initially and is resistant to the antimicrobial therapy chosen. Treatment of the dominant organism unmasks the presence of the second strain. The fourth cause is rapid reintroduction of a new resistant species while the patient is undergoing initial therapy. Rapid reinfection that mimics unresolved bacteriuria should alert the clinician to the possibility of an enterovesical fistula. If the culture obtained on therapy shows that the initial species is still present and susceptible to the antimicrobial chosen to treat the infection, the unresolved infection must be caused by either inability to deliver an adequate concentration of antimicrobial agents into the urinary tract or an excessive number of bacteria that "override" the antimicrobial activity. In patients with azotemia, a determination of urinary antimicrobial concentrations usually shows that the level of the drug is below the minimal inhibitory concentration of the infecting organism.

In patients with papillary necrosis, severe defects in the medullary concentrating ability dilutes the antimicrobial agent. A large mass of bacteria within the urinary tract is most commonly associated with a giant staghorn calculus. Even though adequate urinary levels of bactericidal drugs are present, the concentration is inadequate to sterilize the urine. This occurs because even susceptible bacteria cannot be inhibited once they reach a certain critical density, particularly if attached to a foreign body.

TABLE 4.3. CAUSES OF UNRESOLVED BACTERIURIA IN DESCENDING ORDER OF IMPORTANCE

1. Bacteria resistance to the initial drug selected for treatment[a]
2. Development of resistance from initially susceptible bacteria
3. Bacteriuria caused by two different bacterial species with mutually exclusive susceptibilities
4. Rapid reinfection from a new, resistant species during initial therapy for the original susceptible organism
5. Azotemia
6. Staghorn calculi in which the "critical mass" of the susceptible bacteria is too great for antimicrobial inhibition
7. Papillary necrosis from analgesic abuse

[a]The first four causes are characterized by identification of bacteria resistant to the antimicrobial agent the patient is receiving.
Modified with permission from Stamey TA. *Pathogenesis and treatment of urinary tract infections.* Baltimore: Williams & Wilkins, 1989.

RECURRENT URINARY TRACT INFECTIONS

Recurrent urinary tract infections are caused by either reemergence of bacteria from a site within the urinary tract *(bacterial persistence)* or new infections from bacteria outside the urinary tract *(reinfection)*. Clinical identification of these two types of recurrence is based on the pattern of recurrent infections. Bacterial persistence must be caused by the same organism in each instance, and infections that occur at close intervals are characteristic. Conversely, reinfections usually occur at varying and sometimes long intervals and often are caused by different species. The distinction between bacterial persistence and reinfection is important in management because patients with bacterial persistence can usually be cured of the recurrent infections by identification and surgical removal or correction of the focus of infection. Conversely, women with reinfection usually do not have an alterable urologic abnormality and usually require long-term medical management. Reinfections in men are uncommon and may be associated with an underlying abnormality, such as urethral stricture; therefore, at a minimum, endoscopic evaluation is indicated.

Bacterial Persistence

Although patients with bacterial persistence are relatively uncommon, their identification is important because they represent the only surgically curable cause of recurrent urinary tract infections. A systematic radiologic and endoscopic evaluation of the urinary tract is mandatory. Excretory urography and cystoscopy provide the initial screening. Urea-splitting organisms, such as *P. mirabilis,* cause infection stones that are relatively radiolucent. If such a stone is suspected, plain film tomograms and, if necessary, computed tomographic scans without contrast should be obtained (114). Retrograde urography may be required in selected patients to delineate abnormalities, such as diverticulum or nonrefluxing ureteral stump.

The infection that ultimately leads to an infection stone commonly begins inconspicuously as inadequately treated cystitis. Underlying urinary tract abnormalities are not a prerequisite for this type of infection. However, patients with indwelling catheters, urinary diversions, or other urinary tract abnormalities are particularly susceptible to these infections. Medical management with continued suppressive antimicrobial therapy and acidification temporarily relieves symptoms and retards deterioration of renal function in some patients. Complete removal of the calculus is generally required for bacteriologic cure and to prevent renal damage due to obstruction (319). Percutaneous nephrolithotomy and extracorporeal shock wave lithotripsy (ESWL) are now the preferred treatment for most renal and upper ureteral calculi. Follow-up radiographs are essential to ensure that all the stone fragments are removed, and cultures must demonstrate that the urease-splitting bacteria are eradicated. Most of the other congenital or acquired abnormalities listed in Table 4.4 require surgical removal for eradication of the source of bacterial persistence. Chronic bacterial prostatitis is treated initially with long-term antimicrobial therapy and, in select cases, by radical transurethral resection (222).

In patients in whom the focus of infection cannot be eradicated, long-term, low-dose antimicrobial suppression is necessary to prevent symptoms of infection. The antimicrobial drugs used for low-dose prophylaxis will also be effective for bacterial suppression if the persistent strain is susceptible. These include nitrofurantoin, TMP-SMX, cephalexin, and the fluoroquinolones.

TABLE 4.4. CAUSES OF BACTERIAL PERSISTENCE OF URINARY TRACT INFECTIONS[a]

1. Infection renal stone
2. Chronic bacterial prostatitis
3. Infected pericalyceal diverticulum
4. Infected nonrefluxing ureteral stump following nephrectomy
5. Atrophic, infected kidney
6. Medullary sponge kidney
7. Infected urachal cyst
8. Infected necrotic papilla from papillary necrosis

[a]Although patients with bacterial persistence are relatively uncommon, these circumstances are important because they represent the only surgically curable causes of recurrent urinary tract infections.
Modified with permission from Stamey TA. *Pathogenesis and treatment of urinary tract infections.* Baltimore: Williams & Wilkins, 1980.

Reinfections

Patients with recurrent infections caused by different species or occurring at long intervals almost invariably have reinfections. These reinfections most often occur in women and girls and are associated with ascending colonization from the fecal flora. Reinfections in men are often associated with a urinary tract abnormality. The possibility of a vesicoenteric or vesicovaginal fistula should be considered when the patient has any history of pneumaturia, fecaluria, diverticulitis, obstipation, previous pelvic surgery, or radiation therapy. Evaluation of the patient with presumed reinfections must be individualized.

Failure to recognize and correct abnormalities that reduce formation, transmission, and elimination of urine by the urinary tract increases the incidence of reinfection in susceptible patients and reduces the effectiveness of antimicrobial therapy. Abnormalities should be corrected and urinary tract function restored by medical, pharmacologic, or surgical management. A thorough urologic evaluation is essential in all men and in women with evidence of upper tract infections (fevers, chills, flank pain, hemorrhagic cystitis, or other risk factors, such as history of unexplained hematuria, obstructive symptoms, neurogenic bladder dysfunction, renal calculi, fistula, analgesic abuse, or severe disease such as diabetes mellitus). In women, diaphragm-spermicide use has been associated with an increased risk of urinary tract infection and vaginal colonization with *E. coli* (143). Spermicides containing the active ingredient nonoxynol-9 may provide a selective advantage in colonizing the vagina, perhaps by a reduction in vaginal lactobacilli and through enhancement of adherence of *E. coli* to epithelial cells (116,144). Thus spermicidals should be discontinued in women with recurrent urinary tract infection, and other forms of contraception should be used. In postmenopausal women, the risk of infection is reduced by estrogen replacement (274).

Excretory urography will demonstrate the anatomy of the urinary tract and provide reasonable assessment of its functional status. In healthy women, upper tract abnormalities associated with reinfections are very rare; therefore routine excretory urography is not indicated. Cystoscopy should be performed in men or women who have frequent reinfections and symptoms suggestive of obstruction, bladder dysfunction, and fistula. Dilation of a stenotic urethra to a normal caliber would appear appropriate. There is little evidence, however, that repeated urethral dilation is indicated in the routine management of most women.

Antimicrobial management in women who have had two or more symptomatic urinary tract infections over a 6-month period or three or more episodes within a 12-month period involves one of three regimens: low-dose continuous prophylaxis, self-start intermittent therapy, or postintercourse prophylaxis.

Low-dose Continuous Prophylaxis

Low-dose continuous prophylaxis is indicated when the urine culture shows no growth (usually when a patient has completed antimicrobial therapy). Nightly therapy is then begun with one of the following drugs: (a) nitrofurantoin 50 to 100 mg half-strength (HS) (332), (b) TMP-SMX, 40 to 200 mg (346), (c) TMP 50 mg (346), or (d) Keflex 250 mg (213). Patients will have less than one urinary tract infection per year while taking these regimens. Every-other-night therapy is also effective and is probably practiced by most patients. When breakthrough infections occur, they are not necessarily accompanied by symptoms; therefore we advocate monitoring for infections every 1 to 3 months, even in asymptomatic patients. Breakthrough infections usually respond to full-dose therapy with the drug used for prophylaxis. However, cultures and susceptibility tests may indicate that another drug is indicated. After the infection is cured, prophylaxis may be reinstituted. Low-dose prophylaxis is usually discontinued after about 6 months, and the patient is monitored for reinfection. Approximately 30% of women will have spontaneous remissions that last up to 6 months (183). Unfortunately, many of the remissions are followed by reinfections, and low-dose prophylaxis must be reinstituted. At this point, many patients prefer an alternative form of management.

Self-start Intermittent Therapy

With self-start intermittent therapy, the patient is given a dip-slide device to culture the urine and is instructed to perform a urine culture when symptoms of urinary tract infection occur (294). The patient is also provided a 3-day course of empiric, full-dose antimicrobial therapy to be started immediately after performing the culture. It is important that the antimicrobial agent selected for self-start therapy have a broad spectrum of activity and achieve high urine levels to minimize development of resistant mutants. In addition, there should be minimal or no side effects on the fecal flora. Fluoroquinolones are ideal for self-start therapy because they have a spectrum of activity broader than any of the other oral agents and are superior to many parenteral antimicrobials, including aminoglycosides. Nitrofurantoin and TMP-SMX are acceptable alternatives, although they are somewhat less effective. Antimicrobial agents such as tetracycline, ampicillin, SMX, and cephalexin in full doses should be avoided because they can give rise to resistant bacteria (395).

The culture is brought to the office as soon as possible. If the culture is positive and the patient is asymptomatic, a culture is performed 7 to 10 days after therapy to determine efficacy. In most cases, the therapy is limited to two inexpensive dip-slide cultures and a short course of antimicrobial therapy. If the patient has symptoms that do not respond to initial antimicrobial therapy, a repeat culture and susceptibility testing of the initial culture specimen are performed and therapy adjusted accordingly. If symptoms of infection are not associated with positive cultures, urologic evaluation should be performed to rule out other causes of irritative bladder symptoms, including carcinoma in situ, interstitial cystitis, and neurogenic bladder dysfunction. Our experience with this technique has been very favorable, and we find that it is particularly attractive to patients who have less frequent infections and are willing to play an active role in their diagnosis and management.

Postintercourse Prophylaxis

Antimicrobial management through postintercourse prophylaxis is based on research establishing that sexual intercourse can be an important risk factor for acute cystitis in women (241). Diaphragm users have a significantly greater risk of urinary tract infection than do women who use other contraceptive methods (86). Postintercourse therapy with antimicrobials, such as nitrofurantoin, cephalexin, TMP-SMX, or a fluoroquinolone taken as a single dose, will effectively reduce the incidence of reinfection (224,265).

RENAL INFECTION (BACTERIAL NEPHRITIS)

Although renal infection is less prevalent than bladder infection, it often is a more difficult problem for the patient and his or her physician because of its often varied and morbid presentation and course, the difficulty in establishing a firm microbiologic and pathologic diagnosis, and its potential for significantly impairing renal function. Although the classic symptoms of acute onset of fever, chills, and flank pain are usually indicative of renal infection, some patients with these symptoms do not have renal infection. Conversely, significant renal infection may be associated with an insidious onset of nonspecific local or systemic symptoms, or it may be entirely asymptomatic. Therefore a high clinical index of suspicion and appropriate radiologic and laboratory studies are required to establish the diagnosis of renal infection.

Unfortunately, the relationship between laboratory findings and the presence of renal infection often is poor.

Bacteriuria and pyuria, the hallmarks of urinary tract infection, are not predictive of renal infection. Conversely, patients with significant renal infection may have sterile urine if the ureter draining the kidney is obstructed or the infection is outside of the collecting system.

The pathologic and radiologic criteria for diagnosing renal infection may also be misleading. Interstitial renal inflammation, once thought to be caused predominantly by bacterial infection, is now recognized as a nonspecific histopathologic change associated with a variety of immunologic, congenital, or chemical lesions that usually develop in the absence of bacterial infection. Infectious granulomatous diseases of the kidney often have either radiologic or pathologic characteristics that mimic renal cystic disease, neoplasia, or other renal inflammatory disease.

The effect of renal infection on renal function is varied. Acute or chronic pyelonephritis may transiently or permanently alter renal function, but nonobstructive pyelonephritis is no longer recognized as a major cause of renal failure. However, pyelonephritis, when associated with urinary tract obstruction or granulomatous renal infection, may lead rapidly to significant inflammatory complications, renal failure, or even death.

If urinary tract infection is associated with fever, chills, and flank pain, the infection is judged to be more severe and usually involves the kidneys. Bacterial nephritis, whether isolated or recurrent, may cause acute or chronic renal parenchymal damage and act as the source for recurrent episodes of renal or lower urinary tract infection (13,95).

Interstitial renal inflammation is a nonspecific cellular response of the renal interstitium that may or may not be complicated by fibrosis and varying degrees of tubular or glomerular damage. It generally has been believed that bacterial infection of the kidney, such as pyelonephritis, was the most common cause of interstitial renal inflammation and subsequent development of serious renal disease. More recently, however, the nonspecific nature of the histopathologic changes of interstitial renal inflammation has been appreciated. As a result of urologic evaluations of patients with chronic preexisting interstitial renal inflammation, it is now recognized that interstitial renal inflammation is associated with immunologic reactions, congenital lesions, or papillary damage in the absence of bacterial infection and that bacterial infection is often a secondary event. Thus histologic evidence alone is too often assumed indicative of bacterial nephritis and is not sufficient to establish whether interstitial changes in the kidney are either primary or secondary to bacterial infection or of noninfectious causes.

Pathology

The opportunity for pathologic confirmation of acute bacterial nephritis is rare. The kidney may be edematous. Focal acute suppurative bacterial nephritis caused by hematogenous dissemination of bacteria to the renal cortex is characterized by multiple focal areas of suppuration on the surface of the kidney (Fig. 4.7). Histologic examination of the renal cortex shows focal suppurative destruction of glomeruli and tubules. Adjacent cortical structures and the medulla are not involved in the inflammatory reaction. Acute ascending pyelonephritis is characterized by linear bands of inflammation extending from the medulla to the renal capsule (Fig. 4.8). Histologic examination usually reveals a focal wedge-shaped area of acute interstitial inflammation with the apex of the wedge in the renal medulla. Polymorphonuclear leukocytes or a predominantly lymphocytic and plasma cell response are seen. Bacteria also may be present.

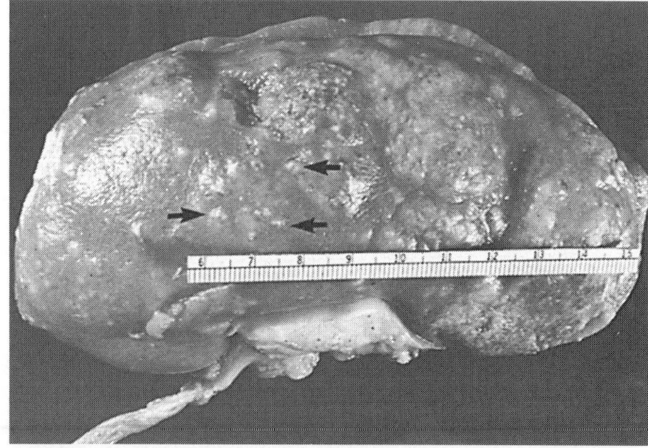
A

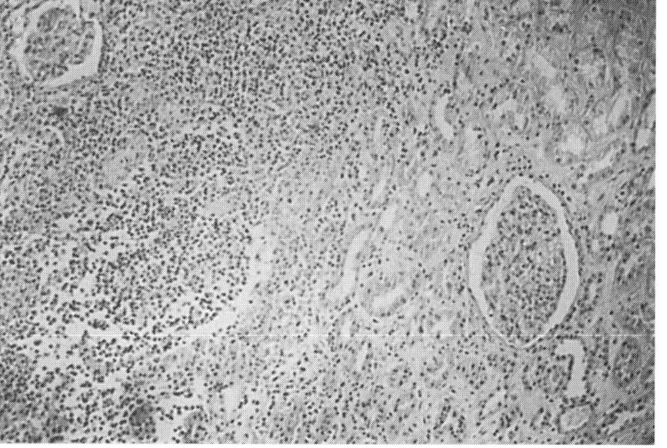
B

FIGURE 4.7. Acute focal suppurative bacterial nephritis. **A:** Surface of kidney. *Arrows* indicate focal areas of suppuration. **B:** Renal cortex showing focal suppuration destruction of glomeruli and tubules.

The changes that appear to be most specific for chronic pyelonephritis are evident on careful gross examination of the kidney and consist of a cortical scar associated with retraction of the corresponding renal papilla (97,131, 135,137). The kidney shows evidence of patchy involvement with numerous chronic inflammatory foci mainly confined to the cortex but also involving the medulla (Fig. 4.9). The scars may be separated by intervening zones of normal parenchyma, causing a grossly irregular renal outline. The microscopic appearance, as with most chronic

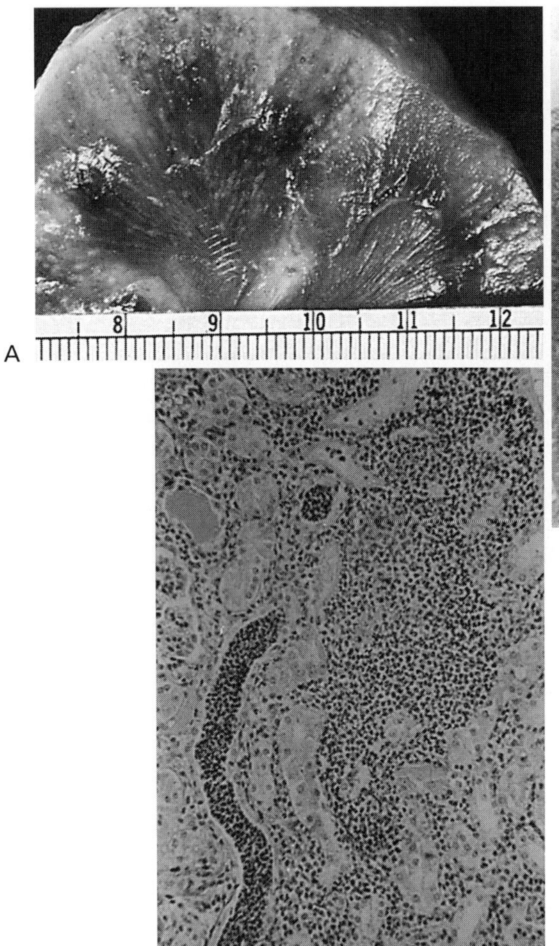

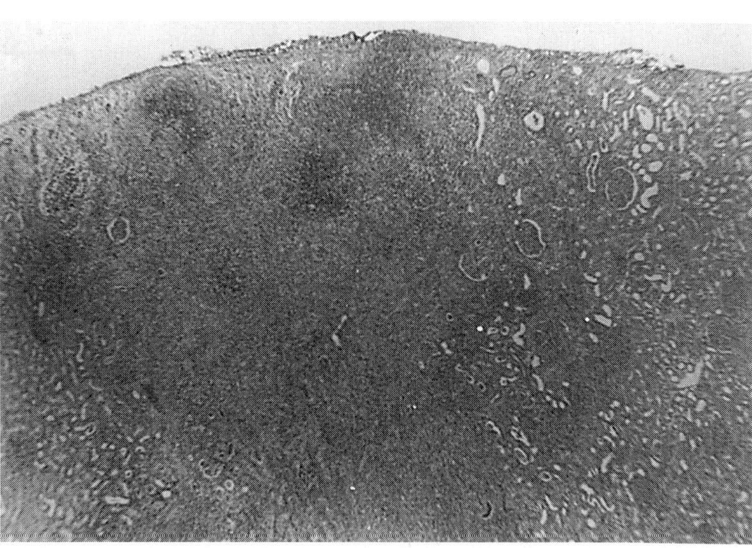

FIGURE 4.8. Acute ascending pyelonephritis. **A:** Cortical structures, tubules, and collecting ducts diffusely infiltrated with inflammatory cells. **B:** Section of the renal cortex showing wedge-shaped destruction of renocortical structures as a result of ascending infiltration with inflammatory cells. **C:** Thickened and inflamed tissue surrounding the collecting ducts in the medulla. A polymorphonuclear cast of segmented neutrophils is clearly visible.

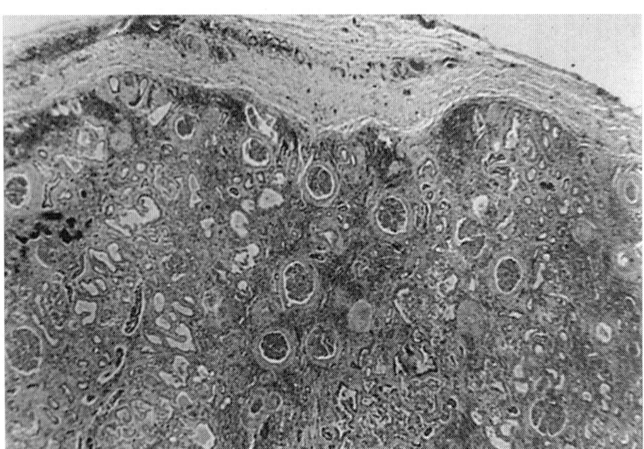

FIGURE 4.9. Chronic pyelonephritis. The renal cortex shows thickened fibrous capsule and focal retracted scar on surface of kidney. Focal destruction of tubules in center of picture is accompanied by periglomerular fibrosis and scarring.

interstitial disease, includes the presence of lymphocytes and plasma cells. Although glomeruli within scars may be surrounded by a cuff of fibrosis or be partially or completely hyalinized, glomeruli outside these severely scarred zones are relatively normal. Vascular involvement is variable, but in patients with hypertension, nephrosclerosis may be found. Papillary abnormalities include deformity, sclerosis, and sometimes necrosis. Studies in animals have clearly indicated the critical role of the papilla in the initiation of pyelonephritis (98). However, these changes are not necessarily specific for bacterial infection and may occur in the absence of infection as a result of other disorders such as analgesic abuse, diabetes, and sickle cell disease.

The classic pathologic description of chronic pyelonephritis has traditionally been that of Weiss and Parker (382); however, their autopsy studies included late stages of the disease, which are often complicated by hypertension and vascular changes and are best referred to as *end-stage kidneys.* They repeatedly emphasized that patients with this form of renal disease did not always have clinical evidence of bacterial infections of the urinary tract sufficient to explain the severe loss of renal tissue. Stamey and Pfau (334) presented a case of pure symptomatic pyelonephritis, incurable with drug therapy and uncomplicated by vascular hypertension. The microscopic sections together with Heptinstall's comments represent an unusual opportunity to study the pathologic characteristics of this disease in its purest form.

Acute Pyelonephritis

Clinical Findings

The onset of acute pyelonephritis is usually abrupt. The classic clinical features are chills, fever (100°F or greater), and costovertebral angle or flank pain accompanied by symptoms of cystitis.

Although some authors regard loin pain and fever in combination with significant bacteriuria as diagnostic of acute pyelonephritis, it is clear from localization studies using ureteral catheterization (335) or the bladder wash-out technique (83) that clinical symptoms correlate poorly with the site of infection (77,80,321,333). In a large study of 201 women and 12 male patients with recurrent urinary tract infection, Busch and Huland (32) showed that fever and flank pain are no more diagnostic of pyelonephritis than they are of cystitis. Of patients with flank pain, fever, or both, more than 50% had lower tract bacteriuria. Patients with bladder symptoms or no symptoms frequently had upper tract bacteriuria. Approximately 75% of patients give a history of previous lower urinary tract infections.

On physical examination, there often is tenderness to deep palpation in the costovertebral angle. Variations of this clinical presentation have been recognized. Acute pyelonephritis may also simulate gastrointestinal tract abnormalities with abdominal pain, nausea, vomiting, and diarrhea. Asymptomatic progression of acute pyelonephritis to chronic pyelonephritis, particularly in compromised hosts, may occur in the absence of overt symptoms.

Laboratory Findings

The patient may have leukocytosis with predominance of neutrophils. Urinalysis usually reveals numerous WBCs, often in clumps, and bacteria. Leukocytes exhibiting brownian motion in the cytoplasm (glitter cells) may be present if the urine is hypotonic, but they are not in themselves diagnostic of pyelonephritis. The presence of large amounts of granular or leukocyte casts in the urinary sediment is suggestive of acute pyelonephritis. A specific type of urinary cast characterized by the presence of bacteria in its matrix has been demonstrated in the urine of patients who have had acute pyelonephritis (Fig. 4.10) (199). Bacteria in the casts were not easily distinguished by simple bright-field microscopy without special staining of the sediment. Staining the sediment with a basic dye such as dilute toluidine blue or KOVA (I.C.L. Scientific, Fountain Valley, California) stain demonstrated the bacteria in casts without difficulty. Urine cultures are invariably positive. Most often, the causative microorganism is *E. coli.* However, more resistant species, such as *Proteus, Klebsiella, Pseudomonas,* or *Serratia,* should be suspected in patients who have recurrent urinary tract infections, are hospitalized, or have indwelling catheters, as well as in those who required recent urinary tract instrumentation. Except for *Enterococcus faecalis* and *S. epidermidis,* Gram-positive bacteria rarely cause pyelonephritis. Blood cultures should be obtained in patients with severe toxicity because bacteremia and sepsis are common.

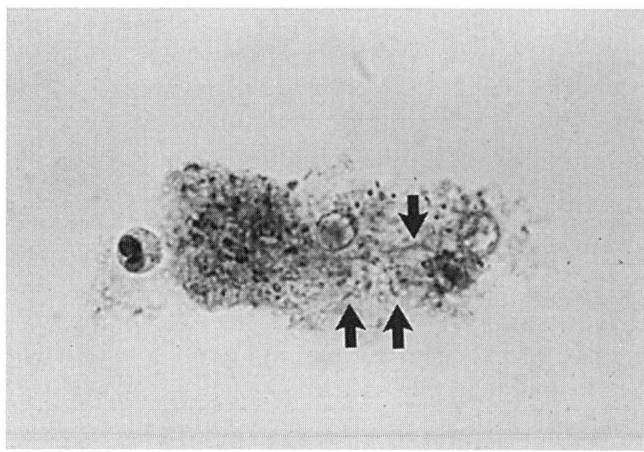

FIGURE 4.10. Bright-field micrograph of a mixed bacterial leukocyte cast from patient with acute pyelonephritis. Only the bacteria and the nucleus of a leukocyte stain strongly. *Arrows* show some bacteria. Many more are clearly demonstrated by through-focusing (toluidine blue O stain, magnification ×640). (Reprinted with permission from Lindner LE, Jones RN, Haber MH. A specific urinary cast in acute pyelonephritis. *Am J Clin Pathol* 1980;73:810.)

Differential Diagnosis

Acute appendicitis, diverticulitis, and pancreatitis can cause a similar degree of pain, but the location of the pain often is different. Results of the urine examination are usually normal. Herpes zoster can cause superficial pain in the region of the kidney but is not associated with symptoms of urinary tract infection; the diagnosis will be apparent when shingles appear.

Initial Management

Hospitalization, initially with complete bed rest, intravenous fluids, and antipyretics, is required for patients with significant toxicity. Patients with less severe disease may be managed as outpatients. Bladder outlet obstruction and associated urinary retention should be relieved by an indwelling urethral or suprapubic catheter. Upper tract obstruction, if suspected, should be ruled out by ultrasonography or intravenous urogram. An obstructed kidney has difficulty concentrating and excreting antimicrobial agents. In addition, obstruction in effect creates a potential abscess, pyonephrosis, which can rapidly destroy the renal parenchyma and endanger the patient's life. Any substantial obstruction must be relieved expediently by the safest and simplest means.

Until the results of the culture and susceptibilities are available, broad-spectrum antimicrobial therapy should be instituted. A Gram stain of the urine sediment is helpful to guide the selection of the initial empiric antimicrobial therapy. Outpatient, single-drug oral therapy with a fluoroquinolone is more effective than TMP-SMX for patients with domiciliary infections (359). Many physicians administer a single parenteral dose of an antimicrobial (ceftriaxone, gentamicin, or a fluoroquinolone) before initiating oral therapy (158,267). If a Gram-positive organism is suspected, amoxicillin or amoxicillin/clavulanic acid is recommended (377). If a patient is sufficiently ill to require hospitalization (high fever, high WBC count, vomiting, dehydration, or evidence of sepsis) or fails to improve during the initial outpatient treatment period, the patient should be admitted and treated with intravenous antimicrobials. A parenteral fluoroquinolone, an aminoglycoside with or without ampicillin, or an extended-spectrum cephalosporin with or without an aminoglycoside is recommended (377). If Gram-positive cocci are causative, ampicillin/sulbactam with or without an aminoglycoside is recommended.

Subsequent Management

Even though the urine usually becomes sterile within a few hours of starting antimicrobial therapy, patients with acute pyelonephritis may continue to have fever, chills, and flank pain for several more days (18). Ambulatory patients should be treated with a fluoroquinolone for 7 days (359). Alterations in antimicrobial therapy may be made depending on the patient's clinical response and the results of the culture and susceptibility tests. Susceptibility tests should also be used to replace potentially toxic drugs, such as aminoglycosides, with less toxic drugs, such as the fluoroquinolones, aztreonam, and cephalosporins. For women with uncomplicated pyelonephritis, 7-day fluoroquinolone therapy is associated with greater bacteriologic and clinical cure rates than 14-day TMP-SMX therapy (359). In hospitalized patients with bacteremia, parenteral therapy should be continued for 7 days. If results of the blood cultures are negative, parenteral therapy can be discontinued after several days. In either case, an appropriate oral antimicrobial drug (fluoroquinolone; TMP, TMP-SMX, or amoxicillin or amoxicillin/clavulanic acid for Gram-positive organisms) should be continued in full dosage for an additional 10 to 14 days.

Excretory urography is usually performed after institution of adequate therapy and resolution of the patient's symptoms; therefore it is not surprising that most patients with pyelonephritis have a normal excretory urogram (317,385). However, if obtained during acute pyelonephritis, the most common radiologic abnormality is renal enlargement, which occurs from generalized renal edema as a consequence of the inflammatory process (Fig. 4.11A). An overall length of 15 cm or a length 1.5 cm greater than the unaffected side has been established as criteria for the diagnosis of renal enlargement in acute pyelonephritis (56,317,385). The inflammatory response may also cause cortical vasoconstriction, which is presumably responsible for the diminished nephrogram and delayed appearance of the pyelogram, as well as compression of the collecting structures, so that the calyces have an attenuated or spidery appearance. In addition to these abnormalities, calyceal and ureteral dilation have occasionally been reported (124). This finding has been commonly attributed to a decrease in ureteral peristalsis caused by bacterial endotoxin. Although ureteral dilation may occur with infection, this diagnosis should not be made until obstruction, either past or present, has been excluded.

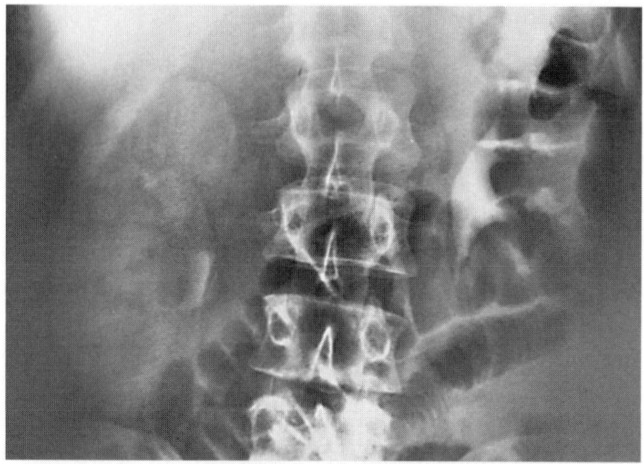
A

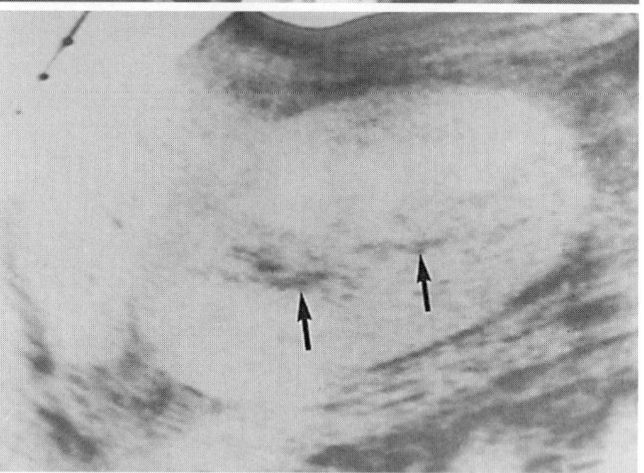
B

FIGURE 4.11. Acute pyelonephritis. **A:** Excretory urogram. Ten-minute film demonstrates enlarged right kidney with minimum function. Findings are consistent with edema. **B:** Ultrasound of the right kidney demonstrates renal enlargement, hypoechoic parenchyma, and compressed central collecting complex *(arrows).*

Ultrasound (Fig. 4.11B) and CT show renal enlargement, hypoechoic or attenuated parenchyma, and a compressed collecting system. In patients with fever greater than 72 hours, these studies are most helpful for ruling out obstruction and identifying complicated renal and perirenal infections (327).

Unfavorable Response to Therapy

When the response to therapy is slow or the urine continues to show infection, an immediate reevaluation is mandatory.

Urine and blood cultures must be repeated and appropriate alterations in antimicrobial therapy made on the basis of susceptibility testing. Radiologic investigation is indicated to attempt to identify unsuspected obstructive uropathy, urolithiasis, or underlying anatomic abnormalities that may have predisposed the patient to infection, prevented a rapid therapeutic response, or caused complications of the infectious process, such as renal or perinephric abscess. Radionuclide imaging may be useful to demonstrate functional changes associated with acute pyelonephritis (decrease in renal blood flow, delay in peak function, and delay in excretion of the radionuclide) (87) and cortical defects associated with vesicoureteral reflux.

Follow-up

Repeat urine cultures should be performed on the fifth to seventh day of therapy and 10 to 14 days and 4 to 6 weeks after discontinuing antimicrobial therapy to ensure that the urinary tract remains free of infections. For the few patients who have recurrent infections that presumably represent "relapse," re-treatment for 6 weeks has been recommended (162).

Depending on the clinical presentation and response and initial urologic evaluation, some patients may require additional evaluation (e.g., voiding cystourethrogram, cystoscopy, bacterial localization studies) and correction of an underlying abnormality of the urinary tract.

Acute Focal or Multifocal Bacterial Nephritis

Acute focal or multifocal bacterial nephritis is an uncommon, severe form of acute renal infection in which a heavy leukocyte infiltrate is confined to a single renal lobe (focal) or multiple lobes (multifocal).

Clinical Findings

The clinical presentation of patients with acute bacterial nephritis is similar to that of patients with acute pyelonephritis but usually is more severe. About half of the patients are diabetic, and sepsis is common. Generally, leukocytosis and urinary tract infection resulting from Gram-negative organisms are found; more than 50% of the patients are bacteremic (385).

Radiologic Findings

The diagnosis must be made by radiologic examination. The urographic findings are those of a mass, most commonly poorly marginated and suggestive of renal abscess or tumor (Fig. 4.12A). The mass has slightly less nephrographic density than the surrounding normal renal parenchyma.

Ultrasonography and CT aid in establishing the diagnosis. On ultrasonography, the lesion is typically poorly marginated and relatively sonolucent with occasional low-amplitude echoes that disrupt the cortical medullary junction (56) (Fig. 4.12B). Contrast enhancement is necessary with CT studies because the lesion is difficult to visualize on the unenhanced study (Fig. 4.12C). Wedge-shaped areas of decreased enhancement are seen. No definite wall is evident, and frank liquefaction is absent. Conversely, abscesses tend to have liquid centers, are usually round, and are present both before and after contrast enhancement. More chronic abscesses may also show a ring-shaped area of increased enhancement surrounding the lesion (56). Gallium scanning reveals uptake that is in the region of and larger than the previously demonstrated mass (284). In patients with multifocal disease, the findings are similar, but multiple lobes are involved.

Management

Acute bacterial nephritis probably represents a relatively early phase of frank abscess formation. In a series of cases reported by Lee and co-workers (195), a patient with acute focal bacterial nephritis progressed to abscess formation. Treatment includes hydration and intravenous antimicrobials for at least 7 days, followed by 7 days of oral antimicrobial therapy. Patients with bacterial nephritis typically respond to medical therapy, and follow-up studies will show resolution of the wedge-shaped zones of diminished attenuation. Failure to respond to antimicrobial therapy is an indication for appropriate studies to rule out obstructive uropathy, renal or perirenal abscess, renal carcinoma, or acute renal vein thrombosis. Long-term follow-up studies performed in a few patients with multifocal disease have demonstrated a decrease in renal size and focal calyceal deformities suggestive of papillary necrosis (62).

Emphysematous Pyelonephritis

Emphysematous pyelonephritis is an acute necrotizing parenchymal and perirenal infection caused by gas-forming uropathogens. The pathogenesis is poorly understood. Because the condition usually occurs in diabetic patients, it has been postulated that the high tissue glucose levels provide the substrate for microorganisms such as *E. coli,* which are able to produce carbon dioxide by the fermentation of sugar (303). Although glucose fermentation may be a factor, the explanation does not account for the rarity of emphysematous pyelonephritis despite the high frequency of Gram-negative urinary tract infection in diabetic patients, nor does it explain the rare occurrence of the condition in nondiabetic patients.

In addition to diabetes, many patients have urinary tract obstruction associated with urinary calculi or papillary necrosis and significant renal functional impairment. It seems

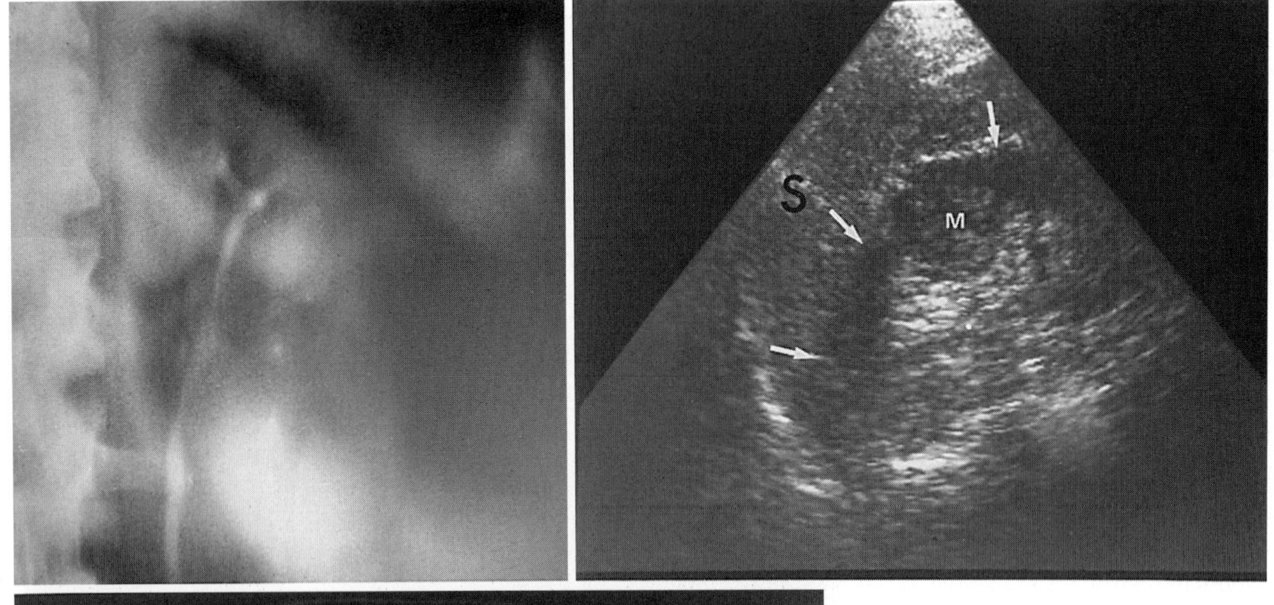

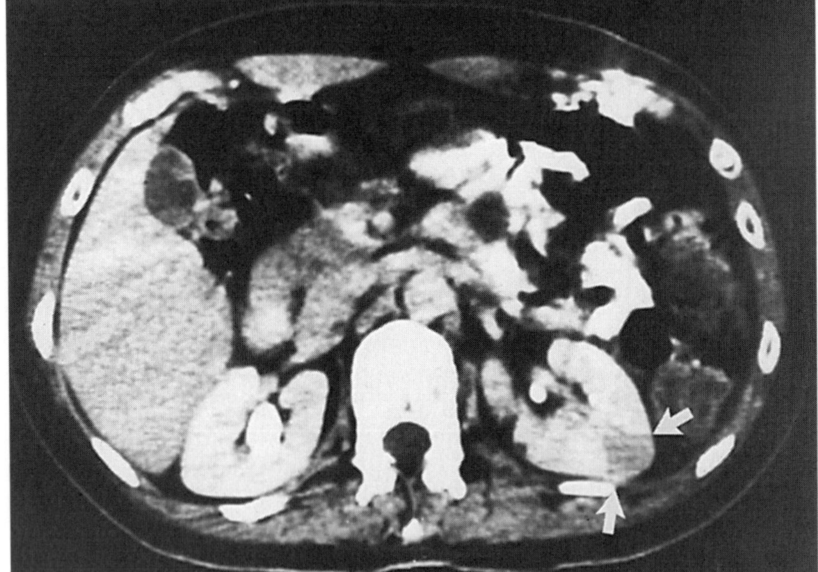

FIGURE 4.12. Acute focal bacterial nephritis. **A:** Excretory urogram. Five-minute tomogram demonstrates normally functioning upper and lower poles and a poorly marginated midrenal mass with poor function and absent collecting system visualization. **B:** Ultrasound; longitudinal view of the left kidney demonstrates spleen *(S)* and left kidney *(arrows).* Note irregular midpole mass *(M)* of slightly higher echo texture than surrounding normal renal parenchyma. **C:** Contrast-enhanced computed tomography scan demonstrates a wedge-shaped area of low density *(arrows)* in the middle portion of the left kidney. The findings resolved after antibiotic therapy.

more reasonable to postulate that impaired host response caused by local factors, such as obstruction, or a systemic condition, such as diabetes, allows organisms with the capability of producing carbon dioxide to use necrotic tissue as a substrate to generate gas *in vivo.* Thus emphysematous pyelonephritis should be considered a complication of severe pyelonephritis rather than a distinct entity.

Clinical Findings

All of the documented cases of emphysematous pyelonephritis have occurred in adults (130). Juvenile diabetic patients do not appear to be at risk. Women are affected more often than men.

The usual clinical presentation is severe, acute pyelonephritis, although in some instances, a chronic infection precedes the acute attack. Almost all patients display the classic triad of fever, vomiting, and flank pain (303). Pneumaturia is absent unless the infection involves the collecting system. Results of urine cultures are invariably positive. *E. coli* is most commonly identified. *Klebsiella* and *Proteus* are less common.

Radiologic Findings

The diagnosis is established radiographically. Tissue gas that is distributed in the parenchyma may appear on abdominal x-ray films as mottled gas shadows over the involved kidney

(Fig. 4.13). This finding is often mistaken for bowel gas. A crescentic collection of gas over the upper pole of the kidney is more distinctive. As the infection progresses, gas extends to the perinephric space and retroperitoneum. This distribution of gas should not be confused with cases of emphysematous pyelitis in which air is in the collecting system of the kidney. Emphysematous pyelitis is secondary to a gas-forming bacterial urinary tract infection, often occurs in nondiabetic patients, is less serious, and usually responds to antimicrobial therapy.

Excretory urography is rarely of value in emphysematous pyelonephritis because the affected kidney usually is nonfunctioning or poorly functioning. Because of the significant risk of contrast nephropathy in critically ill, dehydrated diabetic patients with abnormal renal function, retrograde pyelography rather than excretory urography is advisable to demonstrate obstruction. Obstruction is demonstrated in approximately 25% of the cases. Ultrasonography usually demonstrates strong focal echoes suggesting the presence of intraparenchymal gas (27,53). CT is the imaging procedure of choice in defining the extent of the emphysematous process and guiding management (Fig. 4.14). An absence of fluid in CT images or the presence of streaky or mottled gas with or without bubbly and loculated gas appears to be associated with rapid destruction of renal parenchyma and a 50% to 60% mortality rate (19,376). The presence of renal or perirenal fluid, the presence of bubbly or loculated gas or gas in the collecting system, and the absence of streaky or mottled gas patterns is associated with a less than 20% mortality rate. A nuclear renal scan should be performed to assess the degree of renal function impairment in the involved kidney and the status of the contralateral kidney.

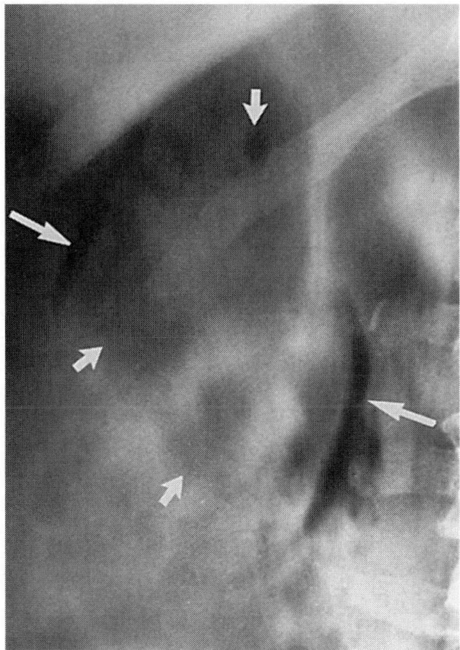

FIGURE 4.13. Emphysematous pyelonephritis; plain film. Extensive perinephric *(long arrows)* and intraparenchymal *(short arrows)* gas secondary to acute bacterial pyelonephritis.

Management

Emphysematous pyelonephritis is a surgical emergency. Most patients are septic, and fluid resuscitation and broad-spectrum antimicrobial therapy are essential. If the kidney is functioning, medical therapy can be considered (19,376). Nephrectomy is recommended for patients who do not improve after a few days of therapy (73). If the affected kidney is nonfunctioning and not obstructed, nephrectomy should be performed because medical treatment alone is usually lethal. If a kidney is obstructed, catheter drainage must be instituted. If the patient's condition improves, nephrectomy may be deferred pending a complete urologic evaluation. Although there are isolated case reports of retention of renal function after medical therapy combined with relief of obstruction, most patients require nephrectomy (149).

Renal Abscess

Renal abscess or carbuncle is a collection of purulent material confined to the renal parenchyma. Before the antimicrobial era, 80% of renal abscesses were attributed to hematogenous seeding by staphylococci (36). Although experimental and clinical data document the facility for abscess formation in normal kidneys after hematogenous inoculation with staphylococci, widespread use of antimicrobials in the past 25 years appears to have diminished the propensity for Gram-positive abscess formation (57,64).

During the past two decades, Gram-negative organisms have been implicated in many adults with renal abscesses. Hematogenous renal seeding by Gram-negative organisms may occur, but this is not likely to be the primary pathway for Gram-negative abscess formation. Clinically, there is no evidence that Gram-negative septicemia antedates most lesions. Furthermore, Gram-negative hematogenous pyelonephritis is virtually impossible to produce in animals unless the kidney is traumatized or completely obstructed (57,362). The partially obstructed kidney rejects blood-borne Gram-negative inocula, as does a normal kidney. Thus ascending infection associated with tubular obstruction from prior infections or calculi appears to be the primary pathway for establishment of Gram-negative abscesses. Two-thirds of Gram-negative abscesses in adults are associated with renal calculi or damaged kidneys (290) (Fig. 4.15). Although the association of pyelonephritis with vesicoureteral reflux is well established, the association of renal abscess with vesicoureteral reflux has rarely been noted in the past (310). However, it has been observed that reflux often is associated with renal abscesses and persists long after sterilization of the urinary tract (362).

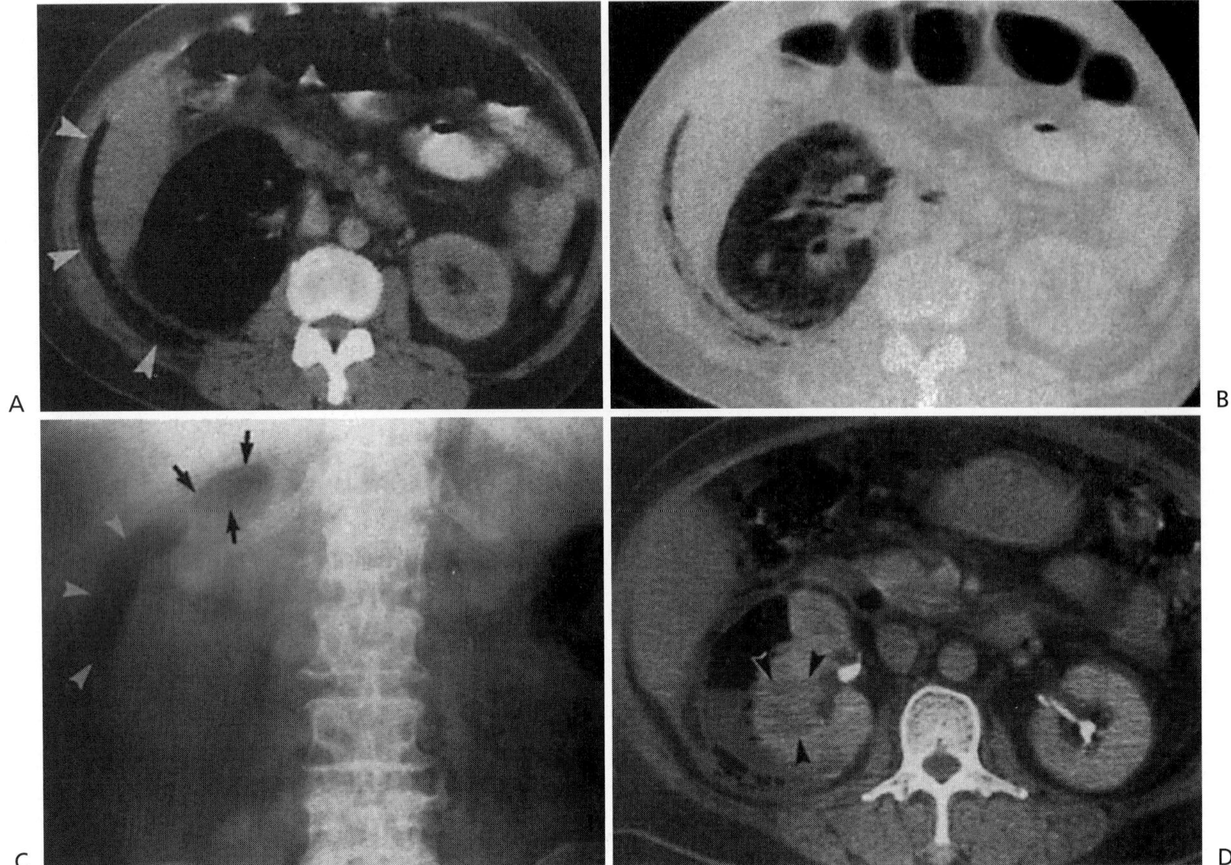

FIGURE 4.14. **A, B:** Type I emphysematous pyelonephritis (EPN) with complete renal destruction in a 49-year-old woman. **A:** Computed tomography (CT) scan of the right kidney shows complete destruction with gas *(arrowheads)* extending beyond the renal fascia. **B:** CT scan with a modified lung window display shows the characteristic streaky gas in the completely destroyed kidney. The patient died on arrival in the emergency department before nephrectomy was attempted. **C, D:** Type II EPN in a 57-year-old woman. **C:** Radiograph shows crescent-shaped *(arrowheads)* and loculated *(arrows)* gas in the right renal area. **D:** CT image obtained after administration of contrast material shows a low-attenuation area *(arrowheads)* in the right kidney due to acute pyelonephritis as well as a subcapsular abscess with fluid, bubbly, and loculated gas. The patient survived after percutaneous drainage was performed.

Clinical Findings

The patient's symptoms may include fever, chills, abdominal or flank pain, and occasionally, weight loss and malaise. Lower urinary tract infections, including cystitis, also usually occur. Occasionally, these symptoms may be vague and delay diagnosis until surgical exploration or, in more severe cases, at autopsy (5). A thorough history may reveal a Gram-positive source of infection 1 to 8 weeks before the onset of urinary tract symptoms. The infection may have occurred in any area of the body. Multiple skin carbuncles and intravenous drug abuse introduce Gram-positive organisms into the bloodstream. Other common sites are the mouth, lungs, and bladder (205). Complicated urinary tract infections associated with stasis, calculi, pregnancy, neurogenic bladder, and diabetes mellitus also appear to predispose the patient to abscess formation (5).

Laboratory Findings

The patient typically has marked leukocytosis. The blood cultures are usually positive. Pyuria and bacteriuria may not be evident unless the abscess communicates with the collecting system. Because Gram-positive organisms are most commonly blood borne, urine cultures in these cases will typically show no growth or a microorganism different from that isolated from the abscess. When the abscess contains Gram-negative organisms, the urine culture usually demonstrates the same organism isolated from the abscess.

Radiologic Findings

The urographic findings depend on both the nature and the duration of the infection. In patients in whom abscess formation has progressed from an episode of acute bacterial nephritis or those in whom the kidney has been seeded by an outside infection, radiologic examination may demonstrate generalized renal enlargement with distortion of the renal contour on the affected side. There also may be renal fixation evident on inspiratory and expiratory films and obliteration of the corresponding psoas shadow. Scoliosis is often present, with a concavity of the curve facing the affected kidney. If renal involvement is diffuse, the nephrogram will be delayed or even absent. When an abscess is more localized, the findings may be similar to those of acute focal bacterial nephritis.

In a more chronic abscess, the predominant urographic abnormalities are those of a renal mass lesion (Fig 4.15). The calyceal system may be poorly defined or show distortion or even amputation. Nephrotomography usually reveals a relative radiolucency in the involved area. Occasionally, the excretory urogram will appear normal despite the presence of a renal abscess, particularly if the abscess involves the anterior or posterior portion of the kidney without impinging on the parenchyma or collecting system.

CT appears to be the diagnostic procedure of choice for renal abscesses because it provides excellent delineation of the tissue. On CT, abscesses are characteristically well defined both before and after contrast enhancement. Initially, CT shows renal enlargement and focal, rounded areas of decreased attenuation (Fig 4.16A). After several days of the onset of the infection, a thick, fibrotic wall begins to form around the abscess. CT of a chronic abscess shows obliteration of adjacent tissue planes, thickening of Gerota's fascia, and a round or oval parenchymal mass of low attenuation that forms a ring when the scan is enhanced with contrast material (Fig 4.17A). The ring sign is caused by the increased vascularity of the abscess wall.

Ultrasonography is the quickest and least expensive method to demonstrate a renal abscess. An echo-free or low-echo-density space-occupying lesion with increased transmission is found on the sonogram. The margins of an abscess are indistinguishable in the acute phase, but the structure contains a few echoes, and the surrounding renal parenchyma is edematous (Fig 4.16B). Subsequently, the appearance tends to be that of a well-defined mass. However, the internal appearance may vary from a virtually solid lucent mass to one with large numbers of low-level internal echoes (Fig 4.17B). The number of echoes depends on the amount of cellular debris within the abscess. Presence of air results in a strong echo with a shadow. Differentiation between an abscess and a chronic tumor is impossible in many cases. Arteriography is used occasionally to demonstrate abscesses. The center of the mass tends to be hypovascular or avascular, with increased vascularity at the cortical margins and lack of vascular displacement and neovascularity.

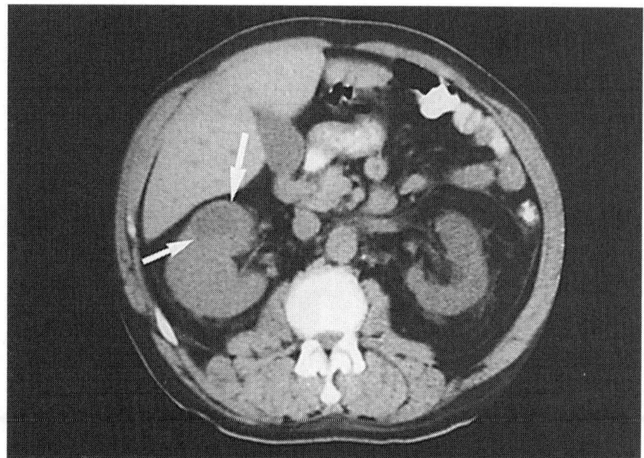

A

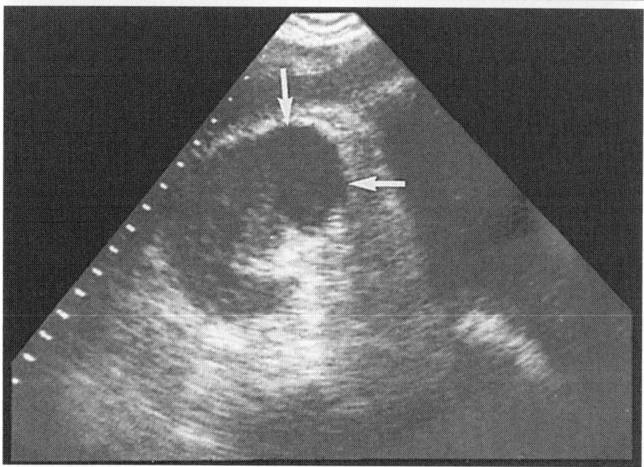

B

FIGURE 4.16. Acute renal abscess. **A:** Nonenhanced computed tomography scan through the midpole of the right kidney demonstrates right renal enlargement and an area of decreased attenuation *(arrows)*. After antimicrobial therapy, follow-up scan showed complete regression of these findings. **B:** Ultrasound. Transverse scan of the right kidney demonstrates a poorly marginated rounded focal hypoechoic mass *(arrows)* in the anterior portion of the kidney.

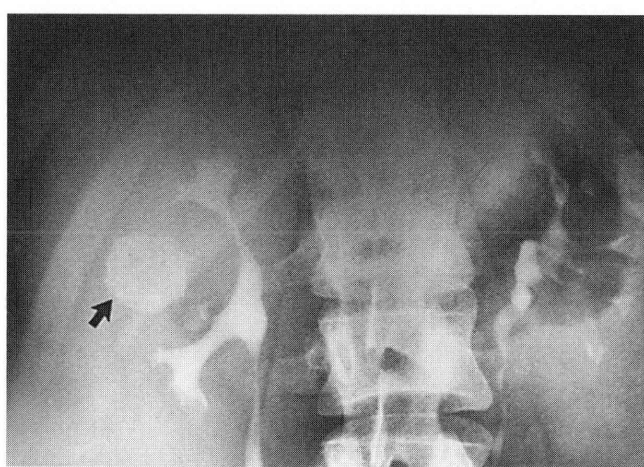

FIGURE 4.15. Renal abscess associated with infection stone. Excretory urogram. Twenty-minute film demonstrates a large, right midpole calculus *(arrow)*. Abscess associated with this infection stone causes displacement of adjacent collecting system.

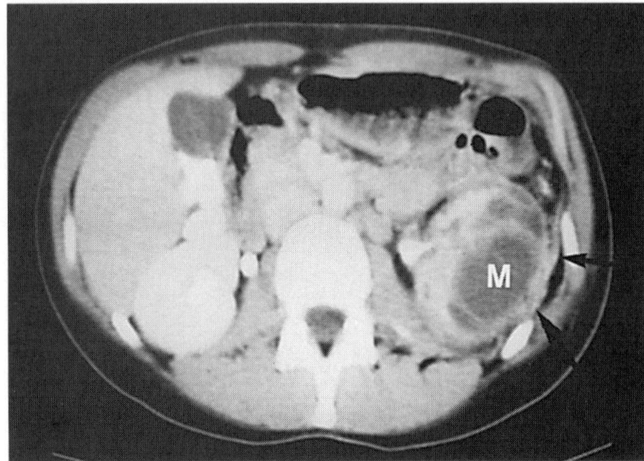

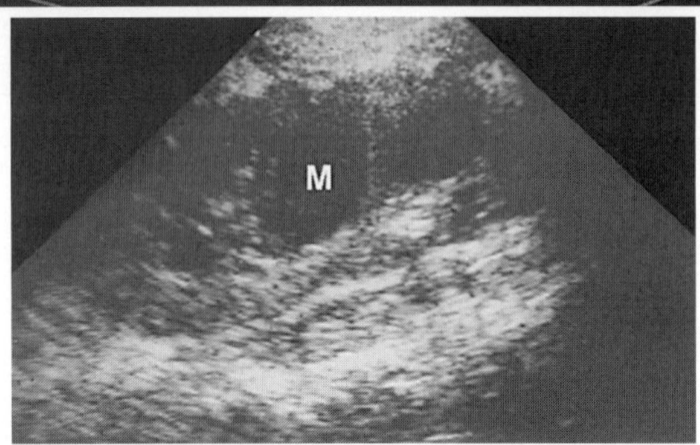

FIGURE 4.17. Chronic renal abscess. **A:** Enhanced computed tomography scan shows irregular septated low-density mass *(M)* extensively involving the left kidney. Note thickening of perinephric fascia *(arrows)* and extensive compression of the renal collecting system. Findings are typical of renal abscess. **B:** Ultrasound. Longitudinal scan demonstrates septated hypoechoic mass *(M)* occupying much of the renal parenchymal volume.

Radionucleotide imaging with gallium or indium is sometimes useful in evaluating patients with renal abscesses. The exact mode of gallium-67 localization in tissues is not clear. Suggested possible mechanisms include concentration within labeled polymorphonuclear leukocytes, leakage of protein-bound gallium through capillaries, and increased vascularity of the lesion. Delayed imaging is often necessary. Gallium is a nonspecific method of identifying an inflammatory lesion; more important, it lacks anatomic detail. In addition, gallium is excreted into the colon and sequestered in postsurgical beds, inflammatory sites, and tumors; therefore the interpretation of gallium scans can be extremely difficult.

Indium-111–labeled leukocyte scanning is a clinically effective method for detecting inflammatory diseases and abscesses. Indium-111–labeled leukocytes accumulate only in sites of inflammation and not in normal kidneys or in tumors. Thus their presence appears highly specific for inflammation. However, the indium scan has limitations. Hyperalimentation and hyperglycemia can prevent the accumulation at the site of inflammation, and the distribution of leukocytes is altered in patients who have had splenectomy or bone marrow radiation. The necessity of high doses of radiation with indium scanning may make it unsuitable for pediatric patients (107).

Ultrasonography and CT identify more than 90% of abscesses (91,316). Ultrasonography demonstrates a hypoechoic mass with irregular walls and acoustic shadowing if gas is present. CT scan findings depend in part on the age and severity of the abscess (16).

Management

Although the classic treatment for an abscess has been incision and drainage, there has been good evidence that the use of intravenous antimicrobials and careful observation of a small abscess less than 3 cm in diameter, if begun early enough in the course of the process, may obviate surgical procedures (198).

When hematogenous dissemination is suspected, the pathogenic organism most commonly is penicillin-resistant *Staphylococcus,* and the antibiotic of choice therefore is a penicillinase-resistant penicillin (305). If a history of penicillin hypersensitivity is present, the recommended drug is either cephalosporin or vancomycin. Cortical abscesses that occur in the abnormal urinary tract are associated with more typical Gram-negative pathogens and should be treated empirically with intravenous third-generation cephalosporins, antipseudomonal penicillins, or aminoglycosides until specific therapy can be instituted. These individuals can have follow-up with ultrasonography or CT until the abscess resolves. A clinical course contrary to this should lead to the suspicion of misdiagnosis or an uncontrolled infection with development of perinephric abscess or infection with an organism resistant to the antimicrobials used in therapy. In these instances, drainage is usually necessary.

CT- or ultrasound-guided needle aspiration may be necessary to differentiate a small abscess from a hypovascular tumor. Aspirated material can be cultured and appropriate antimicrobial therapy instituted on the basis of the findings. Abscesses larger than 3 cm and smaller abscesses in immunocompromised hosts or those that do not respond to antimicrobial therapy should be drained percutaneously (91,316). However, surgical drainage currently remains the procedure of choice for most renal abscesses greater than 5 cm in diameter.

Infected Hydronephrosis and Pyonephrosis

If bacterial infection occurs in a hydronephrotic kidney, a purulent exudate will collect in the renal collecting system. Pyonephrosis refers to infected hydronephrosis associated with suppurative destruction of the parenchyma of the kidney, with total or near-total loss of renal function (Fig.

4.18). The point at which infected hydronephrosis ends and pyonephrosis begins is difficult to determine.

Clinical Findings

The clinical presentation is variable, ranging from no complaints to urosepsis. However, many patients will be ill with fever, chills, and flank pain and tenderness. A history of urinary tract calculi, infection, or surgery is common. Bacteriuria may not be present if the ureter is completely obstructed. Wu and colleagues (398) observed significantly higher erythrocyte sedimentation rates and C-reactive protein levels in patients with infected hydronephrosis or pyonephroses compared with those with simple hydronephrosis. A cutoff of erythrocyte sedimentation rate greater than 100 mm per hour and C-reactive protein of 3 mg/dL yielded a specificity and sensitivity of 89% and 100%, respectively, and a diagnostic accuracy of 97%. Changes in these parameters can be used to evaluate the effectiveness of antimicrobial therapy.

Radiologic Findings

The ultrasonographic diagnosis of infected hydronephrosis depends on demonstration of internal echoes within the dependent portion of a dilated pyelocalyceal system. CT scan is nonspecific but may show thickening of the renal pelvis, stranding of the perirenal fat, and a striated nephrogram. The urographic findings are those of urinary tract obstruction and depend on the degree and duration of obstruction. Typically, the obstruction is longstanding, and excretory urography shows a poorly functioning or nonfunctioning hydronephrotic kidney. Ultrasound demonstrates hydronephrosis and fluid debris levels within the dilated collecting system (56) (Fig 4.19A). The diagnosis of pyonephrosis is suggested if focal areas of decreased echogenicity are seen within the hydronephrotic parenchyma.

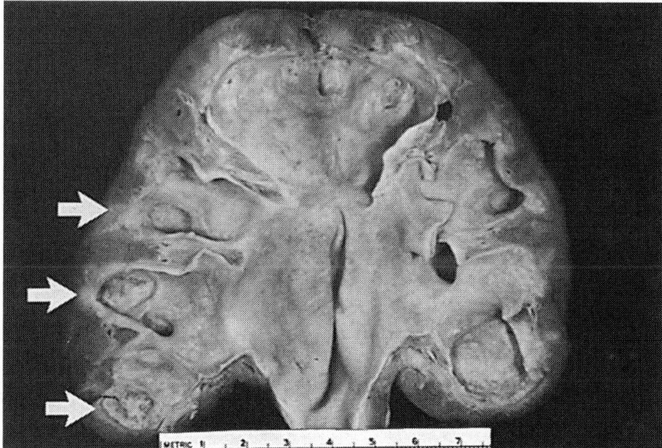

FIGURE 4.18. Pyonephrosis; gross specimen. Kidney shows marked thinning of renal cortex and medulla, suppurative destruction of the parenchyma *(arrows),* and distention of the pelvis and calyces. Previous incision released large quantity of purulent material. Ureter showed obstruction distal to the point of section.

Management

Appropriate intravenous antimicrobial therapy is important, but immediate drainage of the kidney is mandatory. Percutaneous nephrostomy (Fig. 4.19B) or retrograde ureteral catheterization (or, if necessary, open nephrostomy) must be performed. When the patient's condition has stabilized, appropriate corrective surgery or nephrectomy can be performed depending on the patient's age, the cause and type of obstruction, and the degree of renal function impairment.

Perinephric Abscess

Perinephric abscess (PNA) usually results from rupture of an acute cortical abscess into the perinephric space. Patients with pyonephrosis, particularly when a calculus is present in the kidney, are susceptible to perinephric abscess formation. Diabetes mellitus is present in approximately one-third of patients with perinephric abscess (70,361). In about one-third of the cases, perinephric abscess is caused by hematogenous spread, usually from sites of skin infection. A perirenal hematoma can become secondarily infected by the hematogenous route or by direct extension of a primary renal infection. Rarely, perinephric or psoas abscess may be the result of bowel perforation, Crohn's disease, or spread of osteomyelitis from the thoracolumbar spine. *E. coli, Proteus,* and *S. aureus* account for most infections.

Clinical Findings

The onset of symptoms is typically insidious. Symptoms have been present for more than 5 days in most patients with perinephric abscess compared with only about 10% of patients with pyelonephritis. The clinical presentation may be similar to that of pyelonephritis; however, more than one-third of patients may be afebrile. An abdominal or flank mass can be felt in about half of the cases. Psoas abscess should be suspected if the patient has a limp and flexion and external rotation of the ipsilateral hip. Laboratory features include leukocytosis, elevated levels of serum creatinine, and pyuria in more than 75% of cases. Edelstein and McCabe (70) showed that results of urine cultures predicted PNA isolates in only 37% of cases; a blood culture, particularly with multiple organisms, was often indicative of perinephric abscess, but identified all organisms in only 42% of cases. Therefore therapy based on the results of urine and blood cultures often may be inadequate. Pyelonephritis usually responds within 4 to 5 days of appropriate antibiotic therapy; perinephritic abscess does not. Thus perinephric abscess should be suspected in a patient with urinary tract

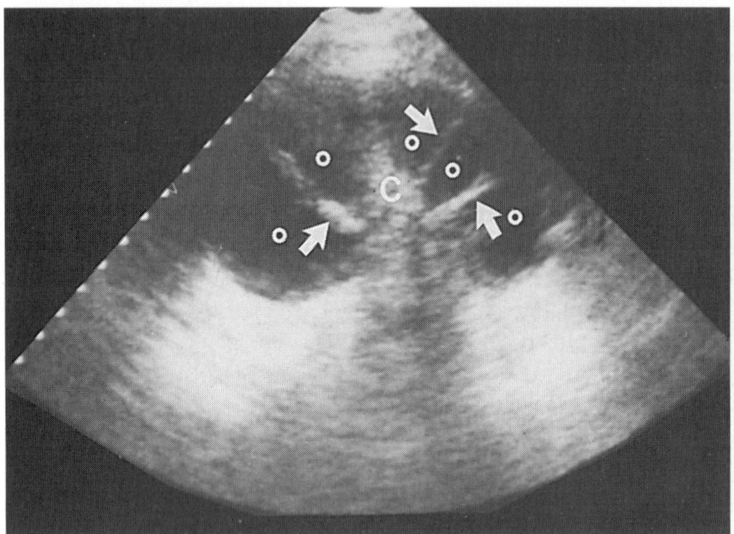

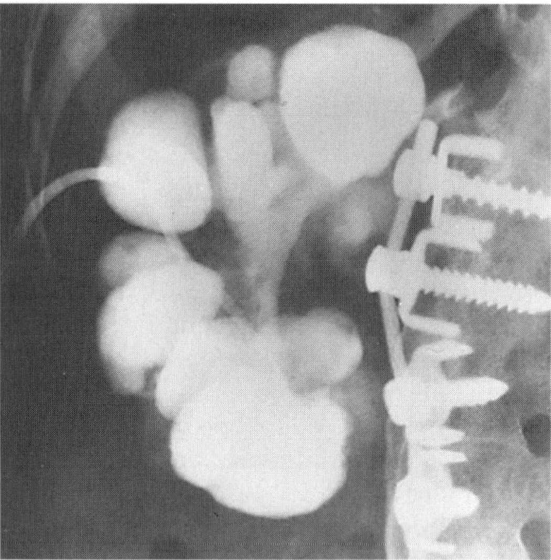

FIGURE 4.19. Pyonephrosis. **A:** Ultrasound. Longitudinal scan of the right kidney demonstrates echogenic central collecting complex *(C)* with radiating echogenic septae *(arrows)* and thinned hypoechoic parenchyma. Multiple dilated calyces *(o)* with diffuse low-level echoes are seen. **B:** Antegrade pyelogram performed through a percutaneous nephrostomy catheter correlates well with the ultrasound image. Dilated pus-filled calyces are demonstrated. The renal pelvis is obliterated by chronic scarring and stone disease. The kidney did not regain function.

infection and abdominal or flank mass or persistent fever after 4 days of antimicrobial therapy.

Radiologic Findings

Excretory urography is abnormal in 80% of cases. However, the abnormalities are not specific. Classically, the radiographic features of perinephric abscess have been the absence of psoas shadow, a mass in the perirenal area often associated with indistinct renal outlines, and an elevated or immobile diaphragm. With large abscesses, the soft tissue density may extend to the pelvis following the renal fascia. In patients with perinephric abscess secondary to gas-forming organisms, bubbled collections of extraluminal gas are seen surrounding the kidney (203). CT is particularly valuable for demonstrating the primary abscess. In some cases, the abscess is confined to the perinephric space; however, extension to the flank or psoas muscle may occur (Fig. 4.20). CT is able to show with exquisite anatomic detail the route of spread of infection into the surrounding tissues. This information may be helpful in planning the approach for surgical drainage. Ultrasound demonstrates a diverse sonographic appearance ranging from a nearly anechoic mass displacing the kidney to an echogenic collection that tends to blend with normally echogenic fat within Gerota's fascia (56).

Occasionally, a retroperitoneal or subdiaphragmatic infection may spread to the paranephric fat that is outside Gerota's fascia. The clinical symptoms of insidious onset of fever, flank mass, and tenderness are indistinguishable from those associated with perinephric abscess. Urinary tract

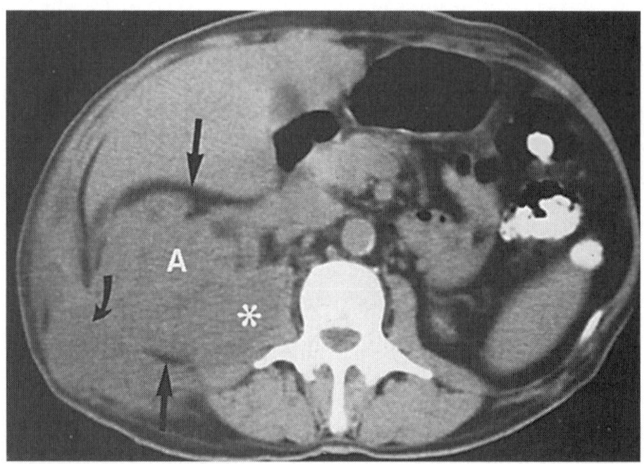

FIGURE 4.20. Extensive perinephric abscess. Nonenhanced computed tomography scan through the lower pole of the right kidney (previous left nephrectomy). Extensive abscess *(A)* distorts and enlarges renal contour, infiltrates perinephric fat *(arrows),* and also extends into the psoas muscle *(asterisk)* and the soft tissues of the flank *(curved arrow).* Also note that normal renal collecting system fat has been obliterated by the process.

infection, however, is absent. Ultrasonography and CT can usually delineate the abscess outside Gerota's fascia (Fig. 4.21).

Management

Once the diagnosis of perinephric or paranephric abscess is established, the primary treatment is surgical drainage. Gram stain identifies the pathogenesis and guides antimi-

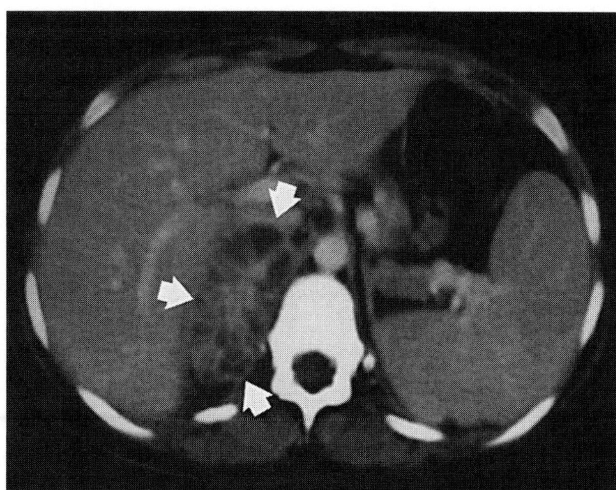

FIGURE 4.21. Perinephric abscess involving the right adrenal gland. Computed tomography scan. Large right pararenal mass *(arrows)* with multiple low-density areas within. At surgery, a large pararenal abscess with extensive involvement of the right adrenal was found.

crobial therapy. An aminoglycoside together with an antistaphylococcal agent, such as methicillin or oxacillin, should be started immediately. If the patient has a penicillin hypersensitivity, cephalothin or vancomycin may be used.

Once the perinephric abscess has been drained, the underlying problem must be dealt with. Some conditions, such as renal cortical abscess or enteric communication, require prompt attention. Nephrectomy for pyonephrosis may be performed concurrent with drainage of the perinephric abscess if the patient's condition is good. In other instances, it is best to drain the perinephric abscess first and correct the underlying problem or perform a nephrectomy when the patient's condition has improved.

Chronic Pyelonephritis

In patients without underlying renal or urinary tract disease, chronic pyelonephritis secondary to urinary tract infection is a rare disease and an even more rare cause of chronic renal failure. In patients with underlying functional or structural urinary tract abnormalities, however, chronic renal infection can cause significant renal impairment. Hence, it is essential that appropriate studies be used to diagnose, localize, and treat chronic renal infection.

The prevalence of chronic pyelonephritis has also been assessed in patients undergoing dialysis for end-stage renal disease. Despite a 2% to 5% prevalence of bacteriuria in women, only 1,000 to 2,000 women have end-stage renal disease as a result of pyelonephritis. Schechter and colleagues (304) analyzed the cause for renal failure in 170 patients referred to them for dialysis. Chronic pyelonephritis was the primary cause of end-stage renal disease in 22 (13%) but was usually associated with an underlying structural defect. Unequivocal nonobstructive chronic pyelonephritis was not found. The authors also observed that symptomatic infections tended to occur before the onset of azotemia in most patients with chronic pyelonephritis. Similarly, Huland and Busch (151) evaluated 161 patients with end-stage renal disease and found that 42 had chronic pyelonephritis. However, in addition to a history of urinary tract infections, these 42 patients had complicating defects, such as vesicoureteral reflux, analgesic abuse, nephrolithiasis, or obstruction. Nonobstructive uncomplicated urinary tract infection alone was never found to be the cause of renal insufficiency. Thus, using end-stage renal disease seen at autopsy or at the dialysis clinic as an indicator, the prevalence of uncomplicated chronic bacterial pyelonephritis is rare.

In addition, the role of bacterial infection in development of chronic renal disease can be assessed in patients with renal interstitial and tubular damage similar to that which has classically been called *chronic pyelonephritis.* The frequency with which various potential causes of interstitial damage are operative in patients with interstitial nephritis was assessed by Murray and Goldberg (234). These investigators not only concluded that urinary tract infection is rarely the sole cause of chronic renal disease in the adult, but they also observed that 89% of their azotemic patients had a readily identifiable primary cause of their interstitial nephritis. Thus, when patients with a clinical diagnosis of chronic interstitial nephritis are selected as the starting point, it is easy to associate many factors with this disease, but urinary tract infection does not seem to be one of them.

Clinical Findings

There are no symptoms of chronic pyelonephritis until it produces renal insufficiency, and then the symptoms are similar to those of any other form of chronic renal failure. If a patient's chronic pyelonephritis is thought to be an end result of many episodes of acute pyelonephritis, a history of intermittent symptoms of fever, flank pain, and dysuria may be elicited. Similarly, urinary findings and the presence of renal infection correlate poorly. Bacteriuria and pyuria, the hallmarks of urinary tract infection, are not predictive of renal infection. Conversely, patients with significant renal infection may have sterile urine if the ureter draining the kidney is obstructed or the infection is outside of the collecting system.

The pathologic and radiologic criteria for diagnosing renal infection may also be misleading. Asscher (7a) has tabulated eight long-term follow-up studies from the literature on kidneys of adults with urinary tract infections. The data from these reports on 901 patients show that bacteriuria present in otherwise healthy adults for long periods may be associated with nonexistent or extremely minimum evidence of kidney damage. Conversely, patients who have chronic pyelonephritis may have negative urine cultures.

Radiologic Findings

The diagnosis of chronic pyelonephritis can be made with the greatest confidence on the basis of pyelographic findings. The essential features are asymmetry and irregularity of the kidney outlines, blunting and dilation of one or more calyces, and cortical scars at the corresponding site (Fig. 4.22). In the absence of stones, obstruction, and tuberculosis, and with the single exception of analgesic nephritis with papillary necrosis (which can be readily excluded by history), chronic pyelonephritis is virtually the only disease that produces a localized scar over a deformed calyx (331). In advanced pyelonephritis, calyceal distortion and irregularity together with cortical scars complete the picture. Hodson (135) pointed out that renal infarction, an extremely rare condition, may closely resemble pyelonephritic scars but that the renal pyramid remains with renal infarction in contradistinction to pyelonephritis.

Management

Management of radiographic evidence of pyelonephritis should be directed at treating infection, if present; preventing future infections; and monitoring and preserving renal function. The treatment of existing infection must be based on careful antimicrobial susceptibility tests and selection of drugs that can achieve bactericidal concentrations in the urine and yet are not nephrotoxic. Achievement of acceptable bactericidal levels of a drug in the urine of a patient with chronic pyelonephritis may be difficult because the diminished concentrating ability of pyelonephritis may impair excretion and concentration of the antimicrobial agent. The duration of antimicrobial therapy is often prolonged to maximize the chance of cure. With patients in whom renal damage develops or progresses in the presence of urinary tract infection, the working hypothesis should be that there is an underlying renal, usually papillary, lesion or underlying urologic condition, such as obstruction or calculus, that has increased susceptibility to renal damage. Appropriate nephrologic and urologic evaluation should be undertaken to identify and, if possible, correct these abnormalities.

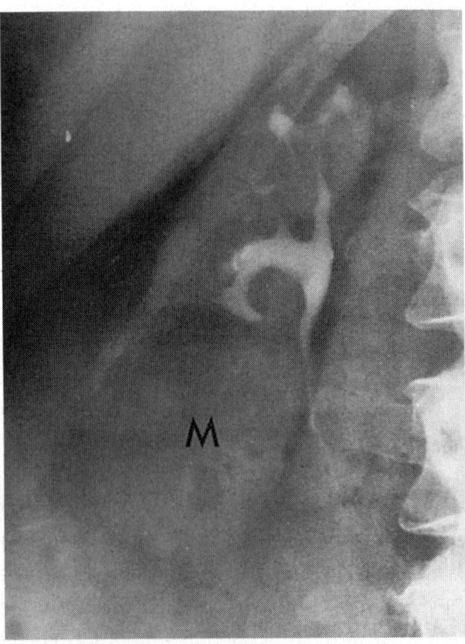

FIGURE 4.22. Chronic pyelonephritis. Excretory urogram. Ten-minute film demonstrates irregular renal outline with upper pole parenchymal atrophy. Note significant loss of renal cortical thickness over blunted and dilated calyces. Lower pole mass *(M)* is a simple cyst.

Bacterial "Relapse" from a Normal Kidney

The concept that bacteria persist in the renal parenchyma between bacteriuric episodes and cause "relapsing" urinary tract infections was based on a study by Turck and colleagues (366) that suggested that bacterial persistence could be recognized by simply identifying two consecutive recurrent infections with the same organism. Unfortunately, this study did not indicate whether the urine was cultured during therapy to ensure that the original infection had actually been eradicated. It is possible that some of these so-called relapses were in fact unresolved initial infections and that ureteral edema associated with catheterization may have impeded clearance of the initial infecting strain.

Subsequent studies summarized by Stamey (331) and Forland and associates (90) have shown that in a normal urinary tract recurrent infections are not caused by relapse from bacterial persistence in the kidney. With ureteral catheterization techniques, Cattell and associates (39) localized the site of bacteriuria in 42 patients who had follow-up for 6 months after therapy. They analyzed the response to antimicrobial therapy of 2 weeks' duration. Of the 26 patients who were cured of their initial infection, 16 had recurrence with the same organism; 8 had upper tract infections, and 8 had bladder bacteriuria.

If bacterial persistence in the kidney is a major problem after therapy, one would expect that patients who have more recurrent infections would also have more relapses than those who have less frequent recurrences. Mabeck (206) analyzed this, however, and found that with an increasing number of recurrences, the relationship among treatment failure, relapse, and reinfection remained unchanged. Thus bacteria do not persist in normal kidneys between recurrent urinary tract infections (331), and recurrences with the same strain are not caused by "relapse" from the kidney.

INFECTIOUS GRANULOMATOUS NEPHRITIS

Renal Tuberculosis

Tuberculosis is an acute or chronic infectious disease that in the United States is usually caused by *Mycobacterium tuberculosis. Mycobacterium bovis, Mycobacterium kansasii,* and *Mycobacterium intracellulare* are rare causes of tuberculosis.

Mycobacteria customarily gain access to the human body by inhalation, although the bovine organisms may be acquired by ingestion of unpasteurized milk. After initiation of the tuberculous infection, a primary pathologic focus develops, which usually heals spontaneously. In addition, the primary infection often results in an initial silent bacillemia that is responsible for systemic spread of *Mycobacterium* with latent infection of many organs. These latent foci of tuberculous infection may break down and result in overt tuberculosis of the kidney or other organs many years later. Bacillemia and seeding of the kidneys or other organs may also occur from a focus of progressive primary or reactivation tuberculosis in the lung or from clinically evident secondary tuberculosis in other organs. Therefore any individual who has previously been infected with tuberculosis is at risk for developing renal involvement.

Renal infection is among the most common sites for extrapulmonary tuberculosis. Approximately 5% of the estimated 250,000 patients with active tuberculosis in the United States have cavitary tuberculosis of the genitourinary tract (236,323,381). Thirty percent to 50% of patients with renal tuberculosis have had previous tuberculous pulmonary disease documented by history or implied from chest roentgenograms (320). However, it is uncommon for pulmonary tuberculosis to be active at the time of diagnosis of renal tuberculosis. Although effective chemotherapy has resulted in a significant decrease in the prevalence of pulmonary tuberculosis, the frequency of renal tuberculosis has not declined significantly in recent decades (197,236).

Pathology and Pathogenesis

In the hematogenous phase that takes place after the primary infection, both kidneys are seeded with tubercle bacilli in 90% of cases. However, clinically apparent renal tuberculosis is usually unilateral. The initial lesions involve the renal cortex with multiple small granulomas in the glomeruli and in the juxtaglomerular regions. With patients in whom acquired cellular immunity develops, there is inhibition of bacterial multiplication and containment of the disease process to the renal cortex. Microscopic examination reveals central caseation necrosis surrounded by pink staining epithelial histiocytes, Langhans' giant cells, and more peripherally, lymphocytes and plasma cells (125). Most patients are asymptomatic and have normal findings on radiologic examination. The asymptomatic cortical disease may be stable for many years and an incidental finding at nephrectomy or autopsy. These early lesions may resolve completely either spontaneously or as a result of treatment.

In untreated patients who fail to heal spontaneously, the lesions may progress slowly and remain asymptomatic for variable periods. In most individuals, the latent period between initial exposure and reactivation of renal disease is 10 to 40 years (320) and may be increased by appropriate therapy (236). The cortical areas of infection may seed the glomerular filtrate, creating lesions in the tubules and Henle's loop, resulting in additional foci in the renal pyramid. As the lesions progress, they produce areas of caseous necrosis, chronic interstitial nephritis with papillary necrosis, and parenchymal cavitation (Fig. 4.23). Large, tumorlike parenchymal lesions or tuberculomas often have a fibrous wall and can resemble a solid mass lesion. Their content may vary from caseous to calcified material (125). Larger blood vessels may show obliterative arteritis.

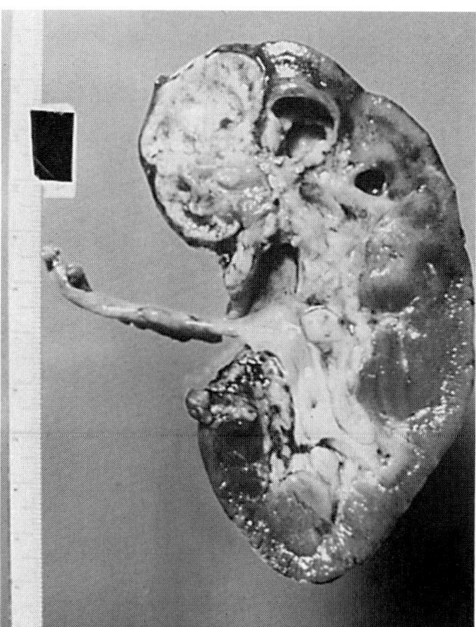

FIGURE 4.23. Tuberculoma, gross specimen. A destructive necrotic mass is present in the upper pole. (Reprinted with permission from Hartman DS. Radiologic pathologic correlation of the infectious granulomatous diseases of the kidney. I and II. *Monogr Urol* 1985;6:3.)

Once cavities form, spontaneous healing is rare and destructive lesions result. With necrotizing papillitis, there is spread of the infection to the renal pelvis, ureter, and bladder. The inflammation and edema produce obstruction of the infundibula and ureter, leading to caliectasis, calyceal clubbing, and ureteral strictures, with consequent pelvic and ureteral dilation. Extensive peripelvic fibrosis may cause a substantial decrease in the pelvic capacity (Fig. 4.24). With extensive renal tuberculosis, parenchymal calcification is often present, varying from faint punctate foci to a complete cast of the kidney. Total destruction of the kidney may occur, resulting in autonephrectomy (Fig. 4.25).

Seeding of the urine may also result in involvement of the bladder and male genital organs. Tuberculous inflammation in the bladder produces necrosis, ulceration, and fibrosis, which result in a thick-walled sac of small capacity.

Clinical Findings

Renal tuberculosis is predominantly a disease of young to middle-aged adults. Approximately 50% of the patients are

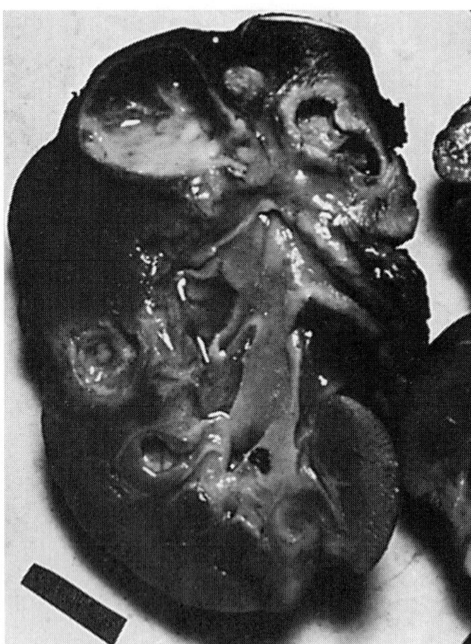

FIGURE 4.24. Tuberculosis with pelvic fibrosis. Gross specimen shows several large necrotic cavities. The peripelvic fibrosis has caused marked diminution in the pelvic volume. (Reprinted with permission from Hartman DS. Radiologic pathologic correlation of the infectious granulomatous diseases of the kidney. I and II. *Monogr Urol* 1985;6:3.)

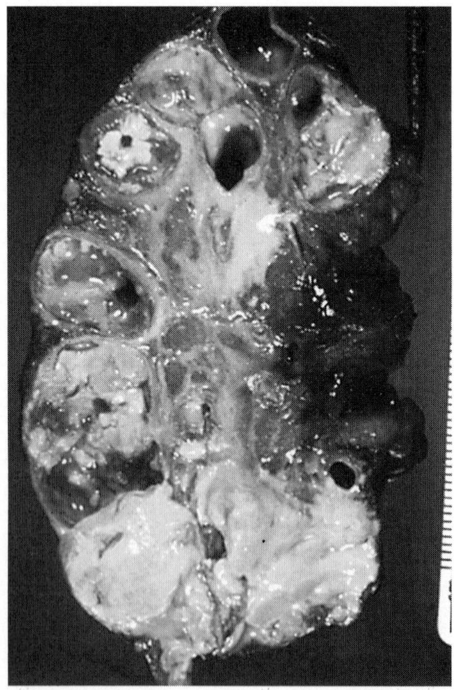

FIGURE 4.25. Tuberculosis, autonephrectomy. Gross specimen shows complete parenchymal destruction by extensive caseous necrosis. (Reprinted with permission from Hartman DS. Radiologic pathologic correlation of the infectious granulomatous diseases of the kidney. I and II. *Monogr Urol* 1985;6:3.)

20 to 40 years of age, and approximately 75% are younger than 50 years of age (247,381).

Because of the slow progression and variable course of the disease, there is no classic presentation. Approximately 20% of patients subsequently found to have tuberculosis will be symptom free. Tuberculous nephropathy is an insidious process that often goes unrecognized for long periods. Up to 70% of patients with even advanced cavitary tuberculosis of the kidney may have few diagnostic renal symptoms (22,193). Gross hematuria; dull, vague flank discomfort; and ureteral colic secondary to passage of clots, debris, or calculi are the most common renal symptoms. Constitutional complaints such as fevers, chills, night sweats, weight loss, and malaise are uncommon. It is only when the bladder is involved that the patients become severely symptomatic. Frequency is the most common presenting symptom and is often progressive and occurs during the day and at night. Pain, urgency, and dysuria are also common with bladder involvement.

The physical examination is usually not helpful diagnostically. A chronic draining fistula tract from previous renal surgery or palpably enlarged, firm seminal vesicles on rectal examination should arouse suspicion. Patients with chronic epididymitis unresponsive to therapy should also be evaluated for tuberculosis.

Patients may also have complications of renal tuberculosis, including draining sinus, hypertension, renal failure, secondary amyloidosis, and adenocarcinoma of the renal pelvis (20,88,187,352,383,392). A draining sinus or abscess cavity can occur many years after completion of chemotherapy even in the presence of sterile organs. Pyelocutaneous fistula is often associated with calculus obstruction of the ureteropelvic junction.

Hypertension is present in approximately 5% to 10% of patients with renal tuberculosis; the incidence in patients with unilateral nonfunctioning or poorly functioning kidneys is approximately 25%. Although some of these individuals have evidence of renal ischemia as determined by renal vein renin studies and normalization of blood pressure after nephrectomy, most patients appear to have hypertension that is not mediated by the renin-angiotensin system and is not cured by nephrectomy (246).

Laboratory Findings

The urinalysis is abnormal in 90% of the patients. The most common finding is sterile, acid pyuria, often accompanied by hematuria and proteinuria. Pyuria in the absence of a positive culture for the usual uropathogens should always warrant consideration of diagnosis of renal tuberculosis. Acid-fast smears of urinary concentrates are usually negative and are not totally reliable if positive because the saprophytic organism *Mycobacterium smegmatis* may contaminate the urine and is morphologically indistinguishable from *M. tuberculosis* on acid-fast smear.

The most important laboratory test is urine culture for

M. tuberculosis. Cultures are positive in approximately 90% of affected individuals (55). First-morning urine specimens are more reliable than 24-hour collections because they are easier to collect and there is much less chance of bacterial contamination. Because discharge of *M. tuberculosis* into the urine may be intermittent, it is advisable to collect morning urine specimens on a total of at least 3 separate days (236). Cultures should be obtained regardless of whether pus is present in the urine because positive cultures have been found in otherwise normal specimens (156). Susceptibility testing should be performed on isolated organisms.

Although the classic finding of renal tuberculosis is sterile pyuria, many patients have a concurrent positive culture for uropathogenic organisms at initial presentation. This finding should not preclude consideration of diagnosis of renal tuberculosis in the proper clinical setting. Such patients continue to demonstrate pyuria after the uropathogenic organism is eradicated by appropriate antimicrobial therapy.

The sealing off of cavitary lesions in chronic infections may in rare cases result in persistently negative findings on urine culture for tuberculosis and may mean that the disease in some patients remains undiagnosed despite repeated cultures (204). The tuberculin test, although not diagnostic, is of value only if positive.

Tuberculosis depresses renal function, but the damage has to be widespread before the serum creatinine level is elevated. Biochemical evidence of renal functional impairment is seen in less than 10% of patients with renal tuberculosis. Renal failure may be accentuated by obstructive uropathy that results from ureteral stricture or by secondary amyloidosis (210). Estimations of renal function are essential to preliminary assessment of patients with renal tuberculosis and determining the dose levels of antituberculous drugs. Wisnia and colleagues (392) showed that 58% of patients with renal tuberculosis had chronic renal failure at the time of diagnosis; 43% had subclinical impairment of creatinine clearance, 10% had compensated renal failure, and 5% had uremia.

It is apparent that the clinical presentation may be subtle, and therefore a high index of suspicion of renal tuberculosis is indicated in patients with a history of past or present tuberculosis, with chronic cystitis that fails to respond to adequate antimicrobial therapy, or with sterile pyuria accompanied by gross or microscopic hematuria.

Radiologic Findings

Approximately 90% of patients with renal tuberculosis will have abnormal excretory urograms. The roentgenographic findings vary according to the severity of the destructive process and the duration of the disease. Early changes in the radiologic appearance of the tuberculous kidney may be subtle and difficult to find; hence, a normal excretory urogram does not rule out renal tuberculosis.

The most suggestive urographic features of renal parenchymal tuberculosis are the presence of cavities that communicate with the collecting system and fill with contrast medium and dilation of part or all of the calyceal system (125,236). Initially, the cavities are small; appear as a slight irregularity of a minor calyx; and show a moth-eaten, feathery, irregular appearance (Fig. 4.26A). Fibrous stenosis may cause amputation of one or more calyces (Fig. 4.26B).

A 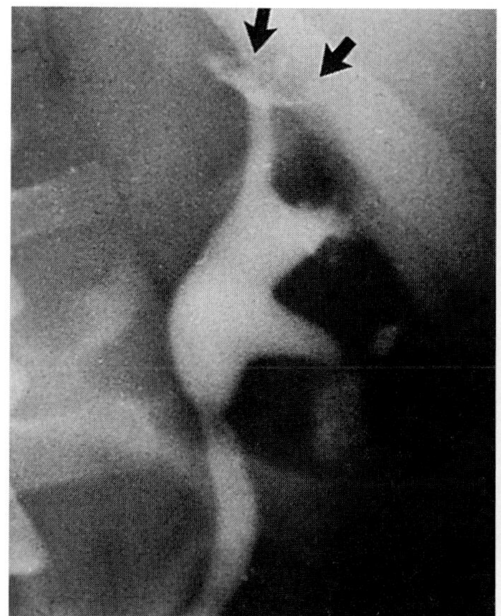

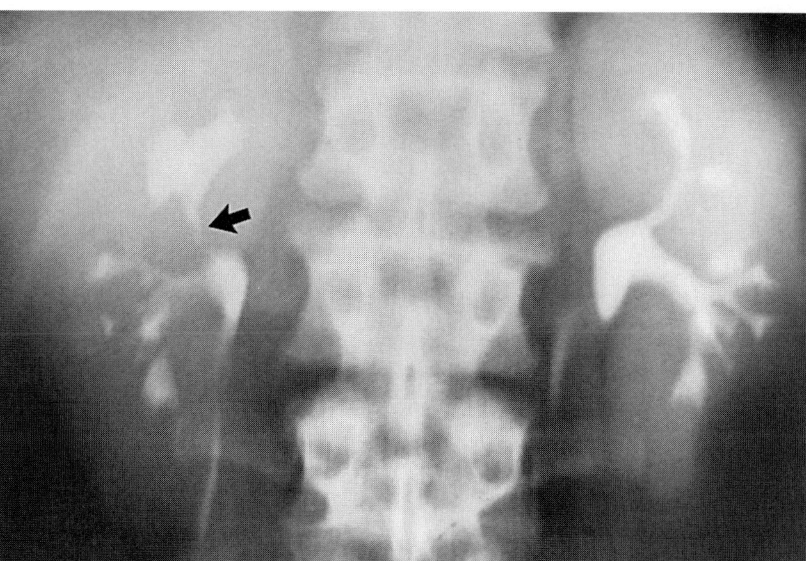 B

FIGURE 4.26. Tuberculosis. Early disease. Excretory urograms. **A:** Calyceal surface is irregular with linear rays of contrast material extending into the medulla *(arrows).* **B:** Tomogram demonstrates upper pole infundibular stenosis *(arrow).* No ureteral involvement is seen. (Reprinted with permission from Hartman DS. Radiologic pathologic correlation of the infectious granulomatous diseases of the kidney. I and II. *Monogr Urol* 1985;6:3.)

As the calyceal system becomes eroded, the parenchyma is destroyed by cavitation and the picture may closely resemble pyelonephritis (Fig. 4.27). The kidney will be either enlarged if caseous sacs are present or atrophic if there is longstanding infection. Parenchymal curvilinear or confluent calcifications in areas of caseous necrosis are common (Fig. 4.28). Autonephrectomy with complete nonvisualization of kidney may result from complete parenchymal destruction or hydronephrosis caused by stenosis of the renal pelvis or ureter (Fig. 4.29).

Fibrosis may cause the volume of the renal pelvis to be markedly reduced (Fig. 4.30). Tuberculous ureteritis is common and results in rigidity and a beading or corkscrew appearance (Fig. 4.31). Ureterovesical junction obstruction is caused by tuberculous cystitis or strictures of the distal third of the ureter. Although not common, mural calcification in the wall of the calyces, pelvis, ureter, or bladder is extremely suggestive of renal tuberculosis (125).

Retrograde urography should be used in cases of nonvisualized or poorly functioning kidneys. A voiding cystogram may show a severely contracted bladder with vesicoureteral reflux in one or both sides.

Sonographic examination has limited diagnostic value. CT has several advantages; it can be used in nonfunctioning kidneys and is very sensitive for detecting calcifications and perinephric extension or perinephric hemorrhage that may complicate renal tuberculosis. CT is also

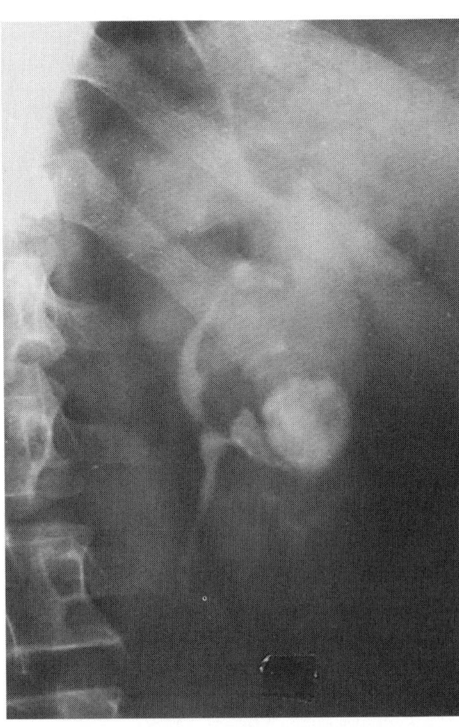

FIGURE 4.27. Tuberculosis, advanced disease. Excretory urogram shows a large cavity communicating with the calyx in the middle portion of the kidney. Note the irregularity and narrowing of the remainder of the collecting system. (Reprinted with permission from Hartman DS. Radiologic pathologic correlation of the infectious granulomatous diseases of the kidney. I and II. *Monogr Urol* 1985;6:3.)

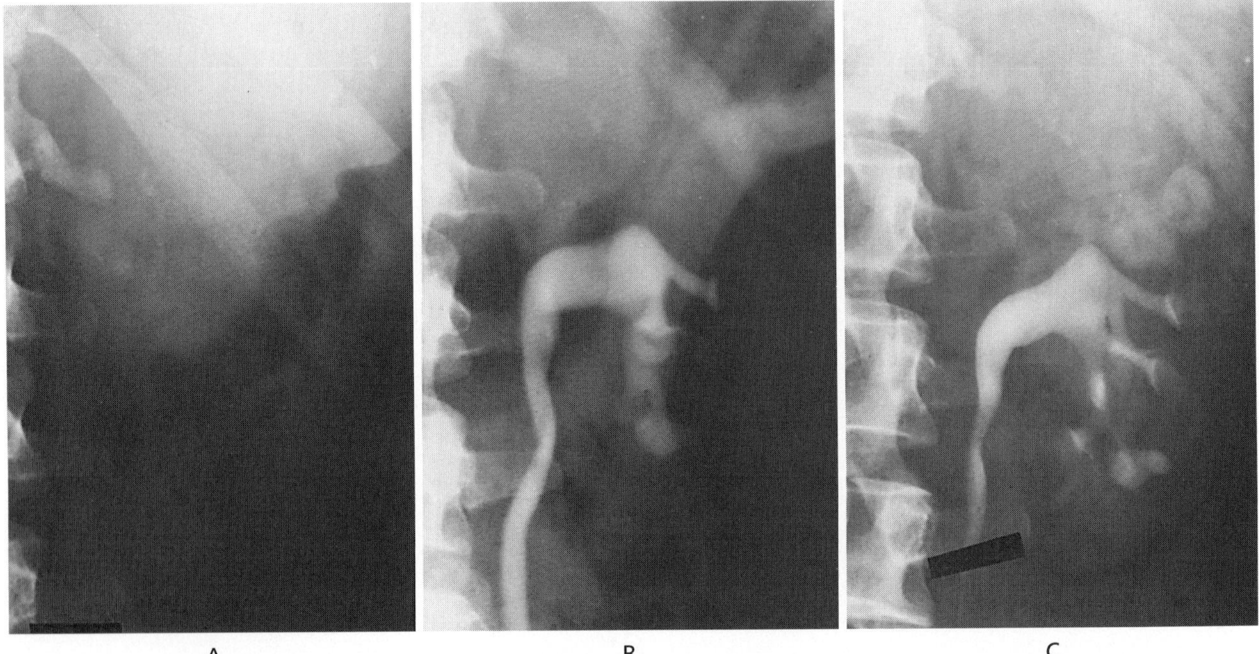

FIGURE 4.28. Tuberculoma. **A:** Faint calcification over the renal fossa. **B:** Fifteen-minute film from an excretory urogram shows "amputation" of the upper pole calyx in the region of calcification. **C:** Delayed film reveals contrast material filling the mass, indicating its communication with the collecting system. (Reprinted with permission from Hartman DS. Radiologic pathologic correlation of the infectious granulomatous diseases of the kidney. I and II. *Monogr Urol* 1985;6:3.)

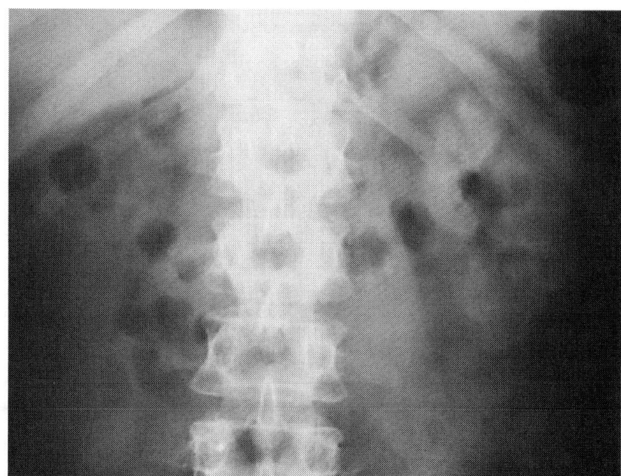

FIGURE 4.29. Tuberculosis, autonephrectomy. Extensive confluent calcifications in the renal fossa. The excretory urogram indicated no function. (Reprinted with permission from Hartman DS. Radiologic pathologic correlation of the infectious granulomatous diseases of the kidney. I and II. *Monogr Urol* 1985;6:3.)

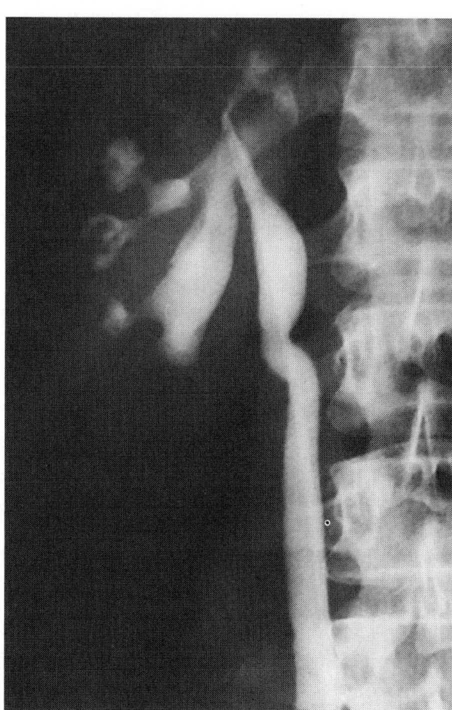

FIGURE 4.30. Tuberculosis with pelvic fibrosis. Retrograde pyelogram shows significant calyceal irregularity. The calyces come together and empty into the proximal ureter. (Reprinted with permission from Hartman DS. Radiologic pathologic correlation of the infectious granulomatous diseases of the kidney. I and II. *Monogr Urol* 1985;6:3.)

the best technique for demonstrating pelvic and ureteral mural thickening. Angiography has limited usefulness in diagnosing renal tuberculosis. Arterial fibrosis results in narrowing or amputation of the small intrarenal arteries (101,125).

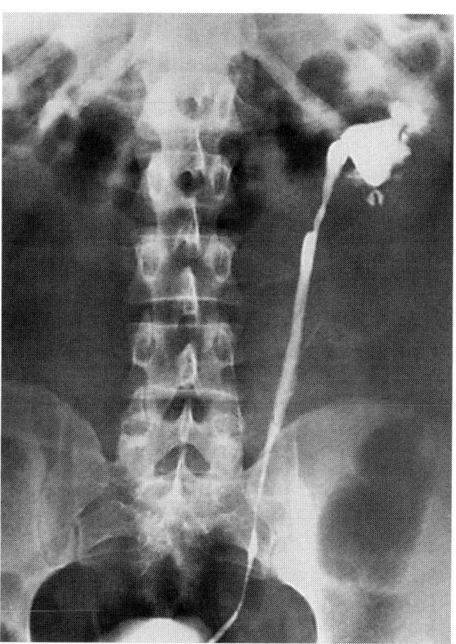

FIGURE 4.31. Tuberculosis, advanced disease. Retrograde pyelogram shows extensive ureteral changes including irregularity and rigidity, giving "pipestem" appearance. Note extensive distortion, irregularity, and amputation of the upper pole calyx.

Differential Diagnosis

If all of the radiographic findings are typical of renal tuberculosis, the diagnosis is straightforward. However, all of the classic findings are often absent, and the radiographs may suggest medullary sponge kidney, papillary necrosis, invasive transitional cell carcinoma, chronic pyelonephritis, or schistosomiasis. The pertinent radiologic discriminators have been summarized by Hartman (125).

Medullary sponge kidney and papillary necrosis demonstrate extracaliceal accumulations of contrast material and medullary nephrocalcinosis, but cortical calcification and parenchymal masses are rare. Ring calcification near a necrotic or sloughed papilla is extremely suggestive of papillary necrosis. Chronic urinary tract infection and pyelonephritis show distortion of the renal cortex and collecting system similar to tuberculosis, but calyceal, pelvic, and ureteral strictures are not commonly associated with typical urinary tract infections. Invasive transitional cell carcinoma may show infundibular narrowing or calyceal amputation and may be difficult to differentiate radiographically from tuberculosis. Transitional cell carcinoma is not associated with communicating cavities or parenchymal calcification. Infundibular narrowing and submucosal calcifications are seen in amyloidosis of the kidney, but amyloidosis is not associated with destructive communicating cavities or parenchymal calcification. *Schistosoma haematobium* infection of the urinary tract may cause ureteral and bladder calcifications. However, schistosomiasis does not involve the renal parenchyma primarily and is not associated with renal calcification. Schistosomiasis affects only the distal ureter, whereas tuberculosis often involves the entire ureteral length.

Cystoscopy

In early cases of tuberculosis, the bladder is diffusely red and extremely sensitive. Bladder wall ulcerations, severe contracture of the bladder, and golf-hole ureteral orifices are seen in more advanced disease. Ulcerated areas in the bladder strongly suggest tuberculosis. Tuberculous ulcers are irregular and shallow with undermined edges, often well circumscribed from adjoining normal-appearing mucosa. Neoplasms may have a similar appearance and must be differentiated by biopsy.

Management

Appropriate management must be based on an accurate bacteriologic diagnosis and initial assessment of the extent of the disease, the level of renal function, and the nature and severity of ureteric obstruction. Renal tuberculosis in the absence of active pulmonary tuberculosis does not represent a significant infectious risk; therefore isolation is not required. Management always includes appropriate chemotherapy and surgery when indicated. With close and long-term follow-up, the overall mortality rate for renal tuberculosis has dropped from approximately 50% to 2%.

Table 4.5 gives an overview of agents available for treatment of tuberculosis. There is no uniformly recommended chemotherapeutic program. Patients with positive urine cultures but negative findings on urinalysis and normal urograms usually are treated with isoniazid and rifampin for 1 year. Patients with clinically manifest renal tuberculosis are usually treated with three antituberculous drugs such as isoniazid, ethambutol, and rifampin for 2 years (381). If the patient's initial urinary isolate is *M. tuberculosis* resistant to isoniazid or is one of the nontuberculous (atypical) mycobacteria, isoniazid therapy should be stopped and two other drugs chosen on the basis of *in vitro* susceptibilities. A short-term regimen of only 4 months' duration has been recommended by Gow (110) and is summarized in Table 4.6. The initial results with this regimen appear promising, but longer follow-up is required.

Usually, tuberculous bacilli disappear from urine immediately after initiating chemotherapy, but to monitor the drug's effect, repeated cultures should be done every 3 to 4 months. All of the antituberculous drugs have toxic effects when used continuously. Renal and hepatic function should be monitored during the treatment. Rifampin and isoniazid appear to be the safest drugs in the presence of impaired renal function (276).

Surgery was once commonly used in the treatment of renal tuberculosis, but since the advent of effective antituberculous chemotherapy, it is reserved primarily for man-

TABLE 4.5. COMMONLY USED AGENTS IN THE TREATMENT OF TUBERCULOSIS

Drug	Usual Dose	Route	Frequency	Adverse Effects
Isoniazid	300 mg/day	p.o.	Once daily	Hepatotoxicity, peripheral neuropathy, asymptomatic transaminase rise
Ethambutol	25 mg/kg/day 15 mg/kg/day	p.o. p.o.	Once daily for 60 days Once daily for remainder of treatment period	Optic neuritis seen at 25-mg/kg dose, less frequent at 15-mg/kg dose; usually reversible if drug is stopped immediately
Rifampin	600 mg/day	p.o.	Once daily	Hepatotoxicity, thrombocytopenia
Pyrazinamide	25 mg/kg/day	p.o.	Once daily	Hepatotoxicity: dose and duration related, hyperuricemia
Ethionamide	750–1,000 mg/day	p.o.	Divided doses, 250 mg each	Nausea, vomiting, anorexia, abdominal pain
Cycloserine	750–1,000 mg/day	p.o.	Divided doses, 250 mg each	Neurotoxicity: headache, drowsiness, convulsions, psychotic disturbance, peripheral neuropathy
Para-aminosalicylic acid	200 mg/kg/day	p.o.	2 divided doses	Gastrointestinal irritation, rash, and fever; hemolysis in glucose-6-phosphate dehydrogenase deficiency
Streptomycin	750–1,000 mg/day	i.m.	Once daily for 60–90 days and twice weekly thereafter	Ototoxicity, especially in older patients; rash and fever, nausea
Capreomycin	750–1,000 mg/day	i.m.	Once daily	Renal toxicity and ototoxicity, especially in older patients

Compiled from Kucers AM, Bennett N. *The use of antibiotics,* ed 3. London: Heinemann Medical Books, 1979, by Corigliano B, Leedom JM. Renal tuberculosis: part 2. In: Massry SG, Glassock RJ, eds. *Textbook of nephrology,* vol 1. Baltimore: Williams & Wilkins, 1983.

TABLE 4.6. GOW'S SHORT-COURSE REGIMEN FOR TREATMENT OF RENAL TUBERCULOSIS

Phase	Drug	Dosage (mg/day)	Frequency
Intensive phase (2 mo)	Isoniazid	300	Daily
	Rifampin	450	Daily
	Pyrazinamide	1,000	Daily
	Ethambutol	1,000	Daily
Continuation phase (2 mo)	Isoniazid	600	3 times/wk at night
	Rifampin	900	3 times/wk at night

Modified with permission from Gow JG. The management of genitourinary tuberculosis. *J Antimicrob Chemother* 1981;7:590.

agement of local complications, such as ureteral stricture or for treatment of nonfunctioning kidneys. If surgery is warranted, it is wise to precede the operation with at least 3 weeks and preferably 3 months of triple-drug chemotherapy.

The incidence of ureteral strictures has been reported to be as high as 10% in centers that treat large numbers of patients with urinary tuberculosis (248). The stricture may be present at the time of diagnosis of renal tuberculosis, but it often develops or progresses during otherwise effective treatment with chemotherapeutic agents (48). Recommended treatment of strictures includes ureteroneocystostomy, construction of a Boari flap, or transluminal balloon ureteral dilation (10,233,375). Success rates with these procedures have been reported at 60% to 90%.

Horne and Tulloch (146) added prednisolone 5 mg four times a day to the standard chemotherapy regimen in all patients with renal tuberculosis who had evidence of stricture formation at presentation or in whom it developed during treatment. No important side effects were noted. Of 29 patients so treated, 72% were relieved of obstruction and only 2 (7%) patients showed recurrence after withdrawal of steroids; both individuals responded to further courses of steroids. Success with steroid therapy has not been universal, however (48).

Removal of a nonfunctioning kidney is usually indicated for advanced unilateral disease complicated by sepsis, hemorrhage, intractable pain, newly developed severe hypertension, suspicion of malignancy, inability to sterilize the urine with drugs alone, abscess formation with development of fistula, or inability to have appropriate follow-up (194,201,236). Prophylactic removal of a nonfunctioning kidney to prevent complications, remove a potential source of viable organisms, and shorten the duration of convalescence and requirement for chemotherapy is advocated by some authors (88,252,394).

Others who have followed up a large series of patients treated with medical therapy alone have concluded that because the frequency of late complications is only 6%, routine nephrectomy should not be performed for every nonfunctioning kidney (194,380). These authors treated patients for 2 years. The merits of short-term therapy and prophylactic nephrectomy versus long-term, 2-year chemotherapy and selected nephrectomy warrant further study.

Xanthogranulomatous Pyelonephritis

Xanthogranulomatous pyelonephritis is a chronic inflammatory disease characterized by accumulation of lipid-laden foamy macrophages. It begins within the pelvis and calyces and subsequently extends into and destroys renal parenchymal and adjacent tissues. In most cases, xanthogranulomatous pyelonephritis is unilateral and results in a nonfunctioning, enlarged kidney associated with obstructive nephropathy secondary to nephrolithiasis. It has been known to imitate virtually every other inflammatory disease of the kidney, as well as renal cell carcinoma, on radiographic examination. In addition, the microscopic appearance of xanthogranulomatous pyelonephritis has been confused with clear cell adenocarcinoma of the kidney on frozen section and has led to radical nephrectomy (33).

Pathology and Pathogenesis

The kidney is usually massively enlarged and has a normal contour. Xanthogranulomatous pyelonephritis may be diffuse, as in approximately 80% of the patients, or segmental. In the diffuse form of the disease, the entire kidney is involved, whereas in segmental xanthogranulomatous pyelonephritis, only the parenchyma surrounding one or more calyces or one pole of a duplicated collecting system is involved. On sectioning, the kidney usually demonstrates nephrolithiasis and peripelvic fibrosis. The calyces are dilated and filled with purulent material, but fibrosis surrounding the pelvis usually prevents dilation. The papillae are often destroyed by papillary necrosis (109). In advanced stages of the disease, multiple parenchymal abscesses are filled with viscous pus and lined by yellowish tissue (Fig. 4.32A). The cortex is often thin and is often replaced by xanthogranulomatous tissue. The capsule is often thickened, and extension of the inflammatory process into the perinephric or paranephric space is common (109,115,219).

On microscopic examination, the yellowish nodules that line the calyces and surround the parenchymal abscesses contain dark sheets of lipid-laden macrophages (foamy histiocytes with small, dark nuclei and clear cytoplasm) intermixed with lymphocytes, giant cells, and plasma cells (Fig. 4.32B). Xanthogranulomatous cells are not specific to xanthogranulomatous pyelonephritis but may be present anywhere inflammation or obstruction coexists. The origin of the fatty substance is disputed. Cholesterol esters that

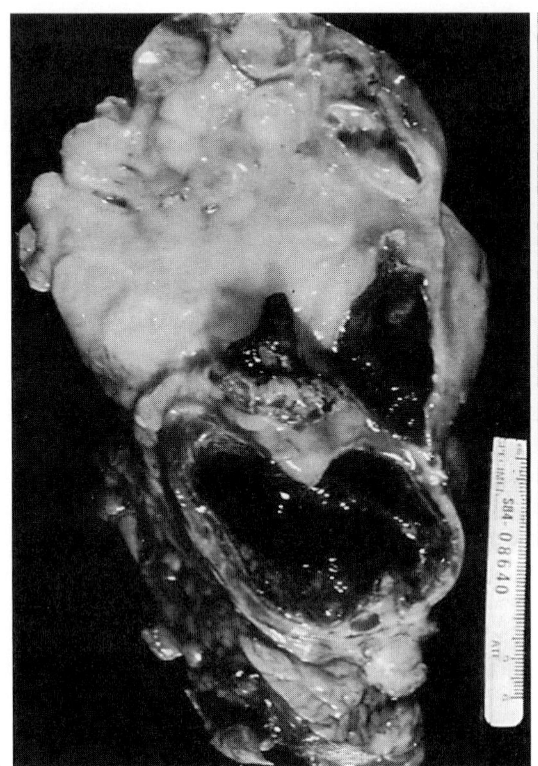

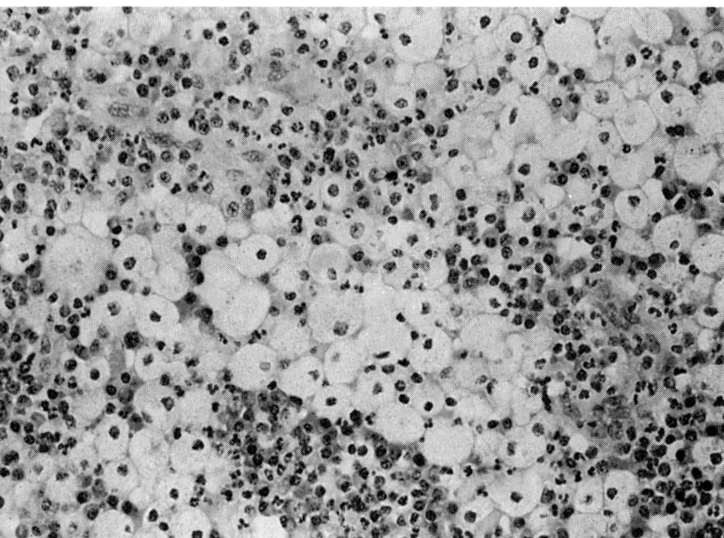

FIGURE 4.32. Xanthogranulomatous pyelonephritis. **A:** Gross specimen. Kidney is massively enlarged, measures 23 by 12 cm; the normal architecture is replaced by a shaggy yellow upper pole mass corresponding to xanthogranulomatous inflammation and numerous distorted and dilated calyces. **B:** Microscopically, the shaggy yellow tissue is composed primarily of lipid-laden histiocytes mixed with other inflammatory cells.

make up a part of the lipid might be derived from lysis of erythrocytes after hemorrhage (286).

The primary factors involved in the pathogenesis of xanthogranulomatous pyelonephritis are nephrolithiasis, obstruction, and infection (115). Nephrolithiasis has been noted in as many as 83% of the patients in various series; approximately half of the renal stones have been of the staghorn type (45,237,255). It has been proposed clinically and demonstrated experimentally that primary obstruction followed by infection with *E. coli* can lead to tissue destruction and collections of lipid material by histiocytes (271). The bacteria appear to be of low virulence because spontaneous bacteremia has rarely been described. Other possible interrelated factors include venous occlusion and hemorrhage, abnormal lipid metabolism, lymphatic blockage, failure of antimicrobial therapy in urinary tract infection, altered immunologic competence, and renal ischemia (99,109,219, 226,363). The concept that xanthogranulomatous pyelonephritis is related to incomplete bacterial degradation and altered host response has received mixed support (176,254). Thus it appears that there is probably no single factor that is instrumental in the pathogenesis of this disease. Rather there is an inadequate host acute inflammatory response within an obstructed, ischemic, or necrotic kidney.

Clinical Findings

Xanthogranulomatous pyelonephritis should be suspected in patients with urinary tract infections and a unilateral enlarged nonfunctioning or poorly functioning kidney with a stone or a mass lesion indistinguishable from malignant tumor. Although it may occur at any age, the peak incidence of xanthogranulomatous pyelonephritis is in the fifth to the seventh decade. Women are more commonly affected than men. There is no predilection for either kidney.

Most patients have multiple, chronic symptoms that are variable and nonspecific. Patients usually have flank pain, fever or chills, malaise, weight loss, symptoms of cystitis, calculi or palpable mass, and a history of recurrent urinary tract infection. Many patients are admitted to the hospital for urosepsis. Less commonly, hypertension, hematuria, or hepatomegaly is the presenting complaint. The medical history is often positive for urinary tract infections and urologic instrumentation (69,89,109,111, 209,237,260,400).

Laboratory Findings

Hematologic evaluation commonly shows anemia and leukocytosis. Diabetes mellitus is present in approximately 15% of the patients. Urinalysis reveals proteinuria and pyuria in nearly all cases. Urine cultures are positive in approximately 70% of patients. Although earlier reports indicated that *P. mirabilis* was the primary pathogen, in recent studies, *E. coli* was cultured in 40% of specimens, and *P. mirabilis* was cultured in approximately 30%. Other pathogens include *Klebsiella, Pseudomonas,* and *Bacteroides* (73). Anaerobes, most often bacteroids, have been isolated in a small number of patients (45,69,111). Approximately 10% of the patients will have mixed cultures. It is noteworthy that about one-third of the patients have sterile urine, probably because many patients receive long-term antimicrobial therapy or are taking antimicrobials when the culture is obtained. The infecting organism may be revealed only by tissue cultures obtained during surgery.

Ballesteros and associates (14) reported accurate preoperative diagnosis of xanthogranulomatous pyelonephritis by serial urinary cytology in 80% of their cases. Subsequent investigators have sought but not found xanthogranuloma cells in the urine (45,69). Thus the diagnostic value of urine cytologic testing remains unclear.

Xanthogranulomatous pyelonephritis is usually unilateral; therefore azotemia or frank renal failure is uncommon (109,115). Reversible hepatic dysfunction has been observed in 20% to 40% of patients with diffuse xanthogranulomatous pyelonephritis (209,363). Liver enzymes return to normal after nephrectomy.

Radiologic Findings

Approximately 50% to 80% of patients show the classic triad of unilateral renal enlargement with little or no function and a large calculus in the renal pelvis (73). At times, the enlargement may be localized and resemble a renal mass. Less commonly, excretory urography demonstrates delayed function and hydronephrosis, which may be massive. Smaller calcifications within the mass are not uncommon but are much less specific (Fig. 4.33A). Although there is abundant intracellular fat, the plane almost never demonstrates significant lucency (126). Retrograde pyelography may show the point of obstruction and dilation of the renal pelvis and calyces. If there is extensive parenchymal damage, contrast studies may demonstrate an ulcerated pyelocalyceal system with multiple irregular filling defects.

Sonography usually demonstrates global enlargement of the kidney (225). The normal renal architecture is replaced by multiple hypoechoic fluid-filled masses that correspond to debris-filled, dilated calyces or foci of parenchymal destruction (78,127). With focal involvement, a solid mass involving a segment of the kidney is demonstrated with an associated calculus in the collecting system or ureter. Renal cell carcinoma and other solid renal lesions must be considered in the differential diagnosis (73).

CT is probably the most useful radiologic technique in evaluating patients with xanthogranulomatous pyelonephritis. CT usually demonstrates a large, reniform mass with the renal pelvis tightly surrounding a central calcification without pelvic dilation (69,108,126,326) (Fig. 4.33B). Renal parenchyma is replaced by multiple water density masses representing dilated calyces and abscess cavities filled with varying amounts of pus and debris. On enhanced scans, the walls of these cavities demonstrate a prominent blush resulting from the abundant vascularity within the granulation tissue. However, the cavities fail to enhance, whereas tumors and other inflammatory lesions usually do. The findings of focal xanthogranulomatous pyelonephritis often mimic

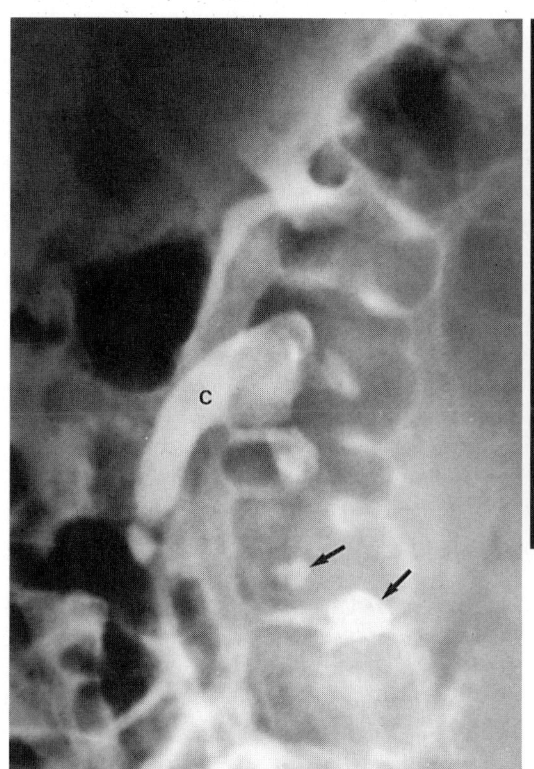

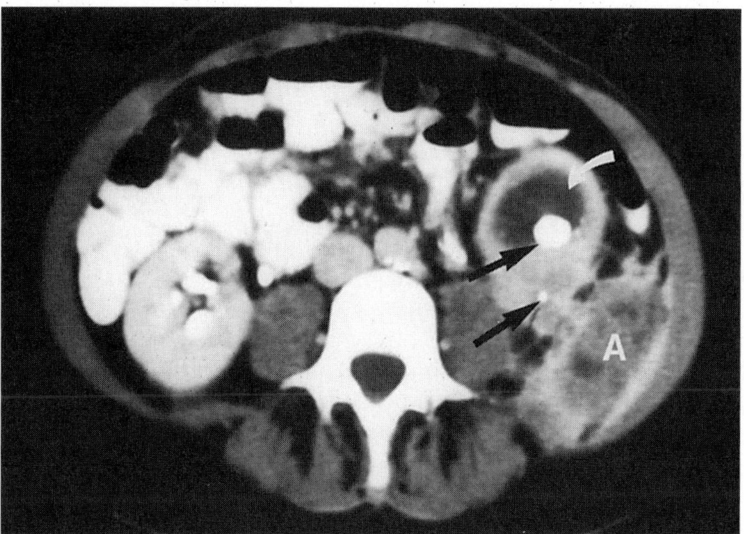

FIGURE 4.33. Xanthogranulomatous pyelonephritis. Excretory urogram. **A:** Ten-minute film shows lower-pole enlargement and nonfunction. Note a large pelvic calculus *(C)* and several smaller parenchymal calculi *(arrows)*. The upper pole of the bifid collecting system functions normally. **B:** Enhanced computed tomography scan shows collecting system and parenchymal calculi *(arrows)* with lower pole pyonephrosis *(curved arrow)* and an irregular, predominantly low-density perinephric abscess *(A)* extending into the soft tissues of the flank.

neoplasm. The CT scan is particularly helpful in demonstrating the extent of renal involvement and may indicate whether adjacent organs or the abdominal wall is involved (69,170).

Radionuclide renal scanning using ^{99}Te dimercaptosuccinic acid (DMSA) is used to confirm and quantify the differential lack of function in the involved kidney (115). Magnetic resonance imaging has not yet superseded CT in the evaluation of renal inflammation, but it provides some advantages in delineating extrarenal extension of inflammation (325). Lesions of xanthogranulomatous pyelonephritis may appear as cystic foci of intermediate intensity signal on T_1-weighted images and hyperintensity on T_2-weighted images. Angiography is seldom required for diagnosing xanthogranulomatous pyelonephritis. Most commonly, there is stretching and attenuation of vessels around avascular masses with an irregular nephrogram (73). Benign neovascularity, absence of irregular vessels, and arterial-venous shunting are also characteristic.

Differential Diagnosis

Diagnosis of segmental xanthogranulomatous pyelonephritis without calculi may be difficult. Xanthogranulomatous pyelonephritis in association with massive pelvic dilation cannot be distinguished from pyonephrosis. When xanthogranulomatous pyelonephritis occurs within a small contracted kidney, the radiographic findings are nonspecific and nondiagnostic. Renal parenchymal malakoplakia may show renal enlargement and multiple inflammatory masses replacing the normal renal parenchyma, but calculi are usually not present. Renal lymphoma may be associated with multiple hypoechoic masses surrounding the contracted, nondilated pelvis, but lymphoma is usually clinically obvious, and renal involvement is usually bilateral and not associated with calculi (126).

Management

The management of xanthogranulomatous pyelonephritis is usually surgical. Antimicrobial therapy may be necessary to stabilize the patient preoperatively; occasionally, long-term antimicrobial therapy will eradicate the infection and restore renal function (230). Nephrectomy is required for diffuse xanthogranulomatous pyelonephritis. Partial nephrectomy is the preferred treatment for focal xanthogranulomatous pyelonephritis if the diagnosis can be established preoperatively or, if necessary, by frozen section at the time of surgery (251,259). However, the lipid-laden macrophages associated with xanthogranulomatous pyelonephritis closely resemble clear cell adenocarcinoma and may be difficult to distinguish solely on the basis of frozen section. Furthermore, xanthogranulomatous pyelonephritis has been associated with renal cell carcinoma, papillary transitional cell carcinoma of the pelvis or bladder, and infiltrating squamous cell carcinoma of the pelvis (268,307,363). Therefore, if malignant renal tumor cannot be excluded, nephrectomy should be performed.

It is important to remove the entire inflammatory mass because in nearly 75% of patients, xanthogranulomatous tissue is infected. If incision and drainage alone are performed rather than nephrectomy, the patient may continue to suffer from protracted debilitating illness and may develop a renocutaneous fistula, and an even more difficult nephrectomy will be necessary (73). Extensive xanthogranulomatous pyelonephritis may make surgical dissection and ligation of the friable vascular pedicle particularly difficult. Extension of the inflammatory reaction to adjacent bowel, diaphragm, and aorta requires tedious dissection and at times resection of the involved tissues.

Renal Parenchymal Malakoplakia

Malakoplakia, from the Greek words meaning "soft plaque," is an uncommon inflammatory lesion described originally by Michaelis and Gutmann (227). It was characterized by Von Hansemann (373) as soft, yellow-brown plaques with granulomatous lesions in which the histiocytes contain distinct basophilic inclusions or Michaelis-Gutmann bodies. Although its exact pathogenesis is unknown, malakoplakia probably results from abnormal macrophage function in response to a bacterial infection, which is most often *E. coli.* The inclusions probably represent calcification around incompletely digested bacteria (1,217).

The disease usually affects the lower urinary tract; only about 50 patients with renal parenchymal malakoplakia have been reported (216). Clinically, radiologically, and at surgery, malakoplakia often mimics a neoplastic growth. The mortality rate can exceed 50%, and morbidity can be substantial (347). Extension of renal parenchymal malakoplakia into the perirenal space is uncommon (6). Renal parenchymal malakoplakia may also be complicated by renal vein thrombosis and inferior vena cava thrombosis (128,216).

Concomitant nonrenal foci of malakoplakia are seen occasionally in patients with renal parenchymal malakoplakia (347). The most common locations of other foci are the bladder and ureter. Less common sites that have been reported include the retroperitoneum, abdominal wall, colon, testis and epididymis, lungs, scrotum, prostate, adrenal gland, lymph nodes, and diaphragm (216).

Pathology and Pathogenesis

Two basic patterns of renal parenchymal malakoplakia have been described: multifocal and unifocal. The multifocal pattern accounts for 75% of the reported cases and is bilateral in about half of the patients (128). The kidney is usually enlarged and contains multiple masses varying from

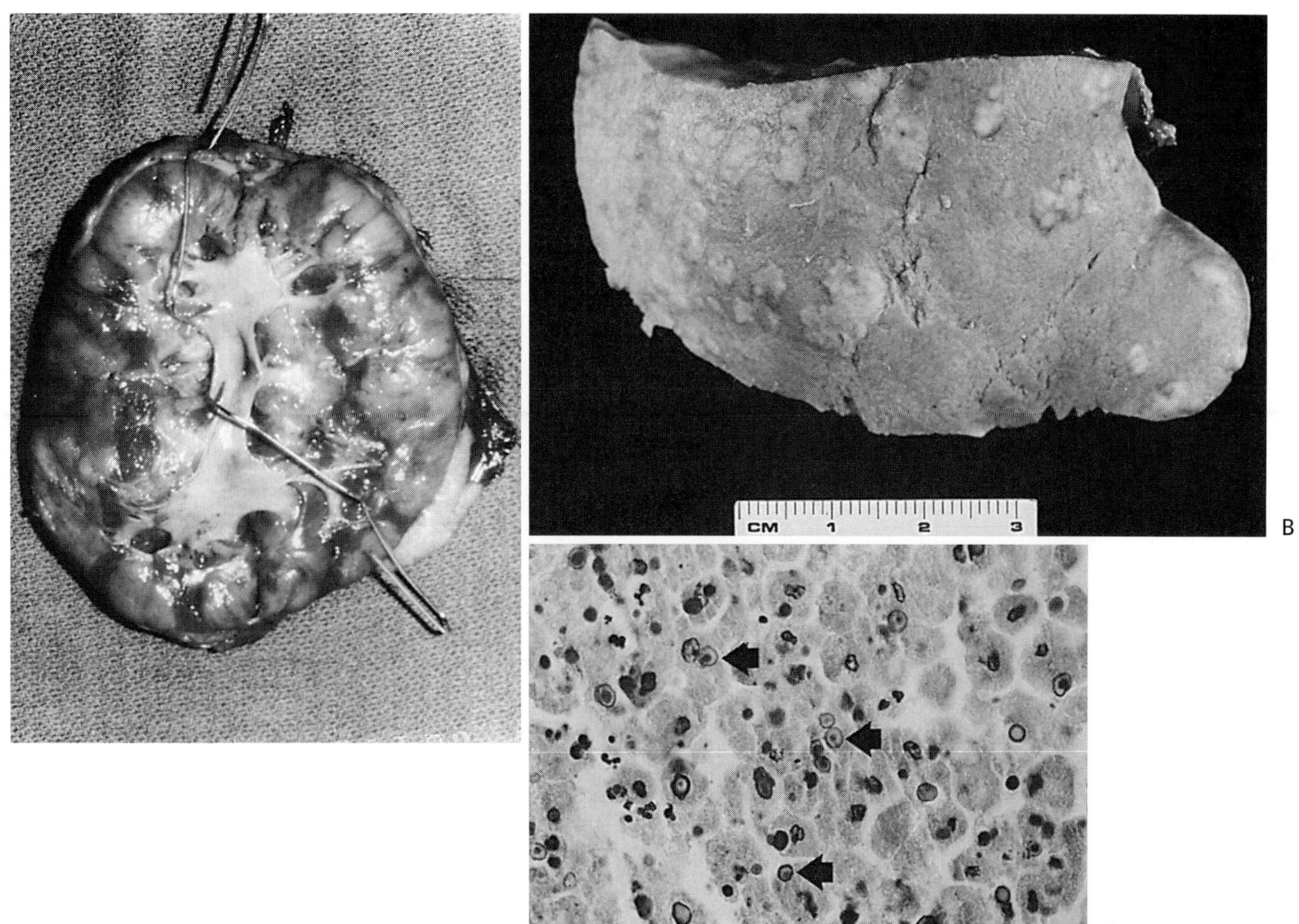

FIGURE 4.34. Renal parenchymal malakoplakia. **A:** Cut surface demonstrates extensive cortical and upper medullary replacement by multifocal, confluent, tumorlike masses. **B:** Cortical surface exhibits multiple, firm, plaquelike lesions. **C:** Hallmark of malakoplakia is demonstration of the Michaelis-Gutmann body *(arrows)*, which represents incompletely destroyed bacteria surrounded by lipoprotein membrane (hematoxylin-eosin stain). (**A, B:** Reprinted with permission from Hartman DS. Radiologic pathologic correlation of the infectious granulomatous diseases of the kidney. I and II. *Monogr Urol* 1985;6:3.)

several millimeters to several centimeters. They are usually yellow, are well demarcated, and may have a focus of hemorrhage or suppuration (Fig. 4.34A and B). The masses often coalesce to form larger nodules. These nodules often project beyond the cortical margin, resulting in an irregular contour. Less commonly, the nodules are limited to the papilla or the medulla and occasionally mimic necrotizing papillitis, in which cases the renal contour is normal (26,66,125).

Unifocal disease usually appears as a large yellow-gray mass, 2.5 to 8 cm in diameter (128). The mass is usually smooth and well marginated, and central necrosis or cyst formation may be present. Calcification of the mass is unusual (309).

Microscopically, malakoplakia is characterized by the Von Hansemann histiocyte, a large polygonal cell with foamy eosinophilic cytoplasm and compact, dark nucleus admixed with intracellular and extracellular Michaelis-Gutmann bodies. The latter contain precipitated calcium phosphate crystals and iron so that both periodic acid–Schiff and von Kossa calcium stains and iron stains are useful in demonstrating the inclusions (202). They are slightly smaller than a red blood cell and are recognized by concentric laminations that impart a targetoid or owl's-eye appearance (102) (Fig. 4.34C). Histochemical and ultrastructural studies have shown that these Michaelis-Gutmann bodies represent incompletely destroyed bacteria surrounded by concentric lipoprotein membranes. Extracytoplasmic Michaelis-Gutmann bodies probably represent debris released from dead cells (216).

It has been shown that macrophages in malakoplakia involving the kidney and bladder contain large amounts of immunoreactive α-antitrypsin (35). The amount of α-antitrypsin remains unchanged during the morphogenetic stages of the pathologic process. Macrophages from other pathologic processes, closely resembling malakoplakia but without Michaelis-Gutmann bodies, do not contain α-antitrypsin except for a few macrophages in tuberculosis and xanthogranulomatous pyelonephritis. Therefore immunohistochemical staining for α-antitrypsin may be a useful test for an early and accurate differential diagnosis of malakoplakia.

Megalocytic interstitial nephritis shows histologic changes that are similar to those of renal parenchymal malakoplakia, but the lesions are usually confined to the renal cortex and Michaelis-Gutmann bodies are less prevalent. Some authors believe that megalocytic interstitial nephritis and renal parenchymal malakoplakia represent two ends of the spectrum of a similar process (102,125,273).

The pathogenesis of malakoplakia is unknown. Almost all reported cases are associated with Gram-negative urinary tract infections, and one of the most popular theories is that malakoplakia results from incomplete resolution of the bacterial infection. Hematogenous dissemination of *E. coli* and subsequent foci of renal parenchymal malakoplakia may explain the finding of lesions limited to the cortex and medulla without renal-pelvic or lower tract disease. Patients with renal malakoplakia limited to the renal papilla or associated with contiguous renal pelvic involvement or obstructive uropathy probably have had an ascending infection (125).

The demonstration of bacteria within phagocytic vacuoles of histiocytes suggests an inability of the histiocyte to digest the bacteria. It is not clear, however, why a histiocyte response is found instead of the usual polymorphonuclear leukocyte response. The association of malakoplakia with debilitating diseases such as sarcoidosis, diabetes mellitus, and tuberculosis suggests an immunologic defect as a prerequisite for its development. Defective monocyte function has been demonstrated in one patient with malakoplakia (1). In this case phagocytosis was normal, but complete degradation of the bacteria was impossible because of low levels of cyclic guanine monophosphate, which may have resulted in decreased lysosomal degradation and inability of the cell to release the lysosomal enzymes. This defect appears to be reversible by cholinergic agonists that cause accumulation of cyclic guanine monophosphate in monocytes and enhance chemotaxis, but this finding has yet to be confirmed. At present, malakoplakia should be considered an unusual inflammatory lesion resulting from altered host macrophage or histiocytic response.

Clinical Findings

The diagnosis of renal parenchymal malakoplakia is difficult but should be suspected if there is substantial enlargement of the kidney in the presence of urinary tract infection. Renal parenchymal malakoplakia usually affects middle-aged women with recurrent urinary tract infections. The most common signs and symptoms are fever, flank pain, or a palpable flank mass (125,347). The most common pathogen is *E. coli,* which accounts for approximately 75% of the cases. *Aerobacter aerogenes, Klebsiella pneumoniae,* and *Proteus* are cultured less commonly (102,216). In addition, *E. coli* cultures have been obtained from the resected kidney, perinephric abscess, or blood or cerebrospinal fluid of affected patients. Renal failure without evidence of obstruction is not uncommon when malakoplakia is bilateral or occurs in a solitary kidney.

The association of some cases of malakoplakia with altered immune states, such as transplantation, sarcoidosis, hemolytic uremic syndrome, tuberculosis, steroid therapy, lymphoma, leukemia, alcoholism, or emaciation, is common (34,125). Nevertheless, many patients in whom malakoplakia occurs have no recognized defects.

Radiologic Findings

Multifocal malakoplakia on excretory urography typically manifests as enlarged kidneys with multiple filling defects (Fig. 4.35A). Renal calcification, lithiasis, and hydronephrosis are absent. The multifocal nature is best appreciated with ultrasonography, CT, or arteriography. Sonographic examination may demonstrate renal enlargement and distortion of the central echo complex. The masses are often confluent, resulting in an overall increase in the echogenicity of the renal parenchyma (128). CT often shows masses or enlargement of the kidneys. On CT, the foci of malakoplakia are less dense than the surrounding enhanced parenchyma (125). Arteriography typically reveals a hypovascular mass with peripheral neovascularity (Fig. 4.35B and C) (41,364).

Intense renal uptake of gallium-67 in the clinical setting of fever, progressive renal failure, and nephromegaly strongly supports a diagnosis of renal parenchyma malakoplakia (147). Unifocal malakoplakia on intravenous urography manifests as a noncalcified mass that is indistinguishable from other inflammatory or neoplastic lesions. Ultrasound and CT may demonstrate a solid or cystic structure depending on the degree of internal necrosis. Angiography may demonstrate neovascularity (364). Extension beyond the kidney, which can occur with either multifocal or unifocal malakoplakia, is best demonstrated by CT.

Differential Diagnosis

The differential diagnosis includes renal cystic disease, neoplasia, and renal inflammatory disease (125). Malakoplakia should be considered when one or more renal masses are observed, particularly in female patients with recurrent urinary tract infections with *E. coli,* altered immune response syndromes, or cystoscopic evidence of malakoplakia or filling defects in the collecting system (43). Malakoplakia should also be suspected when these radiographic findings

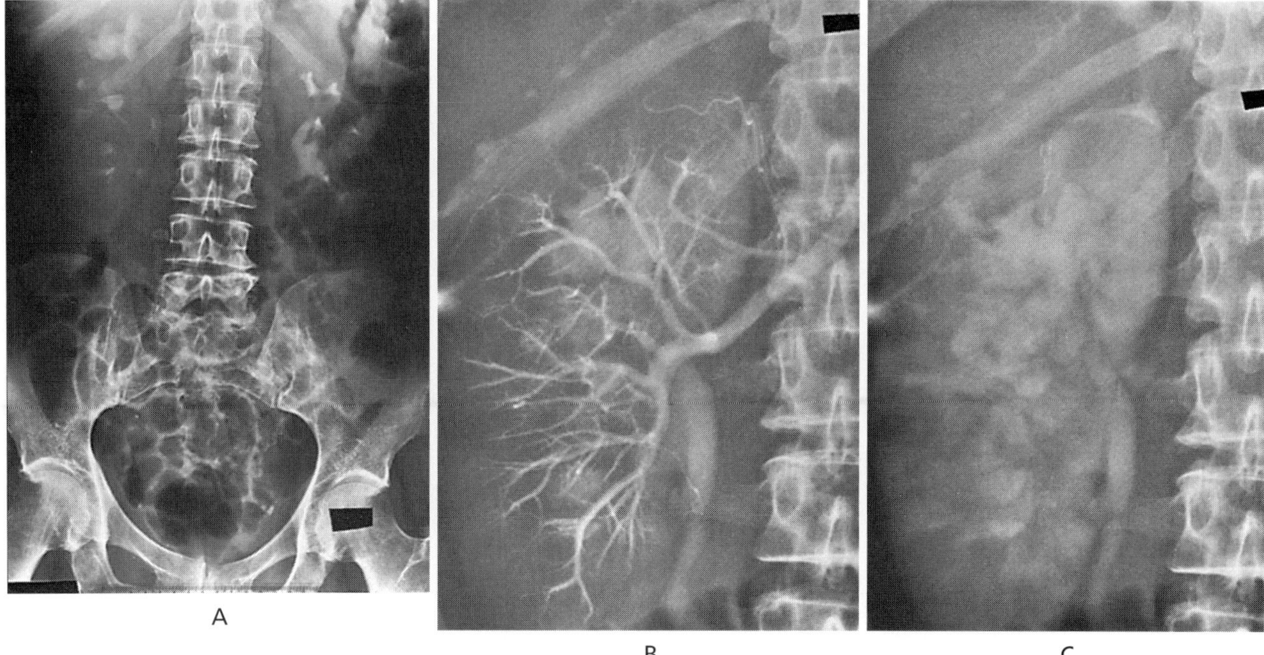

FIGURE 4.35. Multifocal renal parenchymal malakoplakia. **A:** Excretory urogram. The right kidney is enlarged (16.5 cm) with dilation of the upper pole calyces and poor filling of the renal pelvis. **B:** Early angiogram. Separation of the intrarenal vessels without neovascularity. **C:** Angiographic nephrogram. Multiple irregular filling defects located primarily within the cortex. (Courtesy of Charles E. Bickham Jr., MD, Bethesda, MD. Reprinted with permission from Hartman DS, Davis CJ, Lichtenstein JE, et al. Renal parenchymal malakoplakia. *Radiology* 1980;136:33.)

occur in a renal transplant patient who has persistent urinary tract infection despite appropriate antimicrobial therapy. Cystic disease generally can be excluded by careful sonographic and CT evaluations. Renal involvement with metastatic disease or lymphomas usually occurs late in the course of the disease, which is well established. Multifocal renal cell carcinoma is most often seen in the context of von Hippel–Lindau disease with its other clinical manifestations. Patients with xanthogranulomatous pyelonephritis usually have signs and symptoms of urinary tract infection. As with malakoplakia, the involved kidney is enlarged, but renal calculi and obstruction are common. Multiple renal abscesses are often associated with hematogenous dissemination resulting from cardiac disease.

Management

Initial management is directed at controlling the urinary tract infection, correcting the immunologic defect, and improving renal function if necessary (125). Nephrectomy is usually performed for unilateral disease.

Long-term antimicrobial therapy, such as rifampin, TMP-SMX, and doxycycline, has been used successfully in approximately 10% to 15% of patients with renal parenchymal malakoplakia established by biopsy (347). Dramatic improvement has also been reported in patients with intraabdominal malakoplakia treated with cholinergic agents and ascorbic acid (1).

The long-term prognosis appears to be related most directly with the extent of disease. When parenchymal renal malakoplakia is bilateral or occurs in the transplanted kidney, death usually occurs within 6 months (26,66,134). Patients with unilateral disease usually have a long-term survival after nephrectomy.

Renal Echinococcosis

Echinococcosis is a parasitic infection caused by the larval stage of the tapeworm *Echinococcus granulosus.* The disease is prevalent in dogs, sheep, cattle, and humans in South Africa, Australia, New Zealand, Mediterranean countries (especially Greece), and some parts of the former Soviet Union. In the United States, the disease is rare; however, it is found in immigrants from Eastern Europe or other foreign endemic areas or as an indigenous infection among Native Americans in the southwest and Eskimos (269).

Pathology and Pathogenesis

Echinococcosis is produced by the larval form of the tapeworm, which in its adult form resides in the intestine of the dog, the definitive host. The adult worm is 3 to 9 mm long.

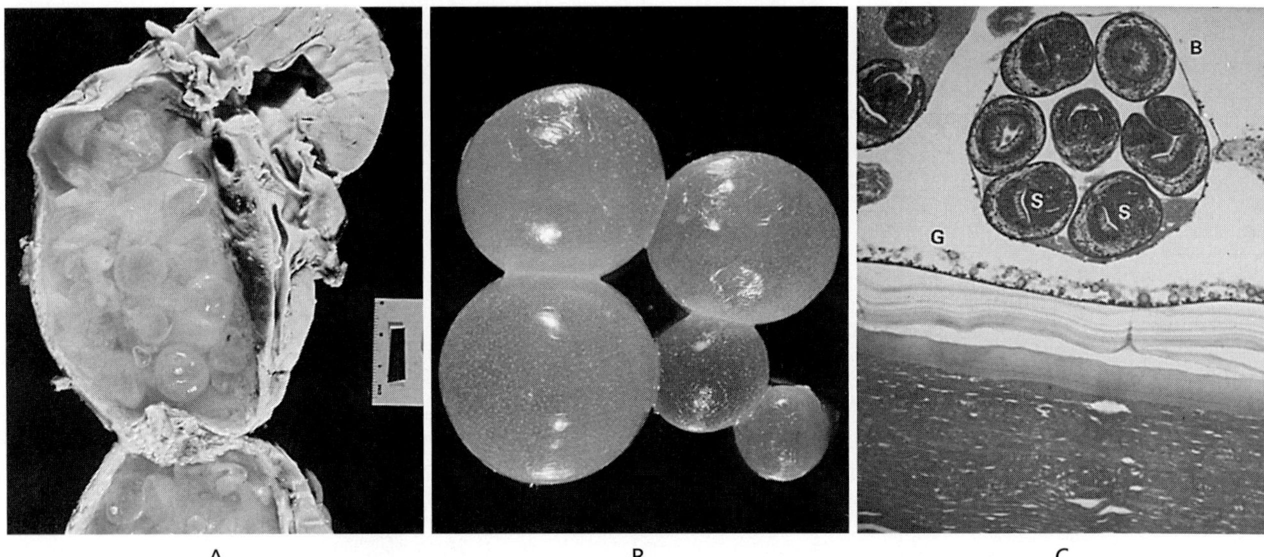

FIGURE 4.36. Echinococcosis. **A:** Gross specimen. A cystic mass 7 by 11 cm in lower pole. Smaller daughter cysts are identified within the larger cystic mass. **B:** Gross specimen. Daughter cysts represent brood capsules that have detached and move freely. **C:** Photomicrograph. Brood capsules *(B)* arising from the germinal layer *(G)* contain viable and degenerating scoleces *(S)*. (Reprinted with permission from Hartman DS. Radiologic pathologic correlation of the infectious granulomatous diseases of the kidney. III and IV. *Monogr Urol* 1985;6:26.)

The ova in the feces of the dog contaminate grass and farmlands and are ingested by sheep, pigs, or humans, the intermediate hosts. Larvae hatch, penetrate venules in the wall of the duodenum, and are carried by the bloodstream to the liver. Those larvae that escape the liver are next filtered by the lungs. Approximately 3% of the organisms that escape entrapment in the liver and lungs may then enter the systemic circulation and infect the kidneys. The larvae undergo vesiculation, and the resultant hydatid cyst gradually develops at a rate of about 1 cm per year. Thus the cyst may take 5 to 10 years to reach pathologic size.

Echinococcosis cysts of the kidney are usually single and located in the cortex (235). The wall of the hydatid cyst has three zones: (a) a peripheral zone of fibroblasts derived from tissues of the host becomes the adventitia and may calcify, (b) an intermediate laminated layer that becomes hyalinized, and (c) a single inner layer that is composed of nucleated epithelium (called the *germinal layer*). The germinal layer gives rise to brood capsules that increase in number, become vacuolated, and remain attached to the germinal membrane by a pedicle. New larvae (scoleces) develop in large numbers from the germinal layer within the brood capsule (Fig. 4.36). The hydatid cyst is also filled with fluid. When brood capsules detach, they enlarge and move freely in the fluid and are then called daughter cysts. Hydatid sand is composed of free larvae and daughter cysts.

Clinical Findings

The symptoms of echinococcosis are those of a slowly growing tumor. Most patients are asymptomatic or have flank mass, dull pain, or hematuria (105,235). Because the cyst is focal, it rarely affects renal function. Rarely, the cyst ruptures into the collecting system, and the patient may experience severe colic and passage of debris resembling grape skins in the urine (hydatiduria). The cyst may also rupture into an adjacent viscus or the peritoneal cavity. The fluid is extremely antigenic (126).

Laboratory Findings

If cyst rupture occurs, the definitive diagnosis can be established by identifying daughter cysts in the urine or by identifying the laminated wall of the cyst (328).

Fewer than half of the patients have eosinophilia. The most reliable diagnostic test uses partially purified hydatid arc 5 antigens in a double diffusion test (51). Complement fixation, hemagglutination, and the Casoni intradermal skin tests are less reliable but, when combined, are positive in approximately 90% of patients (328).

Radiologic Findings

Excretory urography typically shows a thick-walled cystic mass, occasionally calcified (29). If the cyst ruptures into the collecting system, daughter cysts may be outlined in the pelvis as an irregular mass or as multiple solitary lesions (105). Occasionally, direct filling of the cyst with contrast medium occurs.

Ultrasonography and CT are useful in characterizing the mass; CT is more sensitive (314). Ultrasonography usually demonstrates a multicystic or multiloculated mass. A sudden change in position may demonstrate bright falling echoes corresponding to hydatid sand, which can be observed during real-time evaluation of a hydatid cyst (287).

On CT, several patterns of renal echinococcosis may be recognized. The most specific is a cystic mass with discrete round daughter cysts and a well-defined enhancing member (214). The less specific pattern is that of a thick-walled multiloculated cystic mass (105). The presence of daughter cysts within the mother cyst differentiates the lesion from simple renal cyst and from renal abscesses, infected cysts, and necrotic neoplasm.

Both CT and ultrasound are useful in evaluating the liver. Angiography is seldom required. Diagnostic aspiration carries a high risk of rupture and spillage of the highly antigenic cyst contents and risk of fatal anaphylaxis (285). Nevertheless, Baijal and colleagues (11) described a percutaneous management of renal hydatidosis as a minimally invasive diagnostic and therapeutic option.

Management

The prognosis of echinococcosis is good but depends on the site and size of the cysts. Although there have been preliminary reports on the use of mebendazole in the treatment of hydatid disease, the results have been less than satisfactory (71).

Surgery remains the mainstay of treatment of renal echinococcosis (270). The cyst should be removed without rupture to reduce the chance of seeding and recurrence. If the cyst wall is calcified, the larvae are probably dead and the risk of seeding is low, although a daughter cyst may be viable. If the cyst ruptures or cannot be removed and marsupialization is required, the cyst contents initially should be aspirated and the cyst filled with a scolecoidal agent such as 30% sodium chloride, 0.5% silver nitrate, 2% formalin, or 1% iodine for approximately 5 minutes to kill the germinal portions (235,315,328).

BACTERIURIA IN PREGNANCY

Asymptomatic bacteriuria is one of the most common infectious complications of pregnancy. The overall prevalence of bacteriuria in pregnancy ranges from 2% to 7%, and the risk of acquiring bacteriuria during pregnancy increases with duration of pregnancy (37,243,351). Spontaneous resolution of bacteriuria in pregnant women is unlikely unless treated. Nonpregnant patients often clear their asymptomatic bacteriuria, but pregnant women become symptomatic more frequently and tend to remain bacteriuric (74). Pyelonephritis develops in 1% to 4% of all pregnant women (358) and in 20% to 40% of pregnant women with untreated bacteriuria (257,401). Treatment of asymptomatic bacteriuria found early in pregnancy has been shown to decrease the prevalence of subsequent acute pyelonephritis from 28% to less than 3% (358).

Pathogenesis

The anatomic and physiologic changes induced by the gravid state significantly alter the natural history of bacteriuria (256). The significant physiologic changes in pregnancy, which may develop as early as the first trimester, lead to urinary stasis and mild hydroureteronephrosis and contribute to development of pyelonephritis. Recent studies of *E. coli* adhesins and their respective specific tissue receptors have established an adhesin-based mechanism of pyelonephritis-induced preterm births and low birth weights in mice (172). There is a higher incidence of *E. coli* bearing Dr adhesins during the third trimester of pregnancy in women with gestational pyelonephritis (245) and an upregulation of Dr adhesin in the kidney, endometrium, and placenta during the third trimester of pregnancy (212). When infected intravesically with *E. coli*–bearing Dr adhesin, nearly 90% of mice that were hyporesponsive to bacterial lipopolysaccharide and had a deficient immune response delivered preterm, compared with 10% of mice infected with *E. coli* without Dr. Also, there was a significant reduction in fetal birth weight in the Dr-infected group. Bacterial tissue culture showed systemic spread of the Dr *E. coli* to the placentae and fetuses.

Management

In the preantibiotic era, pregnant women with symptomatic urinary tract infections and bacterial pyelonephritis were reported to have a high incidence of prematurity, low birth weight, and death (106). The relationship between asymptomatic bacteriuria and prematurity is less clear. Gilstrap and colleagues (106) found no difference in pregnancy among patients treated for asymptomatic bacteriuria as compared with nonbacteriuric controls. However, because women with asymptomatic bacteriuria are at higher risk for developing a symptomatic urinary tract infection that results in adverse fetal sequelae, all women with asymptomatic bacteriuria should be treated. The pathogens are similar to those seen in nonpregnant women (207).

An initial screening culture should be performed in all pregnant women during the first trimester (351). If the culture shows no growth, repeat cultures are generally unnecessary because patients who have no growth in their urine early in their pregnancy are unlikely to develop bacteriuria later (220,243). Pregnant women with a history of recurrent urinary tract infection or vesicoureteral reflux may benefit from antimicrobial prophylaxis (30).

If the culture is positive, special consideration must be given to the selection of antimicrobial agents chosen to treat infection to prevent fetal toxicity. Table 4.7 lists the antimicrobial agents and dosing for use in pregnancy. The aminopenicillins and cephalosporins are considered safe and generally effective throughout pregnancy. In patients with penicillin allergy, nitrofurantoin is a reasonable alternative. It may be used safely during the first two

TABLE 4.7. ORAL ANTIMICROBIAL AGENTS USED IN PREGNANCY

Drug	Dosage	Comments
Agents Considered Safe		
Penicillins		
Ampicillin	500 mg q.i.d.	Extensively used
Amoxicillin	250 mg t.i.d.	Safe and effective
Penicillin V	500 mg q.i.d.	Used less frequently, but achieves excellent urinary levels
Cephalosporins		
Cephalexin	500 mg q.i.d.	Extensively used
Cefaclor	500 mg q.i.d.	Somewhat more effective against Gram negatives
Agents That May Be Used with Caution		
Nitrofurantoin	100 mg q.i.d.	May result in hemolytic anemia in patients with glucose-6-phosphate dehydrogenase deficiency
Sulfisoxazole	1 g, followed by 500 mg q.i.d.	May cause kernicterus in the newborn; also may cause hemolytic anemia when glucose-6-phosphate dehydrogenase deficiency is present; especially avoid in last few weeks of gestation
Agents That Should Be Avoided		
Fluoroquinolones		Possible damage to immature cartilage
Chloramphenicol		Associated with gray-baby syndrome
Trimethoprim		May cause megaloblastic anemia because of antifolic action
Erythromycin		Associated with maternal cholestatic jaundice
Tetracyclines		May cause acute liver decompensation in the mother and inhibition of new bone growth in the fetus

trimesters in patients without glucose-6-phosphate dehydrogenase deficiency. Given the low efficacy of short-course β-lactam therapy in nonpregnant women, it is prudent to describe a full 7-day course of therapy in pregnant women. Follow-up cultures should be obtained to document absence of infection. Pregnant women with acute pyelonephritis should be hospitalized and treated initially with parenteral antimicrobials. More than 95% of these patients respond within 24 hours using ampicillin and an aminoglycoside (59) or cephalosporins (291). Appropriate oral agents should then be given for at least 14 days (84). After the treatment course is completed, low-dose prophylaxis with nitrofurantoin, amoxicillin, or cephalexin has been shown to be effective in preventing reinfection (292,370). The efficacy of postcoital prophylaxis with either cephalexin (250 mg) or nitrofurantoin (50 mg) has been reported (264).

Drugs that are relatively contraindicated during pregnancy include the fluoroquinolones, TMP, chloramphenicol, erythromycin, tetracycline, sulfonamides, and nitrofurantoin. Fluoroquinolones are contraindicated because of their effects on immature cartilage. TMP may have teratogenic effects and should be avoided, especially in the first trimester. The "gray-baby syndrome" is a toxic effect of chloramphenicol on neonates resulting from the inability of the infant to metabolize or excrete the drug. Erythromycin may cause cholestatic jaundice in the mother. Tetracycline may cause fetal malformations and maternal liver decompensation. Sulfonamides may cause kernicterus and neonatal hyperbilirubinemia and should be avoided in the third trimester. Nitrofurantoin can cause hemolytic anemia in both mother and child when glucose-6-phosphate dehydrogenase deficiency is present.

BACTERIURIA IN THE ELDERLY

Urinary tract infections in the elderly are a common and expanding health problem (174). The prevalence of bacteriuria increases with age, institutionalization, and concurrent diseases and may exceed 50% in selective groups (23,297). Longitudinal studies have clarified the dynamic aspect of bacteriuria in the elderly with frequent, spontaneous alteration between positive and negative urine cultures (231). The incidence of asymptomatic bacteriuria is much more common than is apparent from a single survey, implying that most elderly will eventually have episodes of bacteriuria (24).

Pathogenesis

The pathophysiology of increased susceptibility is multifactorial and poorly understood. Age-related changes include decline in cell-mediated immunity, neurogenic bladder dysfunction, increased perineal soiling as a result of fecal and urinary incontinence, increased incidence of urethral catheter placement, and in women, changes in the vaginal environment associated with estrogen depletion (274,297). Bacteriologic characteristics of infection in the elderly differ from those in younger patients (12). *E. coli* remains the most common uropathogen, but there is a significant increase in the incidence of *Proteus, Klebsiella, Enterobacter, Serratia,* and *Pseudomonas* species, as well as enterococci. *S. saprophyticus* is not seen in this population. Polymicrobial bacteriuria is more common among the elderly (240).

Diagnosis

Diagnosis of urinary tract infections in the elderly can be difficult. Urinary tract symptoms are often absent, and concomitant disease can mask or mimic urinary tract infection. Even severe upper tract infections may not be associated with fever or leukocytosis (12). Therefore a high index of suspicion is warranted, and diagnosis should rely on the results of a carefully obtained urinalysis and culture. The presence of greater than 10^5 CFU/mL of urine remains the standard for diagnosis in these patients. Pyuria alone is not a good predictor of bacteriuria in this population (253). Boscia and associates (25) reported that more than 60% of women with pyuria of 10 WBCs/mm^3 or greater (noted in midstream specimens) did not have a concurrent bacteriuria. However, the absence of pyuria was a good predictor of the absence of bacteriuria. Because urinary tract abnormalities can often predispose and complicate bacteriuria in the elderly, a thorough urologic evaluation is warranted. Commonly used studies include plain radiographs of the abdomen, renal and bladder ultrasonography, excretory urography, and cytoscopy.

Significance of Screening Bacteriuria

The significance of asymptomatic bacteriuria in the elderly is unclear (297). There is no documented relationship between asymptomatic bacteriuria and uncomplicated urinary tract infections and worsening renal function in this population. The treatment of asymptomatic bacteriuria to improve incontinence has not been justified (12). Although studies have demonstrated decreased survival in bacteriuric patients compared with nonbacteriuric control subjects, it is unclear whether increased mortality rates and bacteriuria are causally related (2,12). Nicolle and associates (240) randomized institutionalized women with bacteriuria to treatment or observation and followed these patients for more than 1 year. Treatment did not result in improved survival and was associated with a number of adverse effects.

Management

The exceedingly high prevalence of recurrent bacteriuria in this population, concern over the adverse actions of drugs, and the emergence of resistance associated with antimicrobial use make a universal recommendation to treat asymptomatic bacteriuria in the elderly unwarranted. However, asymptomatic patients with an alkaline pH and cultures indicating that urea-splitting organisms are present should be treated to prevent development of infection stones. When symptomatic infections are being treated, antimicrobial selections should take into account the potential for impaired metabolism and excretion of these drugs, as well as the greater likelihood of drug interactions in this population.

CATHETER-ASSOCIATED BACTERIURIA

Catheter-associated bacteriuria is the most common hospital-acquired infection, with an incidence of more than 1 million per year (121,342). The development of bacteriuria in the presence of an indwelling catheter is inevitable and occurs at an incidence of approximately 10% per day of catheterization. Intermittent catheterization has been associated with rates of bacteriuria of less than 1% in healthy individuals and 15% in elderly hospitalized patients (365). The most important risk factors associated with increased likelihood of developing catheter-associated bacteriuria are duration of catheterization, female gender, absence of systemic antimicrobials, and catheter-care violations (342). Most catheter-associated urinary tract infections are asymptomatic. In patients with short-term catheter placement, only 10% to 30% of bacteriuric episodes produce typical symptoms of acute infection (120,129). Similarly, although patients with long-term catheters are bacteriuric, the incidence of febrile episodes occurs at a rate of only 1 per 100 days of catheterization (378).

Pathogenesis

Bacteria enter the urinary tract of a catheterized patient by several routes. Bacteria can be introduced at the time of initial catheter placement by either mechanical inoculation of urethral bacteria or contamination from poor technique. Subsequently, the bacteria most commonly gain access via a periurethral or intraluminal route (342). In women, periurethral entry is the most prevalent. Daifuku and Stamm (60) found that among 18 women who developed catheter-associated bacteriuria, 12 had antecedent urethral colonization with the infecting strain. Bacteria may also enter the drainage bag and follow the intraluminal route to the bladder. This route is particularly common in patients who are clustered among other patients with indwelling catheters (208).

The urinary catheter system provides a unique environment that allows for two distinct populations of bacteria: those that grow within the urine and another population that grows on the catheter surface. A biofilm represents a microbial environment of bacteria embedded in an extracellular matrix of bacterial products and host proteins that often lead to catheter encrustation (342). Certain bacteria, particularly of the *Pseudomonas* and *Proteus* species, are adept at biofilm growth, which may explain their higher incidence in this clinical setting (229). The uropathogens isolated from the catheterized urinary tract often differ from those found in noncatheterized ambulatory patients. *E. coli* is still the most common organism isolated, but *Pseudomonas, Proteus,* and *Enterococcus* species are very prevalent (378). In patients with long-term catheterization of more than 30 days, the bacteriuria is usually polymicrobial and the presence of four or five pathogens is not uncommon (379). Although certain species may persist for long periods, the bacterial populations in these patients tend to be dynamic.

Significant bacteriuria in patients with catheters is present when greater than 100 CFU/mL is present because even this low level progresses to greater than 10^5 CFU/mL in almost all patients (208,350). Pyuria is not a discriminate indicator of infection in this population.

Management

Careful aseptic insertion of the catheter and maintenance of a closed dependent drainage system are essential to minimize development of bacteriuria. The catheter–meatal junction should be cleaned daily with water, but antimicrobials should be avoided because they lead to colonization with resistant pathogens, such as *Pseudomonas.*

Incorporation of silver oxide (301) or silver alloy (288) into the catheter and hydrogen peroxide into the drainage bag has been reported to decrease the incidence of bacteriuria in some studies (301), but not in other populations (342). Concurrent administration of systemic antimicrobials transiently decreases the incidence of bacteriuria associated with short-term catheterization, but after 3 to 4 days, the incidence of bacteriuria is similar to the rate in catheterized patients not taking systemic antimicrobials, and the prevalence of resistant bacteria and side effects is substantial. The concept of instilling nonvirulent bacteria into the bladder to completely block colonization and infection by pathogens has been tested in patients with spinal cord injuries (152). Patients successfully colonized with the nonvirulent strain had reduced symptomatic urinary tract infection and a subjective improvement in quality of life.

In patients with indwelling catheters, urine cultures should be performed if they become febrile and require antimicrobial therapy. The antimicrobial should be discontinued within 48 hours of resolution of the infection. If the catheter has been indwelling for several weeks, encrustation may shelter bacteria from the antimicrobial; therefore the catheter should be changed.

When a catheter is to be removed and there is a high probability of bacteriuria, a culture should be obtained 24 hours before removal. The patient should be started on empiric antimicrobial therapy such as TMP-SMX just before decatheterization and maintained on therapy for 2 days. A posttherapy culture should be obtained 7 to 10 days later to confirm the eradication of the bacteriuria.

FUNGURIA

Funguria is usually associated with predisposing factors, including indwelling catheters, antimicrobial therapy, diabetes mellitus, hospitalization, and immunosuppressed states (184).

Clinical Findings

Fungi may invade the kidneys as the result of hematogenous spread from other sources of infection or the gastrointestinal tract. *Candida albicans* accounts for approximately 50% of positive fungal cultures. *Candida glabrata* is the second most common fungus, representing approximately 10% to 15% of positive fungal cultures (228). *C. glabrata* is a normal commensal organism of the gastrointestinal tract and vagina and probably colonizes the urinary tract by ascending infection.

Asymptomatic funguria, implying urinary colonization rather than infection, is common. Invasive infection is suggested by the presence of irritative voiding symptoms and pyuria. Renal or perinephric abscesses and fungus balls (also known as bezoars) may result from funguria. These patients may demonstrate symptoms suggestive of pyelonephritis with flank pain and fever. However, fungal balls may develop in the collecting system of asymptomatic patients.

Diagnosis

The criteria for diagnosis are unclear. Particularly in women, vaginal or perineal colonization may contaminate urine specimens. Microscopic examination can reveal fungi budding forms or pseudohyphae. The presence of pyuria does not correlate well with the presence of symptoms or the degree of funguria. Cultures of 10,000 to 15,000 CFU/mL have been suggested as cutoff points for infection (182). Regardless of the count, a positive culture requires evaluation.

Management

A treatment algorithm for genitourinary fungal infection has been presented by Wise (388) (Fig. 4.37). Before antifungal therapy, predisposing factors to funguria should be eliminated. Unnecessary indwelling catheters should be removed and the nutritional status should be optimized. Discontinuation of broad-spectrum antimicrobial agents reduces fungal colonization. If, after removal of the catheter, fungal infection persists, amphotericin B may be instilled intravesically for up to 1 week. Fifty milligrams of amphotericin B dissolved in 1 L of sterile water is introduced into

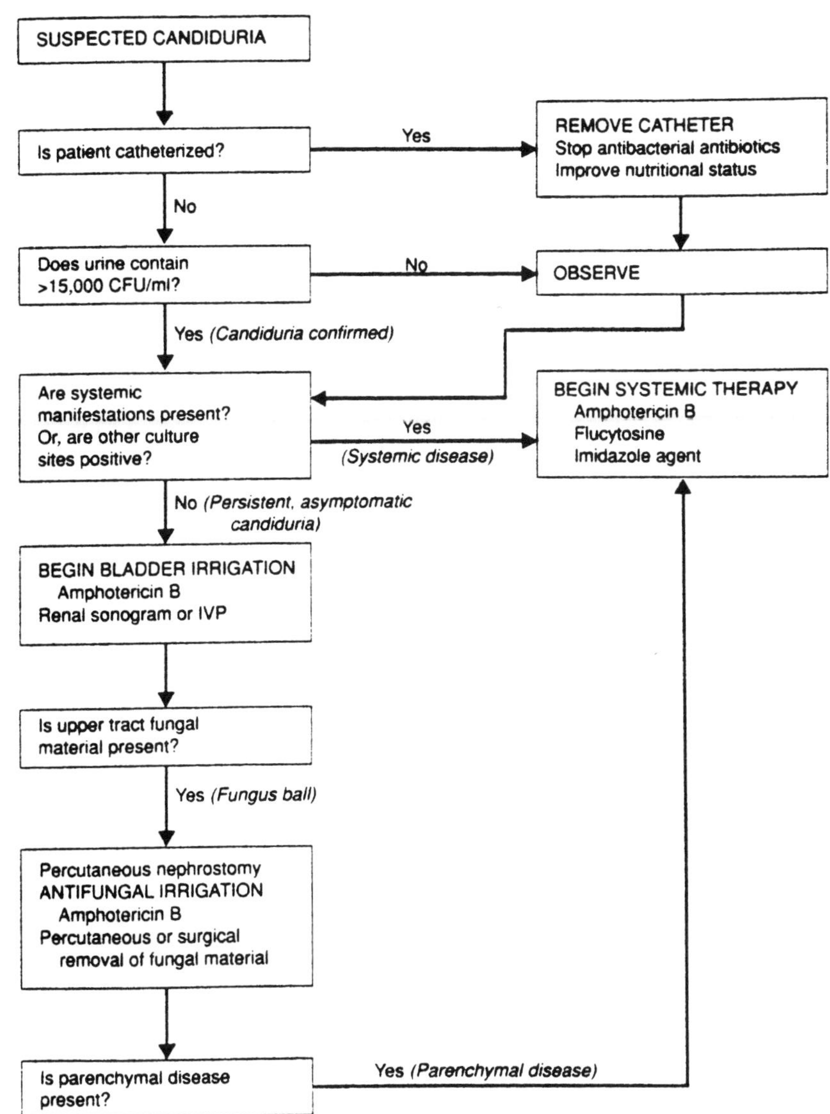

FIGURE 4.37. Treatment algorithm for management of suspected candiduria. IVP, intravenous pyelogram. (Reprinted with permission from Wise GJ. Amphotericin B in urologic practice. *J Urol* 1990;144:215.)

the bladder via a three-way catheter over a 24-hour period (390). Alternatively, 200 to 300 mL of irrigant may be instilled for 1 to 2 hours with clamping of the catheter. Miconazole (50 mg per liter per day) has also been shown to be effective as a bladder irrigant (391). Amphotericin B may also be instilled via nephrostomy tube for upper tract fungal infection. Oral fluconazole has been shown to be as effective and safe as amphotericin B bladder irrigation for treatment of older adults with funguria (160).

Funguria also may be treated effectively with oral agents. Flucytosine is readily absorbed from the gastrointestinal tract and is primarily excreted renally. A dosage of 100 to 200 mg/kg per day in four divided doses for 2 to 3 weeks is recommended. Dosing adjustments should be made for patients with renal insufficiency. Wise and associates (389) reported success (as defined by a decrease in colony counts or clinical improvement) in 212 of 225 patients treated for 21 to 28 days. Fungal resistance was reported in 14 of the patients. Flucytosine may be used in combination with amphotericin B bladder irrigation. Side effects include an elevation in liver function tests, diarrhea, and agranulocytosis.

Fluconazole is a triazole antifungal agent that is readily absorbed from the gastrointestinal tract and is excreted predominantly in unchanged form in the urine. Dosing is typically 200 mg for the first day followed by 100 mg daily for 10 to 14 days. Success rates of greater than 75% to 80% have been reported in studies treating *Candida* species with limited numbers of patients (15,221,242). The most common side effects present in 60% of patients include nausea, headache, skin rash, abdominal pain, vomiting, and diarrhea (113).

Patients with renal candidiasis and disseminated infection are usually treated with intravenous amphotericin B. Amphotericin B acts in a fungicidal fashion by binding to the fungal-cell membranes, eventually resulting in disruption of the internal cellular components. Fungal resistance is uncommon. Because excretion is primarily biliary, amphotericin B may be administered to patients with renal insufficiency with caution because of its nephrotoxic effects, but without need for dosing adjustment. Side effects of significance with amphotericin B include chills, rigors, fevers, phlebitis, bone marrow toxicity, and potassium and magnesium depletion. After an initial dose of 1 mg, the dose may be increased gradually in daily increments of 5 mg to a maintenance dose of 0.3 to 1.2 mg/kg. Daily dosing should not exceed 50 mg. Although strict guidelines for duration of total amount of therapy do not exist, most renal infections require between 500 mg and 1.5 to 2 g over a 6- to 12-week period (223). Fluconazole has not been used extensively for upper tract infections, but when given intravenously, it has been shown to be effective in treating systemic candidiasis in critically ill patients (4,54,112,186).

The presence of fungal balls and accompanying obstruction should be assessed in patients with suspected upper tract funguria. Fungal balls typically involve *Candida* species because of their propensity to develop pseudohyphae. Patients with upper tract obstruction are especially prone to fungemia. The patients often require the placement of percutaneous nephrostomy tubes to relieve the obstruction. This tube may then be used to instill antifungal irrigant or to provide a tract for access for percutaneous endourologic removal of the fungal ball.

REFERENCES

1. Abdou NI et al. Malakoplakia: evidence for monocytic lysosomal abnormality correctable by cholinergic agonist *in vitro* and *in vivo*. *N Engl J Med* 1977;297:1413.
2. Abrutyn E, Mossey J, Berlin JA, et al. Does asymptomatic bacteriuria predict mortality and does antimicrobial treatment reduce mortality in elderly ambulatory women? *Ann Intern Med* 1994;120:827.
3. Ahlering TE et al. Emphysematous pyelonephritis: a 5-year experience with 13 patients. *J Urol* 1985;134:1086.
4. Anaissie E, Brody GP, Kantarjan H, et al. Fluconazole therapy for chronic disseminated candidiasis in patients with leukemia and prior amphotericin B therapy. *Am J Med* 1991;91:142.
5. Anderson KA, McAninch JW. Renal abscesses: classification and review of 40 cases. *Urology* 1980;16:333.
6. Angell JC, Smith I. Renal malakoplakia with perinephric extension. *Br J Urol* 1968;40:429.
7. Aronson M, Medalia O, Schori L, et al. Prevention of colonization of the urinary tract of mice with *Escherichia coli* by blocking of bacteria adherence with methyl-D-mannopyranoside. *J Infect Dis* 1979;139:329.

7a. Asscher AW. *The challenge of urinary tract infection.* New York: Academy Press, 1980.

8. Asscher AW, Sussman M, Weiser R. Bacterial growth in human urine. In: O'Grady F, Brumfitt W, eds. *Urinary tract infection.* Oxford University Press, 1968.
9. Asscher AW, Chick S, Radford N, et al. Natural history of asymptomatic bacteriuria in nonpregnant women. In: Brumfitt W, Asscher AW, eds. *Urinary tract infection.* London: University Press, 1973.
10. Badenock AW. Reparative surgery for tuberculous stricture of the ureter. *X Congress Society International D Urology* 1961; 1:163.
11. Baijal SS, Basarge N, Srinadh ES, et al. Percutaneous management of renal hydatidosis: a minimally invasive therapeutic option. *J Urol* 1995;1199.
12. Baldassarre JS, Kaye D. Special problems of urinary tract infection in the elderly. *Med Clin North Am* 1991;75:375.
13. Bailey RR, Lynn KL, Robson RA, et al. DMSA renal scans in adults with acute pyelonephritis. *Clin Nephrol* 1996;46:99.
14. Ballesteros JJ, Faus R, Gironella J. Preoperative diagnosis of renal xanthogranulomatosis by serial urine cytology: preliminary report. *J Urol* 1980;124:9.
15. Bamberger MH, Fan-Harvard P, Eng R, et al. Role of fluconazole in the management of fungal urinary tract infections. *J Urol* 1992;147[pt 2]:231A (abst).
16. Baumgarten DA, Baumgarten BR. Imaging and radiologic management of upper urinary tract infections. *Uroradiology* 1997;24:545.
17. Beeson PB, Rowley D. The anticomplementary effect of kidney tissue: its association with ammonia production. *J Exp Med* 1959;110:685.
18. Behr MA, Drummond R, Libman MD, et al. Fever duration in hospitalized acute pyelonephritis patients. *Am J Med* 1996; 101: 277.
19. Best CD, Terris MK, Tacker JR, et al. Clinical and radiological findings in patients with gas forming renal abscess treated conservatively. *J Urol* 1999;162:1273.
20. Bhargava BN et al. Pyeloduodenal fistula secondary to renal tuberculosis. *J R Coll Surg Edinb* 1982;27:242.
21. Bjorksten B, Kaijser B. Interaction of human serum and neutrophils with *Escherichia coli* strains: differences between strains isolated from urine or patients with pyelonephritis or asymptomatic bacteriuria. *Infect Immun* 1978;22:308.
22. Borthiwick WM. Genitourinary tuberculosis. *Tubercle* 1956; 37:120.
23. Boscia JA, Kaye D. Asymptomatic bacteriuria in the elderly. *IDCNA* 1987;1:839.
24. Boscia JA, Kobasa WK, Knight RA, et al. Epidemiology of bacteriuria in an elderly ambulatory population. *Am J Med* 1986;80:208.
25. Boscia JA et al. Pyuria and asymptomatic bacteriuria in elderly ambulatory women. *Ann Intern Med* 1989;110:404.
26. Bowers JH, Cathey WJ. Malakoplakia of the kidney with renal failure. *Am J Clin Pathol* 1971;55:765.
27. Brenbridge AN et al. Renal emphysema of the transplanted kidney: sonographic appearance. *AJR Am J Roentgenol* 1979; 132:656.
28. Brumfitt W, Gruneberg RN, Leigh DA. Bacteriuria in pregnancy, with reference to prematurity and long-term effects on the mother. In: *Symposium on pyelonephritis.* Edinburgh: E & S Livingstone, 1967.
29. Buckley RJ et al. Echinococcal disease of the kidney presenting as a renal filling defect. *J Urol* 1985;133:660.
30. Bukowski TP, Betrus GG, Aquilina JW, et al. Urinary tract infections and pregnancy in women who underwent antireflux surgery in childhood. *J Urol* 159:1286.
31. Burman LG. Significance of the sulfonamide component for the clinical efficacy of trimethoprim-sulfonamide combinations. *Scand J Infect Dis* 1986;18:89.
32. Busch R, Huland H. Correlation of symptoms and results of direct bacterial localization in patients with urinary tract infections. *J Urol* 1984;132:282.

33. Butnick R. Xanthogranulomatous pyelonephritis: an unusual case. *J Urol* 1971;106:815.
34. Cadnapaphornchai P et al. Renal parenchymal malakoplakia: an unusual cause of renal failure. *N Engl J Med* 1978;299:1110.
35. Callea F, Van Damme B, Desmet VJ. Alpha-1-antitrypsin in malakoplakia. *Virchows Arch [A]* 1982;395:1.
36. Campbell MF. Perinephric abscess. *Surg Gynecol Obstet* 1930; 51:654.
37. Campbell-Brown M, McFadyen IR, Seal OR, et al. Is screening for bacteriuria in pregnancy worth while? *BMJ Clin Res* 1987; 294:1579.
38. Carlson KJ, Mulley AG. Management of acute dysuria: a decision-analysis model of alternative strategies. *Ann Intern Med* 1985;102:244.
39. Cattell WR et al. *The localization of urinary tract infection and its relationship to relapse, reinfection and treatment.* London: Oxford University Press, 1973.
40. Cattell WR, McSherry MA, Northeast A, et al. Periurethral enterobacterial carriage in pathogenesis of recurrent urinary infections. *BMJ* 1974;4:136.
41. Cavins JA, Goldstein AMB. Renal malakoplakia. *Urology* 1977; 10:155.
42. Chan RCY, Bruce AW, Reid G. Adherence of cervical, vaginal and distal urethral normal microbial flora to human uroepithelial cells and the blockage of adherence of uropathogens by competitive exclusion. *J Urol* 1984;131:596.
43. Charboneau JW et al. Malakoplakia of the urinary tract with renal parenchymal involvement. *Urol Radiol* 1980;2:89.
44. Charlton CAC, Crowther A, Davies JG, et al. Three-day and ten-day chemotherapy for urinary tract infections in general practice. *BMJ* 1976;1:124.
45. Chaung CK, Lai MK, Chang PL, et al. Xanthogranulomatous pyelonephritis: experience in 36 cases. *J Urol* 1992;147:333.
46. Chernow B et al. Measurement of urinary leukocyte esterase activity: a screening test for urinary tract infections. *Ann Emerg Med* 1984;13:150.
47. Christ W, Lehnert T, Ulbrich B. Specific toxicologic aspects to the quinolones. *Rev Infect Dis* 1988;10:141.
48. Claridge M. Ureteric obstruction in tuberculosis. *Urology* 1970; 42:688.
49. Cockerill FR, Edson RS. Trimethoprim-sulfamethoxazole. *Mayo Clin Proc* 1991;66:1249.
50. Cohen ML. Epidemiology of drug resistance: implications for a post-antimicrobial era. *Science* 1992;257:1050.
51. Coltorti EA, Varela-Diaz VM. Detection of antibodies against *Echinococcus granulosus* arc 5 antigens by double diffusion test. *Trans R Soc Trop Med Hyg* 1978;72:226.
52. Connell H, Agace W, Klemm P, et al. Type 1 fimbrial expression enhances *Escherichia coli* virulence for the urinary tract. *Proc Natl Acad Sci USA* 1996;93:9827.
53. Conrad MR, Bregman R, Kilman WJ. Ultrasonic recognition of parenchymal gas. *AJR Am J Roentgenol* 1979;132:395.
54. Corbella X, Carratala J, Castells, M, et al. Fluconazole treatment in *torulopis glabrata* upper urinary tract infection causing ureteral obstruction. *J Urol* 1992;147:1116.
55. Corigliano B, Leedom JM. Renal tuberculosis: part 2. In: Massry SG, Glassock RJ, eds. *Textbook of nephrology,* vol 1. Baltimore: Williams & Wilkins, 1983.
56. Corriere JN, Sandler CM. The diagnosis and immediate therapy of acute renal and perirenal infections. *Urol Clin North Am* 1982;9:219.
57. Cotran RS. Experimental pyelonephritis. In: Rouiller C, Muller AF, eds. *The kidney,* vol 2. New York: Academic Press, 1969.
58. Cox CE, Hinman F Jr. Experiments with induced bacteriuria, vesical emptying and bacterial growth on the mechanism of bladder defense to infection. *J Urol* 1961;86:739.
59. Cunningham FG, Morris GB, Mickal A. Acute pyelonephritis of pregnancy: a clinical review. *Obstet Gynecol* 1973;42:112.
60. Daifuku R, Stamm W. Association of rectal and urethral colonization with urinary tract infection in patients with indwelling catheters. *JAMA* 1984;252:2028.
61. Dalkin BL, Schaeffer AJ. Fluoroquinolone antimicrobial agents: use in the treatment of urinary tract infections and clinical urologic practice. *Probl Urol* 1988;2:476.
62. Davidson AG, Talner LB. Late sequelae of adult onset bacterial nephritis. *Radiology* 1978;127:367.
63. Davies BI, Maesen FPV. Drug interactions with quinolones. *Rev Infect Dis* 1989;11:1083.
64. DeNavasquez S. Experimental pyelonephritis in the rabbit produced by staphylococcal infection. *J Pathol* 1950;62:429.
65. DeRee JM, Van Den Bosch JF. Serological response to the P fimbriae of uropathogenic *Escherichia coli* in pyelonephritis. *Infect Immun* 1987;55:2204.
66. Deridder PA et al. Renal malakoplakia. *J Urol* 1977;117:428.
67. Duguid JP, Clegg S, Wilson MI. The fimbrial and nonfimbrial haemagglutinins of *Escherichia coli. J Med Microbiol* 1979; 12:213.
68. Duncan JL. Differential effect of Tamm-Horsfall protein on adherence of *Escherichia coli* to transitional epithelial cells. *J Infect Dis* 1988;158:1379.
69. Eastham J, Ahlering T, Skinner E. Xanthogranulomatous pyelonephritis: clinical findings and surgical consideration. *Adult Urol* March 1994;43:295.
70. Edelstein H, McCabe RE. Perinephric abscess. *Medicine* 1988; 67:118.
71. Editorial: medical treatment for hydatid disease. *BMJ* 1979; 2:563.
72. Eisenstein BI. Phase variation of type-1 fimbriae in *Escherichia coli* is under transcriptional control. *Science* 1981;214:337.
73. Elder JS. Xanthogranulomatous pyelonephritis and gas forming infections of the urinary tract. *AUA Update* 1984;III.2, lesson 31.
74. Elder JS et al. The natural history of asymptomatic bacteriuria during pregnancy: the effect of tetracycline on the clinical course and the outcome of pregnancy. *Am J Obstet Gynecol* 1971;111:441.
75. Elliott TSJ et al. Bacteriology and ultrastructure of the bladder in patients with urinary tract infections. *J Infect* 1985;11:191.
76. Ena J, Concepcion A, Martinez C, et al. Risk factors for acquisition of urinary tract infections caused by ciprofloxacin resistant *Escherichia coli. J Urol* 1995;153:117.
77. Eykyn S et al. The localization of urinary tract infection by ureteric catheterization. *Invest Urol* 1972;9:271.
78. Fagerholm M. Case of the autumn season. *Semin Ultrasound* 1983;4:145.
79. Fair WR, Timothy MM, Millar MA, et al. Bacteriologic and hormonal observations of urethra and vaginal vestibule in normal, premenopausal women. *J Urol* 1981;104:426.
80. Fairley KF. The routine determination of the site of infection in the investigation of patients with urinary tract infection. In: Kincaid-Smith P, Fairley KF, eds. *Renal infection and renal scarring.* Melbourne: Mercedes, 1972.
81. Fairley KF, Birch DF. Detection of bladder bacteriuria in patients with acute urinary symptoms. *J Infect Dis* 1989; 159: 226.
82. Fairley KF, Bond AG, Adey FD. The site of infection in pregnancy bacteriuria. *Lancet* 1966;1:939.
83. Fairley KF, Bond AG, Brown RB, et al. Simple test to determine the site of urinary tract infection. *Lancet* 1967;2:427.

84. Faro S, Pastorek JG, Plauche WC. Short-course parental antibiotic therapy for pyelonephritis in pregnancy. *South Med* 1984; 77:455.
85. Fihn SD. Single-dose antimicrobial therapy for urinary tract infections: "Less is more"? or "Reductio ad absurdum"? *J Gen Intern Med* 1986;1:62.
86. Fihn SD, Latham RH, Roberts P, et al. Association between diaphragm use and urinary tract infection. *JAMA* 1985; 254:240.
87. Fischman NH, Roberts JA. Clinical studies in acute pyelonephritis: is there a place for renal quantitative camera study? *J Urol* 1982;128:452.
88. Flechner SM, Gow JG. Role of nephrectomy in the treatment of nonfunctioning or very poorly functioning unilateral tuberculous kidney. *J Urol* 1980;123:822.
89. Flynn JT et al. The underestimated hazards of xanthogranulomatous pyelonephritis. *Br J Urol* 1979;51:443.
90. Forland M, Thomas V, Shelokov A. Urinary tract infections in patients with diabetes mellitus: studies on antibody coating of bacteria. *JAMA* 1977;238:1924.
91. Fowler JE, Perkins T. Presentation, diagnosis and treatment of renal abscesses: 1972-1988. *J Urol* 1994;151:847.
92. Fowler JE, Stamey TA. Studies of the introital colonization in women with recurrent urinary tract infections; VII. The role of bacterial adherence. *J Urol* 1977;117:472.
93. Foxman B, Marsh J, Gillespie B, et al. Condom use and first-time urinary tract infection. *Epidemiology* 1997;8: 637.
94. Foxman B, Geiger AM, Palin K, et al. First-time urinary tract infection and sexual behavior. *Epidemiology* 1995;6:162.
95. Fraser IR, Birch D, Fairley KF, et al. A prospective study of cortical scarring in acute febrile pyelonephritis in adults: clinical and bacteriological characteristics. *Clin Nephrol* 1995;43:159.
96. Freedman LR. Natural history of urinary tract infection in adults. *Kidney Int* 1975;8:896.
97. Freedman LR. Interstitial renal inflammation, including pyelonephritis and urinary tract infection. In: Early LE, Gottschalk CW, eds. *Strauss and Welt's diseases of the kidney,* vol 2, ed 3. Boston: Little, Brown, 1979.
98. Freedman LR, Beeson PB. Experimental pyelonephritis. IV. Observations on infections resulting from direct inoculation of bacteria in different zones of the kidney. *Yale J Biol Med* 1958;30:406.
99. Friedenberg MJ, Spjut HJ. Xanthogranulomatous pyelonephritis. *AJR Am J Roentgenol* 1963;90:97.
100. Gaffney RA, Venegas MF, Kanerva C, et al. Effect of vaginal fluid on adherence of type 1 piliated *Escherichia coli* to epithelial cells. *J Infect Dis* 1995;172:1528.
101. Gajaraj A, Victor S. Tuberculous aortoarteritis. *Clin Radiol* 1981;32:461.
102. Garrett IR, McClure J. Renal malakoplakia: experimental production and evidence of a link with interstitial megalocytic nephritis. *J Pathol* 1982;136:111.
103. Gilbert DN. Once daily aminoglycoside therapy. *Antimicrob Agents Chemother* 1991;35:399.
104. Gillenwater JY, Harrison RB, Kunin CM. Natural history of bacteriuria in school girls: a long-term case-control study. *N Engl J Med* 1979;301:396.
105. Gilsanz V, Lozano G, Jimenez J. Renal hydatid cysts: communicating with collecting system. *AJR Am J Roentgenol* 1980; 135:357.
106. Gilstrap et al. Renal infection and pregnancy outcomes. *Am J Obstet Gynecol* 1981;141:709.
107. Godec CJ et al. Diagnostic strategy in evaluation of renal abscess. *Urology* 1981;18:535.
108. Goldman SM et al. CT of xanthogranulomatous pyelonephritis: radiologic-pathologic correlation. *AJR Am J Roentgenol* 1984;141:963.
109. Goodman M, Curry T, Russell T. Xanthogranulomatous pyelonephritis (XGP): a local disease with systemic manifestations: report of 23 patients and review of the literature. *Medicine* 1979;58:171.
110. Gow JG. The management of genitourinary tuberculosis. *J Antimicrob Chemother* 1981;7:590.
111. Grainger RG, Longstaff AJ, Parsons MA. Xanthogranulomatous pyelonephritis: a reappraisal. *Lancet* 1982;1:1398.
112. Graninger W, Presteril E, Schneeweiss B, et al. Treatment of *Candida albicans* fungaemia with fluconazole. *J Infect* 1993; 26:133.
113. Grant SM, Clissold SP. Fluconazole. A review of pharmacodynamic and pharmacokinetic properties and therapeutic potential in superficial and systemic mycoses. *Drugs* 1990;39:877.
114. Greenberg M, Falkowski WS, Sekowicz BA, et al. Use of computerized tomography in the evaluation of filling defects of the renal pelvis. *J Urol* 1982;127:1172.
115. Gregg CR, Rogers TE, Munford RS. Xanthogranulomatous pyelonephritis. *Curr Clin Topics Infect Dis* 1999;19:287.
116. Gupta K, Hillier SL, Hooton TM, et al. Effects of contraceptive method on the vaginal microbial flora: a prospective evaluation. *J Infect Dis* 2000;181:595.
117. Gupta K, Scholes D, Stamm WE. Increasing prevalence of antimicrobial resistance among uropathogens causing acute uncomplicated cystitis in women. *JAMA* 1999;281:736.
118. Gutman LT, Turck M, Peterdorf RG, et al. Significance of bacterial variants in urine of patients with chronic bacteriuria. *J Clin Invest* 1965;44:1945.
119. Guze LB, Beeson PB. Experimental pyelonephritis. I. Effect of ureteral ligation on the course of bacterial infection in the kidney of the rat. *J Exp Med* 1956;104:803.
120. Haley RW et al. Nosocomial infection in U.S. hospitals, 1975-1976: estimated frequency by selected characteristics of patients. *Am J Med* 1981;70:947.
121. Haley R, Culver O, White J, et al. The nationwide nosocomial infection rate: a new need for vital statistics. *Am J Epidemiol* 1985;121:159.
122. Haraoka M, Hang, L, Frendéus B, et al. Neutrophil recruitment and resistance to urinary tract infection. *J Infect Dis* 1999;180:1220.
123. Harbord RB, Gruneberg RN. Treatment of urinary tract infection with a single dose of amoxycillin, cotrimoxazole, or trimethoprim. *BMJ* 1981;283:1301.
124. Harrison RB, Shaffer HA Jr. The roentgenographic findings in acute pyelonephritis. *JAMA* 1979;241:1718.
125. Hartman DS. Radiologic pathologic correlation of the infectious granulomatous diseases of the kidney. Parts I and II. *Monogr Urol* 1985;6:3.
126. Hartman DS. Radiologic pathologic correlations of the infectious granulomatous diseases of the kidney. Parts III and IV. *Monogr Urol* 1985;6:26.
127. Hartman DS, Sanders RC, Davis CJ. Xanthogranulomatous pyelonephritis: sonographic-pathologic correlation of 16 cases. *J Ultrasound Med* 1984;3:481.
128. Hartman DS, Davis CJ, Lichtenstein JE, et al. Renal parenchymal malakoplakia. *Radiology* 1980;136:33.
129. Hartstein AI, Garber SB, Ward TT, et al. Nosocomial urinary tract infection: a prospective evaluation of 108 catheterized patients. *Infect Control* 1981;2:380.
130. Hawes S et al. Emphysematous pyelonephritis. *Infect Surg* 1983;2:191.

131. Heptinstall RH. *Pathology of the kidney,* ed 2. Boston: Little, Brown, 1974.
132. Hicks, RM. The mammalian urinary bladder: an accommodating organ. *Biol Rev* 1975;50: 215.
133. Hjelm EM. Local cellular immune response in ascending urinary tract infection: occurrence of T-cells, immunoglobulin-producing cells, and Ia-expressing cells in rat urinary tract tissue. *Infect Immun* 1984;44:627.
134. Ho Khang-Loon, Rassekh ZA, Nam SH. Bilateral renal malakoplakia. *Urology* 1979;13:321.
135. Hodson CJ. Coarse pyelonephritis scarring of "atrophic pyelonephritis." *Proc R Soc Med* 1965;58:785.
136. Hodson CJ, Edwards D. Chronic pyelonephritis and vesicoureteral reflux. *Clin Radiol* 1960;11:219.
137. Hodson CJ, Wilson S. Natural history of chronic pyelonephritis scarring. *BMJ* 1965;2:191.
138. Hootkins R, Fenzer AZ, Stephens MK. Acute renal failure secondary to oral ciprofloxacin therapy: a presentation of three cases and a review of the literature. *Clin Nephrol* 1989;32:75.
139. Hooton TM, Scholes D, Hughes JP, et al. A prospective study of risk factors for symptomatic urinary tract infection in young women. *N Engl J Med* 1996;335:468.
140. Hooton TM, Stamm WE. Diagnosis and treatment of uncomplicated urinary tract infection. *Infect Dis Clin North Am* 1991;11:551.
141. Hooton TM, Stamm WE. Management of acute uncomplicated urinary tract infection in adults. *Med Clin North Am* 1991;75:339.
142. Hooton TM, Johnson C, Roberts PL, et al. The association of sex, with or without diaphragm and spermicide use, with UTI, abstract 8, p 102. In: *Programs and Abstracts of the 29th Interscience Conference on Antimicrobial Agents and Chemotherapy,* Houston, 1989.
143. Hooton TM et al. *Escherichia coli* bacteriuria and contraceptive method. *JAMA* 1991;265:64.
144. Hooton TM et al. Nonoxynol-9: differential antibacterial activity and enhancement of bacterial adherence to vaginal epithelial cells. *J Infect Dis* 1991;164:1216.
145. Hopkins WJ, Gendron-Fitzpatrick A, Balish E, et al. Time course and host responses to *Escherichia coli* urinary tract infection in genetically distinct mouse strains. *Infect Immun* 1998; 66:2798.
146. Horne NW, Tulloch WS. Conservative management of renal tuberculosis. *Br J Urol* 1975;47:481.
147. Houston T II, Peacock J Jr, Appel RG, et al. Gallium-67-citrate scanning of renal parenchymal malacoplakia. *J Nucl Med* 1998; 39:1454.
148. Hovelius B, Mardh PA. *Staphylococcus saprophyticus* as a common cause of urinary tract infection. *Rev Infect Dis* 1984;6:328.
149. Hudson MA, Weyman PJ, van der Vliet AH, et al. Emphysematous pyelonephritis: successful management by percutaneous drainage. *J Urol* 1986;136:884.
150. Hughes CE, Hacker J, Roberts A, et al. Hemolysin production as a virulence marker in symptomatic and asymptomatic urinary tract infections caused by *Escherichia coli. Infect Immun* 1983;39:546.
151. Huland H, Busch R. Chronic pyelonephritis as a cause of end-stage renal disease. *J Urol* 1982;127:642.
152. Hull R, Rudy D, Donovan W, et al. Urinary tract infection prophylaxis using *Escherichia coli* 83972 in spinal cord injured patients. *J Urol* 1999;163:872.
153. Hultgren SJ et al. Role of type-1 pili and effects of phase variation on lower urinary tract infection produced by *Escherichia coli. Infect Immun* 1985;50:370.
154. Hultgren SJ et al. Regulation of production of type-1 pili among urinary tract isolates of *Escherichia coli. Infect Immun* 1986;54:613.
155. Hurlbut AT, Littenberg B. The diagnostic accuracy of rapid dipstick tests to predict urinary tract infection. *Am J Clin Pathol* 1991;96:582.
156. Innes JA. Nonrespiratory tuberculosis. *J R Coll Physicians (Lond)* 1981;15:227.
157. Iravani A. Advances in the understanding and treatment of urinary tract infections in young women. *Urology* 1991;37:503.
158. Israel RS, Lowenstein SR, Marx JA, et al. Management of acute pyelonephritis in an emergency department observation unit. *Ann Emerg Med* 1991;20:253.
159. Iwahi T, Abe Y, Nakao M, et al. Role of type-1 fimbriae in the pathogenesis of ascending urinary tract infection induced by *Escherichia coli* in mice. *Infect Immun* 1983;39:1307.
160. Jacobs LG, Skidmore EA, Freeman K, et al. Oral fluconazole compared with bladder irrigation with amphotericin B for treatment of fungal urinary tract infections in elderly patients. *Clin Infect Dis* 1995;22:30.
161. Jenkins RD, Fenn JP, Matsen J. Review of urine microscopy for bacteriuria. *JAMA* 1986;255:3397.
162. Johnson JR, Stamm WE. Diagnosis and treatment of acute urinary tract infections. *Infect Dis Clin North Am* 1987;1:907.
163. Johnson JR, Stamm WE. Urinary tract infections in women: diagnosis and treatment. *Ann Intern Med* 1989;111:906.
164. Johnson JR, Mosely SL, Roberts PL, et al. Aerobactin and other virulence factor genes among strains of *Escherichia coli* causing urosepsis: association with patient characteristics. *Infect Immun* 1988;56:405.
165. Jones CH, Pinkner JS, Roth R, et al. FimH adhesin of type 1 pili is assembled into a fibrillar tip structure in the Enterobacteriaceae. *Proc Natl Acad Sci USA* 1995;92:2081.
166. Jordan PA, Iravani A, Richard GA, et al. Urinary tract infection caused by *Staphylococcus saprophyticus. J Infect Dis* 1980; 142:510.
167. Josephson S, Thomason J, Sturino K, et al. *Gardnerella vaginalis* in the urinary tract: incidence and significance in a hospital population. *Obstet Gynecol* 1988;71:245.
168. Kallenius G, Mollby R, Svenson SB, et al. The p^k antigen as receptor for the haemagglutinin of pyelonephritic *Escherichia coli. FEMS Microbiol Lett* 1980;7:297.
169. Kallenius G, Mollby R, Svenson SB, et al. Occurrence of P-fimbriated *Escherichia coli* in urinary tract infections. *Lancet* 1981;2:1369.
170. Kaplan DM, Rosenfield AT, Smith RC. Advances in the imaging of renal infection—helical CT and modern coordinated imaging. *Infect Dis Clin North Am* 1997;11:681.
171. Kass EH, Finland M. Asymptomatic infection of the urinary tract. *Trans Assoc Am Physicians* 1956;69:56.
172. Kaul AK, Khan S, Martens MG, et al. Experimental gestational pyelonephritis induces preterm births and low birth weights in C3H/HeJ mice. *Infect Immun* 1999;67:5958.
173. Kaye D. Antibacterial activity of human urine. *J Clin Invest* 1968;47:2374.
174. Kaye D. Urinary tract infection in the elderly. *Bull N Y Acad Med* 1980;56:209.
175. Kennedy RP, Plorde JJ, Petersdorf RG. Studies on the epidemiology of *Escherichia coli* infections. IV. Evidence for a nosocomial flora. *J Clin Invest* 1965;44:193.
176. Khalyl-Mawad J, Greco MA, Schinella RA. Ultrastructural demonstration of intracellular bacteria in xanthogranulomatous pyelonephritis. *Hum Pathol* 1982;13:41.

177. Kincaid-Smith P, Bullen M. Bacteriuria in pregnancy. *Lancet* 1965;1:395.
178. Kisielius PV, Schwan WR, Amundsen SK, et al. *In vivo* expression and phase variation of type-1 and P pili by *Escherichia coli* in the urine of adults with acute urinary tract infections. *Infect Immun* 1989;57:1656.
179. Klemm P. Fimbrial adhesions of *Escherichia coli. Rev Inf Dis* 1985;7:321.
180. Komaroff AL. Acute dysuria in women. *N Engl J Med* 1984; 310:368.
181. Komaroff AL. Urinalysis and urine culture in women with dysuria. *Ann Intern Med* 1986;104:212.
182. Kozinn PJ, Taschdjian CL, Goldberg PK, et al. Advances in the diagnosis of renal candidiasis. *J Urol* 1978;119:184.
183. Kraft JK, Stamey AT. The natural history of symptomatic recurrent bacteriuria in women. *Medicine* 1977;56:55.
184. Krcmery S, Dubrava M, Krcmery V. Fungal urinary tract infections in patients at risk. *Int J Antimicrob Agents* 1999; 11:289.
185. Krieger JN, Ross SO, Simonsen JM. Urinary tract infections in healthy university men. *J Urol* 1993;149:1046.
186. Kujath P, Lerch K. Secondary mycosis in surgery: treatment with fluconazole. *Infection* 1989;17:111.
187. Kulkarni SH et al. Adenocarcinoma of the renal pelvis with associated tuberculosis of the kidney. *Indiana J Cancer* 1981; 18:229.
188. Kumar S, Muchmore A. Tamm-Horsfall protein—Uromodulin (1950-1990). *Kidney Int* 1990;37:1395.
189. Kunin CM. Use of antimicrobial agents in treating urinary tract infection. *Adv Nephrol* 1985;14:39.
190. Kunin CM. *Detection, prevention and management of urinary tract infections,* ed 4. Philadelphia: Lea & Febiger, 1987.
191. Langermann S, Palaszynski S, Barnhart M, et al. Prevention of mucosal *Escherichia coli* infection by FimH-adhesin-based systemic vaccination. *Science* 1997;276: 607.
192. Latham RH, Running K, Stamm WE. Urinary tract infections in young adult women caused by *Staphylococcus saprophyticus. JAMA* 1983;250:3036.
193. Lattimer JK. Current concepts of renal tuberculosis. *N Engl J Med* 1965;273:208.
194. Lattimer JK, Wechsler MW. Editorial comment: surgical management of nonfunctioning tuberculous kidneys. *J Urol* 1980; 124:191.
195. Lee JKT et al. Acute focal bacterial nephritis: emphasis on gray-scale sonography and computed tomography. *AJR Am J Roentgenol* 1980;135:87.
196. Leffler H, Svanborg Eden C. Chemical identification of glycosphingolipid receptor for *Escherichia coli* attaching to human urinary tract epithelial cells and agglutinating erythrocytes. *FEMS Microbial Lett* 1980;8:127.
197. Lester TW. Extrapulmonary tuberculosis. *Clin Chest Med* 1980;1:219.
198. Levin R et al. The diagnosis and management of renal inflammatory processes in children. *J Urol* 1984;132:718.
199. Lindner LE, Jones RN, Haber MH. A specific urinary cast in acute pyelonephritis. *Am J Clin Pathol* 1980;73:809.
200. Lomberg H, Hanson LA, Jacobsson B, et al. Correlation of P blood group, vesicoureteral reflux, and bacterial attachment in patients with recurrent pyelonephritis. *N Engl J Med* 1983; 308:1189.
201. Lorin MI, Hsu KHF, Jacob SC. Treatment of tuberculosis in children. *Pediatr Clin North Am* 1983;30:333.
202. Lou TY, Teplitz C. Malakoplakia: pathogenesis and ultrastructural morphogenesis: a problem of altered macrophage (phagolysosomal) response. *Hum Pathol* 1974;5:191.
203. Love L, Baker D, Ramsey R. Gas-producing perinephric abscess. *AJR Am J Roentgenol* 1973;119:738.
204. Lowe J, Pfau A, Stein H. Reactivated musculoskeletal tuberculosis with concomitant asymptomatic genitourinary infection. *Isr J Med Sci* 1983;19:262.
205. Lyons RW, Long JM, Lytton B, et al. Arteriography and antibiotic therapy of a renal carbuncle. *J Urol* 1972;107:524.
206. Mabeck CE. Treatment of uncomplicated urinary tract infection in nonpregnant women. *Postgrad Med J* 1972;48:69.
207. MacDonald P, Alexander D, Catz G, et al. Summary of a workshop on maternal genitourinary infections and the outcome of pregnancy. *J Infect Dis* 1983;147:596.
208. Maizels M, Schaeffer AJ. Decreased incidence of bacteriuria associated with periodic instillations of hydrogen peroxide in the urethral catheter drainage bag. *J Urol* 1980;123:841.
209. Malek RS, Elder JS. Xanthogranulomatous pyelonephritis: a critical analysis of 26 cases and of the literature. *J Urol* 1978; 119:589.
210. Mallinson JW et al. Diffuse interstitial renal tuberculosis—an unusual cause of renal failure. *BJM* 1981;198:137.
211. Marrie TJ, Harding GKM, Ronald AR. Anaerobic and aerobic urethral flora in healthy females. *J Clin Microbiol* 1978;8:67.
212. Martens M, Kaul AK, Nowicki S, et al. Presence of receptors for Dr-hemagglutinin of uropathogenic *E. coli* in the uterus of pregnant rats. Poster presented at the Third World Congress for Infectious Diseases in OB/GYN, Acapulco, Mexico, 1993.
213. Martinez FC, Kindrachuk RW, Thomas E, et al. Effect of prophylactic, low dose cephalexin on fecal and vaginal bacteria. *J Urol* 1985;133:994.
214. Martorana G, Gilberti C, Pescatore D. Giant echinococcal cyst of the kidney associated with hypertension evaluated by computerized tomography. *J Urol* 1981;126:99.
215. McCabe WR, Jackson GG. Treatment of pyelonephritis: bacterial drug and host factors in success for failure among 252 patients. *N Engl J Med* 1965;272:1037.
216. McClure J. Malakoplakia. *J Pathol* 1983;140:275.
217. McClurg FV et al. Ultrastructural demonstration of intracellular bacteria in three cases of malakoplakia of the bladder. *Am J Clin Pathol* 1973;60:780.
218. McCue JD. Urinary tract infection and dysuria. Cost-conscious evaluation and antibiotic therapy. *Postgrad Med* 1986;80:133.
219. McDonald GS. Xanthogranulomatous pyelonephritis. *J Pathol* 1981;133:203.
220. McFadyen IR et al. Bacteriuria in pregnancy. *J Obstet Gynaecol Br Commonw* 1973;80:385.
221. McGuire LM, Wise GJ. Fluconazole treatment of urinary fungal infection. *J Urol* 1992;147[pt 2]:231A (abst).
222. Meares EM Jr. *Campbell's urology,* ed 4. Philadelphia: Saunders, 1978.
223. Medoff G, Kobayashi GS. Strategies in the treatment of systemic fungal infections. *N Engl J Med* 1980;302:145.
224. Melekos MD, Asbach HW, Gerharz E, et al. Post-intercourse versus daily ciprofloxacin prophylaxis for recurrent urinary tract infections in premenopausal women. *J Urol* 1997;157:935.
225. Merenich WM, Popky GL. Radiology of renal infection. *Med Clin North Am* 1991;75:425.
226. Mering JH, Kaplan GW, McLaughlin AP. Xanthogranulomatous pyelonephritis. *Urology* 1973;1:338.
227. Michaelis L, Gutmann C. Über Einschlüsse in Blasentumoren. *Z Klin Med* 1902;47:208.
228. Michigan S. Genitourinary fungal infections. *J Urol* 1976; 116:390.
229. Mobley HLT, Warren JW. Urease-positive bacteriuria and obstruction of long-term urinary catheters. *J Clin Microbiol* 1987;25:2216.

230. Mollier S, Descotes JL, Pasquier D, et al. Pseudoneoplastic xanthogranulomatous pyelonephritis—a typical clinical presentation but unusual diagnosis and treatment. *Eur Urol* 1995; 27:170.
231. Monane M, Gurwitz JH, Lipsitz LA, et al. Epidemiologic and diagnostic aspects of bacteriuria: a longitudinal study in older women. *J Am Geriatr Soc* 1995;43:618.
232. Mulvey MA, Lopez-Boado YS, Wilson CL, et al. Induction and evasion of host defenses by type 1 piliated uropathogenic *Escherichia coli. Science* 1998;282:1494.
233. Murphy DM et al. Tuberculous stricture of ureter. *Urology* 1982;20:382.
234. Murray T, Goldberg M. Chronic interstitial nephritis: etiologic factors. *Ann Intern Med* 1975;82:453.
235. Nabizadeh I, Morehouse HT, Freed SZ. Hydatid disease of the kidney. *Urology* 1983;22:176.
236. Narayana AS. Overview of renal tuberculosis. *Urology* 1982; 3:231.
237. Nataluk EA, McCullough DL, Scharling EO. Xanthogranulomatous pyelonephritis, the gatekeeper's dilemma: a contemporary look at an old problem. *Urology* 1995;45:377.
238. Navas EL et al. Blood group antigen expression on vaginal and buccal epithelial cells and mucus in secretor and nonsecretor women. *J Urol* 1993;149:1492.
239. Nicolau DP, Freeman CD, Belliveau PP, et al. Experience with a once-daily aminoglycoside program administered to 2,184 adult patients. *Antimicrob Agents Chemother* 1995; 39:650.
240. Nicolle LE, Mayhew WJ, Bryan L. Prospective, randomized comparison of therapy and no therapy for asymptomatic bacteriuria in institutionalized elderly women. *Am J Med* 1987; 83:27.
241. Nicolle LE, Harding GKM, Preiksaitis J, et al. The association of urinary tract infection with sexual intercourse. *J Infect Dis* 1982;146:579.
242. Nito H. Clinical efficacy of fluconazole in urinary tract fungal infections. *Jpn J Antibiot* 1989;42:171.
243. Norden CW, Kass EH. Bacteriuria of pregnancy: a critical appraisal. *Annu Rev Med* 1968;19:431.
244. Norrby SR. Short-term treatment of uncomplicated lower urinary tract infections in women. *Rev Infect Dis* 1990;12:458.
245. Nowicki BJ, Martens MG, Hart A, et al. Gestational age dependent distribution of *E. coli* fimbriae in pregnant patients with pyelonephritis. *Ann N Y Acad Sci* 1994;730:290.
246. Ocon J et al. Renal tuberculosis and hypertension: value of the renal vein renin ratio. *Eur Urol* 1984;10:114.
247. O'Flynn JD. Surgical treatment of genitourinary tuberculosis. *Eur J Urol* 1970;42:667.
248. O'Flynn JD. Genitourinary tuberculosis. *Urol Dig* 1979;18:25.
249. O'Hanley PD et al. A globoside binding *E. coli* pilus vaccine prevents pyelonephritis. *Clin Res* 1983;31:372A (abst).
250. Ooi BS, Chen NU. Prevalence and site of bacteriuria in diabetes mellitus. *Postgrad Med J* 1974;50:497.
251. Osca JM, Peiro MJ, Rodrigo M, et al. Focal xanthogranulomatous pyelonephritis: partial nephrectomy as definitive treatment. *Eur Urol* 1997;32:375.
252. Osterhage HR, Fischer V, Haubensak K. Positive histological tuberculous findings despite stable sterility of the urine on culture: results of 111 nephrectomies and partial nephrectomies. *Eur Urol* 1980;6:116.
253. Ouslander JG, Shapira M, Schnelle JF, et al. Pyuria among chronically incontinent but otherwise asymptomatic nursing home residents. *J Am Geriatr Soc* 1996;44:420.
254. Overgaard Nielsen H, Lorentzen M. Xanthogranulomatous pyelonephritis: an immunohistochemical and ultrastructural study on the occurrence of bacteria and bacterial antigen. *Urol Int* 1981;36:335.
255. Parsons MA, Harris SC, Longstaff AJ, et al. Xanthogranulomatous pyelonephritis: a pathological, clinical and aetiological analysis of 87 cases. *Diagn Histopathol* 1883;6:203.
256. Patterson TF, Andriole VT. Bacteriuria in pregnancy. *IDCNA* 1987;1:807.
257. Pedler SJ, Bint AJ. Management of bacteriuria in pregnancy. *Drugs* 1987;33:413.
258. Pels RJ et al. Dipstick urinalysis screening of asymptomatic adults for urinary tract disorders. *JAMA* 1989;262:1220.
259. Peréz LM, Thrasher JB, Anderson EE. Successful management of bilateral xanthogranulomatous pyelonephritis by bilateral partial nephrectomy. *J Urol* 1993;149:100.
260. Petronic V, Buturovic J, Isvaneski M. Xanthogranulomatous pyelonephritis. *Br J Urol* 1989;64:336.
261. Pezzlo M. Detection of urinary tract infection by rapid methods. *Clin Microbiol Rev* 1988;1:268.
262. Pfaller MA, Koontz FP. Laboratory evaluation of leukocyte esterase and nitrite tests for the detection of bacteriuria. *J Clin Microbiol* 1985;21:840.
263. Pfau A, Sacks T. The bacteria flora of the vaginal vestibule, urethra and vagina in the normal premenopausal woman. *J Urol* 1977;118:292.
264. Pfau A, Sacks TG. Effective prophylaxis for recurrent urinary tract infections during pregnancy. *Clin Infect Dis* 1992;14:810.
265. Pfau A, Sacks T, Engelstein D. Recurrent urinary tract infections in premenopausal women: prophylaxis based on an understanding of the pathogenesis. *J Urol* 1983;129:1153.
266. Philbrick JT, Bracikowski JP. Single-dose antibiotic treatment for uncomplicated urinary tract infections. *Arch Intern Med* 1985;145:1672.
267. Pinson AG, Philbrick JT, Lindbeck GH, et al. ED management of acute pyelonephritis in women: a cohort study. *Am J Emerg Med* 1994;12: 271.
268. Pitts JC, Peterson NE, Conley MC. Calcified functionless kidney in a 51-year-old man. *J Urol* 1981;125:398.
269. Plorde LL. Echinococciasis. In: *Harrison's principles of internal medicine,* ed 8. New York: McGraw-Hill, 1977.
270. Poulios C. Echinococcal disease of the urinary tract: review of the management of 7 cases. *J Urol* 1991;145:924.
271. Povysil C, Konickova L. Experimental xanthogranulomatous pyelonephritis. *Invest Urol* 1972;9:313.
272. Rajan N, Cao Q, Anderson BE, et al. Roles of glycoproteins and oligosaccharides found in human vaginal fluid in bacterial adherence. *Infect Immun* 1999;67(10):5027.
273. Ravel R. Megalocytic interstitial nephritis: an entity probably related to malakoplakia. *Am J Clin Pathol* 1967;47:781.
274. Raz R, Stamm WE. A controlled trial of intravaginal estriol in postmenopausal women with recurrent urinary tract infections. *N Engl J Med* 1993;329:753.
275. Reid G, Sobel JD. Bacterial adherence in the pathogenesis of urinary tract infection: a review. *Rev Infect Dis* 1987;9:470.
276. Reidenberg MM, Shear L, Cohen RV. Estimation of isoniazid in patients with impaired renal function. *Am Rev Respir Dis* 1973;108:1426.
277. Rene P, Dinolfo M, Silverblatt FJ. Serum and urogenital antibody response to *Escherichia coli* pili in cystitis. *Infect Immun* 1982;37:749.
278. Riedasch G, Heck P, Rautenbug E, et al. Does low urinary SIgA predispose to urinary tract infection? *Kidney Int* 1983; 23:759.

279. Robbins SL, Tucker AW. The cause of death in diabetes. *N Engl J Med* 1944;231:865.
280. Roberts AP, Phillips R. Bacteria causing symptomatic urinary tract infection or bacteriuria. *J Clin Pathol* 1979;32:492.
281. Roberts JA, Kaack MB, Baskin G. Treatment of experimental pyelonephritis in the monkey. *J Urol* 1990;143:150.
282. Romano JM, Kaye D. UTI in the elderly: common yet atypical, *Geriatrics* 1981;36:113.
283. Rosenberg M. Pharmacoeconomics of treating uncomplicated urinary tract infections. *Int J Antimicrobial Agents* 1999;11:247.
284. Rosenfeld AT et al. Acute focal bacterial nephritis (acute lobar nephronia). *Radiology* 1979;132:553.
285. Roylance J, Davies ER, Alexander WD. Translumbar puncture of a renal hydatid cyst. *Br J Radiol* 1973;46:960.
286. Saedd SM, Fine G. Xanthogranulomatous pyelonephritis. *Am J Clin Pathol* 1963;39:616.
287. Saint Martin G, Chiesa JC. "Falling snowflakes": an ultrasound sign of hydatid sand. *J Ultrasound Med* 1984;3:257.
288. Saint S, Elmore JG, Sullivan SD, et al. The efficacy of silver alloy–coated urinary catheters in preventing urinary tract infection: a meta-analysis. *Am J Med* 1998;105:236.
289. Salit IE, Hanley J, Clubb L, et al. The human antibody response to uropathogenic *Escherichia coli:* a review. *Can J Microbiol* 1988;34:312.
290. Salvatierra O Jr, Bucklew WB, Morrow JW. Perinephric abscess: a report of 71 cases. *J Urol* 1967;98:296.
291. Sanchez-Ramos L, McAlpine KJ, Adair CD, et al. Pyelonephritis in pregnancy: once-a-day ceftriaxone versus multiple doses of cefazolin. *Am J Obstet Gynecol* 1995;172:129.
292. Sandberg T, Brorson JE. Efficacy of long-term antimicrobial prophylaxis after acute pyelonephritis in pregnancy. *Scand J Inf Dis* 1991;23:221.
293. Schaeffer AJ, Rajan N, Wright ET, et al. Role of vaginal colonization in urinary tract infections (UTIs). In: Baskin LS, Hayward S, eds. *Advances in bladder research.* New York: Kluwer Academic/Plenum, 1999.
294. Schaeffer AJ, Stuppy BA. Efficacy and safety of self-start therapy in women with recurrent urinary tract infections. *J Urol* 1999;161:207.
295. Schaeffer AJ. Urinary tract infections in urology: a urologist's view of chronic bacteriuria. *ICDNA Urinary Tract Infections* 1987;1:875.
296. Schaeffer AJ. The role of bacterial adherence in urinary tract infection. *Urologe-Ausgabe A* 1993;32:7.
297. Schaeffer AJ. Urinary tract infections in the elderly. *Eur Urol* 1991;19[Suppl 1]:2.
297a. Schaeffer AJ, Amundsen SK, Schmidt LN. Adherence of *E. coli* to human urinary tract epithelial cells. *Infect Immun* 1979;24:753.
298. Schaeffer AJ, Jones JM, Dunn JK. Association of *in vitro Escherichia coli* adherence to vaginal and buccal epithelial cells with susceptibility of women to recurrent urinary-tract infections. *N Engl J Med* 1981;304:1062.
299. Schaeffer AJ, Radvany RM, Chmiel JS. Human leukocyte antigens in women with recurrent urinary tract infections. *J Infect Dis* 1983;148:604.
300. Schaeffer AJ, Stamey AT. Studies of introital colonization in women with recurrent urinary infections. IX. The role of antimicrobial therapy. *J Urol* 1977;118:221.
301. Schaeffer AJ, Stony KO, Johnson SM. Effect of silver oxide/trichloroisocyanuric acid antimicrobial urinary drainage system on catheter-associated bacteriuria. *J Urol* 1988;139:69.
302. Schaeffer AJ et al. Variation of blood group antigen expression of vaginal cells and mucus of secretor and nonsecretor women. *J Urol* 1994;152:859.
303. Schainuck LT, Fouty R, Cutler RE. Emphysematous pyelonephritis: a new case and review of previous observations. *Am J Med* 1968;44:134.
304. Schechter H, Leonard CD, Scribner BH. Chronic pyelonephritis as a cause of renal failure in dialysis candidates: analysis of 173 patients. *JAMA* 1971;216:514.
305. Schiff M Jr, Glickman M, Weiss RM. Antibiotic treatment of renal carbuncle. *Ann Intern Med* 1977;87:305.
306. Schlagenhaufer F. Über eigentümliche Staphylomykosen der Nieven und des pararenalen Bindegewebes. *Frankfurt Z Pathol* 1916;19:139.
307. Schoborg TW et al. Xanthogranulomatous pyelonephritis associated with renal carcinoma. *J Urol* 1980;124:125.
308. Schultz HJ, McCaffrey CA, Keys TF, et al. Acute cystitis: a prospective study of laboratory tests and duration of therapy. *Mayo Clin Proc* 1984;59:391.
309. Scullin DR, Hardy R. Malakoplakia of the urinary tract with spread of the abdominal wall. *J Urol* 1972;107:908.
310. Segura JW, Kelalis PP. Localized renal parenchymal infections in children. *J Urol* 1973;109:1029.
311. Semeniuk H, Church D. Evaluation of the leukocyte esterase and nitrite urine dipstick screening tests for detection of bacteriuria in women with suspected uncomplicated urinary tract infections. *J Clin Microbiol* 1999;37:3051.
312. Sheehan G, Harding GKM, Ronald AR. Advances in the treatment of urinary tract infection. *Am J Med* 1984;76:141.
313. Sheinfeld J, Schaeffer AJ, Cordon-Cardo C, et al. Association of the Lewis blood-group phenotype with recurrent urinary tract infections in women. *N Engl J Med* 1989;320:773.
314. Shetty SD, Al-Saigh AA, Ibrahim IA, et al. Hydatid disease of the urinary tract: evaluation of diagnostic methods. *Br J Urol* 1992;69:476.
315. Shetty SD, Al-Saigh A, Ibrahim IA, et al. Management of hydatid cysts of the urinary tract. *Br J Urol* 1992;70:258.
316. Siegel JF, Smith A, Moldwin R. Minimally invasive treatment of renal abscess. *J Urol* 1996;155:52.
317. Silver TM, Kass EJ, Thornbury JR, et al. The radiological spectrum of acute pyelonephritis in adults and adolescence. *Radiology* 1976;118:65.
318. Silverblatt FJ, Dreyer J, Schauer S. Effect of pili on susceptibility of *Escherichia coli* to phagocytes. *Infect Immun* 1979;24:218.
319. Silverman DE, Stamey AT. Management of infection stones. The Stanford experience. *Medicine* 1983;62:44.
320. Simon MB et al. Genitourinary tuberculosis. Clinical features in a general hospital population. *Am J Med* 1977;63:410.
321. Smeets F, Gower PE. The site of infection in 123 patients with bacteriuria. *Clin Nephrol* 1973;1:290.
322. Smellie JM, Edwards O, Hunter N, et al. Vesicoureteral reflux and renal scarring. *Kidney Int* 1975;8:565.
323. Smith A, Lattimer JK. Genitourinary tract involvement in children with tuberculosis. *N Y Stat J Med* 1973;73:2325.
324. Sobel JD. Pathogenesis of urinary tract infections: host defenses. *IDCNA* 1987;1:751.
325. Soler R, Pombo F, Gayol A, et al. Focal xanthogranulomatous pyelonephritis in a teenager: MR and CT findings. *Eur J Radiol* 1997;24:77.
326. Solomon A et al. Computerized tomography in xanthogranulomatous pyelonephritis. *J Urol* 1983;130:323.
327. Soulen MC et al. Bacterial renal infection: role of CT. *Radiology* 1989;171:703.
328. Sparks AK, Connor DH, Neafie RC. Echinococcosis. In: Binford CH, Connor DH, eds. *Pathology of tropical and extraordinary diseases.* Washington, DC: Armed Forces Institute of Pathology, 1976.

329. Stamey TA. *Urinary infections.* Baltimore: Williams & Wilkins, 1972.
330. Stamey TA. The role of introital enterobacteria in recurrent urinary tract infections. *J Urol* 1973;109:467.
331. Stamey TA. *Pathogenesis and treatment of urinary tract infections.* Baltimore: Williams & Wilkins, 1980.
332. Stamey TA, Condy M, Mihara G. Prophylactic efficacy of nitrofurantoin-macro-crystals and trimethoprim-sulfamethoxazole in urinary infections: biologic effects on the vaginal and rectal flora. *N Engl J Med* 1977;296:780.
333. Stamey TA, Govan DE, Palmer JM. The localization and treatment of urinary tract infections: the role of bactericidal urine levels as opposed to serum levels. *Medicine* 1965;44:1.
334. Stamey TA, Pfau A. Some functional, pathologic, bacteriologic, and chemotherapeutic characteristics of unilateral pyelonephritis in man. I. Fundamental and pathologic characteristics. *Invest Urol* 1963;1:134.
335. Stamey TA, Pfau A. Some functional, pathologic, bacteriologic, and chemotherapeutic characteristics of unilateral pyelonephritis in man. II. Bacteriologic and chemotherapeutic characteristics. *Invest Urol* 1963;1:162.
336. Stamey TA, Timothy MM. Studies of introital colonization in women with recurrent urinary infections. I. The role of vaginal pH. *J Urol* 1975;114:261.
337. Stamey TA, Timothy M, Millar M, et al. Recurrent urinary infections in adult women: the role of introital enterobacteria. *Calif Med* 1971;115:1.
338. Stamey TA, Fair WR, Timothy MM, et al. Serum versus urinary antimicrobial concentrations in cases of urinary tract infections. *N Engl J Med* 1974;291:1159.
339. Stamey TA, Wehner N, Mihara G, et al. The immunologic basis of recurrent bacteriuria: role of cervicovaginal antibody in enterobacterial colonization of the introital mucosa. *Medicine* 1978;57:47.
340. Stamm WE. Recent developments in the diagnosis and treatment of urinary tract infections. *West J Med* 1982;137:213.
341. Stamm WE. When should we use urine culture? *Infect Control* 1986;7:431.
342. Stamm WE. Catheter-associated urinary tract infections: epidemiology, pathogenesis, and prevention. *Am J Med* 1991; 91[Suppl 3B]65S.
343. Stamm WE, Wagner KF, Ainsel R, et al. Causes of the acute urethral syndrome in women. *N Engl J Med* 1980;303:409.
344. Stamm WE, Running K, McKevitt M, et al. Treatment of the acute urethral syndrome. *N Engl J Med* 1981;304:956.
345. Stamm WE, Counts GW, Running KR, et al. Diagnosis of coliform infection in acutely dysuric women. *N Engl J Med* 1982;307:463.
346. Stamm WE, Counts GW, McKevitt M, et al. Urinary prophylaxis with trimethoprim and trimethoprim-sulfamethoxazole: efficacy influence on the natural history of recurrent bacteriuria, and cost control. *Rev Infect Dis* 1982;4:450.
347. Stanton MJ, Maxted W. Malakoplakia: a study of the literature and current concepts of pathogens. *J Urol* 1981;125:139.
348. Stapleton A, Hooton TM, Fennell C, et al. Effect of secretor status on vaginal and rectal colonization with fimbriated *Escherichia coli* in women with and without recurrent urinary tract infection. *J Infect Dis* 1995;171:717.
349. Stapleton A, Nudelman E, Clausen H, et al. Binding of uropathogenic *Esherichia coli* R45 to glycolipids extracted from vaginal epithelial cells is dependent on the histo-blood group secretor status. *J Clin Invest* 1992;90:965.
350. Stark RP, Maki DG. Bacteriuria in the catheterized patient. What quantitative level of bacteriuria is relevant? *N Engl J Med* 1984;311:560.
351. Stenqvist K, Dahlen-Nilsson I, Lidin-Janson G, et al. Bacteriuria in pregnancy. Frequency and risk of acquisition. *Am J Epidemiol* 1989;129:372.
352. Studer UE, Weidmann P. Pathogenesis and treatment in renal tuberculosis. *Eur Urol* 1984;10:164.
353. Sun TT. Epithelial growth and differentiation: an overview. *Mol Biol Rep* 1996;23:1.
354. Svanborg Eden C, Svennerholm AM. Secretory immunoglobulin A and G antibodies prevent adhesion of *Escherichia coli* to human urinary tract epithelial cells. *Infect Immun* 1978;22:790.
355. Svanborg Eden C, Hanson LA, Jodal U, et al. Variable adherence to normal human urinary tract epithelial cells of *Escherichia coli* strains associated with various forms of urinary tract infections. *Lancet* 1976;2:490.
356. Svenson SB et al. P-fimbriae of pyelonephritis *Escherichia coli:* identification and chemical characterization of receptors. *Infection* 1983;11:61.
357. Svenson SB, Kallenius G, Korhonen TK, et al. Initiation of clinical pyelonephritis—the role of P-fimbriae-mediated bacterial adhesion. *Contrib Nephrol* 1984;39:252.
358. Sweet RL. Bacteriuria and pyelonephritis during pregnancy. *Semin Perinatol* 1977;1:25.
359. Talan DA, Stamm WE, Hooton TM, et al. Comparison of ciprofloxacin (7 days) and trimethoprim-sulfamethoxazole (14 days) for acute uncomplicated pyelonephritis in women. *JAMA* 2000;12:1583.
360. Thankavel K, Madison B, Ikeda T, et al. Localization of a domain in the FimH adhesin of *Escherichia coli* type 1 fimbriae capable of receptor recognition and use of domain-specific antibody to confer protection against experimental urinary tract infection. *J Clin Invest* 1997;100:1123.
361. Thorley JD, Jones SR, Sanford JP. Perinephric abscess. *Medicine* 1974;53:441.
362. Timmons JW, Perlmutter AD. Renal abscess: a changing concept. *J Urol* 1976;115:299.
363. Tolia BM et al. Xanthogranulomatous pyelonephritis: detailed analysis of 29 cases and a brief discussion of atypical presentations. *J Urol* 1981;126:437.
364. Trillo A, Lorentz WB, Whitley NO. Malakoplakia of kidneys simulating renal neoplasm. *Urology* 1977;10:472.
365. Turck M, Goffe B, Petersdorf RG. The urethral catheter and urinary tract infection. *J Urol* 1962;88:834.
366. Turck M, Ronald AR, Petersdorf RG. Relapse and reinfection in chronic bacteriuria. II. The correlation between site of infection and pattern of recurrence in chronic bacteriuria. *N Engl J Med* 1968;278:422.
367. Uehling D, Mizutani K, Bolish E. Effect of immunization on bacterial adherence to uroepithelium. *Invest Urol* 1978;16:145.
368. Uehling D, Wolf I. Enhancement of the bladder defense mechanisms by immunization. *Invest Urol* 1969;6:520.
369. Uehling D et al. Vaginal immunization of monkeys against urinary tract infection with a multi-strain vaccine. *J Urol* 1994; 151:214.
370. van Dorsten JP, Lenke RR, Schifrin BS. Pyelonephritis in pregnancy. The role of in-hospital and nitrofurantoin suppression. *J Reprod Med* 1987;32:895.
371. Vejlsgaard R. Studies on urinary infections in diabetes. IV. Significant bacteriuria in pregnancy in relation to age of onset, duration of diabetes, angiopathy and urological symptoms. *Acta Med Scand* 1973;193:337.
372. Venegas MF, Navas EL, Gaffney R, et al. Binding of type 1 piliated *Escherichia coli* to vaginal mucus. *Infect Immun* 1995;63:416.
373. Von Hansemann D. Über Malakoplakie der Harnblase. *Arch Pathol Anat* 1903;173:302.

374. Vromen M, van der Ven AJAM, Knols A, et al. Antimicrobial resistance patterns in urinary isolates from nursing home residents. Fifteen years of data reviewed. *J Antimicrob Chemother* 1999;44:113.
375. Waller RM, Finnerty DP, Casarella WJ. Transluminal balloon dilation of a tuberculous ureteral stricture. *J Urol* 1983;129: 1225.
376. Wan YL, Lee TY, Bullard MJ, et al. Acute gas-producing bacterial renal infection: correlation between imaging findings and clinical outcome. *Radiology* 1996;198:433.
377. Warren JW, Abrutyn E, Hebel JR, et al. Guidelines for antimicrobial treatment of uncomplicated acute bacterial cystitis and acute pyelonephritis in women. *Clin Infect Dis* 1999;29:745.
378. Warren JW. The catheter and urinary tract infection. *Med Clin North Am* 1991;75:481.
379. Warren JW, Terry JW, Hoopes JM, et al. A prospective microbiologic study of bacteriuria in patients with chronic indwelling urethral catheters. *J Infect Dis* 1982;146:719.
380. Wechsler H, Lattimer JK. An evaluation of the current therapeutic regimen for renal tuberculosis. *J Urol* 1975;113:760.
381. Wechsler H, Westfall M, Lattimer JK. The earliest signs and symptoms of 127 male patients with genitourinary tuberculosis. *J Urol* 1960;83:801.
382. Weiss S, Parker F Jr. Pyelonephritis: its relation to vascular lesions and to arterial hypertension. *Medicine* 1939;18:221.
383. Wesson LG. Unilateral renal disease and hypertension. *Nephron* 1982;31:2.
384. Wheat LJ. Infection and diabetes mellitus. *Diabetes Care* 1980; 3:187.
385. Wicks JD, Thornbury JR. Acute renal infections in adults. *Radiol Clin North Am* 1979;17:245.
386. Wigton RS et al. Use of clinical findings in the diagnosis of urinary tract infection in women. *Arch Intern Med* 1985;145: 2222.
387. Wilhelm MP, Edson RS. Antimicrobial agents in urinary tract infections. *Mayo Clin Proc* 1987;62:1025.
388. Wise GJ. Amphotericin B in urologic practice. *J Urol* 1990; 144:215.
389. Wise GJ, Kozinn PJ, Goldberg PE. Flucytosine in the management of genitourinary candidiasis: 5 years of experience. *J Urol* 1980;124:70.
390. Wise GJ, Kozinn PF, Goldberg PE. Amphotericin B as a urologic irrigant in the management of noninvasive candiduria. *J Urol* 1982;128:82.
391. Wise GJ, Goldman WM, Goldberg PE, et al. Miconazole: a cost-effective antifungal genitourinary irrigant. *J Urol* 1987; 138:1413.
392. Wisnia LG et al. Renal function damage in 131 cases of urogenital tuberculosis. *Urology* 1978;11:457.
393. Wong ES, Fennell CL, Stamm WE. Urinary tract infection among women attending a clinic for sexually transmitted diseases. *Sex Transm Dis* 1984;11:18.
394. Wong SH, Lau WY. The surgical management of nonfunctioning tuberculous kidney. *J Urol* 1980;124:187.
395. Wong ES, McKevitt M, Running K, et al. Management of recurrent urinary tract infections with patient-administered self-dose therapy. *Ann Intern Med* 1985;102:302.
396. Wright AJ, Walker RC, Barrett DM. The fluoroquinolones and their appropriate use in treatment of genitourinary tract infections. In: Ball TP, Novicki DE, eds. *AUA update series.* Houston: American Urologic Association, 1993.
397. Wu XR, Sun TT, Medina JJ. *In vitro* binding of type 1–fimbriated *Escherichia coli* to uroplakins Ia and Ib: relation to urinary tract infections. *Proc Natl Acad Sci* 1996;93:9630.
398. Wu TT, Lee YH, Tzeng WS, et al. The role of C-reactive protein and erythrocyte sedimentation rate in the diagnosis of infected hydronephrosis and pyonephrosis. *J Urol* 1994;152:26.
399. Yamamoto S, Tsukamoto T, Terai A, et al. Genetic evidence supporting the fecal-perineal-urethral hypothesis in cystitis caused by *Escherichia coli. J Urol* 1997;157:1127.
400. Yazaki T et al. Xanthogranulomatous pyelonephritis in childhood: case report and review of English and Japanese literature. *J Urol* 1982;127:80.
401. Zhanel GG, Hoban DJ, Harding GKM. The postantibiotic effect: a review of *in vitro* and *in vivo* data. *Ann Pharmocother* 1991;25:153.

5

MANAGEMENT OF UROLOGIC PROBLEMS IN PREGNANCY

JAY Y. GILLENWATER
JEFFREY P. WEISS

The urinary tract in pregnancy is of interest to the urologist because of the interesting physiologic changes that pose challenges in the management of its problems. In caring for patients during pregnancy, the urologist must always consider the effects of treatment on both the mother and the fetus. In this chapter, the marked changes in urinary tract anatomy and function during pregnancy are presented, as well as the clinical problems of urolithiasis, infection, hydronephrosis, coexistent renal diseases, and lower urinary tract dysfunction.

Physiologic changes during pregnancy include (a) an increase in renal blood flow of 60% to 80%; (b) increased glomerular filtration of 40% to 50%, with subsequent lowering of mean serum creatinine to less than 0.5 mg/dL; and (c) increases in cardiac output of 30% to 50%, associated with decreased peripheral resistance and increased stroke volume. Hydronephrosis of pregnancy is caused by both hormonal and mechanical factors. During pregnancy, there is net retention of sodium, potassium, and calcium. Urolithiasis has a similar incidence and causes as for nonpregnant patients, but it creates problems in the last trimester because one cannot safely operate or use shock wave lithotripsy on lower ureteral stones. Hypertension, renal insufficiency, and bacteriuria are major risk factors in fetal outcome. Pregnancy does not affect most renal diseases, and renal function usually increases temporarily in the diseased kidney during pregnancy. Acute renal failure of pregnancy, acute cortical necrosis, and idiopathic postpartum acute renal failure are problems seen in pregnancy. Pregnancy can be a success during dialysis or after renal transplantation. Excellent reviews have been published by Loughlin (148), Dafnis and Sabatini (51), Jungers and co-workers (118), and Weiss and Hanno (269).

J.Y. Gillenwater: Professor of Urology, University of Virginia Medical School, Charlottesville, VA 22908.

J.P. Weiss: Clinical Adjunct Assistant Professor of Urology, Weill/Cornell University Medical College, New York, NY 10595.

RENAL PHYSIOLOGY IN PREGNANCY

Several changes in renal function normally occur owing to the gravid state; the one most relevant to urologists is dilation of the ureters, pelves, and calyces (146). Hydronephrosis of pregnancy may be attributed to a combination of factors, principally hormonal and mechanical. There is evidence that circulating estrogenic and progestational compounds produced by placentas in animals surgically lacking fetuses result in ureterectasis in the absence of mechanical obstruction (208,257,258). Prostaglandin E_2 has smooth muscle–relaxing properties that also contribute to hormonally induced hydronephrosis (217). Probably a greater contributing factor in physiologic hydronephrosis of pregnancy is stasis induced by the dextrorotating and enlarging uterus at midterm, explaining the proclivity for such obstruction to occur on the right. Experimental evidence for what otherwise may be taken as obvious is that differential pressure measurements in the ureter, above and below the pelvic brim, reveal a gradient at the level of the uterus in erect patients that resolves in the knee-chest position (165,219).

During pregnancy, cardiac output is increased. This is associated with decreased peripheral resistance and increased stroke volume. Initially, blood pressure decreases; later in pregnancy, the heart rate increases and stroke volume returns toward normal. Plasma volume increases 40%, and red blood cell volume increases 25% (141). Changes in the respiratory system include a 20% reduction in functional residual capacity by the fifth month of pregnancy (204). This is accompanied by a 15% increase in oxygen consumption, putting the mother at risk for developing hypoxemia during periods of hypoventilation.

There are gestational increases in both glomerular filtration rate (GFR) of 40% to 50% and renal plasma flow (RPF) of 60% to 80% (67). These changes occur in patients with either a solitary (native or transplant) kidney or two functioning kidneys (54,55). Increases in GFR and RPF also occur in the diseased kidney. An explanation for these hemodynamic and physiologic changes likely derives from increased cardiac output and decreased renal vascular resistance (133), as well as increased serum levels of aldosterone, deoxycorticosterone, progesterone, placental lactogen, and chorionic gonadotropin (146). A practical consequence of increased GFR is that plasma creatinine levels are reduced to a mean of 0.46 mg/dL during pregnancy because creatinine production is unchanged. Thus plasma creatinine concentrations that are normal for the general population are abnormally high in gravid patients and should signal a nephrologic evaluation for possible renal functional impairment (146,253). A corollary of increased RPF and glomerular filtration during pregnancy is the increase in urinary excretion of protein, glucose, amino acids, and vitamins (22,146,275).

An increase in renal volume as much as 30% is observed in pregnant patients in the absence of hydronephrosis. This is thought to be due to hemodynamic and hormonal factors, specifically increases in RPF and increased glomerular filtration surface area caused by a growth hormone–like effect of prolactin (38).

It has long been known that pregnancy is associated with hypercalciuria (129), a phenomenon attributed to increased GFR (163), increased calcium filtration (105), and excess intestinal calcium absorption secondary to high plasma levels of calcitriol (83). However, overwhelming evidence suggests that stone formation is not enhanced by pregnancy, and stone-formers who become pregnant do not incur a higher incidence of urolithiasis (103). Thus it may be assumed that pregnancy also occurs within a milieu of factors that mitigate the stone-forming effect of hypercalciuria, such as increased excretion of stone inhibitors (citrate, magnesium, and glycosaminoglycans) (20,80,179,180).

Pregnancy is associated with diminished plasma osmolality (60). A maximum decrease in osmolality of 10 mOsm/kg can be expected from week 10 of gestation until parturition. Although it is tempting to explain this finding in terms of altered vasopressin metabolism, no such evidence exists and the cause for the altered osmoregulation of pregnancy is obscure (56,58,59). On the other hand, renal handling of sodium during pregnancy is better understood.

A small quantity of sodium (950 mEq) is accumulated during pregnancy. Thus there must be factors accounting for this maintenance of sodium homeostasis in that the increase in GFR that normally accompanies pregnancy in and of itself would cause a loss of 5,000 to 10,000 mEq sodium daily as an additional filtered load (146). Tubular reabsorption accounts for preservation of the majority of this increased filtered sodium load (13). However, other factors, including hormonal and physical changes, result in sodium maintenance. Aldosterone production and excretion are known to increase to high levels as an offset to natriuresis during pregnancy (27). Deoxycorticosterone, another potent mineralocorticoid, likewise increases in pregnancy, especially during the third trimester (28,187,272). Further enhancing sodium retention are high levels of circulating estrogens in pregnancy (145,271). The antinatriuretic effect of estrogens is also enhanced by their induction of 21-hydroxylation of progesterone (a salt-wasting hormone), yielding salt-retaining deoxycorticosterone (155). Other potentially salt-retaining hormones of pregnancy include adrenocorticotropic hormone, cortisol, prolactin, growth hormone, and placental lactogen (146). Although circulating catecholamines may result in natriuresis via direct renal effects or indirectly through renal sympathetic innervation, levels of these compounds are variably and only slightly changed; thus their effects on sodium metabolism appear to be minimal (12). Renin and angiotensin II levels are distinctly elevated during gestation (15,106). The influence of the renin-angiotensin axis on sodium homeostasis is indirect, to the extent of its relation to aldosterone metabolism and volume status. It is currently theorized that gestational renin levels may be affected by increases in prostaglandin E_2 and prostacyclin produced by the uterus, resulting in general vasodilation, decreased blood pressure, and augmented vascular volume during pregnancy (75,79).

The physical factors influencing sodium metabolism in pregnancy are increased ureteral pressure and increased uterine blood supply with its arteriovenous shunting characteristics (35,208). These physical factors are greatly influenced by position and levels of ambulation and generally are believed to result in sodium retention in the pregnant subject.

In summary, the tremendous potential for gestational salt loss owing to increased GFR is offset in multiple ways that are both hormonal and physical. These factors combine to the net observation that sodium is retained slightly during pregnancy.

UROLOGIC SYMPTOMS IN PREGNANCY

The most common urologic symptom in pregnancy is frequency of voiding (nearly universal at term in primigravidas), followed by stress incontinence, 35% at term (237). Other symptoms often found include urgency, urge incontinence, poor stream, and incomplete emptying, although these are not typically found to be severe enough to warrant investigation with micturitional studies (49).

Hematuria may occur as a normal concomitant of pregnancy because of microanatomic changes in such (enlarged) kidneys that exhibit renal venous fragility in the collecting tubules or pelvis (264). Recurrent unilateral gross hematuria occurring during consecutive pregnancies has been reported to be related to renal varicosities owing to mechanical (uterine compressive) and hormonal factors causing pelvic venous congestion (52). Another common urologic gestational symptom is flank pain, which can be attributed to multiple underlying processes, such as hydronephrosis, pyelonephritis, urinary calculi, spontaneous renal rupture, or tumors.

USE OF MEDICATIONS DURING PREGNANCY

Urologists often are asked to treat pregnant patients for conditions that require prescriptions, such as pain relievers, antimicrobials, antipyretics, anesthetics, and anticholinergics. The potential for pharmaceutical teratogenicity behooves a detailed knowledge of medications safe for use in pregnancy.

Antibiotics (Table 5.1) and analgesics are the most commonly prescribed medications by urologists for pregnant women. Antimicrobials that are considered safe without reservation (barring allergies) include penicillins, cephalosporins, and erythromycin (133,182,276). Nitrofurantoin is regarded as safe in pregnancy because of low blood levels, although the rare complication of idiosyncratic pulmonopathy should be kept in mind with long-term administration (6,198). The safety of this drug during pregnancy should not be confused with its association with hemolytic anemia in breastfed infants with glucose-6-phosphate dehydrogenase (G6PD) deficiency. Aminoglycosides may be safely administered during pregnancy (44) when used with the usual judicious attention to monitoring of renal function and serum peak and trough levels. Sulfonamides are safe until 28 weeks, after which time there is a risk of fetal kernicterus and

TABLE 5.1. ANTIBIOTIC USE IN PREGNANCY

Antibiotic	Safety Margin (Barring Allergy)
Penicillins	Safe
Cephalosporins	Safe
Erythromycin	Safe
Nitrofurantoin	Safe (hemolytic anemia in breastfed infants with G6PD deficiency)
Aminoglycosides	Potential CNS toxicity, ototoxicity (monitor serum levels, renal function)
Sulfonamides	Safe until 28 weeks (thereafter risk hemolysis, kernicterus if G6PD deficiency)
Trimethoprim/sulfamethoxazole	Contraindicated (teratogenic, fetal folate antagonist)
Tetracyclines	Contraindicated (fetal limb, dental dysgenesis)
Chloramphenicol	Contraindicated near term (fetal bone marrow depression, "gray syndrome")
Isoniazid	May cause congenital defects (e.g., infant encephalopathy)
Metronidazole	Use with caution in second and third trimesters only (possibly mutagenic)
Amoxicillin/clavulanic acid	Formal studies lacking; safety unknown
Quinolones	Bone growth retardation
Ketoconazole	Contraindicated (teratogenic in rats; inhibits steroid synthesis)

CNS, central nervous system; G6PD, glucose-6-phosphate dehydrogenase.

hemolysis in patients with G6PD deficiency (113,133). Trimethoprim/sulfamethoxazole is contraindicated because of possible teratogenicity and fetal folate antagonism (211). Tetracycline should be assiduously avoided to prevent dysgenesis of fetal limbs (weeks 0 to 12) and teeth, which results from competition with calcium for access into sites of bone development (87,113). Chloramphenicol is contraindicated near term because of potential bone marrow depression and fetal gray syndrome (113,267), although it may be used safely throughout most of gestation. Isoniazid may cause a number of congenital defects, such as infant encephalopathy; metronidazole must be used with caution during the second and third trimesters (37) in that rat lung adenomas and increased bacterial mutation rates have been found experimentally (113). Erythromycin and amoxicillin/clavulanic acid are considered safe in pregnancy, although formal human studies of the latter combination are lacking (2,113). Although ketoconazole as an antifungal has not been documented to cause fetal malformation, it is not recommended during pregnancy because of its association with teratogenicity in rats and an inhibitory effect on androgen and corticosteroid synthesis (168). Angiotensin-converting enzyme inhibitors cause neonatal renal failure and hypotension and should thus not be used.

Fortunately, a variety of analgesics may be used with a wide safety margin during pregnancy. Whereas acetaminophen is safe in pregnancy, aspirin is contraindicated, particularly during the third trimester, because of a propensity for causing newborn intracranial (subchoroidal) hemorrhage (41,220,231). However, prospective studies have failed to demonstrate an increased risk of aspirin-induced fetal malformations (231). From the maternal standpoint, aspirin may cause anemia, peripartum uterine hemorrhage, prolonged gestation, or labor (119). Although theoretically nonsteroidal antiinflammatory drugs may be thought to carry the same caveats as aspirin, they should be avoided, especially during the third trimester, to prevent premature closure of the ductus arteriosus, a prostaglandin-dependent phenomenon (144). For more severe pain, narcotic analgesics are considered safe without reservation when used short term before parturition (107). Under these circumstances, the urologist may prescribe appropriate dosages of morphine, meperidine, or oxycodone.

Although an exhaustive discussion of all pharmaceuticals is beyond the scope of this chapter, two specific substances deserve special mention. As surgeons, urologists will often need to use topical sterilizing agents. When administered near term, povidone-iodine may be absorbed vaginally or perineally to the extent that neonatal hypothyroidism and goiter may result (26,134). Hexachlorophene, another common topical antiseptic, is also of concern because of its association with neurotoxicity and white matter vacuolar degeneration (270). These substances should be used judiciously during pregnancy and should be rinsed thoroughly with sterile water where applied.

DECISION MAKING FOR GESTATIONAL URINARY TRACT IMAGING

Paramount in the mind of the physician caring for a pregnant patient in need of roentgenographic imaging studies is radiation-dosage tolerance. Significant pelvic radiation dosages (5 to 15 cGy) during the first trimester increase the risk of teratogenicity from 1% to 3% (244). Putting this into perspective, a standard urogram renders 1.5 cGy to the fetus; however, prudence dictates the standard that limited exposure to two or three "shots" should be taken during a gestational urogram. These images include the plain film, a 30-minute exposure, and a 2- or 3-hour exposure if the diagnosis of obstruction remains in doubt. Because each plain abdominal film yields 0.2 cGy to the fetus, the two- or three-shot urogram is considered safe even during the first trimester (66,103,159). On the other hand, data exist to cause concern with even low doses of roentgen ray exposure to the fetus. Specifically, an average of 1 rad of fetal exposure has been correlated with a net 2.4-fold increase in the incidence of all childhood malignancies (99). However, it is not clear during which trimesters radiation exposure occurred. Although ultrasound is safe under all circumstances of pregnancy, its use in diagnosing obstruction is of limited value because of its suboptimal view of the ureter and presence of hydroureteronephrosis as a physiologic concomitant of pregnancy. Thus, because urography is found to have diagnostic value greatly in excess of sonography during pregnancy (103), it is recommended in the following situations: (a) persistent fever, (b) massive or increasing hydronephrosis as seen during serial urosonography, and (c) pain or emesis refractory to conservative therapy.

The theoretic risk of development of childhood cancer (not necessarily teratogenicity) should at all times be kept in mind when subjecting the fetus to roentgen ray exposure (156,177). In particular, there is no evidence that fetal radiation exposure below 5 rad causes congenital malformation, spontaneous abortion, or growth retardation (25). However, the relative risk of childhood leukemia occasioned by fetal exposure of 1 to 2 rad is increased from 1 in 3,000 (general population) to 1 in 2,000 (229). Put into perspective, the risk of leukemia for a sibling of a leukemic child is 1 in 700 (25).

In view of these data, it is useful to discuss radiation dosages received by the uterus owing to specific imaging studies. For example, cerebral angiography causes less than 10 mrad exposure to the uterus, a negligible dosage, due to the maximum distance of the collimated beam from the brain to the pelvis (262). In contrast, double-vessel coronary angioplasty provides 90 mrad uterine exposure (76,86), and barium enema causes 2 to 4 rad fetal exposure due to proximity of the study to the uterus (16). Other roentgen ray studies may be ordered during pregnancy. Computed tomography causes maximum radiation exposure at the skin level, with a progressive decrease toward the body interior.

Correspondingly, radiation dosage to the fetus diminishes with enlargement of the pregnancy and its investing tissues (48). Specifically, a ten-slice abdominal study causes 2.6 rad fetal exposure at weeks 0 to 14, whereas the same study provides only 1.7 rad to the conceptus at weeks 35 to 42 (48,207,228). Likewise, administration of radiopharmaceuticals may be safely done during pregnancy. Nuclear medicine studies of the brain, biliary system, skeleton, lungs, kidneys, abscesses, and heart may all be accomplished with fetal exposures varying from 40 to 1,100 mrad (48). In general, because radioactive iodine readily crosses the blood-placental barrier, isotopic iodine administration should be avoided during pregnancy (261). Magnetic imaging is thought to be safe during pregnancy because studies of static, gradient, and radiofrequency magnetic fields at strengths lower than 2 tesla have thus far failed to demonstrate mutagenic or other deleterious effects on the fetus (48,81,225,262).

In summary, it is useful to keep in mind the American College of Obstetricians and Gynecologists' guidelines for diagnostic imaging during pregnancy (5):

- X-ray exposure under 5 rad has not been associated with increased fetal anomaly or spontaneous abortion.
- Maternal health should not be compromised by irrational fears of the dangers of ionizing radiation to the fetus. However, alternative imaging procedures such as ultrasonography and magnetic resonance imaging (MRI) should be used instead of x-rays when applicable.
- Although ultrasonography and MRI are unassociated with known adverse fetal effects, MRI to date is not recommended for use in the first trimester.
- Radiologic consultation is advisable if it is deemed necessary to estimate fetal dose when roentgenologic procedures are performed during pregnancy.
- Therapeutic radioactive iodine isotopes are contraindicated during pregnancy.

Ultrasound is the most common modality used in diagnosis of calculous disease in pregnancy. However, because most symptomatic gestational calculi will be in the ureter and hydronephrosis is a normal finding in pregnancy, in most cases, ultrasound and its suboptimal view of the ureter will fail to be diagnostic in this setting. Horowitz and Schmidt (103) performed 11 ultrasound examinations in six gravid patients with calculi and found this modality to be diagnostic only once. In comparison, excretory urography was diagnostic in six of ten pregnant patients. These authors use a two-shot urogram consisting of a plain film and 3-hour postcontrast film with the idea that clearance of contrast from the symptomatic side excludes significant obstruction. They specifically outline the following situations in which urography is indicated: (a) persistent pyrexia or positive urine culture despite 48 hours of intravenous antibiotics, (b) declining renal function, (c) massive hydronephrosis detected by sonography, and (d) unrelenting pain or vomiting. In conclusion, sonography is most useful in evaluating gravid patients thought to have acute symptomatic stone disease requiring further investigation with roentgenographic imaging studies (269).

Renal sonography can be used in serial fashion without concern of radiation-induced fetal injury in the pregnant patient. Muller-Suur and Tyden (178) found that 31 of 35 patients with flank pain had hydronephrosis. In this study, the upper limit of normal pelvic diameter was determined to be 17 mm. In asymptomatic patients, normal renal pelvic diameters during the first, second, and third trimesters were 5 ± 1 mm, 10 ± 3 mm, and 12 ± 2 mm, respectively, on the right side, and 3 ± 1 mm, 4 ± 1 mm, and 5 ± 1 mm, respectively, on the left. These parameters constitute a guide to selection of patients having ureteral colic for further study. Whereas neither parity nor a history of urinary tract problems is found to be related to the degree of dilation, the incidence of hydronephrosis as determined by ultrasound investigation is 90% on the right side and 67% on the left (197). When hydronephrosis is found sonographically during pregnancy, a question may arise as to whether it is caused by obstruction or normal physiologic changes of the gravid state. Such a distinction may be made by determination of internal vascular resistivity indices by use of renal Doppler duplex ultrasound. Statistically significant relation is made between elevation of resistivity index and pathologic upper tract dilation in symptomatic pregnant patients (101). In this fashion, duplex renal ultrasound may be used to attribute hydronephrosis caused by calculus as opposed to nonobstructive physiologic phenomena.

HYDRONEPHROSIS OF PREGNANCY

Obstructive changes in the upper tracts during pregnancy are attributable to evolution of a physiologic process. Stadfeldt (236) reported right hydroureteronephrosis caused by uterine compression of the ureter at the level of the iliac vessels as long ago as 1861. Although their subject matter was autopsies of women dying in late pregnancy, Harrow and colleagues (98) were able to draw the same conclusion 103 years later using data compiled from excretory urography. Further support for the direct compression theory derives from the observation that hydronephrosis tends not to occur in gravid women with either ectopic ureters or those placed ectopically as in patients with urinary diversion; in neither of these two cases do the ureters become compressed between the uterus and iliac great vessels (247). Clark (39) reported an alternative explanation for hydronephrosis of pregnancy; namely, ureteral compression is caused by a dilated right ovarian vein that crosses over the ureter on its way toward the vena cava, as opposed to the left ovarian vein that runs a more parallel course with its ureteral mate. Although both he and others (68) performed resection of the offending ovarian veins plus ureterolysis with good results, this experience largely has not been found to be reproducible (214).

Hydroureterectasis in pregnancy first occurs as a simple consequence of ureteral compression above the pelvic brim by the enlarging, dextrorotating uterus at about midterm (70,269). Such rotation explains why hydronephrosis of pregnancy is usually found on the right. Hormonal factors may also contribute to this "physiologic" hydronephrosis. The elegant experiments in rhesus monkeys of Van Wagenen and Jenkins (257) and Van Wagenen and Newton (258) permitted the conclusion that in these animals, hormonal changes by a functioning placenta lacking a (surgically removed) conceptus induce ureterectasis. Whereas in the past these changes have been thought to be normal concomitants of pregnancy and not necessarily pathologic, current literature is replete with reports of obstructive uropathy in gravid women causing acute renal failure and polyhydramnios (71,102), acute pain (206), hypertension (138), and spontaneous renal rupture (88).

When symptoms of pain or infection are refractory to conventional nonoperative therapy with analgesics or antimicrobials, invasive manipulation of the hydronephrosis of pregnancy is indicated. The most commonly used method of temporary relief of this type of obstruction is placement of a ureteral stent or drainage catheter (19,71,112,138,151, 184,240). Alternatively, for example, when ureteral tortuosity late in pregnancy precludes retrograde stent passage, percutaneous nephrostomy under either fluoroscopic (206) or sonographic (24,31,124,256) guidance may resolve symptomatic hydronephrosis. Indeed, for the tortuous ureter late in pregnancy, the straightening technique described by Pryor and Gillenwater (205) can be helpful in negotiating an otherwise unnavigable channel in stent passage. These authors suggest preliminary passage of a floppy-tip guidewire through a dual-channel cystoscope bridge to straighten the ureter in anticipation of catheter placement through the second channel. Stent passage also can be facilitated without the need for roentgenographic imaging through the use of endoluminal ultrasound (273). Goldfarb and associates (85) caution that pregnant stone-formers are at additional risk for development of concretions on indwelling stents. Thus increased fluid intake should accompany care of hydronephrosis of pregnancy treated with stenting.

Aside from the drainage procedures described previously, other solutions to the symptomatic hydronephrosis of pregnancy include epidural block (209) and delivery of the fetus at or near term, either by labor induction through amniotomy (192) or cesarean section (61). Bed rest in the contralateral position cannot be overemphasized to prevent complications of severe hydronephrosis of pregnancy, especially in patients with a solitary kidney (102).

An uncommon but potentially life-threatening complication of hydronephrosis of pregnancy is spontaneous renal rupture. The pathogenesis of this entity stems from increased hydrostatic pressure within the collecting structures that exceeds the holding capacity of the calyceal–renal capsular junctions resulting in extravasation (172). Kidneys with prior damage through infection, trauma, or surgery are particularly prone to rupture because of increased intracavitary pressure against noncompliant, scarred renal parenchyma. Symptoms occur between 18 weeks of gestation (172,258,278) and 1 day postpartum (61,121, 172). Flank pain, hematuria, flank mass, and hypotension are harbingers of spontaneous renal rupture of pregnancy. Specific diagnosis may be carried out using sonography, limited excretory urography, and retrograde ureteropyelography. In addition, arteriography may be used to identify the source of hemorrhage in ruptured kidneys that have bled and caused hemodynamic instability (114). This technique may prove therapeutic with the addition of angioembolization, although radiation dosage for such a procedure is such that it cannot be recommended during the first trimester. Although most patients with hemorrhagic spontaneous renal rupture of pregnancy have required nephrectomy (172), timely use of rest in the contralateral decubitus position, ureteral stenting, or percutaneous nephrostomy may be expected to prevent this disastrous complication (64,132,162,189).

It should be noted that retroperitoneal hemorrhage may have origins in other than hydronephrosis of pregnancy as evidenced by the report of Plaus (202); he found hemorrhagic necrosis of metastatic renal choriocarcinoma related to a prior pregnancy in a patient with a positive pregnancy test and normal pelvic examination who was clearly not pregnant. A related problem is the rare spontaneous rupture of the ureter in pregnancy due to impacted proximal ureteral calculus (69).

URINARY CALCULOUS DISEASE IN PREGNANCY

Although symptomatic urinary calculi of pregnancy are vexing and pose problems that challenge all who treat them, they are neither more nor less common than their counterparts in the general population (103). This is accounted for in that the many determinants that tend to increase stone formation in pregnancy are offset by opposing factors. Hydronephrosis, decreased ureteral peristalsis, infection, and calcium supersaturation (159) all augment the stone-forming tendency of pregnancy, whereas increased excretion of stone inhibitors (magnesium, citrate, and glycosaminoglycans) works in the reverse (80). Although most researchers have found that calculi of pregnancy tend to occur in multiparas (9,47,170,191,227, 235,241), a more recent study found primiparas to be more commonly afflicted (191).

Diagnosis of calculi in the pregnant patient begins with symptoms of flank or abdominal pain, urinary urgency, nausea, and vomiting. Because any of these symptoms are compatible with normal pregnancy, imaging studies must be done for confirmation. Ultrasound may reveal hydronephrosis, but as discussed earlier, this finding is entirely consistent with physiologic dilation and may lack diagnostic capability. Even demonstration of the presence of a calculus in the renal collecting system may not be definitive because most symptomatic calculi during pregnancy are located in the ureter (269). A diligent sonographer may occasionally demonstrate a calculus in the ureter adjacent to a filled bladder; however, the unreliability of sonography in this setting leads to the conclusion that roentgenography is necessary to diagnose most symptomatic urinary calculi requiring intervention by the urologist, as discussed previously.

Because most symptomatic stones during pregnancy will pass spontaneously, the treatment of these stones is primarily expectant (62,100,103,240). This conservative posture is feasible because most calculi become asymptomatic after the first trimester (137,240), so stones that remain in the urinary tract but become asymptomatic can be "nursed along" until intervention may be undertaken without concerns for fetal health following parturition.

Similar to treatment for symptomatic hydronephrosis of pregnancy, intervention most commonly assumes the form of stent placement (66,103,150,158). It has been suggested that stents be changed monthly to prevent rapid encrustation in patients with chronic recurrent stone disease or in those with persistent infection (216). We consider it axiomatic that asymptomatic stone disease in women of childbearing age be treated prophylactically to preempt the dilemma of diagnosis and treatment of stones during pregnancy. Rittenberg and Bagley (213) recommend flexible ureteroscopy for both diagnosis and extraction of symptomatic calculi in pregnancy; however, narrow-caliber, semirigid fiberoptic telescopes have been useful in our experience, especially because most of these calculi are below the iliac crossover. Ureteroscopy is further facilitated during pregnancy by ureterectasis, both physiologic and obstructive in nature.

Alternative management options of calculi include placement of percutaneous nephrostomy tubes and open lithotomy (47,66,96), both considered safe in pregnancy. However, the position of extracorporeal shock wave lithotripsy (ESWL) in pregnant patients is less clear. Although female fertility is believed to be unaffected by ESWL (259), there is a dearth of information as to the safety of shock waves administered in the vicinity of a fetus. Ultrasound-guided shock waves during early pregnancy in Sprague-Dawley rats were not found to be harmful (232a). Certainly, the small but significant radiation dosage received by many patients from fluoroscopic imaging during ESWL would support the use of devices using ultrasound coupling to the shock wave energy source. Suffice it to say that the lack of mitigating data at present places pregnancy as a relative contraindication to ESWL.

Open surgery can be safely performed for stones in the kidney or upper ureter. Open surgery is *contraindicated* in the last half of pregnancy for lower ureteral stones. There is not enough room in the pelvis to operate, and it would be difficult to correct any surgical complications. In the past, some urologists approached lower ureteral stones through a small vaginal incision.

To continue medications for prophylaxis of stone disease during pregnancy is questionable. Gregory and Mansell (90) reported experience with 46 pregnancies in cystinuric patients. D-Penicillamine was continued during gestation (with the exception of weeks 6 through 20 to prevent mutagenicity) with no congenital defects identified. Sodium bicarbonate and potassium citrate were also continued throughout pregnancy with no ill effects on the fetus. However, thiazides are known to cross the placental barrier, causing fetal or neonatal jaundice and thrombocytopenia, thus creating a relative contraindication for pregnancy (93,269). Calcium-binding agents and low-calcium diets should be replaced with liberal fluid intake alone to prevent nutritional deficiencies in the evolving conceptus.

URINARY INFECTION IN PREGNANCY

Asymptomatic bacteruria is present in 4% to 7% of pregnancies, similar to the incidence in menstruating women generally (127,133,188,246). Thus, although pregnancy does not in and of itself cause bacteruria, the latter's association with pyelonephritis results indirectly in prematurity, low birth weight, and growth retardation (133,135,277, 278). Kass (121,123) demonstrated that 20% to 40% of pregnant women with first trimester bacteruria acquire pyelonephritis in the third trimester. Conversely, successful treatment of bacteruria significantly lessens the progression to pyelonephritis of pregnancy and associated low birth weight, growth retardation, and premature labor (42,122). This is especially true in diabetic patients (176). It is therefore considered axiomatic that bacteruria of pregnancy be both screened for and treated. In a study of 3,254 patients screened for bacteruria of pregnancy (238), it was found that the risk of acquiring bacteruria increased with the duration of pregnancy, from 0.8% at the end of the first trimester to 1.93% at term. Because the risk of onset of bacteruria is highest between weeks 9 and 17 of gestation, it was suggested that week 16 is the optimal time for screening if considerations of economy dictate a single specimen be selected for this purpose. A meticulous, clean-catch midstream urine culture growing greater than 100,000 colony-forming units (CFU)/mm is considered significant for purposes of treatment and antimicrobial prophylaxis during pregnancy (196).

Offending microorganisms in the genesis of urinary tract infections during pregnancy are those causing infection in the general adult female population, primarily Gram-negative rods. *Escherichia coli* is the most common, followed by *Klebsiella, Enterobacter, Proteus,* Gram-positive cocci, and enterococci (in order of frequency) (7,154). Stenqvist and colleagues (239) demonstrated that pregnancy does not diminish the virulence of *E. coli* strains that cause pyelonephritis compared with those causing only asymptomatic bacteruria, suggesting that pregnancy does not enhance host factors for resistance to upper urinary tract infection. Matorras and associates (164) found 20% of pregnant diabetic patients (twice as many as nondiabetic patients) to be colonized rectovaginally with group B streptococcus. However, group B streptococci did not cause more frequent urinary infection in diabetic than in nondiabetic patients. Urethritis caused by *Chlamydia trachomatis* occurs in 50% of women with dysuria, pyuria, and urinary frequency (266). In addition, chlamydial cervicitis was found in 21% of 11,544 women at their first prenatal visit; when untreated, it was associated with premature rupture of membranes, as well as low birth weight and decreased survival (221). Neonatal complications of chlamydial infection included nasopharyngitis, pneumonitis, and conjunctivitis. Thus *Chlamydia* is not "normal flora" and should be treated when discovered during pregnancy with erythromycin 500 mg four times daily for 7 to 10 days (266).

Once urinary tract infection is established in the pregnant patient, it becomes necessary to select both initial treatment and subsequent prophylaxis. Krieger (133) recommends full-dose antibiotic therapy for 7 to 10 days in treatment of gestational bacteruria. In addition, treatment for acute cystitis is the same as for asymptomatic bacteruria of pregnancy (169). However, regimens for initial treatment vary from single-dose to 3-day courses using amoxicillin (82,115), nitrofurantoin (97), and cephalexin (115,167). Angel and co-workers (8) found that in the absence of bacteremia, oral antibiotic therapy was as safe and effective as intravenous treatment for acute pyelonephritis during pregnancy.

Prophylaxis against recurrence of bacteruria for the remainder of pregnancy once the initial positive culture has been treated may be given as a daily or periodic dose of a suppressive antimicrobial agent. Van Dorsten and colleagues (254) used nitrofurantoin 50 mg three times daily as uroprophylaxis unless the initial posttreatment urine culture grew an organism resistant to that drug. Alternatively, Pfau and Sacks (201) use postcoital prophylaxis in the form of either cephalexin (250 mg) or nitrofurantoin (50 mg), similar to the case in nonpregnant patients. An intermediate prophylaxis regimen would be an equivalent dose of any antibiotics known to be safe and effective in pregnancy and for the particular microorganism in question as a nightly dose for the duration of the remainder of gestation (142,196,254). Close bacteriologic follow-up (e.g., semiweekly or monthly urine cultures) should follow initial treatment and be used to determine when additional bursts of full-course antibiotics should be prescribed.

Demonstration of persistent bacteruria during pregnancy is associated with structural urinary tract defects warranting thorough urologic evaluation postpartum (65). Austenfeld and Snow (10) found increased rates of urinary tract infection and miscarriage in women having undergone prior ureteroneocystostomy for childhood vesicoureteral reflux. Evaluation with early and repetitive urine cultures accompanied by prompt intervention with antimicrobials as described previously is appropriate in pregnant patients with any preexisting anatomic urinary anomaly.

RENAL FAILURE IN PREGNANCY

Chronic renal failure can be exacerbated by pregnancy, and acute renal failure (ARF) can be caused by pregnancy. Pregnancy is further complicated by end-stage renal disease (ESRD) treated either by dialysis or transplantation. These parallel management problems and counseling for women with renal disease facing pregnancy are now considered.

Renal failure resulting from pregnancy is classified into three etiologic categories: prerenal, renal, and postrenal. Prerenal states are caused principally by hypovolemia attributable to hyperemesis gravidarum and uterine bleeding (131). Hemorrhage in turn has three primary etiologies: abortion, placenta previa, and abruptio placentae. Unchecked by appropriate replacement of lost fluids, prerenal azotemia deteriorates into acute tubular necrosis (ATN), the most common cause of ARF in pregnancy (55). ATN and its counterpart, renal cortical necrosis (RCN), are the chief causes of ARF of pregnancy (Table 5.2). ATN and RCN are

TABLE 5.2. ACUTE RENAL FAILURE IN PREGNANCY: ACUTE TUBULAR NECROSIS AND RENAL CORTICAL NECROSIS COMPARED

Acute Renal Failure Etiology	Acute Tubular Necrosis	Renal Cortical Necrosis
Predisposing factors	Prerenal azotemia (hyperemesis gravidarum, uterine hemorrhage), preeclampsia, eclampsia, sepsis	Disseminated intravascular coagulation (amniotic fluid embolism, abruptio, intrauterine fetal demise), transfusion reactions, sepsis (chorioamnionitis, septic abortion, pyelonephritis)
Clinical manifestations	Nonoliguric renal failure	Oligoanuric renal failure; may occur as idiopathic postpartum renal failure
Outcome	Resolution of renal insufficiency	Chronic renal failure; renal cortical calcification

distinguished from one another in that ATN occurs in a setting of preeclampsia (hypertension, proteinuria, and edema), eclampsia (preeclampsia plus seizure and coma), sepsis, and hemorrhage (215). In contrast, RCN follows disseminated intravascular coagulation (caused by amniotic fluid embolism, intrauterine fetal demise, or abruptio placentae), transfusion reactions, and sepsis (caused by chorioamnionitis, septic abortion, and pyelonephritis) (92,131). Clinically, ATN may be distinguished from RCN in that, whereas ATN rarely causes anuria and is usually reversible, RCN is manifested by anuria followed by irreversible renal damage accompanied by renal cortical calcification (269). RCN may occur during the puerperium as the syndrome of idiopathic postpartum renal failure. This rare syndrome is clinically characterized by oligoanuric acute renal failure following an otherwise uneventful pregnancy, which often progresses to RCN. [Three of five cases in a series of 57 cases of ARF in pregnancy were reported by Grunfeld and Pertuiset (92).] Although ARF occurs with an incidence of 1 in 2,000 to 5,000 pregnancies, more than 20% of cases of ARF in women are seen during pregnancy (92,131). Fortunately, ARF in females is declining as a result of improved obstetric care in general, and it has nearly disappeared late in the first trimester because of eradication of septic abortion (269).

Whereas pregnancy may be a cause of acute renal disease, it may exacerbate preexisting renal disorders. Imbasciati and associates (109) reported 18 patients with serum creatinines more than 1.6 mg/dL underwent 19 pregnancies resulting in 13 live births, of which 50% were premature. Of the 18 patients, 14 were followed postnatally; 5 of 14 (36%) developed rapidly progressive renal insufficiency. Abe and colleagues (1) described renal deterioration in 25% of women with chronic renal disease in the midst of or following pregnancy. Others have recommended termination of pregnancy if the pregnancy causes progressive decline in renal function (152). Pregnancy does not seem to permanently influence kidneys with diabetic nephropathy, glomerulonephritis, renal transplants, or polycystic kidneys (136). However, manifestations of cystic renal disease, such as hypertension, infection, hematuria, and calculi, may cause management problems in pregnant patients with autosomal-dominant polycystic kidney disease (APCKD). In contrast, reflux nephropathy entails significant risk for acceleration of renal dysfunction during and after pregnancy. Becker and co-workers (14) reviewed 20 patients during a 10-year span and found 4 (20%) developing ESRD within 2 years of parturition, while 4 others who aborted went on to develop hypertension and ESRD. They conclude that patients with a history of reflux nephropathy incur a 50% risk of progression to end-stage renal failure. Patients with renal failure or hypertension are at greater risk for impairing renal function during pregnancy.

Although pregnancy might accelerate the progression of chronic renal disease toward the end stage, pregnancy remains a possibility for the patient with established ESRD. The first term pregnancy in a hemodialysis patient was reported in 1971 (43). A more recent series (210) describes nine births resulting from 14 pregnancies in 13 patients enrolled in dialysis programs (8 patients receiving chronic ambulatory peritoneal dialysis and 6 receiving hemodialysis). Although no congenital anomalies were identified, pregnancies tended to be complicated by exacerbation of hypertension and worsening residual renal function; babies were small for gestational age. These data support the general recommendation for allowing attempt of conception in the dialysis population with close medical surveillance.

If ESRD presents a set of risks to patients contemplating or facing pregnancy, renal transplantation becomes a "double-edged sword" in (to the positive) eliminating the azotemic state and (to the negative) causing fetal exposure to immunosuppressive drugs (63). It is now known that successful renal transplantation improves the likelihood of pregnancy from 1 in 200 (pretransplantation) to 1 in 50 (34). Conversely, pregnancy is unlikely to harm an adequately functioning renal graft (54). Specifically, only 15% of renal transplants will deteriorate as a result of pregnancy (226). However, in those few transplant patients experiencing increasing azotemia during pregnancy, termination has been recommended to prevent irreversible transplant damage (226). An interesting window of opportunity has been observed in transplant patients who become pregnant. That is, pregnancy occurring more than 5 years after transplantation causes permanent renal injury in 75% of cases (57). On the other hand, the outcome of pregnancy itself is superior at least 2 years after transplantation (34). These combined observations yield the conclusion that renal transplant patients should plan their pregnancies between 2 and 5 years after transplantation.

Pregnancy further affects renal transplant function in that the immunologically privileged state of gestation diminishes the incidence of transplant rejection (195). A corollary of this phenomenon is the occasional "rebound" of transplant rejection occurring postpartum. Immunosuppressive drugs (e.g., steroids, azathioprine, cyclosporine), although teratogenic at high dosages, are usually safe at moderate dosages during pregnancy (63,139,186). Although renal transplant patients must be monitored closely throughout pregnancy for development of hypertension, urinary infection, prematurity, and preeclampsia, transplant function is only minimally jeopardized during gestation (30,190).

UROLOGIC CONSIDERATIONS IN THE PREGNANT PATIENT WITH A SPINAL INJURY

Approximately 2,000 women of childbearing age sustain spinal cord injury annually in the United States alone (46). As a result of vastly improved rehabilitative measures, pregnancy has become a real possibility in such patients. Cross and associates (46) reported 25 pregnancies in 16 women with cervical (7 patients) or thoracic (9 patients) spinal injuries. Twenty-two babies, four of whom were delivered via cesarean section, and three abortions resulted from these pregnancies. Eleven patients had symptomatic urinary tract infections, one had removal of a bladder calculus, and seven had autonomic dysreflexia (see also reference 265) related to a number of stimuli, such as a full bladder, enema, bowel movement, Foley catheter change (143), or uterine contraction. Greenspoon and Paul (89) recommend maintenance of a clean perineum to prevent ascent of bacteria from skin to bladder. The usual means of bladder drainage (e.g., intermittent clean catheterization, suprapubic catheterization, Credé maneuver) should be continued intrapartum. All spinal injury patients should be monitored closely and are at increased risk for asymptomatic bacteruria of pregnancy. Because most are managed with some type of catheterization, bacteruria is the rule in pregnant patients with a spinal injury; consequently, most will require antibiotic prophylaxis during pregnancy to reduce attendant complications, such as prematurity or low birth weight.

In the past, many patients with spinal injury or those with congenital spinal anomalies have been managed with extensive urologic surgical procedures to relieve obstruction or stasis in the upper or lower tracts. Such patients requiring delivery via cesarean section especially should be treated with great care, preferably with a team of operating gynecologic and urologic surgeons to avoid injury to bladder, ureter, or diversionary intestinal segment (212).

LOWER URINARY TRACT DYSFUNCTION IN PREGNANCY

Whereas urinary stress incontinence and frequency are common lower tract symptoms during pregnancy, gestational urinary retention is distinctly uncommon (237). The latter is thought to occur as a result of uterine retroversion during early pregnancy, a situation that tends to spontaneously reverse in the second trimester (95). That is, urethral obstruction caused by first trimester uterine retroversion resolves with backward cervical movement and fundal anteversion occurring at week 14 or 15 (84). Thus this form of urinary retention may be resolved by either temporary placement of a pessary or manual repositioning of the fundus (84,183,230). The problem may be circumvented by intermittent catheterization and voiding in the prone position (203).

Urinary retention may occur as a consequence of epidural block preceding delivery by cesarean section. This complication may be avoided by preoperative placement of a Foley catheter that is indwelling for several days postpartum. The incidence of urinary retention in this cohort is thereby reduced from 40% to zero (126). In patients with neurogenic urinary retention treated with indwelling bladder stimulator devices, there have been no adverse effects on the pregnancy or fetus (157,181).

Urinary stress incontinence occurs commonly both during and after pregnancy. The genesis of pregnancy-related stress incontinence remains controversial. It seems likely that myogenic or neurogenic damage to the urethral sphincter may occur after difficult vaginal delivery or that facilitated by application of forceps (245). On the other hand, Van Geelen and associates (255) found that neither functional urethral length nor urethral closure pressure changed significantly during pregnancy, nor was there a notable influence by either the duration of labor or the presence of an episiotomy on postpartum urethral pressure profiles. In the same study of 43 asymptomatic primigravidas, urethral closure response to stress maneuvers did not change during the course of pregnancy, nor did birth weight influence urethral pressure or length parameters postpartum in patients undergoing vaginal delivery. The conclusion was that inherent weakness in the sphincter mechanism rather than pregnancy itself caused stress incontinence.

In contrast, Iosif (110) found that only 4.9% of 1,411 patients developed permanent pregnancy-related stress incontinence, and of this 4.9%, most developed incontinence during their first pregnancy. Moreover, the incidence of stress incontinence in parous patients' mothers was greater by fivefold in incontinent patients as compared with that of controls. It was inferred that pregnancy itself rather than birth trauma was responsible for stress incontinence. The same author has studied stress-incontinent women urodynamically during and after pregnancy and has found that urethral closure pressure progressively diminishes during the course of gestation, as opposed to continent women, who exhibit an increase in both urethral length and urethral closure pressure as pregnancy proceeds (111). This finding supports the concept that physiologic changes in urethral function (or the lack thereof), as opposed to direct trauma to urethral smooth muscle or innervation during parturition, lead to stress incontinence. Petros and Ulmsten (200) propose an effect of relaxin, produced by the corpus luteum of pregnancy, on urethral collagen (depolymerization and resulting tissue softening) as causing reversible stress incontinence in a pregnant patient having had an intravaginal sling operation. Further studies will be necessary to confirm whether relaxin or other hormonal phenomena are responsible for temporary or permanent changes in urethral function during and after pregnancy.

UROLOGIC COMPLICATIONS OF CESAREAN SECTION AND VAGINAL DELIVERY

The incidence of overall injuries to the urinary tract during caesarean section is less than 1%, although it is much higher if associated with cesarean hysterectomy (147). Ureteral injury during cesarean section occurs 0.1% of the time (148). Such injuries are most often repaired using ureteroneocystostomy facilitated by psoas hitch (148). Injury to the urinary bladder is the most commonly reported acute urologic obstetric injury and is often caused by an opening in the bladder dome created during cesarean section (11,72,173). Repair is straightforward owing to the lack of involvement of the trigonal structures. However, low-segment cesarean section may injure the bladder base or ureters, risking vesicovaginal (0.7% incidence) or, more rarely, ureterovaginal fistula (4,104,147). Multilayer closure and omental interposition during repair is prudent in prevention of such complications. Rare urologic obstetric complications include urethral diverticula that may obstruct labor (174), atraumatic bladder or urethral rupture, necrosis of the anterior vaginal wall leading to vesicovaginal fistula secondary to obstructed labor (147), vesicouterine fistula following repeat cesarean section (250), loss of pelvic floor muscle tone after episiotomy and high forceps delivery (94,128,243,249), and trans-serosal invasion of the bladder by placenta percreta (222,232). Recent data suggest that repeat cesarean section has now become the principle cause of vesicouterine fistula due to altered vascularization of the supravaginal septum and distortion of bladder anatomy after primary section (116).

Vesical neck support and mobility are affected by both vaginal delivery and cesarean section, more so with the latter. Forceps delivery in particular may have profound effects on ability of women to contract their pelvic floor musculature. In addition, forceps delivery causes prolonged pudendal nerve terminal latencies as compared with vaginal delivery without forceps. Multiparity with or without forceps delivery results in pudendal nerve dysfunction similar to forceps delivery in primigravidas or in women having had a prolonged second stage of labor or high birth weight (3,233,242). Such pudendal nerve dysfunction may persist and worsen over the years following delivery (234). Cesarean delivery seems to preserve pudendal nerve function and, by extension, pelvic floor muscle tone. Similarly, noninstrumented vaginal delivery leads to transient but reversible pudendal nerve dysfunction (248). Thus it is clear that preservation of pelvic floor neuromuscular integrity is directly related to efforts to minimize the use of forceps and episiotomy in facilitating vaginal delivery, as well as limiting prolongation of the second stage of labor, prevention of third- and fourth-degree lacerations, and judicious application of cesarean delivery (94,250).

URINARY TRACT RECONSTRUCTION AND PREGNANCY

Pregnancy is possible in patients having undergone prior urinary tract reconstruction, whether for neurogenic bladder, tumor, or voiding dysfunction. Fenn and colleagues (74) described 19 pregnancies in 18 women ages 21 to 36 years having undergone clam enterocystoplasty for intractable detrusor instability. Pajor and colleagues (193) advocate lower urinary reconstruction with an ileocecal as opposed to ileal bowel segment to avoid uterine-induced mesenteric compromise during the course of pregnancy. Kennedy and co-workers (125) reported on successful pregnancies in four women with exstrophy having had flap vaginoplasty and creation of subsequent continent right colonic urinary reservoir with an orthotopic perineal stoma (Indiana pouch). The authors performed cesarean section and close monitoring for maternal or fetal distress in all cases. Creagh and colleagues (45) reported 34 pregnancies in 27 women with reconstructed lower urinary tracts who underwent either vaginal or cesarean delivery, indicated by specific obstetric considerations. Most of their patients (28 of 34) underwent successful vaginal delivery. Thus patients having undergone lower urinary reconstruction may safely deliver either vaginally or via cesarean section; attendance of the urologist is essential in all cases.

URINARY TRACT TUMORS DISCOVERED DURING PREGNANCY

Despite pregnancy being an immunologically impaired state, the incidence of malignancy is similar to that in the general population (185). A wide variety of urologic tumors have been reported to occur during pregnancy (149). Specifically, renal cell carcinoma is the most common renal neoplasm of pregnancy; because the latter is a condition of the young, angiomyolipoma occurs next in frequency (263). For the same reason, Wilms' tumor is known in pregnancy (23). Bladder cancer during pregnancy may take the form of adenocarcinoma (78), transitional cell carcinoma (18,19), or squamous cell lesions (120). Because electrical current may induce neighboring uterine contractions, obstetric treatment to diminish uterine smooth muscle reactivity may be helpful in reducing the possibility of premature labor from electroresection and cautery. Similarly, laser phototherapy is useful to treat bladder tumors of pregnancy while eschewing prematurity.

Adrenal tumors such as pseudocyst (251) and pheochromocytoma (29,224) are extant during pregnancy. Key issues in pheochromocytoma of pregnancy include diagnostic conundrum (symptoms and signs resemble those of preeclampsia, leading to mortality rate greater than 50% when undiagnosed), choice of α-blockade (prazosin, to avoid teratogenicity of phenoxybenzamine), means of imaging (MRI is especially useful for localizing pheochromocytoma and is free of ionizing radiation), timing of surgical resection (expeditiously), and route of delivery (vaginal preferred) (29,91,149,160,224,260).

TIMING OF ANESTHESIA DURING PREGNANCY

General anesthesia in and of itself does not entail a risk of adversity to pregnancy (48). This holds especially true when the (nonobstetric) procedure is complication free. A landmark study from Scandinavia evaluated 5,405 incidental surgical procedures performed during all three trimesters of pregnancy. Although the incidence of low birth weight and prematurity was greater in these patients as compared with a large cohort of pregnancies, there was no tendency toward congenital malformation in the operated group. It was concluded that there is an increased risk of prematurity following intragravid surgical procedures requiring general anesthesia, which may be attributed to the underlying condition rather than the procedure or anesthetic itself (40,166).

Other considerations involving anesthesia during pregnancy include timing of semiurgent procedures that may not be postponed until parturition. There is evidence that nonobstetric surgical procedures are most safely performed during the second trimester owing to the increased risk of spontaneous abortion during the first trimester and induction of premature labor when procedures take place near term (108).

A related issue is the diminished requirement for both local and general anesthetics during pregnancy (149). Thus dosages of inhalation anesthetics such as halothane and isoflurane should be reduced in pregnancy to compensate for the sedative effects of progesterone (153,171, 194). Likewise, the requirement for local anesthetics is decreased during the first trimester because of increased cell membrane receptor sensitivity to these agents, again a progestational-mediated phenomenon (53,73).

CONCLUSION

Urologic problems during pregnancy are often undertreated because of unfounded fears of causing fetal harm. An understanding of pathophysiologic changes in the urinary tract, as well as appropriate use of antimicrobials, anesthetics, imaging studies, and invasive procedures, will lead to resolution of most such problems while providing a margin of safety for both mother and child.

REFERENCES

1. Abe S, Amagaski Y, Konishi K, et al. The influence of antecedent renal disease on pregnancy. *Am J Obstet Gynecol* 1985; 153:508.
2. Abramowitz M, ed. *Handbook of antimicrobial therapy.* New Rochelle, NY: Medical Letter, 1988.
3. Allen RE, Hosker GL, Smith ARB, et al. Pelvic floor damage and childbirth: a neurophysiologic study. *Br J Obstet Gynecol* 1990;97:770.
4. Allenby K, Rand RJ. Pregnancies in a woman with a vesicouterine fistula following lower segment caesarean section. *Br J Obstet Gynecol* 1996;103:87.
5. American College of Obstetricians and Gynecologists: Guidelines for diagnostic imaging during pregnancy. Committee opinion no. 158. September 1995.
6. Amon K, Amon I, Huller H. Distribution and kinetics of nitrofurantoin in early pregnancy. *Int J Clin Pharmacol Ther Toxicol* 1972;6:218.
7. Andriole VT, Patterson TF. Epidemiology, natural history, and management of urinary tract infections in pregnancy. *Med Clin North Am* 1991;75:359.
8. Angel JL, O'Brien WF, Finan MA, et al. Acute pyelonephritis in pregnancy: a prospective study of oral versus intravenous antibiotic therapy. *Obstet Gynecol* 1990;76:28.
9. Arnell RE, Getzoff PL. Renal and ureteral calculi in pregnancy. *Am J Obstet Gynecol* 1942;44:34.
10. Austenfeld MS, Snow BW. Complications of pregnancy in women after reimplantation for vesicoureteral reflux. *J Urol* 1988;140:1103.
11. Barclay DL. Cesarean hysterectomy: a thirty year experience. *Obstet Gynecol* 1970;35:120.
12. Barron WM, Mujais SK, Zinaman M, et al. Plasma catecholamine responses to physiologic stimuli in normal human pregnancy. *Am J Obstet Gynecol* 1986;154:80.
13. Baylis C. Glomerular filtration and volume regulation in gravid animal models. *Clin Obstet Gynaecol* 1987;1:789.
14. Becker GJ, Ihle BU, Fairley KF, et al. Effect of pregnancy on moderate renal failure in reflux nephropathy. *BMJ* 1986; 292:796.
15. Becker RA, Hayashi RH, Franks RC, et al. Effects of positional change and sodium balance on the renin-angiotensin-aldosterone system, big renin and prostaglandins in normal pregnancy. *J Clin Endocrinol Metab* 1978;46:467.
16. Bednarek BR, Rudin S, Wong R, et al. Reduction of fluoroscopic exposure: the air-contrast barium enema. *Br J Radiol* 56:823, 1983.
17. Belman AB. A perspective on vesicoureteral reflux. *Urol Clin North Am* 22:139, 1995.
18. Bendsen J, Muller EK, Povey G, et al. Bladder tumor as apparent cause of vaginal bleeding in pregnancy. *Acta Obstet Gynecol Scand* 64:329, 1985.
19. Bennett AH, Adler S. Bilateral ureteral obstruction causing anuria secondary to pregnancy. *Urology* 1982;20:631.
20. Bisaz S, Newman WF, Bleisch H. Quantitative determinations of inhibitors of calcium phosphate precipitation in whole urine. *Miner Electrol Metabol* 1978;17:74.
21. Blackwell AL, Thomas PD, Wareham K, et al. Health gains from screening for infection of the lower genital tract in women attending for termination of pregnancy. *Lancet* 24:342, 1993.
22. Boler L, Zbella EA, Gleicher N, et al. Quantitation of proteinuria in pregnancy by the use of single-voided urine samples. *Obstet Gynecol* 1987;70:99.
23. Bozeman G, Bissada NK, Abboud MR, et al. Adult Wilms' tumor: prognostic and management considerations. *Urology* 1995;45:1055.
24. Bravo RH, Katz M. Ureteral obstruction in a pregnant patient with an ileal loop conduit. *J Reprod Med* 1983;28:427.
25. Brent RL. The effect of embryonic and fetal exposure to x-ray, microwaves and ultrasound: counseling the pregnant and non-pregnant patient about these risks. *Semin Oncol* 16:347, 1989.
26. Briggs GG, Freeman RK, Sumner JY. *Drugs in pregnancy and lactation.* Philadelphia: Williams & Wilkins, 1986.
27. Brown MA, Sinosich MJ, Saunders DM, et al. Potassium regulation and progesterone-aldosterone interrelationships in human pregnancy. A prospective study. *Am J Obstet Gynecol* 1986;155:349.
28. Brown RD, Strott CA, Liddle GW, et al. Plasma deoxycorticosterone in normal and abnormal pregnancy. *J Clin Endocrinol Metab* 1972;35:736.

29. Burgess GE III. Alpha blockade and surgical intervention of pheochromocytoma in pregnancy. *Obstet Gynecol* 1978;53:266.
30. Buszta C, Braun WE, Steimuller DR, et al. Pregnancy and the renal transplant patient. *ANNA J* 1985;12:183.
31. Carey MP, Ihle BU, Woodward CS, et al. Ureteric obstruction by the gravid uterus. *Aust NZ J Obstet Gynaecol* 1989;29:308.
32. Carr LK, Herschorn S. Periurethral collagen injection and pregnancy. *J Urol* 155:1037, 1996.
33. Carringer M, Swartz R, Johansson JE. Management of ureteric calculi during pregnancy by ureteroscopy and laser lithotripsy. *Br J Urol* 77:17, 1996.
34. Casciani CU, Pasetto N, Piccione E, et al. Pregnancy in renal transplantation. *Clin Exp Obstet Gynecol* 1984;11:136.
35. Chesley LC. *Hypertensive disorders in pregnancy.* Norwalk: Appleton Century Crofts, 1978.
36. Choate JW, Thiede HA, Miller HC. Carcinoma of the bladder in pregnancy: Report of three cases. *Am J Obstet Gynecol* 90:526, 1964.
37. Chow AW, Jewesson PJ. Pharmacokinetics and safety of antimicrobial agents during pregnancy. *Rev Infect Dis* 1985;7:674.
38. Christensen T, Klebe JG, Bertelsen V, et al. Changes in renal volume during normal pregnancy. *Acta Obstet Gynecol Scand* 1989;68:541.
39. Clark JC. The right ovarian vein syndrome. In: Emmett JL, Witten DM, eds. *Clinical urography.* Philadelphia: Saunders, 1971.
40. Cohen SE. Nonobstetric surgery during pregnancy. In: Chestnut DH, ed. *Obstetric anesthesia.* St Louis: Mosby, 1994.
41. Collins E, Turner G. Maternal effects of regular salicylate ingestion in pregnancy. *Lancet* 1975;2:335.
42. Condie AP, Williams JD, Reeves DS, et al. Complications of bacteriuria in pregnancy. In: O'Grady F, Brumfitt E, eds. *Urinary tract infection.* London: Oxford University Press, 1968.
43. Confortini P, Galanti G, Ancona G, et al. Full-term pregnancy and successful delivery in a patient on chronic hemodialysis. *Proc Eur Dial Transpl Assoc* 1971;18:74.
44. Cox SM, Cunningham FG. Acute focal pyelonephritis (lobar nephronia) complicating pregnancy. *Obstet Gynecol* 1988;71.
45. Creagh TA, McInerney PD, Thomas PJ, et al. Pregnancy after lower urinary tract reconstruction in women. *J Urol* 154:1323, 1995.
46. Cross LL, Meythaler J, Tuel SM, et al. Pregnancy following spinal cord injury. *West J Med* 1991;154:607.
47. Cumming DC, Taylor PJ. Urologic and obstetric significance of urinary calculi in pregnancy. *Obstet Gynecol* 1979;53:505.
48. Medical and surgical complications in pregnancy. In: Cunningham FG, MacDonald PC, Gant NF, et al, eds. *Williams obstetrics.* Stamford, CT: Appleton & Lange, 1997.
49. Cutner A, Cardozo LD, Benness CJ. Assessment of urinary symptoms in early pregnancy. *Br J Obstet Gynaecol* 1991;98:1283.
50. Cutner A, Cardozo LD, Wise BG. The effects of pregnancy on previous incontinence surgery. Case report. *Br J Obstet Gynecol* 1991;98:1181.
51. Dafnis E, Sabatini S. The effect of pregnancy on renal function: physiology and pathophysiology. *Am J Med Sci* 1992;303:184.
52. Danielli L, Korchazak D, Beyar H, et al. Recurrent hematuria during multiple pregnancies. *Obstet Gynecol* 1987;69:446.
53. Datta S, Lambert DH, Gregus J. Differential sensitivities of mammalian nerve fibers during pregnancy. *Anesth Analg* 1983;62:1070.
54. Davison JM. Changes in renal function in early pregnancy in women with one kidney. *Yale J Med Biol* 1978;51:347.
55. Davison JM. The effect of pregnancy on kidney function in renal allograft recipients. *Kidney Int* 1985;27:74.
56. Davison JM, Barron WA, Lindheimer MD. Metabolic clearance rates of vasopressin increase markedly in late gestation. A possible cause of polyuria in pregnant women. *Trans Assoc Am Phys* 1987;100:91.
57. Davison JM, Lindheimer MD. Pregnancy in renal transplant patients. *J Reprod Med* 1982;27:613.
58. Davison JM, Shiells EA, Barron WM, et al. Changes in the metabolic clearance of vasopressin and of plasma vasopressinase throughout human pregnancy. *J Clin Invest* 1989;83:1313.
59. Davison JM, Shiells EA, Philips PR, et al. Serial evaluation of vasopressin release and thirst in human pregnancy: role of chorionic gonadotropin in the osmoregulatory changes of gestation. *J Clin Invest* 1988;81:798.
60. Davison JM, Vallotton MB, Lindheimer MD. Plasma osmolality and urinary concentrating and dilution during and after pregnancy: evidence that lateral recumbency inhibits maximal urinary concentrating ability. *Br J Obstet Gynaecol* 1981;88:472.
61. D'Elia FL, Brennan RE, Brownstein PK. Acute renal failure secondary to ureteral obstruction by a gravid uterus. *J Urol* 1982;128:803.
62. Denstedt JD, Razvi H. Management of urinary calculi during pregnancy. *J Urol* 1992;148:1072.
63. Derfler K, Schaller A, Herold C, et al. Successful outcome of a complicated pregnancy in a renal transplant recipient taking cyclosporine. *Clin Nephrol* 1988;29:96.
64. Dhabuwala CB, Riehle RA Jr. Spontaneous rupture of hydronephrotic kidney during pregnancy. *Urology* 1984;24:591.
65. Diokno AC, Compton A, Seski J. Urologic evaluation of urinary tract infection in pregnancy. *J Reprod Med* 1986;31:23.
66. Drago JR, Rohner TJ Jr, Chez RA. Management of urinary calculi in pregnancy. *Urology* 1982;20:578.
67. Dunlop W, Davison JM. Renal haemodynamics and tubular function in human pregnancy. *Clin Obstet Gynaecol* 1987;1:769.
68. Dykhuizen RF, Roberts JA. The ovarian vein syndrome. *Surg Gynecol Obstet* 1970;130:443.
69. Eaton A, Martin PC. Ruptured ureter in pregnancy—a unique case? *Br J Urol* 1981;53:78.
70. Eckford SD, Gingell JC. Ureteric obstruction in pregnancy—diagnosis and management. *Br J Obstet Gynaecol* 1991;98:1137.
71. Eika B, Skajaa K. Acute renal failure due to bilateral ureteral obstruction by the pregnant uterus. *Urol Int* 1988;43:315.
72. Eisenkop SM, Richman R, Platt LD, et al. Urinary tract injury during cesarean section. *Obstet Gynecol* 1982;60:591.
73. Fagraeus L, Urban BJ, Bromage PR. Spread of epidural analgesia in early pregnancy. *Anesthesiology* 58:184, 1983.
74. Fenn N, Barrington JW, Stephenson TP. Clam enterocystoplasty and pregnancy. *Br J Urol* 75:85, 1995.
75. Ferris TF. Prostanoids in normal and hypertensive pregnancy. In: Rubin PC, ed. *Handbook of hypertension,* vol 10, *Hypertension in pregnancy.* Amsterdam: Elsevier, 1988.
76. Finci L, Meier B, Steffenino G, et al. Radiation exposure during diagnostic catheterization and single- and double-vessel percutaneous transluminal coronary angioplasty. *Am J Cardiol* 60:1401, 1987.
77. Fishman IJ, Scott FB. Pregnancy in patients with the artificial urinary sphincter. *J Urol* 1993;150(2 pt 1):340.
78. FitzGerald MP, Hernandez E, Hadley C, et al. Bladder adenocarcinoma during pregnancy: a case report. *J Reprod Med* 1996;41:59.
79. Friedman SA. Preeclampsia: a review of the role of prostaglandins. *Obstet Gynecol* 1988;71:122.

80. Gambaro G et al. Increased urinary excretion of glycosaminoglycans in pregnancy and in diabetes mellitus: a protective factor against nephrolithiasis. *Nephron* 1988;50:62.
81. Geard CR, Osmak RS, Hall EJ, et al. Magnetic resonance imaging and ionizing radiation: a comparative evaluation in-vitro of oncogenic and genotoxic potential. *Radiology* 1984; 152:199.
82. Gerstner GJ, Muller G, Nahler G. Amoxicillin in the treatment of asymptomatic bacteriuria in pregnancy: a single dose of 3 g amoxicillin versus a 4-day course of three doses 750 mg amoxicillin. *Gynecol Obstet Invest* 1989;27:84.
83. Gertner JM, Coustan DR, Kliger AS, et al. Pregnancy as state of physiologic absorptive hypercalciuria. *Am J Med* 1986;81:451.
84. Goldberg KA, Kwart AM. Intermittent urinary retention in first trimester of pregnancy. *Urology* 1981;17:270.
85. Goldfarb RA, Neerhut GJ, Lederer E. Management of acute hydronephrosis of pregnancy by ureteral stenting: risk of stone formation. *J Urol* 1989;141:921.
86. Gorson RO, Lassen M, Rosenstein M. Patient dosimetry in diagnostic radiology. In: Waggener RG, Kereiakes JG, Shalek R, eds. *Handbook of medical physics,* vol II. Boca Raton, FL: CRC Press, 1984.
87. Greene G. Tetracycline in pregnancy. *N Engl J Med* 1976; 295:512.
88. Greenspoon JS. Differential diagnosis of spontaneous renal rupture in pregnant women. *Mayo Clin Proc* 1991;66:969.
89. Greenspoon JS, Paul RH. Paraplegia and quadriplegia: special considerations during pregnancy and labor and delivery. *Am J Obstet Gynecol* 1986;155:738.
90. Gregory MC, Mansell MA. Pregnancy and cystinuria. *Lancet* 1983;2:1158.
91. Griffin J, Brooks N, Patricia F. Pheochromocytoma in pregnancy: Diagnosis and collaborative management. *South Med J* 77:1325, 1984.
92. Grunfeld JP, Pertuiset N. Acute renal failure in pregnancy. *Am J Kid Dis* 1987;9:359.
93. Hamar C, Levy G. Serum protein binding of drugs and bilirubin in newborn infants and their mothers. *Clin Pharmacol Ther* 1980;28:58.
94. Handa VL, Harris TA, Ostergard DR. Protecting the pelvic floor: obstetric management to prevent incontinence and pelvic organ prolapse. *Obstet Gynecol* 1996;88:470.
95. Hansen JH, Asmussen M. Acute urinary retention in first trimester of pregnancy. *Acta Obstet Gynecol Scand* 1985;64:279.
96. Harris RE, Dunnihoo DR. The incidence and significance of urinary calculi in pregnancy. *Am J Obstet Gynecol* 1967;99:237.
97. Harris RE, Gilstrap LC, Pretty A. A single-dose antimicrobial therapy for asymptomatic bacteriuria during pregnancy. *Obstet Gynecol* 1982;59:546.
98. Harrow BR, Sloane JA, Salhanick L. Etiology of the hydronephrosis of pregnancy. *Surg Gynecol Obstet* 1964;119:1042.
99. Harvey EB, Boice JD, Honeyman M, et al. Prenatal x-ray exposure and childhood cancer in twins. *N Engl J Med* 1985; 312:541.
100. Hendricks SK, Ross SO, Krieger JN. An algorithm for diagnosis and therapy of management and complications of urolithiasis during pregnancy. *Surg Gynecol Obstet* 1991;172:49.
101. Hertzberg BS, Carroll BA, Bowie JD, et al. Doppler US assessment of maternal kidneys: analysis of intrarenal resistivity indexes in normal pregnancy and physiologic pelvicaliectasis. *Radiology* 1993;186:689.
102. Homans DC, Blake GD, Harrington JT, et al. Acute renal failure caused by ureteral obstruction by a gravid uterus. *JAMA* 1981;246:1230.
103. Horowitz E, Schmidt JD. Renal calculi in pregnancy. *Clin Obstet Gynecol* 1985;28:324.
104. Hosseini SY, Roshan YM, Sararinejad MR, et al. Ureterovaginal fistula after vaginal delivery. *J Urol* 1998;160:829.
105. Howarth AT, Morgan DB, Payne RB. Urinary excretion of calcium in late pregnancy and its relation to creatinine clearance. *Am J Obstet Gynecol* 1977;129:499.
106. Hsueh WA, Luetscher JA, Carlson EJ, et al. Changes in active and inactive renin throughout pregnancy. *J Clin Endocrinol Metab* 1982;54:1010.
107. Huff PS, Bucci KK. Drug use in pregnancy. In: Andolsek KM, ed. *Obstetric care: standards of prenatal, intrapartum and postpartum management.* Philadelphia: Lea & Febiger; 1990.
108. Hull LM, Johnson CE, Lee RA. Cholecystectomy in pregnancy. *Obstet. Gynecol* 9:291, 1975.
109. Imbasciati E, Pardi G, Capetta P, et al. Pregnancy in women with chronic renal failure. *Am J Nephrol* 1986;6:193.
110. Iosif S. Stress incontinence during pregnancy and in puerperium. *Int J Gynaecol Obstet* 1981;19:13.
111. Iosif S, Ulmsten UI. Comparative urodynamic studies of continent and stress incontinent women in pregnancy and in puerperium. *Am J Obstet Gynecol* 1981;140:645.
112. Ismail MA, Cervenka RP. Ureteral stent placement for recurrent hydronephrosis in pregnancy. *J Reprod Med* 1986;31:280.
113. Ives TJ, Tepper RS. Drug use in pregnancy and lactation. *Pharmacother Prim Care Phys* 1990;17:623.
114. Izumoto H, Matsui H, Hayashi H, et al. Spontaneous renal rupture in pregnancy. *Arch Surg* 1989;124:389.
115. Jakobi P, Neiger R, Merzbach D, et al. Single-dose antimicrobial therapy in the treatment of asymptomatic bacteriuria in pregnancy. *Am J Obstet Gynecol* 1987;156:1148.
116. Jozwik M, Jozwik M. A link between vesicouterine fistula and repeat cesarian section continued. Abstracts of the International Continence Society, Ref. 506, 1999.
117. Jungers P, Hovillier P, Chaveau D, et al. Pregnancy in women with reflux nephropathy. *Kidney Int* 1996;50:593.
118. Jungers P, Hovillier P, Forget D, et al. Specific controversies concerning the natural history of renal disease in pregnancy. *Am J Kid Dis* 1991;17:116.
119. Jurecka W, Gebhart W. Drug prescribing during pregnancy. *Semin Dermatol* 1989;8:30.
120. Karim M, Ammar R, Dadawy S. Carcinoma of the bladder with pregnancy. *J Egypt Med Assoc* 1968;51:1037.
121. Kass EH. Asymptomatic infection of urinary tract. *Trans Assoc Am Phys* 1956;69:56.
122. Kass EH. The role of asymptomatic bacteriuria in the pathogenesis of pyelonephritis. In: Quinn EL, Kass EH, eds. *Biology of pyelonephritis.* Boston: Little, Brown, 1960.
123. Kass EH. The role of unsuspected infection in the etiology of prematurity. *Clin Obstet Gynecol* 1973;16:134.
124. Kavoussi LR, Albala DM, Basler JM, et al. Percutaneous management of urolithiasis during pregnancy. *J Urol* 1992;148: 1069.
125. Kennedy WA, Hensle TW, Reiley EA, et al. Pregnancy after orthotopic continent urinary diversion. *Surg Gynecol Obstet* 1993;177:405.
126. Kerr-Wilson RHJ, McNally S. Bladder drainage for caesarean section under epidural analgesia. *Br J Obstet Gynaecol* 1986; 93:28.
127. Kinningham RB. Asymptomatic bacteriuria in pregnancy. *Am Fam Physician* 1993;47:1232.
128. Klein MC, Gauthier RJ, Robbins JM, et al. Relationship of episiotomy to perineal trauma and morbidity, sexual dysfunction, and pelvic floor relaxation. *Am J Obstet Gynecol* 1994; 171:591.

129. Knapp EL. *Studies on the urinary excretion of calcium.* Dissertation thesis for Doctor of Philosophy. Department of Chemistry, State University of Iowa, 1943.
130. Knebel L, Tschada R, Mickisch G, et al. Le drainage interne de l'urine en cas de stase urinaire compliquee provoquee par une grossesse. *Journal d'Urologie* 1993;99:169.
131. Knuppel RA, Montenegro R, O'Brien WF. Acute renal failure in pregnancy. *Clin Obstet Gynecol* 1985;28:288.
132. Kramer RL. Urinoma in pregnancy. *Obstet Gynecol* 1983; 62:26S.
133. Krieger JN. Complications and treatment of urinary tract infections during pregnancy. *Urol Clin North Am* 1986;13:685.
134. L'Allemand D, Gruters A, Heidemann P, et al. Iodine-induced alterations of thyroid function in newborn infants after prenatal and perinatal exposure to povidone iodine. *J Pediatr* 1983; 102:935.
135. Landers DV, Green JR, Sweet RL. Antibiotic use during pregnancy and the postpartum period. *Clin Obstet Gynecol* 1983; 26:391.
136. Lashgari M, Keene ME. Pregnancy in women with adult polycystic kidney disease. *Conn Med* 1986;50:374.
137. Lattanzi DR, Cook WA. Urinary calculi in pregnancy. *Obstet Gynecol* 1980;56:462.
138. Laverson PL, Hankins GDV, Quirk G Jr. Ureteral obstruction during pregnancy. *J Urol* 1984;131:327.
139. Leb DE, Weiskoff B, Kanovitz BS. Chromosome aberrations in the child of a kidney transplant recipient. *Arch Intern Med* 1971;128:441.
140. Lee JG, Wein AJ, Levin RM. Effects of pregnancy on urethral and bladder neck function. *Urology* 42:747, 1993.
141. Lees MM, Taylor SH, Scott DB, et al. A study of cardiac output at rest throughout pregnancy. *J Obstet Gynaecol Br Commonw* 1967;74:319.
142. Lenke RR, Van Dorsten JP, Schifrin BS. Pyelonephritis in pregnancy: a randomized trial to prevent recurrent disease evaluating suppressive therapy with nitrofurantoin and close surveillance. *Am J Obstet Gynecol* 1983;146:953.
143. Letcher JC, Goldfine LJ. Management of a pregnant paraplegic patient in a rehabilitation center. *Arch Phys Med Rehabil* 1988; 67:477.
144. Levin DL. Effects of inhibition of prostaglandin synthesis on fetal development, oxygenation and the fetal circulation. *Semin Perinatol* 1980;4:35.
145. Lindheimer MD, Katz AI. Fluid and electrolyte metabolism in normal and abnormal pregnancy. In: Arieff AI, DeFronzo R, eds. *Fluid electrolyte and acid-base disorders.* New York: Churchill Livingstone, 1985.
146. Lindheimer M, Katz A. The kidney and hypertension in pregnancy. In: Brenner BM, Rector FC, eds. *The kidney,* vol 2. Philadelphia: Saunders, 1991.
147. Lobel RW, Sand PK, Bowen LW, et al. The urinary tract in pregnancy. In: Ostergard DR, Bent AE, eds. *Urogynecology and urodynamics,* ed 4. Baltimore: Williams & Wilkins, 1996.
148. Loughlin KR. Management of urologic problems during pregnancy. *Urology* 1994;44:159.
149. Loughlin KR. Management of urologic problems in the pregnant patient. *AUA Update Series* 16:10, 1997.
150. Loughlin KR, Bailey RB Jr. Internal ureteral stents for conservative management of ureteral calculi during pregnancy. *N Engl J Med* 1986;315:1647.
151. Lowes JJ, Mackenzie JC, Abrams PH, et al. Acute renal failure and acute hydronephrosis in pregnancy: use of the double J-stent. *J Royal Soc Med* 1987;80:524.
152. Lynn KL, Bailey RR. Pregnancy and the nephrologist: a review of one year's experience. *N Z Med J* 1983;96:433.
153. Lyreras S, Nyberg F, Linberg B. Cerebrospinal fluid activity of dynorphin-converting enzyme at term pregnancy. *Obstet Gynecol* 1988;72:54.
154. MacDonald P, Alexander D, Catz C, et al. Summary of a workshop on maternal genitourinary infections and the outcome of pregnancy. *J Infect Dis* 1983;147:596.
155. MacDonald PC, Cutrer S, MacDonald SC, et al. Regulation of extraadrenal steroid 21-hydroxylase activity: increased conversion of plasma progesterone to deoxycorticosterone during estrogen treatment of women pregnant with a dead fetus. *J Clin Invest* 1982;69:469.
156. MacMahon B. Prenatal x-ray exposure and childhood cancer. *J Natl Cancer Inst* 1962;28:1173.
157. Magasi P, Simon Z. Electrical stimulation of the bladder and gravidity. *Urol Int* 1986;41:241.
158. Maggiolo LF, Lockhart JL, Wasmer JM. Palliative treatment of obstructing stone during pregnancy. *Urology* 1987;29:402.
159. Maikranz P, Coe FL, Parks J, et al. Nephrolithiasis in pregnancy. *Am J Kid Dis* 1987;9:354.
160. Manger WM, Gifford RW, Hoffman BB. Pheochromocytoma: a clinical and experimental overview. *Curr Prob Cancer* 1985;9:1.
161. Mansfield JT, Snow BW, Cartwright PC, et al. Complications of pregnancy in women after childhood reimplantation for vesicoureteral reflux: an update with 25 years of followup. *J Urol* 1995;154(2 pt 2):787.
162. Maresca L, Koucky CJ. Spontaneous rupture of the renal pelvis during pregnancy presenting as acute abdomen. *Obstet Gynecol* 1981;58:745.
163. Marya RK, Rathee S, Manrow M. Urinary calcium excretion in pregnancy. *Gynecol Obstet Invest* 1987;23:141.
164. Matorras R, Garcia-Perea A, Usandizaga JA, et al. Recto-vaginal colonization and urinary tract infection by group B streptococcus in the pregnant diabetic patient. *Acta Obstet Gynecol Scand* 1988;67:617.
165. Mattingly RF, Borkowf HI. Clinical implications of ureteral reflux in pregnancy. *Clin Obstet Gynecol* 1978;21:863.
166. Mazze RI, Kallen B. Reproductive outcome after anesthesia and operation during pregnancy: a registry study of 5405 cases. *Obstet Gynecol* 1989;161:1178.
167. McFadyen IR, Campbell-Brown M, Stephenson M, et al. Single-dose treatment of bacteriuria in pregnancy. *Eur Urol* 1987;13(suppl):22.
168. McGregor JA, Pont A. Contraindications of ketoconazole in pregnancy. *Am J Obstet Gynecol* 1984;150:793.
169. McNeeley SG Jr. Treatment of urinary tract infections during pregnancy. *Clin Obstet Gynecol* 1988;31:480.
170. McVann RM. Urinary calculi associated with pregnancy. *Am J Obstet Gynecol* 1964;89:314.
171. Merman W. "Progesterone" anesthesia in human subjects. *J Clin Endocrinol Metab* 1954;14:1567.
172. Meyers SJ, Lee RV, Munschauer RW. Dilatation and nontraumatic rupture of the urinary tract during pregnancy: a review. *Obstet Gynecol* 1985;66:809.
173. Michal A, Begneaud WP, Hawes TP Jr, et al. Pitfalls and complications of cesarean section hysterectomy. *Clin Obstet Gynecol* 1969;12:660.
174. Mikhail MS, Anyaegbunam A. Lower urinary tract dysfunction in pregnancy: a review. *Obstet Gynecol Surv* 1995;50:675.
175. Millar LK, Wing DA, Paul RH, et al. Outpatient treatment of pyelonephritis in pregnancy: a randomized controlled trial. *Obstet Gynecol* 1995;86:560.

176. Mimouni F, Miodovnik M, Siddiqi TA, et al. High spontaneous premature labor rate in insulin-dependent diabetic pregnant women: an association with poor glycemic control and urogenital infection. *Obstet Gynecol* 1988;72:175.
177. Mole R. Antenatal irradiation and childhood cancer: causation or coincidence? *Br J Cancer* 1974;30:199.
178. Muller-Suur R, Tyden O. Evaluation of hydronephrosis in pregnancy using ultrasound and renography. *Scand J Urol Nephrol* 1985;19:267.
179. Nakagawa Y, Abram V, Kezdy FJ, et al. Purification and characterization of the principal inhibitor of calcium oxalate monohydrate crystal growth in human urine. *J Biol Chem* 1983;256:3936.
180. Nakagawa Y, Abram V, Parks JH, et al. Urine glycoprotein crystal growth inhibitors. *J Clin Invest* 1985;76:1455.
181. Nanninga JB, Einhorn C, Deppe F. The effect of sacral nerve stimulation for bladder control during pregnancy: a case report. *J Urol* 1988;139:121.
182. Nation RL. Drug kinetics in childbirth. *Clin Pharmacokinet* 1977;5:340.
183. Nelson MS. Acute urinary retention secondary to an incarcerated gravid uterus. *Am J Emerg Med* 1986;4:231.
184. Nielsen FR, Rasmussen PE. Hydronephrosis during pregnancy: four cases of hydronephrosis causing symptoms during pregnancy. *Eur J Obstet Gynecol Reprod Biol* 1988;27:245.
185. Nieminen N, Remes N. Malignancy during pregnancy. *Acta Obstet Gynecol Scand* 1970;49:315.
186. Nolan GH, Sweet RL, Laros RK, et al. Renal cadaver transplantation followed by successful pregnancies. *Obstet Gynecol* 1974; 43:732.
187. Nolten WE, Lindheimer MD, Oparil S, et al. Deoxycorticosterone in normal pregnancy. I. Sequential studies of the secretory patterns of desoxycorticosterone, aldosterone and cortisol. *Am J Obstet Gynecol* 1978;132:414.
188. Norden CW, Kass EH. Bacteriuria of pregnancy: a critical appraisal. *Annu Rev Med* 1968;19:431.
189. Oesterling JE, Besinger RE, Brendler CB. Spontaneous rupture of the renal collecting system during pregnancy: successful management with a temporary ureteral catheter. *J Urol* 1988; 140:588.
190. Ogburn PL Jr, Kitzmiller JL, Hare JW, et al. Pregnancy following renal transplantation in class T diabetes mellitus. *JAMA* 1986;255:911.
191. O'Regan S, Laberge I, Homsy Y. Urolithiasis in pregnancy. *Eur Urol* 1984;10:40.
192. O'Shaughnessy R, Weprin SA, Zuspan FR. Obstructive renal failure by over distended pregnant uterus. *Obstet Gynecol* 1980; 55:247.
193. Pajor L, Koiss I, Nagy F, et al. Bladder augmentation with detubularized intestinal segment. *Int Urol Nephrol* 1997; 27:387.
194. Palahniuk RJ, Shnider SM, Eger EI. Pregnancy decreases the requirements for inhaled anesthetic agents. *Anesthesiology* 1974; 41:82.
195. Papoff P et al. Pregnancy in renal transplant recipients: report of two successful pregnancies in a patient with impaired renal function. *Can Med Asso J* 1977;117:1288.
196. Patterson TF, Andriole VT. Bacteriuria in pregnancy. *Infect Dis Clin North Am* 1987;1:807.
197. Peake SL, Roxburgh HB, Langlois SLP. Ultrasonic assessment of hydronephrosis of pregnancy. *Radiology* 1983;146:167.
198. Pedler SJ, Bint AJ. Management of bacteruria in pregnancy. *Drugs* 1987;33:413.
199. Petersson C, Hedges S, Stenqvist K, et al. Suppressed antibody and interleukin-6 responses to acute pyelonephritis in pregnancy. *Kidney Int* 1994;45:571.
200. Petros PEP, Ulmsten UI. Pregnancy effects on the intravaginal sling operation. *Acta Obstet Gynecol Scand* 1990;153:77.
201. Pfau A, Sacks TG. Effective prophylaxis for recurrent urinary tract infections during pregnancy. *Clin Infect Dis* 1992;14:810.
202. Plaus WJ. Retroperitoneal hemorrhage presenting as a ruptured ectopic pregnancy. *Ann Emerg Med* 1987;16:1398.
203. Prichard J, MacDonald PC, Gant NF. Abnormalities of the reproductive tract. In: *Williams' obstetrics,* ed 17. Norwalk: Appleton-Century-Crofts, 1985.
204. Prowse CM, Gaensler EA. Respiratory and acid-base changes during pregnancy. *Anesthesiology* 1965;26:381.
205. Pryor JL, Gillenwater JY. A new technique for retrograde stone displacement in the tortuous ureter before extracorporeal shock wave lithotripsy. *J Urol* 1989;142:778.
206. Quinn AD, Kusuda L, Amar AD, et al. Percutaneous nephrostomy for treatment of hydronephrosis of pregnancy. *J Urol* 1988;139:1037.
207. Ragossino MW, Breckle R, Hill LM, et al. Average fetal depth in utero: data for estimation of fetal absorbed radiation dose. *Radiology* 1986;158:513.
208. Rasmussen PE, Nielsen FR. Hydronephrosis during pregnancy: a literature survey. *Eur J Obstet Gynecol Reprod Biol* 1988; 27:249.
209. Ready LB, Johnson ES. Epidural block for treatment of renal colic during pregnancy. *Canad Anaesth Soc J* 1981;28:77.
210. Redrow M, Cherem L, Elliott J, et al. Dialysis in the management of pregnant patients with renal insufficiency. *Medicine* 1988;67:199.
211. Reid DWJ, Caille G, Kaufman NR. Maternal and transplacental kinetics of trimethoprim and sulfamethoxazole, separately and in combination. *Can Med Assoc J* 1975 (suppl 112);13:67S.
212. Richmond D, Zaharievski I, Bond A. Management of pregnancy in mothers with spina bifida. *Eur J Obstet Gynecol Reprod Biol* 1987;25:341.
213. Rittenberg MH, Bagley DH. Ureteroscopic diagnosis and treatment of urinary calculi during pregnancy. *Urology* 1988; 32:427.
214. Roberts JA. The ovarian vein and hydronephrosis of pregnancy. Experimental studies in the rhesus monkey (Macaca mulatta). *Invest Urol* 1971;8:610.
215. Robertson EG. Assessment and treatment of renal disease in pregnancy. *Clin Obstet Gynec* 1985;28:279.
216. Rodriguez PN, Klein AS. Management of urolithiasis during pregnancy. *Surg Gynecol Obstet* 1988;166:103.
217. Rosenfeld JA. Renal disease and pregnancy. *Am Fam Physician* 1989;39:209.
218. Rouse DJ, Andrews WW, Goldenberg RL, et al. Screening and treatment of asymptomatic bacteruria of pregnancy to prevent pyelonephritis: a cost-effectiveness and cost-benefit analysis. *Obstet Gynecol* 1995;86:119.
219. Rubi RA, Sala NL. Ureteral function in pregnant women. III. Effect of different positions and of fetal delivery upon ureteral tonus. *Am J Obstet Gynecol* 1968;101:230.
220. Rudolph AM. Effects of aspirin and acetaminophen in pregnancy and the newborn. *Arch Intern Med* 1981;141:358.
221. Ryan GM Jr, Abdella TN, McNeeley SG, et al. *Chlamydia trachomatis* infection in pregnancy and effect of treatment on outcome. *Am J Obstet Gynecol* 1990;162:34.
222. Sanders RP. Placenta previa percreta invading the urinary bladder. *Aust N Z J Obstet Gynaecol* 1992;32:375.

223. Scarpa RM, De Lisa A, Usai E. Diagnosis and treatment of ureteral calculi during pregnancy with rigid ureteroscopes. *J Urol* 1996;155:875.
224. Schenker JG, Grant M. Pheochromocytoma and pregnancy: an updated appraisal. *Aust N Z J Obstet Gynaecol* 1982;22:1.
225. Schwartz JL, Crooks LE. NMR imaging produces no observable mutations or cytotoxicity in mammalian cells. *Am J Radiol* 1982;139:5.
226. Sciarra JJ, Toledo-Pereyra LH, Bendel RD, et al. Pregnancy following renal transplantation. *Am J Obstet Gynecol* 1975; 123:411.
227. Semmens JP. Major urologic complications in pregnancy. *Obstet Gynecol* 1964;23:561.
228. Shope TG, Gagne RM, Johnson GC. A method for describing the doses delivered by transmission x-ray computed tomography. *Med Phys* 1981;8:488.
229. Shu XO, Jin F, Lnet MS, et al. Diagnostic x-ray and ultrasound exposure and risk of childhood cancer. *Br J Cancer* 1994; 70:531.
230. Silva PD, Berberich W. Retroverted impacted gravid uterus with acute urinary retention: report of two cases and a review of the literature. *Obstet Gynecol* 1986;68:121.
231. Slone D, Siskind V, Heinonen OP, et al. Aspirin and congenital malformation. *Lancet* 1976;1:1373.
232. Smith CS, Ferrar LP. Placenta previa with bladder invasion presenting as incarcerated hernia. *Urology* 1992;39:371.
232a. Smith DP et al. The effects of ultrasound-guided shock waves during early pregnancy in Sprague-Dawley rats. *J Urol* 1992; 147:231.
233. Snooks SJ, Setchell M, Swash M, et al. Injury to innervation of pelvic floor sphincter musculature in childbirth. *Lancet* 1984; 2:546.
234. Snooks SJ, Swash M, Mathers SE, et al. Effect of vaginal delivery on pelvic floor: a 5-year follow-up. *Br J Surg* 1990;77: 1358.
235. Solomon EM. Urinary calculi in pregnancy. *Am J Obstet Gynecol* 1954;67:1351.
236. Stadfeldt A. Bidrag til hydronephroses aetiologi. *Hosp Tid Kjobenh* 1861;4:101.
237. Stanton SL, Kerr-Wilson, R, Grant Harris V. The incidence of urological symptoms in normal pregnancy. *Br J Obstet Gynecol* 1980;87:897.
238. Stenqvist K, Dahlen-Nilsson I, Lidin-Janson G, et al. Bacteriuria in pregnancy. *Am J Epidemiol* 1989;129:372.
239. Stenqvist K, Sandberg T, Lidin-Janson G, et al. Virulence factors in *Escherichia coli* in urinary isolates from pregnant women. *J Infect Dis* 1987;156:870.
240. Stothers L, Lee LM. Renal colic in pregnancy. *J Urol* 1992;148: 1383.
241. Strong DW, Murchison RJ, Lynch DF. The management of ureteral calculi during pregnancy. *Surg Gynecol Obstet* 1978; 146:604.
242. Sultan AH, Kamm MA, Hudson CN, et al. Prudendal nerve damage during labour: propective study before and after childbirth. *Br J Obstet Gynecol* 1994;101:22.
243. Sultan AH, Kamm MA, Hudson CN, et al. Anal-sphincter disruption during vaginal delivery. *N Engl J Med* 1993;329: 1905.
244. Swartz HM, Reichling BA. Hazards of radiation exposure for pregnant women. *JAMA* 1978;239:1907.
245. Swash M. Childbirth and incontinence. *Midwifery* 1988;4:13.
246. Sweet RL. Bacteriuria and pyelonephritis during pregnancy. *Semin Perinatol* 1977;1:25.
247. TeLinde RW. Urological aspects of gynecology. *Am J Obstet Gynecol* 1950;60:273.
248. Tetzschner T, Sorensen M, Lose G, et al. Pudendal nerve recovery after a non-instrumental vaginal delivery. *Int Urogynecol J* 1996;7:102.
249. Thorp JM, Jones LG, Bowes WA, et al. Electromyography with acrylic plug surface electrodes after delivery. *Am J Perinatol* 1995;12:125.
250. Tomezsko JE, Sand PK. Pregnancy and intercurrent diseases of the urogenital tract. *Clin Perinatol* 1997;24(2):343.
251. Trauffer PM, Malee MP. Adrenal pseudocyst in pregnancy. A case report. *J Reprod Med* 1996;41:195.
252. Ulvik NM, Bakke A, Hoisaeter PA. Ureteroscopy in pregnancy. *J Urol* 1995;154:1660.
253. Uttendorfsky OT, Veersema D, Mooij PN, et al. Protein/creatinine ratio in the assessment of proteinuria during pregnancy. *Eur J Obstet Gynecol Reprod Biol* 1988;27:221.
254. Van Dorsten JP, Lenke RR, Schifrin BS. Pyelonephritis in pregnancy: the role of in-hospital management and nitrofurantoin suppression. *J Reprod Med* 1987;32:895.
255. Van Geelen JM, Lemmens WA, Eskes TK, et al. The urethral pressure profile in pregnancy and after delivery in healthy nulliparous women. *Am J Obstet Gynecol* 1982;144:636.
256. Van Sonnenberg E, Casola G, Talner LB, et al. Symptomatic renal obstruction or urosepsis during pregnancy: treatment by sonographically guided percutaneous nephrostomy. *Am J Radiol* 1992;158:91.
257. Van Wagenen G, Jenkins RH. An experimental examination of factors causing ureteral dilatation of pregnancy. *J Urol* 1939;42: 1010.
258. Van Wagenen G, Newton WH. Pregnancy in the monkey after removal of the fetus. *Surg Gynecol Obstet* 1943;77:539.
259. Vieweg J, Weber HM, Miller K, et al. Female fertility following extracorporeal shock wave lithotripsy of distal ureteral calculi. *J Urol* 1992;148:1007.
260. Wagener GW, Van Rendborg LC, Schaetzing A. Pheochromocytoma in pregnancy. A case report and review. *S Afr J Surg* 1981;19:251.
261. Wagner LK, Fabrikant JI, Fry RJM. *Radiation bioeffects and management test and syllabus.* Reston, VA: American College of Radiology, 1991.
262. Wagner LK, Lester RG, Saldana LR. *Exposure of the pregnant patient to diagnostic radiation.* Philadelphia: Lippincott, 1985.
263. Walker JL, Knight EL. Renal cell carcinoma in pregnancy. *Cancer* 1986;58:2343.
264. Waltzer WC. The urinary tract in pregnancy. *J Urol* 1981; 125:271.
265. Wanner MB, Rageth CJ, Zach GA. Pregnancy and autonomic hyperreflexia in patients with spinal cord lesions. *Paraplegia* 1987;25:482.
266. Watts DH, Eschenbach DA. Treatment of chlamydia, mycoplasma, and group B streptococcal infections. *Clin Obstet Gynecol* 1988;31:435.
267. Weiss CR, Glazka AJ, Weston JK. Chloramphenicol in the newborn infant: a physiological explanation of its toxicity when given in excessive doses. *N Engl J Med* 1960;262:787.
268. Weiss JP, Gillenwater JY. Management of urologic problems in pregnancy. In: Gillenwater JY et al, editors. *Adult and pediatric urology.* St Louis: Mosby, 1996.
269. Weiss JP, Hanno PM. Pregnancy and the urologist. *AUA Update Series* 1990;9:266.
270. Wiggins RC. Myelination: a critical stage in development. *Neurotoxicology* 1986;7:103.
271. Wilson M, Morganti AA, Zervoudakis I, et al. Blood pressure, the renin-aldosterone system and sex steroids throughout normal pregnancy. *Am J Med* 1980;68:97.

272. Wintour EM, Coghlan JP, Oddie CJ, et al. A sequential study of adrenocorticosteroid level in human pregnancy. *Clin Exp Pharm Physiol* 1978;5:399.
273. Wolf MC, Hollander JB, Salisz JA, et al. A new technique for ureteral stent placement during pregnancy using endoluminal ultrasound. *Surg Gynecol Obstet* 1992;175:575.
274. Wolff JM, Jung PK, Adam G, et al. Non-traumatic rupture of the urinary tract during pregnancy. *Br J Urol* 1995;76:645.
275. Wright A, Steele P, Bennett JR, et al. The urinary excretion of albumin in normal pregnancy. *Br J Obstet Gynaecol* 1987; 94:408.
276. Yamada N, Kido K, Uchida H, et al. Application of cephalosporins to obstetrics and gynecology: transfer of cefazolin and cephalothin to uterine tissue. *Am J Obstet Gynecol* 1980;136: 1036.
277. Zinner SH, Kass EH. Long-term (10 to 14 years) follow-up of bacteriuria of pregnancy. *N Engl J Med* 1971;285:820.
278. Zinner SH, Kass EH. Bacteriuria and babies revisited. *N Engl J Med* 1979;300:853.
279. Zwergel T, Lindenmeir T, Wullich B. Management of acute hydronephrosis in pregnancy by ureteral stenting. *Eur Urol* 1996;29:292.

6

UROLOGIC LASER SURGERY

DOUGLAS F. MILAM
JOSEPH A. SMITH, JR.

The usefulness of an individual surgical laser is predicated by the unique tissue effect generated by thermal transformation of light energy. Lasers can be used to coagulate, incise, or vaporize tissue and, under certain circumstances, provide a combination of these processes. Selective absorption of laser energy by the target tissue is possible, thereby increasing the efficiency of therapy and decreasing the risk of side effects. The transmission of laser energy by small, flexible optical fibers facilitates energy delivery either directly or through an endoscope. Adaptations allowing side firing and diffuser tip emission of laser energy have further expanded the therapeutic capabilities for surgical lasers.

This chapter reviews the pertinent aspects of laser history, physics, and tissue interaction. To safely use laser energy, the surgeon must have an adequate understanding of methods to manipulate and influence tissue effects. Specific urologic applications of laser surgery are discussed in detail. No written document can be all-inclusive; nevertheless, detailed recommendations are provided for individual urologic problems in an effort to be a practical reference for the clinical surgeon.

D.F. Milam and J.A. Smith, Jr.: Department of Urologic Surgery, Vanderbilt University Medical Center, Nashville, TN 37232-2765.

LASER PHYSICS

Although the concept of stimulated emission of radiation was hypothesized by Einstein in 1917, the first beam of laser light was not generated until 1960 (69). Mulvaney and Beck used ruby laser and carbon dioxide (CO_2) lasers in urology and found them to have minimal value in destroying kidney stones but projected possible use for tumor ablation (91). It was not until the development of the neodymium:yttrium-aluminum-garnet (Nd:YAG) laser and a suitable fiber delivery system that lasers began to play a role in urologic surgery.

To safely and effectively apply laser energy as a surgical tool, a basic understanding of laser physics and tissue effects is essential. The tissue-destructive properties of a laser beam can be therapeutically beneficial if properly used, but they can also produce unique complications if misdirected or applied with inadequate knowledge or experience.

The word *laser* is an acronym for "light amplification by stimulated emission of radiation." White light from an incandescent bulb is a divergent mix of multiple wavelengths (colors). In contrast, laser light consists of nearly a single wavelength (monochromatic) that travels in a unidirectional manner (collimated) and can be deflected for projection onto tissue surfaces. In theory, the beam is nondivergent, although the angle of divergence from surgical laser fibers is at least 5 degrees and often much greater.

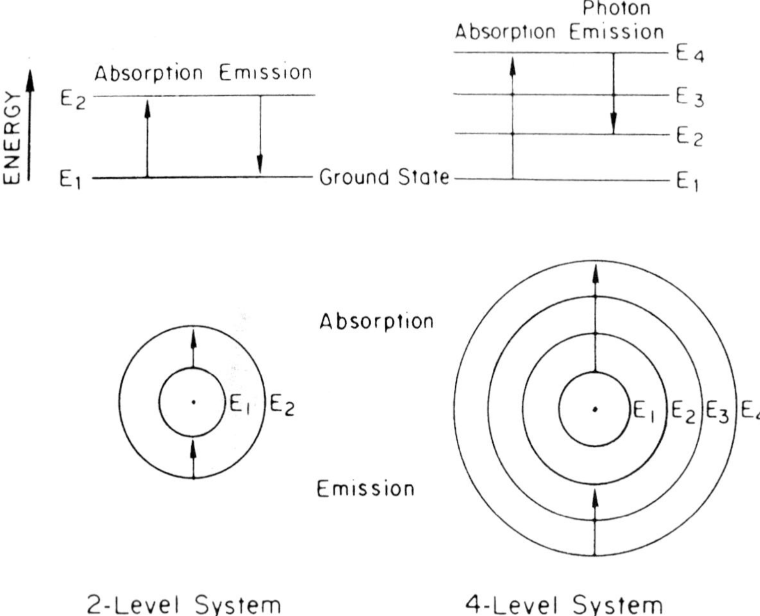

FIGURE 6.1. Diagram of energy states corresponding to electron energy levels. Laser wavelength is directly related to the energy released by electron decay from the excited to the ground state.

Surgical lasers are powered by electricity, which is used to ignite a flashlamp. Atoms of the active medium in the laser resonator are energized from the ground state to an excited state by photons produced by the flashlamp. When the atoms spontaneously decay to the ground state, a photon of specific wavelength is emitted (Fig. 6.1). The spontaneously emitted photon interacts with an excited-state atom, stimulating it to decay, and emits a second monochromatic photon. Because the original incident photon is also released, stimulated emission of radiation involves a factor of two energy gain with each atomic interaction (Fig. 6.2). A totally reflecting mirror at one end of the laser cavity and a partially reflecting mirror at the other preserve photons within the resonator. Photon reflection through the laser resonator substantially increases laser output because photons have greater opportunity to stimulate excited-state atoms to decay. Photons exit the resonator as a nearly nondivergent beam through the partially reflecting mirror at one end. The laser beam may pass directly from the laser or be coupled to a flexible, fused-silica glass optical fiber.

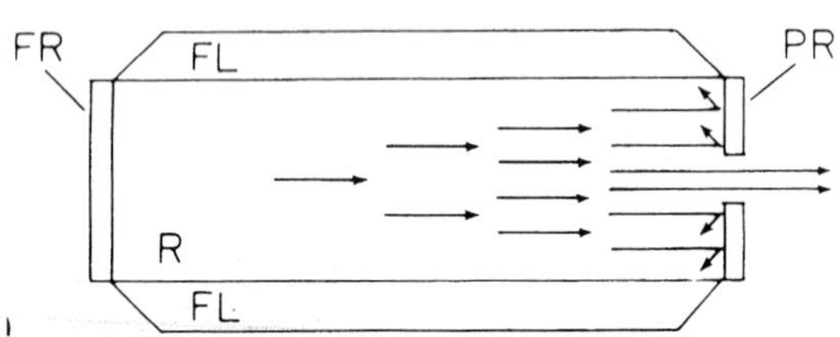

FIGURE 6.2. Laser design and energy gain. FL, flash lamp; FR, fully reflective mirror; PR, partially reflective mirror; R, laser resonator rod.

The active medium, that is, the source from which the photons are emitted, determines the wavelength of a particular laser. It may be a gas (CO_2, argon), a liquid (rhodamine-B, coumarin green), or a solid [neodymium, potassium titanyl phosphate (KTP)].

In general, minimum modifications are necessary to prepare an operating room or cystoscopic area for laser use. Electrical outlets [220 V (three-phase), 50 amp], ideally with isolated transformers, are required for argon and some older or high-energy Nd:YAG lasers. A 206-V (single-phase), 50-amp wall power source is optimal for most Nd:YAG, holmium, and KTP lasers. A few lower-power devices such as diode lasers, CO_2 lasers, and some newer Nd:YAG lasers require only a 110-V power source. When planning an operating room for laser surgery, one should have all three of the power outlets near each other in a convenient location. This includes a high-amperage 110-V power source; a three-phase 220-V, 50-amp power source; and a single-phase 206-V, 50-amp power source.

Lasers generate a large amount of waste heat that must be removed from the resonator cavity to prevent overheating. All currently available urologic lasers use an internal radiator and fan for cooling. Very-high-energy systems and older medical lasers may require cooling water obtained through a hose connected to a running water source. A wastewater drain is also required if external cooling water is used. Externally cooled systems are cumbersome and have limited portability.

Access to the operating room should be controlled to prevent accidental entry during laser use. Protective shades should cover all windows. As with any procedure using electrically powered equipment, the operating room floor should be kept as dry as possible. Deflection of the laser beam into the eye can produce retinal injury with the Nd:YAG, argon, and KTP lasers and a corneal burn with the CO_2 or holmium laser. Therefore eye protection is mandatory for all persons in the operating room during laser use. Typically, glasses or goggles with green-tinted lenses are used for the Nd:YAG laser, amber lenses for the argon and KTP lasers, and clear lenses for the CO_2 and holmium lasers. Newer, more expensive clear lenses are available to protect the eye from Nd:YAG and KTP laser energy. During endoscopic laser surgery, the use of either a solid-state CCD camera or a wavelength-specific lens cap over the eyepiece of the telescope may suffice once the fiber is inserted into the cystoscope or laparoscope. One should never underestimate the amount of laser light that can be reflected backward from the end of the fiber through the cystoscope toward the surgeon's eye.

TISSUE EFFECTS OF LASER ENERGY

Tissue Optical Properties

Tissue optical properties control the transformation of laser light energy into heat (124). Cellular destruction generally is not evident when tissue temperatures less than 60°C are maintained for only a few seconds. Above 60°C, protein denaturation ensues, although minimum volatilization and tissue vaporization occur below 100°C. Above 100°C, cellular water evaporates and charring and tissue vaporization are observed.

Several important factors influence the extent of thermal destruction that occurs when a laser beam is projected onto tissue surfaces. The most easily controlled factor is laser wavelength. Body tissues contain chromophores, such as hemoglobin, that preferentially absorb certain wavelengths of light. The absorption characteristics of a particular laser wavelength depend on the relative tissue absorption and can vary significantly from one wavelength to another.

Absorption and scattering of laser light are important in determining the extent of tissue injury during laser surgery. As tissue is irradiated, light traveling through the tissue is attenuated by absorption and scattering. The proportionality constant describing the amount of light attenuated by absorption is the absorption coefficient (μ_a). The constant describing the attenuation of light due to scattering away from the direction of propagation is the scattering coefficient (μ_s). A third parameter, the anisotropy coefficient (g), describes the fraction of light scattered into any given direction and is assumed to be the average cosine of the scattering angle. These three coefficients are referred to as the *optical properties.* The propagation of light in tissue depends on three dimensionless parameters, one of which has already been discussed (g); the other two are based on the absorption and scattering coefficients. These are the albedo (a) and the optical depth (τ), defined as follows:

$$a = \mu_s/(\mu_a + \mu_s)$$

and

$$\tau = d(\mu_a + \mu_s)$$

where d is the sample thickness.

Because the distribution of light in tissue depends on tissue optics, much research on measuring the optical properties of tissues has been conducted and several methods have been introduced (98,123,127,130). A study of the optical properties of rat prostate tumor revealed values of 0.05 mm^{-1}, 27.0 mm^{-1}, and 0.98 for μ_a, μ_s, and g, respectively (4). Scientific studies into the tissue effects of various laser treatments must consider these factors.

Energy Density

In addition to wavelength and angle of incidence, other parameters can be used to predict and, to some extent, control the tissue effects and depth of penetration of a particular laser, including energy density. Stated simply, energy density is the amount of energy delivered to a given area of tissue. It is determined by the following formula:

$$\text{Power (Watts)} \times \text{Duration (seconds)}/\text{Area}^2\ (\text{cm}^2)$$

The power output of a particular laser is controlled from the instrument panel. Duration can be modified by controlling the time length of a particular pulse or by varying the speed with which the beam is moved across the tissue surface.

An influential component of the formula for energy density is the size of the treatment area. Treatment area is a function of offset distance and divergence angle:

$$\text{Area} = \pi \times [\text{Offset distance} \times \tan(\text{Divergence angle}/2)]^2$$

Surgical laser fibers with a wide angle of divergence produce a lower energy density than nondivergent fibers by treating a larger surface area or spot size with the same amount of energy. The distance between the fiber tip and the tissue surface also influences the energy density by markedly changing the treated surface area. Contact techniques increase energy density by limiting the treatment surface area.

The angle of divergence from the fiber tip is unique to each device. The end-fire probes used over the last decade have an angle of divergence of only 5 to 15 degrees. Tissue injury from short-duration (2 to 3 seconds), high-energy density exposure may extend for several centimeters. Widely divergent beams (up to 90 degrees) produce a much lower energy density. Long-duration (60 to 90 seconds), low-power (40 to 60 W) exposure with these fibers can coagulate a large volume of tissue with coagulation depths of over 1 cm.

Optical properties of tissue have been shown to be temperature dependent. This is of concern because an increase in the absorption or scattering coefficient prevents light from penetrating deeper into the tissue, thus compromising laser treatment. Chambettaz and colleagues (21) measured temperature-dependent changes in total reflectance and transmittance while irradiating excised arterial wall specimens at 383 W/cm^2 and 191 W/cm^2. They found that with the higher irradiance, transmittance decreases rapidly with increasing temperature up to 51.4°C, followed by a rapid increase in transmittance as temperatures continued to increase. Reflectance measurements showed inverse responses. When the tissues were irradiated at 191 W/cm^2, changes in transmittance and reflectance occurred more slowly with their extrema occurring at 44.1°C. Another study reported a fourfold increase in the scattering coefficient (0.43 to 1.74 mm^{-1}) of porcine myocardium during coagulation, whereas the absorption coefficient remained relatively unchanged (0.04 to 0.05 mm^{-1}) (31). Splinter and colleagues (123) also demonstrated a twofold to threefold increase in the reduced scattering coefficient in canine and human coagulated myocardial tissue. Pickering and colleagues (99) found that the scattering coefficient of rat liver increased while the absorption and anisotropy coefficients decreased during tissue heating. They also noted that the rates of change in these properties were proportional to the amount of energy used to heat the samples.

Coagulation

When tissues are heated to less than 60°C for only a few seconds, tissue warming without irreversible damage is observed. Between 60° and 100°C, permanent protein denaturation occurs, causing tissue coagulation. Although this is irreversible and destructive, immediate tissue removal does not occur. The thermally injured tissue either sloughs or is reabsorbed by the body's inflammatory mechanism. Transurethral laser treatment of the prostate causes coagulation and delayed slough of tissue for 4 to 8 weeks (75). Tissue sloughed from the urinary tract is amorphous and does not cause urinary retention. Hemostasis both during and after treatment usually is excellent because the coagulation process extends to blood vessels within the volume of treated tissue. Poorly absorbed wavelengths, such as the 1,064-nm light produced by the Nd:YAG laser, primarily cause tissue coagulation. Coagulation rather than vaporization may be favored when using a given wavelength by lowering the energy density. In general, low-power, long-duration laser exposure through a large irradiated area such as that produced by diode lasers for interstitial laser prostatectomy increases the amount of coagulation and the depth of tissue injury compared with higher-power laser sources used for a short duration.

Vaporization

When high tissue temperatures (generally above 100°C) are achieved, immediate tissue vaporization ensues. Surface carbonization may be observed and a smoke plume generated. Some degree of coagulation accompanies carbonization, so hemostasis is usually adequate, although less than that observed with pure coagulation techniques. Carbonization significantly increases the tissue absorption coefficient, leading to further marked tissue heating in the small area of carbonized tissue. The total coagulation depth may actually be decreased by absorption of nearly all the laser light at the tissue surface.

Vaporization is more difficult to achieve under water than in an air environment. This is particularly pertinent for urologic endoscopic use because the irrigating fluid causes surface cooling. If desired, vaporization is facilitated by using highly absorbed wavelengths (CO_2 or holmium lasers), using a high laser power output, applying the energy pulse over a very brief period, or decreasing the treated surface area (as with contact tips).

Physics of Laser Prostatectomy

Side-firing Laser Prostatectomy

Side-firing laser coagulation prostatectomy involves disposition of laser light into tissue. The prostate, like other bodily tissues, is somewhat transparent to incident light. Photons of laser light experience three possible interactions during passage through tissue. Initially, photons pass through tissue in the original incident direction. This is termed *through transmission.* Interaction with tissue causes photons to be extensively scattered in directions other than the original incident direction. This process is wavelength dependent and causes the beam to form a plume with lateral width. Once a photon is *absorbed* by tissue, its energy is liberated as heat. Thermocoagulation will occur if enough laser energy is used to achieve tissue temperatures of 60° to 70°C for more than a few seconds.

Many factors affect tissue temperature distribution, including laser, optical, and thermal parameters. Laser parameters consist of wavelength, power, spot size, beam profile, and scanning velocity. The optical parameters of importance are surface reflection and the tissue absorption and scattering coefficients. Thermal parameters are the characteristics of the tissue, such as thermal conductivity, specific heat, tissue density, and convective heat transfer coefficient. Of these, thermal and optical properties depend on temperature and wavelength.

Tissue optical characteristics define the effect of a specific laser delivery system. Three parameters are most important: energy loss caused by urethral reflection, tissue absorption, and scattering coefficients. Loss caused by urethral reflection is largely unavoidable, although there is some evidence that incident beams normal to the tissue surface transmit a higher portion of their energy into tissue-oblique beams.

Tissue absorption for a given wavelength is estimated by the Lambert-Beers law: $I_x = I_0\, e^{-ax}$, where

I_0 = Incident beam intensity
I_x = Beam intensity at tissue depth × centimeters
a = Tissue absorption coefficient (μ_a)
x = Depth (cm)

The relatively low absorption coefficient at the 1,064-nm wavelength (Nd:YAG) permits deep tissue penetration and therefore deeper tissue heating and coagulation (Fig. 6.3). The greater absorption coefficient at the 532-nm (KTP) or the 633-nm wavelength (helium:neon) causes rapid tissue absorption. Absorption of most incident energy in a relatively small volume of tissue will cause rapid heating of superficial tissues. Several studies have demonstrated the wavelength dependency of the absorption coefficient in a typical biologic tissue (22,49). This is the principal mechanism causing differing tissue effects of lasers with different wavelengths. Rapid superficial vaporization seen with the CO_2 laser is a consequence of the tissue absorption coefficient being greater than 1,000 times that of the Nd:YAG laser operating at 1,064 nm.

Surface carbonization is one clinically important factor that markedly affects the tissue absorption coefficient. Carbon black is a near-perfect absorber of all visible and infrared wavelengths. Surface charring increases the absorption coefficient (μ_a) by several orders of magnitude. During Nd:YAG laser prostatectomy, surface char can alter the treatment session producing a superficial effect similar to the CO_2 laser. Surface charring should be avoided if possible during a side-firing coagulative treatment session. This has been theorized to be the causative mechanism of why, in one series, exposure at 40 W proved clinically superior to exposure at 60 W (54).

Tissue heating is also influenced by the light-scattering coefficient described previously (22,49,95). Scattering measures the propensity of the laser photons to reflect within tissue (Fig. 6.4). This process causes divergence from the original beam path and therefore increases the width of tissue injury from a given incident beam (100). Both laser wavelength and tissue temperature increase the scattering coefficient. The initial importance of light scattering at physiologic temperature during Nd:YAG lasing is limited. However, increasing tissue temperature during a treatment session greatly increases the scattering effect (94). Coagulated tissue volume is substantially increased because of tissue scatter when using the Nd:YAG laser.

Laser parameters, such as wavelength, power, spot size, beam profile, and scanning velocity, also substantially affect tissue treatment (102). The importance of wavelength is largely determined by tissue absorption and scattering coefficients as discussed earlier. Although near-infrared light

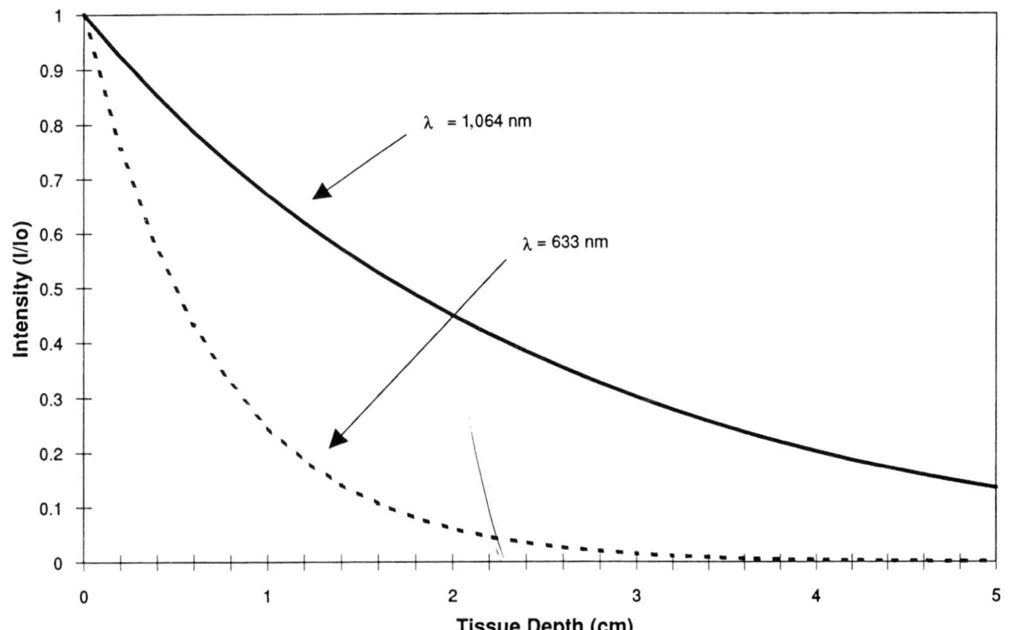

FIGURE 6.3. Relative intensity of light passing through tissue in canine prostatic tissue from two clinically important laser sources. Only the effect of the absorption coefficient (μ_a) is considered here.

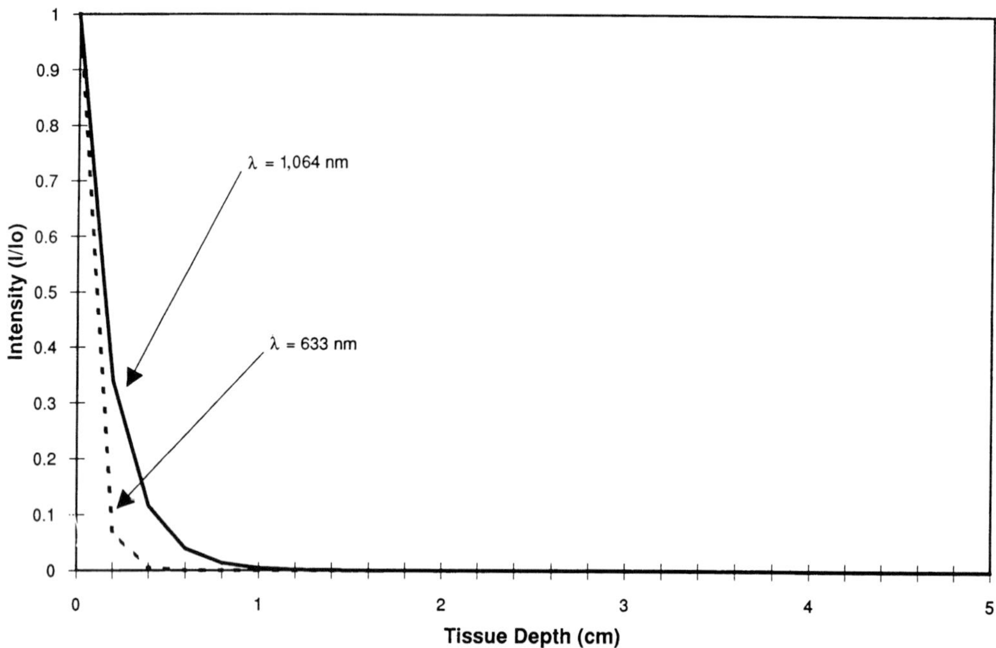

FIGURE 6.4. Laser scattering plays a critical role in depth-dependent attenuation of laser light. This figure describes light passage through canine prostatic tissue of two clinically important laser sources. Comparison with Fig. 6.3 clearly demonstrates the importance of light scattering.

from the Nd:YAG (1,064 nm) laser provides good results, other sources in the range of 800 to 1,000 nm may also be used. High-power (25 to 50 W) diode lasers are competitive alternatives to the continuous-wave Nd:YAG laser source. Although diode lasers may achieve results comparable to the volume of prostatic coagulation achieved using the Nd:YAG laser, exposure at these wavelengths may not achieve superior clinical or experimental results. Other commonly available medical laser sources (CO_2, holmium, alexandrite, KTP, and argon) are too strongly absorbed by tissue (high μ_a) to be useful for side-firing, noncontact coagulation prostatectomy.

Laser power is an important determinant of the extent of tissue injury. Coagulation prostatectomy requires tissue temperatures of 60° to 70°C for about 3 seconds to effect reliable protein denaturation. It is important to differentiate between temperature and heat. The relationship between heat, or enthalpy, and tissue temperature is described by the following equation:

$$\Delta H = \text{(Enthalpy) the amount of heat in tissue} = (Cp)(\Delta T)$$

where Cp is the tissue heat capacity and ΔT is the tissue temperature change. From this equation, one could conclude that increased power would yield increased tissue coagulation. Surface effects negate this relationship, however. Extreme surface heating, as seen in high-power applications, causes surface charring. In the presence of char, laser light transmission deep into tissue is limited because of surface absorption. To overcome this effect, laser power must be increased substantially.

The extent of surface heating at a given power is also a function of spot size. Indeed, power density (power divided by spot size) and the prostatic optical absorption coefficient are the critical determinants of surface tissue heating. Side-fire laser beam profile is often considered analogous to spot size. This is an oversimplification based on the assumption that laser power is uniformly spread throughout the incident spot (25). Data have shown marked variations in visible laser beam profile between different side-firing devices. These data are useful for determination of optimal exposure techniques. Narrow beam–profile devices require different exposure techniques than those with widely divergent beams.

The importance of movement of the laser beam during prostatectomy is only now being understood. Initial laser prostatectomy studies were performed with a static exposure technique using a divergent laser fiber (low power density) (33,54). This technique treated a large volume of tissue, minimized surface charring, and facilitated laser scattering. Static treatment is clearly not appropriate for many of the newer fibers with a narrow divergence angle and, consequently, smaller spot size.

Several devices with narrow divergence angles have less than a 3-mm spot size. Laser light scattering at 1,064 nm throughout prostate tissue is not sufficient to ensure thorough coverage of an entire prostate without probe movement. Analytic and finite element mathematical models for predicting optimum tissue exposure (94) predicted the volume of coagulated tissue (greater than 70°C) to be 36% to 109% greater with a laser scanning rate of 1 mm per second than an identically powered laser source where the beam is stationary for 60 seconds. Intuitively, the optimal scanning-rate speed would be as slow as possible without causing tissue charring.

In addition to a slow scan rate, optimal treatment depends on the initial static "dwell" period. During probe movement, tissue ahead of the probe is heated because of forward scatter of the laser light. Tissue treated at the beginning of a laser pass is not exposed to energy from prior forward scatter. Undertreatment of the initial region may occur unless the fiber is held static for 2 to 4 seconds before initiating movement. Mathematical modeling techniques have predicted the optimal dwell period (90). These data indicate that a dwell period of approximately 4 seconds is optimal. Intuitively, however, one should dwell for as long a period as possible without creating tissue carbonization.

Contact Vaporization Prostatectomy

Contact vaporization prostatectomy differs considerably from the coagulation procedures described previously and from techniques that use a holmium laser to resect the prostatic adenoma. During contact vaporization, ablation occurs in real time creating an open prostatic fossa similar to transurethral resection of the prostate (TURP). During vaporization prostatectomy, the structural components of tissue are carbonized and much of the water component is vaporized. Equipment unique to contact laser prostatectomy is required for the procedure.

Contact vaporization prostatectomy is most commonly performed using the Contact Laser system (SLT, Inc., Valley Forge, Pennsylvania). When using this system, a 7-mm diameter, round contact probe is threaded onto a 600-μm optical fiber (Fig. 6.5). A black, absorbent coating is deposited onto the probe surface during manufacture. This coating absorbs approximately 30% of the laser energy, causing intense probe heating. Contact between the hot probe and tissue produces tissue vaporization. Passage of laser energy through the probe into tissue further enhances vaporization and facilitates hemostasis because of subsurface tissue coagulation. The advantage of true tissue vaporization is not without cost. Contact prostatectomy requires considerably more time than coagulation techniques.

Other Vaporization Techniques

Durable, side-firing laser fibers may also be used for tissue vaporization. Nonmetallic refractive fibers having a narrow divergence angle are used both in contact and slightly offset from tissue. Fournier and Narayan (35) have reported using the Ultraline fiber for contact and noncontact vaporization in the clinical and laboratory setting. These investigators reported superior vaporization when the fiber was used in contact with tissue because of the markedly increased power density during contact treatment. Fiber durability is an issue. The same authors reported consistent fiber tip etching at approximately 50,000 Joules (J) and recommended increasing laser output from 60 to 80 W to compensate for transmission loss at that point. Total device failure occurred after 150,000 J. Other nonmetallic fibers have not been tested as extensively in this application, but they may be useful. These data are particularly important in confirming the appropriateness of side-firing fibers for laser-vaporization prostatectomy. Physical laws involving the heat of vaporization of prostatic tissue apply to both the contact-probe and side-firing devices. Total energy requirements should be similar. Side-firing devices must be able to withstand at least 100,000 J to be useful for vaporization prostatectomy.

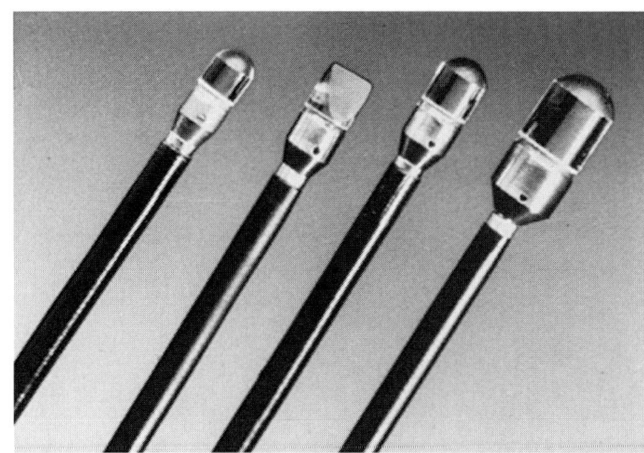

FIGURE 6.5. Contact laser prostatectomy devices. Reusable, fused-silica glass contact probes are threaded onto a semirigid, coaxial optical fiber. Several probe sizes are available; however, the larger probes produce more efficient tissue vaporization during contact laser prostatectomy.

CHOICE OF LASER WAVELENGTH

Laser instruments differ primarily in the wavelength and pulse duration of the emitted light. Wavelength is a function of the chemical composition of the active medium in the resonator cavity, which may be a solid, liquid, or gas as described previously. In addition, a frequency-doubling crystal may be used to modify the wavelength of an existing laser source. An example of this is the KTP laser, which is a frequency-doubled Nd:YAG laser.

Argon Laser

Argon has several potential lasing lines between 488 and 514 nm. Light at this wavelength is poorly absorbed by water but strongly absorbed by body pigments, such as melanin and hemoglobin, and chromophores, such as hematoporphyrins. Consequently, tissue absorption is intermediate between that of the poorly absorbed Nd:YAG and the strongly absorbed CO_2 laser. The selective absorption of argon energy by hemoglobin has led to its use for treatment of hemangioma. Commercially available surgical argon lasers have a relatively limited power output and generally can only be used for small (less than 1 cm in size) lesions. Use of argon lasers has been largely abandoned for treatment of superficial transitional cell carcinoma of the bladder. Other devices such as continuous-wave Nd:YAG, KTP, and holmium lasers are better suited for this application.

Argon Dye Laser

Dye lasers can be used to produce coherent monochromatic laser light over a wide range of wavelengths depending on the type of dye used. The argon-pumped dye laser uses an argon laser instead of a flashlamp to power a dye laser. By selecting the proper wavelength (choosing the proper dye), one can selectively excite a tissue chromophore. Hematoporphyrin derivative has been used in several studies because of selective uptake by carcinoma *in situ* in the bladder (15–17,42,101). Hematoporphyrin derivative is activated by wavelength-specific (630-nm) argon-pumped dye laser light. The use of an inefficient laser to pump another inefficient laser causes tremendous energy loss. For this reason, energy output of the argon-pumped dye laser is limited to 5 to 10 W. Most treatment protocols require bladder illumination time to be 1 hour or more. Research into selective absorption of chromophores by tumor cells and preferential laser destruction of those cells continues; however, these techniques have yet to find widespread acceptance.

Carbon Dioxide Laser

The 10,600-nm wavelength of a carbon dioxide laser is strongly absorbed by water. Thus the energy is rapidly absorbed at the tissue surface, creating high-temperature vaporization. The depth of CO_2 laser light penetration is limited, less than 1 mm. High-intensity vaporization coupled with superficial penetration can produce a scalpel-like effect. Carbonization will occur if the energy is applied to a cutaneous surface for more than a few seconds. A smoke plume is produced, and a dedicated smoke evacuator should be used if infectious material such as condyloma is being treated.

The relatively long wavelength of the carbon dioxide laser creates problems for transmission via flexible fibers. Wavelengths in the far-infrared position of the electromagnetic spectrum are absorbed by optical and most fiberoptic glass. Attempts have been made to develop cystoscopes using a series of reflecting mirrors. So far, however, a practical CO_2 laser cystoscope has not been developed, although specific optical devices to redirect the CO_2 laser beam have been designed for otolaryngologic applications. In urologic applications, the beam is delivered to tissue via a series of articulating arms and reflecting mirrors. CO_2 lasers have proven useful for first-line therapy of various lesions of the external genitalia and with open surgical applications.

Diode Laser

Diode lasers operate differently than the previously described lasers that generate laser light by illuminating a resonator cavity with a flashlamp. Monochromatic coherent light can be generated directly by semiconducting laser diodes. Low-power diode lasers are commonly used to read information from computer and audio discs. Diode lasers designed for urologic applications produce greater power than those found in consumer applications; however, maximum power output is less than that produced by most other laser sources. Current urologic diode lasers weigh less than 20 pounds, fit in a briefcase, and require only a 110-V electrical source. The most commonly used urologic application of the diode laser is transurethral interstitial laser therapy of the prostate. In this application, the laser is coupled to a fused silica glass fiber that incorporates a diffuser tip onto the distal end.

Holmium:Yttrium-Aluminum-Garnet Laser

The holmium:YAG laser emits light in the midinfrared region of the electromagnetic spectrum (2,100 nm). Unlike the continuous-wave lasers described previously, energy emission occurs in a rapid pulse over a few milliseconds. Holmium:YAG laser light is highly absorbed by water and produces explosive vaporization and cutting.

Several companies produce holmium lasers. All have pulse repetition rates of about 5 to 20 Hz, 3 to 5 J per pulse, each of which is delivered over approximately 500 microseconds. The light, invisible to the human eye, is readily transmitted through a flexible optical fiber. All manufacturers provide a range of optical fibers from 200 to 1,000 microns. The smaller fibers are particularly useful for ureteroscopic applications.

Unlike an electrohydraulic lithotripsy probe, the holmium laser fiber tip should be held in close approximation to the stone or tissue surface being treated. Otherwise, rapid attenuation of the laser light will occur because of absorption by water. When treating ureteral or renal stones, the clinician must take care to keep the fiber tip away from urothelial tissue. Unlike coumarin green-pulse dye lasers that were widely used in the 1990s, holmium laser light will cut ureteral tissue as well as fragment stones.

The hemostatic abilities of the holmium laser are less than a continuous-wave Nd:YAG laser because there is more vaporization of tissue. One should keep this in mind because once started, bleeding may be difficult to stop without switching to electrocoagulation. The holmium:YAG laser has been extensively used for urinary tract stone fragmentation in addition to cutting and coagulation of soft tissue. Most urologists would agree that the holmium laser is the most used and most versatile laser for a wide range of urologic applications.

Potassium Titanyl Phosphate Laser

KTP lasers use a potassium titanyl phosphate crystal to double the frequency of Nd:YAG lasers, thereby producing 532-nm wavelength green light. Interaction of Nd:YAG light with the KTP crystal causes substantial energy loss. Therefore the energy output of the typical dual-wavelength laser in KTP mode is only approximately half that of the Nd:YAG mode. The 532-nm wavelength provides an intermediate level of vaporization and coagulation. The energy can be transmitted by the same standard optical fiber used for Nd:YAG treatment. Tissue effects are similar to those achieved with an argon laser, although greater power can be produced than with most surgical argon lasers. KTP lasers have been used for treatment of superficial transitional cell cancer in the bladder, ureter, and renal pelvis. In some circumstances, KTP lasers provide an increased safety margin compared with Nd:YAG lasers because of limited coagulation depth. However, treatment is slower than with Nd:YAG lasers, and treatment for large tumors may be more difficult. KTP lasers have also been used for treatment of external genital and urethral lesions.

Combined techniques for treatment of benign prostatic hyperplasia (BPH) using coagulating energy followed by vaporization of prostate tissue with a KTP laser have been described. Early studies clearly demonstrated the feasibility of this method; however, widespread acceptance of the technique did not occur because of the increased operative time and the need to use more than one modality. Higher-energy KTP lasers are now available that address these concerns.

Nd:YAG Laser

For many years since its introduction into clinical practice in 1979, the Nd:YAG laser was the most commonly used laser in urologic surgery. This continuous-wave laser produces an invisible 1,064-nm light that is nearly ideal for deep tissue coagulation. When used in a noncontact mode, tissue coagulation is complete and hemostasis is total. The Nd:YAG is the preferred laser source for coagulative destruction of vascular lesions of the urogenital tract. Because of this great utility, the Nd:YAG laser can be purchased coupled with a holmium laser source. Most urologic surgical laser applications can be performed using a single dual-wavelength Nd:YAG/holmium laser.

The active medium within the resonator cavity consists of neodymium atoms contained within a YAG lattice. The Nd:YAG laser emits invisible infrared 1,064-nm wavelength light. Light at this wavelength is poorly absorbed by water and body pigments. Because of poor absorption, the light penetrates deeper into tissue than other commonly used urologic lasers.

In a fluid environment, the poor absorption of the laser energy results in thermal coagulation of both surface and subsurface tissue. Structural and architectural integrity of the tissue is maintained. A certain percentage of the energy is transmitted through the target organ. Thus the thermal effects may extend to adjacent organs. After noncontact Nd:YAG laser treatment, hemostasis is usually total. The coagulated tissue takes on a white, fluffy appearance. The tissue sloughs secondarily over a several-week period, although complete healing may take up to 3 months (75).

CLINICAL APPLICATIONS OF LASER SURGERY

The thermal effects of laser energy have been used for the treatment of a variety of urologic lesions. In certain situations, lasers do not appear to be as effective as standard therapy or offer no particular advantages. In other circumstances, lasers provide substantial practical and therapeutic improvements over other treatment methods. The unique physics and tissue effects of laser energy have created new treatment opportunities for selected problems in urologic surgery. Table 6.1 indicates which lasers are used for various problems in urologic surgery.

Urinary Tract Stones

Successful treatment of urinary tract stones is the single largest reason for the popularity of the holmium laser. The holmium laser improved on the previously available coumarin green-pulse dye laser by producing more rapid and complete stone fragmentation. The coumarin green laser had the important limitation of frequently not fragmenting the hardest calcium oxalate monohydrate stones. With the holmium laser, this limitation has been overcome.

One group of investigators examined the end products of stone fragmentation (129). These authors found that after holmium laser treatment, calcium oxylate monohydrate produced calcium carbonate, cystine yielded cysteine and free sulfur, calcium phosphate produced calcium pyrophosphate, magnesium ammonium phosphate produced ammonium carbonate and magnesium carbonate, and uric acid yielded cyanide. The same group later examined in detail the conversion of uric acid to cyanide (126). No reports of adverse health consequences of cyanide exposure have been reported to this date.

Tissue cutting in addition to stone fragmentation is the principle disadvantage of the holmium laser for work in the ureter. Ureteral injury is avoided by careful placement of the optical fiber tip onto the stone surface and away from

TABLE 6.1. UROLOGIC LASER APPLICATIONS

	CO_2 Laser	KTP Laser	Nd:YAG Laser	Pulse Dye Laser	Holmium Laser
Genital condylomata	***	**			
Urethral/bladder condylomata		**	***		*
Penile carcinoma	*	**	***		
Urethral stricture		**	**		***
TUIP		**	**		***
Coagulation prostatectomy			***		
Prostatic resection		**	**		***
Urothelial hemangioma			***		
Bladder calculus				**	***
Bladder carcinoma		*	***		**
Ureteral/renal calculus				***	***
Ureteral carcinoma		***	**		*
Renal pelvic carcinoma		**	***		*
Calyceal diverticulum		*	***		*

Most frequently (***), frequently (**), and less frequently (*) used applications of urologic lasers.

the ureteral wall. Although laser energy settings for stone fragmentation are less than those used for transurethral incision of the prostate (TUIP) or most other cutting procedures, energy at these settings can do considerable damage to the ureteral wall if placed in direct contact. Laser energy settings for ureteral stone fragmentation typically range between 1 and 2 J with pulse repetition rates of between 5 and 15 Hz. Even the hardest stones fragment successfully with this amount of energy (65).

Some care should be taken to avoid head-on holmium laser exposure to ureteroscopic guidewires. Freiha and colleagues (36) demonstrated that it is possible to cut a guidewire with holmium laser energy. However, the authors found that the energy had to be applied directly and from a distance of less than 1 mm.

Renal and bladder stones are also effectively fragmented with the holmium laser. Given the larger size of those stones and the more open operative space, energy settings are often increased when treating renal and bladder stones. Treatment is more time efficient if peripheral stone tissue is treated first. One should avoid the temptation to break large stones into several pieces early in the treatment session. By staying on the periphery of a stone, one can continuously break off the superficial layers into dust or sand. Treatment continues until the stone has been completely ablated. Further details of stone management with the holmium laser are presented elsewhere in this text.

External Genitalia

Laser treatment of lesions of the external genitalia usually uses the CO_2, Nd:YAG, or KTP laser. Direct application of CO_2 laser energy to lesions of the external genitalia is performed either with a hand piece and a series of articulating arms and mirrors or a coupling microscope. Fiber-conducted light from a KTP or Nd:YAG laser can be directed using a hand piece. The choice of laser is based on the desired depth of tissue destruction. CO_2 lasers produce only superficial vaporization, KTP lasers produce a moderate level of coagulation, and Nd:YAG lasers produce the greatest depth of coagulation for tumor treatment.

Condyloma Acuminatum

Lasers are well established as effective treatment for condyloma acuminatum. CO_2, Nd:YAG, argon, and KTP lasers can be used, although most clinical experience is with CO_2 and Nd:YAG lasers (37,47). With a CO_2 laser the lesion is vaporized, and large amounts of smoke are produced. Proper smoke evacuation equipment must be available to prevent inhalation of viral particles that may be in the smoke plume. Application of laser energy to the skin is painful, and local anesthetics are injected subcutaneously before treatment. For large or more extensive lesions, a penile block may be preferable. The skin is cleansed with an iodine-based or equivalent compound. The power output chosen is based to some extent on the size of the lesion, but the lowest output that successfully vaporizes the condyloma is desirable. Usually, 5 to 10 W of power will suffice. Rosemberg and colleagues (105) described a technique of vertical, horizontal, and oblique application of the beam to ensure complete removal. As successive portions of the condyloma are treated, the carbonized surface is removed by wiping with a saline-soaked sponge. Bleeding does not occur until the deeper layers of the dermis are reached. Care should be taken to avoid a full-thickness skin injury. The white dermal layer underlying the condyloma should be left intact. An antibacterial cream may be applied topically after treatment, but analgesics are usually unnecessary. Lesions of the urethral meatus can be treated satisfactorily with a CO_2 laser and nasal speculum, but the lack of a fiber delivery system has precluded treatment of more proximal urethral lesions.

Very large lesions should be treated in stages to prevent a large area of full-thickness burn. Bridges of either normal or pathologic tissue should remain intact between large treatment areas even if this commits the patient to a second treatment session. Untreated tissue bridges will hasten the healing process and lessen the chance that skin grafting of a large area will be required. In most patients, excellent cosmetic results can be anticipated.

Using the CO_2 laser, Lundquist and Lindstedt (68) treated more than 150 patients with condyloma resistant to podophyllin therapy. Ninety-five percent of patients were reported cured, although some required a second treatment. Similar results have been reported by Bellina (13). Rosemberg (103) found an 88% cure rate in 61 patients undergoing only a single treatment. More recently, others have used erbium and pulse dye lasers for condylomata (48). Tissue ablation with the erbium laser is extremely superficial, more so than the CO_2 laser. This laser offers a potential benefit relative to existing therapy. One other benefit is that the plume from erbium laser treatment apparently does not contain viable viral particles (48).

The Nd:YAG laser also has been shown to be effective in the treatment of condyloma acuminatum (72). Unlike after CO_2 laser treatment, the lesions do not undergo vaporization. Rather, they are coagulated and may be removed with forceps or allowed to slough secondarily. Treatment depth may be more difficult to control than with the CO_2 laser, but a treatment session proceeds more rapidly when large lesions are encountered.

Nd:YAG laser energy is applied with a power of 10 to 15 W until the lesion turns a pale white color. The epithelium surrounding the lesion should be treated for a distance of 2 to 3 mm to destroy the virus in adjacent areas. Care should be taken to avoid excessive energy density, which can result in third-degree thermal injury and full-thickness skin slough. One must also consider the location of the dorsal neurovascular bundles and underlying corporal bodies when using the Nd:YAG laser.

The oncogenic potential of certain subtypes of the human papillomavirus has been reported. Microscopic lesions can often be detected on the penis of sexual partners of women with carcinoma or carcinoma *in situ* of the cervix (6,8). Five percent acetic acid applied to the penis for 5 minutes on a soaked gauze wrap produces a white discoloration of small human papillomavirus lesions that can then be detected by examination with magnifying loupes (34). Carpiniello and associates (20) found a high recurrence rate of these lesions after CO_2 laser treatment despite the use of topical 5-fluorouracil cream after laser treatment. This and other studies have demonstrated that condylomata are difficult to eradicate. Previous studies probably overstated the cure rate by a substantial margin.

Carcinoma of the Penis

Laser treatment of selective carcinomas of the penis may avoid the need for partial penectomy in some patients. Although topical application of 5-fluorouracil cream seems to be the preferred initial treatment for erythroplasia of Queyrat, lasers have been effective in eliminating resistant lesions (70). Because this is a premalignant lesion that does not invade deeply into tissue, lasers with superficial penetration produce sufficient treatment. Good results have been achieved with the CO_2 laser.

For an invasive carcinoma, a greater depth of coagulation is advisable (Fig. 6.6). Appropriate patient selection is the key element determining success. Pretreatment biopsies of the lesion should be taken in order to assess tumor depth. In most situations, the Nd:YAG laser is preferable. Energy should be applied to the entire lesion, as well as the surrounding, more normal-appearing skin. Generally, 25 to 35 W of energy is used with the Nd:YAG laser. Iced saline applied to the surface of the lesion during treatment helps cool the superficial tissues and prevent carbonization. This avoids a smoke plume and increases the effective energy penetration because char at the tissue surface absorbs laser light. Treatment should continue until all areas of the lesion are coagulated. The tissue surface will remain intact.

After treatment with the Nd:YAG laser using these energy parameters, a third-degree thermal injury is created. The lesion is usually painless, but slough of necrotic tissue and drainage may persist for up to 2 months. Eventually, reepithelialization will occur unless residual cancer is present. The necrotic lesion may result in secondary adenopathy, making the assessment of the inguinal lymph nodes during the healing process more difficult. Cosmetic results are good considering the other options. Most patients are left with a shallow divot and normal epithelial covering.

Results of laser treatment of carcinoma of the penis indicate that treatment generally can be successful in properly selected patients. Malloy and colleagues (73) have treated 23 patients with the Nd:YAG laser for carcinoma of the penis. Six patients had T_{is} and no evidence of recurrent cancer an average of 34 months after treatment. Of 15 men with T_1 tumors, 12 were cancer free with a mean follow-up of 31 months. Two men with T_2 cancer had reduction of the tumor mass but were not cured. Hofstetter (44) treated 17 patients with T_1 and T_2 tumors. With follow-up of 3 to 6 years, only one patient had died from metastatic disease.

The obvious advantage of laser treatment of penile cancer is preservation of the phallus. Although efforts to avoid partial or total penectomy ultimately should not compro-

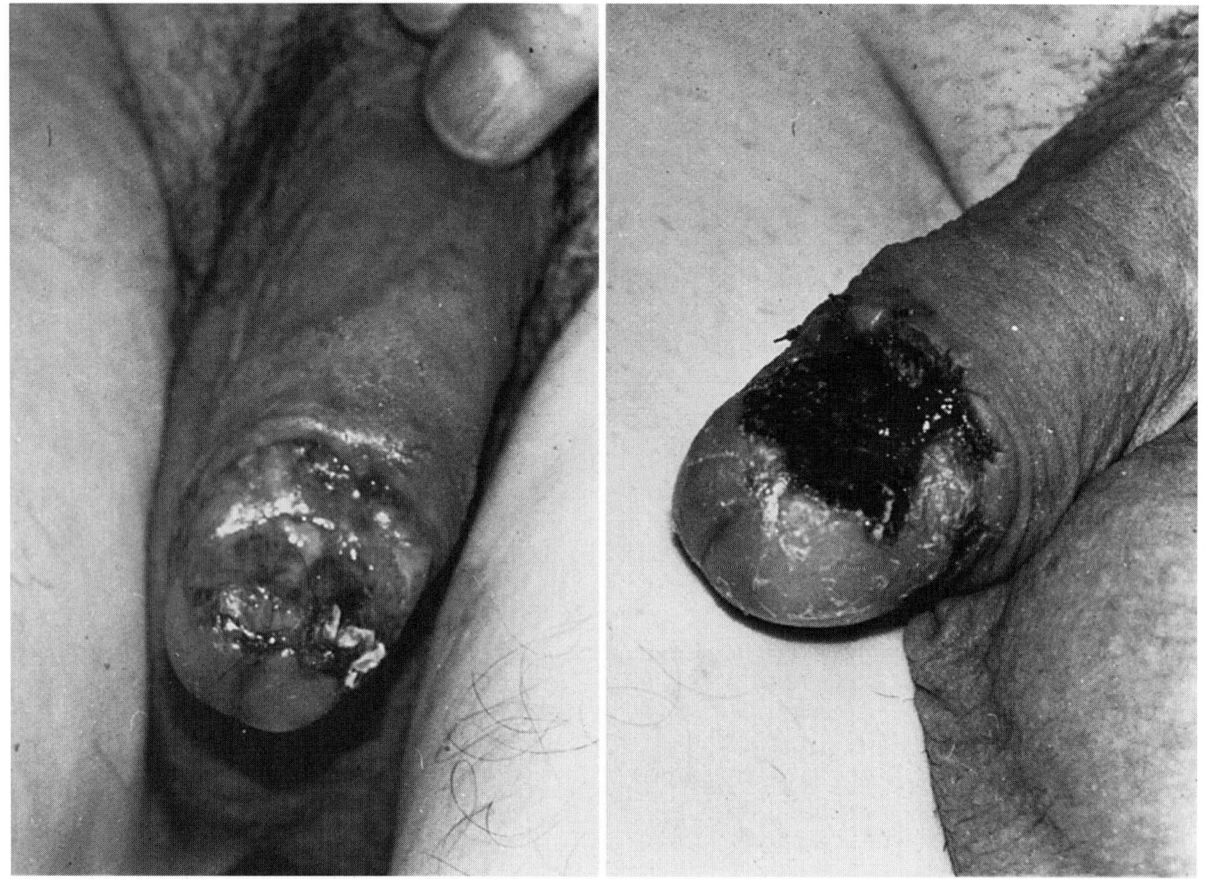

FIGURE 6.6. **A:** Invasive squamous cell carcinoma of the penis. **B:** After Nd:YAG laser treatment, the lesion has a coagulation eschar that may take up to 6 weeks for complete healing.

mise the chances for cure, not all patients with squamous cell cancer require amputation. Laser therapy plays an important role in the management of properly selected patients with carcinoma of the penis.

Urethral Stricture Disease

Lasers have been extensively used for incision and coagulation of urethral scar tissue. The Nd:YAG laser has been used with or without contact tips. More recently, the holmium laser has been extensively used for both incision and ablation of urethral stricture tissue.

Animal data suggest that tissue treated with Nd:YAG laser light heals with more elastic fibers and less collagen deposition than comparable electrosurgical injury. In addition, there is less bleeding into the tissues, with possibly less secondary scarring. These ideas have formed the basis for laser treatment of benign urethral strictures. There is no doubt that laser energy can cut urethral strictures, but delayed results have been mixed.

Holmium:YAG laser properties are nearly optimal for urethral stricture incision. Under direct vision, the fiber tip is placed immediately adjacent to the scar. One should not push the optical fiber tip into tissue because that maneuver may result in deep bleeding that cannot be stopped with further laser energy. Laser power is set at 1 to 3 J per pulse and the pulse rate at about 5 Hz. Absorption of holmium laser light by superficial scar tissue results in cellular disruption and cutting. Given appropriate power, tissue injury is limited to a 1- to 2-mm coagulation zone below the cleavage zone. Cutting proceeds until the appropriate depth is reached. Holmium laser urethrotomy produces less deep tissue injury than Nd:YAG laser urethrotomy.

Several techniques for Nd:YAG laser treatment of urethral strictures have been described. A metal guidewire is inserted through the urethral lumen to maintain orientation. Circumferential laser energy may be delivered to the entire stricture in anticipation of secondary slough of this tissue and normal healing (Fig. 6.7). With this technique and no postoperative Foley catheter, Smith and Dixon (120) reported a recurrence rate of 56% at 6 months and considered this method generally to offer no advantages over standard therapy. Shanberg and Tansey (113) described radial incisions through the stricture with direct contact between the fiber and the tissue. Results in five patients with bladder neck contractures were good. How-

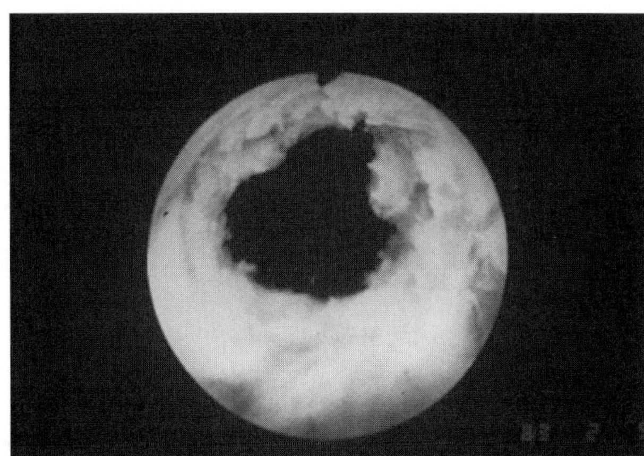

FIGURE 6.7. Urethral stricture after circumferential Nd:YAG laser application. The coagulated tissue sloughs secondarily.

ever, recurrences were noted in 58% of the patients with urethral strictures.

Merkle (87) described short-duration (0.2-second) pulses of 25 W placed at multiple sites of the stricture. A catheter was left indwelling for 2 weeks. Successful results (no recurrence of the stricture) were reported in 90% of patients, but others have not reproduced this experience.

Tips for laser fibers may be designed for direct contact between the tissue and the fiber tip. These can be constructed of various materials in differing geometric configurations. By concentrating the energy density, they increase the cutting effect. Smith (118) conducted a prospective study with sapphire contact-tip Nd:YAG laser fibers in 20 men with benign urethral strictures. The cutting effect was unsatisfactory in half of the patients, and recurrence was seen in 13.

The argon laser has been used in other series (1). Rothauge and colleagues (107) treated 41 patients, but long-term results were not reported. The coagulative effects on the tissue would be similar to those obtained with a KTP laser (111,128), but the limited power output of an argon laser appears to make the procedure tedious and technically unsatisfactory for strictures with dense scar tissue.

On the basis of physics and tissue effects, a CO_2 laser is the most appealing laser for the treatment of urethral strictures. Theoretically, the scar could be vaporized with little effect on the underlying urethra. However, until a contact CO_2 laser fiber or cystoscope is perfected, treatment requires gaseous distention of the urethra, a setting in which fatal air embolus has been reported.

Benign Lesions of the Bladder

Lasers are the preferred treatment for patients with bladder hemangioma (121). Although this is an unusual lesion, it can be a particularly debilitating and difficult problem, especially in patients with various congenital venous anomalies such as the Klippel-Trenaunay-Weber syndrome. Nd:YAG laser treatment has been performed in these patients with excellent results, and there have been no reported instances of serious bleeding induced by the laser (Fig. 6.8).

Laser treatment for control of chronic bleeding from radiation cystitis or Cytoxan-induced cystitis has been less successful. Nd:YAG lasers are capable of ablating focal areas of bleeding from cystitis, but the diffuse nature of these diseases is the primary limitation of therapy. Unlike hemangioma or arterial venous malformations, hemorrhagic cystitis is a diffuse condition that is not well treated by local methods.

The success that some have reported with Nd:YAG laser treatment of interstitial cystitis is intriguing but somewhat difficult to explain. In some series, 60% to 70% of patients experience significant pain relief and improvement in their irritative voiding symptoms after laser treatment of active Hunner's ulcers and areas of the bladder most intensely involved with the process (110). Virtually all patients treated had failed multiple alternative treatments. Symptomatic recurrence is common some 8 to 10 months after laser treatment, but successful results can be achieved with a second laser treatment. At this point, laser therapy for interstitial cystitis has not been shown to be more effective than more conventional therapy or placebo.

Bladder Cancer

Since they were first introduced into clinical practice almost 15 years ago, lasers have been used for ablation of transitional cell carcinoma of the bladder. Justification for the use of lasers as an alternative to standard methods of electrocautery resection has been based on theoretic therapeutic advantages, as well as an observed decrease in

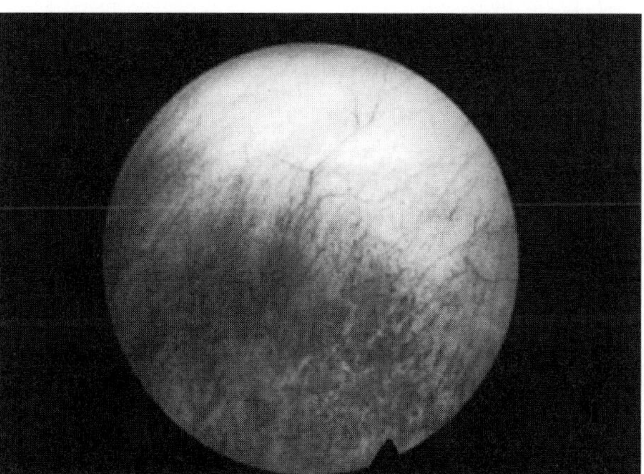

FIGURE 6.8. Hemangioma of the bladder 3 months after Nd:YAG laser application contrasting the treated area *(upper right)* with the nontreated region.

treatment-related morbidity. The development of new laser wavelengths and instrumentation has facilitated and expanded the use of lasers in a number of areas of urologic surgery, including treatment of bladder cancer.

Patient Selection

Although some investigators maintain that tumor recurrence rate is decreased after laser treatment compared with electrocautery resection (43), laser therapy of superficial bladder cancer is performed most often to decrease or eliminate the need for inpatient hospitalization. Commonly, patients with bladder cancer of low invasive potential undergoing laser treatment have previously undergone resection or biopsy of recurrent, low-grade papillary transitional cell carcinoma. When papillary tumors of low invasive potential are seen on routine surveillance cystoscopy, laser treatment can be an effective, low-morbidity treatment.

Laser vaporization or coagulation results in tumor destruction that does not allow retrieval of tissue for adequate histologic examination. Preoperative, cold-cup biopsies can partially address this issue and allow pathologic examination to determine tumor grade and give some staging information. In general, though, sessile-appearing tumors or those with broad stalks should be treated by electrocautery resection with biopsies of the underlying bladder muscle wall. Some investigators believe that first-time tumors should be treated by electrocautery resection rather than laser treatment so that adequate histologic material is available (116).

Tumor size is another consideration. Lesions greater than 1 to 2 cm in size are difficult to treat with laser alone and may require a debulking electrocautery resection before a laser treatment of the tumor base. However, this may obviate many of the practical advantages of laser if electrocautery resection is required anyway.

Tumor location is a relatively minor issue. Virtually all parts of the bladder are accessible for laser treatment. Extra caution is appropriate for tumors on the bladder dome where loops of small bowel may be adjacent. Small bowel thermal injury and perforation with intact bladder wall has occurred. Treatment of tumors overlying the ureteral orifice appears to be associated with a very low risk of stricture and ureteral obstruction.

Treatment Technique

A number of different treatment techniques have been described for laser destruction of bladder tumors. Differences exist depending on the laser wavelength. The amount and manner of energy delivery depend on the preoperative assessment of tumor stage.

Superficial Tumors of Low Invasive Potential

Laser treatment of superficial transitional cell carcinoma of the bladder (stages T_a to T_1) is usually performed on an outpatient or ambulatory surgery basis. When treatment is performed without anesthesia, the patient is able to perceive the laser energy and often describes it as a burning type of discomfort. However, treatment is tolerated better than electrocautery resection. The exact reason for this is uncertain. However, laser energy probably results in rapid heating and destruction of nerve fibers in a well-defined volume of tissue. Electrocautery resection is associated with more irregular propagation of the energy along nerve and muscle bundles. The decision to perform laser therapy with general or regional anesthesia is based primarily on the surgeon's experience; the patient's personality; and the size, number, and location of the tumors.

When a rigid cystoscope is used, the patient is placed in a standard lithotomy position. Most cystoscope instrument companies offer a laser bridge that adapts to the standard cystoscope with either a 19- or 21-Fr sheath. The laser insert allows stabilization of the fiber tip and a watertight entry port. The optical fiber is inserted through the channel, and the tip of the laser fiber is positioned just beyond the end of the visualizing telescope. Fiber tip placement is especially important when using the holmium:YAG laser because treatment energy may destroy the telescope lens if the two are in close proximity.

Nd:YAG and holmium lasers are the most commonly used lasers for treatment of bladder carcinoma. Both lasers can be used satisfactorily. One needs to know the relative merits of each laser, however. Noncontact treatment with the Nd:YAG laser results in tumor coagulation and preservation of the underlying bladder wall. As mentioned, underlying small bowel injury may occur, but the mechanical integrity of the bladder wall is almost always preserved. The holmium laser, on the other hand, produces tissue cutting at even moderate settings. Aggressive resection may result in bladder wall perforation.

For a noncontact technique with the Nd:YAG laser, a standard 400- or 600-micron end-fire optical fiber is used. The fiber tip is positioned 3 to 5 mm from the tumor surface with the aiming beam illuminating the region of intended treatment. With the Nd:YAG laser, 20 to 30 W of energy usually is sufficient for complete tumor coagulation. The duration of the treatment usually is controlled by the speed with which the aiming beam is moved across the tumor surface. The laser can be operated in a continuous mode whereby energy is emitted whenever the foot pedal is depressed. An aiming beam, either from a flashlamp or a helium neon laser, marks the point of impact (the Nd:YAG laser beam is invisible to the human eye). Sterile water, normal saline, or amino acid solutions can be used for irrigation. A continuous-flow system is not required; the irrigant usually can be turned off during treatment because bleeding is usually nonexistent.

Laser treatment is best performed as a dynamic process rather than a series of adjacent, static impulses. The beam is slowly moved across the surface of the tumor in a "painting"

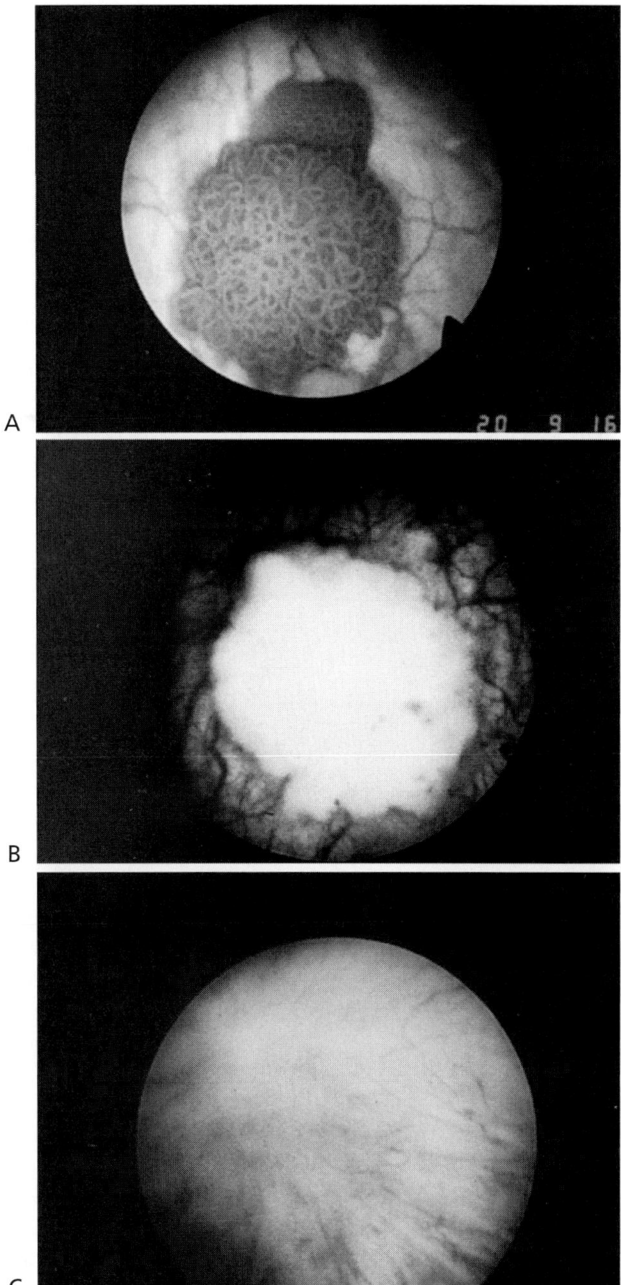

FIGURE 6.9. **A:** Papillary transitional cell carcinoma of the bladder. **B:** After Nd:YAG laser treatment, the lesion undergoes a white discoloration indicative of adequate thermal necrosis. **C:** Six weeks later, complete bladder healing is evident.

fashion. The tumor undergoes a white discoloration indicative of adequate thermal coagulation (Fig. 6.9). Care should be taken to avoid excessive laser energy application in any given area. Usually 2 to 3 seconds of duration is required in a given area for complete thermal coagulation to be evident. Techniques have been described wherein a ring of coagulated tissue is created around the tumor base to seal blood and lymphatic vessels. In practice, this is unnecessary because bleeding does not occur even if the energy is applied initially to the center of the exophytic portion of the tumor.

It is not necessary to treat the tumor base initially, but it is important to make certain that all aspects of the lesion have been thermally coagulated. After the papillary frondular tissue is coagulated, it usually can be dislodged with the tip of the fiber or the cystoscope to expose deeper portions and the tumor base. Treatment is best performed with the bladder as empty as possible to avoid excessive thinning of the bladder wall. This allows an added margin of safety for underlying small bowel. If the tumor is located in the air bubble, either the air can be evacuated or the patient can be tilted to remove the tumor from the air bubble. If this proves to be difficult, treatment can be performed through the air bubble itself, but there is usually some surface carbonization and smoke production. The temperature of the irrigating fluid does not seem to be a major factor in determining tissue or treatment effect.

Subsurface boiling may be observed during treatment, producing a popcornlike effect. These microexplosions, although sometimes dramatic, carry no particular significance. If the fiber tip inadvertently touches the bladder wall, there usually is some superficial carbonization and a cratering effect. The foot pedal is released and the fiber withdrawn from the tissue surface. If there is any tissue adherent to the fiber tip, it should be wiped away with a moist sponge before proceeding with therapy. If necessary, cleavage of the fiber tip and stripping of the outer sheath will restore the fiber to original condition.

The depth of coagulation cannot be monitored satisfactorily intraoperatively. In general, coagulation depth is predicted preoperatively based on known characteristics of the wavelength, power, duration of laser output, and spot size. In most circumstances, 3 to 5 mm of complete tissue coagulation can be anticipated.

If a small amount of bleeding occurs, especially after a cold-cup biopsy, hemostasis usually is accomplished in the course of laser treatment. However, even a relatively small amount of blood undergoes rapid carbonization and can both obscure and prevent effective energy delivery to the tumor surface.

Superficial tumors in bladder diverticula can be treated satisfactorily with a laser. Even though, by definition, there is no muscular backing to a diverticulum, actual free perforation of the diverticulum and bladder wall is uncommon. Usually, there is some shriveling of the mucosa of the diverticulum as the coagulation process occurs. The iliac blood vessels and obturator nerve are often adjacent to diverticula, but if appropriate energy densities are used, direct injury is unlikely. The obturator nerve is not stimulated by laser energy. Obturator spasm and a leg jerk, as may be observed with electrocautery, do not occur.

Treatment of tumors directly overlying the ureteral orifices is performed in the same manner as if the tumor were located elsewhere in the bladder. Stents should be removed from the ureteral orifice before treatment is performed because the laser energy may melt the stent itself. Metal guidewires can be used alternatively. After an extensive treatment overlying the ureteral orifice, postoperative management with a stent may be advisable because of temporary edema. However, the long-term risk of ureteral stenosis appears to be low.

A postoperative Foley catheter is usually not necessary because of the lack of bleeding. The thermally coagulated tissue either sloughs as imperceptible particles or is resorbed. If the treatment is thought to be adequate, follow-up cystoscopy can be performed as per the routine for a particular patient depending on tumor grade, stage, and prior history.

Intravesical drugs can be used after laser treatment, and the indications for their use should be the same as after electrocautery resection. However, because raw surfaces of the bladder wall are not exposed after laser treatment, intravesical drugs, such as bacille Calmette-Guérin (BCG) or chemotherapy, can be introduced more rapidly after treatment with an apparent decreased risk of systemic absorption (24).

Muscle-invasive Tumors

The ability of Nd:YAG lasers to produce transmural coagulation without perforation has allowed laser treatment of some invasive bladder cancers. Even in a controlled setting, however, the treatment depth is variable (122). However, application of energy to both the inner and outer bladder wall through both a cystoscope and a laparoscope allows overlapping zones of thermal necrosis and complete transmural coagulation (108). When treated with this technique, the bladder wall maintains structural integrity because of rapid fibroblast infiltration and collagen deposition (108). The location of most invasive bladder tumors near the trigone makes laparoscopic visualization and energy application somewhat difficult.

Patients being considered for laser treatment of invasive bladder cancer should first undergo a standard transurethral electrocautery resection. This accomplishes two purposes. First, it allows accurate histologic examination for tumor staging. Second, resection debulks the surface of the tumor. Logically, if laser therapy is considered a method for extending the margin of resection, the electrocautery resection should extend deeply into the bladder muscle.

Under most circumstances, it is best to delay laser treatment for at least 3 to 5 days after an electrocautery resection. This allows any bleeding to cease and any overlying clot to lyse. Active bleeding or blood clot interferes with delivery of energy. General or regional anesthesia is required because relatively large amounts of laser energy are needed. The irregular appearance of the resection crater does not allow visual determination of treatment adequacy. Therefore systematic application of laser energy to the entire resection crater, as well as an adequate surrounding margin, should be performed.

Because the goal of treatment is transmural necrosis, energy output up to 45 or 50 W may be appropriate. When an end-fire fiber with a 5- to 15-degree angle of divergence is used, the energy is maintained in a given area for 2 to 3 seconds. If a laparoscope has been inserted, the small bowel can be displaced from the treatment area. After adequate energy has been applied through the cystoscope, the Nd:YAG laser fiber can be inserted through the laparoscope and energy can be applied to the intraperitoneal surface of the bladder in the same region, if visualization is adequate. Steaming or subtle coagulation of the intraperitoneal bladder surface behind the tumor can often be seen laparoscopically during cystoscopic Nd:YAG laser therapy. Otherwise, the intended treatment site may be difficult to determine.

The most appropriate patients for laser treatment of invasive bladder cancer are those with minimally invasive lesions (11,117). Lasers have been used to treat bulky, invasive bladder cancers. However, the surface effect that is obtained in this circumstance usually offers no demonstrable benefit compared with electrocautery debulking and cauterization of the tumor surface.

A catheter is not required postoperatively but may be used depending on the amount of the bladder surface area requiring treatment. Follow-up cystoscopy is performed after 1 month to assess healing and to detect any obvious residual tumor. Reepithelialization of the bladder surface overlying residual cancer is feasible, but most often, there is no residual tumor present when complete reepithelialization occurs within 2 to 3 months of treatment.

Complications of Bladder Treatment

Laser treatment of bladder cancer is used because of the observed decrease in patient morbidity and treatment-related complications. Usually, there is minimal discomfort after treatment. A distinct advantage is the almost complete lack of bleeding that occurs with coagulative procedures. Bleeding that may be present from a preoperative biopsy usually is coagulated adequately during the course of energy application. The coagulation that occurs from the laser energy itself causes virtually no bleeding either as an immediate or a delayed phenomenon.

The most feared complication of laser treatment of bladder cancer is perforation of an adjacent viscus. The small bowel or colon may lie in direct approximation with the peritoneal surface of the bladder. Thus the risk for bowel perforation is greatest with laser treatment on the posterior bladder wall or dome. Hofstetter and colleagues (43) treated more than 500 tumors and reported only two incidences of small bowel perforation, in at least one of which excessive energy levels were used inadvertently. Smith (116) has had no cases of small bowel perforation in over 150 laser treatments of superficial bladder tumors.

Most patients with bowel perforation develop signs and symptoms within 8 to 24 hours of treatment, but symptomatic presentation has been delayed for as long as 2 weeks. Abdominal pain, physical examination findings consistent with an acute abdomen, and free intraperitoneal air are all associated with bowel perforation from laser therapy. It is important to recognize that bowel perforation may occur in the absence of bladder perforation. A cystogram may be normal. The thicker muscle wall of the bladder makes it less prone to perforation, and forward scatter of the energy can place the bowel at risk.

Immediate laparotomy is indicated if small bowel or colon perforation is suspected. The site of laser energy is identified. The zone of tissue injury may be far greater than is visibly evident, so resection of the affected site is indicated.

Results

Initially, laser treatment of superficial bladder cancer was promoted as a means to decrease the recurrence rate (45,74). Indeed, both Nd:YAG and holmium laser treatments have low local recurrence rates at the site of prior resection. Modern thinking about urothelial field change disease has produced serious questions about whether any therapy directed toward specific lesions can affect the eventual rate of recurrence, however.

Both prospective and retrospective clinical series have, in general, failed to support a favorable effect of laser treatment on recurrence rate of bladder cancer (12,50). In most retrospective series, the patient population under study is one of the most influential factors in determining recurrence rate. This complicates comparisons of laser-treated patients to historical series of those undergoing electrocautery resection. Prospective studies have shown no apparent salutary effect of laser treatment on the overall recurrence of superficial bladder cancer.

On the other hand, there is good evidence attesting to the effectiveness of laser therapy in eradicating existing and visible superficial bladder tumors. Multiple series have shown a local recurrence rate of around 5% to 10%, a figure that compares favorably with electrocautery resection. In a randomized, prospective study, Beisland and Seland (12) found a local recurrence rate of 43% for stage T_1 transitional cell carcinoma treated with electrocautery resection alone compared with only 7% for Nd:YAG laser treatment.

There are no studies comparing various laser fibers, wavelengths, or contact versus noncontact treatment of superficial bladder tumors. There have been published reports of holmium:YAG treatment of bladder tumors (50). If adequate vaporization or coagulation of the lesion occurs, good results can be anticipated in terms of local eradication of visible tumors with any of the laser wavelengths. Overall, though, the Nd:YAG laser has proven to be the most versatile and produces the most complete hemostasis. There is no evidence that other laser treatment techniques offer an increased margin of safety.

Laser therapy is firmly established as an effective treatment for superficial bladder cancer of low malignant potential. The ability to eradicate existing, visible tumors is comparable or, perhaps, superior to results obtained with electrocautery resection. Overall, though, there is no demonstrable favorable effect on tumor recurrence. Therefore the indications for adjuvant intravesical treatment with either BCG or cytotoxic drugs are unchanged after laser therapy compared with standard treatment recommendations.

Laser treatment of superficial bladder cancer has been associated with an observed decrease in treatment-related morbidity. Bleeding is almost nonexistent, and catheter drainage of the bladder is not required. Treatment can be performed on an ambulatory basis. A complication unique to laser therapy, perforation of an adjacent viscus, is unusual if appropriate treatment parameters are used. A number of laser wavelengths and fibers have been used successfully to treat superficial bladder cancer. One has not been proven to be inherently superior to another, although the Nd:YAG laser used in a noncontact manner produces optimum coagulation. Holmium laser energy may also be safely used to cut and coagulate bladder tumors. The primary limitations of laser treatment of superficial bladder cancer are the lack of tissue available for histologic examination and the difficulty in treating tumors that are larger than 2 cm with laser alone. Laser treatment of invasive bladder cancer is limited by difficulties and inaccuracies with clinical staging of invasive transitional cell carcinoma and by the inability to predict and control the depth of coagulation.

Benign Prostatic Hyperplasia

Lasers exert their therapeutic effects on tissue through transformation of light energy into heat. Contemporary BPH treatment methods rely on various modifications of laser parameters to produce a desired therapeutic effect. Modifications in instruments for delivery of energy have facilitated treatments that rely on coagulation (e.g., side-firing refractive, reflective free-beam techniques), vaporization (e.g., contact tips, holmium desiccation), or cutting (e.g., holmium laser resection of the prostate). Coagulation is associated with superb hemostasis but results in minimal immediate tissue removal. Obstructive voiding symptoms usually worsen for several days because of postoperative tissue edema. Irritative voiding symptoms also may be prolonged and problematic in some patients. Cystoscopy as long as 3 months after coagulation laser prostatectomy may show residual shaggy gray necrotic tissue (75). On the other hand, vaporization techniques with current instrumentation are slow, and hemostasis is less secure.

The techniques and results that have been reported for laser treatment of BPH are discussed next. Despite the considerable differences between some techniques, similar satisfactory results have been reported. Laser prostatectomy is a compromise procedure in which one attempts to achieve most of the benefits of TURP with decreased morbidity.

Historical Perspective

Early attempts at laser treatment of the prostate met with some anticipated limitations because of difficulty in energy delivery. We and others observed that noncontact laser coagulation of prostatic tissue using conventional end-fire probes resulted in unsatisfactory removal of prostatic tissue (83,119). There was no immediate relief of obstructive symptoms. In fact, some of the edema that occurred secondary to the laser treatment resulted in a temporary increase in symptoms and often urinary retention.

In 1982, McPhee and colleagues developed a modified cautery resectoscope that enabled the simultaneous availability of both electrical (cautery resection/coagulation) and Nd:YAG laser energy. Eleven patients (five with prostatic cancer and six with BPH) underwent transurethral resections using laser irradiation alone for hemostatic control. From 12 to 45 g of tissue was resected using 9,600 to 17,200 J of laser energy at dose ranges of 60 to 90 W for a duration of 1 to 3 seconds. All patients had a satisfactory postoperative voiding pattern, although one patient had bleeding on the third postoperative day, requiring a 3-unit transfusion. The technique was cumbersome, and difficulty was encountered in controlling bleeding of large vessels at the bladder neck when an exaggerated oblique angle of laser application was required (82).

When an end-fire probe is used, obtaining hemostasis on actively bleeding vessels often is difficult. Hemoglobin absorbs Nd:YAG laser energy and effectively diminishes penetration of the laser beam into the tissue. Direction of the beam to the end of the bleeding vessel can be problematic. Thus, although the Nd:YAG laser is an excellent device for coagulating tissue with virtually complete hemostasis during treatment, it is less useful as an instrument to stop active bleeding.

Littrup and colleagues (67) performed percutaneous ablation of the canine prostate using transrectal ultrasound guidance, ethanol injection, and Nd:YAG laser ablation. Transrectal ultrasound guidance was used to direct treatment. Ethanol injections produced an intraglandular hemorrhagic necrosis that extended in some animals to the external prostatic sphincter and the mucosa of the urethra and bladder. Ninety-two percent (11 of 12) of the laser ablations produced intraglandular foci of thermal tissue damage that had distinct margins of transition between necrotic and viable cells. Ultrasound visualized the areas of ablation well, and it was believed that ultrasound could be used as a real-time, intraoperative monitor of treatment effects. However, no follow-up clinical trials have been published.

Although limited success was reported in some of these series, historically laser treatment achieved a very minor role in the management of prostatic obstruction. End-fire probes created access difficulty, tissue coagulation and vaporization was suboptimal, and laser treatment was inferior to electrocautery in gaining hemostasis of actively bleeding vessels. The side-firing laser device altered significantly the methodology for laser treatment of the prostate and improved clinical results.

One of the earliest side-firing techniques to report the results of a controlled study was the transurethral laser-induced prostatectomy (TULIP) (IntraSonix, Burlington, Massachusetts) (106). The system combined a real-time ultrasound transducer and Nd:YAG laser delivery system contained within a 22-Fr urethral probe (5). The laser energy was delivered through a 600-micron, fused-silica fiber that, at the distal end, was coupled to a novel, right-angle microprism integrated into a probe. A 2.8-mm spot size was produced on the tissue surface when the probe was centered inside a 36-Fr balloon. The ultrasound scanner produced a 90-degree real-time sector scan using a 7.5-MHz transducer. Angular resolution was approximately 2 mm, and the depth of view could be set from 2 to 5 cm. A sweep rate of 2 Hz was used in initial studies. A polymer balloon transparent to Nd:YAG laser frequency light encloses the fiber tip and the deflecting prism. This allows the prism to be surrounded by pure degassed water and prevented fouling of the tip by contact with surrounding tissue. The procedure was performed by imaging the bladder neck with ultrasound and slowly withdrawing the laser beam from the bladder neck to the apex of the prostatic urethra using ultrasound guidance. Multiple passes are made depending on the size of the prostate. Laser power in the 20- to 40-W range at a pull rate of approximately 1 mm per second was used in most treatments (77).

Takahashi and colleagues (125) followed 30 patients after a TULIP procedure for symptomatic BPH. At 3 months, flow rate increased from 7.9 to 14.5 mL and remained at 14.7 mL at 1 year. Prostate volume was not significantly different than the pretreatment value when examined at 1 year. Using a modified Boyarsky Symptom Score, there was a mean decrease from 18.4 preoperatively to 7.6 at 3 months after treatment, 6.2 at 6 months, and 6.2 at 12 months. The changes at all three of these intervals are statistically significant ($P < .05$). Peak flow rates did not improve immediately, but they improved progressively over time. The mean peak flow rate increased from a preoperative level of 7.2 mL per second to 12.4 mL per second at 3 months, 13.1 mL per second at 6 months, and 11.1 mL per second at 12 months. Again, all of these changes are statistically significant ($P < .05$).

None of the patients undergoing the TULIP procedure in the clinical trial required a blood transfusion, although

1.5% required cystoscopy after treatment for irrigation of bladder clots (78). Urethral strictures were observed in 9.8% of patients and impotence in 4.6%. Only 5.2% of patients reported retrograde ejaculation. Persistent problems with incontinence have been observed in 4.6% of the patients undergoing the TULIP procedure. Most of these complications or adverse treatment effects are well within the ranges reported for series of patients undergoing electrosurgical transurethral prostatectomy. The mean blood loss of less than 16 mL for the procedure clearly is less than that observed after comparable patient groups undergoing transurethral prostatectomy.

The primary limitation of the TULIP procedure was the delayed time until optimal treatment results were achieved. In fact, most patients had aggravation of symptoms during the first several weeks after treatment until laser-induced edema and tissue effects resolved. Although the duration of hospitalization was short, most patients required bladder drainage via a urethral catheter or suprapubic tube for 1 to 2 weeks, and irritative voiding symptoms often persisted for 6 weeks or longer. The TULIP device never was marketed in the United States. Nevertheless, the clinical trial was one of the most carefully conducted multicenter trials of laser BPH therapy.

Contemporary Techniques

Technologic improvement and methodologic changes have altered significantly the manner in which laser treatment of the prostate is performed. The theoretic basis for treatment is more substantially founded than with the techniques described previously. Promising clinical results have emerged.

It is important to recognize that the term *laser prostatectomy* encompasses a wide variety of instruments, laser wavelengths, and techniques. Often, the described methodology bears little resemblance to alternative techniques. Therefore it is invalid to discard all methods of laser prostatectomy simply because one described technique may not achieve satisfactory clinical results. Likewise, promising results or advantages with one particular method of laser prostatectomy may not be applicable to other techniques.

Each of the various methods of laser prostatectomy is described categorically. Clinical techniques and postoperative results are discussed in detail. Laser prostatectomy methods are continuously evolving, and it is not possible to define the optimal method, if any, for laser treatment of the prostate.

Clinical and Laboratory Studies

Right-angle Delivery Systems

The Urolase fiber (C.R. Bard, Covington, Georgia) was the first side-firing optical fiber to experience widespread use for laser prostatectomy. Although it is no longer available, a large part of the total laser prostatectomy literature describes results using this device. This fiber originally was developed for use in gynecology to ablate the endometrium. However, Johnson and associates (52) performed laboratory dosimetry studies and canine experimentation for potential use in the prostate. They found no evidence of tissue penetration beyond the prostatic capsule in their initial study.

In a follow-up study, Johnson and associates (53) performed serial gross and histopathologic examinations of the prostate following transurethral laser prostatectomy in the canine model. Gross examination of the prostate immediately after treatment showed acute swelling of the prostate, causing an overall increase in size of 25% to 35%. The acute swelling regressed rapidly as evidenced by an increase in the size of the urethral lumen at 3 hours. A urethral catheter was left indwelling for 7 to 10 days following the laser treatment to prevent postoperative urinary retention. Within 24 hours, the well-demarcated sphere of thermal necrosis measuring 2.7 cm in diameter had begun liquefaction and cavitation. By the end of 1 week, a central cavity had been formed with a peripheral rim of viable tissue. Within 5 weeks, reepithelialization of the central cavity was observed. The findings were reproducible despite variability in the flow of irrigation and difficulty maintaining a consistent distance between the fiber tip and the prostatic urethral lumen.

Various methods are used to create angled or side-firing laser fibers. Many fibers have a wide angle of divergence, allowing noncontact coagulation of large volumes of prostate tissue. In general, low-power, prolonged-duration exposure generates deeper tissue coagulation than high-power, shorter-duration exposure (19). Using a Urolase fiber, Kabalin and Gill (55) found maximum tissue coagulation with 40 W applied for 90 seconds in both a canine model and an *in vivo* human prostate model. The mean depth of tissue ablation was 16 mm with a mean volume of tissue ablation of 5.5 mL. A plateau effect was observed wherein longer exposure or higher power did not appreciably extend the depth of injury.

Shanberg and associates (112) applied laser energy transurethrally before radical prostatectomy with a Prolase II fiber. Sixty Watts applied for 60 seconds had the greatest treatment depth, and coagulation necrosis extended a mean of 1.75 cm into tissue.

Most of the clinical and laboratory studies using side-firing lasers have involved noncontact application resulting in coagulation necrosis. When placed in direct contact with tissue, energy density is increased. Using high power output and tissue contact, Fournier and Narayan (35) evaporated canine prostate tissue with an Ultraline fiber (Hereaus, LaserSonics, Milpitas, California) (Fig. 6.10). This potentially allows bulk tissue removal for immediate voiding.

It is important to recognize that differences exist between various fibers, and the optimal energy parameters for one fiber may not apply to others. Furthermore, laser tissue

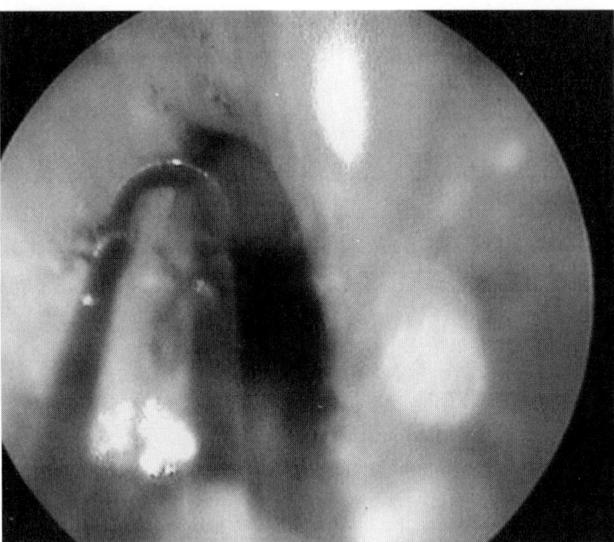

FIGURE 6.10. Side-firing refractive laser prostatectomy.

effects in dog prostates are different and, usually, exaggerated compared with a human prostate. Differences in the stromal-to-epithelial ratio may account partly for the lack of direct comparability (32).

Costello and associates (26,27) initially published results of small, clinical series of patients undergoing laser prostatectomy with a Urolase fiber (visual laser ablation of the prostate [VLAP]). The patients underwent epidural anesthesia; a 23-Fr cystoscope with a deflecting mechanism was used. The fiber was positioned approximately 5 mm beyond the end of the telescope just proximal to the verumontanum. Either glycine or water was used for irrigation. The metal alloy tip of the laser delivery system was placed approximately 1 mm away from the prostatic urethra.

In the initial pilot study, energy was delivered at 60 W continuous wave for 1 minute in each of four quadrants, including the roof of the prostatic fossa, the floor, and both lateral lobes. However, subsequent improvements in the reflectivity of the fiber tip decreased the treatment time to 15 to 30 seconds in four quadrants (27). For patients with significant median lobe enlargement, laser energy was applied for approximately 30 seconds to the bladder neck. Treatment was continued until the circular fibers of the bladder neck were visually apparent. Visible vaporization of the lateral lobes was observed.

Subsequent clinical trials generally used longer treatment times than the 15 to 30 seconds reported in this study. An average of 18,000 J of laser energy was delivered per patient with a mean treatment time of 4.2 minutes. Six weeks after treatment, the mean symptom score fell from 15 to 4, and the mean peak flow increased from 5 to 9 mL per second. Of 12 patients treated, postoperative urinary retention developed in one patient; 2 subsequently required TURP because of persistent symptoms; and one underwent a bladder neck incision. A Foley catheter was left indwelling postoperatively for 2 to 3 days.

Norris and associates (97) reported results in 108 patients treated on an outpatient basis using a Urolase fiber with energy parameters of 60 W for 60 seconds. An average of 19,457 J of energy was applied. Preoperative American Urological Association (AUA) symptom score was a mean of 22.3 compared with 9.2 postoperatively. The peak flow rate increased from a mean of 7.56 to 12 mL per second. No blood transfusions were required, and none of the patients developed a urethral stricture. Seventeen percent of patients required reinsertion of a Foley catheter for urinary retention, and four subsequently required a TURP. Visually, the prostatic fossa eventually resembles a post-TURP appearance (75).

Kabalin (54) reported his initial experience using 40 W of power for 30 to 60 seconds. Total energy ranged from 7,200 to 19,200 J. In 25 patients, peak urine flow rates increased 120% and 141% at 3 and 6 months, respectively, and symptom scores decreased 66% and 78%, respectively. Treatment modifications occurred, and subsequent experience in more than 250 patients has shown no transfusion requirement. Re-treatment has been required in only 5 of the last 150 patients (3.3%). A power of 40 W for 90 seconds has been used with a total energy of a mean of 44,000 J. Peak flow increased from 6.7 mL per second preoperatively to a mean of 18.5 mL after 1 year of follow-up (55).

Dixon and colleagues (33) reported the initial results of a randomized, prospective double-blind study of TURP versus laser prostatectomy using a side-firing, noncontact technique. At 12 months, 16% of the laser group had failed and required an additional procedure compared with 4% for TURP. This re-treatment rate is higher than that reported in comparable series. Symptom score was decreased 30% for laser and 59% for TURP, whereas flow rate increased 82% in the laser group and 147% for TURP. The number of patients randomized at the time of the report (56) was too small for a meaningful comparison of side effects.

A common theme throughout these clinical series is objective and subjective treatment response that approaches that of TURP. However, laser-treated patients have a higher rate of recatheterization, prolonged voiding symptoms, and repeat procedures. In turn, bleeding is almost nonexistent with laser, the risk of urethral stricture is diminished because of the use of smaller instruments, and antegrade ejaculation is preserved in many patients. Coagulative side-firing laser prostatectomy can be performed safely in anticoagulated patients (18). Furthermore, the lack of bleeding facilitates performance of laser prostatectomy on an outpatient basis (66), although TURP also can be performed successfully without hospitalization (63).

Other Side-firing Devices

Numerous side-firing devices have been produced for laser prostatectomy. The number of such devices changes frequently and precludes complete listing. All major urologic laser manufacturers offer side-firing fibers that can be used for laser prostatectomy.

Most practitioners use a scanning technique. Probe movement occurs at the slowest possible rate while avoiding carbonization. A methodical, cylindric treatment pattern satisfactorily ensures thorough exposure of the entire prostate. Each pass through the prostate begins with a dwell period as long as possible while avoiding carbonization.

Other investigators have used high-power exposure. These techniques involve a combination of both coagulation and vaporization. Slow fiber movement allows surface heating sufficient to ablate superficial tissue. With sufficient energy input, the Nd:YAG laser may be used to bore cavities into the prostate. This technique requires far greater energy use and therefore longer treatment time than pure coagulation prostatectomy. Decreased postoperative obstruction is a potential benefit, however.

Clinical results from other side-firing devices are similar to those achieved with the Urolase device. Patients experience symptom score decreases similar to those of TURP, uroflow increases about two-thirds those of TURP, frequent urinary retention, and decreased procedure-related morbidity (23).

Contact Vaporization

Contact laser systems use a conventional fiberoptic waveguide with a fused-silica glass or synthetic-sapphire contact tip coupled to the fiber. Because energy density is inversely related to the square of the radius of the spot size, contact fibers greatly increase the energy delivered for a given volume of tissue. This facilitates tissue vaporization. The contact probes initially developed could tolerate only limited power output without melting. In addition, these devices proved to be relatively inefficient for incising or vaporizing large tissue volumes as is required for treatment of prostatic enlargement (118). Recent advances in contact-probe development have increased efficiency, however. Absorptive coatings added to the contact-probe surface increase direct thermal heating.

Similar to TURP, contact prostatectomy demands considerable understanding of the treatment procedure. The procedure begins using the Nd:YAG laser in continuous-wave mode at 40- to 80-W output. Under cystoscopic visualization, the hot contact probe is pushed into prostatic tissue. Knowledge of anatomic landmarks is critical for efficient tissue vaporization. For that reason, the procedure begins at the bladder neck (Fig. 6.11). Initial short passes are repeated over 360 degrees to open the bladder neck. Subsequent longer passes vaporize progressively more distal tissue (Fig. 6.12). The procedure is repeated until an open prostatic fossa is created to the verumontanum. Contact vaporization prostatectomy causes minimal bleeding but is not bloodless. It is important to vaporize tissue in a methodical fashion to maintain adequate visualization. As discussed previously, increased vaporization sometimes implies decreased coagulation and hemostasis. However, this has not been a practical problem with contact laser treatment of the prostate. Adequate hemostasis occurs during treatment. The primary limitation has been that, even with some of the design changes and improvements, vaporization of the prostate is relatively slow and tedious. Milam (88) has calculated that nearly 50,000 J of energy must be converted to heat and effectively transferred to the prostate in order to vaporize 20 g of tissue. Considering inefficiencies in the system that result in loss of nearly 50% to 90% of the energy before

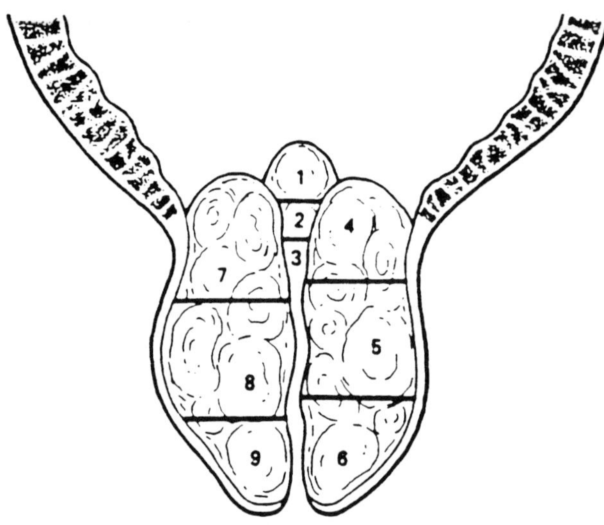

FIGURE 6.11. The sequence for contact laser vaporization of the prostate. Initial vaporization of the median lobe and bladder neck region facilitates improved visualization during the procedure. The procedure extends distally until the entire prostate is vaporized.

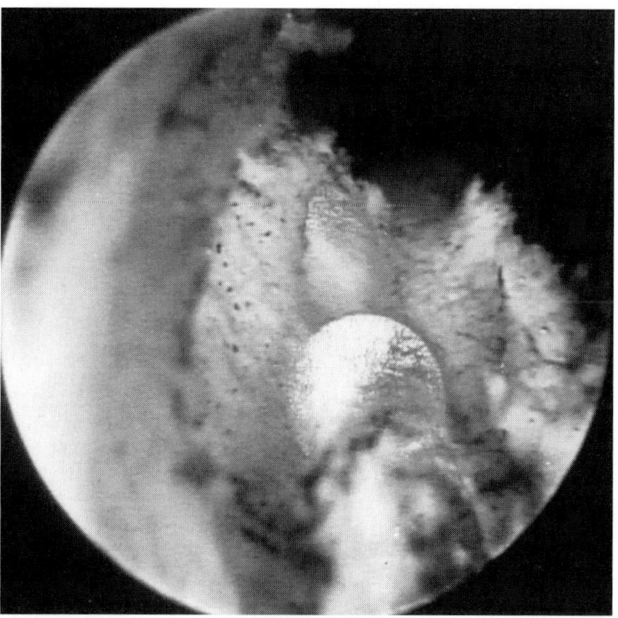

FIGURE 6.12. Contact vaporization of prostatic tissue.

reaching the prostate, total laser outputs of over 100,000 J may be necessary to completely vaporize 20 g of prostatic tissue. Thus further improvements in energy delivery are necessary.

Contact laser treatment of the prostate theoretically is appealing because the technique results in immediate tissue vaporization. Thus therapeutic results do not depend on secondary tissue slough. The immediate voiding problems experienced by some patients after noncontact laser treatment methods may be avoided with contact lasers. This, coupled with the excellent hemostasis observed during treatment, minimizes the need for postoperative Foley catheter drainage of the bladder. Most investigators routinely remove the catheter on the morning of the first postoperative day. Although hemostasis is good, the procedure is not bloodless. Unlike side-firing coagulation prostatectomy, contact prostatectomy should not be performed on anticoagulated patients.

Anson and associates (3) found earlier voiding in their patients compared with noncontact treatment. Aleida (2) used contact laser tips as an adjunct to electrocautery and thought that the combination allowed earlier hospital discharge (29).

Narayan and co-workers (93) performed prostatectomy using direct contact with a side-firing Ultraline fiber. The fiber has a beam divergence of only 17 degrees. Tissue vaporization was achieved using 60 to 80 W of power and dragging the fiber tip through tissue. Mean total energy for glands 20 to 40 g in size was 42,024 J and 95,732 J for those more than 40 g. The prostatic fossa healed completely by 6 months with a decrease in ultrasound-measured prostate volume of 34%. Only 2 of 61 patients subsequently required a TURP, and no significant bleeding occurred. Peak flow was increased 164% at 12 months.

Interstitial Fiber Placement

It has been known for many years that application of low-power laser energy to a given location within a solid organ over several minutes will induce a 1- to 2-cm zone of coagulation necrosis. By using several fiber placements, nearly the entire prostate can be treated while preserving the urethral lining. This principle is used in interstitial laser coagulation (ILC) of the prostate.

ILC has become popular due to the technical ease of treatment, low morbidity, outpatient nature of therapy, and relatively low cost of equipment acquisition. Most described laser treatments of the prostate involve transurethral application of the laser energy. Just as with transurethral electrocautery resection of the prostate, laser injury to the urethral mucosa accounts for some of the treatment-related morbidity. A procedure that preserves the integrity of the prostatic urethra conceivably could decrease or eliminate any treatment-related bleeding, as well as postoperative, irritative voiding symptoms.

As discussed previously, Littrup and colleagues (67) performed interstitial treatment of the canine prostate using the Nd:YAG laser. Placement of the laser fiber was monitored by transurethral-ultrasound guidance. They observed pathologically a homogeneous zone of thermal necrosis and concluded that this technique may be useful for treatment of benign prostatic hypertrophy. However, no follow-up clinical studies have been reported.

McPhee and associates (85) performed studies on interstitial application of laser irradiation using hematoporphyrin-derivative photosensitized Dunning R-3327 prostate cancers. They showed a beneficial effect of treatment on tumors, with either arrest of tumor growth or a decrease in tumor size in most animals. However, the photosensitizers currently available are retained in malignant or dysplastic cells and require systemic administration. Therefore this technique would have no utility for treatment of benign prostatic hypertrophy. Nonetheless, there is at least the potential for the future development of photodynamic therapy of the benign prostate using locally administered photosensitizers.

Johnson and associates (51) placed a frosted Nd:YAG laser fiber interstitially in dog prostates and delivered 10 W of power for 5 minutes to each lobe. Coagulation necrosis followed by interstitial cysts 6 weeks later was observed. A subsequent study using a cylindrically diffusing tip and 25 W for 10 minutes showed large areas of liquefaction necrosis followed by cystic cavitation (28).

McNicholas and associates (81) used interstitial Nd:YAG laser fibers placed percutaneously with low-power (1 to 2 W), long-duration (400 to 1,500 seconds) exposure in dogs. Coagulation necrosis followed by liquefaction and cystic degeneration was observed. Muschter and colleagues (92) reported 15 patients with symptomatic BPH treated with interstitial Nd:YAG laser application and subsequently have accumulated a much larger experience. Five Watts of energy was applied for up to 10 minutes, creating tissue temperatures exceeding 100°C. By 2 months, prostate size measured by ultrasound had decreased from an average of 63 to 44 g and peak flow had increased from 6.6 to 15.2 mL per second. A follow-up report of 42 patients from the same group showed a 30% decrease in prostate size 3 months after treatment (92). The same authors went on to investigate diffuser tip probes coupled to a lightweight diode laser source. This device is now known as the Indigo Laser System (Johnson and Johnson, Superior, Colorado). Many practitioners have used this device with good results. One group found that symptom scores using the AUA symptom index fell from 20.2 to 9.8 at 9 months after treatment and that the uroflow rate increased from 4.4 to 6.2 mL per second over the same period (40). An indwelling catheter was used in all patients postoperatively and was removed between day 3 and day 7. Interstitial laser coagulation appears to produce results similar to those reported with noncontact techniques. One potential advantage is urethral preservation, although urinary retention remains a problem.

Holmium Laser Resection

Holmium laser resection of the prostate (HoLRP) differs substantially from the techniques described previously in this chapter. As noted, the holmium:YAG laser at greater than 1 J per pulse is an excellent cutting laser. HoLRP uses this property to cut and resect rather than coagulate or desiccate tissue. Much like TURP, there is a substantial learning curve. With experience, however, the urologist can learn to resect a volume of tissue similar to that removed during TURP (57,58,64). Unlike coagulation prostatectomy with a side-firing device, tissue is immediately removed, symptom scores drop rapidly, and postoperative urinary retention due to tissue edema is not a problem. Properly performed, HoLRP results in immediate tissue resection similar to TURP with improved hemostasis. Unlike coagulation techniques, though, HoLRP is not bloodless.

HoLRP has been compared with VLAP in a small multicenter study of experienced investigators (39). Forty-four men were randomized to either HoLRP or VLAP. There were no significant differences between the preoperative patient groups. Mean total operative time was longer with HoLRP than with VLAP, 52 versus 41 minutes, respectively. Catheterization time differed considerably, 1.4 days for HoLRP versus 11.6 days for VLAP. There were no significant differences in postrecovery AUA symptom score; however, PdetQmax and Schafer grade measurements at 3 months showed greater relief of obstruction in the HoLRP group. The Qmax did not differ statistically.

Matsuoka and associates (76) evaluated 103 patients treated with HoLRP. They used a high-power laser and a forward-firing 550-micron optical fiber. Symptom score, Qmax, and quality of life were significantly improved at the 1-week visit. Similar results were maintained for up to 36 months postoperatively.

Carcinoma of the Prostate

Laser therapy has never been proved effective for curative treatment of adenocarcinoma of the prostate and is not advocated. An investigative method for endoscopic laser treatment of carcinoma of the prostate has been described, and initial clinical results are available (9,10). An "extended" or "radical" transurethral resection with electrocautery was performed with the intent of removing all prostatic tissue (80). Six to ten weeks after the resection, laser treatment was performed with the Nd:YAG laser. A power output of up to 70 W was used and applied to the entire prostatic capsule. The laser fiber tip was positioned 1 to 2 mm from the tissue surface.

McNicholas (79) has treated 30 patients by this method. Ultrasound follow-up has shown a nearly 75% reduction in the overall volume of the prostate, but it is uncertain how much of the reduction in size is secondary to the transurethral resection as opposed to the laser therapy. Fifty-four percent of patients had an undetectable postoperative prostate-specific antigen (PSA) level, whereas 14% of patients had a PSA level outside the normal range. Undoubtedly, further follow-up will be necessary to assess the efficacy of this technique. The multifocal nature of prostatic adenocarcinoma makes one question whether this type of ablative therapy has promise.

Ureter

The small diameter and flexibility of laser fibers allow their use through either rigid or flexible ureteroscopes (115). Flexible 200- to 400-micron fibers are particularly suited for ureteroscopic application. Larger-diameter fibers may pass through the working ports of several small ureteroscopes, but the rigidity of a 400- to 600-micron fiber inhibits active deflection of the ureteroscope tip. Nd:YAG, KTP, and holmium lasers may all be used on the ureter for soft tissue ablation. KTP and holmium lasers have a theoretic advantage over the Nd:YAG laser for treatment in the thin-walled ureter. Both lasers produce more superficial zones of tissue injury than the Nd:YAG laser.

In highly selected patients with low-grade transitional cell carcinoma of the ureter, successful treatment can be achieved with endoscopic Nd:YAG, KTP, or holmium laser therapy (62,72) (Fig. 6.13). Several authors have reported extensive single-institution experience.

Schmeller (109) treated 18 patients using the Nd:YAG laser. Treatment was not feasible in three patients because of tumor size or location. Of the remaining 15 patients, 14 had no evidence of recurrence with a variable but generally

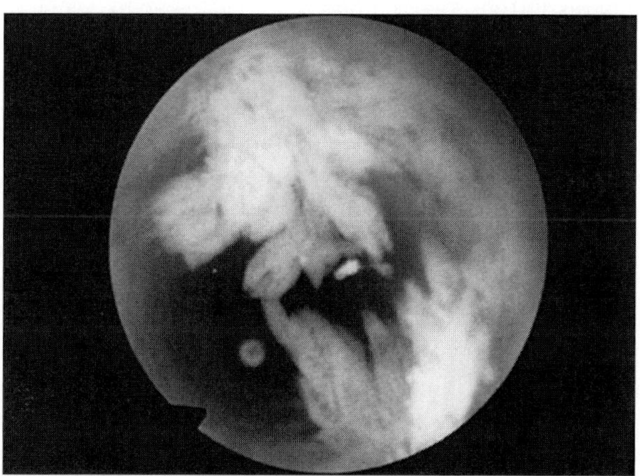

FIGURE 6.13. Papillary transitional cell carcinoma of the ureter. Nd:YAG laser energy can be applied via a small fiber inserted through either a flexible or rigid ureteroscope.

adequate length of follow-up after laser treatment. Ureteral strictures developed in three patients in whom circumferential treatment was performed.

Kaufman and Carson (61) reported nine patients with ureteral tumors treated with the Nd:YAG laser. No patient had a recurrence, and no strictures were observed. Gaboardi and colleagues (38) treated 18 patients with biopsy-confirmed ureteral tumors with Nd:YAG laser energy applied through a ureteroscope (25 to 30 W for 3 seconds). Eight patients developed a recurrence that was subsequently treated with a repeat Nd:YAG laser application. Nephroureterectomy was required in one patient for tumor control.

Thirty-eight patients with upper tract transitional cell carcinoma were treated in one series using both Nd:YAG and holmium lasers (62). Patients underwent ureterorenoscopy every 6 to 12 weeks until they were proven to be tumor free. Seventy-five percent of recurrent tumors were not identified radiographically. Patients were treated with the Nd:YAG laser or later with the holmium laser. Median follow-up was 35.1 and 26 months, respectively. High tumor grade, size, and multifocality were associated with tumor persistence and recurrence. The authors concluded that endoscopic management of upper tract transitional cell carcinoma is reasonable in selected patients. No significant difference was noted between the Nd:YAG and holmium laser–treated groups.

Kidney

Lasers have not proven to be particularly beneficial for partial nephrectomy. The hemostasis achieved with the CO_2 laser is suboptimal (7,104). The Nd:YAG laser is a poor cutting instrument and is not useful for incising the renal parenchyma (14). When combined with an ultrasonic surgical aspirator, the Nd:YAG laser does appear to be capable of decreasing the blood loss associated with partial nephrectomy (86). However, this technique requires the combination of two cumbersome instruments, and the inconvenience may outweigh the benefits.

The Nd:YAG laser has been useful when the surgical margins are precarious after treatment of a renal cell carcinoma. After enucleation of a renal tumor or a compromised partial nephrectomy, Nd:YAG laser energy can be applied to further extend the margin some 5 mm and help gain hemostasis (71). Virtually no patient morbidity is involved in this technique, and it seems to be a potentially beneficial use of the Nd:YAG laser.

The Nd:YAG laser has been used for percutaneous thermoablation of inoperative renal tumors. The investigators treated three patients using real-time guidance in an open-access interventional magnetic resonance imaging (MRI) scanner (30). Ablation and necrosis of target tissue was confirmed by follow-up gadolinium-enhanced MRI. Whether this type of treatment affects patient outcome remains to be seen. Nevertheless, the authors have demonstrated the concept of percutaneous ablation of malignant renal tissue with the Nd:YAG laser.

REFERENCES

1. Adkins WC. Argon laser treatment of urethral stricture and vesical neck contracture. *Lasers Surg Med* 1988;8:600.
2. Aleida FT. Contact laser assisted TURP: a 5-year follow-up. *J Laser Med Surg* 1994;14:68A.
3. Anson KM, Watson GM, Shah TK, et al. Laser prostatectomy: our initial experience of a technique in evolution. *J Endourol* 1993;7:333.
4. Arnfield M, Tulip J, McPhee M. Optical propagation in tissue with anisotropic scattering. *IEEE Trans Biomed Eng* 1998; 35:372.
5. Artez HT, Roth RA. Acute and chronic tissue effects of the transurethral ultrasound guided laser induced prostatectomy (TULIP) system in the canine prostate. *Lasers Surg Med* 1991; 3[Suppl]:76.
6. Baggish MS, Poiesz BJ, Joret D, et al. HIV virus DNA in laser plume. *Lasers Surg Med* 1991;11:197.
7. Barzilay B, Lijovetzky G, Shapiro A, et al. The clinical use of CO_2 laser beam in the surgery of kidney parenchyma. *Lasers Surg Med* 1982;2:81.
8. Bauer HM, Ting Y, Greer CE, et al. Genital papillomavirus infection in female university students as determined by a PCR-based method. *JAMA* 1991;265:472.
9. Beisland HO. Neodymium:YAG laser in the treatment of localized prostatic cancer. *Ann Chir Gynaecol* 1990;79:200.
10. Beisland HO, Sander S. First clinical experiences on neodymium:YAG laser irradiation of localized prostatic carcinoma. *Scand J Urol Nephrol* 1986;20:113.
11. Beisland HO, Sander S. Neodymium:YAG laser irradiation of stage T_2 muscle-invasive bladder cancer: long-term results. *Br J Urol* 1990;65:24.
12. Beisland HO, Seland O. A prospective randomized study on neodymium:YAG laser irradiation versus TUR in the treatment of urinary bladder cancer. *Scand J Urol Nephrol* 1986; 20:209.
13. Bellina JH. Lasers in gynecology. *World J Surg* 1983;7:692.
14. Benderev TV, Schaeffer AJ. Efficacy and safety of the Nd:YAG laser in canine partial nephrectomy. *J Urol* 1985;133:108.
15. Benson RC Jr. Endoscopic management of bladder cancer with hematoporphorin derivative phototherapy. *Urol Clin North Am* 1984;11:637.
16. Benson RC Jr, Farrow GM, Kensey KH, et al. Detection and localization of in situ carcinoma of the bladder with hematoporphorin derivative. *Mayo Clin Proc* 1982;57:548.
17. Benson RC Jr, Kensey JH, Cortese DA, et al. Treatment of transitional cell carcinoma of the bladder with hematoporphorin derivative phototherapy. *J Urol* 1983;130:1090.
18. Bolton DM, Costello AJ. Management of benign prostatic hyperplasia by transurethral laser ablation in patients treated with warfarin anticoagulation. *J Urol* 1994;151:79.
19. Cammack JT, Motamedi IM, Torres JH, et al. Endoscopic Nd:YAG laser coagulation of the prostate: comparison of low power versus high power. *J Urol* 1993;149:215A.
20. Carpiniello VL, Malloy TR, Sedlacek TV, et al. Results of CO_2 laser therapy and topical 5-fluorouracil treatment for subclinical condyloma found by magnified penile surface scanning. *J Urol* 1988;140:53.

21. Chambettaz F, Weible M, Salathe R. Temperature dependence of reflectance and transmittance of the artery exposed to air during laser irradiation. *IEEE Trans Biomed Eng* 1993;40:105.
22. Cheong W, Prahl S, Welch A. A review of the optical properties of biological tissues. *IEEE J Quantum Electronics* 1990;26:2166.
23. Chertin B, Moriel EZ, Hadas-Halpern I, et al. Laser prostatectomy. Long term follow-up of 303 patients. *Eur Urol* 1999; 35:285.
24. Cho YH, Chi SH, Hernandez AD, et al. Adriamycin absorption after Nd:YAG laser coagulation compared to electrosurgical resection of the bladder wall. *J Urol* 1992;147:1139.
25. van Swol CF, Verdaasdonk RM, Mooibroek J, et al. Physical evaluation of laser prostatectomy devices. *Proc SPIE* 1994; 2129:25.
26. Costello AJ, Bowsher WG, Bolton DM, et al. Laser ablation of the prostate in patients with benign prostatic hypertrophy. *Br J Urol* 1992;69:603.
27. Costello AJ, Johnson DE, Bolton DM. Nd:YAG laser ablation of the prostate as a treatment for benign prostatic hypertrophy. *Lasers Surg Med* 1992;12:121.
28. Cromeens DM, Price RE, Johnson DE. Pathologic changes following transurethral canine prostatectomy with a cylindrically diffusing fiber. *Lasers Surg Med* 1994;14:306.
29. Daughtry JD, Rodin BA. Transurethral resection of the prostate. *J Clin Lasers Med Surg* 1992;10:269.
30. de Jode MG, Vale JA, Gedroyc WM. MR-guided laser thermoablation of inoperable renal tumors in open-configuration interventional MR scanner: preliminary clinical experience in three cases. *J Magn Reson Imaging* 1999;10:545.
31. Derbyshire G, Bogen D, Unga M. Thermally induced optical property changes in myocardium at 1.06 m. *Lasers Surg Med* 1990;10:28.
32. Dixon CM, Lepor H. Laser ablation of the prostate. *Semin Urol* 1992;10:273.
33. Dixon CM, Machi G, Theune C, et al. A preoperative, double-blind, randomized study comparing the safety, efficacy, and cost of laser ablation of the prostate to TURP in the treatment of BPH. *J Urol* 1994;151:229A.
34. Ferenczy A. Strategies to eradicate genital HPV infection in men. *Contemp Urol* 1990;2:19.
35. Fournier GR Jr, Narayan P. Factors affecting size and configuration of neodymium:YAG laser lesions in the prostate. *Lasers Surg Med* 1994;14:314.
36. Freiha GS, Glickman RD, Teichman JM. Holmium:YAG laser-induced damage to guidewires: experimental study. *J Endourol* 1997;11:331.
37. Fuselier H Jr, McBurney EI, Brannan W, et al. Treatment of condylomata acuminata with carbon dioxide laser. *Urology* 1980;15:265.
38. Gaboardi F, Bozzola A, Dotti E, et al. Conservative treatment of upper urinary tract tumor with Nd:YAG laser. *J Endourol* 1994;8:37.
39. Gilling PJ, Cass CB, Malcolm A, et al. Holmium laser resection of the prostate versus neodymium:yttrium-aluminum-garnet visual laser ablation of the prostate: a randomized prospective comparison of two techniques for laser prostatectomy. *Urology* 1998;51:573.
40. Greenberger M, Steiner MS. The University of Tennessee experience with the Indigo 830e laser device for the minimally invasive treatment of benign prostatic hyperplasia: interim analysis. *World J Urol* 1998;16:386.
41. Hardie EM, Stone EA, Spaulding FA, et al. Subtotal canine prostatectomy with the neodymium:yttrium-aluminum-garnet laser. *Vet Surg* 1990;19:348.
42. Hisazumi H, Misahi T, Myoshi N. Photoradiation of bladder tumors. *J Urol* 1983;130:685.
43. Hofstetter A, Frank K, Keiditsch E. Laser treatment of the bladder. Experimental and clinical results. In: Smith JA Jr, ed. *Lasers in urologic surgery.* St. Louis: Mosby, 1985.
44. Hofstetter A. Lasers in urology. *Lasers Surg Med* 1986;5:412.
45. Hofstetter A. Treatment of urological tumors by neodymium: YAG laser. *Eur Urol* 1986;12[Suppl]:21.
46. Hofstetter A. Interstitial laser-assisted thermocoagulation for the treatment of prostatic tumors. *Curr Opin Urol* 1993;3:14.
47. Hruza GJ. Laser treatment of warts and other epidermal and dermal lesions. *Dermatol Clin* 1997;15:487.
48. Hughes PS, Hughes AP. Absence of human papillomavirus DNA in the plume of erbium:YAG laser-treated warts. *J Am Acad Derm* 1998;38:426.
49. Jacques S, Prahl S. Modelling optical and thermal distributions in tissue during laser or radiation. *Lasers Surg Med* 1987;6:494.
50. Johnson DE. Use of the holmium:YAG laser for treatment of superficial bladder carcinoma. 1994;14:213.
51. Johnson DE, Cromeens DM, Price RE. Interstitial laser prostatectomy. *Lasers Surg Med* 1994;14:299.
52. Johnson DE, Levinson AK, Greskovich FJ, et al. Transurethral laser prostatectomy using a right-angle laser delivery system. *Lasers Urol Laparoscopy Gen Surg* 1991;1421:36.
53. Johnson DE, Price RE, Gromeens DM. Pathologic changes occurring in the prostate following transurethral laser prostatectomy. *Lasers Surg Med* 1992;12:254.
54. Kabalin JN. Laser prostatectomy performed with a right angle firing Nd:YAG laser at 40 watts power setting. *J Urol* 1993;150:95.
55. Kabalin JN, Gill HS. Dosimetry studies utilizing the Urolase right angle firing neodymium:YAG laser fiber. *Lasers Surg Med* 1994;14:145.
56. Kabalin JN, Gill HS, Bite G. Laser prostatectomy performed with a right-angle firing Nd:YAG laser fiber at 60 watts power setting. *J Urol* 1995;153(5):1502.
57. Kabalin JN, Gilling PJ, Fraundorfer MR. Holmium:yttrium-aluminum-garnet laser prostatectomy. *Mayo Clin Proc* 1998; 73:792.
58. Kabalin JN, Gilling PJ, Fraundorfer MR. Application of the holmium:YAG laser for prostatectomy. *J Clin Laser Med Surg* 1998;16:21.
59. Kandel LB, Harrison LH, McCullough DL, et al. Transurethral laser prostatectomy: creation of a technique for using the neodymium:yttrium-aluminum-garnet (YAG) laser in the canine model. *J Urol* 1986;135:110A (abst).
60. Kandel LB, Harrison LH, McCullough DL, et al. Transurethral laser prostatectomy in the canine model. *Lasers Surg Med* 1992;12:33.
61. Kaufman RF, Carson CC. Ureteroscopic management of transitional cell carcinoma of the ureter using the Nd:YAG laser. *Lasers Surg Med* 1993;13:625.
62. Keeley FX Jr, Bibbo M, Bagley DH. Ureteroscopic treatment and surveillance of upper urinary tract transitional cell carcinoma. *J Urol* 1997;157:1560.
63. Klimberg IW, Locke DR, Leonard E, et al. Outpatient transurethral resection of the prostate at a urological ambulatory surgery center. *J Urol* 1994;151:1547.
64. Le Duc A, Gilling PJ. Holmium laser resection of the prostate. *Eur Urol* 1999;35:155.
65. Juo Rl, Aslan P, Zhong P, et al. Impact of holmium laser settings and fiber diameter on stone fragmentation and endoscope deflection. *J Endourol* 1998;12:523.

66. Leach GE, Sirls L, Ganabathi K, et al. Outpatient visual laser assisted prostatectomy under local anesthesia. *Urology* 1994; 42:149.
67. Littrup PJ, Lee F, Borlaza GS, et al. Percutaneous ablation of canine prostate using transrectal ultrasound guidance. Absolute ethanol and Nd:YAG laser. *Invest Radiol* 1988;23:734.
68. Lundquist SG, Lindstedt EM. Laser treatment of condylomata acuminata, abstracted. *Lasers Surg Med* 1983;3:152.
69. Maiman TH. Stimulated optical radiation in ruby. *Nature* 1960;187:493.
70. Malek RS. Laser treatment of premalignant and malignant squamous cell lesions of the penis. *Lasers Surg Med* 1992; 12:246.
71. Malloy TS, Schultz RE, Wern AJ, et al. Renal preservation utilizing neodymium:YAG laser. *Urology* 1986;27:99.
72. Malloy TR. Treatment of lesions of external genitalia. In: Smith JA Jr, ed. *Lasers in urologic surgery.* Chicago: Year Book Medical Publishers, 1985.
73. Malloy TR, Wein AJ, Carpiniello VL. Carcinoma of the penis treated with the neodymium:YAG laser. *Urology* 1988;31:26.
74. Malloy TR, Wein AJ, Shanberg A. Superficial transitional cell carcinoma of the bladder treated with neodymium:YAG laser. A study of the recurrence rate within the first year. *J Urol* 1984;131:251-A (abst).
75. Marks LS. Serial endoscopy following visual laser ablation of prostate. *Urology* 1993;42:66.
76. Matsuoka K, Iida S, Tomiyasu K, et al. Transurethral holmium laser resection of the prostate. *J Urol* 2000;163:515.
77. McCullough DL. This month in investigative urology: transurethral laser treatment of benign prostatic hyperplasia. *J Urol* 1991;146:1126 (comment).
78. McCullough DL, Roth RA, Babayan RK, et al. Transurethral ultrasound guided laser induced prostatectomy: national human cooperative study results. *J Urol* 1993;150:1607.
79. McNicholas TA. Prostate cancer. In: Smith JA Jr, ed. *Lasers in urologic surgery,* ed 3. Chicago: Mosby, 1994.
80. McNicholas TA, Carter SStC, Wickham JEA, et al. YAG laser treatment of early carcinoma of the prostate. *Br J Urol* 1988; 61:239.
81. McNicholas TA, Steger AC, Bown SG. Interstitial laser coagulation of the prostate: an experimental study. *Br J Urol* 1993; 7:439.
82. McPhee MS. Lasers in the treatment of cancer of the prostate, an overview. *Biomed Pharmacother* 1986;40:321.
83. McPhee MS. Prostate. In: Smith JA Jr, ed. *Lasers in urologic surgery.* Chicago: Year Book Medical Publishers, 1989.
84. McPhee MS, Mador D, Tulip J. Segmental irradiation of the bladder with neodymium:YAG laser irradiation. *J Urol* 1982; 128:1101.
85. McPhee MS, Thorndyke CW, Thomas G, et al. Interstitial applications of laser irradiation in hematoporphyrin-derivative photosensitized Dunning R-3327 prostate cancers. *Lasers Surg Med* 1984;4:93.
86. Melzer RB, Wood TW, Landau ST, et al. Combination of CUSA and Nd:YAG laser for canine partial nephrectomy. *J Urol* 1985;134:620.
87. Merkle W. Urethral stricture. In: Smith JA Jr, ed. *Lasers in urologic surgery,* ed 3. Chicago: Mosby, 1994.
88. Milam DF. Unpublished data.
89. Milam DF, Nau WH, Roselli R. Quantitative canine laser prostatectomy model. *Abstracts of the Southeastern Section, American Urologic Association,* New Orleans, La, March 1994.
90. Milam DF, Roselli RJ, Nau WH. Evaluation of optimal laser prostatectomy dwell and scanning rates. Unpublished data.
91. Mulvaney WP, Beck CW. The laser beam in urology. *J Urol* 1968;99:112.
92. Muschter R, Hessel S, Hofstetter A, et al. Die Interstitielle Laserkoagulation der benignen Prostatahyperplasie. *Urologe A* 1993;32:273.
93. Narayan P, Fournier G, Indudharo R, et al. Transurethral evaporation of prostate (TUEP) with Nd:YAG laser using a contact-free beam technique: result in 61 patients with benign prostate hyperplasia. *Urology* 1994;43:813.
94. Nau WH. Modeling photocoagulation of the prostate during exposure to laser radiation. Ph.D. dissertation. Nashville: Vanderbilt University, 1996.
95. Nau WH, Roselli RJ, Milam DF. Finite element modeling of laser prostatectomy, vol 2129. *Abstracts of the International Society for Optical Engineering,* Los Angeles, Jan 1994, p 34.
96. Newman CT, Wishnow KI, von Eschenbach AC. Real-time ultrasonic changes associated with laser photoirradiation of the canine prostate. *J Urol* 1991;145:395A (abst).
97. Norris JP, Norris DM, Lee RD, et al. Visual laser ablation of the prostate: clinical experience in 108 patients. *J Urol* 1993; 150:1612.
98. Patterson M, Chanee B, Wilson B. Time resolved reflectance and transmittance for the non-invasive measurement of tissue optical properties. *Applied Optics* 1989;28:2331.
99. Pickering J, Posthumes P, van Gemert M. Continuous measurement of the head-induced changes in the optical properties (at 1064 nm) of rat liver. *Lasers Surg Med* 1994;15:200.
100. Pickering J, Prahl S, van Wieringen N, et al. Double integrating sphere system for measuring the optical properties of tissue. *Applied Optics* 1993;32:399.
101. Prout GR Jr, Linn CW, Benson RC Jr, et al. Photodynamic therapy with hematoporphorin derivative in the treatment of superficial transitional cell carcinoma of the bladder. *N Engl J Med* 1987;317:251.
102. Roselli RJ, Milam DF, Nau WH. Determination of tissue temperature distribution during laser prostatectomy with an analytic model. *Abstracts of the Biomedical Engineering Society,* Tempe, Arizona, Oct 1994.
103. Rosemberg SK. The use of the CO_2 laser in urology. *Lasers Surg Med* 1983;3:114 (abst).
104. Rosemberg SK. Clinical experience with CO_2 laser in renal surgery. *Urology* 1985;25:115.
105. Rosemberg SK, Fuller T, Jacobs H. Continuous wave carbon dioxide laser treatment of giant condylomata acuminata of the distal urethra and perineum: technique. *J Urol* 1981;126:827.
106. Roth RA, Aretz HT. Transurethral ultrasound-guided laser-induced prostatectomy. *J Urol* 1991;146:1128.
107. Rothauge CF, Noske HD, Kraushaar J. Erfahrungen mit der argon-laser Applikation bei urologischen Erkrankungen. *Urologe A* 1981;20:333.
108. Scaletscky R, Milam DF, Smith JA. Combined laparoscopic and cystoscopic Nd:YAG laser photocoagulation of the porcine bladder wall. *J Urol* 1993;149:411A.
109. Schmeller NT. Laser treatment of the ureter. In: Smith JA Jr, ed. *Lasers in urologic surgery.* Chicago: Year Book Medical Publishers, 1988.
110. Shanberg A, Baghdassarian R, Tansey LA. Treatment of interstitial cystitis with the neodymium:YAG laser. *J Urol* 1985; 134:885.
111. Shanberg A, Baghdassarian R, Tansey L, et al. KTP-532 laser in treatment of urethral strictures. *Urology* 1988;23:517.
112. Shanberg AM, Lee IS, Tansey LA, et al. Depth of penetration of the Nd:YAG laser in the human prostate at various dosimetry. *Urology* 1994;43:809.

113. Shanberg AM, Tansey LA. Laser treatment of urethral strictures. In: Smith JA Jr, ed. *Urologic surgery.* Chicago: Mosby, 1985.
114. Shanberg AM, Tansey CA, Baghdassarian R. The use of the Nd:YAG laser in prostatectomy. *J Urol* 1985;133:331A.
115. Smith JA Jr. Neodymium:YAG laser photoradiation of canine ureters: an analysis of penetration depth and subsequent healing. *Surg Forum* 1983;34:696.
116. Smith JA Jr. Endoscopic applications of laser energy. *Urol Clin North Am* 1986;13:405.
117. Smith JA Jr. Treatment of invasive bladder cancer with a neodymium:YAG laser. *J Urol* 1986;135:55.
118. Smith JA Jr. Treatment of benign urethral strictures using a sapphire tipped neodymium:YAG laser. *J Urol* 1989;142: 1221.
119. Smith JA Jr. Laser treatment of the urethra and prostate. *Semin Urol* 1991;3:180.
120. Smith JA Jr, Dixon JA. Neodymium:YAG laser treatment of benign urethral strictures. *J Urol* 1984;131:1080.
121. Smith JA Jr, Dixon JA. Neodymium:YAG laser irradiation of bladder hemangioma. *Urology* 1984;24:134.
122. Smith JA Jr, Landau S. Neodymium:YAG laser specifications for safe intravesical use. *J Urol* 1989;141:1238.
123. Splinter R, Svenson R, Littman L, et al. Optical properties of normal, diseased, and laser photocoagulated myocardium at Nd:YAG wavelength. *Lasers Surg Med* 1991;11:117.
124. Stein BS. Laser physics and tissue interaction. *Urol Clin North Am* 1986;3:365.
125. Takahashi S, Homma Y, Minowada S, et al. Transurethral ultrasound-guided laser-induced prostatectomy for benign prostatic hyperplasia: clinical utility at one year follow-up and imaging analysis. *Urology* 1994;43:802.
126. Teichman JM, Vassar GJ, Glickman RD, et al. Holmium: YAG lithotripsy: photothermal mechanism converts uric acid calculi to cyanide. *J Urol* 1998;160:320.
127. Thomsen S. Medical lasers: how they work and how they affect tissue. *Cancer Bulletin* 1989;41:203.
128. Turek PJ, Malloy TR, Cendron M, et al. KTP-532 laser ablation of urethral strictures. *Urology* 1992;40:330.
129. Vassar GJ, Chan KF, Teichman JM, et al. Holmium:YAG lithotripsy: photothermal mechanism. *J Endourol* 1999;13:181.
130. Wilson B, Jacques S. Optical reflectance and transmittance of tissues, principles, and applications. *IEEE Journal of Quantum Electronics* 1990;26:2186.

Adult and Pediatric Urology, 4/e, edited by Jay Y. Gillenwater, John T. Grayhack, Stuart S. Howards, and Michael E. Mitchell.
Lippincott Williams & Wilkins, Philadelphia © 2002

7

GENITOURINARY MALIGNANCY: ETIOLOGY AND MOLECULAR GENETICS, NATURAL HISTORY, AND TREATMENT

McCLELLAN M. WALTHER
FREDRICK LEACH
DAVID K.ORNSTEIN
NORMAN ZAMBRANO
W. MARSTON LINEHAN

M.M. Walther, F. Leach, D.K. Ornstein, and W.M. Linehan: Urologic Oncology Branch, National Cancer Institute, Bethesda, MD 20892.

N. Zambrano: Department of Urology, Catholic University of Chile, Santiago, Chile; Urology Service, Sotero Del Rio Hospital, Puente Alto, Santiago, Chile.

Kidney cancer, prostate cancer, and bladder cancer affect more than 250,000 people annually in the United States, and nearly 56,000 die from these diseases each year. Significant and dramatic improvements have been made in the last decade in both the diagnosis and the treatment of these malignancies. However, despite these remarkable advances, most patients with advanced renal, prostate, or bladder cancer still die from these diseases. We have witnessed a dramatic biotechnologic revolution over the past two decades, which has provided significant opportunities for the development of better methods for diagnosis, prevention, and treatment of these genitourinary malignancies. Many scientists and clinicians believe that the key to the development of rational and effective forms of therapy for patients with advanced genitourinary malignancies lies in the understanding of the fundamental basis of these cancers, that is, in identification of the genes that cause these cancers and elucidation of the molecular genetic basis for their progression. Examples of molecular therapeutics have proven this principle, and it is the hope of scientists and clinicians that understanding the molecular genetic basis of genitourinary cancers and their molecular pathways will lead to even better methods for diagnosis, prevention, and treatment of these cancers.

RENAL CELL CARCINOMA: ETIOLOGY, NATURAL HISTORY, AND MOLECULAR GENETICS

Renal cell carcinoma is a historical term that has been applied to a number of renal parenchymal tumors of different histopathologic types. An attempt to classify renal cell carcinomas was begun by Grawitz (160) in 1883, when the origin of renal tumors was attributed to an ectopic adrenal rest and named "hypernephroma." Understanding of the genetic abnormalities found in renal tumors has led to a recognition of distinctive histologic types of tumors. Kovacs (245) classified genetically similar renal cell tumors and divided them clinically into four groups: those with papillary growth or nonpapillary pattern, chromophobe renal cell carcinomas, and renal oncocytomas. Papillary renal cell carcinomas were defined by the presence of at least 75% of the tumor with a papillary pattern (245).

Recently, a division of renal cell tumors into benign and malignant categories has been proposed (462). Benign tumors were subclassified into oncocytoma, papillary renal adenoma, and metanephric adenoma. Malignant tumors were subclassified into conventional (clear-cell) renal carcinoma; papillary renal carcinoma; chromophobe renal carcinoma; collecting duct carcinoma; and renal cell carcinoma, unclassified.

Incidence and Time Trends

Malignant tumors of the kidney account for about 3% of cancer incidence in the United States. Approximately 30,800 new cases of renal cancer were estimated to occur in the United States in the year 2001, and 12,100 patients were predicted to die of their disease (163a). Generally, renal cancers occur at a median age of 65 years, and men are affected 1.5 times as frequently as women (163).

The incidence of renal cancer in the United States has been increasing over the last 65 years (69). The age-adjusted incidence rates for renal cancer over approximately the last 20 years have been 9.6 per 100,000 person-years for Caucasian men, 11.1 for African-American men, 4.4 for Caucasian women, and 4.9 for African-American women (69). Annual incidence rates in these groups have risen from 2.3% to 4.3% per year. Increases occurred in all stages, the largest occurring in patients with localized renal tumors (rising from 3.8% to 5.6% per year during the same period). The development of new imaging technologies has not accounted for all of these changes (69). Trends in 5-year relative cancer survival rates have been increasing for both Caucasians and African-Americans (163).

Etiology

Environmental and hereditary genetic factors have been associated with the development of the renal cell carcinomas, although individual toxins have not been linked to specific histologies. Environmental factors thought to confer risk include cigarette smoking, petrochemicals, cadmium, and thorium dioxide. Other related factors include obesity and long-term renal dialysis for the treatment of end-stage renal disease. Hereditary forms of most of the histologic types of renal cell carcinoma have also been described.

The increasing incidence of renal cell carcinoma in the United States has been attributed to increased obesity and protein intake, rising incidence of hypertension in the increasing obese and elderly populations, and increasing exposure to toxic environmental agents. Smoking has been on the decline, and this may contribute to a smaller proportion of patients developing renal cancer in the future.

Cigarette Smoking

Case-control studies generally report an association between cigarette smoking and the development of renal cancer (relative risk of 1.35 to 2.2) (255,289,299,300,415,458, 461) with risk related to duration of exposure (300,317). The risk attributed to cigarette smoking has been shown to increase with increasing number of cigarettes smoked per day (461). The dose-response relation observed further substantiates this association (48,255,289,300). The lack of association in some studies has been attributed to lack of power secondary to small sample size or biased samples with a high prevalence of smoking in the control group, such as hospital controls (413). With cessation of smoking, the risk of renal cell carcinoma decreases, as much as 30% to 50% at 10 to 25 years (299,461). Gender and presence of a filter on the cigarette have not been found to alter risk. It has been estimated that 24% of female and 30% of male renal cell carcinomas (24) to approximately 18% overall may be caused by cigarette smoking (300a).

In patients with renal cancer, it has been suggested that patients who smoke have more advanced disease at diagnosis and shorter survival than nonsmokers (411).

Obesity

The presence of obesity has been highly correlated with the development of renal cell carcinoma in case-control studies (317,415). The question of whether the risk of renal cell carcinoma is attributed to obesity alone or obesity-related food pattern remains to be answered. Obesity is linked to dietary intake. The incidence of renal cell carcinoma has been positively correlated with intake of fat-containing foods (fats, oil, meat, milk, sugar) and negatively correlated with cereals and vegetables (36,289).

Case-control studies and cohort studies have shown increased risk of developing renal cancer related to high caloric intake (relative risk of 1.7), high intake of fatty foods (relative risk of 1.90), and high protein intake (relative risk of 1.71) (11,36,289,456). Decreasing risk was seen with increasing intake of fruit (relative risk of 0.4 to 0.85) and vitamin C (relative risk of 0.62) (36,456). Studies controlling for caloric intake, body mass, and smoking show protein intake as an independent risk factor (11). It has been estimated that 21% of renal cell carcinoma in the general population is attributed to excess body weight (24).

Hypertension

Cohort studies have been performed to evaluate the association of hypertension and associated medical treatment with the development of renal cancer (186,373,415). Hypertension alone does not appear to be associated with such a risk (186). Although not entirely consistent, the accumulated data suggest that diuretics may increase the risk of renal cancer, especially among women. Increase usage or duration of use was associated with greater risk. The use of β-adrenergic blockers has also been suggested to be associated with the development of renal carcinoma (odds ratio of 1.5 to 3.0) (415). It has been estimated that 18% of renal cell carcinoma is attributable to hypertension (24).

Occupation

Case-control and cohort studies have shown that exposure to various chemicals is significantly linked to the development of renal cancer (294,301,433). Significant associations have been reported in the blast-furnace and coke-oven industries (odds ratio of 1.7 to 2.0); in the iron and steel industry (odds ratio of 1.6 to 2.5); among firefighters (odds ratio of 3.5), glassworkers (odds ratio of 3.5), chemical processors (odds ratio of 2.6), photographers (odds ratio of 2.1), and painters (odds ratio of 1.6); and for exposure to asbestos (odds ratio of 1.4 to 1.6), cadmium (odds ratio of 2.0), dry cleaning solvents (odds ratio of 1.4 to 1.5), gasoline (odds ratio of 1.6 to 2.1), petroleum products (odds ratio of 1.6), carbon tetrachloride (odds ratio of 2.5), and tetrachlorethene (odds ratio of 10.8) (98,294,301,433).

Carcinogenesis is thought to occur secondary to exposure to toxic metabolites of the environmental agents. A common mechanism of metabolism is enzymatic conjugation with glutathione, which facilitates further processing. Further conjugation with cysteine adducts allows acetylation to mercaptic acids, which are excreted in the urine, or cleavage by kidney tubular epithelium to highly reactive chlorinated thioketenes. *In vitro* and *in vivo* studies suggest that these metabolites are highly genotoxic (171,229).

End-stage Renal Disease

The development of cystic disease in kidneys of patients undergoing hemodialysis was first observed by Dunnill (108) in an autopsy study in 1977. Cystic disease has subsequently been found in patients with chronic renal failure and undergoing dialysis. Patients with end-stage renal disease maintained by dialysis have an 18% to 88% incidence of acquired renal cystic disease and a 1% to 7% incidence of renal cancer (187,348,364). Risk of cystic disease appears to increase with duration of dialysis (364,432). The renal cancer histology that is clinically apparent has most frequently been clear cell. Clinically inapparent cancers, that is, microscopic papillary renal cancers, have also been reported with some frequency (187,348).

Male patients may be more frequently affected (187, 348). Patient survival appears to be related to tumor stage (348). Overall survival in patients reviewed in the literature was 70% at 1 year, 35% at 5 years, and 10% at 10 years (298).

Medical and Family History

A single first-degree relative affected with renal cancer is associated with an increased familial risk of developing renal cancer (relative risk of 1.6) (373). Thyroid disease was also associated with the development of renal cancer (relative risk of 1.6) (373). A significant trend in risk was reported with number of childbirths in women (272). Use of oral contraceptives has also been associated with a reduced risk of renal cancer in nonsmoking women (272). No association has been reported with estrogen replacement therapy in women (272).

Polymorphic Xenobiotic-metabolizing Enzymes

Environmental toxins may be directly toxic, or they may require metabolic activation by oxidative (phase I) enzymes, such as members of the cytochrome P450 family (CYP), to be transformed into toxic metabolites. Removal of most carcinogens starts with the conjugation action of phase II enzymes, such as the glutathione-S-transferase (GST) and arylamine *N*-acetyltransferases (NAT) families of enzymes.

A wide range of metabolizer enzyme activity in each gene family has been described, ranging from a polymophism associated with loss of the involved gene to a gene with full enzymatic activity. These naturally occurring genetic polymorphisms could infer great interindividual variation in susceptibility to develop cancer after exposure to environmental toxins. Polymorphisms of these types have been shown to be associated with development of bladder and head and neck cancers in patients who smoke (195,256).

The ability to metabolize environmental toxins may be protective for the development of renal cancer. Presence of the 1A1 allele of CYP has been associated with an increased risk of developing renal cancer (283). Presence of the CYP1A1allele with either the TT1 or TP1 alleles of GST or the NAT2 (slow acetylator) polymorphism has been reported to further increase this risk (283). Patients with loss of the Mu1 allele of GST (null polymorphism) and presence of π1 GST polymorphism have even higher risk if the CYP1A1 or NAT2 (slow acetylator) is also present (283).

Hereditary Forms of Renal Cancer

Renal cell carcinoma can occur in an inherited form, similar to retinoblastoma, breast cancer, prostate cancer, and colon cancer. As many as 4% of renal cancers may be inherited (275). Inherited renal cancers are characterized by early age of onset of bilateral, multifocal renal tumors. Two forms of clear-cell renal cancer have been described. Von Hippel–Lindau disease (VHL) is an autosomal dominant inherited multiorgan tumor syndrome in which 40% to 45% of affected individuals develop clear-cell renal tumors (Fig. 7.1) (150,349). Its incidence has been estimated as 1:36,000 (291). Individual families have also been described with reciprocal germline chromosome 3 translocations that are associated with the development of clear-cell renal tumors (35,74,240,248,271,449).

Hereditary basophilic papillary renal cell carcinoma (Fig. 7.2) (463,464) and hereditary renal oncocytoma (453) have also been described, both manifesting with autosomal dominant inheritance of bilateral, multifocal renal tumors.

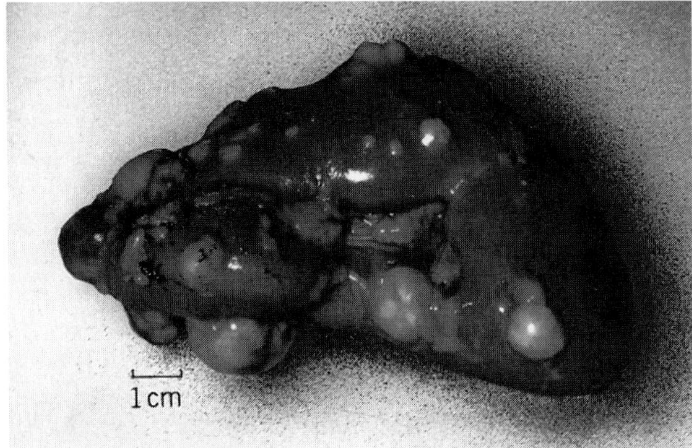

FIGURE 7.1. Von Hippel–Lindau (VHL) disease is characterized by the development of multiple bilateral clear-cell renal cancers and cysts over the course of the patient's life. A typical VHL kidney is shown here.

Birt-Hogg-Dubé syndrome (BHD) is characterized by the clinical manifestations of skin fibrofolliculomas and pulmonary cysts leading to spontaneous pneumothorax. Recently, it has been observed that renal tumors of several histologic tumor types can develop in these patients. This syndrome is currently being characterized (428).

Natural History

Patient survival is strongly associated with tumor stage. Five-year disease-specific survival has been reported as 91%, 74%, 67%, and 32% for tumor, node, metastasis (TNM) stages I, II, III, and IV lesions (69,430). Tumor characteristics similarly correlated with a 5-year survival rate of 83% for stage T_1, 57% for stage T_2, 42% for stage T_3, and 28% for stage T_4 disease. Tumor grade is also associated with

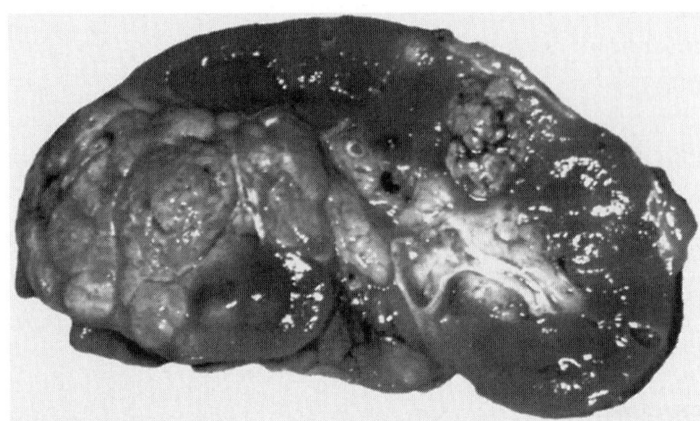

FIGURE 7.2. Hereditary papillary renal cancer is characterized by the development of bilateral basophilic (type 1) papillary renal cell cancers over the course of the patient's life. Cystic disease does not occur as part of HPRC. A typical HPRC kidney is shown here (463).

patient survival: 89% 5-year survival for grade 1, 65% for grade 2, and 46% for grades 3 and 4. Overall, TNM stage and tumor grade were the most important prognostic indicators, whereas the Eastern Cooperative Oncology Group (ECOG) performance status was a less significant predictor and tumor stage was not an independent predictor (209,216,316,430).

Evaluation of prognosis associated with different tumor histopathologies suggests that some renal cancer types may be more aggressive than others. In patients with similar size renal tumors, those with clear-cell renal cancer had metastases at the time of diagnosis more frequently than patients with papillary or chromophobe renal tumors (37% versus 16% versus 8%, p = .044 and .048, respectively) (280). Patients with papillary and chromophobe renal cancer also had longer survival.

Clinical parameters at initial presentation have also been correlated with survival. Symptomatic presentation and significant weight loss have been associated with decreased survival (144). Shortened survival has been associated with the laboratory findings of elevated serum lactate dehydrogenase, C-reactive protein, erythrocyte sedimentation rate, and alkaline phosphatase; low hemoglobin; and hypercalcemia (144,297,316).

Molecular Genetics

Renal carcinoma may occur in both inherited and noninherited forms. As many as 4% patients with renal carcinoma may carry an inherited factor (275). Inherited renal cancer gives special insight into the earliest genetic changes required for the different histologic types of renal cancer to develop. Clinically, patients with familial renal cancer are characterized by early age at presentation of multiple, bilateral renal tumors. New renal tumors can develop over the course of the patient's life.

The best-characterized hereditary renal cancer is VHL (151), in which as many as 45% of affected individuals develop clear-cell renal carcinoma (151,349). Individual families have also been described with hereditary clear-cell renal cancer associated with the reciprocal germline translocation of chromosome 3 to 8 (74,271,449), chromosome 3 to 6 (248), or chromosome 3 to 2 (35,240). Hereditary papillary renal cell carcinoma is a familial form with autosomal dominant transmission, but at a reduced penetrance in comparison with VHL and familial clear-cell cancer (463). Hereditary renal oncocytoma has been described in a number of families (453) BHD is a hereditary renal syndrome characterized by autosomal dominant inheritance of multiple bilateral chromophobe renal tumors, spontaneous pneumothorax, and characteristic cutaneous trichofolliculoma (34,362,428).

The study of inherited forms of renal tumors allows the use of the powerful tools of linkage analysis to localize and identify the initial genetic abnormality leading to a specific histologic subtype of renal cancer. Identification of these genes may be useful clinically in the diagnosis of renal tumors and their metastases.

TABLE 7.1. UICC CLASSIFICATION OF RENAL TUMORS

Malignant Neoplasms
1. Conventional (clear-cell) carcinoma
2. Papillary renal carcinoma
3. Chromophobe renal carcinoma
4. Collecting duct carcinoma
5. Renal cell carcinoma, unclassified

Benign Neoplasms
1. Oncocytoma
2. Papillary adenoma
3. Metanephric adenoma

Histologic classification of renal tumors by the Union Internationale Contre le Cancer (UICC) and the American Joint Committee on Cancer.

HISTOPATHOLOGIC CLASSIFICATION OF RENAL TUMORS

Renal tumors have been classified based on cytomorphologic characteristics and presumed cellular origin. Thoenes and colleagues (422) developed one of the first modern classifications of benign and malignant renal tumors based on these features. Renal tumors were categorized as (a) clear cell, (b) chromophil, (c) chromophobe, (d) spindle shaped or pleomorphic, or (e) oncocytoma. The study of tumor genetics has led to the recognition of distinctive types of renal tumors: carcinoma with papillary morphologic pattern, carcinoma with nonpapillary pattern, chromophobe renal cell carcinoma, and renal oncocytoma (245).

Storkel and colleagues (406) and Kovacs and colleagues (243) proposed a histopathologic classification of renal tumors based on the underlying genetic abnormalities of the different subtypes. Both classifications recognize benign and malignant renal neoplasms. Malignant tumors were classified into conventional or clear-cell, papillary, chromophobe, collecting duct, and unclassified renal cancer. Benign tumors were classified into metanephric adenoma and adenofibroma, papillary renal cell adenoma, and renal oncocytoma. A European and American joint working group adopted a similar histologic classification system in 1997 (Table 7.1) (406,462).

GENETIC CLASSIFICATION OF RENAL NEOPLASMS

Hereditary Conventional Renal Cancer

Germline mutations in the VHL gene (chromosome 3p25) lead to conventional (clear-cell) renal cancer, the most common form of inherited renal cancer. Single families with reciprocal germline translocations involving chromosome 3 have also been described to develop a hereditary form of conventional renal cancer (35,74,240,248,271,449). Evaluation of tumors from these patients reveals both copies of the VHL gene to be inactivated. One copy of the gene has the germline mutation and the second copy has a somatic (acquired) mutation (35,154,271,377). Inactivation of both copies of a gene in this fashion is characteristic of a tumor-suppressor gene. These findings support mutation of the VHL gene as the initial genetic event in the development of clear-cell renal cancer.

Clear-cell Renal Carcinoma

Conventional, or clear-cell, renal carcinoma makes up 70% to 80% of renal tumors (462) and is the most studied renal tumor. Conventional renal carcinoma is believed to derive from proximal renal tubular epithelial cells (25,129). These tumors consist predominantly of cells with clear cytoplasm, although foci of cells with eosinophilic cytoplasm are common. Tumor architecture is usually solid and cystic, and tumors have a characteristic delicate branching vasculature. Approximately 5% of these tumors develop high-grade, sarcomatoid changes (406,462).

Sporadic Clear-cell Renal Cancer

Similar to inherited conventional (clear-cell) renal cancer, sporadic conventional renal cancer is thought to arise from loss of function of both copies of the VHL gene. In sporadic tumors, both mutations occur as somatic events. Ninety-eight localized and advanced conventional renal tumors analyzed by Gnarra and colleagues (154) had loss of one copy of the VHL gene [loss of heterozygosity (LOH)]. The second copy of the VHL gene was mutated in 57% of the tumors. These findings have been confirmed by other reports of chromosome 3p LOH and by cytogenetic studies (10,154,227).

An alternative mechanism of inactivation to LOH, hypermethylation, has also been described. Chromosomal regions rich in groups of CpG, termed *CpG islands,* are often found in the 5′ regulatory areas of genes, where hypermethylation could render the genes inactive (33). Hypermethylation of the VHL gene was reported in 11% (149) to 19% (191) of sporadic conventional renal tumors. Hypermethylation of the VHL gene has been associated with loss of expression of the VHL gene by Northern blot analysis (191).

These data show a very high degree of loss of one copy of the VHL gene by LOH, and at least 53% to 76% inactivation of the second copy, in conventional renal cancers (154,191,227,410). Inactivation of the VHL gene has been associated specifically with conventional renal cancers (154,227) and suggests the requirement of inactivation of both copies of the VHL gene for the development of conventional renal cancer.

Other Early Genetic Changes

Loss of function of the VHL tumor-suppressor gene has been associated with increased expression of transforming growth factor-α (TGF-α) (234). Northern blot mRNA expression of TGF-α and TGF-β_1 has been reported elevated in 60% of undefined sporadic renal cancers when compared with normal kidney (156). As many as 75% of undefined sporadic renal cancers have increased expression of the *myc* oncogene (232,452).

Late Events or Progression

Higher clinical stage, higher tumor grade, and poor prognosis have been associated with the expression of specific genetic abnormalities. The best-characterized changes have been in the p53 (chromosome 17p13) tumor-suppressor gene. P53 is the most commonly mutated gene in human cancer and is linked to control of cell cycling from G_1 to S phase. Oda and colleagues (329) studied both carcinomatous and high-grade sarcomatous portions of 14 sarcomatoid renal cancers by polymerase chain reaction, subcloning and sequencing the p53 gene. Sarcomatoid tumors had a high mutation rate for the p53 gene (78.6%), compared with a low p53 mutation rate (14.3%) in carcinomatous tumors. Immunohistochemical studies of p53 in these tumor types has demonstrated similar findings (196).

Thirty-seven percent of conventional renal cancers examined with dual-color fluorescence in situ hybridization had loss of chromosomes 14q (457). This loss was significantly correlated with higher stage, higher histologic grade, and worse patient outcome. Similar studies have shown loss of chromosome 14q correlated with higher nuclear grade and advanced tumor stage (379). Smaller studies have shown loss of genetic material on chromosome 2 (351) correlated with higher tumor stage and gain of chromosomes 12 and 20 (102) with higher nuclear grade. Increased expression of type IV collagenase in renal cancer cell lines from patients with metastatic renal cancer has correlated with shortened survival (445) Larger studies are required to corroborate these findings.

Loss and mutations of the VHL gene in all stages of conventional renal carcinoma, as well as in familial forms, indicates that the VHL gene is central to the origin of this tumor (154,259).

Papillary Renal Cell Carcinoma

The second most common cancer of the kidney is papillary renal cancer, accounting for 10% to 15% of renal neoplasms

(245,422). Papillary renal cancer has distinct morphologic and cytogenetic features that distinguish it from conventional (clear-cell) and chromophobe renal cancer (99, 245,422).

Papillary renal cancer is defined by the presence of at least 75% of the tumor composed of papillary or tubulopapillary architectural pattern (6,99,422). Papillary tumors are chromophilic, describing their characteristic uptake of dyes, and are subdivided into eosinophil, basophil, and duophil tumors (422). Basophilic tumors contain small cells with scanty amphophilic cytoplasm and small, low-grade nuclei (244,422). Eosinophilic tumors are characterized by large cells with abundant eosinophilic cytoplasm and large nuclei. Delahunt and Eble (99) proposed to classify papillary renal cancer into type I and type II, corresponding to chromophil-basophilic and chromophil-eosinophilic tumors (422).

Papillary renal cancer occurs more often in men, with a 5:1 to 8:1 preponderance (245,247). Basophilic papillary renal cancer occurs about twice as frequently as the eosinophil variant (99). The incidence of eosinophil papillary renal cancer is higher in patients with end-stage renal disease than in the general population (203,250). Survival rates for patients with all types of papillary renal cancer are higher than those for patients with conventional renal cancer (6,172,358).

Hereditary Papillary Renal Cancer

A hereditary form of basophilic papillary (type I) renal cancer has been described, characterized by multiple bilateral renal tumors inherited in an autosomal dominant fashion (376). The hereditary papillary renal cell carcinoma gene is the protooncogene, *c-met,* located on chromosome 7q31.1-34 (374). Missense mutations in the tyrosine kinase domain of the *c-met* gene have been identified in the germline of affected family members.

Sporadic Papillary Renal Cancer

Approximately 80% of sporadic papillary renal cancers contain multiple copies of genes. Trisomy or tetrasomy of chromosome 7 and trisomy of chromosome 17 have been found in 45% to 100% and in 64% to 100% of papillary renal cancers, respectively (27,101,203,246,462). Sporadic papillary renal carcinomas have been shown to contain mutations of the *c-met* gene (374,375). Introduction of mutant *c-met* will transform cells *in vitro* and is tumorigenic in nude mice (217), findings typical of a tumor oncogene. The chromosome 7 mutations have been observed in all stage and grade tumors, suggesting that *c-met* oncogene expression is an initial event in the development of basophilic papillary renal cancer. Early molecular events in eosinophilic papillary renal cancers are not well described, although there has been an associated with the 1:X translocation (221,390,454).

Trisomy of chromosome 17 may occur as a later abnormality (27,101). No p53 mutations have been reported in these tumors, suggesting that other genes in this chromosome are involved in tumor progression (78,101). Other DNA losses described include LOH on chromosomes 9p, 11q, 14q, 21q, and 6p in 43%, 43%, 37%, 37%, and 33% of the tumors, respectively (425). In addition, Y chromosome loss has been observed in 80% to 90% of papillary renal cancers from males (101,202,252).

Mutations in the *c-met* oncogene differentiate papillary renal tumors from conventional tumors on a genetic basis. Chromosome 3p and VHL gene abnormalities are not important in the development of this neoplasm (10, 132,425).

Chromophobe Renal Cell Carcinoma

Chromophobe renal cancer accounts for approximately 5% of renal neoplasms (90,422). Chromophobe renal cancer is characterized histologically by compact growth pattern of large polygonal cells with pale reticular cytoplasm and prominent cell membranes (423). Chromophobe cells often have numerous cytoplasmic vesicles by electron microscopic analysis (31,90). Compared with conventional renal cancer, these cells have low glycogen content. Another diagnostic finding in chromophobe renal cancer is lack of cytoplasmic staining with routine dyes. A diffuse, strong cytoplasmic staining with Hale's colloid iron stain has been suggested to be characteristic for chromophobe renal cancer (427). This tumor, however, may be composed of so-called eosinophilic chromophobe cells, which have a large number of mitochondria and few cytoplasmic vesicles (421). The presumed progenitor cells for chromophobe renal cancer are the intercalated cells of the collecting duct (337,420).

Five-year survival has been reported as 92% for chromophobe and 62% for conventional renal cancer of equal nuclear grade (423). Other studies, however, demonstrated similar 5-year survival rates between chromophobe and conventional renal cancers of nuclear grade II and Robson clinical stage I (85% and 84%, respectively), perhaps because most chromophobe renal cancers were stage I (86%) or were discovered incidentally (53%) (90).

Karyotypic changes in chromophobe renal cancers included monosomies of chromosomes 1, 2, 6, 10, 13, and 17 (211,242,251). Molecular genetic studies have confirmed these findings, with loss in 54% to 95% of tumors (50,382,398). Chromosome 3p loss of heterozygosity was observed in 25% of chromophobe tumors, with only rare mutations in the VHL gene (227,389).

Mutations in the p53 gene were identified in 30% of chromophobe renal cancers studied, whereas LOH on chromosome 17p was detected in 78% of tumors. The lack of correlation of p53 mutations with LOH suggested the presence of a second genetic abnormality on chromosome 17 (78).

No genetic change has been observed to occur in all tumor nuclear grades or clinical or pathologic stages, suggesting the initial genetic occurrence characteristic of this tumor type.

Collecting Duct Carcinoma (Bellini Duct Carcinoma)

Collecting duct carcinoma (CDC) makes up approximately 0.4% to 2.6% of renal cancers (243,406,462) and is thought to arise from the medullary collecting ducts (420). Collecting duct carcinomas are usually centrally located, arising in the renal medulla, are white-gray in color, and demonstrate a tubulopapillary growth pattern and a microcystic and solid pattern. Microscopic findings are high-grade cytologic atypia and stromal desmoplasia with dysplastic changes in the neighboring medullary renal tubules. Strong positivity for intracytoplasmic mucin is seen on appropriate stains (228). Collecting duct cancer may be more aggressive in clinical behavior than other renal cancers (14,103). Local invasion or lymph node metastases are common (228).

Few chromosomal studies have been performed on CDC. The most frequently described karyotypic abnormalities have been monosomy of chromosomes 18, 21, and Y (57,165). Other findings include gain of chromosomes 7, 12, 17, and 20. Loss of heterozygosity has been found on chromosome 1q in 57% to 69% of CDC, especially in the region of 1q32 (346,405). LOH has also been detected on chromosomes 8p (48%), 6p (45%), 21q (40%), and 13q (50%). Forty-five percent of tumors have amplification of the oncogene *c-erbB* (383). All patients with this finding died within 1 year, whereas half of patients without amplification were alive after a mean follow-up of 42 months (383).

Renal medullary carcinoma (RMC) may be a variant of CDC (243,406) first described by Davis and colleagues (93) in 1995. RMC has been reported only in African-American patients with sickle cell trait or hemoglobin–sickle cell disease (92,93). Karyotypic findings were loss of chromosome 11 in four of six tumors examined (13). This finding is noteworthy for the presence of the β-globin gene on chromosome 11p (97).

Renal medullary cancer manifests in the second or third decade of life, usually with metastatic disease (92,93). Mean patient survival has been reported as 3.5 months after diagnosis (135,194).

Mean tumor size at presentation has been 7 cm in diameter, located primarily in the renal medulla (92,93). There is a characteristic infiltrative growth pattern (92) with peripheral satellite tumors in the renal cortex and venous and lymphatic invasion. RMC demonstrated a reticular, yolk sac–like, or adenoid cystic appearance, frequently with poorly differentiated areas in a highly desmoplastic stroma.

Renal Oncocytoma

Renal oncocytomas make up 3% to 5% of renal tumors and are thought to originate from the distal renal tubule (7,420). Renal oncocytomas are predominantly composed of eosinophilic cells arranged in a characteristic nested or organoid fashion (7,341). Oncocytomas are usually well circumscribed, beige or mahogany brown tumors that lack areas of necrosis. A gross or microscopic central scar may be present. Renal oncocytomas have nuclei that are round with uniform contours. About half of tumors have prominent nucleoli. A high content of cytoplasmic mitochondria is characteristic of oncocytoma (115). Renal oncocytoma lack significant necrosis, mitosis, or conspicuous papillary formations (7). The eosinophilic (granular) cytoplasm of oncocytomas may appear similar to that found in other renal neoplasms such as chromophobe, conventional, and papillary renal cancer (341). Typical renal oncocytomas are considered a benign neoplasm (7,304,406).

Three types of genetic abnormalities of oncocytoma have been observed: (a) numerical anomalies, including loss of chromosomes Y and 1 (46,188,426); (b) translocations involving the breakpoint region 11q13 [t(5;11)(q35;q13) and t(9;11)(p23;q13)] (323,393); and (c) a variety of other genetic abnormalities, including chromosomal monosomies (164), trisomy 1, 7, 12, and 14 (434), and loss of heterozygosity of chromosomes 17p, 17q, 10q, and 3p (414). Genetic abnormalities in patients with hereditary forms of renal oncocytoma have not been described (453) (Fig. 7.3).

Papillary Adenoma

The most common renal neoplasm is papillary adenoma, occurring in as many as 20% of patients (166). Papillary adenomas are solid-tubular-papillary structures consisting of small "blue" cells (basophilic) or large eosinophilic cells, similar to low-grade papillary renal cancers. Papillary adenomas are usually less than 5 mm in diameter (246,406). There are no cytologic criteria to distinguish papillary adenomas from small papillary renal cancers, suggesting that papillary adenoma could represent early papillary renal cancer (45). Genetic findings are trisomy or tetrasomy 7, trisomy 17, and loss of the Y chromosome (246,249).

Metanephric Adenoma

Renal metanephric adenomas are rare, benign, well-circumscribed tumors that may represent the benign counterpart of Wilms' tumor (143,356). Histologically, metanephric adenomas are composed of uniformly small epithelial cells forming tubules or tubulopapillary structures. They are characterized by an unusual degree of cell

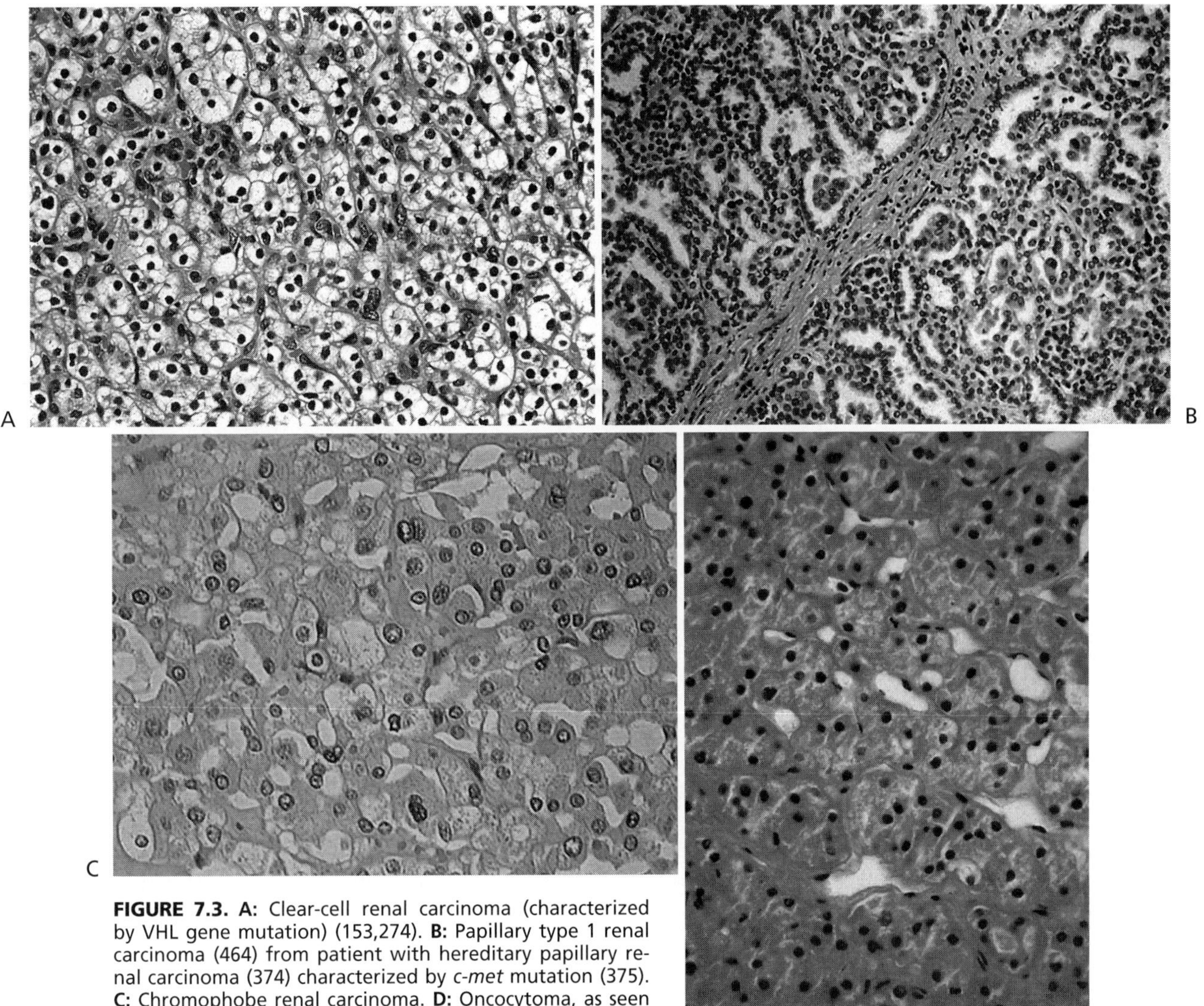

FIGURE 7.3. A: Clear-cell renal carcinoma (characterized by VHL gene mutation) (153,274). **B:** Papillary type 1 renal carcinoma (464) from patient with hereditary papillary renal carcinoma (374) characterized by *c-met* mutation (375). **C:** Chromophobe renal carcinoma. **D:** Oncocytoma, as seen in patients affected with Birt-Hogg-Dubé syndrome (428).

maturation and differentiation. Rosette-like configurations with no evidence of necrosis or cellular atypia can be present. The cell nuclei are oval, smooth, and without mitosis. Only rare cytogenetic studies have been reported (143,356).

OVERVIEW

The initial genetic changes important for the development of each histologic tumor subtype appear to be unique to each tumor type and may be useful in molecular diagnosis of renal tumors or their metastases (Table 7.2). Characterization of these genetic anomalies will allow more accurate diagnosis and prognostic evaluation and may help in planning therapy. The identification of familial forms of these tumors is an important tool in the identification of hereditary forms of renal cancer. Identification of germline mutations in these families allows earlier diagnosis with an associated wider range of treatment options. The identification of secondary genetic markers, such as mutations of p53, duplication of chromosome 5q22, loss of chromosome 14q, and overexpression of collagenase type IV, will contribute to prognostic planning of individual patients' tumors in the future.

CLINICAL MANAGEMENT OF HEREDITARY RENAL CANCER

Types of Hereditary Renal Cancer

The best-characterized form of hereditary renal cancer is von Hippel–Lindau disease (VHL). VHL is an autosomal dominant inherited disorder caused by a defect in the VHL gene, located on chromosome 3p25, resulting in the development of clear-cell tumors (259). Mutations in the VHL

TABLE 7.2. COMMON GENETIC FINDINGS IN PATHOLOGIC SUBTYPES OF RENAL TUMORS

Pathologic Subtype Findings	Initial Findings	Later Findings
Conventional (clear-cell) carcinoma	3p LOH VHL gene mutation	+5q −8p, −9p, −14q p53 mutation C-erbB-1 oncogene expression
Papillary renal carcinoma	+7, +17 −Y Met gene mutation	+12, +16, +20 −9p, −11q, −14q, −17p, −21q PRCC-TFE3 gene fusion
Chromophobe renal carcinoma	−1	−1p, −2p, −6p, −13q, −21q, −Y p53 mutation
Collecting duct carcinoma	−18, −Y	−1q, −6p, −8p, −11, −13q, −21q C-erbB-1 oncogene expression
Oncocytoma	−1, −Y, 11q rearrangement*	
Papillary adenoma	+7, +17 −Y	—

Genetic findings and pathologic subtypes of renal tumors. Common genetic abnormalities, or abnormalities not associated with stage, were assumed to occur early. Other abnormalities were assumed to occur later, possibly associated with progression. −, Loss of chromosomal segment; +, gain of chromosomal segment; LOH, loss of heterozygosity. Unclassified renal cell carcinoma and metanephric adenoma are not characterized sufficiently to identify common genetic abnormalities.
*Not enough data to assign abnormality as an early or late event.

gene predispose patients to develop retinal angiomas, central nervous system hemangioblastomas, endolymphatic sac tumors, renal cysts and cancers, pancreatic cysts and islet cell tumors, pheochromocytomas, and epididymal cystadenomas (32,257,295,447). Patients with VHL demonstrate variable clinical penetrance of these tumors.

From 24% to 45% of patients with VHL have been reported to develop renal cell carcinoma (64,257,292). However, of patients in the 60- to 70-year-old age group, 90% to 95% develop cystic or solid renal lesions (64). Affected patients with VHL usually develop multiple, bilateral clear-cell renal tumors and can develop new tumors over the course of their life. Patients develop VHL and renal cancer at a mean age of 39 years, 10 to 20 years younger than patients with sporadic renal cancer (151) (Fig. 7.4).

A hereditary form of basophilic papillary renal cancer (type 1) has been also been described. Hereditary papillary renal cancer (HPRC) is inherited in an autosomal dominant fashion and, like all other forms of hereditary renal tumors, is characterized by multiple, bilateral renal tumors. Other associated tumors are not known to occur in patients with HPRC. HPRC is caused by germline mutations in the *met* gene, located on chromosome 7q31 (463,464).

Familial renal oncocytoma (FRO) is characterized by multifocal, bilateral renal oncocytoma (453). Few FRO families have been identified, and the clinical manifestations of this entity are not well characterized. Familial linkage and tumor loss of heterozygosity studies have not suggested the location of a responsible gene. Affected patients have a lifelong risk of recurrent tumors (453).

BHD comprises characteristic skin lesions (fibrofolliculomas), renal tumors, and pulmonary cysts predisposing patients to spontaneous pneumothorax. Renal tumors in BHD are usually chromophobe tumors. A unique aspect of this form of hereditary renal tumor syndrome is the development of other histologic tumor types, although at a low frequency (428).

Treatment Options in Patients with Hereditary Renal Cancer

Patients with hereditary forms of renal cancer are predisposed to develop multiple bilateral renal tumors over the course of their lives. Although radical nephrectomy will cure patients with localized disease, there are quality-of-life issues associated with renal replacement therapy. The largest experience in treating patients with hereditary renal cancer is in patients with clear-cell renal cancer associated with VHL. Management approaches used in VHL patients with renal tumors have ranged from observation to bilateral nephrectomy with renal replacement therapy to renal-sparing operations (80,137,155,200,327,339).

Although observation of patients with renal cancer is not traditionally recommended, there is historical experience with this approach. In the era before the use of abdominal computed tomography imaging, patients were followed with intravenous pyelogram (IVP) imaging studies. IVP

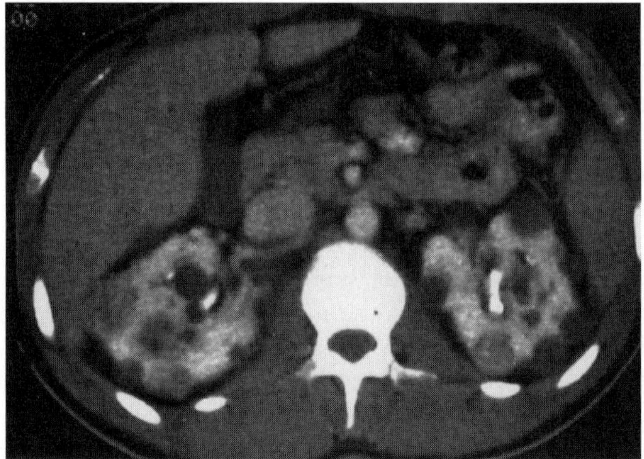

FIGURE 7.4. Abdominal computed tomography of renal masses in a patient with Von Hippel–Lindau disease.

studies do not detect small tumors and even some larger tumors. During this era, 23% to 45% of patients with VHL were reported to develop renal cell carcinoma, similar to recent reports, and about one-third of these patients died of metastatic disease (70,126,151,257).

A second approach has been to perform bilateral nephrectomy, removing all renal tumors and their associated risk of metastases (80,155,200). Unfortunately, there is little experience in treating VHL patients with renal replacement therapy. Survival of non-VHL patients managed with dialysis or transplant is only 65% at 2 years (1). Similar treatments of small groups of patients with VHL have had a similar outcome (343). Some transplant centers, however, consider the presence of or potential for VHL-related tumors (renal and extrarenal) a contraindication for renal transplantation.

A third treatment option is renal parenchymal-sparing surgery. Patients with hereditary forms of renal tumors have been predicted to have hundreds or thousands of microscopic tumors present in the normal renal parenchyma (336,446). Surgery in these patients is not thought of as being curative, but rather as "resetting the clock" until small microscopic tumors grow to become clinically detectable. The decision of when to operate can be somewhat arbitrary in these patients.

In patients with sporadic renal tumors, the risk of metastases has been correlated with size of the primary tumor (22,116,133). Small renal cancers were even historically termed *adenomas* to emphasize their benign clinical course (26). Based on these observations, the management of patients with hereditary renal cancer has evolved to use size criteria as an indication for surgery. A French group follows renal tumors in patients with VHL until they reach 2.5 cm in diameter before recommending surgery (63,72); the National Cancer Institute (NCI) group uses 3 cm (193); and a German group uses 6 cm (324).

The large numbers of tumors that are often present in these patients do not allow traditional partial nephrectomy with margin of 1 cm or more of normal renal tissue. Rather, simple enucleation is used to remove the many tumors present (448). Small tumors are easily removed by this technique, but even tumors larger than 3 cm in diameter have been managed in this fashion. The NCI has reported the largest follow-up of patients with VHL treated in this fashion (193).

At the NCI, VHL patients with solid renal tumors were followed with serial imaging studies until the largest solid tumor reached 3 cm in size. At that time, surgery was recommended to remove all solid lesions and all accessible cystic lesions in the kidney. Renal cystic disease was not included in a patient's evaluation for surgery. In addition, the cystic component of solid renal masses was subtracted out when measuring tumor growth toward the 3-cm cutoff.

VHL patients with renal tumors less than 3 cm in diameter followed for a median of 60 months did not develop metastases or require renal replacement therapy (443). VHL patients with larger renal tumors had a risk of developing metastases related to tumor size (Table 7.3) (443). Similar management strategy has been used in patients with other hereditary forms of renal cancer.

TABLE 7.3. COMPARISON OF TUMOR SIZE AND THE DEVELOPMENT OF METASTASES IN PATIENTS WITH VHL

Frequency of Metastases	Tumor Diameter (cm)
0/52 (0%)	≤3.0
1/17 (6%)	3.2–4.0
2/10 (20%)	4.1–5.5
4/12 (33%)	6.0–10.0
4/5 (80%)	≥11.0

Comparison of tumor size and the development of metastases in patients with von Hippel–Lindau (VHL). VHL patients with renal tumors larger than 3 cm had an increased risk of developing metastases with increasing tumor size.

Planning Surgery in Patients with Hereditary Renal Cancer

Patients with VHL develop multiple tumor types, which can cause problems during an operation. Pheochromocytoma can be associated with hypertensive crisis, retinal angioma can bleed during periods of hypertension or with the use of anticoagulation, and central nervous system (CNS) hemangioblastomas can be at risk for bleeding or CNS herniation. Preoperative evaluation of all VHL manifestations is performed to identify tumors in the brain, eye, pancreas, and adrenal. CNS tumors may require treatment before abdominal surgery can be safely performed. Medical blockade of pheochromocytoma is necessary before surgery. Once the patient is cleared for abdominal surgery, a multispecialty approach can allow simultaneous treatment of renal, adrenal, and pancreatic tumors.

Renal angiography has not been helpful for diagnosis of renal tumors, with identification of only 16% of the multiple, small renal tumors present (308). Renal angiography is helpful in defining renal arterial anatomy, including small polar branches, which could be damaged during initial or repeat renal operations.

The multiple tumors found in patients with hereditary renal cancer syndromes do not allow partial nephrectomy with a wide resection of normal tissue around each tumor. Pathologic evaluation of renal tumors in patients with VHL consistently reveals a fibrous pseudocapsule margin (349). The multiple renal tumors and fibrous pseudocapsule lend these tumors well to enucleation (448). Patients with other hereditary tumor syndromes have been well managed with similar surgical treatment (193).

Patients with VHL also develop multiple simple and complex renal cysts. Although these lesions behave in a benign fashion, microscopic examination reveals that at least 21% contain foci of renal cell carcinoma (349). Based on these findings, surgical removal of cystic lesions has been recommended when extensive injury of normal renal parenchyma is not necessary to remove the cysts.

Color Doppler intraoperative ultrasound has been an important contribution to the management of patients with hereditary renal cancer. Additional tumors were found in 25% of patients with intraoperative ultrasound, contributing to a more thorough evaluation and treatment of each kidney (71).

Results of Surgery in Patients with Hereditary Renal Cancer

The largest single-institution experience treating patients with hereditary renal cancer is at the NCI. There, 28 men and 22 women were reported undergoing a total of 71 surgical procedures (193). Affected patients were identified by screening affected families. Sixty-eight patients had pathologic stage T_1, one had stage T_2, and two had stage T_{3b}. Two patients with pathologic stage T_1 renal cancer had tumor thrombus in minor renal veins. No patient had lymph node or other metastases.

Fifty-three kidneys were treated with enucleation, five with partial nephrectomy, six with enucleation plus partial nephrectomy, and nine with nephrectomy. Patients underwent a median of one renal operation (range of one to four). During a median overall follow-up of 80 months, eight kidneys underwent repeat renal parenchymal-sparing surgery a median of 31 months after the first operation. Forty percent of renal parenchymal-sparing operations were performed with cold renal ischemia (Table 7.4). Eight patients with VHL underwent resection of VHL-associated tumors at the same time, including enucleation of pancreatic neuroendocrine tumors (n = 4), bilateral adrenalectomy for pheochromocytoma (n = 2), and unilateral adrenalectomy for pheochromocytoma (n = 2). The most notable complications were renal atrophy in 3 of 65 kidneys (4.6%) treated with renal parenchymal-sparing surgery and a single intraoperative myocardial infarction resulting in postoperative death. Urinary leakage persisting longer than 30 days occurred in three patients. Similar complications have been encountered in previous series, with the exception of renal failure, which was lower in the NCI series (64,403). No patient in the NCI series treated with renal parenchymal-sparing surgery has required dialysis. Thirty-five percent of kidneys undergoing renal parenchymal-sparing surgery developed a recurrence during the 80-month follow-up.

TABLE 7.4. THE NCI RENAL PARENCHYMAL-SPARING SURGICAL EXPERIENCE IN PATIENTS WITH HEREDITARY FORMS OF RENAL CELL CARCINOMA

Surgical Characteristics			
Parameter	N	Mean	Range
Lesions resected per kidney	65	14.7 ± 1.3 lesions	1–51 lesions
Cold renal ischemic time	26	51.1 ± 5.6 minutes	10–120 min
Operative time	71	354.5 ± 19.0 minutes	117–830 min
Estimated blood loss	71	2885.1 ± 494.5 mL	150–23,000 mL
Blood units transfused	71	4.3 ± 0.9 units	0–34 units

The use of nephrectomy was reduced in the NCI experience. Seven nephrectomies were performed in the first 5 years, with only two in the second 5 years (444). The use of nephrectomy in this series was lower than previously reported (12% versus 26%) in multiinstitutional reports, even accounting for differences in stage (403). This lower rate of nephrectomy may be related to the broad use of the enucleation technique, regardless of number of tumors or location of renal tumors.

Follow-up After Renal Parenchymal-sparing Surgery

Among 65 kidneys managed primarily using enucleation techniques, 35% developed recurrent tumors during 80 months of follow-up, similar to previous studies (403). This high recurrence rate is not surprising, because there are reports of many microscopic tumors in normal renal parenchyma of VHL and HPRC patients (336,446). Evaluation of normal VHL renal tissue predicts 600 microscopic clear-cell renal tumors and 1,100 clear-cell cysts in the average VHL kidney undergoing surgery. Similar evaluation of HPRC patients predicts 3,400 microscopic papillary renal tumors per kidney. These findings support the strategy of watching renal tumors grow to a predetermined size because renal surgery in these patients is not curative in the traditional sense. They also emphasize the need to search for the smallest tumors present during exploration to best treat these patients. Intraoperative ultrasound has been extremely useful for maximizing the number of lesions identified at the time of surgery (71,444). Disease-specific survival in these patients was excellent and may reflect the early detection of small tumors by periodic screening.

The treatment strategy applied to these patients with hereditary renal tumor syndromes is not curative, but is designed to "reset the clock" relative to the time required for microscopic tumors to grow to a size at which they present a significant metastatic risk. This management approach balances the goals of minimizing the risk of renal cell carcinoma metastasis while preserving renal function. Additionally, this approach attempts to minimize the total number of surgeries a patient will require in a lifetime.

MOLECULAR GENETICS OF PROSTATE CANCER

Despite significant improvements in early detection and local curative therapies, carcinoma of the prostate remains a major public health issue. Prostate cancer is now the most common noncutaneous malignancy in the United States and is the cause of more cancer-related deaths in men than any human malignancy other than lung cancer (162). Because of this, we must strive to improve the accuracy of diagnostic tests and prognostic measures. We must improve efficacy while reducing morbidity of local therapies, and we must devise methods to effectively prevent or treat hormone-refractory prostate cancer. A better understanding of the underlying molecular genetic events responsible for prostate cancer initiation and progression will enhance our chances for achieving these goals. This basic knowledge should allow us to develop better diagnostic tests that will eliminate false-positive results of prostate-specific antigen (PSA) screening. In the future, molecular pathology should also be able to accurately distinguish between "clinically indolent" and potentially lethal prostate cancers so that aggressive treatment is prescribed only to those who require it. We should be able to use this knowledge to design therapies that prevent progression of androgen-dependent to androgen-independent disease. Ultimately, we should be able to custom design effective treatments and prevention strategies based on a man's specific genetic makeup, the molecular abnormalities of his tumor, or both.

Currently, our understanding of the molecular genetics of prostate cancer is in its infancy. There is compelling evidence that a small proportion of prostate cancers (approximately 10%) is inherited but that the remaining 90% is caused by a complex interplay between environmental factors and somatic genetic molecular events (56). Several known tumor-suppressor genes (TSGs) are thought to play a role in a subset of prostate cancers, and alterations in various oncogenes, growth factors, and apoptotic pathways have been implicated as well. Recent advances in molecular technology that enable accurate, high-throughput analysis of genomic structure, as well as gene expression profiles, will almost certainly facilitate efforts to understand prostate cancer biology. This section reviews what we currently know about potential genomic and somatic events that may be responsible for prostate cancer development and then discusses the application of genomics and proteomics to prostate cancer investigation.

Hereditary Prostate Cancer

Several epidemiologic studies have demonstrated a familial clustering of a subset of prostate cancer cases, and some investigators have suggested that patterns of affected men can be explained by dominant inheritance of a rare high-risk allele (55,56,169,404). Studies suggest that hereditary cases account for 40% of cases of early-onset prostate cancer (i.e., age less than 55 years) but only 9% of other cases (56,168). There is a familial aggregation of prostate cancer, and an individual man's risk increases with the number of affected family members. Prostate cancer risk is increased twofold to threefold for men with one affected first-degree relative and elevenfold for men with three affected first-degree relatives (442).

TABLE 7.5. HEREDITARY PROSTATE CANCER SUSCEPTIBILITY LOCI

Chromosomal Band	Locus
1q24-25	HPC1
1q42-43	PCAP
Xq27-18	HPCX
1p36	CAPB

To date, linkage analysis has identified four separate prostate cancer susceptibility loci (HPC1 on 1q24-25, PCAP on 1q42-43, CAPB on 1p36, and HPC on Xq27-28) (Table 7.5) (30,146,395,459). Positional cloning efforts are currently underway to identify these specific genes. Although it appears that each one of the genes will only be responsible for a subset of hereditary prostate cancers, their identification will provide important information regarding the underlying biologic mechanism of prostate cancer development.

Genetic Polymorphisms

It has been estimated that 1 in every 300 to 500 bases in the human genome is a single nucleotide polymorphism and that some of these single-base pair differences may alter protein function, contributing directly to a trait or disease phenotype (77). One of the must highly characterized polymorphisms in prostate cancer is within a gene in the chromosomal Xq11-12 region encoding the androgen receptor. Androgen responsiveness of prostate cancer is well documented, and circulating androgens are necessary for prostate cancer development (96). It has been suggested that the length of the highly polymorphic region of the CAG repeat coding for the polyglutamine chain in the androgen receptor inversely correlates with an individual's prostate cancer risk (147,378,401). Data from two separate large, population-based, case-controlled studies have demonstrated this relationship. In the Physicians Health Study, men with an androgen-receptor CAG repeat length of less than 18 had a 50% increased risk of developing prostate cancer compared with those men with CAG repeat lengths greater than 26 (147). A study using a population identified from the Surveillance, Epidemiology, and End Results (SEER) program showed that men with two short repeat lengths (CAG less than 22 and GGN less than 16) had a twofold higher prostate cancer risk than men with longer repeat lengths (401). Epidemiologic studies of CAG repeat lengths in different racial populations support these findings. That is, African-American men (the racial group with the highest prostate cancer incidence) have on average the shortest CAG repeat length, whereas Asian-American men (the racial group with the lowest prostate cancer incidence) have on average the longest CAG repeat length. Caucasians as a group have an intermediate prostate cancer incidence and have an intermediate CAG repeat length (73,368). Studies have also shown that among prostate cancer patients, those with shorter CAG repeat lengths are more likely to develop prostate cancer at a younger age (180) and are more likely to have aggressive prostate cancer with unfavorable pathologic features compared to those with longer CAG repeats (147). The underlying biologic mechanism for this relationship is not known. *In vitro* studies have demonstrated that transactivation of the androgen receptor is inversely related to its polyglutamine length, and some have hypothesized that increased androgen responsiveness predisposes prostate epithelium to malignant transformation. More study is needed to determine whether a short polyglutamine length directly increases prostate cancer risk or is merely associated with this phenotype.

There is epidemiologic evidence suggesting that decreased vitamin D levels, either from reduced exposure to sunlight or conversion of 7-dehydrocholestrol to vitamin D, may predispose to prostate cancer development (81,179). Several *in vitro* studies have also suggested that vitamin D may act as a tumor inhibitor for prostate cancer. Interestingly, different polymorphisms in the vitamin D receptor gene have been reported to be associated with either an increased or a decreased prostate cancer risk (176,208).

Other potentially important genetic polymorphisms associated with prostate cancer development have been observed in members of the glutathione S-transferase family. It has been shown that a single nucleotide polymorphism (SNP) in the glutathione S-transferase Pi gene, resulting in an amino acid change, alters prostate cancer risk by an odds ratio of 0.4 (182). In addition to SNPs, homozygous deletions within the human genome are also commonly observed (354). One of these, at the glutathione S-transferase-0 (GSTT1) locus on chromosome 22q11.2, occurs in 20% to 30% of Caucasian men in the United States. Studies have shown that men who do not have a homozygous deletion at GSTT1 are at increased risk of developing prostate cancer (354).

In the near future, molecular epidemiologic studies will define many more genetic polymorphisms that either predispose to or protect from the development of prostate cancer. It is likely that a man's prostate cancer risk will ultimately be determined by a panel of different genetic polymorphisms and that this information will be critical for designing and executing effective prostate cancer prevention strategies.

Chromosomal Abnormalities

Alterations in chromosomal number and structure are common findings in all human cancers. Cytogenetic studies of prostate cancer have demonstrated alterations on multiple different chromosomes, but the most common finding is loss or rearrangement of sequences on the short arm of chromosome 8 and gain of sequences on the long arm of chromosome 8 (67,290,438). In fact, studies have shown that 8p loss and 8q gain are associated with more aggressive disease (437). PSCA and c-*myc* are two genes located on 8q whose amplification may play a role in prostate cancer progression. The responsible genes on 8p have yet to be determined. Microsatellite-based LOH analysis is a powerful molecular tool used to define regions of genetic loss in attempts to discover TSGs. LOH studies of nonmetastatic prostate cancer revealed a deletion frequency of as high as 86% on the short arm of chromosome 8 and have suggested the presence of at least three separate TSGs located on this chromosome (438). Chromosomal bands 8p21-12, 8p22, 8p23, and 8q12-13 are regions with high rates of LOH (28,342,438). LOH at chromosomal bands 13q, 6q, 16q, 18q, 9p, and 7q31 have been observed less frequently (260,437).

Researchers have found a homozygous deletion in a metastatic tumor focus that maps to 12p12-13, suggesting that there is a prostate cancer metastasis suppressor gene in this region (230). One intriguing candidate gene in this region is p27. This gene encodes a cyclin kinase inhibitor that induces cell cycle arrest in the G_1 phase. This mechanism prevents DNA replication in cells with substantial DNA damage (15). Several studies have shown that reduced levels of p27 are associated with aggressive and metastatic prostate cancers (84,174,460). Other studies have shown that LOH at 8p22 is a common finding in metastatic prostate cancer, suggesting that this region also contains a metastasis suppressor gene (269).

Contemporary scientific data suggest that there are multiple genes responsible for development and progression of prostate cancer and that multiple different genetic pathways for this common human malignancy exist. Defining any of these genetic defects will provide researchers tremendously important insight into the underlying biology of prostate cancer. Examples of some potential candidate genes on chromosome band 8p include FEZ1 (212), NKX3.1 (185), N33 (429), and Dematin (286), among many others. Currently, efforts to determine which genes have tumor-suppressor function in prostate cancer now focus on further defining areas of minimal deletion and sequence analysis of candidate genes within regions of high LOH.

Promoter Methylation

Methylation of cytosine bases in CpG-rich promoter regions is an important mechanism to regulate tissue-specific gene expression. Alterations in methylation patterns are commonly observed in multiple different human malignancies. Reduction in gene expression can be the result of promoter hypermethylation, whereas promoter hypometh-

TABLE 7.6. GENES WHOSE EXPRESSION IS ALTERED BY METHYLATION IN PROSTATE CANCER

GSTP1	E-cadherin
CD44	Endothelin B
P16	Androgen receptor
PTEN	Loci D17S5 on 17p

ylation can cause increases in gene expression. In fact, extensive methylation of the glutathione S-transferase Pi (GSTP1) promoter region is the most common somatic genomic alteration described in prostate cancer to date (265). Immunohistochemical analysis of GSTP1 expression has demonstrated that promoter methylation does in fact correlate with reduced protein expression. Studies of radical prostatectomy specimens have demonstrated loss of GSTP1 expression in the vast majority of invasive prostatic carcinomas and high-grade prostatic intraepithelial neoplasia lesions (44). Researchers have proposed that because GSTP1 functions as a detoxification enzyme, loss of GSTP1 activity can predispose prostate cells to accumulate damaged DNA, leading to malignant transformation. If loss of GSTP1 is an important event leading to prostate carcinogenesis, medication or dietary supplements with detoxification functions may be effective prostate cancer prevention strategies.

It appears that prostate cancer is associated with methylation changes within promoter regions of several other genes as well (Table 7.6). For example, it has been shown that hypermethylation of the CD44 promoter region is a common finding in high-grade localized and metastatic human prostate cancer (284). CD44 is a transmembrane glycoprotein involved in cell-cell and cell-matrix interactions that suppresses metastasis in a highly metastatic prostate cancer model (Dunning rat) (142). Hypermethylation of the p16/CDKN2 gene, which encodes an inhibitor of cyclin-dependent kinase 4, has been observed in a limited number of prostate cancers (189,190,305). It has been shown that inactivation of the p16/Rb pathway can result in cellular immortalization (215). Methylation of the endothelin B receptor gene in prostate cancer has also been reported, and it has been suggested that this event may be responsible for endothelin-1 secretion (215). It has been shown that exposing androgen receptor–negative prostate cancer cell lines to a demethylating agent increases androgen receptor expression. It has been suggested that promoter methylation may be a cause of heterogeneous androgen receptor expression observed with hormone-refractory prostate cancer (214). It is clear that altered promoter methylation of a variety of genes is a common event in prostate cancer, but it remains to be seen which gene alterations are responsible for prostate cancer development and progression and which merely are associated with the malignant phenotype.

Tumor-suppressor Genes

A tumor-suppressor gene responsible for early prostate cancer development has yet to be discovered. However, there are several known TSGs that may play a role in prostate cancer progression. The gene for PTEN maps to chromosomal band 10q23.3. The protein product of the PTEN gene is a dual-specific phosphatase with documented tumor-suppressor function in some cultured cells and nude mice (141). Within cancerous prostate cells, PTEN can be inactivated by multiple different mechanisms, including genomic deletions, point mutation, and hypermethylation (53,161, 409,450). In general, PTEN inactivation is far more common among high-grade or advanced prostate cancers than in lower-grade and earlier-stage disease (105,161). In fact, the vast majority of PTEN mutations have been found in patients without organ-confined prostate cancer (105, 161). Collectively, these data suggest that PTEN may be an important metastasis-suppressor gene, but it probably does not play an important role in prostate cancer initiation.

Likewise, p53 mutations are far more common in high-grade metastatic prostate cancer than in earlier lesions (110,307). Clinical studies have shown that the presence of p53 mutations in prostate cancer correlates with poorer cure rates for both radiotherapy and radical prostatectomy (65,66,320).

The WAF1 gene is the primary target of the transcription activation by P53 and is also an important regulator of cell cycle kinetics (111). P21, the product of the WAF1 gene, inhibits the activity of cyclin E and cyclin D, which prevent cells from entering the S phase of the cell cycle (181). A few small preliminary studies suggest that overexpression of the P21 or cyclin D1 protein is associated with higher tumor grade and adverse clinical outcome (2,365).

Growth Factors

Alterations in a variety of growth factors and their receptors have been implicated in prostate cancer growth and progression. Among the most widely studied growth factor in prostate cancer are members of the epidermal growth factor family, epidermal growth factor (EGF) and TGF-α. Within normal prostates, EGF expression is restricted to stromal cells (134), and epidermal growth factor receptor (EGFR) expression is restricted to basal cells of prostatic epithelium (305). Immunohistochemical analysis of benign prostatic hyperplasia demonstrates overexpression of EGF in hyperplastic glands. In contrast, immunohistochemistry has demonstrated that both EGF and EGFR levels are upregulated in malignant prostate epithelium (95). Studies of prostate cancer cells suggest that EGF and TGF-α play a role in upregulation of EGFR mRNA and protein (384). Furthermore, there is evidence that a variant EGFR (EGFRvIII), lacking the external domain of the native receptor, is overexpressed in prostate cancer cells, and that aberrant expression of EGFRvIII is associated with more aggressive disease

(330). Collectively, these studies suggest that autocrine expression of EGF and TGF-α signaling through the EGFR may contribute to the autonomous growth and invasiveness of human prostate cancer cells (231).

The HER-2/neu (erbB-2) gene encodes for another tyrosine growth factor receptor that is a member of the EGFR family. Interestingly, gains in genomic content of the HER-2/neu gene are observed in 40% to 60% of high-grade prostate cancers (361,381). It has been demonstrated that overexpression of HER-2/neu restores androgen-receptor functions in androgen-independent prostate cancer xenograft model (88).

Overexpression of several fibroblast growth factor (FGF) family members has been associated with prostate cancer progression. Studies have shown that FGF8 mRNA expression is increased in prostate cancer (266) and that overexpression correlates with higher Gleason grade and advanced tumor stage (106). Overexpression of growth factors by prostatic stromal cells may also play a role in prostate cancer progression. For example, expression of FGF2 is restricted to stromal fibroblasts and endothelial cells, and expression levels are greatly enhanced within cancerous glands (148). Interestingly, the receptor for FGF2 is overexpressed in malignant prostate epithelium (148).

Insulin growth factor (IGF) may also play a role in prostate cancer development and progression. IGF-II mRNA is expressed by some prostate cancer cells, and it has been suggested that it may function as an autocrine growth factor (167). All studies have suggested that alteration in the IGF binding proteins may alter bioavailability of IGF and play a role in prostate cancer progression (125). Results of a large retrospective study demonstrated a correlation between higher serum IGF levels and increased prostate cancer risk (61). In this study, men with serum IGF levels in the highest quartile had a 2.4 times greater chance of being diagnosed with prostate cancer compared with age-matched men with lower IGF levels. Prospective studies are needed to determine whether elevated serum IGF levels predispose to prostate cancer development and whether lower serum IGF levels could be an effective prostate cancer prevention strategy.

Other growth factors that have been implicated to play a role in prostate cancer include transforming growth factor-β (TGF-β) (54), hepatocyte growth factor (HGF) (326), nerve growth factor (NGF) (9,397), bone morphogenetic proteins (BMPs) (12,207,424), and platelet-derived growth factor (PDGF) (394), among others. The role of TGF-β in prostate cancer is not entirely clear, because TGF-β inhibits prostate cancer growth *in vitro* (407) but promotes growth and metastasis *in vivo* (18). This paradoxic response may be explained by data suggesting that prostate cancer cells downregulate TGF-β receptors so that increased expression of TGF-β induces host effects that facilitate cancer progression and metastasis (173). Among the metastasis-promoting effects attributed to TGF-β are immunosuppression, angiogenesis, and extracellular matrix deposition (455). HGF ("scatter factor") is secreted almost exclusively by prostatic stromal cells and binds to the product of the *c-met* protooncogene expressed on prostate epithelium (205). Preliminary data suggest that expression of *c-met* is elevated in prostate cancer and increases with increasing grade, thereby enhancing mobility and cellular scattering (344). BMP and NGF have been implicated in development of bony metastasis and hormone-independent growth, respectively (12,91).

The realization that alterations in growth factors and growth factor receptors may play a role in prostate cancer progression has led to development of novel therapeutic strategies. A recombinant anti–HER-2/neu antibody (Herceptin) that inhibits growth of breast cancer cells that overexpress HER-2/neu has been developed (122,201) and is now approved for the treatment of human breast cancer (39). Studies of two prostate cancer xenograft models have shown that Herceptin provides synergistic antitumor activity when combined with paclitaxel chemotherapy (5). Another potential therapeutic strategy explored by researchers relies on EGFR blockade. Interestingly, *in vitro* studies have shown that blockade of the EGFR not only attenuates the actions of EGF, but also IGF-I (352). This suggests that it may be possible to reverse several functional autocrine growth factor pathways by blocking a single receptor site. Although the efficacy for human prostate cancer therapy remains to be seen, both Herceptin and EGFR receptor blockade are good examples of how understanding alterations in growth factors and their receptors can lead to the design of novel targeted prostate cancer therapies. Therapeutic approaches directed at physiologic pathways altered in cancer will likely provide the cornerstone for treatment of hormone-refractory prostate cancer in the future.

Apoptosis

Programmed cell death (apoptosis) is an important regulator of cellular hemostasis, and alterations in apoptotic pathways have been implicated in prostate carcinogenesis. Bcl-2, Bcl-x, and Mcl-1 are proteins that inhibit apoptosis, and Bax is a protein that induces apoptosis (19). Immunohistochemical studies have demonstrated overexpression of Bcl-2 in 25% and Mcl-1 in 81% of prostate cancers (253). Studies have shown that overexpression of Bcl-2 is a predictor of poor clinical outcome in patients undergoing radical prostatectomy or radiation therapy for clinically localized prostate cancer (41,372,400). It has also been suggested that the ratio of Bcl-2/Bax immunohistochemical staining correlates with poor response to radiotherapy (288).

Animal studies have shown that overexpression of Bcl-2 protein augments growth of LnCaP tumors (21), and these findings have been used to design a novel prostate cancer therapy. In preclinical studies, researchers have shown that antisense Bcl-2 oligonucleotides inhibited growth of LnCaP and Shinogi and prevented PSA progression both *in vitro* and in castrated mice with subcutaneously implanted tumors (309). Chemosensitivity to taxol and mitoxanthrone was also enhanced. A phase I clinical trial using antisense Bcl-2 alone or in combination with mitoxanthrone is currently in progress (335).

Angiogenesis

Angiogenesis may play an important role in prostate cancer progression. Both *in vitro* and *in vivo* studies of LnCaP cells demonstrate that cells expressing higher levels of vascular endothelial growth factor (VEGF) exhibit enhanced metastatic potential (17). VEGF is the best-characterized angiogenesis factor to date (109,123), and one immunohistochemical study demonstrated positive staining for VEGF in 80% of prostate cancers compared with only 18% of benign glands (123,124). Some studies of human prostate cancer have shown that increased microvascular density in localized prostate cancer specimens predicts advanced pathologic stage and treatment failure (408), but other studies have failed to demonstrate this relationship (145,363).

Blocking tumor angiogenesis is a potentially exciting new approach to cancer therapy (131). The discovery and characterization of two potent endogenous angiogenesis inhibitors, angiostatin and endostantin, will facilitate the development of prostate cancer therapies targeting angiogenesis (37,119,396). Animal studies using these agents are currently underway (335).

Cell Adhesion Molecules

Alterations in cell adhesion molecules may also play a role in prostate cancer progression. The genes encoding two important cell adhesion molecules, E-cadherin and KAI-a, map to chromosomal bands 16q24 and 11p11.2, respectively. Both regions are frequently deleted in metastatic prostate cancer (104,270), and expression levels of E-cadherin can also be reduced in prostate cancer by promoter methylation (159). Animal studies suggest that KAI-1 can suppress prostate cancer metastasis (206). Likewise, E-cadherin plays an important role in establishing and maintaining ordered intercellular connections and morphogenesis (311). *In vivo* studies of the Dunning rat prostate tumor showed that transfecting tumor cells with E-cadherin downregulates matrix metalloproteinase 2 expression (another factor implicated in prostate cancer progression) and reduces cellular invasiveness (285). Immunohistochemical studies of human prostate cancer tissue have suggested that reduced levels of E-cadherin expression correlate with higher Gleason score and advanced pathologic stage (94). Restoring functional cell adhesion molecules to prostate cancer cells may be one possible strategy that could be used to prevent tumor progression and metastasis.

New Frontiers in Molecular Profiling of Human Malignancies

By the year 2003, the complete map and sequence of the entire human genome will be known, and sequencing of cDNA's coding for all human genes will be completed shortly thereafter (77). This information will provide us with the "periodic table of life" and will be the foundation for understanding both normal and diseased cellular functions. Over the past several years, we have witnessed tremendous advances in gene expression technology. In the near future, it will be possible to rapidly assess expression patterns of virtually all genes and proteins within a particular population of human cells. Advances in microdissection and cell-sorting technology allow one to isolate pure populations of cells from human tissue sections and then extract DNA, RNA, and protein. Differential display and cDNA microarrays are evolving technologies that facilitate high-throughput mRNA expression analysis. Advances in proteomic techniques have also made it possible to assess expression patterns of a large number of proteins simultaneously. Combining new approaches for "molecular profiling" with the complete human genome sequence will provide new opportunities to understand the underlying mechanism responsible for human malignancy. This knowledge should ultimately revolutionize diagnosis and treatment of men and women with cancer.

Tissue Processing and Procurement of Pure Populations of Cells

One of the major limitations to the direct study of molecular changes in human malignancy has been the challenge to obtain pure populations of malignant and benign cells. This difficulty arises because of cellular heterogeneity such as is seen in prostate cancer or the presence of inflammatory cells that infiltrate certain tumors such as renal cell carcinoma. To overcome this investigative hurdle, different microdissection techniques have been developed for the purpose of procuring pure or semipure populations of cells from human tissue sections. One methodology relies on ablating all the unwanted tissue with a laser and then isolating the macromolecules from the remaining tissue. Another methodology, laser capture microdissection (LCM), is currently the most widely used technique (113). LCM allows researchers to visualize a tissue section via light microscopy and then procure the desired cells by activating a 7.5- to 30-micron-diameter infrared laser beam. The laser beam melts an ethyl-vinyl-acetate film in contact with the tissue section, thereby capturing the cells of interest. Lifting up the cap pulls these cells out of the tissue sections. Intact DNA, RNA, and protein can then be extracted from the cap using various lysing buffers and analyzed by conventional methods. The advantage of this technology is that it allows for simple, fast, and reliable microdissection of human tissue sections. This technology facilitates *in vivo* molecular analysis of defined populations of human cells.

High-throughput Gene Expression Analysis

Rapid advances in high-throughput gene expression analysis technology are making it possible to analyze expression patterns of a large number of human genes simultaneously and to study how these patterns are altered in different stages of malignancy. Currently, the most widely used method to analyze gene expression patterns in cancer is through cDNA microarrays (47,100). This technology involves labeling a sample of cDNA, representing the expressed genes from a population of cells, with a radioactive or fluorescent probe. The probe is then hybridized to a nylon filter or glass array slide containing cDNA fragments representing several thousand human genes of interest. Analysis of these experiments allows one to determine relative expression levels for different genes within the same population of cells or different genes within different populations of cells. Researchers have begun to apply this technology to the study of prostate cancer. Using cDNA microarrays to compare gene expression in the androgen-independent and androgen-dependent tumors in CWR22 xenograft model yielded 37 candidate genes that were upregulated by more than twofold in the androgen-independent state (49). Although the biologic relevance of these differentially expressed genes remains to be determined, the use of cDNA microarray will be an important approach to the study of prostate cancer progression. One important caveat to this study and many others is that they use xenograft or cell culture models that may not accurately represent *in vivo* gene expression in human prostate cancer. This is a particularly important problem when it comes to the study of premalignant lesions and early-stage prostate cancer because few good animal models or cell lines are available. The recent development of LCM technology and the ability to isolate RNA from specific populations of LCM-procured cells should facilitate the *in vivo* study of gene expression in human prostate cancer. In fact, preliminary data suggest that this approach can be used to identify several (approximately 40 genes in one experiment) differentially expressed candidate genes (75). Limitations of cDNA microarray technology include potential for artifacts (particularly if using PCR amplification) and the fact that the only genes that will be studied are those that have been placed on the array filter.

Another technique used to determine genes that are important in prostate cancer development and progression rely on generating cDNA libraries from defined populations of cells (279,321,322). This strategy allows one, in theory, to study all genes (both known and unknown) expressed by a particular population of cells. The NCI-sponsored Cancer Genome Anatomy Project (CGAP) has used both bulk tissue and microdissected procured cells to create cDNA libraries from several common human cancers and corresponding normal tissue (www.ncbi.nih.gov//ncicgap/) (112). The primary goals of the project are twofold: (a) aid in discovering new human genes and (b) profile gene expression patterns for particular human cancers and tissue types. It has been estimated that more than 50% of the approximately 100,000 human genes will have been discovered through this initiative (112). This information will be a critical foundation for future prostate cancer studies. The use of microdissected-derived samples has been the cornerstone of the gene-profiling aspect of the CGAP project. In regard to prostate cancer, twelve microdissected-based libraries have been produced from epithelial components of radical prostatectomy specimens, including normal epithelium, premalignant foci, locally invasive cancers, and metastatic lesions (112). This will allow us to define all of the genes that are expressed in normal prostate (prostate unigene set) and those genes whose expression is altered in different stages of malignancy. Research efforts will focus on correlating gene expression profiles with pathologic and clinical outcomes. Ultimately, this strategy will allow us to understand how alteration in a complex network of genes leads to prostate cancer development and progression.

Although gene expression analysis holds great promise for understanding the molecular events underlying prostate cancer progression, the malignant phenotype is ultimately the reflection of quantitative and qualitative changes in cellular proteins. Therefore many researchers believe that proteomic analysis of human cancers provides unique and complementary information to genomic DNA and gene expression studies (8,107). Two-dimensional gel electrophoresis (2D-PAGE) is a highly effective and widely used means of separating a large number of proteins. Advances in 2D-PAGE technology and protein staining methods have greatly improved the reproducibility and sensitivity of protein analysis. It is now possible to separate as many as 10,000 different protein forms with high-resolution 2D-PAGE, and computer software can be used to compare spot patterns between different gels (59,60,441). One of the major advantages of 2D-PAGE protein analysis is that it allows for relatively easy identification of specific protein spots. Unknown proteins can be identified by utilization of an electrospray that can be used to generate additional partial-sequence information. One major limitation with proteomic studies of prostate cancer has resulted from difficulty in obtaining enough material from pure populations of cells. Cell lines are a good source of pure populations of cells, but recent studies suggest that protein expression patterns of cultured tumor cells may differ substantially from those of the same cells *in vivo* (58). One potential strategy to overcome these problems is to analyze proteins isolated from microdissected populations of cells. In fact, researchers have shown that highly reproducible protein profiles can be generated using cellular lysates from populations of benign and malignant prostate epithelium procured by LCM, and that differentially expressed proteins can be identified by this approach.

Although significant technologic advances have been made, the major shortcoming of 2D-PAGE protein analysis remains sensitivity. Therefore cancer researchers should combine these robust proteomic techniques with more sensitive mRNA expression analysis. In the future, advances in technology may allow proteomic analysis of all cellular proteins, even the least abundant ones.

Conclusions

Although current understanding of the underlying biologic mechanisms responsible for prostate cancer development and progression is at a relatively rudimentary stage, there is overwhelming hope and optimism for the future. There has been tremendous progress in the search for genomic alteration associated with prostate cancer development, and it is likely that in the very near future, several specific "prostate cancer genes" for both hereditary and sporadic prostate cancer will be identified. As more genetic polymorphisms are linked with prostate cancer, there will be new opportunities to assess prostate cancer risk with more certainty, and to design rational and effective prevention strategies. The completion of the human genome sequence combined with the revolution in gene and protein expression analysis technology should allow us to classify different prostate cancers more accurately based on molecular and histopathologic features. Ultimately, an improved understanding of prostate cancer biology should be used to improve quality of life for all men with prostate cancer, as well as those at risk for this disease.

MOLECULAR GENETICS OF BLADDER CANCER

Bladder cancer is the second most common urologic cancer and fifth most common malignancy in the United States (163a). Furthermore, bladder cancer is 2.5 times more common in men than women and is the second most prevalent malignancy in older men (130). More than 50,000 patients were diagnosed with bladder cancer in the year 2000, and although the mortality rate from bladder cancer is declining, more than 10,000 deaths were expected (163a). In the United States, urologists are the primary referral for patients with unspecified microscopic and gross hematuria. As a result, the diagnosis and treatment of most bladder cancers is left almost exclusively to the practicing urologist. Our current diagnostic algorithm and treatment options for bladder cancer result in very few cases of undiagnosed and untreated bladder cancers found at autopsy (233). Fortunately, most patients (70% to 80%) have superficial (non–muscle-invasive) tumors that can be managed with bladder-sparing procedures, intravesical agents, and surveillance cystoscopy and cytology. As a result, the majority of patients treated for bladder cancer survive but require diligent follow-up because more than two-thirds of superficial tumors recur and a large percentage of high-grade tumors progress to muscle-invasive disease (192).

In contrast to superficial involvement of the bladder wall, the presence of muscle invasion makes bladder cancer a life-threatening condition. Approximately 50% of patients with muscle-invasive disease will have occult or overt metastases at the time of presentation, and the majority of these patients will die from their disease. Patients with muscle-invasive bladder cancer are managed aggressively with radical cystectomy alone or with adjuvant chemotherapy, radiation, or both for patients with advanced disease. Patients with localized muscle-invasive bladder cancer can enjoy long-term survival, and the use of orthotopic neobladders and nerve-sparing approaches has improved quality of life in appropriate surgical candidates (183). Still, approximately half of patients with muscle-invasive bladder cancer will develop overt metastases within 2 years of treatment. Metastatic bladder cancer is always associated with a high mortality rate despite aggressive chemotherapeutic regimens, and the urologic management of patients with metastatic transitional cell carcinoma usually consists of palliative procedures with or without cystectomy. Although new chemotherapeutic regimens are being investigated (435,439), treatment of metastatic transitional cell carcinoma is clearly an opportunity for molecular biologists and physicians to develop novel treatment regimens based on genetic changes that occur in these highly aggressive and lethal tumors.

Urothelial malignancies have diverse clinical and histologic presentations (114,314). Some patients have large, solitary, noninvasive papillary lesions (pTa); others have multiple noninvasive tumors. Some patients have low- or high-grade papillary or sessile lesions invading into the lamnia propria (pT_1) but not into the detrusor muscle layer of the bladder. Still others have diffuse high-grade flat lesions, carcinoma in situ (CIS, pTIS), confined to the urothelium that are associated with synchronous muscle-invasive lesions ($pT_{2\text{-}4}$) or progression to muscle-invasive lesions. Although the majority (60% to 70%) of patients with low-grade papillary urothelial malignancies experience a recurrence, a significant percentage do not. Some tumors respond to intravesical agents such as bacille Calmette-Guérin (BCG) or mitomycin C; others are resistant. Many patients are treated for years for multiple recurrent tumors that do not progress, but a significant percentage of patients with superficial high-grade disease progress to muscle-invasive or metastatic disease (192).

Transitional cell carcinoma (TCC) of the bladder is the most common histologic type and location of urothelial malignancy in the United States. However, squamous cell carcinoma (SCC) of the bladder is more common in areas inhabited by the microorganism *Schistosoma haematobium*

(313). In these areas, bladder cancer is the most common malignancy and provides clues to the importance of inflammation and chronic infection in the etiology of bladder cancer (359). Other tumors, such as adenocarcinomas, neuroendocrine tumors, lymphomas, and pheochromocytomas, are rare primary bladder malignancies. The genetic abnormalities responsible for the histologic diversity in bladder cancer are not clearly defined, and molecular studies have not demonstrated consistent genetic differences between the common histologic types (177,385). Urothelial malignancies affecting the upper tracts of the urinary system (renal pelvis and ureter) are comparatively rare and assumed to have similar genetic changes as bladder cancer. TCC of the renal pelvis accounts for only 10% of renal tumors, and TCC of the ureter is uncommon (4% of urothelial malignancies). However, a hereditary cancer predisposition syndrome known as hereditary nonpolyposis colon cancer (HNPCC) or the Lynch II syndrome is associated with an increased incidence of upper tract urothelial malignancy (287,451). This syndrome and the association with upper tract TCC are discussed later in this chapter.

Oncogenes and Urothelial Cancer

Oncogenes are altered human genes that dominantly transform cells. Unaltered oncogenes (protooncogenes) are involved in important cellular functions such as cell surface signaling, apoptosis, cell cycle regulation, and gene expression or function as growth factors or growth factor receptors. Many protooncogenes were first described in their altered form as part of an oncogenic retrovirus that caused tumors in rodents or birds. The human homologs were subsequently isolated and the corresponding oncogene identified in human malignancies, including bladder cancer. Oncogenes often belong to families of homologous genes, and the three oncogenes to be discussed in urothelial malignancy, ras, myc, and bcl-2, are no exceptions. The genetic alterations in some oncogenes are tumor specific. For instance, c-myc is a DNA-binding nuclear protein associated with chromosome 8q amplifications and overexpression in bladder tumors (278,370), n-myc is associated with amplification on chromosome 2 in neuroblastomas (380), and l-myc is amplified in lung cancer (319). In contrast, mutations in all members of the ras gene family have been described in bladder cancer (121,139,355,387).

Unlike TSGs (described in the following section), alterations in oncogenes usually involve point mutations or chromosomal amplifications associated with increased transcription, increased stability, or increased activity. Inactivating point mutations, intragenic deletions, or gross chromosomal alterations generally do not occur in protooncogenes unless they result in increased stability or increased expression. Two classic examples of gross chromosomal alterations resulting in the protooncogene activation are bcl-2 located on chromosome 18q and c-myc on chromosome 8q. A translocation event between chromosomes 14 and 18 t (14,18) in follicular B cell lymphomas causes deregulation of bcl-2 due to approximation of an immunoglobulin heavy chain enhancer and the bcl-2 transcription unit (431). A similar type of translocation event has been described for c-myc in Burkitt's lymphoma (89). Therefore gross chromosomal alterations are an apparently common mechanism for oncogene activation in lymphoma.

The Harvey ras gene (H-ras) and other members of the ras gene family are involved in cell surface signaling through a variety of pathways including growth factor and growth factor receptor interactions (306). Ras proteins are activated by binding to guanosine triphosphate (GTP) and inactivated when GTP is dephosphorylated by GTPases. Characteristic ras point mutations at codons 12, 13, and 61 in bladder cancer and other malignancies are associated with unregulated activation of ras proteins potentially causing unregulated signaling for cell proliferation via growth factors (417). Mutations in H-ras were initially described in the bladder cancer cell line T-24 (355) and subsequently shown to be mutated in primary bladder tumors (121). Mutations in Kirsten ras (K-ras) and n-ras have also been described in bladder cancer, but K-ras mutations are more common in colon cancer and n-ras mutations in lymphoid malignancies. The ras protooncogenes are highly homologous, and activation of any ras protein is likely to cause a similar mechanism of cellular transformation. H-ras activation commonly occurs due to point mutations in codon 12 (38), and mutations affecting any ras codon have been described in up to 40% of bladder tumors (128,139,140).

The c-myc, n-myc, and l-myc protooncogenes are well studied and have contributed extensively to our understanding of DNA binding proteins and protein-protein interactions (76). The importance of c-myc in a variety of human malignancies has been reported and usually involves gene amplification or rearrangements as described previously. The c-myc gene is expressed in proliferating cells (226). The myc proteins are transcription factors associated with increased expression of genes involved in DNA replication and cell growth (76,241). Amplification and alterations of the c-myc locus in cancer have been described (29,370); however, the role of c-myc in bladder cancer is not well understood. Although overexpression and amplification of the homologous n-myc gene in neuroblastoma has prognostic implications (380), a similar role for c-myc in TCC has not been demonstrated (278). However, low-level amplification and overexpression of c-myc in TCC has been described and correlated with progression in one study (370).

Overexpression of the bcl-2 protooncogene prevents apoptosis, a form of programmed cell death that involves activation of cellular proteases known as caspases (328). Inhibition of cell death is important in tumorigenesis for several reasons. First, the homeostatic balance is shifted toward cellular accumulation; second, apoptosis removes genetically defective cells that may become malignant if allowed to expand; and third, the toxic effect of chemotherapeutic agents on malignant cells may be abrogated. Bcl-2 is normally located in mitochondrial membranes, where it regulates pore formation. Mitochondrial pores are important in regulating free radical formation and ion fluxes and maintaining membrane potentials within the cell. Intracellular fluxes mediated by these pores can signal caspase activation and initiate the cascade of proteolytic events leading to DNA fragmentation and irreversible cell death. Some caspases are specific for cleavage of bcl-2 whereas others have a more general proteolytic spectrum. Bcl-2 prevents the initiation of these events by blocking the transduction of apoptotic signals to trigger the caspase proteolytic cascade. Therefore decreased bcl-2 expression would be associated with apoptosis and increased expression with resistance to apoptosis.

Expression of bcl-2 has been investigated in bladder as a prognostic marker and as a target for apoptotic directed therapy for bladder cancer (152,225). The tumor-suppressor protein, p53 (discussed later), is an important negative regulator of bcl-2 expression, and molecular studies demonstrate increased expression of bcl-2 in the absence of wild type p53 (223). Other members of the bcl-2 family of genes have apoptotic promoting and apoptotic preventive effects. One example, bax, binds to bcl-2, preventing it from functioning and thereby promoting apoptosis. Bax is transcriptionally activated by p53 and is therefore an effector of p53 regulated apoptosis (223). Other bcl-2–related proteins such as bcl-xL prevent apoptosis, and bcl-xs, bad, and others promote apoptosis. The mechanism of action of bcl-2 and related proteins is incompletely understood, but its location in mitochondrial membranes and regulation of pore formation are important aspects of function.

Tumor-suppressor Genes and Urothelial Cancer

Oncogenes were the first human cancer genes discovered and investigated in detail, but genetic alterations in TSGs appear to be the more common mechanism leading to human malignancies (392). Oncogenes promote tumorigenesis in a dominant fashion, and TSGs prevent or slow tumorigenesis in a dominant fashion. Classically, one allele of a protooncogene acquires an activating mutation, whereas both alleles of a TSG must be inactivated for tumorigenesis (120,239). Unlike protooncogenes, large deletions and chromosomal alterations are common events leading to TSG inactivation. One TSG allele may be completely lost while a point mutation inactivates the remaining allele (16). This phenomenon can be detected through the use of polymorphic markers and is known as loss of heterozygosity (LOH) because one allele of a marker is missing when tumor DNA is compared to normal (germline) DNA in the same patient.

TSGs can be artificially classified into two groups. The first group consists of TSGs associated with hereditary cancer predisposition syndromes and in these kindreds are associated with an inherited mutation in one allele (238). Group one TSGs were initially suspected because of increased occurrence and autosomal dominant inheritance of tumors such as retinoblastomas in affected families. Linkage analysis confirmed the presence of a cancer-predisposing gene and resulted in cloning of the inherited mutated allele (136). Once identified, TSGs are often found to be mutated in sporadic tumors, as was the case for retinoblastoma. Other TSGs were identified as mutated genes in sporadic malignancies and subsequently identified as the altered gene in a cancer predisposition syndrome (293). Investigation of these genes in transgenic mice with homozygous inactivation of the target gene confirmed importance in cell growth and tumorigenesis. The second group consists of candidate TSGs that are located in areas of LOH in sporadic cancers. Members of this second group have not yet been linked with inherited mutations in familial cancer syndromes. These TSGs are located within a common genetically altered region but have not been conclusively shown to be the target of complete inactivation in tumor cells. Several genes in this group are being investigated in bladder cancer (235,236).

TSGs that belong to the first group are retinoblastoma (Rb), p53, adenomatous polyposis coli (APC), VHL, neurofibromatosis type 1 (NF-1), neurofibromatosis type 2 (NF-2), Wilms' tumor (WT-1), tuberous sclerosis complex–1 (TSC-1), and tuberous sclerosis complex–2 (TSC-2). The first TSG products identified in this group were p53 and Rb. Rb was identified by its association with inherited retinoblastoma and subsequently shown to be inactivated in bladder cancer (213,412). The p53 TSG was shown to be mutated in colon cancer (16) and then identified as the inherited and mutated gene in the Li-Fraumeni cancer predisposition syndrome (293). Although these two important TSGs were identified by different approaches, Rb and p53 are functionally linked in suppression of cell growth by blocking the progression through the cell cycle.

Unphosphorylated Rb suppresses tumorigenesis by sequestering a transcription factor known as E2F-1 (236). E2F-1 causes transcriptional activation of genes involved in DNA synthesis and progression through the cell cycle (219,281). When RB is phosphorylated by an assembly of proteins that includes cyclins and cyclin dependent kinases (cdk), it can no longer sequester E2F-1. The result is progression of cells into the DNA synthesis (S) phase of the cell cycle from a growth or gap (G_1) phase. This block in the cell cycle at G_1 is known as a cell cycle checkpoint, and Rb is an important effector of G_1 cell cycle arrest. Cyclin D1 (CCND1) is also important at this checkpoint by its ability to regulate Rb phosphorylation through its association with cdk-4 and -6 (315). Amplification and overexpression of CCND1 has been described in cancers such as bladder (42,264,318,465) and has prognostic significance. CCND1 overexpression can overcome the G_1 cell cycle checkpoint by promoting unregulated phosphorylation of RB and causing increased bioavailability of E2F-1. The ability of cyclin D1 and other cyclins to dominantly promote tumor formation by promoting cell proliferation makes them potential oncogenes in bladder carcinogenesis (315,353,388).

The important and versatile TSG, p53, is mutated in over 50% of human malignancies, including TCC (4,197). The normal or wild type p53 protein has many important functions in suppressing tumorigenesis, such as growth arrest and apoptosis (267,268). Transactivation of a gene known as p21/waf-1/cip-1 by p53 causes inhibition of cdk-dependent phosphorylation of RB and thereby causes inhibition of E2F-1–mediated cell cycle progression (111). As mentioned previously, p53 transcriptionally activates genes such as bax that promote apoptosis and transcriptionally represses bcl-2 that prevents apoptosis (223). Other genes transcriptionally activated by p53 such as GADD45 and FAS/Apo1 also play a role in growth arrest or apoptosis (223). An important signal for many p53 functions is DNA damage from a variety of causes such as chemotherapy or radiation. These agents can block progression through cell cycle checkpoints influenced by DNA repair (222).

Another protein, p14ARF (called p19ARF in mouse) on chromosome 9p and within the same transcription unit as p16 (discussed in the next section), is transcriptionally activated by E2F-1 (20,347). The p14ARF protein interacts with a protein known as mouse double minute–2 (mdm-2), causing it to be degraded (254,347,466). The mdm-2 gene on chromosome 12 is transcriptionally activated by p53 but negatively regulates p53 by binding and targeting p53 for ubiquitin-mediated degradation (184). Mdm-2 is often amplified and overexpressed in tumors (175,262,331) and has oncogenic properties through its physical interaction with the tumor-suppressor properties of p53 (175,332). The interaction of p14ARF with mdm-2 allows increased activity of p53 and negatively regulates progression through the G_1 checkpoint. This entire process serves as a negative feedback loop for E2F-1–mediated cell cycle progression and potentiates the action of other cdk inhibitors such as p21/waf-1/cip-1. Therefore p53 and Rb are functionally related through their effects on the cell cycle. Inactivating mutations that affect either p53 or Rb promote unregulated cell growth, and mutations in both may be synergistic (83,86,170).

The role of Rb and p53 expression in bladder cancer has been a very active area of research. The p53 gene is often mutated in bladder cancer and associated with high-grade invasive lesions (117,118,138,333). Other studies have investigated the role of p53 in tumor recurrence, progression, and response to treatment such as radical cystectomy, radiation, chemotherapy, or intravesical therapy (85,263,276, 366,367). Using immunohistochemistry, p53 expression generally correlates with poor outcome in terms of recurrence, progression, resistance, and survival. However, immunohistochemical analysis of p53 has caused some discrepancies when used as the sole assay for p53 mutational analysis in these studies.

Immunohistochemistry correlates with mutations that increase stability of the altered p53 protein product (118). Mutations in p53 correlated with immunohistochemistry when 20% of cells demonstrated nuclear staining in one large bladder cancer series (276). However, a positive immunohistochemical result may not be specific for the mutant protein due to biologic factors (178). This observation, combined with the technical limitations of immunohistochemistry, has led to different results using p53 as an independent variable for clinical outcome in bladder cancer (402). The clinical response of bladder cancer patients to chemotherapy is one recent example. In one study, mutant p53 (as determined by immunohistochemical analysis) was associated with favorable outcome when cystectomy was combined with adjuvant chemotherapy (87), while in another study immunohistochemical staining of p53 was associated with decreased response to neoadjuvant chemotherapy (367).

The underlying hypotheses for each result is the ability of wild type p53 to induce apoptosis when using agents such as MVAC that cause DNA damage. Tumors with increased p53 staining (mutant p53) cannot undergo p53-mediated apoptosis induced by the chemotherapeutic agents and are therefore resistant. Alternatively, the absence of p53-mediated G_1 arrest may allow tumor cells with damaged DNA to proceed through S phase but arrest at mitosis and subsequently undergo apoptosis (440). Tumor cells with normal p53 presumably repair DNA damage before entering S-phase and then undergo mitosis. The true mechanism is currently unknown and may be dependent on the status of other proteins such as Rb, mdm-2, p21, or proteins involved in DNA repair. In addition, experimental and study design differences may prove to be the most important factor. Although p53 mutation is independently associated with higher grade, stage, and progression in most studies and may have clinical applications in the future, the practicality of using p53 immunohistochemistry instead of routine pathologic staging and grading has not been definitively proven (436).

Immunohistochemical analysis of Rb expression has also been extensively investigated in bladder cancer (82,282). Although mutations in Rb have not been associated with increased reactivity using immunohistochemistry, increased expression has been observed in some tumors (86). Absent or altered Rb staining is associated with muscle-invasive disease, and studies have associated abnormal Rb expression with poor outcome (82,86). Moreover, loss or abnormal expression of Rb combined with p53 immunoreactivity has independent and prognostic value in some studies (83,170).

Investigation of p53 and Rb proves that development of bladder cancer is complex and dependent on accumulation of mutations in multiple targets. Mutations in parallel pathways may be important for development and progression of high-grade malignancy, whereas single pathway alterations are necessary for low-grade tumors.

Many chromosomal regions are associated with high rates of LOH in bladder cancer (40,52,199,236,237,310, 345,350,360). However, most common and consistent area of LOH in bladder cancer are the long and short arms of chromosome 9 (224,236). At least three genes in this region are important in tumor suppression via their effect on progression through the cell cycle. The ink4a (p16, mts-1, ckn2a), and ink4b (p15, mts-2) genes encode inhibitors of cyclin-dependent kinases, and ink4a/ARF encodes a peptide that regulates p53 activity, as discussed previously. This region has a high rate of homozygous deletions in cell lines and primary tumors (51,220). Methylation and transcriptional repression may also be an important mechanism of inactivation of these genes (158). Moreover, these genes are associated with hereditary melanomas fulfilling the criteria as group one TSGs described previously.

LOH on the short and long arms of chromosome 9 is common in bladder cancer. Over 50% of superficial and invasive TCCs have LOH on chromosome 9 (235). Unlike p53 and RB, where LOH on chromosomes 17p and 13q, respectively, usually occur in high-grade lesions (52,333), chromosome 9p losses occur early and are associated with low-grade superficial TCC in addition to high-grade lesions. These findings suggest that 9p genes are important initiators in TCC, allowing growth advantage until other genetic events select more aggressive clones. Genetic alterations affecting Ink4a appear to be common in tumorigenesis (51,158,334), but the mechanism of inactivation implies that all genes in this region are important TSGs. Both p15 and p16 proteins are cdk inhibitors that function in G_1 (68). By inhibiting cdks, p16 prevents RB phosphorylation, E2F-1 remains sequestered and cells are prevented from entering S-phase. Loss of p16 and p15 activity by homozygous deletion of ink4a and ink4b allows unregulated phosphorylation of Rb and increased E2F-1 activity. Furthermore, loss of ink4a/ARF results in increased mdm-2 (due to the lack of ink4a/ARF-mediated mdm-2 degradation) and increased ubiquinin-mediated degradation of p53. Therefore homozygous deletion of these three genes affects Rb and p53 regulation of the cell cycle.

Regions on chromosomes 3p, 4q, 9q, 8p, 11q, 14q, and 18q are also associated with high rates of LOH in bladder cancer and are undoubtedly locations of group two TSGs (40,52,62,199,236,237,345,350,360). In addition, candidate TSGs on chromosomes 4 and 9 have been identified and are currently being investigated (23,198,236,345,386). The pattern of LOH and gene mutations in bladder cancer suggests a model of tumorigenesis in which inactivation of genes on chromosome 9p and 9q are early events and associated with low-grade papillary lesions (357,399). These tumors have a growth advantage but tend to remain localized to the urothelial mucosa. High-grade lesions such as CIS are associated with early 13q and 17p losses, and progression may be associated with these and other TSGs (310). The important role of TSGs in bladder cancer is well established, and the discovery of other TSGs will most likely enhance our understanding of bladder cancer pathogenesis.

Growth Factors and Growth Factor Receptors

Growth factors and their receptors have been investigated in human bladder cancer (306,392). The met gene (chromosome 7) and its ligand hepatocyte growth factor were described in another section. Trisomy of chromosome 7 in bladder tumors has been described, and therefore met gene alterations may play a role in these tumors. However, the factors most extensively studied in bladder cancer are EGF, EGFR, and ERB-B2 (a 185-kD transmembrane protein homologous to the EGFR) also known as HER-2/neu. Growth factors and their receptors have a normal role in promoting growth, and therefore most alterations cause increased expression by increasing copy number or transcription similar to oncogenes. In addition, alterations in growth factor receptors can affect intracellular signaling (418).

EGF has been studied extensively in bladder cancer and normal urothelium (306,391). Studies have shown increased expression of EGF in the basal layers of normal urothelium and increased expression in TCC. Increased levels of EGF have been detected in the urine of patients with TCC but do not correlate with tumor grade or stage (402). The EGF receptor is an independent predictor of poor survival when overexpressed in TCC (277,303). ErbB-2 is amplified and often overexpressed in bladder tumors (72,302,369). In breast cancer, erbB-2 amplification has been well documented and shown to have prognostic implications (29). Conflicting results have been reported as to the importance of amplification of this gene in bladder cancer progression (371,416).

Hereditary Predisposition and Urothelial Cancer

Although environmental agents such as smoking, organic compounds, and phenacetin have been implicated in the development of bladder cancer, hereditary bladder cancer syndromes have not been clearly defined. Clustering of TCC in families has been described, but linkage to a specific gene(s) had not been described until recently (273,340). Lynch and colleagues (287,451) described an increased incidence of upper tract TCC in an inherited cancer predisposition syndrome known as hereditary nonpolyposis colon cancer (HNPCC). Although colon cancer is the predominant malignancy found in these kindreds, extracolonic tumors, including upper tract TCC, are also prevalent in a subset of families.

The mutated genes responsible for HNPCC are highly conserved genes involved in mismatch repair (MMR) (43,127,261,325,338). At least nine human MMR genes have been identified, and several have been shown to be mutated in families with hereditary predisposition to cancer (hMSH2, hMSH6, hMLH1, PMS-1, and PMS-2); however, the most commonly mutated MMR genes in hereditary and sporadic tumors are hMSH2 and hMLH1 (338). MMR-deficient tumors have a characteristic phenotype referred to as microsatellite instablility (MSI) due to alterations in dinucleotide and trinucleotide repeats (3,210,419).

Several features of MMR in urologic malignancies deserve special attention. As mentioned previously, HNPCC is the only well-characterized hereditary cancer predisposition syndrome with increased risk of TCC. The absence of increased bladder TCC risk in HNPCC is surprising but may reflect subtle differences in cell biology of upper tract and bladder urothelium. Alternatively, the association of an increased incidence of upper tract TCC with HNPCC may have been more easily established due to the low incidence of upper tract TCC in the general population. HNPCC patients develop bladder cancer, and it would be interesting to determine if bladder tumors in HNPCC patients exhibit MSI due to inactivation of the wild type MMR gene allele.

Approximately 10% to 15% of sporadic colon cancers have MMR mutations (3). However, only about 3% of superficial bladder tumors showed MSI (157). An immunohistochemical analysis of hMSH2 expression identified 25% of TCC with reduced expression of hMSH2 and complete absence of expression in 2% (218). Decreased hMSH2 expression was predominantly found in high-grade and recurrent tumors, suggesting that alterations in MMR activity may be involved in recurrence and progression. In addition, cell lines deficient for MMR are resistant to DNA alkylating agents (204). This finding may be important for urothelial malignancies because alkylating agents are sometimes used in the treatment of superficial bladder tumors and MMR deficiency may be important for resistance to other chemotherapeutics.

INFECTIOUS AGENTS AND UROTHELIAL CANCER

Bladder cancer associated with chronic irritation, inflammation, and certain infections usually has the histologic appearance of SCC. The schistosome *S. haematobium* is one of four schistosome species that infects humans (312) and the only schistosomal infection associated with development of bladder cancer. The etiology of the SCC is related to the intense inflammatory response to the *S. haematobium* eggs deposited within the bladder wall. Molecular analysis of SCC from individuals infected with *S. haematobium* suggests that the genetic alterations are similar to nonbilharzial tumors (385). SCC development using *S. haematobium* as a model system could be useful for investigation of immune response initiation of these tumors and response to treatment.

Markers in Urothelial Cancer

An important area in bladder cancer research is development of markers for early detection of primary or recurrent tumors, progression, and prognosis. Currently, cystoscopy with cytology is an essential component for diagnosis of urothelial malignancies. Insufficient sensitivity for low-grade cancer does not allow cytology to be used independent of cystoscopy. As a result, a number of markers have been developed and assessed for detection of urothelial malignancies (402). Currently, no single marker or test has sufficient sensitivity and specificity to replace cystoscopy and cytology in diagnosis or surveillance of bladder cancer patients.

A novel approach to detection of urothelial malignancies uses the detection of genetic alterations in the form of LOH and MSI (296). The clonal nature of tumors expands and propagates genetic alterations that can be detected using a panel of molecular markers. High sensitivity and specificity has been achieved using this technique in urothelial malignancies. However, sensitivity is achieved by screening large numbers of markers and may be impractical for routine clinical use. Similar approaches using gene expression may prove less cumbersome, but these tests have not been proven useful in a large series. In addition, tests that can predict or direct responses to standard or novel anticancer agents will need further investigation.

Conclusion

Urothelial malignancies are common due to environmental, infectious, and genetic factors. Bladder cancer is the most common manifestation of urothelial malignancy and usually exists as two histologic and pathologic diseases. Superficial disease is easily treated, but recurrence and progression are of major importance. Invasive disease is aggressive and potentially lethal because of high metastatic potential. However, the natural history of bladder cancer and its treatment makes this disease an excellent model for cancer recurrence, progression, and response to treatment. Urologists should be instrumental in the investigation of bladder cancer because management of localized disease is completely within the field of urology. Our goals as urologists, molecular biologists, and physician scientists are to develop better treatment options for advanced and metastatic urothelial malignancies and develop markers for recurrence and progression.

REFERENCES

1. United States Renal Data System. *1994 annual data report.* Washington, DC: US Department of Health and Human Services, 1994.
2. Aaltomaa S. Expression of cyclin A and D proteins in prostate cancer and their relation to clinicopathological variables and patient survival. *Prostate* 1999;38:175.
3. Aaltonen LA et al. Clues to the pathogenesis of familial colorectal cancer. *Science* 1993;260:812.
4. Abdel-Fattah R et al. Alterations of TP53 in microdissected transitional cell carcinoma of the human urinary bladder: high frequency of TP53 accumulation in the absence of detected mutations is associated with poor prognosis. *Br J Cancer* 1998; 77:2230.
5. Agus DB. Response of prostate cancer to anti-Her-2/neu antibody in androgen-dependent and -independent human xenograft models. *Cancer Res* 1999;59:4761.
6. Amin MB et al. Papillary (chromophil) renal cell carcinoma: histomorphologic characteristics and evaluation of conventional pathologic prognostic parameters in 62 cases. *Am J Surg Pathol* 1997;21:621.
7. Amin MB et al. Renal oncocytoma: a reappraisal of morphologic features with clinicopathologic findings in 80 cases. *Am J Surg Pathol* 1997;21:1.
8. Anderson NL, Anderson NG. Proteome and proteomics: new technologies, new concepts, and new words. *Electrophoresis* 1998;19:1853.
9. Angelsen A. NGF-beta, NE-cells and prostatic cancer cell lines. A study of neuroendocrine expression in the human prostatic cancer cell lines DU-145, PC-3, LNCaP, and TSU-pr1 following stimulation of the nerve growth factor–beta. *Scand J Urol Nephrol* 1998;32:7.
10. Anglard P et al. Molecular analysis of genetic changes in the origin and development of renal cell carcinoma. *Cancer Res* 1991;51:1071.
11. Auperin A et al. Occupational risk factors for renal cell carcinoma: a case-control study. *Occup Environ Med* 1994;51:426.
12. Autzen P. Bone morphogenetic protein 6 in skeletal metastases from prostate cancer and other common human malignancies. *Br J Cancer* 1998;78:1219.
13. Avery RA et al. Renal medullary carcinoma: clinical and therapeutic aspects of a newly described tumor. *Cancer* 1996;78:128.
14. Baer SC et al. Sarcomatoid collecting duct carcinoma: a clinicopathologic and immunohistochemical study of five cases. *Hum Pathol* 1993;24:1017.
15. Bai C et al. SKPI connects cell cycle regulators to the ubiquitin proteolysis machinery through a novel motif, the F-box. *Cell* 1996;86:263.
16. Baker SJ et al. Chromosome 17 deletions and p53 gene mutations in colorectal carcinomas. *Science* 1989;244:217.
17. Balbay PCK. Highly metastatic human prostate cancer growing within the prostate of athymic mice overexpresses vascular endothelial growth factor. *Clin Cancer Res* 1999;5:783.
18. Barrack ER. TGF beta in prostate cancer: a growth inhibitor that can enhance tumorigenicity. *Prostate* 1997;31:61.
19. Basu A. The relationship between Bc12, Bax and p53: consequences for cell cycle progression and cell death. *Mol Hum Reprod* 1998;4:1099.
20. Bates S et al. p14ARF links the tumor suppressors RB and p53 [letter]. *Nature* 1998;395:124.
21. Beham AW. Molecular correlates of bcl-2-enhanced growth following androgen-ablation in prostate carcinoma cells in vivo. *Int J Mol Med* 1998;1:953.
22. Bell ETA. Classification of renal tumors with observations on the frequency of the various types. *J Urol* 1938;39:238.
23. Bell SM et al: Identification and characterization of the human homologue of SH3BP2, an SH3 binding domain protein within a common region of deletion at 4p16.3 involved in bladder cancer. *Genom* 1997;44:163.
24. Benichou J et al. Population attributable risk of renal cell cancer in Minnesota. *Am J Epidemiol* 1998;148:424.
25. Bennington JL. Proceedings: cancer of the kidney—etiology, epidemiology, and pathology. *Cancer* 1973;32:1017.
26. Bennington KL. Renal adenoma. *World J Urol* 1987;5:66.
27. Bentz M et al. Chromosome imbalances in papillary renal cell carcinoma and first cytogenetic data of familial cases analyzed by comparative genomic hybridization. *Cytogenet Cell Genet* 1996;75:17.
28. Bergerheim US et al. Deletion mapping of chromosomes 8, 10, and 16 in human prostatic carcinoma. *Genes Chromosomes Cancer* 1991;3:215.
29. Berns EM et al. C-myc amplification is a better prognostic factor than HER2/neu amplification in primary breast cancer. *Cancer Res* 1992;52:1107.
30. Berthon P et al. Predisposing gene for early-onset prostate cancer, localized on chromosome 1q42.2-43. *Am J Hum Genet* 1998;62:1416.
31. Billis A et al. Chromophobe renal cell carcinoma: clinicopathological study of 7 cases. *Ultrastruct Pathol* 1998;22:19.
32. Binkovitz LA, Johnson CD, Stephens DH. Islet cell tumours in von Hippel-Lindau disease: increased prevalence and relationship to the multiple endocrine neoplasias. *AJR Am J Roentgenol* 1990;155:501.
33. Bird AP. CpG-rich islands and the function of DNA methylation. *Nature* 1986;321:209.
34. Birt AR, Hogg GR, Dube WJ. Hereditary multiple fibrofolliculomas with trichodiscomas and acrochordons. *Arch Dermatol* 1977;113:1674.
35. Bodmer D et al. An alternative route for multistep tumorigenesis in a novel case of hereditary renal cell cancer and a t(2;3)(q35;q21) chromosome translocation. *Am J Hum Genet* 1998; 62:1475.
36. Boeing H, Schlehofer B, Wahrendorf J. Diet, obesity and risk for renal cell carcinoma: results from a case control-study in Germany. *Z Ernahrungswiss* 1997;36:3.
37. Borgstrom P. Neutralizing anti-vascular endothelial growth factor antibody completely inhibits angiogenesis and growth of human prostate carcinoma micro tumors in vivo. *Prostate* 1998;35:1.
38. Bos JL. Ras oncogene in human cancer: a review. *Cancer Res* 1989;49:4682.
39. Brenner TL. First MAb approved for treatment of metastatic breast cancer. *J Am Pharm Assoc (Wash)* 1999;39:236.
40. Brewster SF et al. Loss of heterozygosity on chromosome 18q is associated with muscle-invasive transitional cell carcinoma of the bladder. *Br J Cancer* 1994;70:697.
41. Brewster SF et al. Preoperative p53, bcl-2, CD44 and E-cadherin immunohistochemistry as predictors of biochemical relapse after radical prostatectomy. *J Urol* 1999;161:1238.
42. Bringuier PP et al. Expression of cyclin DI and EMSI in bladder tumours; relationship with chromosome 11q13 amplification. *Oncogene* 1996;12:1747.
43. Bronner CE et al. Mutation in the DNA mismatch repair gene homologue hMLH1 is associated with hereditary non-polyposis colon cancer. *Nature* 1994;368:258.
44. Brooks JD et al. CG island methylation changes near the GSTP1 gene in prostatic intraepithelial neoplasia. *Cancer Epidemiol Biomarkers Prev* 1998;7:531.

45. Brown JA et al. Simultaneous chromosome 7 and 17 gain and sex chromosome loss provide evidence that renal metanephric adenoma is related to papillary renal cell carcinoma. *J Urol* 1997;158:370.
46. Brown JA et al. Fluorescence in situ hybridization analysis of renal oncocytoma reveals frequent loss of chromosomes Y and 1. *J Urol* 1996;156:31.
47. Brown PO, Botstein D. Exploring the new world of the genome with DNA microarrays. *Nat Genet* 1999;21:33.
48. Brownson RC. A case-control study of renal cell carcinoma in relation to occupation, smoking, and alcohol consumption. *Arch Environ Health* 1988;43:238.
49. Bubendorf L et al. Hormone therapy failure in human prostate cancer: analysis by complementary DNA and tissue microarrays. *J Natl Cancer Inst* 1999;91:1758.
50. Bugert P et al. Specific genetic changes of diagnostic importance in chromophobe renal cell carcinoma. *Lab Invest* 1997; 76:203.
51. Cairns P et al. Frequency of homozygous deletion at p16/ CDKN2 in primary human tumours. *Nat Genet* 1995;11:210.
52. Cairns P, Proctor AJ, Knowles MA. Loss of heterozygosity at the RB locus in frequent and correlates with muscle invasion in bladder carcinoma. *Oncogene* 1991.
53. Cairns P. Frequent inactivation of PTEN/MMAC1 in primary prostate cancer. *Cancer Res* 1997;57:4997.
54. Cardillo MR. Transforming growth factor–beta expression in prostate neoplasia. *Anal Quant Cytol Histol* 2000;22-1.
55. Carter BS, Carter HB, Isaacs JT. Epidemiologic evidence regarding predisposing factors to prostate cancer. *Prostate* 1990; 16:187.
56. Carter BS et al. Familial risk factors for prostate cancer. *Cancer Surv* 1991;11:5.
57. Cavazzana AO et al. Bellini duct carcinoma. A clinical and in vitro study. *Eur Urol* 1996;30:340.
58. Celis A et al. Short-term culturing of low-grade superficial bladder transitional cell carcinomas leads to changes in the expression levels of several proteins involved in key cellular activities [In Process Citation]. *Electrophoresis* 1999;20:355.
59. Celis JE et al. Human and mouse proteomic databases: novel resources in the protein universe. *FEBS Lett* 1998;430:64.
60. Celis JE et al. A comprehensive protein resource for the study of bladder cancer: http://biobase.dk/cgi-bin/celis [In Process Citation]. *Electrophoresis* 1999;20:300.
61. Chan JM et al. Plasma insulin-like growth factor–I and prostate cancer risk: a prospective study [see comments]. *Science* 1998; 279:563.
62. Chang WY et al. Novel suppressor loci on chromosome 14q in primary bladder cancer. *Cancer Res* 1995;55:3246.
63. Chassagne S et al. Renal and adrenal involvement in von Hippel-Lindau disease: clinical features and therapeutic strategies. *Prog Urol* 1996;6:878.
64. Chauveau D et al. Renal involvement in von Hippel-Lindau disease. *Kidney Int* 1996;50:944.
65. Cheng L et al. p53 alteration in regional lymph node metastases from prostate carcinoma: a marker for progression? *Cancer* 1999;85:2455.
66. Cheng L et al. p53 protein overexpression is associated with increased cell proliferation in patients with locally recurrent prostate carcinoma after radiation therapy. *Cancer* 1999;85: 1293.
67. Cher ML et al. Genetic alterations in untreated metastases and androgen-independent prostate cancer detected by comparative genomic hybridization and allelotyping. *Cancer Res* 1996;56: 3091.
68. Chin L, Pomerantz J, DePinho RA. The INK4a/ARF tumor suppressor: one gene—two products—two pathways. *Trends Biochem Sci* 1998;23:291.
69. Chow WH et al. Rising incidence of renal cell cancer in the United States. *JAMA* 1999;281:1628.
70. Choyke PL et al. Von Hippel-Lindau disease: radiologic screening for visceral manifestations. *Radiology* 1990;174:815.
71. Choyke PL et al. Intra-operative ultrasound during renal parenchymal-sparing surgery in hereditary renal cancers: a ten year experience. *J Urol* 2001;165:777.
72. Chretien Y et al. Treatment of von Hippel-Lindau disease with renal involvement. *Prog Urol* 1997;7:939.
73. Coetzee GA. Re: prostate cancer and the androgen receptor. *J Natl Cancer Inst* 1994;86:872.
74. Cohen AJ et al. Hereditary renal-cell carcinoma associated with a chromosomal translocation. *N Engl J Med* 1979;301:592.
75. Cole KA. The genetics of cancer—a 3D model. *Nat Genet* 1999;21:38.
76. Cole MD. The myc oncogene: its role in transformation and differentiation. *Annu Rev Genet* 1986;20:361.
77. Collins FS. Stattuck lecture—medical and societal consequences of the Human Genome Project. *N Engl J Med* 1999; 341:28.
78. Contractor H et al. Mutation of the p53 tumour suppressor gene occurs preferentially in the chromophobe type of renal cell tumour. *J Pathol* 1997;181:136.
79. Coombs LM et al. Immunocytochemical localization of c-erbB-2 protein in transitional cell carcinoma of the urinary bladder. *J Pathol* 1993;169:35.
80. Cooper JD, Arieff AI. Lindau disease treated by bilateral nephrectomy and hemodialysis. *West J Med* 1979;130:456.
81. Corder EH et al. Vitamin D and prostate cancer: a prediagnostic study with stored sera [see comments]. *Cancer Epidemiol Biomarkers Prev* 1993;2:467.
82. Cordon-Cardo C et al. Altered expression of the retinoblastoma gene product is a prognostic indicator in bladder cancer. *J Natl Cancer Inst* 1992;84:1251.
83. Cordon-Cardo C et al. Cooperative effects of p53 and pRB alterations in primary superficial bladder tumors. *Cancer Res* 1997;57:1217.
84. Cote RJ. Association of p27Kipl levels with recurrence and survival in patients with stage C prostate carcinoma. *J Natl Cancer Inst* 1998;90:916.
85. Cote RJ, Chatterjee SJ. Molecular determinants of outcome in bladder cancer. *Cancer J Sci Am* 1999;5:2.
86. Cote RJ. Elevated and absent pRb expression is associated with bladder cancer progression and has cooperative effects with p53. *Cancer Res* 1998;58:1090.
87. Cote RJ et al. p53 and treatment of bladder cancer [letter; comment]. *Nature* 1997;385:123.
88. Craft N et al. A mechanism for hormone-independent prostate cancer through modulation of androgen receptor signaling by the HER-2/neu tyrosine kinase [see comments]. *Nat Med* 1999;5:280.
89. Croce CM, Nowell PC. Molecular basis of human B cell neoplasia. *Blood* 1985;65:1.
90. Crotty TB, Farrow GM, Lieber MM. Chromophobe cell renal carcinoma: clinicopathological features of 50 cases. *J Urol* 1995; 154:964.
91. Dalal R. Molecular characterization of neurotrophin expression and the corresponding tropomyosin receptor kinases (trks) in epithelial and stromal cells of the human prostate. *Mol Cell Endocrinol* 1997;134:15.
92. Davidson AJ et al. Renal medullary carcinoma associated with sickle cell trait: radiologic findings. *Radiology* 1995;195:83.

93. Davis CJ Jr, Mostofi FK, Sesterhenn IA. Renal medullary carcinoma. The seventh sickle cell nephropathy. *Am J Surg Pathol* 1995;19:1.
94. De Marzo AM. E-cadherin expression as a marker of tumor aggressiveness in routinely processed radical prostatectomy specimens. *Urology* 1999;53:707.
95. De Miguel P. Immunohistochemical comparative analysis of transforming growth factor alpha, epidermal growth factor, and epidermal growth factor receptor in normal, hyperplastic and neoplastic human prostates. *Cytokine* 1999;11:722.
96. de Vere W. Human androgen receptor expression in prostate cancer following androgen ablation. *Eur Urol* 1997;31:1.
97. Deisseroth A et al. Chromosomal localization of human beta globin gene on human chromosome 11 in somatic cell hybrids. *Proc Natl Acad Sci USA* 1978;75:1456.
98. Delahunt B, Bethwaite PB, Nacey JN. Occupational risk for renal cell carcinoma. A case-control study based on the New Zealand Cancer Registry. *Br J Urol* 1995;75:578.
99. Delahunt B, Eble JN. Papillary renal cell carcinoma: a clinicopathologic and immunohistochemical study of 105 tumors. *Mod Pathol* 1997;10:537.
100. DeRisi J. Use of a cDNA microarray to analyze gene expression patterns in human cancer. *Nat Genet* 1996;14:457.
101. Dijkhuizen T et al. Chromosomal findings and p53-mutation analysis in chromophilic renal-cell carcinomas. *Int J Cancer* 1996;68:47.
102. Dijkhuizen T et al. Genetics as a diagnostic tool in sarcomatoid renal-cell cancer. *Int J Cancer* 1997;72:265.
103. Dimopoulos MA et al. Collecting duct carcinoma of the kidney. *Br J Urol* 1993;71:388.
104. Dong JT. KAI1, a metastasis suppressor gene for prostate cancer on human chromosome 11p11.2. *Science* 1995;268:884.
105. Dong JT et al. PTEN/MMAC1 is infrequently mutated in pT2 and pT3 carcinomas of the prostate. *Oncogene* 1998;17:1979.
106. Dorkin TJ. FGF8 over-expression in prostate cancer is associated with decreased patient survival and persists in androgen independent disease. *Oncogene* 1999;18:2755.
107. Dove A. Proteomics: translating genomics into products? *Nat Biotechnol* 1999;17:233.
108. Dunnill MS, Millard PR, Oliver D. Acquired cystic disease of the kidneys: a hazard of long-term intermittent maintenance haemodialysis. *J Clin Pathol* 1977;30:868.
109. Dvorak HF. Vascular permeability factor/vascular endothelial growth factor, microvascular hyperpermeability, and angiogenesis. *Am J Pathol* 1995;146:1029.
110. Eastham JA et al. Association of p53 mutations with metastatic prostate cancer. *Clin Cancer Res* 1995;1:1111.
111. el-Deiry WS. WAF1, a potential mediator of p53 tumor suppression. *Cell* 1993;75:817.
112. Emmert-Buck MR. Molecular profiling of clinical tissue specimens: feasibility and applications. *Am J Pathol* 2000;156(4):1109.
113. Emmert-Buck MR et al. Laser capture microdissection [see comments]. *Science* 1996;274:998.
114. Epstein JI et al. The World Health Organization/International Society of Urological Pathology consensus classification of urothelial (transitional cell) neoplasms of the urinary bladder. Bladder Consensus Conference Committee. *Am J Surg Pathol* 1998;22:1435.
115. Erlandson RA, Shek TW, Reuter VE. Diagnostic significance of mitochondria in four types of renal epithelial neoplasms: an ultrastructural study of 60 tumors. *Ultrastruct Pathol* 1997;21:409.
116. Eschwege P et al. Radical nephrectomy for renal cell carcinoma 30 mm or less: long-term follow results. *J Urol* 1996;155:1196.
117. Esrig D et al. Accumulation of nuclear p53 and tumor progression in bladder cancer. *N Engl J Med* 1994;331:1259.
118. Esrig D et al. p53 nuclear protein accumulation correlates with mutations in the p53 gene, tumor grade, and stage in bladder cancer. *Am J Pathol* 1993;143:1389.
119. Evans CP. Inhibition of prostate cancer neovascularization and growth by urokinase-plasminogen activator receptor blockade. *Cancer Res* 1997;57:3594.
120. Fearon ER, Vogelstein B. A genetic model for colorectal tumorigenesis. *Cell* 1990;61:759.
121. Feinberg AP et al. Mutation affecting the 12th amino acid of the c-Ha-ras oncogene product occurs infrequently in human cancer. *Science* 1983;220:1175.
122. Fendly BM. Characterization of murine monoclonal antibodies reactive to either the human epidermal growth factor receptor or HER2/neu gene product. *Cancer Res* 1990;50:1550.
123. Ferrer FA. Vascular endothelial growth factor (VEGF) expression in human prostate cancer: in situ and in vitro expression of VEGF by human prostate cancer cells. *J Urol* 1997;157:2329.
124. Ferrer FA. Angiogenesis and prostate cancer: in vivo and in vitro expression of angiogenesis factors by prostate cancer cells. *Urology* 1998;51:161.
125. Figueroa JA. Differential expression of insulin-like growth factor binding proteins in high versus low Gleason score prostate cancer. *J Urol* 1998;159:1379.
126. Fill WL, Lamiell JM, Polk NO. The radiographic manifestations of von Hippel-Lindau disease. *Radiology* 1979;133:289.
127. Fishel R et al. The human mutator gene homolog MSH2 and its association with hereditary nonpolyposis colon cancer. *Cell* 1993;75:1027.
128. Fitzgerald JM et al. Identification of H-ras mutations in urine sediments complements cytology in the detection of bladder tumors. *J Natl Cancer Inst* 1995;87:129.
129. Fleming S, Lindop GB, Gibson AA. The distribution of epithelial membrane antigen in the kidney and its tumours. *Histopathology* 1985;9:729.
130. Fleshner NE et al. The National Cancer Data Base report on bladder carcinoma. The American College of Surgeons Commission on Cancer and the American Cancer Society. *Cancer* 1996;78:1505.
131. Folkman J. Seminars in medicine of the Beth Israel Hospital, Boston. Clinical applications of research on angiogenesis. *N Engl J Med* 1995;333:1757.
132. Foster K et al. Molecular genetic investigation of sporadic renal cell carcinoma: analysis of allele loss on chromosomes 3p, 5q, 11p, 17 and 22. *Br J Cancer* 1994;69:230.
133. Frank W et al. Renal cell carcinoma: the size variable. *J Surg Oncol* 1993;54:163.
134. Freeman MR. Heparin-binding EGF-like growth factor in the human prostate: synthesis predominantly by interstitial and vascular smooth muscle cells and action as a carcinoma cell mitogen. *J Cell Biochem* 1998;68:328.
135. Friedrichs P et al. Renal medullary carcinoma and sickle cell trait. *J Urol* 1997;157:1349.
136. Friend SH et al. A human DNA segment with properties of the gene that predisposes to retinoblastoma and osteosarcoma. *Nature* 1986;323:643.
137. Frydenberg M, Malek RS, Zincke H. Conservative renal surgery for renal cell carcinoma in von Hippel-Lindau's disease. *J Urol* 1993;194:461.
138. Fujimoto K et al. Frequent association of p53 gene mutations in invasive bladder cancer. *Cancer Res* 1992;52:1393.
139. Fujita J, Srivastava SK, Kraus MH. Frequency of molecular alterations affecting ras protooncogenes in human urinary tract tumors. *Proc Natl Acad Sci USA* 1985;82:3849.

140. Fujita J et al. Ha-ras oncogenes are activated by somatic alterations in human urinary tract tumours. *Nature* 1984;309:464.
141. Furnari FB. Growth suppression of glioma cells by PTEN requires a functional phosphatase catalytic domain. *Proc Natl Acad Sci USA* 1997;94:12479.
142. Gao AC. CD44 is a metastasis suppressor gene for prostatic cancer located on human chromosome 11p13. *Cancer Res* 1997;57:846.
143. Gatalica Z et al. Metanephric adenoma: histology, immunophenotype, cytogenetics, ultrastructure. *Mod Pathol* 1996; 9:329.
144. Gelb AB. Renal cell carcinoma: current prognostic factors. Union Internationale Contre le Cancer (UICC) and the American Joint Committee on Cancer. *Cancer* 1997;80:981.
145. Gettman MT. Role of microvessel density in predicting recurrence in pathologic stage T3 prostatic adenocarcinoma. *Urology* 1999;54:479.
146. Gibbs M. Evidence for a rare prostate cancer-susceptibility locus at a chromosome 1p36. *Am J Hum Genet* 1999;64:776.
147. Giovannucci E et al. The CAG repeat within the androgen receptor gene and its relationship to prostate cancer [published erratum appears in *Proc Natl Acad Sci USA* 1997;94(15):8272]. *Proc Natl Acad Sci USA* 1997;94:3320.
148. Giri D. Alterations in expression of basic fibroblast growth factor (FGF) 2 and its receptor FGFR-1 in human prostate cancer. *Clin Cancer Res* 1999;5:1063.
149. Glavac D et al. Genetic changes in the origin and development of renal cell carcinoma (RCC). *Pflugers Arch* 1996;431:R193.
150. Glenn GM et al. Von Hippel-Lindau disease. *Prob Urol* 1990; 4:312.
151. Glenn GM et al. Von Hippel-Lindau disease: clinical review and molecular genetics. In: Anderson EE, ed. *Problems in urologic surgery: benign and malignant tumors of the kidney.* Philadelphia: JB Lippincott, 1990.
152. Glick SH, Howell LP, White RW. Relationship of p53 and bcl-2 to prognosis in muscle-invasive transitional cell carcinoma of the bladder. *J Urol* 1996;155:1754.
153. Gnarra JR et al. Mutations of the VHL tumor suppressor gene in renal carcinoma. *Nat Genet* 1994;7:85.
154. Reference deleted in proofs.
155. Goldfarb DA. Nephron-sparing surgery and renal transplantation in patients with renal cell carcinoma and von Hippel-Lindau disease. *J Intern Med* 1998;243:563.
156. Gomella LG et al. Expression of transforming growth factor alpha in normal human adult kidney and enhanced expression of transforming growth factors alpha and beta 1 in renal cell carcinoma. *Cancer Res* 1989;49:6972.
157. Gonzalez-Zulueta M et al. Microsatellite instability in bladder cancer. *Cancer Res* 1993;53:5620.
158. Gonzalgo ML et al. The role of DNA methylation in expression of the p19/p16 locus in human bladder cancer cell lines. *Cancer Res* 1998;58:1245.
159. Graff JR et al. E-cadherin expression is silenced by DNA hypermethylation in human breast and prostate carcinomas. *Cancer Res* 1995;55:5195.
160. Grawitz VP. Die Sogenannten lipome der niere. *Pathol Anat* 1883;93:39.
161. Gray IC et al. Mutation and expression analysis of the putative prostate tumour-suppressor gene PTEN. *Br J Cancer* 1998;78: 1296.
162. Greenlee RT et al. Cancer statistics, 2000. *CA Cancer J Clin* 2000;50:7.
163. Greenlee RT et al. Cancer statistics, 2000. *CA Cancer J Clin* 2000;50:10.
163a. Greenlee RT et al. Cancer statistics, 2001. *CA Cancer J Clin* 2001;51:15.
164. Gregori-Romero MA, Morell-Quadreny L, Llombart-Bosch A. A singular case of near-haploid stemline karyotype in a renal oncocytoma. *Cancer Genet Cytogenet* 1996;92:28.
165. Gregori-Romero MA, Morell-Quadreny L, Llombart-Bosch A. Cytogenetic analysis of three primary Bellini duct carcinomas. *Genes Chromosomes Cancer* 1996;15:170.
166. Grignon DJ, Eble JN. Papillary and metanephric adenomas of the kidney. *Semin Diagn Pathol* 1998;15:41.
167. Grimberg A. Role of insulin-like growth factors and their binding proteins in growth control and carcinogenesis. *J Cell Physiol* 2000;183:1.
168. Gronberg H. Characteristics of prostate cancer in families potentially linked to the hereditary prostate cancer 1 (HPC1) locus. *JAMA* 1997;278:1251.
169. Gronberg H. Segregation analysis of prostate cancer in Sweden: support for dominant inheritance. *Am J Epidemiol* 1997; 146:552.
170. Grossman HB et al. p53 and RB expression predict progression in T1 bladder cancer. *Clin Cancer Res* 1998;4:829.
171. Guengerich FP et al. Conjugation of carcinogens by theta class glutathione S-transferases: mechanisms and relevance to variations in human risk. *Pharmacogenetics* 1995;5:S103.
172. Guinan PD et al. Renal cell carcinoma: tumor size, stage and survival. Members of the Cancer Incidence and End Results Committee. *J Urol* 1995;153:901.
173. Guo Y. Down-regulation of protein and mRNA expression for transforming growth factor–beta (TGF-betal) type I and type II receptors in human prostate cancer. *Int J Cancer* 1997;71:573.
174. Guo Y et al. Loss of the cyclin-dependent kinase inhibitor p27(Kip1) protein in human prostate cancer correlates with tumor grade. *Clin Cancer Res* 1997;3:2269.
175. Habuchi T et al. Oncogene amplification in urothelial cancers with p53 gene mutation or MDM2 amplification [see comments]. *J Natl Cancer Inst* 1994;86:1331.
176. Habuchi T et al. Association of vitamin D receptor gene polymorphism with prostate cancer and benign prostatic hyperplasia in a Japanese population. *Cancer Res* 2000;60:305.
177. Habuchi T et al. Influence of cigarette smoking and schistosomiasis on p53 gene mutation in urothelial cancer. *Cancer Res* 1993;53:3795.
178. Hall PA, Lane DP. p53 in tumour pathology: can we trust immunohistochemistry? Revisited! [editorial] [see comments]. *J Pathol* 1994;172:1.
179. Hanchette CL, Schwartz GG. Geographic patterns of prostate cancer mortality. Evidence for a protective effect of ultraviolet radiation. *Cancer* 1992;70:2861.
180. Hardy DO et al. Androgen receptor CAG repeat lengths in prostate cancer: correlation with age of onset. *J Clin Endocrinol Metab* 1996;81:4400.
181. Harper JW. The p21 cdk-interacting protein cip1 is a potent inhibitor of G1 cyclin-dependent kinases. *Cell* 1993;75:805.
182. Harries LW et al. Identification of genetic polymorphisms at the glutathione S-transferase Pi locus and association with susceptibility to bladder, testicular and prostate cancer. *Carcinogenesis* 1997;18:641.
183. Hart S et al. Quality of life after radical cystectomy for bladder cancer in patients with an ileal conduit, cutaneous or urethral Kock pouch. *J Urol* 1999;162:77.
184. Haupt Y et al. Mdm2 promotes the rapid degradation of p53. *Nature* 1997;387:296.
185. He WW et al. A novel human prostate-specific, androgen-regulated homeobox gene (NKX3.1) that maps to 8p21, a region frequently deleted in prostate cancer. *Genomics* 1997; 43:69.

186. Heath CW Jr et al. Hypertension, diuretics, and antihypertensive medications as possible risk factors for renal cell cancer. *Am J Epidemiol* 1997;145:607.
187. Heinz-Peer G et al. Prevalence of acquired cystic kidney disease and tumors in native kidneys of renal transplant recipients: a prospective US study. *Radiology* 1995;195:667.
188. Herbers J et al. Lack of genetic changes at specific genomic sites separates renal oncocytomas from renal cell carcinomas. *J Pathol* 1998;184:58.
189. Herman JG. Inactivation of the CDKN2/p16/MTS1 gene is frequently associated with aberrant DNA methylation in all common human cancers. *Cancer Res* 1995;55:4525.
190. Herman JG. Hypermethylation-associated inactivation indicates a tumor suppressor role for P15INK4B. *Cancer Res* 1996; 56:722.
191. Herman JG et al. Silencing of the VHL tumor suppressor gene by DNA methylation in renal carcinoma. *Proc Natl Acad Sci USA* 1994;91:9700.
192. Herr HW. Tumor progression and survival of patients with high grade, noninvasive papillary (TaG3) bladder tumor: 15-year outcome [see comments]. *J Urol* 2000;163:60.
193. Herring J et al. Parenchymal sparing surgery in patients with hereditary renal cell carcinoma—ten year experience. *J Urol* 2001;165:1623.
194. Herring JC et al. Renal medullary carcinoma: a recently described highly aggressive renal tumor in young black patients. *J Urol* 1997;157:2246.
195. Hirvonen A et al. The GSTM1 null genotype as a potential risk modifier for squamous cell carcinoma of the lung. *Carcinogenesis* 1993;14:1479.
196. Hofmockel G et al. Expression of p53 and bcl-2 in primary locally confined renal cell carcinomas: no evidence for prognostic significance. *Anticancer Res* 1996;16:3807.
197. Hollstein M et al. p53 mutations in human cancers. *Science* 1991;253:49.
198. Hornigold N et al. Mutation of the 9q34 gene TSC1 in sporadic bladder cancer. *Oncogene* 1999;18:2657.
199. Hovey RM et al. Genetic alterations in primary bladder cancers and their metastases. *Cancer Res* 1998;58:3555.
200. Hudson HC, Wilson CE. Bilateral renal cell carcinoma in von Hippel-Lindau disease: treatment with staged bilateral nephrectomy and hemodialysis. *South Med J* 1979;72:363.
201. Hudziak RM. p185HER2 monoclonal antibody has antiproliferative effects in vitro and sensitizes human breast tumor cells to tumor necrosis factor. *Mol Cell Biol* 1989;9:1165.
202. Hughson MD et al. Nonpapillary and papillary renal cell carcinoma: a cytogenetic and phenotypic study. *Mod Pathol* 1993;6:449.
203. Hughson MD et al. Renal cell carcinoma of end-stage renal disease: a histopathologic and molecular genetic study. *J Am Soc Nephrol* 1996;7:2461.
204. Humbert O et al. Mismatch repair and differential sensitivity of mouse and human cells to methylating agents. *Carcinogenesis* 1999;20:205.
205. Humphrey PA. Hepatocyte growth factor and its receptor (c-met) in prostatic carcinoma. *Am J Pathol* 1995;147:386.
206. Ichikawa T. Localization of metastasis suppressor gene(s) for prostatic cancer to the short arm of human chromosome 11. *Cancer Res* 1992;52:3486.
207. Ide H. Growth regulation of human prostate cancer cells by bone morphogenetic protein-2. *Cancer Res* 1997;57:5022.
208. Ingles SA et al. Association of prostate cancer risk with genetic polymorphisms in vitamin D receptor and androgen receptor [see comments]. *J Natl Cancer Inst* 1997;89:166.
209. Inoue T et al. Multivariate analysis of prognostic determinants after surgery for renal cell carcinoma at Himeji National Hospital. *Hinyokika Kiyo* 2000;46:229.
210. Ionov Y et al. Ubiquitous somatic mutations in simple repeated sequences reveal a new mechanism for colonic carcinogenesis. *Nature* 1993;363:558.
211. Iqbal MA, Akhtar M, Ali MA. Cytogenetic findings in renal cell carcinoma. *Hum Pathol* 1996;27:949.
212. Ishii H. The FEZ1 gene at chromosome 8p22 encodes a leucine-zipper protein, and its expression is altered in multiple human tumors. *Proc Natl Acad Sci USA* 1999;96:3928.
213. Ishikawa J et al. Inactivation of the retinoblastoma gene in human bladder and renal cell carcinoma. *Cancer Res* 1991;51: 5736.
214. Jarrard DF et al. Methylation of the androgen receptor promoter CpG island is associated with loss of androgen receptor expression in prostate cancer cells. *Cancer Res* 1998;58:5310.
215. Jarrard DF et al. p16/pRb pathway alterations are required for bypassing senescence in human prostate epithelial cells. *Cancer Res* 1999;59:2957.
216. Javidan J et al. Prognostic significance of the 1997 TNM classification of renal cell carcinoma. *J Urol* 1999;162:1277.
217. Jeffers M et al. Activating mutations for the met tyrosine kinase receptor in human cancer. *Proc Natl Acad Sci USA* 1997;94: 11445.
218. Jin TX et al. Human mismatch repair gene (hMSH2) product expression in relation to recurrence of transitional cell carcinoma of the urinary bladder. *Cancer* 1999;85:478.
219. Johnson DG et al. Expression of transcription factor E2F1 induces quiescent cells to enter S phase. *Nature* 1993;365:349.
220. Kamb A et al. A cell cycle regulator potentially involved in genesis of many tumor types. *Science* 1994;264:436.
221. Kardas I et al. Translocation (X;1)(p11.2;q21) in a papillary renal cell carcinoma in a 14-year-old girl. *Cancer Genet Cytogenet* 1998;101:159.
222. Kastan MB et al. A mammalian cell cycle checkpoint pathway utilizing p53 and GADD45 is defective in ataxia-telangiectasia. *Cell* 1992;71:587.
223. Keegan PE, Lunec J, Neal DE. p53 and p53-regulated genes in bladder cancer [see comments]. *Br J Urol* 1998;82:710.
224. Keen AJ, Knowles MA. Definition of two regions of deletion on chromosome 9 in carcinoma of the bladder. *Oncogene* 1994;9: 2083.
225. Kelly JD et al. Apoptosis and its clinical significance for bladder cancer therapy. *BJU Int* 1999;83:1.
226. Kelly K et al. Cell-specific regulation of the c-myc gene by lymphocyte mitogens and platelet-derived growth factor. *Cell* 1983;35:603.
227. Kenck C et al. Mutation of the VHL gene is associated exclusively with the development of non-papillary renal cell carcinomas. *J Pathol* 1996;179:157.
228. Kennedy SM et al. Collecting duct carcinoma of the kidney. *Hum Pathol* 1990;21:449.
229. Ketterer B. Glutathione S-transferases and prevention of cellular free radical damage. *Free Radic Res* 1998;28:647.
230. Kibel AS et al. Identification of 12p as a region of frequent deletion in advanced prostate cancer [In Process Citation]. *Cancer Res* 1998;58:5652.
231. Kim HG et al. EGF receptor signaling in prostate morphogenesis and tumorigenesis. *Histol Histopathol* 1999;14:1175.
232. Kinouchi T, Saiki S, Maoe T. Correlation of c-myc expression with nuclear pleomorphism in human renal cell carcinoma. *Cancer Res* 1989;49:3627.
233. Kishi K et al. Carcinoma of the bladder: a clinical and pathological analysis of 87 autopsy cases. *J Urol* 1981;125:36.

234. Knebelmann B et al. Transforming growth factor α is a target for the von Hippel-Lindau tumor suppressor. *Cancer Res* 1998; 58:226.
235. Knowles MA. Identification of novel bladder tumour suppressor genes. *Electrophoresis* 1999;20:269.
236. Knowles MA. The genetics of transitional cell carcinoma: progress and potential clinical application. *BJU Int* 1999;84:412.
237. Knowles MA et al. Allelotype of human bladder cancer. *Cancer Res* 1994;54:531.
238. Knudson AG. All in the (cancer) family [news]. *Nat Genet* 1993;5:103.
239. Knudson AGJ. Hereditary cancer, oncogenes, and antioncogenes. *Cancer Res* 1985;45:1437.
240. Koolen MI et al. A familial case of renal cell carcinoma and a t(2;3) chromosome translocation. *Kidney Int* 1998;53:273.
241. Koskinen PJ, Alitalo K. Role of myc amplification and overexpression in cell growth, differentiation and death. *Semin Cancer Biol* 1993;4:3.
242. Kovacs A. Mitochondrial and chromosomal DNA alterations in human chromophobe renal cell carcinomas. *J Pathol* 1992; 167:273.
243. Kovacs G et al. The Heidelberg classification of renal cell tumors. *J Pathol* 1997;183:131.
244. Kovacs G. Papillary renal cell carcinoma. A morphologic and cytogenetic study of 11 cases. *Am J Pathol* 1989;134:27.
245. Kovacs G. Molecular differential pathology of renal cell tumours. *Histopathology* 1993;22:1.
246. Kovacs G. Molecular cytogenetics of renal cell tumors. In: Vande WG, Klein G, eds. *Advances in cancer research.* Frederick, Md: Academic Press, 1994.
247. Kovacs G. The value of molecular genetic analysis in the diagnosis and prognosis of renal cell tumours. *World J Urol* 1994;12:64.
248. Kovacs G, Brusa P, de Riese W. Tissue-specific expression of a constitutional 3;6 translocation: development of multiple bilateral renal-cell carcinomas. *Int J Cancer* 1989;43:422.
249. Kovacs G et al. Cytogenetics of papillary renal cell tumors. *Genes Chromosom Cancer* 1991;3:249.
250. Kovacs G, Ishikawa I. High incidence of papillary renal cell tumours in patients on chronic haemodialysis. *Histopathology* 1993;22:135.
251. Kovacs G, Soudah B, Hoene E. Binucleated cells in a human renal cell carcinoma with 34 chromosomes. *Cancer Genet Cytogenet* 1988;31:211.
252. Kovacs G, Tory K, Kovacs A. Development of papillary renal cell tumours is associated with loss of Y-chromosome-specific DNA sequences. *J Pathol* 1994;173:39.
253. Krajewska M. Immunohistochemical analysis of bcl-2 family proteins in adenocarcinomas of the stomach. *Am J Pathol* 1996;149:1449.
254. Kubbutat MH, Jones SN, Vousden KH. Regulation of p53 stability by Mdm2. *Nature* 1997;387:299.
255. La Vecchia C et al. Smoking and renal cell carcinoma. *Cancer Res* 1990;50:5231.
256. Lafuente A et al. Human glutathione S-transferase mu (GST mu) deficiency as a marker for the susceptibility to bladder and larynx cancer among smokers. *Cancer Lett* 1993;68:49.
257. Lamiell JM, Salazar FG, Hsia YE. Von Hippel-Lindau disease affecting 43 members of a single kindred. *Medicine* 1989;68:1.
258. Landis SH et al. Cancer statistics, 1999 [see comments]. *CA Cancer J Clin* 1999;49:8.
259. Latif F et al. Identification of the von Hippel-Lindau disease tumor suppressor gene. *Science* 1993;260:1317.
260. Latil A et al. Infrequent allelic imbalance at the major susceptibility HPC1 locus in sporadic prostate tumours [letter]. *Int J Cancer* 1997;71:1118.
261. Leach FS et al. Mutations of a mutS homolog in hereditary nonpolyposis colorectal cancer. *Cell* 1993;75:1215.
262. Reference deleted in proofs.
263. Lebret T et al. Correlation between p53 over expression and response to bacillus Calmette-Guérin therapy in a high risk select population of patients with T1G3 bladder cancer. *J Urol* 1998;159:788.
264. Lee CC et al. Significance of cyclin D1 overexpression in transitional cell carcinomas of the urinary bladder and its correlation with histopathologic features. *Cancer* 1997;79:780.
265. Lee WH et al. Cytidine methylation of regulatory sequences near the pi-class glutathione S-transferase gene accompanies human prostatic carcinogenesis. *Proc Natl Acad Sci USA* 1994; 91:11733.
266. Leung HY. Over-expression of fibroblast growth factor-8 in human prostate cancer. *Oncogene* 1996;12:1833.
267. Levine AJ. p53, the cellular gatekeeper for growth and division. *Cell* 1997;88:323.
268. Levine AJ, Momand J, Finlay CA. The p53 tumour suppressor gene. *Nature* 1991;351:453.
269. Levy A, Dang UC, Bookstein R. High-density screen of human tumor cell lines for homozygous deletions of loci on chromosome arm 8p. *Genes Chromosomes Cancer* 1999;24:42.
270. Li C. Distinct deleted regions on chromosome segment 16q23-24 associated with metastases in prostate cancer. *Genes Chromosomes Cancer* 1999;24:175.
271. Li FP et al. Clinical and genetic studies of renal cell carcinomas in a family with a constitutional chromosome 3;8 translocation: genetics of familial renal carcinoma. *Ann Intern Med* 1993;118:106.
272. Lindblad P et al. International renal-cell cancer study. V. Reproductive factors, gynecologic operations and exogenous hormones. *Int J Cancer* 1995;61:192.
273. Lindblom A et al. Genetic mapping of a second locus predisposing to hereditary non-polyposis colon cancer. *Nat Genet* 1993;5:279.
274. Linehan WM, Klausner RD. Renal carcinoma. In: Vogelstein B, Kinzler K, eds. The genetic basis of human cancer. Baltimore: Williams & Wilkins, 1998.
275. Linehan WM, Lerman MI, Zbar B. Identification of the VHL gene: its role in renal carcinoma. *JAMA* 1995;273:564.
276. Lipponen PK. Over-expression of p53 nuclear oncoprotein in transitional cell bladder cancer and its prognostic value. *Int J Cancer* 1993;53:365.
277. Lipponen P, Eskelinen M. Expression of epidermal growth factor receptor in bladder cancer as related to established prognostic factors, oncoprotein (c-erbB-2, p53) expression and long-term prognosis. *Br J Cancer* 1994;69:1120.
278. Lipponen PK. Expression of c-myc protein is related to cell proliferation and expression of growth factor receptors in transitional cell bladder cancer. *J Pathol* 1995;175:203.
279. Liu AY. Analysis and sorting of prostate cancer cell types by flow cytometry. *Prostate* 1999;40:192.
280. Ljungberg B et al. Prognostic significance of the Heidelberg classification of renal cell carcinoma. *Eur Urol* 1999;36:565.
281. Lloyd RV et al. p27kip1: a multifunctional cyclin-dependent kinase inhibitor with prognostic significance in human cancers. *Am J Pathol* 1999;154:313.
282. Logothetis CJ et al. Altered retinoblastoma protein expression and known prognostic variables in locally advanced bladder cancer. *J Natl Cancer Inst* 1992;84:1257.

283. Longuemaux S et al. Candidate genetic modifiers of individual susceptibility to renal cell carcinoma: a study of polymorphic human xenobiotic-metabolizing enzymes. *Cancer Res* 1999;59: 2903.
284. Lou W. Methylation of the CD44 metastasis suppressor gene in human prostate cancer. *Cancer Res* 1999;59:2329.
285. Luo J. Suppression of prostate cancer invasive potential and matrix metalloproteinase activity by E-cadherin transfection. *Cancer Res* 1999;59:3552.
286. Lutchman M. Loss of heterozygosity on 8p in prostate cancer implicates a role for dematin in tumor progression. *Cancer Genet Cytogenet* 1999;115:65.
287. Lynch HT, Ens JA, Lynch JF. The Lynch syndrome II and urological malignancies. *J Urol* 1990;143:24.
288. Mackey TJ. bcl-2/bax ratio as a predictive marker for therapeutic response to radiotherapy in patients with prostate cancer. *Urology* 1998;52:1085.
289. Maclure M, Willett W. A case-control study of diet and risk of renal adenocarcinoma. *Epidemiology* 1990;1:430.
290. Macoska JA et al. Evidence for three tumor suppressor gene loci on chromosome 8p in human prostate cancer. *Cancer Res* 1995;55:5390.
291. Maher ER, Kaelin WG Jr. Von Hippel-Lindau disease. *Medicine (Baltimore),* 1997;76:381.
292. Maher ER et al. Clinical features and natural history of von Hippel-Lindau disease. *Q J Med* 1990;77:1151.
293. Malkin D et al. Germ line p53 mutations in a familial syndrome of breast cancer, sarcomas, and other neoplasms. *Science* 1990;250:1233.
294. Mandel JS et al. International renal-cell cancer study. IV. Occupation. *Int J Cancer* 1995;61:601.
295. Manski TJ et al. Endolymphatic sac tumors: a source of morbid hearing loss in von Hippel-Lindau Disease. *JAMA* 1997;277: 1461.
296. Mao L et al. Molecular detection of primary bladder cancer by microsatellite analysis. *Science* 1996;271:659.
297. Masuda H et al. Significant prognostic factors for 5-year survival after curative resection of renal cell carcinoma. *Int J Urol* 1998;5:418.
298. Matson MA, Cohen EP. Acquired cystic kidney disease: occurrence, prevalence, and renal cancers. *Medicine (Baltimore)* 1990;69:217.
299. McCredie M, Stewart JH. Risk factors for kidney cancer in New South Wales—I. Cigarette smoking. *Eur J Cancer* 1992; 28A:2050.
300. McLaughlin JK et al. International renal-cell cancer study. I. Tobacco use. *Int J Cancer* 1995;60:194.
300a. McLauglin JK et al. A population-based case-control study of renal cell carcinoma. *J Natl Cancer Inst* 1984;72:275.
301. Mellemgaard A et al. Occupational risk factors for renal-cell carcinoma in Denmark. *Scand J Work Environ Health* 1994; 20:160.
302. Mellon JK et al. C-erbB-2 in bladder cancer: molecular biology, correlation with epidermal growth factor receptors and prognostic value [see comments]. *J Urol* 1996;155:321.
303. Mellon K et al. Long-term outcome related to epidermal growth factor receptor status in bladder cancer. *J Urol* 1995;153:919.
304. Merino MJ, Livolsi VA. Oncocytomas of the kidney. *Cancer* 1982;50:1852.
305. Merlo A. 5′ CpG island methylation is associated with transcriptional silencing of the tumor suppressor p16/CDKN2/MTS1 in human cancers. *Nat Med* 1995;1:686.
306. Messing EM. Growth factors and bladder cancer: clinical implications of the interactions between growth factors and their urothelial receptors. *Semin Surg Oncol* 1992;8:285.
307. Meyers FJ et al. Very frequent p53 mutations in metastatic prostate carcinoma and in matched primary tumors. *Cancer* 1998;83:2534.
308. Miller DL et al. Von Hippel-Lindau disease: inadequacy of angiography for identification of renal cancers. *Radiology* 1991; 179:833.
309. Miyake H. Inhibition of progression to androgen-independence by combined adjuvant treatment with antisense BCL-XL and antisense bcl-2 oligonucleotides plus taxol after castration in the shionogi tumor model. *Int J Cancer* 2000; 86:855.
310. Miyamoto H et al. Loss of heterozygosity at the p53, RB, DCC and APC tumor suppressor gene loci in human bladder cancer. *J Urol* 1996;155:1444.
311. Morita N. E-cadherin and alpha-, beta- and gamma-catenin expression in prostate cancers: correlation with tumour invasion. *Br J Cancer* 1999;79:1879.
312. Mostafa MH, Sheweita SA, O'Connor PJ. Relationship between schistosomiasis and bladder cancer. *Clin Microbiol Rev* 1999;12:97.
313. Reference deleted in proofs.
314. Mostofi FK, Sobin LH, Torloni H. *Histologic typing of urinary bladder tumours. International histological classification of tumors.* Geneva: World Health Organization, 1973.
315. Motokura T, Arnold A. Cyclin D and oncogenesis. *Curr Opin Genet Dev* 1993;3:5.
316. Motzer RJ et al. Survival and prognostic stratification of 670 patients with advanced renal cell carcinoma. *J Clin Oncol* 1999;17:2530.
317. Muscat JE, Hoffmann D, Wynder EL. The epidemiology of renal cell carcinoma. A second look. *Cancer* 1995;75:2552.
318. Naitoh H et al. Overexpression and localization of cyclin D1 mRNA and antigen in esophageal cancer. *Am J Pathol* 1995; 146:1161.
319. Nau MM et al. L-myc, a new myc-related gene amplified and expressed in human small cell lung cancer. *Nature* 1985;318:69.
320. Navone NM et al. p53 mutations in prostate cancer bone metastases suggest that selected p53 mutants in the primary site define foci with metastatic potential. *J Urol* 1999;161:304.
321. Nelson PS et al. The prostate expression database (PEDB): status and enhancements in 2000. *Nucleic Acids Res* 2000; 28:212.
322. Nelson PS et al. Negative selection: a method for obtaining low-abundance cDNAs using high-density cDNA clone arrays. *Genet Anal* 1999;15:209.
323. Neuhaus C et al. Involvement of the chromosomal region 11q13 in renal oncocytoma: case report and literature review. *Cancer Genet Cytogenet* 1997;94:95.
324. Neumann HP et al. Prevalence, morphology and biology of renal cell carcinoma in von Hippel-Lindau disease compared to sporadic renal cell carcinoma. *J Urol* 1998;160:1248.
325. Nicolaides NC et al. Mutations of two PMS homologous in hereditary nonpolyposis colon cancer. *Nature* 1994;371:75.
326. Nishimura K. Prostate stromal cell-derived hepatocyte growth factor induces invasion of prostate cancer cell line DU145 through tumor-stromal interaction. *Prostate* 1999;41:145.
327. Novick AC, Streem SB. Long-term followup after nephron sparing surgery for renal cell carcinoma in von Hippel-Lindau disease. *J Urol* 1992;147:1488.
328. Nunez G et al. Caspases: the proteases of the apoptotic pathway. *Oncogene* 1998;17:3237.

329. Oda T et al. Mutation pattern of the p53 gene as a diagnostic marker for multiple hepatocellular carcinoma. *Cancer Res* 1992; 52:3674.
330. Olapade-Olaopa EO et al. Evidence for the differential expression of a variant EGF receptor protein in human prostate cancer. *Br J Cancer* 2000;82:186.
331. Oliner JD et al. Amplification of a gene encoding a p53-associated protein in human sarcomas. *Nature* 1992;358:80.
332. Oliner JD et al. Oncoprotein MDM2 conceals the activation domain of tumour suppressor p53. *Nature* 1993;362:857.
333. Olumi AF et al. Allelic loss of chromosomes 17p distinguishes high grade from low grade transitional cell carcinoma of the bladder. *Cancer Res* 1990;50:7081.
334. Orlow I et al. Deletions of the INK4A gene in superficial bladder tumors. Association with recurrence. *Am J Pathol* 1999; 155:105.
335. Ornstein DK et al. Review of the AACR meeting: new research approaches in the prevention and cure of prostate cancer, 2-6 December 1998, Indian Wells, CA. *Biochim Biophys Acta* 1999; 1424:R11.
336. Ornstein DK et al. Prevalence of microscopic tumors in normal appearing renal parenchyma from patients with hereditary papillary renal cancer. *J Urol* 2000;163:431.
337. Ortmann M, Vierbuchen M, Fischer R. Sialylated glycoconjugates in chromophobe cell renal carcinoma compared with other renal cell tumors. Indication of its development from the collecting duct epithelium. *Virchows Arch B Cell Pathol Incl Mol Pathol* 1991;61:123.
338. Papadopoulos N et al. Mutation of a mutL homolog in hereditary colon cancer [see comments]. *Science* 1994;263:1625.
339. Pearson JC, Weiss J, Tanagho EA. A plea for conservation of kidney in renal adenocarcinoma associated with von Hippel-Lindau disease. *J Urol* 1980;124:910.
340. Peltomaki P et al. Genetic mapping of a locus predisposing to human colorectal cancer. *Science* 1993;260:810.
341. Perez-Ordonez B et al. Renal oncocytoma: a clinicopathologic study of 70 cases. *Am J Surg Pathol* 1997;21:871.
342. Perinchery G et al. Loss of two new loci on chromosome 8 (8p23 and 8q12-13) in human prostate cancer. *Int J Oncol* 1999;14:495.
343. Peterson GJ et al. Renal transplantation in Lindau-von Hippel disease. *Arch Surg* 1977;112:841.
344. Pisters LL. c-met proto-oncogene expression in benign and malignant human prostate tissues. *J Urol* 1995;154:293.
345. Polascik TJ et al. Distinct regions of allelic loss on chromosome 4 in human primary bladder carcinoma. *Cancer Res* 1995;55: 5396.
346. Polascik TJ et al. Distal nephron renal tumors: microsatellite allelotype. *Cancer Res* 1996;56:1892.
347. Pomerantz J et al. The Ink4a tumor suppressor gene product, p19Arf, interacts with MDM2 and neutralizes MDM2's inhibition of p53. *Cell* 1998;92:713.
348. Pope JC, Koch MO, Bluth RF. Renal cell carcinoma in patients with end-stage renal disease: a comparison of clinical significance in patients receiving hemodialysis and those with renal transplants. *Urology* 1994;44:497.
349. Poston CD et al. Characterization of the renal pathology of a familial form of renal cell carcinoma associated with von Hippel-Lindau disease: clinical and molecular genetic implications. *J Urol* 1995;153:22.
350. Presti JC et al. Molecular genetic alterations in superficial and locally advanced human bladder cancer. *Cancer Res* 1991;51: 5405.
351. Presti JC et al. Renal cell carcinoma genetic analysis by comparative genomic hybridization and restriction fragment length polymorphism analysis. *J Urol* 1996;156:281.
352. Putz T et al. Epidermal growth factor (EGF) receptor blockade inhibits the action of EGF, insulin-like growth factor I, and a protein kinase A activator on the mitogen-activated protein kinase pathway in prostate cancer cell lines. *Cancer Res* 1999; 59:227.
353. Rabbani F, Cordon-Cardo C. Mutation of cell cycle regulators and their impact on superficial bladder cancer. *Urol Clin North Am* 2000;27:83.
354. Rebbeck TR et al. Glutathione S-transferase-mu (GSTM1) and -theta (GSTT1) genotypes in the etiology of prostate cancer. *Cancer Epidemiol Biomarkers Prev* 1999;8:283.
355. Reddy EP et al. A point mutation is responsible for the acquisition of transforming properties by the T24 bladder carcinoma oncogene. *Nature* 1982;300:149.
356. Renshaw AA, Maurici D, Fletcher JA. Cytologic and fluorescence in situ hybridization (FISH) examination of metanephric adenoma. *Diagn Cytopathol* 1997;16:107.
357. Reznikoff CA et al. A molecular genetic model of human bladder cancer pathogenesis. *Semin Oncol* 1996;23:571.
358. Robson CJ, Churchill BM, Anderson W. The results of radical nephrectomy for renal cell carcinoma. *J Urol* 1969;101:297.
359. Rosin MP, Anwar WA, Ward AJ. Inflammation, chromosomal instability, and cancer: the schistosomiasis model. *Cancer Res* 1994;54:1929s.
360. Rosin MP et al. Partial allelotype of carcinoma in situ of the human bladder. *Cancer Res* 1995;55:5213.
361. Ross JS. HER-2/neu gene amplification status in prostate cancer by fluorescence in situ hybridization. *Hum Pathol* 1997; 28:827.
362. Roth JS et al. Bilateral renal cell carcinoma in the Birt-Hogg-Dubé syndrome. *J Am Acad Dermatol* 1993;29:1055.
363. Rubin MA. Microvessel density in prostate cancer: lack of correlation with tumor grade, pathologic stage, and clinical outcome. *Urology* 1999;53:542.
364. Sarasin FP et al. Screening for acquired cystic kidney disease: a decision analytic perspective. *Kidney Int* 1995;48:207.
365. Sarkar FH. Relationship of P21(WAF1) expression with disease-free survival and biochemical recurrence in prostate adenocarcinomas (PCa). *Prostate* 1999;40:256.
366. Sarkis AS et al. Nuclear overexpression of p53 protein in transitional cell bladder carcinoma: a marker for disease progression. *J Natl Cancer Inst* 1993;85:53.
367. Sarkis AS et al. Prognostic value of p53 nuclear overexpression in patients with invasive bladder cancer treated with neoadjuvant MVAC. *J Clin Oncol* 1995;13:1384.
368. Sartor O, Zheng Q, Eastham JA. Androgen receptor gene CAG repeat length varies in a race-specific fashion in men without prostate cancer. *Urology* 1999;53:378.
369. Sato K et al. An immunohistologic evaluation of c-erbB-2 gene product in patients with urinary bladder carcinoma. *Cancer* 1992;70:2493.
370. Sauter G et al. c-myc copy number gains in bladder cancer detected by fluorescence in situ hybridization. *Am J Pathol* 1995;146:1131.
371. Sauter G et al. Heterogeneity of erbB-2 gene amplification in bladder cancer. *Cancer Res* 1993;53:2199.
372. Scherr DS et al. BCL-2 and p53 expression in clinically localized prostate cancer predicts response to external beam radiotherapy [published erratum appears in *J Urol* 1999;162(2): 503]. *J Urol* 1999;162:12.

373. Schlehofer B et al. International renal-cell-cancer study. VI. The role of medical and family history. *Int J Cancer* 1996; 66:723.
374. Schmidt L et al. Germline and somatic mutations in the tyrosine kinase domain of the MET proto-oncogene in papillary renal carcinomas. *Nat Genet* 1997;16:68.
375. Schmidt L et al. Novel mutations of the MET proto-oncogene in papillary renal carcinomas. *Oncogene* 1999;18:2343.
376. Schmidt L et al. Two North American families with hereditary papillary renal carcinoma and identical novel mutations in the MET proto-oncogene. *Cancer Res* 1998;58:1719.
377. Schmidt L et al. Mechanism of tumorigenesis of renal carcinomas associated with the constitutional chromosome 3;8 translocation. *Cancer J Sci Am* 1995;1:191.
378. Schoenberg MP et al. Microsatellite mutation (CAG24—>18) in the androgen receptor gene in human prostate cancer. *Biochem Biophys Res Commun* 1994;198:74.
379. Schullerus D et al. Loss of heterozygosity at chromosomes 8p, 9p, and 14q is associated with stage and grade of non-papillary renal cell carcinomas. *J Pathol* 1997;183:151.
380. Schwab M. Amplification of n-nyc as a prognostic marker for patients with neuroblastoma. *Semin Cancer Biol* 1993;4:13.
381. Schwartz SJ. Gains of the relative genomic content of erbB-1 and erbB-2 in prostate carcinoma and their association with metastasis. *Int J Oncol* 1999;14:367.
382. Schwerdtle RF et al. Allelic losses at chromosome 1p, 2p, 6p, 10p, 13q, 17p, and 21q significantly correlate with the chromophobe subtype of renal cell carcinoma. *Cancer Res* 1996;56: 2927.
383. Selli C et al. Retrospective evaluation of c-erbB-2 oncogene amplification using competitive PCR in collecting duct carcinoma of the kidney. *J Urol* 1997;158:245.
384. Seth D. Complex post-transcriptional regulation of EGF-receptor expression by EGF and TGF-alpha in human prostate cancer cells. *Br J Cancer* 1999;80:657.
385. Shaw ME et al. Partial allelotype of schistosomiasis-associated bladder cancer. *Int J Cancer* 1999;80:656.
386. Shaw ME, Knowles MA. Deletion mapping of chromosome 11 in carcinoma of the bladder. *Genes Chromosomes Cancer* 1995;13:1.
387. Shimizu E et al. Phase II study of oral administration of 5′-deoxy-5-fluorouridine (5′-DFUR) for solid tumors. *Jpn J Clin Oncol* 1984;14:679.
388. Shin KY et al. Overexpression of cyclin D1 correlates with early recurrence in superficial bladder cancers. *Br J Cancer* 1997;75: 1788.
389. Shuin T et al. Frequent somatic mutations and loss of heterozygosity of the von Hippel-Lindau tumor suppressor gene in primary human renal cell carcinomas. *Cancer Res* 1994;54: 2852.
390. Sidhar SK et al. The t(X;1)(p11.2;q21.2) translocation in papillary renal cell carcinoma fuses anovel gene PRCC to the TFE3 transcription factor gene. *Hum Mol Genet* 1996;5:1333.
391. Sidransky D et al. Clonal origin of bladder cancer. *N Engl J Med* 1992;326:737.
392. Sidransky D, Messing E. Molecular genetics and biochemical mechanisms in bladder cancer. Oncogenes, tumor suppressor genes, and growth factors. *Urol Clin North Am* 1992;19:629.
393. Sinke RJ et al. Fine mapping of the human renal oncocytoma-associated translocation (5;11)(q35;q13) breakpoint. *Cancer Genet Cytogenet* 1997;96:95.
394. Sintich SM. Transforming growth factor-beta1-induced proliferation of the prostate cancer cell line, TSU-Pr1: the role of platelet-derived growth factor. *Endocrinology* 1999;140:3411.
395. Smith JR et al. Major susceptibility locus for prostate cancer on chromosome 1 suggested by a genome-wide search [see comments]. *Science* 1996;274:1371.
396. Sokoloff MH. Targeting angiogenic pathways involving tumor-stromal interaction to treat advanced human prostate cancer. *Cancer Metastasis Rev* 1998;17:307.
397. Sortino MA. Mitogenic effect of nerve growth factor (NGF) in LNCaP prostate adenocarcinoma cells: role of the high- and low-affinity NGF receptors. *Mol Endocrinol* 2000;14:124.
398. Speicher MR et al. Specific loss of chromosomes 1, 2, 6, 10, 13, 17, and 21 in chromophobe renal cell carcinomas revealed by comparative genomic hybridization. *Am J Pathol* 1994; 145:356.
399. Spruck CH et al. Two molecular pathways to transitional cell carcinoma of the bladder. *Cancer Res* 1994;54:784.
400. Stackhouse GB et al. p53 and bcl-2 immunohistochemistry in pretreatment prostate needle biopsies to predict recurrence of prostate cancer after radical prostatectomy [see comments]. *J Urol* 1999;162:2040.
401. Stanford JL et al. Polymorphic repeats in the androgen receptor gene: molecular markers of prostate cancer risk. *Cancer Res* 1997;57:1194.
402. Stein JP et al. Prognostic markers in bladder cancer: a contemporary review of the literature. *J Urol* 1998;160:645.
403. Steinbach F et al. Treatment of renal cell carcinoma in von Hippel-Lindau disease: a multicenter study. *J Urol* 1995;153: 1812.
404. Steinberg GD et al. Family history and the risk of prostate cancer. *Prostate* 1990;17:337.
405. Steiner G et al. High-density mapping of chromosomal arm 1q in renal collecting carcinoma: region of minimal deletion at 1q32.1-32.2. *Cancer Res* 1996;56:5044.
406. Storkel S et al. Classification of renal cell carcinoma: workgroup no. 1. Union Internationale Contre le Cancer (UICC) and the American Joint Committee on Cancer (AJCC). *Cancer* 1997; 80:987.
407. Story MT. Expression of transforming growth factor beta 1 (TGF beta 1), -beta 2, and -beta 3 by cultured human prostate cells. *J Cell Physiol* 1996;169:97.
408. Strohmeyer D. Tumor angiogenesis is associated with progression after radical prostatectomy in pT2/pT3 prostate cancer. *Prostate* 2000;42:26.
409. Suzuki H. Interfocal heterogeneity of PTEN/MMAC1 gene alterations in multiple metastatic prostate cancer tissues. *Cancer Res* 1998;58:204.
410. Suzuki H et al. Mutational state of von Hippel-Lindau and adenomatous polyposis coli genes in renal tumors. *Oncology* 1997;54:252.
411. Sweeney C, Farrow DC. Differential survival related to smoking among patients with renal cell carcinoma. *Epidemiology* 2000;11:344.
412. Takahashi R et al. The retinoblastoma gene functions as a growth and tumor suppressor in human bladder carcinoma cells. *Proc Natl Acad Sci USA* 1991;88:5257.
413. Talamini R et al. A case-control study of risk factor for renal cell cancer in northern Italy. *Cancer Causes Control* 1990;1:125.
414. Tallini G et al. Analysis of nuclear and mitochondrial DNA alterations in thyroid and renal oncocytic tumors. *Cytogenet Cell Genet* 1994;66:253.
415. Tavani A, La Vecchia C. Epidemiology of renal-cell carcinoma. *J Nephrol* 1997;10:93.
416. Tetu B et al. Prevalence and clinical significance of HER/2neu, p53 and Rb expression in primary superficial bladder cancer. *J Urol* 1996;155:1784.

417. Theodorescu D et al. Ha-ras induction of the invasive phenotype results in up-regulation of epidermal growth factor receptors and altered responsiveness to epidermal growth factor in human papillary transitional cell carcinoma cells. *Cancer Res* 1991;51:4486.
418. Reference deleted in proofs.
419. Thibodeau SN, Bren G, Schaid D. Microsatellite instability in cancer of the proximal colon. *Science* 1993;260:816.
420. Thoenes W, Rumpelt HJ, Storkel S. Classification of renal cell carcinoma/tumors and their relationship to the nephron-collecting tubules system. *Klin Wochenschr* 1990;68:1102.
421. Thoenes W, Storkel S, Rumpelt HJ. Human chromophobe renal cell carcinoma. *Virchows Archiv B Cell Pathol* 1985; 48:207.
422. Thoenes W, Storkel S, Rumpelt HJ. Histopathology and classification of renal cell tumors (adenomas, oncocytoma and carcinomas). The basic cytological and histological elements and their use for diagnosis. *Path Res Pract* 1986;181:125.
423. Thoenes W et al. Chromophobe cell renal carcinoma and its variants—a report on 32 cases. *J Pathol* 1988;155:277.
424. Thomas R. Androgen-dependent gene expression of bone morphogenetic protein 7 in mouse prostate. *Prostate* 1998; 37:236.
425. Thrash-Bingham CA et al. Genomic alterations and instabilities in renal cell carcinomas and their relationship to tumor pathology. *Cancer Res* 1995;55:6189.
426. Thrash-Bingham CA et al. Loss of heterozygosity studies indicate that chromosome arm 1p harbors a tumor suppressor gene for renal oncocytomas. *Genes Chromosomes Cancer* 1996; 16:64.
427. Tickoo SK, Amin MB, Zarbo RJ. Colloidal iron staining in renal epithelial neoplasms, including chromophobe renal cell carcinoma: emphasis on technique and patterns of staining. *Am J Surg Pathol* 1998;22:419.
428. Toro J et al. Birt-Hogg-Dubé syndrome: a novel marker of kidney neoplasia. *Arch Dermatol* 1999;135:1195.
429. Trapman J. Loss of heterozygosity of chromosome 8 microsatellite loci implicates a candidate tumor suppressor gene between the loci D8S87 and D8S133 in human prostate cancer. *Cancer Res* 1994;54:6061.
430. Tsui KH et al. Prognostic indicators for renal cell carcinoma: a multivariate analysis of 643 patients using the revised 1997 TNM staging criteria. *J Urol* 2000;163:1090.
431. Tsujimoto Y et al. Cloning of the chromosome breakpoint of neoplastic B cells with the t(14;18) chromosome translocation. *Science* 1984;226:1097.
432. Uchida T. Developmental process of acquired renal cysts and neoplasms in patients receiving chronic hemodialysis: ultrasonographic, morphometric and histopathological studies. *Nippon Jinzo Gakkai Shi* 1991;33:889.
433. Vamvakas S et al. Renal cell cancer correlated with occupational exposure to trichloroethene. *J Cancer Res Clin Oncol* 1998;124:374.
434. Van Den BE et al. Chromosomal changes in renal oncocytomas. Evidence that t(5;11)(q35;q13) may characterize a second subgroup of oncocytomas. *Cancer Genet Cytogenet* 1995; 79:164.
435. Vaughn DJ. Review and outlook for the role of paclitaxel in urothelial carcinoma. *Semin Oncol* 1999;26:117.
436. Vet JA et al. p53 mutations have no additional prognostic value over stage in bladder cancer. *Br J Cancer* 1994;70:496.
437. Visakorpi T et al. Genetic changes in primary and recurrent prostate cancer by comparative genomic hybridization. *Cancer Res* 1995;55:342.
438. Vocke CD et al. Analysis of 99 microdissected prostate carcinomas reveals a high frequency of allelic loss on chromosome 8p12-21. *Cancer Res* 1996;56:2411.
439. Vogelzang NJ, Stadler WM. Gemcitabine and other new chemotherapeutic agents for the treatment of metastatic bladder cancer. *Urology* 1999;53:243.
440. Waldman T et al. Uncoupling of S phase and mitosis induced by anticancer agents in cells lacking p21 [see comments]. *Nature* 1996;20:713.
441. Walsh BJ. The Australian Proteome Analysis Facility (APAF): assembling large scale proteomics through integration and automation. *Electrophoresis.* 1998;19:1883.
442. Walsh PC. Early age at diagnosis in families providing evidence of linkage to the hereditary prostate cancer locus (HPC1) on chromosome 1. *J Urol* 1998;160:265.
443. Walther MM et al. Renal cancer in families with hereditary renal cancer: prospective analysis of a tumor size threshold for renal parenchymal sparing surgery. *J Urol* 1999;161:1475.
444. Walther MM et al. Parenchymal sparing surgery in patients with hereditary renal cell carcinoma. *J Urol* 1995;153:913.
445. Walther MM et al. Progelatinase A mRNA expression in cell lines derived from tumors in patients with metastatic renal cell carcinoma correlates inversely with survival. *Urology* 1997; 50:295.
446. Walther MM et al. Prevalence of microsocpic lesions in grossly normal renal parenchyma from patients with von Hippel-Lindau disease, sporadic renal cell carcinoma, and no renal disease: clinical implications. *J Urol* 1995;154:2010.
447. Walther MM et al. A clinical and genetic characterization of pheochromocytoma in von Hippel-Lindau disease. Comparison with sporadic pheochromocytoma gives insight into natural history of pheochromocytoma. *J Urol* 1999;162:659.
448. Walther MM, Thompson N, Linehan WM. Enucleation procedures in patients with multiple hereditary renal tumors. *World J Urol* 1995;13:248.
449. Wang N, Perkins KL. Involvement of band 3p14 in t(3;8) hereditary renal carcinoma. *Cancer Genet Cytogenet* 1984; 11:479.
450. Wang SI. Homozygous deletion of the PTEN tumor suppressor gene in a subset of prostate adenocarcinomas. *Clin Cancer Res* 1998;4:811.
451. Watson P, Lynch HT. Extracolonic cancer in hereditary nonpolyposis colorectal cancer. *Cancer* 1993;71:677.
452. Weidner U, Strohmeyer T. Inverse relationship of epidermal growth factor receptor and HER2/neu gene expression in human renal cell carcinoma. *Cancer Res* 1990;50:4504.
453. Weirich G et al. Familial renal oncocytoma: clinicopathologic study of 5 families. *J Urol* 1998;160:335.
454. Weterman MAJ et al. Fusion of the transcription factor TFE3 gene to a novel gene, PRCC, in t(X;1)(p11;q21)-positive papillary renal cell carcinomas. *Proc Natl Acad Sci USA* 1996;93: 15294.
455. Wilding G. Response of prostate cancer cells to peptide growth factors: transforming growth factor–beta. *Cancer Surv* 1991; 11:147.
456. Wolk A et al. International renal cell cancer study. VII. Role of diet. *Int J Cancer* 1996;65:67.

457. Wu SQ et al. The correlation between the loss of chromosome 14q with histologic tumor grade, pathologic stage, and outcome of patients with nonpapillary renal cell carcinoma. *Cancer* 1996;77:1154.
458. Wynder EL, Mabuchi K, Whitmore WF Jr. Epidemiology of adenocarcinoma of the kidney. *J Natl Cancer Inst* 1974;53:1619.
459. Xu J et al. Evidence for a prostate cancer susceptibility locus on the X chromosome. *Nat Genet* 1998;20:175.
460. Yang RM. Low p27 expression predicts poor disease-free survival in patients with prostate cancer. *J Urol* 1998;159:941.
461. Yuan JM et al. Tobacco use in relation to renal cell carcinoma. *Cancer Epidemiol Biomarkers Prev* 1998;7:429.
462. Zambrano NR et al. Histopathology and molecular genetics of renal tumors: toward unification of a classification system. *J Urol* 1999;162:1246.
463. Zbar B et al. Hereditary papillary renal cell carcinoma: clinical studies in 10 families. *J Urol* 1995;153:907.
464. Zbar B et al. Hereditary papillary renal cell carcinoma. *J Urol* 1994;151:561.
465. Zhang SY et al. Immunohistochemistry of cyclin D1 in human breast cancer. *Am J Clin Pathol* 1994;102:695.
466. Zhang Y, Xiong Y, Yarbrough WG. ARF promotes MDM2 degradation and stabilizes p53: ARF-INK4a locus deletion impairs both the Rb and p53 tumor suppression pathways. *Cell* 1998;92:725.

Adult and Pediatric Urology, 4/e, edited by Jay Y. Gillenwater, John T. Grayhack, Stuart S. Howards, and Michael E. Mitchell.
Lippincott Williams & Wilkins, Philadelphia © 2002

8

CALCULUS FORMATION

ALAN D. JENKINS

Most patients who have passed a kidney stone do not understand the nature of their disease and want to know why they form kidney stones. Other patients may have an easily identifiable cause such as cystinuria or renal tubular acidosis (RTA) for their stone formation. Specific and effective medical treatment programs exist for these patients. Other patients may benefit from simple measures such as increased fluid intake and dietary moderation. Patients with recurrent stone formation require a medical regimen that is designed to correct any physicochemical abnormalities.

This chapter imparts an understanding of the basic pathophysiology of urinary tract stone formation and enables the urologic practitioner to blend the medical and surgical management of urolithiasis patients.

A.D. Jenkins: Department of Urology, University of Virginia, Charlottesville, VA 22908.

BASIC PRINCIPLES

Biologic mineralization involves the precipitation of a poorly soluble salt, usually in association with an organic matrix. Supersaturation (SS) of the precipitating phase must be present before crystallization can occur. If at least local SS is not present, then crystallization is thermodynamically impossible. Most medical treatment programs depend on a reduction of SS to prevent further stone formation. The solubility concept is one of the most important aspects of biologic mineralization (262).

The physical chemistry of ions in an aqueous solution involves four basic concepts: ion activity, ion pairing, solubility, and relative supersaturation (RSS). The effective concentration of an ion, such as calcium (Ca^{2+}), in solution is different from its actual concentration. This effective concentration, the chemical activity, depends on the ionic strength of the solution. Through electrical field effects, the other ions in the solution affect the true chemical activity of a particular ion. The ionic strength is a measure of the magnitude of this electrical field and increases as the concentration of ions increases and their valence or charge increases. The activity of an ionic species decreases as the ionic strength increases. For a given total calcium concentration, the activity of Ca^{2+} would be greater in distilled water, which contains only the Ca^{2+} and its accompanying anions, than in urine, which contains many different ions.

The relation between ion activity, $\{Na^+\}$, and ion concentration, $[Na^+]$, is given by the following equation:

$$\{Na^+\} = [Na^+] \times a_1$$

where a_1 is the activity coefficient for Na^+. Activity coefficients are always less than 1 and approach unity as the concentration of the solution decreases. The ionic strength of a physiologic salt solution, such as urine, is approximately 0.15 M. The corresponding activity coefficients for the divalent ions Ca^{2+} and $C_2O_4^{2-}$ (oxalate) are approximately 0.3. The activity of each of these ions is less than one-third of the concentration.

Specific ions of opposite charge, such as Ca^{2+} and sulfate (SO_4^{2-}), can interact to form soluble ion pairs or complexes. These interactions effectively reduce the "ionized" concentrations of the ions involved. Many such interactions are possible in urine. Ionized calcium can be measured directly with an ion-selective electrode, but no satisfactory method has been developed to measure the free ion concentrations of those anions (especially oxalate) that participate in urinary tract mineralization.

Computer programs have been written to calculate the free ion concentrations of the major ionic species in urine, given the total concentrations of the ions, the pH, and the stability constants of the various ion pairs (94,361). (The stability constant is a measure of the strength of the association between the ions forming an ion pair.) These algorithms also permit the calculation of ionic strength, activity coefficients, and activity products. The activity product of a salt such as sodium chloride (NaCl) is given by the product of the activities of Na^+ and Cl^-: $\{Na^+\} \times \{Cl^-\}$. An estimate of SS can be made if the activity product is compared with the thermodynamic solubility product.

A solid salt added to an aqueous solution dissolves to an extent determined by the thermodynamic solubility product of the particular compound. If the solution is at equilibrium with the solid phase, the numeric value of the solubility product is equal to the product of the activities of the constituent ions of the salt. The equation for NaCl solubility is as follows:

$$K_{sp} = \{Na^+\} \times \{Cl^-\}$$

where $\{Na^+\}$ and $\{Cl^-\}$ are the activities of Na^+ and Cl^- in equilibrium with pure, solid NaCl. Potassium (K_{sp}) is a constant at a given temperature and pH.

Within the range of physiologic urine pH, the solubilities of two common stone salts, calcium phosphate and uric acid, are pH sensitive. The equation for calcium phosphate solubility is as follows:

$$Ca_5(PO_4)_3OH = 5Ca^{2+} + 3PO_4^{3-} + OH^-$$
$$K_{sp} = \{Ca^{2+}\}^5 \times \{PO_4^{3-}\}^3 \times \{OH^-\}$$
$$H_2PO_4 = HPO_4^{2-} + H^+$$
$$HPO_4^{2-} = PO_4^{3-} + H^+$$

As the pH increases, $\{OH^-\}$ increases and hydrogen ion activity (H^+), decreases. More phosphate exists as PO_4^{3-}, and the solubility of $Ca_5(PO_4)_3OH$ decreases. Clinically, calcium phosphate urolithiasis tends to occur in alkaline urine.

The pKa at 38°C of the first dissociable proton in uric acid is 5.5 (98). In an aqueous solution of uric acid at pH 5.5 and 38°C, half exists as dissolved uric acid (HU) and half exists as urate ion (U^-): $HU = H^+ + U^-$. This physicochemical property of uric acid is responsible for the sensitive pH dependence of uric acid solubility in urine. As urinary pH increases, more of the uric acid exists as urate ion, and urate is more soluble than uric acid. The solubility of uric acid as a function of pH is shown in Table 8.1. The dramatic increase of uric acid solubility with increasing pH is the cornerstone of the medical treatment of uric acid lithiasis.

The ratio of the calculated activity product *(AP)* to

TABLE 8.1. SOLUBILITY OF URIC ACID AS A FUNCTION OF pH

pH	Solubility (mg/L)
5.0	60
6.0	200
7.0	1,600

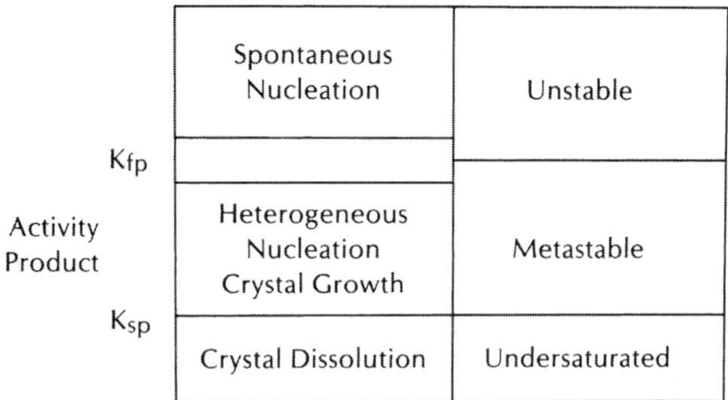

FIGURE 8.1. Schematic representation of states of saturation. K_{sp}, solubility product; K_{tp}, formation product (range).

the thermodynamic solubility product *(K_{sp})* is the relative supersaturation *(RSS or SS):*

$$RSS = AP \div K_{sp}$$

If solid crystals of a salt are added to a solution of the salt, they will dissolve if SS is less than 1 and will grow if SS is more than 1. If SS is 1, the crystals will not grow or dissolve. SS (RSS ratio more than 1) of the precipitating salt must be present for stones to form and grow.

The initial step in the actual formation of a crystal is nucleation or the birth of crystals from solution (356). If the supersaturated solution is pure, nucleation may occur homogeneously at a critical level of SS. However, urine contains many foreign surfaces, such as cell membranes, that can act as heterogeneous nuclei. Heterogeneous nucleation occurs at a lower level of SS than does homogeneous nucleation and is the most common, if not the only, type of nucleation that occurs in biologic systems (104). The level of SS at which nucleation occurs often is referred to as the *formation product.* The formation product is not as precisely defined as the solubility product and is most accurately described as a range of SS that permits nucleation.

The range of SS between the solubility product and the formation product is called the *metastable zone* (Fig. 8.1). Spontaneous nucleation does not occur in this zone, but preformed crystals grow until the RSS is reduced to 1.

Ideal crystals are composed of identical units arranged in a repetitive pattern. These units may be atoms, molecules, ions, or groups of these particles. In real crystals, these units are not always identical, and the pattern is not strictly repetitive. Deviations from periodicity, called *dislocations,* commonly occur in crystals formed in biologic systems. However, all crystalline substances have an approximate periodic structure, or lattice, that can be characterized with x-ray diffraction. If the lattice structure of one crystal is similar to that of a different crystal, the second crystal may be able to nucleate and grow on the first crystal. This oriented overgrowth is called *epitaxy* (179,203). The concept of epitaxy was offered several years ago as a possible explanation for the growth of mixed urinary stones. The clinical association of disorders of uric acid metabolism (hyperuricosuria and hyperuricemia) with calcium oxalate urolithiasis motivated the intensive study of a possible epitaxial relation between urate crystallization and calcium oxalate crystallization (56,164,225). Other investigators have questioned the specific importance of epitaxial crystal growth in clinical urolithiasis (33,195,196). It is likely that mixed stone formation in the urinary tract occurs by heterogeneous nucleation and overgrowth, not by the highly specific mechanism of epitaxy.

More recent *in vitro* studies have shown that the promotion of calcium oxalate crystallization by dissolved urate is not caused by the epitaxial nucleation of calcium oxalate or by the inactivation of urinary glycosaminoglycans (119). A "salting out" mechanism may be responsible for the promotion of calcium oxalate crystallization by dissolved urate (279).

Nuclei will grow to form larger crystals if the urine remains supersaturated for the precipitating phase. The growth units of the crystal are added to growth sites on the crystal surface (216). Available evidence suggests that the growth sites of urinary crystals are screw dislocations (Fig. 8.2). As the crystal grows, the step winds itself into a spiral with the center fixed at the dislocation. Because the step does not disappear during growth, the crystal can grow continuously at a low SS. The crystal grows as long as the bathing solution remains supersaturated for the precipitating phase.

Many collisions occur between the small crystals in an aqueous solution. Some of these crystals may stick together to form larger crystalline masses. This process is called *aggregation* or *agglomeration;* it is another mechanism by which crystals can increase in size to form a stone. Crystal growth produces a more dense particle than does aggregation (95). The density of actual uroliths is similar to that of pure stone crystals. This implies that urinary tract stones increase in size primarily through crystal growth, not aggregation. However, initial particle retention could still involve crystal aggregation.

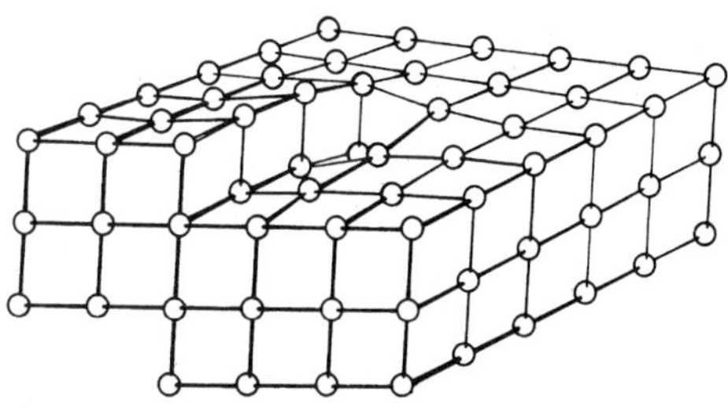

FIGURE 8.2. Schematic representation of a crystal with a screw dislocation.

CLINICAL STONE FORMATION

Why do some people form many kidney stones? Four factors are involved: urinary SS, inhibition and promotion, particle retention, and matrix (34). Our understanding of the pathophysiology and effective treatment of urolithiasis is based on these four factors.

Supersaturation

Urinary SS for the precipitating stone salt is a necessary condition for stone formation. It is thermodynamically impossible for a stone to grow if the urine is not supersaturated for the particular salt, but continuous SS does not have to be present. Urine may become supersaturated after meals. This effect may be accentuated after the evening meal, because the lack of fluid consumption during sleep permits a decrease in overnight urine volume. Stone growth can occur only at night, even though daytime fluid intake is sufficient to prevent SS.

Inhibitors and Promotors

Urinary SS alone does not explain the presence of stone disease in some individuals and its absence in others. Urine commonly is supersaturated for stone salts, especially calcium oxalate (110,270). Small urinary crystals often are passed by individuals who have never formed a stone (271,359). One explanation for this apparent paradox is the presence of crystallization inhibitors in urine (100). Inhibitors of crystal growth and aggregation have been isolated from human urine, and inhibitors of nucleation may exist (272,280); inhibitors of crystal growth have received the most attention (101). Inhibitors usually are classified according to their ability to inhibit the growth of calcium phosphate or calcium oxalate. Pyrophosphate, citrate, and magnesium are known inhibitors of calcium phosphate crystal growth. Pyrophosphate and citrate also inhibit calcium oxalate crystal growth (299), but most of the calcium oxalate crystal growth inhibition in urine is provided by larger-molecular-weight polyanions: glycosaminoglycans and RNA fragments (21,37,197,293). Heparin, although not found in urine, is a potent inhibitor of *in vitro* calcium oxalate crystal growth.

Acidic glycoproteins have been isolated from human urine and human kidney tissue culture medium (141, 212,213). Evidence shows that patients with calcium oxalate nephrolithiasis have intrinsically abnormal acidic glycoproteins (210). These glycoproteins from healthy persons contain γ-carboxyglutamic acid and are strong inhibitors of calcium oxalate crystal growth at low concentrations (10 to 7 M). Glycoprotein crystal growth inhibitor from patients does not contain γ-carboxyglutamic acid and is a functionally poor inhibitor.

This glycoprotein inhibitor of calcium oxalate crystal growth has been named *nephrocalcin* (209). Nephrocalcin has been isolated from human calcium oxalate renal stones (211) and appears to localize to the proximal tubule cells of the human kidney (312). The γ-carboxyglutamic acid residues of nephrocalcin are synthesized by the addition of a carboxyl group to the γ-carbon of glutamic acid residues after messenger RNA translation. The same investigators have reported that nephrocalcin and Tamm-Horsfall glycoprotein inhibit calcium oxalate crystal aggregation at concentrations as low as 2×10^{-9} M and 1×10^{-8} M (132).

Tamm-Horsfall protein is a glycoprotein that is produced in the thick ascending limb of Henle's loop. It inhibits calcium oxalate monohydrate crystal aggregation at a low ionic strength and a high urinary pH (131). In highly concentrated urine, Tamm-Horsfall protein readily polymerizes, thereby overwhelming other urinary inhibitors and promoting the agglomeration of calcium oxalate monohydrate crystals (118,294).

Uronic acid–rich protein, another glycoprotein that has been isolated from human urine, also exhibits inhibitory activity against crystal growth (8). It appears to be a more potent inhibitor than nephrocalcin.

Patients who form stones appear to excrete more lipids or acid phospholipids than normal individuals. Urinary excretion of glycolipid, cholesterol, and cholesterol esters also was higher in stone-formers (154). The greater excretion of lipids may reflect sloughing of tubular cells in response to a challenge by oxalate or calcium oxalate crystals. Acid phospholipids from cellular membranes may be involved with crystal nucleation and retention.

Citrate, through its ability to complex calcium and inhibit the growth of calcium salts, may play a role in the pathogenesis of calcium urolithiasis. Citrate is a tricarboxylic acid that, when totally ionized above pH 6.5 at 37°C, has a charge of minus 3:

```
        COO⁻
         |
        CH2
         |
   HO — C — COO⁻
         |
        CH2
         |
        COO⁻
```

The following reactions occur with calcium in urine at a physiologic pH:

$$Ca_3Cit_2 \rightarrow Ca^{2+} + 2CaCit^{2-}$$
$$CaCit^{-} \rightarrow Ca^{2+} + Cit^{3-}$$

As the concentration of citrate increases, the reaction is shifted toward the left with increased complexation of calcium. This effect decreases calcium oxalate SS and the potential for crystallization. Citrate weakly inhibits the growth of preformed calcium oxalate crystals, but this action is not as important as complexation.

Citrate is filtered at the glomerulus and reabsorbed primarily in the proximal tubule (309). The ability of renal mitochondria to metabolize citrate by means of the tricarboxylic acid cycle is thought to control the renal clearance of citrate. Metabolic acidosis increases the entry of citrate into the matrix space of mitochondria and decreases the exit of citrate from mitochondria, thereby allowing mitochondrial oxidation of citrate. Cytoplasmic citrate levels decline, reabsorption of citrate from tubular fluid is enhanced, and less citrate appears in the final urine. Metabolic alkalosis has an opposite effect.

The luminal membrane of the proximal tubules (brush border membrane) is equipped with a Na^+-gradient–dependent transport system that is highly specific for intermediates of the tricarboxylic acid cycle, including citrate (157). Metabolic acidosis caused by dietary acid loading increases the intrinsic capacity of proximal tubular brush border membrane to transport citrate from the tubular lumen into the cell interior (143). A corresponding decrease in urinary citrate excretion was seen. A dramatic increase in urinary citrate excretion was seen with dietary alkali loading (with $NaHCO_3$), but brush border membrane transport of citrate was unchanged. These studies demonstrate that urinary citrate excretion is exquisitely sensitive to manipulation of systemic acid–base balance through effects on renal cellular function.

Urine from patients with recurrent calcium oxalate nephrolithiasis tends to have greater calcium oxalate SS and lower inhibitor levels than urine from healthy individuals (76,271), but considerable overlap exists. It is impossible to predict consistently on the basis of SS or inhibition alone who will and who will not recurrently form calcium oxalate stones. A combination of these two factors, the saturation-inhibition index, has discriminated between healthy individuals and patients with recurrent stone formation (269). The saturation-inhibition index is a mathematic combination of relative calcium oxalate and inhibition of crystal growth and aggregation (as measured by the change in particle-size distribution in an *in vitro* crystal growth system). Patients with the greatest saturation-inhibition indexes had the highest recurrence rates. Because SS and inhibition are difficult to measure, this method has not had widespread clinical application.

The concept of urinary risk factors is an extension of the saturation-inhibition index. This concept attempts to account for the multifactoral nature of calcium urolithiasis by considering six factors (236,266,267): urine volume, urine pH, urinary excretion of oxalate, uric acid, calcium, and alcian blue precipitable polyanions (a measure of acid mucopolysaccharides or large-molecular-weight inhibitors). Although no solitary abnormality may distinguish a stone-former, clear discrimination can be made by the presence of several risk factors. A low urine volume has the greatest risk, followed by a high urinary oxalate excretion. A high urine pH or uric acid excretion is associated with a higher probability of forming stones. Hypercalciuria is the least important risk factor.

Crystal Retention

Freshly voided urine samples from most healthy persons intermittently contain small crystals (usually calcium oxalate dihydrate), but only 5% to 10% of such persons will ever develop an actual kidney stone. These crystals probably form in the papillary collecting ducts and are flushed out with the urine before they grow large enough to become lodged in the lumen. Anatomic abnormalities or adherence to the epithelium may prevent these particles from leaving the kidney. This increased particle retention permits the crystals to grow larger, further reducing the likelihood that they will be passed spontaneously (35). This condition could easily predispose an individual to the formation of kidney stones. An attractive hypothesis is that patients with stone disease may have an increased particle retention time, possibly resulting from an abnormal tendency for small crystals to adhere to the epithelial lining of the upper urinary tract.

Two theoretical mechanisms have been proposed for crystal retention: free particle or fixed particle. The free particle mechanism assumes that nucleation and initial crystal growth occur in the tubular lumen. The crystalline particles grow with such sufficient rapidity that they become trapped in the papillary collecting ducts, where they grow to form a macroscopic stone (350). Estimates of calcium oxalate crystal growth rates in the distal tubule have cast doubt on the ability of these crystals to grow rapidly enough to occlude the lumen before they are washed out of the collecting ducts (97). Some investigations have suggested that rapid aggregation of small crystals would permit free particle trapping to occur.

More support exists for the second theory, a fixed particle mechanism. Rats with magnesium deficiency develop nephrocalcinosis and stone formation (219). Small stones were found attached to normal-appearing tubular epithelium near the bend of Henle's loop. This intranephronic calculosis may have occurred by crystal nucleation on the luminal membrane or attachment of a passing crystalline particle. Carr (38) suggested that crystals floating in the renal pelvis could be trapped in forniceal lymphatic vessels and grow to macroscopic size. Papillary tip stones could originate from crystals that had become attached to the epithelial lining of the distal collecting ducts and had grown out of the lumen to form a papillary cup (351). Randall's plaques (254) are macroscopic subepithelial deposits of calcium crystals. Although older studies found a poor correlation between the incidence of stone disease and the incidence of Randall's plaques, it was still hypothesized that the epithelium over the plaque could erode, and a calyceal stone could develop from crystal growth on the plaque (252). More recent studies of Randall's plaques have found that they are not just subepithelial deposits (326); they appear to extend deep into the papilla and are intimately associated with collecting tubules and vasa recta. These same investigators found that papillary plaques were more common in patients with calcium oxalate and calcium phosphate stones than in patients without a history of stone disease (180). Endoscopic examinations found that most patients with calcium stone disease had Randall's plaques.

Investigators have induced calcium oxalate nephrolithiasis in rats with intraperitoneal injections of oxalate (146,151). Calcium oxalate crystals were found in the tubular lumina, in the intercellular spaces between cells, and attached to the tubular epithelial basal lamina. Necrosis of tubular cells was responsible for exposure of the tubular basal lamina. Oxalate itself may be toxic to renal epithelium (166,331), and renal tubular epithelial damage can result in the shedding of membranous cellular debris, thereby providing a substrate for heterogeneous nucleation (153).

The attachment of crystals to the kidney epithelium may involve a specific molecular interaction between stone crystals and the epithelial membrane. Rat renal inner-papillary collecting tubule cells have been isolated in primary cultures and used as a model for the study of crystal-membrane interactions (358). Riese and colleagues (258) developed a mathematic model of the binding of calcium oxalate crystals to these cells. This binding is location specific, saturable, and inhibitable. Calcium oxalate crystal binding appears to be related to cell membrane polarity (259). This binding is enhanced if a monolayer of cultured cells is depolarized by disrupting the normal intercellular tight junctions. These results suggest that the crystals preferentially attach to a basolateral cell membrane component. Renal epithelial cells also can endocytose calcium monohydrate crystals (175). Other studies continue to confirm the ability of calcium oxalate monohydrate crystals to specifically bind to cultured renal epithelial cells (22,163,176).

The most provocative hypothesis regarding stone formation involves nanobacteria (147). Nanobacteria are sterile-filterable, Gram-negative, atypical bacteria that have been detected in bovine and human blood. They produce carbonate apatite on their cell walls and could potentially act as nidi for the precipitation of other stone salts, such as calcium oxalate. The smallest apatite units in kidney stones resemble the site and morphology of nanobacteria by scanning electron microscopy (48). One investigator has isolated nanobacteria from more than 90% of nonstruvite kidney stones.

Meticulous work by Delatte and associates (72) revealed that small calcium oxalate stones are not uniformly round but have one surface with a concave depression. A small crystalline aggregate of calcium phosphate sometimes was found in this depression. Clinically significant growth of calcium oxalate stones may be initiated by epithelial precipitation of calcium phosphate that subsequently is overgrown with calcium oxalate (114,124,341).

Matrix

Kidney stones contain a variable amount of organic material called *matrix*. The matrix content of most urinary calculi is 2.5% by weight (25). Cystine stones contain approximately 10% matrix. The rare matrix calculus is a soft, radiolucent body that occurs in patients whose upper urinary tracts are infected with urea-splitting bacterial organisms (253). The matrix content of these calculi averages 62%.

Macroscopic examination of whole renal calculi reveals concentric laminations and radial striations (25). Scanning electron microscopic studies of fractured calcium oxalate calculi demonstrate fibrous material bridging adjacent crystals (321). These findings support the proposal that matrix acts as a ground substance (153).

Other investigators believe that the presence of matrix in urinary stones is serendipitous (99). Nonspecific physical adsorption of organic compounds on growing crystals may account for at least some of the matrix found in calculi (169). Electron microscopic examination of calcium oxalate crystals incubated with γ-globulin or albumin has revealed an amorphous coat of material covering the crystals (146). This continuous coat is consistent with simple adsorption.

Few studies have attempted to isolate and precisely identify the chemical composition of matrix. The best known investigations found similarities between urinary mucoproteins and matrix material that was extracted from renal stones with ethylenediaminetetra-acetic acid (EDTA). A mucoprotein material, matrix substance A, was identified in urine from patients with recurrent stone disease (27). This organic compound constituted approximately 85% of the total organic matrix of kidney stones. One-third of matrix substance A was carbohydrate and two-thirds was protein. Aspartic and glutamic acids were the most common amino acids found in the protein component. The carbohydrate component contained galactose, mannose, methylpentose, glucosamine, and galactosamine (24). Studies of dialyzed ultrafiltrates of matrix also found aspartic and glutamic acids. Alkaline hydrolysis revealed the presence of γ-carboxyglutamic acid (174). Proteins containing this amino acid have a strong affinity for calcium ions.

Urinary stone protein, or uropontin, is an aspartic acid–rich glycoprotein that is found in stone matrix (161). It binds calcium and has the same structure as osteopontin, which is found in bone and other mineralized tissue (36). Increased staining of distal renal tubular cells for this glycoprotein is seen in rats that have been induced to form stones by the administration of glyoxylic acid (160).

Uropontin also has been isolated from urine and is a potent inhibitor of the nucleation, growth, and aggregation of calcium oxalate crystals and the binding of these crystals to renal epithelial cells (202). Uropontin concentration in urine appears to vary inversely with urine volume. Its ability to prevent calcium oxalate crystallization would increase as urinary concentration increases.

EPIDEMIOLOGY

In the United States and in other technologically developed countries, urolithiasis commonly occurs as upper tract stones. Bladder stones are more common in less-developed countries (7). Epidemiologic data suggest that climate, geography, and diet are important factors in the pathogenesis of urolithiasis (261). The best-known example of this influence is the apparent existence of "stone belts." These are geographic areas that are associated with a high prevalence of stone formation (134). A questionnaire survey of hospitals estimated that, during 1952, 0.95 persons per 1,000 population were admitted to a hospital with a diagnosis of urinary calculi (26). A rate of 1.93 per 1,000 population in South Carolina and 0.43 per 1,000 in Missouri provided evidence of geographic variability. Each of the southeastern states had a high rate of urinary calculi. A more recent study found that 1.64 persons per 1,000 population were admitted to a hospital with the diagnosis of urolithiasis, an increase of 75% over the 22-year period (303). High rates were again found in the southeastern states, especially in the Carolinas (North Carolina, 3.0 per 1,000 population; South Carolina, 2.7 per 1,000 population), but the differences were not statistically significant.

Studies of hospitalization rates may underestimate the number of patients with urolithiasis because not all patients with stones are hospitalized (145). A study of residents of Rochester, Minnesota, found that 51% of patients with stone disease were seen only as outpatients. These investigators precisely defined their epidemiologic terms and the population under study. *Incidence* was defined as the first symptomatic and diagnosed episode in a person's life. The *incidence rate* was the ratio of the number of persons who experienced such initial episodes during a specified period to the size of the population at the midpoint of the period. *Prevalence* was the number of people who had had at least one symptomatic episode, whereas *recurrence* referred to episodes that followed the initial episode. Patients with asymptomatic stones, urinary tract infections, or struvite calculi were excluded from this study.

Six hundred seventy-two persons had their first episode of symptomatic urolithiasis while a resident of Rochester, Minnesota: 468 (70%) men and 204 (30%) women. The first episode tended to occur between the ages of 30 and 60 years. The annual age-adjusted incidence rate for males was 1.1 per 1,000 population and for females it was 0.36 per 1,000 population. The incidence rates for females were stable over the 25-year study period (1950 to 1974), but the male rate per 1,000 population increased from 0.8 to 1.24. This increase was statistically significant and most apparent in the group of men aged 50 to 70 years. Prevalence was estimated to increase to a peak of approximately 12% in males older than age 70 years. Prevalence in females was less than 5%. Recurrences tended to occur during the first year: 15.9% in males and 12.4% in females. Annual recurrence rates for subsequent years was 3.7% for males and 2.0% for females.

Studies of racial differences in the incidence of urolithiasis have been inconsistent. A retrospective review found that the frequency of urinary stones in Caucasian patients was three to four times that in African American patients (289). More African American women than African American men formed stones, and the most common type of stone formation in African American patients was struvite and carbonate apatite. Stones tended to occur at a younger age in African American males.

Normal pregnancy causes hypercalciuria, but pregnancy is not a stone-forming condition (57,182). Abnormal crystalluria is not seen in pregnant patients, and more frequent stone production is not seen in stone-formers who become pregnant. A prospective study of 11 women revealed no change in urine volume (183). Although citrate excretion increased during pregnancy, this increase was not proportional to the increase in urinary calcium. Citrate failed to increase in parallel with calcium excretion, even though the urine pH rose. SS for calcium oxalate and brushite was as high in pregnancy as in patients with proven calcium nephrolithiasis. One explanation for the lack of clinical stone formation is the relatively short duration of pregnancy. Another explanation is an increase of protective mechanisms, such as crystal growth inhibition. Nephrocalcin excretion may increase during pregnancy.

Many explanations have been offered for the increasing incidence of kidney stones in the world population. These include increased dietary protein intake, increased intake of refined sugar, decreased dietary fiber, and increased affluence. Recurrent stone formation is associated with a greater expenditure on food (378). There is a positive correlation between monthly income and urinary excretion of calcium, uric acid, and inorganic phosphorus. Stone-forming patients may consume less dietary fiber than those who do not form stones (260). One explanation is that fiber, possibly through its phytate content, binds calcium in the gastrointestinal (GI) tract and prevents its absorption. The relationship between stone disease and sugar consumption is more controversial. Increased dietary sugar can increase urinary calcium excretion (338), but epidemiologic data show an inverse relationship between sugar consumption and hospitalization rates for stone disease (260).

High consumption of animal protein seems to correlate best with affluence and stone disease (266,268). Individuals on a high-protein diet excrete more urinary calcium, cyclic adenosine monophosphate, and hydroxyproline (93). The increased fixed acid load provided by a high-protein diet may cause mild resorption of bone and reduced renal tubular reabsorption of calcium. GI absorption of calcium is not affected. Calculated urinary SS for calcium oxalate does not change, but urinary citrate excretion and pH decrease. The reduced effectiveness of crystal growth inhibitors at the lower urinary pH would allow the growth of larger crystals.

Salt abuse also is a risk factor for kidney stone formation (111). A high sodium intake significantly increases urinary sodium, calcium, and pH, and decreases urinary citrate (283). Urinary saturation of calcium phosphate and monosodium urate increases, and inhibitor activity against calcium oxalate crystallization increases. The net effect is a higher likelihood for the precipitation of calcium salts in urine.

The relation between the composition of drinking water and urolithiasis has been examined in several studies. Dissolved calcium and magnesium are responsible for the hardness of water. The incidence of urolithiasis tends to be higher in areas of the United States that have softer drinking water (44,304). Another study examined two specific geographic regions: North and South Carolina, which had soft water and a high stone incidence, and the Rockies (Colorado, Idaho, Montana, Nevada, Utah, and Wyoming), which had hard water and a low stone incidence (300). No significant differences were found for the concentration of calcium, magnesium, or sodium in home tap water. An incidental finding was that individuals drinking private well water had a greater risk of stone formation than those drinking public water. The authors concluded that water hardness should be a minor concern with respect to stone formation.

Patients with calcium stone formation often are advised to limit their intake of dietary calcium. This advice is based on the presence of hypercalciuria in up to half of patients with idiopathic calcium urolithiasis (ICU). However, restriction of dietary calcium may increase the risk of stone formation by enhancing dietary oxalate absorption and urinary oxalate excretion (188). A prospective study in a cohort of 45,619 men without a history of kidney stones found an inverse relationship between the relative risk of kidney stone formation and dietary calcium intake (62). Stone formation was negatively correlated with fluid intake but positively correlated with intake of animal protein.

The inverse relationship between stone formation and dietary calcium content is consistent with the hypothesis that mild hyperoxaluria is more important than hypercalciuria in the pathogenesis of urolithiasis (263). One of the determinants of urinary oxalate excretion is intestinal oxalate absorption. Intestinal oxalate absorption is influenced by the oxalate-to-calcium ratio of the diet, because oxalate that is bound to calcium is not absorbed. Enhanced absorption of "free" oxalate could occur if dietary calcium is restricted or intestinal absorption of calcium is enhanced (108).

Oxalobacter formigenes is a specific oxalate-degrading, anaerobic bacterium that colonizes the GI tracts of vertebrates, including humans. It appears to maintain a symbiotic relationship with its host by regulating oxalate absorption (2). It catabolizes free oxalic acid, thereby preventing absorption, and also enhances oxalate secretion from plasma. Fecal samples from patients with Crohn's and other inflammatory bowel diseases lack *O. formigenes* and have a low rate of oxalate degradation (3). When noncolonized laboratory rats were colonized with live bacteria or treated with a preparation of oxalate-degrading enzymes derived from *O. formigenes,* they developed increased resistance to a subsequent high oxalate challenge, excreted far lower levels of oxalate, and did not develop crystalluria, as seen in control animals (302).

Excessive sweating also may contribute to stone formation. Moderate physical exercise lowers urinary pH and citrate excretion due to a mild metabolic acidosis (285). Although the total excretion of stone-forming salts decreases, the greater decrease in urine volume results in an increase in urinary calcium oxalate SS and the concentration of undissociated uric acid (secondary to an increase in total uric acid concentration and a fall in urinary pH). Nephrolithiasis is more prevalent in machinists chronically exposed to a hot environment (e.g., a glass plant) (23). These individuals had higher urinary uric acid concentrations than individuals who worked in an environment with a normal temperature. This biochemical difference was clinically expressed by uric acid stone formation in 39%.

Another study found a positive association between urinary stone disease and consumption of carbonated beverages (e.g., sugared cola) (301). A negative association existed between coffee and beer consumption and stone disease in the Rockies. Primary intake of milk, water, or tea was not associated with urinary stone disease.

The widespread consumption of iced tea has been suggested as a reason for the high incidence of urolithiasis in the southeastern United States. Although dietary oxalate is responsible for only 10% to 15% of total urinary oxalate (138), urinary oxalate excretion increases after the ingestion of oxalate-rich foods such as spinach (330). A case-control study from Newfoundland examined tea consumption in stone-formers but found no evidence to support the suggestion that tea drinking is a risk factor for calcium oxalate urolithiasis (46). These investigators calculated that 1 cup of tea would add only 0.5 mg of oxalate to total urinary excretion.

ETIOLOGY

A classification of causes of urolithiasis is given in Table 8.2. The syndrome of ICU accounts for 70% to 80% of stone disease in industrialized nations. Inherited enzyme disorders or renal tubular syndromes are found in fewer than 1% of stone-forming patients. Primary hyperparathyroidism is the most common hypercalcemic condition associated with

TABLE 8.2. CAUSES OF UROLITHIASIS

Renal tubular syndromes	Enzyme disorders
Renal tubular acidosis	Primary hyperoxaluria
Cystinuria	Xanthinuria
	2,8-Dihydroxyadeninuria
Hypercalcemic disorders	
Primary hyperparathyroidism	Secondary urolithiasis
Immobilization	Enteric hyperoxaluria
Milk-alkali syndrome	Infection
Sarcoidosis	Obstruction
Hypervitaminosis D	Medullary sponge kidney
Neoplastic diseases	Urinary diversion
Cushing's syndrome	Drugs
Hyperthyroidism	
	Idiopathic calcium urolithiasis
Uric acid lithiasis	Hypercalciuria
Idiopathic	Normocalciuria
Gout	
Low urine output states	
Myeloproliferative diseases	

urolithiasis and is responsible for stone formation in 5% of patients.

Renal Tubular Acidosis

RTA is a syndrome of disordered renal acidification that causes a hypokalemic hyperchloremic metabolic acidosis (156). The inability to excrete normal amounts of acid into the urine may be responsible for the entire syndrome, because the administration of sodium bicarbonate corrects the hyperchloremic acidosis and the excessive urinary losses of potassium, calcium, and phosphorus (297).

Two basic types of defective urinary acidification have been identified in these patients. Patients with type 2 RTA (proximal) have a defect in the reabsorption of filtered bicarbonate, a process that occurs in the proximal tubule (204). When the plasma bicarbonate is reduced only moderately, the urinary pH is inappropriately high, but with the development of a more severe systemic acidosis the bicarbonaturia disappears and the urinary pH decreases to a normal minimum. Patients with the most frequently studied disorder, type 1, or classic, RTA (distal) have a normal capacity to reabsorb filtered bicarbonate but cannot lower the urine pH below 6.0, regardless of the severity of the systemic acidosis (325).

Classic RTA may exist as a primary or secondary form. The primary form may be subdivided into infantile or adult types. Adult, or persistent, primary RTA occurs predominantly in females. Most of the cases are sporadic, but the disease may be inherited as an autosomal-dominant trait (32). The reclamation of filtered bicarbonate is intact in the proximal tubules, but the distal tubule is unable to generate or maintain steep lumen-peritubular hydrogen ion gradients.

The electrolyte abnormalities are responsible for the symptoms. Chronic acidosis may contribute to the impaired growth of children with type 1 RTA (191), because the retained acid is buffered in bone (86). Although urinary wasting of calcium and phosphorus may lead to osteomalacia, the hyperchloremic acidosis is so readily detected that patients rarely are left untreated long enough to develop this complication. Urinary potassium wasting may result in severe hypokalemia and a flaccid paralysis.

Nephrolithiasis occurs in 70% of patients with distal RTA (142,347). Multiple calculi usually are present in both kidneys. Nephrocalcinosis is found in approximately three-fourths of adults with type 1 RTA (28). Stone formation is related to hypercalciuria, relatively alkaline urine, and low urinary citrate excretion. Reduced urinary excretion of pyrophosphate, sulfate, and inhibitors of hydroxyapatite and of crystal growth also may contribute to clinical stone formation.

The diagnosis of distal RTA is made when systemic acidosis (serum bicarbonate less than 20 mEq/L) is present and urine pH is greater than 5.5 (42,167). An ammonium chloride (NH_4Cl) load often is used as a stress test to confirm the diagnosis. Liquid NH_4Cl (100 mg/kg as a 5% solution) is given in the evening; the patient voids at 6 AM on the following day, drinks three 8-ounce glasses of water, and voids again at 7:30 AM. The pH of this latter urine specimen is measured with a pH meter. The pH of this urine sample is between 5.0 and 5.5 in a healthy individual. If the pH is greater than 5.5 and the serum bicarbonate is greater than 20 mEq/L, the NH_4Cl load is repeated. The urinary pH measurement is repeated in 4 hours.

The distal tubular acidification mechanism is intact in type 2 or proximal RTA, but the reabsorption of filtered bicarbonate is reduced in the proximal tubule (205). Proximal RTA usually is associated with an underlying disorder of proximal tubular function, such as Fanconi's syndrome, hereditary fructose intolerance, Wilson's disease, or multiple myeloma. The most common cause of proximal RTA in adults is intestinal malabsorption that leads to vitamin D deficiency, hypocalcemia, secondary hyperparathyroidism, and hypophosphatemia (207). Proximal RTA is not associated with stone formation.

Previously, infants and children with a distal acidification defect and bicarbonate wasting were believed to have had type 3 RTA. This term is no longer used because the bicarbonate wasting is thought to reflect the same defect in renal acid excretion that causes type 1 RTA in adults (192). The reduction in acid excretion is secondary to the renal bicarbonate wasting as a cause of the acidosis. Adults with type 1 RTA excrete 1% to 3% of filtered bicarbonate, whereas infants and children with this disorder excrete 6% to 14% of filtered bicarbonate.

The term *type 4 RTA* has been applied to an acidification defect that may accompany a reduction in the renal clearance of potassium. This disorder is thought to involve the cation-exchange segment of the distal nephron, where aldosterone stimulates hydrogen ion secretion. Type 4 RTA may be the most common form of RTA, and often is associated with the syndrome of hyporeninemic hypoaldosteronism (18). Hyperkalemic distal RTA also has been found in patients with obstructive uropathy (18). Type 4 RTA is not associated with nephrolithiasis.

Some patients with recurrent calcium urolithiasis are not systemically acidotic but are unable to lower their urine pH after an NH_4Cl load (31). Both proximal and distal acidification defects have been identified in stone-formers with the syndrome of incomplete RTA (10,221,337). Patients with these disorders tend to develop stone disease at an earlier age, have more frequent recurrences, and grow larger stones. Hypocitruria and hypercalciuria usually are present. The hypercalciuria is unexplained because these patients do not have systemic acidosis. Serum electrolyte concentrations are normal, and a standardized acid loading study is required for the diagnosis of incomplete RTA.

Urolithiasis is a complication of long-term treatment with carbonic anhydrase inhibitors (241,336). Carbonic anhydrase, which catalyzes the hydration of carbon dioxide, is present in both the proximal and distal nephrons. Because carbonic anhydrase aids the proximal reclamation of filtered bicarbonate and the distal secretion of hydrogen ions, the administration of an inhibitor of the enzyme, such as acetazolamide, causes a proximal and distal RTA. Treatment with acetazolamide produces alterations in the ionic composition of urine, such as a low citrate concentration, which closely resemble those found in untreated distal RTA (126,308). All of the changes can be reversed by stopping administration of the carbonic anhydrase inhibitor.

Cystinuria

Cystine is a disulfide composed of two cysteine molecules (Fig. 8.3), and its pKa is 8.0. Cystinuria is an inherited disorder of amino acid metabolism in which transport of *c*ystine, *o*rnithine, *l*ysine, and *a*rginine in the renal tubule and GI tract is defective. (The mnemonic "COLA" or "COAL" can be used to remember these four amino acids.) The defect is transmitted as an autosomal-recessive trait. This disorder would be a metabolic curiosity if it were not for the relative insolubility of cystine in urine (61,63). Approximately 300 mg of cystine is soluble in 1 L of urine at a pH of 7.0; the solubility of cystine more than doubles as

```
   S              S ———————— S
   |              |          |
  CH2            CH2        CH2
   |              |          |
H–C–NH2       H–C–NH2    H–C–NH2
   |              |          |
  COOH           COOH       COOH

Cysteine            Cystine
```

FIGURE 8.3. Structures of cysteine and cystine (a disulfide).

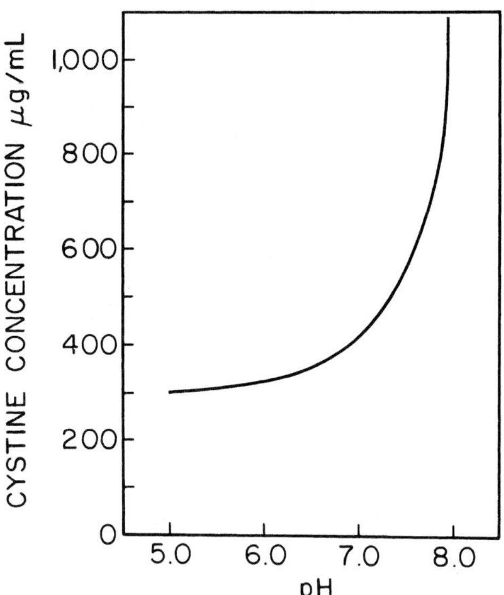

FIGURE 8.4. The pH dependence of the solubility of cystine. (Modified from Dent CE, Senior B. Studies on the treatment of cystinuria. *Br J Urol* 1955;27:317, with permisison.)

the pH rises above 7.5 (Fig. 8.4). Homozygotes excrete large amounts of cystine, lysine, arginine, and ornithine in their urine.

Cystinosis, another recessively inherited metabolic disorder, may be confused with cystinuria. Cystinosis is characterized by the intracellular accumulation of excessive quantities of cystine (291). Crystal deposition occurs in the cornea, conjunctiva, bone marrow, lymph nodes, leukocytes, and internal organs. All patients with nephropathic cystinosis have a generalized amino aciduria, but the daily excretion of cystine is only 5% to 10% of that found in patients with cystinuria. Children with cystinosis tend to produce a relatively alkaline urine, and stone formation rarely occurs.

Cystinuria is manifested clinically by the formation of homogeneous radiodense calculi that may have a branched configuration. Multiple small satellite stones may accompany a large stone. The stones have the gross appearance of maple sugar and tend to be hard and tough. Hexagonal cystine crystals may be present in a voided urine sample, especially one that is concentrated and acidified. The diagnosis is confirmed by the analysis of a stone and the finding of increased urinary cystine on an amino acid analysis. Urine can be screened with the cyanide-nitroprusside test, which is positive if more than 75 to 125 mg of cystine per gram of creatinine is present (63). This test does not differentiate homozygotes from heterozygotes. A new test kit based on the reaction of cystine with nickel ion and sodium hyposulfite has been marketed by Mission Pharmacal Company (107). This convenient method can be used to screen patients who are interested in extracorporeal shock wave lithotripsy (ESWL), but whose stones have a radiographic appearance strongly suggestive of cystine.

Urinary excretion of cystine is less than 30 mg per day in healthy adults. Heterozygous adults excrete less than 400 mg of cystine per day and usually do not form stones. Daily urinary cystine excretion is usually greater than 400 mg in homozygous cystine stone-formers. No overlap in cystine excretion has been demonstrated between well-confirmed homozygotes and heterozygotes (60).

Hypercalcemic Disorders

Primary hyperparathyroidism is the most common disorder associated with hypercalcemia and urolithiasis. It is found in approximately 5% of patients with stone disease (6). The diagnosis is based on the presence of hypercalcemia with an inappropriately elevated parathyroid hormone (PTH) level.

PTH is synthesized in the chief cells of the parathyroid gland and is split into at least two major fragments after being secreted into the circulation (148). The N-terminal fragment is responsible for the biologic activity and has a short half-life. The C-terminal fragments have longer half-lives but no biologic activity. PTH increases bone resorption, increases renal reabsorption of calcium, decreases renal absorption of phosphate, and augments renal conversion of 25-hydroxyvitamin D to 1,25-dihydroxyvitamin D, thereby increasing intestinal absorption of calcium (177,320). All of the effects of PTH tend to increase the serum concentration of calcium, which exerts negative feedback control over the secretion of PTH. The phosphaturia in patients with primary hyperparathyroidism may lead to hypophosphatemia, but most patients have normal serum phosphate concentrations. A liberal dietary phosphate intake may compensate for the phosphaturia.

A single adenoma, usually chief cell, is responsible for the disease in 80% of patients (113). Chief cell hyperplasia is found in most of the remaining 20%. The hypercalcemia and inappropriately high PTH levels found in patients with primary hyperparathyroidism are caused by the relatively autonomous function of the adenomatous or hyperplastic tissue.

The clinical presentation of primary hyperparathyroidism has changed over the past 20 years. Generalized osteitis fibrosa cystica is extremely rare, and the incidence of urolithiasis has decreased. A population study in Rochester, Minnesota, from 1965 through 1976, found that the average annual incidence of cases of primary hyperparathyroidism increased from 7.8 persons per 100,000 population to 51 per 100,000 population (127). This dramatic increase in the apparent incidence occurred immediately after routine measurement of serum calcium was begun in 1974. The frequency of urolithiasis decreased from 51% to 4%. The proportion of patients without symptoms or complications increased from 18% to 51%. A more recent study found that fewer than 2% of patients with renal stones had primary hyperparathyroidism (295). Bone demineralization occurs with a similar frequency in patients with and without stone disease (306).

The reason for stone formation in patients with hyperparathyroidism and urolithiasis is not known. Patients have urine that is supersaturated with respect to calcium stone salts whether or not stone disease is present (233), and the magnitude of SS is not greater for patients with stones. Patients with hyperparathyroid-induced stone formation may have been predisposed to form stones. One study found that hyperparathyroid stone-formers excreted less citrate than non—stone-formers (4).

Immobilization may be complicated by hypercalcemia, hypercalciuria, and stone formation. The hypercalcemia and hypercalciuria may be especially severe in adolescents with active bone growth. Approximately 10% of patients with traumatic spinal cord injuries develop renal calculi (77). The risk of stone formation is greatest during the first 3 months after injury. Urinary calcium excretion exceeds normal levels at approximately the fourth week of immobilization and reaches maximum levels at 16 weeks. The hypercalciuria may persist for 12 months but resolves by 18 months. Resorption of bone appears to be the primary process. Serum calcium levels are elevated or in the high-normal range. Hypercalcemia and nephrolithiasis also have been reported in patients with multiple fractures (218).

Hypercalciuria and hyperphosphaturia occur during the weightlessness of space travel, but there has been no evidence of clinical stone formation (181). Long-term bed rest is used as a model to study the effects of weightlessness on metabolism. Such studies at simulated high altitudes disclosed that urinary losses of calcium were significantly smaller at a higher altitude. Exercise does not prevent hypercalciuria (140).

Nephrocalcinosis and renal insufficiency may occur with the milk-alkali syndrome and vitamin D intoxication. Stone formation also occurs in sarcoidosis, where there is increased intestinal calcium absorption, hypercalcemia, and hypercalciuria (39,128). Hypercalcemic patients with sarcoidosis have elevated serum levels of 1,25-dihydroxyvitamin D. Healthy persons produce this active metabolite of vitamin D only in the renal tubule. There is evidence that patients with sarcoidosis convert 25-hydroxyvitamin D to the active compound in the granulomas (171). Hypercalcemia also occurs in patients with other granulomatous diseases, such as tuberculosis, berylliosis, and coccidioidomycosis.

Uric Acid Lithiasis

Uric acid is the endproduct of purine metabolism in humans. Uric acid has two dissociable protons (Fig. 8.5), the first with a pKa of 5.5 and the second with a pKa of 10.3 (98). The limited solubility of this weak acid accounts for its propensity to form renal calculi (Fig. 8.6). Uric acid solubility is approximately 15 mg/dL at a pH of 5, but is 200 mg/dL at a pH of 7.

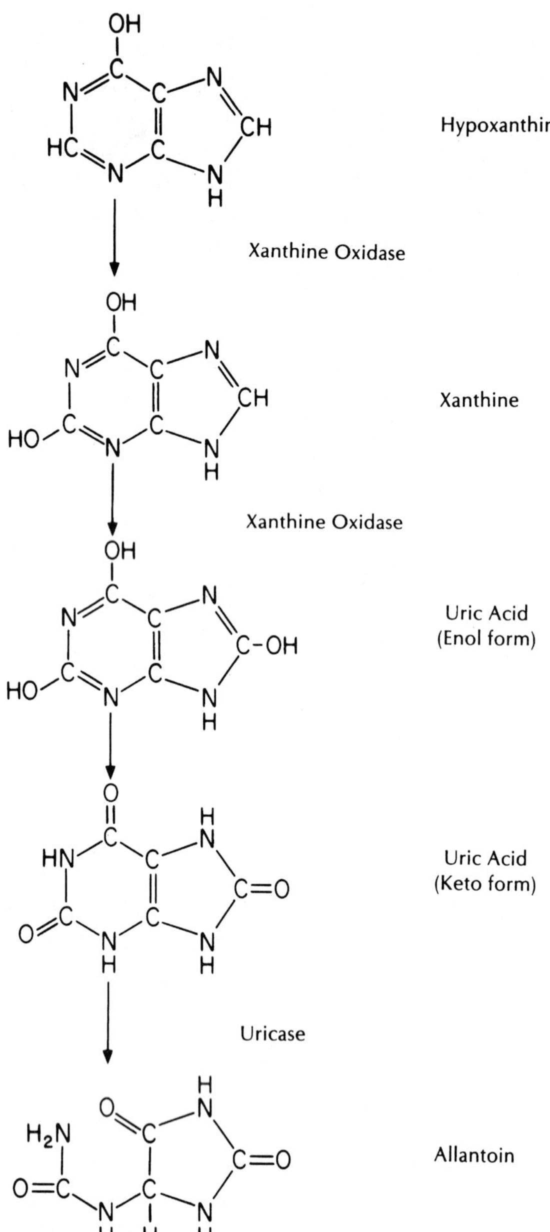

FIGURE 8.5. Metabolic pathway for conversion of hypoxanthine to xanthine and uric acid. Most ureotelic mammals, except humans, have hepatic uricase that converts uric acid into the more soluble allantoin.

Uric acid excretion depends on the biosynthesis of new purines and, to a lesser extent, on preformed dietary purines (90,121). A series of enzymatic reactions leads to the formation of the mononucleotide, inosine monophosphate. Dietary nucleic acids can be catabolized to form two other mononucleotides: adenosine monophosphate and guanine monophosphate. Cleavage of the phosphate group by nucleotidases forms the corresponding nucleosides: inosine, guanosine, and adenosine. The action of nucleoside phosphorylases forms the purine bases: hypoxanthine (from inosine), guanine, and adenine. Xanthine oxidase converts hypoxanthine to xanthine and uric acid (Fig. 8.5). The purine salvage enzymes, hypoxanthine-guanine-phosphoribosyltransferase (HGPRT) and adenine phosphoribosyltransferase, can reconvert the purine bases to the mononucleotides. This is the purine salvage pathway.

An X-linked deficiency of HGPRT is responsible for two clinical syndromes (370). Enzyme activity is virtually absent in the Lesch-Nyhan syndrome, a disease characterized by uric acid overproduction and a central nervous system disorder (e.g., mental retardation, spasticity, choreoathetosis, self-mutilation). HGPRT activity is partially deficient in the second syndrome, which is characterized by uric acid overproduction and severe gout, but no neurologic abnormality. Uric acid lithiasis may occur in both syndromes.

Biosynthesis of purines from amino acids also provides a way to eliminate waste nitrogen as uric acid (121). This is the major pathway of waste nitrogen disposal in birds and uricotelic reptiles. Loss of water and electrolytes is minimized by discharging a semisolid uric acid mass through a cloaca. In most ureotelic mammals, except humans, urate that enters the glomerular filtrate is reabsorbed in the proximal tubule and recycled through the liver for conversion to water-soluble allantoin by hepatic uricase. Allantoin is freely excreted by the kidney. Uricase is not present in humans, and uric acid cannot be converted to the more soluble allantoin. Plasma and urine uric acid levels in humans are an order of magnitude greater than those in most mammals. The high concentrations of uric acid are precariously held in solution, a situation that predisposes humans to gout and uric acid lithiasis.

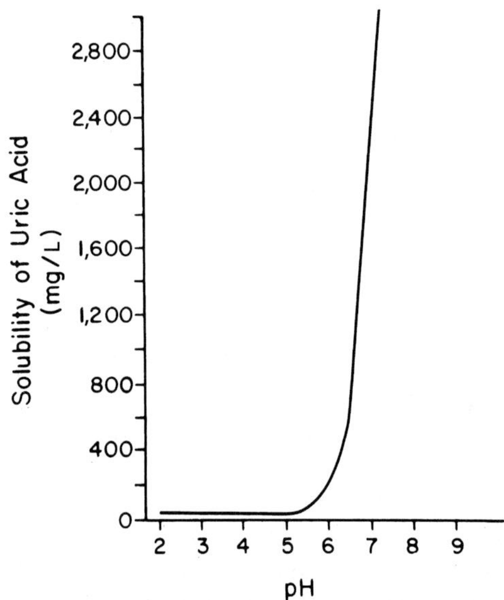

FIGURE 8.6. The pH dependence of the solubility of uric acid at 38°C. (Modified from Finlayson B, Smith A. Stability of first dissociable proton of uric acid. *J Chem Eng Data* 1974;19:94, with permission.)

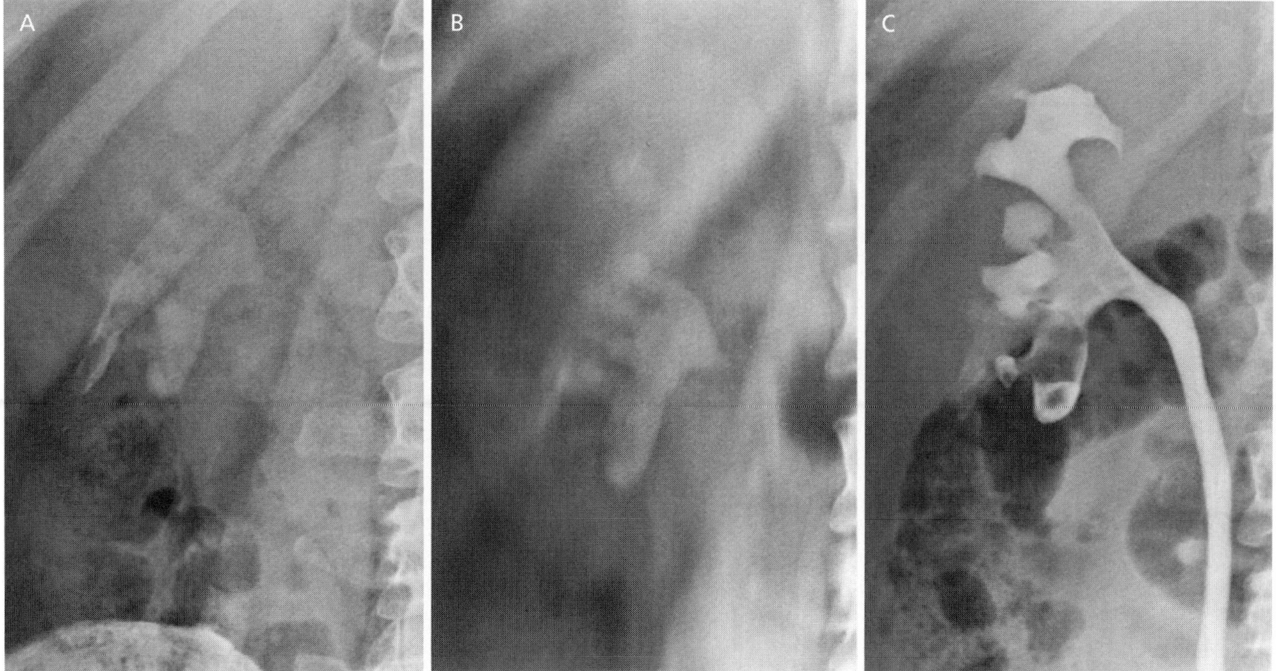

FIGURE 8.7. A: Plain abdominal radiograph that demonstrates a large branched right renal calculus. **B:** Plain tomographic film. **C:** Retrograde pyelogram that demonstrates a filling defect. Analysis of the removed stone material revealed 98% uric acid.

The dalmatian coach hound also is predisposed to uric acid urolithiasis (377). Normal quantities of uricase are present in the liver, but uric acid conversion to allantoin is slow and incomplete. This, together with defective tubular reabsorption of urates, leads to hyperuricosuria and stone formation.

Uric acid lithiasis accounts for 5% to 10% of stones formed in the United States. Approximately one-fourth of patients with primary gout develop uric acid stones. Uric acid lithiasis is found in approximately 40% of stone-forming persons in Israel (9). Uric acid bladder calculi are a common problem in children of rural Southeast Asia.

Patients with uric acid lithiasis may excrete too much uric acid or excessively acidic urine (259). Overproduction of uric acid, as occurs in some patients with gout, may be responsible for the hyperuricosuria. Purine and protein gluttony also may increase uric acid excretion. Most patients with uric acid lithiasis do not have gout or any recognizable disorder of purine metabolism. Serum and urine uric acid levels are usually normal in patients with idiopathic uric acid urolithiasis. Many of these patients have a persistently low urine pH. Although some investigators have found an isolated defect in renal tubular ammonia secretion, the mechanism of the low urinary pH is still poorly understood. Urinary pH also tends to be low in gout (120).

Gouty patients who are treated with uricosuric agents may be at risk for uric acid stone formation. This can be prevented with an increased fluid intake and urinary alkalinization. Patients with myeloproliferative disorders are also at risk for uric acid stone formation, especially with the initiation of chemotherapy or radiotherapy. The increased purine load may even lead to intratubular precipitation of uric acid and anuria.

Disorders that reduce urine volume are associated with uric acid precipitation in an acid urine. Patients with ileostomies or chronic diarrhea can lose large amounts of fluid and bicarbonate. Maintenance of an adequately dilute urine can be difficult for these patients because oral fluids and electrolytes are not well absorbed. The diarrhea or ileostomy output may increase as fluid intake increases. Small bladder calculi composed of uric acid may be found in men with prostatism. These patients reduce their urinary frequency by reducing their fluid intake. Pure uric acid is radiolucent, but gradual incorporation of impurities (usually metals such as calcium) makes larger stones (more than 2 cm diameter) faintly radiopaque. Identification of smaller stones can be accomplished with excretory urography, sonography, or computed tomography (CT). Large uric acid stones may have a branched configuration (Fig. 8.7).

Xanthinuria

Xanthine is less soluble than uric acid (Fig. 8.4). Its solubility increases with rising urine pH, but the effect is not as great as that with uric acid. The pKa of the first dissociable proton of xanthine is 7.7. Like uric acid, xanthine is radiolucent. Xanthine calculi have been reported to occur in xanthinuria, a rare, inherited deficiency of xanthine oxidase (75). Serum and urine uric acid levels are low, but urinary excretion of hypoxanthine and xanthine is elevated. Stone formation has occurred in approximately one-third of patients.

Urinary excretion of hypoxanthine and xanthine is more commonly elevated in patients who are being treated with a xanthine oxidase inhibitor such as allopurinol (Fig. 8.8). Xanthine stone formation during allopurinol administration has been reported in patients with Lesch-Nyhan syndrome and in patients with myeloproliferative disorders who are receiving chemotherapy (29).

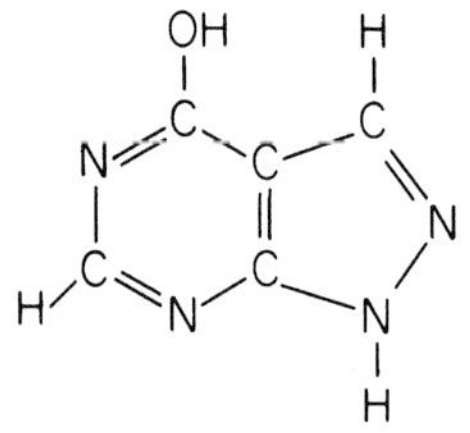

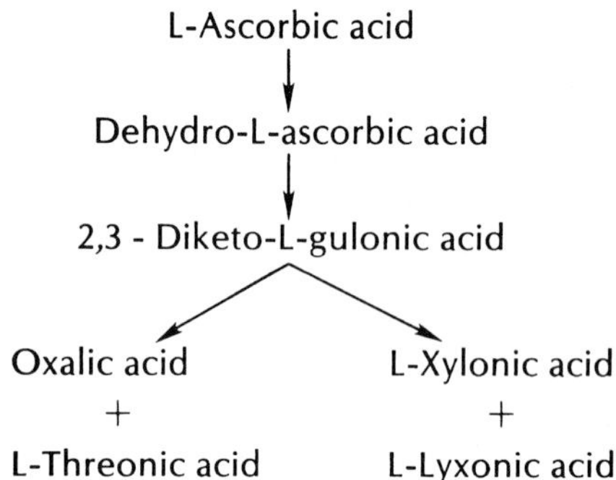

FIGURE 8.8. Structure of allopurinol, an analog of hypoxanthine and xanthine.

L-Ascorbic acid

↓

Dehydro-L-ascorbic acid

↓

2,3 - Diketo-L-gulonic acid

↙ ↘

Oxalic acid + L-Threonic acid | L-Xylonic acid + L-Lyxonic acid

FIGURE 8.9. Oxidative metabolism of ascorbic acid leads to the production of oxalate.

2,8-Dihydroxyadeninuria

2,8-Dihydroxyadeninuria is an inherited disorder caused by a defect of the purine salvage enzyme, adenine phosphoribosyltransferase (105,372). Adenine is converted to 2,8-dihydroxyadenine (2,8-DHA), which is insoluble over a wide range of urinary pH. Stone formation and renal failure have been described, usually in children (102). Like uric acid, 2,8-DHA stones are radiolucent. Uric acid stones are hard and yellowish, whereas 2,8-DHA stones are friable and brown or gray. Enzymatic analysis with uricase avoids mistaken identification as uric acid, and infrared spectroscopy or x-ray crystallography confirms the diagnosis. "Uric acid" stones in children must always be suspect and subjected to a sophisticated analysis. The failure to diagnose this disorder can lead to needless recurrent stone formation and even renal failure (40).

Primary Hyperoxaluria

Primary hyperoxaluria is a rare, inherited disorder of glyoxylate metabolism. Clinical manifestations include recurrent calcium oxalate nephrolithiasis, nephrocalcinosis, and chronic renal failure. Extrarenal deposits of oxalate, or oxalosis, develop in the presence of renal failure.

Approximately 10% of oxalate excreted in urine is absorbed from the GI tract. The remainder is derived from endogenous metabolism. Oxalate is produced in mammals as an endproduct of the oxidative metabolism of ascorbic acid (Fig. 8.9) and by oxidation of glyoxylic acid (Fig. 8.10). The major precursor of oxalate in humans is glyoxylate.

Type 1 primary hyperoxaluria, or glycolic aciduria, was thought to be caused by deficiency of the cytoplasmic enzyme α-ketoglutarate-glyoxylate carboligase (367). More recent investigations have shown that this disorder is caused by a deficiency or functional abnormality of peroxisomal alanine-glyoxylate aminotransferase in the liver (Fig. 8.10) (67–69). This enzyme acts on glyoxalate and alanine in peroxisomes to produce pyruvate and glycine. Glutamate-glyoxylate aminotransferase is a cytoplasmic enzyme that

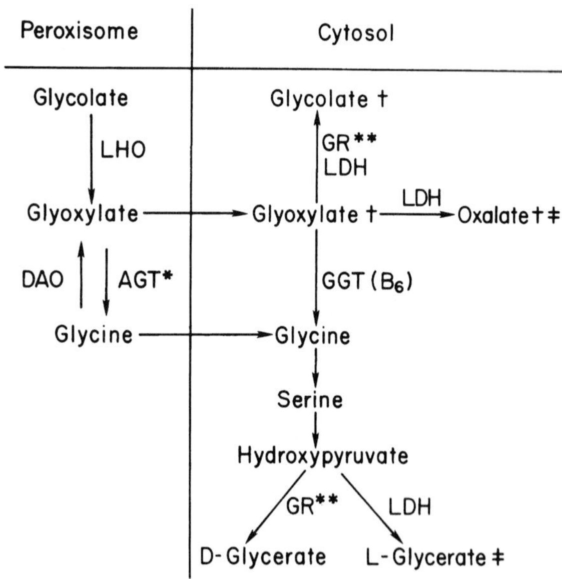

FIGURE 8.10. Pathways of oxalate metabolism in humans. A deficiency of peroxisomal AGT* is responsible for primary hyperoxaluria type 1 (67,68) and results in elevated urinary levels of glycolate†, glyoxylate†, and oxalate†. A deficiency of cytoplasmic GR** is responsible for primary hyperoxaluria type 2 and results in elevated urinary levels of L—glycerate‡ but normal levels of glycolate and glyoxylate. *Peroxisomal enzymes:* LHO, L-α-hydroxy acid oxidase/glycolate oxidase; DAO, D-amino acid oxidase/glycine oxidase; AGT, alanine: glyoxylate aminotransferase/serine: pyruvate aminotransferase. *Cytosolic enzymes:* GGT, glutamate: glyoxyl aminotransferase/alanine:2-oxoglutarate aminotransferase (pyridoxine is a cofactor); GR, glyoxylate reductase/D-glycerate dehydrogenase; LDH, lactate dehydrogenase.

acts on cytoplasmic glyoxylate and glutamate to form glycine and 2-oxoglutarate. Pyridoxine (vitamin B_6) is a cofactor in this latter reaction. Urinary excretion of oxalate, glyoxalate, and glycolate is elevated in type 1 primary hyperoxaluria, which is the most common form of the disease.

Type 2 primary hyperoxaluria, or L-glyceric aciduria, is caused by a deficiency of the enzyme glyoxylate reductase/D-glycerate dehydrogenase (Fig 8.10) (43,366). Urinary excretion of oxalate and L-glyceric acid is elevated, but glycolate excretion is normal, as is that of glyoxylate.

Primary hyperoxaluria is a rare disorder. An extensive review in 1964 reported on 63 typical and 47 atypical cases (137). The disease had become clinically manifest in more than half of the patients by age 4 years. Almost half had died of renal failure by 20 years of age.

The disease should be suspected in patients who are young, have a family history of urolithiasis, and have nephrocalcinosis or large, radiodense calculi on plain abdominal radiographs. Urinary oxalate excretion generally is greater than 100 mg per 24 hours, except in the presence of renal failure. Differentiation between types 1 and 2 is made with urinary glycolate measurements. Glycolate excretion is normal in type 2 but elevated in type 1.

Secondary Urolithiasis

Stone formation may be associated with a group of unrelated conditions: small bowel dysfunction; urinary tract infection with bacterial organisms that produce urease; obstructive uropathy; structural anomalies such as medullary sponge kidney; urinary diversion; and pharmacologic agents. Although all of these disorders may be associated with stone formation, they may not be its primary cause. It is important to search for underlying disorders, such as primary hyperparathyroidism, cystinuria, RTA, or idiopathic hypercalciuria. Prevention of further stone formation requires treatment of any underlying metabolic disorder and the immediate cause of stone formation.

Enteric Hyperoxaluria

Dietary oxalate is a relatively minor source of urinary oxalate in healthy persons, but patients with small bowel disorders may develop hyperoxaluria and recurrent calcium oxalate stone disease. GI absorption of dietary oxalate is more avid in these patients. Enteric hyperoxaluria was first described in the early 1970s and was partly responsible for the abandonment of jejunoileal bypass surgery as a means to control obesity (217,317). Major sources of dietary oxalate are the green leafy vegetables such as rhubarb, spinach, and kale. Tea, cocoa, chocolate, and pepper also have a high oxalate content. The average daily diet contains 100 to 900 mg of oxalate (365).

The acid medium in the stomach releases oxalate from foodstuffs. After combining with free dietary calcium in the alkaline medium of the small intestine, most of the oxalate exists as insoluble calcium oxalate. The small amount of free oxalate that does exist can be absorbed. The colon seems to be the major absorptive area. Patients with ileostomies rarely develop hyperoxaluria (83). The reaction between intestinal calcium and oxalate prevents the absorption of no more than 10% of dietary oxalate by healthy persons.

Patients with a variety of chronic GI disorders such as small bowel resection, inflammatory small bowel disease, chronic pancreatitis, or a jejunoileal bypass may malabsorb fat. The intraluminal concentration of fatty acids increases and calcium is bound to form calcium–fatty acid soaps (85). Less calcium is available to bind oxalate, and more free oxalate is available for absorption. Evidence also shows that malabsorbed fatty acids or bile acids increase colonic permeability to oxalate (82). Patients with enteric hyperoxaluria may absorb up to one-third of their dietary oxalate.

The incidence of nephrolithiasis in inflammatory bowel disease is 2% to 3%, but ileal resection increases the risk to 10% (81). The primary risk factor is increased urinary excretion of oxalate. In comparison with the primary hyperoxalurias, excretion of L-glyceric acid and glycolic acid is normal.

Elevated urinary oxalate is not the only risk factor in these patients (319). The multiple risk factors are shown in Table 8.3. All factors increase the propensity for calcium oxalate precipitation. Reduced urinary volume and pH may promote uric acid stone formation.

Another form of enteric hyperoxaluria is that possibly associated with ascorbic acid (310,344). The metabolic pathway for *in vivo* conversion of ascorbate to oxalate is shown in Fig. 8.6. *In vitro* conversion of ascorbate to oxalate may occur in saline solutions or pooled urine samples, especially those that have not been acidified (278). This may produce a factitious hyperoxaluria in patients who are

TABLE 8.3. ENTERIC HYPEROXALURIA RISK FACTORS FOR UROLITHIASIS

Malabsorbed Component	Urine Composition
Fatty acids, bile acids	Increased oxalate
Water	Decreased volume
Electrolytes	Decreased ionic strength
Bicarbonate	Decreased pH, decreased citrate
Magnesium	Decreased magnesium
Protein	Decreased sulfate, decreased phosphate, decreased pyrophosphate

Modified from Smith LH, Werness PG, Wilson DM. Enteric hyperoxaluria: associated abnormalities that promote formation of renal calculi. In: Rose GA, Robertson WG, Watts RWE, eds. *Oxalate in human biochemistry and clinical pathology.* London: Wellcome Foundation, 1979:224, with permission.

consuming large quantities of vitamin C. A further confounding factor is that some methods used to measure oxalate may not be able to distinguish ascorbate metabolites from oxalate (122). Patients should be advised not to take large amounts of vitamin C when they are collecting a 24-hour urine specimen for chemical analysis.

Infected Renal Lithiasis

Infected renal lithiasis refers to the pathologic occurrence of stones composed of magnesium ammonium phosphate ($MgNH_4PO_4 \cdot 6H_2O$, or struvite). Stones caused by infection are not pure struvite—careful crystallographic analysis of infected stone material from humans has revealed a mixture of struvite, carbonate apatite [$Ca_{10}(PO_4)_6 \cdot CO_3$], and hydroxyapatite [$Ca_{10}(PO_4)_6(OH)_2$] (116).

Infection of the urinary tract with urease-producing bacterial organisms is a necessary prerequisite for the formation and growth of struvite stones (117). The enzyme urease catalyzes the formation of ammonia and carbon dioxide (CO_2) from urea:

$$(NH_2)_2CO + H_2O \rightarrow 2NH_3 + CO_2$$

The formation of ammonia leads to an increase in urinary pH:

$$NH_3 + H_2O \rightarrow NH_4^+ + OH^-(pK = 9.0)$$

When urine is physiologically alkaline, ammonia levels are low, but when urease is present, the urine is alkaline and ammonia levels are high.

The higher pH also leads to the further dissociation of phosphate:

$$H_2PO_4^- \rightarrow H^+ + HPO_4^{2-}(pK = 7.2)$$

$$HPO_4^{2-} \rightarrow H^+ + PO_4^{3-}(pK = 12.4)$$

Under these conditions, urine is supersaturated for magnesium ammonium phosphate, and precipitation of this material occurs.

Because all of the reactions occur in aqueous solution, CO_2 exists as carbonic acid:

$$CO_2 + H_2O \rightarrow H_2CO_3$$

In the presence of an alkaline pH, the carbonic acid dissociates to form bicarbonate:

$$H_2CO_3 \rightarrow H^+ + HCO_3^-(pKa = 6.3)$$

and the bicarbonate dissociates to form carbonate:

$$HCO_3^- \rightarrow H^+ + CO_3^{2-}(pKa = 10.2)$$

The CO_3^{2-} can precipitate with $PO_4^{3-}$and Ca^{2+} to form carbonate apatite.

Proteus species most commonly are associated with infection stones, but some species of *Klebsiella, Pseudomonas* and *Staphylococcus* may produce urease (116). Virtually all *Proteus* species produce urease, whereas *Escherichia coli* never produces urease. *Ureaplasma urealyticum* will induce alkalinization and crystallization of magnesium ammonium phosphate and calcium phosphates in synthetic urine, and a recent clinical review found this organism in 25% of patients with infection stones (19). Even some anaerobic bacterial organisms produce urease.

Infection stones account for 15% to 20% of all urinary stones. Struvite stones frequently have a branched or staghorn configuration, but not all branched calculi are infection induced. Cystine and uric acid stones also may have a branched configuration.

Some patients with metabolic stone disease may have urinary tract infections with bacteria that do not produce urease. The stones do not contain struvite, and the infection is not responsible for the stone formation. The infection can be treated successfully with antibiotics alone in half of these patients.

Some patients with metabolic stone disease may develop recurrent urinary tract infections with urease-producing bacterial organisms. Struvite may then precipitate on a core of calcium oxalate or cystine. Some investigators have found an underlying metabolic disorder in more than 50% of patients with struvite stone formation (256,296). Prevention of further stone formation requires the identification and treatment of any such metabolic disorder. Other investigators found that recurrent stone formation was negligible in a group of patients who had operative removal of their stone material, specific antimicrobial therapy, and postoperative irrigation of the collecting system with hemiacidrin solution (307). This study implies that metabolic disorders are relatively unimportant in the pathogens of struvite urolithiasis.

Obstruction

Stone formation may be associated with obstructive uropathy. The most common example is uric acid bladder stone formation with bladder outlet obstruction, usually from prostatic hyperplasia. Upper urinary tract obstruction may delay the normal washout of crystal aggregates and gravel. These particles may continue to grow and form macroscopic stones. Persistent infection with urease-producing bacterial organisms may occur in the presence of urinary stasis and result in struvite stone formation. Most patients with obstruction do not form kidney stones.

Medullary Sponge Kidney

Medullary sponge kidney is characterized by dilated collecting tubules in one or more renal papillae. In the absence of complications, it is an asymptomatic and benign condition, but urinary tract infection and nephrolithiasis are frequent complications (373). The diagnosis is made by excretory urography; linear or spherical tubules in the renal papillae are filled with contrast medium.

The role of medullary sponge kidney in the pathogenesis of nephrolithiasis has not been clarified, but 20% of patients with calcium urolithiasis may have this disorder (373). Other investigators found medullary sponge kidney in fewer than 5% of their calcium stone–forming patients (220). Medullary sponge kidney is found more commonly in women than in men. Patients with medullary sponge kidney and nephrolithiasis have the same spectrum of metabolic abnormalities as the overall population of calcium stone-formers (220,243). Calcium oxalate is the most common stone salt found in patients with medullary sponge kidney (125).

Polycystic Kidney Disease

Nephrolithiasis occurs in approximately 20% of patients with autosomal-dominant polycystic kidney disease (ADPKD). Approximately half of the patients are symptomatic, even though most of the stones are in calices or attached to the papillary tips. Careful intravenous urography or CT is required to distinguish stones from parenchymal or cyst wall calcification. Tubular ectasia is found in 15%, but the relationship of this radiographic finding to the pathogenesis of the stone formation is unknown.

Most of the calculi are composed of uric acid, often in association with calcium oxalate. The distorted renal anatomy and urinary stasis may contribute to stone formation, but most patients have concurrent metabolic abnormalities. A retrospective review at the Mayo Clinic found hypocitraturia in 67% of patients, hyperuricemia in 19%, hyperoxaluria in 19%, hyperuricosuria in 15%, hypercalciuria in 11%, and primary hyperparathyroidism in 5% (342). A defect in the transfer of ammonium to the final urine may prevent patients with ADPKD from responding appropriately to acidosis. This would explain the hypocitraturia found in a majority of patients.

Urinary Diversion

Stone formation and recurrent infections may be associated with urinary tract diversion. Urease-producing bacterial infections may lead to struvite stone formation. The diversionary procedure also may produce metabolic abnormalities that encourage stone formation. GI bicarbonate loss and hyperchloremic acidosis are known side effects of ureterosigmoid anastomoses (189). The systemic acidosis may lead to hypercalciuria and hypocitruria. Osteomalacia has been reported to develop in patients with ureterosigmoidostomies and a metabolic acidosis (305). Occasional patients with ileal conduits develop a hyperchloremic acidosis (84,159). Most stones form in the presence of *Proteus* infections and are composed of struvite. Because excess conduit length may contribute to the bicarbonate loss and chloride absorption, these metabolic derangements may occur more frequently with the new continent diversionary procedures. The use of nicotinamide to block intestinal chloride transport may be a useful preventive measure (158).

The incidence of calculus formation after augmentation cystoplasty has been reported to be as high as 50% (239). Urinary tract infection, mucus production, foreign bodies, and hypocitraturia have been identified as potential risk factors (155). The acidic environment provided by gastrocystoplasty retards mucous production and bacterial overgrowth (240). As expected, stone formation occurs less frequently than after enterocystoplasty.

Drugs

The metabolic effects of some drugs lead to stone formation. Acetazolamide, a carbonic anhydrase inhibitor, produces changes in urine composition that are similar to those found in distal RTA. Kidney stones have formed in patients who have received this drug for the treatment of glaucoma. Nephrolithiasis also has been reported in patients who have received long-term acetazolamide for the treatment of periodic paralysis and myotonia (336).

Drugs or their metabolites may have limited solubility in urine. These compounds may be absorbed onto calculi already present in the urinary tract or may precipitate to form new stones. Approximately 50% of an ingested dose of allopurinol is excreted as oxypurinol, an oxidative metabolite. Oxypurinol, like xanthine, is less soluble than allopurinol or hypoxanthine. The solubility of oxypurinol decreases with a decrease in pH. Radiolucent oxypurinol stone formation has been reported in a patient with regional enteritis who was receiving allopurinol for the prevention of recurrent uric acid lithiasis (327). Persistent oliguria and aciduria contributed to the precipitation of oxypurinol. Rarely, xanthine stones have formed in patients treated with allopurinol.

Triamterene and its metabolites have been identified in renal calculi. Some investigators have suggested that their precipitation may be a causative factor in the formation of calcium stones (364). Other investigators found that triamterene and its metabolites adsorb to stone matrix (360). Because stones that contain triamterene have an unusually high matrix content, triamterene and its metabolites may be a passive constituent of renal calculi. Clinical studies of patients receiving a combination of triamterene and hydrochlorothiazide (Dyazide) suggest that nephrolithiasis is not a clinically significant side effect (144).

Sulfonamides were one of the first classes of drugs to precipitate in the urinary tract, but numerous other drugs and their metabolites have been identified in renal calculi (70). Sulfadiazine urolithiasis has been reported in patients with AIDS who have received this drug for the treatment of toxoplasmosis (41,199). Another example is the report of several ceftriaxone stones in a 13-year-old boy treated for acute bacterial meningitis (51). Infrared spectrophotometry found that 92% of the stone material was ceftriaxone disodium; calcium oxalate monohydrate and protein comprised the remaining 8%.

Indinavir is a protease inhibitor used for treating HIV-1 (288). Indinavir was the third such drug introduced into the United States and is the most widely prescribed drug in this class of retroviral agents. Indinavir therapy has been associated with a 4% incidence of nephrolithiasis. Indinavir crystalluria (platelike rectangles and fan-shaped or starburst forms) can be found in 20% of patients and often is associated with irritative voiding symptoms (162).

Pure indinavir stones cannot be seen with CT scanning unless intravenous contrast is used (332). Symptomatic urolithiasis usually can be treated with hydration alone.

Several factors can predispose an individual to the urinary precipitation of a drug: a high renal excretion rate, a low solubility of a drug or its metabolites, a low urine volume, and prolonged treatment at a high dose. The appearance of synthetic compounds in renal calculi is to be expected as new drugs are introduced and analytic methods of stone analysis become more sophisticated.

Urinary calculi also may form on foreign bodies in the urinary tract (65). Foreign-body stones in the upper urinary tract have been associated with ureteral catheters, nephrostomy tubes, sutures, biliary calculi, shrapnel, and acupuncture needles. Renal papillary necrosis with calcification of the sloughed papillae may mimic nephrolithiasis (Fig. 8.11).

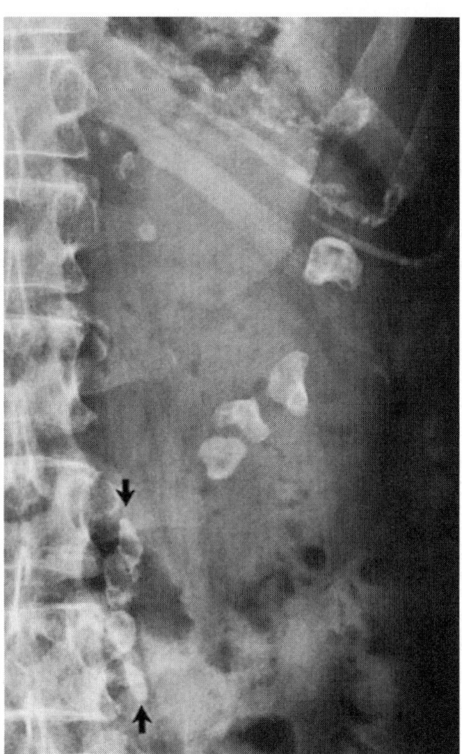

FIGURE 8.11. Multiple calcified bodies in left kidney and ureter *(between arrows).* The radiolucent centers could represent uric acid or necrotic renal papillae *(arrows).* Histologic examination revealed necrotic calcified renal papillae.

Ammonium acid urate calculus formation has been reported in women with a history of laxative abuse (79). Urinary volume over 24 hours and excretion of sodium, potassium, and citrate were low. GI loss of fluid and electrolytes led to chronic extracellular volume depletion and intracellular acidosis (low urinary citrate and potassium).

Idiopathic Calcium Urolithiasis

The diagnosis of ICU is one of exclusion and is applicable in 70% to 80% of North American and Western European patients with urolithiasis. If pure uric acid lithiasis, cystinuria, RTA, primary and secondary hyperoxaluria, and hypercalcemia have been excluded in a patient with calcium oxalate or mixed calcium oxalate and/or calcium phosphate stone formation, this diagnosis may be applied. However, a patient may have more than one disorder. Primary hyperparathyroidism and ICU or cystinuria and ICU may occur in the same patient.

Careful metabolic studies of patients with ICU reveal a multiplicity of abnormalities: hypercalciuria, mild hyperoxaluria, hyperuricosuria, crystal growth–inhibitor deficiencies, hypocitruria, and "incomplete" RTA. One or more of these abnormalities may be found in the same patient, and some of the abnormalities may be related to the others, such as hypocitruria to incomplete RTA. Some patients with ICU may have no clearly recognizable disorder other than calcium stone formation.

Between 50% and 70% of these patients have hypercalciuria (264). Most healthy men receiving a 1-g calcium diet excrete less than 275 mg of calcium over 24 hours. The corresponding figure for women is 250 mg per 24 hours. A more convenient way to remember is that urinary calcium excretion should not exceed 4 mg/kg per 24 hours. Most patients with ICU and hypercalciuria are thought to have primary intestinal hyperabsorption of dietary calcium (234). Increased absorption of dietary calcium may slightly increase the serum calcium concentration and suppress PTH secretion. The increased filtered load of calcium and decreased tubular reabsorption results in hypercalciuria. The urinary calcium loss compensates for the enhanced intestinal absorption, thereby maintaining serum calcium within a normal range. In the past, patients with absorptive hypercalciuria have been separated into three categories that depended on the serum phosphorous level and the level of dietary calcium at which hypercalciuria ensued.

A positive correlation exists between urinary calcium excretion and sodium excretion (255). Another study found that a group of hypercalciuric subjects on a 200-mEq sodium diet converted to normocalciuria on an 80-mEq sodium diet (208). The sensitive relationship between urinary calcium and sodium and the normal day-to-day variation of sodium intake may confound the results of standard 24-hour urine collections.

It is not known if absorptive hypercalciuria is caused by a primary intestinal defect or by a more complex metabolic disorder. Several investigators have found elevated vitamin D metabolites in one-third to one-half of patients with absorptive hypercalciuria (298). Some patients with absorptive hypercalciuria have low serum phosphorus levels. The stimulation of 1,25-dihydroxyvitamin D synthesis in the kidney by hypophosphatemia could lead to increased intestinal calcium absorption (115); the primary event would be a "renal leak" of phosphate. However, other investigators do not think that vitamin D and its metabolites play a critical role in the pathogenesis of absorptive hypercalciuria (215,222).

Two sources exist for calcium that appears in urine: GI absorption and bone resorption (172). Augmentation of intestinal absorption of dietary calcium is responsible for most of the increase in urinary calcium. Increased bone resorption is an unlikely primary source because the magnitude and duration of the hypercalciuria would lead to overt bone disease. Nevertheless, calcium balances are slightly but significantly negative in patients with idiopathic hypercalciuria. The existence of a generalized disorder of calcium homeostasis is further supported by an elevation of urinary hydroxyproline excretion that is seen in some patients. This reflects bone resorption. Lumbar bone density is significantly lower in patients with absorptive or fasting hypercalciuria compared with normocalciuric stone-formers (246). Bone loss in these patients also may be related to environmental factors such as intake of sodium or animal protein.

A familial basis of some types of hypercalciuria is supported by a high frequency of calcium stone disease and hypercalciuria in first-degree relatives of stone-formers (89). Most family studies of idiopathic hypercalciuria are broadly consistent with an autosomal-dominant mode of inheritance. However, the complexity and high variability of the inheritance patterns suggest that idiopathic hypercalciuria is a polygenic trait and involves alleles at several loci.

A smaller group of patients with hypercalciuria may have impaired renal tubular reabsorption of calcium (53,222). Fasting urinary calcium excretion is elevated, the serum concentration of calcium is reduced, and parathyroid function is stimulated. The elevated PTH level tends to restore serum calcium to normal levels by mobilizing bone calcium and enhancing intestinal absorption. Renal hypercalciuria and absorptive hypercalciuria are differentiated by measuring PTH levels and fasting urinary calcium excretion. PTH levels should be elevated in renal hypercalciuria but normal in absorptive hypercalciuria. Fasting urinary calcium excretion should be high in renal hypercalciuria but normal in absorptive hypercalciuria.

Early studies found renal hypercalciuria in more than 50% of patients with hypercalciuria, but this proportion decreased to 10% with later studies. This discrepancy may have been the result of differences in the specific immunoassays used to measure PTH. More intensive fasting tends to reduce the proportion of patients with renal hypercalciuria. Renal and absorptive hypercalciuria may represent extremes of a variable disorder rather than distinct clinical entities. A uniform elevation of intestinal calcium reabsorption may better explain the data than separate absorptive and renal forms of hypercalciuria (54).

Many studies have examined calcium metabolism in nephrolithiasis, but relatively few have investigated the role of oxalate in ICU. The paucity of such studies is related to the difficult nature of oxalate measurement in urine. Several investigators have found a mild but definite increase in urinary oxalate excretion in a subset of patients with ICU (12,265). A mildly elevated urinary oxalate is a greater risk factor for the precipitation of calcium oxalate than is a mildly elevated urinary calcium, because normal urinary oxalate levels are tenfold lower than normal urinary calcium levels. A small increase in urinary oxalate leads to the precipitation of a greater volume of crystals than does a comparable increase in urinary calcium.

Patients with mild hyperoxaluria do not appear to have a specific disturbance of glyoxylate metabolism. The hyperoxaluria is thought to be secondary to intestinal hyperabsorption of oxalate and calcium (186). The mechanism is analogous to that for enteric hyperoxaluria, but intraluminal intestinal calcium is reduced by hyperabsorption, not by complexation with fatty acids. Less calcium is available to bind oxalate, thereby permitting more avid absorption of free oxalate. A similar situation may occur when patients with recurrent calcium lithiasis are instructed to limit their dietary intake of foods that contain calcium. Isolated dietary calcium restriction may increase the risk of stone formation by allowing oxalate excretion to increase without a commensurate decrease in calcium excretion (17).

Intestinal hyperabsorption of oxalate may not be solely secondary to calcium hyperabsorption and reduced complexation. A more widespread defect in cellular transport of oxalate may exist. Transport of oxalate across red blood cell membranes differs in healthy persons and patients with recurrent calcium oxalate nephrolithiasis (13,14,103). The mean transmembrane oxalate flux rate in stone-forming patients was triple that in healthy control subjects. This meant that oxalate could cross the red blood cell membrane faster in patients with ICU. A similar situation in the luminal membrane of the GI tract could provide another mechanism for oxalate hyperabsorption.

Some patients with ICU have a concurrent disorder of uric acid metabolism. These patients tend to have a more severe form of stone disease, manifested by more frequent stone formation and a greater need for surgical intervention (52). Specific epitaxial overgrowth of calcium oxalate on uric acid or monosodium urate has been suggested as a possible explanation, but it is doubtful that this occurs in the urinary tract. Heterogeneous nucleation could occur, but freshly voided urine specimens from patients with ICU rarely contain uric acid or urate crystals (359). The binding of macromolecular inhibitors by another form of urate (colloidal) was proposed and has been supported by some studies (281). The reduction of hyperuricosuria with allopurinol also increased calcium oxalate–crystal growth inhibition (226), and hyperuricosuric calcium oxalate nephrolithiasis has been treated successfully with alkalizing agents (235).

A quantitative or qualitative disorder of crystal growth inhibition has been proposed as a possible reason for stone formation in patients with ICU. As discussed in the section on clinical stone formation, citrate is a complexor of calcium and a weak inhibitor of calcium oxalate crystal growth. Some investigators have found a subgroup of patients with ICU who have low urinary citrate levels (194,277). Hypocitnaturia in patients with distal RTA may enhance stone growth. Although the most beneficial action of citrate is through complexation of calcium, its weak inhibitory effects would help prevent further stone formation. Pharmacologic citrate preparations, through their alkalizing property, have successfully prevented further stone formation in patients with hypocitraturic calcium lithiasis (236).

Persistently alkaline urine has been found in another subset of patients with ICU but no clearly identifiable acid–base disorder (273). Careful analysis of stone material formed by patients with ICU reveals the presence of calcium phosphate, albeit in small amounts, in most of the stones. Because calcium phosphate preferentially precipitates at an alkaline pH, small calcium phosphate crystals may provide heterogeneous nuclei for the overgrowth of calcium oxalate. This mechanism may become more important as alkalizing agents are more commonly used to treat patients with ICU.

Patients with incomplete RTA are not systemically acidotic, but they have an impaired ability to acidify their urine after an ammonium chloride load. This implies the presence of a renal tubular defect in hydrogen ion secretion. The hypocitruria found in some patients with ICU may be the result of a subtle intracellular acidosis.

Defective tubular reabsorption of calcium is thought to be the cause of renal hypercalciuria. All of these disorders may be different manifestations of a more widespread tubular dysfunction. Evidence for this was provided by a study of the effects of hydrochlorothiazide and acetazolamide on the urinary excretions of calcium, sodium, and magnesium (334). These diuretic agents were chosen for their known actions at different sites in the nephron. Hydrochlorothiazide augmented sodium, calcium, and magnesium excretion to a greater extent in patients with ICU than in control subjects. With acetazolamide, the increase in sodium excretion was less in the patients than in the control subjects. The abnormal responses to both diuretics were most significant in patients with hypercalciuria during fasting. Such studies implicate a disorder of renal tubular transport as the primary abnormality in ICU. GI hyperabsorption of calcium would be a secondary phenomenon.

EVALUATION

The goal of a metabolic evaluation is to identify any physiologic or environmental factors that could be responsible for or exacerbate clinically active stone formation. No single approach is universally accepted, but it is possible to provide the general principles of a practical and efficient evaluation. The specifics of three different approaches were presented at a recent National Institutes of Health Consensus Development Conference on Prevention and Treatment of Kidney Stones (247,369,376).

History

The clinical history may help determine the cause of stone formation. The important elements in the history are outlined in Table 8.4. Inherited disorders, such as primary hyperoxaluria, cystinuria, and RTA, are clearly associated with urolithiasis, but even ICU tends to occur within families. Idiopathic stone formation and uric acid lithiasis are more common in males, whereas primary hyperparathyroidism and RTA are more common in females. Although ICU is the most common type of stone disease in children and adults, the classic inherited disorders associated with stone formation are more common in children than in adults.

Residence in a geographic area with a high incidence of stone disease, such as the southeastern United States, may have some epidemiologic importance, but temporary residence in an arid climate may be more pertinent. People who are not acclimated to these conditions may have a low urine-output state as a result of large fluid losses from perspiration and respiration. Long-distance runners may have the same problem. Evidence suggests that stone formation may be more common in marathon runners than in the general population (201). Urine volume tends to be low in patients who must perform manual labor in a hot environment. Easy access to fluids and bathroom facilities may not be possible with some occupations. A low urine-output state is a byproduct of many occupations.

TABLE 8.4. CLINICAL HISTORY

Age at onset	Diet
Sex	Medications
Family history	Previous stone passage
Geographic residence	Interventional procedures
Occupation	Previous stone composition
Fluid intake	Urinary tract infections

Excess dietary intake of calcium, oxalate, or protein and a low fluid intake may encourage the formation of stones. Stone formation also is associated with certain medications: vitamin D, absorbable alkali (calcium carbonate), and carbonic anhydrase inhibitors (acetazolamide). Patients need not consistently overindulge to form a stone. Brief periods of dietary indiscretion or poor fluid intake may initiate crystallization. A similar consideration applies to medications, particularly those associated with a nutritional fad.

A patient's past experience with stone formation and passage may provide clues about the cause of the stone disease and the patient's motivation to pursue a lifelong treatment program. A history of multiple stone passages and rapid recurrent stone formation may indicate a fundamental metabolic cause such as primary hyperparathyroidism or RTA. The necessity for multiple interventional procedures implies the growth of larger stones. Struvite lithiasis should be suspected if the patient has a history of infection with urease-producing bacterial organisms. The composition of previously analyzed stones should be sought. If old stones have not been analyzed, they should be examined and sent for formal analysis. It often is possible to determine a stone's composition just by looking at it. Cystine and uric acid stones are good examples.

Physical Examination

Recognizable physical abnormalities may be present in a few disorders associated with urolithiasis (Table 8.2): sarcoidosis, Cushing's syndrome, hyperthyroidism, and gout. Patients with neurogenic bladder dysfunction may be at risk for recurrent urinary tract infections and infected stone formation. Calcium stones may form in a recently immobilized patient. Extensive abdominal scarring is seen in some patients with small bowel disorders and should raise the possibility of enteric hyperoxaluria. Most patients do not have physical findings related to their stone disease, and laboratory studies are required to uncover the cause.

Laboratory Evaluation

The extent of the laboratory evaluation of a particular patient depends on the severity of the stone disease. A 40-year-old man who has passed several dozen calculi over the past 10 years needs a more extensive metabolic evaluation than a 60-year-old woman who has a 1-cm asymptomatic renal pelvic stone but no previous history of stone disease. Patients who have formed a single calcium stone have the same range of metabolic abnormalities as do patients with recurrent stone formation (224,328). Hypercalciuria was present in 50% to 75% of patients; approximately 5% had primary hyperparathyroidism, and 20% to 30% had no identifiable metabolic disorder. The patients with single stones were older when they passed their stones, had a higher incidence of urinary tract infection, and were more likely to have had surgical or endoscopic intervention. These authors recommended that single-stone-formers have the same evaluation and be treated no differently from other patients with stone disease.

TABLE 8.5. LABORATORY EVALUATION

Serum	Urine chemistry (24-hr volume)
Calcium	Calcium
Phosphorus	Phosphorus
Uric acid	Uric acid
Creatinine	Oxalate
Alkaline phosphatase	Cystine
Urine	Citrate
Urinalysis	Sodium
Culture	Magnesium
Fasting pH	Stone analysis
24-hr volume	

Patients who have formed a single stone may be willing to modify their diet and increase their intake of fluids, but are unwilling to take a medication for several years. The benefit of an extensive metabolic evaluation in such a patient is not readily apparent. A utilitarian evaluation of a single-stone-former would include an assessment of calcium metabolism and renal function (usually obtained as a multichannel chemical analysis of serum), a urinalysis and culture, and a stone analysis. These studies should detect obvious hyperparathyroidism, infected stone formation, and most of the disorders for which specific therapy is especially beneficial (e.g., uric acid lithiasis and cystinuria). A more extensive evaluation usually is reserved for those patients who prove to have metabolically active stone disease.

A complete metabolic workup should include the studies listed in Table 8.5. An isolated elevated serum calcium level should be confirmed on two or three separate occasions. The normal range varies among laboratories, but one should be suspicious of a serum calcium level greater than 10.1 mg/dL. Total serum calcium includes ultrafilterable calcium and protein-bound calcium. Ultrafilterable calcium, that which enters the glomerular filtrate, is composed of ionized calcium and a small amount of complexed calcium. Approximately half of total serum calcium is protein bound, primarily to albumin. The critical fraction that is controlled by the homeostatic mechanisms of the body is ionized calcium, but it is difficult to measure reliably ionized calcium. Total serum calcium usually is measured and corrected for serum albumin.

Serum phosphorus varies with age, sex, renal function, and diet, but may be low in patients with primary hyperparathyroidism and some patients with ICU. Serum alkaline phosphatase activity may be elevated in patients with hyperparathyroidism. Elevated serum uric acid levels are found in some patients with uric acid lithiasis, but calcium stone-formers also may have hyperuricemia. A serum bicarbonate measurement usually is included in a multichannel analysis and may be decreased in patients with RTA or with small bowel disorders associated with malabsorption.

A urinalysis should be performed promptly after collection. The pH is best measured in a morning urine specimen after an overnight fast. A pH less than 5.5 eliminates distal RTA. A short urinary acidification test can be performed if the pH is not less than 5.5. Uric acid stone-formers may have a persistently low pH. A high urine pH (more than 8.0) is found if the urine is infected with a urease-producing bacterial organism. The infection must be eliminated to accurately assess the pH. Ingestion of alkali or citrate preparations also raises the pH.

Red blood cells and white blood cells usually are seen with urolithiasis, and bacteria may be visible if an infection is present. A urine culture will confirm the presence of an infection, but some patients with struvite stone formation will have negative bladder urine and even renal pelvic urine cultures. Bipyramidal-shaped calcium oxalate dihydrate crystals can be found in healthy persons. Multiple small, platelike or dumbbell-shaped calcium oxalate monohydrate crystals often are found in patients with hyperoxaluria, usually the primary disorder. Calcium oxalate monohydrate crystals are birefringent and will appear as bright specks with polarized microscopy. The presence of hexagonal cystine crystals is virtually diagnostic of cystinuria. A 24-hour urine collection is the traditional mainstay of a metabolic stone evaluation. The most important and often most neglected measurement is the volume. Many patients with recurrent calcium stone formation have a 24-hour urine volume that is approximately 1 L. The basic principles of the medical treatment of urolithiasis are dietary moderation and a consistently high urine volume. Patients can easily monitor their progress by measuring their 24-hour urine volume at home.

Urinary excretion of calcium, phosphorus, oxalate, and uric acid is a function of dietary intake. Increased urinary oxalate is found in patients with primary or secondary hyperoxaluria. Dietary oxalate content has its greatest impact in patients with enteric hyperoxaluria. Uric acid excretion may be elevated in uric acid or calcium oxalate stone-forming patients. Urinary calcium excretion has received much attention. Elaborate protocols have been devised to differentiate the renal and absorptive hypercalciurias and the various types of absorptive hypercalciuria (231). The goal has been to institute specific pharmacologic therapy, but these calcium tolerance tests have achieved limited clinical utility (170).

Urinary cystine excretion can be screened with the traditional cyanide-nitroprusside reaction or newer spot tests (107). A positive reaction should be followed by a quantitative amino acid analysis. Urinary citrate excretion is decreased in patients with distal RTA and intestinal malabsorption. Citrate is low in the presence of a urinary tract infection because bacteria metabolize citrate. Urinary magnesium excretion is of some interest to investigators but is not clinically useful. Urinary sodium excretion may be elevated in some patients with hypercalciuria.

Computer programs have been written to calculate urinary saturations for the major stone-forming salts (94,262) and are available commercially (237). These programs are useful in research, but their widespread clinical utility has not been demonstrated. Examination of the 24-hour urine volume and the total excretions of the major ions should provide enough information to make sound clinical decisions.

Stone material that has been passed or removed should be analyzed. Many different crystalline components have been identified in urinary calculi (Table 8.6), and several methods have been used to identify accurately these constituents (333). The composition of some calculi, such as cystine, can be identified with simple macroscopic or microscopic analysis. Whole stones covered with calcium oxalate dihydrate crystals have a burr or "hair-on-end" appearance. If the whole stone is available, an attempt should be made to separate the nucleus from the rest of the stone because the composition of the nucleus may differ from that of the outer layers. Optical properties (i.e., crystal system, optical sign, refractive index, angle of extinction, and birefringence) can be measured with polarization microscopy (251). The limited number of crystalline components in urinary calculi can be identified from these optical properties. X-ray powder diffraction has been the standard method for stone analysis because it enables almost absolute identification of crystalline materials and mixtures of these materials (206). The equipment is expensive, and the procedure is time-consuming.

Infrared spectroscopy is becoming the most widely used method of stone analysis (20,133,363). Finely powdered stone material is pressed into a transparent tablet with optically pure potassium bromide. The infrared spectrum is recorded and compared with a library of standard spectra. Infrared spectroscopy is rapid and relatively inexpensive, and it permits the identification of noncrystalline components and artifacts. This method is especially useful for identifying drugs and their metabolites. Other methods of stone analysis such as thermogravimetric technique (275), scanning electron microscopy with energy dispersive x-ray analysis (150), and CT (136) have been proposed, but they appear to have limited applicability.

Activity

The propensity to form stones varies from patient to patient as well as in a particular patient over time. An arbitrary method for assessing activity was developed at the Mayo Clinic (315). The concept of stone activity enables one to evaluate the need for long-term pharmacologic therapy and the response to such therapy. Two basic categories of activity are defined: surgical and metabolic. A patient with

TABLE 8.6. CRYSTALLINE CONSTITUENTS OF HUMAN URINARY CALCULI

Substance	Mineralogic Name	Formula
Calcium oxalate monohydrate	Whewellite	$CaC_2O_4 \cdot H_2O$
Calcium oxalate dihydrate	Weddellite	$CaC_2O_4 \cdot 2H_2O$ (to $2.5H_2O$)
Magnesium hydrogen phosphate trihydrate	Newberyite	$MgHPO_4 \cdot 3H_2O$
Magnesium ammonium phosphate hexahydrate	Struvite	$MgNH_4PO_4 \cdot 6H_2O$
Hydroxyapatite	Hydroxyapatite	$Ca_{10}(PO_4)_6(OH)_2$
Carbonate-apatite	Carbonate-apatite	$Ca_{10}(PO_4)_{6-x}(OH)_{2-y}(CO_3)_{x+y}$
Calcium hydrogen phosphate dihydrate	Brushite	$CaHPO_4 \cdot 2H_2O$
Tricalcium phosphate	Whitlockite	β-$Ca_3(PO_4)_2$
Octacalcium phosphate		$Ca_4H(PO_4)_3 \cdot 2.5H_2O$
Uric acid		$C_5H_4N_4O_3$
Uric acid dihydrate		$C_5H_4N_4O_3 \cdot 2H_2O$
Ammonium acid urate		$C_5H_3N_4O_3NH_4$
Sodium acid urate monohydrate		$C_5H_3N_4O_3Na \cdot H_2O$
Cystine		$[-SCH_2CHNH_2COOH]_2$
Xanthine		$C_5H_4N_4O_2$
Calcium sulphate dihydrate	Gypsum	$CaSO_4 \cdot 2H_2O$

Modified from Sutor DJ, Scheidt S. Identification standards for human urinary calculus components, using crystallographic methods. *Br J Urol* 1968;40:22, with permission.

renal colic, obstruction, or infection associated with a stone has surgically active urolithiasis.

Metabolic activity refers to the precipitation of stone material. Urolithiasis is metabolically active in patients who have had growth of old stones, formation of new stones, or the passage of gravel within the past year. These criteria must be documented radiographically. If a patient's stone disease meets none of these criteria, the urolithiasis is metabolically inactive. If previous radiographs are unavailable or of poor quality, the metabolic activity is said to be indeterminate. Such patients are instructed to increase their fluid intake and avoid dietary excesses. They receive follow-up until the metabolic activity can be determined.

The distinction between surgical and metabolic activity is important because a symptomatic stone may have formed several years before. No specific medical treatment may be needed after the immediate surgical problem is resolved. Metabolically active urolithiasis may exist without symptoms. No surgical intervention may be needed, but specific medical therapy may be required to prevent further stone formation.

One of the goals of urolithiasis research has been the development of a method to predict stone activity when a patient is first evaluated (123). Several measures have been proposed, including the previously discussed saturation-inhibition index, but none has had greater utility than this simple, time-dependent method of assessing activity. Recurrent stone formation is common, but it cannot be predicted from standard laboratory evaluations in individual patients (178).

Radiographic Evaluation

The assessment of metabolic activity depends on the availability of high-quality radiographs. Tomographic views provide more detail than standard radiographs because the overshadowing effects of bowel gas and intestinal contents are lessened. Spiral CT scans have virtually replaced intravenous pyelography in the evaluation of patients with ureteral calculi (64,352). Renal calculi can be seen easily on such studies, but plain or tomographic radiographs usually are easier to use for longitudinal follow-up. Relatively radiolucent stones such as uric acid or cystine are best monitored with ultrasonography or CT scanning.

The radiographic appearance of a stone depends on the composition of the stone, its thickness and orientation, surrounding tissues or bowel contents, and radiographic technique. A stone may rotate and give the illusion of a change in size. This rotation cannot be prevented, but its possible occurrence should be remembered when radiographs are examined. All stones, except uric acid, are clinically radiopaque. Even large uric acid stones appear faintly radiopaque from incorporated impurities. Small cystine and struvite stones may be difficult to see on plain radiographs. Relative radiodensities of the common stone salts have been measured and, in decreasing order, are apatite, whitlockite, brushite, whewellite, weddellite, cystine, struvite, and uric acid (276).

MEDICAL MANAGEMENT

With few exceptions (dissolution of uric acid and cystine stones), the goal of medical treatment is to prevent the formation of new stones or the further growth of old stones. This prophylaxis must be effective and continuous. Patients must understand that prevention of further stone formation probably will require lifetime treatment.

The therapy of urolithiasis is based on two principles: a reduction of urinary SS, and an increase in net inhibitory activity. The latter can be achieved by increasing the quantity of inhibitors, by increasing the potency of inhibitors, or by corresponding decreases in promoter activity.

The purpose of a high fluid intake is to lower urinary SS. The dilution reduces ionic strength, complexation, and the concentration of inhibitors, but these side effects are more than offset by the reduction of SS. It is impossible for stone formation to occur in urine that is undersaturated for the particular stone salt. All patients with renal calculi should be counseled to increase their fluid intake. An 8-ounce glass of fluid should be consumed hourly while awake, and 8 to 16 ounces of fluid should be consumed if the patient is up at night. Approximately half of the fluid should be water. The patient should produce at least 2,500 mL of urine per 24 hours. The fluid intake should be consistent. A liberal intake of fluids during the day but poor intake during the night does not uniformly lower SS, especially after a heavy evening meal. Patients can use a container of known volume to inexpensively monitor their 24-hour urine output. A fixed numeric goal is helpful because most patients are poor estimators of their fluid intake and urine output.

A dietary history should be taken and dietary excesses eliminated (238). The traditional recommendation has been a low-calcium diet, but this may increase urinary oxalate excretion. Urinary SS can be lowered with a low-calcium, low-oxalate diet, but patients are less likely to adhere to a more complex program. The same criticism applies to a low-carbohydrate diet, a high-fiber diet, and a low–animal protein diet, although the last may be useful in the treatment of idiopathic uric acid lithiasis. Because dietary therapy requires long-term patient compliance, the encouragement of dietary moderation may be the best advice (135).

Fluid and dietary therapy should be used in all patients with urolithiasis and should be the only initial therapy in patients with ICU. One hundred eight patients with ICU of indeterminate metabolic activity were treated initially with fluid and dietary therapy at the Mayo Clinic (139). No stone growth or new stone formation was seen in 58% of these patients during a mean follow-up period of more than 5 years. Of those patients with hypercalciuria alone, 70% proved to have metabolically inactive stone disease. The existence of metabolically active stone formation should be proved before a patient is committed to lifelong pharmacologic therapy (314).

Renal Tubular Acidosis

The metabolic abnormalities of patients with distal RTA are corrected with replacement of sodium, potassium, and bicarbonate. Daily, 90 to 150 mEq of base usually is required and may be given as sodium bicarbonate or citrate (Bicitra, Polycitra, or Urocit-K). Total body potassium levels are low in untreated patients, and the serum potassium level may decrease as the acidosis is corrected. Potassium should be replaced while monitoring serum levels. Urinary calcium excretion decreases, and urinary citrate increases to a normal level with correction of the systemic acidosis.

Sodium bicarbonate, sodium citrate, potassium bicarbonate, and potassium citrate are equally effective in increasing urinary citrate (30). The advantage of citrate is that it produces a more even and longer-lasting effect on renal citrate excretion than bicarbonate. The advantage of potassium citrate over sodium citrate is that a long-term reduction of urinary calcium is seen with the former but not the latter (249,250).

Cystinuria

The goal of therapy is to reduce the urinary SS of cystine (130). Urine volume over 24 hours should be maintained at 3 to 4 L. The solubility of cystine in normal urine is approximately 300 mg/L but increases as the pH increases (Fig. 8.4). If the 24-hour urinary cystine excretion of a patient is known, the information in Fig. 8.4 can be used to calculate the urine volume and pH required to solubilize adequately all of the cystine. The pH usually must be increased to 7.5 to 7.8. This degree of alkalinization may be difficult to maintain and can promote the coprecipitation of calcium phosphate.

A carbonic anhydrase inhibitor such as acetazolamide can be used to maintain urinary alkalinity throughout the night, but these agents probably should be avoided because they induce changes in urinary composition that favor the precipitation of calcium phosphate. If a cystine stone becomes covered with a layer of calcium phosphate, further attempts at dissolution will be fruitless.

Cystine is two cysteine molecules linked by a disulfide bond (Fig. 8.3). The drug D-penicillamine (Cuprimine) reacts with cystine to form penicillamine-cysteine, a mixed disulfide that is more soluble than cystine in urine. The dose of D-penicillamine is 250 to 500 mg four times daily. It is given 30 minutes before meals and at bedtime. D-penicillamine is a potentially toxic drug that should be used for attempted stone dissolution or in patients whose disease cannot be controlled with hydration and alkalization. Adverse reactions include skin rashes, fever, arthralgias, and lymphadenopathy. A potential pyridoxine deficiency can be avoided with prophylactic pyridoxine (50 mg twice daily) therapy. Stone dissolution may require several months to 1 or 2 years.

Urinary cystine excretion also can be lowered by limiting dietary methionine. This therapy severely limits protein intake and is rarely, if ever, used.

α-Mercaptopropionyglycine (α-MPG, or Thiola) shares chemical properties with D-penicillamine but appears to have fewer adverse effects (230). A multicenter study of 66 patients with cystinuria found that the effectiveness of α-MPG in reducing cystine excretion was equal to that of D-penicillamine. A mean dose of 1,193 mg of α-MPG per day maintained daily cystine excretion at 350 to 560 mg. In 59 patients who had taken both drugs, adverse reactions forced 31% to stop taking α-MPG and 60% to stop taking D-penicillamine.

Captopril, an angiotensin-converting enzyme inhibitor, contains a sulfhydryl group that can participate in a thiol exchange reaction to form captopril-cysteine that has a 200-fold greater solubility than cystine (313). Captopril further lowers urinary cystine excretion by a mechanism other than thiol exchange. Captopril may be a useful drug for the treatment of cystinuria (245,329), but a sufficient dose may cause orthostatic hypotension. Other physicians question the clinical utility of captopril (59).

Other metabolic disturbances may occur in patients with cystinuria. A comprehensive metabolic evaluation of 27 patients with homozygous cystinuria revealed that 19% had hypercalciuria and 22% had hyperuricosuria (286). Hypocitruria was found in 44%. Recurrent stones in cystinuric patients may be composed of calcium or uric acid, not cystine. It is important to remember that multiple metabolic abnormalities may exist in a single patient.

Hypercalcemic Disorders

The primary cause of hypercalcemia determines the therapy. If surgical treatment of a stone is contemplated in a patient with primary hyperparathyroidism, a parathyroidectomy should be the first procedure, although concomitant parathyroidectomy and ESWL, ureteroscopic stone removal, or percutaneous stone removal have been performed safely (349). Patients should have careful follow-up after parathyroidectomy to ensure that the hypercalcemia has been corrected and stone formation has ceased. Persistent stone growth may be caused by another disorder.

An adequate intake of fluids should be encouraged in all immobilized patients. Oral orthophosphates decrease urinary calcium excretion in immobilized patients and may be used if fluid therapy is unsuccessful (112). Corticosteroids should reduce the hypercalciuria in patients with sarcoidosis.

Uric Acid Lithiasis

The medical treatment of uric acid lithiasis is satisfying because uric acid stones can be dissolved. Fluid intake should be increased to achieve a 24-hour urine output of 3 L. The solubility of uric acid can be increased 10-fold by raising the urine pH to 6.5 (Fig. 8.6). A sodium bicarbonate or citrate preparation can be used to accomplish this (130). A daily dose of 300 mg of allopurinol, a xanthine oxidase inhibitor (Figs. 8.5 and 8.8), reduces the amount of uric acid excreted in the urine.

When all three elements of this program are used, most uric acid stones can be dissolved within 3 months. The allopurinol can be stopped after the stones are dissolved. New stone formation usually can be prevented by maintaining an alkaline urine. Overexuberant alkalization may precipitate a layer of calcium phosphate over the stone. Dissolution then becomes impossible. Use of carbonic anhydrase inhibitors should be avoided for the same reason.

Xanthinuria

Patients who form xanthine calculi while taking allopurinol should discontinue the drug. Patients with xanthinuria secondary to an inherited deficiency of xanthine oxidase should maintain a high urine volume and restrict their dietary intake of foods that contain purine. Because the pKa of the first dissociable proton of xanthine is 7.7, the solubility of xanthine cannot be increased significantly by physiologic alkalization.

2,8-Dihydroxyadeninuria

Xanthine oxidase is responsible for the oxidation of adenine to 2,8-DHA (40,102,106). Treatment consists of fluids and allopurinol without urinary alkalization. The solubility of 2,8-DHA is not affected by urinary pH. Dietary adenine may contribute to stone formation and should be reduced. Lentils and other grains have a high adenine content (50).

Primary Hyperoxaluria

Large doses of pyridoxine (50 mg four times daily) reduce oxalate excretion in 20% to 50% of patients (109). Neutral orthophosphate (1.5 to 2.0 g per 24 hours of elemental phosphorus in four divided doses) may halt the growth of existing stones and prevent the formation of new stones (318). Sodium citrate increases urinary citrate excretion, reduces calcium oxalate saturation, and reduces stone formation in patients with primary hyperoxaluria (173).

Renal transplantation has been attempted in patients with primary hyperoxaluria and renal failure, but oxalate mobilization from preexistent oxalosis may lead to deposition of oxalate in the transplanted kidney (71). Transplantation should be performed soon after the onset of renal failure, because oxalate is not removed efficiently by hemodialysis (73,185).

Hepatic or combined hepatic-renal transplantation has been performed for the treatment of primary hyperoxaluria (190,357). This aggressive approach corrects the enzymatic defect. Urinary oxalate and glycolate return to normal levels, and extrarenal deposits of oxalate are mobilized.

Enteric Hyperoxaluria

Dietary intake of oxalate and fat should be restricted. An additional advantage of a low-fat (50 g) diet is that bothersome steatorrhea is reduced. Dietary calcium supplementation has been used to increase precipitation of calcium oxalate within the GI lumen (324), but this may increase urinary calcium. Stone disease usually can be controlled without resorting to calcium supplementation. Cholestyramine (12 g daily in three or four divided doses) binds acidic compounds, including oxalate, in the colonic lumen. Oxalate absorption decreases, steatorrhea decreases, and water absorption and urine volume may increase. Intestinal bicarbonate loss reduces urinary pH and citrate excretion. Some patients may even have a mild metabolic acidosis. These abnormalities can be corrected with base replacement. If metabolically active stone formation persists in patients with an ileal bypass, the normal anatomy of the GI tract should be restored (80).

Infection Stones

Surgical removal of a struvite stone generally is necessary to preserve renal function and reduce long-term morbidity and potential mortality (256). Urine cultures should be obtained and specific bactericidal therapy should be started 48 hours before surgery. All infected stone material should be removed. Antibiotic treatment should be continued for 10 to 14 days after surgery. Postoperative irrigation of the collecting system with hemiacidrin has been advocated to dissolve any minute retained stone fragments (5,214).

The patients should be maintained on antibacterial prophylaxis for 3 to 12 months. Adjunctive urinary acidification with ammonium chloride (2 g per day) has been used in conjunction with long-term antimicrobial therapy (379). Small retained fragments may dissolve with this regimen. The proper antibacterial agents suppress bacterial growth, and because of the decrease in urease production, urinary acidification can be achieved with ammonium chloride. Ammonium chloride (1.5 to 3 g per day) is a more effective urinary acidifier than either methenamine hippurate (2 g per day) or ascorbic acid (1.8 g per day) (355).

Acetohydroxamic acid, a urease inhibitor, may prevent the further growth of struvite stones and rarely may lead to dissolution of the stone material (368). Up to 50% of patients may experience side effects from the drug, including tremulousness, headache, or deep vein thrombosis.

The Shorr regimen combines a low-phosphorus diet with aluminum hydroxide capsules to achieve selective dietary phosphorus depletion (168). A few uncontrolled studies suggest that the Shorr regimen is an effective therapy for struvite urolithiasis, but the diet is difficult to follow. Low-phosphorus diets also increase urinary calcium excretion and promote crystalluria (362).

Most investigators report recurrent stone growth in 25% to 30% of patients (116). If recurrent metabolic stone formation is excluded, recurrent struvite stone formation occurs in 10% to 15% of patients. The lowest reported recurrence rate was only 2% (307).

Idiopathic Calcium Urolithiasis

Patients who consume adequate amounts of fluid and in whom dietary excesses have been eliminated may continue to have metabolically active stone formation. Several effective treatment programs are available.

Thiazide Diuretics

Thiazide diuretics are particularly effective when significant hypercalciuria is present. Hydrochlorothiazide 50 mg twice daily or trichlormethiazide 2 mg twice daily will reduce urinary calcium excretion, crystalluria, and urinary SS for calcium oxalate and calcium phosphate (374). The mechanism of action is thought to be stimulation of renal tubular calcium reabsorption, possibly by extracellular volume contraction (165). A high-sodium diet can blunt or prevent the hypocalciuric effect of thiazides. Moderate sodium restriction may be needed to reduce urinary calcium excretion. Up to 90% of patients who are treated with thiazides cease further stone formation.

Thiazides also may prevent stone formation in normocalciuric persons. This is a controversial finding, but may be related to a reported reduction in oxalate excretion after long-term thiazide therapy (58,375). Another study found that hydrochlorothizide did not reduce oxalate excretion, at least in patients with renal leak hypercalciuria (343). Side effects, including fatigue unrelated to the hypokalemia; hypomagnesemia; muscle weakness and cramping; decreased libido; impotence; and abnormalities in serum calcium, glucose, and uric acid, occur in up to 10% of patients.

There is some evidence that the treatment of all hypercalciuric patients with thiazide diuretics may be inappropriate (248). These investigators examined the effect of hydrochlorothiazide in 12 patients with absorptive hypercalciuria and in 10 patients with renal hypercalciuria. At short-term (3 to 6 months) follow-up, urinary calcium was significantly decreased in both groups. At long-term (30 to 120 months) follow-up, half of the patients with absorptive hypercalciuria were again hypercalciuric. The increased long-term stone formation seen in those patients with absorptive hypercalciuria was not statistically significant.

Yet another study found that chlorthalidone at a daily dose of 25 or 50 mg reduced the predicted rate of calculous events by 90% (87). This was a double-blind, randomized study that did not differentiate the mechanism of the hypercalciuria.

Orthophosphate

Orthophosphate has been the treatment of choice in patients with normocalciuria (314). It also may be effective in patients with hypercalciuria. Orthophosphate decreases urinary calcium excretion and increases inhibitor activity (371). Increased calcium complexation and decreased free calcium ion activity are a result of increased urinary phosphate, citrate, and pH. Calcium oxalate SS decreases, but the SS of hydroxyapatite or brushite does not change. Excretion of the inhibitors, pyrophosphate and citrate, increases, and the more alkaline pH increases the potency of pyrophosphate as a crystal growth inhibitor. Orthophosphate also may reduce 1,25-dihydroxyvitamin D synthesis (348).

Orthophosphate usually is given as the neutral or mildly alkaline salt. The total daily dose should provide 1.5 to 2.0 g of elemental phosphorus. Patients may lose previously formed stone material during the first 3 to 6 months of therapy. If radiographs document that stone mass is being lost and no new stone material is precipitating, patients should be reassured that the medication is preventing further stone growth and that the troublesome stones were formed before drug therapy was started. Calcium stone formation ceases in 90% of patients taking orthophosphate (339).

Diarrhea is the most common complication of orthophosphate therapy. The dose may be halved until the diarrhea subsides, and then gradually increased to a therapeutic level. Orthophosphates should not be used in the presence of secondary urolithiasis resulting from infection or obstruction or in the presence of renal failure (glomerular filtration rate, less than 30 mL per minute).

Cellulose Phosphate

The purpose of cellulose phosphate therapy, unlike orthophosphate therapy, is not to provide absorbable phosphate. Cellulose phosphate binds calcium in the intestinal lumen and decreases calcium absorption (227). Cellulose phosphate should be used only in patients with absorptive hypercalciuria, because it may result in a negative calcium balance in those patients with normal intestinal calcium absorption or renal hypercalciuria. The usual dose is 5 g two or three times daily.

When given alone, cellulose phosphate may be ineffective or even increase calcium oxalate crystalluria (10). Urinary oxalate excretion increases with cellulose phosphate therapy alone, probably because intestinal absorption increases. Less calcium is available to complex dietary oxalate in the intestinal lumen. Cellulose phosphate also binds magnesium and decreases urinary magnesium excretion. Supplementation of cellulose phosphate therapy with magnesium (1 to 1.5 g magnesium gluconate per day), a low-oxalate diet, and a high fluid intake will effectively halt stone formation in almost 80% of patients (223).

Magnesium

Magnesium oxide (193) and magnesium hydroxide (66) have been advocated for the treatment of ICU, but the effectiveness of this therapy has not been demonstrated systematically. [The same criticism may be applied to clinical trials of thiazides and orthophosphates (45).] Anticipated benefits of increased magnesium excretion are increased complexation of oxalate and phosphate and a slight increase in crystal growth inhibition. Some investigators have reported prevention of recurrent stone formation in 80% of treated patients. Approximately 1 g of magnesium oxide or 250 to 750 mg of magnesium hydroxide have been given in two or three divided daily doses.

Ettinger and colleagues (87) used a prospective, double-blind, randomized clinical trial to examine the effectiveness of chlorthalidone or magnesium hydroxide in the prevention of recurrent calcium oxalate stone formation. The duration of the study was 3 years. Compared with historic control subjects (pretreatment rates of stone formation), all of the treatments, including placebo, appeared to prevent recurrent stone formation. With appropriate controls, chlorthalidone was more effective than placebo or magnesium hydroxide. The placebo groups had 56% fewer stones than predicted; the low-dose magnesium hydroxide group had 62% fewer stones. Both low-dose and high-dose chlorthalidone reduced the predicted rate of new stone formation by 90%.

The pitfalls of clinical trials of thiazides have been reviewed by Churchill and Taylor (47). Without a control group, it is difficult to determine how much of a decrease in new stone formation is caused by regression to the mean and how much is a result of treatment.

Allopurinol

The use of allopurinol in patients with hyperuricosuric calcium urolithiasis has been controversial (96). Early reports were encouraging (55), but later reports were less optimistic (198). Two adverse effects of hyperuricosuria have been proposed: heterogeneous nucleation of calcium oxalate on urate crystals and binding of large-molecular-weight calcium oxalate–crystal growth inhibitors to colloidal urate (91). An allopurinol-induced reduction of urate excretion could preclude either mechanism. Allopurinol has even been reported to decrease urinary oxalate excretion (292). Allopurinol does not appear to have a direct effect on calcium oxalate precipitation. The most conservative approach may be to use allopurinol as a secondary drug in those patients who have abnormal uric acid metabolism. Tiselius and colleagues (340) concluded that empiric allopurinol is ineffective in the treatment of recurrent calcium oxalate stone disease in the absence of hyperuricosuria or hyperuricemia.

Between 10% and 20% of patients with idiopathic calcium urolithiasis have hyperuricosuria as an isolated metabolic abnormality. Ettinger and colleagues (88) found that allopurinol effectively prevented recurrent stone formation in this subset of patients. They recommended allopurinol instead of thiazides for patients with isolated hyperuricosuria, even though thiazides can be as effective. The risk of allergic reactions is increased with the simultaneous administration of thiazides and allopurinol.

Potassium Citrate

Potassium citrate has been used to treat patients with ICU and hypocitruria (228). The alkalizing effects of citrate increase urinary pH and urinary citrate excretion. Complexation of calcium with citrate increases, and ionized calcium and calcium oxalate SS decrease. Inhibition and calcium oxalate crystal growth increases slightly (increased citrate excretion and greater potency of pyrophosphate at a more alkaline urinary pH). In a study by Pak and Fuller, further stone formation ceased in almost 90% of ICU patients with hypocitruria. Citrate excretion increased to the normal range, whereas urinary pH was maintained at 6.5 to 7.0.

Several liquid preparations of citrate contain sodium. The effects of sodium citrate and potassium citrate on urine composition have been compared (284). Urinary pH and citrate excretion increased with both compounds, but calcium excretion decreased only with potassium citrate. The higher urinary pH increased brushite (calcium phosphate) saturation in both groups of patients, but a supersaturated condition was obtained only in those patients treated with sodium citrate. The failure to reduce urinary calcium excretion may have contributed to this latter effect.

In a trial by Pak and associates, long-term treatment with potassium citrate (20 mEq three times daily) reduced stone formation in 98% of patients, and stone formation ceased in 80% (236). Minor GI complaints were the most common side effects. No patients had melena or occult fecal blood. Although potassium citrate therapy of ICU is becoming more popular, not all investigators think that it is more beneficial than thiazides or even a placebo (242).

Pak and Fuller (228) studied 37 adults with a history of recurrent calcium oxalate stone formation. Seventeen had hypocitruria as an isolated abnormality, 18 had absorptive hypercalciuria, and 2 had hyperuricosuria. Potassium citrate (30 to 80 mEq per day) was administered to 25 patients. Twelve patients took thiazide, allopurinol, or both. Sustained increases in urinary citrate, potassium, and pH were seen with potassium citrate therapy. Only 4 patients continued to form stones, for a remission rate of 89%.

In spite of some early skepticism, studies continue to support the clinical effectiveness of potassium citrate (1,129). A randomized, double-blind study in patients with idiopathic hypocitraturic calcium nephrolithiasis found that, compared with a placebo, potassium citrate (30 to 60 mEq daily in wax matrix tablets) significantly reduced stone formation (16). This reduction in clinical stone formation was accompanied by increases in urinary citrate, pH, and potassium. Citrate has even been used to prevent the deposition of calcium oxalate on fragments that remain after ESWL (335).

Potassium citrate may be useful in patients who do not respond to thiazides (236). Thirteen patients had hypercalciuria that was corrected by thiazide treatment, but stones continued to form. The addition of potassium citrate to thiazide therapy prevented the development of hypokalemia and caused a sustained increase in urinary citrate and pH. Urinary calcium, oxalate, sodium, or volume did not change. Stone formation was reduced in all patients, and a complete remission occurred in 77%.

Citrus fruit juices are rich sources of potassium and citrate. The ingestion of these juices potentially represents an alternative to potassium citrate in the management of hypocitraturia calcium and uric acid nephrolithiasis. A study of eight healthy men and three men with hypocitraturic nephrolithiasis found that, compared with potassium citrate, orange juice delivered an equivalent alkali load and caused a similar increase in urinary pH (354). Orange juice increased urinary oxalate without altering calcium excretion, whereas potassium citrate decreased urinary calcium without altering urinary oxalate. Orange juice lacked the ability of potassium citrate to reduce calcium oxalate saturation. Nevertheless, orange juice should be beneficial in the treatment of calcium and uric acid lithiasis.

Other Agents

Some patients with ICU and mild hyperoxaluria have been treated with pharmacologic doses of pyridoxine (200 to 400 mg per day) (15). Oxalate excretion decreased by approximately one-third. The proposed mechanism is stimulation of pyridoxal-5-phosphate–dependent transaminases that are responsible for the conversion of glyoxalate to glycine (Fig. 8.10). Less glyoxalate would be available for conversion to oxalate. Pyridoxine also decreased urinary glycolate excretion and increased erythrocyte glutamic oxaloacetic transaminase activity. Individuals who consume large quantities of pyridoxine (2 to 6 g per day) may develop a sensory neuropathy (290).

Pentosan polysulfate is a structural analog of heparin but has little anticoagulant activity (282). Up to 4% of an oral dose is excreted in the urine. This agent was used initially to treat patients with interstitial cystitis (244). Pentosan polysulfate is also a potent inhibitor of calcium oxalate crystal growth (187). A 50% reduction in the rate of calcium oxalate crystal growth was achieved with a concentration of 2.4×10^{-9} M. A daily dose of 300 mg should provide a urinary concentration of 10 mg/L and increase inhibition by one-third. A recent clinical trial of this compound found no difference in the rate of stone formation before and during treatment, although patients who continued to form stones reported that they were smaller and more easily passed spontaneously (92).

Potassium-magnesium citrate is similar to potassium citrate, but the magnesium may lower urinary oxalate by binding oxalate in the intestinal tract (232). It also causes a greater rise in urinary citrate and pH. Consequently, it may be more effective than potassium citrate in inhibiting the crystallization of uric acid and calcium oxalate in urine.

BLADDER CALCULI

Bladder calculi commonly are found in children who live in lesser developed countries and in men with bladder outlet obstruction. Bladder stones usually are freely movable in the bladder, but may be fixed to a bladder wall suture placed during a previous surgical procedure. The usual symptoms of bladder outlet obstruction may be present: urinary hesitancy, frequency, and nocturia. Patients also may have hematuria, dysuria, suprapubic pain that often radiates to the tip of the penis, and an interrupted urinary stream.

The diagnosis of a bladder stone usually is confirmed by radiographic examination, ultrasonography, or cystoscopy. Because many bladder stones are composed of radiolucent uric acid, the absence of a radiopaque shadow on a plain abdominal radiograph does not exclude the presence of a stone.

PROSTATIC CALCULI

Most prostatic calculi are found in men aged 50 to 65 years. Prostatic calculi are formed by the deposition of calcium salts on corpora amylacea. Corpora amylacea are laminated organic structures that are thought to form around desquamated epithelial cells in prostatic alveoli. Prostatic calculi may be associated with prostatic hyperplasia or prostatitis or may be asymptomatic. They may be seen on a plain roentgenogram of the pelvis and frequently can be palpated by rectal examination. Asymptomatic prostatic calculi require no treatment, but they often are removed during a transurethral prostatectomy for benign prostatic hyperplasia.

URETHRAL CALCULI

Urethral stones may form in the urethra or may migrate from the bladder or upper urinary tract. Primary or native urethral calculi usually are associated with chronic stasis and infection. Virtually all urethral calculi in women have been found in a urethral diverticulum. Men with urethral stones often have urethral strictures, a history of prostatic surgery, or coexistent bladder stones. Calcium phosphate and calcium carbonate are the most common chemical constituents.

Primary urethral calculi may be asymptomatic because they grow slowly with the urethral lumen or a diverticulum. Migrant stones may become symptomatic when they drop into the prostatic urethra. Patients may have dysuria, a weak urinary stream, or retention. Two-thirds of urethral stones are found in the posterior urethra, and one-third are found in the anterior urethra.

Fewer than half of urethral stones are diagnosed radiographically. Retrograde urethrography can define urethral anatomy in men but usually does not reveal a urethral diverticulum in women. Cystourethroscopy confirms the diagnosis.

CHILDHOOD UROLITHIASIS

Bladder stone disease was common in children in 18th century Europe (274). Boys younger than 10 years of age typically were affected. The prevalence of pediatric bladder stone disease became less common as Europe became industrialized. The occurrence of bladder stones in children was virtually unknown in Norway by 1831 (287). The disappearance of this disease is probably related to the concurrent improvement in nutrition. The disease still exists in less well-developed nations in Asia and the Middle East.

Bladder stone disease has been studied extensively in Thailand (78,346). Boys younger than age 10 years usually are affected. The stones are composed of a mixture of calcium oxalate and ammonium acid urate. Concurrent renal lithiasis typically is not present. A low intake of breast milk and early rice supplementation provide a diet low in protein and minerals. Urinary excretion of phosphate, sulfate, sodium, potassium, and magnesium is low. Urinary excretion of oxalate, calcium, uric acid, and ammonia is high. The high oxalate excretion is thought to be caused by consumption of local vegetables and plant leaves that have a high oxalate content. The hot climate and low fluid intake also contribute to crystallization.

Of patients with urinary calculi, 2% to 3% are children (345). Bladder stone disease is now uncommon in Europe and the United States. Most children with urolithiasis present with renal or ureteral calculi. Most patients have stones composed of calcium oxalate, calcium phosphate, or mixtures of these stone salts (184,311). Most children with urolithiasis have bacteriuria that is secondary to stone formation, but most of these organisms do not produce urease. One study found struvite stone formation in one-third of the patients (184). All had a history of multiple urologic procedures, diversionary procedures, or indwelling drainage devices. *Proteus* was the most common bacterial organism. Other investigators found a lower incidence of infection-induced stone formation.

The spectrum of causes is the same in children as it is in adults. One-third to one-half of patients have ICU. One study reported finding primary hyperparathyroidism in 6% of the pediatric patients (184), but most authors think that hyperparathyroidism as a cause of urinary stone formation in children is extremely rare. Some of the discrepancy may be explained by the rarity of any kind of urolithiasis in children. Other metabolic causes of stone formation in children are distal RTA, cystinuria, and primary hyperoxaluria. Inflammatory bowel disease also is responsible for recurrent calcium oxalate stone formation in children (49). The pathophysiology is the same as that for enteric hyperoxaluria in adults.

A subsequent review of 221 pediatric patients referred to the Mayo Clinic found an almost even split between boys and girls (108 versus 113, respectively) (200). Analysis of stone material from 122 of the patients revealed calcium oxalate in 45%, calcium phosphate in 24%, cystine in 8%, struvite in 17%, and uric acid in 2%. A metabolic predisposition to form stones was found in 52%: hypercalciuria in 34% and hyperoxaluria in 20%. Other factors predisposing to stone formation were structural abnormalities or chronic infection.

Episodic gross hematuria may precede overt urolithiasis in children with hypercalciuria (323). Hypercalciuria was present in approximately 40% of children with gross hematuria but without urinary infection or proteinuria. Many children had concurrent abdominal or suprapubic pain, dysuria, and urinary frequency. Three-fourths of the children with hypercalciuria had a family history of urolithiasis. The hematuria resolved during anticalciuric therapy with hydrochlorothiazide or dietary calcium restriction.

The frequency and prognostic importance of hypercalciuria in children with hematuria were examined in a prospective multicenter study (322). Hypercalciuria was found in 76 (35%) of 215 patients (aged 3 to 18 years) who had unexplained isolated hematuria. No patient had proteinuria, urolithiasis, infection, or a systemic disorder. The children with hypercalciuria tended to be white males, have a family history of urolithiasis, and have gross hematuria with calcium oxalate crystalluria. Oral calcium loading tests showed renal hypercalciuria in 26 patients, showed absorptive hypercalciuria in 15 patients, and were not diagnostic in 35 patients. One week of dietary calcium restriction normalized urinary calcium excretion in those patients without renal hypercalciuria. During the follow-up period of 1 to 4 years, more hypercalciuric than normocalciuric children developed urolithiasis or renal colic. The authors also concluded that oral calcium loading tests offered little diagnostic benefit over 24-hour urinary calcium excretion measurement after dietary calcium restriction. Hydrochlorothiazide will correct the hypercalciuria (353).

REFERENCES

1. Abdulhadi MH, Hall PM, Streem SB. Can citrate therapy prevent nephrolithiasis? *Urology* 1993;41:221.
2. Allison M, Dawson K, Mayberry W, et al. Oxalobacter formigenes gen. nov., sp. nov.: oxalate degrading anaerobes that inhabit the gastrointestinal tract. *Arch Microbiol* 1985;141:1.
3. Alliston M, Cook H, Milne D, et al. Oxalate degradation by gastrointestinal bacteria from humans. *J Nutr* 1986;116:455.
4. Alvarez-Arroyo MV, Traba ML, Rapado A, et al. Role of citric acid in primary hyperparathyroidism with renal lithiasis. *Urol Res* 1992;20:88.
5. Angermeier K, Streem SB, Yost A. Simplified infusion method for 10% hemiacidrin irrigation of renal pelvis. *Endourol* 1993; 41:243.
6. Arnaud CD, Wilson DM, Smith LH. Primary hyperparathyroidism, renal lithiasis and the measurement of parathyroid hormone serum by radioimmunossay. In: Cifuentes Delatte L, Rapado A, Hodgkinson A, eds. *Urinary calculi—recent advances in aetiology, stone structure and treatment.* Basel, Switzerland: S Karger AG, 1973:346.
7. Asper R, Schmucki O. Socio-economic aspects of urinary stone disease in Eurasia in the 19th and 20th century. In: Ryall Rik Brockis JG, Marshall V, et al., eds. *Urinary stone.* New York: Churchill Livingstone, 1984:18.
8. Atmani F, Lacour B, Driieke T, et al. Isolation and purification of a new glycoprotein from human urine inhibiting calcium oxalate crystallization. *Urol Res* 1993;21:61.
9. Atsmon A, deVries A, Frank M. *Uric acid lithiasis.* Amsterdam: Elsevier, 1963.
10. Backman U, Danielson BG, Johansson G, et al. Incidence and clinical importance of renal tubular defects in recurrent renal stone formers. *Nephron* 1980;25:96.
11. Backman U, Danielson BG, Johansson G, et al. Treatment of recurrent calcium stone formation with cellulose phosphate. *J Urol* 1980;123:9.
12. Baggio B, Gambaro G, Favaro S, et al. Prevalence of hyperoxaluria in idiopathic calcium oxalate kidney stone disease. *Nephron* 1983;35:11.
13. Baggio B, Gambaro G, Marchini F, et al. An inheritable anomaly of red-cell oxalate transport in "primary" calcium nephrolithiasis correctable with diuretics. *N Engl J Med* 1986; 314:599.
14. Baggio B, Gambaro G, Marchini G, et al. Raised transmembrane oxalate flux in red blood cells in idiopathic calcium oxalate nephrolithiasis. *Lancet* 1984;2:12.
15. Balcke P, Schmidt P, Zazgornik J, et al. Pyridoxine therapy in patients with renal calcium oxalate calculi. *Pro Eur Dial Transplant Assoc* 1983;20:417.
16. Barcelo P, Wuhl O, Servitage E, et al. Randomized double-blind study of potassium citrate in idiopathic hypocitraturic calcium nephrolithiasis. *J Urol* 1993;150:1761.
17. Bataille P, Pruna A, Gregoire I, et al. Critical role of oxalate restriction in association with calcium restriction to decrease the probability of being a stone former: insufficient effect in idiopathic hypercalciuria. *Nephron* 1985;39:321.
18. Batlle DC, Shey JT, Roseman MK, et al. Clinical and pathophysiologic spectrum of acquired distal renal tubular acidosis. *Kidney Int* 1981;20:389.
19. Becopoulos T, Tsagatakis E, Constantinides C, et al. Ureaplasma urealyticum and infected renal calculi. *J Chemother* 1991;3:39.
20. Beischer DE. Analysis of renal calculi by infrared spectroscopy. *J Urol* 1955;73:653.
21. Bek-Jensen H, Tiselius HG. Inhibition of calcium oxalate crystallization by urinary macromolecules. *Urol Res* 1991; 19:165.
22. Bigelow M, Wiessner J, Kleinman J, et al. Calcium oxalate crystal attachment to cultured kidney epithelial cell lines. *J Urol* 1998;160:1528.
23. Borghi L, Meschi T, Amato F, et al. Hot occupation and nephrolithiasis. *J Urol* 1993;150:1757.
24. Boyce WH. Organic matrix of human urinary concretions. *Am J Med* 1985;45:673.

25. Boyce WH. Proteinuria in kidney calculous disease. In: Manuel Y, Revillard JP, Betuel H, eds. *Proteins in normal and pathological urine.* Baltimore: University Park Press, 1970:235.
26. Boyce WH, Garvey FK, Strauscutter HE. Incidence of urinary calculi among patients in general hospitals, 1948 to 1952. *JAMA* 1956;161:1437.
27. Boyce WH, King JS Jr, Fielden ML. Total nondialyzable solids (TNDS) in human urine: XIII. Immunological detection of a component peculiar to renal calculous matrix and to urine of calculous patients. *J Clin Invest* 1962;41:1180.
28. Brennan RJ, Spring DB, Sebastian A, et al. Incidence of radiographically evident bone disease, nephrocalcinosis, and nephrolithiasis in various types of renal acidosis. *N Engl J Med* 1982;307:217.
29. Brock WA, Golden J, Kaplan GW. Xanthine calculi in the Lesch-Nyhan syndrome. *J Urol* 1983;130:157.
30. Buckalew VM Jr. Nephrolithiasis in renal tubular acidosis. *J Urol* 1989;141:731.
31. Buckalew VM Jr, McCurdy DK, Ludwig GD, et al. Incomplete renal tubular acidosis. *Am J Med* 1968;45:32.
32. Buckalew VM Jr, Purvis ML, Shulman MG, et al. Hereditary renal tubular acidosis. *Medicine* 1974;53:229.
33. Burns JR, Finlayson B. The effect of seed crystals on calcium oxalate nucleation. *Invest Urol* 1980;18:133.
34. Burns JR, Finlayson B. Why some people have stone disease and others do not. In: Roth RA, Finlayson B, eds. *Stones: clinical management of urolithiasis.* Baltimore: Williams & Wilkins, 1983:3.
35. Burns JR, Finlayson B, Gauthier J. Calcium oxalate retention in subjects with crystalluria. In: Ryall R, Brockis JG, Marshall V, et al., eds. *Urinary stone.* New York: Churchill Livingstone, 1984:253.
36. Butler WT. The nature and significance of osteopontin. *Conn Tissue Res* 1989;23:123.
37. Carlotti ME, Morel S, Cavalli R. Inhibition of crystal growth of calcium oxalate by glycosaminoglycanes. *J Disp Sci Tech* 1993; 14:35.
38. Carr RJ. Aetiology of renal calculi: micro-radiographic studies. In: Hodgkinson A, Nordin BEC, eds. *Renal stone research symposium.* London: J & A Churchill, 1969:123.
39. Casella FJ, Allon M. The kidney in sarcoidosis. *J Am Soc Nephrol* 1993;3:1555.
40. Ceballos-Picot I, Perignon JL, Hamet M, et al. 2,8-dihydroxyadenine urolithiasis, an underdiagnosed disease. *Lancet* 1992; 339:1050.
41. Cendron M, Garber BB. Sulfadiazine urolithiasis in a patient with AIDS. *Inf Urol* 1993;Mar/Apr:60.
42. Chafe L, Gault MH. First morning urine pH in the diagnosis of renal tubular acidosis with nephrolithiasis. *Clin Nephrol* 1994; 41:159.
43. Chlebeck PT, Milliner DS, Smith LH. Long-term prognosis in primary hyperoxaluria type II. *Am J Kidney Dis* 1994;23:255.
44. Churchill D, Bryant D, Fodor G, et al. Drinking water hardness and urolithiasis. *Ann Intern Med* 1978;88:513.
45. Churchill DN. Appraisal of methodology in studies of either thiazide or orthophosphate therapy for recurrent calcium urolithiasis. In: Schwille PO, Smith LH, Robertson WG, et al., eds. *Urolithiasis and related clinical research.* New York: Plenum Publishing, 1985:479.
46. Churchill DN, Morgan J, Gault MH. Tea drinking—a risk factor for urolithiasis? In: Schwille PO, Smith LH, Robertson WG, et al., eds. *Urolithiasis and related clinical research.* New York: Plenum Publishing, 1985:789.
47. Churchill DN, Taylor DW. Thiazides for patients with recurrent calcium stones: still an open question. *J Urol* 1985; 133:749.
48. Ciftcioglu N, Bjorklund M, Kuorikoski K, et al. Nanobacteria: an infectious cause for kidney stone formation. *Kidney Int* 1999;56:1893.
49. Clark JH, Fitzgerald JF, Bergstein JM. Nephrolithiasis in childhood inflammatory bowel disease. *J Pediatr Gastroenterol Nutr* 1985;4(5):829.
50. Clifford AJ, Story DL. Levels of purines in foods and their metabolic effects in rats. *J Nutr* 1976;106:435.
51. Cochat P, Cochat N, Jouvenet M, et al. Ceftriaxone-associated nephro-lithiasis. *Nephrol Dial Transplant* 1990;5:974.
52. Coe F. Uric acid and calcium oxalate nephrolithiasis. *Kidney Int* 1983;24:392.
53. Coe FL, Canterbury JM, Firpo JJ, et al. Evidence for secondary hyperparathyroidism in idiopathic hypercalciuria. *J Clin Invest* 1973;52:134.
54. Coe FL, Favus MJ, Crockett T, et al. Effects of low-calcium diet on urine calcium excretion, parathyroid function and serum 1,24(OH)2D3 levels in patients with idiopathic hypercalciuria and in normal subjects. *Am J Med* 1982;72:25.
55. Coe FL, Kavalach AG. Hypercalciuria and hyperuricosuria in patients with calcium nephrolithiasis. *N Engl J Med* 1974;291: 1344.
56. Coe FL, Lawton RL, Goldstein RB, et al. Sodium urate accelerates precipitation of calcium oxalate in vitro. *Proc Soc Exp Biol Med* 1975;149:926.
57. Coe FL, Parks JH, Lindheimer MD. Nephrolithiasis during pregnancy. *N Engl J Med* 1978;298:324.
58. Cohanim M, Yendt ER. Reduction of urine oxalate during therapy in patients with calcium urolithiasis. *Invest Urol* 1980; 18:170.
59. Coulthard M, Richardson J, Fleetwood A. Captopril is not clinically useful in reducing the cystine load in cystinuria or cystinosis. *Pediatr Nephol* 1991;5:98.
60. Crawhall JC, Purkiss P, Watts RWE, et al. The excretion of amino acids by cystinuric patients and their relatives. *Ann Hum Genet* 1969;33:149.
61. Crawhall JC, Watts RWE. Cystinuria. *Am J Med* 1968;45:736.
62. Curhan G, Willett W, Rimm EB. A prospective study of dietary calcium and other nutrients and the risk of symptomatic kidney stones. *N Engl J Med* 1993;328:833.
63. Dahlberg PJ, Van den Berg CJ, Kurtz SB, et al. Clinical features and management of cystinuria. *Mayo Clin Proc* 1977; 52:533.
64. Dalrymple N, Verga M, Anderson K, et al. The value of unenhanced helical computerized tomography in the management of acute flank pain. *J Urol* 1998;159:735.
65. Dalton DL, Hughes J, Glenn JF. Foreign bodies and urinary stones. *Urology* 1975;6:1.
66. Danielson BG. Drugs against kidney stones: effects of magnesium and alkali. In: Schwille PO, Smith LH, Robertson WG, et al., eds. *Urolithiasis and related clinical research.* New York: Plenum Publishing, 1985:525.
67. Danpure C. Molecular and clinical heterogeneity in primary hyperoxaluria type 1. *Am J Kidney Dis* 1991;17:366.
68. Danpure CJ, Jennings PR. Peroxisomal alanine: glyoxylate aminotransferase deficiency in primary hyperoxaluria type I. *FEBS Letters* 1986;201:20.
69. Danpure CJ, Jennings PR, Watts RWE. Enzymological diagnosis of primary hyperoxaluria type I by measurement of hepatic alanine: glyoxylate aminotransferase activity. *Lancet* 1987; 7:289.

70. Daudon M, Reveillalud RJ. Drug nephrolithiasis: an unrecognized pathology. In: Schwille PO, Smith LH, Robertson WG, et al., eds. *Urolithiasis and related clinical research.* New York: Plenum Publishing, 1985:371.
71. David DS, Cheigh JS, Stenzel KH, et al. Successful renal transplantation in a patient with primary hyperoxaluria. *Transplant Proc* 1983;15:2168.
72. Delatte CF, Minon-Cifuentes J, Medina JA. New studies on papillary calculi. *J Urol* 1987;137:1024.
73. Dell'Aquila R, Feriano M, Mascalzoni E, et al. Oxalate removal by differing dialysis techniques. *ASAIO J* 1992;38:797.
74. Dent CE, Senior B. Studies on the treatment of cystinuria. *Br J Urol* 1955;27:317.
75. Dent CE, Philpot GR. Xanthinuria: an inborn error (or deviation) of metabolism. *Lancet* 1954;1:182.
76. Dent DF, Sutor DJ. Presence or absence of inhibitor of calcium-oxalate crystal growth in urine of normals and of stone formers. *Lancet* 1971;2:775.
77. DeVivo MJ, Fine PR, Cutler GR, et al. The risk of renal calculi in spinal cord injury patients. *J Urol* 1984;131:857.
78. Dhanamitta S, Valyasevi A, Susilavorn B. Research report on bladder stone disease, Thailand. In van Reem R, ed. *Idiopathic urinary bladder stone disease.* Washington, DC: Department of Health, Education, and Welfare, Publication DHEW No. 77-1063, 1977:151.
79. Dick WH, Lingeman JE Preminger GM, et al. Laxative abuse as a cause for ammonium urate renal calculi. *J Urol* 1990;143:244.
80. Dickstein SS, Frame B. Urinary tract calculi after intestinal shunt operations for the treatment of obesity. *Surg Gynecol Obstet* 1973;136:257.
81. Dobbins JW. Nephrolithiasis and intestinal disease. *J Clin Gastroenterol* 1985;7:21.
82. Dobbins JW, Binder HJ. Effect of bile salts and fatty acids on the colonic absorption of oxalate. *Gastroenterol* 1976;70:1096.
83. Dobbins JW, Binder HJ. Importance of the colon in enteric hyperoxaluria. *N Engl J Med* 1977;296(6):298.
84. Dretler SP. The pathogenesis of urinary tract calculi occurring after ileal conduit diversion: I. Clinical study, II. Conduit study. III. Prevention. *J Urol* 1973;109:204.
85. Earnest KL, Johnson G, Williams HE, et al. Hyperoxaluria in patients with ileal resection: an abnormality in dietary oxalate absorption. *Gastroenterol* 1974;66:1114.
86. Eiam-ong S, Kurtzman N. Metabolic acidosis and bone disease. *Miner Electrolyte Metab* 1994;20:72.
87. Ettinger B, Citron JT, Livermore B, et al. Chlorthalidone reduces calcium oxalate calculous recurrence but magnesium hydroxide does not. *J Urol* 1988;139:679.
88. Ettinger B, Tang A, Citron JT, et al. Randomized trial of allopurinol in the prevention of calcium oxalate calculi. *N Engl J Med* 1986;315:1386.
89. Favus MJ. Familial forms of hypercalciuria. *J Urol* 1989; 141:719.
90. Fellstrom B. Allopurinol treatment in urolithiasis. In: Schwille PO, Smith OH, Robertson WG, et al., eds. *Urolithiasis and related clinical research.* New York: Plenum Publishing, 1985:505.
91. Fellstrom B. Urate metabolism and renal calcium stone disease [Suppl]. *Scand J Urol Nephrol* 1981;62:1.
92. Fellstrom B, Backman U, Danielson B, et al. Treatment of renal calcium stone disease with the synthetic glycosaminoglycan pentosan polysulphate. *World J Urol* 1994;12:52.
93. Fellstrom B, Danielson BG, Karlstrom B, et al. Effects of high intake of dietary animal protein on mineral metabolism and urinary supersaturation of calcium oxalate in renal stone formers. *Br J Urol* 1984;56:263.
94. Finlayson B. Calcium stones: some physical aspects. In: David DS, ed. *Calcium metabolism in renal failure and nephrolithiasis.* New York: John Wiley & Sons, 1977:337.
95. Finlayson B. Physicochemical aspects of urolithiasis. *Kidney Int* 1978;13:344.
96. Finlayson B, Newman RC, Hunter PT. The role of urate and allopurinol in stone disease. In: Schwille PO, Smith LH, Robertson WG, et al., eds. *Urolithiasis and related clinical research.* New York: Plenum Publishing, 1985:499.
97. Finlayson B, Reid F. The expectation of free and fixed particles in urinary stone disease. *Invest Urol* 1978;15:442.
98. Finlayson B, Smith A. Stability of first dissociable proton of uric acid. *J Chem Eng Data* 1974;19:94.
99. Finlayson B, Vermeulen CW, Stewart EJ. Stone matrix and mucoprotein from urine. *J Urol* 1961;86:355.
100. Fleisch H. Inhibitors and promoters of stone formation. *Kidney Int* 1978;13:361.
101. Fleisch H. Round table discussion on the comparison of models for the study of inhibitory activity in urine. In: Schwille PO, Smith LH, Robertson WG, et al., eds. *Urolithiasis and related clinical research.* New York: Plenum Publishing, 1985:903.
102. Fye KH, Sahota A, Hancock DC. Adenine phosphoribosyltransferase deficiency with renal deposition of 2,8-dihydroxyadenine leading to nephrolithiasis and chronic renal failure. *Arch Int Med* 1993;153:767.
103. Gambaro G, Bruno B. Idiopathic calcium oxalate nephrolithiasis: a cellular disease. *Scanning Microsc* 1992;6:247.
104. Garside J. Nucleation. In: Nancollas GH, ed. *Biological mineralization and demineralization.* New York: Springer-Verlag, 1982:23.
105. Gault MH, O'Toole T, Wilson JM, et al. Urolithiasis in a large kindred deficient in adenine phosphoribosyl transferase (APRT). In: Schwille PO, Smith LH, Robertson WG, et al., eds. *Urolithiasis and related clinical research.* New York: Plenum Publishing, 1985:9.
106. Gault MH, Simmonds HA, Sneeden W, et al. Urolithiasis due to 2,8- dihydroxyadenine in an adult. *N Engl J Med* 1981;305: 1570.
107. George RJ, Politzer WM. A new method for the detection of cystine and its mechanism. *Clin Chim Acta* 1979;30:737.
108. Giannini S, Nobile M, Castrignano R, et al. Possible link between vitamin D and hyperoxaluria in patients with renal stone disease. *Clin Sci* 1993;84:51.
109. Gibbs DA, Watts RWE. The action of pyridoxine in primary hyperoxaluria. *Clin Sci* 1970;38:277.
110. Gill WB, Silvert MA, Roma MJ. Supersaturation levels and crystallization rates from urines of normal humans and stoneformers determined by a 14C-oxalate technique. *Invest Urol* 1974;12:203.
111. Goldfarb S. Diet and nephrolithiasis. *Ann Rev Med* 1994; 45:235.
112. Goldsmith RS, Killian P, Ingbar SH, et al. Effect of phosphate supplementation during immobilization of normal men. *Metabolism* 1969;18:349.
113. Granberg PO, Cedermark B, Farnebo LO, et al. Parathyroid tumors. *Curr Prob Cancer* 1985;9:1.
114. Grases F, Costa-Bauzá A, Conte A. Studies on structure of calcium oxalate monohydrate renal papillary calculi. Mechanism of formation. *Scanning Microsc* 1993;7:1067.

115. Gray RW, Wilz DR, Caldas AE, et al. The importance of phosphate in regulating plasma 1,25-(OH)-vitamin D levels in humans: studies in healthy subjects, in calcium-stone formers and in patients with primary hyperparathyroidism. *J Clin Endocrinol Metab* 1977;45:299.
116. Griffith DP. Struvite stones. *Kidney Int* 1978;13:372.
117. Griffith DP, Musher DM, Itin C. Urease: the primary cause of infection-induced urinary stones. *Invest Urol* 1976;13:346.
118. Grover PK, Ryall RL, Marshall VR. Dissolved urate promotes calcium oxalate crystallization: epitaxy is not the cause. *Clin Sci* 1993;85:303.
119. Grover PK, Ryall RL, Marshall VR. Does Tamm-Horsfall mucoprotein inhibit or promote calcium oxalate crystallization in human urine? *Clin Chim Acta* 1990;190:223.
120. Gutman AB, Yu TF. Uric acid nephrolithiasis. *Am J Med* 1968;45:756.
121. Gutman AB, Yu TF. Urinary ammonia excretion in primary gout. *J Clin Invest* 1965;44:1474.
122. Hagen L, Walker VR, Sutton RA. Plasma and urinary oxalate and glycolate in healthy subjects. *Clin Chem* 1993;39:134.
123. Hallson PC, Rose GA. A new urinary test for stone "activity." *Br J Urol* 1978;50:442.
124. Hallson PC, Rose GA. Measurement of calcium phosphate crystalluria: Influence of pH and osmolality and invariable presence of oxalate. *Br J Urol* 1989;64:458.
125. Harrison AR, Rose GA. Medullary sponge kidney. *Urol Res* 1979;7:197.
126. Harrison HE, Harrison HC. Inhibition of urine citrate excretion and the production of renal calcinosis in the rat by acetazolamide (Diamox) administration. *J Clin Invest* 1955;34: 1662.
127. Heath H III, Hodgson SF, Kennedy MA. Primary hyperparathyroidism: Incidence, morbidity, and potential impact in a community. *N Engl J Med* 1980;302:189.
128. Heneman PH, Dempsey EF, Carroll EL, et al. The cause of hypercalciuria in sarcoid and its treatment with cortisone and sodium phytate. *J Clin Invest* 1956;35:1229.
129. Herrmann U, Schwille PO, Schwarzlaender H, et al. Citrate and recurrent idiopathic calcium urolithiasis. *Urol Res* 1992; 20:347.
130. Hess B. Prophylaxis of uric acid and cystine stones. *Urol Res* 1990;18:S41.
131. Hess B. The role of Tamm-Horsfall glycoprotein and nephrocalcin in calcium oxalate monohydrate crystallization processes. *Scanning Microsc* 1991;5:689.
132. Hess B, Nakagawa Y, Coe FL. Inhibition of calcium oxalate monohydrate crystal aggregation by urine proteins. *Am J Physiol* 1989;257:F99.
133. Hesse A, Bach D. Stone analysis by infrared spectroscopy. In: Rose GA, ed. *Urinary stones—clinical and laboratory aspects.* Baltimore: University Park Press, 1982:87.
134. Higgins CC. Urolithiasis. In: Campbell M, ed. *Urology.* Philadelphia: WB Saunders, 1954:767.
135. Hill JM, Harvey PWJ, Fleming SJ. Dietary treatment of idiopathic calcium urolithiasis. *Med J Aust* 1993;159:366.
136. Hillman BJ, Drach GW, Tracey P, et al. Computed tomographic analysis of renal calculi. *Am J Radiol* 1984;142:549.
137. Hockaday TDR, Calyton JE, Frederick EW, et al. Primary hyperoxaluria. *Medicine* 1964;43:315.
138. Hodgkinson A. *Oxalic acid in biology and medicine.* London: Academic Press, 1977.
139. Hosking DH, Erickson SB, Van den Berg C, et al. The stone clinic effect in patients with idiopathic calcium urolithiasis. *J Urol* 1983;130:1115.
140. Issekutz B Jr, Blizzard JJ, Birkhead NC, et al. Effect of prolonged bed rest on urinary calcium output. *J Appl Physiol* 1966;21:1013.
141. Ito H, Coe FL. Acidic peptide and polyribonucleotide crystal growth inhibitors in human urine. *Am J Physiol* 1977;233: F455.
142. Ito H, Kotake T, Suzuki F. Incidence and clinical features of renal tubular acidosis-1 in urolithiasis. *Urol Int* 1993;50:82.
143. Jenkins AD, Dousa TP, Smith LH. Transport of citrate across renal brush border membrane: effects of dietary acid and alkali loading. *Am J Physiol* 1985;249:F590.
144. Jick H, Dinan BJ, Hunter JR. Triamterene and renal stones. *J Urol* 1982;127:224.
145. Johnson CM, Wilson DM, O'Fallon WM, et al. Renal stone epidemiology: a 25-year study in Rochester, Minnesota. *Kidney Int* 1979;16:624.
146. Kahn SR, Finlayson B, Hackett RL. Experimental calcium oxalate nephrolithiasis in the rat—role of the renal papilla. *Am J Pathol* 1982;107:59.
147. Kajander E, Ciftcioglu N. Nanobacteria: an alternative mechanism for pathogenic intra- and extracellular calcification and stone formation. *Proc Natl Acad Sci USA* 1998;95:8274.
148. Khan SR, Hackett RL. Hyperoxaluria, enzymuria and nephrolithiasis. *Contrib Nephrol* 1993;101:190.
149. Khan SR, Hackett RL. Role of organic matrix in urinary stone formation: an ultrastructural study of crystal matrix interface of calcium oxalate monohydrate stones. *J Urol* 1993;150:239.
150. Kao PC. Parathyroid hormone assay. *Mayo Clin Proc* 1982; 57:596.
151. Khan SR, Hackett RL. Stone matrix as proteins absorbed on crystal surfaces: a microscopic study. *Scan Electron Microscopy 1983;1:379.*
152. Khan SR, Hackett RL. Identification of urinary stone and sediment crystals by scanning electron microscopy and x-ray microanalysis. *J Urol* 1986;135:818.
153. Khan SR, Hackett RL. Retention of calcium oxalate crystals in renal tubules. *Scanning Microsc* 1991;5:707.
154. Khan S, Glenton P. Increased urinary excretion of lipids by patients with kidney stones. *Br J Urol* 1996;77:506.
155. Khoury A, Salomon M, Doche R, et al. Stone formation after augmentation cystoplasty: the role of intestinal mucus. *J Urol* 1997;158:1133.
156. Kinkead TM, Tan FSJ, Menon M. The varied forms of RTA and how to treat them. *Contemp Urol* 1991;Apr:33.
157. Kippen I, Hirayama B, Klinenberg JR, et al. Transport of tricarboxylic acid cycle intermediates by membrane vesicles from renal brush border. *Proc Natl Acad Sci USA* 1979;76: 3397.
158. Koch MO, McDougal WS. Nicotinic acid: treatment for the hyperchloremic acidosis following urinary diversion through intestinal segments. *J Urol* 1985;134:162.
159. Koff SA. Mechanism of electrolyte imbalance following urointestinal anastomosis. *Urology* 1975;5:109.
160. Kohri K, Nomura S, Kitamura Y, et al. Structure and expression of the MRNA encoding urinary stone protein (osteopontin). *J Biol Chem* 1993;268:15180.
161. Kohri K, Suzuki Y, Yoshida K, et al. Molecular cloning and sequencing of cDNA encoding urinary stone protein, which is identical to osteopontin. *Biochem Biophys Res Comm* 1992; 184:859.
162. Kopp J, Miller K, Mican J, et al. Crystalluria and urinary tract abnormalities associated with indinavir. *Ann Int Med* 1997; 127:119.
163. Koul H, Koul S, Fu S, et al. Oxalate: from crystal formation to crystal retention. *J Am Soc Nephrol* 1999;10:S417.

164. Koutsoukos PD, Lan-Erwin CY, Nancollas GH. Epitaxial considerations in urinary stone formation: I. The urate-oxalate-phosphate system. *Invest Urol* 1980;18:178.
165. Krause U, Zielke A, Schmidt-Gayk H, et al. Direct tubular effect on calcium retention by hydrochlorothiazide. *J Endocrinol Invest* 1989;12:531.
166. Kumar S, Sigmon D, Miller T, et al. A new model of nephrolithiasis involving tubular dysfunction/injury. *J Urol* 1991;146:1384.
167. Lash JP, Arruda JAL. Laboratory evaluation of renal tubular acidosis. *Clin Lab Med* 1993;13:117.
168. Lavengood RW, Marshall VF. The prevention of urinary phosphatic calculi by the Shorr regimen. *J Urol* 1972;108:368.
169. Leal JJ, Finlayson B. Adsorption of naturally occurring polymers onto calcium oxalate crystal surfaces. *Invest Urol* 1977;14:278.
170. Lein JW, Keane PM. Limitations of the oral calcium loading test in the management of the recurrent calcareous renal stone former. *Am J Kidney Dis* 1983;3:76.
171. Lemann J Jr, Gray RW. Calcitriol, calcium, and granulomatous disease. *N Engl J Med* 1984;311:1115.
172. Lemann J Jr, Gray RW. Idiopathic hypercalciuria. *J Urol* 1989;141:715.
173. Leumann E, Hoppe B, Neuhaus T. Management of primary hyperoxaluria: efficacy of oral citrate administration. *Pediatr Nephrol* 1993;7:207.
174. Lian JB, Prien EF Jr, Glincher MJ, et al. The presence of protein-bound gamma-carboxyglutamic acid in calcium-containing renal calculi. *J Clin Invest* 1977;59:1151.
175. Lieske JC, Toback FG. Regulation of renal epithelial cell endocytosis of calcium oxalate monohydrate crystals. *Am J Physiol* 1993;264:F800.
176. Lieske J, Huang E, Toback F. Regulation of renal epithelial cell affinity for calcium oxalate monohydrate crystals. *Am J Physiol Renal Physiol* 2000;278:F130.
177. Lindsjö M, Danielson BG, Fellström B, et al. Parathyroid function in relation to intestinal function and renal calcium reabsorption in patients with nephrolithiasis. *Scand J Urol Nephrol* 1992;26:55.
178. Ljunghall S, Danielson BG. A prospective study of renal stone recurrences. *Br J Urol* 1984;56:122.
179. Lonsdale K. Epitaxy as a growth factor in urinary calculi and gallstones. *Nature* 1968;217:56.
180. Low R, Stoller M. Endoscopic mapping of renal papillae for Randall's plaques in patient with urinary stone disease. *J Urol* 1997;158:2062.
181. Lutwak L, Whedon GD, Lachance PA, et al. Mineral, electrolyte and nitrogen balance studies of the Gemini-VII fourteen day orbital space flight. *J Clin Endocrinol* 1969;29:1140.
182. Maikranz P, Coe FL, Parks J, et al. Nephrolithiasis in pregnancy. *Am J Kidney Dis* 1987;9:354.
183. Maikranz P, Holley JL, Parks JH, et al. Gestational hypercalciuria causes pathological urine calcium oxalate supersaturations. *Kidney Int* 1989;36:108.
184. Malek RS, Kelalis PP. Pediatric nephrolithiasis. *J Urol* 1975;113:545.
185. Marangella M, Bagnis C, Bruno M, et al. Determinants of oxalate balance in patients on chronic peritoneal dialysis. *Am J Kidney Dis* 1993;21:419.
186. Marangella M, Fruttero B, Bruno M, et al. Hyperoxaluria in idiopathic calcium stone disease: further evidence of intestinal hyperabsorption of oxalate. *Clin Sci* 1982;63:381.
187. Martin X, Werness PG, Bergert JH, et al. Pentosan polysulfate as an inhibitor of calcium oxalate crystal growth. *J Urol* 1984;132:786.
188. Massey LK, Roman-Smith H, Sutton RAL. Effect of dietary oxalate and calcium on urinary oxalate and risk of formation of calcium oxalate kidney stones. *J Am Diet Assoc* 1993;93:901.
189. McConnel JB, Murison J, Stewart WK. The role of the colon in the pathogenesis of hyperchloraemic acidosis in ureterosigmoid anastomosis. *Clin Sci* 1979;57:305.
190. McDonald JC, Landreneau MD, Rohr MS, et al. Reversal by liver transplantation of the complications of primary hyperoxaluria as well as the metabolic defect. *N Engl J Med* 1989;321:1100.
191. McSherry E. Acidosis and growth in nonuremic renal disease. *Kidney Int* 1978;14:349.
192. McSherry E, Sebastian A, Morris RC Jr. Renal tubular acidosis in infants: the several kinds, including bicarbonate-wasting, classic renal tubular acidosis. *J Clin Invest* 1972;51:499.
193. Melnick I, Landes RR, Hoffman AA, et al. Magnesium therapy for recurring calcium oxalate urinary calculi. *J Urol* 1971;105:119.
194. Menon M, Mahle CJ. Urinary citrate excretion in patients with renal calculi. *J Urol* 1983;129:1158.
195. Meyer JL. Nucleation kinetics in the calcium oxalate-sodium urate monohydrate system. *Invest Urol* 1981;19:197.
196. Meyer JL, Bergert JH, Smith LH. The epitaxially induced crystal growth of calcium oxalate by crystalline uric acid. *Invest Urol* 1976;14:115.
197. Meyer JL, Smith LH. Growth of calcium oxalate crystals: II. Inhibition by natural urinary crystal growth inhibitors. *Invest Urol* 1975;13:36.
198. Miano L, Petta S, Galatioto GP, et al. A placebo controlled double-blind study of allopurinol in severe recurrent idiopathic renal lithiasis—preliminary results. In: Schwille PO, Smith LH, Robertson WG, et al., eds. *Urolithiasis and related clinical research.* New York: Plenum Publishing, 1985:521.
199. Miller MA, Gallicano K, Dascal A, et al. Sulfadiazine urolithiasis during antitoxoplasma therapy. *Drug Invest* 1993;5:334.
200. Milliner DS, Murphy ME. Urolithiasis in pediatric patients. *Mayo Clin Proc* 1993;68:241.
201. Milvy P, Colt E, Thornton J. A high incidence of urolithiasis in male marathon runners. *J Sports Med* 1981;21:295.
202. Min W, Shinaga H, Chalko C, et al. Quantitative studies of human urinary excretion of uropontin. *Kidney Int* 1998;53:189.
203. Modlin M. The aetiology of renal stone: a new concept arising from studies on a stone-free population. *Ann R Coll Surg Engl* 1967;40:155.
204. Morris RC Jr. Renal tubular acidosis. *N Engl J Med* 1981;304:418.
205. Morris RC Jr. Renal tubular acidosis. *N Engl J Med* 1969;281:1405.
206. Morriss RH, Beeler MF. X-ray diffraction analysis of 464 urinary calculi. *Am J Clin Pathol* 1967;48:413.
207. Muldowney FP, Donohoe JP, Freaney R, et al. Parathormone-induced renal bicarbonate wastage in intestinal malabsorption and in chronic renal failure. *Ir J Med Sci* 1970;3:221.
208. Muldowney FP, Freaney R, Moloney MF. Importance of dietary sodium in the hypercalciuria syndrome. *Kidney Int* 1982;22:292.
209. Nakagawa Y, Kaiser ET, Coe FL. Isolation and characterization of calcium oxalate crystal growth inhibitors from human urine. *Biochem Biophys Res Commun* 1978;84:1038.
210. Nakagawa Y, Margolis HC, Yokoyama S, et al. Purification and characterization of a calcium oxlate monohydrate crystal growth inhibitor from human kidney tissue culture medium. *J Biol Chem* 1981;256:3936.

211. Nakagawa Y, Abram V, Parks JH, et al. Urine glycoprotein crystal growth inhibitors: Evidence for a molecular abnormality in calcium oxalate nephrolithiasis. *Clin Invest* 1985;76:1455.
212. Nakagawa Y, Ahmed M, Hall SL, et al. Isolation from human calciumoxalate renal stones of nephrocalcin, a glycoprotein inhibitor of calcium oxalate crystal growth: evidence that nephrocalcin from patients with calcium oxalate nephrolithiasis is deficient in gamma-carboxyglutamic acid. *J Clin Invest* 1987; 79:1782.
213. Nakagawa Y. Properties and function of nephrocalcin: mechanism of kidney stone inhibition or promotion. *Keio J Med* 1997;46:1.
214. Nemoy NJ, Stamey TA. Surgical, bacteriological, and biochemical management of "infection stones." *JAMA* 1971;215:1470.
215. Netelenbos JC, Jongen MJM, van der Vijgh WJF, et al. Vitamin D status in urinary calcium stone formation. *Arch Intern Med* 1985;145:681.
216. Nielsen AE, Christoffersen J. The mechanisms of crystal growth and dissolution. In: Nancollas GH, ed. *Biological mineralization and demineralization.* New York: Springer-Verlag, 1982:36.
217. Obialo CI, Clayman RV, Matts JP, et al. Pathogenesis of nephrolithiasis post-partial ileal bypass surgery: case-control study. *Kidney Int* 1991;39:1249.
218. O'Donnell D, Gunn J. Hypercalcaemia and nephrolithiasis following multiple fractures. *J Bone Joint Surg* 1991;73:174.
219. Oliver J, MacDowell M, Whang R, et al. The renal lesions of electrolyte imbalance: IV. The intranephronic calculosis of experimental magnesium depletion. *J Exp Med* 1966;124:263.
220. O'Neill M, Breslau NA, Pak CYC. Metabolic evaluation of nephrolithiasis in patients with medullary sponge kidney. *JAMA* 1981;245:1233.
221. Osther PJ, Bollerslev J, Hansen AB, et al. Pathophysiology of incomplete renal tubular acidosis in recurrent renal stone formers: evidence of disturbed calcium, bone and citrate metabolism. *Urol Res* 1993;21:169.
222. Pak CYC. A cautious use of sodium cellulose phosphate in the management of calcium nephrolithiasis. *J Urol* 1981;19:187.
223. Pak CYC. Physiological basis for absorptive and renal hypercalciurias. *Am J Physiol* 1979;237:F415.
224. Pak CYC. Should patients with single renal stone occurrence undergo diagnostic evaluation? *J Urol* 1982;127:855.
225. Pak CYC, Arnold LH. Heterogeneous nucleation of calcium oxalate by seeds of monosodium urate. *Proc Soc Exp Biol Med* 1975;149:930.
226. Pak CYC, Barilla DE, Holt K, et al. Effect of oral purine load and allopurinol on the crystallization of calcium salts in urine of patients with hyperuricosuric calcium urolithiasis. *Am J Med* 1978;65:593.
227. Pak CYC, Delea CS, Bartter FC. Successful treatment of recurrent nephrolithiasis (calcium stones) with cellulose phosphate. *N Engl J Med* 1974a;290:175.
228. Pak CYC, Fuller C. Idiopathic hypocitraturic calcium-oxalate nephrolithiasis successfully treated with potassium citrate. *Ann Intern Med* 1986;104:33.
229. Pak CYC, Fuller C, Sakhaee K, et al. Long-term treatment of calcium nephrolithiasis with potassium citrate. *J Urol* 1985; 134:11.
230. Pak CYC, Fuller C, Sakhaee K, et al. Management of cystine nephrolithiasis with alpha-mercaptopropionylglycine. *J Urol* 1986;136:1003.
231. Pak CYC, Kaplan R, Bone H, et al. A simple test for the diagnosis of absorptive, resorptive and renal hypercalciurias. *N Engl J Med* 1975;292:497.
232. Pak CYC, Koenig K, Khan R, et al. Physicochemical action of potassium-magnesium citrate in nephrolithiasis. *J Bone Min Res* 1992;7:281.
233. Pak CYC, Nicar MJ, Peterson R, et al. A lack of unique pathophysiologic background for nephrolithiasis of primary hyperparathyroidism. *J Clin Endocrinol Metab* 1981;53:536.
234. Pak CYC, Ohata M, Lawrence EC, et al. The hypercalciurias—causes, parathyroid functions, and diagnostic criteria. *J Clin Invest* 1974;54:387.
235. Pak CYC, Peterson R. Successful treatment of hyperuricosuric calcium oxalate nephrolithiasis with potassium citrate. *Arch Intern Med* 1986;146:863.
236. Pak CYC, Peterson R, Sakhaee K, et al. Correction of hypocitraturia and prevention of stone formation by combined thiazide and potassium citrate therapy in thiazide-unresponsive hypercalciuric nephrolithiasis. *Am J Med* 1985a;79:284.
237. Pak CYC, Skurla C, Harvey J. Graphic display of urinary risk factors for renal stone formation. *J Urol* 1985b;134:867.
238. Pak CYC, Smith LH, Resnick MI, et al. Dietary management of idiopathic calcium urolithiasis. *J Urol* 1984;131:850.
239. Palmer L, Franco I, Kogan S, et al. Urolithiasis in children following augmentation cystoplasty. *J Urol* 1993;150:726.
240. Palmer L, Palmer J, Firlit B, et al. Recurrent urolithiasis after augmentation cystoplasty. *J Urol* 1998;159:1331.
241. Parfitt AM. Acetazolamide and sodium bicarbonate induced nephrocalcinosis and nephrolithiasis. *Arch Intern Med* 1969; 124:736.
242. Park GD, Spector R. Hypocitraturic calcium-oxalate nephrolithiasis [Letter]. *Ann Intern Med* 1986;104:723.
243. Parks JH, Coe FL, Strauss AL. Calcium nephrolithiasis and medullary sponge kidney in women. *N Engl J Med* 1982;306: 1088.
244. Parsons CL, Schmidt JD, Pollen JJ. Successful treatment of interstitial cystitis with sodium pentosan polysulfate. *J Urol* 1983;130:51.
245. Perazella MA, Buller GK. Susccessful treatment of cystinuria with captopril. *Am J Kidney Dis* 1993;21:504.
246. Pietschmann F, Breslau NA, Pak CYC. Reduced vertebral bone density in hypercalciuric nephrolithiasis. *J Bone Min Res* 1992; 7:1383.
247. Preminger GM. The metabolic evaluation of patients with recurrent nephrolithiasis: a review of comprehensive and simplified approaches. *J Urol* 1989;141:760.
248. Preminger GM, Pak CYC. Eventual attenuation of hypocalciuric response to hydrochlorothiazide in absorptive hypercalciuria. *J Urol* 1987;137:1104.
249. Preminger GM, Sakhaee K, Pak CYC. Alkali action on the urinary crystallization of calcium salts: contrasting responses to sodium citrate and potassium citrate. *J Urol* 1988;139:240.
250. Preminger GM, Sakhaee K, Skurla C, et al. Prevention of recurrent calcium stone formation with potassium citrate therapy in patients with distal renal tubular acidosis. *J Urol* 1985; 134:20.
251. Prien EL. The riddle of Randall's plaques. *J Urol* 1975; 114:500.
252. Prien EL. Use of polarized light in analyses of calculi and study of crystals in tissue. *J Urol* 1941;45:765.
253. Pyrah LN. *Renal calculus.* New York: Springer-Verlag, 1979.
254. Randall A. The origin and growth of renal calculi. *Ann Surg* 1937;105:1009.
255. Rao PN, Faraghar EB, Buxton A, et al. Is salt restriction necessary to reduce the risk of stone formation? In: Schwille FO, Smith LH, Robertson WG, et al., eds. *Urolithiasis and related clinical research.* New York: Plenum Publishing, 1985:429.

256. Resnick MI. Evaluation and management of infection stones. *Urol Clin North Am* 1981;8:265.
257. Riese RJ, Mandel NS, Wiessner JH. Cell polarity and calcium oxalate crystal adherence to cultured collecting duct cells. *Am J Physiol* 1992;262:F177.
258. Riese RJ, Riese JW, Kleinman JG, et al. Specificity in calcium oxalate adherence to papillary epithelial cells in culture. *Am J Physiol* 1988;255:F1025.
259. Riese RJ, Sakhaee K. Uric acid nephrolithiasis: pathogenesis and treatment. *J Urol* 1992;148:765.
260. Robertson WG. Dietary factors important in calcium stone formation. In: Schwille PO, Smith LH, Robertson WG, et al., eds. *Urolithiasis and related clinical research.* New York, Plenum Publishing Corp, 1985:61.
261. Robertson WG. Epidemiology of urinary stone disease. *Urol Res* 1990;S18:S3.
262. Robertson WG. The solubility concept. In: Nancollas GN, ed. *Biological mineralization and demineralization.* New York: Springer-Verlag, 1982:5.
263. Robertson WG, Hughes H. Importance of mild hyperoxaluria in the pathogenesis of urolithiasis—new evidence from studies in the Arabian Peninsula. *Scanning Microsc* 1993;7:391.
264. Robertson WG, Morgan DB. The distribution of urinary calcium excretions in normal persons and stone-formers. *Clin Chim Acta* 1972;37:503.
265. Robertson WG, Peacock M. The cause of idiopathic calcium stone disease: hypercalciuria or hyperoxaluria? *Nephron* 1980; 26:105.
266. Robertson WG, Peacock M, Heyburn PJ, et al. A risk factor model of stone formation: application to the study of epidemiological factors in the genesis of calcium stones. In: Smith LH, Robertson WG, Finlayson B, eds. *Urolithiasis—clinical and basic research.* New York: Plenum Publishing, 1981b:303.
267. Robertson WG, Peacock M, Heyburn PJ, et al. Risk factors in calcium stone disease of the urinary tract. *Br J Urol* 1978; 50:449.
268. Robertson WG, Peacock M, Heyburn PJ et al. The risk of calcium stone formation in relation to affluence and dietary animal protein. In: Brockis JG, Finlayson B, eds. *Urinary calculus.* Littleton, MA: PSG Publishing, 1981a:3.
269. Robertson WG, Peacock M, Marshall RW, et al. Saturation-inhibition index as a measure of the risk of calcium oxalate stone formation in the urinary tract. *N Engl J Med* 1976; 294:249.
270. Robertson WG, Peacock M, Nordin BEC. Activity products in stone-forming and non-stone–forming urine. *Clin Sci* 1968; 34:579.
271. Robertson WG, Peacock M, Nordin BEC. Calcium oxalate crystalluria and urine saturation in recurrent renal stone formers. *Clin Sci* 1971;40:365.
272. Robertson WG, Peacock M, Nordin BEC. Inhibitors of the growth and aggregation of calcium oxalate crystals in vitro. *Clin Chim Acta* 1973;43:31.
273. Robertson WG, Peacock M, Nordin BEC. Measurement of activity products in urine from stone-formers and normal subjects. In: Finlagson B, Hench LL, Smith LH, eds. *Urolithiasis: physical aspects.* Washington, DC: National Academy of Sciences, 1972:79.
274. Rose GA. An overview of some problems in urolithiasis. In: Rose GA, ed. *Urinary stones—clinical and laboratory aspects.* Baltimore: University Park Press, 1982:1.
275. Rose GA. Stone analysis by thermogravimetric technique. In: Rose GA, ed. *Urinary stones—clinical and laboratory aspects.* Baltimore: University Park Press, 1982:77.
276. Roth R, Finlayson B. Observations on the radiopacity of stone substances with special reference to cystine. *Invest Urol* 1973; 11:186.
277. Rudman D, Kutner MH, Redd SC II, et al. Hypocitraturia in calcium nephrolithiasis. *J Clin Endocrinol Metab* 1982;55: 1052.
278. Rundquist RT, Smith LH, Werness PG. Factitious hyperoxaluria from ascorbic acid [Abstract]. Central Society for Clinical Research, Midwest Meeting, Chicago, 1981.
279. Ryall RL, Grover PK, Marshall VR. Urate and calcium stones—picking up a drop of mercury with one's fingers? *Am J Kidney Dis* 1991;17:426.
280. Ryall RL, Harnett RM, Marshall VR. The effect of uric acid on the inhibitory activity of glycosaminoglycans and urine. In: Schwille PO, Smith LH, Robertson WG, et al., eds. *Urolithiasis and related clinical research.* New York: Plenum Publishing, 1985:855.
281. Ryall RL, Harnett RM, Marshall VR. The effect of urine, pyrophosphate, citrate, magnesium and glycosaminoglycans on the growth and aggregation of calcium oxalate crystals in vitro. *Clin Chim Acta* 1981;12:349.
282. Ryde M, Eriksson H, Tangen O. Studies on the different mechanisms by which heparin and polysulfated xylan (PZ 68) inhibit blood coagulation in man. *Thromb Res* 1981;23:435.
283. Sakhaee K, Harvey JA, Padalino PK, et al. The potential role of salt abuse on the risk for kidney stone formation. *J Urol* 1993;150:310.
284. Sakhaee K, Nicar M, Hill K, et al. Contrasting effects of potassium citrate and sodium citrate therapies on urinary chemistries and crystallization of stone-forming salts. *Kidney Int* 1983;24:348.
285. Sakhaee K, Nigam S, Snell P, et al. Assessment of the pathogenetic role of physical exercise in renal stone formation. *J Clin Endocrinol Metab* 1987;65:974.
286. Sakhaee K, Poindexter JR, Pak CYC. The spectrum of metabolic abnormalities in patients with cystine nephrolithiasis. *J Urol* 1989;141:819.
287. Salliner A. Some aspects of urolithiasis in Finland. *Acta Chim Scand* 1959/1960;118:479.
288. Saltel E, Angel J, Futter N, et al. Increased prevalence and analysis of risk factors for indinavir nephrolithiasis. *J Urol* 2000;164:1895.
289. Sarmina I, Sprinak JP, Resnick MI. Urinary lithiasis in the black population: an epidemiological study and review of the literature. *J Urol* 1987;138:14.
290. Schaumburg H, Kaplan J, Windebank A, et al. Sensory neuropathy from pyridoxine abuse—a new megavitamin syndrome. *N Engl J Med* 1983;309:445.
291. Schneider JA, Schulman JD, Seegmiller JE. Cystinosis and the Fanconi syndrome. In: Stanbury JB, Wyngaarden JB, Fredrickson DS, eds. *The metabolic basis of inherited disease.* New York: McGraw-Hill, 1978:1660.
292. Scott R, Paterson PJ, Mathieson A, et al. The effect of allopurinol on urinary oxalate excretion in stone formers. *Br J Urol* 1978;50:455.
293. Scurr DS, Robertson WG. Modifiers of calcium oxalate crystallization found in urine. III. Studies on the role of Tamm-Horsfall mucoprotein and of ionic strength. *J Urol* 1986; 136:505.
294. Scurr DS, Robertson WG. Studies on the mode of action of polyanionic inhibitors of calcium oxalate crystallization in urine. In: Schwille PO, Smith LH, Robertson WG, et al., eds. *Urolithiasis and related clinical research.* New York: Plenum Publishing, 1985:835.

295. Sedlack JD, Kenkel J, Czarapata BJR. Primary hyperparathyroidism in patients with renal stones. *Surg Gynecol Obstet* 1990;171:206.
296. Segura JW, Erickson SB, Wilson DM, et al. Infected renal lithiasis: results of long-term surgical and medical management. In: Smith LH, Robertson WG, Finlayson B, eds. *Urolithiasis—basic and clinical research.* New York: Plenum Publishing, 1981:195.
297. Seldin DW, Wilson JD. Renal tubular acidosis. In: Stanbury JB, Wyngaarden JB, Fredrickson DS, eds. *The metabolic basis of inherited disease.* New York: McGraw-Hill, 1978:1618.
298. Shen FH, Baylink DJ, Nielson RL, et al. Increased serum 1,25-dihydroxyvitamin D in idiopathic hypercalciuria. *J Lab Clin Med* 1977;90:955.
299. Shirane Y, Kagawa S. Scanning electron microscopic study of the effect of citrate and pyrophosphate on calcium oxalate crystal morphology. *J Urol* 1993;150:1980.
300. Shuster J, Finlayson B, Schaeffer R, et al. Water hardness and urinary stone disease. *J Urol* 1962;128:422.
301. Shuster J, Finlayson B, Schaeffer RL, et al. Primary liquid intake and urinary stone disease. *J Chronic Dis* 1985;38:907.
302. Sidhu H, Schmidt M, Cornelius J, et al. Direct correlation beetween hyperoxaluria/oxalate stone disease and the absence of the gastrointestinal tract-dwelling bacterium *Oxalobacter formigenes:* possible prevention by gut recolonization or enzyme replacement. *J Am Soc Nephrol* 1999;10:S334.
303. Sierakowski R, Finlayson B, Landes R. Stone incidence as related to water hardness in different geographical regions of the United States. *Urol Res* 1979;7:157.
304. Sierakowski R, Finlayson B, Landes RR, et al. The frequency of urolithiasis in hospital discharge diagnoses in the United States. *Invest Urol* 1978; 15:438.
305. Siklos P, Davie M, Jung RT, et al. Osteomalacia in ureterosigmoidostomy: healing by correction of the acidosis. *Br J Urol* 1980;52:61.
306. Silverberg SJ, Shane E, Jacobs TP, et al. Nephrolithiasis and bone involvement in primary hyperparathyroidism. *Am J Med* 1990;89:327.
307. Silverman DE, Stamey TA. Management of infection stones: the Stanford experience. *Medicine* 1983;62:44.
308. Simpson DP. Citrate excretion: a window on renal metabolism. *Am J Physiol* 1982;244:F2323.
309. Simpson DP. Effect of acetazolamide on citrate excretion in the dog. *Am J Physiol* 1964;206:883.
310. Singh PP, Kiran R, Pendse AK, et al. Ascorbic acid is an abettor in calcium urolithiasis: an experimental study. *Scanning Microsc* 1993;7:1041.
311. Sinno K, Boyce WH, Resnick MI. Childhood urolithiasis. *J Urol* 1979;121:662.
312. Sirivongs D, Nakagawa Y, Vishny WK, et al. Evidence that mouse renal proximal tubule cells produce nephrocalcin. *Am J Physiol* 1989;257:F390.
313. Sloand JA, Izzo JL Jr. Captopril reduces urinary cystine excretion in cystinuria. *Arch Intern Med* 1987;147:1409.
314. Smith LH. Medical treatment of idiopathic calcium urolithiasis. *Kidney* 1983;16:9.
315. Smith LH. New treatment for struvite urinary stones. *N Engl J Med* 1984;311:792.
316. Smith LH. Stone activity. In: Roth RA, Finlayson B, eds. *Stones: clinical management of urolithiasis.* Baltimore: Williams & Wilkins, 1983:183.
317. Smith LH, Fromm H, Hoffman AF. Acquired hyperoxaluria, nephrolithiasis, and intestinal disease: description of a syndrome. *N Engl J Med* 1972;286:1371.
318. Smith LH, Jones SD, Keating KR Jr. Primary hyperoxaluria. In: Hodgkinson A, Nordin BEC, eds. Proceedings of the Renal Stone Research Symposium held in Leeds, April, 1968. London: Churchill, 1969:297.
319. Smith LH, Werness PG, Wilson DM. Enteric hyperoxaluria: associated abnormalities that promote formation of renal calculi. In: Rose GA, Robertson WG, Watts RWE, eds. *Oxalate in human biochemistry and clinical pathology.* London: Wellcome Foundation, 1979:224.
320. Spiegel AM. Pathophysiology of primary hyperparathyroidism. *J Bone Min Res* 1991;6:S15.
321. Stacholy J, Goldberg EP. Mirostructural matrix-crystal interactions in calcium oxalate monohydrate kidney stones. *Scan Electron Microscopy* 1985;2:781.
322. Stapleton FB, The Southwest Pediatric Nephrology Study Group. Idiopathic hypercalciuria: association with isolated hematuria and risk for urolithiasis in children. *Kidney Int* 1990; 37:807.
323. Stapleton FM, Roy S III, Noe HN, et al. Hypercalciuria in children with hematuria. *N Engl J Med* 1984;310:1345.
324. Stauffer JQ, Stewart RJ, Bertrand G. Acquired hyperoxaluria: relationship to dietary calcium content with severity of steatorrhea. *Gastroenterology* 1974;66:783.
325. Stinebaugh BJ, Schloeder FX, Tan SC, et al. Pathogenesis of distal renal tubular acidosis. *Kidney Int* 1981;19:1.
326. Stoller M, Low R, Shami G, et al. High resolution radiography of cadaveric kidneys: unraveling the mystery of Randall's plaque formation. *J Urol* 1996;156:1263.
327. Stote RM, Smith LH, Budd JW, et al. Oxypurinol nephrolithiasis in regional enteritis secondary to allopurinol therapy. *Ann Intern Med* 1980;92:384.
328. Stauss AL, Coe FL, Parks JH. Formation of a single calcium stone of renal origin—clinical and laboratory characteristics of patients. *Arch Intern Med* 1982;142:504.
329. Streem SB, Hall P. Effect of captopril on urinary cystine excretion in homozygous cystinuria. *J Urol* 1989;142:1522.
330. Strenge A, Hess A, Bach D, et al. Excretion of oxalic acid following the ingestion of various amounts of oxalic acid-rich foods. In: Smith LH, Robertson WG, Finlayson B, eds. *Urolithiasis—clinical and basic research.* New York: Plenum Publishing, 1981:789.
331. Strzelecki T, McGraw BR, Scheid CR, et al. Effect of oxalate on function of kidney mitochondria. *J Urol* 1989;141:423.
332. Sundaram C, Saltzman B. Urolithiasis associated with protease inhibitors. *J Endourol* 1999;13:309.
333. Sutor DJ, Scheidt S. Identification standards for human urinary calculus components, using crystallographic methods. *Br J Urol* 1968;40:22.
334. Sutton RAL, Walker VR. Responses to hydrochlorothiazide and acetazolamide in patients with calcium stones. *N Engl J Med* 1980;302:709.
335. Suzuki K, Tsugawa R, Ryall RL. Inhibition by sodium-potassium citrate (CG-120) of calcium oxalate crystal growth on to kidney stone fragments obtained from extracorporeal shock wave lithotripsy. *Br J Urol* 1991;68:132.
336. Tawil R, Moxley RT, Griggs RC. Acetazolamide-induced nephrolithiasis. *Neurology* 1993;43:1105.
337. Tessitore N, Ortalda V, Fabris A, et al. Renal acidification defects in patients with recurrent calcium nephrolithiasis. *Nephron* 1985;41:325.
338. Thom JA, Morris JE, Bishop A, et al. The influence of refined carbohydrate on urinary calcium excretion. *Br J Urol* 1978; 50:459.
339. Thomas WC Jr. Use of phosphates in patients with calcareous renal calculi. *Kidney Int* 1978;13:390.

340. Tiselius HG, Larsson L. Calcium phosphate: an important crystal phase in patients with recurrent calcium stone formation? *Urol Res* 1993;21:175.
341. Tiselius HG, Larsson L, Hellgren E. Clinical results of allopurinol treatment in prevention of calcium oxalate stone formation. *J Urol* 1986;138:50.
342. Torres VE, Wilson DM, Hattery RR, et al. Renal stone disease in autosomal dominant polycystic kidney disease. *Am J Kidney Dis* 1993;22:513.
343. Urivetzky M, Braverman S, Motola JA, et al. Uinary excretion of oxalate by patients with renal hypercalciuric stone disease. *Urology* 1991;37:327.
344. Urivetzky M, Kessaris D, Smith AD. Ascorbic acid overdosing: a risk factor for calcium oxalate nephrolithiasis. *J Urol* 1992; 147:1215.
345. Vahlensieck W, Bastian HP. Clinical features and treatment of urinary calculi in childhood. *Eur Urol* 1976;2:129.
346. Valyasevi A, Dhanamitta S. A general hypothesis concerning the etiological factors in bladder stone disease. In: van Reem R, ed. *Idiopathic urinary bladder stone disease.* Washington, DC: Department of Health, Education, and Welfare, 1977:135.
347. Van den Berg CJ, Harrington TM, Bunch TW, et al. Treatment of renal lithiasis associated with renal tubular acidosis. *Proc Eur Dial Transplant Assoc* 1983;20:473.
348. Van den Berg CJ, Kumar R, Wilson DM, et al. Orthophosphate therapy decreases urinary calcium excretion and serum 1,25-dihydroxyvitamin D concentrations in idiopathic hypercalciuria. *J Clin Endocrinol Metab* 1980;51:998.
349. van Heerden JA, Segura JW, Grant CS. Primary hyperparathyroidism and urolithiasis: concomitant surgical management. *Surgery* 1989;106:992.
350. Vermeulen CW, Lyon ES. Mechanisms of genesis and growth of calculi. *Am J Med* 1968;45:684.
351. Vermeulen CW, Lyon ES, Ellis JE, et al. The renal papilla and calculogenesis. *J Urol* 1967;97:573.
352. Vieweg J, The C, Freed K. Unenhanced helical computerized tomography for the evaluation of patients with acute flank pain. *J Urol* 1998;160:679.
353. Voskaki I, Al Qadreh A, Mengreli Ch, et al. Effect of hydrochlorothiazide on renal hypercalciuria. *Child Nephrol Urol* 1992;12:6.
354. Wabner C, Pak C. Effect of orange juice consumption on urinary stone risk factors. *J Urol* 1993;149:1405.
355. Wall I, Tiselius H. Long-term acidification of urine in patients treated for infected renal stones. *Urol Int* 1990;45:336.
356. Walton AG. *The formation and properties of precipitates.* Huntington, NY: Robert E. Krieger, 1979.
357. Watts RWE, Mansell MA. Oxalate, livers, and kidneys. *BMJ* 1990;301:772.
358. Weissner JH, Kleinman JG, Blumenthal SS, et al. Calcium oxalate crystal interaction with rat renal inner papillary collecting tubule cells. *J Urol* 1987;138:640.
359. Werness PG, Bergert JH, Smith LH. Crystalluria. *J Crystal Growth* 1981;53:166.
360. Werness PG, Bergert JH, Smith LH. Triamterene urolithiasis: solubility, pK, effect on crystal formation, and matrix binding of triamterene and its metabolites. *J Lab Clin Med* 1982; 99:254.
361. Werness PG, Brown CM, Smith LH, et al. Equil 2: a basic computer program for the calculation of urinary saturation. *J Urol* 1985;134:1242.
362. Werness PG, Knox FG, Smith LH. Low phosphate diet in rats: a model for calcium oxalate urolithiasis. In: Smith LH, Robertson WG, Finlayson B, eds. *Urolithiasis—clinical and related research.* New York: Plenum Publishing, 1981:731.
363. Westbury EJ. A chemist's view of the history of urinary stone analysis. *Br J Urol* 1989;64:445.
364. White DJ, Nancollas GH. Triamterene and renal stone formation. *J Urol* 1982;127:593.
365. Williams HE. Oxalic acid: absorption, excretion, and metabolism. In: Fleisch H, Robertson WG, Smith LH, et al., eds. *Urolithiasis research.* New York: Plenum Publishing, 1976:181.
366. Williams HE, Smith LH Jr. L-Glyceric aciduria. A new genetic variant of primary hyperoxaluria. *N Engl J Med* 1968;278:233.
367. Williams HE, Smith LH Jr. Primary hyperoxaluria. In: Stanbury JB, Wyngaarden JB, Fredrickson DS, eds. *The metabolic basis of inherited disease.* New York: McGraw-Hill, 1978:182.
368. Williams JJ, Rodman JS, Peterson CM. A randomized double-blind study of acetohydroxamic acid in struvite nephrolithiasis. *N Engl J Med* 1984;311:760.
369. Wilson DM. Clinical and laboratory approaches for evaluation of nephrolithiasis. *J Urol* 1989;141:770.
370. Wilson JM, Young AB, Kelley WN. Hypoxanthine-guanine phosphoribosyl transferase deficiency. *N Engl J Med* 1983; 309:900.
371. Wilson JWL, Werness PG, Smith LH. Effect of orthophosphate treatment on urine composition in idiopathic calcium urolithiasis. In: Schwille PO, Smith LH, Robertson WG, et al., eds. *Urolithiasis and related clinical research.* New York: Plenum Publishing, 1985:491.
372. Winter P, Hesse A, Klocke K, et al. Scanning electron microscopy of 2,8-dihydroxyadenine crystals and stones. *Scanning Microsc* 1993;7:1075.
373. Yendt ER. Medullary sponge kidney and nephrolithiasis. *N Engl J Med* 1982;306:1106.
374. Yendt ER, Cohanim M. Absorptive hyperoxaluria: a new clinical entity—successful treatment with hydrochlorothiazide. *Clin Invest Med* 1986;9:44.
375. Yendt ER, Cohanim M. Clinical and laboratory approaches for evaluation of nephrolithiasis. *J Urol* 1989;141:764.
376. Yendt ER, Cohanim M. The prevention of calcium stones with thiazides. In: Schwille PO, Smith LH, Robertson WG, et al., eds. *Urolithiasis and related clinical research.* New York: Plenum Publishing, 1985:463.
377. Yu TF, Berger L, Gutman AB. Defective conversion of uric acid to allantoin in the Dalmatian dog. *Arthritis Rheum* 1966;9:552.
378. Zechner O, Scheiber V. The role of affluence in recurrent stone formation. In: Smith LH, Robertson WG, Finlayson B, eds. *Urolithiasis—clinical and basic research.* New York: Plenum Publishing, 1981:309.
379. Zinsser HH, Seneca H, Light I, et al. Management of infected stones with acidifying agents. *N Y State J Med* 1968; 68:3001.

Adult and Pediatric Urology, 4/e, edited by Jay Y. Gillenwater, John T. Grayhack, Stuart S. Howards, and Michael E. Mitchell.
Lippincott Williams & Wilkins, Philadelphia © 2002

9

SURGICAL MANAGEMENT OF CALCULUS DISEASE

STEVAN B. STREEM
GLENN M. PREMINGER

The surgical management of urinary calculus disease has evolved considerably over the past two decades. Twenty years ago, open procedures for stones were some of the most frequently performed urologic operations. Since then, however, stone management has been at the forefront of "minimally invasive" intervention. Specifically, the introduction and refinement of percutaneous and ureteroscopic access to the upper tracts, along with the nearly simultaneous development of both extracorporeal and intracorporeal lithotripsy, has relegated the role of open surgery to less than 1% of patients undergoing intervention for their stone disease.

S.B. Streem: Urological Institute, The Cleveland Clinic Foundation, Cleveland, OH 44195.
G.M. Preminger: Division of Urologic Surgery, Duke University Medical Center, Durham, NC 27710.

This chapter reviews the indications to intervene for urinary calculi, the basic physics of the most frequently used devices for both extracorporeal and intracorporeal lithotripsy, and the respective roles of extracorporeal and intracorporeal lithotripsy with percutaneous or ureteroscopic access and open surgery. The results and complications associated with each of these forms of intervention are reviewed as well.

PATIENT EVALUATION

Radiographic Evaluation

A thorough radiologic evaluation is one of the most important aspects of the overall investigation of urinary stone disease. These studies are invaluable aids in assessing three major issues that must be addressed before selecting appropriate treatment: stone burden and location, urinary tract anatomy, and overall and ipsilateral renal function.

Plain Abdominal Radiography

More than 90% of stones within the urinary tract are radiopaque, and a plain film of the kidney, ureter, and bladder (KUB) is often the initial radiographic examination obtained in patients with nephrolithiasis. The KUB should be performed before any subsequent films that use contrast media because contrast may prevent the visualization of any calculi.

It is important not to overlook stones that may be obscured when they overlie bony structures, such as the sacrum or transverse processes of the lumbar vertebrae. These stones can be more easily identified using oblique views in addition to those obtained in the anteroposterior position. In addition, nephrotomograms can also be used to assist in the identification of small, less radiopaque calculi within the kidneys.

Intravenous Pyelography

An intravenous pyelogram (IVP) can be instrumental in defining the relationship of calculi to the pyelocalyceal system and ureter. The exact location of the stones, the presence or absence of obstruction, and renal or ureteral anomalies are important pieces of information that can be gleaned from the IVP. In addition, the IVP can approximate renal function in both the affected and the contralateral kidney as suggested by the promptness of contrast excretion, thickness of renal parenchyma, and amount of pyelocaliectasis. However, for more precise information on renal function, a differential renal scan should be obtained.

For patients with an apparent ureteral calculus, delayed films are obtained for as long as necessary to specifically identify their location and to prove their presence within the urinary tract. An IVP may also suggest the presence of radiolucent stones, and it may also identify anatomic abnormalities that contribute to stone formation such as a ureteropelvic junction obstruction or calyceal diverticula.

Renal Ultrasonography

Ultrasonography (US) can be used as a screening tool for hydronephrosis or stones within the collecting system. Additional information provided by sonographic examination of the kidneys includes an estimate of the amount of renal parenchyma present and identification of otherwise radiolucent calculi, because a classic "sonographic shadow" will often clearly identify stones that may not be visualized on standard plain films. However, the middle ureter and distal ureter are often not satisfactorily visualized on US due to the presence of bowel gas anteriorly and the bony pelvis posteriorly. US may also be useful in the acute setting to rule out other causes of abdominal pain and during follow-up of patients with recurrent nephrolithiasis because its use avoids x-ray exposure.

Computed Tomography

Computed tomography (CT) scanning is particularly useful in helping identify the etiology of otherwise radiolucent filling defects within the renal pelvis or ureter. In addition, obstruction, anatomic anomalies, or other urologic problems such as a vascular insult that can mimic ureteral colic can also be easily identified.

Nonenhanced spiral CT is currently the preferred diagnostic tool in the assessment of patients with acute flank pain (182). This technique is more sensitive than either simple radiography or US. All stones, with the exception of certain drug-related crystals, are visualized by this method, which is also fast and cost-effective. Moreover, other manifestations of obstruction, such as periureteric and perinephric stranding, and periureteric edema and hydronephrosis are easily identified (Fig. 9.1). Finally, spiral CT scan has the advantage of being able to definitively identify other causes of acute flank or abdominal pain such as appendicitis, diverticulitis, cholecystitis, or abdominal aneurysmal disease.

Radionuclide Evaluation

Renal radionuclide studies provide rapid and safe information about total and differential renal function. These tests are specifically advantageous because they are noninvasive, require no bowel or other specific preoperative preparation, subject the patient to only minimal radiation exposure, and are apparently free of allergic complications. A differential renal scan should be performed in those patients in whom an obstructing stone might have resulted in a permanent and significant reduction in renal function, because nephrectomy may be the procedure of choice for kidneys that, after relief of obstruction, will supply less than 10% to 15% of overall function.

THE ACUTE STONE EPISODE

Classic symptoms associated with an acutely obstructing urinary stone include colicky flank pain with or without nausea or vomiting. The pain may radiate anteriorly or even to the groin, ipsilateral testicle, or labia. Stones in the distal ureter may also result in frequency, urgency, and dysuria. If the obstruction is associated with infection, high-grade fever or even sepsis may ensue. If a patient demonstrates these classic findings and has a previous history of recurrent radiopaque nephrolithiasis, further studies are warranted to address the size and location of the stone to determine the appropriate course of treatment. Stones 4 mm or smaller in

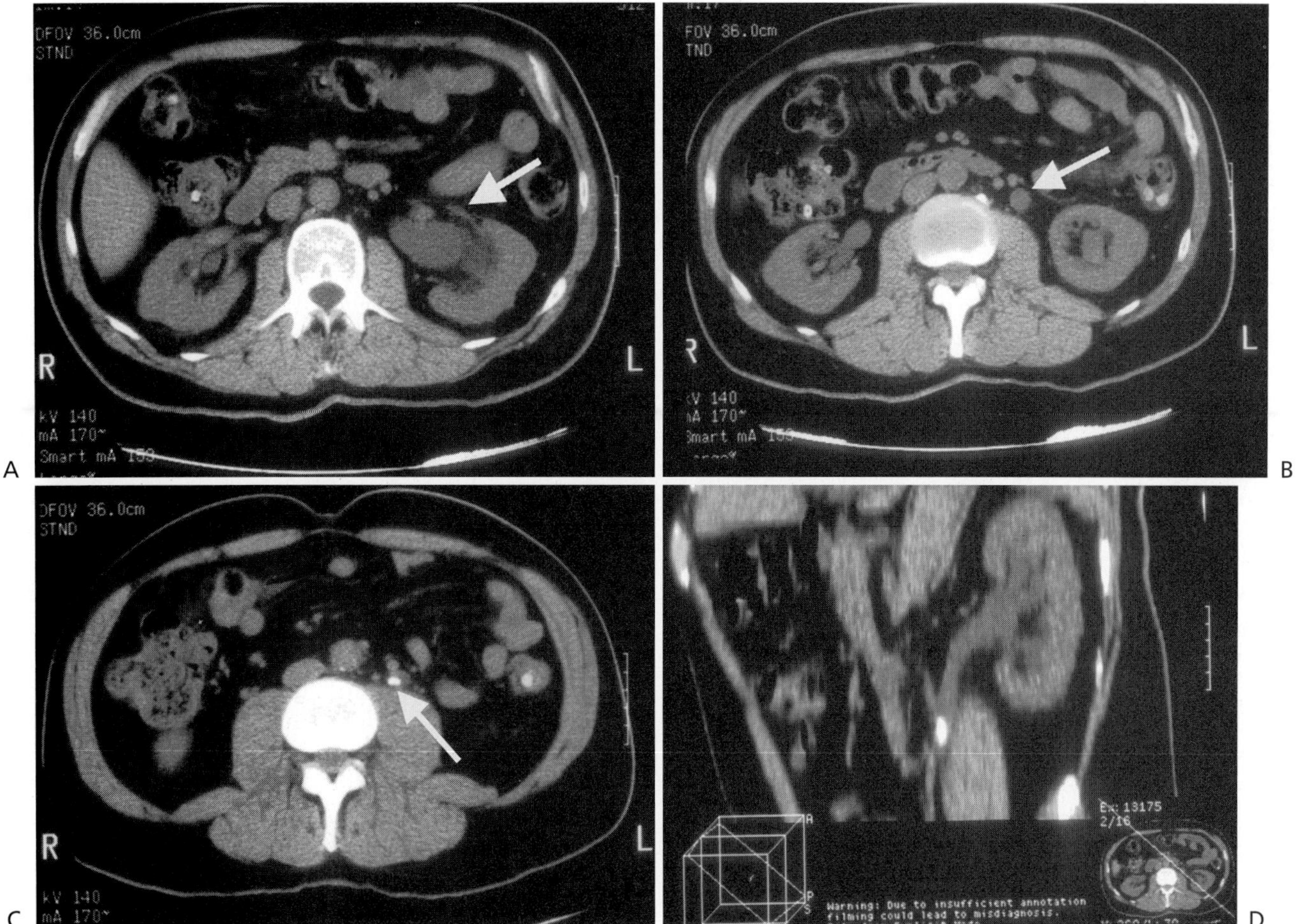

FIGURE 9.1. **A:** Dilation of left renal collecting system *(arrow)*. **B:** Dilated left ureter overlying psoas muscle *(arrow)*. **C:** Calculus in proximal ureter *(arrow)*. **D:** Reconstructed computed tomography imaging confirms partially obstructing proximal ureteral calculus.

largest diameter have a greater than 90% rate of spontaneous passage with conservative measures alone; however, stones 6 mm or larger have only a 10% rate of spontaneous passage (121).

For patients who lack classic symptoms and are experiencing their first stone episode or who are known to form radiolucent stones, either a nonenhanced spiral CT or an IVP should be performed. Sonography may be used to assess hydronephrosis and intrarenal calculi, but it may be especially insensitive for the diagnosis of ureteral stones.

If the patient is clinically stable and has no evidence of systemic infection, progressive obstruction, or obstruction of a solitary kidney, conservative management may be offered with pain medications alone such as nonsteroidal antiinflammatory drugs or narcotic analgesics. However, in the presence of obstruction with infection, unrelenting pain, or significantly compromised renal function, urinary drainage should be instituted on an emergent basis, either as ureteral stent placement or as percutaneous nephrostomy drainage.

INDICATIONS FOR INTERVENTION

Although the use of newer, less invasive modalities has become the standard of management for nearly all patients requiring intervention for stones, the indications to intervene have remained essentially unchanged. These include chronic or progressive obstruction from the stone; pain, infection, or hematuria associated with the stone; or active stone growth despite appropriate medical management (Table 9.1). In addition, even in the absence of an otherwise clear indication, stone removal should be considered for any "high-risk" patient, such as an airplane pilot, who cannot afford to experience an inopportune episode of renal colic.

TABLE 9.1. INDICATIONS FOR INTERVENTION

Chronic or progressive obstruction from the stone
Pain, infection, or hematuria associated with the stone
Active stone growth despite appropriate medical management

SHOCK WAVE LITHOTRIPSY

Since the first patient was successfully treated with shock wave lithotripsy (SWL) in 1980, rapid acceptance and widespread use have made this form of stone therapy the treatment of choice for more than 80% of all patients undergoing intervention for renal and ureteral calculi. Although the basic principles of SWL remain unchanged, a number of technologic advances and modifications in currently available lithotripters have significantly expanded the clinical applications of lithotripsy. The rapid acceptance and widespread application of SWL have also led to many advances in lithotripsy technology and have stimulated numerous studies to better understand the basic physics and the bioeffects of this modality.

Following the initial success of the first-generation lithotripter (Dornier HM-3), more than 20 different models of second-generation lithotripters were developed, utilizing various energy sources, focusing schemes, coupling media, and stone localization techniques (135,144). Moreover, several "third-generation" lithotripters, characterized by their dual imaging and variable power capabilities, have recently been developed and are either commercially available or undergoing clinical trials both in Europe and the United States (14,92,104,152). Although the fundamental principles of SWL remain unchanged, these advances in lithotripsy technologies have generally led to improved safety and, in some cases, improved cost-effectiveness of urolithiasis treatment.

Basic physics and animal studies performed in the past two decades have greatly advanced our understanding of the mechanisms of stone fragmentation, as well as tissue injury and renal functional alterations, induced by SWL. A basic understanding of the physical and biologic effects of high-intensity shock waves is important to ensure the safety and efficacy of SWL treatment. This knowledge is essential for the optimization of SWL technology to achieve maximal efficacy of stone fragmentation while minimizing adverse effects on renal tissue.

Not all stones are amenable to SWL, and clinical studies have demonstrated that the size and composition of the calculi, along with location and renal and ureteral anatomy, all significantly affect successful stone fragmentation and clearance. This section provides a critical review of our current understanding of SWL and offers insights into the future of this innovative technology.

Historical Aspects

Physicists at Dornier Systems, Ltd., and Friedrich Shafen, Germany, began experimenting with shock waves and their travel through water and tissue in 1963. Throughout the 1970s, numerous experimental lithotripters were developed that used new methods of transmitting shock waves, as well as different techniques of stone localization. In addition, experimental studies were being performed both *in vitro* and *in vivo* examining the effects of shock waves on various organs and tissues.

In 1980, Chaussy and associates successfully treated the first human patient, and they then reported their initial series of 72 patients in 1982 (25). Subsequently, nearly 2,000 articles have been published in the peer-reviewed literature detailing the use of SWL for the management of renal and ureteral calculi. Moreover, numerous second- and third-generation devices have been introduced and are currently being used throughout the world. Enhancements in these newer lithotripters may ultimately prove to facilitate stone fragmentation while reducing tissue injury.

Lithotripsy Design

All lithotripters share four main features: an energy source, a focusing device, a coupling medium, and a stone localization system (Table 9.2). The original Dornier HM-3 design uses a spark plug energy generator with an elliptical reflector for focusing the shock waves. A water bath transmits the shock waves to the patient with stone localization provided by biplanar fluoroscopy. Modification of the four basic components of this first-generation lithotripter has provided the development of second- and third-generation devices, of which more than ten machines are currently either available commercially or undergoing clinical trials (136).

Shock Wave Generation

All lithotripters share the four aforementioned features, but it is the mode of shock wave generation that determines the actual physical characteristics of that particular lithotripter. The objectives for using different types of energy sources include maximum efficacy (the overall stone-free rate) and maximum efficiency (cost-effectiveness, including need for secondary treatments). The two basic types of energy sources for generating shock waves are point sources and extended sources. The electrohydraulic machines use point sources for energy generation, whereas extended sources are incorporated into the piezoelectric and the electromagnetic devices.

Electrohydraulic Generators

The electrohydraulic generator is located at the base of a water bath and produces shock waves by an electric spark gap of 15,000 to 25,000 volts and 1 μs duration. This high-voltage spark discharge results in the rapid evaporation of water, which generates a shock wave by expanding the

TABLE 9.2. MAIN LITHOTRIPTER COMPONENTS

Shock wave generator	Coupling medium
Shock wave focusing	Stone localization

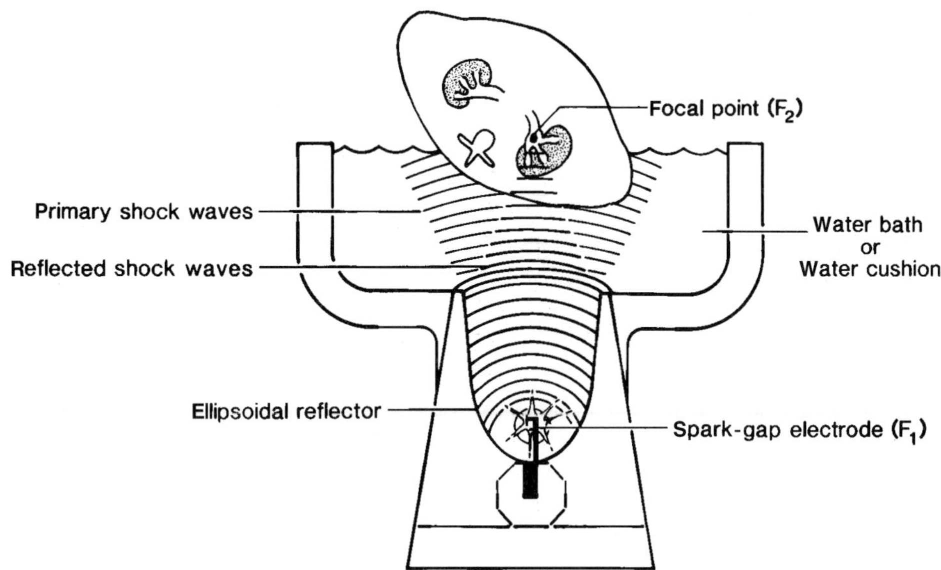

FIGURE 9.2. Schematic of electrohydraulic shock wave generator.

surrounding fluid. The spark plug is located in an ellipsoidal reflector that concentrates the reflected shock waves at a second focal point, F_2, with F_1 being the origin of the primary shock waves (Fig. 9.2). The spark-gap method of shock wave generation was pioneered by the first-generation Dornier HM-3 lithotripter and is also used in the Direx, Medstone, Northgate, and Technomed machines, among others.

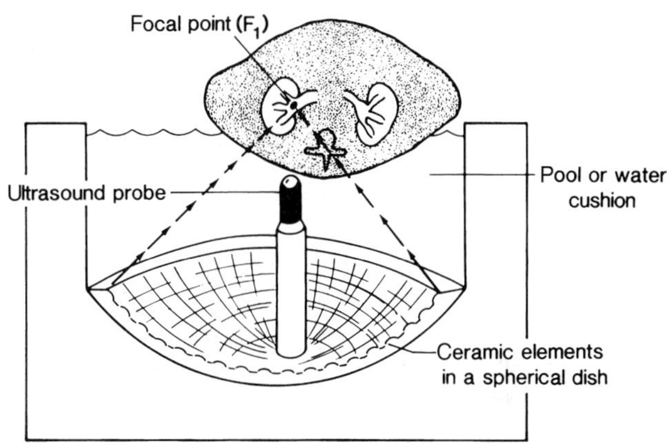

FIGURE 9.3. Schematic of piezoelectric shock wave generator.

Piezoelectric Generators

Piezoelectric shock waves are generated by the sudden expansion of ceramic elements excited by a high-frequency, high-voltage pulse. Thousands of these tiny elements are placed along the inner surface of a hemisphere at the base of a pool of water. Although each of these ceramic elements moves only slightly in response to a pulse of electrical energy, the summation of the simultaneous expansion of multiple elements results in a high-energy shock wave directed to the focal point at the center of the sphere. The shock wave is propagated through either a small water basin or a water-filled bag to the focal point, F_1 (Fig. 9.3). The spherical focusing mechanism of the piezoelectric lithotripters provides a wide point of shock wave entry at the skin surface and a very small focal point.

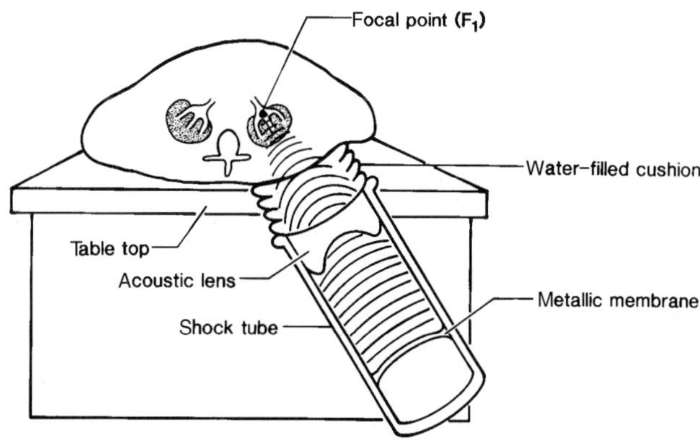

FIGURE 9.4. Schematic of electromagnetic shock wave generator.

Electromagnetic Generators

In electromagnetic devices, shock waves are generated when an electrical impulse moves a thin, circular metallic membrane, which is housed within a cylindric "shock tube." The resulting shock wave, produced in the water-filled shock tube, passes through an acoustic lens and is thereby directed to the focal point, F_1 (Fig. 9.4). The shock wave is coupled to the body surface with a moveable water cushion and coupling gel.

Shock Wave Focusing

Shock waves must be focused to concentrate their energy on a target such as a calculus. The type of shock wave generation dictates the method of focusing used. Machines that use point sources, such as spark-gap electrodes, generate shock waves that travel in an expanding circular pattern. All of these machines use ellipsoid reflectors for focusing the shock waves at the second focal point, F_2.

Because a single piezoelectric element produces a very small amount of energy, larger transducers with multiple ceramic elements are required for piezoelectric lithotripters. The array of ceramic elements is positioned in a spherical dish that allows focusing in a very small focal region, F_1. The vibrating metal membranes of the electromechanical lithotripters produce an acoustic plane wave that uses an acoustic lens for focusing the shock wave at F_1.

Coupling Medium

The original Dornier HM-3 machine uses a 1,000-L water bath to transmit the shock waves to the patient. This method of coupling requires unique positioning of the patient, because the anesthetized subject has to be lowered into the tub and the calculus accurately positioned at the second focal point. Remote monitoring and the physiologic effects of almost total body immersion thus produced unique challenges for the anesthesiologist. Second-generation lithotripters were designed to alleviate the physiologic, functional, and economic problems of the large water bath, and current models use an enclosed water cushion, or a totally contained shock tube, to allow simplified positioning and "dry" lithotripsy.

Stone Localization

Stone localization during lithotripsy is accomplished with either fluoroscopy or US. Fluoroscopy provides the urologist with a familiar modality and has the added benefits of effective ureteral stone localization. Moreover, fluoroscopy allows the use of contrast material to help delineate the anatomy of the collecting system. However, fluoroscopy requires more space, carries the inherent risk of ionizing radiation to both the patient and medical staff, and is not useful, without adjunctive contrast injection, in localizing radiolucent calculi.

Sonography-based lithotripters offer the advantages of stone localization with continuous monitoring and effective identification of even radiolucent stones, without radiation exposure (135). In addition, US has been documented to be effective in localizing stone fragments as small as 2 to 3 mm and is as good as or better than routine KUB to assess patients for residual stone fragments following lithotripsy (1). The major disadvantages of US stone localization include the basic mastery of the use of ultrasonic techniques by the urologist and difficulty in localizing minimally obstructing or nonobstructing ureteral stones.

Anesthesia Requirements

Three factors contribute to the need for anesthesia during SWL: shock wave pressure (power), area of the shock wave at its skin entry site, and size of the shock wave focal point. The intensity of the shock wave is determined by the type of generator used and the amount of power (usually electrical charge) supplied to the shock wave generator. The original electrohydraulic design delivers the most powerful shock waves but also causes the greatest amount of discomfort for the patient. Therefore either general, regional, or local anesthesia is used in the original spark-gap machines. Recent studies have demonstrated the ability to reduce anesthesia requirements with the first-generation electrohydraulic devices (123).

The size of the focal point and the area of shock wave entry at the skin are both determined by the configuration of the focusing device (Fig. 9.5). The increased area of skin entry and diminished focal size have lessened the need for general or regional anesthesia in patients treated with second- or third-generation lithotripters. Currently, variable-power electrohydraulic lithotripters provide the advantage of a wide range of shock wave intensities to allow for either a reduction in anesthesia requirements or increased fragmentation efficacy with higher power under general or regional anesthesia. Using the lower power setting, however, causes the overall stone-free rate to decrease, while increasing the number of shocks required per treatment and the re-treatment rate. Therefore, to achieve an anesthesia-free status, one must expect the number of secondary treatments to increase. Therefore the efficiency of that lithotripter will be diminished.

Shock waves generated by a piezoelectric source tend to be less powerful than those from an electrohydraulic source. This leads to a higher re-treatment rate, but when combined with other design modifications, it allows treatment of stones without anesthesia (135). The wide aperture of the focusing sphere, the larger skin entry zone, and the small focal point combined with lower peak pressures make piezoelectric machines truly anesthesia free.

Design characteristics of the electromechanical lithotripters tend to place them between the other two machine types in terms of anesthesia requirements. The electromagnetic devices have a relatively small skin entry site and a large focal area. Electromagnetic lithotripsy is usually performed with intravenous or oral sedation, with or without the use of local anesthesia at the skin entry site. A transcutaneous electrical nerve stimulator may provide adequate analgesia during lithotripsy with electromagnetic lithotripsy (31).

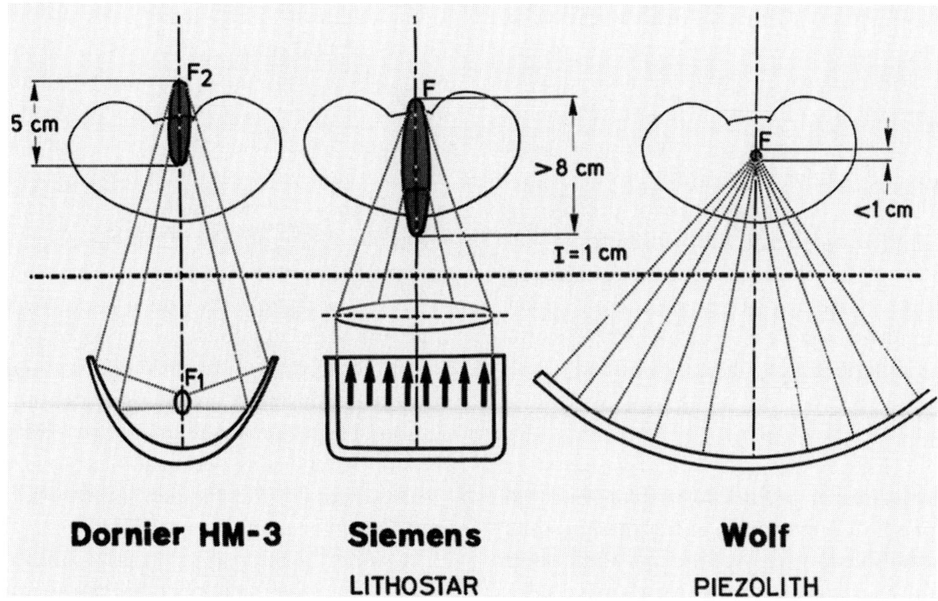

FIGURE 9.5. Configuration of focal regions for three types of shock wave generators.

Indications and Contraindications

Indications for SWL in urinary tract stone management are the same as the indications for surgical intervention. These include renal colic or chronic pain, urinary obstruction, infection, or decreasing renal function. Relative contraindications to SWL include large stone size (i.e., calcium oxalate stones greater than 2.5 cm in diameter or struvite stones greater than 5.0 cm in diameter), most cystine stones, active infection, proximate calcified abdominal aortic or renal artery aneurysms, distal obstruction, pregnancy, and poorly informed patients (167) (Table 9.3).

Results: Clinical Considerations

Efficiency Quotient

The determination of lithotripter efficiency with regard to adequate stone fragmentation requires a delicate balance between the completeness of stone fragmentation and the need for anesthesia or analgesia. As the shock wave intensity is decreased to allow for "anesthesia-free" lithotripsy, the ability to adequately fragment stones is also reduced, thereby decreasing lithotripter efficiency. Diminished efficiency can be seen as an increase in the number of treatments needed to render a patient stone free or as an increased need for auxiliary procedures before or following lithotripsy. Auxiliary procedures would include placement of a percutaneous nephrostomy tube, formal percutaneous nephrostolithotomy, ureteropyeloscopy, or placement of a ureteral stent.

An "efficiency quotient" can be calculated by determining the stone-free rate obtained by various lithotripters in relation to the need for repeat lithotripsy, as well as the number of auxiliary procedures performed to render patients stone free (40). Using this efficiency quotient, one can make more valid comparisons between different types of first- and later-generation lithotripters.

Reports for many second-generation lithotripters have revealed stone-free rates similar to those obtained from the original electrohydraulic lithotripsy devices. If one also considers the need for repeat lithotripsy as well as the number of auxiliary procedures performed, however, the efficiency quotients of the lower-power, second-generation devices and the original electrohydraulic machines might not be equivalent. The efficiency quotient offers the urologist a more reliable gauge for comparing the effectiveness of individual lithotripters than does the stone-free rate alone (144).

With their higher re-treatment rate, second-generation lithotripters increase the time commitment necessary for both patient and treating physician. However, the decrease in stone fragmentation efficiency may be compensated by the fact that many of the second-generation devices allow

TABLE 9.3. RELATIVE CONTRAINDICATIONS TO SHOCK WAVE LITHOTRIPSY

Large stone	Active infection
Calcium oxalate >1.5 cm	Proximate calcified abnormal aortic or renal artery aneurysm
Struvite >3 cm	Pregnancy
Significant dilation of collecting system	Poorly informed patient
Distal ureteral obstruction	
Untreated coagulopathy	

for office-based lithotripsy and require no hospitalization or intravenous lines, no anesthesia or analgesia, and no recovery room charges. Therefore some physicians and patients may accept the inconvenience of multiple repeat treatments if the safety and ease of operation of the second-generation machines outweighs the disadvantage of diminished lithotripsy "efficiency." In fact, it is probably not possible to have true anesthesia-free capability with a lithotripsy device that rates high on an efficiency quotient scale. To achieve anesthesia-free status, one has to expect the number of secondary treatments to increase, and therefore the efficiency quotient of that lithotripter will be diminished.

"Small" Calculi

The first-generation Dornier HM-3 represents the gold standard in terms of efficacy (overall stone-free rate) in stone fragmentation. As the shock wave pressure and focal point area of second- and third-generation machines have been reduced, so has the requirement for anesthesia or analgesia. However, the price paid for anesthesia-free lithotripsy is an increase in the secondary treatment rates and a subsequent reduction in efficiency. Although there is a compromise in efficiency with the piezoelectric lithotripters, the decreased efficiency may be balanced by the fact that each treatment can be performed as an "office" procedure, without anesthesia or analgesia. Electromagnetic lithotripsy, usually performed with intravenous or oral sedation, has been found to require a mean of approximately 3,600 shock waves per treatment, with stone-free rates of 69% to 80% and retreatment rates of 7% to 21%.

"Large" Calculi

With increased stone volume, the efficacy of all lithotripters decreases significantly. With a Dornier HM-3, the stone-free rate may be as low as 30% for patients with a dilated collecting system and a stone or group of stones with total volume greater than 3 cm (105). Although the stone-free rate for large calculi is approximately 70% for patients with normal collecting system anatomy, many clinicians advocate the use of percutaneous nephrolithotripsy as the initial form of therapy in this setting (120,158).

In some situations, the combination of percutaneous nephrolithotripsy and SWL can be more effective than SWL alone. With this type of combination therapy, stone-free rates approaching 85% to 90% have been reported, even for large calculi (168).

Stone Location

Stone location in the collecting system is another important determinant of the outcome of SWL. Treatment of renal pelvic and upper ureteral stones may result in stone-free rates of 85% to 92% (91). In contrast, stone-free rates for patients with lower calyceal calculi are less than 60%, compared with 75% to 80% for those with middle and upper calyceal stones (106). Recent studies have also documented the importance of lower pole renal anatomy and its impact on stone clearance following SWL (49).

Stone-free rates of 65% to 70% for lower ureteral calculi (below the pelvic brim) have been achieved through various modifications in patient positioning and lithotripter design. However, ureteroscopy for the management of calculi in a similar location is successful in 95% to 100% of patients, and ureteroscopic extraction is now generally considered the first line of therapy for stones in the distal ureter (190).

Stones in calyceal diverticula have long been a source of treatment controversy. SWL provides improvement or resolution of symptoms in many patients but is generally unsuccessful in rendering such patients stone free. Percutaneous management of these stones, by contrast, produces significantly higher stone-free rates (12,87). These data suggest that stones in calyceal diverticula should be managed with SWL only when specific criteria regarding stone size and diverticular emptying are met (169).

Stone Composition

As the stone composition varies, so does the efficacy of SWL. "Harder" stones such as calcium oxalate monohydrate and cystine require an increased number of shock waves at higher intensity levels to achieve adequate fragmentation. Even at these higher settings, however, results with cystine calculi have been inferior to those with calcium oxalate stones (30). Most investigators advocate the use of percutaneous or "combination" therapy for large cystine calculi (27).

Auxiliary Procedures

Another area of controversy has been the efficacy of, and indications for, the use of ureteral stenting before SWL. Although some reports advocate the liberal use of ureteral stents before lithotripsy, the benefits of anesthesia-free lithotripsy would be diminished if an anesthetic or analgesia were required for stent placement. In fact, a recent clinical series evaluating the use of ureteral stents with lithotripsy found no improvement in stone-free rates or postlithotripsy complications in patients with ureteral stents. However, use of stents was associated with a significantly higher incidence of patient morbidity, including discomfort, frequency, urgency, and hematuria (109,137). Urologists generally exercise their own judgment regarding the merit of ureteral stenting in individual patients, and patients with large calculi or those requiring general or regional anesthesia for lithotripsy are more likely to undergo stent placement.

Current Lithotripters: Limitations

In the two decades since the first clinical application of SWL by Chaussy and associates (25), technical refinements have produced more than 15 second- and third-generation devices. These designs have concentrated on altering the methods of shock wave generation, focusing, coupling, and localization, with the primary goal of equaling the stone-free rate of the Dornier HM-3 while increasing the safety, convenience, and cost-effectiveness of treatment. The new devices are designed to offer equivalent or better stone fragmentation, to decrease or eliminate anesthesia requirements, and to decrease radiation exposure from x-rays. Despite great technical progress, however, these new machines still have important shortcomings.

In general, second-generation lithotripters can be divided into a higher-power electrohydraulic and electromagnetic group and a lower-power piezoelectric group. Disadvantages of the first group include pain and attendant anesthesia requirements and as yet poorly quantified renal tissue damage. Disadvantages of the second group include a small focal size of the shock wave, with the need for a greater total number of shock waves, and a higher retreatment rate.

The apertures of the electrohydraulic and electromechanical lithotripters are relatively small, leading to a smaller skin entry site and larger focal zone. This creates the need for general or regional anesthesia or heavy intravenous sedation. The larger aperture of the treatment dish of the piezoelectric lithotripters results in a large area of skin entry and a small focal zone. The discomfort produced by treatments with these machines is minimal enough to allow for anesthesia-free lithotripsy (135).

The relatively large focal region of electrohydraulic lithotripters exposes a larger amount of normal renal tissue to maximal shock wave pressures, and both animal and clinical studies have demonstrated more acute renal parenchymal injury from electrohydraulic and electromagnetic lithotripters when compared with piezoelectric units. However, one drawback of the small focal region in the piezoelectric machines is that it mandates constant monitoring of the effects of treatment on the targeted calculus. Accurate focusing of the shock wave is mandatory, because there is a rapid dropoff in pressure outside the small focal zone. The requirement of exact focusing is not necessary with the electrohydraulic or electromagnetic machines, which have a much larger area of maximal shock wave energy. As noted previously, for the advantage gained by performing anesthesia-free lithotripsy, one loses efficiency of stone fragmentation. Currently, it appears that it is not possible to have true anesthesia-free capabilities with a very "efficient" lithotripter.

Additional limitations of current lithotripsy devices relate to the method of stone localization. Although lithotripters using fluoroscopy can visualize the entire urinary system, they have the disadvantage of exposing the patient to a significant amount of radiation. In addition, it is often difficult, if not impossible, to identify small calculi within the kidney or ureter, or any radiolucent stones without the aid of contrast injection.

The devices that use sonography for stone localization potentially can be used for both renal and biliary lithotripsy, and they pose no risk of radiation exposure. Their main disadvantage is that they offer poor visualization of middle and lower ureteral stones. Efforts to develop echogenic ureteral stents, as well as new modes of sonography to aid in ureteral stone localization, are now in progress.

The Ideal Lithotripter

SWL can be used effectively to treat most renal and ureteral calculi with minimal morbidity and convalescence. Research in lithotripter design is ongoing, however, with attempts to improve performance and ultimately to design the "ideal lithotripter." Such a device should be physically compact and portable, thereby allowing a lithotripter to be transported or shared between smaller institutions. In fact, a number of mobile lithotripsy units are currently in operation. The ideal lithotripter should also be adaptable for other endourologic procedures, as well as for biliary lithotripsy. Many of the current machines that use fluoroscopic stone localization can be used for percutaneous or ureteroscopic stone removal, and the US-based machines can easily be used for both urinary and biliary calculi.

By having an adjustable energy source, the ideal lithotripter would allow for anesthesia-free treatment of smaller or "routine" calculi, yet would have the potential power required to fragment either very hard or large renal or ureteral stones. This capability would allow for effective and efficient lithotripsy treatments, with the knowledge that in some cases, sedation or anesthesia must be administered to allow the use of the more powerful shock wave energy.

Finally, the ideal lithotripter should be economical to install and operate. This would entail minimal site renovations before installation of the lithotripter and little or no daily operating costs once the machine is on-line and running.

New-generation Lithotripters

A number of new-generation lithotripters have incorporated many of the characteristics of the ideal lithotripter (28). The basic design of these third-generation machines includes dual imaging capabilities, as well as variable shock wave power (Table 9.4). Currently, a number of third-generation lithotripters are currently in use across the globe. These include the Dornier MFL 5000 (HM5), Dornier Compact S, Siemens Lithostar Plus, Storz Modu-

TABLE 9.4. NEW-GENERATION LITHOTRIPTERS

Dual imaging	Ultrasonography
Fluoroscopy	Variable power

lith SL20 and SLX, and Wolf Piezolith 2500 (77,93,107, 118,138,177).

Dual Imaging

Dual imaging capability entails having both fluoroscopic and sonographic localization systems available in the same machine. Such a design has the advantage of using fluoroscopy for imaging stones within the kidney and the ureter, while having the option to use sonography for the identification of radiolucent renal or biliary calculi. Another advantage of a sonographic localization system is that it allows the operator to target a stone using fluoroscopy initially, and then to switch to sonography to avoid excessive use of ionizing radiation.

Interestingly, while the Dornier, Siemens, and Storz machines have all added US capabilities to provide dual imaging, none of these systems provides "in-line" imaging for both the fluoroscopic and sonographic localization devices. For example, with the Dornier and Siemens devices, one can use sonography to target a radiolucent or biliary tract calculus, yet the patient must be moved "blindly" to the fluoroscopy unit, which is in line with the shock wave generator. Alternatively, one can use the fluoroscopic localization system with the Storz machine, yet only the US is in line with the shock wave generator. The Wolf Piezolith 2500 is currently the only third-generation device that has both fluoroscopy and sonography in line with the piezoelectric shock wave generator (Fig. 9.6). This permits rapidly changing from fluoroscopic to sonographic stone localization, without moving the patient off the treatment dish.

Variable Power

All of the third-generation devices discussed here have variable-power shock wave generators. This capability allows the shock wave energy to be tailored to the requirements of a particular stone. The operator can turn down the generator power to provide significantly reduced anesthesia and analgesia requirements with the Dornier, Siemens, and Storz machines, as well as to provide totally anesthesia- and analgesia-free lithotripsy with the Wolf device. Moreover, the shock wave intensity can be increased with all these machines to allow adequate fragmentation of extremely hard or large calculi. However, when used in the high-power mode, these lithotripters will require some form of anesthesia or analgesia.

The ideal shock wave machine that allows anesthesia-free lithotripsy with maximum efficiency has yet to be developed. However, by varying the shock wave energy, a highly efficient shock wave can be administered, with the understanding that anesthesia or analgesia will be required when high shock wave pressures are used. Alternatively, with a

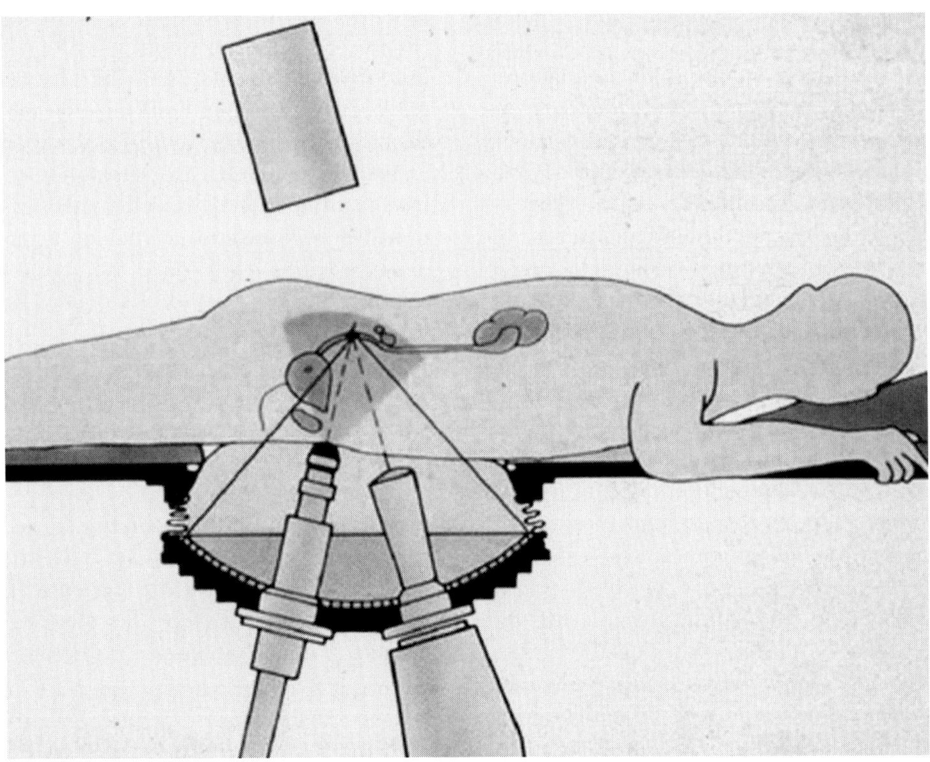

FIGURE 9.6. Illustration of dual imaging capabilities (fluoroscopy and ultrasonography) in newer-generation lithotripters.

small or fragile stone, the shock wave energy can be significantly decreased to allow the use of minimal analgesia or even anesthesia-free lithotripsy. With the availability of variable-powered lithotripters that use electrohydraulic, electromagnetic, or piezoelectric energy sources, urologists must continue to monitor the amount of energy delivered to limit the incidence of potentially significant renal injury.

Conclusions

SWL has revolutionized the treatment of urinary calculi, and this technology can be considered the treatment of choice for almost any renal calculus smaller than 2 cm and for most nonimpacted ureteral calculi. Under these circumstances, stone-free rates approaching 90% can be expected, although for larger renal stones or impacted ureteral calculi, endoscopic technique should probably be considered first-line therapy.

Whereas the original lithotripter design requires general anesthesia, requires a 1,000-L water bath, and subjects patients to fairly high doses of ionizing radiation, second-generation devices incorporate technical refinements that increase the safety and convenience of this procedure. Although a decrease in shock wave pressure and focal point size has diminished or eliminated anesthesia requirements, this development has been associated with a rise in the re-treatment rate. An efficiency quotient can be used to compare the relative benefits and disadvantages of various second-generation machines. Current lithotripters do not seem to have the ability to rate high on the efficiency quotient scale while still maintaining anesthesia-free capabilities. Third-generation machines, however, with modifications to allow variable shock wave power and dual imaging capabilities, may represent a step toward achieving this goal. As research continues and new devices become adaptable to multiple tasks, we will come closer to making the "ideal lithotripter" a reality.

In the past decade, significant progress has also been made in the realm of basic SWL physics research. The majority of this effort has been devoted to further characterization and better understanding of the dynamics of cavitation bubbles induced by SWL, as well as the role of cavitation in both stone fragmentation and tissue injury. There is now increasing evidence to suggest that appropriate control of cavitation during SWL can lead to significantly improved stone fragmentation or reduced tissue injury, and this topic should be a major focus of SWL research in the near future. In addition, several new competing mechanisms of tissue injury have been proposed, and their validity will be tested by carefully designed experiments both *in vitro* and *in vivo*. For improved SWL therapy, it is also important to understand the stress wave propagation and the corresponding dynamic fatigue process of both stones and tissue during SWL. Knowledge gained from SWL basic research will become indispensable for the improvement of SWL technology and for the design of better clinical treatment protocols for SWL.

PERCUTANEOUS STONE EXTRACTION

Historical Aspects

Rupel and Brown (151) used an operatively established nephrostomy tract to extract an obstructing renal calculus in 1941. Nearly 15 years later, Goodwin and associates (63) reported the use of percutaneous nephrostomy drainage to provide relief of obstruction and infection. However, removal of a renal calculus via a percutaneous tract established specifically for that purpose was not performed until Fernstrom and Johansson (54) used such a technique successfully in three patients 20 years later. Subsequently, safe and effective means to fragment even large calculi were introduced, and percutaneous stone extraction gained acceptance as the procedure of choice for management of most patients with upper tract calculi in the late 1970s and early 1980s. As such, during that era, any patient who would have otherwise required open stone extraction was instead considered a potential candidate for percutaneous management, and the indications for this procedure were essentially identical to the indications to intervene for any stone.

Contemporary Indications and Contraindications

SWL has significantly affected the general indications for percutaneous stone management. These indications are now well defined and are nearly identical to the contraindications to SWL. As such, most of these indications are more relative than absolute. As the twenty-first century begins, the indications for percutaneous management of upper tract calculi include unusual body habitus precluding SWL, obstruction distal to the stone, cystine stones, stones associated with upper tract foreign bodies, and large or otherwise complex stones. Relative indications for percutaneous management rather than SWL may include the presence of an implanted cardiac pacemaker or defibrillator and a proximate calcified aortic or renal artery aneurysm. Another important indication for percutaneous management is failure of SWL. Currently, the only absolute contraindication to percutaneous stone extraction is an irreversible coagulopathy.

In 1987, Leroy and associates (103) at the Mayo Clinic reported a contemporary experience with percutaneous stone management in the era of SWL. During 1 year at their tertiary care center, 854 patients were managed with SWL while 143 with renal or upper ureteral calculi were managed percutaneously. In regard to their current indications and results for percutaneous management, the authors concluded that despite the increased complexity of patients undergoing percutaneous management, excellent results could still be achieved with acceptably low morbidity.

Patient Preparation

As with any intervention, the patient should be apprised of the potential risks and benefits of percutaneous lithotomy as compared with the applicable alternatives. In these often complex cases, this should include the risks of requiring secondary intervention, transfusion of blood products, infection, or rarely, emergent open operative intervention. Although complications can occur, most patients will ultimately benefit from a percutaneous procedure by experiencing a relatively short hospital stay and period of convalescence, especially compared with open operative intervention (17,19,20,139).

Standard preoperative preparation includes assurance of the availability of blood for possible transfusion with a blood type and screen, although formal crossmatching is generally not necessary. Patients with urinary tract infection are treated for approximately 1 week with sensitivity-specific antibiotics on an outpatient basis and are then intravenously "on call" to the procedure. The need for prophylactic antibiotic in the face of a sterile urine is unproven (24), although we generally use a "short course" protocol in this setting that consists of a first-generation cephalosporin given just before percutaneous access and continued for 24 hours following stone extraction.

Technique

The exact technique of percutaneous stone extraction used is specific to the size, location, configuration, and presumed composition of the stone. However, the procedure is always performed with the same four sequential steps: establishment of percutaneous access, dilation of the tract, stone manipulation with fragmentation and extraction, and post-extraction drainage and tamponade of the tract. Techniques of percutaneous access are addressed elsewhere in this volume. As such, the percutaneous procedures described herein start with the assumption that access has been established.

The patient is in a prone or slightly oblique position with the ipsilateral side elevated to approximately 20 degrees (Fig. 9.7). For patients with rotational anomalies such as horseshoe kidneys, the contralateral side is elevated instead to allow a more medial rotation of the otherwise anteriorly projected renal pelvis. This allows the posterior infundibula and calices to project more laterally, thus fluoroscopically simulating a more orthotopic position of the kidney. At this point, before percutaneous stone manipulation, a second wire should be placed as a safety wire using a 9- or 10-Fr introducer set. Over the remaining "working" wire, the tract is dilated to 30 Fr using either sequential fascial dilators or, preferably, a 10-Fr, 12-cm balloon over which is back-loaded a 30-Fr working sheath (Fig. 9.8). At this point, then, a 30-Fr working sheath will be in place with a safety wire alongside.

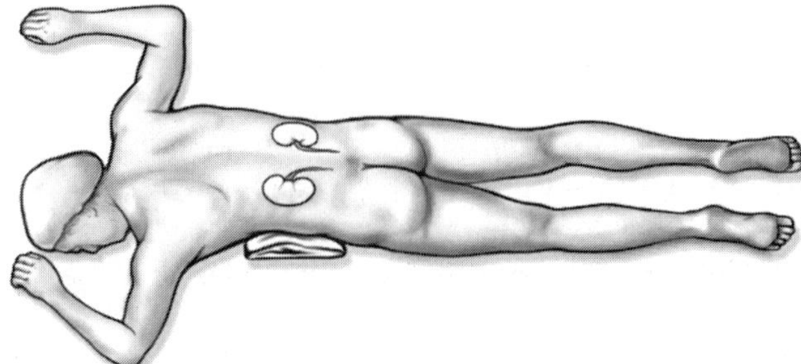

FIGURE 9.7. A prone-oblique position is standard for percutaneous procedures.

Stone extraction itself can be accomplished with a variety of techniques using direct vision through a nephroscope along with fluoroscopic guidance. At most centers, percutaneous stone extraction is accomplished using ultrasonic lithotripsy guided by direct vision through a rigid nephroscope. This approach was first described by Alken and colleagues (2) in Germany and Marberger and colleagues (115) in Austria, and it was subsequently popularized in the United States by Segura and associates at the Mayo Clinic (159) and Clayman and associates at the University of Minnesota (32).

The nephroscope is readied by attaching the light, suction, and irrigation, and it is then inserted through the working sheath. Once proper positioning in the pyelocalyceal system is ensured, the working wire, which is still within the sheath, is removed, taking care to keep a safety wire in place alongside the sheath. The irrigant of choice for percutaneous nephroscopy is normal saline. This prevents

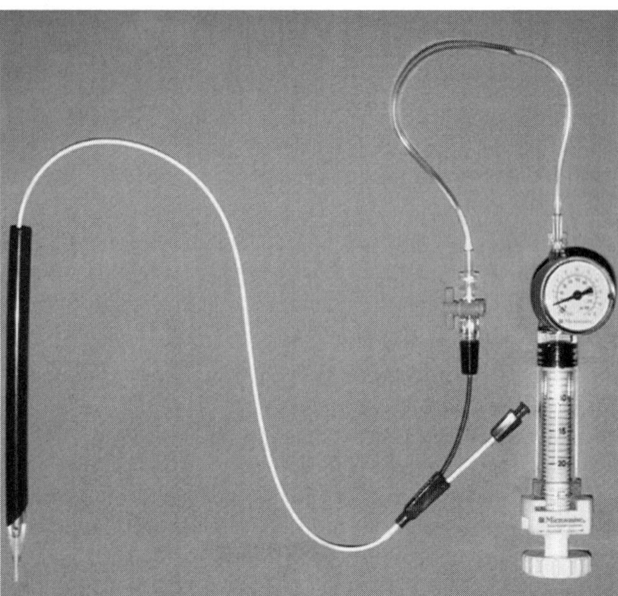

FIGURE 9.8. A 30-Fr working sheath back-loaded over a 10-Fr, 12-cm balloon dilator.

the possibility of hyponatremia that might result from intravascular absorption if hyposmotic solutions are used (155). At the outset of nephroscopy, vision may be obscured by blood clots, which are easily evacuated by adjusting the irrigation and suction from the nephroscope sheath or by using suction through the US wand while ultrasonic energy is being applied to the clot.

Stones with a smallest diameter less than 9 or 10 mm are small enough to extract intact through an appropriate-size working sheath. Such stones are simply grasped under direct vision using rigid graspers or endoscopic forceps passed via the working port of the nephroscope (Fig. 9.9). However, most stones managed percutaneously are too large to be extracted intact, and intracorporeal lithotripsy will be required. The most commonly used modality for this has been ultrasonic lithotripsy (33). The US wand (Sonotrode) with its own suction attachment is introduced via the working channel of a rigid nephroscope (Fig. 9.10). Under direct vision, the tip of the Sonotrode is pressed against the stone while suction is applied through the hollow Sonotrode, holding the stone in place. This allows the stone pieces to be evacuated via the Sonotrode as fragmentation proceeds. Fragments that are too large to pass through the Sonotrode, but now measure less than 9 mm, are easily extracted using grasping techniques via the nephroscope under direct vision, bringing the pieces out through the working sheath that remains in place. The process of ultrasonic fragmentation with suctioning of fragments or forceps extraction continues until all visible stone has been removed.

Although ultrasonic lithotripsy can reliably fragment most stones, some stones are physically too hard to fragment with this modality. For the most part, this includes large calcium oxalate monohydrate stones, which often appear extremely dense and homogenous on plain radiographs, and some mixed calcium oxalate–uric acid stones. In such patients, intracorporeal lithotripsy can be performed effectively with several alternative modalities, including electrohydraulic lithotripsy (EHL), which has proven both safe and effective in this setting (116,141). The EHL probe is passed through the working port of the nephroscope under direct vision, and the stone is fragmented into smaller pieces, which are individually grasped and removed, or further fragmented and suctioned out with a US wand. Newer, even more contemporary alternatives to both electrohydraulic lithotripsy and ultrasonic lithotripsy include the holmium

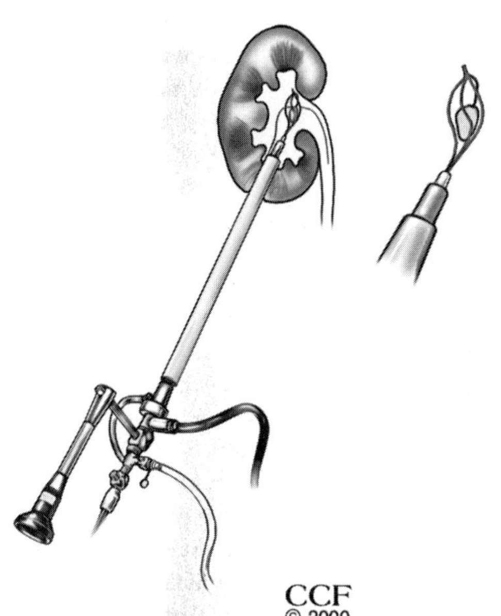

FIGURE 9.9. Small stones—those less than 10 mm—can often be extracted intact using graspers or baskets passed via the working port of the nephroscope under direct vision.

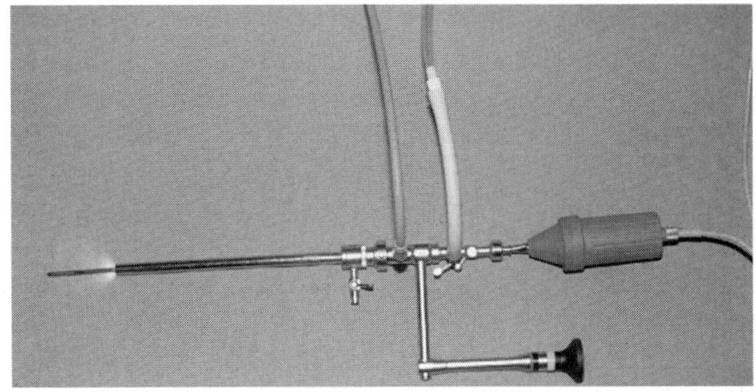

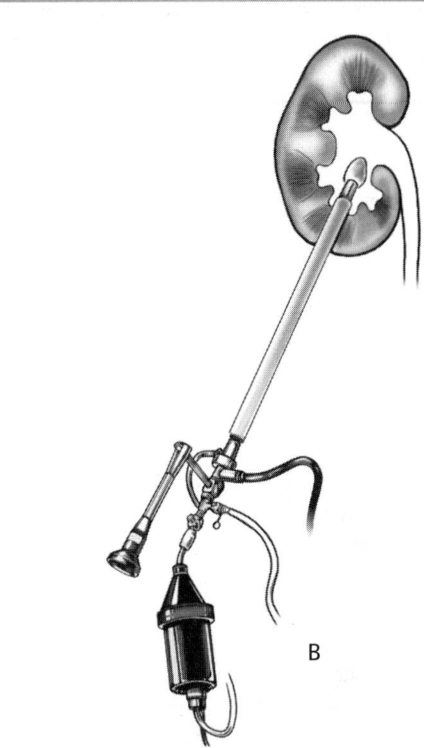

FIGURE 9.10. **A:** Rigid nephroscope with offset lens allows passage of a rigid Sonotrode. **B:** The nephroscope and ultrasound wand are placed through the working sheath. The ultrasound wand is abutted against the stone and ultrasonic energy applied, with simultaneous suction of fragments through the hollow Sonotrode.

laser (175) and variations of electromechanical lithotripsy such as the Lithoclast (41).

For infundibular or calyceal calculi lying at acute angles to the percutaneous tract, visualization, fragmentation, and extraction often require flexible nephroscopy (101,146). Although flexible nephroscopy can be successful when used during the initial percutaneous procedure, even a moderate amount of bleeding may obscure vision. As such, flexible nephroscopy will often be even more successful when performed via a mature tract. In either case, a working sheath is again in place and the flexible nephroscope is passed through this under direct vision (Fig. 9.11). Fluoroscopic guidance is even more important during flexible nephroscopy than rigid nephroscopy to ensure proper orientation. When the stone is visualized, a grasping forceps, prongs, or basket can be passed through the working port of the flexible scope and the stone engaged and withdrawn intact. Alternatively, larger stones can be fragmented with either the holmium laser or EHL, both of which allow intracorporeal lithotripsy via these flexible instruments.

When visual and radiographic control ensure that all accessible stone has been extracted, nephrostomy drainage is instituted. Our preference is to pass a 24-Fr nephrostomy tube through the working sheath and position it fluoroscopically with its tip in the renal pelvis, at which time the working sheath is removed. The remaining safety wire is then used to pass a pyeloureteral catheter with its distal tip in the distal one-third of the ureter and the proximal end coiled at skin level (Fig. 9.12). This pyeloureteral catheter is secured in place and acts as a precautionary measure that allows rapid access back to the pyelocalyceal system should that be required before elective removal of the nephrostomy tube.

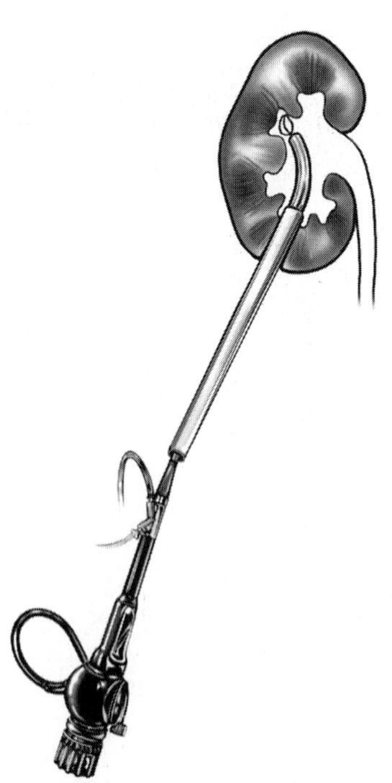

FIGURE 9.11. Flexible nephroscopy performed through a working sheath allows access to stones lying in otherwise inaccessible infundibulocalyces.

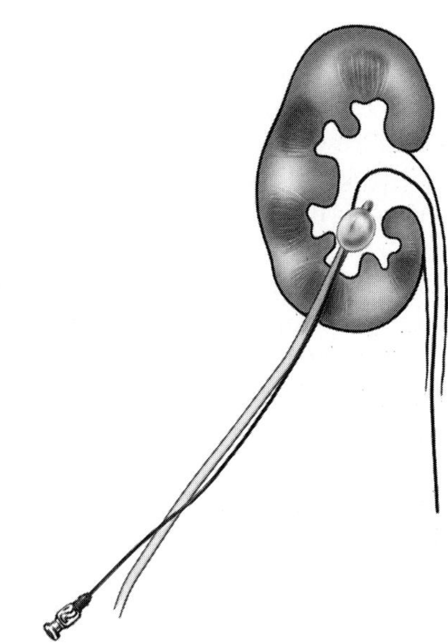

FIGURE 9.12. At the completion of the procedure, a 24-Fr nephrostomy tube is positioned in the renal pelvis, and a 6-Fr pyeloureteral catheter is left in place alongside.

Specific Indications

Body Habitus Precluding Shock Wave Lithotripsy

Patients in whom an unusual body habitus precludes SWL provide some of the most challenging indications for percutaneous stone extraction. This indication occurs most frequently in patients with morbid obesity to the extent that the stone cannot be positioned at the focal point or within the "power path" of an extracorporeally generated shock wave (179). In these patients, both the percutaneous access and tract dilation are more difficult, at least in part because fluoroscopic imaging is compromised. Furthermore, once an adequate tract has been established, stone fragmentation and extraction can be severely hampered by limitations in the length of available instrumentation.

In many cases, the limitations in length of instrumentation can be overcome by allowing the tract to mature for several days following the initial dilation and placement of a large-caliber nephrostomy tube. During this time, the kidney tends to fall back posteriorly toward skin level such that access with standard nephroscopic instrumentation can then be accomplished. Furthermore, a mature tract can be used to pass readily available alternative instruments such as standard flexible cystoscopes or even rigid cystoscopes, which are longer than most available nephroscopes. Working laparoscopes may also be of value in this setting because of their length (60).

Kerbl and associates (89) have proposed using a flank position for percutaneous management of patients with morbid obesity. A suggested advantage of this position is that it may result in less restriction of pulmonary dependent chest wall movement, which then facilitates both anesthesiologic access and ventilation. Furthermore, the flank position allows the abdominal pannus to fall anteriorly, which may result in a decrease in the amount of tissue to be traversed to access the kidney. Overall, although there are clearly difficulties inherent in percutaneous stone management in morbidly obese patients, there may be little difference in overall success rates and ultimate morbidity compared with nonobese patients, at least when the procedure is performed by those experienced in these techniques (22,129).

Another contraindication to SWL regarding body habitus is occasionally seen in patients with severe scoliosis or body contractures preventing adequate positioning of the stone. In these patients, access may be difficult because of the altered anatomy. In some, the kidney may be located in a relatively anterior position, such that prevention of injury to adjacent solid or hollow viscera becomes an important consideration. Skoog and associates (164) have suggested using CT guidance to obtain access in patients with horseshoe kidneys or other fusion anomalies, and we have also found CT or US guidance valuable in preventing injury to adjacent organs in patient with severe scoliosis or other related anatomic abnormalities (Fig. 9.13).

Cystine Stones

Although small cystine stones can at times be managed successfully with SWL, in our experience, most cystinuric patients requiring intervention have larger stones at the time of presentation, and these tend to respond poorly to that modality. Fortunately, however, cystine stones are very amenable to most forms of intracorporeal management, including ultrasonic and holmium laser lithotripsy. At our center, percutaneous ultrasonic nephrolithotomy remains the preferred approach for the majority of cystinuric patients requiring intervention (27), although at a few centers, a ureteroscopic approach is being used with increasing frequency, even for pyelocalyceal cystine stones (64).

Upper Tract Foreign Bodies

Urologic practice has seen an increasingly frequent use of self-retaining stents, nephrostomy tubes, and dilating balloons, and this has led to a corresponding increase in the number of patients requiring management of "retained" upper tract foreign bodies. In many cases, these foreign bodies can be managed with retrograde endoscopy using standard ureteroscopic instrumentation. However, a ureteroscopic approach may be precluded by a prior urinary diversion, making access difficult if not impossible or by the formation of calculi on the foreign body that are too large for ureteroscopic management. When ureteroscopic management has failed or is contraindicated for any of these reasons, a percutaneous approach is indicated (Fig. 9.14) (180). For these patients, the site of the access to the foreign body is chosen as for any stone, and this then depends on its size and location within the pyelocalyceal system. Standard nephroscopic instrumentation, including forceps, graspers,

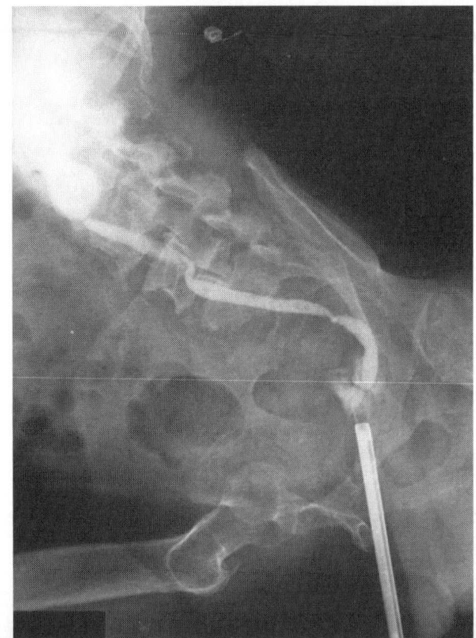

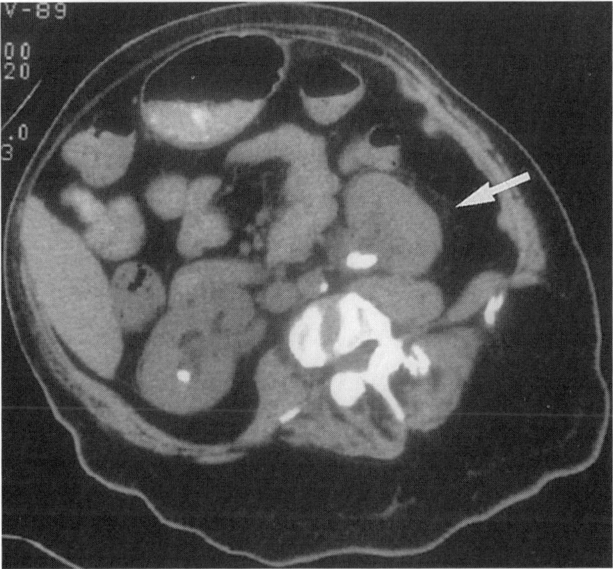

FIGURE 9.13. A: Retrograde study reveals renal pelvic stones that are difficult to see because they overlie the spine in this patient with severe body contractors. **B:** Computed tomography scan without contrast shows bilateral renal pelvic calculi and suggests an appropriate "window" *(arrow)* for safe percutaneous access.

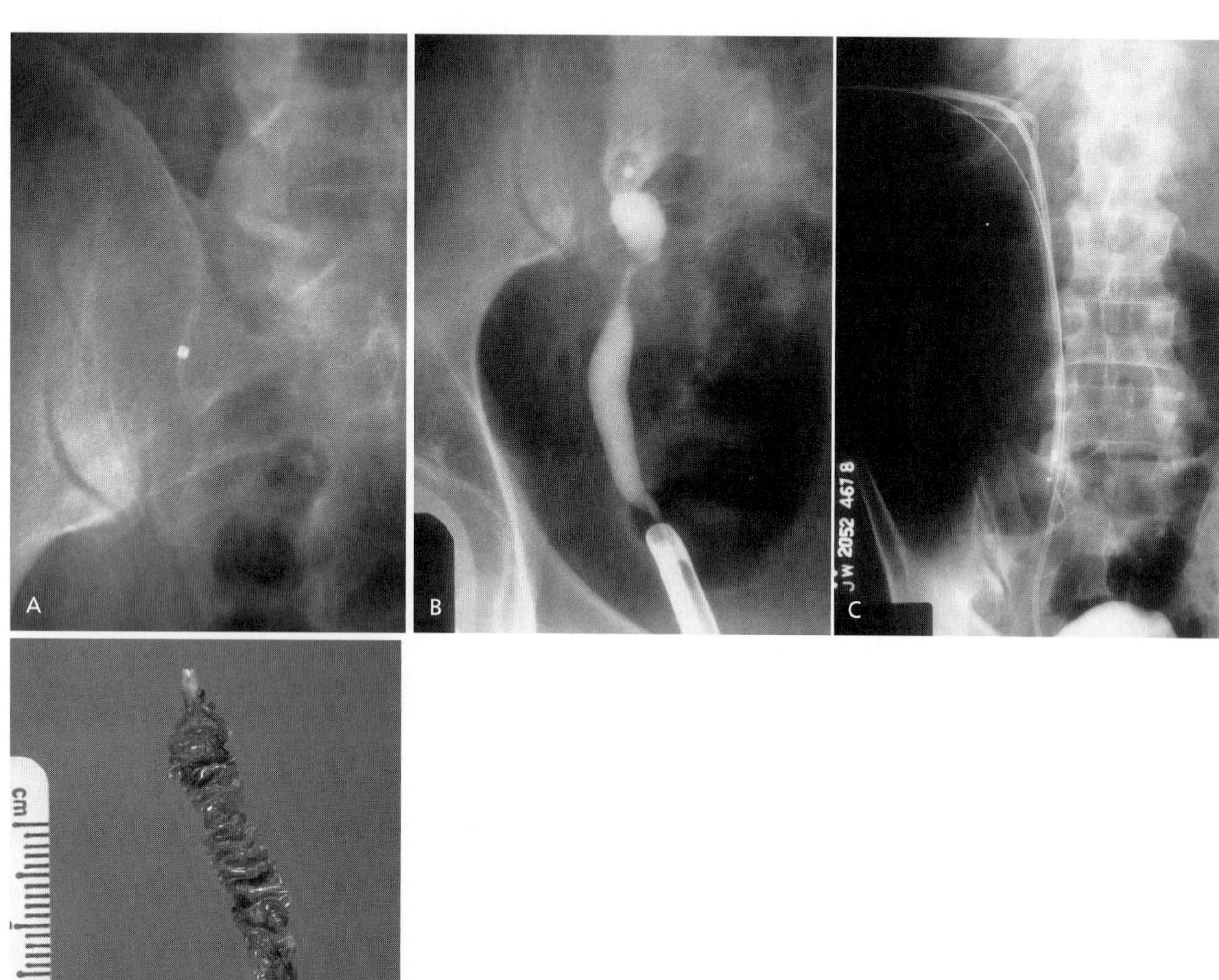

FIGURE 9.14. **A:** Plain radiograph reveals a metallic foreign body over the iliac bone. This represents the tip of a balloon catheter that became dislodged during an attempted balloon dilation for a ureteral stricture. **B:** Retrograde study confirms ureteral stricture below the level of the foreign body, which precludes its removal via retrograde ureteroscopic access. **C:** Antegrade approach using flexible instrumentation. **D:** The foreign body was extracted intact via an antegrade approach. The ureteral stricture was subsequently managed in an antegrade endourologic fashion.

or baskets, may be used in conjunction with any form of currently available intracorporeal lithotripsy.

Distal Obstruction

Successful SWL requires spontaneous passage of the resulting stone fragments. As such, obstruction distal to the targeted stone is a contraindication to SWL as primary treatment. For most affected patients, the distal obstruction will relate to the ureter or ureteropelvic junction (UPJ), although the same principle applies to stones in calyceal diverticula or those in calices associated with true infundibular stenosis. In these patients, percutaneous management is ideal because it provides an opportunity both to remove the stone and provide permanent relief of obstruction as described herein.

Calyceal Diverticular Calculi

Stones in calyceal diverticula are often amenable to a percutaneous approach (11,13,85,162). Ideally, the access should involve direct puncture of the diverticulum containing the stone (Fig. 9.15). Working and safety wires can either be coiled within the diverticulum or occasionally, under fluoroscopic control, passed through the diverticular neck, into the main pyelocalyceal system, and down the ureter. The tract is dilated and a working sheath placed. Nephroscopic

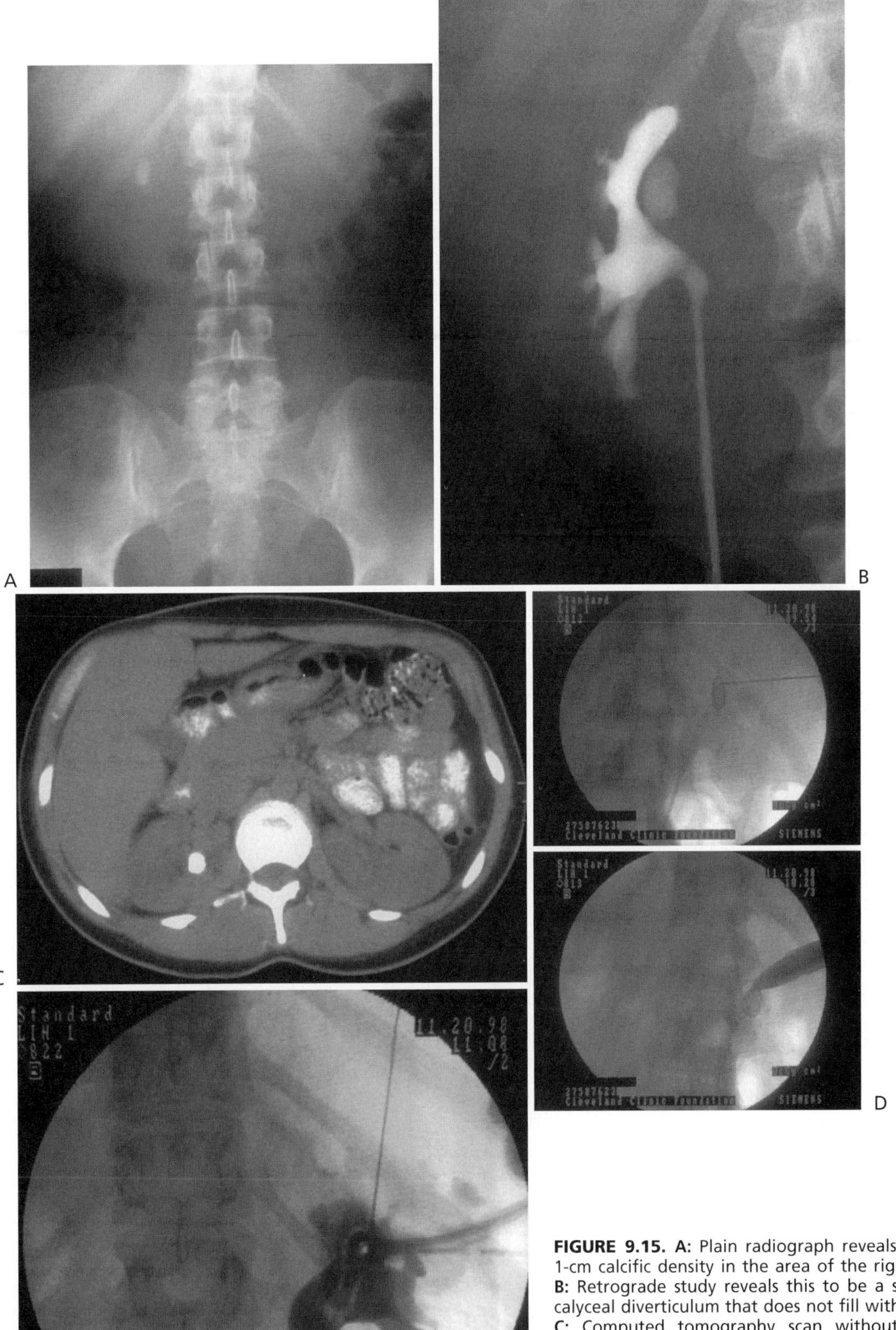

FIGURE 9.15. A: Plain radiograph reveals a 1.5-by-1-cm calcific density in the area of the right kidney. **B:** Retrograde study reveals this to be a stone in a calyceal diverticulum that does not fill with contrast. **C:** Computed tomography scan without contrast reveals a somewhat posteromedial location of the diverticulum, which as such can be managed percutaneously. **D:** Fluoroscopic control of direct percutaneous access to the diverticulum and dilation of the tract. **E:** Diverticular neck has been dilated and a 24-Fr nephrostomy tube left across it with its tip in the renal pelvis.

stone removal proceeds in a standard fashion following which the diverticular neck is often better visualized. If a wire has not already been passed across the neck, it can often be done at this time and the diverticular neck subsequently dilated. When the neck has been managed with dilation, a nephrostomy tube is left across it into the main pyelocalyceal system for several days. An adjunct to help identify the diverticular neck in these patients is cystoscopic placement of an open-end ureteral catheter up to the renal pelvis at the outset of the procedure. During nephroscopic visualization of the calyceal diverticulum, dilute methylene blue can be injected in a retrograde fashion through the ureteral catheter, and this often allows ready identification of the diverticular neck.

An alternative to dilation of the diverticular neck, especially when it cannot be visualized directly or intubated fluoroscopically, is simple fulguration (122). A nephrostomy tube is left in place in the diverticulum, but not across the neck. This acts to "marsupialize" the diverticulum, which does not have secretory urothelium.

Infundibular Stenosis

Stones located in calices drained by long, narrow infundibula or those in calices associated with true infundibular stenosis often require percutaneous management, and the best approach is again a direct one to the involved calyx (Fig. 9.16). In a situation analogous to stones in calyceal diverticula, subsequent access through the involved infundibulum at times cannot be obtained until the stone is extracted. Therefore the working and safety wires may be coiled in the involved calyx and then passed under direct vision once the nephroscope has been introduced.

In contrast to management of calyceal diverticular necks, a stenotic infundibulum should always be dilated rather than fulgurated because the calyx contains secretory urothelium. The infundibulum can be dilated using sequential fascial dilators or a balloon catheter under direct vision, fluoroscopic control, or both. Following stone extraction and dilation of the infundibulum, a large-caliber nephrostomy tube is left indwelling across the infundibulum into the renal pelvis.

Ureteropelvic Junction Obstruction

The association of upper tract stones with ureteropelvic junction obstruction provides an ideal setting for percutaneous management because this allows simultaneous extraction of the stones and relief of obstruction (126). Percutaneous management of the stones is performed in a standard manner with the caveat that for this procedure, percutaneous access is best accomplished via a more superolateral calyx or infundibulum that will allow direct endoscopic access to the ureteropelvic junction with rigid instrumentation (Fig. 9.17). However, stone extraction should precede the actual endopyelotomy incision to prevent extravasation of irrigant or stone particles during stone fragmentation and removal. At completion of the stone removal and endopyelotomy, a relatively large-caliber stent is left indwelling for approximately 4 weeks.

Transplanted and Pelvic Kidneys

Stones in renal allografts or autografts require several management considerations, including the facts that they are generally solitary kidneys and that retrograde access to the ureter may be impossible following the requisite ureteral reimplantation. Relatively small stones (less than 1 cm) may often be treated with SWL, but consideration should be given to percutaneous management for even moderate-size stones. This is because of the inherent difficulty of obtaining retrograde access in the face of potential obstruction from post-SWL fragments and the need to ensure a stone-free result.

Percutaneous access to transplanted kidneys is generally straightforward because the kidney lies at near skin level. The only real difference from the procedure performed in native kidneys is that the patient is in a supine rather than prone position. When renal function is adequate, access can be obtained with standard fluoroscopic imaging after intravenous contrast injection, although US or CT guidance may otherwise be necessary. Once the tract is established, the procedure proceeds as for native kidneys with standard tract dilation, stone manipulation, and nephrostomy drainage (Fig. 9.18).

Management of stones in congenital pelvic kidneys poses different problems. In contrast to transplanted kidneys, congenitally pelvic kidneys are deeper within the pelvis, and peritoneal contents, including small and large intestines, may be interposed. In such cases, percutaneous access may safely be obtained using laparoscopic control.

Proximate Calcified Arterial Aneurysms: Cardiac Pacemakers and Defibrillators

A cardiac pacemaker or implanted defibrillator is no longer an absolute contraindication to SWL (29,36). However, the presence of an implanted cardiac defibrillator may preclude such treatment because the stone is often obscured from vision in at least one plane by the defibrillator. In such cases, percutaneous management often becomes the primary modality of choice for these patients. Likewise, the presence of a proximate calcified aortic or renal artery aneurysm is at times considered a contraindication to SWL, and therefore an indication for percutaneous management (21). When SWL is considered inappropriate in any of these circumstances, percutaneous management is accomplished in a straightforward fashion using standard techniques as described earlier.

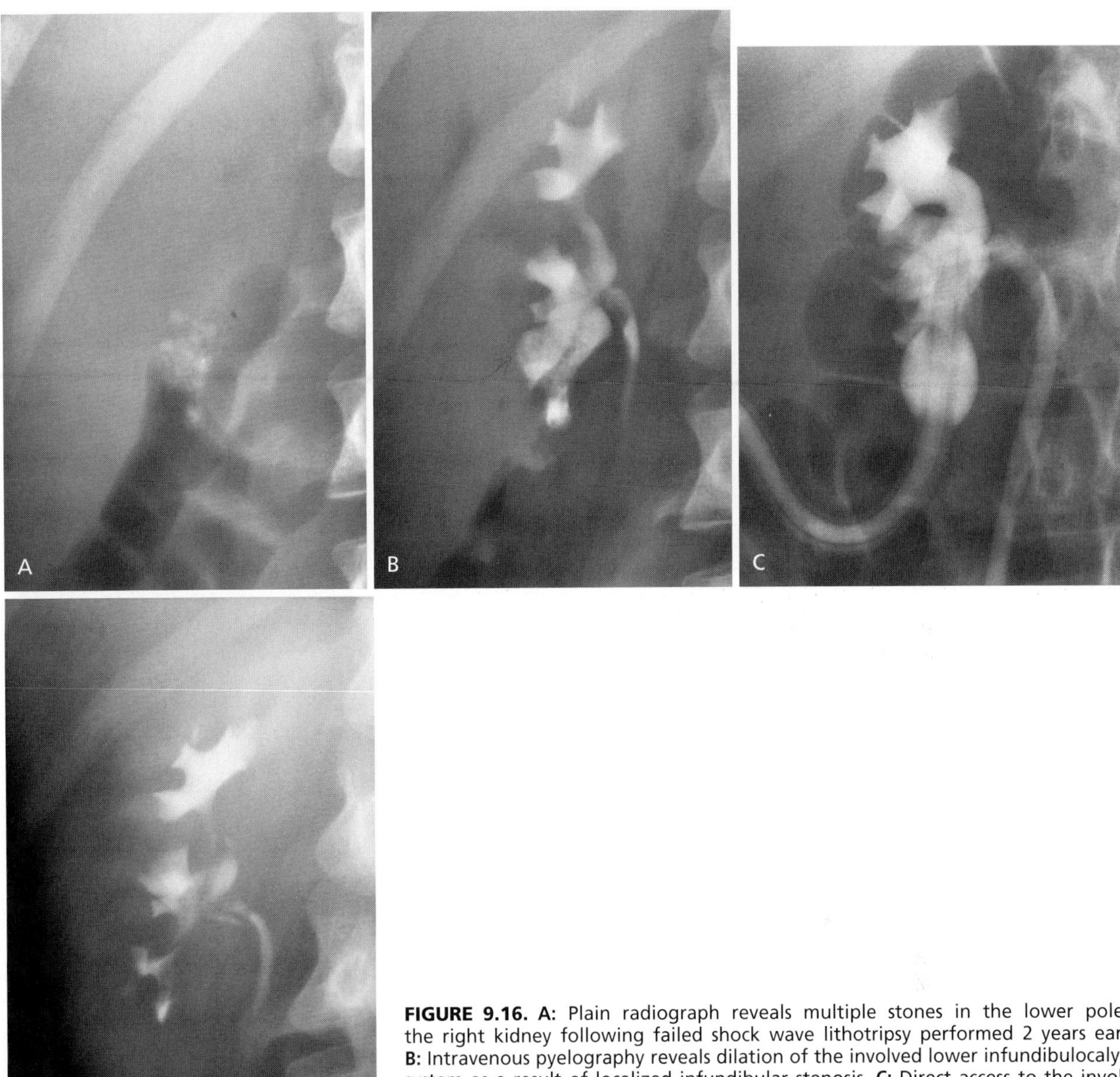

FIGURE 9.16. A: Plain radiograph reveals multiple stones in the lower pole of the right kidney following failed shock wave lithotripsy performed 2 years earlier. **B:** Intravenous pyelography reveals dilation of the involved lower infundibulocalyceal system as a result of localized infundibular stenosis. **C:** Direct access to the involved infundibulum allows direct stone removal. The infundibulum was then dilated percutaneously and a nephrostomy tube left across the infundibulum into the renal pelvis. **D:** Follow-up urogram reveals complete resolution of the localized hydrocalices following percutaneous dilation of the infundibular stenosis.

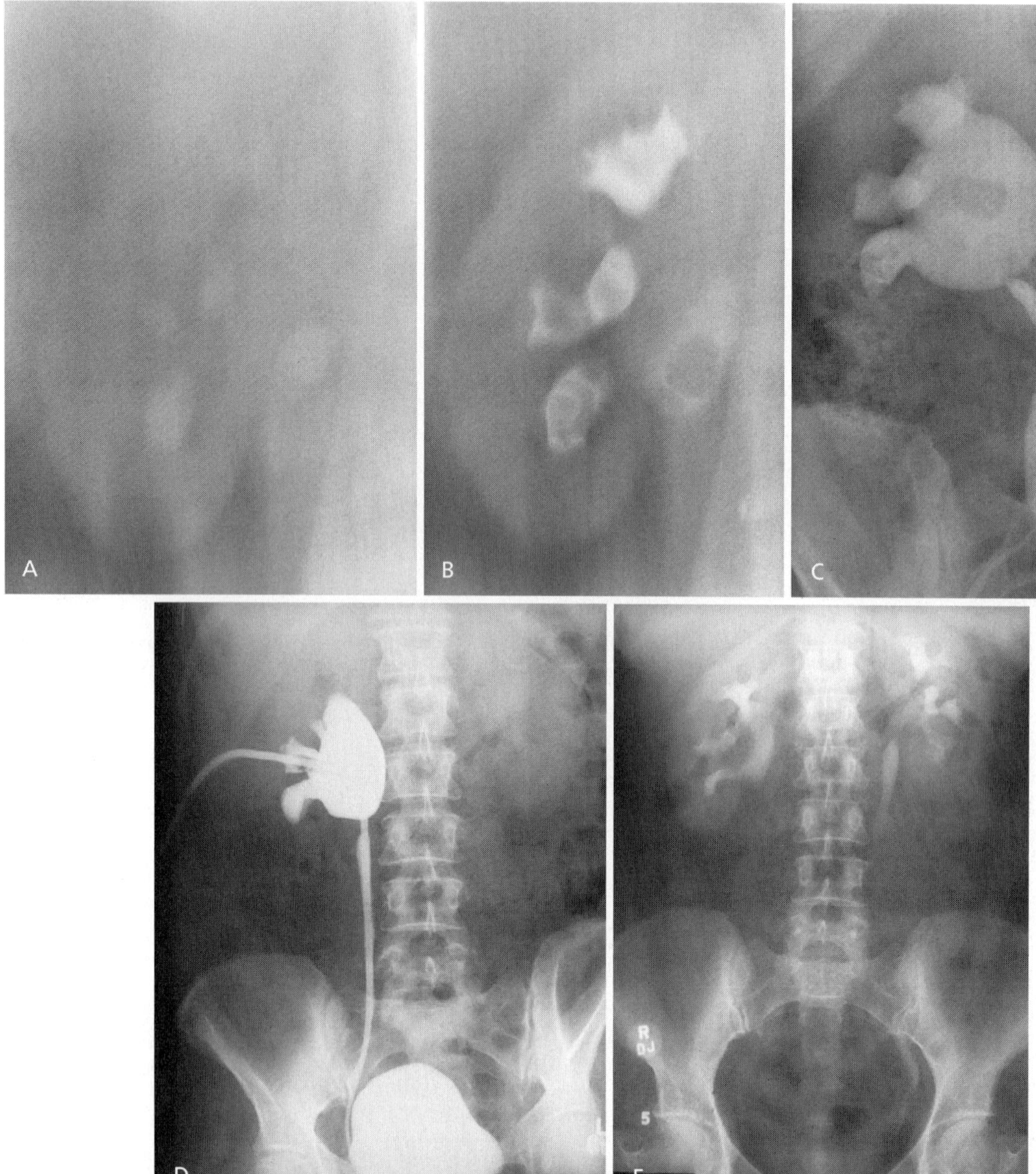

FIGURE 9.17. A: Opaque radiodensities overlying the right renal outline. **B:** Following intravenous contrast injection, dilated calices are visualized with the stones appearing as relatively radiolucent filling defects. **C:** Retrograde study confirms the stones to be associated with primary ureteropelvic junction obstruction. **D:** Percutaneous management of the stones has been performed via superolateral access, which allows direct visualization of the ureteropelvic junction for simultaneous percutaneous endopyelotomy. This follow-up nephrostogram shows resolution of the stones and patency of the endopyelotomy stent such that the nephrostomy tube is removed at this time. **E:** Follow-up intravenous pyelogram performed 1 month after stent removal confirms resolution of the stones and the obstruction.

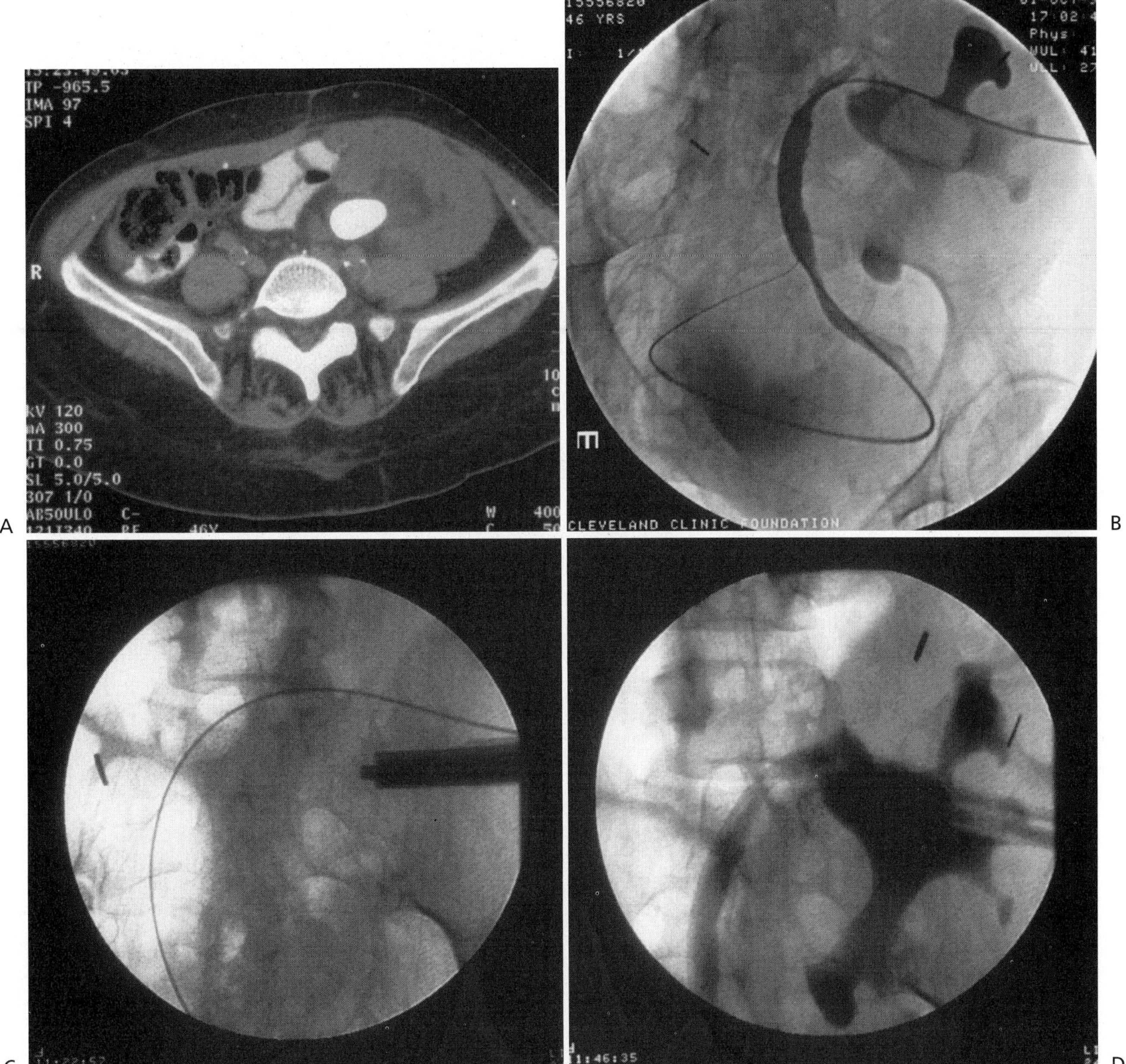

FIGURE 9.18. A: Computed tomography scan without contrast in this combined pancreas-kidney transplant patient reveals a large stone in the transplant renal pelvis on the left side. **B:** Percutaneous access is straightforward, although the patient is in the supine rather than prone position. **C:** As for native kidneys, rigid nephroscopy with ultrasonic fragmentation and suction is generally the preferred form of management. **D:** Follow-up nephrostogram shows resolution of the stone without any obstruction or extravasation.

Large or Complex Calculi

Some patients with large, extensively branched, or otherwise complex stones may be managed definitively with a percutaneous approach alone (Fig. 9.19) (35,59,165,188). The best candidates are those in whom the stone burden is primarily central rather than peripheral, and our preference is to use percutaneous monotherapy for those patients in whom the stone can be safely accessed via one or two tracts. For patients with more extensively branched and peripherally located stones in whom complete extraction would require more than two or three tracts, percutaneous management can be used as a primary approach for "debulking" before adjunctive SWL as part of a planned, combination "sandwich" approach (Fig. 9.20) (88,156,170). In such cases, the initial percutaneous debulking reduces the stone burden for subsequent SWL. Furthermore, the placement of a large-caliber nephrostomy tube at completion of the primary percutaneous procedure allows proximal diversion with prevention of obstruction and subsequent bacteremia or sepsis from passage of fragments subsequent to SWL. A secondary percutaneous procedure can then be done via the mature tract or tracts within 24 to 48 hours of the shock wave procedure to hasten clearance of stone fragments and allow early nephrostomy tube removal (171).

Failed Shock Wave Lithotripsy

Percutaneous management can be used as a "salvage" procedure for essentially any patient who has failed SWL. When failure of SWL has led to obstruction resulting from ureteral stone fragments, initial percutaneous drainage allows recovery of function and treatment of any associated infection. When the patient is stable, tract dilation and stone manipulation can proceed in a standard fashion. Following percutaneous management of any pyelocalyceal stones, remaining ureteral fragments can be extracted in an antegrade or retrograde fashion ureteroscopically using flexible or semi-rigid instrumentation.

Postoperative Care

An estimate of the volume of irrigation and output should be kept during stone extraction. Generally, furosemide 20 mg is given intravenous at termination of the percutaneous procedure. Vital signs are monitored closely, and serial blood counts are obtained as determined by the clinical course. For the first 24 hours postoperatively, intravenous fluids are administered at a rate fast enough to ensure a sustained diuresis. For patients with documented urinary infection associated with the stone disease, sensitivity-specific antibiotics are continued intravenously for at least 48 to 72 hours while the patient is in the hospital and then orally until the first follow-up visit, at which time the need for chronic antibiotic prophylaxis is determined. In patients without a history of infection, prophylactic antibiotic coverage can be discontinued within 48 hours of an uncomplicated percutaneous stone extraction.

One to two days after stone removal, a nephrostogram is obtained and any residual fragments seen on this study

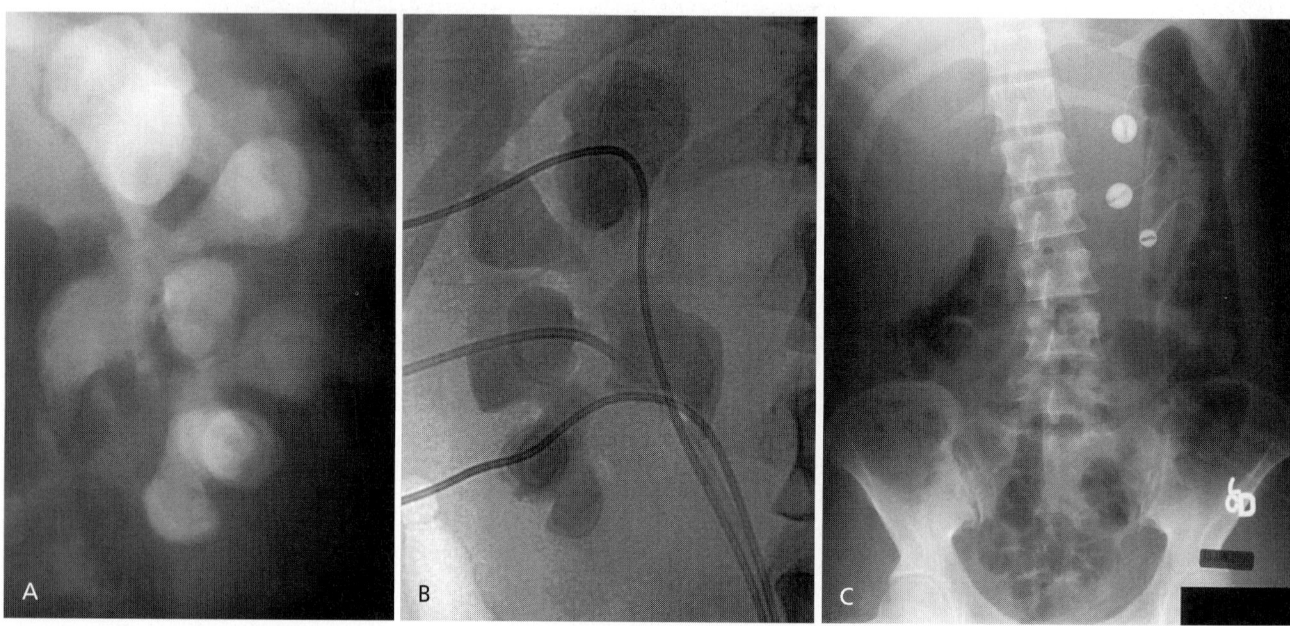

FIGURE 9.19. A: Plain film in this 22-year-old woman with recurrent proteus urinary infection reveals a complete, fully branched staghorn calculus overlying the left kidney. **B:** Reverse fluoroscopic view of percutaneous access via three tracts. **C:** Plain film from follow-up nephrostogram shows complete resolution of the stones.

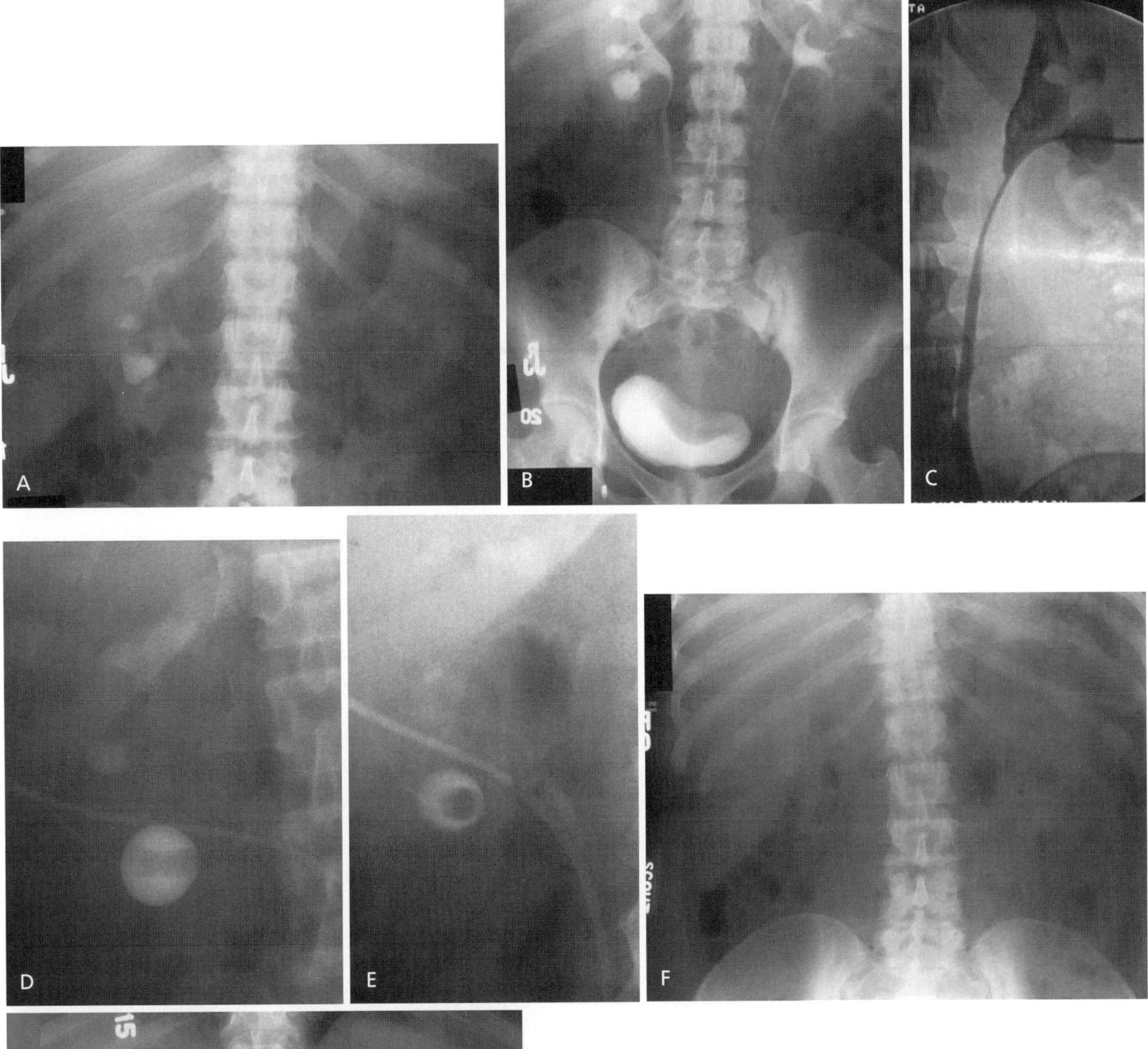

FIGURE 9.20. **A:** Plain film reveals a complete staghorn calculus filling the collecting system of the right kidney. **B:** Intravenous urography confirms an otherwise well-functioning kidney. Note that the kidney is "high riding" such that percutaneous access to the upper infundibulocalyceal portion of the stone would require access above the eleventh rib with subsequent risk of hydrothorax or pneumothorax. **C:** As an alternative, percutaneous debulking is performed via a lower infundibulocalix allowing access to the pelvic and lower infundibulocalyceal portions of the stone. **D:** Scout film from initial nephrostogram reveals mid and upper infundibulocalyceal fragments remaining that are inaccessible to rigid access via the lower-pole percutaneous tract. These inaccessible residual fragments are treated with shock wave lithotripsy. **E:** Twenty-four hours following shock wave lithotripsy, the previously inaccessible upper infundibulocalyceal fragments have migrated to the renal pelvis, where they are easily managed with second-look nephroscopy. **F:** Scout film from follow-up intravenous pyelogram 6 weeks later reveals no residual stone fragments. **G:** Following contrast injection, the kidney is seen to be well functioning.

that appear accessible to the percutaneous tract are managed with repeat rigid or flexible nephroscopy, often performed with light intravenous sedation. If there are no residual stones and no obstruction or extravasation is noted on the nephrostogram, the pyeloureteral catheter is removed and the nephrostomy tube clamped for approximately 12 hours. The tube is removed if there has been no flank pain, fever, or increased drainage around the tube during that time. The patient is then discharged home and allowed to return to full prehospitalization activity 7 to 10 days later.

If extravasation or obstruction is noted on the initial nephrostogram, the nephrostomy tube is left to provide drainage and serial studies are obtained. Ureteral obstruction found at this time usually results from blood clots or edema, either of which should resolve spontaneously within 24 to 48 hours. Occasionally, obstruction results from small stone fragments in the ureter that often pass spontaneously, or they may be managed with antegrade or retrograde manipulation.

Complications of Percutaneous Stone Removal

Hemorrhage

Bleeding is one of the most significant complications associated with percutaneous stone removal. At least some bleeding is apparent in all cases, and it can become evident at any time during or after the procedure. Management then depends on timing and severity of the bleeding.

Bleeding during access or tract dilation generally responds to placement of the next size dilator, which effectively tamponades the tract. The more recent use of balloon dilation, rather than sequential fascial dilation, may decrease the incidence of bleeding during this step. If significant bleeding occurs during stone manipulation, the procedure should be temporarily halted and nephrostomy drainage instituted for a couple of days.

Bleeding through the nephrostomy tube is often evident at the completion of even a relatively uncomplicated procedure. Successful management in almost all such cases can be achieved by temporarily plugging the nephrostomy tube and allowing the collecting system to tamponade. Generally, the nephrostomy tube can be unplugged several hours later, at which time effluent will be markedly clearer. Bleeding that occurs during removal of the nephrostomy tube is best managed by immediate reinsertion. When the tract has matured for even 24 hours, fluoroscopic control is generally not required for this. Delayed hemorrhage (bleeding occurring several days following removal of the nephrostomy tube) is best managed conservatively, that is, with close monitoring of vital signs, bed rest, hydration, and transfusion as necessary.

Bleeding at any time that does not respond to conservative measures that include transfusion is best managed by renal angiography and selective or even superselective arterial embolization. Open operative exploration should be reserved only for failure of all other modalities because such surgery generally leads to partial, or more likely total, nephrectomy (90).

Extravasation

Extravasation of irrigating solution, contrast, or urine is perhaps the most frequent complication of percutaneous technology. Obviously, some degree of extravasation of all of these occurs during any percutaneous procedure; fortunately, in a control setting, this is generally a benign and self-limiting problem. Extravasation does imply urothelial disruption, which may be minor or more severe. However, the ability of the collecting system to repair itself in the setting of proximal diversion and drainage is remarkable.

Obviously, the collecting system is purposely perforated to obtain access to the pyelocalyceal system. Unplanned perforation generally occurs at the medial pelvic wall or ureteropelvic junction and may be the result of access, tract dilation, or stone manipulation. Potential adverse effects of this injury can be minimized by maintaining a sterile urine, carefully monitoring irrigation input and output during the procedure, use of a safety wire at all times to ensure access back to the collecting system, and perhaps most important, use of normal saline as the irrigant of choice rather than distilled water. In that way, the potential complicating effects of hyponatremia are essentially obviated; otherwise, large amounts of hypotonic solution may be absorbed.

Essentially all minor degrees of extravasation and even some major ones can be managed with nephrostomy drainage alone as long as the nephrostomy tube is confirmed to be in the collecting system, urine is aggressing, and the patient is clinically stable. In such cases, especially when the injury occurs in the renal pelvis or at the ureteropelvic junction, it is preferable to have a stent across the ureteropelvic junction either as a percutaneous pyeloureteral catheter or as an indwelling ureteral stent in addition to the nephrostomy tube. Again, as long as the patient is stable, serial nephrostograms can be obtained and the nephrostomy tube removed as soon as the extravasation is no longer radiographically evident and distal patency is ensured. When satisfactory drainage cannot be ensured, or when the patient is clinically unstable, open operative exploration and repair is indicated.

Extrarenal Organ Injury

Injury to a hollow or solid organ other than the kidney occurs in 1% to 5% of patients. Intraperitoneal extravasation can occur from breaching the peritoneum, and the treatment is generally conservative, although paracentesis may be required. On the right side, injury to the liver can occur; this will usually respond to conservative measures because analogous percutaneous intervention is often performed purposely for such procedures as percutaneous biliary drainage. On the left side, splenic injury can occur, and although initial management is again conservative, open operative exploration and repair may be required.

With the recent increasing use of upper pole and supracostal access, hydrothorax, hemothorax, and pneumothorax are becoming more frequent. Management depends on the patient's clinical picture. If the patient is completely stable with no ventilatory or respiratory embarrassment, observation alone may allow spontaneous resolution. Alternatively, simple aspiration on a one-time basis may be adequate, although placement of a chest tube for a few days may be required.

Duodenal or colonic injury may also occur (191). In many cases, even when such injury involves the colon, conservative management may again be successful and consists of withdrawing the nephrostomy tube back to the colon to provide percutaneous colostomy drainage. An internal stent should also be placed into the involved collecting system to separate the colonic and urinary streams. In all cases, conservative management should also include the use of intravenous antibiotics. The patient should initially be placed on nothing-by-mouth status, and this should be followed by a low-residue diet.

Another important consideration in determining whether the patient is a candidate for further conservative management versus open operative repair is whether the injury is intraperitoneal or extraperitoneal. In most cases, this can be determined on the radiographic study used to initially make the diagnosis, whether it is a nephrostogram or a CT scan. Generally, extraperitoneal injuries can be managed using these nonoperative techniques. However, injuries that are intraperitoneal should be given careful consideration for immediate open operative repair.

Results

Percutaneous nephrolithotomy has been documented to be both safe and efficacious. In a community setting, approximately 90% of targeted stones can be removed successfully, and at experienced subspecialty care centers, this rate can approach 100% (9,102,147,160). Furthermore, morbidity for the procedure is acceptably low, even in patients with comorbid medical conditions and complex stones (22,103), and early return to prehospitalization employment and recreational activities can be expected for most patients, especially in comparison with open operative intervention (17,19,20,139). Most important, both functional and morphologic studies have repeatedly shown that percutaneous nephrolithotomy has little if any clinically significant adverse effect on renal function (58,117,119,154,184), even in patients with preexisting renal insufficiency or anatomically solitary kidneys (23,172).

URETEROSCOPY

The advent of ureteroscopy has significantly affected the management of ureteral calculi. Semirigid ureteroscopy can be used in conjunction with pneumatic, laser, and electrohydraulic lithotripsy probes to successfully fragment ureteral calculi (81,112,132), and flexible, actively deflectable ureteropyeloscopes have made access to the upper ureter and intrarenal collecting system a safer, and at times less tedious, procedure (4,6,140). These instruments can be advanced under direct vision or fluoroscopic guidance directly to the level of the stone, which may be fragmented or, when especially small, extracted intact.

Ureteroscopy is a versatile technique that can be used to treat stones throughout the urinary tract (52,161), although a small working channel (2.4 to 4.0 Fr) often limits the size and usefulness of the adjunctive instrumentation that is used for actual stone retrieval. This limitation on available instrumentation has necessitated the use of intracorporeal lithotripsy for the management of most ureteral and intrarenal calculi, and various modalities for intracorporeal stone fragmentation such as the holmium laser, pneumatic lithotripter, and electrohydraulic lithotripter can be used to fragment stones. Although the choice of intracorporeal fragmentation technique is often based on the location and composition of the stone, the experience of the physician and availability of equipment more often dictate this decision (173).

The major advantage of ureteroscopy compared with open operative or percutaneous intervention is decreased morbidity and trauma for the patient because most ureteroscopic cases are performed as an ambulatory surgical procedure with the patient returning to work within 1 to 2 days (78).

Semirigid Ureteroscopy

The technique of rigid transurethral ureteroscopy has undergone significant refinements. Early ureteroscopes were large, fixed-lens systems that, although smaller than the cystoscopes of the day, were still cumbersome to use due to their large (11- to 13-Fr) size, and ureteral dilation was often required for instrument insertion (15). The current generation of semirigid ureteroscopes incorporates fiberoptic light and image bundles into small metal frames (Fig. 9.21) (46,55,82). This miniaturization of the ureteroscope often obviates the need for ureteral dilation, which saves time and allows the visualization of ureteral mucosa unaltered by the trauma of dilation.

Semirigid ureteroscopes using fiberoptic image and light bundles were introduced in the late 1980s. These mini-

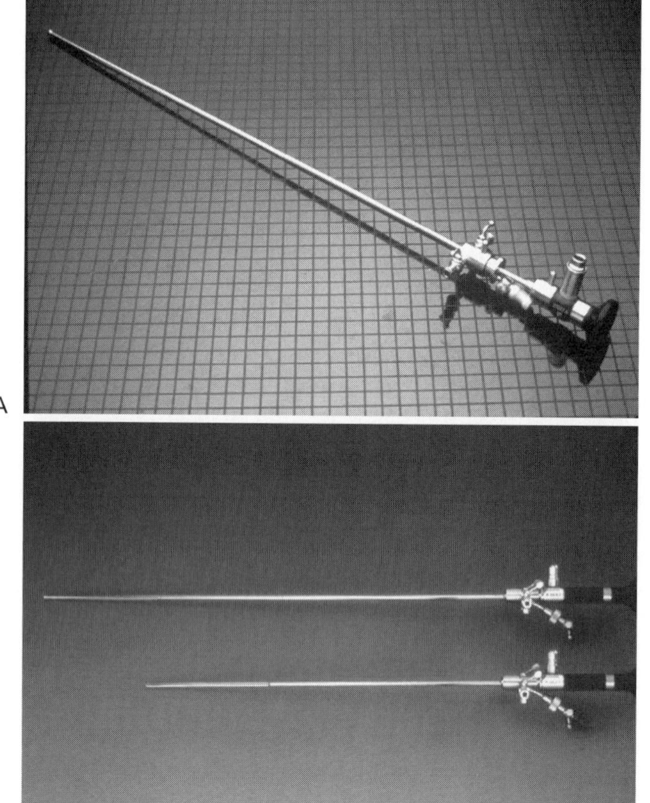

FIGURE 9.21. A: Semirigid ureteroscope. (Karl Storz Endoscopy, Inc., Culver City, California.) **B:** Semirigid ureteroscopes. (Richard Wolf Medical Instruments, Vernon Hills, Illinois.)

ureteroscopes were initially designed for use with laser lithotripsy of ureteral calculi. Initial ureteroscope design used two 2.1-Fr channels for both irrigation and instrument passage. Although these channels were too small to allow use of standard 3-Fr ureteroscopic accessories, they would easily accept laser lithotripsy fibers and guidewires. Since the first mini-ureteroscope was introduced, a number of other semirigid fiberoptic ureteroscopes have been developed that use either one or two working channels. All share the benefits of significantly reduced outer diameter and increased ease of passage (Fig. 9.22).

Indications

Semirigid mini-scopes are ideally suited for both diagnostic and therapeutic maneuvers performed in the lower half of the ureter. The semirigid mini-scopes are somewhat easier to manipulate in the distal portion of the ureter and therefore allow more rapid ureteroscopic procedures. However, the flexible ureterorenoscope is the ideal instrument to access the proximal half of the ureter, as well as lesions within the renal collecting system. Therefore a combination approach with both instruments is thought to allow easy and safe access to the entire upper urinary tract.

Technique

The standard technique involves passage of a 0.038-inch floppy-tipped guidewire under both cystoscopic and fluoroscopic guidance at the outset of the procedure. The semirigid ureteroscope is then passed under direct vision alongside the guidewire to the level of interest. If the ureteral orifice will not accept the ureteroscope, ureteral dilation is performed with a 10-Fr introducing catheter or, if necessary, a standard 15- to 18-Fr ureteral dilating balloon (34,83,86). Instruments used with the semirigid mini-ureteroscopes include stone baskets, grasping forceps, electrohydraulic lithotripsy probes, laser lithotripsy fibers, Bugbee electrodes, biopsy forceps, and brushes.

The most common indication for use of semirigid ureteroscopy is for the management of symptomatic ureteral stones. However, further refinements in the semirigid endoscope and holmium laser technologies now allow management of other forms of ureteral pathology, including ureteral obstruction and urothelial tumors (55,57,65,127,163).

Complications

Complications of semirigid ureteroscopy are usually minor and in most cases can be treated with placement of an indwelling ureteral stent (71). The most common complication developing during ureteroscopy is ureteral perforation, which has been reported in 2% to 6% of contemporary cases (97). The perforation is usually a result of stone fragmentation (EHL or laser lithotripsy) as opposed to passage of the ureteroscope. Occasionally, stone material may migrate through a ureteral perforation. Several studies have suggested that there are no long-term sequelae if a non–infection-related stone has migrated completely through the wall of the ureter (51,98,109,124). However, if stone fragments remain within the wall of the ureter, a ureteral

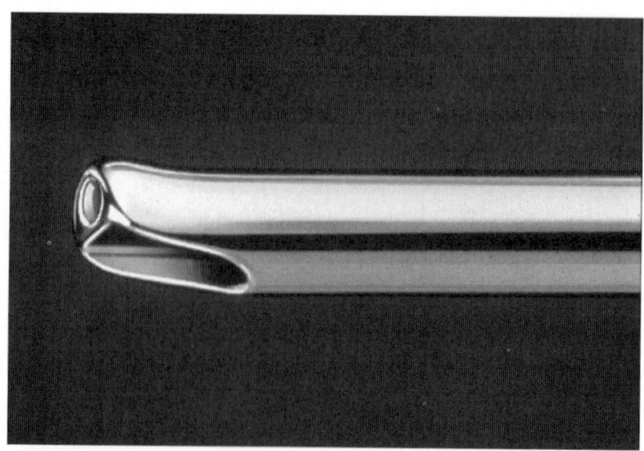

FIGURE 9.22. Distal tip of semirigid ureteroscope. (Richard Wolf Medical Instruments, Vernon Hills, Illinois.)

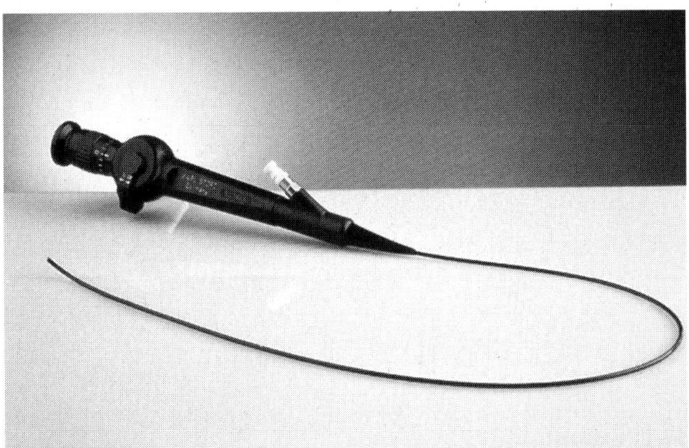

FIGURE 9.23. A 7.5-Fr flexible ureterorenoscope. (Karl Storz Endoscopy, Inc., Culver City, California.)

granuloma with subsequent stricture formation may result (45,66,148).

The most significant complication of ureteroscopic stone retrieval is ureteral avulsion. This complication is usually a result of basketing a stone that is too large to be extracted intact. When in doubt, intracorporeal stone fragmentation should obviate the possibility of avulsion. Although endourologic techniques have been used to manage ureteral avulsion, essentially all of these significant complications will require ureteral reconstruction (113,134,189).

Flexible Deflectable Ureterorenoscopy

Innovations in fiberoptic technology have propelled the further development of flexible ureteropyeloscopes. The widespread use of these new instruments has enabled diagnostic and therapeutic procedures to be performed routinely within the upper ureter and kidney. With the addition of active deflection capabilities, these newer endoscopes are often able to access the entire upper urinary tract, including all of the intrarenal collecting system (7,8,67) (Fig. 9.23), and even lesions or stones located in the lower pole or extremely lateral calyces can now be reached.

In addition to the more conventional uses of flexible deflectable ureteropyeloscopes, many special applications of these instruments have and will be used to take advantage of their unique capabilities. However, many of the attributes that make flexible ureteropyeloscopy a useful and effective tool can lead to potential complications, as discussed later in this chapter.

Technique

Perhaps the most difficult aspect of flexible ureteropyeloscopy is introducing the instrument into the distal ureter, because the flexibility of these small instruments, which allows their manipulation throughout the entire upper tract, may also act as an impediment to their passage. Appropriate dilation of the intramural ureter and introduction of the instrument are integral factors for the performance of flexible ureteropyeloscopy (Table 9.5).

Dilation of the Intramural Ureter

The majority of actively deflectable, flexible ureteropyeloscopes measure between 7.5 and 9.0 Fr in diameter, thus requiring some dilation of the intramural ureter. Dilation can be accomplished successfully with metal cone-tipped bougies, graduated flexible dilators, flexible olive-tipped metal dilators passed over a guidewire, or a ureteral dilating balloon. Currently, balloon dilators are the quickest, most effective, and potentially safest method to perform dilation of the intramural ureter (48).

Introduction of the Flexible Ureterorenoscope

Several techniques can be used to pass the flexible ureterorenoscope into the distal ureter. Most of these scopes can be passed directly over a guidewire that has been placed in the collecting system. This procedure is similar to other endourologic or radiologic techniques that use a guidewire for instrument passage. Care must be taken to follow the instrument fluoroscopically, prevent kinking of the wire, and avoid coiling of the flexible scope in the bladder.

Our current procedure for passage of an actively deflectable, flexible ureteropyeloscope entails initial placement of a 0.038-inch floppy-tipped wire up to the renal pelvis, usually using a 6-Fr open-end ureteral catheter to help guide the floppy guidewire into the ureteral meatus. Intermittent fluoroscopic monitoring during the entire case is an integral part of the procedure that allows confirmation of ureteroscopic position at any time. After the ureteral catheter has been removed, a second guidewire, or safety guidewire, is passed alongside the original (working) guidewire. Fluoroscopy should again be used to confirm that both wires are coiled within the renal pelvis.

If necessary, a 10-Fr introducing catheter or a 5-mm balloon dilator is passed over the working guidewire. Again, fluoroscopic visualization combined with direct view through the cystoscope will confirm inflation of the balloon with adequate dilation of the intramural ureter.

After removal of the balloon dilator, the flexible ureterorenoscope is passed directly over the working guidewire. Using both direct vision through the ureteropyeloscope

TABLE 9.5. PASSAGE OF FLEXIBLE URETEROSCOPE

Initial retrograde pyelogram
Passage of two 0.038-inch guidewires (safety and working wire)
Dilation of intramural ureter
Passage of flexible ureteroscope over working wire
Passage alongside wire if using access sheath
Use of fluoroscopic monitoring to confirm position of wires and scope

and fluoroscopic monitoring, the flexible ureteropyeloscope is passed up to the area of interest either in the ureter or renal collecting system. Once the area of interest has been reached, the working guidewire can be removed and the working port used either for irrigation or passage of adjunctive diagnostic or therapeutic instruments. The safety guidewire remains coiled within the renal pelvis at all times.

Flexible guide tubes made of Teflon or similar materials are also available to assist in passage of flexible ureteropyeloscopes. These guide tubes can be easily placed over a flexible dilator similar to the placement of a nephroscopy sheath during percutaneous endoscopic procedures (3,166). Early versions of these flexible guide tubes were limited by kinking in the bulbar urethra. However, newer ureteral access sheaths may further facilitate passage of the flexible ureteropyeloscope (Fig. 9.24) (94).

Whatever method is used, it is strongly recommended that fluoroscopy and a safety guidewire be used in every case. These two modalities will allow continuous monitoring of the procedure and provide access to the renal pelvis should a problem occur during passage of the telescope. As long as safety guidewire access is maintained, a ureteral stent can usually be placed in the event of a complication.

Current Applications

The most common indication for flexible ureteropyeloscopy is for removal of symptomatic calculi located throughout the ureter or within the intrarenal collecting system. Under direct vision, various intracorporeal lithotripsy devices, stone baskets, grasping forceps, or snares can be manipulated to fragment or entrap ureteral or renal calculi or fragments under direct vision with fluoroscopic monitoring. During withdrawal, distal progression of the scope is monitored fluoroscopically and with visual documentation of the moving ureteral mucosa. This helps ensure that the ureter is not entrapped as the stone or fragment is being extracted.

Limitations

With the development of flexible deflectable ureteropyeloscopes, ureteral and renal calculi can often be accessed successfully. However, a major limiting factor in using these

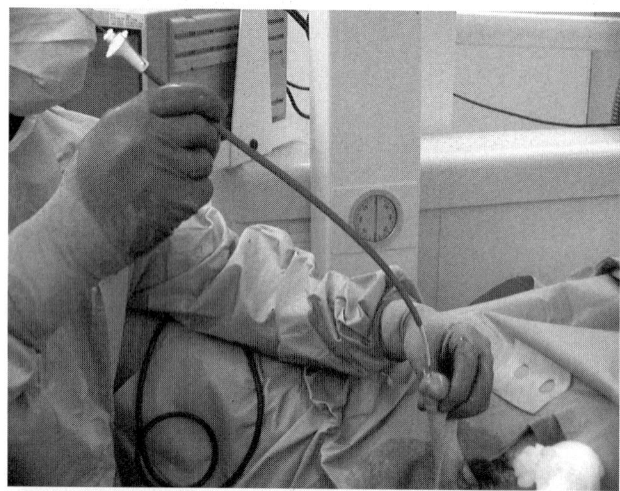
A

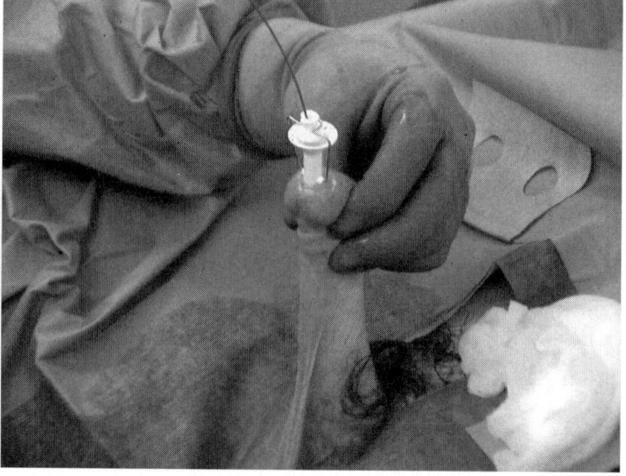
B

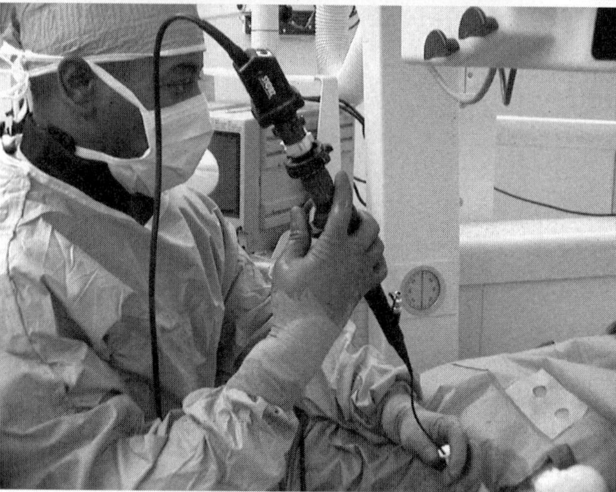
C

FIGURE 9.24. A: Ureteral access sheath passed over safety guidewire. (Applied Medical Resources, Laguna Hills, California.) **B:** Ureteral access sheath in place. **C:** Flexible ureteroscope passed alongside guidewire within access sheath.

smaller endoscopes to manage urinary stones is the small size of the working channel; the currently available flexible deflectable ureteropyeloscopes have working ports ranging from only 3.6 to 4.0 Fr in diameter. Current instrumentation to be used through the working ports of these instruments includes a vast number of baskets, graspers, electrodes, and laser fibers. Unfortunately, not all urologists have access to the myriad number of accessories that are available for use through the flexible deflectable ureteropyeloscope.

The limited size of the working channels of these flexible deflectable ureteropyeloscopes not only limits the instrumentation that can be used but also severely restricts irrigant flow, and this will have a negative impact on visualization during the actual therapeutic procedure. Studies have demonstrated that irrigant flow through a flexible deflectable ureteropyeloscope with a 3.6-Fr working channel is only 32 mL per minute with gravity irrigation, which is only 40% of the total flow that can be achieved through a 13-Fr rigid ureteroscope (186). Moreover, when placing a 3-Fr instrument through the 3.6-Fr working channel, the gravity irrigant flow will be reduced to only 2 mL per minute, which will significantly affect visualization.

Two potential ways to augment irrigant flow, and thereby enhance visualization during flexible ureteropyeloscopic procedures, would be to either limit the size of the instrument used through the working channel or to forcefully inject irrigant fluids. By reducing the instrument size to approximately 1 Fr (about the size of a laser fiber or small electrohydraulic lithotripsy probe), one can increase irrigant flow to 24 mL per minute with gravity irrigation, a 1,200-fold increase (187).

Raising the irrigant pressure, either by using a mechanical pump or forceful hand irrigation, can also significantly increase irrigant flow. However, one should be aware of the potential deleterious effects that can be induced by forceful hand irrigation because studies have demonstrated that this maneuver can raise intrarenal pressures to more than 400 mm Hg, and these pressures have been demonstrated to cause rupture of the intrarenal collecting system in animal studies (157). One must be cognizant of the potential deleterious effects of such high intrarenal pressures generated by forceful hand irrigation, and consider using a "pop-off" valve or, alternatively, a mechanical irrigator that will limit the amount of irrigant pressure (50,187).

Intracorporeal Lithotripsy

The extremely small working channels of the semirigid and flexible endoscopes, which range from 2.4 to 4.0 Fr, has limited the size and usefulness of instruments that can be passed and used for stone removal. For larger stones, baskets or grasping forceps are often inadequate and potentially dangerous to accomplish successful stone extraction. This limitation of available instrumentation has prompted the use of intracorporeal lithotripsy for the management of most larger ureteral and intrarenal calculi.

TABLE 9.6. INTRACORPOREAL LITHOTRIPSY MODALITIES

Electrohydraulic lithotripsy	Laser lithotripsy
Ultrasonic lithotripsy	Pneumatic lithotripsy

Even with the availability of SWL for the management of urinary tract stones, intracorporeal lithotripsy still provides significant advantages in select cases. Because fragmentation is performed under direct vision, the stone can be entirely removed and there is no need to wait for fragments to pass, as with SWL (Table 9.6). Although the choice of intracorporeal fragmentation is often based on the location and composition of the stone to be treated, the experience of the clinician and availability of equipment often dictate this decision.

Selection of Modality

A number of modalities can be used for intracorporeal lithotripsy of both urinary and biliary tract calculi. Although there is no "best" device, considerations for choosing a specific technology include efficacy, safety, and cost. Electrohydraulic lithotripsy, using the small EHL probes, offers a combination of low cost and flexible endoscopic delivery. However, if a holmium laser is available, this multipurpose laser offers perhaps the best option. Both ultrasonic and pneumatic lithotripsy offer the advantage of rapid fragmentation, even with very large or hard stones, but use is limited to rigid or semirigid delivery systems.

Modalities

Electrohydraulic Lithotripsy

The principles of electrohydraulic lithotripsy were initially described and developed by a Russian engineer in 1950 (147). This technology had been used extensively for the destruction of bladder stones, and in 1975, reports were published on its use for the fragmentation of ureteral stones (142,143). The EHL unit consists of a probe, a power generator, and a foot pedal. The probe is made up of a central metal core and two layers of insulation with another metal layer between them. Probes are flexible and available in varying sizes. Commercially available EHL units are manufactured with power up to 120 volts. The electrical discharge is transmitted to the probe where a spark is generated at the tip. The intense heat production in the immediate area surrounding the tip of the probe results in a cavitation bubble, which produces a shock wave that radiates spherically in all directions (193). Collapse of the bubble causes a second shock wave. These shock waves, repeated at a frequency of 50 to 100 per second, result in destruction of the stone.

EHL will effectively fragment all kinds of urinary calculi, including cystine, uric acid, and calcium oxalate monohydrate stones (178). Because the probes are small and flexible, they can be used through flexible endoscopes to fragment stones that are inaccessible for ultrasonic lithotripsy through a rigid instrument. The primary disadvantage of EHL is that in general, the resultant fragments have to be either washed out during intraoperative irrigation, or grasped with forceps or baskets.

The first experience with electrohydraulic lithotripsy in the ureter entailed a 6-Fr EHL probe that was fluoroscopically guided to the obstructing calculus. The most common cause of failure in this early experience was the operator's inability to pass the probe to the level of the stone. Additional early experience with EHL in the ureter described the use of a 9-Fr probe that provided excellent fragmentation of the stone, although 40% of the patients had ureteral extravasation following the procedure. This high complication rate was believed to be mainly attributable to the large probe size. The use of a smaller 5-Fr EHL probe through a rigid ureteroscope was compromised by decreased stone visualization because the probe occupied the majority of the working channel of the rigid ureteroscope (70).

The development of an even smaller 3-Fr EHL probe used through a flexible endoscope was first reported in 1988 (10,42,53). Recently, 1.2- to 1.9-Fr EHL probes have been developed that have been effective in fragmenting ureteral, intrarenal, and biliary tract stones. An additional benefit of these small-caliber probes is that they allow improved visualization through the flexible endoscope because a larger portion of the working channel is available for irrigation (80,133).

Power settings of the EHL unit normally range from 60 to 90 volts, and normal saline irrigation can be used with modern units. Excellent fragmentation of most ureteral calculi is to be expected, and intracorporeal lithotripsy with EHL for both urinary tract and biliary calculi offers a safe, effective, and cost-efficient modality when small-caliber, flexible lithotripsy probes are used.

Ultrasonic Lithotripsy

Ultrasonic energy was first used to fragment kidney stones in 1979. Commercially available units consist of a power generator combined with a US transducer and a probe that form the Sonotrode. A piezoceramic element in the handle of the Sonotrode is stimulated to resonate, and this converts electrical energy into US waves (23,000 to 27,000 Hz), which are transmitted along the hollow metal probe creating a vibrating action at its tip. When the vibrating tip is brought in contact with the surface of a stone, the stone can be disintegrated. The probe must be rigid because sound waves cannot be transmitted without energy loss along flexible probes. The probes come in varying sizes and are passed through the straight working channel of a rigid endoscope with a 30- or 90-degree-offset lens. Suction tubing can be connected to the end of the Sonotrode probe, thus converting the unit into a "vacuum cleaner" for stone fragments (62,84,185). Smaller 2.5-Fr solid US probes are available for use through rigid ureteroscopes (26), and these can be used for rare cases in which fragmentation of large, distal ureteral calculi with EHL or laser lithotripsy has been ineffective. In all cases, normal saline at body temperature should be used as irrigant.

We continue to use US mainly for the fragmentation of large renal calculi during percutaneous nephrolithotripsy procedures. The large, hollow US probes offer the advantage of effective stone fragmentation while allowing simultaneous aspiration of the fragments. This is especially useful when treating renal calculi in which a large volume of stone must be removed. US is now used only rarely via a ureteroscopic approach.

Laser Lithotripsy

The development of the pulsed dye laser for fragmentation of ureteral calculi was initiated in 1986 (47,183). Significant advances in laser fibers and power generation systems have propelled laser lithotripsy to the treatment of choice for fragmentation of most ureteral stones. The pulsed dye laser delivers short, 1-μs energy pulsations at 5 to 10 Hz produced from a coumarin green dye. Instantaneous fluid evaporation causes a plasma at the stone surface, resulting in a highly localized shock wave. The 504-nm wavelength produced by the pulsed dye laser is selectively absorbed by the stone, but not the surrounding ureteral wall. Because the energy is delivered in short pulses, minimal heat is generated, again protecting the ureteral mucosa. Initial experience yielded stone fragmentation rates ranging from 64% to 95% (68,80).

Failures are often related to equipment malfunction (4% to 19%) or to resistant stone composition. As such, the use of EHL had often been necessary as an adjunctive measure with the pulsed dye laser. However, use of the pulsed dye laser in the ureter appears to be safe, because no significant intraoperative or postoperative complications have been noted from the laser energy alone.

The primary advantages of laser fragmentation were initially thought to be its increased safety during stone fragmentation and increased irrigant flow through the flexible endoscope due to the small diameter of the laser probes. However, the smaller electrohydraulic lithotripsy probes have been proven to be just as safe and almost as small in diameter as some laser fibers. The major drawback of pulsed dye laser lithotripsy had been the high purchase price of the laser, as well as the need for relatively expensive ongoing maintenance and regular dye changes.

Recently, new solid-state lasers have been developed (Q-switched yttrium-aluminum-garnet, alexandrite, and holmium lasers) for the fragmentation of ureteral calculi.

These solid-state systems offer better efficacy rates than the pulsed dye lasers and are significantly less expensive to acquire and to maintain (130).

The holmium laser is the newest laser to be introduced for stone fragmentation. The holmium wavelength is not selectively absorbed and works equally well to fragment stones of varying color and composition (153,176,194). Moreover, the holmium laser has the advantage of being a multipurpose laser system. Not only can it be used for stone fragmentation, but it can also be used for its hemostatic and tissue effects, including incision of urinary tract strictures and prostatic resection (99,145). One potential limitation of the holmium device is its "drilling action" on hard stones. This can often be particularly time consuming when using the smaller holmium fibers (100,181). Moreover, the tissue effects demand a greater degree of caution because injury to the urothelium or damage to the guidewire or endoscope can occur during stone fragmentation.

Our own experience with the holmium laser shows it to be ideal for use through all kinds of flexible endoscopes, and we now use it almost exclusively as our fragmentation modality of choice with both semirigid and flexible ureteroscopes.

Pneumatic Lithotripsy

Another new technique developed for the fragmentation of ureteral, renal, and bladder calculi is pneumatic lithotripsy. The first pneumatic device, the Lithoclast, consists of a pneumatically driven piston that fragments stones by direct contact (Fig. 9.25) (43,74). A major advantage of this device is its efficiency in breaking up calculi of all composition. Pneumatic lithotripters use a semirigid probe and therefore can only be passed through instrumentation with a straight working channel (Fig. 9.26). At present, the smallest pneumatic probe is 0.8 mm, which can be used with the small semirigid ureteroscopes.

A number of basic science and clinical studies have demonstrated the safety and efficacy of the pneumatic device (44,72). In a randomized, prospective trial, Hofbauer and colleagues (75) compared the fragmentation of distal ureteral calculi with both EHL and pneumatic lithotripsy. Although the fragmentation rates for both devices were similar (85% fragmentation for EHL and 90% fragmentation for pneumatic lithotripsy), ureteral perforation was noted in only 2.6% of the patients undergoing pneumatic lithotripsy, and there was a 17% incidence of perforation in the EHL group. In a clinical experience using pneumatic lithotripsy, successful fragmentation of stones of varying composition located in the kidney, ureter, and bladder was achieved, although ureteral stone migration was a problem in a limited number of patients who had significantly dilated proximal ureters (178).

Two recent innovations have expanded the use of pneumatic lithotripsy for the intracorporeal fragmentation of ureteral calculi. A suction device (Lithovac) has been de-

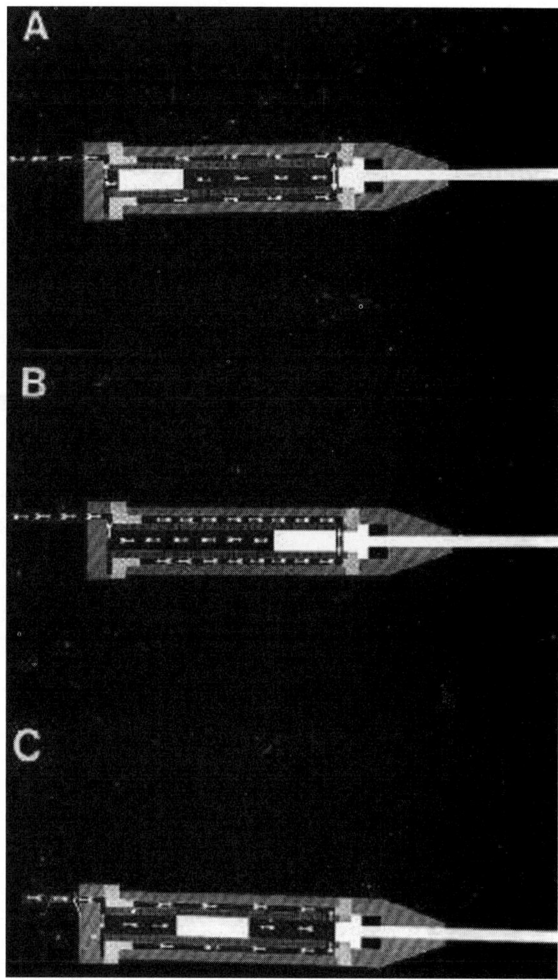

FIGURE 9.25. A–C: Schematic of projectile within handle of pneumatic lithotripsy probe.

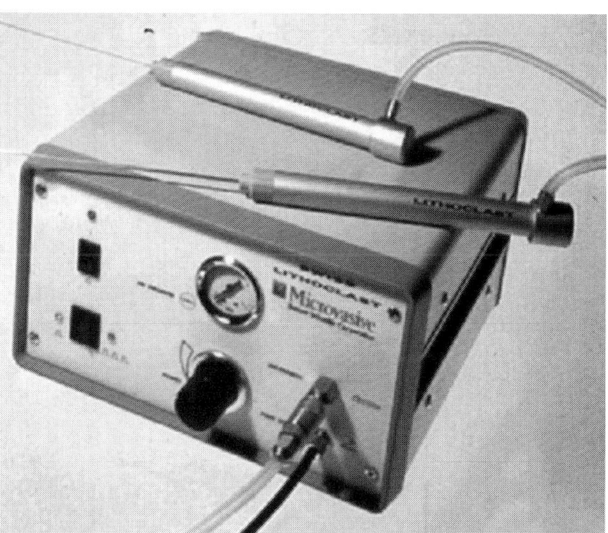

FIGURE 9.26. Pneumatic lithotripter. (Lithoclast, Microvasive Urology, Natick, Massachusetts.)

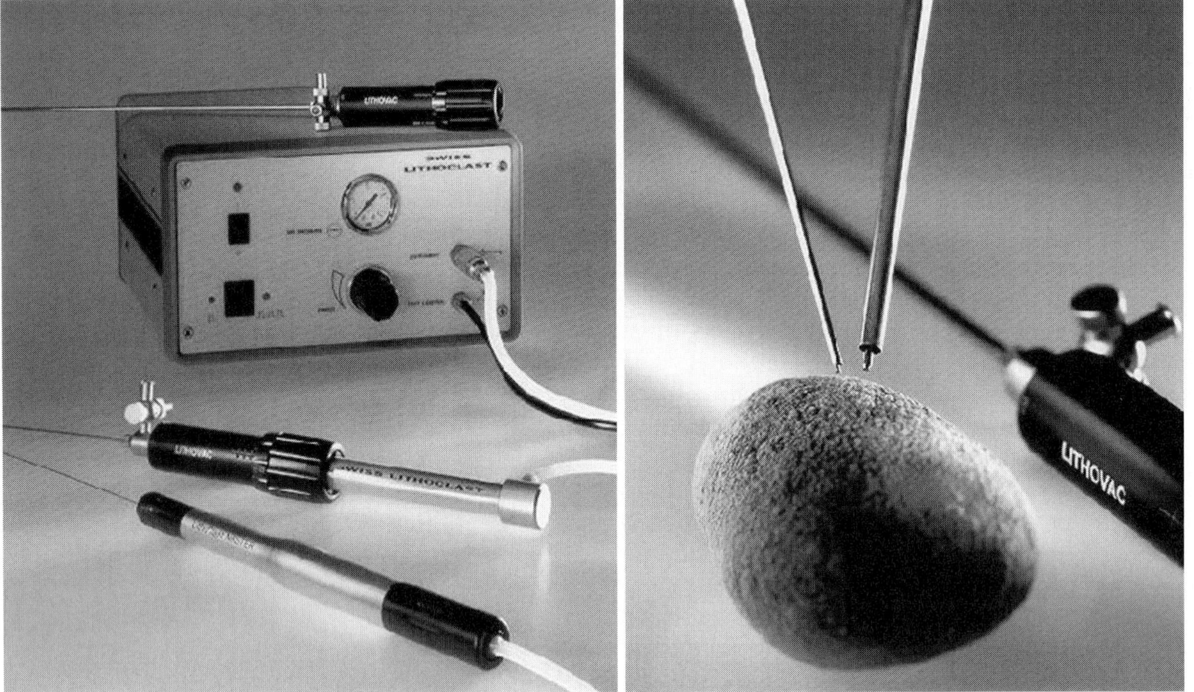

A B

FIGURE 9.27. A: Lithovac suction device with Lithoclast. (Microvasive Urology, Natick, Massachusetts.) **B:** Close-up view of pneumatic probe within 5-Fr Lithovac and 9-Fr Lithovac. (Microvasive Urology, Natick, Massachusetts.)

veloped to aid in removal of stone fragments during pneumatic lithotripsy (Fig. 9.27) and limit the proximal migration of ureteral calculi (39,73). In addition, flexible pneumatic probes are under development that will allow the use of pneumatic lithotripsy with flexible ureteroscopes (108,174,195).

Ureteroscopic Management of Renal Calculi

Most renal calculi are currently treated with SWL. However, certain predictors of inadequate fragmentation or clearance of residual fragments preclude successful treatment with this modality. The factors that may predict a poor outcome of SWL for management of renal calculi include large stone size (greater than 1.5 cm), "hard" stone composition (calcium oxalate monohydrate or cystine), distal ureteral obstruction, and "adverse" intrarenal anatomy.

Limitations of Shock Wave Lithotripsy

The size and composition of renal calculi are obvious predictors of SWL success or failure, but the impact of renal anatomy combined with stone location is less well defined. Recent studies have suggested that for larger stones located in lower pole calices or calyceal diverticula, or for those associated with significant dilation of the intrarenal collecting system, clearance of fragments will be less predictable. For most of these conditions, percutaneous nephrolithotomy is often the best alternative to both access the stone and achieve complete clearance of all fragments. However, certain instances may preclude the use of percutaneous stone removal, and thus favor ureteroscopic management. These factors include the coexistence of ureteral calculi or strictures in addition to the renal calculi, irreversible bleeding diatheses, renal anomalies, or morbid obesity (Fig. 9.28).

A major factor that now allows for routine ureteroscopic access and management of intrarenal calculi has been the introduction of holmium:yttrium-aluminum-garnet (Ho:YAG) laser lithotripsy. The holmium laser is an efficient and relatively safe device that will fragment stones of any composition. The major advantage of the holmium laser is that these small fibers can be placed through small, flexible ureteropyeloscopes. Both the 200- and 365-micron fibers can be placed through a flexible ureterorenoscope, although the 200-micron fiber is preferred when managing intrarenal calculi because the smaller fiber diameter allows for greater ureteroscopic deflection (100,194). However, the smallest EHL probes are even more flexible, and they may be beneficial in some instances

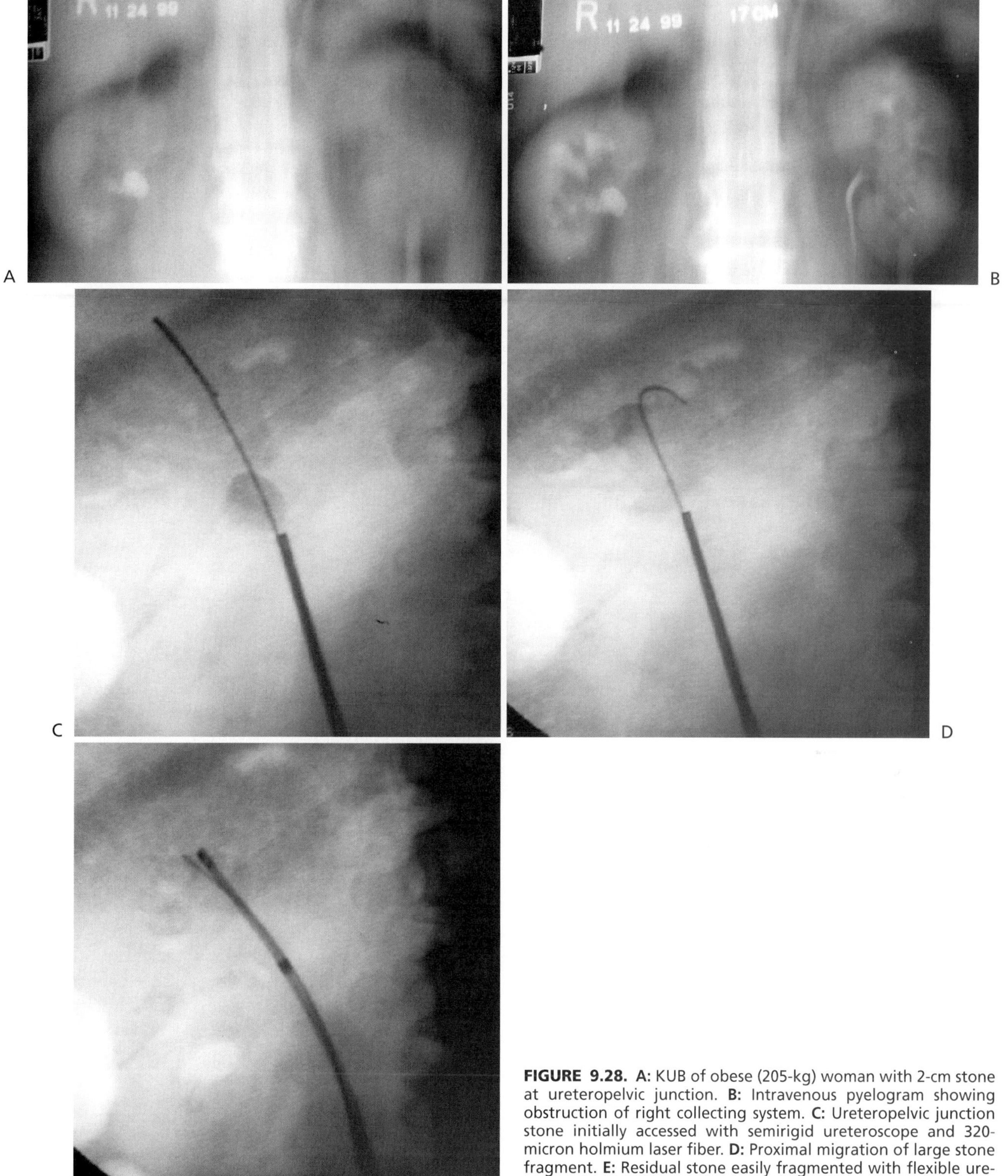

FIGURE 9.28. **A:** KUB of obese (205-kg) woman with 2-cm stone at ureteropelvic junction. **B:** Intravenous pyelogram showing obstruction of right collecting system. **C:** Ureteropelvic junction stone initially accessed with semirigid ureteroscope and 320-micron holmium laser fiber. **D:** Proximal migration of large stone fragment. **E:** Residual stone easily fragmented with flexible ureterorenoscope and 200-micron holmium laser fiber.

requiring very acute ureteroscopic flexion for stone visualization.

Our preferred settings for the holmium laser are 0.6 to 0.8 joules at 6 to 8 Hz. Studies have demonstrated that increasing the power to more than 1 joule will rapidly damage the small-caliber 200-micron fiber. Moreover, the relatively low power required to fragment calculi also allows the use of low-power holmium lasers. These low-power units provide 25 to 30 W of power, at a significantly reduced cost as compared with the high-power, 80-W lasers (95).

As mentioned, even though the 200-micron fiber is highly flexible, one can still lose anywhere from 10 to 45 degrees of tip deflection of a 7.5-Fr flexible ureteroscope when a 200-micron laser fiber is placed through the working channel (100,133). Another recent innovation, in the form of nitinol baskets and graspers, now allows for virtually full deflection of the flexible ureteroscopes such that a 3-Fr nitinol basket or grasper can be passed through a deflected endoscope with minimal loss of tip deflection (Fig. 9.29) (76,96).

One useful technique for stones that are difficult to access is utilization of a nitinol basket or grasper to reposition them. For example, lower pole calyceal stones can be brought back up to a less dependent portion of the collecting system, such as the renal pelvis or an upper pole calyx, and this then allows for easier fragmentation with a holmium fiber.

OPEN OPERATIVE INTERVENTION

Contemporary Indications

Whereas the indications to intervene for stones have not changed significantly with the advent of new technology, the indications for open operative intervention have narrowed considerably (128). Currently, these indications include an associated anatomic abnormality that would best be managed with open operative intervention at the time of stone extirpation, a failure of or a contraindication to both SWL and percutaneous management, or in the urologist's judgement, a stone so large and complex that a single open operative procedure would more likely render the patient stone free, with less risk, than would the option of a complicated percutaneous procedure with or without adjunctive SWL.

The type of open operative intervention planned takes into consideration several factors, the most important of which are stone size, configuration, and location relative to the pyelocalyceal system. The approaches to be discussed in this section include standard and extended pyelolithotomy, simple nephrolithotomy, coagulum pyelolithotomy, calyceal diverticulolithotomy, anatrophic nephrolithotomy, partial nephrectomy, and nephrectomy.

Specific Techniques

Pyelolithotomy

A pyelolithotomy had been perhaps the most commonly performed open operative procedure for patients with renal calculi, but this was supplanted almost 20 years ago by the advent of percutaneous and shock wave technology. Currently, the only indications for this procedure are a failure of or contraindication to both SWL and percutaneous nephrolithotomy or the presence of an associated abnormality such as ureteropelvic junction obstruction, which could then be managed simultaneously. However, even in that setting, open pyelolithotomy is performed less often today because percutaneous stone management can be combined with percutaneous endopyelotomy.

Czerny (37) is credited with performing the first removal of a stone via an incision in the renal pelvis in 1880. However, that approach remained controversial because most surgeons of the time favored nephrolithotomy. In 1913, Lower (111), at The Cleveland Clinic, popularized a vertical pyelolithotomy, which remained the preferred approach to uncomplicated renal pelvic calculi for many years. In 1965, Gil-Vernet (61) advocated a transverse rather than a vertical pyelolithotomy based on his studies of the functional anatomy of the renal pelvic musculature.

Standard Pyelolithotomy

Today, almost any patient whose stone could be managed via a pyelotomy incision can and should be managed with either percutaneous or shock wave technology such that the role of pyelolithotomy is now extremely limited. Currently, then, the indications for a standard pyelolithotomy, within the context of the limited indications for open operative intervention, include stones limited to the renal pelvis with minimal or no branching (Fig. 9.30). The procedure is performed through a standard flank incision, generally with twelfth-rib resection, or through a dorsal lumbotomy. Either of these approaches allows rapid access to the renal pelvis posteriorly.

The retroperitoneum is entered and Gerota's fascia opened posteriorly at the lower pole of the kidney. The proximal ureter is identified and surrounded with a vessel loop. This aids dissection and prevents distal stone migration during the subsequent procedure. The dissection is then carried proximally along the posterior aspect of the ureter, up toward the renal pelvis. Once the pelvis is exposed posteriorly, stay sutures are placed in preparation for the transverse pyelotomy. This incision is made well away from the ureteropelvic junction itself, and it is carried as far laterally on the pelvis as is necessary to extract the stone under direct vision (Fig. 9.31A). The stone is removed with a Randall's forceps and the vessel loop on the ureter is relaxed (Fig. 9.31B). An 8-Fr red rubber catheter is then passed antegrade down the ureter to the bladder to ensure

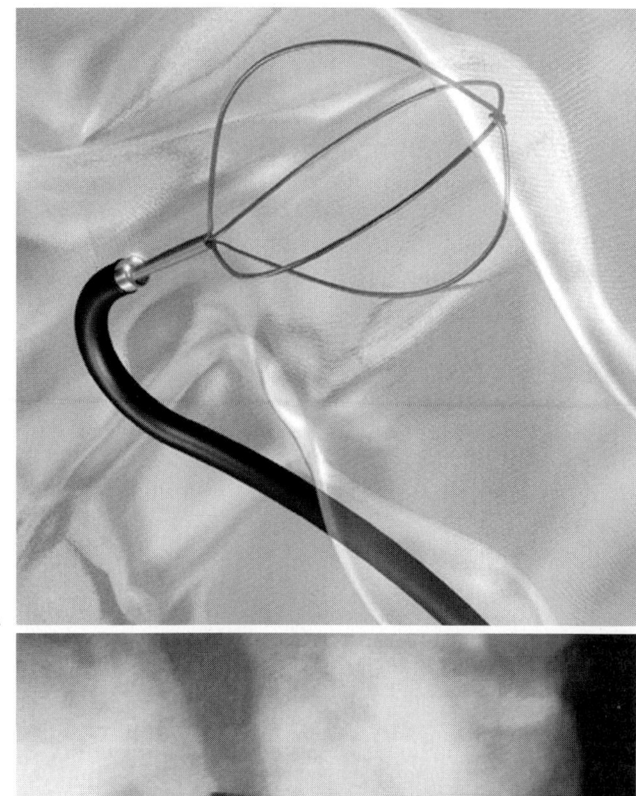
A

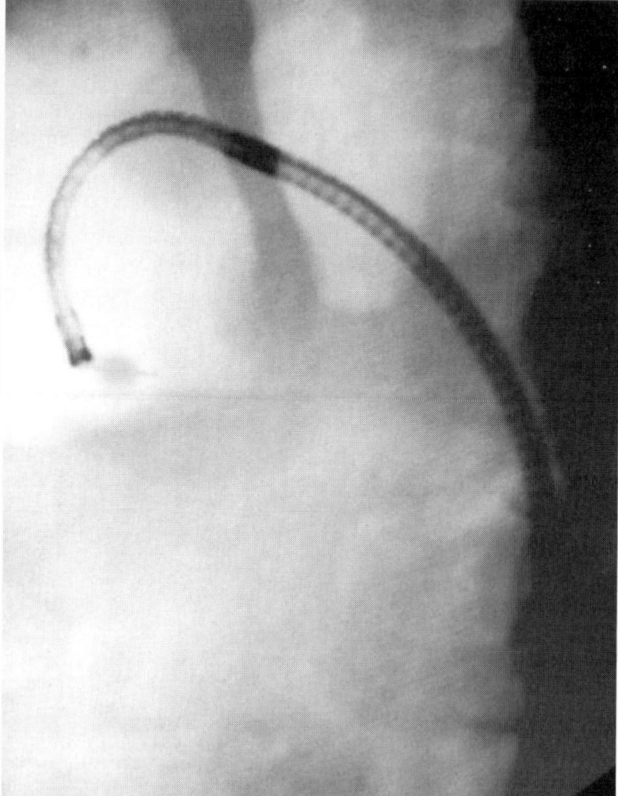
B

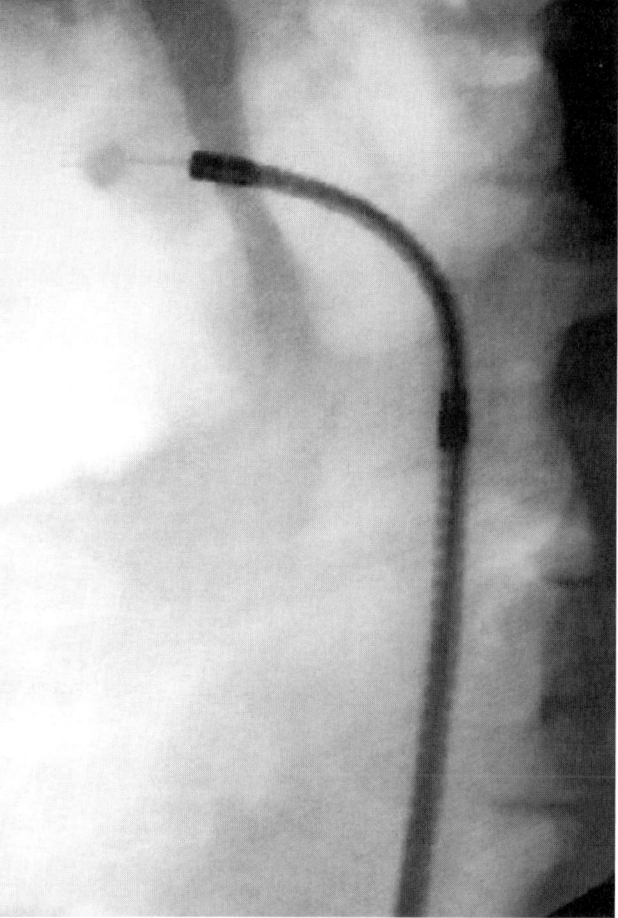
C

FIGURE 9.29. A: Nitinol stone grasper. (Microvasive Urology, Natick, Massachusetts.) **B:** Nitinol grasper can be passed through a fully flexed flexible ureteroscope to access lower pole renal calculus. **C:** Lower pole calculus repositioned into lateral calyx to allow for laser fragmentation with a 200-micron holmium laser fiber.

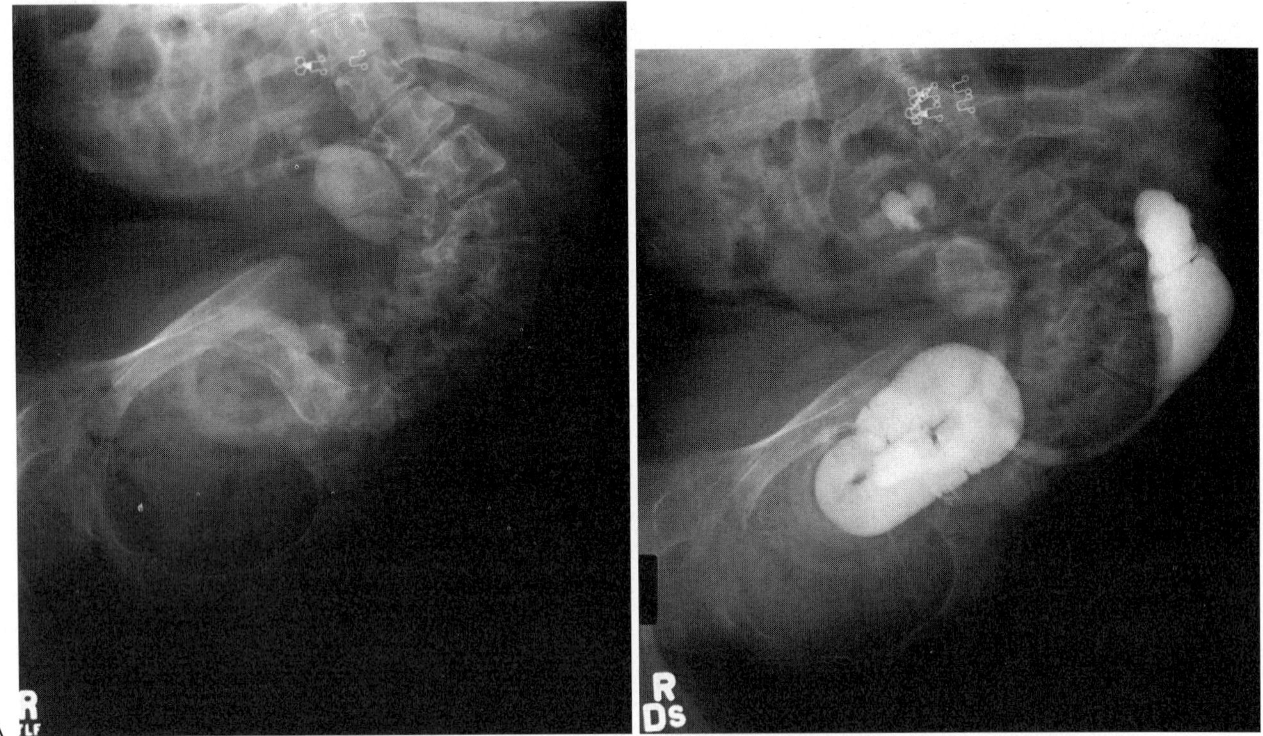

FIGURE 9.30. **A:** Plain film in this myelodysplasia patient status post–urinary diversion reveals a large calcification filling the right upper quadrant. **B:** Loopogram reveals free reflux into a nonfunctioning shell of a left kidney and hydronephrosis on the right associated with the large renal pelvic calculus. Percutaneous access to this stone is hindered by the severe scoliosis and would require supracostal puncture with risk of injury to the pleura or liver on the right. Open pyelolithotomy was indicated with consideration for simultaneous left nephrectomy.

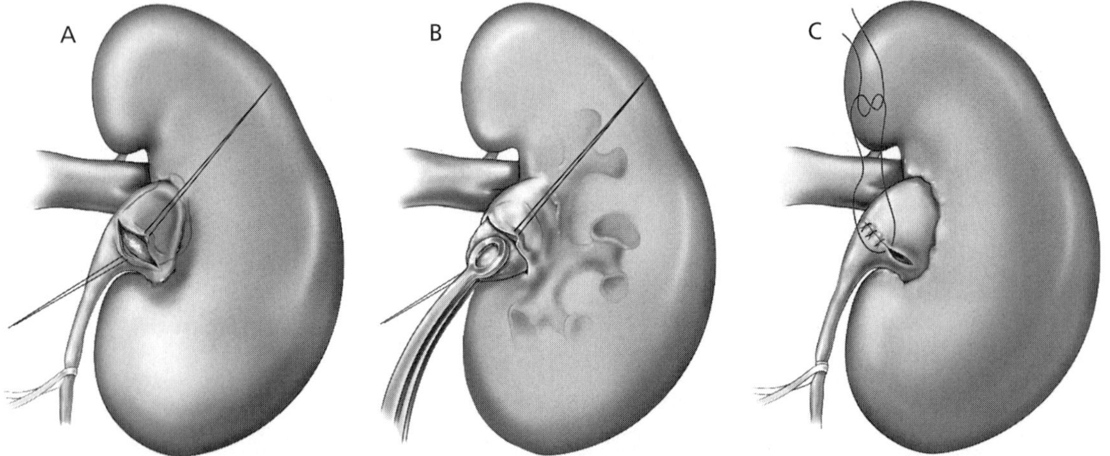

FIGURE 9.31. **A:** The pyelotomy incision is performed horizontally on the renal pelvis between stay sutures, taking care to avoid the ureteropelvic junction. **B:** The stone is extracted under direct vision with standard stone forceps. **C:** The pyelotomy incision is closed with full-thickness, interrupted, absorbable suture.

ureteral patency. The renal pelvis is thoroughly irrigated and the catheter removed. The pyelotomy is then closed in a single layer using running or interrupted 4-0 absorbable suture placed full thickness through the posterior renal pelvic wall such that peripelvic adventitia, musculature, and mucosa are all encompassed with each bite (Fig. 9.31C). In all cases, external drainage is provided with a Penrose or closed-suction drain placed near but not on the pyelotomy incision.

In uncomplicated cases, there is no need for an internal stent, although this should be considered in the presence of recent infection or if there is any question of residual calculi. Nephrostomy tubes are indicated only in the most complicated cases, such as in the setting of previous surgery with intense inflammation and scarring or if there is a question of ureteral patency or residual calculi. This allows excellent access for antegrade radiographic studies in the postoperative period.

Extended Pyelolithotomy

In 1891, Disse described fibrous extensions from the renal capsule that extended to the posterior renal pelvis and normally acted to separate the renal sinus from the retroperitoneal space. An extended pyelolithotomy, as advocated by Gil-Vernet in 1965 (61), takes advantage of dissection into the renal sinus to gain access to the intrarenal collecting system. This approach gained favor in Europe even for management of some extensive staghorn calculi. In general, though, its use had been limited to management of relatively large renal pelvic stones with or without extension into one or more infundibula, but without dumbbell-shaped calyceal extensions or associated infundibular stenosis (Fig. 9.32). However, these indications are now considered only within the narrower context of current indications for open operative intervention.

The posterior aspect of the renal pelvis is exposed as described for a standard pyelolithotomy. Dissection is then carried into the renal sinus by incising the fibrous tissue between the posterior hilar lip of renal parenchyma and the renal pelvis itself, and the plane between the renal pelvis and peripelvic fat is entered. Further exposure of the intrarenal collecting system can then be accomplished using vein retractors, or specifically designed Gil-Vernet renal sinus retractors, to elevate the posterior parenchymal lip. Dissection into the sinus then continues using a moist gauze or Kittner sponge (Fig. 9.33A). As described by Wulfsohn (192), temporary occlusion of the renal artery done in association with local hypothermia can serve to soften the renal parenchyma and allow further exposure of the intrarenal collecting system, which may be necessary in select cases.

A curvilinear transverse pyelotomy is then performed between stay sutures, taking care to keep well away from the ureteropelvic junction. The pyelotomy is then extended along both the upper and lower infundibula, thus creating a renal pelvic flap, which affords access to even large calculi with early branch formation (Fig. 9.33B). Any infundibular extensions that remain after extraction of the renal pelvic stone can be removed using Randall's forceps.

For more extensive stones, this approach can be combined with a simple or lower pole nephrotomy. For dumbbell-shaped calyceal extensions near the mid or superior poles that cannot be withdrawn via the infundibulum, a nephrotomy incision is made directly over the stone. This approach is best reserved for those patients in whom the stone is associated with cortical loss and local cortical thinning.

Lower pole infundibulocalyceal extensions of pelvic calculi can be managed by extending the inferior aspect of the pyelotomy incision onto the posterior renal parenchyma itself as a pyeloinfundibulotomy, directly over the involved lower infundibulum (Fig. 9.34). The infundibulonephrotomy incision thus performed is in an avascular plane between the junction of the posterior and basilar segments of the kidney.

As for a simple pyelolithotomy, on removal of all visible and palpable stone material, a catheter is passed antegrade down the ureter and the intrarenal collecting system is thoroughly irrigated. If multiple stones have been present, intraoperative radiography, fluoroscopy, US, or pyeloscopy should be performed to exclude the presence of residual calculi.

The pyelotomy incision is closed as for a standard pyelolithotomy. For cases requiring extensive dissection, placement of an internal stent may be desirable. External drainage is routinely provided.

Coagulum Pyelolithotomy

In 1943, Dees (38) combined human fibrinogen and clotting globulin to form an extractable cast of the upper collecting system, which he used to remove multiple renal calculi. Several authors have since reported their own modifications of the coagulum "recipe" to both simplify the procedure and reduce the risk of complications. At the authors' institution, we have used the technique described by Fischer and associates in 1980 (56). In that protocol, cryoprecipitate is the fibrinogen source and is converted to fibrin using thrombin as the active catalyst. Calcium chloride in the mixture serves to increase the tensile strength of the coagulum by neutralizing the citrate already present in the cryoprecipitate and by acting as a cofactor in the conversion of prothrombin to thrombin. To further obviate the risk of transmission of blood-borne disease, McVary and O'Conor (114), in 1989, reported the use of autologous cryoprecipitate in this setting.

The contemporary indication for a coagulum pyelolithotomy is the presence of multiple stones scattered throughout the collecting system, again in context of the otherwise limited contemporary indications for open operative intervention. Stones in calices drained by relatively narrow infundibula cannot be extracted with this method because the dumbbell-shaped calyceal extensions of the coagulum would simply break off as the pelvic portion is removed. However, any residual coagulum left within the collecting system is of no consequence because it will dissolve spontaneously in 24 to 48 hours in response to urokinase normally present in the urine.

Exposure of the renal pelvis is accomplished as described for pyelolithotomy. Again, an occluding vessel loop is placed about the proximal ureter to prevent distal migration of either stone fragments or the coagulum itself. The volume of the pyelocalyceal system is now estimated by puncturing and draining the renal pelvis with a 14-gauge angiocatheter. The pelvis is filled to capacity with a measured amount of saline, and the volume of coagulum prepared is then based on the amount of saline required for gentle distention. The estimated amount of required cryoprecipitate is then drawn up into one large syringe while the requisite volume of thrombin and calcium chloride is combined together in a second syringe. The amount of each constituent required is based on a ratio of 1 mL of cryoprecipitate to 2 units of thrombin and 1 mg of calcium chloride.

At this time, the angiocatheter that had been left in place in the renal pelvis is used to again completely drain the pyelocalyceal system. The thrombin and calcium chloride are then injected into the syringe containing the cryoprecipitate, and the complete mixture is injected into the renal

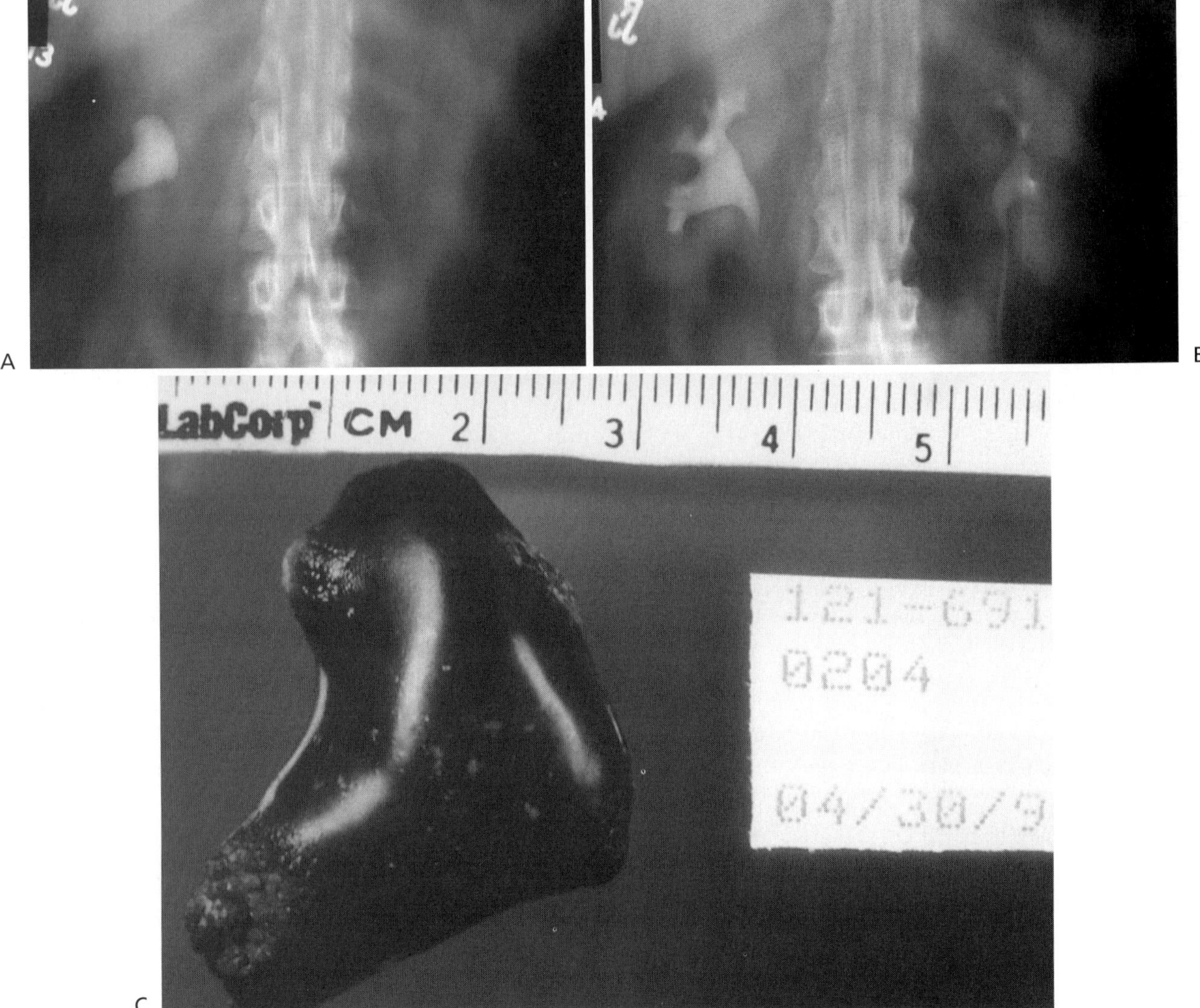

FIGURE 9.32. Intravenous urogram. **A:** Scout film. **B:** Following contrast injection, a large renal pelvic calculus is revealed extending from the upper to the lower infundibula. The patient had failed percutaneous management elsewhere and was adamant in her request for open operative intervention. Anatomically, this patient is a good candidate for an extended pyelolithotomy. **C:** Stone removed from this patient with an extended pyelolithotomy incision.

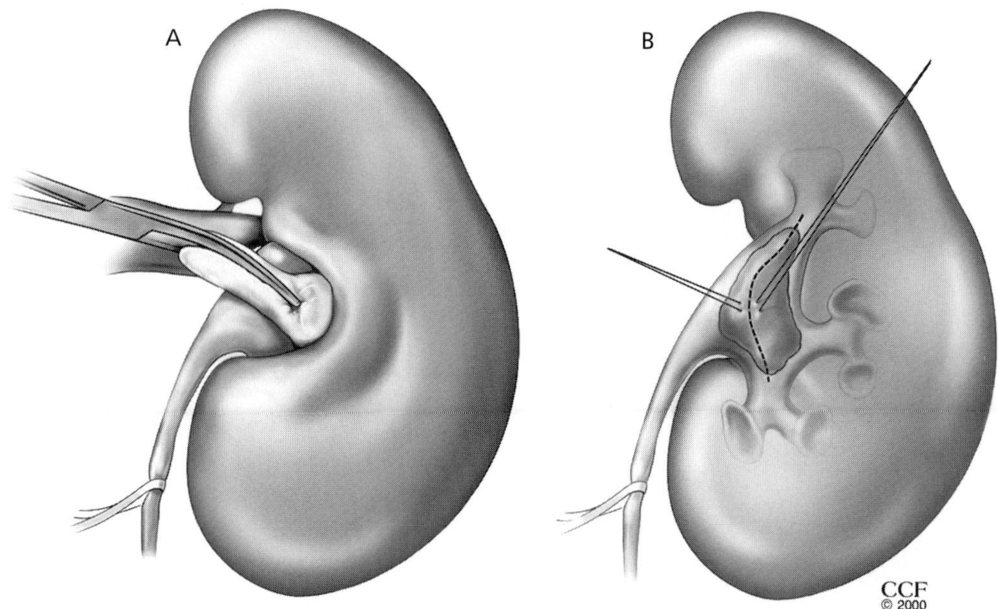

FIGURE 9.33. **A:** A moist gauze or sponge is used to develop the avascular plane posteriorly between the renal pelvis and parenchyma. **B:** An extended pyelolithotomy requires a curvilinear incision that extends from the upper infundibulum across the renal pelvis and into the lower infundibulum.

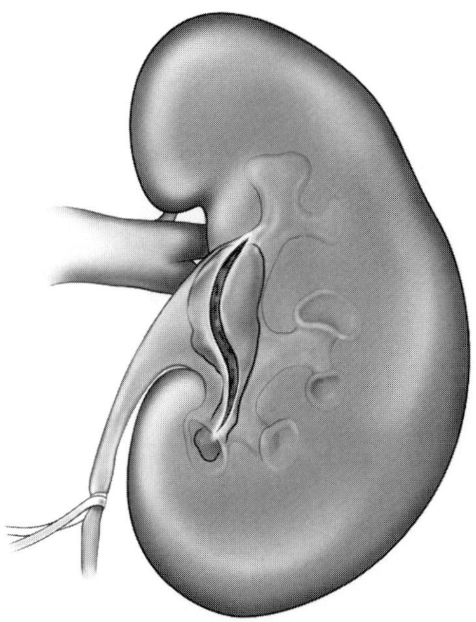

FIGURE 9.34. A pyeloinfundibulonephrotomy incision can be made on the anterior aspect of the kidney through a relatively avascular plane between the junction of the posterior and basilar segments of the kidney. Such an incision can be used to manage renal pelvic calculi extending into the lower infundibulocalyceal system.

pelvis within 45 seconds (Fig. 9.35A), after which time clotting will have irreversibly begun. At this point, assuming the measured capacity was correct, there will be complete filling and gentle distention of the renal pelvis. Care should be taken not to overdistend the system because this could result in pyelovenous backflow of the cryoprecipitate, and rarely, a pulmonary embolus can develop in this setting as reported by Pence and colleagues in 1981 (131).

After 5 to 10 minutes, the coagulum should be well established. A standard or extended pyelotomy incision is made and the coagulum extracted (Fig. 9.35B). If the procedure has been performed correctly, the coagulum has formed a cast of the collecting system and multiple stones will be trapped within the substance of the coagulum (Fig. 9.36).

As for any procedure involving a patient with multiple stones, intraoperative radiographs, fluoroscopy, US, or pyeloscopy is then performed as necessary to exclude the presence of residual calculi. Because the procedure is always performed in patients with multiple calculi, it is generally prudent to leave an internal stent at this time to prevent migration of any potentially unrecognized residual stones in the early postoperative period. External drainage is routinely provided with a Penrose or closed-suction drain.

Calyceal Diverticulolithotomy

Calyceal diverticula are transitional epithelium-lined cavities in the renal parenchyma. Communication with a calix or infundibulum is implied by definition, although that communication may not be demonstrable at the time the patient is initially examined. Because some calyceal diverticula are associated with localized urinary stasis, they may be a source of stone formation, although as reported by Hsu and Streem (79), metabolic factors also play a role. The indications to intervene for calyceal diverticular stones are the

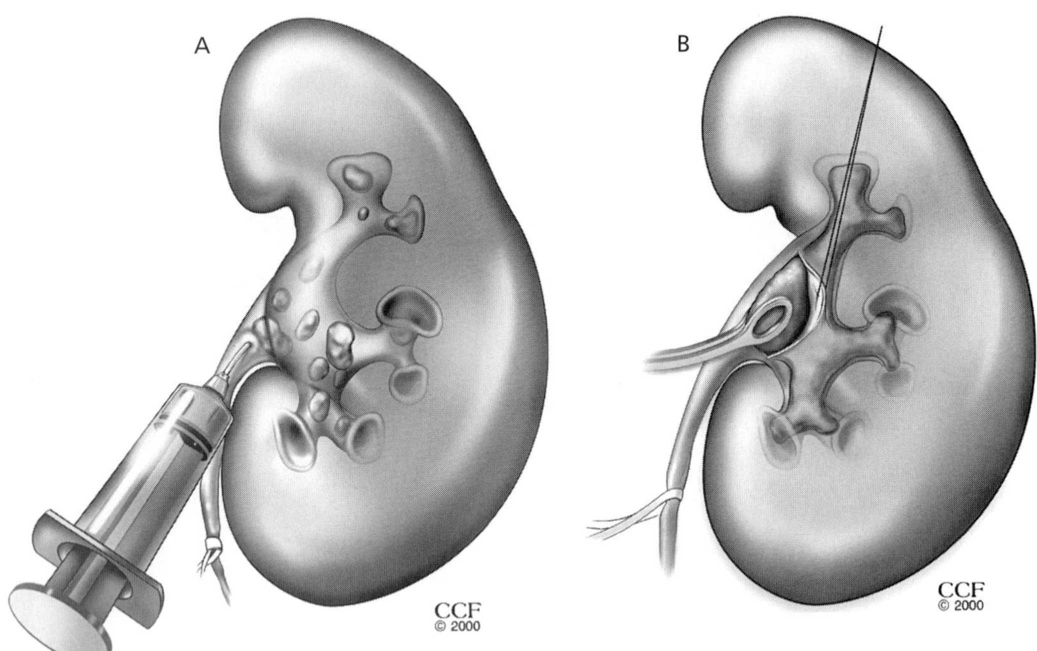

FIGURE 9.35. **A:** The proximal ureter is secured with a vascular tape as the coagulum, consisting of cryoprecipitate, bovine thrombin, and calcium chloride, is injected into the collecting system. **B:** A pyelotomy incision is made and the coagulum is extracted.

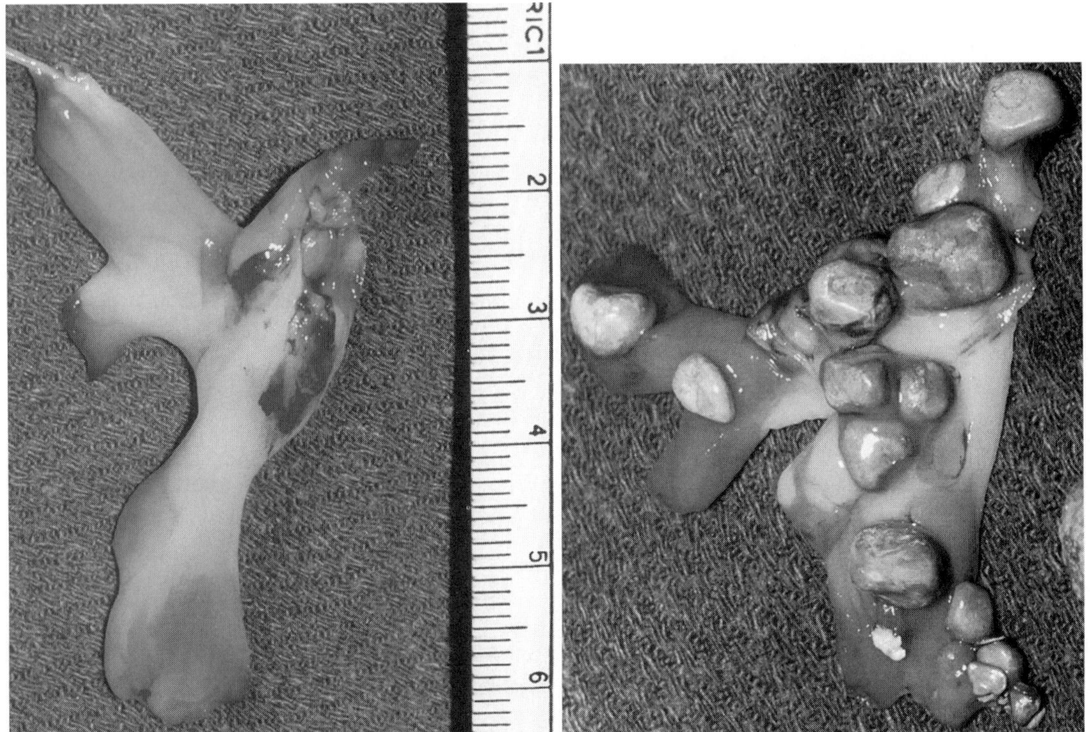

FIGURE 9.36. **A:** The coagulum has assumed the shape of the pyelocalyceal system. **B:** Multiple stones entrapped within the substance of the coagulum.

same as for any upper tract stones, although the indications for open operative intervention are considerably narrower. In highly select patients, SWL can be successful (169), although ureteroscopic and percutaneous techniques are generally considered more definitive (11,13,85,162). When these techniques are contraindicated or have failed, open operative intervention may be considered.

Preoperative planning generally includes a CT scan for three-dimensional radiographic localization (Fig. 9.37). The kidney is exposed via a standard flank incision. Generally, the diverticulum is readily apparent by inspection and palpation, although intraoperative localization can be performed when necessary with intraoperative fluoroscopy or US. In all cases, confirmation that the suspicious area represents the diverticulum can be performed by using a small-gauge needle to aspirate urine from the diverticulum or to "sound" the calculus.

When the diverticulum is associated with thinning of the overlying parenchyma, appropriate management is marsupialization. The thin parenchyma overlying the diverticulum is excised, and the calculi are removed. The diverticular neck can then be identified and is oversewn with absorbable suture or simply fulgurated. The lining of the diverticulum may also be fulgurated either with electrofulguration or an argon beam coagulator. The rim of remaining parenchyma is then oversewn with absorbable suture or simply fulgurated.

Occasionally, identification of the diverticular neck may be difficult. This can be circumvented with placement of a ureteral catheter at the outset of the procedure. Dilute methylene blue can then be injected retrograde via the ureteral catheter, and the diverticular neck is identified as the methylene blue flows into the diverticulum.

In some cases, the diverticulum may be located deep within the renal parenchyma. With the aid of intraoperative US, the area containing the diverticulum can easily be identified. In such cases, however, rather than unroofing, a local wedge resection is more appropriate. In all cases, a Penrose or closed-suction drain is placed near the site of excision, and the wound is irrigated and closed in a standard fashion.

Although open calyceal diverticulolithotomy and diverticulectomy should be a part of the urologic armamentarium, many patients who otherwise would have required open operative intervention because of a failure of or contraindication to less invasive techniques can and should be managed with a laparoscopic approach as described by Ruckle and Segura in 1994 (150).

Anatrophic Nephrolithotomy

Most opaque staghorn calculi are composed of magnesium-ammonium-calcium phosphate and are associated with urinary infection that will always recur as long as the stone is present. In 1994, the American Urological Association (AUA) Nephrolithiasis Clinical Guidelines Panel made recommendations regarding the management of these branched, infection-related stones (158). The AUA Nephrolithiasis Clinical Guidelines Panel stressed that left untreated, these stones are invariably associated with recurrent infection, loss of renal function, and high rates of renal-related morbidity and even death. In reviewing outcome probabilities for management of such stones, the AUA Nephrolithiasis Clinical Guidelines Panel concluded that any newly diagnosed struvite staghorn calculus was an indication for intervention. The AUA Nephrolithiasis Clinical Guidelines Panel further recommended that most such stones could be managed with percutaneous nephrolithotomy or SWL, either alone or in combination. However, open operative intervention was recommended as an appropriate option in cases where the stone was so extensive that an unreasonable number of percutaneous or shock wave procedures would be required to achieve a stone-free result.

In affected patients, the most common relative indication for open operative intervention is the finding of a massively sized, complete, fully branched staghorn calculus with multiple dumbbell-shaped infundibulocalyceal extensions associated with relatively narrow infundibula (Fig. 9.38). Multiple areas of true infundibular stenosis would also be a relative indication for open operative intervention so that this anatomic abnormality could be managed simultaneously. In such cases, the most appropriate open operative approach is generally anatrophic nephrolithotomy as initially described by Boyce and Smith in 1967 (16). With this procedure, the stones are removed through an incision that is least traumatic to overall renal function, that is, an incision through a relatively avascular plane in the kidney. The renal artery will temporarily be occluded during the procedure to provide a bloodless field in which to work, and the kidney must therefore be protected from the resulting ischemic insult. Finally, areas of true, functionally significant infundibular stenosis are addressed such that adequate drainage is provided from all parts of the collecting system.

Our preference is a flank approach with resection of the eleventh or twelfth rib, with medial extension of the incision to the lateral border of the rectus muscle. The peritoneum is reflected medially, and access to the retroperitoneum is attained. The proximal ureter is surrounded with a vessel loop to prevent distal migration of stone fragments during the subsequent procedure. The kidney is then completely mobilized and the renal pedicle isolated. The renal artery is surrounded with a vessel loop and mannitol, 12.5 g, is given intravenously for protection during the subsequent renal ischemic episode (Fig. 9.39). Further dissection of the renal artery is accomplished until the anterior and posterior divisional branches are identified. The first major branch of the renal artery generally represents the posterior division (Fig. 9.40).

As described by Brodell in 1901 (18) and subsequently by Graves in 1954 (69), there is an avascular plane between

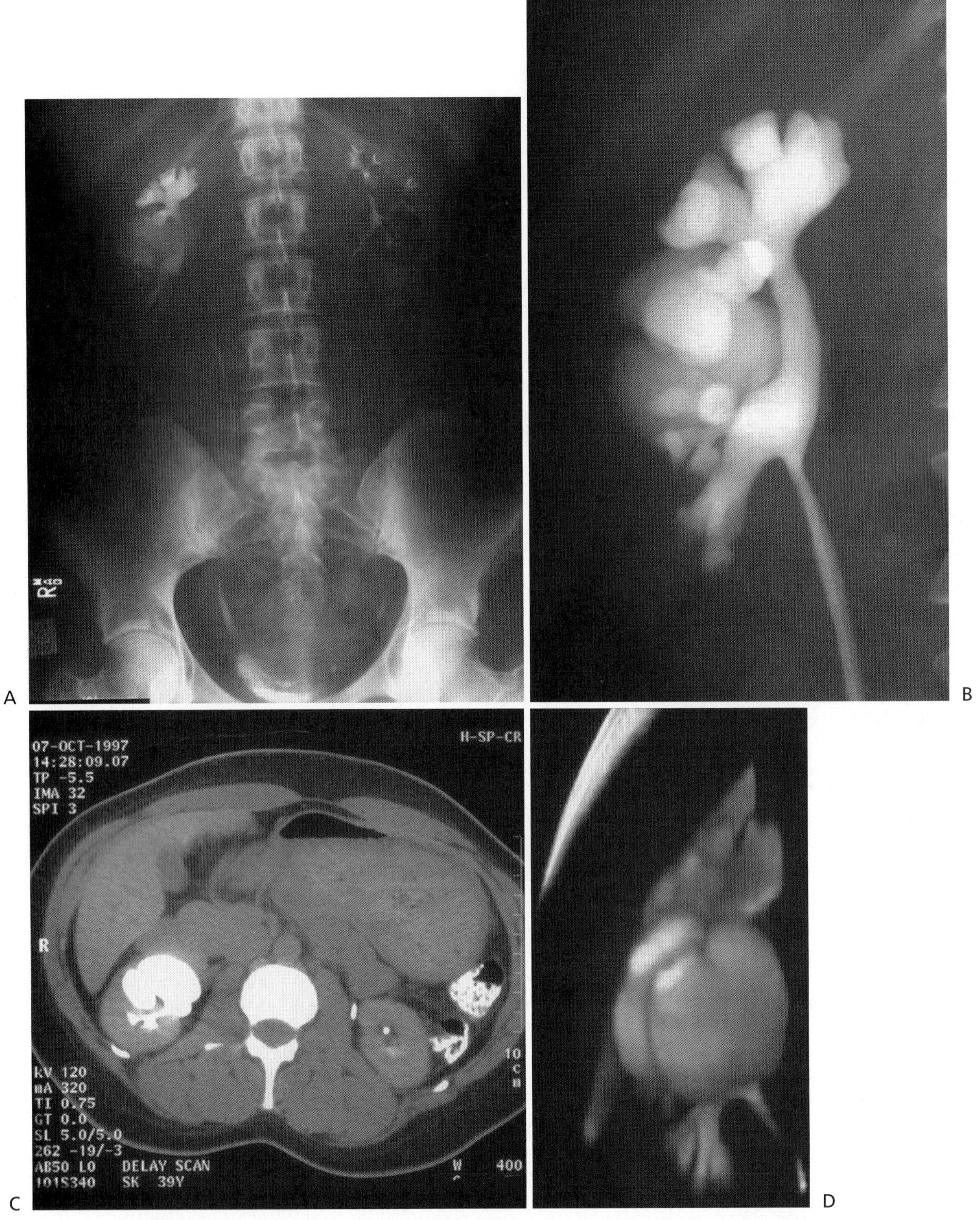

FIGURE 9.37. A: Intravenous urogram in this patient with chronic right flank pain suggests the presence of a large calyceal diverticulum in the central aspect of the kidney. **B:** Retrograde study confirms filling of a central calyceal diverticulum. **C:** Computed tomography reveals the diverticulum to be located anteriorly with thinning of the overlying parenchyma. **D:** Three-dimensional reconstruction confirms the anterior location of the diverticulum and allows better evaluation of the relationship to the collecting system. The anterior location of this diverticulum and the thin overlying parenchyma suggest that the best approach is either open or laparoscopic diverticulolithotomy.

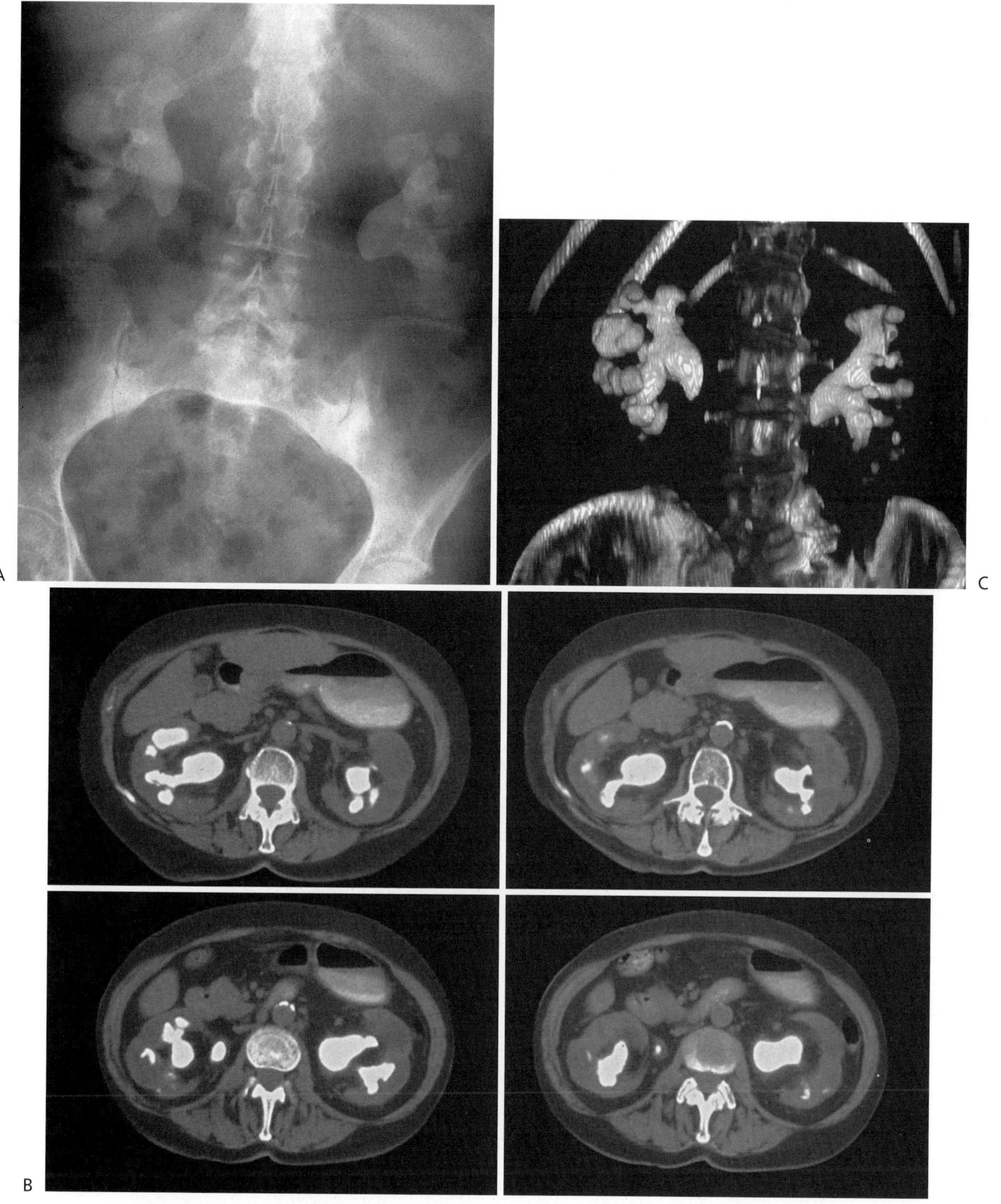

FIGURE 9.38. A: Plain abdominal film in this patient with significant renal insufficiency and proteus urinary infection reveals extensive, fully mature staghorn calculi bilaterally. Anatrophic nephrolithotomy is a reasonable approach compared with the option of multiple percutaneous and shock wave procedures. **B:** Standard computed tomography scan without contrast helps delineate the stone and the thickness of the overlying parenchyma. **C:** More recently, three-dimensional reconstruction has been used for more precise anatomic definition.

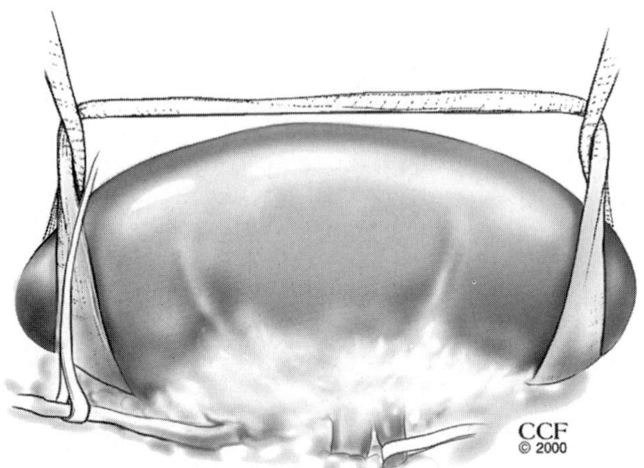

FIGURE 9.39. The kidney is mobilized and the renal artery identified and surrounded with a vessel loop. The kidney may be elevated into the wound using a Jones roll as a sling.

the junction of the blood supply to the anterior and posterior segments of the kidney. At the surface of the kidney, this generally lies on the posterior aspect approximately two-thirds of the way from the renal hilum to the true lateral border of the kidney. When desired, this can be further delineated by temporarily placing a vascular clamp on the anterior division of the renal artery (Fig. 9.41). Ten milliliters of methylene blue is then injected intravenously into the systemic circulation. This will stain the posterior renal segment and thus help identify the appropriate line of incision and further dissection into the renal parenchyma. Although delineation of the arterial blood supply in this manner may be useful, it may not be a requisite for a successful nephron-sparing result (125).

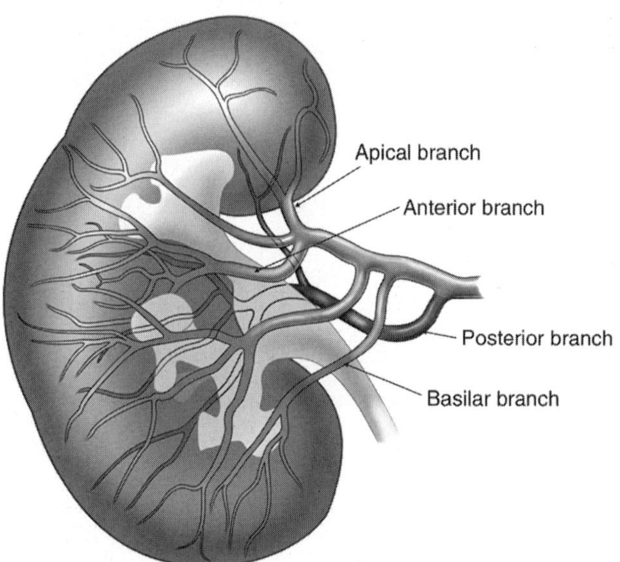

FIGURE 9.40. The first major branch of the renal artery generally represents the posterior division.

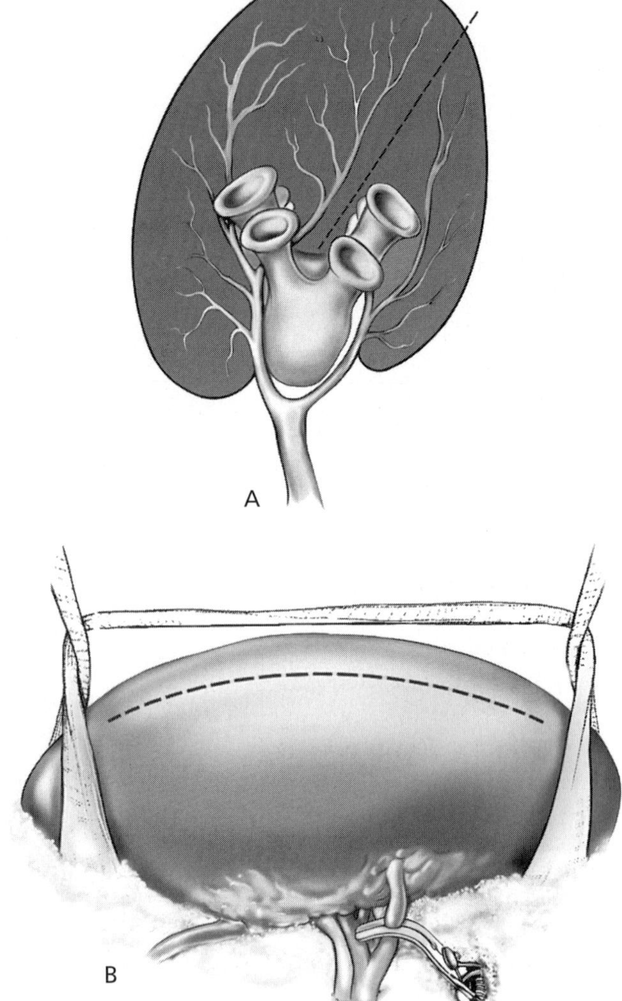

FIGURE 9.41. A: An avascular plane exists between the junction of the blood supply to the anterior and posterior segments of the kidney, and this plane generally provides the correct line of dissection for anatrophic nephrolithotomy. **B:** Temporary occlusion of the posterior branch of the renal artery can help delineate the optimal line of incision in this plane.

A bowel bag is the placed beneath the kidney and wrapped around the pedicle as a reservoir for ice slush. An additional 12.5 g of mannitol is given, and the main renal artery is subsequently occluded with a vascular clamp. At this point, the renal vein may also be occluded to ensure a blood-free surgical field. The kidney is packed with slush with a goal of obtaining a core temperature of 10°C as protection from the subsequent renal ischemic insult.

Once the kidney has reached core temperature, the capsule is incised longitudinally between the anterior and posterior segments, but extended only to the apical and basilar renal segments. The incision through parenchyma continues in a plane along the line of demarcation between the anterior and posterior arterial segments, down toward the renal pelvis. The correct plane generally runs

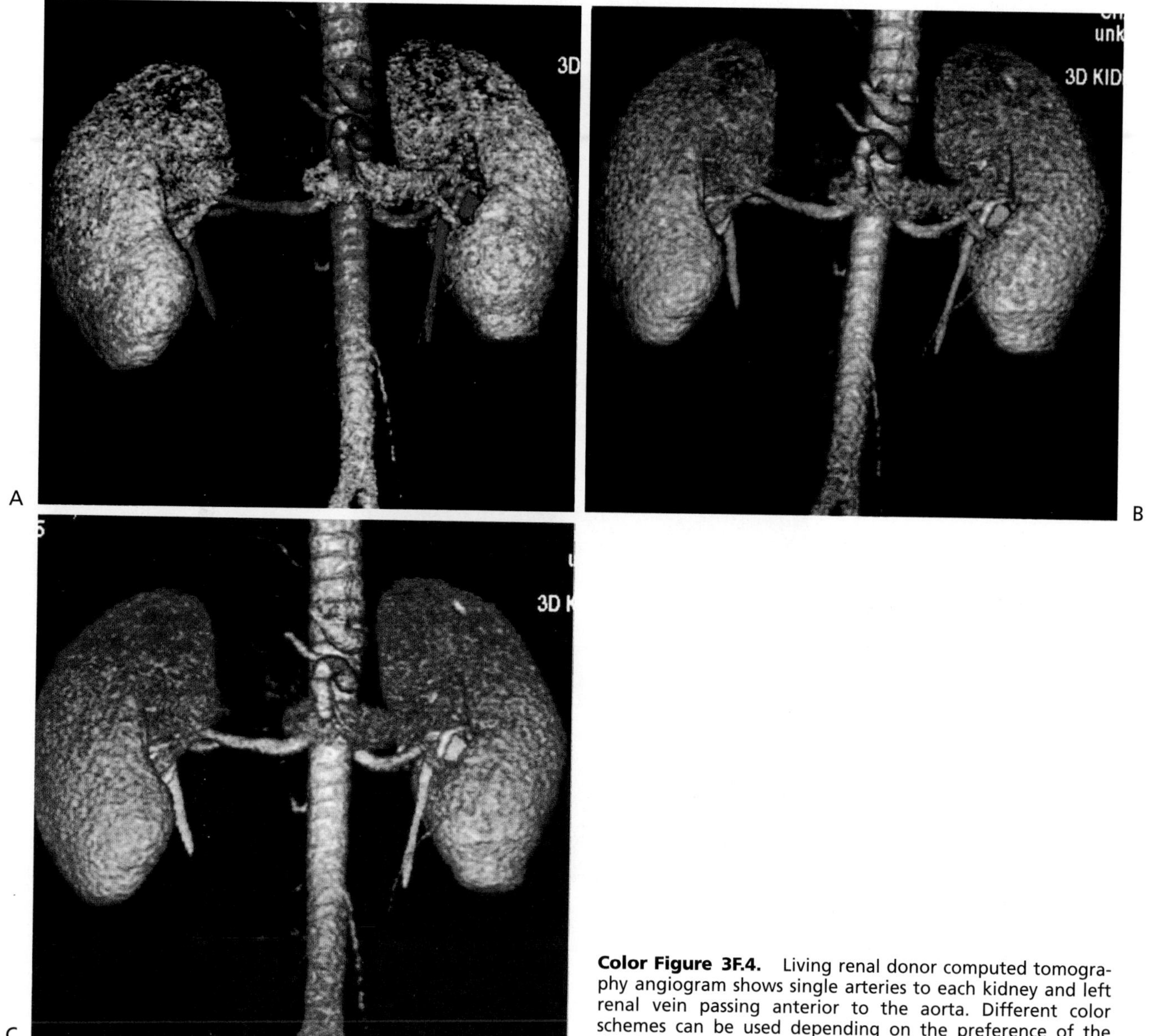

Color Figure 3F.4. Living renal donor computed tomography angiogram shows single arteries to each kidney and left renal vein passing anterior to the aorta. Different color schemes can be used depending on the preference of the viewing physicians. See also Figure 3F.4, page 178.

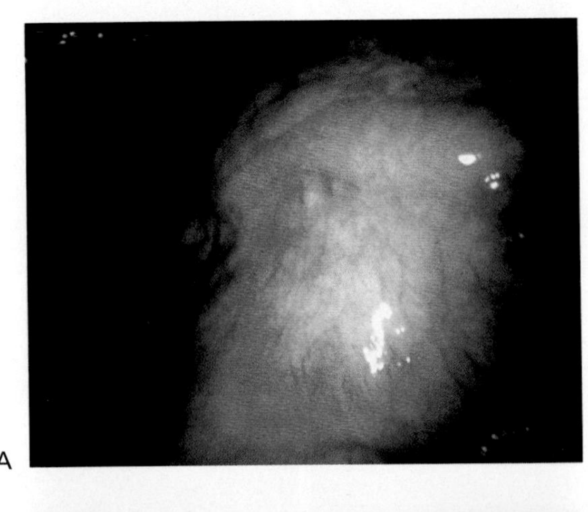

A

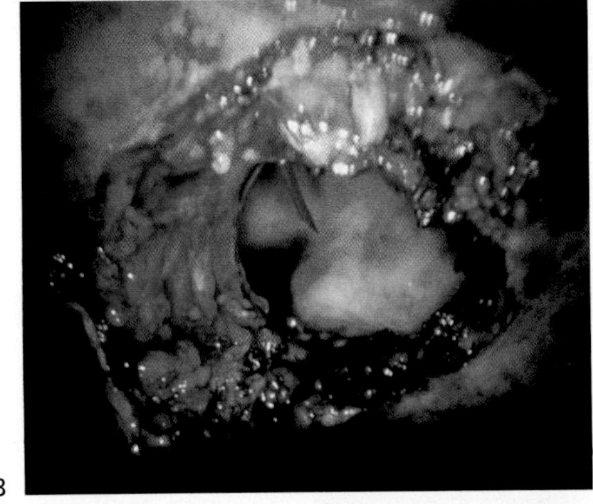

B

Color Figure 18.12. A: Laparoscopic inspection revealing the bluish-gray bulge of the lymphocele in the pelvis. **B:** Unroofed lymphocele with percutaneously placed needle visible within. See also Figure 18.12, page 685.

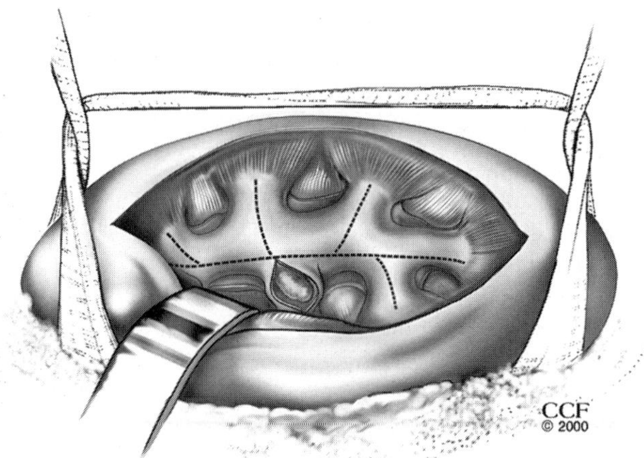

FIGURE 9.42. The collecting system is entered with an incision into one of the involved posterior infundibulocalyces containing stone.

just anterior to the posterior row of infundibula and calices. If small arterioles or venules are cut and identified during this incision or during the subsequent dissection, these are managed using fine chromic figure-of-eight absorbable suture.

The stone is now identified either by palpation in one of the involved posterior infundibula or calyceals or by direct visualization. Once the initial stone-bearing infundibulocalix is open, a longitudinal infundibulotomy is performed and extended down to the renal pelvis (Fig. 9.42). Similarly, each involved posterior infundibulocalix is subsequently opened longitudinally as far as necessary to extract any stone, and the infundibulotomy is carried down its anterior aspect toward the renal pelvis.

Once the pelvic and posterior infundibulocalyceal aspects of the stone are identified, the anterior and polar portions are exposed, again with sequential longitudinal infundibulotomies. However, these are performed on the posterior aspect of the anterior segmental infundibula and central aspects of the polar infundibula. The infundibulotomies should begin at each infundibulopelvic junction and extend outward toward the calix as far as necessary to provide adequate exposure for stone removal.

Eventually, the entire staghorn calculus is exposed and ready for removal (Fig. 9.43). In some cases, the entire stone can be delivered intact, but piecemeal extraction is usually required. Infundibulocalyceal extensions may break off due to a relatively soft and friable intrinsic nature of the stone, or alternatively, the entire stone may not have been in continuity to start. If infundibulocalyceal extensions of the stone are not extracted with the main portion, the involved infundibulum should be dilated or further incised out toward the calix to ensure complete visualization and stone removal.

Once the bulk of the stone is removed (Fig. 9.44), each infundibulocalix is individually explored both visually and with palpation to exclude residual fragments. Occasionally, residual fragment can be palpated through thin parenchyma, but the infundibulum leading to the stone cannot be visualized. In such cases, a small nephrotomy made directly over the palpable stone is acceptable. The stone is extracted, and the nephrotomy is closed with absorbable sutures. The entire collecting system should now be thoroughly lavaged with iced saline using appropriately sized red rubber catheters placed sequentially into each infundibulocalix.

Because an optimal result requires removal of all stone fragments, several adjunctive maneuvers can be performed to identify and remove any potential residual stones, including intraoperative static radiography (Fig. 9.45A), fluoroscopy (Fig. 9.45B), US, and intraoperative pyeloscopy using flexible instrumentation (Fig. 9.45C).

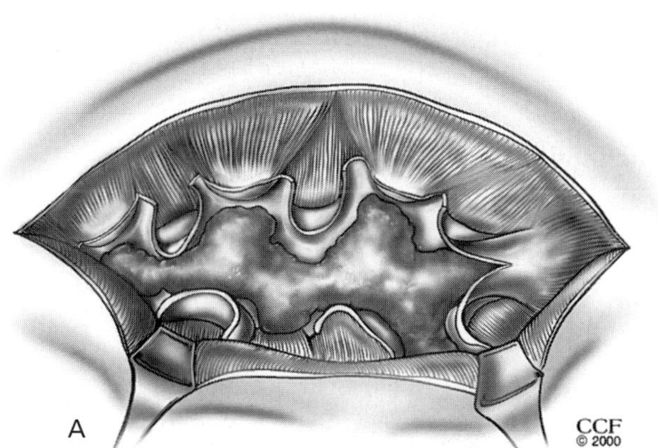

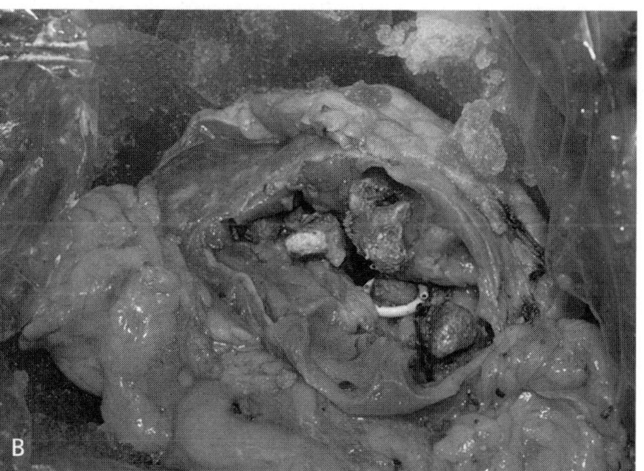

FIGURE 9.43. A: The entire stone is now exposed after performing sequential longitudinal infundibulotomies and opening the lateral portion of the renal pelvis. **B:** Intraoperative view of completed anatrophic incision with entire collecting system exposed. Note the bloodless field availed by clamping of the renal artery. The kidney is packed in ice slush to minimize the adverse effect of renal ischemic injury.

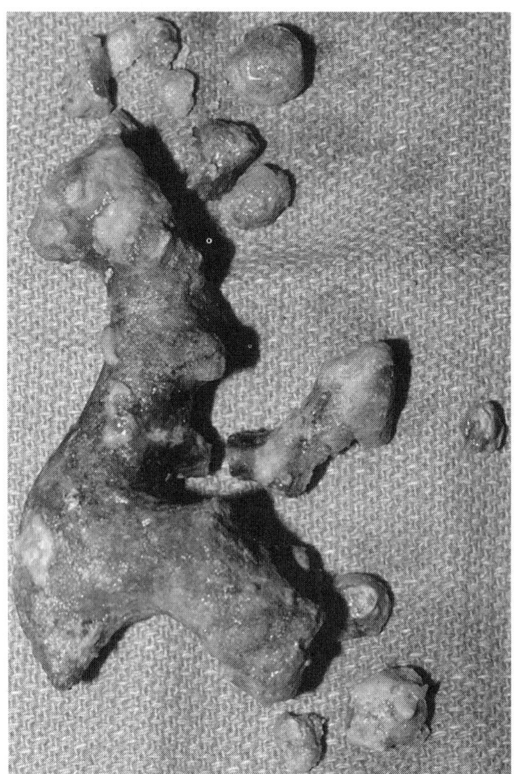

FIGURE 9.44. Staghorn calculus removed with anatrophic nephrolithotomy.

When all identifiable stone has been removed, a red rubber catheter is passed antegrade down the ureter, and the ureter is irrigated with saline. An internal stent may be placed at this time, and although this is not mandatory, it should be considered in those patients who may have residual fragments and in patients with compromised renal function. Nephrostomy tubes are used even less frequently and generally only for patients with severely compromised renal function and thinned parenchyma.

The collecting system is now reconstructed using fine absorbable suture (Fig. 9.46A). In areas of significant infundibular stenosis, infundibulorrhaphy is performed by suturing the adjacent borders of involved infundibula on their mirror-image sides, thus converting two or more stenotic infundibulocalyceal systems into one larger portion of the renal pelvis (Fig. 9.46B). Alternatively, isolated infundibular stenosis or polar infundibular stenosis can be managed with an individual infundibulorrhaphy that involves horizontal closure of the initial vertical infundibulotomy in a Heineke-Mikulicz fashion (Fig. 9.46C). However, when no infundibular stenosis is present, separate closure of the collecting system may not be necessary (125).

The renal capsule is now approximated with running or interrupted 3-0 chromic sutures incorporating only a very small bite of renal parenchyma (Fig. 9.46D). At this time, an additional 12.5 g of mannitol is given intravenously and the vascular clamps are removed. Perirenal fat can be reapproximated over the nephrotomy incision, and external drainage is provided with a Penrose or closed-suction drain placed near, but not directly on, the nephrotomy incision itself.

Partial Nephrectomy

A partial nephrectomy is considered when stone disease is associated with a localized area of irrevocably poor renal function as can occur in the setting of chronic obstruction, especially with infection (Fig. 9.47). In such cases, removal of the diseased portion of the kidney along with the stone may be the best option, especially when localized xanthogranulomatous pyelonephritis may be present.

Nephrectomy

Nephrectomy is indicated only rarely for management of renal calculi. The specific indication is stone disease associated with a nonfunctioning or poorly functioning kidney that is irrevocably damaged and would be unlikely to support life off dialysis should it be the sole kidney (Fig. 9.48). This generally implies renal function less than 10% to 15% of overall function, or a glomerular filtration rate of less than 15 mL per minute. In these cases, salvageability of the kidney is best determined preoperatively with radiographic evaluation that includes a differential nuclear scan. We have also found CT scanning to be especially useful in determining the residual cortical thickness and to search for evidence of xanthogranulomatous pyelonephritis, which is best managed by nephrectomy. If there is any question as to recoverability of function in the setting of chronic obstruction, placement of percutaneous nephrostomy provides temporary relief of obstruction and allows follow-up differential renal functional studies.

Ureterolithotomy

Open ureterolithotomy is rarely performed in contemporary practice. Essentially, the only indication today is a failure of, or a contraindication to, all less invasive procedures, including SWL, retrograde ureteroscopic management, and percutaneous antegrade management. In such cases, an extraperitoneal approach is used with the incision positioned at the level of the stone. The peritoneum is reflected medially, the ureter is identified, and the stone is palpated. Generally, extensive ureteral mobilization is not necessary and should be avoided whenever possible. The ureter proximal to the stone is controlled by placement of a vascular tape (Fig. 9.49A). This prevents proximal migration of the stone up into the dilated ureter during the subsequent procedure. A longitudinal ureterotomy is then made directly over the stone using a "banana blade." The stone is extracted with an appropriate-size stone forceps (Fig. 9.49B). The ureter is then thoroughly irrigated distally and proximally with a small-caliber red rubber catheter, and distal patency is ensured by passage of the catheter all of the

Text continued on page 443

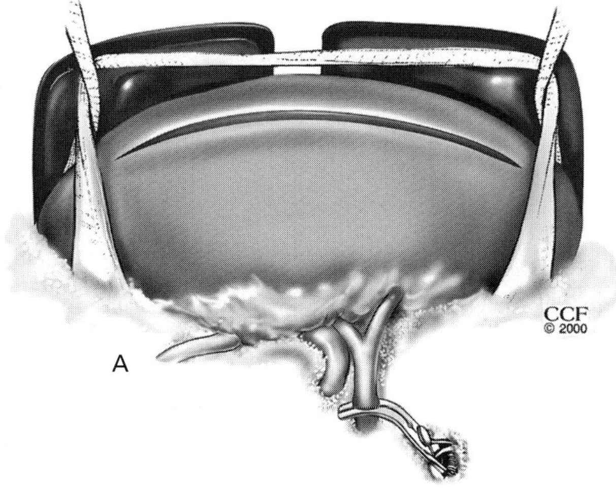

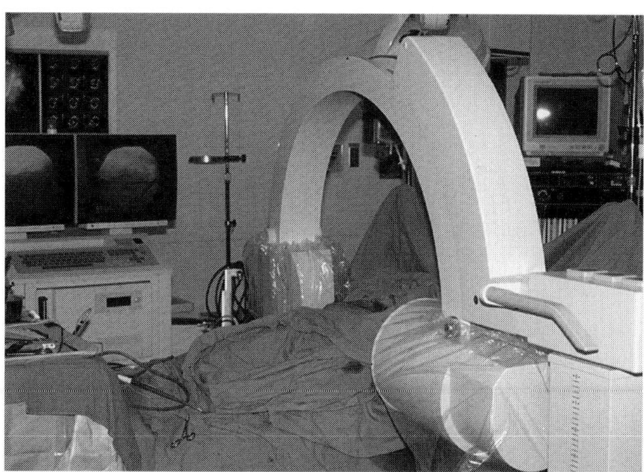

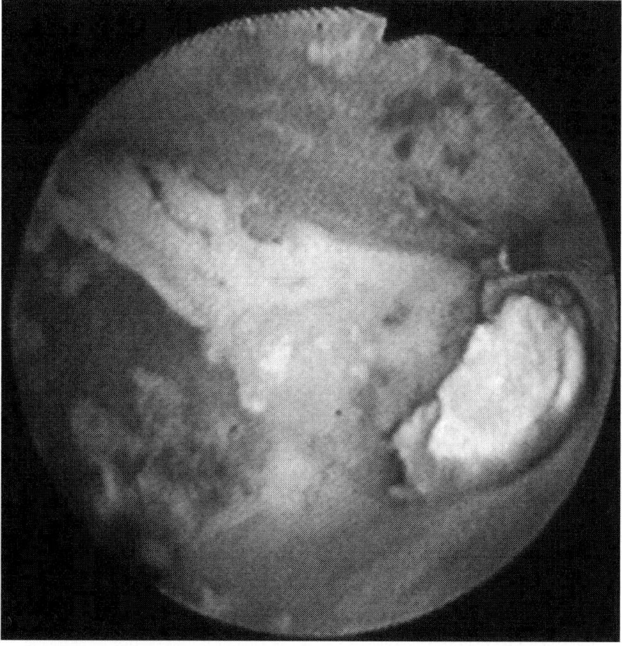

FIGURE 9.45. A: Intraoperative organ films had been a standard part of the procedure to exclude the presence of residual fragments. In general, such static radiography has been replaced with more contemporary adjunctive techniques such as intraoperative real-time fluoroscopy, ultrasound, or pyeloscopy. **B:** Intraoperative fluoroscopy has become a standard part of these stone procedures to exclude the presence of residual fragments and to help locate them for removal. **C:** Residual calyceal stone identified during intraoperative flexible pyeloscopy.

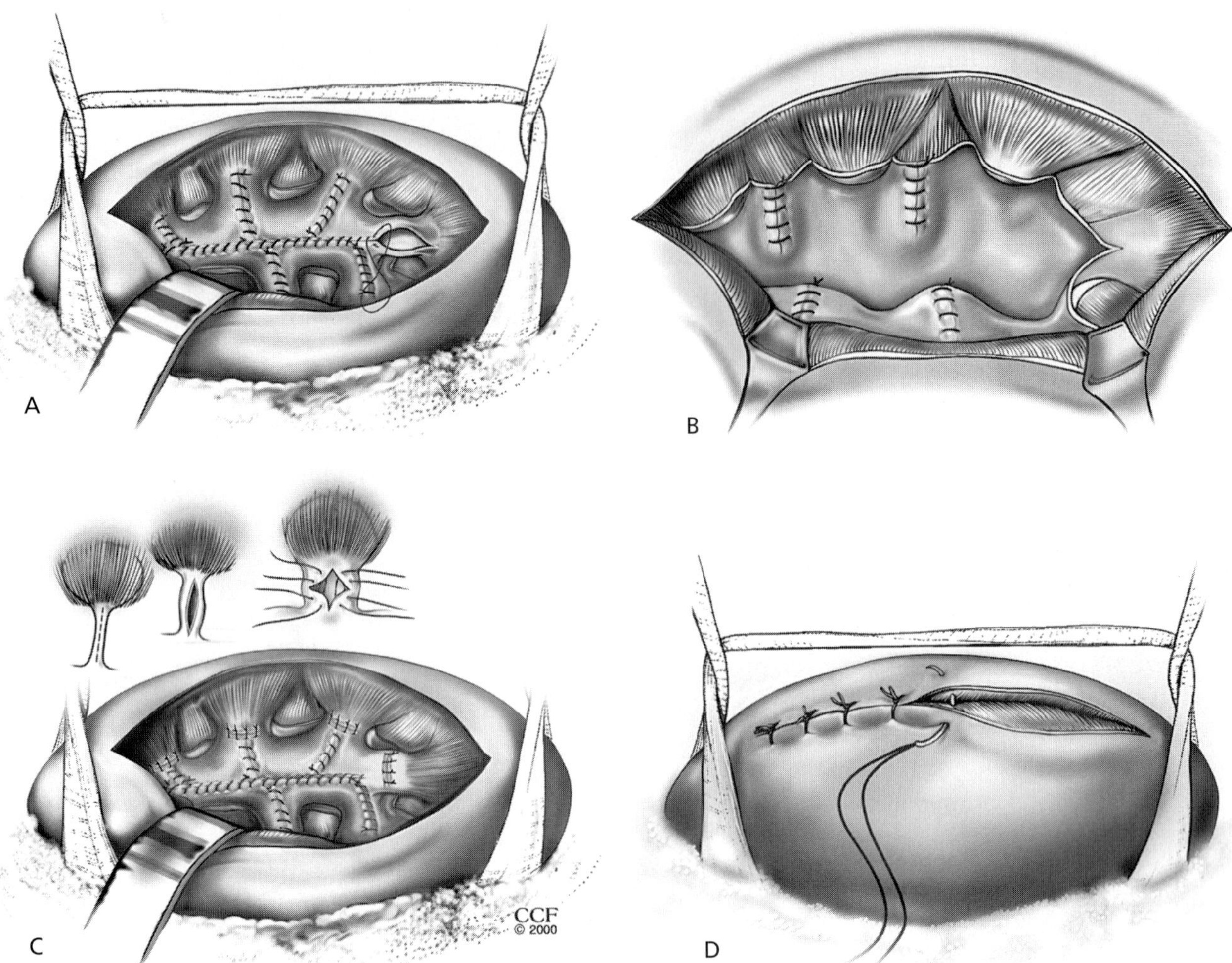

FIGURE 9.46. A: Closure of the collecting system begins with reconstruction of the incised infundibula and continues until the pelvis has been reapproximated. **B:** Infundibular stenosis is managed with infundibulorrhaphy. The lateral aspects of two adjacent infundibula are sutured to one another, creating widely patent, compound infundibulocalyces. **C:** Isolated polar infundibular stenosis is managed with a Heineke-Mikulicz infundibulorrhaphy. **D:** The renal capsule is approximated using running or interrupted mattress 3-0 chromic sutures taking a small bite of renal parenchyma.

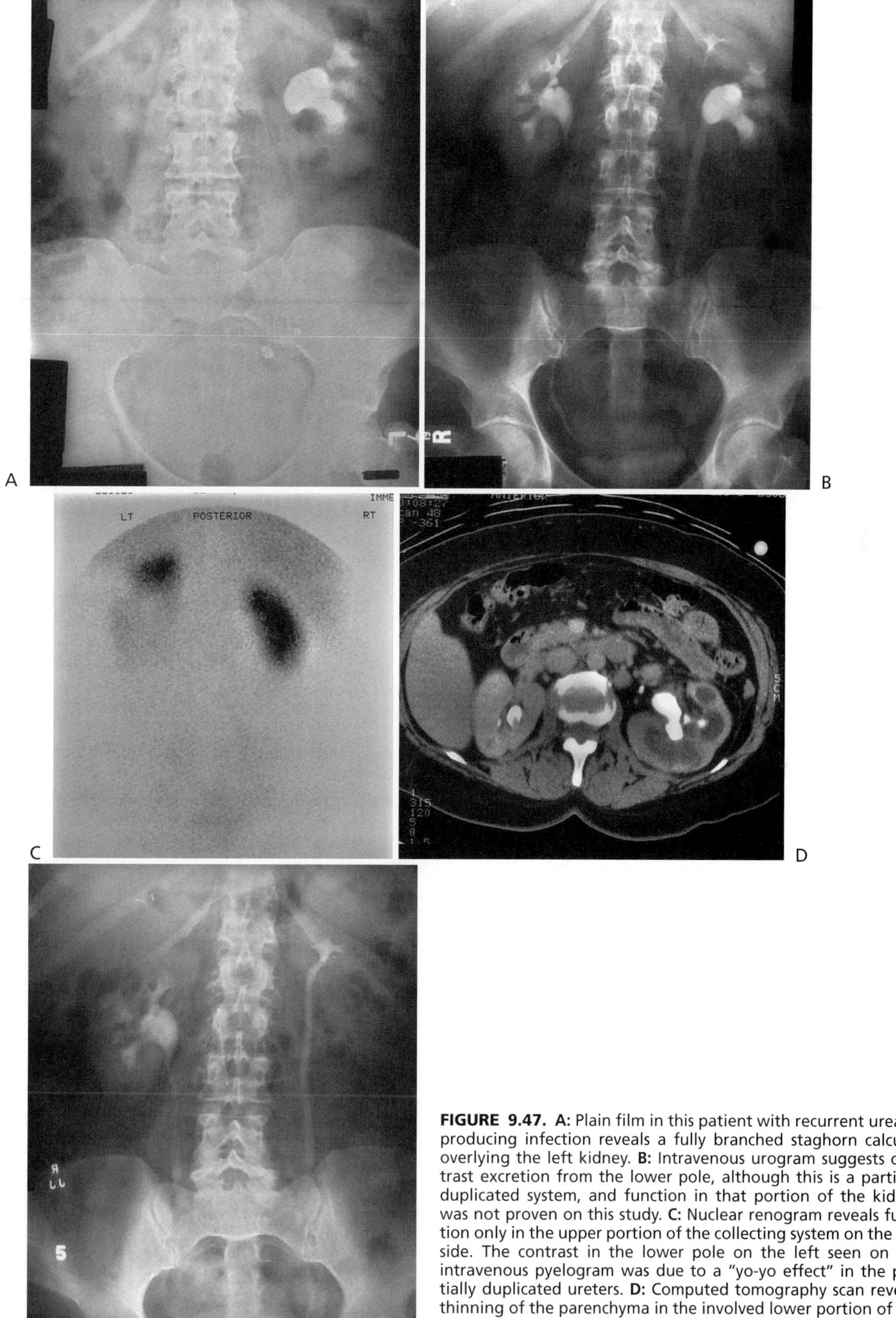

FIGURE 9.47. A: Plain film in this patient with recurrent urease-producing infection reveals a fully branched staghorn calculus overlying the left kidney. **B:** Intravenous urogram suggests contrast excretion from the lower pole, although this is a partially duplicated system, and function in that portion of the kidney was not proven on this study. **C:** Nuclear renogram reveals function only in the upper portion of the collecting system on the left side. The contrast in the lower pole on the left seen on the intravenous pyelogram was due to a "yo-yo effect" in the partially duplicated ureters. **D:** Computed tomography scan reveals thinning of the parenchyma in the involved lower portion of the collecting system. **E:** Following lower-pole partial nephrectomy, a well-functioning upper-pole system remains, as seen on this postoperative pyelogram.

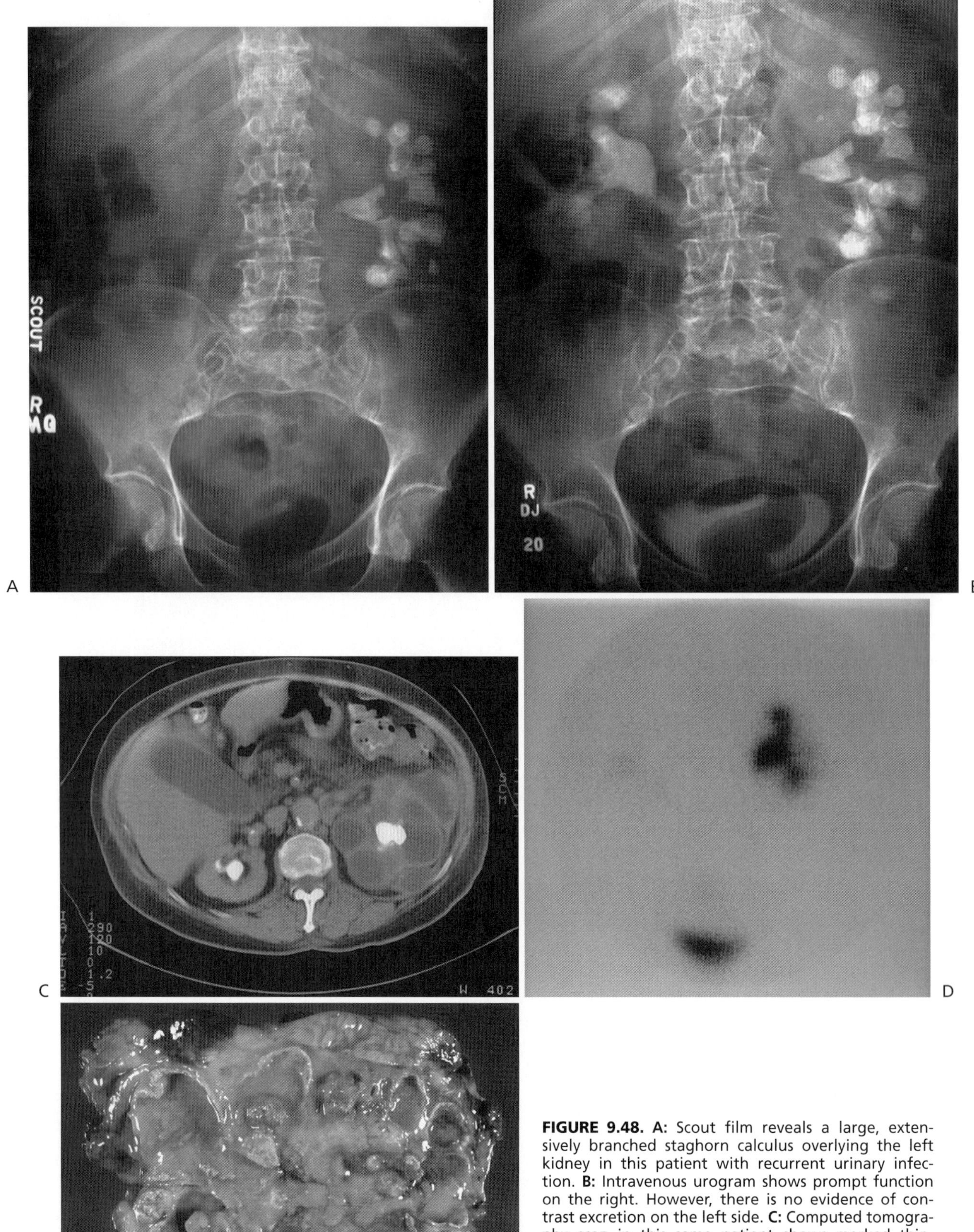

FIGURE 9.48. A: Scout film reveals a large, extensively branched staghorn calculus overlying the left kidney in this patient with recurrent urinary infection. **B:** Intravenous urogram shows prompt function on the right. However, there is no evidence of contrast excretion on the left side. **C:** Computed tomography scan in this same patient shows marked thinning of parenchyma and multiple cystic areas in the kidney consistent with local hydrocalices, and suggestive of xanthogranulomatous pyelonephritis. **D:** Renal scan shows essentially no function in the left kidney (posterior view). **E:** Nephrectomy specimen reveals chronic pyohydronephrosis. Pathologic examination confirmed xanthogranulomatous pyelonephritis.

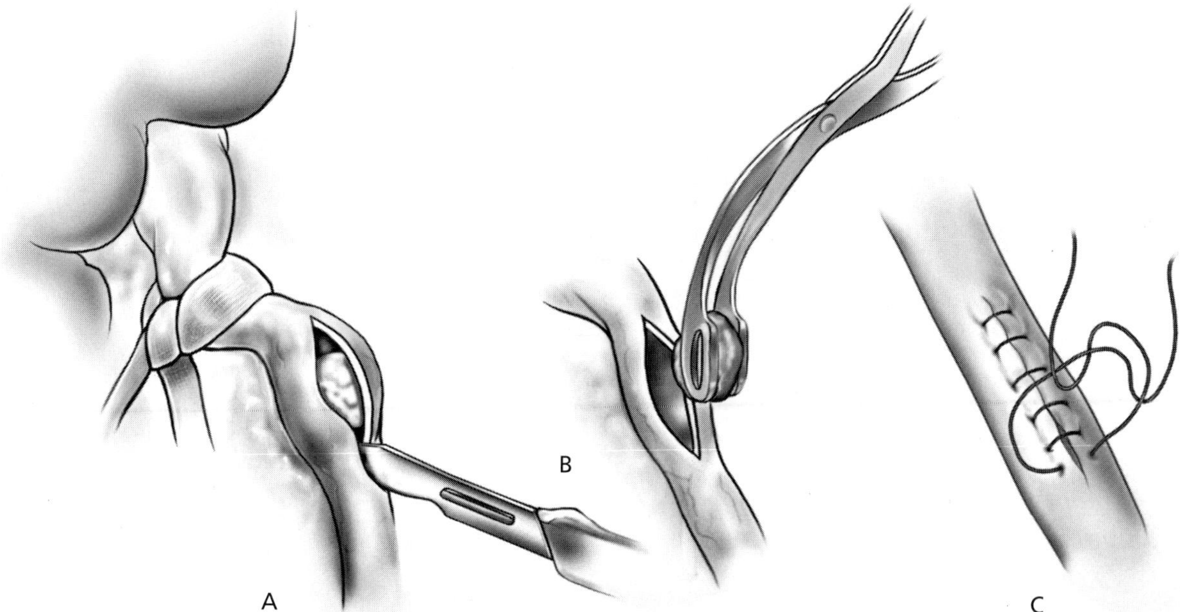

FIGURE 9.49. A: The ureter is isolated and controlled proximal to the stone using a vessel loop. **B:** A longitudinal ureterotomy is made directly over the stone, and the stone is extracted. **C:** The ureterotomy is closed using fine, absorbable interrupted suture to approximate the seromuscular layer.

way into the bladder. The ureterotomy is closed with interrupted fine absorbable suture (Fig. 9.49C) and the area drained with a Penrose drain. In the face of extensive ureteral edema or infection, strong consideration should be given to leaving an internal stent placed intraoperatively before closure of the ureterotomy.

Complications

Retained calculi can occur in up to 20% of patients, and when such retained stones are symptomatic or associated with infection or obstruction, further intervention is required. Fortunately, today, almost all such retained stones can be managed with SWL or percutaneous techniques, although these procedures should be delayed at least 4 to 6 weeks after the initial open operative intervention.

Persistent urinary drainage is uncommon and generally implies a local area of devascularization or distal obstruction. In most cases, such fistulae resolve spontaneously with conservative measures, including provision of local drainage and assurance of distal patency, at times with placement of an internal stent.

Bleeding into the collecting system or around the kidney almost always resolves spontaneously, and conservative, supportive measures are the initial treatment. When bleeding results in the need for multiple transfusions or an unstable cardiovascular status, intervention is indicated. In most cases, the treatment of choice is selective angiographic embolization because open surgical exploration generally results in nephrectomy (5).

REFERENCES

1. Abernathy BB, Morris JS, Wilson WT, et al. Evaluation of residual stone fragments following lithotripsy: sonography versus KUB. In: Lingeman JE, Newman DM, eds. *Shock wave lithotripsy II.* New York: Plenum Press, 1989.
2. Alken P, Hutschenreiter G, Gunther R, et al. Percutaneous stone manipulation. *J Urol* 1981;125:463.
3. Aslan P, Malloy B, Preminger GM. Access to the distal ureter after failure of direct visual ureteroscopy. *Br J Urol* 1998; 82:290.
4. Aso Y, Ohtawara Y, Fukuta K, et al. Operative fiberoptic nephroureteroscopy: removal of upper ureteral and renal calculi. *J Urol* 1987;137:629.
5. Assimos DG, Boyce WH, Harrison LH, et al. Postoperative anatrophic nephrolithotomy bleeding. *J Urol* 1986;135:1153.
6. Bagley DH, Huffman JL, Lyon ES. Combined rigid and flexible ureteropyeloscopy. *J Urol* 1983;130:243.
7. Bagley DH. Removal of upper urinary tract calculi with flexible ureteropyeloscopy. *Urology* 1990;35:412.
8. Bagley DH. Active versus passive deflection in flexible ureteroscopy. *J Endourol* 1987;1:15.
9. Bass RB Jr, Beard JH, Looner WH, et al. Percutaneous ultrasonic lithotripsy in the community hospital. *J Urol* 1985; 133:586.
10. Begun FP, Jacobs SC, Lawson RK. Use of a prototype 3F electrohydraulic electrode with ureteroscopy for treatment of ureteral calculous disease. *J Urol* 1988;139:1188.
11. Bellman GC, Silverstein JI, Blickensderfer S, et al. Technique and follow-up of percutaneous management of caliceal diverticula. *Urology* 1993;42:21.
12. Bellman GC, Silverstein JI, Blickensderfer S, et al. Technique and follow-up of percutaneous management of caliceal diverticula. *Urology* 1993;42:21.

13. Bennett JD, Broan TC, Kozak RI, et al. Transdiverticular percutaneous nephrostomy for caliceal diverticular stones. *J Endourol* 1992;6:55.
14. Bierkens AF, Hendrikx AJ, de Kort VJ, et al. Efficacy of second generation lithotriptors: a multicenter comparative study of 2,206 extracorporeal shock wave lithotripsy treatments with the Siemens Lithostar, Dornier HM4, Wolf Piezolith 2300, Direx Tripter X-1 and Breakstone lithotriptors. *J Urol* 1992;148: 1052.
15. Blute ML, Segura JW, Patterson DE. Ureteroscopy. *J Urol* 1988;139:510.
16. Boyce WH, Smith MGV. Anatrophic nephrotomy and plastic calyorrhaphy. *Trans Am Assoc Genitourin Surg* 1967;59:18.
17. Brannen GE, Bush WH, Correa RJ, et al. Kidney stone removal: percutaneous versus surgical lithotomy. *J Urol* 1985; 133:6.
18. Brodell M. The intrinsic blood vessels of the kidney and their significance in nephrotomy. *Bull Johns Hopkins Hosp* 1901;12:10.
19. Brown MW, Culley CC III, Dunnick NR, et al. Comparison of the costs and morbidity of percutaneous and open flank procedures. *J Urol* 1986;135:1150.
20. Burns JR, Hamrick LC, Keller FS. Percutaneous nephrolithotomy in 86 patients: analysis of results and costs. *South Med J* 1986;79:975.
21. Carey SW, Streem SB. Extracorporeal shock wave lithotripsy for patients with calcified ipsilateral renal arterial or abdominal aortic aneurysms. *J Urol* 1992;148:18.
22. Carson CC, Danneberger JE, Weinerth JL. Percutaneous lithotripsy in morbid obesity. *J Urol* 1988;139:243.
23. Chandhoke PS, Albala DM, Clayman RV. Long-term comparison of renal function in patients with solitary kidneys and/or moderate renal insufficiency undergoing ESWL or percutaneous nephrolithotomy. *J Urol* 1992;147:1226.
24. Charton M, Vallancien G, Veillon B, et al. Urinary tract infection in percutaneous surgery for renal calculi. *J Urol* 1986; 135:15.
25. Chaussy C, Schmiedt E, Jocham D, et al. First clinical experience with extracorporeally induced destruction of kidney stones by shock waves. *J Urol* 1982;127:417.
26. Chaussy C, Fuchs G, Kahn R, et al. Transurethral ultrasonic ureterolithotripsy using a solid-wire probe. *Urology* 1987; 29:531.
27. Chow GK, Streem SB. Contemporary urologic intervention for cystinuric patients: immediate and long term impact and implications. *J Urol* 1998;160:341.
28. Chow GK, Streem SB. Extracorporeal lithotripsy: update on new technology. *Urol Clin North Am* 2000;27:315.
29. Chung MK, Streem SB, Ching E, et al. Effects of extracorporeal shock wave lithotripsy on tiered therapy implantable cardioverter defibrillators. *PACE Pacing Clin Electrophysiol* 1999; 22:738.
30. Chuong CJ, Zhong P, Preminger GM. Acoustic and mechanical properties of renal calculi: implications in shock wave lithotripsy. *J Endourol* 1993;7:437.
31. Clayman RV, McClennan BL, Garvin TJ, et al. Lithostar: an electromagnetic acoustic shock wave unit for extracorporeal lithotripsy. *J Endourol* 1989;3:307.
32. Clayman RV, Surya V, Miller RP, et al. Percutaneous nephrolithotomy: Extraction of renal and ureteral calculi from 100 patients. *J Urol* 1984;131:868.
33. Clayman RV. Techniques in percutaneous removal of renal calculi: mechanical extraction and electrohydraulic lithotripsy. *Urology* 1984;23:11.
34. Clayman RV, Elbers J, Palmer JO, et al. Experimental extensive balloon dilation of the distal ureter: immediate and long-term effects. *J Endourol* 1987;1:19.
35. Clayman RV, Surya V, Miller RP, et al. Percutaneous nephrolithotomy: an approach to branched and staghorn renal calculi. *JAMA* 1983;250:73.
36. Cooper D, Wilkoff B, Masterson M, et al. Effects of extracorporeal shock wave lithotripsy on cardiac pacemakers and its safety in patients with implanted cardiac pacemakers. *PACE Pacing Clin Electrophysiol* 1988;22:1607.
37. Czerny V. Veber Nierenextripation. *Zentralbl Chir* 1897;6:737.
38. Dees JE. The use of intrapelvic coagulum in pyelolithotomy: preliminary report. *South Med J* 1943;36:167.
39. Delvecchio FC, Kuo RL, Preminger GM. Combination lithoclast and lithovac stone removal during ureteroscopy. *J Urol* 2000;164:40.
40. Denstedt JD, Clayman RV, Preminger GM. Efficiency quotient as a means of comparing lithotripters. *J Urol* 1990;143: 376A.
41. Denstedt JD, Razvi HA, Rowe E, et al. Investigation of the tissue effects of a new device for intracorporeal lithotripsy: the Swiss Lithoclast. *J Urol* 1995;153:535.
42. Denstedt JD, Clayman RV. Electrohydraulic lithotripsy of renal and ureteral calculi. *J Urol* 1990;143:13.
43. Denstedt JD, Eberwein PM, Singh RR. The Swiss Lithoclast: a new device for intracorporeal lithotripsy. *J Urol* 1992;148: 1088.
44. Denstedt JD, Razvi HA, Rowe E, et al. Investigation of the tissue effects of a new device for intracorporeal lithotripsy—the Swiss Lithoclast. *J Urol* 1995;153:535.
45. Dretler SP, Young RH. Stone granuloma: a cause of ureteral stricture. *J Urol* 1993;150:1800.
46. Dretler SP, Cho G. Semirigid ureteroscopy: a new genre. *J Urol* 1989;141:1314.
47. Dretler SP, Watson G, Parrish JA, et al. Pulsed dye laser fragmentation of ureteral calculi: initial clinical experience. *J Urol* 1987;137:386.
48. Elashry OM, Elbahnasy AM, Rao GS, et al. Flexible ureteroscopy: Washington University experience with the 9.3F and 7.5F flexible ureteroscopes. *J Urol* 1997;157:2074.
49. Elbahnasy AM, Clayman RV, Shalhav AL, et al. Lower-pole caliceal stone clearance after shockwave lithotripsy, percutaneous nephrolithotomy, and flexible ureteroscopy: impact of radiographic spatial anatomy. *J Endourol* 1998;12:113.
50. Eshghi M, Addonizio JC. Renal pelvic decompression during ureterorenoscopy. *Urology* 1987;29:398.
51. Evans CP, Stoller ML. The fate of the iatrogenic retroperitoneal stone. *J Urol* 1993;150:827.
52. Fabrizio MD, Behari A, Bagley DH. Ureteroscopic management of intrarenal calculi. *J Urol* 1998;159:1139.
53. Feagins BA, Wilson WT, Preminger GM. Intracorporeal electrohydraulic lithotripsy with flexible ureterorenoscopy. *J Endourol* 1990;4:347.
54. Fernstrom I, Johansson B. Percutaneous pyelolithotomy: a new extraction technique. *Scand J Urol Nephrol* 1976;10:257.
55. Ferraro RF, Abraham VE, Cohen TD, et al. A new generation of semirigid fiberoptic ureteroscopes. *J Endourol* 1999;13:35.
56. Fischer GP, Sonda LP, Diokno AC. Use of cryoprecipitate coagulum in extracting renal calculi. *Urology* 1980;15:6.
57. Gerber GS, Steinberg GD. Endourologic treatment of renal pelvic and ureteral transitional cell carcinoma. *Techniques in Urology* 1999;5:77.
58. Geterud K, Henriksson CH, Pettersson S, et al. Computed tomography after percutaneous stone extraction. *Acta Radiol* 1987;28:55.
59. Gettman MT, Segura JW. Struvite stones: diagnosis and current treatment concepts. *J Endourol* 1999;135:653.
60. Giblin JG, Lossef S, Pahira JJ. A modification of standard percutaneous nephrolithotripsy technique for the morbidly obese patient. *Urology* 1995;46:491.

61. Gil-Vernet J. New surgical concepts in removing renal calculi. *Urol Int* 1965;20:255.
62. Goodfriend R. Ultrasonic and electrohydraulic lithotripsy of ureteral calculi. *Urology* 1984;23:5.
63. Goodwin WE, Casey WC, Woolf W. Percutaneous trocar (needle) nephrostomy in hydronephrosis. *JAMA* 1955;157:891.
64. Grasso M, Corlin M, Bagley D. Retrograde ureteropyeloscopic treatment of 2 cm or greater upper urinary tract and minor staghorn calculi. *J Urol* 1998;160:346.
65. Grasso M, Fraiman M, Levine M. Ureteropyeloscopic diagnosis and treatment of upper urinary tract urothelial malignancies. *Urology* 1999;54:240.
66. Grasso M, Liu JB, Goldberg B, et al. Submucosal calculi: endoscopic and intraluminal sonographic diagnosis and treatment options. *J Urol* 1995;153:1384.
67. Grasso M, Bagley D. Small diameter, actively deflectable, flexible ureteropyeloscopy. *J Urol* 1998;160:1648.
68. Grasso M, Bagley DH. Endoscopic pulsed-dye laser lithotripsy: 159 consecutive cases. *J Endourol* 1994;8:25.
69. Graves FT. The anatomy of the intrarenal arteries and its application to segmental resection of the kidney. *Br J Surg* 1954;42:132.
70. Green DF, Lytton B. Early experience with direct vision electrohydraulic lithotripsy of ureteral calculi. *J Urol* 1985; 133:767.
71. Harmon WJ, Sershon PD, Blute ML, et al. Ureteroscopy: current practice and long-term complications. *J Urol* 1997; 157:28.
72. Haupt G, van Ophoven A, Pannek J, et al. *In vitro* comparison of two ballistic systems for endoscopic stone disintegration. *J Endourol* 1996;10:417.
73. Haupt G, Pannek J, Herde T, et al. The Lithovac: new suction device for the Swiss Lithoclast. *J Endourol* 1995;9:375.
74. Hofbauer J, Hobarth K, Marberger M. Lithoclast: new and inexpensive mode of intracorporeal lithotripsy. *J Endourol* 1992;6:429.
75. Hofbauer J, Hobarth K, Marberger M. Electrohydraulic versus pneumatic disintegration in the treatment of ureteral stones: a randomized, prospective trial. *J Urol* 1995;153:623.
76. Honey RJ. Assessment of a new tipless nitinol stone basket and comparison with an existing flat-wire basket. *J Endourol* 1998; 12:529.
77. Hosking MP, Morris SA, Klein FA, et al. Anesthetic management of patients receiving calculus therapy with a third-generation extracorporeal lithotripsy machine. *J Endourol* 1997; 11:309.
78. Hosking DH, Bard RJ. Ureteroscopy with intravenous sedation for treatment of distal ureteral calculi: a safe and effective alternative to shock wave lithotripsy. *J Urol* 1996; 156:899.
79. Hsu THS, Streem SB. Metabolic abnormalities in patients with caliceal diverticular calculi. *J Urol* 1998;160:1640.
80. Huang S, Patel H, Bellman GC. Cost effectiveness of electrohydraulic lithotripsy v Candela pulsed-dye laser in management of the distal ureteral stone. *J Endourol* 1998;12:237.
81. Huffman JL, Bagley DH, Lyon ES. Treatment of distal ureteral calculi using rigid ureteroscope. *Urology* 1982;20:574.
82. Huffman JL. Experience with the 8.5 French compact rigid ureteroscope. *Semin Urol* 1989;7:3.
83. Huffman JL, Bagley DH. Balloon dilation of the ureter for ureteroscopy. *J Urol* 1988;140:954.
84. Huffman JL, Bagley DH, Schoenberg HW, et al. Transurethral removal of large ureteral and renal pelvic calculi using ureteroscopic ultrasonic lithotripsy. *J Urol* 1983;130:31.
85. Hulbert JC, Reddy PK, Hunter DW, et al. Percutaneous techniques for the management of caliceal diverticula containing calculi. *J Urol* 1986;135:225.
86. Jarrett TW, Lee CK, Pardalidis NP, et al. Extensive dilation of distal ureter for endoscopic treatment of large volume ureteral disease. *J Urol* 1995;153:1214.
87. Jones JA, Lingeman JE, Steidle CP. The roles of extracorporeal shock wave lithotripsy and percutaneous nephrostolithotomy in the management of pyelocaliceal diverticula. *J Urol* 1991; 146:724.
88. Kahnoski RJ, Lingeman JE, Coury TA, et al. Combined percutaneous and extracorporeal shock wave lithotripsy for staghorn calculi: an alternative to anatrophic nephrolithotomy. *J Urol* 1986;135:679.
89. Kerbl K, Clayman RV, Chandhoke PS, et al. Percutaneous stone removal with the patient in a flank position. *J Urol* 1994;151:686.
90. Kessaris DN, Bellman GC, Pardalidis NP, et al. Management of hemorrhage after percutaneous renal surgery. *J Urol* 1995; 153:604.
91. Kim HH, Lee JH, Park MS, et al. In situ extracorporeal shockwave lithotripsy for ureteral calculi: investigation of factors influencing stone fragmentation and appropriate number of sessions for changing treatment modality. *J Endourol* 1996; 10:501.
92. Klein FA. Storz Modulith SL-20: the new optimal acoustic source for extracorporeal lithotripsy. *Semin Urol* 1991; 9:269.
93. Kohrmann KU, Rassweiler JJ, Manning M, et al. The clinical introduction of a third generation lithotriptor: Modulith SL 20. *J Urol* 1995;153:1379.
94. Kourambas J, Byrne RR, Preminger GM. Does a ureteral access sheath facilitate ureteroscopy? *J Urol* 2000;163(4S):66.
95. Kourambas J, Delvecchio FC, Preminger GM. Low power holmium laser for the management of urinary tract calculi, tumors and strictures. *J Endourol (in press).*
96. Kourambas J, Delvecchio FC, Preminger GM. Nitinol stone retrieval-assisted ureteroscopic management of lower pole renal calculi. *Urology* 2000;56:935.
97. Kramolowsky EV. Ureteral perforation during ureterorenoscopy: treatment and management. *J Urol* 1987;138:36.
98. Kriegmair M, Schmeller N. Paraureteral calculi caused by ureteroscopic perforation. *Urology* 1995;45:578.
99. Kuo RL, Aslan P, Fitzgerald KB, et al. Use of ureteroscopy and holmium:YAG laser in patients with bleeding diatheses. *Urology* 1998;52:609.
100. Kuo RL, Aslan P, Zhong P, et al. Impact of holmium laser settings and fiber diameter on stone fragmentation and endoscope deflection. *J Endourol* 1998;12:523.
101. Lange PH, Reddy PK, Hulbert JC, et al. Percutaneous removal of caliceal and other "inaccessible" stones: instruments and techniques. *J Urol* 1984;132:439.
102. Lee WJ, Smith AD, Cubelli V, et al. Percutaneous nephrolithotomy: analysis of 500 consecutive cases. *Urol Radiol* 1986; 8:61.
103. Leroy AJ, Segura JW, Williams HJ Jr, et al. Percutaneous renal calculus removal in an extracorporeal shock wave lithotripsy practice. *J Urol* 1987;138:703.
104. Lingeman JE, Newman DM. Dornier MFL 5000 and compact lithotriptors. *Semin Urol* 1991;9:225.
105. Lingeman JE, Coury TA, Newman DM, et al. Comparison of results and morbidity of percutaneous nephrostolithotomy and extracorporeal shock wave lithotripsy. *J Urol* 1987;138:485.
106. Lingeman JE, Lower Pole Study Group. Prospective randomized trial of extracorporeal shock wave lithotripsy and percutaneous nephrostolithotomy for lower pole nephrolithiasis: initial long-term follow-up. *J Endourol* 1997;11:S95.
107. Lingeman JE, Newman DM, Siegel YI, et al. Shock wave lithotripsy with the Dornier MFL 5000 lithotriptor using an external fixed rate signal. *J Urol* 1995;154:951.

108. Loisides P, Grasso M, Bagley DH. Mechanical impactor employing nitinol probes to fragment human calculi: fragmentation efficiency with flexible endoscope deflection. *J Endourol* 1995;9:371.
109. Lopez-Alcina E, Broseta E, Oliver F, et al. Paraureteral extrusion of calculi after endoscopic pulsed-dye laser lithotripsy. *J Endourol* 1998;12:517.
110. Low RK, Stoller ML, Irby P, et al. Outcome assessment of double-J stents during extracorporeal shockwave lithotripsy of small solitary renal calculi. *J Endourol* 1996;10:341.
111. Lower WE. Conservative surgical methods in operating for stone in the kidney. *Cleve Med J* 1913;12:260.
112. Lyon ES, Kyker JS, Schoenberg HW. Transurethral ureteroscopy in women: a ready addition to the urological armamentarium. *J Urol* 1978;119:35.
113. McQuitty DA, Boone TB, Preminger GM. Lower pole calicostomy for the management of iatrogenic ureteropelvic junction obstruction. *J Urol* 1995;153:142.
114. McVary KT, O'Conor VJ. Transmission of non-A non-B hepatitis during coagulum pyelolithotomy. *J Urol* 1989;141:923.
115. Marberger M, Stackl W, Hruby W. Percutaneous litholapaxy of renal calculi with ultrasound. *Eur Urol* 1982;8:236.
116. Marberger M. Disintegration of renal and ureteral calculi with ultrasound. *Urol Clin North Am* 1983;10:729.
117. Marberger M, Stackl W, Hruby W, et al. Late sequelae of ultrasonic lithotripsy of renal calculi. *J Urol* 1985;133:170.
118. Mathes GL Jr, Mathes LT. High-energy v low-energy shockwave lithotripsy in treatment of ureteral calculi. *J Endourol* 1997;11:319.
119. Mayo ME, Krieger JN, Rudd TG. Effect of percutaneous nephrostolithotomy on renal function. *J Urol* 1985;133:167.
120. Meretyk S, Gofrit ON, Gafni O, et al. Complete staghorn calculi: random prospective comparison between extracorporeal shock wave lithotripsy monotherapy and combined with percutaneous nephrostolithotomy. *J Urol* 1997;157:780.
121. Miller OF, Kane CJ. Time to stone passage for observed ureteral calculi: a guide for patient education. *J Urol* 1999; 162:688.
122. Monga M, Smith R, Ferral H, et al. Percutaneous ablation of caliceal diverticulum: long-term follow-up. *J Urol* 2000;163:28.
123. Monk TG, Boure B, White PF, et al. Comparison of intravenous sedative-analgesic techniques for outpatient immersion lithotripsy. *Anesth Analg* 1991;72:616.
124. Moretti KL, Miller RA, Kellett MJ, et al. Extrusion of calculi from upper urinary tract into perinephric and periureteric tissues during endourologic stone surgery. *Urology* 1991;38:447.
125. Morey AF, Nitahara KS, McAninch JW. Modified anatrophic nephrolithotomy for management of staghorn calculi: is renal function preserved? *J Urol* 1999;162:670.
126. Motola JA, Badlani GH, Smith AD. Results of 212 consecutive endopyelotomies: an 8-year follow-up. *J Urol* 1993;149:453.
127. Mugiya S, Ohhira T, Un-No T, et al. Endoscopic management of upper urinary tract disease using a 200-micron holmium laser fiber: initial experience in Japan. *Urology* 1999;53:60.
128. Paik ML, Wainstein MA, Spirnak JP, et al. Current indications for open stone surgery in the treatment of renal and ureteral calculi. *J Urol* 1998;159:374.
129. Pearle MS, Nakada SY, Womack JS, et al. Outcomes of contemporary percutaneous nephrostolithotomy in morbidly obese patients. *J Urol* 1998;160:669.
130. Pearle MS, Sech SM, Cobb CG, et al. Safety and efficacy of the Alexandrite laser for the treatment of renal and ureteral calculi. *Urology* 1998;51:33.
131. Pence JR, Airhart RA, Novicki DE. Coagulum pyelolithotomy [Letter]. *J Urol* 1981;125:134.
132. Perez-Castro Ellendt E, Martinez-Pineiro JA. Ureteral and renal endoscopy. A new approach. *Eur Urol* 1982;8:117.
133. Poon M, Beaghler M, Baldwin D. Flexible endoscope deflectability: changes using a variety of working instruments and laser fibers. *J Endourol* 1997;11:247.
134. Postoak D, Simon JM, Monga M, et al. Combined percutaneous antegrade and cystoscopic retrograde ureteral stent placement: an alternative technique in cases of ureteral discontinuity. *Urology* 1997;50:113.
135. Preminger GM. Sonographic piezoelectric lithotripsy: more bang for your buck. *J Endourol* 1989;3:321.
136. Preminger GM. Shock wave physics. *Am J Kidney Dis* 1991; 17:431.
137. Preminger GM, Kettelhut MC, Elkins SL, et al. Ureteral stenting during extracorporeal shock wave lithotripsy: help or hindrance? *J Urol* 1989;142:32.
138. Preminger GM. Richard Wolf piezoelectric lithotripters: Piezolith 2300 and 2500. *Semin Urol* 1991;9:288.
139. Preminger GM, Clayman RV, Hardeman SW, et al. Percutaneous nephrostolithotomy vs. open surgery for renal calculi: a comparative study. *JAMA* 1985;254:1054.
140. Preminger GM, Kennedy TJ. Ureteral stone extraction utilizing nondeflectable flexible fiberoptic ureteroscopes. *J Endourol* 1987;1:31.
141. Raney AM, Handler J. Electrohydraulic nephrolithotripsy. *Urology* 1975;6:439.
142. Raney AM. Electrohydraulic lithotripsy: experimental study and case reports with the stone disintegrator. *J Urol* 1975; 113:345.
143. Raney AM, Handler J. Electrohydraulic nephrolithotripsy. *Urology* 1975;6:439.
144. Rassweiler J, Henkel TO, Kohrmann KU, et al. Lithotripter technology: present and future. *J Endourol* 1992;6:1.
145. Razvi HA, Chun SS, Denstedt JD, et al. Soft-tissue applications of the holmium:YAG laser in urology. *J Endourol* 1995;9:387.
146. Reddy PK, Hulbert JC, Lange PH, et al. Percutaneous removal of renal and ureteral calculi: experience with 400 cases. *J Urol* 1985;134:662.
147. Reddy PK, Lange PH, Hulbert JC, et al. Percutaneous removal of caliceal and other "inaccessible" stones: results. *J Urol* 1984; 132:443.
148. Roberts WW, Cadeddu JA, Micali S, et al. Ureteral stricture formation after removal of impacted calculi. *J Urol* 1998; 159:723.
149. Rouvalis P. Electronic lithotripsy for vesical calculus with "Urat-1." An experience of 100 cases and an experimental application of the method to stones in the upper urinary tract. *Br J Urol* 1970;42:486.
150. Ruckle HC, Segura JW. Laparoscopic treatment of a stone-filled caliceal diverticulum: a definitive, minimally invasive therapeutic option. *J Urol* 1994;151:122.
151. Rupel E, Brown R. Nephroscopy with removal of stone following nephrostomy for obstructive calculous anuria. *J Urol* 1941; 46:177.
152. Saltzman B. Direx Tripter X-1. *Semin Urol* 1991;9:222.
153. Santa-Cruz RW, Leveillee RJ, Krongrad A. *Ex vivo* comparison of four lithotripters commonly used in the ureter: what does it take to perforate? *J Endourol* 1998;12:417.
154. Schiff RG, Lee WJ, Esghi M, et al. Morphologic and functional changes in the kidney after percutaneous stone extraction. *AJR Am J Roentgenol* 1986;147:283.
155. Schultz RE, Hanno PM, Wein AJ, et al. Percutaneous ultrasonic lithotripsy: choice of irrigant. *J Urol* 1953;130:858.

156. Schulze H, Hertle L, Graff J, et al. Combined treatment of branched calculi by percutaneous nephrolithotomy and extracorporeal shock wave lithotripsy. *J Urol* 1986;135:1138.
157. Schwalb DM, Eshghi M, Davidian M, et al. Morphological and physiological changes in the urinary tract associated with ureteral dilation and ureteropyeloscopy: an experimental study. *J Urol* 1993;149:1576.
158. Segura JW, Preminger GM, Assimos DG, et al. Nephrolithiasis Clinical Guidelines Panel summary report on the management of staghorn calculi. The American Urological Association Nephrolithiasis Clinical Guidelines Panel. *J Urol* 1994;151: 1648.
159. Segura JW, Patterson DE, LeRoy AJ, et al. Percutaneous stone removal of kidney stones: preliminary report. *Mayo Clin Proc* 1982;57:615.
160. Segura JH, Patterson DE, LeRoy AJ, et al. Percutaneous removal of kidney stones: review of 1000 cases. *J Urol* 1985;134: 1077.
161. Segura JW, Preminger GM, Assimos DG, et al. Ureteral Stones Clinical Guidelines Panel summary report on the management of ureteral calculi. *J Urol* 1997;158:1915.
162. Shalhav AL, Soble JJ, Nakada SY, et al. Long-term outcome of caliceal diverticula following percutaneous endosurgical management. *J Urol* 1998;160:1635.
163. Singal RK, Denstedt JD, Razvi HA, et al. Holmium:YAG laser endoureterotomy for treatment of ureteral stricture. *Urology* 1997;50:875.
164. Skoog SJ, Reed MD, Gaudier FA Jr, et al. The posterolateral and the retrorenal colon: implication in percutaneous stone extraction. *J Urol* 1985;134:110.
165. Snyder JA, Smith AD. Staghorn calculi: percutaneous extraction versus anatrophic nephrolithotomy. *J Urol* 1986;136:351.
166. Spirnak JP, Fleischmann JD. Finlayson ureteral access system: review of 32 cases. *J Endourol* 1991;5:237.
167. Streem SB. Contemporary clinical practice of shock wave lithotripsy: a re-evaluation of contraindication. *J Urol* 1997;157: 1197.
168. Streem SB, Yost A, Dolmatch B. Combination "sandwich" therapy for extensive renal calculi in 100 consecutive patients: immediate, long-term and stratified results from a 10-year experience. *J Urol* 1997;158:342.
169. Streem SB, Yost A. Treatment of caliceal diverticular calculi with ESWL. Patient selection and extended follow-up. *J Urol* 1992;148:1043.
170. Streem SB, Geisinger MA, Risius B, et al. Endourologic "sandwich" therapy for extensive staghorn calculi. *J Endourol* 1987; 1:253.
171. Streem SB, Yost A, Dolmatch B. Combination "sandwich" therapy for extensive renal calculi in 100 consecutive patients: immediate, long-term and stratified results from a 10-year experience. *J Urol* 1997;158:342.
172. Streem SB, Zelch MG, Risius B, et al. Percutaneous extraction of renal calculi in patients with solitary kidneys. *Urology* 1986; 27:247.
173. Tawfiek ER, Bagley DH. Management of upper urinary tract calculi with ureteroscopic techniques. *Urology* 1999;53:25.
174. Tawfiek ER, Grasso M, Bagley DH. Initial use of Browne Pneumatic Impactor. *J Endourol* 1997;11:121.
175. Teichman JMH, Rao RD, Glickman RD, et al. Holmium: YAG percutaneous nephrolithotomy: the laser incident angle matters. *J Urol* 1998;159:690.
176. Teichman JM, Rao RD, Rogenes VJ, et al. Ureteroscopic management of ureteral calculi: electrohydraulic versus holmium:YAG lithotripsy. *J Urol* 1997;158:1357.
177. Teh CL, Aslan P, Preminger GM. What's new in shock wave lithotripsy? *Contemporay Urology* 1997;9:26.
178. Teh CL, Zhong P, Preminger GM. Laboratory and clinical assessment of pneumatically driven intracorporeal lithotripsy. *J Endourol* 1998;12:163.
179. Thomas R, Cass AS. Extracorporeal shock wave lithotripsy in morbidly obese patients. *J Urol* 1993;150:30.
180. Troy RB, Streem SB, Zelch MG. Percutaneous management of upper tract foreign bodies. *J Endourol* 1994;8:43.
181. Vassar GJ, Chan KF, Teichman JM, et al. Holmium:YAG lithotripsy: photothermal mechanism. *J Endourol* 1999;13:181.
182. Vieweg J, Teh C, Freed K, et al. Unenhanced helical computerized tomography for the evaluation of patients with acute flank pain. *J Urol* 1998;160:679.
183. Watson G, Murray S, Dretler SP, et al. The pulsed dye laser for fragmenting urinary calculi. *J Urol* 1987;138:195.
184. Webb DR, Fitzpatrick JM. Percutaneous nephrostolithotomy: a functional and morphological study. *J Urol* 1985;134:587.
185. Weinerth JL, Flatt JA, Carson CC III. Lessons learned in patients with large steinstrasse. *J Urol* 1989;142:1425.
186. Wilson TW, Eberhart RC, Preminger GM. Flow, pressure, and deflection characteristics of flexible deflectable ureterorenoscopes. *J Endourol* 1990;4:283.
187. Wilson WT, Preminger GM. Intrarenal pressures generated during flexible deflectable ureterorenoscopy. *J Endourol* 1990; 4:135.
188. Winfield HN, Clayman RV, Chaussy CG, et al. Monotherapy of staghorn renal calculi: a comparative study between percutaneous nephrolithotomy and extracorporeal shock wave lithotripsy. *J Urol* 1988;139:895.
189. Wise KL, Carson CC. Ileocecal substitution in the treatment of severe ureteroscopy-related ureteral trauma: report of three cases. *J Endourol* 1990;4:143.
190. Wolf JS Jr, Carroll PR, Stoller ML. Cost-effectiveness v patient preference in the choice of treatment for distal ureteral calculi: a literature-based decision analysis. *J Endourol* 1995;9:243.
191. Wolf JW. Management of intra-operatively diagnosed colonic injury during percutaneous nephrostolithotomy. *Tech Urol* 1998;4:160.
192. Wulfsohn MA. Extended pyelolithotomy: the use of renal artery clamping and regional hypothermia. *J Urol* 1981; 125:467.
193. Zhong P, Tong HL, Cocks FH, et al. Transient oscillation of cavitation bubbles near stone surface during electrohydraulic lithotripsy. *J Endourol* 1997;11:55.
194. Zhong P, Tong HL, Cocks FH, et al. Transient cavitation and acoustic emission produced by different laser lithotripters. *J Endourol* 1998;12:371.
195. Zhu S, Kourambas J, Munver R, et al. Characterization of tip movement of the lithoclast flexible probe. *J Urol* 2000; 163(4S):318.

10

PERIOPERATIVE CARE

W. SCOTT McDOUGAL

The risk of an operative procedure must be weighed against its benefit so that the patient can be given a realistic view of the probable outcomes of both the nonoperative and the operative approaches. Although determining risk is simple in theory, it is extremely difficult in practice. Because of the wide variety of surgical procedures performed and the uniqueness of each patient, attempts to quantitate the risk factor have not met with great success. Many investigations have been unable to correlate accurately risk with any specific factor; however, a loose association has been shown with poor general health, advanced

W.S. McDougal: Department of Urology, Harvard Medical School; Department of Urology, Massachusetts General Hospital, Boston, MA 02111.

age, emergency operation, and the site of the surgical procedure (41).

In an attempt to quantitate the risk associated with an anesthetic, irrespective of procedure performed, the American Society of Anesthesiologists (ASA) has proposed a classification of physical status: Class I is a normal healthy person, class II is used for patients with mild to moderate systemic disease, class III represents patients with severe systemic diseases that are not incapacitating, class IV indicates an incapacitating systemic disease that is a constant threat to the patient's life, and class V denotes a moribund patient not expected to survive more than 24 hours without an operation. This classification allows a general assessment but is not specific enough to accurately quantitate risk.

The most important factor in evaluating the risk of an operation is the functional status of the cardiovascular system. Pulmonary function also significantly affects the risk of anesthesia; perhaps the most common postoperative complication involves the respiratory tract. Hypoxemia secondary to respiratory dysfunction, when combined with myocardial disease, significantly increases the risk of myocardial infarction and death following the procedure.

The death rate from anesthesia, taking into account all operative procedures, has been estimated to be approximately 0.3%. Of patients who die as a result of the anesthetic and operative procedure, approximately 10% die in the period of induction, approximately 33% during the operative procedure, and the remainder within the first 48 hours after operation (32). The death rate attributed to anesthesia in patients who are ASA class I or II is much less and is estimated to be about 1 in 500,000 (27).

Preoperative assessment is undertaken to determine the risk of the proposed procedures and to identify abnormalities that can be corrected to reduce morbidity and mortality. The assessment should include an evaluation of the blood count and blood volume; the integrity of the hemostatic mechanisms; an evaluation of the cardiac function; an assessment of pulmonary function; and a review of the metabolic status, which should include an assessment of the liver, the kidneys, the immune system, the patient's nutritional status, the integrity of the adrenal glands, and an evaluation of any systemic diseases, such as diabetes, obesity, and thyroid disease.

BLOOD COUNT

All preoperative patients in whom a significant blood loss is anticipated or who are suspected of having an abnormal blood count require determination of a packed cell volume or hematocrit level. A value between 30% and 50% is acceptable. As the hematocrit level falls below 30%, the viscosity of the blood is reduced and flow characteristics through the small vessels improve. However, this is offset by the decreased oxygen-carrying capacity of the blood. Patients with chronic renal failure often have hematocrit levels of 20% to 24% and tolerate surgery well, provided there has not been a recent short-term change in the hematocrit level. The disadvantage is that there is little margin for error in terms of major blood loss. Patients with hematocrit levels above 55% have marked increased viscosity in their blood and are prone to thrombosis during periods of major fluid shifts. Therefore, except under extenuating circumstances, a hematocrit level between 30% and 50% should be sought in the preoperative preparation of the patient.

BLOOD VOLUME

The status of the patient's blood volume also must be assessed. Hypovolemia may be a consequence of secondary hyperaldosteronism, Addison's disease, acute blood loss, vomiting, diarrhea, pancreatic fistula, ileostomy, intestinal obstruction, pheochromocytoma, and neuroblastoma, among others. When these disorders are present, the blood volume must be restored through preoperative fluid administration and/or pharmacologic manipulation. α-Adrenergic blockade allows for volume expansion through relaxation of peripheral vasoconstriction with homeostatic volume restoration over a several-week period in patients with a pheochromocytoma and in hypertensive patients with a neuroblastoma. Fluid loss into the bowel, as occurs in bowel obstruction, diarrhea, or hemorrhagic blood loss, is not appropriately corrected by pharmacologic means; however, drugs may be used as temporary blood pressure stabilizers—intravenously (IV) when such losses are sufficient to cause cardiovascular instability—until fluid volumes can be restored generally.

The central venous pressure (CVP) is an indirect measure of the blood volume and competency of the heart to receive and propel blood. Provided heart disease is not significant, it is an accurate measure of volume status. A normal CVP ranges between 4 and 8 cm H_2O with reference to the left atrium (4 cm below the angle of the sternum). A low CVP suggests hypovolemia, and an elevated CVP suggests volume overload. A pulmonary artery catheter (right sided, Swan-Ganz) is necessary to determine accurately the volume status in patients with cardiac disease, those with chronic obstructive pulmonary disease, and patients in whom the CVP does not correlate with the clinical status (a high CVP in the presence of hypoperfusion). Although the CVP is adequate, a pulmonary artery catheter may be preferred in the patient with multisystem trauma, septic shock, decompensated cirrhosis, severe pancreatitis, or peritonitis, as well as in those receiving massive transfusions. In these circumstances, major fluid shifts can be more accurately titrated with a right-sided heart catheter. A normal pulmonary wedge pressure ranges between 12 and 15 cm of H_2O. This catheter also allows for the measurement of cardiac output and peripheral vascular resistance. Restoration of circulating volume and correction of metabolic disorders may require several weeks of proper fluid and pharmacologic manipulation. The use of right-sided heart catheterization to monitor fluid administration in critically ill patients has been questioned recently. In one study in which similarly critically ill patients were compared, those who had right-sided heart catheterization had a higher mortality and greater utilization of resources than those who were managed without a cannula in the pulmonary artery (16).

A kidney in the diuretic state is less prone to injury; therefore patients who have operations on their urinary tract should be volume replete before and during surgery. The usual practice of nothing by mouth past midnight requires an intraoperative catch-up of fluids. Most patients tolerate this quite well; however, in the critically ill or those who are severely compromised, maintenance of normal fluid balance minimizes postoperative complications. This can be accomplished by beginning the IV fluid administration the night before surgery and giving the patient normal replacement fluids (see Fluids and Electrolytes).

HEMOSTASIS

The competency of the hemostatic mechanisms is assessed by history that addresses bleeding tendencies, bruisability, or a family history of bleeding disorders and serum studies. *A platelet count, a prothrombin time (PT), and a partial thromboplastin time (PTT) serve as good screening tests for major surgery.* PT and PTT are thought by many to be unnecessary in patients when there is no reason to suspect a coagulation problem. It is important to remember that there may be a qualitative platelet defect such as occurs in uremic patients and those taking aspirin, which would not be picked up by a routine platelet count.

RENAL FUNCTION

It has long been known that the onset of acute renal failure in the critically ill patient is a poor prognostic sign with an excessively high mortality. Many believed that acute renal failure was merely an indication of systemic organ failure accounting for the increased mortality. However, more recent data suggest that renal failure alone increases mortality, even if the degree of insufficiency is not enough to require dialysis. This makes it imperative to aggressively treat patients who have even modest elevations of their serum creatinine (5).

CARDIAC FUNCTION

Cardiac function is evaluated by history, physical examination, an electrocardiogram (ECG), and in select cases, a gated blood pool scan to provide ejection fraction. A previous myocardial infarction is of particular significance. *As a group, patients with a history of a myocardial infarction have a tenfold increase in the probability of having a subsequent postoperative infarction. A further analysis reveals that the time elapsed since the infarction is of prime importance.* One-third of patients who have operations within 3 months of their myocardial infarction will have another. Patients who have operations 6 months or longer after their myocardial insult have their risk of postoperative infarction reduced to approximately 6% to 8%. A postoperative infarction generally occurs within the first 7 postoperative days and has a 50% to 75% mortality (91). Other factors that appear to be particularly important in predicting myocardial dysfunction in the operative and perioperative period include (a) an S_3 gallop and/or jugular venous distention; (b) a preoperative cardiac rhythm other than sinus; (c) more than five premature ventricular contractions per minute; (d) an intraperitoneal, intrathoracic, or aortic operation; (e) an age greater than 70 years; (f) aortic valvular heart disease; (g) the necessity for an emergency operation; and (h) a poor general medical condition as reflected by an arterial blood gas abnormality, decreased renal function, and/or evidence of hepatic disease (40). Clearly, the most important predictors are the presence of congestive heart failure with jugular venous distention and/or an S_3 gallop and a history of a myocardial infarction within the preceding 6 months. These two findings carry with them a significant risk of death from the anesthetic.

Hypertension also increases the risk of an operative procedure, particularly if associated with coronary artery disease. Hypertensive patients have wider and more frequent blood pressure swings during anesthesia and are more likely to have associated cerebral vascular and coronary artery blood flow compromise.

Patients should continue antihypertensive medicine if they are normotensive, or the dosages should be adjusted to achieve a normal blood pressure. In general, medications should not be discontinued in the preoperative period. The monoamine oxidase (MAO) inhibitors may be an exception because they can interfere with anesthetic management.

Patients thought to have severe cardiac disease are best prepared preoperatively with a right-sided heart catheter placed in the pulmonary artery, inotropics or antiarrhythmics given as needed, and careful fluid resuscitation. An evaluation of cardiac and respiratory status can be performed by noting the patient's resting pulse, having him or her walk briskly a short distance, and then rechecking the pulse. If the pulse rate does not rise to twice the resting level, the patient is probably not at significant risk.

An excellent assessment of cardiac reserve can be accomplished by the determination of the ejection fraction. This may be performed by an isotopic method or by ultrasound. If the ejection fraction exceeds 50%, it is likely that the patient's heart will tolerate the procedure well. If the ejection fraction is between 40% and 50%, the patient is at increased risk for myocardial dysfunction but is still acceptable from a cardiac standpoint. If the ejection fraction is less than 40%, the patient is at an increased risk and requires exceedingly close monitoring for cardiac malfunction, which is likely.

The need for sufficient cardiac reserve is made apparent by the fact that in the critically injured patient, a high normal or moderately increased cardiac output and oxygen consumption portends a much better prognosis with significantly reduced mortality compared with those in whom little increase is noted (5).

RESPIRATORY FUNCTION

Respiratory status is evaluated by history and determination of exercise tolerance. A smoking history of more than 20 pack-years is particularly significant. If the respiratory status is at all questionable, simple spirometry is an excellent screen. If the forced expiratory volume in 1 second (FEV_1) is under 15 mL/kg and the vital capacity is less than 1.5 L or the maximum voluntary ventilation is under 50%, further pulmonary function tests and additional preoperative preparation are in order.

METABOLIC STATUS

The metabolic status of the patient is assessed with regard to the hepatic, renal, and immune function, as well as the nutritional and adrenal status. If indicated by history, hepatic function is determined by evaluation of liver enzymes, PT, and albumin. In patients with compromised hepatic function, preoperative preparation includes improving the nutritional status (see Nutrition) and, in those with an impaired clotting mechanism, the administration of fresh-frozen plasma and vitamin K. Cirrhotic patients with ascites are prepared preoperatively by improving nutritional status, limiting sodium intake to 1 to 2 g per day, and reducing ascitic fluid by judicious use of spironolactone with or without other diuretics. Renal dysfunction is addressed in another chapter; however, renal function abnormalities generally do not significantly impair the operation, provided fluid and electrolyte balance is corrected. It still has a significant impact on postoperative survival in the critically ill though (5).

The patient's immune status, if in question, may be examined by determining whether the patient is allergic to cutaneous skin tests. Unfortunately, little can be done to alter the immune status unless it is caused by nutritional deficiency. A nutritional assessment also should be performed (see Nutrition). Medications of particular significance include antihypertensives and steroids. Adrenal insufficiency resulting from intrinsic disease or suppression secondary to exogenous steroid administration demands administration of preoperative, intraoperative, and postoperative steroids. The dose should be approximately ten times the resting nonstressed level and administered in three equally divided doses. Because the normal basal production of cortisol is about 35 mg per day, a replacement of an equivalent of approximately 300 mg of cortisone is indicated. Cortisol equivalent (100 mg) is administered several hours before the operation, 100 mg intraoperatively and 100 mg 8 hours postoperatively. The dosage is gradually tapered to maintenance levels over several days, or if the adrenal glands function normally, it may be discontinued altogether. If postoperative complications occur, however, the ten-times basal level dosage should be continued until the complications have resolved. All patients who have taken steroids preoperatively do not of necessity require preoperative, high-dose steroid replacement. In one study, patients who received less than 5 mg of prednisolone per day had a normal pituitary-adrenal axis. If the adrenal gland's ability to respond to stress is at all questionable, an adrenocorticotropic hormone (ACTH) stimulation test may be performed.

SYSTEMIC DISEASE

The evaluation of systemic disease generally involves a determination of the carbohydrate (diabetes) and thyroid status. In diabetic patients, it is important to avoid hypoglycemic ketosis or hyperosmolarity. This is best accomplished if the blood glucose level is maintained between 125 and 250 mg/dL. If the patient is taking insulin, half the usual dose is given on the morning of surgery and an IV dextrose-containing solution is begun. During the operative procedure, blood glucose levels are determined and regular insulin administered as necessary. In the postoperative period, blood glucose levels must be determined every 4 hours and regular insulin administered IV or subcutaneously for diabetic patients with major alterations in glucose metabolism. For patients who are particularly labile, an insulin infusion pump may be used in the postoperative period. Continuous monitoring of blood glucose levels must be performed throughout the period of administration, particularly when metabolic aberrations, sepsis, and trauma coexist, because these can significantly alter glucose utilization and cause wide fluctuations in serum levels.

METABOLIC RESPONSE TO INJURY

Basal Metabolic Rate

Uninjured humans at rest expend a definable amount of energy to perform physiologic work—the work required to maintain cardiac output, endocrine function, body temperature, hepatic function, respiration, renal function, and so on. The amount of energy required to maintain these functions at rest is called *basal metabolic rate* and is expressed in calories per hour per square meter of body surface. Basal metabolism is the energy expended by the cells that constitute the active mass of the body; fat, extracellular fluid, and bone make no direct contribution to the metabolic rate. The energy used in physiologic work is derived from chemical energy, which in the course of the performance of the work is converted to heat and lost from the body. Therefore the basal metabolic rate, or energy expenditure, may be determined by direct calorimetry in which the heat lost from the body is directly measured. Direct calorimetry is difficult to perform and often impractical in the critically ill. Thus indirect methods of estimating the basal metabolic rate are more commonly used. The heat lost may be indirectly estimated from (a) oxygen consumption, carbon dioxide (CO_2) production, and nitrogen excretion; (b) measurement of energy intake and losses, coupled with the measurement of changes in body composition; or (c) measurement of insensible water loss, assuming that this represents 25% of the total heat loss. The basal metabolic energy requirement depends on patient age, sex, and lean body mass. A 1-month-old infant requires about 40 kcal/kg body weight per day. The requirement increases with age and body mass, so boys between the ages of 15 and 18 years consume 1,700 kcal per day and girls between the ages of 12 and 18 years require 1,400 kcal per day. The energy requirement remains relatively stable during the active years of life. With progressive aging, however, it decreases to 1,300 kcal per day for men and 1,100 kcal per day for women (74). The difference in metabolic rate between men and women probably relates to the fact that women have a larger proportion of fat per unit body weight. Indeed, if basal metabolic rate is expressed per unit fat-free body weight, it is remarkably similar for both males and females over an age span of 20 to 60 years (1.3 kcal/kg per hour).

Hypermetabolism

The response to injury is characterized by an increase in the basal metabolic rate, even though the patient remains at rest. The intensity of this hypermetabolic response depends on the severity of the injury, the patient's nutritional status, and the presence or absence of infection. Patients in good nutritional balance undergoing an elective operation will have a change in metabolic rate of no more than 10% in the postoperative period, provided there are no complications. In contrast, patients with multiple fractures have an increase of their resting energy expenditure by 10% to 25%, those with major infections by 20% to 50%, and those with major thermal burns by 50% to 125%. In the early posttraumatic period, satisfaction of these energy demands results in degradation of body protein (manifested by a negative nitrogen balance), depletion of energy reserves, and loss of body weight. The initial catabolic response in which body protein, fat, and carbohydrate are depleted is gradually reduced and reversed later in the recovery period. An anabolic phase ensues, provided adequate nutritional intake occurs, in which new protein is laid down and carbohydrate and fat reserves are repleted. The hypermetabolic response also gradually diminishes as the wounds heal and as infection is eradicated.

In the early postinjury period, energy requirements are satisfied by glucose, derived mainly from liver and muscle glycogen and by fatty acids released from adipose tissue. Glycogen reserves are rapidly depleted (usually within 48 hours). Fat stores, however, which supply the bulk of the energy requirement during this period, continue to supply fatty acids for many days. Protein catabolism also occurs, even though it may not serve as a primary energy source. Amino acids are released primarily from skeletal muscle at rates three to four times normal and are essential for maintenance of cellular metabolism. Moreover, the gluconeogenic amino acids serve as a source of new glucose and provide the basic glucose structure that is necessary for normal metabolism. Alanine is the most important gluconeogenic amino acid, and its principal site of uptake is the liver. It is part of the glucose-alanine cycle in which its deamination in the liver results in new glucose formation. When glucose undergoes anaerobic glycolysis in muscle, the resultant pyruvate is transaminated, producing alanine and completing the cycle. Rapid depletion of glucose stores coupled with the inability of the two carbon fragments of the fatty acids to serve as a source for gluconeogenesis make protein the only available substrate from which new glucose can be synthesized. Protein catabolism can be reduced but not eliminated by providing exogenous glucose (nitrogen-sparing effect of glucose). Also, certain amino acids can be used as energy sources thus sparing glucose. For example, glutamine from muscle is taken up by the intestine where it is used as respiratory fuel (94).

Catecholamines and Glucocorticoids

Posttraumatic catecholamine levels are elevated and promote hepatic glycogenolysis, inhibition of insulin release, stimulation of glucagon production, and stimulation of fat hydrolysis with the release of free fatty acids. This hormone is produced almost exclusively by the adrenal medulla and has been implicated as the mediator of the hypermetabolic response in injured patients (94).

Glucocorticoid levels are also characteristically elevated and remain so throughout the recovery period. The increased production is the direct result of an increased ACTH secretion by the anterior pituitary. It is presumed that the pituitary is stimulated to release ACTH by the action of the nerves from the periphery responding to the traumatic injury and perhaps by a direct effect of the elevated epinephrine levels. Patients who have sustained severe trauma that requires a prolonged period of convalescence, such as thermal burns, often have marked adrenal hyperplasia. Glucocorticoids promote gluconeogenesis and inhibit the action of insulin.

Insulin

Immediately after injury, circulating levels of insulin and glucose are elevated. Insulin facilitates glucose transport across cell membranes and inhibits both the release of amino acids from muscle and the release of free fatty acids from adipose tissue. In the posttraumatic period, hyperglycemia is common, possibly as a result of the development of insulin resistance. Glucose tolerance curves performed during this period simulate those observed in diabetes and have led many to refer to this state as the *diabetes of injury* (49).

However, the mechanism of the hyperglycemia may not be one of insulin resistance. More recent evidence indicates that glucose oxidation is unimpaired and that the hyperglycemia is caused by an increase in gluconeogenesis rather than a reduction in peripheral utilization. Moreover, glucose flow studies have clearly demonstrated that glucose turnover rate is increased above normal (59,95). Others suggest that the amount of circulating insulin is inadequate for the concentration of glucose.

Glucagon

The increased production of catecholamines after injury is known to stimulate the α-cell of the pancreatic islets, resulting in increased circulating levels of glucagon, a hormone that promotes glycogenolysis and gluconeogenesis. The relation between the concentration of insulin and glucagon (the insulin-to-glucagon molar ratio) determines whether the major influence is toward glucose breakdown or glucose formation. Early after injury, although the level of insulin is elevated, glucagon is disproportionately increased, and the ratio of the two favors gluconeogenesis at the expense of protein formation. As healing occurs, the molar ratio reverses, favoring glycolysis and protein formation. After injury, the hypermetabolic response and hormonal balance direct the metabolism and utilization of carbohydrate, fat, and protein. They set the stage for a negative nitrogen balance and weight loss, both of which are related to the extent of injury. The protein that is catabolized to satisfy energy and substrate requirements is derived mainly from skeletal muscle. Alanine and glutamine released from the muscle are transported to the liver, where they are converted to glucose (gluconeogenesis). With protein breakdown, urinary excretion of nitrogen (predominantly as urea), potassium, phosphate, creatinine, magnesium, zinc, and sulfate are greatly increased, reflecting catabolism of protoplasmic mass.

NUTRITION

The metabolic response to the trauma of operation or injury is characterized by hypermetabolism, which if left unchecked, results in increased tissue breakdown, loss of lean body mass, and depletion of essential intracellular constituents. The prevalence of malnutrition in hospitalized patients has been said to range between 30% and 50%. Protein-calorie malnutrition is characterized by (a) weight loss, (b) hypoalbuminemia, (c) decreased skeletal muscle mass, (d) reduced fat stores, and (e) decreased total lymphocytes (92).

Malnutrition has increased the incidence of clean-wound infections, prolonged postoperative ileus, impaired wound healing, depressed immunocompetence, increased the patient's susceptibility to sepsis, inhibited vital organ function, and increased the risk of respiratory infections and respiratory insufficiency (56,64,89). Moreover, severe malnutrition results in loss or malfunction of various intestinal enzymes. Lactase seems to be particularly sensitive to variations in nutritional status. Thus a patient who develops a lactase deficiency because of malnutrition will be incapable of absorbing supplements that contain milk or milk byproducts. This greatly limits the type of supplements that can be administered orally.

If malnutrition is allowed to persist, morbidity and mortality significantly increase. Loss of body protein appears to be the critical factor determining the point at which the nutritional depletion compromises the ability of the host to respond appropriately to the injury. Mortality and morbidity associated with weight loss and starvation are directly related to the loss of essential protein stores: Death occurs with the loss of 25% of body nitrogen or 33% total body weight (68). Therefore it is essential to limit and ultimately reverse the loss of body protein to promote early recovery and reduce the incidence of life-threatening complications.

Nutritional Requirements

The daily caloric requirement for resting humans is approximately 25 kcal/kg body weight. Hypometabolic, starved humans may require somewhat less, but it is generally at the expense of limited organ function. Most surgical patients are hypermetabolic and require an additional 5 to 60 kcal/kg body weight. *Thus, when the total caloric requirement in the average surgical patient are calculated, 30 to 35 kcal/kg body weight is used.* Daily protein intake requirements are normally about 0.8 g/kg body weight per day, but under conditions of acute stress, they may be as high as 2.5 to 3.5 g/kg body weight per day. Although protein provides only 4 kcal/g, it is the number of grams of protein that is important, with satisfaction of caloric requirements being provided by the addition of carbohydrate or fat. For each gram of protein administered, 25 kcal (carbohydrate or fat) should be provided. Protein consists of amino acids that are either essential or nonessential. The former cannot be manufactured by the body, whereas the latter can.

In selected circumstances, it may be important to limit the total intake of protein or to alter the protein composition of the infusion. In patients with renal and hepatic failure, excessive amounts of protein may result in an excessively elevated blood urea nitrogen (BUN) and/or serum ammonia level with systemic manifestations of uremia in the former or hepatic encephalopathy in the latter. In these cases, 0.5 to 1.0 g protein/kg body weight may be appropriate.

Alteration of the composition of the protein infusion also may be helpful. Essential amino acid infusions without their nonessential counterparts may lessen the rise in serum urea in patients with acute renal failure, and branched-chain amino acids, which are metabolized by muscle and do not require the liver for metabolism, may be more appropriate in patients with hepatic disease. Certain amino acids also have been added to nutritional regimens because they appear to play a more central role during injury than their counterparts. Glutamine serves as a vehicle for nitrogen transfer between tissues; it is also the most important substrate for renal ammoniagenesis, a regulator of protein synthesis, and an essential precursor in nucleic acid biosynthesis (76,93). Glutamine-supplemented nutritional regimens improve nitrogen balance (88). Glutamine may be administered in its more stable form as the dipeptide alanyl-glutamine or glycyl-glutamine. Arginine has potent secretagogue activity, and its administration may have trophic effects in the immune system and, when given, has been shown to improve weight gain and wound healing (4).

Fats have a high caloric value and provide 9 kcal/g. They also are classified as either nonessential or essential, depending on whether the body can manufacture them. Fats that cannot be manufactured by the body include linoleic, arachidonic, and linolenic. Only linolenic is absolutely essential because a fatty acid deficiency will not develop if it alone is provided. Vitamins must be provided daily, particularly the water-soluble vitamins, because they are depleted rapidly. Sodium, potassium, calcium, magnesium, and phosphate also must be provided in sufficient quantities on a daily basis. Trace elements, such as zinc, copper, iodine, manganese, and selenium, must be provided regularly over long-term periods.

A stable weight is often a good indication that basal needs are being met, provided that loss of lean body mass is not hidden by an increase in extracellular water. If the patient is incorporating exogenous protein into endogenous stores, he or she is said to be in a positive nitrogen balance. Nitrogen balance may be grossly calculated by assuming that 1 g per day of nitrogen is lost in the feces, if the patient is stooling, and about a quarter of a gram of nitrogen is lost through the skin. The remaining nitrogen loss occurs in the urine. Approximately 80% of the nitrogen lost in the urine is lost as urea nitrogen. Therefore it becomes apparent that the nitrogen balance of any patient may be calculated quickly by measuring the 24-hour urine and its urea content. The amount of urea nitrogen excreted is multiplied by 1.25 to give the total nitrogen excreted in the urine. If an additional 1 to 2 g is added for skin and stool loss and this quantity is subtracted from the protein nitrogen intake, a positive or negative number is obtained. These urine collections are appropriate for patients in whom bowel is not interposed in the urinary tract. Patients with bowel interpositions alter urea excretion so that this measurement cannot be performed accurately. If the nitrogen balance is positive, the patient is lying down or retaining protein (anabolism); if negative, body protein is being broken down for energy requirements (catabolism).

Nutritional Status

Several modalities have been used to determine whether the patient is malnourished and, if so, to quantitate the degree of nutritional deprivation. Among the indices most often used are weight loss, reactivity to skin-test antigens, creatinine excretion index, middle-arm circumference measurement, tricep skinfold thickness, the measurement of lymphocyte count, serum albumin, serum transferrin, retinal-binding protein, and thyroxine-binding prealbumin. A history of a recent weight loss is particularly important in determining current nutritional status. It must be remembered, however, that this may underestimate loss of lean body mass, because when body protein is metabolized, there is an obligate increase in extracellular fluid. Therefore the weight loss may not accurately reflect the loss of lean body mass. A patient who has lost fewer than 10 pounds in the preceding 3 months is said to be mildly malnourished; between 10 and 20 pounds moderately malnourished; and more than 20 pounds, severely malnourished. A patient's current weight can be compared with height/weight tables and a percentage deviation from normal obtained.

Reactivity to skin-test antigens has been used frequently to determine a patient's immune status. Indirectly, the response to these antigens reflects the patient's nutritional status. If a patient is known to be allergic to one of the antigens and is anergic when tested or if anergic to agents that normally cause a response, severe malnutrition is present. Antigens commonly used are dermatophytin, mumps, purified protein derivative (PPD), streptokinase, and streptodornase. The importance of this index is illustrated by the fact that in several series, cancer patients did not respond effectively to chemotherapy or surgery if their skin-test antigens were negative. However, if the patients were nutritionally repleted, approximately half converted to a positive status and then responded to either chemotherapy or surgery (18,22). More recent data have called into question the reliability of skin-test antigens in critically ill patients. The creatinine excretion index measures the lean body mass or muscle protein stores as does a measurement of middle-arm circumference. Triceps skinfold measurements indicate the status of fat stores. Lymphocyte count is a measure of visceral protein status and should normally be above 2,000 cells/mm^3. If the lymphocyte count is between 1,200 and 2,000 cells/mm^3, the patient is said to be mildly nutritionally depleted; between 800 and 1,200 cells/mm^3, moderately nutritionally depleted; lower than 800 cells/mm^3, severely nutritionally depleted.

Albumin levels are another measure of visceral protein status. Serum albumin has been demonstrated to accurately reflect the patient's nutritional status. In one series, the only parameter that correlated with an increased hospital stay in nutritionally depleted patients was their albumin status (2). Others have found it to be an accurate predictor of the success of a nutritional regimen and an indicator of the degree of nutritional repletion (12). There is a 20% increase in wound infections if the serum albumin concentration is less than 2.9 g/dL (78). If the albumin level is between 3 and 3.5 g/dL, the patient is said to be mildly nutritionally depleted; between 2.5 and 3.0 g/dL, moderately nutritionally depleted; less than 2.5 g/dL, severely nutritionally depleted.

Serum transferrin levels also have been used as an indicator of visceral protein status. Transferrin determinations may not be readily available but can be calculated if one obtains a total iron-binding capacity (TIBC). The formula for calculation is as follows:

$$\text{Serum transferrin} = (0.8 \times \text{TIBC}) - 43$$

If the level is between 150 and 200 mg/dL, the patient is mildly nutritionally depleted; between 100 and 150 mg/dL, moderately nutritionally depleted; less than 100 mg/dL, severely nutritionally depleted. Retinal-binding protein and thyroxine-binding prealbumin are also measures of visceral protein status and are helpful in select cases.

In practice, it is often difficult for the busy clinician to seek out the various tables required for a complete nutritional assessment. *Three modalities are conveniently used to assess the patient's status: weight loss, lymphocyte count, and albumin level.* With these indices, the patient can be placed into one of four categories: normal nutritional status or mildly, moderately, or severely nutritionally depleted. If one is still unsure, skin-test antigens may be used. If the patient is anergic to a battery of skin-test antigens, he or she is considered severely malnourished irrespective of the previously mentioned indices (Table 10.1).

TABLE 10.1. NUTRITIONAL ASSESSMENT: THE CATEGORIZATION OF PATIENTS INTO MILD, MODERATE, OR SEVERELY NUTRITIONALLY DEPLETED

Measurement	Mild	Moderate	Severe
Weight loss (lb)	<10	10–20	>20
Lymphocyte count (cells/mm^3)	1,200–2,000	800–1,200	<800
Albumin (g/dL)	3.0–3.5	2.5–3.0	<2.5
Serum transferrin (mg/dL)	150–200	100–150	<100
Skin-test antigens	+	+	Anergy

TABLE 10.2. BASIC CALORIC REQUIREMENTS OF UNINJURED HUMANS AT REST

	Body Weight (kcal/kg)
Children	
First 10 kg (0–10)	100
Second 10 kg (10–20)	50
Each additional kg >20	20
Adults	25

The amount of calories required per day for repletion also must be calculated so that appropriate amounts may be administered. The patient's weight times 25 gives the basal metabolic requirement of the patient. Depending on the severity of the insult, an additional 5 to 60 kcal/kg is added. In children, the amount of kilocalories metabolized varies according to weight. For the first 10 kg, 100 kcal/kg is metabolized; for the second 10 kg, 50 kcal per kg; and for each kilogram over 20, 20 kcal/kg (Table 10.2). The success of the regimen is determined by the return of the serum values to normal; the return of an allergic response to the skin-test antigens, if previously anergic; and weight gain. Moreover, periodic, crude measurements of nitrogen balance as previously described, if positive, will confirm that the amount and composition of the calorie load are appropriate. Having determined how much the patient requires, one must determine the route of administration: enteral, IV, or a combination.

Enteral Feedings

Enteral feedings are preferred if possible because complications are decreased and a more balanced, physiologic diet can be provided. Enteral diets are either nonelemental or elemental. Nonelemental enteral feedings consist of undigested and minimally digested protein hydrolysates, fat, and carbohydrates, whereas elemental diets consist of medium-chain triglycerides, glucose, and amino acids. *Enteral feedings can be provided either by a small feeding tube, a gastrostomy, or a feeding jejunostomy. Generally, nonelemental enteral feedings are preferred, provided the gut is not diseased, because they have lower osmolality and are cheaper.* The advantages of an elemental diet include its bulk-free and lactose-free composition (30). Therefore patients with severely diseased bowels or patients who have been chronically starved are probably better served with an elemental diet—at least at the outset.

One should begin with the enteral feeding diluted to half strength at a rate of 50 to 75 mL per hour in the adult. If this is tolerated, the volume is increased to 2,500 to 3,000 mL per 24 hours, and if tolerated, osmolality is increased to full osmotic content (i.e., approximately 1 kcal/mL will be administered at 500 to 1,000 mOsm/kg). Complications include abdominal cramps, diarrhea, and diaphoresis. If any of these symptoms occur, the infusion is slowed, the osmolality is reduced, or both. Once the symptoms disappear, a gradual return to the strength and rate desired is begun. If diarrhea continues to be poorly controlled, the administration of paregoric 5 mL in divided doses may be helpful.

Isosmotic Intravenous Nutrition

Carbohydrate, protein, and fat substrates may be infused individually or in combination in near-isosmotic concentrations. Because of their isosmotic character, not only may they be administered by peripheral vein but also the rate of administration may be rapidly changed to satisfy a change in fluid requirements or even stopped so that medications, colloid, and blood may be administered. These properties make such solutions advantageous during periods of critical care when instability of the patient is not uncommon.

An understanding of the metabolic effects of each type of caloric source with respect to energy provision and its potential for endogenous protein preservation and maintenance of optimum organ function is essential if the proper substrate or combination of substrates is to be administered to acutely ill patients. The provision of glucose in dosages up to 100 g per day decreases protein loss as measured by the loss of urinary nitrogen. This protein-sparing effect is directly proportional to the quantity of calories administered. Infusion of larger quantities of glucose results in disproportionately lesser reductions in nitrogen losses. Supplying 700 protein-free calories to fasting normal humans results in maximum reduction of protein losses. Increasing the nonprotein caloric intake is without further effect in the sparing of body protein. Indeed, positive nitrogen balance cannot be achieved even with high-dose glucose infusions. Starved, unstressed humans given approximately 700 g of glucose maintain a negative nitrogen balance of about 1.5 g/m^2 per day. If the same total caloric load is given, however, but part of the glucose calories are replaced by an equivalent amount of amino acid calories, the negative balance is eliminated (96). Supplying dietary protein with calories further improves nitrogen balance. Thus, on a fixed adequate protein intake, energy level is the deciding factor in nitrogen balance, and at a fixed adequate caloric intake, nitrogen intake is the determinant of nitrogen balance (9). Similarly, in critically ill, traumatized patients and in those with superimposed bacteremia, at low-dose levels (or those that can be easily achieved employing isosmotic solutions), glucose has the same effect on nitrogen sparing as does an equivalent caloric load of amino acids (63). Thus, at low-dose levels, total caloric load, whether derived from protein or carbohydrate, determines the degree of nitrogen sparing, whereas when the caloric load is increased, amino acid intake becomes a more dominant determinant of nitrogen balance.

Fat emulsions also may be administered by peripheral vein and have the advantage of providing high caloric loads in relatively small volumes because fat provides 9 kcal/g, whereas glucose and protein provide a little less than 4 kcal/g. The effect of fat emulsion on nitrogen sparing, however, is not equivalent to equal caloric amounts of glucose or amino acids. In normal unstressed humans, equivalent caloric amounts of infused fat emulsion and glucose result in a lesser degree of nitrogen sparing for the former. When amino acids are added to equivalent caloric amounts of fat emulsion or glucose, the latter combination results in a less negative nitrogen balance. In severely injured humans some investigators failed to observe any reduction in nitrogen sparing with the infusion of large doses of soybean fat emulsions. Conversely, more recent studies have demonstrated adequate utilization of fat calories in the immediate posttraumatic and postoperative period. In view of the degree of nitrogen sparing observed in normal and injured humans, when used in combination with amino acids, fat emulsions seem helpful in sparing nitrogen, but glucose and amino acids are more effective than fat, calorie for calorie.

Although there are no distinct differences in nitrogen balance in comparing low-dose isosmotic administration of glucose and amino acids, there are clear advantages to infusing a medium-dose combination of the two substrates. First, their effect is augmentative, and the impact on calories is not limited when protein is provided. Second, amino acids administered alone cause a constant rise in BUN that is not observed when glucose is added. Third, altered hepatic and renal transport occur in critically ill patients who are given amino acids as their sole caloric source. The altered transport properties may be restored to normal by the addition of glucose. An appropriate combination that provides maximum nitrogen sparing per gram of nutrient administered while maintaining optimal hepatic, renal, and cardiac function consists of a liter solution in which half is provided as 10% dextrose and the other half as a 7% to 8% amino acid solution. Fat emulsions given in 500-mL amounts once or twice a day provide additional calories. Because these solutions may be administered by peripheral vein and because alterations in infusion rate and even abrupt cessation of infusion can be accomplished without untoward effects so that blood, antibiotics, and other medications can be given, these infusates are an ideal means of preserving normal metabolic function of vital organs while limiting nitrogen loss in early posttraumatic, postoperative, and unstable critically ill patients. Unfortunately, it is generally not possible to achieve positive nitrogen balance with isosmotic solutions because the amount of calories required would necessitate excessive fluid administration. If illness is protracted and oral alimentation is not possible, positive nitrogen balance is achieved by administration of hyperosmotic solutions (hyperalimentation).

Hyperosmotic Intravenous Nutrition

Hyperosmotic IV solutions, which are capable of providing enough nitrogen and calories in an acceptable volume, are made up of equivalent amounts of a 50% dextrose and 7% to 8% amino acid solution, providing approximately 1 kcal/mL

TABLE 10.3. COMPOSITION OF HYPERALIMENTATION SOLUTIONS

Ingredient	Concentration
Amino acid (7%–8%)	500 mL
Dextrose (50%)	500 mL
Potassium (KCl)	60–150 mEq
Sodium (NaCl)	60–180 mEq
Calcium (Ca gluconate)	5–15 mEq
Magnesium ($MgSO_4$)	8–24 mEq
Phosphate (K_2HPO_4)	15–20 mmol
Trace elements	—
Multiple vitamins	—

of solution. Electrolytes including potassium, sodium, calcium, magnesium, and phosphate are added as required (Table 10.3). Trace elements (zinc, copper, manganese, chromium) and multivitamins also are added as required. In addition, essential fatty acids are provided by the administration of 500 mL of fat emulsion two to three times a week.

Because the hyperalimentation solution is hyperosmotic, it must be administered through a central venous line and its rate of administration rigidly controlled. If long-term or home hyperalimentation is to be administered, the solution should be given through a long-term indwelling catheter, such as a Broviac or Hickman catheter. The catheters are placed in the superior vena cava, tunneled subcutaneously under the skin beneath the anterior chest wall, and brought out at about the level of the nipple—between it and the sternum. We have kept catheters functional as long as 21 months in adults and 14 months in children. In most cases, hyperalimentation will be administered for limited periods, and a percutaneous central line is placed. The central venous line must be placed and maintained with an assiduously sterile technique; otherwise, infection will invariably follow. The IV line is placed in the superior vena cava, either by a subclavian or internal jugular puncture. A sterile dressing is applied with an antibiotic ointment placed over the catheter entrance site. On alternate days, the dressing is changed and a new sterile dressing, iodophor preparation, and iodophor ointment are applied. A millipore filter is placed in line. The filter is changed and cultured every 24 hours. The IV tubing is changed with each bottle. The hyperalimentation solutions are made fresh daily and stored refrigerated. No medications, blood, or other fluid should be administered through the hyperalimentation line, nor should CVP measurements be made using the catheter through which the hyperalimentation solution is being administered. Fluid should be administered initially at low rates (50 mL per hour) until tolerance has been achieved (blood glucose remains below 200 mg/dL), after which the rate of infusion may be gradually increased until the proper caloric load is achieved. Usually, 3 to 4 L per day is given, providing 3,000 to 4,000 kcal per 24 hours. Blood must be monitored for glucose concentration periodically, when high, either the infusion rate must be reduced or insulin administered.

Blood glucose levels may be particularly difficult to control in the immediate postoperative and posttraumatic period. Insulin given IV every 4 hours, adjusting it to blood glucose levels, usually suffices. Occasionally, blood glucose levels can be better controlled with a continuous insulin infusion. Two to three units of regular insulin are administered per hour in a concentration of 1 U/mL of saline solution. If these simple measures do not control the glucose level or large amounts of insulin are required, the solution should be tapered or fat should be substituted for the glucose. It is apparent that high-dose insulin can lower serum glucose, but it is probable that under these conditions abnormal metabolism at the mitochondrial level occurs, obviating any beneficial effect of lowering the serum glucose.

Similarly, after IV fat administration, the serum must be observed for clearance. Normally, immediately after the infusion of IV lipid, the serum is lipemic. It should be totally clear approximately 8 hours after infusion. This may be checked by obtaining serum cholesterol and triglyceride levels, or grossly, at the bedside by drawing a blood sample, spinning it down, and observing the serum for lipemia. Plasma osmolality and sodium, potassium, chloride, CO_2, BUN, creatinine, calcium, phosphate, and glucose also should be monitored on a frequent periodic basis—initially daily. Magnesium levels should be monitored regularly, but somewhat less frequently.

When discontinuing the infusion, the clinician should gradually taper the rate over 24 to 36 hours. A prolonged infusion should never be stopped abruptly because severe hypoglycemia may ensue. On the other hand, many patients with home hyperalimentation tolerate abrupt cessation of the infusion well. These patients generally infuse their hyperalimentation solution over a 12-hour period while sleeping and immediately cease infusion when ambulatory. Critically ill and hospitalized patients are generally better served by tapering rather than abrupt cessation. Complications are not uncommon with hyperalimentation and can be life-threatening. Placement of the central venous catheter has resulted in pneumothorax, hemothorax, hydrothorax, brachial plexus injury, venous thrombosis, and embolism. Because of the nature of the solution infused and the central venous location of the catheter, infectious complications have been reported and must be recognized and immediately corrected. Alterations in glucose metabolism may result in hyperglycemia, glucosuria with an osmotic diuresis, and in severe cases, hyperosmolar nonketotic dehydration and coma. The mortality in the last situation can be as high as 50%.

Early recognition of hyperglycemia and its treatment by reducing the rate of infusion and/or administration of insulin correct these complications. A sudden change in glucose concentration in a patient who is receiving hyperalimentation should suggest sepsis. Patients with nonketotic hyperosmolar coma characteristically have blood glucose levels in excess of 500 mg/dL and must be treated aggressively, often with large doses of insulin and fluid. Ketoacids in diabetic patients given inadequate insulin for the additional carbohydrate load and postinfusion hypoglycemia resulting from rapid withdrawal of glucose in the face of persistently elevated endogenous insulin levels also may occur and are treated by increasing insulin and glucose infusions, respectively. Rarely, the complete metabolism of glucose for energy needs results in an elevated partial pressure of CO_2 (P_{CO_2}) and CO_2 narcosis with respiratory insufficiency. Blood gas determinations confirm the diagnosis. Treatment is directed at reducing the amount of CO_2 produced for energy requirements by providing a greater share of the caloric load as fat. Alterations in amino acid metabolism may result in hyperchloremic metabolic acidosis, plasma and amino acid imbalances, hyperammonemia, and elevated BUN levels (26). Alterations in the content of the infusion or rate of infusion must be made. Hypophosphatemia and hypercalcemia and hypocalcemia are corrected by addition or removal from the infusate of the appropriate inorganic ion. Vitamin deficiencies; essential fatty acid deficiencies; trace mineral deficiencies; and abnormal plasma potassium, sodium, and magnesium levels have been reported and are corrected by appropriate addition or removal of the particular substance. Trace minerals and essential fatty acid deficiencies are not encountered when fresh-frozen plasma and fat emulsions are administered as previously described. Finally, alterations in liver enzymes, cholestatic jaundice, and fatty infiltration of the liver complicate long-term administration. Indeed, the administration of more calories than required results in lipogenesis and fatty infiltration of the liver. This may be eliminated in patients receiving long-term hyperalimentation by administering it in a cyclic manner. Glucose is periodically withheld, and only amino acids and fats are infused for an 8-hour period. This has reduced and, in fact, cleared fatty livers.

Once the amount of calories for maintenance of basal needs and restitution of adequate nutrition is determined, the route may be chosen. If the amount of calculated calories can be administered by oral or tube feedings, this is preferred. It appears that patients require fewer calories to maintain body functions and normal weight status if they are given orally rather than IV. If the gut cannot be used and the total caloric requirements must be replaced, IV hyperosmolar solutions must be used. If the gut is temporarily unavailable and will be functional soon, isosmotic IV solutions may be used to limit catabolism until the gut is functional.

Perioperative Total Parenteral Nutrition

The benefits of perioperative nutrition have been difficult to assess in properly controlled studies. It has been shown conclusively to be of benefit only in severely malnourished patients. For all others, it seems to add risk rather than benefit. Indeed, overfeeding can be detrimental because it increases septic complications and compromises immune and hepatic function. In the severely malnourished patient who cannot take oral alimentation, total parenteral nutrition should be administered 7 to 10 days preoperatively. This reduces complications by 10%. The enteral route is preferred, if possible, because it reduces septic complications and maintains structure and functional integrity of the gastrointestinal tract (92).

Intravenous Nutrition for Specific Organ Malfunction

Surgical patients who have sustained acute renal failure have been successfully managed by providing them with hyperalimentation solutions. Providing adequate amounts of calories in these patients can be difficult because fluid administration may be limited. This can be obviated by either frequent dialyses or continuous plasma filtration. Unfortunately, dialysis and plasma filtration result in 6 to 10 g of amino acids lost per day. This amount must be added to the usual requirement to attain optimum balance. Mortality in surgical patients with acute renal failure is exceedingly high. According to some reports, mortality may be reduced significantly by the provision of adequate calories and essential amino acids (1). Hyperalimentation in patients with acute renal failure unfortunately does not reduce the frequency of dialyses, although it may have some effect on lessening the duration of renal failure. Essential amino acids have been found to be more efficacious than a combination of essential and nonessential regimens by some groups. It appears that those given essential amino acids have a less rapid rise in BUN and reduced mortality compared with a similar group given essential and nonessential amino acids in the hyperalimentation solution (36).

Patients who have hepatic failure or hepatic encephalopathy are often nutritionally depleted. Straight-chain amino acids are metabolized by the liver, whereas branched-chain amino acids are metabolized by muscle. Amino acid profiles examined in patients with hepatic failure reveal that the concentrations of straight-chain amino acids are elevated, whereas the branched-chain amino acids are diminished. The assumption is that of the two major sites of amino acid metabolism, liver and muscle, the liver is incapable of metabolizing amino acids. Moreover, it has been proposed that if the amino acids the liver metabolizes are withheld while those metabolized by muscle are given, the nutritional status of the patient might be improved. In one series, patients with cirrhosis given branched-chain amino acids had an 87% improvement in their condition, and 75% of those with hepatitis were improved after the administration of branched-chain amino acids (37). Patients with significant hepatic disease probably should have a limited protein intake, ranging between 0.5 and 1 g/kg body weight. Simultaneous administration of oral neomycin and lactulose, by reducing gut flora and ammonia metabolism, may enhance protein tolerance.

More directed use of nutrients are currently being studied. L-Arginine and L-glutamine stimulate host defenses and increased wound healing. Glutamine may preserve the intestinal barrier in stressed patients and essential fatty acids and polyribonucleotides may enhance immune function in cancer patients. Thus in the future, it may be possible to assess a patient's specific needs and provide a selected nutrient regimen to meet these needs (78).

FLUIDS AND ELECTROLYTES

Body Fluid Compartments

The treatment of many fluid and electrolyte disorders requires a knowledge of the body fluid compartments and the ability to calculate them in a given individual. Specific therapy of postobstructive diuresis, dehydration, hypovolemia, and water intoxication requires that knowledge for appropriate therapy. *Total body water constitutes approximately 60% of the body weight in males and 50% in females.* For a lean person, 10% is added; for an obese person, 10% is subtracted because muscle cells contain the greatest fraction of water. *The total body water is divided into compartments: extracellular, intracellular, and transcellular* (Table 10.4). *The extracellular fluid compartment composes approximately 20% of the body weight and is divided into plasma (4.5%), interstitial fluid (16%), and lymph (2%). Because the blood volume is made up of solids and plasma, it can be calculated by multiplying the body weight by 7%.* Intracellular fluid composes 30% to 40% of the total body weight and is accessible only by freely diffusible molecules. Transcellular fluid constitutes 1% to 3% of the total body weight and is composed of pleural, peritoneal, cerebrospinal, intraocular, salivary, and digestive secretions. It is in equilibrium with the extracellular fluid and in disease conditions may increase in amount, particularly during trauma. This is the so-called third space, fluid that is unavailable to the intravascular compartment in situations of injury.

The osmolality of the plasma is an indication of the endogenous substances contained in that compartment and is helpful clinically in situations of dehydration and hypervolemia. The osmolality is generally measured by freezing-point depression but can be calculated conveniently by doubling the sum of the sodium and potassium concentrations and adding to that quantity the blood glucose level divided by 20 plus the blood urea level divided by three. These latter two substances are osmotically active and may contribute significantly to the total osmotic content.

The amount of fluid necessary to maintain homeostasis is equivalent to the urine output plus insensible loss plus abnormal losses minus the water produced by the metabolism of fat, carbohydrate, and protein (Table 10.5). Each of these entities must be calculated for the individual patient if optimum fluid balance is to be achieved.

The amount of urine necessary to maintain proper balance is dictated by the physiologic limits of the kidney for solute and water excretion. *In resting humans, the products of normal metabolism produce a solute load that requires a minimum of 400 to 600 mL of urine for excretion.* Traumatized and critically ill patients are hypermetabolic and may produce twice the normal solute load, necessitating a minimum of 800 to 1,200 mL of urine excretion per day. Conversely, excessive output may lead to a washout of the renal medullary osmotic gradient, resulting in impaired concentrating capabilities of the kidney. The fluid intake required to produce large urine outputs also may result in fluid retention and vascular overload. Thus there are limits between which urine output should be maintained. The adult kidney is most efficient in maintaining balance when fluid intake is sufficient to produce a urine output of 800 to 1,200 mL per day, or 30 to 50 mL per hour. Urine output in children should be maintained between 1 and 2 mL/kg body weight per hour.

Insensible loss refers to the water lost from the respiratory tract and skin. The amount lost depends on the ambient temperature and humidity, as well as the patient's body surface area and body temperature. *The normothermic adult in a comfortable environment loses 800 to 1,000 mL per day (10 to 15 mL/kg of body weight per 24 hours).* Insensible losses

TABLE 10.4. BODY FLUID COMPARTMENTS

Compartment	%
Total body water	50–60
? Extracellular fluid	20–22
?? Blood plasma	4.5
?? Interstitial fluid	16
?? Lymph	2
? Intracellular fluid	30–40
? Transcellular fluid	1–3

TABLE 10.5. FLUID REQUIREMENTS

	Requirement
Urine output (UO)	= 30–50 mL/hr (adult) 1–2 mL/kg/hr (child)
Insensible loss	= 10–15 mL/kg/24 hr (adult) 25–45 mL/100 kcal (child)
Abnormal loss	= Measured external or estimated third-space loss
Water of metabolism	= 0.1 × 25 × body weight (adult) 0.1 × kcal met (child)

Note: Basic fluid requirement = (UO + Insensible loss + Abnormal loss) – H_2O metabolism.

in children are conveniently related to caloric consumption. A child will lose 25 to 45 mL of H_2O for each 100 kcal metabolized. The amount of calories consumed per day may be calculated by multiplying the body weight by 100 for each of the first 10 kg, by 50 for each of the second 10 kg, and by 20 for each additional kg body weight in excess of 20 kg (Table 10.2). Therefore a 10-kg child loses about 350 mL per day and a 20-kg child about 420 mL. Insensible losses increase by about 10% for each degree centigrade of temperature elevation above normal.

The water produced by metabolism is calculated from the caloric expenditure of the patient. The amount of water produced in milliliters is numerically equal to 10% of the total amount of kilocalories consumed. The resting adult metabolizes approximately 25 kcal/kg of body weight per 24 hours, whereas the child's caloric expenditure is calculated on a graduated basis as previously described. *An 80-kg adult who consumes 2,000 kcal (25 kcal/kg × 80 kg) produces 200 mL of H_2O, whereas a 12-kg child who consumes 1,100 kcal (10 kg × 100 kcal/kg + 2 kg × 50 kcal/kg) produces 110 mL of H_2O.* Because these volumes are small, the water of metabolism is often disregarded in total fluid calculations in patients with functioning kidneys.

Abnormal losses refer to fluids lost from the body by nasogastric suction, fistula drainage, vomiting and diarrhea, or the vascular system by third-space sequestration (e.g., retroperitoneal edema, operative trauma, ascites, bowel obstruction). The volumes of these losses are measured when external drainage occurs or estimated when sequestration is present and added to the total daily fluid requirements.

The total daily fluid requirement in an adult is calculated by adding the desired urine output, the insensible loss adjusted for temperature elevations, and measured or estimated abnormal losses. By monitoring the patient's urine output and weight, the clinician can determine the appropriateness of the calculated fluid requirement. The patient who is not receiving total caloric replacement should lose approximately 1 pound per day unless, as in the immediate postoperative period, obligate third-space sequestration of fluid is occurring. If the urine output or weight status is inappropriate, the fluid administered is adjusted accordingly. An example of total fluid replacement calculation follows: an 80-kg febrile (38°C) adult with a nasogastric tube draining 400 mL per day would require 1,200 mL urine output (50 mL per hour × 24 hours) plus 1,320 mL insensible loss (15 mL per kg of body weight per 24 hours × 80 kg + 10% of this quantity for the 1° temperature elevation) plus 400 mL abnormal loss (nasal gastric output) for a total of 2,920 mL per 24 hours.

Total fluid replacement in children may be calculated from the calories metabolized. One milliliter of fluid is administered for each kilocalorie metabolized. *Thus a 25-kg child would require 1,000 mL for the first 10 kg, 500 mL for the second 10 kg, and 100 mL for the final 5 kg, for a total of 1,600 mL per day* (Table 10.2).

TABLE 10.6. AVERAGE ELECTROLYTE CONTENT OF GASTROINTESTINAL LOSSES (mEq/L)

	Sodium	Potassium	Chloride
Gastric	60	10.0	90
Jejunum	105	5.0	100
Ileum	120	10.0	105
Cecum	80	20.0	50
Bile	175	5.0	100
Pancreas	170	4.5	75

Basic Electrolyte Requirements

The average young adult eating a regular diet receives approximately 70 to 120 mEq of sodium, 60 to 80 mEq potassium, 15 to 24 mEq of magnesium, and 80 to 140 mEq of chloride per day. Although the kidney is extremely effective in conserving sodium because it can reabsorb in excess of 99% of that filtered, total renal function is better preserved if enough sodium is administered so that maximum conservation of that filtered is unnecessary. Potassium, on the other hand, is not as efficiently conserved and therefore must be provided to avoid potassium depletion. Because magnesium is stored, patients who are in good nutritional balance before their illness do not require replacement, provided the period of IV therapy is limited. Patients whose nutritional status is marginal or who have alcoholic cirrhosis often require magnesium replacement at a rate of 5 to 20 mEq per day. IV sodium, potassium, and chloride requirements may be satisfied by providing the adult with about 75 mEq of sodium chloride and 40 mEq of potassium chloride per day.

Baseline electrolyte requirements for children are best calculated on the basis of caloric expenditure. Minimum 24-hour requirements are 3 mEq of sodium per 100 kcal, 2 mEq of chloride per 100 kcal, and 2 mEq of potassium per 100 kcal. Thus the 30-kg child would require 1,700 kcal. The sodium requirement is 17 × 3 = 51 mEq, the chloride requirement is 17 × 2 = 34 mEq, and the potassium requirement is 17 × 2 = 34 mEq.

Abnormal losses must be added to these basic requirements. The fluid lost from the body may be analyzed for its electrolyte content to determine accurate replacement (Table 10.6). Fluid sequestered in a third space generally mimics the electrolyte content of plasma and therefore can be replaced accordingly.

Anuria

The fluid and electrolyte requirements for patients who are anephric or anuric are calculated from insensible and abnormal losses. *With insensible loss, an adult should receive 10 to 15 mL/kg of body weight per 24 hours, whereas a child should receive 25 mL of fluid per 100 kcal expended.* The caloric expenditure is estimated on the basis of weight as previously described. Half of the fluid is administered as 10% dextrose in water and the other half as 5% dextrose in 0.2N saline solution. Potassium is generally not administered unless serum studies indicate the need for replacement. Abnormal losses are added to these basic requirements. These calculations are merely estimates of the patient's needs; therefore fluid and electrolyte therapy must be continuously adjusted according to serum electrolyte analyses, patient weight, and when appropriate, urine output.

Volume and Sodium Disturbances

Dehydration

When the patient's minimum fluid requirements are not met, a water deficit accompanied by weight loss occurs. A 4% loss of body weight resulting from a water deficit requires emergent rehydration. A 6% loss of body weight caused by lack of hydration results in a life-threatening condition often manifested by signs and symptoms of shock. The water lost may be relatively isotonic, in which case the dehydration is normonatremic, or hypotonic, which causes hypernatremia to occur.

Dehydration in urologic patients may be caused by postobstructive diuresis, prolonged vomiting and diarrhea, and diabetes insipidus. Postobstructive diuresis may be either physiologic or pathologic. Physiologic diuresis occurs when volume overload precedes the relief of the obstruction or when serum urea is elevated. The kidney responds appropriately when it is unobstructed by excreting the excess volume in the former circumstance or undergoing an osmotic diuresis as a result of the excess urea in the latter situation. The diuresis is self-limited because it ceases when the kidney has returned the body to a homeostatic condition. Rarely, a pathologic diuresis is superimposed on the physiologic diuresis and occurs as a result of specific defects that cause a decreased proximal and distal tubule sodium reabsorption and lack of concentrating capabilities of the kidney, resulting from a reduced medullary osmotic gradient (65). Such patients do not respond to antidiuretic hormone (ADH) or mineralocorticoid administration. Appropriate therapy consists of replacing insensible losses as previously outlined in addition to measured losses. Because the sodium content in the urine usually ranges between 50 and 70 mEq/L, urine output is replaced with 0.5N saline solution. It is important not to overhydrate these patients because such therapy often perpetuates the pathologic diuresis and prevents reestablishment of the medullary osmotic gradient, prolonging the concentrating defect. As the concentrating ability of the kidney returns, fluid therapy is reduced accordingly. It is often helpful in patients who have severe diuresis to follow serum osmolalities and daily weights, adjusting therapy accordingly.

Gastric losses are repleted with 0.5N saline or normal saline solution to which potassium chloride is added. Diarrheic losses are replaced with lactated Ringer's solution. Diabetes insipidus may occur as a result of a lack of ADH, collecting duct unresponsiveness to endogenous ADH, or lack of a medullary osmotic gradient. Patients are often slightly hypernatremic and mildly dehydrated. The urinary sodium content is generally low. Fluid administered should have a relatively modest sodium content until results of urinary electrolytes become available. The diagnosis should be sought expeditiously because specific therapy will often correct the disorder.

Volume Excess

Volume overload may be the result of either hypotonic or isotonic fluid excess. Hypotonic fluid excess results in the water intoxication syndrome manifested by clouded sensorium, irrational behavior, changing neurologic signs, stupor, seizures, and coma. Water intoxication most commonly occurs as a result of hypotonic irrigant absorption through the prostatic bed in patients undergoing transurethral resections. The first signs of volume overload are usually a rising CVP and mental confusion. Blood pressure changes are not often noted initially. If a minimum amount of water is absorbed and central nervous system (CNS) symptoms are not present, fluid restriction with judicious use of diuretics will suffice. In more severe cases in which significant hyponatremia and CNS disorders occur, the treatment should include fluid restriction coupled with hypertonic sodium chloride (3%) administration. Diuretics are not effective in the presence of significant hyponatremia and should be used sparingly until the serum sodium is returning to normal. Inappropriate secretion of ADH, often as a consequence of malignant tumors, is another cause of hypotonic fluid excess and also may result in hyponatremic fluid overload. These patients are often successfully managed by fluid restriction.

Isotonic fluid excesses are usually iatrogenic and are a consequence of excessive administration of fluids that contain sodium. The development of congestive heart failure, inappropriate weight gain, or peripheral edema depends on the severity of the overload. Such patients are treated with diuretics and fluid restriction.

Potassium Disorders

Hyperkalemia usually occurs in urologic patients as a result of acute renal insufficiency, addisonian crisis, trauma, shock, and diabetic acidosis. Life-threatening elevations in serum potassium often produce significant ECG alterations. *Peaking of the T wave, lengthening of the PR interval, prolongation of the QRS complex, and loss of the P wave occur with progressive hyperkalemia.* As potassium continues to rise, the ECG may ultimately resemble a sine wave. Calcium gluconate protects the heart from the adverse effects of potassium and may be administered in severe cases of hyperkalemia. *Treatment consists of IV administration of hypertonic sodium bicarbonate, which results in a shift of hydrogen ion out of the cell and concomitant movement of potassium into the cell, causing a temporary lowering of serum potassium.* Glucose and insulin therapy (10 units of regular insulin plus 50 g of glucose) are recommended only in extremely urgent situations. Potassium is temporarily bound during glucose transport, thus effectively removing it from the serum. Because these measures are only temporary, simultaneous institution of therapy to lower the serum potassium permanently is mandatory. This may be accomplished with ion exchange resins (Kayexalate given by mouth or by rectum), peritoneal dialysis, or hemodialysis.

Hypokalemia usually results from excessive upper gastrointestinal losses, diuretic therapy, steroid administration, and hyperaldosteronism. Metabolic alkalosis is often associated. Therapy is directed at eliminating the disorder and replacing the loss. Administration of solutions that contain sodium in the face of hypokalemia may promote renal potassium loss, particularly in patients with primary hyperaldosteronism. When sodium losses occur concomitantly with potassium deficits, both must be replaced simultaneously. If rapid replacement therapy is required, the ECG should be continuously monitored. If ECG changes occur, the infusion must be slowed or stopped until the abnormalities resolve.

Hypercalcemia

Hypercalcemia in urologic practice is generally the result of metastatic tumor to bone, hydrochlorothiazide therapy, or hyperparathyroidism. The symptoms of hypercalcemia include anorexia, weakness, somnolence, polyuria, and coma. Initial therapy involves the establishment of a sodium diuresis by administering IV saline solution and nonthiazide diuretics. If the diuresis must be prolonged, careful monitoring of serum potassium and magnesium concentrations is essential to prevent deficiencies.

Inorganic phosphate administration will rapidly lower serum calcium but results in metastatic calcification of soft tissues. Ethylenediamine tetraacetic acid (EDTA), a chelating agent, also rapidly lowers serum calcium but has many associated complications. These two agents should not be used unless life-threatening hypercalcemia occurs. On rare occasions, emergency therapy is required in patients with hyperparathyroidism who have uncontrollable serum calcium levels.

Mithramycin and steroids also have been used to control hypercalcemia. With both agents a decrease in serum calcium does not usually occur for 24 to 48 hours. Mithramycin, a cytotoxic agent used in the treatment of malignancies, has many serious side effects including bone marrow depression, renal failure, and hepatic toxicity. It should be used only in patients with neoplasms and then only when more conventional methods fail. The dosage is 1 to 2.5 mg per day for 3 days. Steroids are somewhat less effective and are best used in disorders in which vitamin D sensitivity is etiologic. Dialysis also may be used, particularly in patients with associated renal failure.

Bone resorption and release of calcium may be controlled by the oral or IV administration of etidronate disodium. This drug is useful for controlling hypercalcemia in patients with metastatic disease. It is not useful for treating an acute hypercalcemic crisis. In this situation, saline infusion and diuretics are indicated. Etidronate disodium may be added to the regimen to allay the recurrence of hypercalcemia. If used, adequate renal function and urine output must be present because the drug is excreted in the urine.

A saline diuresis should be the first modality tried, reserving the other forms of therapy for specific indications. It is important that diagnostic studies be instituted early to define the cause of hypercalcemia so that definitive therapy may proceed without delay.

Hypermagnesemia

Hypermagnesemia interferes with neuromuscular transmission both peripherally and centrally. The signs and symptoms include deterioration of mental function, drowsiness, muscular paralysis, and in severe cases, coma. Nausea, vomiting, peripheral vasodilation, and hypotension also may occur. The ECG shows prolongation of the QT interval. Persistent hypermagnesemia may cause soft tissue calcification and interfere with bone mineralization. Hypermagnesemia rarely occurs with normal renal function. Patients with decreased renal function who ingest medications that contain magnesium may be particularly prone to the disorder. Urologic patients in whom magnesium-containing solutions are used to irrigate the urinary system for dissolution of stones also may manifest hypermagnesemia. This is particularly true when the irrigant, such as Suby's solution G or citric acid, glucono-delta-lactone magnesium carbonate (Renacidin), is used at increased pressures in areas where vascular beds are exposed. When the symptoms are severe, emergency treatment with calcium gluconate may be necessary. In patients with normal renal function, however, hydration and furosemide administration generally suffice. Rarely, patients with decreased renal function or those with severe neurologic symptoms require hemodialysis to return magnesium levels to normal.

Hypomagnesemia may be a complication of aminoglycoside therapy, hepatic disease, or nutritional deficiency. Symptoms include somnolence and weakness.

Anion Gap

The anion gap is the difference between the sum of the major cations, sodium and potassium, minus the sum of the major anions, bicarbonate and chloride, and is normally about

16 mEq/L. The anion gap is of considerable importance in distinguishing among several types of acid–base disturbances. Most of the acidoses commonly found in urologic practice do not have an increased anion gap: hyperchloremic metabolic acidosis, renal tubular acidosis, uremic acidosis, and the acidosis accompanying diarrhea or excessive ileostomy drainage. An increased anion gap is most commonly associated with ketoacidosis; lactic acidosis; hyperosmolar, hyperglycemic, and nonketotic coma; and occasionally, uremic acidosis. Rarely, hyperchloremic metabolic acidosis caused by enteric urinary absorption may present with an anion gap.

Acid–Base Disturbances

Acid–Base Balance

Under normal dietary conditions, humans generate acid at 70 to 100 mEq per day, equal to 1 mEq/kg of body weight per 24 hours. This acid load is buffered by both extracellular and intracellular buffers that include hemoglobin, protein, inorganic phosphate, organic phosphate, and the bicarbonic–carbonic acid buffer system. Organic phosphate represents the principal intracellular buffer, whereas the bicarbonic–carbonic acid buffer system constitutes the major extracellular buffer. Under normal circumstances, these buffers can accommodate approximately 15 mEq/kg of body weight of hydrogen ion without causing major shifts in systemic pH. *Acid–base disturbances are classified into one of four basic types: (a) metabolic acidosis, (b) metabolic alkalosis, (c) respiratory acidosis, and (d) respiratory alkalosis.* Irrespective of the primary cause of the acid–base abnormality, the body compensates by establishing an acid–base disturbance. Thus, in patients with metabolic acidosis, there is compensatory respiratory alkalosis, and in those with respiratory alkalosis, there is compensatory metabolic acidosis, and so on. The compensatory mechanisms are generally incomplete, so despite compensation, the pH generally remains on the side of the primary disturbance. Therefore, if the pH is below 7.38, the primary disorder is acidosis; if above 7.42, the primary disorder is alkalosis. The $Paco_2$ distinguishes between respiratory and metabolic. A patient with a pH of 7.44 and a Pco_2 of 48 would have a primary alkalosis, which would be metabolic in view of the elevated Pco_2. The disturbance is a primary metabolic alkalosis with a secondary compensatory respiratory acidosis. The lungs are the primary mediator of the respiratory compensation and the kidneys the mediator of metabolic compensation. Clinically, the four types of acid–base disturbances are not classified as pure and are generally compensated as described. For illustrative purposes, however, each is discussed individually.

Metabolic Acidosis

Metabolic acidosis may be caused by a decreased extracellular bicarbonate concentration or may be a consequence of an increased extracellular volume without a proportional increase in bicarbonate content. The latter explains the acidosis of dilutional hyponatremia and water intoxication. A shift in hydrogen ion from the cell to the extracellular fluid compartment and net loss of body bicarbonate account for the acidosis. Decreased extracellular bicarbonate concentration may be caused by either a decrease in renal bicarbonate reclamation or by the consumption of serum bicarbonate resulting from an excessive acid load to the systemic circulation. In the former, the acidosis develops slowly, whereas in the latter it has an acute onset. Decreased generation of bicarbonate by the kidney occurs in uremic acidosis, renal tubular acidosis, and aldosterone deficiency. An increased production of metabolic acid may occur because of increased protein intake or an increased rate of tissue catabolism; increased production of endogenous organic acids, such as lactic acid (shock) and ketoacids (diabetes); the administration of exogenous acids, such as ammonium chloride; and finally, extrarenal losses, such as gastrointestinal losses of bicarbonate in patients with diarrhea or an ileostomy.

Excessive drug ingestion (salicylate intoxication) also may cause an acidosis. The effects of an acute acidosis include dilation of arterioles, impairment of cardiac contractility, and systemic venous constriction, whereas chronic acidosis results in depletion of bone alkaline stores caused by the buffering capacity of the bone. The bone generally buffers 30 to 40 mEq of acid per day in chronic acidotic states. The differential between a renal or extrarenal cause can conveniently be made by checking the urinary pH. If the acidosis is caused by exogenous or nonrenal mechanisms, the urinary pH is acidic. Conversely, if the mechanism is caused by a lack of bicarbonate generation and reclamation, the urinary pH is persistently alkaline.

Metabolic Alkalosis

When metabolic alkalosis occurs, there is a net addition or increase in extracellular bicarbonate concentration. Because the kidney has a great capacity to excrete bicarbonate, two conditions must be met for metabolic alkalosis to occur. First, there must be a mechanism for increasing extracellular bicarbonate concentration, and second, there must be a mechanism to prevent the kidney from excreting the excess bicarbonate. This may occur as a result of increased loss of hydrochloric acid from the stomach after vomiting or nasogastric tube drainage; increased loss of hydrochloric acid in the stool of patients who have a defect in chloride reabsorption in the ileum and colon (congenital chloridorrhea); potassium depletion, which results in a shift of hydrogen ion into the cell; contraction of the extracellular volume without a proportional decrease in bicarbonate content; an increased renal production of bicarbonate resulting from the use of a diuretic; respiratory acidosis; primary hyperaldosteronism; and hypoparathyroidism. Excessive ingestion of alkali, such as the milk alkali syndrome, also may be causative.

Respiratory Alkalosis

Hyperventilation results in respiratory alkalosis and is always caused by stimulation of the respiratory center. This may be the result of hypoxia, drugs, toxins, CNS disorders, or psychogenic causes, or hyperventilation may occur as a compensatory mechanism for metabolic acidosis. When primary, sepsis always must be suspected.

Respiratory Acidosis

Respiratory acidosis results from hypoventilation and may be caused by depression of the respiratory center from CNS disease, drugs, defects in nerves and muscles of the respiratory center as a result of disease or injury, thoracic cage disorders, airway obstruction, or chronic pulmonary disease.

FLUID AND ELECTROLYTE ABNORMALITIES ASSOCIATED WITH GENITOURINARY IRRIGANTS

Water Intoxication

Water intoxication in urologic practice is generally a result of excessive nonelectrolyte irrigant absorption during endoscopic or endourologic procedures. As the nonelectrolyte fluid is absorbed, volume expansion and dilutional hyponatremia occur. The clinical manifestations of this syndrome (TUR syndrome) were first described in 1946 after a transurethral resection (TUR) of the prostate in which the patient was noted to become restless. There was dark red discoloration of the serum, progressive oliguria, azotemia, and pulmonary edema, followed by death. The development of the syndrome was associated with an 18.5% mortality (20). As more experience has been gained with TURs, this syndrome has become better defined. After substantial volume expansion with resultant hyponatremia, patients generally complain of nausea, become mentally confused or restless, and have sensory disturbances; if allowed to progress, blindness, convulsions, hypotension, coma, oliguria, and death supervene.

During a TUR, some fluid is invariably absorbed; however, the amount is usually insufficient to cause the clinical manifestations of water intoxication. The amount of fluid absorbed is directly related to (a) the pressure of the irrigant, which is a function of the height the bag is placed above the prostatic fossa; (b) the intravesical pressure; (c) the intraprostatic pressure; and (d) the CVP. The duration of the resection, the size of the gland, the quality of resection, and the type of resection equipment used also play a role. Blood loss, like volume absorption, has been correlated with the time of resection. As a rule, 20 mL per minute of fluid are absorbed and 2 mL per minute of blood are lost during resection. A continuous-flow resectoscope is more likely to produce significant water intoxication than the inflow–outflow method. Perhaps most important is the quality of resection because frequent capsular penetration and entrance into venous sinuses predispose the patient to the development of water intoxication. The first sign that should arouse suspicion is an increase in CVP or left atrial pressure (Swan-Ganz). A change in blood pressure is generally not an early sign and in fact may not be noted, even when the syndrome is severe enough to cause blindness.

The pathophysiology of the TUR syndrome has been reasonably well elaborated. After nonelectrolyte irrigant absorption, serum sodium and chloride fall as volume overload occurs. Tachypnea, hypertension, and subsequent bradycardia resulting from the carotid reflex may occur. As electrolyte changes occur from dilution, cardiac output falls, plasma volume is variable, and body weight increases. As the extracellular osmolality decreases, cerebral edema occurs, causing confusion, seizures, and blindness. Pulmonary edema also may occur with hypoxemia, cyanosis, and acidosis, and alteration of the clotting factors may occur with hemorrhage, hemolysis, anemia, and shock. Patients at increased risk for development of this syndrome are those who have cardiac disease and have been on a low-salt diet with diuretic supplementation and patients with hydronephrosis, salt-losing nephritis, urinary retention, or chronic illness and malnutrition.

Treatment of Water Intoxication Syndrome

Patients who are symptomatic and manifest severe neurologic abnormalities require rapid correction of their electrolyte status. This may be accomplished by the simultaneous administration of a potent diuretic, such as furosemide, with the restoration of serum sodium content by the infusion of hypertonic saline solution. The sodium deficit is calculated by subtracting the current serum sodium from the desired serum concentration and multiplying the value by the quantity 0.2 × body weight in kilograms (extracellular fluid volume). This gives the milliequivalent amount required to return the serum sodium to the desired value. Half of this amount is administered rapidly, after which a second serum sodium concentration is obtained and the therapy modified accordingly. If the patient has neurologic symptoms or signs, 3% sodium chloride is used. On the other hand, if neurologic abnormalities are absent, normal saline may be used. The volume is determined by the number of milliequivalents calculated. For example, an 80-kg man whose serum sodium is 110 mEq/L would require 400 mEq to return serum sodium to 135 mEq/L. Half, or 200 mEq (about 400 mL of 3% sodium chloride), would be given rapidly, monitoring the neurologic, pulmonary, and cardiac status. The remainder would be given as needed, depending on a repeated serum measurement and clinical status. For patients who are less symptomatic and have a less severe hyponatremia, the administration of a potent diuretic and the infusion of normal saline solution may suffice.

Other Problems with Irrigants

If the area of instrumentation is infected, the irrigant may carry bacteria with it, resulting in bacteremia occasionally followed by sepsis. Other electrolyte abnormalities depend on the specific irrigant used. Currently, five types of isotonic fluids are in general use: sorbitol, 3.3%; glucose, 5.4%; glycine, 1.5%; mannitol, 3.0%; and urea, 1.8%. Water is also used; however, it is not isotonic.

Water

Because water is not isotonic, it can result in significant hemolysis of red blood cells when it enters the systemic circulation. This hemolysis results in an increased level of serum potassium and, during a typical TUR, elevated serum levels of free hemoglobin. However, it has been shown that hemoglobin is not toxic in levels up to 600 mg, provided it is not combined with abnormal serum proteins. In the latter case, it may in fact be nephrotoxic.

Sorbitol (3.3%)

Sorbitol is metabolized completely either to carbon dioxide and water or to dextrose. It also may be excreted by the kidneys. The use of this solution may result in an elevated level of serum glucose, which may be particularly severe in noncompensated diabetic patients. The same propensity to water intoxication occurs with this fluid as with any other urologic nonelectrolyte irrigant fluid. Rarely, sorbitol may result in an osmotic diuresis with dehydration and a hyperosmolar state. This solution should be used with caution in diabetic patients.

Glucose

Glucose solutions are no longer generally used because they are sticky and are not comfortably handled in the urologic suite. If used, however, they have the same complications as sorbitol.

Glycine (1.5%)

Ammonia intoxication has been reported after the use of glycine. Patients particularly prone to this complication are those with impaired hepatic function who presumably are unable to clear the ammonia generated from glycine metabolism. If the patient receives large doses of glycine, it may also cause salivation, nausea, and light-headedness.

Mannitol (5%)

The main side effect of mannitol is an osmotic diuresis that can result in dehydration and hyperosmolality. Occasionally, this solution may cause systemic acidosis.

Urea

Urea is no longer conventionally used because of its permeability to the intracellular and extracellular space. Its use results in elevated serum urea concentrations and also may cause an osmotic diuresis.

Volume Deficits

With significant loss of body fluids, dehydration, hyperosmolality, and neurologic disturbances occur. If allowed to persist, hypotension and death supervene. With a 4% loss of body weight caused by a water deficit, emergency rehydration is in order. These patients are generally symptomatic. A 6% loss of body weight caused by a water deficit results in shock and often death. Common urologic disorders that lead to dehydration include postobstructive diuresis, which results in a urine with a sodium content of 50 to 70 mEq/L and a potassium content of 10 to 40 mEq/L. These patients' urinary fluid losses may be replaced accurately with 0.5N saline solution. Prolonged vomiting or diarrhea also may result in significant dehydration. The former is replaced with 0.5N saline solution plus 40 mEq/L of potassium chloride if renal function is normal, and the latter is replaced with Ringer's lactate. Finally, diabetes insipidus may result in significant dehydration. This syndrome is discussed in detail in the section on polyuria. During replacement therapy and in the follow-up period, daily body weight, serum sodium, and serum osmolality are measured to determine the efficacy of therapy.

FLUID AND ELECTROLYTE ABNORMALITIES ASSOCIATED WITH URINARY INTESTINAL DIVERSION

Intestinal Conduits

The intestine's primary function is to selectively absorb electrolytes and nutrients. This function makes it less than an ideal structure as a urinary conduit or storage vehicle. Urine exposed to its surface is altered because some constituents are reabsorbed and others are diluted as a result of intestinal secretion. The extent to which the fluid is altered depends on the surface area to which it is exposed, the time of exposure, and the composition of the urine.

Electrolyte transport occurs throughout all segments of the bowel. In the jejunum, sodium absorption is coupled with glucose transport, whereas in the ileum and colon, sodium and chloride are actively absorbed. In these segments of bowel, there may be an exchange between sodium and hydrogen and chloride and bicarbonate. Thus with hydrogen absorption, sodium is secreted; with chloride absorption, bicarbonate is secreted. The movement of these ions depends on cyclic adenosine monophosphate (cAMP), and therefore blocking this enzyme alters transport properties (45). Metabolic disorders of intestinal urine transport are treated by choosing specific drugs that block this enzyme system. Water moves according to its concentration gradient; thus hyperosmotic urine results in the movement of water into the conduit from the systemic circulation. Hypoosmotic urine, on the other hand, may result in a net movement of water into the extracellular space. The flux of water is particularly prominent in the jejunum, less so in the ileum, and least in the colon. Metabolic abnormalities brought about by intestinal alteration of urine are often compensated for by the kidney's ability to increase and alter its excretion rates of unwanted solutes. Severe metabolic disturbances often manifest themselves only when renal function is compromised, particularly when the serum creatinine concentration exceeds 2 mg/dL.

Syndrome of Hyperchloremic Metabolic Acidosis

The ingestion of acetazolamide (or acid), diarrhea, and intestinal fistulae can cause hyperchloremic acidosis; however, the most common cause in urologic practice is intestinal interposition. *This syndrome occurs in patients who have ileum or colon interposed in the urinary tract; is most common in patients in whom the urine remains in contact with the intestinal mucosa for extended periods, particularly those with ureterosigmoidostomies; and is most severe with compromised renal function.* The acidosis usually does not manifest an anion gap; however, recent evidence suggests that an anion gap may occur rarely in those patients with rectal bladders, continent diversions, and other bowel substitutes in which the urine remains in contact with the intestinal mucosa for extended periods. This anion gap is most likely caused by an increased absorption of phosphate, sulfate, and ammonium, resulting in decreased total body elimination of these anions.

Four hypotheses have been proposed to explain the acidosis: (a) renal tubule acidification defect, (b) intestinal absorption of ammonium, (c) intestinal bicarbonate secretion, and (d) active intestinal chloride transport. A renal tubule acidification defect seemed likely because many of these patients had ascending pyelonephritis. Pyelonephritis affects the distal tubule, and it was proposed that this interfered with the kidneys' ability to acidify (55). It is clear that a distal tubule acidification defect will make the acidosis worse, but it is unlikely that it is the primary mechanism because many patients with normal renal function also manifest the acidosis (87).

The second hypothesis proposed that the urea excreted in the urine is split to ammonium by intestinal bacteria, thereby increasing ammonium absorption, which accounts for the acidosis (7,80). Because ammonia derived from urea is not an acid (when hydrated with water, it is a base), this mechanism does not explain proton addition (hydrogen ion) to the systemic circulation. It may be, however, that ammonia serves as a proton acceptor from acid secreted in the urine and then is actively reabsorbed. Data from our laboratory suggest that ammonium is transported and results in significant proton loads to the patient.

The third mechanism proposed is bicarbonate secretion by the intestine. Clearly, the ileum and large bowel are capable of significant bicarbonate losses because patients with ileostomies and those with severe diarrhea can lose enough bicarbonate to become acidotic. Several experiments also have demonstrated bicarbonate loss in measurable quantities in patients with ureterosigmoidostomies (21). However, the amount of bicarbonate lost to the body in most cases of intestinal interposition seems insufficient to explain the severity of the acidosis. Experimental evidence in animals suggests that this plays only a minor role in most cases (52).

The final mechanism proposed is that active chloride transport is the primary cause of the acidosis (31). The hypothesis is that chloride is actively transported and then requires a cation to preserve electrical neutrality to diffuse across the membrane. The cation may be either hydrogen or ammonium, whichever is most available. Thus in effect hydrochloric acid and/or ammonium chloride enter the systemic circulation in sufficient quantities to account for the acidosis. The evidence to support this hypothesis comes from experiments that showed that when ion fluxes are measured across the intestinal segment exposed to urine, net hydrogen uptake is directly proportional to chloride transport. Moreover, chlorpromazine (Thorazine) and niacin, two drugs known to block chloride transport through their effect on cAMP, limit this acidosis (50,51).

From intestinal vesicle experiments it appears that the primary mechanism for the acidosis is the transport of ammonium across the intestinal epithelium in exchange for a proton. Chloride is absorbed to maintain electrical neutrality in exchange for bicarbonate. The net effect is absorption of ammonium chloride in exchange for carbon dioxide and water (60).

Other electrolyte abnormalities associated with hyperchloremic metabolic acidosis include hypokalemia, hyperkalemia, hypocalcemia, hypomagnesemia, and hypersulfatemia. Hypokalemia may be severe because the chronic acidosis falsely elevates the serum potassium and therefore obscures the severity of the total body potassium deficiency. On correction of the acidosis, these patients often require considerable replacement of potassium to replenish body content. The intestinal loss of potassium can be reduced by the administration of spironolactone.

The mechanism of hypocalcemia and hypomagnesemia is not clear. It has been suggested that chronic acidosis results in depletion of bicarbonate stores in the skeleton with release and loss of calcium initially through the urinary tract. The hypocalcemia is merely a reflection of total body depletion. Reports of rickets and growth retardation in some of these patients (8) suggest that abnormal calcium metabolism may be clinically significant. Large losses of calcium in the urine with stimulation of calcium reabsorption by the tubule through the mechanism of parathormone would result in magnesium excretion by the binding of all available transport sites for calcium under maximum parathormone stimulation. Thus excessive magnesium loss through the urinary tract results in hypomagnesemia. Initial experiments in our laboratory suggest that the increased intestinal absorption of sulfate results in its blocking renal reabsorption of calcium and magnesium (62). Whatever the mechanism, it is clear that hypocalcemia and hypomagnesemia occur most commonly when renal function is significantly impaired. In patients with normal renal function, serum concentrations of these two ions are rarely more than slightly depressed.

Urea and creatinine also are reabsorbed by the bowel and may result in elevated serum levels that do not accurately reflect renal function. Because transport properties vary somewhat for various portions of the bowel, electrolyte abnormalities specific for each segment are described subsequently.

Jejunum

The jejunum is seldom used for intestinal diversion because of the severe fluid and electrolyte abnormalities that occur when it is used as a conduit or storage vehicle for urine. *These segments lose large quantities of sodium chloride and absorb significant amounts of potassium and urea.* With the extensive sodium and chloride loss into the lumen of the intestine, the osmotic gradient this creates necessitates the movement of water from the systemic circulation into the lumen of the intestine. This results in substantial fluid losses to the body. Some hydrogen absorption and bicarbonate loss also may occur. These patients become hyponatremic, hypochloremic, hypovolemic, hyperkalemic, and azotemic. They also may have a mild acidosis and an associated serum hyperosmolality (13,46). In response to these abnormalities, there is an increased secretion of aldosterone and renin, thus further reducing urine sodium concentration and thereby increasing the concentration gradient of sodium between serum and lumen, enhancing secretion by the jejunum. When short segments are employed for conduits and drainage is unimpeded, recent reports suggest that severe electrolyte abnormalities occur in fewer than 10% of patients (33).

Ileum

The ileum is perhaps the most commonly employed segment for urinary diversion. *Chloride is absorbed and bicarbonate secreted and ammonium absorbed in exchange for hydrogen ion by this segment.* Although rarely a clinical problem, these patients may develop hypokalemia associated with the hyperchloremic metabolic acidosis (19). The metabolic abnormality is more common in patients with compromised renal function. Although water does move into the conduit if urine flowing through it is hypertonic, because the ileum does not secrete large amounts of osmotically active agents such as sodium and chloride, the amount of fluid lost is not as extensive as for the jejunum.

Colon

The colon also transports chloride in exchange for bicarbonate, so patients with colon segments are prone to develop hyperchloremic metabolic acidosis. These patients are more likely to become hypokalemic, hypomagnesemic, and hypocalcemic than patients with ileal segments. However, they are less likely to become hypovolemic because fluid fluxes are less prominent in the colon than in ileal or jejunal segments. Indeed, patients with colon conduits can actually concentrate to about 400 mOsm/kg, as opposed to ileal segments in which the gradient generally does not exceed 350 mOsm/kg(61).

Treatment

The treatment of hyponatremic, hypochloremic, hyperkalemic, metabolic acidosis found in jejunal segment patients consists of oral sodium chloride, bicarbonate, and fluids. When severe, IV administration of saline solution in large volumes and the establishment of a diuresis correct both the hyponatremia and hyperkalemia, as well as the hypovolemia.

Hyperchloremic metabolic acidosis is treated by oral chloride restriction, bicarbonate replacement (either in the form of sodium bicarbonate or Polycitra), and drainage of the area of storage. In patients with a Koch pouch, rectal bladder, or ureterosigmoidostomy, this requires catheterization of the segment. Studies have shown that chlorpromazine and niacin may be effective. These drugs block active chloride transport in the intestine, thereby limiting the acidosis. This has been demonstrated in experimental animals and in patients (50). The advantage to these drugs is that a sodium or potassium load is not given as when bicarbonate or Polycitra is used. This may be particularly useful in patients who have congestive heart failure or those with severely compromised renal function in whom an excessive sodium or potassium load would be inappropriate. High dosages and prolonged use of chlorpromazine may result in the development of extrapyramidal symptoms including tardive dyskinesia. The side effects of niacin are usually minimal but may consist of agitation and flushing. Because of the CNS effects of chlorpromazine, we prefer to use niacin in children and chlorpromazine in adults.

BOWEL PREPARATION

Urologic operations in which bowel is used as a conduit or storage vehicle for urine are invariably elective; therefore

TABLE 10.7. MECHANICAL BOWEL PREPARATION

	Conventional		PEG + Electrolytes	
Preoperative Day	**Diet**	**Cathartic**	**Diet**	**PEG**
3	Low-residue plus supplements		Regular plus supplements	—
2	Clear liquids		Low-residue plus supplements	—
1	Clear liquids	30–60 mL Fleets Phospho-Soda	Clear liquids	2–4 L PEG + electrolytes

PEG, polyethylene glycol.

proper preparation of the bowel may be planned preoperatively. The major risks involved in operating on the bowel include wound infection, anastomotic breakdown, and peritoneal infections. *In unprepared bowel, the wound infection rate varies between 32% and 58%. This incidence may be reduced to 6% to 9% if mechanical and antibiotic bowel preparation are used* (14). Breakdown of the intestinal anastomosis is more common when performed on unprepared bowel. Antibiotics appear to have a protective effect on the anastomosis, particularly if the blood supply is compromised. In experimental animals, an unprepared bowel that is devascularized results in perforation and death, whereas an antibiotically prepared bowel that is devascularized heals. In a clinical study comparing colon anastomoses in prepared and unprepared bowel, the total number of complications and the number of anastomotic breakdowns were increased in the unprepared group. In this study, if the patients were steroid dependent, had peritonitis, received prior irradiation, or had diabetes mellitus or chronic renal failure, the chance of anastomotic breakdown was significantly increased (3). Finally, intraperitoneal abscesses are more common when unprepared bowel is operated on.

In mechanical preparation of the bowel, the enteric content is reduced, and in antibiotic preparation, the bacterial organisms are reduced. The mechanical bowel preparation reduces the amount of bacteria but not the number of bacteria per milliliter of feces. Spillage of enteric contents is less likely because there is less of it to spill; however, with a spill, the inoculum is the same as if the spill occurred in unprepared bowel. More recent evidence indicates that excessive mechanical bowel preparations are unnecessary. Two to four liters of polyethyleneglycol may be given orally the day before surgery, or 2 days before surgery, clear liquids are begun and 30 to 60 mL Phospho-Soda is given orally. On the day before the operation, 30 mL of Phospho-Soda is given (Table 10.7).

The mechanical preparation reduces the amount of enteric contents, not the number of bacteria in a single inoculum. Therefore the mechanical bowel preparation is supplemented with an antibiotic bowel preparation (Table 10.8). The risk of wound infection and other infectious complications is reduced from 30% to 6% when antibiotics are combined with the mechanical preparation. Antibiotics also protect vulnerable and ischemic bowel. The disadvantage to giving antibiotics in preparation for bowel surgery is that it increases the incidence of tumor implantation on the anastomosis, and it might play a role in the development of pseudomembranous enterocolitis (15). The former is generally of little consequence to the urologist; however, the latter can be a significantly morbid and sometimes fatal complication. It seems unlikely, however, that antibiotics are solely responsible for the development of the latter syndrome because there has been no change in its incidence in the preantibiotic and postantibiotic eras. It was originally

TABLE 10.8. ANTIBIOTIC BOWEL PREPARATION

Preoperative Day	Kanamycin	Neomycin + Erythromycin	Neomycin + Metronidazole	Tinidazole + Doxycycline
3	1 g kanamycin p.o. q.h. × 4, then q.i.d.	—	—	—
2	1 g kanamycin p.o. q.i.d.	—	1 g neomycin q.i.d. + 750 mg metronidazole q.i.d.	—
1	1 g kanamycin p.o. q.i.d.	1 g erythromycin + 1 g neomycin at 1, 2, and 11 PM	1 g neomycin q.i.d. + 750 mg metronidazole q.i.d.	2 hr preoperatively: 1,600 mg tinidazole + 400 mg doxycycline infused IV over 2 hr

thought to be caused by a staphylococci but recently, *Clostridium difficile* and the endotoxin that it elaborates have been implicated. The most important factor in its initiation is intestinal ischemia. Other risk factors include bowel preparation, nasogastric tubes, gastrointestinal surgery, narcotics, advanced age, cancer chemotherapy, and renal disorders. The diagnosis is made by identifying the cytopathic toxin of *C. difficile* in the stool. Treatment is directed at repopulating the bowel surface with normal enteric flora and the administration of antibiotics to which the organism is sensitive: vancomycin, aminoglycosides, metronidazole, and ciprofloxacin.

SHOCK

An all-encompassing definition of shock is impairment of cellular function caused by either a reduction in effective delivery of oxygen and nutrients to the cell or inability of the cell to use these substrates. Shock may be classified as hypovolemic, neurogenic, endocrine, anaphylactic, cardiogenic, and septic.

Hypovolemic Shock

When loss of blood, loss of fluid, or sequestration of fluid is etiologic, cardiac output and blood pressure fall while plasma renin and ADH levels rise. The sympathetic nervous system is stimulated, which results in the constriction of arterioles and major veins, an increase in heart rate and strength of contraction, a reduction in microcirculatory flow and sludging, and mobilization of glucose for energy production. If hypotension and peripheral vasoconstriction continue, a decrease in transmembrane potential occurs, membrane permeability increases, and fluid is sequestered, particularly in muscle cells. If the perfusion defect continues, cellular death supervenes.

Hypovolemic shock is generally divided into three phases. The first phase occurs with volume deficits between 0% and 10% and begins with a sequestration of fluid resulting in cellular edema. During this phase, the blood volume deficit is counteracted by stimulation of the sympathetic nervous system, which results in peripheral vasoconstriction and increased heart rate in an attempt to maintain blood pressure. ADH, renin, and aldosterone also contribute to the vasoconstriction and reduced urinary excretion in an attempt to restore extracellular fluid volume. The second stage occurs with a blood volume deficit of 15% to 20%. Cardiac output and arterial pressure are significantly reduced, despite the compensatory mechanisms previously described. The low blood pressure and the intense adrenergic discharge result in tachycardia, tachypnea, cutaneous vasoconstriction, pallor, diaphoresis, piloerection, apprehension, and restlessness. The third stage occurs when the deficit exceeds 25%. During this stage, tissue perfusion is inadequate, and if it persists for long periods, cellular death occurs. Vital organ function is severely impaired, capillary membrane integrity is lost, and disseminated intravascular coagulation may occur. It is at this point that irreversible shock follows.

Treatment

Hypovolemic shock caused by third-space fluid loss, as occurs in burns and retroperitoneal dissections, is treated with isotonic fluid replacement. Many advocate partial replacement with 5% albumin, suggesting that the total fluid requirement is less with a smaller amount extravasating into the third space and pulmonary interstitium. Other studies suggest that crystalloid is more likely to produce pulmonary edema than solutions of 5% albumin, hetastarch, or dextran. Others disagree, stating that colloid is unnecessary and that only crystalloid should be used in the initial phases of resuscitation. *When blood loss is the cause, whole blood is administered, which is appropriately typed and crossmatched.* Dextran may be used as a blood substitute for volume expansion; however, it carries the risk of creating clotting abnormalities through antigen–antibody reactions. Prolonged use of dextran also may engender renal failure. Hetastarch is a polysaccharide that is available in a 6% solution. It has replaced dextran as the drug of choice for volume expansion when blood and albumin are unavailable because renal and bleeding complications are less common. If after adequate volume resuscitation cardiac output is insufficient, ionotrophes and vasoconstrictors may be in order (see Cardiogenic Shock).

Attention also must be paid to the patient's ventilatory status. Hypoventilation with hypoxemia severely augments the deleterious effects of underperfusion.

In the successfully treated patient, there are three phases of fluid dynamics. The first phase follows the insult and is characterized by sequestration of fluid and cellular edema. This accounts for the major initial pathophysiologic problems encountered in hypovolemic shock. The sequestration generally ceases between 24 and 36 hours, provided the patient has been adequately resuscitated. In the ensuing 2 to 3 days, a homeostatic period occurs in which the sequestered fluid remains unavailable to the intravascular space. At approximately 4 to 7 days after the insult, the third phase is initiated in which the fluid is mobilized. It is during this phase that patients with limited cardiac reserve may develop congestive heart failure as the fluid is mobilized from the third space into the intravascular space. The judicious use of diuretics may be necessary to rapidly restore intravascular volume to normal.

Neurogenic, Endocrine, and Anaphylactic Shock

Neurogenic shock results from a sudden loss of vasomotor tone caused by a neural injury. This commonly occurs in traumatic injuries to the CNS.

Endocrine deficiencies resulting from a lack of function of the adrenal glands or pituitary result in circulatory failure. Uncontrollable diabetes may result in an osmotic diuresis with resultant hypotension.

Anaphylactic shock is the result of an acute systemic autoimmune reaction that causes a marked increase in vascular permeability with sequestration of edema fluid, bronchospasm, and laryngospasm. This sequestered fluid leaves the intravascular space, resulting in hypotension. Of patients who develop intraoperative anaphylaxis, 5% to 10% die (90). Agents that have been implicated in triggering the response include neuromuscular blocking agents, IV anesthetics, antibiotics, radiocontrast, blood products, protamine, and latex. Latex allergy may result in an anaphylactic-like reaction with symptoms as mild as nausea and flushing to angioedema, bronchospasm, and cardiovascular collapse. Three groups of patients appear to be at high risk: (a) myelodysplastic patients, (b) those with congenital urologic abnormalities, and (c) health care workers. In high-risk patients, consideration should be given to prophylactic administration of prednisone, diphenhydramine, and ranitidine (47).

Treatment

Neurogenic shock is treated with isotonic fluid administration until blood pressure returns to normal levels. Patients with adrenal insufficiency or pituitary insufficiency are treated with replacement corticosteroids and fluids that contain sodium. Anaphylactic shock is treated with epinephrine, fluids, antihistamines, and corticosteroids.

Cardiogenic Shock

Cardiogenic shock occurs when the heart fails to act effectively as a pump. This may be brought about by a myocardial infarction, cardiac arrhythmia, or depression of myocardial contractility resulting from a metabolic aberration. Rare causes include mechanical blockage that may occur in a tension pneumothorax, vena caval obstruction, and cardiac tamponade. The most common cause of the disorder is clearly myocardial infarction. Approximately 10% to 15% of patients with an acute myocardial infarction will develop cardiogenic shock. Mortality in this group is exceedingly high, approaching 75% (38). These patients present with cold, clammy skin; hypotension; tachycardia; anuria; and oliguria and are often confused and agitated. The pathophysiologic process includes a decreased cardiac output, decreased ejection fraction, normal or increased CVP, increased pulmonary capillary wedge pressure, and increased left ventricular end-diastolic pressure.

Treatment

Because hypotension results in decreased coronary artery perfusion with a propensity toward limiting the amount of oxygen delivered, one of the first hallmarks of therapy is to provide the patient with oxygen. Decreased oxygenation of the injured myocardium will result in progression of the infarction. Oxygen is administered by face mask, nasal prongs, or rebreathing bag. Patients with chronic pulmonary disease need to be monitored carefully if their respiratory drive is secondary to hypercapnia. These patients may require intubation. It is during the initial postmyocardial infarction period that life-threatening cardiac arrhythmias often occur. Therefore these patients need to be continuously monitored, and a large-bore IV line must be available to administer antiarrhythmogenic drugs. Often, these patients have a slight metabolic acidosis, which must be corrected with bicarbonate administration. The placement of a pulmonary artery catheter is generally indicated because the diagnosis can be conveniently made using this device, and treatment is often dictated by measurements performed. With the pulmonary artery catheter, cardiac output, preload, and afterload can be determined and will verify the diagnosis by revealing a decreased cardiac output. Preload is determined by pulmonary capillary wedge pressure measurement and afterload by peripheral resistance calculation. When the peripheral resistance is normal, an agent is chosen that will improve the cardiac output by increasing myocardial contractility. Dobutamine or isoproterenol is the drug of choice. When there is an increase in peripheral resistance, therapy is directed at increasing cardiac output and decreasing afterload. The afterload may be reduced with nitroprusside, and cardiac output can be increased with either dobutamine or isoproterenol. The dosage of nitroprusside must be monitored carefully because it may result in thiocyanate intoxication. When peripheral resistance and cardiac performance are decreased, the use of vasopressors, such as dopamine and epinephrine, is useful (44).

Septic Shock

Septic shock, unlike hypovolemic shock, does not necessarily result in a perfusion deficit to the tissues. Rather, it results in an inability of the body cell mass to effectively use substrate delivered to it. Septic shock is an important cause of morbidity and mortality among hospitalized patients. Approximately 25% to 40% of patients who sustain a bacteremia develop septic shock (72). In most cases, it originates from an infection with Gram-negative enteric bacilli. *Escherichia coli* is the most common pathogen followed by *Klebsiella, Enterobacter, Serratia,* and *Pseudomonas* species. Gram-positive organisms occasionally cause sepsis, and rarely, viruses, fungi, rickettsia, and protozoa, have been implicated. The genitourinary tract is the most common source, followed, in decreasing order of frequency, by the gastrointestinal tract, the respiratory tract, wound infections, infected IV catheters, and pelvic infections. Urosepsis in the critical care setting carries with it a 25% mortality (71). Patients at increased risk for the development of septic shock include those who have cirrhosis, diabetes mellitus, and neoplastic diseases (67). Radiotherapy and/or chemotherapy particularly predispose the latter group of patients to sepsis. Mortality ranges between 40% and 90%.

Endotoxin, a lipopolysaccharide protein complex, which is part of the cell wall of Gram-negative bacteria, has been implicated as the initiating agent in the pathophysiologic process. Because other than Gram-negative organisms also cause the syndrome, it is clear that if endotoxin is an initiating agent, it is not the only one. The infecting organism activates proinflammatory cytokines. Prominent among these cytokines are tumor necrosis factor-α, interleukin-1 and interleukin-6, among others (10). Other cytokines that have been implicated include interleukin-6 and interleukin-8, a platelet-activating factor, interferon-γ, macrophage-derived proteins, and arachidonic acid metabolites. As a result of the production of these substances and the presence of bacteria, many biochemical and immunologic pathways are activated. The complement, kinin, and clotting systems are stimulated and activation of polymorphonuclear leukocytes occurs, and the release of the β-endorphin histamine and prostaglandins is facilitated.

There are two phases of septic shock: the hyperdynamic and the hypodynamic. In the first phase, patients are hypotensive and have warm, dry skin. Arterial vasodilation, an increase in body temperature, hyperventilation with respiratory alkalosis, and an increase in pulse pressure and cardiac output occur. Although the absolute value of cardiac output in patients with septic shock is generally increased, it cannot achieve adequate perfusion of essential organs. These events may be heralded by a shaking chill, which is followed by a rapid rise in temperature. Lactic acidosis may supervene, indicating the cell's inability to utilize or obtain oxygen and substrate. However, the degree of lactic acidemia does not correlate with the lack of oxygenation in septic shock, nor is it of any prognostic significance (79). The vasoactive kinins, histamine, and prostaglandins result in vasodilation and perhaps some vasoconstriction in various vascular beds. β-Endorphin produces cardiovascular depression, vasodilation, capillary leakage, and hypotension (43).

As sepsis continues, myocardial depression occurs, with a reduced ejection fraction and left ventricular dilation. The activation of the kinin system results in the release of bradykinin, an agent known to produce vasodilation of arterioles. Activation of the complement system results in depletion of the C3 and C5 components (72). The white blood cell count is elevated with a shift to the left; rarely, however, sepsis may result in a depressed count—a poor prognostic sign. Blood glucose is elevated as a result of the increased levels of glucagon, growth hormone, and catecholamines. Progression of the disease leads to leukocyte aggregation with development of disseminated intravascular coagulation, vascular endothelial damage producing capillary leak with interstitial edema, and depression of myocardial function. Platelet aggregation results in the release of vasoactive substances. Pulmonary platelet aggregation has been suggested as the initiating event in the adult respiratory distress syndrome (ARDS). Myocardial depression increases capillary permeability, and impaired cellular function leads to the second phase of septic shock, a hypodynamic state in which unresponsive hypotension and death occur.

Treatment

Treatment is directed at supporting the patient and defining the source of infection so that it can be eliminated. *Initially, blood, urine, sputum, and wound drainage, if present, are sent for culture. IV administration of bactericidal antibiotics is begun immediately.* The choice of antibiotics is dictated by the suspected source of the sepsis. An aminoglycoside at full dosage is administered initially. Dosage level subsequently is adjusted to the renal function. If an intraabdominal source is suspected, anaerobic coverage is added: clindamycin, chloramphenicol, or metronidazole. If a pulmonary source seems likely, a cephalosporin is added; if the urinary tract is suspect, ampicillin is given. *Blood pressure is supported with crystalloid and/or colloid infusions, the rate dictated by the blood pressure, CVP or right atrial filling pressure, and urine output. Crystalloid resuscitation is begun, but if it is inadequate to return filling pressure to normal, colloid is added.* It has been suggested that colloid infusion results in less capillary leakage with less subsequent interstitial edema formation. Corticosteroid administration is generally not recommended, except for specific circumstances of adrenal insufficiency. Recent studies show no benefit to their administration (73,81). Indeed, their administration may even be harmful.

The use of antiendotoxin antibodies has improved survival in some studies. Gram-negative bacilli share a common core lipopolysaccharide. In a series in which antiserum to this antigen from human volunteers was given to septic patients, mortality was reduced by 50% (97). Most subsequent studies have not confirmed these findings (81). In select cases, continuous intraperitoneal lavage also may be helpful. This therapy is particularly amenable to patients who are septic as a result of pelvic inflammation and abscesses. Dialysis catheters placed into the depths of the pelvis and irrigated with saline and antibiotic solutions are particularly helpful in these patients (69).

If hypotension occurs after adequate fluid resuscitation or if it persists, blood pressure may be supported with dopamine. In addition to its inotropic effect, the advantage of dopamine over other agents is that it increases renal blood flow. However, dopamine increases intrapulmonary shunting; therefore dobutamine may be preferable in patients with pulmonary complications. Although dobutamine does support blood pressure, it does not improve renal blood flow. In dopamine-resistant situations, norepinephrine (Levarterenol) may be particularly effective because of both its α- and β-effects. However, neonates and young children have a diminished response to both dobutamine and dopamine and therefore epinephrine is more useful in the immediate resuscitative period (10). β-Endorphins released in response to the stress of shock may be partially responsible for the hypotension. It is clear that pituitary endorphins play a role in the pathophysiology of shock, but their exact role is somewhat controversial. The cardiodepressant effect of endorphins is mediated by opiate receptors in the CNS (29). Naloxone, an inhibitor of β-endorphin binding, may result in significant improvement in the blood pressure and reversal of myocardial depression (75). Others have found that naloxone administration is not associated with an improvement in blood pressure or survival (24). Thyrotropin-releasing hormone also has been used effectively in patients with persistent hypotension. This drug apparently acts centrally, as does naloxone, and like naloxone, it requires an intact sympathoadrenal-medullary axis to be effective. Thyrotropin-releasing hormone and naloxone have an additive effect (24). The prostaglandins PGI and thromboxane A_2 may mediate some of the cardiovascular changes in shock but are not solely responsible for myocardial depression (11). They contribute locally to vasodilation, and it has been found experimentally that blocking the vasoconstrictor thromboxane A_2 in animals improves survival (17).

Antitumor necrosis factor antibodies, anti–interleukin-1 antibodies, and other inhibitors of cytokines have been used with mixed results. Some of the cytokines appear to be protective and thus indiscriminate blockade can be detrimental (81). Other forms of therapy directed at specific pathophysiologic mechanisms such as antiendothelium–leukocyte adhesion antibodies have been developed and may have promise. At this time their clinical role is undefined.

When afterload or ventricular wall tension is increased, cardiac output may be limited. Afterload can be reduced by selective use of vasodilators. Phentolamine (Regitine), an α-blocker, dilates both veins and arteries. It is particularly useful in patients with increased sympathetic tone. Nitroprusside is a short-acting vasodilator whose predominant effect is on the smooth muscle of the arteries. It is an excellent agent for titrating blood pressure in the short-term situation. Nitroglycerin is particularly useful in patients with an associated ischemic myocardium because it improves collateral flow to the heart while dilating the peripheral vasculature.

Sinus rhythm is the most effective rhythm for optimum cardiac output. When supraventricular and ventricular arrhythmias occur in association with a diminished cardiac output, restoration of normal sinus rhythm may be all that is required.

VENOUS THROMBOEMBOLISM

Pelvic operations have a high propensity for thromboembolic disease. Its prevention in the urologic patient is of particular importance because many operations are performed in the pelvic area. Urologic patients are often placed in lithotomy position, which impairs venous return. Because most thrombi develop in venous plexus along the calf and usually begin during the operation, it is easy to appreciate the significance of impaired venous return that is promoted by positioning.

Risk factors that increase the likelihood of thromboembolic disease may be grouped into three categories: stasis, intimal injury, and hypercoagulability. Stasis includes immobility, congestive heart failure, obesity, and varicose veins. Intimal injury is manifested in vascular disease, previous thrombosis, trauma, and surgery. Hypercoagulable states are associated with advanced age, postoperative state, malignancy, and myocardial infarction.

The prevention of thromboembolic disease has been a subject of considerable controversy. Elevation of the foot of the bed, avoidance of extremity compression, early ambulation, physical therapy, and leg wraps all have been used in an effort to prevent the sequelae of thromboembolic disease. Unfortunately, none of these devices has been shown to be of particular efficacy in the prevention of the disorder. More recently, the development of an alternating pressure cuff on the lower extremities, which facilitates venous return, has been shown to be effective (82). Intermittent compression boots have undergone many modifications, the most recent of which is asymmetric compression rather than circumferential, with the intention of being more effective prophylaxis (which is unproven). The role of excellent nursing care is emphasized when one considers the improvement in venous flow as a function of the various methods advocated. Moving the legs is as effective in promoting venous return as any of the aforementioned methods.

In several studies, the use of mini-dose heparin, that is, 5,000 units administered subcutaneously every 12 hours, has been suggested to decrease the incidence of pulmonary emboli. One study found a substantial reduction in pulmonary emboli as diagnosed by routine postoperative scans (54). Other studies have failed to show any significant difference with and without the use of mini-dose heparin. It is clear, however, that in patients undergoing pelvic lymphadenectomy, administration of preoperative and postoperative mini-dose heparin results in a greatly increased incidence of lymphocele formation (53). Therefore, in urologic practice, prophylactic mini-dose heparinization in the preoperative and postoperative periods has not been successful; consequently, it rarely has been used. Low-dose warfarin therapy also has been used for prophylaxis of deep venous thrombosis. In one study, it was as effective as alternate compression stockings; complications were minimal (34).

Pulmonary emboli may occur silently and be an incidental finding on a chest roentgenogram, or they may suggest their presence by causing dyspnea; chest pain; hemoptysis; and rarely, when massive, circulatory collapse. On physical examination, the pulmonic portion of the second heart sound may be increased, a parasternal heave may occur, on occasion a friction rub can be heard, and the ECG often shows right-sided heart strain as evidenced by right-axis deviation. The chest radiograph, when positive, reveals a lucent area that lacks vascular markings. Later a wedge-shaped infiltrate develops. Pulmonary scans may be used to support the diagnosis, but the definitive study is a pulmonary angiogram or magnetic resonance angiogram (MRA). Therapy is directed at identifying the source and treating it while administering anticoagulants to the patient, initially with a continuous heparin infusion. If the pulmonary embolus is large or saddle-type and is causing circulatory collapse that is unresponsive to supportive measures, a pulmonary embolectomy is indicated. In select circumstances, the use of thrombolytic therapy is most effective in dissolving emboli. Urokinase, streptokinase, and recombinant tissue plasminogen activator (rtPA) have all been used. Although rtPA results in a more rapid thrombolysis than the other two drugs, it has not shown increased efficacy, because at 24 hours, the resolution is similar no matter what agent is used (43). It should be noted, however, that in postoperative patients, vascular suture lines and puncture sites are likely to bleed with the use of these drugs. Because thrombolytic therapy increases the risk of hemorrhage without significantly affecting long-term outcome, it is useful in very limited circumstances, such as in nonoperative patients with renal artery emboli or massive pulmonary emboli.

Patients who have had a pulmonary embolus documented by one of the aforementioned studies or those in whom the clinical suspicion is high should be treated preferably by anticoagulation. Patients who have pulmonary emboli and are not treated have a 50% chance of another embolus—half of whom die from the event (48). Thus treatment should be instituted without delay. Heparin is the initial drug of choice. Low-molecular-weight heparin is as safe and effective as unfractionated heparin in preventing pulmonary emboli (23). The advantage of the former is that it can be given twice daily subcutaneously (57). The activated partial thromboplastin time (aPTT) should be kept between 2.0 and 3.0 times control [International Normalized Ratio (INR)]. After stabilization, the patient may be given warfarin and the heparin tapered. Following heparin therapy, oral anticoagulants should be administered according to the risk of recurrent pulmonary emboli. In patients who have an initial episode and no ongoing risk factors, 4 weeks of therapy is required. For those with continuing risk factors, at least 3 months of therapy is required (58). Thrombolytic therapy for acute deep venous thrombosis has been used in an attempt to reduce recurrent deep venous thrombosis and the postthrombotic syndrome. Generally, urokinase is given in repeated boluses. However, its usefulness may be limited because it may be successful only if the agent is infused directly into the thrombus, making it difficult to administer (42).

Vena Cava Filters

Anticoagulants are occasionally contraindicated, in which case a vena cava filter inserted percutaneously should be considered. Complications include malposition, migration, arrhythmia, wound infection, recurrent pulmonary emboli, and recurrent deep venous thrombosis (83). Rarely, a massive saddle pulmonary embolus may require a pulmonary embolectomy when the aforementioned measures are unsuccessful in maintaining the patient's blood pressure.

The efficacy of vena cava filters in patients who have thrombophlebitis and are at risk for pulmonary emboli has been evaluated in a large multiinstitutional study. The use of heparin alone or heparin plus a filter was compared in these patients. Those who had filters had a decreased occurrence of symptomatic and asymptomatic pulmonary emboli. However, no effect was observed in immediate or long-term mortality. Moreover, the initial beneficial affect of filters was offset by a significant increase in deep vein thrombosis—related to thrombosis at the filter site (23).

RESPIRATORY DYSFUNCTION

Respiratory Insufficiency

Inadequate ventilation in the posttraumatic and postoperative periods results in hypercapnia, hypoxemia, or both. The primary goal of therapy is to provide the patient with the capability of maintaining an arterial oxygen partial pressure of at least 60 mm Hg on an inspired oxygen content as close to room air as possible. To achieve this goal, oxygen delivered by nasal prongs, rebreathing mask, a face mask, or an endotracheal tube with respiratory support may be required. However, there are constraints to the amount of oxygen that can be delivered. Limitation of the amount may be a consequence of the device used for delivery, but more commonly, the amount that can be safely delivered is limited by the fact that inhalation of high oxygen concentrations results in pulmonary toxicity. The hazards of high concentrations include suppression of the respiratory drive in patients with chronic pulmonary disease, retrolental fibroplasia (primarily a disease of the newborn but also described in adults), segmental atelectasis caused by the greater solubility of oxygen compared with nitrogen, impairment of respiratory ciliary function, a decrease in pulmonary surfactant, and direct injury to capillary endothelial cells.

The $Paco_2$*, which is normally 40 mm Hg, is a primary indication of the adequacy of ventilation.* Common causes of hypercapnia include obstructive pulmonary disease, ARDS, metabolic alkalosis, and respiratory depression resulting from sedation or CNS trauma. Hypocapnia may be a result of hypoxia, anxiety, pulmonary embolism, sepsis, and pulmonary insufficiency. Although an indicator of ventilatory adequacy, alteration of Pco_2 is rarely an indication for respiratory support. Of more importance is the partial pressure of oxygen (Po_2), which should be maintained above 60 mm Hg. A Po_2 less than 60 mm Hg requires a change in respiratory management. A normal Po_2 for a particular patient breathing room air before injury may be

TABLE 10.9. INDICATIONS FOR ENDOTRACHEAL INTUBATION

Facilitation of pulmonary toilet
Prevention of upper airway occlusion
Protection against aspiration
Need for mechanical ventilation as determined by the following:
1. VC <15 mL/kg body weight
2. Inspiratory force <–25 cm H_2O
3. Respiratory rate >35 breaths/min
4. Po_2 <60 mm Hg despite high ambient O_2 concentration
5. Excessive, prolonged increase in the work of breathing

VC, vital capacity.

estimated by subtracting half the individual's age from 100. If impending airway obstruction is not a problem, initial support of the Po_2 may be obtained by the use of nasal prongs or face masks. Humidified oxygen should be used when possible to prevent drying the nasotracheal mucosa. Oxygen delivered by nasal prongs generally cannot provide an inspired concentration much above 50%. Even though humidified, high-flows have a drying effect on the mucosa; Venturi masks provide constant flows of oxygen ranging between 24% and 40%, depending on the mask. Partial rebreathing masks can deliver in excess of 80% oxygen; however, humidity cannot be added to the system.

On occasion, posttraumatic patients require endotracheal intubation, preferably by the nasotracheal route with a prestretched low-pressure cuff and respiratory support (Table 10.9). Indications for intubation include (a) the facilitation of pulmonary toilet, (b) the prevention of upper airway occlusion, (c) protection against aspiration, and (d) the need for mechanical ventilation. The requirement for mechanical ventilation is assessed by vital capacity, inspiratory force, respiratory rate, arterial oxygen content, and work of breathing. Vital capacity, or the volume of a maximum inspiration after a maximum expiration, is normally 60 to 70 mL/kg body weight. If it is less than 15 mL/kg, ventilatory support is indicated. *The inspiratory force, or amount of pressure that the patient is able to generate against a closed airway, is normally −75 to −100 cm H_2O. Patients who can achieve no more than -25 cm H_2O require mechanical support.* The normal respiratory rate is 12 to 20 breaths per minute. A rate that exceeds 35 breaths per minute suggests the need for ventilatory assistance. The arterial oxygen partial pressure should exceed 60 mm Hg. If this cannot be accomplished by raising the oxygen content of inspired air through the use of face masks and nasal prongs, intubation should be performed. Severe intercostal retractions and a tracheal tug indicate an increased work of breathing and are forerunners of respiratory insufficiency. Initially, the respirator is adjusted to deliver 12 to 15 mL/kg of body weight at a frequency of 8 to 14 times per minute for the adult and 15 to 30 times per minute for the child. Inspired oxygen content (Fio_2) should be the lowest needed to maintain the Po_2 above 60 mm Hg (an Fio_2 of 40% is a good level to begin with, adjusting it as required). Not only must blood gas levels be monitored, adjusting the respirator accordingly, but also the circulatory status must be carefully followed, because occasionally institution of mechanical ventilation will cause a decrease in the cardiac output with lowering of the blood pressure.

When the Po_2 cannot be maintained by an acceptable Fio_2 (less than 60%), the addition of positive end-expiratory pressure (PEEP) may be helpful. This technique maintains a specified pressure at the end of each respiration rather than allowing end-expiratory pressure to fall to zero. It is particularly useful in ARDS. Initially, 5 cm H_2O pressure is used. If the desired response is not achieved, it is increased in increments of 5 cm H_2O, carefully monitoring the blood pressure for signs of a significant reduction in cardiac output. Usually, no more than 15 cm H_2O is required. On rare occasions, however, as much as 25 cm H_2O pressure may be needed. With the use of PEEP, Po_2 can be maintained at acceptable levels with reduced Fio_2. Other advantages include a decrease in pulmonary shunting and an increase in functional residual capacity. A proposed advantage is that it drives pulmonary edema fluid from the alveoli and the interstitium into the pulmonary capillaries. Its major disadvantages are a reduction in cardiac output and a diminished urine output. The latter effect is perhaps the result of an increased release of ADH.

One method of anticipating future respiratory difficulties and determining how the patient is progressing on the respirator is by sequentially determining the arterial oxygen gradient, $P(A\text{-}a)o_2$. This gradient is a sensitive indicator of early respiratory impairment. To calculate the $P(A\text{-}a)o_2$, the patient receives 100% oxygen for 20 to 30 minutes, arterial blood gases are drawn, and the barometric pressure is recorded. The calculation is as follows: barometric pressure minus water vapor pressure (47 mm Hg) minus the partial pressure of alveolar CO_2. Because alveolar CO_2 rapidly equilibrates with arterial CO_2, the Pco_2 obtained from the blood gas analysis may be substituted. This quantity minus the Po_2 is equal to the arterial alveolar oxygen gradient.

Acute posttraumatic pulmonary insufficiency occurs after major trauma, burns, hypoproteinemia, or inadequate fluid resuscitation during shock, severe sepsis, pancreatitis, or transplant rejection crisis (antigen–antibody reaction). The cause of ARDS is unclear. It appears that neutrophils contribute because the lungs of patients with ARDS are populated by large numbers of them. They release oxygen-free radicals and elastase, two substances that injure tissues. Macrophages release oxygen-free radicals, proteases, prostaglandins, leukotrienes, and cytokines and also have been implicated. Moreover, the cytokine tumor necrosis factor has been shown to play a role experimentally. Finally, defects in surfactant may be etiologic or merely perpetuate the disease (77).

After the initiating event, platelet microaggregates form in the pulmonary capillaries and injure the alveolar capillary endothelium. Vasoactive substances are released, resulting in increased capillary permeability (6). Peribronchiolar edema follows, which causes an increase in small airway resistance and a reduction in pulmonary compliance, making aeration of the lungs difficult. Pulmonary shunting also occurs. The Po_2 falls and the Pco_2 rises, often despite increases in the Fio_2. Clinically, the patient becomes dyspneic, tachypneic, and hypoxemic. Functional residual capacity and lung compliance are reduced, and bilateral pulmonary infiltrates are often present on the chest film. The syndrome should be suspected in the septic or traumatized patient when the Po_2 falls despite efforts to increase the Fio_2.

Treatment involves nasotracheal intubation and mechanical ventilation. PEEP is often necessary. If PEEP results in a reduced cardiac output, inotropic agents may be required to return blood pressure to acceptable levels. The use of colloid to increase intravascular oncotic pressure and thereby draw fluid from the pulmonary perivascular space into the capillaries is controversial, as is the use of steroids. Prophylactic antibiotics administered either by the parenteral route or by inhalation have little to recommend them. Infections are treated when they occur with the antibiotic to which the bacteria are sensitive. Unfortunately, none of the newer pharmacologic therapies has produced impressive results. Methylprednisolone, prostaglandin E, and *N*-acetylcysteine have not been shown convincingly to lessen mortality.

REFERENCES

1. Abel RM, Beck CH Jr, Abbott WM, et al. Improved survival from acute renal failure after treatment with intravenous essential L-amino acids and glucose. *N Engl J Med* 1973;288:695.
2. Anderson CF, Wochos DN. The utility of serum albumin values in the nutritional assessment of hospitalized patients. *Mayo Clin Proc* 1982;57:181.
3. Arnspiger RC, Helling TS. An evaluation of results of colon anastomosis in prepared and unprepared bowel. *J Clin Gastroenterol* 1988;10:638.
4. Barbul A. Arginine and immune function. *Nutrition* 1990;6:53.
5. Bessey PQ. What's new in critical care and metabolism. *J Am Coll Surg* 1997;184:115.
6. Blaisdell FW. Pathophysiology of the respiratory distress syndrome. *Arch Surg* 1974;108:44.
7. Boyce WH, Vest SA. The role of ammonia reabsorption in the acid base imbalance following ureterosigmoidostomy. *J Urol* 1952;67:169.
8. Boyd JD. Chronic acidosis secondary to ureteral transplantation. *Am J Dis Child* 1931;42:366.
9. Calloway DH, Spector H. Nitrogen balance as related to calorie and protein intake in active young men. *Am J Clin Nutr* 1954; 2:405.
10. Carcillo JA, Cunnion RE. Septic shock. *Crit Care Clin* 1997; 13:553.
11. Carmona RH, Tsao TC, Trunkey DD. The role of prostacyclin and thromboxane in sepsis and septic shock. *Arch Surg* 1984; 119:189.
12. Ching N, Grossi CE, Angers J, et al. The outcome of surgical treatment as related to the response of the serum albumin level to nutritional support. *Surg Gynecol Obstet* 1980;151:199.
13. Clark SS. Electrolyte disturbance associated with jejunal conduit. *J Urol* 1974;112:42.
14. Clarke JS, Condon RE, Barlett JG, et al. Preoperative oral antibiotics reduce septic complications of colon operations. *Ann Surg* 1977;186:251.
15. Cohn I Jr, Nance FC. Intestinal antisepsis and peritonitis from perforation. In: Sabiston DC Jr, ed. *Textbook of surgery*. Philadelphia: WB Saunders, 1972:948.
16. Connors Jr AF, Speroff T, Dawson NV, et al. The effectiveness of right heart catheterization in the initial care of critically ill patients. *JAMA* 1996;276:889.
17. Cook JA, Wise WC, Halushka PV. Elevated thromboxane levels in the rat during endotoxin shock: protective effects of imidazole, 13-azaprostanoic acid, or essential fatty acid deficiency. *J Clin Invest* 1980;65:227.
18. Copeland EM, MacFadyen BV, Dudrick SJ. Effect of intravenous hyperalimentation on established delayed hypersensitivity in the cancer patient. *Ann Surg* 1976;184:60.
19. Creevy CD. Renal complications after ileal diversion of urine in non-neoplastic disorders. *J Urol* 1960;83:394.
20. Creevy CD, Webb EA. A fatal hemolytic reaction following transurethral resection of the prostate gland. *Surgery* 1947;21:56.
21. D'Agostino A, Leadbetter WF, Schwartz WB. Alterations in the ionic composition of isotonic saline solution instilled into the colon. *J Clin Invest* 1953;32:444.
22. Daly JM, Dudrick SJ, Copeland EM. Intravenous hyperalimentation: effect in delayed cutaneous hypersensitivity in cancer patients. *Ann Surg* 1980;192:587.
23. Decousus H, Leizorovicz A, Parent F, et al. A clinical trial of vena caval filters in the prevention of pulmonary embolism in patients with proximal deep-vein thrombosis. *N Engl J Med* 1998;338:409.
24. DeMaria A, Craven DE, Hefferman JJ, et al. Naloxone versus placebo in treatment of septic shock. *Lancet* 1985;1:1363.
25. Dion YM, Richards GK, Prentis JJ, et al. The influence of oral versus parenteral preoperative metronidazole on sepsis following colon surgery. *Ann Surg* 1980;192:221.
26. Dudrick SJ, MacFadyen BV, Van Buren CT, et al. Parenteral hyperalimentation: metabolic problems and solutions. *Ann Surg* 1972;176:259.
27. Eichhorn JH. Prevention of intraoperative anesthetic accident related to severe injury through safety monitoring. *Anesthesia* 1989;70:572.
28. Eykyn SJ, Jackson BT, Lockhart-Mummery HE, et al. Prophylactic preoperative intravenous metronidazole in elective colorectal surgery. *Lancet* 1979;2:761.
29. Faden AI. Opiate antagonists and thyrotropin-releasing hormone. *JAMA* 1984;252:1177.
30. Fairfull-Smith R, Abunassar R, Freeman JB, et al. Rational use of elemental and nonelemental diets in hospitalized patients. *Ann Surg* 1980;192:600.
31. Farris DO, Odel HM. Electrolyte pattern of the blood after bilateral ureterosigmoidostomy. *JAMA* 1950;142:634.
32. Feigal D, Blaisdell W. The estimation of surgical risk. *Med Clin North Am* 1979;63:1131.
33. Fontaine E, Barthelemy Y, Houlgatte A, et al. Twenty-year experience with jejunal conduits. *Urology* 1997;50:207.
34. Frances CW, Marder CM, Evart S, et al. Warfarin therapy: prevention of post operative venous thrombosis without excessive bleeding. *JAMA* 1993;249:374.

35. Frazee RC, Roberts J, Symmonds R, et al. Prospective randomized trial of inpatient vs outpatient bowel preparation for elective colorectal surgery. *Dis Colon Rectum* 1992;35(3):223.
36. Freund H, Atarmain S, Fischer J. Comparative study of parenteral nutrition in renal failure using essential and nonessential amino acid containing solutions. *Surg Gynecol Obstet* 1980; 151:652.
37. Freund H, Dienstag J, Lehrich J, et al. Infusion of branched-chain enriched amino acid solution in patients with hepatic encephalopathy. *Ann Surg* 1982;196:209.
38. Geddes JS, Adgey AAJ, Pantridge JF. Prevention of cardiogenic shock. *Am Heart J* 1980;99:243.
39. Giercksky KE, Danielson S, Garberg O, et al. A single dose tinidazole and doxycycline prophylaxis in elective surgery of colon and rectum. *Ann Surg* 1982;195:227.
40. Goldman L, Caldera DL, Nussbaum SR, et al. Multifactorial index of cardiac risk in noncardiac surgical procedures. *N Engl J Med* 1977;297:845.
41. Goldman L, Caldera DL, Southwick FS, et al. Cardiac risk factors and complications in noncardiac surgery. *Medicine* 1978; 57:357.
42. Haas SK. Treatment of deep venous thrombosis and pulmonary embolism. *Med Clin North Am* 1998;82:495.
43. Holaday JW. Cardiovascular effects of endogenous opiate systems. *Ann Rev Pharmacol Toxicol* 1983;23:541.
44. Houston MC, Thompson WL, Robertson D. Shock diagnosis and management. *Arch Intern Med* 1984;144:1433.
45. Johnson LR. *Physiology of the gastrointestinal tract.* New York: Raven Press, 1981, vol 2.
46. Jolinbur M, Morales P. Jejunal conduits: technique and complications. *J Urol* 1975;113:787.
47. Kelly KJ. Complications of latex allergy: a pediatric allergist's perspective. *Dialog Pediatr Urol* 1992;15:3.
48. Kinasewitz GJ. Thrombophlebitis and pulmonary embolism in the elderly patient. *Clin Chest Med* 1993;14:523.
49. Kinney JM. The metabolic response to injury. In: Richards JR, Kinney JM, eds. *Nutritional aspects of care in the critically ill.* London: Churchill-Livingstone, 1977.
50. Koch MO, McDougal WS. Chlorpromazine: adjuvant therapy for the metabolic derangements created by urinary diversion through intestinal segments. *J Urol* 1985a;134:165.
51. Koch MO, McDougal WS. Nicotinic acid treatment for the hyperchloremic acidosis following urinary diversion through intestinal segments. *J Urol* 1985b;134:162.
52. Koch MO, McDougal WS. The pathophysiology of hyperchloremic metabolic acidosis following urinary diversion through intestinal segments. *Surgery* 1985c;98:561.
53. Koonce J, Selikowitz S, McDougal WS. Complications of low-dose heparin prophylaxis following pelvic lymphadenectomy. *Urology* 1986;28:21.
54. Lahnborg G, Friman L, Bergstrom K, et al. Effect of low-dose heparin on incidence of post-operative pulmonary embolism detected by photoscanning. *Lancet* 1974;1:329.
55. Lapides J. Mechanism of electrolyte imbalance following ureterosigmoid transplantation. *Surg Gynecol Obstet* 1951;93:691.
56. Law DK, Dudrick SJ, Abdon NI. Immunocompetence of patients with protein-calorie malnutrition: the effects of nutritional repletion. *Ann Intern Med* 1973;79:545.
57. Leizorovicz A. Comparison of the efficacy and safety of low molecular weight heparins and unfractionated heparins in the initial treatment of deep venous thrombosis: an updated meta-analysis. *Drugs* 1996;52[Suppl]:30.
58. Levine MN, Hirsh J, Gent M, et al. Optimal duration of oral anticoagulant therapy: a randomized trial comparing four weeks with three months of warfarin in patients with proximal deep vein thrombosis. *Thromb Haemost* 1995;74:606.
59. Long CL, Spencer JL, Kinney JM, et al. Carbohydrate metabolism in normal man and effect of glucose infusion. *J Appl Physiol* 1971;31:102.
60. McDougal WS. The mechanism of ionized ammonia transport in the acidosis of urinary diversion [Abstract]. *Am Assoc GU Surg* 1993;107:1.
61. McDougal WS, Koch MO. Accurate determination of renal function in patients with intestinal urinary diversions. *J Urol* 1986;135:1175.
62. McDougal WS, Koch MO. Effect of sulfate on calcium and magnesium homeostasis following urinary diversion. *Kidney Int* 1989;35:105.
63. McDougal WS, Wilmore DW, Pruitt BA Jr. Effect of near isosmotic intravenous nutrient infusions on nitrogen balance in critically ill injured patients. *Surg Gynecol Obstet* 1977a;145:408.
64. McDougal WS, Wilmore DW, Pruitt BA Jr. Glucose dependent hepatic membrane transport in non-bacteremic and bacteremic thermally injured patients. *J Surg Res* 1977b;22:697.
65. McDougal WS, Wright FS. Defect in proximal and distal sodium transport in post-obstructive diuresis. *Kidney Int* 1972; 2:304.
66. Menaker GJ, Litvak S, Bendix R, et al. Operations on the colon without preoperative oral antibiotic therapy. *Surg Gynecol Obstet* 1981;152:36.
67. Mizock B. Septic shock: a metabolic perspective. *Arch Intern Med* 1984;144:579.
68. Montemurro DG, Stevenson JA. Survival and body composition of normal and hypothalamic obese rats in acute starvation. *Am J Physiol* 1960;198:757.
69. Moukhtar M, Romney S. Continuous intraperitoneal antibiotic lavage in the management of purulent sepsis of the pelvis. *Surg Gynecol Obstet* 1980;150:548.
70. Nichols RL, Broido P, Condo RE, et al. Effect of preoperative neomycin-erythromycin intestinal preparation on the incidence of infectious complications following colon surgery. *Ann Surg* 1973;178:453.
71. Paradisi F, Corti G, Mangani V. Urosepsis in the critical care unit. *Crit Care Clin* 1998;14:165.
72. Parker MM, Parrillo JE. Septic shock: hemodynamics and pathogenesis. *JAMA* 1983;250:3324.
73. Parrillo JE. Pathogenetic mechanisms of septic shock. *N Engl J Med* 1993;328:1471.
74. Passmore R. Recommended intakes of nutrients for the United Kingdom. *Reports on Public Health and Medical Subjects,* no. 120:34. London: Her Majesty's Stationery Office, 1969.
75. Peters WP, Johnson MW, Friedman PA, et al. Pressor effect of naloxone in septic shock. *Lancet* 1981;1:529.
76. Rennie MJ, MacLennan PA, Hundal HS, et al. Skeletal muscle glutamine transport, intramuscular glutamine concentration, and muscle protein turnover. *Metabolism* 1989;38:47.
77. Repine JE. Scientific perspectives on adult respiratory distress syndrome. *Lancet* 1992;339:466.
78. Rombeau JL, McClane J. Perioperative care of the colorectal patient. *Dis Colon Rectum* 1999;42:845.
79. Rosenberg JC, Rush BF. Lethal endotoxin shock. *JAMA* 1966; 196:767.
80. Rosenberg ML. The physiology of hyperchloremic acidosis following ureterosigmoidostomy: a study of urinary reabsorption with radioactive isotopes. *J Urol* 1953;70:569.

81. Saez-Llorens X, McCracken GH. Sepsis syndrome and septic shock in pediatrics: current concepts of terminology, pathophysiology, and management. *J Pediatr* 1993;123:497.
82. Salzman EW, Ploetz J, Bettman M, et al. Intraoperative external pneumatic calf compression to afford long-term prophylaxis against deep venous thrombosis in urologic patients. *Surgery* 1980;87:239.
83. Schwarz RE, Marrero AM, Conlon KC, et al. Inferior vena cava filters in cancer patients: indications and outcome. *J Clin Oncol* 1996;14:652.
84. Sheagren JN. Septic shock and corticosteroids. *N Engl J Med* 1981;305:456.
85. Solla JA, Rothenberger DA. Preoperative bowel preparation: a survey of colon and rectal surgeons. *Dis Colon Rectum* 1990; 33:154.
86. Souba WW, Smith RJ, Wilmore DW. Glutamine metabolism by the intestinal tract. *JPEN J Parenter Enteral Nutr* 1985;9:608.
87. Stamey TA. The pathogenesis and implications of electrolyte imbalance in ureterosigmoidostomy. *Surg Gynecol Obstet* 1956; 103:736.
88. Stehle P, Zander J, Mertes N, et al. Effect of parenteral glutamine peptide supplements on muscle glutamine loss and nitrogen balance after major surgery. *Lancet* 1989;1:231.
89. Steiger E, Daly JM, Allen JR, et al. Postoperative intravenous nutrition: effects on body weight, protein, regeneration, wound healing and liver morphology. *Surgery* 1973;73:686.
90. Swartz J, Braude B, Gilmour R. Intra-operative anaphylaxis to latex. *Can J Anaesth* 1990;37:589.
91. Tarhan S, Moffitt EA, Taylor WF, et al. Myocardial infarction after general anesthesia. *JAMA* 1972;220:1451.
92. Torosian MH. Perioperative nutrition support for patients undergoing gastrointestinal surgery: critical analysis and recommendations. *World J Surg* 1999;23:565.
93. Welbourne TC, Childress D, Givens G. Renal regulation of interorgan glutamine flow in metabolic acidosis. *Am J Physiol* 1987;251:R858.
94. Wilmore DW, Long JM, Mason AD Jr, et al. Catecholamines: mediator of the hypermetabolic response to thermal injury. *Ann Surg* 1974;180:653.
95. Wilmore DW, Mason AD Jr, Pruitt BA Jr. Insulin response to glucose in hypermetabolic burn patients. *Ann Surg* 1976; 183:314.
96. Wolfe BM, Culebras JM, Sim AJW, et al. Substrate interaction in intravenous feeding: comparative effects of carbohydrate and fat on amino acid utilization in fasting man. *Ann Surg* 1977;186:518.
97. Ziegler EJ. Treatment of gram-negative bacteremia and shock with human antiserum to a mutant *Escherichia coli*. *N Engl J Med* 1982;307:1125.

Adult and Pediatric Urology, 4/e, edited by Jay Y. Gillenwater, John T. Grayhack, Stuart S. Howards, and Michael E. Mitchell.
Lippincott Williams & Wilkins, Philadelphia © 2002

11

RENAL AND URETERAL INJURIES

11A

RENAL INJURIES

JACK W. McANINCH
RICHARD A. SANTUCCI

Trauma is the leading cause of death for persons between 1 and 44 years of age. In addition, each year, millions of dollars are spent to rehabilitate trauma victims. The team approach to management provides the highest level of expertise in reducing morbidity and preventing mortality. The trauma surgeon relies on the urologic surgeon to deal with the complex injuries of the urogenital system. The urologic surgeon may not become involved in the initial resuscitation phases of trauma care because most injuries to the urogenital system are not life-threatening; however, he or she may become the most important member of the team 2 weeks later when urinary extravasation, abscess formation, and septic complications develop secondarily.

The kidney is the most commonly injured organ in the urogenital system (61), and renal injuries are still subject to controversy in diagnosis and management. Despite the current refined approach, many questions remain unanswered regarding when and for what patients a study should be done to evaluate a renal injury. Even when the diagnosis has been established, there is great controversy over operative versus nonoperative management. The urologic and surgical literature is replete with articles debating the merits of the respective approaches (18,22,80). No simple answers exist. One must review the literature critically and become familiar with the variety of approaches in renal trauma care to apply this information to an individual patient.

The following quotation from Erickson's 1860 *Textbook of Surgery* indicates the importance of careful clinical evaluation in patients with major renal injuries:

> If the kidneys are injured, the patient will commonly experience a frequent desire to pass water, and this will be tinged

J.W. McAninch and R.A. Santucci: Department of Urology, Wayne State University, Detroit, MI 48201.

> with blood, often to a considerable extent. The absence of blood in the urine must not, however, be taken as an indication that the kidney is not injured; it may be so disorganized as to be totally incapable of secreting, and subsequently no bloody urine finds its way into the bladder. A man was admitted into the hospital under my care for a buffer injury of the back; he passed water untinged with blood, but after death his right kidney was found completely smashed by the blow, with an extensive extravasation of blood in the celluloadipose tissue around it. Here it was evident that the disorganization was so sudden and complete that no bloody urine had found its way into the bladder.

This clinical picture continues to be reported today.

Approximately 8% to 10% of blunt and penetrating abdominal injuries involve the kidneys. In rural settings, blunt trauma accounts for the largest percentage of renal injuries (90% to 95%) (52); in urban settings, the percentage of penetrating renal injuries increases to 20% (85).

This chapter is intended to provide a logical diagnostic approach to the patient with renal injury and to establish a rationale for management that will ultimately preserve the largest amount of functioning renal tissue, while safely managing the patient's other injuries.

MODE OF INJURY AND PRESENTATION

The mechanism of injury to the kidney is broadly classified as blunt or penetrating. Blunt trauma is more common in most centers, accounting for 80% to 90% of injuries, and results from automobile accidents, auto–pedestrian accidents, falls, contact sports, and assaults (1,2,17,47,59). Gunshot and stab wounds cause 10% to 20% of renal injuries and represent the most common causes of penetrating injury. In 1968, Carlton and co-workers (12) reported associated intraabdominal injuries in 80% of their patients with penetrating renal injury. This observation was supported by Sagalowsky and colleagues (85): Of 122 patients with gunshot wounds, all had associated intraabdominal injury. Liver, small intestine, stomach, and colon were the most commonly injured organs. Stab wounds less frequently have associated intraabdominal injury, with reports ranging from 30% to 70% (42,85). This wide variation may be based on the location of the stab wound. Bernath and others (5) noted that stab wounds posterior to the anterior axillary line were associated with intraabdominal injury in fewer than 12% of cases.

Renal injuries from blunt trauma occur consequent to upper abdominal injury and rapid deceleration. Gross or microscopic hematuria is usually present (8,70). These patients often have profuse abdominal tenderness, lower rib fractures, vertebral body fractures, and flank contusions. A palpable abdominal mass with associated shock may be indicative of a rapidly developing retroperitoneal hematoma from a major renal parenchymal or renal vascular injury. Rapid-deceleration injuries usually involve multiple organ systems, and patients are often unconscious and in shock. Head-on automobile collisions and falls from great heights account for the majority of such injuries. Multiple bony fractures usually are present, as are injuries to the abdominal viscera, vascular system, chest, and head. The renal injury seen in such cases is often a renal pedicle avulsion or acute thrombosis of the main renal artery or one of the segmental arterial branches. Hematuria may not be present, and the diagnosis must be established by radiographic imaging prompted by a high index of suspicion (38,91).

Stab wounds to the kidneys generally have their entrance points in the lower thorax, flank area, or upper abdomen. The size of the entrance wound has little correlation with the extent of injury and the depth of penetration. Hematuria, most often gross, is usually present with major parenchymal injuries. The incidence of associated intraabdominal injuries varies greatly and may be related to the entrance site (5). Careful abdominal examination may reveal marked tenderness and generalized rigidity, indicating bowel perforation. Peritoneal lavage is useful for evaluating intraabdominal injury after stab wounds to the torso (27). Hemorrhagic shock is a common presenting sign, and reestablishment of circulatory volume is of prime importance in the initial treatment. Renal imaging should be done in all patients with stab wounds in the upper abdomen, flank, back, or lower chest, whether hematuria is present or not.

Patients with gunshot wounds to the torso that penetrate the kidney often are in a state of hemorrhagic shock with multiple organ injury. Rapid resuscitation is of prime importance, and immediate surgery may be required before diagnostic studies can be performed. The type of weapon—and of the bullet if known—should be ascertained, but the prevailing wisdom is to "treat the wound and not the weapon" (56). The damage that a missile can inflict is related to the kinetic energy expended, determined from the following formula:

$$KE = \frac{MV^2}{2}$$

where *KE* is kinetic energy, *M* is the mass of the missile, and *V* is the muzzle velocity of the weapon.

In general, the higher the muzzle velocity, the greater the tissue damage, although experimentally the actual wounding effect varies from MV1.5 to MV2.5 (56). Figure 11A.1 demonstrates the method by which bullets of high velocity cause extensive tissue damage: On entering the soft tissue of the body, the bullet creates a temporary pulsatile cavity that can be up to 40 times wider than the diameter of the bullet; a small permanent core of tissue is vaporized; and finally the bullet can tumble or fragment, further widening the area of tissue damage (21). [Many high-

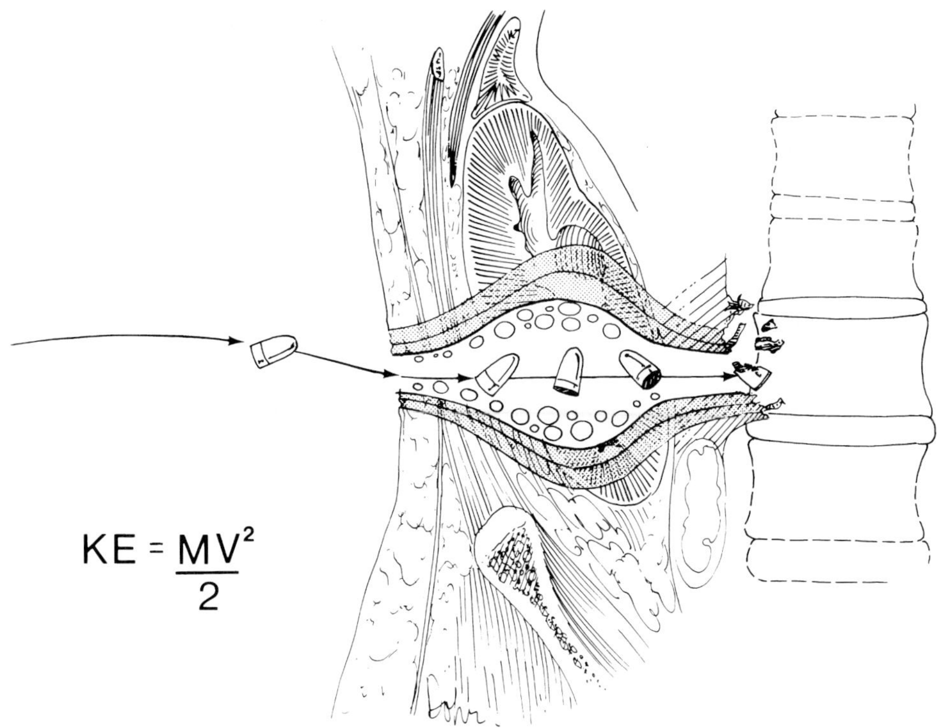

FIGURE 11A.1. Dynamics of missile soft tissue injury. (From McAninch JW. Renal injuries. In: McAninch JW, guest ed. *Urogenital trauma,* vol 2 of Blaisdell WF, Trunkey DD, series eds. *Trauma management*. New York: Thieme Stratton, 1985a:27–49, with permission.)

velocity projectiles such as the M-16 yaw after penetrating some distance into tissue, causing an enlarged permanent cavity from bullet tumbling (33).] Temporary cavitation and vaporization can cause extensive damage (the "blast effect"), which may not be appreciated at operation. However, experts point out that the relationship between the volume of the temporary cavity and tissue damage is not absolute and that many so-called high-velocity wounds from assault weapons can leave a clean track with little devitalization (33). Intensive debridement may be required to remove the nonviable tissue created by such injuries, but some researchers have suggested that only a few millimeters of debridement may be required in cases of gunshot through muscle, whereas more extensive tissue excision may be needed in solid organs like the kidney and liver (56). This is borne out in analysis of gunshot wounds to the kidney: Injuries from high-velocity weapons require nephrectomy more often than those from low-velocity weapons (31).

Most common handguns and many rifles are low-velocity weapons (muzzle velocity of less than 2,000 feet per second), and less extensive debridement may be needed. However, these weapons can cause extensive damage via a number of mechanisms, such as unintentional and intentional bullet fragmentation (34). Increasingly, specialty ammunition is available that is designed to maximize tissue damage after impact, by either intentional fragmentation (Dum-Dum, Devastator, exploding, and other "frangible" ammunition) or an increase in projectile diameter by flattening (hollow-point bullets). The effect of this specialty ammunition, in some cases, is that lower velocity missiles, as from a common handgun, can rival the tissue damage caused even by high-velocity rifles (93). Table 11A.1 lists muzzle velocities of common weapons.

TABLE 11A.1. MUZZLE VELOCITY OF COMMON WEAPONS

Weapon	Velocity (ft/sec)
0.22 short	1,045
0.22 magnum	2,000
0.38 caliber	1,330
0.45 caliber	1,320
AK-47	1,950
Carbine (0.30 caliber)	1,970
7.62 mm (M-14)	2,400–2,800
5.56 mm (M-16)	3,250

From McAninch JW. Renal injuries. In McAninch JW, guest ed. *Urogenital trauma,* vol 2 of Blaisdell WF, Trunkey DD, series eds. *Trauma management.* New York: Thieme Stratton, 1985:27–49, with permission.

HEMATURIA

The presence of blood in the urine is usually the first indicator of renal injury. In most reported series, more than 95% of patients had microscopic or gross hematuria (8,78,82,87,99). However, Bright and co-workers (8) first noted that the degree of hematuria does not correlate with the severity of injury. For example, a renal contusion is diagnosed in a patient with gross hematuria after blunt abdominal trauma, but results on excretory urography are normal. A patient with microscopic hematuria after a rapid-deceleration injury may demonstrate a major renal vascular injury. Guerriero and associates (38) noted gross hematuria in only 10 of 33 patients with renal vascular injuries, and Stables and colleagues (91) found no hematuria in 24% of patients with traumatic renal artery occlusion. In our recent series of 113 grade IV renal injuries, gross hematuria was noted in only 63%, and even microhematuria was absent in 4% (86). All series note the importance of hematuria as an indicator of injury but emphasize that it is a nonspecific finding and does not correlate with the seriousness of the renal damage.

The patient should be evaluated in the emergency room and urine should be obtained for study. Unconscious patients with serious injuries should be catheterized for dipstick urinalysis. If the results are positive, a finding of more than 5 red blood cells per high-power field (RBCs/HPF) would be expected (20). When time permits, microscopic urinary examination should be done.

Nicolaisen and colleagues (78) noted that adult patients sustaining blunt trauma had significant renal injury (defined as minor or major lacerations and vascular injuries) in the presence of gross hematuria or shock (systolic blood pressure less than 90 mm Hg) with microscopic hematuria. Mee and associates (70) subsequently reported a 10-year prospective study of patient selection for radiographic assessment after renal injury. The study included 1,146 patients (1,007 with blunt trauma and 139 with penetrating trauma). Significant injuries were found in 44 patients (4.4%) with blunt trauma, each of whom had either gross hematuria or microscopic hematuria associated with shock. Microscopic hematuria without shock was present in 812 patients with blunt trauma in whom there was no evidence of significant renal injury. Hardeman and associates (41) had similar findings.

Shock is defined as a systolic blood pressure less than 90 mm Hg, and any one measurement at or below this level from the time of evaluation by paramedics in the field satisfies this criterion. This requires careful inspection of paramedic and emergency room records before the determination is made that radiographic assessment is not indicated.

On the basis of available data, the following recommendations apply to the adult patient with blunt trauma: In the presence of gross hematuria or microscopic hematuria associated with shock, radiographic assessment should be done; patients with microscopic hematuria without shock do not require radiographic assessment. However, if physical examination or associated injuries prompt reasonable suspicion of a renal injury, renal imaging should be undertaken. This is especially true for patients with rapid-deceleration injuries, although in the studies of Mee and associates (70) and Hardeman and associates (41) vascular injuries were not missed when the preceding criteria were used.

Renal imaging is required in all patients with microscopic (more than 5 RBCs/HPF) or gross hematuria sustaining penetrating trauma or in pediatric patients. None of the previously mentioned studies found criteria to select patients for imaging who were in the pediatric age group or had penetrating injury.

CLASSIFICATION OF RENAL INJURIES

Categorizing renal injuries according to severity helps in selecting appropriate therapy and predicting results of treatment. Renal injuries can be classified according to the American Association for Surgery of Trauma (75) into five large groups: (a) renal contusions—bruises or subcapsular hematomas associated with an intact renal capsule and collecting system; (b) minor lacerations—superficial cortical disruptions less than 1.0 cm in depth that do not involve the deep renal medulla or collecting system; (c) parenchymal lacerations greater than 1.0 cm in depth without collecting system rupture or urinary extravasation; (d) parenchymal laceration extending through the renal cortex, medulla, and collecting system; or main renal artery or vein injury with contained hemorrhage; and (e) completely shattered kidney or avulsion of main renal artery or vein that devascularizes the kidney (Fig. 11A.2).

Vascular injuries and major and minor lacerations constitute significant trauma. These patients should have complete radiographic assessment to determine the full extent of injury and select appropriate management. Categorization does not mandate operation, but it does aid the surgeon in directing the care of these patients. Review of more than 2,500 renal injuries indicates, for instance, that no grade I injuries require operative repair, while nearly 100% of grade V injuries require speedy nephrectomy or repair (87). Those in between (grades II to IV) require individualized therapy, with a general trend for more serious intervention (renorrhaphy or nephrectomy) as the grade increases (Fig. 11A.3).

STAGING AND ASSESSMENT OF INJURY

Staging is the orderly process by which a renal injury is completely defined by history, physical examination, and radiographic or other imaging techniques. For instance, for

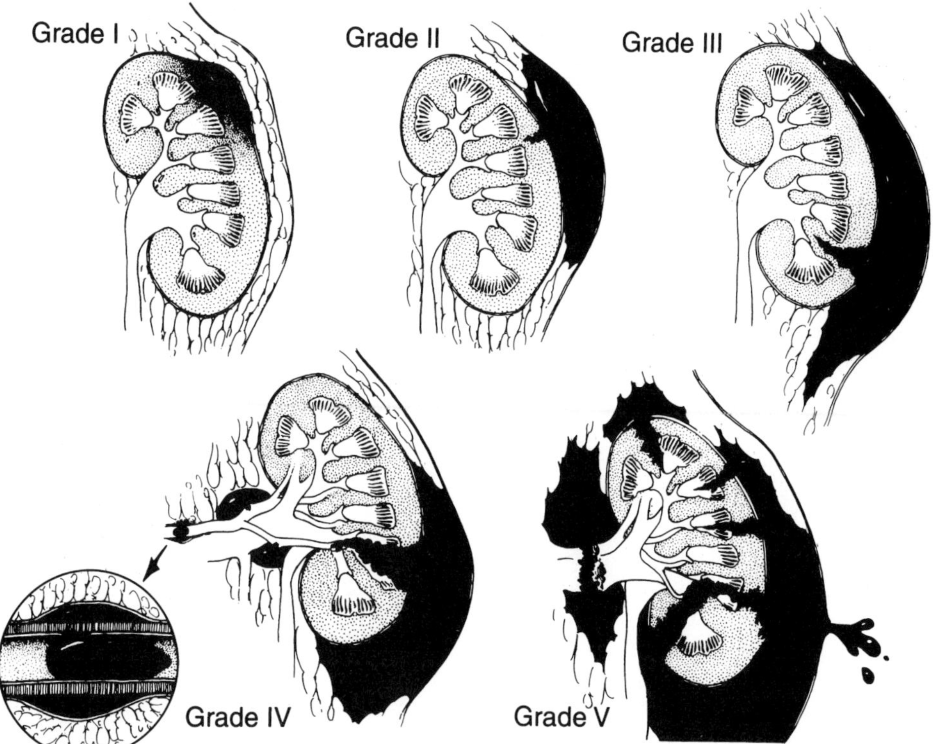

FIGURE 11A.2. Artist's rendition of the Renal Injury Severity Scale of the American Association for the Surgery of Trauma (AAST). Note that grade IV injuries represent parenchymal lacerations extending into the collecting system and injury to the main renal artery or vein with contained hemorrhage. These vascular injuries include traumatic renal artery thrombosis *(inset).* (From Moore EE, et al. Organ injury scaling: spleen, liver, and kidney. *J Trauma* 1989;29:1664, with permission.)

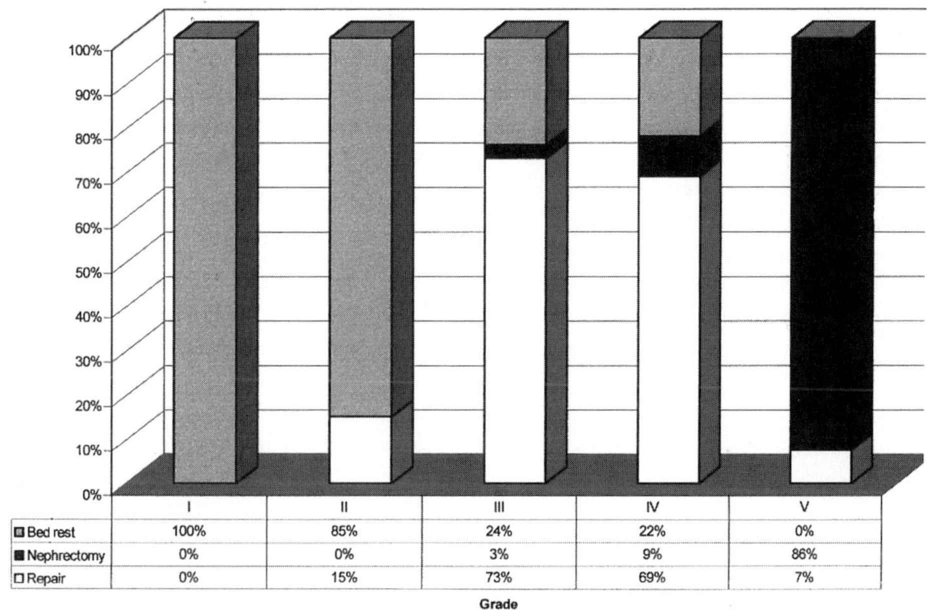

	I	II	III	IV	V
Bed rest	100%	85%	24%	22%	0%
Nephrectomy	0%	0%	3%	9%	86%
Repair	0%	15%	73%	69%	7%

FIGURE 11A.3. Injury scale and treatment of renal injury in 2,500 patients with renal trauma. (From Santucci RA, Mario LA, Segal MR, et al. Classification trees are highly predictive of need for surgery in renal trauma patients. *J Urol* 2000;163[Suppl]:4, with permission.)

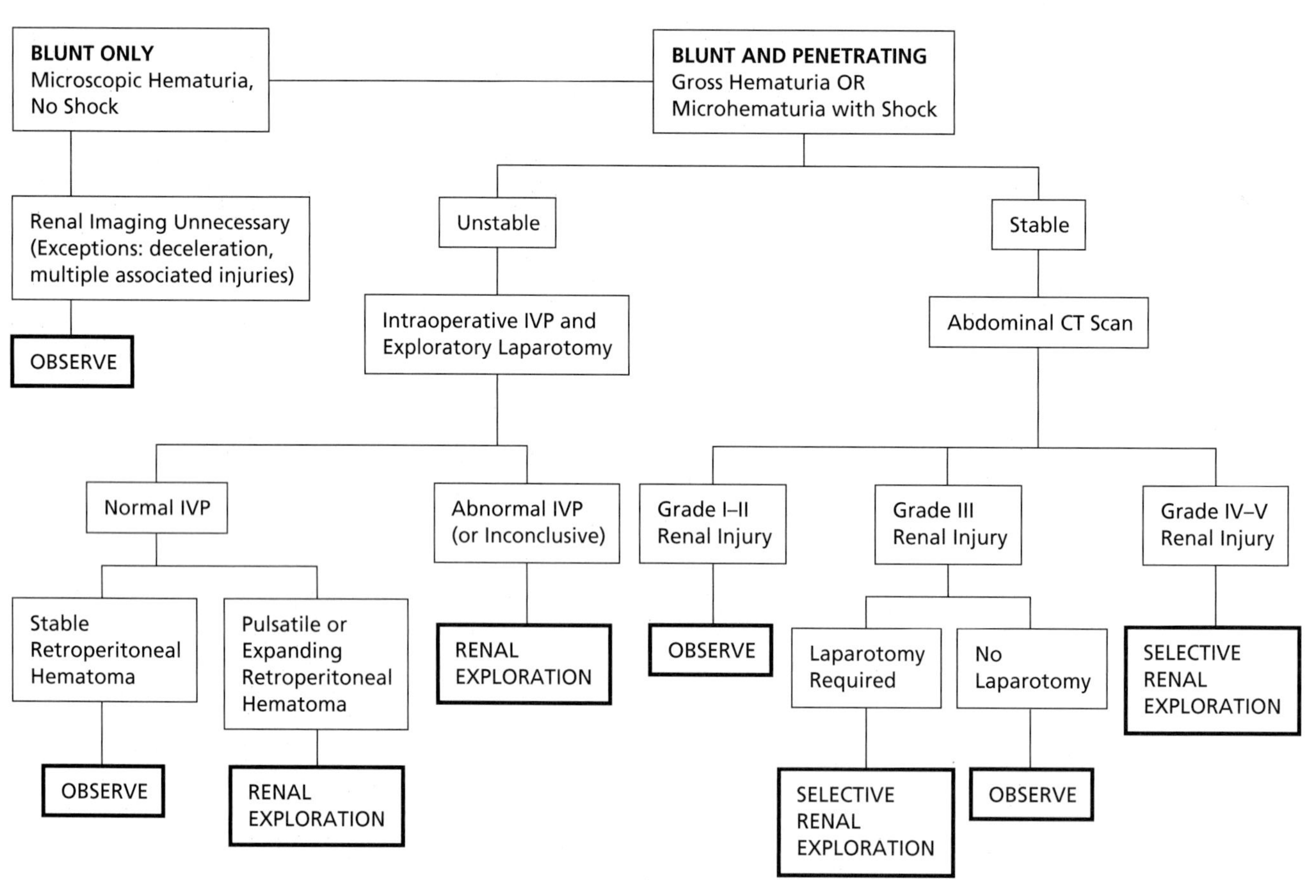

FIGURE 11A.4. Algorithm for the approach to the initial diagnosis and management of renal trauma. CT, computed tomography; IVP, intravenous pyelogram. (Modified from Meng MV, Brandes SB, McAninch JW. Renal trauma: indications and techniques for surgical exploration. *World J Urol* 1999;17:71, with permission.)

a patient with blunt trauma from an automobile accident who has gross hematuria, and in whom renal imaging shows the kidneys to be normal, the injury is categorized as a renal contusion, and no additional studies are necessary. However, if the results of renal imaging are indeterminate or abnormal, additional information will be needed to complete the staging and document the full extent of the injury. Increasing use of computed tomography (CT) scanning has allowed more accurate determination of injury severity than has been available in the past (7,66).

History, physical examination, and the determination of hematuria are the initial evaluative measures. The presence of gross or microscopic hematuria (more than 5 RBCs/HPF) continues to be the best indicator of injury. All patients sustaining penetrating trauma or pediatric patients with positive findings should have radiographic staging. Adult patients with blunt trauma can be selectively imaged. Figure 11A.4 shows a staging algorithm that is a useful systematic approach for renal trauma patients. Patients with gross hematuria or microscopic hematuria associated with shock (systolic blood pressure less than 90 mm Hg) should have radiographic staging studies. If physical examination or extensive associated injuries suggest renal injury, staging studies should be done.

Computed Tomography

We aggressively pursue CT scanning in all patients stable enough to allow it (7). Because modern helical CT scanners can produce images before intravenous contrast is excreted in the urine, we obtain delayed scans (5 to 20 minutes after contrast injection) in all cases of suspected renal injury to allow contrast material to extravasate from the injured collecting system, renal pelvis, or ureter (10,49). For staging renal injuries, CT has several advantages: noninvasiveness, clear delineation of parenchymal lacerations, sensitive detection of urinary extravasation, outlining of nonviable tissue, definition of the extent and size of the surrounding hematoma, detection of associated injury, and provision of three-dimensional views of the kidney and retroperitoneum.

CT also has been useful in detecting arterial injury to the kidney (83,92).

In 85 patients in whom incomplete visualization on excretory urography or nephrotomography prompted suspicion of major renal injury (Table 11A.2), CT clearly differentiated major lacerations and detected extravasation more sensitively than excretory urography (Figs. 11A.5 and 11A.6) (7,32). As a result, CT enabled proper management in all instances. Fifty-two patients were managed nonoperatively, and thirty-three underwent surgery. The renal findings at operation confirmed the observations on CT in all surgical cases. In addition, CT detected major injuries to the liver, spleen, and bowel in seventeen patients.

CT can indirectly detect major vascular injuries (79) and segmental artery injuries. In the patient shown in Fig. 11A.6, in whom excretory urography failed to visualize the kidney after a rapid-deceleration injury, CT demonstrated a nonenhancing soft tissue shadow of a normal-sized kidney on the involved side. One can use angiography to confirm the diagnosis. The major limitation of CT is the lack of detection of venous injuries to the main renal vein or its segmental branches.

Recent innovations in CT technology have shown potential for further improvement in diagnostic accuracy. Techniques such as calculating the volume of perirenal hematoma with CT, then roughly calculating the rate of renal blood loss, have improved the scan's accuracy in small studies (95). The feasibility of using three-dimensional CT reconstruction of renal injuries has also been demonstrated in a small number of patients (73). Although this appears to be a promising enhancement of standard CT, larger studies are required to determine whether it will improve the utility of standard CT imaging enough to enjoy wide use.

Intravenous Pyelography

In patients without a preoperative abdominal CT scan, an intraoperative "one-shot" intravenous pyelogram (IVP) is obtained. This requires 2 mg/kg of intravenous contrast (hypaque sodium 50% [Diatrizoate], Nycomed) given 10 minutes before a plain abdominal film is exposed (76). Standard IVP with multiple images, as would be done to evaluate nontraumatic upper tract disease, is not done. Intraoperative IVP can usually be performed with minimal disruption to the surgical team's efforts to stabilize the patient and is used not only to identify injuries, but also to confirm a functional renal unit on the uninjured side and to determine the presence of urinary extravasation, which can be difficult to detect intraoperatively. It also can exclude the need for renal surgery if findings are absolutely normal and there is only a nonpulsatile/nonexpanding hematoma (i.e., no absolute indication for exploration).

At our institution, intraoperative IVP has safely obviated renal exploration in 32% of patients (76). Although it can at times be insensitive for parenchymal injury, IVP is highly specific for urinary extravasation (14), and some reports have in fact shown it to be highly accurate in staging renal trauma (25,29,53).

TABLE 11A.2. COMPUTED TOMOGRAPHY IN 85 PATIENTS WITH SUSPECTED MAJOR RENAL TRAUMA

		Computed Tomography Findings				
	No. of Patients	Intrarenal Hematoma	Subcapsular Extravasation	Perirenal Hematoma	Parenchymal Disruption	Extracapsular Extravasation
Intravenous Pyelogram						
Subcapsular extravasation	1	0	1	1	0	1
Extracapsular extravasation	2	0	1	2	0	2
Filling defect	3	2	1	2	1	1
Displaced kidney	5	1	1	5	2	0
Irregular cortical margins	6	1	1	3	1	0
Delayed opacification	2	2	1	1	0	1
Diminished opacification	17	10	2	7	8	2
Nonfunction or nonvisualization	2	1	1	1	1	1
Angiography						
Subcapsular extravasation	1	1	1	1	1	1
Extracapsular extravasation	1	1	1	1	1	1
Parenchymal disruption	1	1	1	1	1	1
Vascular obstruction	2	0	0	1	0	0
Surgical Therapy						
Primary closure	4	1	1	4	2	2
Partial nephrectomy	4	1	3	4	4	2
Nephrectomy	3	0	0	3	1	0

From Bretan PN Jr, McAninch JW, Federle MP. Computed tomographic staging of renal trauma: 85 consecutive cases. *J Urol* 1986;136:561, with permission.

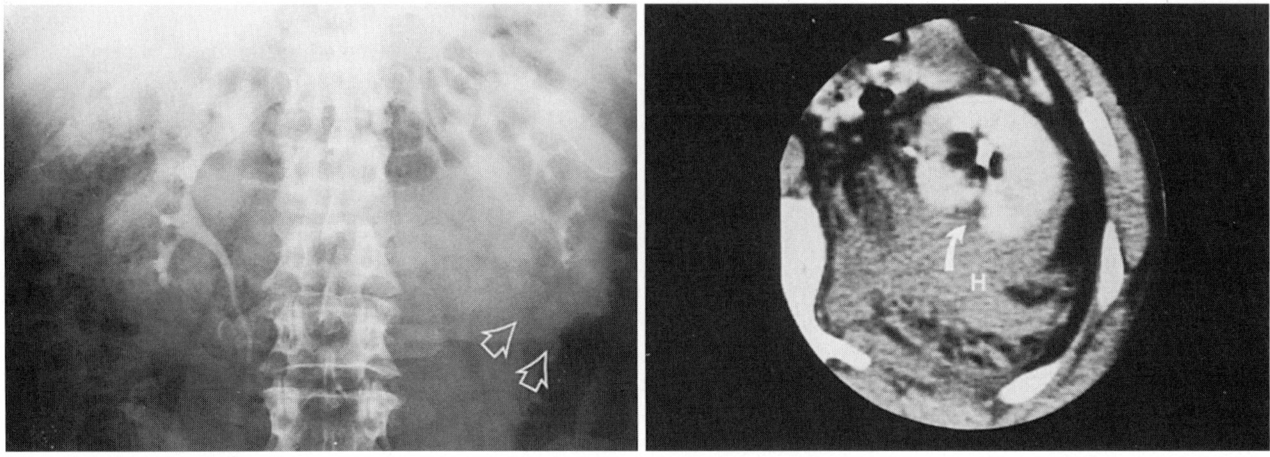

FIGURE 11A.5. **A:** Excretory urogram in a young man with abdominal pain and gross hematuria after blunt trauma reveals poor visualization of the lower pole of the left kidney and lateral deviation *(arrows).* **B:** Computed tomography scan shows retroperitoneal hematoma *(H)* and a minor laceration of the renal parenchyma *(arrow).* Nonoperative management was successful.

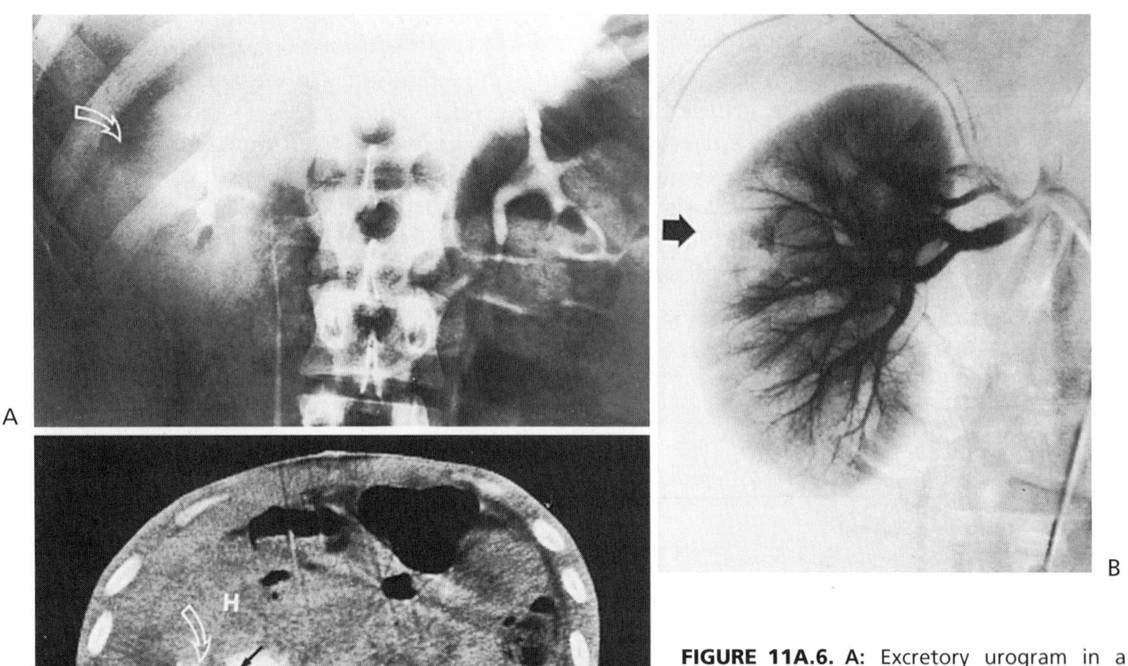

FIGURE 11A.6. **A:** Excretory urogram in a patient with a right flank stab wound and microscopic hematuria suggests a defect in the upper lateral border of the right renal parenchyma *(arrow).* **B:** Arteriography shows a minimum defect in the renal cortex *(arrow)* and no extravasation. **C:** Computed tomography scan reveals a large right renal laceration *(black arrows)* with extensive extravasation of opacified urine *(white arrow).* A large retroperitoneal hematoma is also noted *(H).* Operative repair resulted in renal salvage.

Angiography

In the past, arteriography was the definitive study for staging major renal injuries. With the advent of CT, arteriography has been supplanted. However, it can still provide adequate information for management (54,102). It defines parenchymal lacerations and vascular injuries and is recommended when CT is unavailable. The most common indication for arteriography is nonvisualization of a kidney on excretory urography after major blunt abdominal trauma. Several causes for nonvisualization exist and should be considered: total avulsion of the renal artery and vein; renal artery thrombosis; absence of the kidney, either congenital or from surgical removal; and severe contusion causing major vascular spasm. Either digital subtraction arteriography or conventional arteriography may be used to evaluate vascular injuries. CT can detect vascular injuries (19), but arteriography gives more detailed information and defines the exact anatomic area of vascular injury.

When injuries to the segmental veins, main renal vein, and vena cava are suspected, venography can be used if the patient is stable enough (81). In these injuries, immediate operative intervention may be required to control bleeding and maintain the patient's hemodynamic stability.

Other Imaging Techniques

Although sonography has been used to evaluate and stage renal injuries (4,50,88), it provides less information than CT or arteriography and is unlikely ever to rival the near-100% accuracy of CT. Sonography can detect renal lacerations, but it cannot definitively assess their depth and extent and in one recent study performed very poorly: Experienced sonographers missed renal injuries 78% of the time (69). Furthermore, it cannot accurately detect vascular injuries. Sonographic techniques are improving, however, and it is possible that future use of newer ultrasound modes or contrast agents might improve diagnostic accuracy (44).

The use of radionuclide scanning has been limited. In 24 patients, Chopp and associates (23) combined this method with high-dose excretory urography and found that the number of arteriograms required for further staging was significantly reduced. This technique appears to provide less information than arteriography or CT (35,101).

Retrograde pyelography is of little benefit in evaluating renal injuries but is most useful in detecting associated ureteral or renal pelvic disruptions and perforations (71).

Although CT is still the imaging mode of choice, magnetic resonance imaging (MRI) may play a complementary role in the evaluation of renal trauma. MRI can be used in cases of severe CT contrast allergy, renal insufficiency when intravenous contrast cannot be given, and when CT scan is unavailable (55).

With an orderly approach to the staging of renal trauma, the full extent of the injury can be defined to allow intelligent and accurate management decisions. The ultimate goal of completed staging is to provide sufficient information for management that results in the preservation of renal parenchyma and the salvage of injured kidneys.

INDICATIONS FOR OPERATION

Blunt Trauma

The indications for operative intervention after renal injury vary greatly from one center to another. Blunt traumatic injuries create the most controversy. Contusions, corresponding to grade I injuries, represent 85% to 90% of blunt renal injuries, and in general, series results indicate that they can be managed nonoperatively. The remaining 10% to 15% of blunt injuries constitute minor and major lacerations and vascular injuries, which correspond to grades II to V. Most vascular injuries, when recognized early, call for operation and reconstruction when possible. Need for renorrhaphy or nephrectomy in our last 2,500 renal injury patients is documented in Fig. 11A.7. Management of minor and major lacerations, however, is highly variable. Peterson (80) suggests avoiding renal operation unless bleeding is life-threatening; in most cases, when an operation is required, a nephrectomy should be performed. Cass (17) takes the opposite view and recommends immediate surgical management of major lacerations with or without extravasation. It is difficult to assess individual series because no group has directly compared operative and nonoperative management in a controlled fashion at one institution. The lack of a uniform classification system also makes comparison between series extremely difficult, although more uniform use of the AAST organ injury severity scale should obviate this problem.

Selecting the patient in whom complications are unlikely to develop with nonoperative management is difficult. Delayed bleeding, persistent extravasation with hematoma, and the potential for infection cause concern. Carlton (11) reported that, in his experience, 90% of the complications from expectant treatment occurred in the 10% to 15% of patients with blunt injuries more serious than contusions. Three studies in which nonoperative management was attempted for major renal injuries reported a threefold increase in complications over prompt operative management (46,53,100). Others have noted that when delayed operation is required to manage a complication, total nephrectomy commonly results (45,47).

We take an aggressive approach to staging the injury and thereby obtain adequate information to select the appropriate management, whether it is operative or nonoperative.

Indications for surgical exploration of the kidney can be categorized as absolute and relative. Absolute indications include expanding or uncontained hematoma and pulsatile hematoma, which might indicate the presence of grade V injury. Relative indications include urinary extravasation,

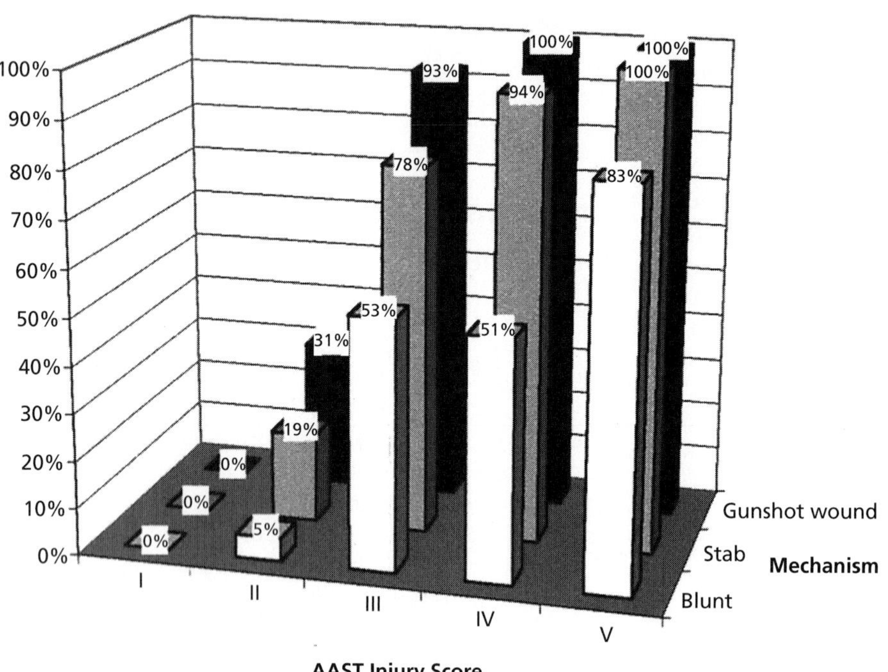

FIGURE 11A.7. The need for renal repair or nephrectomy classified by injury severity (AAST scale) and mechanism of injury (blunt trauma, stab wound, gunshot wound) for 2,500 renal injury patients.

vascular injury, nonviable parenchyma, and incomplete staging. When the degree of urinary extravasation is minor, operation is not required, assuming that no other indication necessitates surgical intervention. Nonviable parenchyma secondary to segmental artery thrombosis without a parenchymal laceration can be followed expectantly with little risk of untoward problems. However, the patient with nonviable tissue involving 20% or more of the kidney in association with a deep parenchymal laceration should have renal exploration and repair to prevent delayed complications. The incompletely staged patient, perhaps already undergoing abdominal exploration for associated injuries, should have renal exploration and repair if necessary (64,68).

In a series of 1,193 patients with blunt renal trauma (68), the preceding indications mandated renal exploration in 31 (2.5%) (Table 11A.3). This experience indicates the high renal salvage rate (87%) that can be achieved in patients who require renal exploration after blunt trauma. With these indications and improved staging techniques, only approximately 2.5% of patients with blunt renal trauma now require renal exploration at our trauma center.

TABLE 11A.3. RENAL INJURIES AT SAN FRANCISCO GENERAL HOSPITAL

	No. of Operations		
Type of Injury	Repair	Nephrectomy	Total Operations
Blunt (1,193 patients)	27	4	31 (2.5%)
Stab wounds (106 patients)	45	4	49 (45%)
Gunshot wounds	46	7	53 (80%)

From McAninch JW, et al. Renal reconstruction after injury. *J Urol* 1991;145:932, with permission.

Penetrating Trauma

Most penetrating renal injuries require operative exploration. Only when preoperative staging clearly indicates that the extent of injury is minor can a nonoperative approach be used successfully. Approximately 70% of patients with penetrating renal injuries at San Francisco General Hospital require operative renal intervention (Table 11A.3). The indications for operative exploration are the same as those listed earlier when careful preoperative staging has been accomplished. Recently, Carroll and McAninch (14) reported that CT provided accurate preoperative assessment in 11 patients with penetrating renal injury and allowed nonoperative management in 8 patients. Associated intraabdominal injuries occur in 80% of patients with penetrating renal injury, and these patients often require immediate surgical intervention with no time allowed for careful preoperative staging (Table 11A.4). In such circumstances, bleeding and life-threatening conditions should be controlled in the operating room, and a "one-shot" excretory urogram should be obtained on the operating table to make certain that at least one normally functioning kidney is present and to gain information regarding the potentially injured kidney. If findings on excretory urography are abnormal, exploration of the ipsilateral kidney should be

TABLE 11A.4. ASSOCIATED ABDOMINAL INJURIES NOTED IN 109 OF 127 PATIENTS

Site of Injury	Number of Patients
Liver	36
Spleen	29
Small bowel	28
Colon	27
Mesentery	20
Stomach	20
Pancreas	19

From McAninch JW, et al. Renal reconstruction after injury. *J Urol* 1991;145:932, with permission.

performed. This careful, selective approach to penetrating renal injuries has not resulted in delayed renal operation at our institution.

Bernath and colleagues (5) and Heyns (42) advocate a nonoperative approach for stab wounds. From their data, it appears that when the entrance site is dorsal to the posterior axillary line, the incidence of associated abdominal injury requiring renal exploration is low.

Heyns and van Vollenhoven (43) have unsuccessfully shown that angiography with selective arterial embolization can control complications of delayed bleeding, which occurred in 15% of their patients initially managed expectantly.

Vascular Injury

Vascular injury of major renal vessels has been reported in 1% to 3% of patients with blunt renal injuries (38,58). Total avulsion of the renal artery and vein, seen after rapid deceleration, is the most serious injury because of acute hemorrhage. Acute renal artery thrombosis also is seen in rapid-deceleration injuries and is difficult to diagnose. The degree of hematuria, if present, is often insignificant (91). Many centers recommend that all patients known to be involved in rapid-deceleration accidents undergo excretory urography, whether hematuria is present or not. However, Mee and colleagues (70) noted that gross hematuria or microhematuria was present in all vascular injuries resulting from blunt trauma in their series, and they recommend selective imaging. When nonvisualization is found on excretory urography, immediate arteriography or CT is indicated.

The free movement of the kidneys in the retroperitoneum results in sudden stretch of the renal artery. The arterial intima, having little elasticity, tears, which produces thrombosis within the vessel lumen (Figs. 11A.8 and 11A.9). This quickly reduces blood flow to the kidney, which may then be viable for only a limited time. Rapid diagnosis and immediate operation are necessary to salvage the kidney (15,60).

Venous injuries of the main renal vein or segmental renal branches constitute a serious, possibly lethal, condition. These injuries can result from blunt or penetrating trauma, and massive blood loss can be expected. Preoperative staging for an accurate diagnosis is difficult because excretory urog-

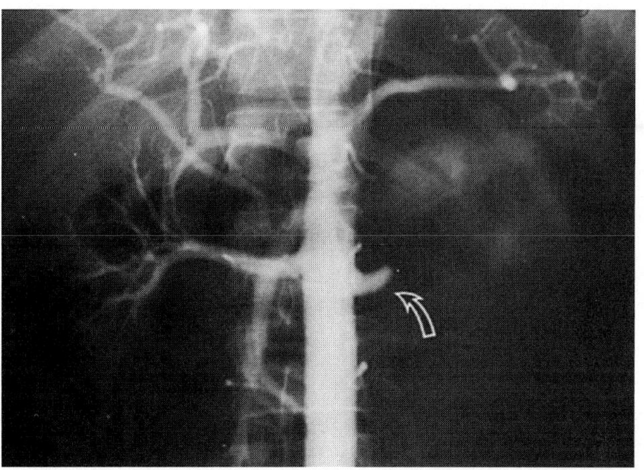

FIGURE 11A.8. In a 29-year-old man with blunt trauma, arteriography demonstrates acute left renal arterial thrombosis. (From McAninch JW. Renal injuries. In: McAninch JW, guest ed. *Urogenital trauma,* vol 2 of Blaisdell WF, Trunkey DD, series eds. *Trauma management*. New York: Thieme Stratton, 1985a:27–49, with permission.)

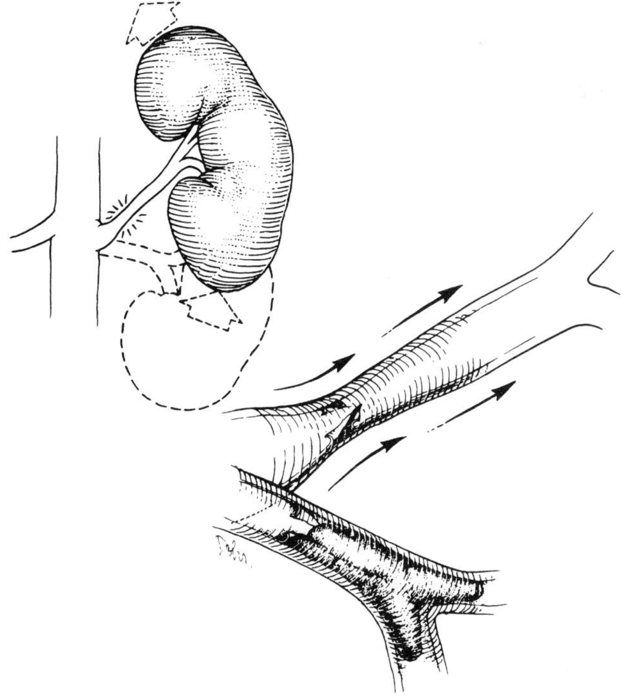

FIGURE 11A.9. Mechanism of arterial thrombosis from blunt trauma. (From McAninch JW. Renal injuries. In: McAninch JW, guest ed. *Urogenital trauma,* vol 2 of Blaisdell WF, Trunkey DD, series eds. *Trauma management*. New York: Thieme Stratton, 1985a:27–49, with permission.)

raphy, nephrotomography, CT, and arteriography do not adequately image venous injuries. Often, particularly on the right side, renal and vena caval injuries coexist (81), and resulting mortality can be as high as 50%.

RETROPERITONEAL HEMATOMA

The general surgeon is often confronted with the unexpected finding of a large retroperitoneal hematoma during exploration for an abdominal injury. Such a hematoma may be found in blunt or penetrating injuries. Historically, exploring the kidney that is surrounded by hematoma has been regarded as hazardous, and complete nephrectomy often has followed (94,99). The urologic surgeon who is called in for consultation should have a systematic approach to evaluating these hematomas. High-dose excretory urography should be performed on the operating room table to evaluate the status of the potentially injured kidney and to confirm the presence of a functioning contralateral renal unit. If the excretory urogram appears normal and no continued expansion of the hematoma is noted, surgical exploration can be avoided. However, when the excretory urogram is indeterminate or abnormal, surgical exploration of the hematoma should be performed. It is imperative to isolate the renal artery and vein before entering the hematoma to control the heavy bleeding that may develop during exploration. In cases of bilateral retroperitoneal hematomas requiring exploration, we choose to explore the kidney suspected of having the lesser injury first, assuming the patient's hemodynamic stability is maintained.

OPERATIVE EXPLORATION AND RENAL EXPOSURE

Once the decision for operative exploration is made, the preferred approach is a midline, transabdominal incision (12,64,89). This allows assessment of other intraabdominal visceral organs and major abdominal vessels. Repair of major vascular, spleen, liver, and bowel injuries should generally be performed before renal exploration and repair. However, if renal bleeding is massive and persistent, renal exploration takes precedence.

To control massive bleeding before renal exploration, it is important to isolate the renal artery and vein individually (Fig. 11A.10A) (9,13,68). The surgeon must be careful to

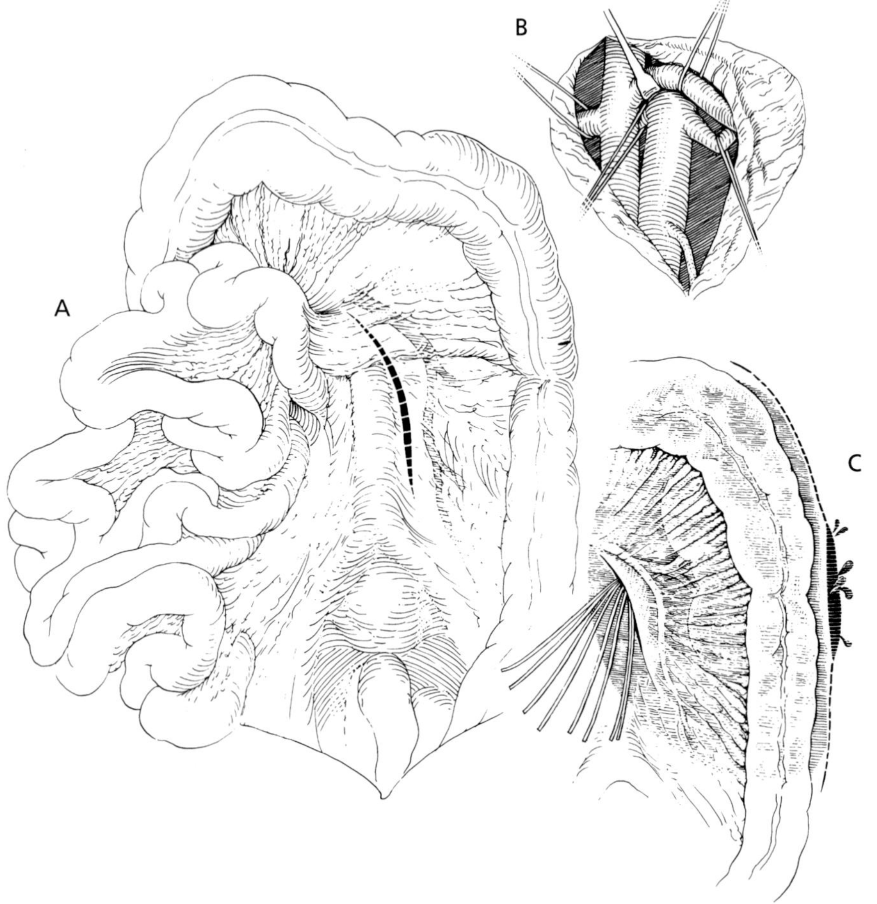

FIGURE 11A.10. Operative approach to renal vessels. **A:** Bowel is retracted superiorly to expose the retroperitoneum, where an incision is made medial to the inferior mesenteric vein over the aorta. **B:** Renal vessels are exposed, and vessel loops are placed. **C:** Hematoma is then entered from a lateral approach. (From McAninch JW, Carroll PR. Renal trauma: kidney preservation through improved vascular control—a refined approach. *J Trauma* 1982;22:285, with permission.)

examine the anatomic relationships within the posterior abdomen and posterior parietal peritoneum before beginning vascular isolation. In many cases, the surgical landmarks are distorted by urinary extravasation and massive hematomas. The transverse colon is lifted from the abdomen and placed on the anterior chest. This allows the small bowel to be lifted free from the abdomen superiorly to the right to expose the small bowel mesentery and the posterior parietal peritoneum.

Anatomic landmarks to be identified at this point are the inferior mesenteric vein and the aorta. If the aorta is covered by large hematoma, an incision can be made in the retroperitoneum just medial to the inferior mesenteric vein; by palpation through the hematoma, the aorta will be found. At this level, the aorta is free of major branches on its anterior surface and is usually easily and safely identified. The aorta is dissected superiorly on the anterior surface up to the area of the ligament of Treitz, where the left renal vein is found crossing anterior to the aorta. This is a major anatomic landmark because the left renal artery originates from the aorta just lateral and superior to the left renal vein, and the right renal artery lies medial and superior as it originates from the aorta (Fig. 11A.10B). Vessel loops of soft silicone can be placed around the individual vessels for retraction and occlusion. In most circumstances, it is unnecessary to occlude the vessels at the time of initial isolation. The right renal vein ordinarily can be isolated through the retroperitoneal incision; however, if it is difficult, mobilization of the second portion of the duodenum readily exposes the right renal vein and vena cava to make the vessel more accessible. Only vessels to the injured kidney need to be isolated.

Once vessel isolation is complete, an incision is made in the peritoneum just lateral to the colon, and the colon is reflected medially to expose the retroperitoneal hematoma in its entirety (Fig. 11A.10C). The kidney should then be totally exposed and mobilized for complete inspection. This can be done quickly and safely without concern for great blood loss because of the vascular control that has been obtained. If heavy bleeding is encountered, vascular clamps or vessel clamps can be used—in our experience, required in 12% of cases. In most circumstances, occlusion of the renal artery beyond 30 minutes is not required, and the kidney tolerates this amount of warm ischemia time well (16). If the time extends beyond this limit, renal cooling is advised during the continued reconstruction process.

Scott and Selzman (89) originally described this technique of early vascular control when exposing a traumatized kidney. Renal bleeding can be prevented and nephrectomy rates reduced. McAninch and Carroll (64) compared a series of patients in whom early vascular control was achieved with another group in whom vascular control was inconsistent (Table 11A.5). The nephrectomy rate in the former group was 18%, and all patients who required nephrectomy had sustained penetrating injuries. In the group with poor vascular control, the nephrectomy rate was 56%—a statistically significant difference. Clearly, when nephrectomy resulting from hemorrhage is prevented, as it can be by this technique, the renal salvage rate is greatly improved.

TABLE 11A.5. NEPHRECTOMY RATES IN PATIENT SERIES WITH AND WITHOUT EARLY VASCULAR CONTROL

Procedure	Early Vascular Control (Series II; 39 Patients), Number (%)	Poor Vascular Control (Series I; 34 Patients), Number (%)
Nephrectomy (n = 26)	7 (18)[a]	19 (56)[a]
Repair (n = 47)	32 (82)	15 (44)

[a] $p < .001$.
Data from McAninch JW, Carroll PR: Renal trauma: kidney preservation through improved vascular control—a refined approach. *J Trauma* 1982;22:285, with permission

Some authors do not advocate isolation of the renal vessels before exploration. Gonzalez and others (37) found no difference in the nephrectomy rate in 56 patients undergoing renal exploration with or without vessel isolation. However, the nephrectomy rate they report is notably higher than that of groups advocating isolation of renal vessels before opening Gerota's fascia. We believe the maneuver, which can be achieved in less than 15 minutes in most cases, is worthwhile and facilitates complex renal reconstruction.

OPERATIVE FINDINGS AND RENAL RECONSTRUCTION

Parenchymal Injuries

Complete renal exposure is of primary importance (Fig. 11A.11). The kidney is often surrounded by large hematoma, which should be completely swept away so that the entire surface area of the kidney and the hilar vessels is available for inspection. If massive bleeding is encountered from a vascular injury or a parenchymal laceration, temporary occlusion of the renal artery may be necessary to control hemorrhage. This is required in 12% of cases (13). Large intrarenal hematomas that reside in lacerations should be completely evaluated and the margins of the laceration inspected (68). All nonviable tissue should be completely removed. Hemostasis should be obtained on the laceration margins with 4-0 chromic sutures on a fine-tapered needle placed in a figure-of-eight over individual bleeding points (Fig. 11A.12). Chromic suture is preferred because its monofilament characteristics allow it to slide through the

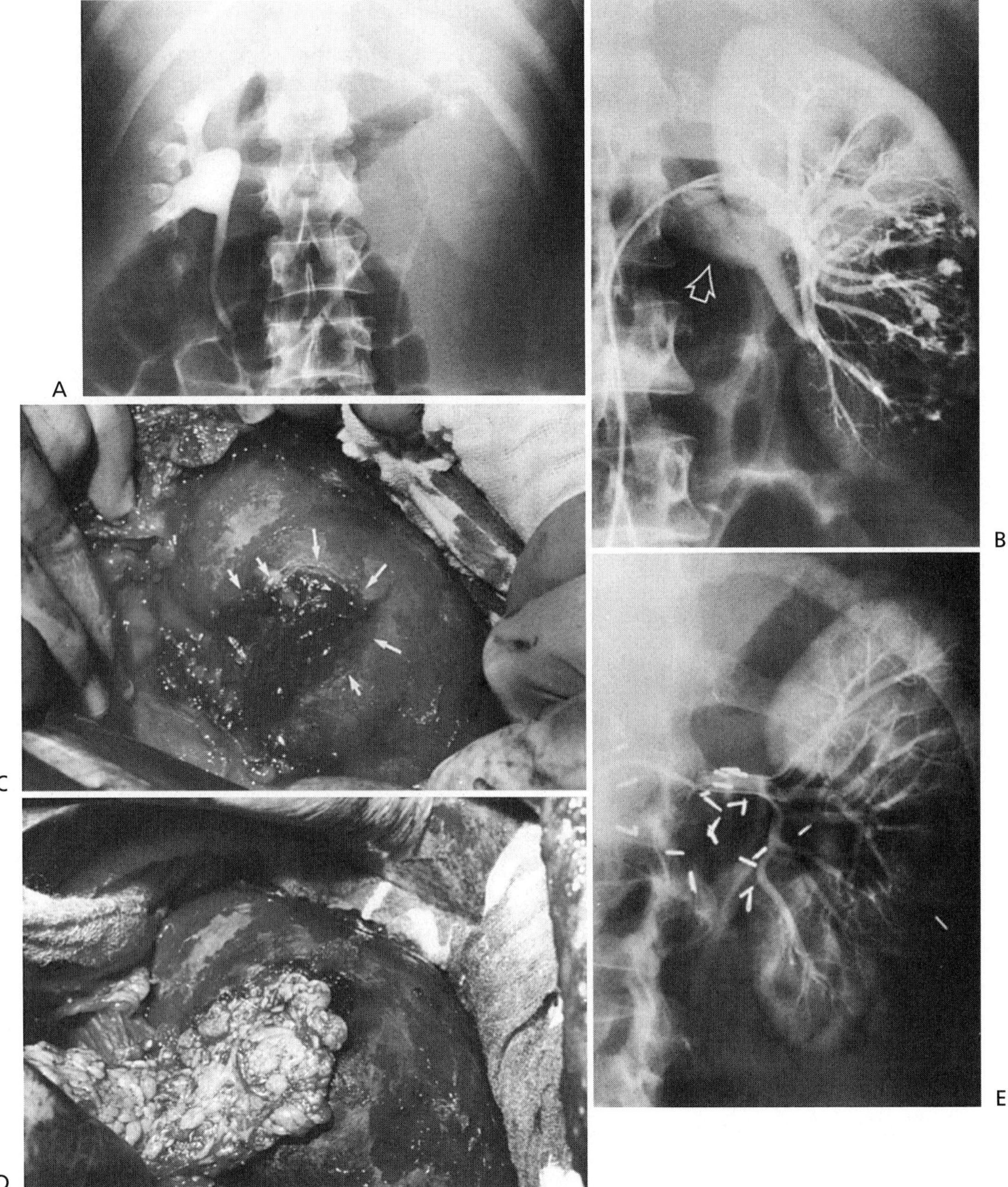

FIGURE 11A.11. **A:** Excretory urogram in a 19-year-old patient with blunt abdominal trauma and gross hematuria demonstrates poor visualization of the left kidney. **B:** Arteriogram shows numerous areas of vascular extravasation in the middle and lower left kidney. The prompt filling of the renal vein indicates massive arteriovenous shunting *(arrow).* **C:** At operation, a deep parenchymal laceration *(arrows)* was noted on the medial aspect of the kidney near the renal hilum. **D:** The laceration was debrided and the bleeding vessels suture ligated. The defect was covered with an omental pedicle flap. **E:** Selective left renal arteriography 6 months after injury demonstrates complete resolution of arteriovenous shunting and healing of the renal laceration. (From McAninch JW, Carroll PR. Renal trauma: kidney preservation through improved vascular control—a refined approach. *J Trauma* 1982;22:285, with permission.)

tissue without tearing or cutting the renal parenchyma. Larger sutures often cause increasing amounts of tissue ischemia and are unnecessary.

As bleeding within the laceration comes under control, inspection should be directed to the collecting system in the depth of the renal laceration. It may be obvious that the collecting system is open; if so, interrupted sutures of 4-0 chromic or 4-0 polydioxanone should be used. Running sutures of the same material may be used to ensure a watertight closure if the collecting system is wide open. Closure of the renal parenchyma over the repaired collecting system provides another barrier to urinary leakage. Between the margins of the lacerated parenchyma, topical absorbable hemostat such as microfibrillar collagen hemostat is placed (Avitene; Bard). The capsule of the kidney is then closed with multiple 3-0 absorbable sutures such as Vicryl on a small taper needle (Fig. 11A.12C). The sutures are tied carefully over a bolster of absorbable gelatin sponge (Gelfoam; Pharmacia/Upjohn; Kalamazoo, Michigan), assisted by hand approximation of the kidney to achieve apposition (Fig. 11A.12D). This technique provides excellent hemostasis and is an aid in any delayed urinary extravasation or delayed bleeding (65). The gelatin sponge is absorbed within 3 weeks; the risk of future infection or calculus formation from its use is minimal (67). To identify the suture line on postoperative CT scans, we place titanium surgical clips (Autosuture Premium Surgiclip II; US Surgical; Norwalk, Connecticut) on the tied sutures. Ureteral stents are not routinely placed unless a renal pelvis injury is identified and repaired.

Often, the capsule will have been destroyed by the traumatic injury and is not available for use in closure. In such cases, we prefer a pedicle flap of omentum to cover the defect and to aid in hemostasis and prevention of urinary extravasation. The omentum has the advantage of being viable tissue, rich in lymphatic vessels and blood supply, which promotes healing of the injured area. When, as is often the case, omentum is not available and fragments of the capsule remain, a patch of perirenal fat or Vicryl mesh (polyglactin) can be placed over the defect and secured with interrupted sutures that catch the margins of the remaining capsule (without extending into the parenchyma), and these can be tied over an absorbable gelatin sponge bolster. In severe cases of renal injury without preservation of capsule, the entire kidney can be wrapped in a polyglycolic acid (Vicryl) mesh bag. This technique holds the injured kidney together until it heals (77).

Multiple lacerations may coexist, and each laceration can be reconstructed similarly. Occasionally after reconstruction and control of hemorrhage within each laceration, the entire

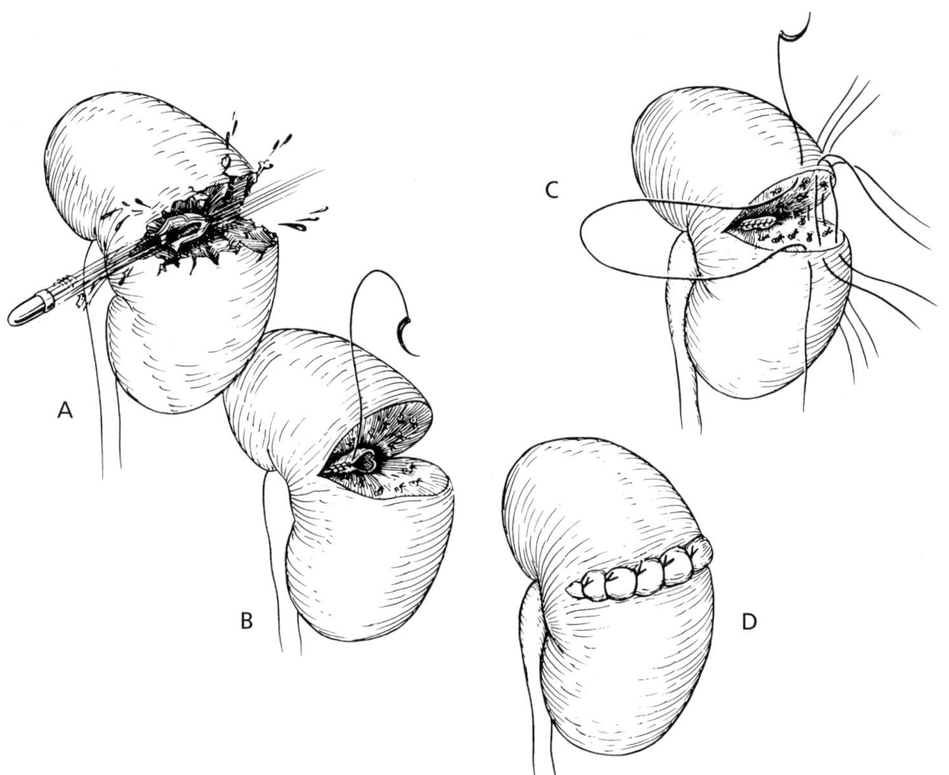

FIGURE 11A.12. Technique of renorrhaphy. **A:** Grade IV injury by gunshot. **B:** Closure of collecting system and ligation of individual bleeding parenchymal vessels. **C:** Closure of the renal defect with multiple interrupted sutures through the renal capsule over gelatin sponge bolster. **D:** Final appearance after repair.

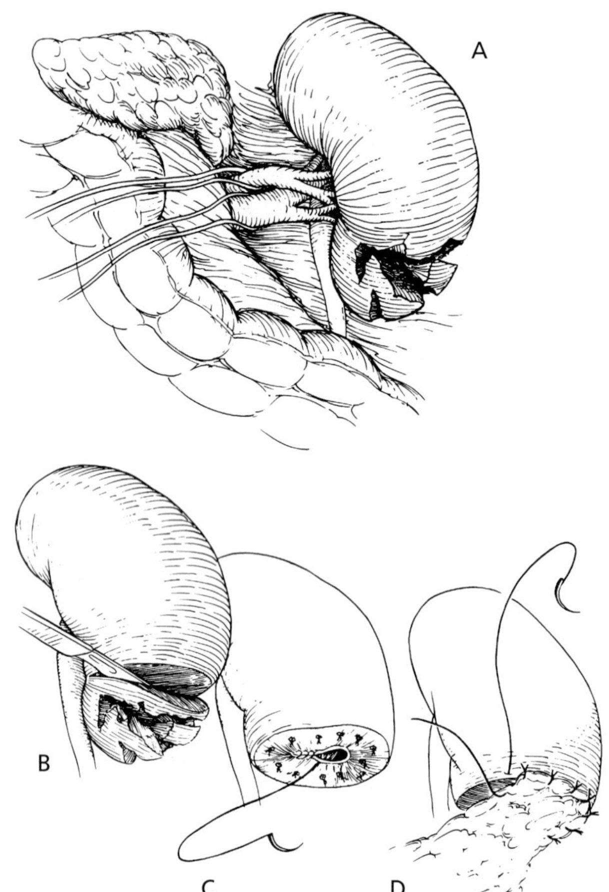

FIGURE 11A.13. Technique of polar nephrectomy for renal injury. **A:** Exposure of kidney with significant lower pole injury. **B:** Sharp amputation of the injured pole. **C:** Ligation of bleeding points with 4-0 chromic suture and watertight closure of the collecting system. **D:** Coverage of the renal defect with omental pedicle flap. (Modified from McAninch JW. Surgery for renal trauma. In: Novick AC, Streem SB, Pontes JE, eds. *Stewart's operative urology.* Baltimore: Williams & Wilkins, 1989:234–239, with permission.)

kidney can be wrapped in omentum to protect it against future problems and to promote wound healing.

Deep lacerations through the upper or lower pole of the kidney may devascularize a large segment of tissue, and a partial nephrectomy may be indicated (Fig. 11A.13A). The capsule should be preserved, and the segmental artery supplying the involved area may require ligation. In most cases, we have been able to spare the segmental vessel, which often supplies additional surrounding tissue, and remove only the nonviable area (Fig. 11A.13B). Hemostasis on the margins of the parenchyma should be achieved with the interrupted suture technique described previously, and the collecting system should be closed carefully (Fig. 11A.13C). To be certain that the closure is watertight, we often occlude the ureter and inject 2 to 3 mL of indigo carmine into the renal pelvis. Any extravasation becomes obvious. Coverage of the renal parenchyma after partial nephrectomy is important. We use any remaining capsule or, if this is unavailable, a pedicle flap of viable omentum (Fig. 11A.13D). If neither of these is available, a free peritoneal graft can be sutured into place over the defect.

Retroperitoneal drains are left in place when there is a question of urinary leakage, but careful management is obligatory to prevent infection that may ascend along a drain tract. The drain is removed on postoperative day 3 if analysis of the drain fluid shows it is not urine. In situations in which urinary extravasation does not occur, drains are unnecessary. They should not be left in place in an attempt to drain retroperitoneal hematoma because they are not effective and only provide an avenue for potential infection. Cefazolin (Kefzol) or similarly appropriate prophylactic antimicrobial coverage is given while the drain is in.

Venous Injuries

Venous injuries cause massive bleeding, and repair on the right is complicated by the shortness of the renal vein and the frequent involvement of the vena cava. Complete occlusion of the vena cava above and below the area of injury temporarily controls bleeding until vascular clamps can be applied to the exact areas of damage. Good results can be expected in a majority of renal vein injuries requiring repair (96). Fine 5-0 vascular sutures should be used to close these defects. The severely injured left renal vein can be ligated if necessary because venous collaterals will adequately drain the kidney (9). Segmental renal vein injuries are best managed by ligation of the vessel. This does not cause ischemic damage because of the inner communication of the veins within the renal parenchyma.

Renal Artery Occlusion

Controversy surrounds the treatment of traumatic total renal artery occlusion. Some authors claim that acceptable success rates can be achieved by prompt revascularization (within 4 to 12 hours) (3,57). However, in multiple studies, the success of revascularization has been poor, approaching 0% (24,40,51,96). Current recommendations are to perform nephrectomy in most cases of traumatic renal artery occlusion, except in patients with solitary kidney or bilateral renal artery injury. Percutaneous placement of an endoluminal stent may be the best method of treatment (97).

Renal Artery Laceration

All patients with renal artery injuries must be treated individually in light of recent evidence that renal salvage is often not achieved in this population (51). Only those patients who can safely undergo several hours of operation in the periinjury period are candidates for renal artery repair. Patients with vascular injuries to the main renal artery occurring from blunt trauma who have delayed diagnosis (more than 8 hours) or who are older (seven decades) have little chance of successful arterial reconstruction. In large series, renal lacerations have required nephrectomy in many cases (76%) (9); when vascular repair was attempted, it was successful in only 60%.

Renal branch injuries, on the other hand, are much less significant lesions that can be managed nonoperatively or, when they are discovered intraoperatively, treated by ligation (6). Angiographic embolization of branch artery injuries after stab wounds (30,36) or blunt trauma (28) also has been advocated.

Renal Pedicle Avulsion

Total renal pedicle avulsion, which involves complete laceration of the renal artery and vein from their attachments, requires immediate surgical intervention and does not allow time for diagnostic studies. Authors have suggested renal salvage in these patients only under extreme circumstances: A stable patient who can undergo lengthy operation, solitary kidney, and bilateral injury. If repair is attempted, autotransplantation appears to be the most successful approach (39).

POSTOPERATIVE CARE AND FOLLOW-UP

The postoperative care of the patient with renal trauma is similar to that for any major transabdominal surgical procedure, with nasogastric suction or gastrostomy as needed for bowel decompression and urethral catheter drainage until the patient is stable enough to void. Antibiotics should be given for bowel perforation or severely contaminated wounds. If the urine is infected, preoperative and postoperative antibiotics should be continued through a full 10-day course.

In most circumstances, the urine becomes free of clots within the first 12 to 24 hours and free of gross blood within 48 hours. Serial hematocrit readings should be obtained to make certain that continued bleeding does not occur. When drains are left in place, significant drainage is often noted, although this is commonly intraperitoneal fluid and not urine. One should check the creatinine content of the fluid, which will be many times the serum concentration if urine is present. Intravenous injection of methylene blue also may be used to evaluate possible urinary extravasation. Blood pressure should be followed closely in the early postoperative period as well as later on, for at least 1 year.

Patients can be discharged as soon as retroperitoneal drains are out and they are stable and eating. At the time of discharge, patients are allowed free ambulation without restriction and should be encouraged to return to normal physical activity as soon as the incisional pain subsides.

The patient should be seen in follow-up every 1 to 2 weeks for the first 6 weeks to monitor blood pressure and evaluate the urine for the presence of blood. Hypertension is uncommon, and microscopic hematuria should gradually subside. Approximately 3 weeks after injury, the patient should have a follow-up CT scan of the kidneys to evaluate the anatomic configuration of the kidney and to verify that no obstruction has resulted from perirenal scarring. Renal radionuclide scans are often helpful in evaluating the functional status of the injured kidney.

COMPLICATIONS

Early complications occur within the first 4 weeks of injury and include delayed bleeding, abscess, sepsis, urinary fistula, urinary extravasation and urinoma, and hypertension (48,90,98). Delayed bleeding can occur from the immediate postoperative period until several weeks later. The greatest risk of delayed heavy retroperitoneal bleeding occurs within the first 2 weeks of injury. Angioembolization is the primary treatment for delayed renal bleeding after trauma (43), but speedy nephrectomy may be required if bleeding is brisk. Abscess may develop in the perinephric space and in most circumstances is noted within the first 7 days. This may be associated with sepsis and is manifested by increasing temperature that may reach 41°C. Prompt surgical exploration and drainage are usually required; however, after appropriate diagnostic procedures, localized abscesses may be drained percutaneously. Symptoms of urinary extravasation in the first 4 weeks of injury may be manifested by a low-grade fever and continued pain in the area of the kidney. CT can aid in establishing the diagnosis and extent of extravasation. Retrograde ureterography should be performed if missed ureteral injury is a possibility. Percutaneous drainage has successfully managed extensive extravasation, but small amounts of urine in the retroperitoneal space appear to be of no particular consequence if they remain uninfected; these often resolve spontaneously without intervention. Hypertension in the postoperative period is uncommon; however, its presence and duration are extremely variable (98). In most circumstances, the hypertension does not require treatment; when indicated, medical therapy usually controls the problem. The hypertension appears to be renin mediated in most cases and is usually transient when it occurs in the early postinjury period.

Late complications include arteriovenous fistula, hydronephrosis, hypertension, calculus formation, and chronic pyelonephritis. Delayed hypertension has been noted by several authors. In a group of patients who had careful follow-up, Jakse and colleagues (48) noted the onset of hypertension some 15 years after renal trauma. Longstanding hypertension persists because of partial renal ischemia, resulting in a renin-mediated type of hypertension (90). Most cases can be managed medically, but surgical intervention may be necessary in unresponsive patients. Montgomery and others (74) have described a cohort of renal trauma patients in whom initial evaluation (CT or IVP) was normal, yet who developed severe renovascular hypertension 2 weeks to 8 months after injury. Subsequent arteriography revealed unappreciated renal artery occlusion, arterial stenosis, segmental artery injuries, or extraparenchymal compression from scarring (Page kidney). Although all were young, these patients presented with complaints, including headaches, chest pain, nosebleeds and fatigue. Vigilance for hypertension is necessary in this population, even when severe renal injury is not expected. Arteriovenous fistulae are caused by both blunt and penetrating injuries but mainly by stab wounds (26). Delayed urinary bleeding is the usual presenting symptom, and many patients have associated hypertension. Angioembolization is the treatment of choice (84), but large fistulae require surgical correction and perhaps nephrectomy. Hydronephrosis can develop in the late postoperative period because of surrounding fibrosis and obstruction to the upper ureter or ureteropelvic junction. This condition may lead to calculus formation or recurrent pyelonephritis or both.

To detect many of these developing delayed complications, a CT scan is strongly recommended within 3 months of major renal injury. Additional follow-up should be done in these patients when persistent problems or suspicion of abnormalities exists.

REFERENCES

1. Ahmed S, Morris LL. Renal parenchymal injuries secondary to blunt abdominal trauma in childhood: a 10-year review. *Br J Urol* 1982;54:470.
2. Banowsky LH, Wolfel DA, Lackner LH. Considerations in diagnosis and management of renal trauma. *J Trauma* 1970; 10:587.
3. Barlow B, Gandhi R. Renal artery thrombosis following blunt trauma. *J Trauma* 1980;20:614.
4. Berger PE, Munschauer RW, Kuhn JP. Computed tomography and ultrasound of renal and perirenal diseases in infants and children: relationship to excretory urography in renal cystic disease, trauma and neoplasm. *Pediatr Radiol* 1980;9:91.
5. Bernath AS, Schutte H, Fernandes RRD, et al. Stab wounds of the kidney: conservative management in flank penetration. *J Urol* 1983;129:468.
6. Bertini JE Jr, Flechner SM, Miller P, et al. The natural history of traumatic branch renal artery injury. *J Urol* 1986;135:228.
7. Bretan PN Jr, McAninch JW, Federle MP, et al. Computed tomographic staging of renal trauma: 85 consecutive cases. *J Urol* 1986;136:561.
8. Bright TC, White K, Peters PC. Significance of hematuria after trauma. *J Urol* 1978;120:455.
9. Brown MF, Graham JM, Mattox KL, et al. Renovascular trauma. *Am J Surg* 1980;140:802.
10. Brown SL, Hoffman DM, Spirnak JP. Limitations of routine spiral computerized tomography in the evaluation of blunt renal trauma. *J Urol* 1998;160:1979.
11. Carlton CE Jr. Injuries of the kidney and ureter. In: Harrison JH, et al., eds. *Campbell's urology.* Philadelphia: WB Saunders, 1978:881–905.
12. Carlton CE Jr, Scott R Jr, Goldman M. The management of penetrating injuries of the kidney. *J Trauma* 1968;8:1071.
13. Carroll PR, Klosterman P, McAninch JW. Early vascular control for renal trauma: a critical review. *J Urol* 1989;141:826.
14. Carroll PR, McAninch JW. Operative indications in penetrating renal trauma. *J Trauma* 1985;25:587.
15. Carroll PR, et al. Renovascular trauma: risk assessment, surgical management, and outcome. *J Trauma* 1990;30:547.
16. Carroll PR, et al. Outcome after temporary vascular occlusion for management of renal trauma. *J Urol* 1994;151:1171.
17. Cass AS. Blunt renal trauma in children. *J Trauma* 1983; 23:123.
18. Cass AS, Luxenberg M. Conservative or immediate surgical management of blunt renal injuries. *J Urol* 1983;130:11.
19. Cass AS, Luxenberg M. Accuracy of computed tomography in diagnosing renal artery injuries. *Urology* 1989;34:249.
20. Chandhoke PS, McAninch JW. Detection and significance of microscopic hematuria in patients with blunt abdominal trauma. *J Urol* 1987;140:16.
21. Charters AC III, Charters AC. Wounding mechanisms of very high velocity projectiles. *J Trauma* 1976;16:464.
22. Chen DL, Lazan D, Stone N. Conservative treatment of type III renal trauma. *J Trauma* 1994;36:491.
23. Chopp RT, Hekmat-Ravan H, Mendez R. Technetium-99m glucoheptonate renal scan in diagnosis of acute renal injury. *Urology* 1980;15:201.
24. Clark DE, Georgitis JW, Ray FS. Renal arterial injuries caused by blunt trauma. *Surgery* 1981;90:87.
25. Coppa GF, Davalle M, Pachter HL, et al. Management of penetrating wounds to the back and flank. *Surg Gynecol Obstet* 1984;159:514.
26. Cosgrove MD, Mendez R, Morrow JW. Traumatic renal arteriovenous fistula: report of 12 cases. *J Urol* 1973;110:627.
27. Danto LA. Paracentesis and diagnostic peritoneal lavage. In: Blaisdell WF, Trunkey DD, eds. *Trauma management,* vol 1. New York: Thieme Stratton, 1982.
28. DeBock L, Verhagen PF. Selective embolization in the treatment of severe blunt renal injury. *Neth J Surg* 1989;41:31.
29. Eastham JA, Wilson TG, Ahlering TE. Urological evaluation and management of renal-proximity stab wounds. *J Urol* 1993; 150:1771.
30. Eastham JA, Wilson TG, Larsen DW, et al. Angiographic embolization of renal stab wounds. *J Urol* 1992;148:268.
31. Ersay A, Akgun Y. Experience with renal gunshot injuries in a rural setting. *Urology* 1999;54:972.
32. Erturk E, Sheinfeld J, DiMarco PL, et al. Renal trauma: evaluation by computerized tomography. *J Urol* 1985;133:946.
33. Fackler ML. Gunshot wound review. *Ann Emerg Med* 1996; 28:194.
34. Fackler ML, Surinchak JS, Malinowski JA, et al. Bullet fragmentation: a major cause of tissue disruption. *J Trauma* 1984; 24:35.
35. Federle MP, Kaiser JA, McAninch JW, et al. The role of computed tomography in renal trauma. *Radiology* 1981; 141:455.
36. Fisher RG, Ben-Menachem Y, Whigham C. Stab wounds of the renal artery branches: angiographic diagnosis and treatment by embolization. *AJR Am J Roentgenol* 1989;152:1231.
37. Gonzalez RP, Falimirksi M, Holevar MR, et al. Surgical management of renal trauma: Is vascular control necessary? *J Trauma* 1999;47:1039.
38. Guerriero WG, Carlton CE Jr, Scott R Jr, et al. Renal pedicle injuries. *J Trauma* 1971;11:53.

39. Guttman FM, Homsy Y, Schmidt E. Avulsion injury to the renal pedicle: successful autotransplantation after "bench surgery." *J Trauma* 1978;18:469.
40. Haas CA, Dinchman KH, Nasrallah PF, et al. Traumatic renal artery occlusion: a 15-year review. *J Trauma* 1998;45:557.
41. Hardeman SW, Husmann DA, Chinn HK, et al. Blunt urinary tract trauma: identifying those patients who require radiologic diagnostic studies. *J Urol* 1987;138:99.
42. Heyns CF, de Klerk DP, de Kock MLS. Stab wounds associated with hematuria—a review of 67 cases. *J Urol* 1983;130:228.
43. Heyns CF, von Hollenhoven P. Increasing role of angiography and segmental artery embolization in management of renal stab wounds. *J Urol* 1992;147:1231.
44. Hochmuth A, Fleck M, Hauff P, et al. First experiences in using a new ultrasound mode and ultrasound contrast agent in the diagnosis of blunt renal trauma: a feasibility study in an animal model. *Invest Radiol* 2000;35:205.
45. Holcroft JW, Trunkey DD, Minagi H, et al. Renal trauma and retroperitoneal hematomas—indications for exploration. *J Trauma* 1975;15:1045.
46. Husmann DA, Gilling PJ, Perry MO, et al. Major renal lacerations with a devitalized fragment following blunt abdominal trauma: a comparison between nonoperative (expectant) versus surgical management. *J Urol* 1993;150:1774.
47. Husmann DA, Morris JS. Attempt at nonoperative management of blunt renal lacerations extending through the corticomedullary junction: short-term and long-term sequelae. *J Urol* 1990;143:682.
48. Jakse G, Putz A, Gassner I, et al. Early surgery in the management of pediatric blunt renal trauma. *J Urol* 1984;131:920.
49. Kawashima A, Sandler CM, Corriere JN Jr, et al. Ureteropelvic junction injuries secondary to blunt abdominal trauma. *Radiology* 1997;205:487.
50. Kay CJ, Rosenfield AT, Armm M. Gray-scale ultrasonography in the evaluation of renal trauma. *Radiology* 1980;134:461.
51. Knudson M, Harrison P, Hoyt D, et al. Outcome following major renovascular injuries: a WTA multi-center report. *J Trauma* 2000;48:191.
52. Krieger JN, Algood CB, Mason JT, et al. Urological trauma in Pacific Northwest: etiology, distribution, management and outcome. *J Urol* 1984;132:70.
53. Kristjansson A, Pedersen J. Management of blunt renal trauma. *Br J Urol* 1993;72:692.
54. Lang EK. Arteriography in the assessment of renal trauma: the impact of arteriographic diagnosis on preservation of renal function and parenchyma. *J Trauma* 1975;15:553.
55. Lappaniemi A, Lamminen A, Tervahartiala P, et al. MRI and CT in blunt renal trauma: an update. *Semin Ultrasound CT MRI* 1997;18:129.
56. Lindsey D. The idolatry of velocity, or lies, damn lies, and ballistics. *J Trauma* 1980;20: 1068.
57. Lock JS, Carraway RP, Hudson HC Jr, et al. Proper management of renal artery injury from blunt trauma. *South Med J* 1985;78:406.
58. Lohse JR, Botham RJ, Waters RF. Traumatic bilateral renal artery thrombosis: case report and review of literature. *J Urol* 1982;127:522.
59. Matthews LA, Smith EM, Spirnak JP. Nonoperative treatment of major blunt renal lacerations with urinary extravasation. *J Urol* 1997;157:2056.
60. McAninch JW. Acute renal artery thrombosis following blunt trauma. *Urology* 1975;6:74.
61. McAninch JW. Renal injuries. In: McAninch JW, guest ed. *Urogenital trauma,* vol 2 of Blaisdell WF, Trunkey DD, series eds. *Trauma management.* New York: Thieme Stratton, 1985a: 27–49.
62. McAninch JW. Renal trauma. In: Resnick MI, ed. *Current trends in urology,* vol 3. Baltimore: Williams & Wilkins, 1985b.
63. McAninch JW. Surgery for renal trauma. In: Novick AC, Streem SB, Pontes JE, eds. *Stewart's operative urology.* Baltimore: Williams & Wilkins, 1989:234–239.
64. McAninch JW, Carroll PR. Renal trauma: kidney preservation through improved vascular control—a refined approach. *J Trauma* 1982;22:285.
65. McAninch JW, Carroll PR. Renal exploration after trauma: indications and reconstructive techniques. *Urol Clin North Am* 1989;16:203.
66. McAninch JW, Federle MP. Evaluation of renal injuries with computerized tomography. *J Urol* 1982;128:456.
67. McAninch JW, Rodkey WG, Stutzman RE, et al. Experimental penetrating renal trauma: a comparison of bench and in situ repair. *Invest Urol* 1979;17:33.
68. McAninch JW, et al. Renal reconstruction after injury. *J Urol* 1991;145:932.
69. McGahan JP, Richards JR, Jones CD, et al. Use of ultrasonography in the patient with acute renal trauma. *J Ultrasound Med* 1999;18:207.
70. Mee SL, McAninch JW, Robinson AL, et al. Radiographic assessment of renal trauma: a 10-year prospective study of patient selection. *J Urol* 1989;141:1095.
71. Mendez R. Renal trauma. *J Urol* 1977;118:698.
72. Meng MV, Brandes SB, McAninch JW. Renal trauma: indications and techniques for surgical exploration. *World J Urol* 1999;17:71.
73. Michel LA, Lacrosse M, Decanniere L, et al. Blunt renal traumas: contribution of spiral CT with three dimensional reconstruction to the surgical decision process? *Int Surg* 1996; 81:377.
74. Montgomery RC, Richardson JD, Harty JI. Posttraumatic renovascular hypertension after occult renal injury. *J Trauma* 1998;45:106.
75. Moore EE, et al. Organ injury scaling: spleen, liver, and kidney. *J Trauma* 1989;29:1664.
76. Morey AF, McAninch JW, Tiller BK, et al. Single shot intraoperative excretory urography for the immediate evaluation of renal trauma. *J Urol* 1999;161:1088.
77. Mounzer AM, McAninch JW, Schmidt RA. Polyglycolic acid mesh in repair of renal injury. *Urology* 1986;28:127.
78. Nicolaisen GS, McAninch JW, Marshall GA, et al. Renal trauma: reevaluation of the indications for radiographic assessment. *J Urol* 1985;133:183.
79. Nunez D Jr, Becerra JL, Fuentes D, et al. Traumatic occlusion of the renal artery: helical CT diagnosis. *AJR Am J Roentgenol* 1996;167:777.
80. Peterson NE. Intermediate-degree blunt renal trauma. *J Trauma* 1977;17:425.
81. Peterson NE, Millikan JS, Moore EE. Combined renal and vena caval trauma: a review of personal and recorded experience. *J Urol* 1985;133:567.
82. Radwin HM, Fitch WP, Robison JR. A unified concept of renal trauma. *J Urol* 1976;116:20.
83. Reagan K, Beckmann CF, Larsen CR, et al. Renal infarction: computerized tomographic appearance with angiographic correlation. *J Urol* 1984;132:331.
84. Reilly KJ, Shapiro MB, Haskal ZJ. Angiographic embolization of a penetrating traumatic renal arteriovenous fistula. *J Trauma* 1996;41:763.

85. Sagalowsky AI, McConnell JD, Peters PC. Renal trauma requiring surgery: an analysis of 185 cases. *J Trauma* 1983; 23:128.
86. Santucci RA, Mario LA, McAninch JW. Grade IV renal injuries: evaluation, treatment and outcome. *World J Surg* 2000 (in press).
87. Santucci RA, Mario LA, Segal MR, et al. Classification trees are highly predictive of need for surgery in renal trauma patients. *J Urol* 2000;163[Suppl]:4 (abst14).
88. Schmoller H, Kunit G, Frick J. Sonography in blunt renal trauma. *Eur Urol* 1981;7:11.
89. Scott RF Jr, Selzman HM. Complications of nephrectomy: review of 450 patients and a description of a modification of the transperitoneal approach. *J Urol* 1965;95:307.
90. Spark RF, Berg S. Renal trauma and hypertension: the role of renin. *Arch Intern Med* 1976;136:1097.
91. Stables DP, Fouche RF, de Villiers van Niekerk JP, et al. Traumatic renal artery occlusion: 21 cases. *J Urol* 1976;115:229.
92. Steinberg DL, Jeffrey RB, Federle MP, et al. The computerized tomography appearance of renal pedicle injury. *J Urol* 1984; 132:1163.
93. Sykes LN Jr, Champion HR, Fouty WJ. Dum-dums, hollow-points, and devastators: techniques designed to increase wounding potential of bullets. *J Trauma* 1988;28:618.
94. Thompson IM, Latourette H, Montie JE, et al. Results of nonoperative management of blunt renal trauma. *J Urol* 1977; 118:522.
95. Tong YC, Chun JS, Tsai HM, et al. Use of hematoma size on computerized tomography and calculated average bleeding rate as indications for immediate surgical intervention in blunt renal trauma. *J Urol* 1992;147:984.
96. Turner WW Jr, Snyder WH, Fry WJ. Mortality and renal salvage after renovascular trauma. A review of 94 patients treated in a 20 year period. *Am J Surg* 1983;146:848.
97. Villas PA, Cohen G, Putnam SG III, et al. Wallstent placement in a renal artery after blunt abdominal trauma. *J Trauma* 1999;46:1137.
98. von Knorring J, Fyhrquist P, Ahonen J. Varying course of hypertension following renal trauma. *Radiology* 1980; 131:461.
99. Wein AJ, Murphy JJ, Mulholland SG, et al. A conservative approach to the management of blunt renal trauma. *J Urol* 1977;117:425.
100. Wilson RF, Ziegler DW. Diagnostic and treatment problems in renal injuries. *Am Surg* 1987;53:399.
101. Woodruff JH Jr, Cockett ATK, Cannon R, et al. Radiologic aspects of renal trauma with the emphasis on arteriography and renal isotope scanning. *J Urol* 1967;97:184.
102. Wynn WW, Ricketts HJ, McRoberts JW, et al. Comparison of arteriography, venography, and pyelography in experimental renal trauma. *Invest Urol* 1978;16:62.

11B

URETERAL INJURIES

JOSEPH N. CORRIERE, JR.

The sole function of the ureter is to transport urine from the kidney to the bladder. When the ureter is injured, it may become obstructed, creating hydroureteronephrosis and loss of renal function, or a fistula may occur, leading to urinary extravasation into the retroperitoneum or peritoneal cavity. If injury to another structure has occurred at the time of the ureteral injury, a fistula may develop. Most fistulae are to the vagina, skin, or bowel.

Extravasated urine can induce an intense inflammatory reaction, resulting in secondary fibrosis and ureteral obstruction. If the urine is infected, phlegmon and possibly life-threatening sepsis may develop, necessitating emergency surgical intervention.

In the past few years, the use of percutaneous and endourologic techniques has decreased the complications from ureteral injuries and prevented many patients from having to undergo open surgical procedures that once were standard therapy for these distressing problems.

ETIOLOGY

There are two major types of ureteral injuries: those caused by external violence, usually penetrating missiles, and the more common injuries resulting from surgical misadventure. The late complications of radiotherapy or migrating foreign bodies also can cause injury to the ureter. Table 11B.1 lists the various causes of ureteral injury.

Injury Caused by External Violence

The most common cause of ureteral injury from external violence is gunshot wounds. These wounds account for more than 95% of the lesions (7,8,22,32,38,40–42,45,54). Knife wounds are the next most common agent, and very rarely, people fall and become impaled on a spike. Uncommonly, the wound from a crushing blow that damages bone involves the ureter. Finally, a well-described but rare injury occurs when the ureter is avulsed from the renal pelvis (Fig. 11B.1) (3,28). This injury is usually seen in a child who has a hyperextensible spinal column. The child is usually struck from behind, and the ureter tenses and snaps against the twelfth rib and transverse processes of the upper lumbar vertebrae. This injury as well as lower ureteral rupture secondary to blunt trauma can be seen in adults as well as children (13,24,26).

Surgical Injury

Ureteral injury may complicate 0.5% to 1.0% of all pelvic operations. Most of these are gynecologic procedures, but urinary tract procedures commonly account for 30%. The most common procedures are hysterectomy, salpingo-oophorectomy, vesicourethral suspension, ureteroscopy, endopyelotomy, and ureterolithotomy (5,9,14–16,34,47, 51,52).

J.N. Corriere, Jr.: Department of Surgery, Division of Urology, The University of Texas, Houston, TX 77030.

Surgical procedures on the great vessels and colon as well as retroperitoneal tumor excision are the next most common procedures leading to ureteral injury (4,6,31,46,48). As listed in Table 11B.1, many other procedures have been implicated infrequently (2,27). In the last few years, laparoscopic procedures have become a common cause of ureteral injuries (17,55,57).

Radiation Injury

Although radiation injury is often considered when a patient with a previously treated pelvic tumor is found to have ureteral obstruction, the incidence of radiation damage to the ureter is only 0.04%, whereas the incidence of ureteral obstruction caused by recurrent tumor in these patients is more than 95% (12,59).

TABLE 11B.1. CAUSES OF URETERAL INJURIES

External Violence	***Urinary Tract Procedures (continued)***
Penetrating Injuries	Transurethral resection of the prostate
Gunshot wound	Radical prostatectomy
Knife wound	***Vascular Surgery***
Impalement on spike	Vena cava ligation
Blunt Injuries	Aortic aneurysmectomy
Avulsion	Bypass procedures
Crushing injury	Lumbar sympathectomy
Surgical Injuries	***Abdominal Procedures***
Gynecologic Procedures	Colectomy
Abdominal hysterectomy	Colostomy
Vaginal hysterectomy	Colostomy closure
Salpingo-oophorectomy	Abdominoperineal resection
Vesicovaginal fistula repair	Appendectomy
Dilation and curettage	Exploratory laparotomy
Excision of cervical stump	Enterolysis
Cystocele repair	Duodenal resection
Colpocleisis	Pancreatic surgery
Endometrioma resection	Herniorrhaphy
Obstetric Procedures	Biliary surgery
Forceps delivery	***Retroperitoneal Procedures***
Precipitous delivery	Retroperitoneal fibrosis surgery
Cesarean section	Retroperitoneal lymphadenectomy
Therapeutic abortion	Retroperitoneal tumor resection
Urinary Tract Procedures	***Laparoscopic Procedures***
Retrograde pyelogram	***Neurosurgical Procedures***
Ureteroscopy	Laminectomy
Endopyelotomy	Paravertebral nerve block
Ureterolithotomy	**Radiation Injury**
Renal pelvic surgery	**Migrating Foreign Bodies**
Vesicourethral suspension	Urinary calculi
Vesicocolic fistula repair	Bullets
Suprapubic excision of bladder tumor	Swallowed objects
Bladder diverticulectomy	
Stone basket manipulation	
Transurethral resection of a bladder tumor	

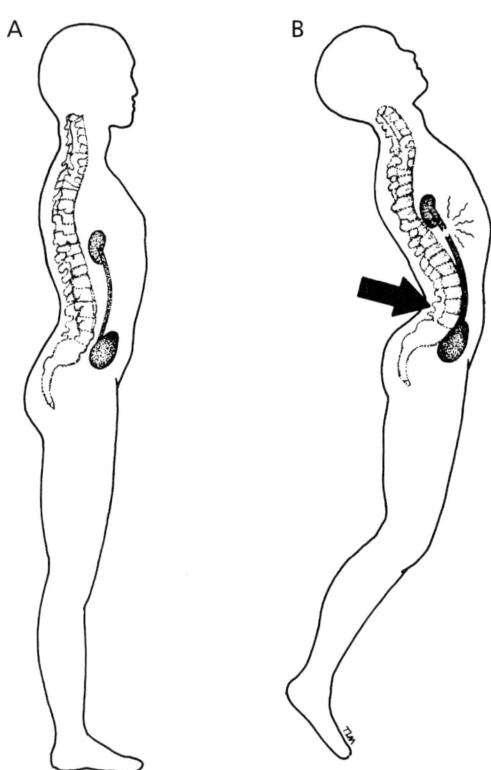

FIGURE 11B.1. A: Normal relation of urinary tract to spine in child. **B:** With a sudden blow to back, the ureter tenses against the hyperextended vertebral column and avulses at the ureteropelvic junction.

Migratory Foreign Bodies

The most common migratory foreign bodies that perforate or obstruct the ureter are urinary calculi, bullets, and swallowed objects (18,43).

DIAGNOSIS

External Violence Injury

An excretory urogram or computed tomography (CT) scan with contrast must be performed when a patient has had a penetrating injury of the abdomen, retroperitoneum, or pelvis in the area of the urinary tract; a fracture of the eleventh or twelfth rib; or a transverse lumbar process or the bony pelvis is present. Such a test should also be performed if hematuria is present in a patient who has had significant abdominal or pelvic trauma.

The excretory urogram and CT scan with contrast are the best methods of diagnosing a ureteral injury. In the presence of such an injury, urinary extravasation will be seen on the study as well as some decrease in collecting system visualization (Fig. 11B.2). If a spiral CT scan is performed, the ureter must be seen in its entirety. If it is not, a delayed CT scan must be done or an injury may be missed because of the rapid time of the spiral study (37,50).

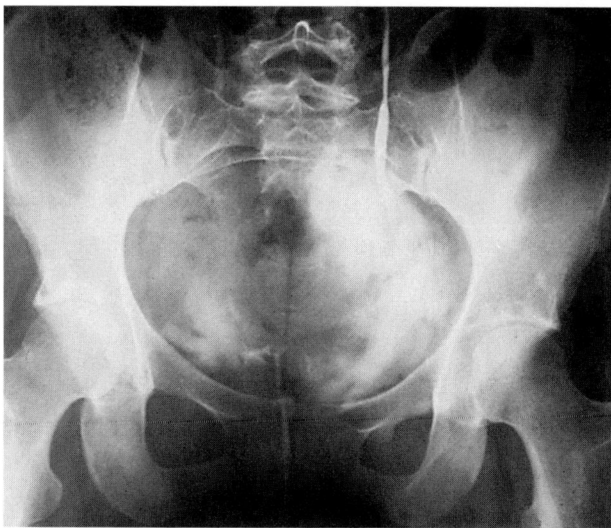

FIGURE 11B.2. Woman, aged 26 years, with lacerated left ureter secondary to stab wound of the abdomen. Intravenous pyelogram on the day of injury shows contrast extravasation in the left lower retroperitoneal area.

If the patient is to undergo surgical exploration, the ureter should be dissected from its bed and examined where it lies in proximity to the missile track. If whether an injury is present cannot be determined positively, one vial (5 mL) of indigo carmine should be injected intravenously (IV). Within 7 to 10 minutes, the dye should leak into the periureteral tissues if the ureter has been injured.

If the patient is not going to undergo exploration and the presence of an injury remains questionable, the most definitive study is a retrograde ureterogram. Often, this is not feasible in the trauma patient with multiple injuries. In such a case, ultrasound examination or, preferably, a CT scan may demonstrate the presence of extravasation (25,37).

Surgical Injury

If the urologist is confronted in the operating room with a possible ureteral injury, *the use of IV indigo carmine, as previously described, helps determine whether urinary extravasation is present.* Unfortunately, there is no good way to determine whether ureteral devascularization from the surgical procedure or the blast effect of a high-velocity missile has occurred other than by cutting the ureter and seeing whether it bleeds. Some surgeons advocate the use of IV fluorescein and a Wood's lamp. If there is fluorescence of the ureter, the vasculature is presumed to be intact. The presence of ureteral peristalsis is not helpful in the diagnosis because peristaltic movement may continue in the ureter for hours after it has been removed from the body.

The diagnosis of a ureteral injury generally is not made until many days after the injury has occurred. Table 11B.2 lists the most common signs and symptoms seen in these patients. If a ureteral injury is suspected, an excretory urogram or CT scan is mandatory. If the imaging study shows extravasation, delayed function, or hydroureteronephrosis, a retrograde ureterogram should be done to confirm the type of injury if it is not well delineated in the imaging study. This should be done just before institution of treatment to prevent sepsis from instrumenting a closed space.

TABLE 11B.2. SIGNS AND SYMPTOMS OF URETERAL INJURIES

Flank pain	1–21 days
Fever	>100°F
Anuria	Bilateral only
Ureterovaginal fistula	1–30 days
Ureterocutaneous fistula	1–30 days

In some patients, it may be determined that a percutaneous nephrostomy and possibly antegrade ureteral stent should be placed as therapy (i.e., an ileal diversion patient). In this instance, an antegrade rather than a retrograde ureterogram should be done.

The proper retrograde study is performed with a Braasch bulb or a cone-tipped catheter and contrast material injected at the level of the ureteral orifice. Passing a whistle-tip catheter into the renal pelvis does not rule out an obstructed ureter and is to be discouraged as a diagnostic study. As discussed later, this may, however, become part of the therapy.

CLASSIFICATION

A useful classification of ureteral injuries is presented in Table 11B.3. An alternative system is that proposed by the American Association for the Surgery of Trauma (AAST) as presented in Table 11B.4 (36).

External Violence Injury

If a missile passes close to but does not penetrate the ureter, a contusion is present. If the ureter is penetrated, either a partial laceration or complete laceration is present. Rarely, a

TABLE 11B.3. CLASSIFICATION OF URETERAL INJURIES

External Violence	**Surgical Injury (continued)**
Contusion	Transection
Partial laceration	Ligation
Complete laceration	Perforation
Crush	Devascularization
Avulsion	Fistula formation
Surgical Injury	**Radiation Injury**
Crush	
Avulsion	

TABLE 11B.4. AAST CLASSIFICATION OF URETERAL INJURIES

Grade I	Hematoma: contusion or hematoma without devascularization
Grade II	Laceration: <50% transection
Grade III	Laceration: >50% transection
Grade IV	Laceration: complete transection with 2 cm of devascularization
Grade V	Laceration: avulsion with >2 cm of devascularization

ureter will be crushed, usually in association with a nearby bony injury of the same type, or avulsed from the ureteropelvic junction by a hyperextension injury.

Surgical Injury

A surgeon may crush a ureter with a clamp, avulse a ureter with a retractor, transect the ureter with a knife or scissors, or ligate the ureter inadvertently. A common endoscopic injury is ureteral perforation with a wire, ureteroscope, or other ureteroscopic tool (e.g., basket, laser). If the ureter is stripped of its adventitia and hence blood vessels, it becomes devascularized and necrosis usually occurs in approximately 10 to 14 days. This may lead to fistula formation, as can any of the other aforementioned injuries.

Radiation Injury

Uncommonly, ureteral injury occurs secondary to irradiation of the organ. These lesions may not be seen for months to years after therapy and usually result in ureteral obstruction.

THERAPY

External Violence Injury

Contusion

A contusion may be discovered during exploration in a patient who has had a missile pass close to the ureter, but the structure has remained intact. No therapy is necessary in these patients. If a high-velocity bullet (more than 2,500 feet per second) is implicated, there is always the danger of late necrosis of the ureter. In this instance, placement of an internal stent and drain in the area of the injury should be considered. This problem is seen more often in military conflicts than in civilian life (1,11,44,56).

Laceration

If a partial laceration is present and the ureter that is still in continuity is viable, placement of an indwelling double-J stent and closure of the wound with interrupted 4-0 or 5-0 absorbable sutures gives the best results (49,54,58). Some authors advocate running closure of the wound and elimination of all stents (9). Before the advent of the totally indwelling stent, this was clearly a better way to handle minor lesions because the placement of a transcutaneous stent and formal nephrostomy may increase the complication rate and extend the scope of the procedure (60). With the use of the indwelling stent, drainage is minimal and the patient can be discharged at an early date. All of the devitalized tissue must be debrided, with a Penrose drain placed at the site of the repair and brought out through a separate stab wound.

However, if the remaining intact ureter is of questionable viability or if there is a complete laceration of the ureter, all devitalized tissue must be excised before the decision on a repair is made.

Clearly, the procedure with the lowest complication rate is the ureteroneocystostomy (Fig. 11B.3). This repair can be performed only on a patient with an injury below the level of the iliac vessels. The kidney can usually be mobilized and lowered so that the gap between the ureter and bladder can be decreased a few centimeters. The use of a bladder flap also can help bring the bladder closer to the ureter (Fig. 11B.4) (10). Sometimes merely suturing the bladder to the psoas fascia (psoas hitch) can ensure that there will not be tension on the repair. A nonrefluxing reimplantation is most desirable but cannot always be performed. Because adults, especially women, usually have little trouble with vesicoureteral reflux, this should not result in major problems later in life.

If the injury is too high for a ureteroneocystostomy to be performed, however, a ureteroureterostomy should be done (Fig. 11B.5). Traditionally, this was performed with a running suture of 4-0 or 5-0 absorbable material without stenting. The use of a stent and nephrostomy added major surgical time and complications to the procedure. If the wound was contaminated by bowel contents, stenting was mandatory.

The use of an indwelling stent and interrupted sutures has become popular with the introduction of the double-J stent. The surgical time is shorter and the margin of

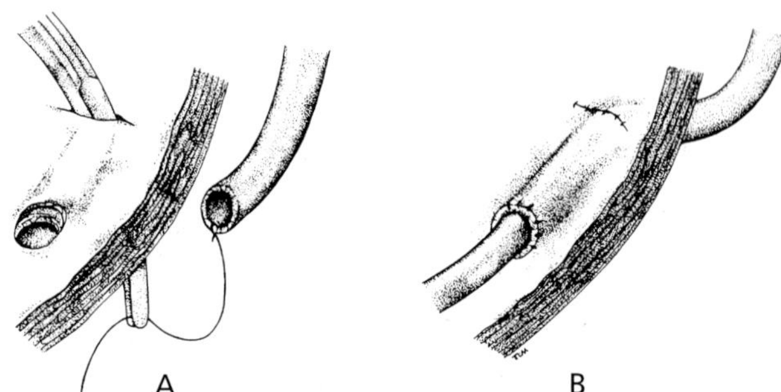

FIGURE 11B.3. Ureteroneocystostomy. **A:** Clamp through bladder wall from mucosa to serosa where ureter will enter bladder. Neo-orifice is created in mucosa of bladder. Submucosal tunnel is created from neo-orifice to entrance of ureter into bladder. **B:** Ureter enters bladder, runs into submucosal tunnel to neo-orifice, and is sewn in place. Stent is in ureter.

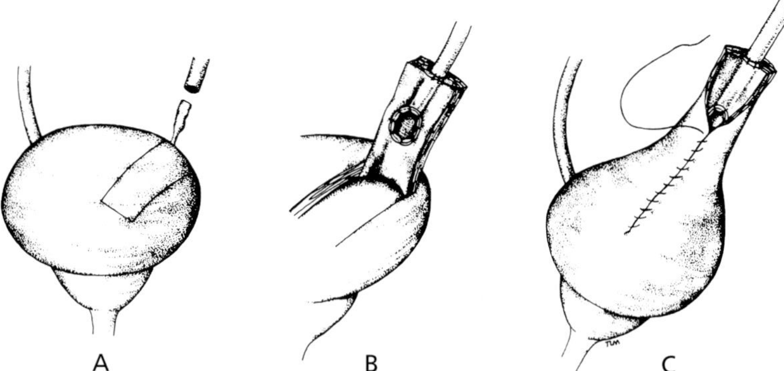

FIGURE 11B.4. **A:** Bladder flap to be created is outlined on bladder. **B:** Flap is created and ureter sewn in place by means of submucosal tunnel. **C:** Flap is sewn into tube to close bladder defect.

safety increased. No matter which technique is used, a Penrose drain should be placed as described previously. If a major length of ureter is lost, consideration should be given to a transureteroureterostomy or merely bringing the cut end of the ureter to the skin as a cutaneous ureterostomy for later definitive repair. Autotransplantation of the kidney to the hypogastric vessels plus ureteroneocystostomy also should be considered (1). This adds major operative time and increases risk to the patient, but in the patient with a solitary kidney it can be lifesaving. There are reports of using the appendix to replace lost segments of the ureter but not with long-term follow-up (33). If immediate reconstruction is impossible, consideration should be given to placement of a nephrostomy and delayed repair.

Crush Injury

When the ureter has been crushed along with other, adjacent tissues, debridement and usually ureteroureterostomy must be performed. All of the previously described techniques should be considered, and whichever seems appropriate should be used.

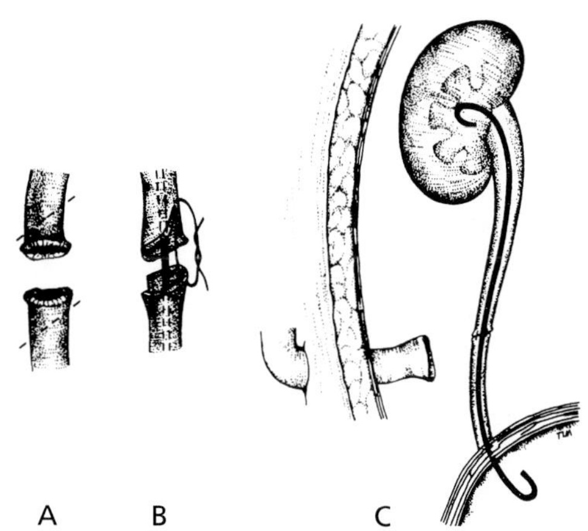

FIGURE 11B.5. **A:** Traumatized and severed ureter. *Dashed lines* show where spatulated edges will be trimmed. **B:** Ureter is spatulated and suturing begun, with stent in place. **C:** Anastomosis complete, double-J catheter in ureter, placement of Penrose drain by means of stab wound to area of anastomosis.

Avulsion Injury

Avulsion injury is essentially a complete laceration and requires debridement and definitive repair with stenting as described earlier.

Surgical Injury

Before a discussion of the types of repairs that should be used for a surgical injury of the ureter, some comments should be made about the prophylactic preoperative placement of ureteral catheters to identify the ureters at the time of exploration. Before performing a surgical procedure—especially when it is clear that the dissection will be difficult because of prior surgery, inflammation, or an inflammatory disease process such as endometriosis—many physicians place retrograde ureteral catheters into the ureters. It is difficult to verify that this technique actually decreases the incidence of ureteral injury in these patients. Perhaps the best that can be said is that it helps identify an injured ureter when the catheter is seen in the operative field.

Crush Injury

During a surgical procedure, a surgeon may inadvertently crush a ureter by placing a clamp on the structure or ligating it and then removing the clamp or ligature. In such a case, a decision must be made. Has the crushed ureteral segment been devascularized enough that it will eventually necrose and develop either a stricture or, more likely, a fistula? Unfortunately, there is no good intraoperative test to resolve this dilemma.

If there is good evidence that major injury has occurred, the ureteral segment should be excised and either a ureteroneocystostomy or ureteroureterostomy with internal stenting performed as described previously. If the surgeon chooses not to resect the segment, an indwelling stent placed either by opening the bladder or transurethrally at the end of the procedure is a good safety measure. Placement of a drain in this instance is probably not mandatory.

Laceration Injury

When the ureter has been completely severed either by avulsion or transection and this is recognized intraoperatively, repair by any of the techniques outlined in the section on lacerations associated with external violence should be used. If a laceration is not recognized until after the surgery has been completed, however, various therapeutic decisions will have to be made. *Initially, retrograde ureteral catheterization should be attempted.* Unfortunately, most of the time the catheter cannot be negotiated past the laceration into the proximal ureter. Obviously, this technique is applicable only for a partial laceration. If it is successful, however, a double-J stent should be placed and the patient observed for resolution of the extravasated urine. At the first sign of deterioration, the patient should have a percutaneous or formally placed drain inserted to remove the extravasation.

If the retrograde catheterization is unsuccessful, a percutaneous nephrostomy should be placed and an antegrade stent passed into the bladder. After the extravasation resolves, a double-J stent can be placed for long-term drainage (15,30,39,53).

If drainage of the kidney cannot be established by the percutaneous route, surgical exploration must be performed (21,35). In the first few postoperative days, primary repair should be considered as discussed previously, but if the injury is discovered later in the postoperative period, nephrostomy tube placement and drainage of the extravasation should be done, with delayed repair planned for many months in the future. When large segments of the ureter have been lost, an ileal ureter can be used when primary repair is planned and not done in an emergency situation. Since autotransplantation has gained in popularity, however, this procedure has been used less. Often, in the seriously ill patient with a normal opposite renal unit, nephrectomy is the best choice.

Ligation Injury

When complete obstruction of the ureter is discovered, it is always tempting to return to the operating room and deligate the ureter. Except for ureters ligated at the time of vesicourethropexy, this may be a hazardous procedure and may lead to delayed necrosis and fistula formation. Probably the reason it works so well with vesicourethral suspension is that during this procedure large amounts of tissue are caught in the suture, so devascularization is less of a problem than is mechanical obstruction from angulation. Perhaps if the ureter is loosely ligated and a stent is placed after deligation, this procedure has some merit (19).

The more conservative approach is to place a percutaneous nephrostomy tube in the kidney and attempt to pass a stent antegrade past the obstruction (15,20,30,35,39,53). Retrograde stenting fails almost all of the time. If stenting is successful, balloon dilation, in an effort to disrupt the suture, may be tried but is unnecessary (23). If the ureter has been ligated with chromic suture material, the obstruction will usually resolve in 3 to 4 weeks (20). If it has been ligated with polyglycolic acid suture, it may take 6 to 8 weeks to resolve (Fig. 11B.6). If it has not resolved in 4 to 6 months, formal repair will be necessary by one of the previously described techniques. Once again, the patient who cannot withstand the complications associated with reconstructive procedures may best be handled by nephrectomy.

Fistula Formation

If necrosis occurs from any of the injuries listed in Table 11B.3 and the urine either collects in the retroperitoneum or abdomen or tracts to the skin, bowel, or vagina, a percutaneous nephrostomy and ureteral stent should be placed. As with ureteral lacerations, if the procedure is successful, in time the ureter will heal and the fistula will usually close. If a stent cannot be passed, the ureter will

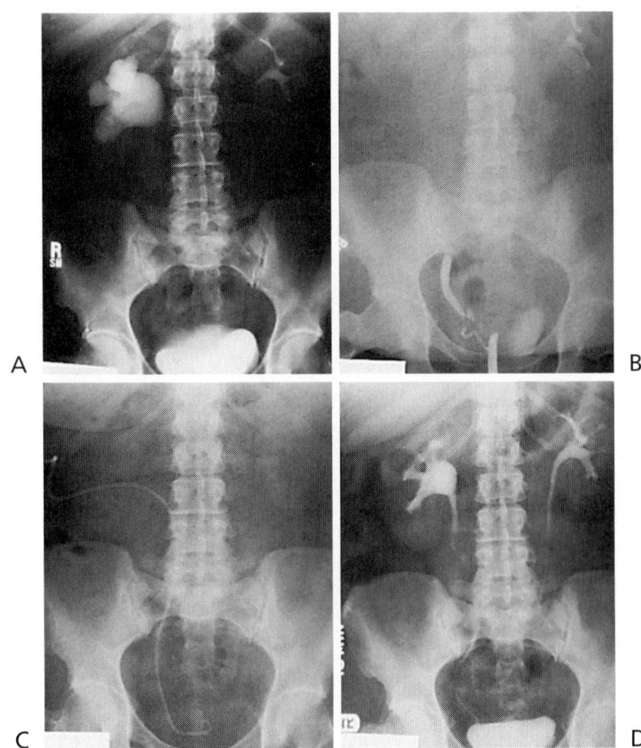

FIGURE 11B.6. Woman, aged 46 years, who developed a ureterovaginal fistula after an abdominal hysterectomy. **A:** Intravenous pyelography done on postoperative day 10 demonstrates obstruction of the right ureter. **B:** Retrograde ureterogram demonstrates the area of obstruction and some extravasation. **C:** An antegrade ureteral stent was placed beyond the fistula the following day and left in place 9 weeks. **D:** Intravenous pyelography done 6 months later demonstrates resolution of the hydronephrosis and a normal collecting system.

usually stricture at the site of the fistula and formal repair will have to be performed 4 to 6 months after the injury with one of the previously described procedures (15,29,30).

Radiation Injury

Radiation injury, although uncommon, is usually discovered months to years after the therapy has been completed. Ureteral stricture formation is usually present. Repair is difficult because irradiated tissue heals poorly. Permanent internal stent diversion is one approach, as is nephrectomy or diversion of the urine into an isolated bowel conduit with both ureter and bowel outside the field of treatment. Occasionally, reconstructive procedures using irradiated tissue wrapped in omentum are successful (59).

POSTOPERATIVE CARE AND COMPLICATIONS

Indwelling ureteral stents can be left in place for up to 6 months without fear of complications. Although many have been in place for more than a year with little difficulty, after 2 months some of them develop calculi and may cause obstruction of the ureter (15). If a drain has been placed, it can usually be removed in a week, even if the stent is left for a longer period. Most patients can be promptly discharged from the hospital and have these items removed in the outpatient setting.

Patients with percutaneous nephrostomy tubes should be taught to irrigate the tubes and to change dressings. A nephrostogram should be done at 3-week intervals to see if the obstruction has been relieved. When the ureter is again draining, the tube can be removed on an outpatient basis.

Stents placed across fistulae should be left in place for at least 4 to 6 weeks and a pull-out ureterogram performed to ensure that the fistula has closed. If the fistula site can be seen (skin or vagina), it should be inspected every 2 weeks until the site has sealed. The stent should not be removed until the opening is completely closed and the overlying skin or mucosa is intact.

Once all foreign materials have been removed, the patient should be treated with antibiotics to ensure that the urinary tract is sterile. Repeated cultures are recommended.

An excretory urogram or ultrasound should be performed 3 to 6 months after the repair and again a year later. Delayed obstruction is rare but can occur.

With formal surgical repairs, return to full activity takes 4 to 6 weeks. With the use of indwelling stents or percutaneous tubes, time to recovery is no longer than that usually seen with the primary surgical procedure.

The major complications from indwelling tubes, either totally indwelling or exiting from the kidney, are infection, tube obstruction, and calculus formation (15). If patients are instructed in how to irrigate the tubes at home, many trips to the emergency room or office can be avoided. Tubes may have to be changed if they obstruct, and pyelonephritis must be treated with appropriate antibiotics. Calculi must be handled at the time of tube removal.

REFERENCES

1. Al-Ali M, Haddad LF. The late treatment of 63 overlooked or complicated ureteral missile injuries: the promise of nephrostomy and role of autotransplantation. *J Urol* 1996;156:1918.
2. Altebarmakian VK, Davis RS, Khuri FJ. Ureteral injury associated with lumbar disk surgery. *Urology* 1981;17:462.
3. Ambiavagar R, Nambiar R. Traumatic closed avulsion of the upper ureter. *Injury* 1979;11:71.
4. Andersson A, Bergdahl L. Urologic complications following abdominoperineal resection of the rectum. *Arch Surg* 1976; 111:969.
5. Assimos DG, Patterson LC, Taylor CL. Changing incidence and etiology of iatrogenic ureteral injuries. *J Urol* 1994;152: 2240.
6. Beahrs JR, Beahrs OH, Beahrs MM, et al. Urinary tract complications with rectal surgery. *Ann Surg* 1978;187:542.
7. Brandes SB, Chelsky MJ, Buckman RF, et al. Ureteral injuries from penetrating trauma. *J Trauma* 1994;36:766.
8. Campbell EW Jr, Filderman PS, Jacobs SC. Ureteral injury due to blunt and penetrating trauma. *Urology* 1992;40:216.
9. Carlton CE Jr, Scott R Jr, Guthrie AG. The initial management of ureteral injuries: a report of 78 cases. *J Urol* 1971;105:335.
10. Chang SS, Koch MO. The use of an extended spiral bladder flap for treatment of upper ureteral loss. *J Urol* 1996;156:1981.
11. Christenson PJ, O'Connell KJ, Clark M, et al. Ballistic ureteral trauma: a comparison of high and low velocity weapons. *Contemp Surg* 1983;23:45.
12. Corriere JN Jr. The obstructed ureter in the patient with cancer. In: Miller TJ, Dudrick SJ, eds. *The management of difficult surgical problems.* Austin: University of Texas Press, 1978:109.
13. Cross JJL, Wong V, Irving HC, et al. Ureteric rupture in an elderly patient following minor trauma: case report. *J Trauma* 1994;36:594.
14. Daly JW, Higgins KA. Injury to the ureter during gynecologic surgical procedures. *Surg Gynecol Obstet* 1988;167:19.
15. Dowling RA, Corriere JN Jr, Sandler CM. Iatrogenic ureteral injury. *J Urol* 1986;135:912.
16. Dwyer PL, Carey MP, Rosamilia A. Suture injury to the urinary tract in urethral suspension procedures for stress incontinence. *Int Urogynecol J* 1999;10:15.
17. Fahlenkamp D, Rassweiler J, Fornara P, et al. Complications of laparoscopic procedures in urology: experience with 2,407 procedures at 4 German centers. *J Urol* 1999;162:765.
18. Fildes JJ, Betlej TM, Barrett JA. Buckshot colic. Case report and review of the literature. *J Trauma* 1995;39:1181.
19. Gurin JI, Garcia RL, Melman A, et al. The pathologic effect of ureteral ligation, with clinical implications. *J Urol* 1982;128: 1404.
20. Harshman MW, Pollack HM, Banner MP, et al. Conservative management of ureteral obstruction secondary to suture entrapment. *J Urol* 1982;127:121.
21. Hoch WH, Kursh ED, Persky L. Early aggressive management of intraoperative ureteral injuries. *J Urol* 1975;114:530.
22. Holden S, Hicks CC, O'Brien DP III, et al. Gunshot wounds of the ureter: a 15 year review of 63 consecutive cases. *J Urol* 1976;116:562.

23. Kaplan JO, Winslow OP Jr, Sneider SE, et al. Dilatation of a surgically ligated ureter through a percutaneous nephrostomy. *AJR Am J Roentgenol* 1982;139:188.
24. Kawashima A, Sandler CM, Corriere JN, et al. Ureteropelvic junction injuries secondary to blunt abdominal trauma. *Radiology* 1997;205:487.
25. Kenney PJ, Panicek DM, Witanowski LS. Computed tomography of ureteral disruption. *J Comput Assist Tomogr* 1987;11:480.
26. Kotkin L, Brock JW. Isolated ureteral injury caused by blunt trauma. *Urology* 1996;47:111.
27. Kuzmorov IW, MacIsaac SG, Sioufi J, et al. Iatrogenic ureteral injury secondary to lumbar sympathetic ganglion blockade. *Urology* 1980;16:617.
28. LaBerge I, Homsy YL, Dadour G, et al. Avulsion of ureter by blunt trauma. *Urology* 1979;13:172.
29. Lang EK. Diagnosis and management of ureteral fistulas by percutaneous nephrostomy and antegrade stent catheter. *Radiology* 1981;138:311.
30. Lask D, Abarbanel J, Luttwak Z, et al. Changing trends in the management of iatrogenic ureteral injuries. *J Urol* 1995;154:1693.
31. Leff EI, Groff W, Rubin RJ, et al. Use of ureteral catheters in colonic and rectal surgery. *Dis Colon Rectum* 1982;25:457.
32. Liroff SA, Pontes JES, Pierce JM Jr. Gunshot wounds of the ureter: 5 years of experience. *J Urol* 1977;118:551.
33. Medina JJ, Cummings JM, Parra RO. Repair of ureteral gunshot injury with appendiceal interposition. *J Urol* 1999;161:1563.
34. Meirow D, Moriel EZ, Zilberman M, et al. Evaluation and treatment of iatrogenic ureteral injuries during obstetric and gynecologic operations for nonmalignant conditions. *J Am Coll Surg* 1994;178:144.
35. Mendez R, McGinty DM. The management of delayed recognized ureteral injuries. *J Urol* 1978;119:192.
36. Moore EE, Logvill TH, Junkovich GV, et al. Organ injury scaling. III Chest wall, abdominal vascular, ureter, bladder and urethra. *J Trauma* 1992;33:337.
37. Mulligan JM, Cagiannos I, Collins JP, et al. Ureteropelvic junction disruption secondary to blunt trauma: Excretory phase imaging (delayed films) should help prevent a missed diagnosis. *J Urol* 1998;159:67.
38. Palmer LS, Rosenbaum RR, Geershbaum MD, et al. Penetrating ureteral trauma at an urban trauma center: 10-year experience. *Urology* 1999;54:34.
39. Persky L, Hampel N, Kedia K. Percutaneous nephrostomy and ureteral injury. *J Urol* 1981;125:298.
40. Pitts JC III, Peterson NE. Penetrating injuries of the ureter. *J Trauma* 1981;21:978.
41. Presti JC Jr, Carroll PR, McAninch JW. Ureteral and renal pelvic injuries from external trauma: diagnosis and management. *J Trauma* 1989;29:370.
42. Rober PE, Smith JB, Pierce JM Jr. Gunshot injuries of the ureter. *J Trauma* 1990;30:83.
43. Roberts BJ, Giblin JG, Tehan TJ, et al. Ureteroduodenal fistula. *Urology* 1996;48:301.
44. Rohner TJ Jr. Delayed ureteral fistula from high velocity missiles: report of 3 cases. *J Urol* 1971;105:63.
45. Rusche CF. Injury of the ureter due to gunshot wounds. *J Urol* 1948;60:63.
46. Sacks D, Miller J. Ureteral leak around an aortic bifurcation graft: complication of ureteral stenting. *J Urol* 1988;140:1526.
47. Schwartz BF, Stoller ML. Complications of retrograde balloon cautery endopyelotomy. *J Urol* 1999;162:1594.
48. Selzman AA, Spirnak JP. Iatrogenic ureteral injuries: a 20-year experience in treating 165 injuries. *J Urol* 1996;155:878.
49. Sieben DM, Howerton L, Amin M, et al. The role of ureteral stenting in the management of surgical injury of the ureter. *J Urol* 1978;119:330.
50. Siegel MJ, Balfe DM. Blunt renal and ureteral trauma in childhood: CT patterns of fluid collections. *AJR Am J Roentgenol* 1989;152:1043.
51. Silverstein JI, Libby C, Smith AD. Management of ureteroscopic ureteral injuries. *Urol Clin North Am* 1988;15:515.
52. Smith AD. Management of iatrogenic ureteral strictures after urological procedures. *J Urol* 1988;140:1372.
53. Stables DP, Ginsburg NJ, Johnson ML. Percutaneous nephrostomy: a series and review of the literature. *AJR Am J Roentgenol* 1978;130:75.
54. Steers WD, Corriere JN Jr, Benson GS, et al. The use of indwelling stents in managing ureteral injuries due to external violence. *J Trauma* 1985;25:1001.
55. Stengel JN, Felderman ES, Zamora D. Ureteral injury: complication of laparoscopic sterilization. *Urology* 1974;4:341.
56. Stutzman RE. Ballistics and the management of ureteral injuries from high velocity missiles. *J Urol* 1977;118:947.
57. Tamussino KF, Lang PFJ, Breinl E. Ureteral complications with operative gynecologic laparoscopy. *Am J Obstet Gynecol* 1998;967.
58. Toporoff B, Sclafawi S, Scalea T, et al. Percutaneous antegrade ureteral stenting as an adjunct for treatment of complicated ureteral injuries. *J Trauma* 1992;32:534.
59. Underwood PB Jr, Lutz MH, Smoak DL. Ureteral injury following irradiation therapy for carcinoma of the cervix. *Obstet Gynecol* 1977;49:663.
60. Weaver RG. The effect of large caliber splints on ureteral healing. *Surg Gynecol Obstet* 1956;103:590.

Adult and Pediatric Urology, 4/e, edited by Jay Y. Gillenwater, John T. Grayhack, Stuart S. Howards, and Michael E. Mitchell.
Lippincott Williams & Wilkins, Philadelphia © 2002

12

TRAUMA TO THE LOWER URINARY TRACT

JOSEPH N. CORRIERE, JR.

BLADDER INJURIES

In the child, the bladder is an abdominal organ and as such is vulnerable to external trauma. As the bony pelvis grows, the bladder becomes protected from injury, especially if it is empty of urine. The bladder is located extraperitoneally in the space of Retzius. Laterally, it is bound by the internal obturator muscles and the lateral umbilical ligaments. Its base is attached to the urogenital diaphragm, and Denonvilliers' fascia, or the rectovesical fascia, binds it loosely posteriorly. Unlike the rest of the organ, however, the dome of the bladder is mobile and distensible.

When the bladder is distended or the pelvis is fractured, the normal protective influence of the intact pelvic ring is lost, and in fact, the shearing force of a pelvic fracture commonly tears the bladder at its moorings. A spicule of bone may lacerate the organ, or it may rupture at the dome by a direct blow to the abdomen without bony injury. Conversely, missiles from an outside force, from internal migration, or in the hands of a well-meaning surgeon, may find the bladder despite its position.

J.N. Corriere, Jr.: Department of Surgery, Division of Urology, The University of Texas, Houston, TX 77030.

Etiology

Penetrating Injuries

In usual civilian practice, the most common penetrating injuries of the bladder occur from surgical misadventure. Table 12.1 lists the types of procedures and instruments that have been associated with operative injury to the bladder (33,37,41,54,55,69,70,77,97,123,124). Trauma from external violence is most commonly caused by gunshot wounds (23,33,145).

Rarely, injury may occur from migration and erosion of internally placed foreign materials or swallowed objects, most commonly surgical drains, intrauterine or sterilization devices, hip prostheses, penile prosthesis, toothpicks, pins, knife blades, or bones (5,14,21,29,58,67,101,117, 131,149). Finally, long-term Foley catheters have been known to erode through the bladder, usually at the dome, where it sits at the tip of the catheter (10).

Blunt Injuries

The most common cause of bladder injuries resulting from external violence is blunt trauma to the abdomen, mostly from motor vehicle accidents but also from falls, crushing injuries to the bony pelvis, or blows to the abdomen (Table

TABLE 12.1. CAUSE OF PENETRATING INJURIES OF THE BLADDER

Operative Injury	External Violence
Transurethral Procedures	Gunshot wound
Resectoscope	Knife wound
Lithotrite	Spike impalement
Cystoscope	**Internal Migration**
Urethral instrumentation	***Surgical Drains***
Gynecologic Procedures	Penrose
Abdominal hysterectomy	Saratoga sump
Vaginal hysterectomy	Foley catheter
Removal of cervical stump	***Intrauterine or Sterilization Devices***
Salpingo-oophorectomy	Lippes loop
Cesarean section	Dalkon Shield
Laparoscopy	Copper-7
Vesicourethral suture suspension	Copper-T
Dilation and curettage	Filshie clip
Suction curettage	***Hip Prosthesis***
Neovaginal construction	Pins
Abdominal Procedures	Trochanteric plate
Herniorrhaphy	***Penile Prosthesis***
Abdominoperineal resection	***Neurosurgical Shunts***
Anterior colon resection	***Swallowed Objects***
Neonatal umbilical artery catheterization	Pins
Laparoscopy	Toothpicks
Aortic bypass grafts	Knife blades
Tenckhoff catheter placement	Bones
Orthopedic Procedures	**Long-dwelling Foley Catheter**
Pelvic fracture manipulation	
Bone screw placement	

12.2). The full bladder is especially vulnerable to a deceleration injury (23).

In motor vehicle accidents, injuries are seen in passengers wearing seat belts when the force of the collision may focus on the abdomen and thus the full bladder, in the unrestrained child (or, less commonly, the adult) who is thrown by the impact against an unyielding object, or secondary to a pelvic fracture (129).

In our experience with 111 bladder injuries over a 7-year period, 86% were caused by blunt trauma and 90% of the blunt injuries were secondary to motor vehicle accidents (33). A total of 89% of the blunt injuries were associated with pelvic fractures. On the other hand, 9% of patients with pelvic fractures had a concomitant injury to the bladder.

TABLE 12.2. CAUSE OF BLUNT INJURIES OF THE BLADDER

Motor vehicle accident	Crush of bony pelvis
Fall	Abdominal blow

Spontaneous Rupture

It is difficult to understand how a bladder can rupture "spontaneously" as is reported in most large series of these injuries. It is usually seen in the patient with preexisting bladder disease, usually in chronic retention, and is most likely associated with minor blunt trauma or unrecognized trauma in an obtunded patient (1,100).

Diagnosis

Signs and Symptoms

The signs and symptoms of rupture of the bladder are usually nonspecific. The patient may complain of suprapubic pain or relate that he attempted to urinate and could not. The discomfort of a concomitant fractured pelvis or other organ system injury often overshadows the pain from the damaged urinary tract.

Tenderness is present in the suprapubic area and bowel sounds absent, especially if it is an intraperitoneal rupture. Shock is rarely caused by an isolated bladder rupture. When it is present, another cause for the hypotension should be sought.

Bladder perforation during a transurethral surgical procedure with the patient under spinal anesthesia is commonly associated with acute symptoms on the operating table. Extraperitoneal injuries will cause lower abdominal pain, and the patient's blood pressure may begin to rise. Intraperitoneal injuries with extravasation of large quantities of fluid lead to abdominal distention and referred pain to the tip of the shoulder if the fluid irritates the diaphragm.

If recognition of an intraperitoneal injury is delayed, uroascites may develop and cause significant abdominal distention. This may cause respiratory distress and even lower limb venous occlusion, especially in the neonate (37). Peritoneal signs of tenderness and rebound will develop, and if the urine is infected, frank peritonitis may eventually be seen.

Hematuria is a hallmark finding with bladder injuries. In our experience and that of others, *gross hematuria occurs more than 95% of the time, with microscopic hematuria present in the remaining cases* (23,33).

Radiographic Examination

The static cystogram is the only study that will definitely diagnose a ruptured bladder (22,126). *If a urethral injury is suspected because of a pelvic fracture; the presence of blood at the urethral meatus; a high-riding prostate on rectal examination; or marked ecchymosis and edema of the perineum, scrotum, and/or penis, a retrograde urethrogram must be done before attempted urethral catheterization.*

If a ruptured urethra is found, urethral catheterization is usually contraindicated and a suprapubic cystotomy should be performed. If the tube is placed percutaneously, a static cystogram must still be done to rule out a concomitant bladder injury. If the cystotomy tube is placed surgically, the bladder can be inspected at the time of the exploration and the cystogram eliminated.

It is best to perform this examination with fixed equipment in the radiology suite. A satisfactory study can be done in the emergency room with portable equipment and grid cassettes if absolutely necessary. A Foley catheter is placed in the bladder and the bladder emptied of urine. A 300-mL bottle of standard infusion contrast material (25% to 30%) and a similar amount of saline solution are attached to a Y connector and then to the catheter to obtain a 50-50 mixture.

A scout radiograph is taken and then 100 mL of the mixture infused. A second film is exposed to check for gross extravasation. If a bladder rupture is seen, the catheter is immediately placed to straight drainage. If extravasation is not seen, the remainder of the solution is instilled and films are obtained in the anteroposterior, oblique, and lateral projections.

The bladder is then drained of all contrast material and an additional film taken. This is especially important in patients in whom the oblique and lateral films may have been omitted because of concomitant injuries or the patient's clinical state. Small amounts of extravasation may be present behind a contrast-filled bladder and may only be seen on this view. The bladder should also be drained before proceeding with studies of the upper urinary tract. An excretory urogram or computed tomography (CT) scan with contrast should then be performed.

It cannot be overemphasized that *a normal cystogram on a urogram is not sufficient evidence to rule out bladder injury.* Often, a blood clot or omentum temporarily seals a small rent and the bladder will appear intact. Only the static cystogram with full vesical distention and a film taken after drainage can verify that a bladder rupture is not present. Similarly, the bladder image on a CT is limited because, like the cystogram on the urogram, it may not show a leak because it is not forcibly distended (51,57,87,108,128). On the other hand, the CT scanner can be used to image the bladder instead of the conventional radiograph in conjunction with a retrograde cystogram, and a proper diagnosis can be made. Ultrasound diagnosis is still not at the level of accuracy of retrograde contrast injection (40).

Classification

As can be seen in Table 12.3, bladder injuries secondary to blunt trauma are subclassified regarding the extent and location of the injury, whereas penetrating injuries are usually grouped together. However, as discussed in the section on therapy, when considering the treatment of iatrogenic penetrating injuries, extent and location become critical and must be differentiated. The American Association for the Surgery of Trauma (AAST) organ scoring system is presented in Table 12.4 (92).

TABLE 12.3. CLASSIFICATION OF BLADDER INJURIES

Blunt Trauma
Contusion
Interstitial rupture
Intraperitoneal rupture
Extraperitoneal rupture
Intraperitoneal and extraperitoneal rupture
Penetrating Trauma

Bladder Contusion

A bladder contusion results from damage to the bladder mucosa or muscularis without loss of wall continuity. Extravasation is not seen on cystogram, but the bladder outline may be distorted (Fig. 12.1). The exact incidence of this injury is difficult to determine because often the diagnosis is made by exclusion in the patient with trauma to the lower abdomen and hematuria. The best overall estimate is that this injury accounts for approximately one-third of all bladder injuries.

Interstitial Rupture

Occasionally, an incomplete tear (non–full-thickness tear) of the bladder wall is seen secondary to blunt trauma. As with the bladder contusion, no extravasation is seen on the cystogram (Fig. 12.2). It is important to distinguish this injury from a bladder contusion because the therapy requires a longer period of catheterization because it may represent a full-thickness injury that has sealed with clots or

TABLE 12.4. AAST CLASSIFICATION OF BLADDER INJURIES

Grade I	Hematoma: contusion, intramural hematoma Laceration: partial thickness
Grade II	Laceration: extraperitoneal bladder wall laceration <2 cm
Grade III	Laceration: extraperitoneal (>2 cm) or intraperitoneal (<2 cm) bladder wall lacerations
Grade IV	Laceration: intraperitoneal bladder wall laceration >2 cm
Grade V	Laceration: intraperitoneal or extraperitoneal bladder wall laceration extending into the bladder neck or ureteral orifice (trigone)

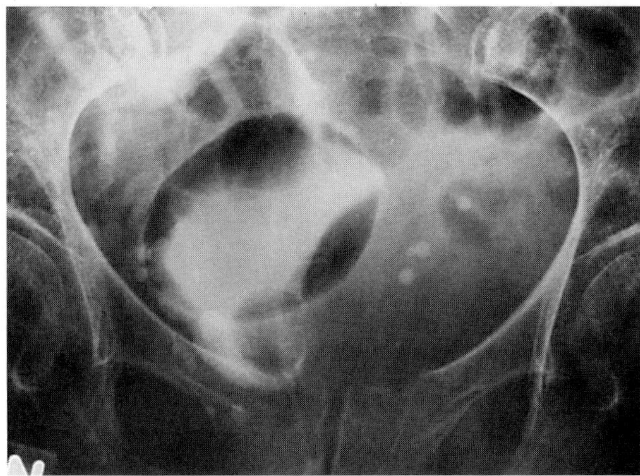

FIGURE 12.1. Bladder contusion secondary to a pelvic hematoma and pelvic fracture. (From Sandler CM, Phillips JM, Harris JD, et al. Radiology of the bladder and urethra in blunt pelvic trauma. *Radiol Clin North Am* 1981;19:195, with permission.)

at least needs a longer time to heal as a result of the extent of the damage to the bladder wall.

Intraperitoneal Rupture

As mentioned, intraperitoneal rupture of the bladder occurs when there is a sudden rise in intravesicular pressure secondary to a blow to the pelvis or lower abdomen. This increased pressure results in rupture of the dome, the weakest and most mobile part of the bladder. Contrast material will fill the cul-de-sac, outline loops of bowel, and eventually extend into the paracolic gutter (Fig. 12.3). This injury is common in children because of the intraperitoneal position of the bladder. Intraperitoneal bladder ruptures probably account for one-third of all bladder injuries and are approximately equal in incidence to extraperitoneal ruptures.

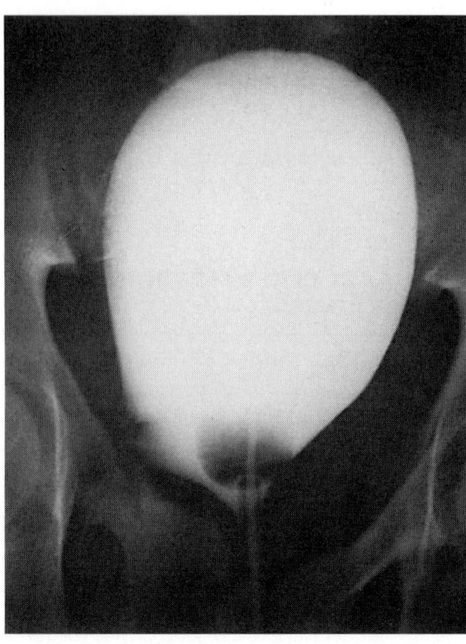

FIGURE 12.2. Interstitial bladder rupture secondary to a pelvic fracture.

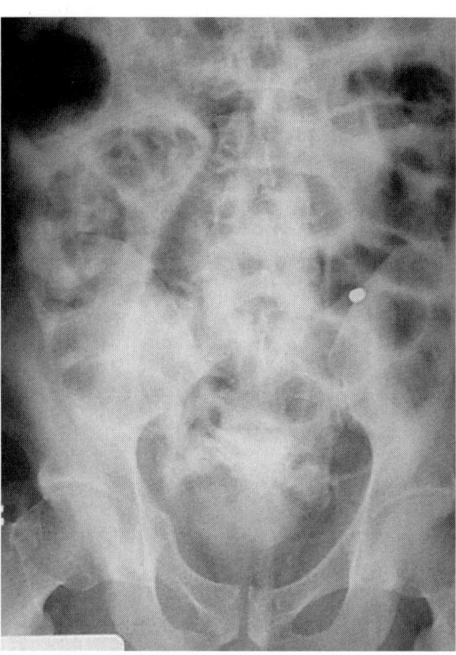

FIGURE 12.3. Intraperitoneal bladder rupture secondary to blunt abdominal trauma.

Extraperitoneal Rupture

Extraperitoneal bladder ruptures are seen almost exclusively with pelvic fractures. The bladder usually is sheared on the anterior lateral wall near the bladder base by the distortion of the pelvic ring disruption. Occasionally, the bladder is lacerated by a sharp, bony spicule. On cystography, flame-shaped areas of extravasation that are usually confined to the perivesical soft tissues are visualized (Fig. 12.4). If there is a large pelvic hematoma, the bladder will often be compressed into the "teardrop deformity." Urinary extravasation may extend to the thigh by means of the obturator foramen to the scrotum by means of the inguinal canal, up the anterior abdominal wall, or retroperitoneally as high as the kidneys (Fig. 12.5). Sixty percent of the time a contracoup bursting rupture opposite the area of fracture is seen as well as an injury near the fracture site (23,33).

Intraperitoneal and Extraperitoneal Bladder Rupture

Occasionally, the bladder is ruptured both intraperitoneally and extraperitoneally. These injuries are caused by penetrating trauma or pelvic fractures. The radiologic find-

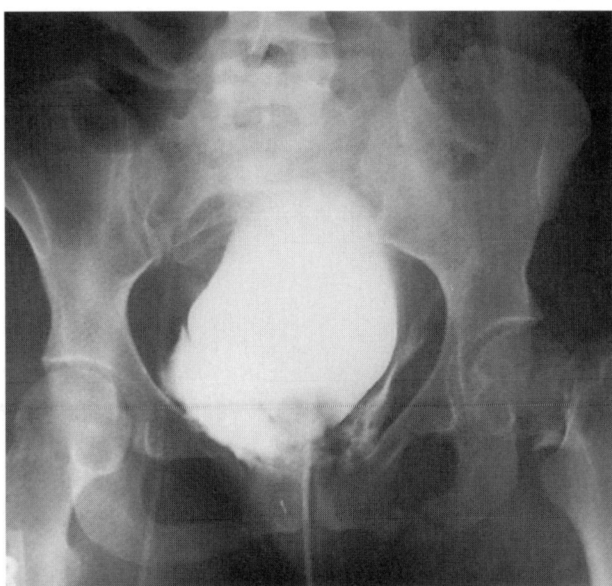

FIGURE 12.4. Extraperitoneal bladder rupture secondary to pelvic fracture.

ings are a mixture of the previous descriptions of the single injuries.

Therapy

Penetrating Injuries from External Violence

All patients with penetrating injuries from external violence should undergo exploration of the abdomen and of the track the missile followed from its entrance wound to its exit wound. The peritoneal cavity should be opened through a midline incision, even if the injury is thought to be entirely extraperitoneal, and the intraabdominal viscera and major vasculature should be examined for damage. All devitalized tissue and debris (e.g., bullets, bone spicules, clothing) should be removed from the bladder and abdomen (23).

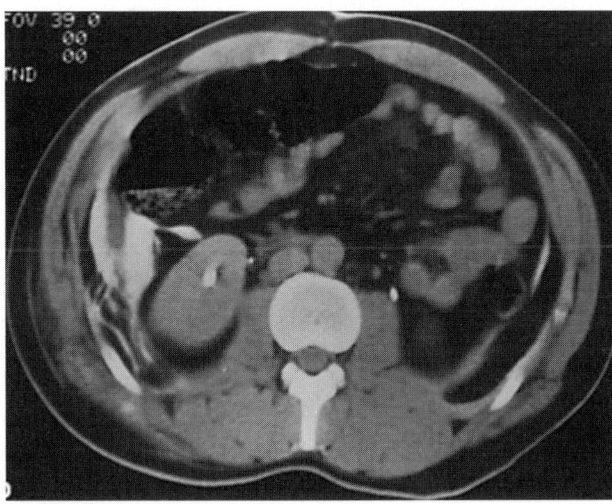

FIGURE 12.5. Computed tomography scan of patient with an extravesical bladder rupture. Note extravasation as high as kidneys.

If the ureteral orifices are involved in the injury or there is concern about the integrity of the ureters, 5 mL of indigo carmine should be injected intravenously. In 7 to 10 minutes, the blue dye should appear in the bladder. A search for extravasation should be made and the ureters intubated with 5-Fr whistle-tip catheters if there is any concern that they have been damaged.

If a large pelvic hematoma is present, it is best left undisturbed if one can be sure by radiography (plain film, cystogram, urogram, and/or arteriogram) that there is no major disruption of the bladder neck, ureters, or vasculature. The bladder is then entered through its peritoneal surface at the dome and thoroughly inspected.

After debridement, the extraperitoneal vesical defect should be closed with a single-layer running 3-0 chromic or polyglycolic suture through the interior of the bladder. Extensive mobilization of the bladder to ensure a watertight closure or to place the knots on the outside of the bladder will usually only increase bleeding. If it is impossible to close the extraperitoneal defects, they should not be disturbed. With adequate bladder drainage, they will eventually heal without difficulty. Only injuries to the bladder neck must undergo reconstruction.

A suprapubic cystotomy tube may then be inserted in the bladder through a separate stab wound. At least a 24-Fr size should be used to ensure egress of blood clots. Either a Malecot or mushroom tube is recommended. The mushroom style has a firmer flange and is less likely to become dislodged, but the sideholes are small. If the tip of the catheter is excised before insertion, this drawback is overcome.

The tube should be sewn in place with an 0 chromic or polyglycolic purse-string suture, which is then used to fix the bladder to the wall at the site where it crosses the abdomen, again through a separate stab wound. This will ensure a controlled fistula if leakage occurs at the time of tube removal. The catheter should not be brought through the bladder wound because removal may disrupt the suture line, nor should it come through the abdominal incision because this increases the chance for wound infection.

The intraperitoneal bladder incision is closed with a double layer of 3-0 chromic or polyglycolic suture in a running watertight fashion. This is best done after the suprapubic tube is sewn into the bladder but before the tube is brought through and fixed to the abdominal wall. If bleeding and clot formation are not excessive, a Foley catheter may be used instead of a suprapubic tube (139).

One-inch Penrose drains are placed near the suture lines and brought through separate stab wounds. The drains and suprapubic tubes are sutured to the skin with 3-0 nonabsorbable suture material. The wound is closed in a standard fashion, and a sterile dressing is applied. If the orthopedic surgeon repairs a pelvic fracture at the same time using internal plates, drains and suprapubic tubes should not be used if at all possible to prevent infection near the foreign material.

Iatrogenic Penetrating Injuries

When the bladder is inadvertently injured during a surgical procedure, prompt repair with a double layer of 3-0 absorbable suture material and tube drainage with a Foley catheter or suprapubic tube usually ensures an excellent result. The most common mistake made is not thoroughly inspecting the entire bladder when the injury is discovered, thereby overlooking a second rent in the organ. This is especially disturbing during gynecologic surgery when a lesion of the dome is seen and repaired, but one at the base that also involves the vagina is missed.

Delayed recognition of operative injuries requires individualized attention. *If recognized in the first few days after surgery, immediate correction usually will be successful. Although some reports advocate repair of bladder injuries at the time of diagnosis despite the age of the injury, after 1 or 2 weeks, tissue edema impedes proper wound healing, increasing the failure rate of the repair. The success rate is improved by delaying repair for months. Only intraperitoneal injuries and uroascites demand prompt repair when they are discovered.*

Injury to the bladder by an endoscope (cystoscope, resectoscope, or laparoscope)—especially if the injury is extraperitoneal and properly recognized, the procedure immediately terminated, and the rent small—can be handled with large-caliber urethral catheter drainage and expectant therapy. These patients must be observed closely, and at the least sign of deterioration, abdominal exploration and repair of the bladder should be performed. If there is any evidence of uroascites or if the urine is infected, formal repair is mandatory.

Internal Migrating Objects

Internal migrating objects are rare injuries that necessitate removal of the foreign material and use of a urethral catheter or suprapubic tube drainage. Formal repair performed as exploration is usually necessary to remove most of these objects and must be done if the injury is intraperitoneal (29,101,131).

Bladder Contusions

Bladder contusions necessitate Foley catheter drainage for a few days or, if minor, no therapy at all. If there is a large pelvic hematoma and marked bladder neck distortion, the patient may have difficulty voiding. These patients may require prolonged catheter drainage. If there is a major injury to the sacrum and the patient cannot urinate, a cystometrogram should be performed to be sure there has not been damage to the sacral nerve roots that innervate the bladder. If no detrusor contraction is seen and the patient continues to be unable to void after multiple trials, intermittent self-catheterization should be instituted. Most of these problems are temporary unless accompanied by major neurologic deficit.

Interstitial Ruptures

As stated in the section on classification, interstitial ruptures are incomplete bladder wall ruptures, or they may represent a small full-thickness rupture that has sealed itself with clot or possibly omentum. They should probably be treated by 10 days of catheter drainage, just as the complete but unrepaired rupture, and followed up closely for a change in clinical status. A cystogram should be performed before catheter removal.

Intraperitoneal Ruptures

All intraperitoneal bladder ruptures caused by blunt abdominal trauma should undergo formal repair. The peritoneal cavity should be opened, all urine and blood evacuated, the viscera and vasculature inspected for injury, and appropriate therapy instituted. The bladder will usually have a large 5-cm or greater rent at the dome. If necessary, it should be widened thoroughly to inspect the interior of the organ. Any concomitant extraperitoneal rents should be closed with a single running 3-0 chromic or polyglycolic suture from inside the bladder. Devitalized tissue should be excised, and after a suprapubic tube has been placed as previously described, the dome wound should be closed with absorbable suture material. The suprapubic tube is brought through a separate stab wound, and a peritoneal drain is placed and brought out through a second stab wound. If the urine is relatively clear, a Foley catheter may be used instead of a suprapubic tube (139). The peritoneal cavity cannot and should not be drained. Closure of the abdomen is as previously described (23).

A few scattered reports indicate that intraperitoneal bladder injuries can be treated with simple Foley catheter drainage (99,121,122). When the literature is carefully reviewed, however, it is clear that most of these authors are discussing iatrogenic transurethral bladder perforations and not wounds caused by external violence. Most patients with intraperitoneal bladder ruptures caused by abdominal blows or a fractured pelvis have large gaping rents and marked uroascites when first seen. These patients must undergo prompt surgical repair because they rapidly deteriorate if not treated in a timely fashion (23). Finally, reports of laparoscopic repair are now appearing in the literature (9).

Extraperitoneal Ruptures

Isolated uncomplicated extraperitoneal bladder ruptures can be handled easily by 10 days of Foley catheter drainage (20,33,99,121,122). As some authors state, one cannot decide to treat only small extraperitoneal ruptures with catheter drainage and formally close large ruptures because it is difficult to relate the amount of contrast extravasation to the extent of the injury (20,23). Extravasation is related to the amount of contrast instilled and to the size of the injury. In our experience, however, extravasation into the pelvis, down the inguinal canal to the scrotum, and up the retroperitoneum as high as the kidneys can be successfully treated with catheter drainage. If the patient has uninfected urine and appropriate catheter care is used, the urine will quickly absorb and the bladder rent will heal.

However, it cannot be stressed enough that the nonoperative catheter drainage therapy is exactly that: No exploration for any reason is being performed, and the catheter is draining well, not poorly and intermittently, being obstructed with clots (76). *If the catheter will not drain easily and the urine does not clear properly, formal repair is best.*

If the patient with an extraperitoneal bladder rupture is to be explored for associated injuries and is not gravely ill, it is best to open the dome of the bladder, not disturb the pelvic hematoma, repair the rupture intravesically, close the bladder, and insert a suprapubic tube or Foley catheter as previously described. If the pelvic hematoma is opened for another reason, a drain should be placed. If it is not opened, no drain is necessary.

Intraperitoneal and Extraperitoneal Ruptures

Intraperitoneal and extraperitoneal ruptures need to be formally repaired as previously described. Most of these patients have major pelvic fractures and often have injured their urethra, bladder neck, or in the female, vagina as well. Prompt reconstruction, even in the face of a marked pelvic disruption, is usually necessary for a good long-term result. These cases all need to be individualized, especially those with major tissue destruction.

Postoperative Care and Follow-up

Postoperatively, if no other injuries are present, oral alimentation may be resumed when gastrointestinal peristalsis returns to normal, usually within 3 to 7 days of the injury. The bladder heals remarkably quickly, and if a good repair was achieved, the suprapubic tube or Foley catheter may be removed within a week. If there is any question about the closure, a cystogram should be performed before tube removal. If extravasation is present, the catheter should be left in place for further drainage and the cystogram repeated on the tenth postoperative day.

When the patient is voiding normally and there is no leakage of urine from the drainage site for 24 hours, the drain may be removed. Routine antibiotics are not necessary, but once the catheter has been removed, the urine should be cultured and appropriate antibiotics given if bacteriuria is present. If the urine is infected at the time of the injury and subsequent extravasation, antibiotics should be begun preoperatively and continued for at least a week. Frequent urine cultures should be obtained to avoid serious complications.

If the patient had an extraperitoneal injury that was treated with Foley catheter drainage alone, a cystogram should be done on the tenth postoperative day. In our experience, more than 85% of bladders are healed by that time, and the catheter can then be removed. Virtually all injuries treated in this manner are healed with less than 3 weeks of catheter drainage. In the rare male patient who has persistent extravasation, a punch suprapubic tube should be placed in the bladder to prevent urethral complications.

Full activity may be resumed within 3 to 4 weeks of surgery unless other injuries or complications dictate further therapy or rest. Other than urine cultures if indicated, no long-term follow-up is necessary.

Complications

The most serious complications for bladder ruptures are secondary to delay in diagnosis. When urine leaks into the peritoneal cavity, it equilibrates with serum, so peritoneal fluid analysis for creatinine and urea will not be helpful in diagnosis. If uroascites becomes marked, respiratory difficulty will develop, especially in infants. Emergency paracentesis may be lifesaving.

Sepsis from infected urine is a major threat. In the unrecognized intraperitoneal rupture, generalized peritonitis or loculated abscesses may develop. The bladder rent must be closed, the urine diverted, and all purulent collections drained surgically. Appropriate antibiotics must be given.

The mortality of patients with bladder ruptures is approximately 12% (23,33). The cause of death in these patients should never be secondary to the bladder wound if it is properly diagnosed and treated but will be caused by associated visceral or vascular injuries.

Injuries to the bladder neck, urethra, and vagina, if not promptly and properly repaired at the time of the injury, may result in incontinence, fistula, or stricture formation (88). In these cases, reconstruction will have to be delayed for months to allow edema, infection, and induration to disappear. In some patients, a neuropathic bladder may accompany the injury, and voiding may be impossible. Intermittent self-catheterization is a good way to overcome this problem.

URETHRAL INJURIES

Anatomically, the male urethra is traditionally divided into (a) the prostatic urethra; (b) the membranous urethra; (c) the bulbous urethra; and (d) the penile, or pendulous, urethra. When considering injuries to the male urethra, most surgeons use a classification that helps determine appropriate therapy such as (a) *posterior urethral injuries*—those of the prostatic and membranous urethra, above and including the urogenital diaphragm and (b) *anterior urethral injuries*—those of the bulbous and penile, or pendulous, urethra, below the urogenital diaphragm.

Because proper diagnosis is so critical to subsequent management and because both of these anatomic and mechanistic classifications can cause confusion, unified classifications have been developed that may help in the proper evaluation and therapy of these injuries [Table 12.5 (49) and Table 12.6 (92)]. These work best for blunt trauma but can be used for penetrating lesions as well.

The female urethra is rarely injured (24,138). When it is damaged, however, it is usually accompanied by a severe bony pelvic disruption with concomitant injury to the bladder neck and vagina. It is usually more common in children than adults (2,56,73,88,113,134).

Etiology

Posterior Urethral Injuries

Almost all injuries of the posterior urethra in the male occur in conjunction with fracture of the bony pelvis (35,89,90,105). In modern civilian society, 90% of these injuries are caused by motor vehicle accidents involving automobiles, motorcycle riders, or pedestrians. Falls from a height, industrial crushing injuries, and sporting accidents make up the other 10% of the pelvic fracture patients (25).

This injury is most commonly caused by the shearing force of the bone disruption, with the prostate, attached by the puboprostatic ligaments, being pulled in one direction while the membranous urethra, attached to the urogenital diaphragm, is pulled in another direction.

Penetrating wounds of the posterior urethra from external violence are uncommon but do occur. Urethral instrumentation with perforation of the prostatic urethra, on the other hand, is more frequently seen (Table 12.7). There are two cases in the literature in which a lateral blow to the pelvis and thigh resulted in rupture of the posterior urethra at the junction of the prostatic and membranous urethra with probable concomitant rupture of the puboprostatic ligaments without fracture of the pelvis (34,119).

TABLE 12.5. CLASSIFICATION OF URETHRAL INJURIES

Type I	Posterior urethra intact but stretched by pelvic hematoma
Type II	Partial or complete prostatomembranous urethral rupture above intact urogenital diaphragm
Type III	Partial or complete combined anterior/posterior urethral rupture with rupture of urogenital diaphragm
Type IV	Bladder neck injury with extension into posterior urethra
Type IVA	Base of bladder injury with periurethral extravasation (simulates type IV injury)
Type V	Partial or complete anterior urethral injury

TABLE 12.6. AAST CLASSIFICATION OF URETHRAL INJURIES

Grade I	Contusion: blood at urethral meatus; urethrography normal
Grade II	Stretch injury: elongation of urethra without extravasation on urethrography
Grade III	Partial disruption: extravasation on urethrography, contrast at injury site with contrast visualization in the bladder
Grade IV	Complete disruption: extravasation on urethrography, contrast at injury site without visualization in the bladder; <2 cm of urethral separation
Grade V	Complete disruption: complete transection with >2 cm urethral separation, or extension into the prostate or vagina

TABLE 12.7. CAUSE OF URETHRAL INJURIES

Posterior Urethral Injuries	***Straddle Injury (continued)***
Fracture of the Pelvis	Kick
Motor vehicle accidents	Bicycle
Fall, crush	***Penetrating Injury***
Sporting accidents	Gunshot
Penetrating Injuries	Machine injury
External Violence	Knife wound
Gunshot	***Urethral Instrumentation***
Stab	Catheters
Urethral Instrumentation	Cystoscope
Resectoscope	Sounds
Sounds	Filiforms, followers
Filiforms, followers	Self-instrumentation
Catheters	***Penile Surgery***
Lateral Pelvic Blow	Prosthesis placement, erosion
Anterior Urethral Injuries	Circumcision
Straddle Injury	***Sexual Intercourse***
Fall	Urethral laceration
Fence, ladder	Fracture of the penis

Anterior Urethral Injuries

Similarly, most injuries to the anterior urethra caused by external violence are the result of blunt trauma to the perineum (15,25,89,115). The bulbous urethra is usually crushed against the pelvic arch, generally when the patient falls astride an object. This may be while falling from a height, straddling a fence, or having a foot slip from the rung of a ladder. It is sometimes caused by a kick to the perineum or hitting a bump in the road while riding a bicycle and coming down hard on the seat or the crossbar.

Penetrating injuries of the anterior urethra caused by external objects are less common, but iatrogenic damage resulting from urethral instrumentation, especially inflation of a Foley catheter balloon in the bulbous urethra, occurs frequently (Table 12.7) (127). Surgery of the penis, most notably for penile prosthesis placement—or, later, prosthesis erosion—and circumcision can inadvertently damage the urethra.

Accidents secondary to sexual activity, either intercourse with urethral laceration or fracture of the penis, masturbation by urethral instrumentation, or genital mutilation by a mentally disturbed patient, also have been reported.

Diagnosis

Signs and Symptoms

Patients with a history of trauma to the perineum or who have a fracture of the bony pelvis should be suspected of having a urethral injury. If the patient has attempted to void, he may find he cannot or he may relate that he had the sensation of voiding but no urine came out of his urethra. This patient may have voided into his tissues.

Most patients with a ruptured urethra will have blood at the urethral meatus, and many of them will have swelling and ecchymosis of the penis, scrotum, and/or perineum. This is caused by urine and/or blood leaking into these structures. If the edema is only in the penis, it is probably contained within Buck's fascia. If it extends to the scrotum, perineum, or anterior abdominal wall, it will be contained by Colles' fascia.

In the patient with a fractured pelvis, rectal examination may reveal the prostate to be in a higher position than usual. This "high-riding prostate" is caused by disruption of the urethra with the prostate elevated from its normal position by a large pelvic hematoma, although the prostate also can be high-riding in the absence of a tear (type I injury, see later discussion). If the puboprostatic ligaments did not rupture, the prostate may have been lifted from its bed attached to a comminuted bone fragment. The soft, boggy hematoma will be felt where the prostate is normally found.

If the patient can urinate, he will usually have gross hematuria. It may be grossly bloody only at the beginning of the stream and/or at the end of the stream if the injury is a partial rupture.

Radiographic Examination

Any patient with a suspected urethral injury must have a retrograde urethrogram performed (32,126). Under no circumstances should an attempt be made to catheterize the urethra until this study delineates the anatomy and any damage done to that organ. Injudicious catheterization of the injured urethra carries the risk of converting a partial urethral rupture into a complete urethral rupture and possibly infecting a sterile periurethral or pelvic hematoma.

Trauma surgeons occasionally comment that placement of a urethral catheter is one of the first maneuvers that should be done in a multiple trauma patient, especially one who is hypotensive. They argue that urine output monitoring is critical in determining organ perfusion and proper fluid infusion rates. The urologic specialist should first counter with the point that blood pressure measurements also give the physician an idea of the level of organ perfusion. Second, the specialist should comment that virtually all multiple trauma patients will be sent to the radiology department to undergo appropriate studies within minutes of emergency room evaluation. At that time, a urethrogram can be performed along with other indicated x-ray films.

Some desperately ill patients who may have urethral injuries must be taken directly to the operating room for abdominal exploration before radiographic examination. At the time of surgery in these patients, a suprapubic tube should be inserted into the dome of the bladder for drainage. The lower tract may then be studied in the postoperative period and indicated therapy instituted. If the tube is not needed, it may be removed easily. As is discussed under complications of urethral ruptures, the long-term problems of incontinence, stricture formation, and erectile dysfunction, which seem unimportant at the time of injury, loom large in the postoperative period of these unfortunate men. The less urethral damage done, the more the patient will recover free of these complications.

Ideally, the urethrogram should be performed under fluoroscopic monitoring. If necessary, it may be obtained with fixed or even portable equipment in the emergency room. An easy technique that does not require special equipment is to insert a number 14- or 16-Fr Foley catheter into the urethra so that the balloon of the catheter is just 2 to 3 cm proximal to the meatus. One to two millimeters of saline solution is injected into the balloon to seat it in the fossa navicularis. No lubricant should be used or the catheter may slide out of the urethra.

The patient is then moved to a 25- to 30-degree oblique position, and approximately 25 mL of 25% to 30% contrast media is injected with a Toomey syringe into the urethra. An exposure is taken during the active injection of the

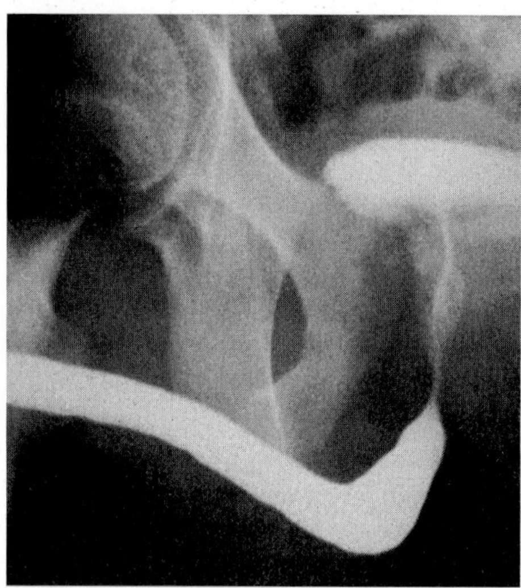

FIGURE 12.6. Normal retrograde urethrogram.

contrast medium to distend the urethra and produce a dynamic urethrogram (Fig. 12.6).

A penile clamp (i.e., Brodney or Knudson) also may be used but is cumbersome and may not always be available. Inserting the tip of the syringe directly into the urethra should not be done because the examiner's hand will be exposed to the x-ray beam.

The oblique position is best for demonstrating the entire anterior and posterior urethra. In the anteroposterior position, the bulbous urethra is foreshortened and the urethra, as well as areas of extravasation, will overlap, making the study uninterpretable.

If the urethra is normal, the balloon should be deflated, the catheter advanced into the bladder, the balloon reinflated, and a cystogram performed as previously discussed to rule out a bladder rupture. If a catheter has already been inserted into the bladder, it should not be removed. If a urethral injury is suspected, a urethrogram should be done around the indwelling catheter to rule out urethral damage. This can be done by inserting a 16-gauge Intracath alongside the Foley catheter and compressing the urethra while injecting contrast material.

Finally, an excretory urogram or CT scan should be performed to evaluate the kidneys and ureters. If a large pelvic hematoma is present, the bladder will have a "teardrop" appearance and ride high out of the pelvis (Fig. 12.7). This is commonly called a "pie-in-the-sky" bladder.

POSTERIOR URETHRAL INJURIES

Classification

As previously stated, virtually all posterior urethral injuries are secondary to fracture of the bony pelvis. Table 12.5 lists the classification of these injuries, which is helpful in planning their management (30,49,125).

Type I Injury

The posterior urethra and proximal bulbous urethra are stretched because the moorings of the prostate to the urogenital diaphragm have been ruptured and a hematoma has collected in the perivesical space (Fig. 12.8). Although stretched, the urethra is not ruptured. This injury accounts for 17% of posterior urethral ruptures.

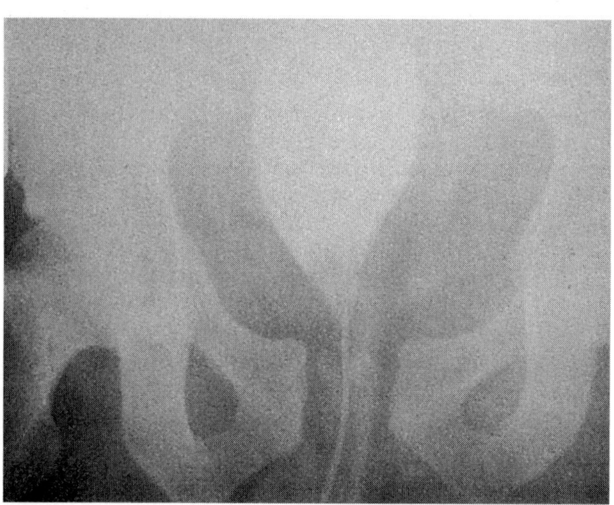

FIGURE 12.7. "Teardrop" or "pie-in-the-sky" bladder from a pelvic hematoma in a patient with a pelvic fracture.

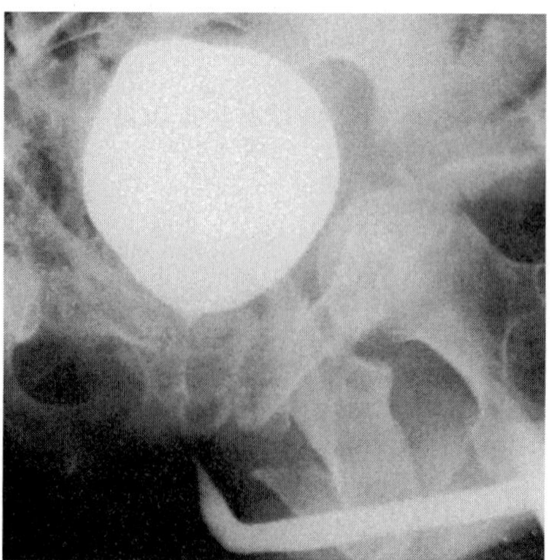

FIGURE 12.8. Type I urethral injury. Posterior urethra is compressed by hematoma. (From Sandler CM, Phillips JM, Harris JD, et al. Radiology of the bladder and urethra in blunt pelvic trauma. *Radiol Clin North Am* 1981;19:195, with permission.)

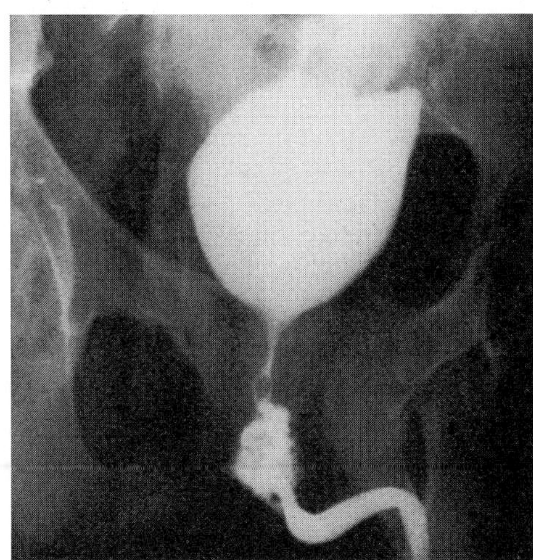

FIGURE 12.9. Type II partial urethral injury. All extravasation is in pelvis. Also note intraperitoneal rupture. (From Sandler CM, Harris JH Jr, Corriere JN Jr, et al. Posterior urethral injuries after pelvic fracture. *AJR Am J Roentgenol* 1981;137:1233, with permission.)

Type II Injury

Until recently, a type II injury was thought to be the most common type of posterior urethral injury. The classic description is rupture of the prostatomembranous urethra at the apex of the prostate above the urogenital diaphragm. Extravasation of contrast occurs superiorly into the pelvis but is limited inferiorly by an intact urogenital diaphragm (Figs. 12.9 and 12.10). The rupture may be complete or incomplete. Recent work has shown that this injury is present only 17% of the time.

Type III Injury (Posterior/Anterior)

Type III is the most common injury seen; it is present 66% of the time. The prostatomembranous urethra is either partially or completely ruptured, and contrast extends into the pelvis. In this injury, however, the urogenital diaphragm and anterior or bulbous urethra also are injured, and contrast material will be seen extending into the perineum and into the bulbous urethra (Fig. 12.11).

Type IV Injury

Many times, an injury of the bladder neck will extend into the proximal urethra. As has been discussed under injuries of the bladder, these must have immediate repair to prevent incontinence and/or stricture formation (Fig. 12.12).

Type IVA Injury

A confusing diagnostic problem occurs in patients with an injury near the bladder base. Contrast may extravasate around the urethra and what is really an extraperitoneal bladder injury can be confused with an injury of the proximal urethra. If the urethrogram is repeated under fluoroscopy, the true site of the injury can be determined (Fig. 12.13).

Penetrating Injuries

When the posterior urethra has been damaged by an external missile or intraurethral instrument, extravasation will follow the track of the injury. The extent and location of the injury are variable, and when caused by a gunshot wound, the bladder neck also is commonly damaged.

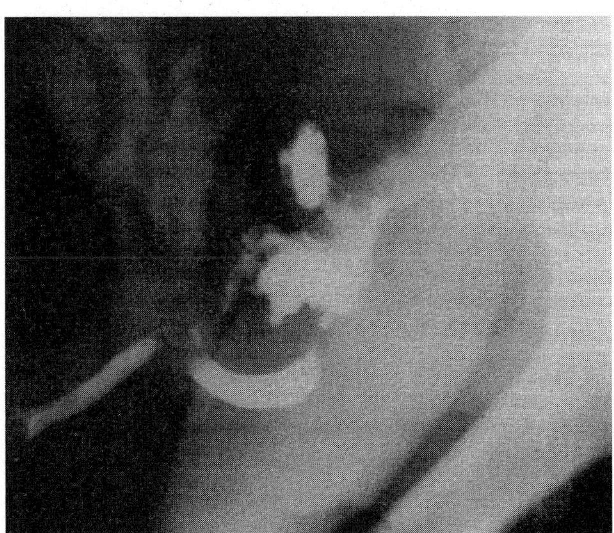

FIGURE 12.10. Type II complete urethral injury. All extravasation is in pelvis.

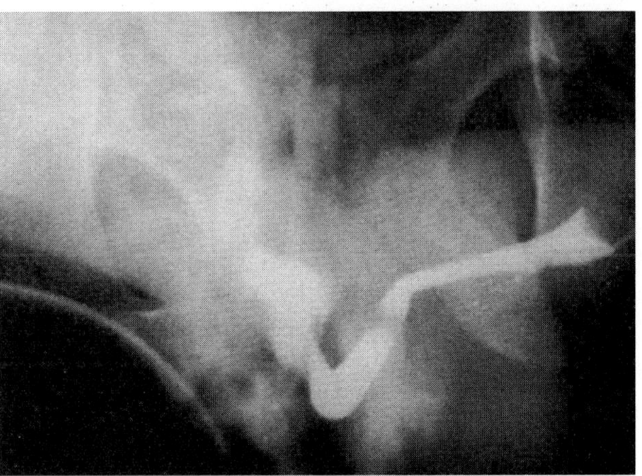

FIGURE 12.11. Type III complete urethral injury. Extravasation extends into perineum as urogenital diaphragm is ruptured. (From Sandler CM, Harris JH Jr, Corriere JN Jr, et al. Posterior urethral injuries after pelvic fracture. *AJR Am J Roentgenol* 1981;137:1233, with permission.)

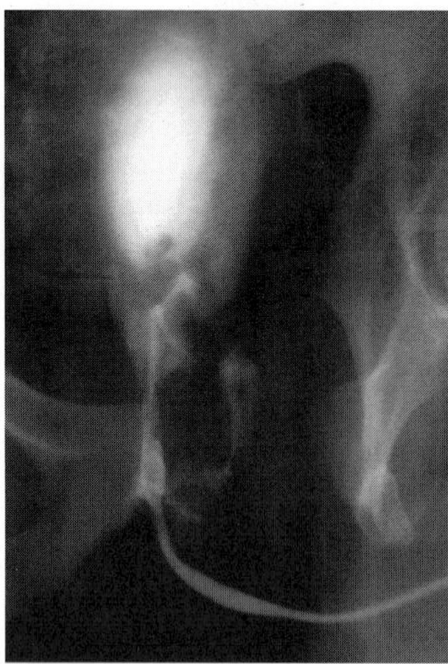

FIGURE 12.12. Type IV injury. Bladder neck injury with extension into the urethra.

Therapy

Type I Injury

The patient with a pelvic hematoma compressing the urethra often will have difficulty voiding, so a urethral catheter should be left indwelling for a few days. However, once the patient has recovered sufficiently from the injuries to discontinue urine output monitoring and is alert enough to attempt to void, the catheter should be removed. Patients with a severe pelvic disruption, especially if the sacrum is damaged, may have some neurologic deficit and be unable to urinate. A cystometrogram should help determine the status of the bladder. If multiple trials of voiding fail, the patient should be taught clean intermittent self-catheterization while awaiting return of detrusor function. There are reports of delayed rupture of these injuries and some authors recommend suprapubic tube drainage instead of urethral catheter drainage (65).

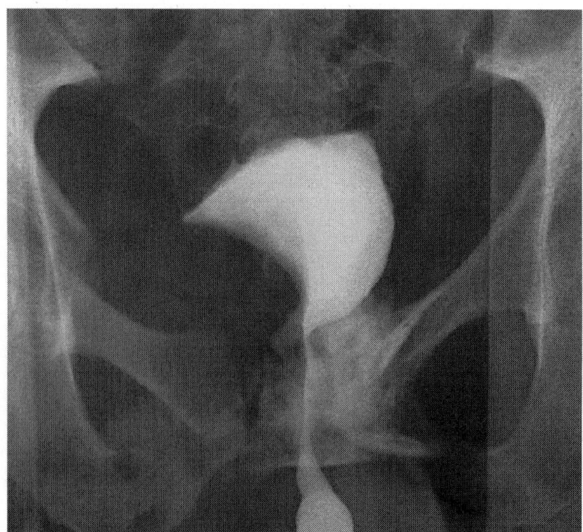

FIGURE 12.13. Type IVA injury. Extraperitoneal bladder rupture with periurethral extravasation simulating a true type IV urethral injury.

Partial Urethral Rupture

The patient with minimum partial urethral rupture may be treated with urethral catheter drainage for 14 to 21 days, followed by a voiding cystourethrogram to ensure healing of the injury. If the catheter does not pass easily into the bladder or if the injury is extensive, urethral catheterization should not be done for fear that the partial rupture may be converted to a complete rupture. The patient should undergo suprapubic cystotomy by either the trochar technique or formal surgical placement. A cystogram must then be done in these patients to rule out a concomitant bladder rupture.

Clearly, the most conservative way to handle all of these injuries is to place a suprapubic cystotomy and not attempt urethral instrumentation. A voiding cystourethrogram through the cystotomy tube should be performed 14 to 21 days after the injury. If extravasation is no longer present and the urethra is of normal caliber or there is only a minimum stricture at the site of the injury, the tube should be removed and the patient allowed to void (32).

If there is a marked narrowing or total occlusion of the urethra at the area of previous extravasation, panendoscopy and a few days of urethral catheter drainage should be performed. The visual urethrotome should be available to incise any strictures that may be present.

If the strictured area cannot be successfully negotiated with the panendoscope, the patient should be left on suprapubic drainage for 6 months and delayed repair by one of the reconstructive procedures discussed later should be performed. Partial urethral ruptures account for approximately one-third of the posterior urethral ruptures.

Complete Urethral Rupture

There are three ways to treat a complete rupture of the posterior urethra: immediate surgical realignment, suprapubic cystotomy and delayed surgical repair, or endoscopic realignment. Immediate surgical realignment is the procedure of choice in the stable patient who (a) is going to have immediate pelvic exploration for a concomitant vascular or rectal injury, (b) has a severe prostatourethral dislocation with perhaps fixation of a "pie-in-the-sky" bladder and prostate to a displaced comminuted bone fragment by the puboprostatic ligaments, or (c) has major bladder neck lacerations or prostatic fragmentation (commonly seen in children) (4,44,47,81,111,135,147).

The procedure is performed through a lower abdominal midline incision. The hematoma is evacuated and a regular or fenestrated 16- or 18-Fr catheter is passed per the urethra

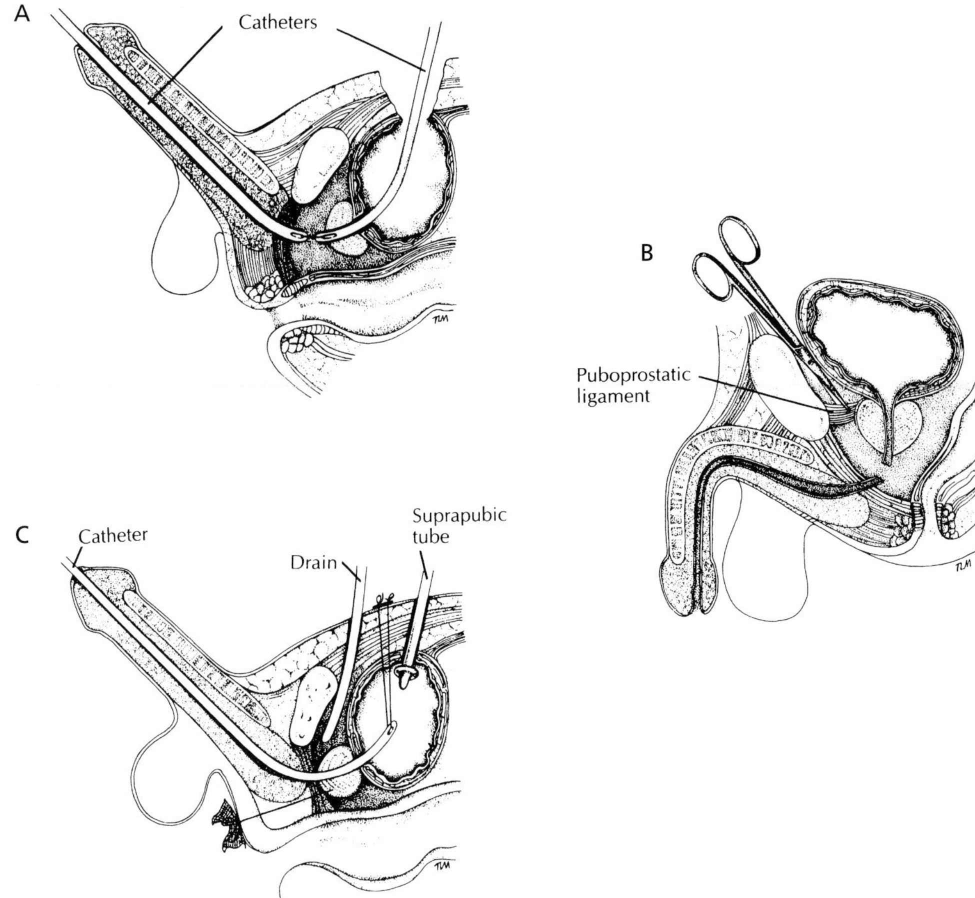

FIGURE 12.14. **A:** Catheter introduced into urethral meatus and by means of surgically opened bladder into bladder neck, then tied together in prevesical space. **B:** Unruptured puboprostatic ligament cut before repositioning of bladder and prostate. **C:** Urethral catheter lock-stitched to abdominal wall. Prostate kept in position against urogenital diaphragm by vest sutures.

through the urogenital diaphragm into the prevesical space. The catheter is identified by sight or feel and brought into the surgical field. The anterior bladder wall is opened and the interior of the organ inspected. Lacerations are repaired with 3-0 absorbable suture. Another catheter is then passed out the bladder neck, through the prostatic urethra, and brought into the surgical field by sight. A single 0 nylon suture is used to tie the tips of the catheters together through their distal most eyes, and the bladder catheter is used to guide the urethral catheter into the bladder (Fig. 12.14A). The bladder catheter is removed, a second 0 nylon catheter is placed through the eye of the urethral catheter, and the suture eventually is brought out through the bladder and abdominal wall as a lock stitch to fix this catheter in place. Some authors have used interlocking sounds or magnetic catheters (116) to effect this alignment, but the high incidence of false passages with this technique has led to its virtual abandonment.

It is now important to verify whether the puboprostatic ligaments have ruptured. If not, they must be transected, freeing the bladder and prostate from their bony attachments. If this is not done and there is severe distortion of the anterior pelvic arch, the bladder and prostate will never be able to be brought down to their normal position alongside the urogenital diaphragm (Fig. 12.14B).

One of the older techniques used to attempt realignment of the prostate was to insert a Foley catheter into the urethra and place it on traction. The idea was to pull the catheter's balloon snugly against the bladder neck and prostate to bring the organ into position. Unfortunately, to effect such a maneuver, if the prostate was still attached to the pubis, the Foley catheter would have to realign the pelvic bone as well. The procedure usually failed to accomplish this, and unfortunately, the force of the balloon on the base of the bladder often caused pressure necrosis of the bladder neck and an irreparable injury followed.

The prostate and bladder should now easily and without tension be repositioned against the urogenital diaphragm. Although some surgeons would attempt directly to anastomose the severed ends of the urethra, an easier and equally effective repair can be effected by placing 0 nylon (Vest) traction sutures through the distal prostate, through the urogenital diaphragm, and onto the perineum, where they are tied snugly over a bolster (Fig. 12.14C). A suprapubic tube is placed in the bladder, a drain in the prevesical space, and the wounds closed.

The Vest sutures and drain can be removed in 14 days, but the urethral catheter should be left in place for 3 weeks. A retrograde urethrogram should then be done around the tube, and if there is no extravasation, it can be removed. A voiding cystourethrogram is then performed, and if the patient voids normally, the suprapubic tube is removed.

Delayed surgical repair is the procedure of choice if (a) the patient is medically unstable or (b) the surgeon is unskilled in performing major urethral reconstructive surgery. In the past few years, more and more urologists have made the delayed repair their procedure of choice for almost all patients with posterior urethral ruptures because the long-term results and complications of the various techniques have become available. As is later discussed, there is evidence that the incidence of stricture incontinence and erectile dysfunction may be lower with the delayed approach to the repair of this injury (59,95,98).

Once the diagnosis of a complete posterior urethral disruption has been made, a suprapubic tube is placed into the bladder either by trocar or formal cystotomy. A cystogram is then performed to ensure that there is no bladder rupture, and nothing more is done about the urethral injury at that time. A cystotomy tube is changed at monthly intervals and the patient has follow-up clinically until the pelvic hematoma has completely reabsorbed, all scar tissue has softened, the pelvic injury has healed, and the patient has been otherwise rehabilitated. This usually takes from 6 to 9 months after the accident.

Before the repair, a cystometrogram is performed to see whether the patient has normal bladder function, as is a combined cystogram and/or retrograde urethrogram x-ray film to determine the length of the urethral defect (Fig. 12.15). Most high-riding prostates and bladders spontaneously return to the pelvis during the delay, as the pelvic hematoma reabsorbs. With this information, a procedure for definitive repair can be made. Broadly the repairs that have been described are (a) a two-stage reconstruction, (b) a one-stage reconstruction, and (3) endoscopic reestablishment.

The two-stage urethroplasty has been used since the early 1950s as a way to repair posterior urethral strictures (64,71,93,95,96). At the first stage, either through a perineal midline or pedicled flap incision, the urethra is incised ventrally through the entire stricture as proximal as the verumontanum. A scrotal or perineal skin inlay flap is then sutured to the cut edges of the urethra with interrupted absorbable suture material (Fig. 12.16). In essence, these techniques cause the strictured urethra to undergo marsupialization. A catheter is placed through the proximal ostium into the bladder, and a pressure dressing is applied to the wound. The previously placed suprapubic tube is removed on the day of surgery and the Foley catheter and dressing a few days later. The patient should void spontaneously.

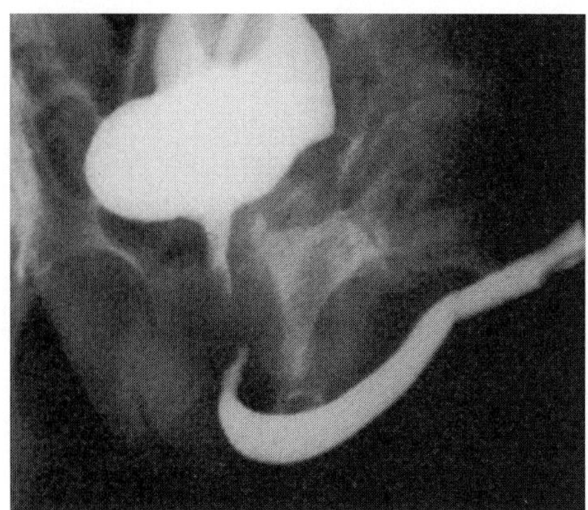

FIGURE 12.15. Combined cystogram and retrograde urethrogram in patient with a complete urethral rupture 6 months after injury.

Between the first and second stages the ostia, both proximally and distally, must be periodically calibrated. Once all the scar has softened and the wounds have healed, the second stage may be performed. The ostia must remain at least a 26-Fr size. It takes 4 to 6 months to be sure that the urethra is ready for closure.

During the second stage, the inlay is circumcised along with the underlying urethra to form an even tube of at least a 24-Fr caliber. The urethra is closed with interrupted or running absorbable sutures, as are the bulbocavernous muscles, subcutaneous tissues, and skin (Fig. 12.17). Some surgeons prefer nonabsorbable running pullout sutures for closure.

Urethral catheter and/or suprapubic tube drainage is used for 10 to 14 days, and a voiding cystourethrogram is

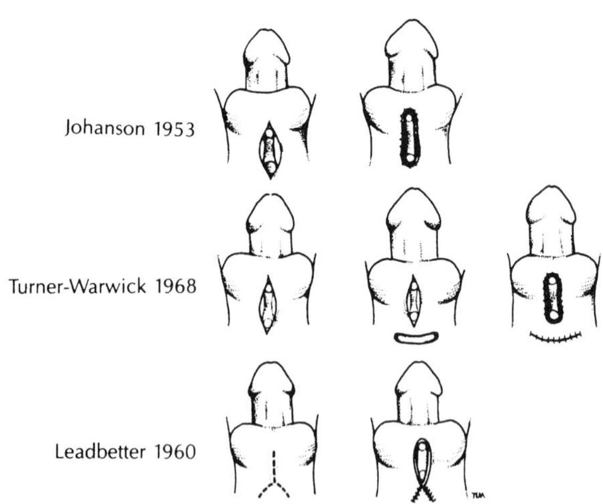

FIGURE 12.16. Various types of first-stage procedures of a two-stage urethroplasty.

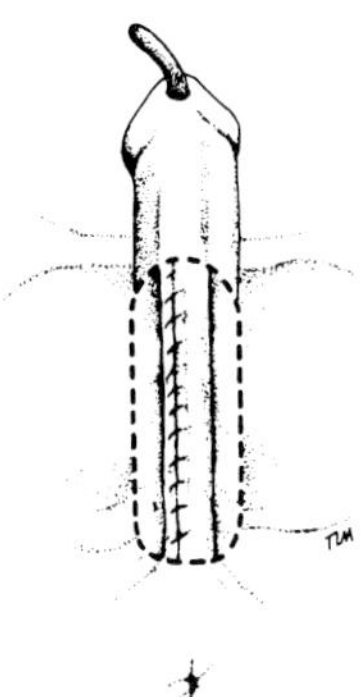

FIGURE 12.17. Second stage of a two-stage urethroplasty. Inlay circumcised *(dotted line)* and neourethra formed and closed. Bulbocavernosus muscles, skin, and subcutaneous tissue will then be closed in layers.

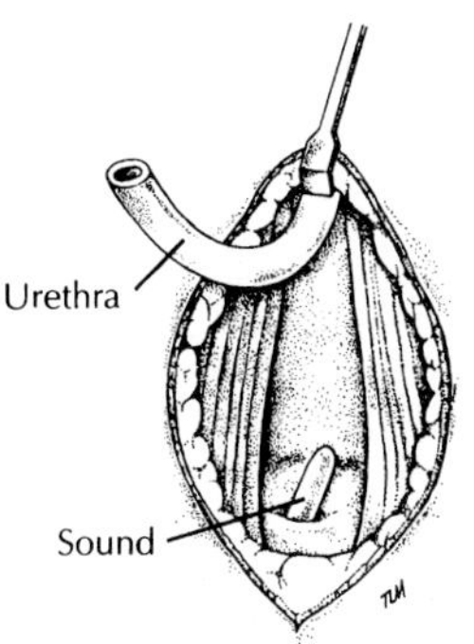

FIGURE 12.18. Urethra severed distal to stricture and retracted. Sound passed by means of bladder into bladder neck and prostatic urethra. Incision over tip of sound allows extrusion of sound into wound.

performed when the tube is removed. Catheter drainage should be continued for another week if extravasation is present.

There are basically three techniques described for one-stage reconstruction of posterior urethral strictures. *The original technique was an intussusception of the distal normal urethra into the proximal scarred urethra and prostate* (13,38,102,112). More recently, this procedure has been refined by performing a direct urethroprostatic anastomosis by either bypassing or excising the scarred area (6,31a,68,71,98,102,112,136,137,141,143,146,150). Resection of the symphysis pubis to attain access to the distal prostate is sometimes helpful (110,142).

With all of these procedures, a midline perineal incision is made and carried through the bulbocavernosus muscle to expose the urethra. The urethra with its corpus spongiosum is then dissected free in both directions to obtain adequate length. It is then divided just distal to the stricture, which means almost flush with the urogenital diaphragm.

If the intussusception technique is to be used, a curved sound is now passed by means of the suprapubic sinus tract, where the suprapubic tube has been in place, and guided into the internal urethral meatus. The tip of the sound is felt in the perineal wound at the site of the stricture. An incision is made with a scalpel onto the sound, which is then forced through into the wound. This tract is dilated to 30 Fr (13,102,112).

A small sound is now placed into the suprapubic sinus and out the distal tract and its tip is firmly invaginated into the open end of a 16-Fr red rubber catheter. The sound and catheter are drawn into the bladder and out the suprapubic sinus, and the free end of the catheter is inserted into the distal urethra for a distance of 5 to 8 cm (Fig. 12.18). The edges of the urethra are sewn to the catheter with 3-0 chromic catgut, and the catheter, with the urethra attached, is pulled through the opening in the prostate into the bladder (Fig. 12.19). The cut end of the urethra should be made to rest approximately 1 cm proximal to the verumontanum. A marking suture on the urethra before invagination is helpful to ensure this position. The outer wall of the urethra is now sewn with a few absorbable sutures to the area where it enters the tract.

The catheter, which is now exiting the suprapubic sinus, is fixed with tension to the abdominal wall. A suprapubic tube is inserted into the bladder and placed to straight drainage. The bulbocavernous muscles, subcutaneous tissues, and skin are closed in layers, and a pressure dressing is applied to the wound.

The dressing is removed on the third day. The red rubber catheter will loosen and can be removed in approximately a week. A voiding cystourethrogram should be done on the fourteenth day and the patient allowed to void. A Foley catheter should be placed into the urethra if voiding is difficult and voiding trials should begin. The suprapubic tube can be removed. These patients may need periodic urethral dilation for a few months if voiding becomes difficult.

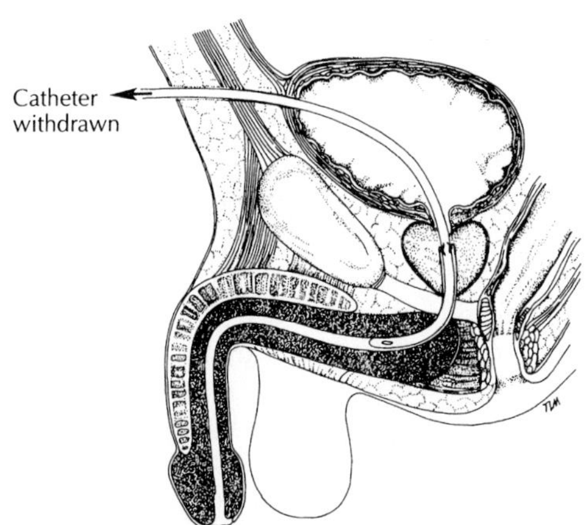

FIGURE 12.19. Catheter previously sewn to cut end of urethra drawn into bladder, intussuscepting bulbous urethra into prostatic urethra.

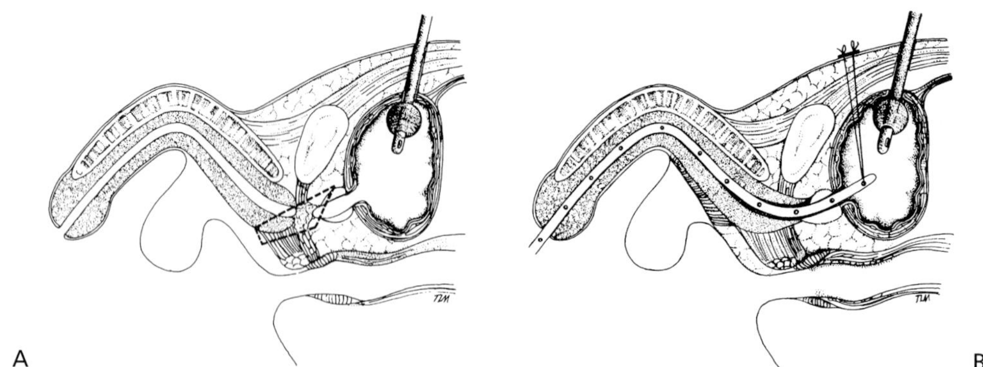

FIGURE 12.20. **A:** Preoperative status. Suprapubic tube in place. Area bounded by *dotted line* will be excised (includes scar). Prostate and urethra beveled. **B:** Urethra sewn to prostate end to end. Fenestrated urethral stent and suprapubic tube in place.

If an end-to-end prostatourethral anastomosis is to be performed after the urethra has been transected distal to the stricture, it should be spatulated (31a,68,71,98,102,112,135, 136,146,150). A curved sound is now passed through the suprapubic sinus into the prostatic urethra. If negotiation of the internal urethral meatus is difficult, a panendoscope can be passed through the suprapubic sinus into the prostatic urethra. Palpation of the tip of the sound or panendoscope in the wound acts as a guide to identify the prostate. Similarly, the light in the panendoscope may shine through the tissues in the perineal wound and help identify the prostate by sight. Now the scar is excised with a scalpel and the prostate beveled from the verumontanum posteriorly to the midprostate anteriorly.

A 16-Fr fenestrated catheter is placed by means of the urethral meatus and drawn into the wound. A 0 nylon suture is tied to the distal eye of the catheter and the suture is drawn out the suprapubic sinus by the sound or panendoscope onto the abdominal wall. The catheter is now pulled into the bladder by the suture to be eventually anchored with the suture to the abdominal wall over a button. The spatulated end of the urethra is now sutured with four 3-0 absorbable quadrant sutures to the beveled-cut end of the prostate. The wound is closed in layers and a suprapubic tube is inserted and placed to straight drainage. A pressure dressing is applied to the wound (Fig. 12.20).

The dressing is removed on the third postoperative day. The urethral stent is removed in 3 weeks and a voiding cystourethrogram is performed. If the urethra is well healed, the suprapubic tube is removed. If extravasation is present, the patient is kept on suprapubic drainage for another week and the voiding cystourethrogram is repeated. By this time, the urethra should be healed, the patient should void normally, and the suprapubic catheter can be removed.

Occasionally, the prostate and bladder will not descend far enough to allow the anastomosis to be made perineally. If this occurs, a midline abdominal incision should be made and the bladder and prostate freed from above. Many times, gouges will have to be used to remove the underside of the pubis to obtain adequate mobilization. The anastomosis, stenting, and closure are still carried out as previously described in these cases, and a prevesical drain is placed. Because of the increased amount of dead space created when the prostate is dissected from above, the omentum should be freed, brought into the pelvis, and wrapped around the anastomosis to fill in this area. Postoperative management is similar to that described above, except the patient cannot be fed orally until his gastrointestinal tract recovers from the abdominal exploration. The drain can be removed in 1 week.

Transpubic urethroprostatic anastomosis without resection of the scarred area is performed through a lower midline abdominal incision (141,143). A Gigli saw is then passed beneath the pubis on either side of the midline and a trapezoidal piece of pubic bone is removed. This gives access to the anterior surface of the prostate, which is entered. The previously perineally mobilized and spatulated distal urethra is brought through the crura and anastomosed to the prostatic incision with 3-0 quadrant absorbable sutures over a 22-Fr Foley catheter. With this procedure, the prostate is not mobilized nor is the stricture excised. A suprapubic tube and prevesical drain are brought out through the abdomen. The wounds are closed as described previously (Fig. 12.20). The timing of urethral catheter, suprapubic tube, and drain removal is essentially identical to the end-to-end anastomosis procedure.

Some urologists have advocated merely reestablishing urethral continuity by *endoscopic realignment* (3,42,50,61, 63,80,118,130). With this technique, a panendoscope is passed by means of the suprapubic sinus into the proximal urethra by one surgeon, and either a visual urethrotome or a resectoscope fitted with a Colling's knife is passed into the distal urethra by a second surgeon. With the light from the panendoscope as a guide, the distal operator cuts through the scar and into the prostatic urethra. A laser also has been used to create an opening (39). A 22-Fr urethral catheter is then placed into the bladder, removed 1 week later, and the patient is allowed to void. Periodic dilations are usually necessary in these patients (7). Recently, the use of an indwelling metal stent also has been advocated (12,107).

ANTERIOR URETHRAL INJURIES

Classification—Type V Injury

Most anterior urethral injuries caused by blunt trauma are secondary to straddle injuries (15,115). In these instances, the pelvis is usually not fractured and the overlying skin remains intact. Perhaps today there is a greater volume of iatrogenic injuries to the anterior urethra as a result of urethral instrumentation. The following subclassification of these injuries is useful when planning appropriate therapy.

Urethral Contusion

When a patient has undergone a straddle injury and has initial or terminal hematuria but has a normal urethrogram, a urethral contusion has occurred.

Partial Urethral Rupture

When a urethral injury is either caused by external blunt trauma or urethral instrumentation and a retrograde urethrogram demonstrates extravasation of contrast material but the urethra is in continuity and contrast material goes freely into the bladder, the patient is said to have a partial urethral rupture (Fig. 12.21).

Complete Urethral Rupture

If after blunt trauma extravasation is demonstrated on a retrograde urethrogram and urethral continuity is lost, a complete urethral rupture is present (Fig. 12.22).

Penetrating Urethral Injury

If the urethra has been injured by an external missile, urethral instrumentation, or migration of a penile prosthesis, a partial or complete disruption of the urethra may result. Only major lacerations or those associated with extensive tissue destruction are handled in a unique way from blunt injuries. Because of these therapeutic decisions, however, penetrating injuries are best placed into a separate category.

Therapy

Urethral Contusions

No special therapy is necessary for patients with anterior urethral contusions from blunt trauma. They usually are able to void normally, and their hematuria promptly clears. If necessary, a urethral catheter can be placed for a short period. In the absence of extravasation, there are probably no long-term sequelae of this injury.

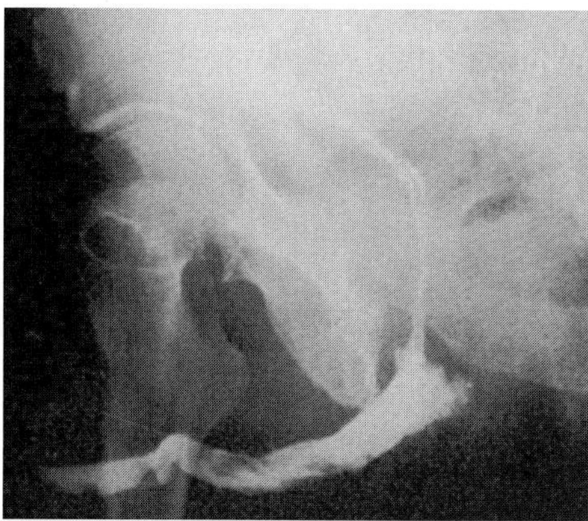

FIGURE 12.21. Partial anterior urethral rupture secondary to Foley catheter balloon blown up in bulbous urethra.

Partial Urethral Rupture

If the extravasation on urethrogram is minimal, contained by Buck's fascia, and urethral continuity is good, patients with partial urethral rupture secondary to blunt trauma may be allowed to void or a urethral catheter can be placed into their bladder for a few days. If the injury is extensive and extends outside Buck's fascia, a suprapubic tube should be placed into the bladder and a voiding cystourethrogram repeated in 10 to 14 days. If the urethra is normal or there is only a large-caliber stricture, the

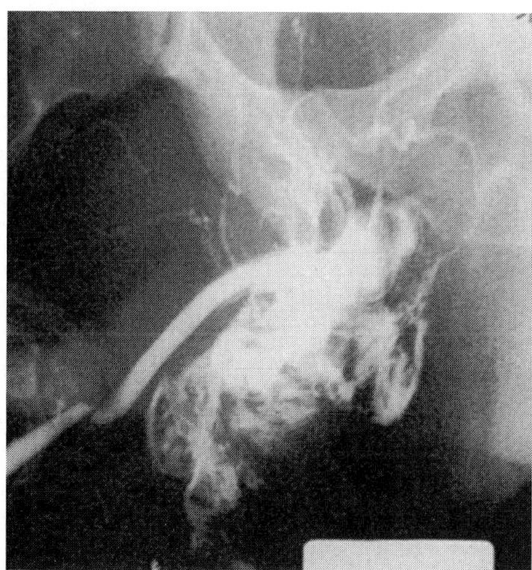

FIGURE 12.22. Complete anterior urethral rupture secondary to a straddle injury. Note the venous extravasation. (From Sandler CM, Phillips JM, Harris JD, et al. Radiology of the bladder and urethra in blunt pelvic trauma. *Radiol Clin North Am* 1981;19:195, with permission.)

tube can be removed and the patient is allowed to void. Periodic urinary flow rates and urethrograms should be done to be sure a stricture does not develop at the site of the injury.

If a significant narrowing has developed, the patient should undergo panendoscopy and visual urethrotomy of the strictured area. A urethral catheter should be left in the urethra for 24 hours and the suprapubic tube removed. When the urethral catheter is removed, the patient should be allowed to void. Periodic urinary flow rates and urethrograms are critical follow-up measures in these patients (17).

Complete Urethral Rupture

Patients with complete urethral rupture from a blunt injury do not do well with primary repair and should have a suprapubic tube placed into their bladders. If extensive perineal extravasation of blood and urine is present, these patients will need close follow-up to determine whether these collections properly reabsorb or need surgical drainage. Occasionally, patients with extensive extravasation delay in presenting to the physician, and erythema, purulence, and frank necrosis may be present in the penis, scrotum, or perineum. These patients need subcutaneous drains placed, debridement and suprapubic urinary diversion performed, and antibiotics prescribed.

When the skin of the genitalia and perineum become normal and at least 14 days have elapsed from the injury, a voiding cystourethrogram and possibly a combined voiding cystourethrogram and retrograde urethrogram should be done to delineate the injury. A stricture of some magnitude will probably have developed. If urethral continuity is intact, panendoscopy and a visual urethrotomy may be all that is needed to incise the stricture (66,144). If this is successful, a urethral catheter should be placed for 24 hours and the suprapubic tube removed. These patients must have careful follow-up with voiding flow rates and retrograde urethrograms for recurrence of their stricture.

Most of these patients, however, will have developed complete occlusion of their urethra. If infection did not supervene on the extravasation of blood and urine, it will commonly be short. The patient should be left on suprapubic drainage until the perineum is well healed before reconstruction. This will usually take 4 to 6 months. A combined voiding cystourethrogram and retrograde urethrogram will delineate the extent of the stricture to be repaired, as was described in posterior urethral ruptures.

The two-stage urethroplasties previously discussed and illustrated in Figs. 12.16 and 12.17 have been used to repair strictures of the anterior and posterior urethra (64,78, 132,133). Because the strictured area is usually at the penoscrotal junction, a simple midline incision rather than the scrotal or perineal inlay flaps is usually adequate for the first stage.

However, if a short stricture is present, a one-stage end-to-end urethroplasty plus or minus a ventral wall skin patch should be performed (36,84). In this procedure, a midline incision is made over the area of the stricture, which is identified with a urethral sound, and the urethra is mobilized in both directions. The strictured area is then excised and the dorsal wall of the urethra is reanastomosed. A full-thickness skin graft may be taken from the shaft of the penis, defatted, and used to widen the anastomosis. It is sutured in place with 4-0 absorbable sutures (Fig. 12.23). This needs to be done only if there is tension on the anastomosis or the lumen is compromised. A pedicle procedure as later described also can be used for this purpose.

The bulbocavernous muscles, subcutaneous tissue, and skin are closed in layers. A urethral catheter is left in place for 3 to 5 days and the suprapubic tube continued on drainage for 14 days. A voiding cystourethrogram is performed at that time, and if no extravasation is seen, the suprapubic tube is removed. If extravasation is seen, suprapubic drainage is continued for another week and the study repeated.

If the stricture is long, a one-stage patch graft urethroplasty or pedicled urethroplasty can be performed (16,36, 85,86,104). In these procedures, the stricture is identified as previously described for the end-to-end urethroplasty, but the urethra is not mobilized. Instead, the stricture is incised ventrally in the manner of a first-stage procedure of the two-stage technique, and then a free graft may be taken from the skin of the penis, defatted, and the entire incised urethra "patched" open (Fig. 12.24). Buccal mucosa also has been used in these repairs (43). In the pedicled technique, instead of a free graft, a suitable length of skin is freed next to the urethral incision but is left attached to its underlying blood supply. This pedicled graft is then inverted and sewn into the urethral defect (Fig. 12.25). A circular skin flap taken from the distal penis may have a

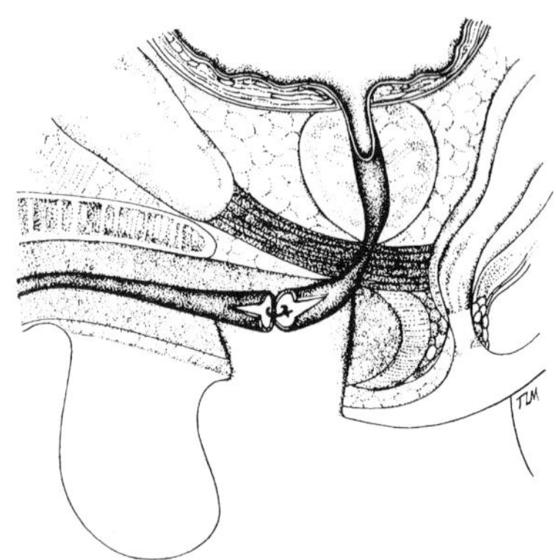

FIGURE 12.23. Strictured area was removed. Cut ends of urethra were spatulated ventrally. Dorsal walls were anastomosed. Ventral defect will be "patched open" with a full-thickness skin graft (see Fig. 12.24).

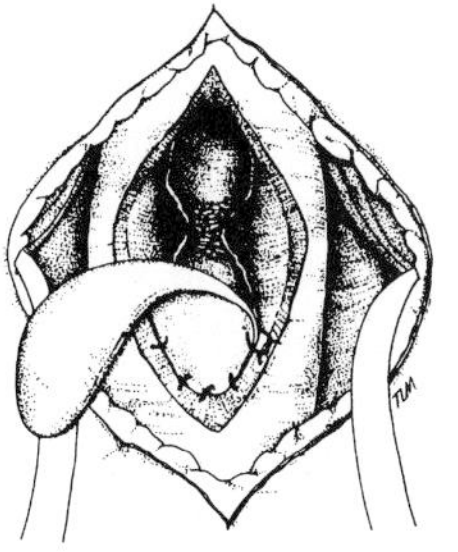

FIGURE 12.24. Free full-thickness skin graft sewn into incised urethra at area of stricture to widen stenotic section.

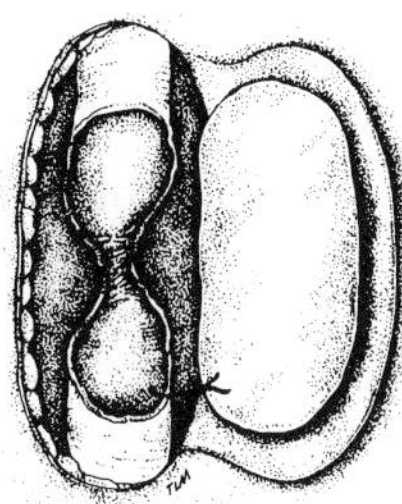

FIGURE 12.25. Pedicled skin graft sutured into area of stricture to widen stenotic section.

higher success rate than the use of local skin (86) (Fig. 12.26). Postoperative care is similar to that of the end-to-end technique with appropriate attention being given to the donor site.

Penetrating Urethral Injury

The most common penetrating injuries of the anterior urethra are secondary to urethral instrumentation. Most of these injuries are minor, and patients are usually allowed to void or a Foley catheter is placed in their bladder for a few days. Occasionally, a sound or filiform and follower is forced through the urethral wall and into the rectum. These patients need a suprapubic tube placed in their bladders for a few weeks, and their wounds will usually heal without sequelae. A retrograde urethrogram and/or voiding cystourethrogram should be done to ensure that the injury has healed before the patient is allowed to void.

During dilation of the corpus cavernosum for placement of a penile prosthesis, the urethra may be ruptured. If the prosthesis is not inserted and a Foley catheter is placed into the bladder for a few days, the perforation will heal. Sometimes, a prosthesis will spontaneously erode through the urethra, especially in patients with decreased sensation from neurologic disease, or if a Foley catheter is left in the urethra

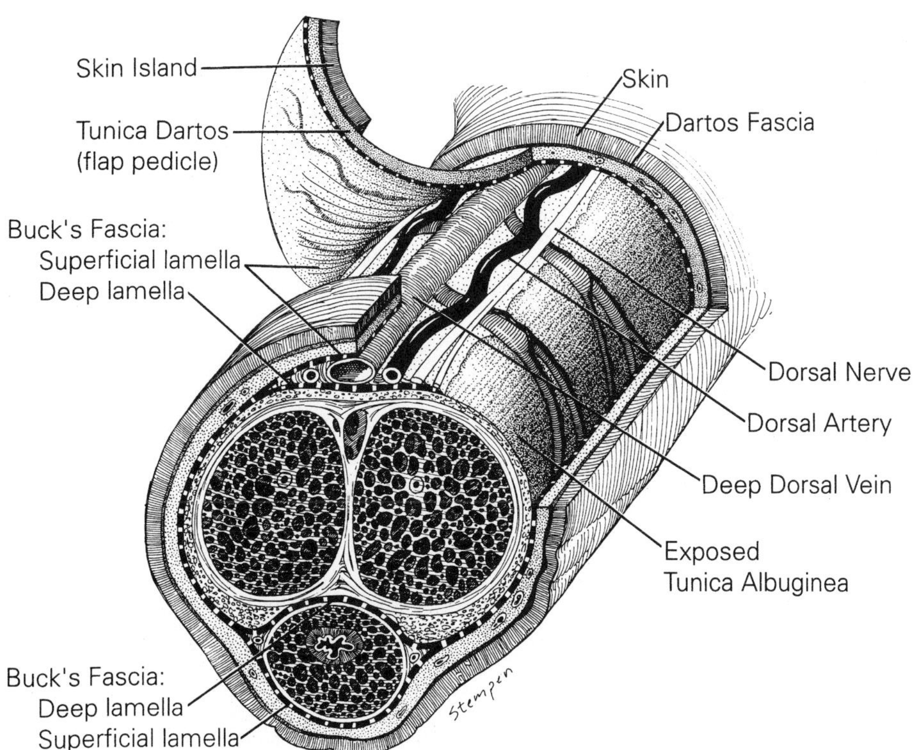

FIGURE 12.26. Flap pedicle with blood supply via tunica dartos. (From McAninch JW, Morey AF. Penile circular fasciocutaneous skin flap in 1-stage reconstruction of complex anterior urethral strictures. *J Urol* 1998;159:1209, with permission.)

for a long time in patients with penile prostheses. Merely removing the prosthesis will allow the urethral lacerations to heal. A Foley catheter may be placed for a few days to facilitate the process.

Penetrating injuries that need prompt surgical attention are those caused by external violence. Clean knife or bullet wounds merely need minimum debridement, closure of the defect with absorbable sutures, and suprapubic catheter drainage for 2 to 3 weeks (52). A voiding cystourethrogram and/or retrograde urethrogram should be done before removal of the suprapubic tube.

Dirty wounds with extensive tissue destruction and foreign material in the wound (e.g., metal pellets, oil, grease, hair, clothing) need to be cleansed thoroughly with antiseptic solutions and copious irrigation. Although debridement of devitalized tissue is important, it must be stressed that contused corpus spongiosum tissue is hemorrhagic and ecchymotic and may appear necrotic when it is only badly bruised. If debridement is vigorous, more urethra than is necessary may be removed and discarded, making eventual repair a formidable task. If a large section of urethra is lost, however, the ends of the urethra that are left should be sutured to the skin in the manner of a first-stage urethroplasty. Skin will have to be brought between the ostia to close the wound (Fig. 12.27).

Suprapubic diversion should be done until the perineum has healed. This may take weeks to months. Radiographic studies will demonstrate residual stricture, which can be handled by one of the previously described urethroplasty techniques.

POSTOPERATIVE CARE AND FOLLOW-UP

A discussion of when the stents, drains, and catheters should be removed is included with each of the previously discussed procedures. Antibiotics should be withheld in these patients until they have all tubes removed from their urinary tracts. At that time, they should receive appropriate antibiotics, and eventually urinalysis and urine cultures should be performed to ensure sterilization has been accomplished.

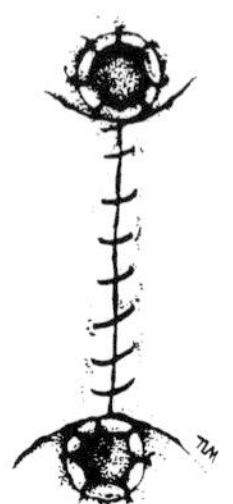

FIGURE 12.27. Damaged urethra has been discarded. Freshened edges of severed urethra sewn to skin. Normal skin brought between ostia to cover defect.

Periodic voiding flow rates should be done at 3-month intervals for at least a year. If flow decreases, a retrograde urethrogram should be performed. Patients with neurologic damage may not be able to void and may have to be taught intermittent self-catheterization. Those with bladder neck damage may be incontinent and need α-adrenergic drugs or collagen injections to become dry (60). Complete neurologic evaluation is imperative in these patients.

RESULTS AND COMPLICATIONS

When the literature is reviewed for the results and complications of these various techniques, it is well established that *the primary realignment patients may have a higher long-term complication rate than do patients treated with delayed repair, despite the technique used* (11,32,44,72,75,83,98,150). The persistent restricture rate with primary repair is approximately 50% (38% to 53%), the erectile dysfunction rate is 36% (20% to 50%), and the major/moderate incontinence rate 14% (3.7% to 21%).

With the delayed procedures, it should be noted that although virtually all partial ruptures heal without stricture, almost all patients with complete ruptures initially develop strictures. After definitive repair, however, it is the rare patient who has a long-term stricture problem. However, the erectile dysfunction rate is similar at approximately 33% (17.6% to 62%) but the major to moderate incontinence rate is lower at 2% (1% to 4%) in well-reported series. It appears to be well worth the trade-off of wearing a suprapubic catheter for 6 or more months when compared with the long-term problems associated with early repair.

There is considerable concern that patients who undergo a transsphincteric urethroplasty and in essence have their internal urethral mechanism destroyed by the procedure, are later at risk for incontinence if a transurethral resection of the prostate is performed. This risk is certainly real. However, when one considers that these are usually young men with 40 to 50 years of life ahead of them and that only 10% of males will need a prostatectomy as they get older, the argument becomes thin for withholding the procedure.

However, when faced with an elderly patient with complete obstruction caused by a posterior urethral rupture who has previously had a transurethral prostatectomy and therefore has no bladder neck continence mechanism, the use of the intussusception procedure should be chosen. With this technique the stricture and sphincter (if it is still intact) are not resected but merely dilated. If the sphincter is intact and the stricture can be kept open with periodic dilations, the patient should be continent and able to void. If the sphincter has been irreparably damaged, the stricture, if not dilated, will recur.

The long-term results reported with endoscopic realignment are poor when compared to the open procedures (3,7,42,63,80,116,130). Although the incidence of erectile dysfunction is approximately 30% (14% to 42%), which is comparable to the other techniques, it is now fairly well accepted that erectile dysfunction in patients with posterior urethral rupture is most likely caused by the injury and is not aggravated by the repair, no matter what procedure is used.

Similarly, the average major to moderate incontinence rate is 5.5% (0% to 12.5%), which is slightly higher than reported with the delayed repairs (2%) but lower than reported with primary realignment (14%).

The major objection to the endoscopic realignment is the persistent stricture rate of 54% (25% to 100%) and the need to continue with prolonged (possibly lifetime) urethral dilations in approximately 56% (25% to 100%) of the patients. Some authors even recommend leaving an indwelling catheter in the urethra after surgery for up to 3 months to keep the scar dilated and permit epithelization of the tract (3).

This high rate of restricture is because the mucosal edges of the disrupted urethra have been separated by scar and even if reepithelization of the tract does occur, the surrounding scar will persistently contract. Only a proper mucosa-to-mucosa anastomosis, with removal of all surrounding scar, can give the repair a high degree of long-term success without need for continued instrumentation.

INJURIES IN FEMALES

There are few reports of rupture of the female urethra in the literature (2,24,56,88,138). Most of them are in children, and most of them also involve the bladder neck and vagina (88,109,134). These injuries need immediate reconstruction of the bladder neck and repair of all vaginal lacerations to ensure that the continence mechanism will be intact after injury as well as to prevent the formation of vesicovaginal fistulae. Retropubic repair over a stenting urethral catheter and use of a suprapubic tube usually produces a good result. Occasionally, a urethrovaginal fistula will develop and require secondary closure.

INJURIES IN CHILDREN

As previously mentioned, most urethral injuries in females are in children and need immediate repair to prevent long-term complications (2,56,88,120,138). Males are treated by any of the previously described procedures but seem to do best when treated with the delayed technique (48,53,73,113). If the patient has an anterior stricture that can be incised with a visual urethrotome, this is preferable. If restricturing occurs, the child should be taught intermittent self-catheterization to keep the stricture dilated. Eventually, a formal urethroplasty should be performed (73,91,113, 140). Transurethral resection of the scar with stenting also has been advocated (148).

FRACTURE OF THE BONY PELVIS

Most patients that have fractures of the bony pelvis have multisystem injuries secondary to high-speed motor vehicle accidents (8,26,31,45,46,62,79,82,94,114). When an anterior arch fracture is present, the probability of a urinary tract injury is high. With a single break of the pelvic ring, 12.5% of patients will have an injury to the lower urinary tract, and with two breaks in the ring, 22% of patients will have such an injury (74,105).

Bladder ruptures, mostly extraperitoneal in nature, are seen 9% of the time, urethral injuries 3.5% of the time, and both a bladder and urethral injury 1% of the time. Aside from the urinary tract complications of stricture and incontinence, in the male, complete or relative erectile dysfunction can be seen in up to 65% of these patients (11,32,83). As previously discussed, there is a wide range of variation in the long-term complication rate depending on the initial care and the reconstructive procedure chosen for the repair of the injury. It must be stressed to emergency room and trauma team personnel that injudicious instrumentation of the urethra in the patient with a fractured pelvis and possible urethral injury may lead to a lifetime of chronic debilitation because of a momentary lapse in the proper management of this injury.

REFERENCES

1. Addar MH, Stuart GCE, et al. Spontaneous rupture of the urinary bladder: a late complication of radiotherapy—case report and review of the literature. *Gynecol Oncol* 1996;62:314.
2. Ahmed S, Neel KF. Urethral injury in girls with fractured pelvis following blunt abdominal trauma. *Br J Urol* 1996; 78:450.
3. Al-Ali M, Al-Shukry M. Endoscopic repair in 154 cases of urethral occlusion: the promise of guided optical urethral reconstruction. *J Urol* 1997;157:129.
4. Al-Ali IH, Husain I. Disrupting injuries of the membranous urethra—the case for early surgery and catheter splinting. *Br J Urol* 1983;55:716.
5. Alagiri M, Rabinovitch HH. Toothpick migration into bladder presents as abdominal pain and hematuria. *Urology* 1998;52: 1130.
6. Allen TD. The transpubic approach for strictures of membranous urethra. *J Urol* 1975;114:63.
7. Alzimaity MFA, Mosli HA, Farsi HMA, et al. Endourethrotomy of posterior urethral obliterations and severe strictures: improved outcome with urethral self-dilatation. *J Endourol* 1996;10:385.
8. Antoci JP, Schiff J Jr. Bladder and urethral injuries in patients with pelvic fracture. *J Urol* 1982;128:25.
9. Appeltans BMG, Schapmans S, et al. Urinary bladder rupture: laparoscopic repair. *Br J Urol* 1998;81:764.
10. Arun N, Kekre NS, et al. Indwelling catheter causing perforation of the bladder. *Br J Urol* 1997;80:675.
11. Aşci R, Sarikaya S, Büyükalpelli R, et al. Voiding and sexual dysfunctions after pelvic fracture urethral injuries treated with either initial cystostomy and delayed urethroplasty or immediate primary urethral realignment. *Scand J Urol Nephrol* 1999; 33:228.

12. Askhen MH, Coulange C, Milroy EJ, et al. European experience with the urethral Wallstent for urethral strictures. *Eur Urol* 1991;19:181.
13. Badenoch AW. A pull-through operation for impassable traumatic stricture of the urethra. *Br J Urol* 1950;22:404.
14. Bingham S, King PA. Sewing-pin perforation of the appendix into the bladder. *Pediatr Surg Int* 1999;15:66.
15. Blandy J. Injuries of the urethra in the male. *Injury* 1975;7:77.
16. Blandy JP, Singh M, Tresidder GC. Urethroplasty by scrotal flap for large urethral strictures. *Br J Urol* 1960;40:261.
17. Bødker A, Ostri P, Rye-Andersen J, et al. Treatment of recurrent urethral stricture by internal urethrotomy and intermittent self-catheterization: a controlled study of a new therapy. *J Urol* 1992;148:308.
18. Bolgar GC, Duncan RE, Evans AT. Primary repair of completely transected female urethra by advancement. *J Urol* 1977; 118:118.
19. Bredael JJ, Kramer SA, Cleeve LK, et al. Traumatic rupture of the female urethra. *J Urol* 1979;122:560.
20. Brosman SA, Paul JG. Trauma of the bladder. *Surg Gynecol Obstet* 1976;143:605.
21. Burnette DG Jr. Bladder perforation and urethral catheter extrusion: an unusual complication of cerebrospinal fluid-peritoneal shunting. *J Urol* 1982;127:543.
22. Carroll PR, McAninch JW. Major bladder trauma: the accuracy of cystography. *J Urol* 1983;130:887.
23. Carroll PR, McAninch JW. Major bladder trauma: mechanisms of injury and a unified method of diagnosis and repair. *J Urol* 1984;132:254.
24. Carter CT, Schafer N. Incidence of urethral disruption in females with traumatic pelvic fractures. *Am J Emerg Med* 1993; 11:218.
25. Cass AS, Godec CJ. Urethral injury due to external trauma. *Urology* 1978;11:607.
26. Cass AS, Ireland GW. Bladder trauma associated with pelvic fractures in severely injured patients. *J Trauma* 1973;13:205.
27. Cass AS, Johnson CP, Khan AU, et al. Nonoperative management of bladder rupture from external trauma. *Urology* 1983; 22:27.
28. Casselman RC, Schillinger JF. Fractured pelvis with avulsion of the female urethra. *J Urol* 1977;117:385.
29. Cohen MS, Warner RS, Fish L, et al. Bladder perforation after orthopaedic hip surgery. *Urology* 1977;9:291.
30. Colapinto V, McCallum RW. Injury to the male posterior urethra in fractured pelvis: a new classification. *J Urol* 1977; 118:575.
31. Conolly WB, Hedberg EA. Observations on fractures of the pelvis. *J Trauma* 1969;9:104.
31a. Corriere JN Jr. 1-stage delayed bulboprostatic anastomotic repair of posterior urethral rupture: 60 patients with 1 year followup. *J Urol* 2001;165:404.
32. Corriere JN Jr, Rudy DC, Benson GS. Voiding and erectile function after delayed one stage repair of posterior urethral disruptions in 50 men with a fractured pelvis. *J Trauma* 1994; 37(4):587.
33. Corriere JN Jr, Sandler CM. Management of the ruptured bladder: 7 years experience with 111 cases. *J Trauma* 1986; 26:830.
34. Das S. Complete rupture of the posterior urethra without fractured pelvis. *J Urol* 1977;118:116.
35. Devine PC, Devine CJ Jr. Posterior urethral injuries associated with pelvic fractures. *Urology* 1982;20:467.
36. Devine PC, Fallon B, Devine CJ Jr. Free full-thickness skin graft urethroplasty. *J Urol* 1976;116:444.
37. Dmochowski RR, Crandell SS, Corriere JN Jr. Bladder injury and uroascites from umbilical artery catheterization. *Pediatrics* 1986;77:421.
38. Dobrowolski Z. Long-term results of surgical treatment of posttraumatic posterior urethral strictures by Solovov's method. *J Urol* 1982;128:700.
39. Dogra PN, Aron M, Rajeev TP. Core through urethrotomy with the neodymium: yag laser for posttraumatic obliterative strictures of the bulbomembranous urethra. *J Urol* 1999; 161:81.
40. Dubinsky TJ, Deck A, et al. Sonographic diagnosis of a traumatic intraperitoneal bladder rupture. *AJR Am J Roentgenol* 1999;172:770.
41. Dwyer PL, Carey MP, Rosamilia A. Suture injury to the urinary tract in urethral suspension procedures for stress incontinence. *Int Urogyn* 1999;10:15.
42. El-Abd SA. Endoscopic treatment of posttraumatic urethral obliteration: experience in 396 patients. *J Urol* 1995;153:67.
43. El-Kasaby AW, Fath-Alla M, Noweir AM, et al. The use of buccal mucosa patch graft in the management of anterior urethral strictures. *J Urol* 1993;149:276.
44. Elliot DS, Barrett DM. Long-term follow-up and evaluation of primary realignment of posterior urethral disruptions. *J Urol* 1997;157:816.
45. Fallon B, Wendt JC, Hawtrey CE. Urological injury and assessment in patients with fractured pelvis. *J Urol* 1984; 131:712.
46. Flaherty JJ, Kelly R, Bradford B, et al. Relationship of pelvic bone fracture patients to injuries of urethra and bladder. *J Urol* 1968;99:297.
47. Follis HW, Koch MO, McDougal WS. Immediate management of prostatomembranous urethral disruptions. *J Urol* 1992;147:1259.
48. Glassberg KI, Talete-Velcek F, Ashley R, et al. Partial tears of prostatomembranous urethra in children. *Urology* 1979;13:500.
49. Goldman SM, Sandler CM, Corriere Jr JN, et al. Blunt urethral trauma: a unified, anatomical mechanical classification. *J Urol* 1997;157:85.
50. Gonzalez R, Chiou R, Hekmat K, et al. Endoscopic reestablishment of urethral continuity after traumatic disruption of the membranous urethra. *J Urol* 1983;130:785.
51. Haas CA, Brown SL, Spirnak JP. Limitations of routine spiral computerized tomography in the evaluation of bladder trauma. *J Urol* 1999;162:51.
52. Hall SJ, Wagner JR, Edelstein RA, et al. Management of gunshot injuries to the penis and anterior urethra. *J Trauma* 1995;38:439.
53. Haller JC, Kassner EG, Waterhouse K, et al. Traumatic strictures of the prostatomembranous urethra in children: radiologic evaluation before and after urethral reconstruction. *Urol Radiol* 1979;1:43.
54. Härkki-Siren P, Sjöberg J, Kurki T. Major complications of laparoscopy: a follow-up Finnish study. *Obstet Gynecol* 1999; 94:94.
55. Härkki-Siren P, Sjöberg J, Tiitinen A. Urinary tract injuries after hysterectomy. *Obstet Gynecol* 1998;92:113.
56. Hemal AK, Dorairajan LN, Gupta NP. Posttraumatic complete and partial loss of urethra with pelvic fracture in girls: an appraisal of management. *J Urol* 2000;163:282.
57. Horstman WG, McClennan BL, Heiken JP. Comparison of computed tomography and conventional cystography for detection of traumatic bladder rupture. *Urol Radiol* 1991;12:188.
58. Hubbard JG, Amin M, Polk HC Jr. Bladder perforations secondary to surgical drains. *J Urol* 1979;121:521.

59. Husmann DA, Wilson WT, Boone TB, et al. Prostatomembranous urethral disruption: management of suprapubic cystostomy and delayed urethroplasty. *J Urol* 1990;144:76.
60. Iselin CE, Webster GD. The significance of the open bladder neck associated with pelvic fracture urethral distraction defects. *J Urol* 1999;162:347.
61. Islam M. Posterior urethral trauma and strictures: an attempt to solve a controversy. *J Urol* 1978;119:418.
62. Iversen HG, Jessing P. Urinary tract lesions associated with fractures of the pelvis. *Acta Chir Scand* 1973;139:201.
63. Jepson BR, Boullier JA, Moore RG, et al. Traumatic posterior urethral injury and early primary endoscopic realignment: evaluation of long-term follow-up. *Urology* 1999;53:1205.
64. Johanson B. Reconstruction of the male urethra in strictures: application of the buried intact epithelium technic. *Acta Chir Scand* 1953[Suppl];176:1.
65. Jones JS, Koch MD. Delayed rupture of type I posterior urethral injury: case report. *J Urol* 1993;149:1132.
66. Katz AS, Waterhouse K. Treatment of urethral strictures in men by internal urethrotomy: a study of 61 patients. *J Urol* 1971;105:807.
67. Kesby GJ, Korda AR. Migration of a Filshie clip into the urinary bladder seven years after laparoscopic sterilisation. *Br J Obstet Gynaecol* 1997;104:379.
68. Khan AU, Furlow WL. Transpubic urethroplasty. *J Urol* 1976; 116:447.
69. Kinmont JC. Penetrating bladder injury caused by a medially placed acetabular screw. *J Southern Orthopaedic Assoc* 1999; 8:98.
70. Kluge A. Inconspicuous path of an aortic bypass straight through the urinary bladder. *AJR Am J Roentgenol* 1999; 173:246.
71. Koraitim MM. The lessons of 145 posttraumatic posterior urethral strictures treated in 17 years. *J Urol* 1995;153:63.
72. Koraitim MM. Pelvic fracture urethral injuries: evaluation of various methods of management. *J Urol* 1996;156:1288.
73. Koraitim MM. Posttraumatic posterior urethral strictures in children: a 20-year experience. *J Urol* 1997;157:641.
74. Koraitim MM, Marzouk ME, Atta MA, et al. Risk factors and mechanism of urethral injury in pelvic fractures. *Br J Urol* 1996;77:876.
75. Kotkin L, Koch MO. Impotence and incontinence after immediate realignment of posterior urethral trauma: result of injury or management? *J Urol* 1996;155:1600.
76. Kotkin L, Koch, MO. Morbidity associated with nonoperative management of extraperitoneal bladder injuries. *J Trauma* 1995;38:895.
77. Kovachev LS. Subtotal cystectomy as a complication of hernia repair in infants. *Eur J Surg* 1999;165.
78. Leadbetter GW Jr. A simplified urethroplasty for strictures of the bulbous urethra. *J Urol* 1960;83:54.
79. Levine JI, Crampton RS. Major abdominal injuries associated with pelvic fractures. *Surg Gynecol Obstet* 1963;116:223.
80. Lieberman SF, Barry JM. Retreat from transpubic urethroplasty for obliterated membranous urethral strictures. *J Urol* 1982; 128:379.
81. Lim PH, Chng HC. Initial management of acute urethral injuries. *Br J Urol* 1989;64:165.
82. Looser KG, Crombie HD Jr. Pelvic fractures: an anatomic guide to severity of injury. *Am J Surg* 1976;132:638.
83. Mark SD, Keane TE, Vandemark RM, et al. Impotence following pelvic fracture urethral injury: incidence, aetiology and management. *Br J Urol* 1995;75:62.
84. Martinez-Piñeiro JA, Cárcamo P, Garcia Matres MJ, et al. Excision and anastomotic repair for urethral stricture disease: Experience with 150 cases. *Eur Urol* 1997;32:433.
85. McAninch JW. Reconstruction of extensive urethral strictures: circular fasciacutaneous penile flap. *J Urol* 1993;149:488.
86. McAninch JW, Morey AF. Penile circular fasciocutaneous skin flap in 1-stage reconstruction of complex anterior urethral strictures. *J Urol* 1998;159:1209.
87. Mee SL, McAninch JW, Federele MP. Computerized tomography in bladder rupture: diagnostic limitations. *J Urol* 1987; 137:207.
88. Merchant WC, Gibbons MD, Gonzales ET. Trauma to the bladder neck, trigone and vagina in children. *J Urol* 1984; 131:747.
89. Mitchell JP. Injuries to the urethra. *Br J Urol* 1968;40:649.
90. Mitchell JP. Trauma to the urethra. *Injury* 1975;7:84.
91. Montfort G, Bretheau D, Di Benedetto V, et al. Urethral stricture in children: treatment by urethroplasty with bladder mucosa graft. *J Urol* 1992;148:1504.
92. Moore EE, Cogbill TH, Jurkovich GJ, et al. Organ injury scaling III: chest wall, abdominal vascular, ureter, bladder and urethra. *J Trauma* 1992;33:337.
93. Morehouse DD, Belitsky P, MacKinnon KJ. Rupture of posterior urethra. *J Urol* 1972;107:255.
94. Morehouse DD, MacKinnon KJ. Urologic injuries associated with pelvic fractures. *J Trauma* 1969;9:479.
95. Morehouse DD, MacKinnon KJ. Posterior urethral injury: etiology, diagnosis, initial management. *Urol Clin North Am* 1977;4:69.
96. Morehouse DD, MacKinnon KJ. Management of prostatomembranous urethral disruption: 13-year experience. *J Urol* 1980;123:173.
97. Moreiras M, Cuiña L, Goyanes GR, et al. Inadvertent placement of a Tenckhoff catheter into the urinary bladder. *Nephrol Dial Transplant* 1997;12:818.
98. Morey AF, McAninch JW. Reconstruction of posterior urethral disruption injuries: outcome analysis in 82 patients. *J Urol* 1997;157:506.
99. Mulkey AP Jr, Witherington R. Conservative management of vesical rupture. *Urology* 1974;4:426.
100. Munshi I, Hong JJ, Mueller CM, et al. Spontaneous rupture of the urinary bladder in the alcoholic patient. *J Trauma* 1999; 46:1133.
101. Napier-Hemy R, Thampuran S, Elem B. Case report. Colovesical fistula after ingestion of a modelling-knife blade. *Br J Urol Int* 1999;83:350.
102. Netto NR Jr. The surgical repair of posterior urethral strictures by the transpubic urethroplasty or pull-through technique. *J Urol* 1985;133:411.
103. Netto NR Jr, Ikari O, Zuppo VP. Traumatic rupture of female urethra. *Urology* 1983;22:601.
104. Orandi A. One-stage urethroplasty. *Br J Urol* 1968;40:717.
105. Palmer JK, Benson GS, Corriere JN Jr. Diagnosis and initial management of urological injuries associated with 200 consecutive pelvic fractures. *J Urol* 1983;130:712.
106. Parkhurst JD, Coker JE, Halverstadt DB. Traumatic avulsion of the lower urinary tract in the female child. *J Urol* 1981; 126:265.
107. Parra RO. Treatment of posterior urethral strictures with a titanium urethral stent. *J Urol* 1991;146:997.
108. Peng MY, Parisky YR, Cornwell EE, et al. CT cystography versus conventional cystography in evaluation of bladder injury. *AJR Am J Roentgenol* 1999;173:1269.
109. Persky L. Childhood urethral trauma. *Urology* 1978;9:603.

110. Pierce JM Jr. Exposure of the membranous and posterior urethra by total pubectomy. *J Urol* 1962;88:256.
111. Pierce JM. Management of dismemberment of the prostatic membranous urethra and ensuing stricture disease. *J Urol* 1972; 107:259.
112. Pierce JM Jr. Posterior urethral stricture repair. *J Urol* 1979; 121:739.
113. Podestá ML, Medel R, Castera R, et al. Immediate management of posterior urethral disruptions due to pelvic fracture: therapeutic alternatives. *J Urol* 1997;157:1444.
114. Pokorny M, Pontes JE, Pierce JM Jr. Urological injuries associated with pelvic trauma. *J Urol* 1979;121:455.
115. Pontes JE, Pierce JM Jr. Anterior urethral injuries: four years of experience at the Detroit General Hospital. *J Urol* 1978; 120:563.
116. Porter JR, Takayama TK, Defalco AJ. Traumatic posterior urethral injury and early realignment using magnetic urethral catheters. *J Urol* 1997;158:425.
117. Puranen J, Koivisto E. Perforation of the urinary bladder and small intestine caused by a trochanteric plate. *Acta Orthop Scand* 1978;49:65.
118. Quint HJ, Stanisic TH. Above and below delayed endoscopic treatment of traumatic posterior urethral disruptions. *J Urol* 1993;149:484.
119. Redman JF, O'Donnell PD. Traumatic severance of prostatomembranous urethra without associated fractured pelvis. *Urology* 1980;16:292.
120. Reinberg O, Yazbeck S. Major perineal trauma in children. *J Pediatr Surg* 1989;24:982.
121. Richardson JR Jr, Leadbetter GW Jr. Nonoperative treatment of the ruptured bladder. *J Urol* 1975;114:213.
122. Robards VL Jr, Haglund RV, Lubin EN, et al. Treatment of rupture of the bladder. *J Urol* 1976;116:178.
123. Saidi MH, Sadler RK, Vancaillie TG, et al. Diagnosis and management of serious urinary complications after major operative laparoscopy. *Obstet Gynecol* 1996;87:272.
124. Salomé F, Cazaux P, Setton D, et al. Bladder entrapment during internal fixation of a pelvic fracture. *J Urol* 1999; 161:213.
125. Sandler CM, Harris JH Jr, Corriere JN Jr, et al. Posterior urethral injuries after pelvic fracture. *Am J Radiol* 1981a;137: 1233.
126. Sandler CM, Phillips JM, Harris JD, et al. Radiology of the bladder and urethra in blunt pelvic trauma. *Radiol Clin North Am* 1981b;19:195.
127. Sellett T. Iatrogenic urethral injury due to preinflation of a Foley catheter. *JAMA* 1971;217:1548.
128. Sivit CJ, Cutting JP, Eichelberger MR. CT Diagnosis and localization of rupture of the bladder in children with blunt abdominal trauma: significance of contrast material extravasation in the pelvis. *AJR Am J Roentgenol* 1995;164:1243.
129. Sivit CJ, Taylor GA, Newman KD, et al. Safety belt injuries in children with lap belt ecchymosis: CT findings in 61 patients. *AJR Am J Roentgenol* 1991;157:111.
130. Spirnak JP, Smith EM, Elder JS. Posterior urethral obliteration treated by endoscopic reconstitution, internal urethrotomy and temporary self-dilation. *J Urol* 1993;149:766.
131. Swana HS, Foster HE: Erosion of malleable penile prosthesis into bladder. *J Urol* 1997;157:2259.
132. Swinney J. Reconstruction of the urethra in the male. *Br J Urol* 1952;24:229.
133. Swinney J. Urethroplasty: an assessment after seven years experience. *Br J Urol* 1957;29:293.
134. Thambi-Dorai CR, Boucaut HA, Dewan PA. Urethral injuries in girls with pelvic trauma. *Eur Urol* 1993;24:371.
135. Turner-Warwick R. Complex traumatic posterior urethral injuries. *J Urol* 1977a;118:564.
136. Turner-Warwick R. A personal view of the management of traumatic posterior urethral strictures. *Urol Clin North Am* 1977b;4:111.
137. Turner-Warwick R. The repair of urethral strictures in the region of the membranous urethra. *J Urol* 1968;100:303.
138. Venn SN, Greenwell TJ, Mundy AR. Pelvic fracture injuries of the female urethra. *Br J Urol Int* 1999;83:626.
139. Volpe MA, Pachter EM, Scalea TM, et al. Is there a difference in outcome when treating traumatic intraperitoneal bladder rupture with or without a suprapubic tube? *J Urol* 1999;161: 1103.
140. Waterhouse K. The surgical repair of membranous urethral strictures in children. *J Urol* 1976;116:363.
141. Waterhouse K, Abrahams JI, Caponegro P, et al. The transpubic repair of membranous urethral strictures. *J Urol* 1974; 111:188.
142. Waterhouse K, Abrahams JI, Gruber H, et al. The transpubic approach to the lower urinary tract. *J Urol* 1973;109:486.
143. Waterhouse K, Laungani G, Patel U. The surgical repair of membranous urethral strictures: experience with 105 consecutive cases. *J Urol* 1980;123:500.
144. Waterhouse K, Selli C. Technique of optical internal urethrotomy. *Urology* 1978;11:407.
145. Weber S, Mauch W, Kalayoglu M, et al. Intraperitoneal and extraperitoneal bladder rupture secondary to rectal impalement. *J Trauma* 1995;38:818.
146. Webster GD, Mathes GL, Selli C. Prostatomembranous urethral injuries: a review of the literature and a rational approach to their management. *J Urol* 1983;130:898.
147. Webster GD, Selli C. Management of traumatic posterior urethral stricture by one stage perineal repair. *Surg Gynecol Obstet* 1983;156:620.
148. Wu YA, Huang CH, Liu JH. Transurethral resection in children with urethral stricture and occlusion. *J Endourol* 1994; 8:69.
149. Yalçin V, Demirkesen O, Alici B, et al. An unusual presentation of a foreign body in the urinary bladder: a migrant intrauterine device. *Urol Int* 1998;61:240.
150. Zincke H, Furlow WL. Long-term results with transpubic urethroplasty. *J Urol* 1985;133:605.

13

THE ADRENALS

ANDREW C. NOVICK
STUART S. HOWARDS

ANATOMY

The adrenal glands are a pair of retroperitoneal organs embedded in perirenal adipose tissue. They lie superior and medial to the upper poles of the kidneys within Gerota's fascia. Their lowest extent, particularly on the left, is close to the renal vessel; thus care must be taken to avoid injury to the renal blood supply during adrenalectomy. Computed tomography (CT) scanning has made it clear that the adrenal glands are anterior to the kidney. The cortex has a characteristic yellow color, which makes it easy to recognize during surgery. The medulla, which is usually not visualized, is brown or red. The glands are flattened with distinct edges and measure approximately 5 cm by 3 cm by 1 cm. The normal human gland weighs 4 to 5 g *in vivo* and 6 g in death (65). The terminal weight increase is caused by adrenocorticotropic hormone (ACTH) release during stress. The shape and size of the glands are variable.

The cortex has a mesodermal origin, arising in utero from the dorsal mesentery near the cranial pole of the mesonephros. The gland differentiates into an outer zone,

A.C. Novick: Urological Institute, The Cleveland Clinic, Cleveland, OH 44106.

S.S. Howards: Departments of Urology and Physiology, University of Virginia, Charlottesville, VA 22908.

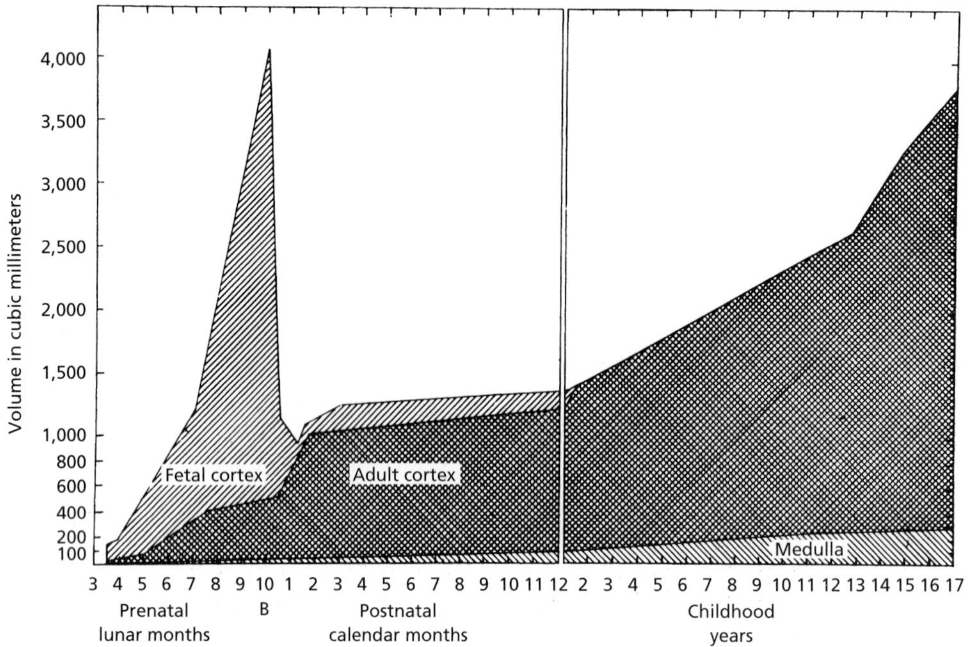

FIGURE 13.1. Growth of the adrenal cortex including the fetal cortex *in utero* and after birth. There is a striking decrease in the size of the fetal cortex after birth and a gradual increase in the adult cortex with aging. (From Bethune JE. *The adrenal cortex. A scope monograph.* Kalamazoo MI: Upjohn Co., 1974.)

which will form the adult cortex, and a much larger inner fetal zone,which will be 80% of the gland at birth but rapidly degenerates while the outer portion grows (Fig. 13.1). The net result is that the gland at birth is twice as large as it is a few weeks later. The medulla arises from ectodermal neural crest tissue, which also generates sympathetic ganglion cells. Strands of this chromaffin tissue migrate to the adrenal cortex on its medial side and become centrally located in the gland.

Each adrenal gland is supplied with blood from three arteries that are branches of the aorta, renal, and inferior phrenic arteries (Fig. 13.2). These arteries form a plexus in the capsule that gives rise to cortical arteries, which in turn supply sinusoids surrounding the cords of cells in the cortex. There are no veins in the cortex. The medulla has a dual blood supply from major capsular arteries that pass directly through the cortex without branching and from the cortical sinusoids that connect to medullary capillaries. Thus the medullary cells are exposed to the cortical effluent with high concentrations of cortical steroids. The medulla and cortex drain into a large central medullary vein, the adrenal vein, which inserts directly into the vena cava on the right and into the renal vein on the left.

The cortical cells have sparse, possibly adrenergic innervation. The medullary cells are innervated by preganglionic sympathetic nerve fibers arising from the intermediolateral column of the lower thoracic spinal cord. These fibers travel with the splanchnic nerves and synapse with a group of medullary cells to form a functional unit. The medullary pheochromocytes are the equivalents of sympathetic ganglion cells.

The adrenal cortex contains three concentric zones: a thin outer zona glomerulosa, a thick zona fasciculata, and a thin zona reticularis (Fig. 13.3). The zona glomerulosa is composed of small (12 to 15 mm) columnar cells with sparse cytoplasm. The cells are packed in clusters and arcades. In humans, the zona glomerulosa may be absent in some areas of the cortex. Aldosterone synthesis occurs in steps in the smooth endoplasmic reticulum and mitochondria where the essential enzymes are located (48).

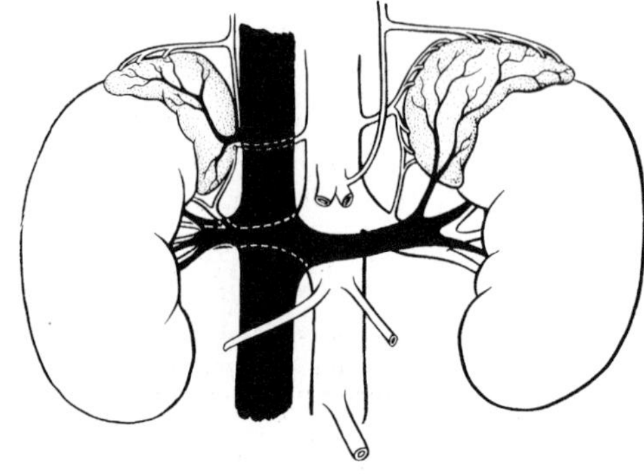

FIGURE 13.2. Blood supply to the adrenal gland. The gland is supplied by three major arteries, the superior, middle, and inferior adrenal arteries, which are branches of the inferior phrenic artery, the aorta, and renal artery. One major vein drains into the renal vein on the left and the vena cava on the right.

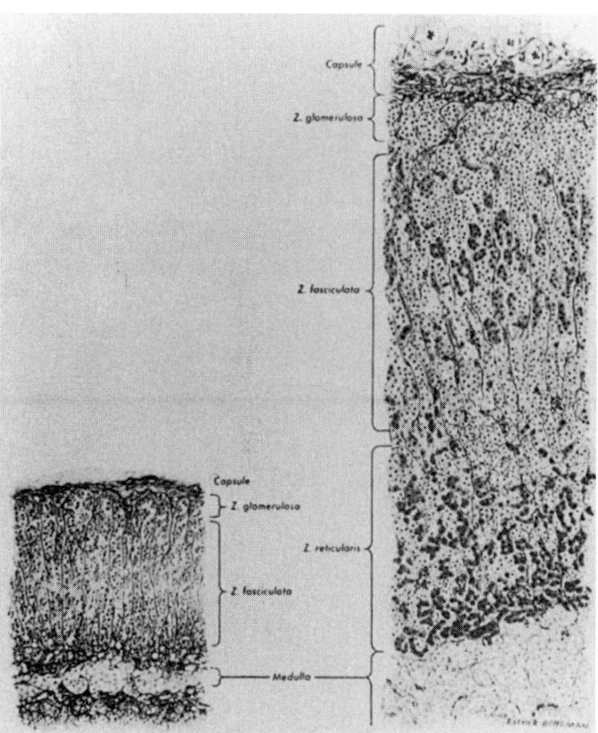

FIGURE 13.3. Histology of the adrenal gland. Note the cortex has three major components: the zona glomerulosis, zona fasciculata, and zona reticularis.

The zona fasciculata consists of polyhedral large (20 mm) cells arranged in straight cords one to two cells thick and filled with lipid droplets. The zona reticularis consists of smaller cells with few lipid droplets. The cells are arranged in now parallel anastomosing cords (Fig. 13.3).

The adrenal medullary consists of chromaffin cells generously supplied with cortex and blood vessels. They are polyhedral and arranged in cords with close association to the vascular spaces. Epinephrine- and norepinephrine-secreting cells are distinct; each contains a specific type of granule (48).

Ectopic adrenal tissue can be found in many locations, particularly near the adrenal glands, kidneys, celiac axis, or testis and spermatic cord. Unilateral congenital absence of an adrenal gland is a rare anomaly. When the kidney is absent, the adrenal is present in its normal position but is more disklike than triangular.

PHYSIOLOGY

The adrenal cortex synthesizes cholesterol and also takes it from the circulation. The first and rate-limiting process in the synthesis of adrenal steroids is the conversion of cholesterol to pregnenolone (Fig. 13.4). The hormones critical to life that are produced by the cortex are (a) the glucocoste-

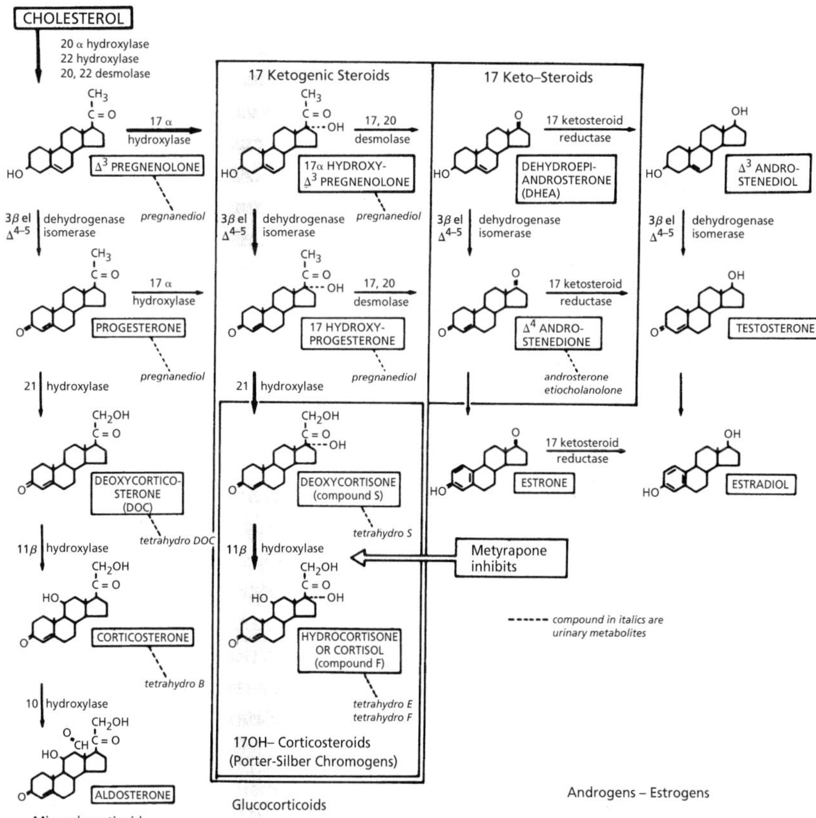

FIGURE 13.4. Biosynthetic pathways for the synthesis of adrenocortical steroids—also the site of metyrapone, urinary metabolites, and the Porter-Silber chromogens.

roids, particularly cortisol, which affect carbohydrate and protein metabolism, and (b) a mineralocorticoid, aldosterone, which regulates sodium and potassium balance. These hormones must be replaced after bilateral adrenalectomy. The adrenal cortex also synthesizes androgens and estrogens, which in normal individuals are not as important in sexual development and function as their counterparts produced by the testis and ovaries. In certain disease states, these sex steroids have dramatic virilizing or feminizing effects.

Steroidogenesis

All adrenal steroid hormones have the same steroid nucleus (Fig. 13.5). A ketone at the 3 position and hydroxyl groups at the 11 and 21 positions are required for potent glucocorticoid activity. An oxygenated carbon at the 18 position results in powerful mineralocorticoid activity. Elimination of the $C_{20\text{-}21}$ side chain and incorporation of an oxygenated carbon at the 18 position create a potent androgen. Aromatization of the A ring generates an estrogen.

The synthesis of glucocorticoids and sex steroids occurs primarily, although not exclusively, in the zona fasciculata and reticularis, respectively. Aldosterone is synthesized exclusively in the zona glomerulosa. The synthesis pathways for production of these hormones are presented in Fig. 13.4. In certain situations, alternative pathways may become important; for example, if cortisol synthesis is specifically blocked, corticosterone synthesis may be increased to provide the necessary glucocorticoid.

Iatrogenic interruption of these pathways may be useful in diagnosis and treatment. Metyrapone decreases the conversion of cholesterol to pregnenolone. Thus, when the drug is used preoperatively, the levels of all adrenal steroids may be reduced. Metyrapone also inhibits 11-hydroxylation, the last step in cortisol synthesis (Fig. 13.4), resulting in an increase in ACTH and thus cortisol precursor production in the normal individual. Therefore metyrapone can be administered to test the hypothalamic-pituitary-ACTH axis and in the treatment of Cushing's syndrome, especially before surgical therapy. Aminoglutethimide inhibits the desmolase and the aromatase reactions, thus decreasing steroid synthesis. This property has been used in the treatment of hypersecretion of adrenal steroids, prostate cancer, and breast cancer.

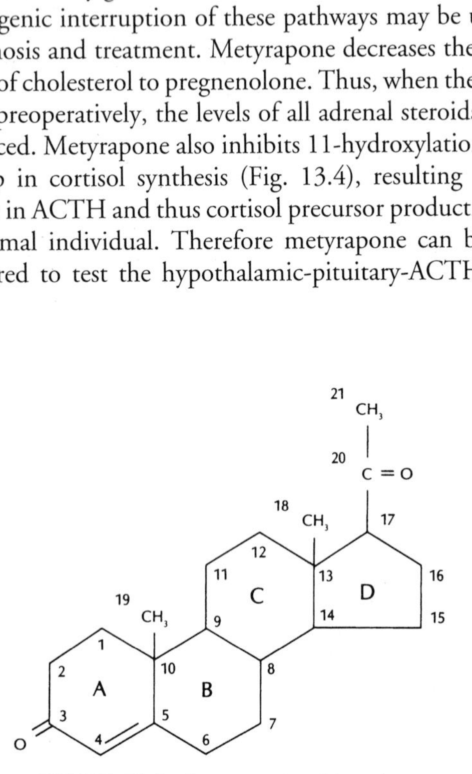

FIGURE 13.5. Common steroid nucleus.

Metabolism

Circulating cortisol is 75% to 80% bound to an α_2-globulin, transcortin; 15% is bound to albumin; and only 5% to 10% is unbound. The biologically active factor is the free hormone; thus alterations in the level of transcortin can have physiologic significance. The half-life of cortisol is approximately 70 minutes. Most of the hormone is metabolized in the liver, conjugated, and excreted as glucuronides in the urine. A small fraction of the cortisol (approximately 50 mg) is excreted unaltered in urine. Measurement of the urinary metabolites and free cortisol can be used to evaluate adrenal function.

Plasma aldosterone is weakly bound to a specific binding globulin and albumin. Ninety percent of the circulating aldosterone is cleared in one pass through the liver and then is reduced and excreted in the urine as the 3 and 18 glucuronides. Less than 1% of the aldosterone is excreted as the free hormone. Because of its rapid metabolism, the half-life of plasma aldosterone is only 20 minutes.

Adrenal androgens are excreted in the urine as dehydroepiandrosterone sulfate (DHEAS) and two reduced isomers, androsterone and etiocholanolone (Fig. 13.4). These compounds make most of the urinary 17-ketosteroids. Two-thirds of the 17-ketosteroids come from the adrenal and one-third from the gonad in normal individuals. Elevation of the urinary 17-ketosteroids generally indicates adrenal hyperfunction.

Regulation

ACTH is the regulator of glucocorticoid secretion and is also the primary determinant of the secretion of adrenal sex steroids. It is derived from a 31,000-Da glycoprotein, proopiomelanocortin, which is cleaved in corticotropic cells into ACTH, β-lipotropin, and a glycopeptide (87). ACTH is a single-chain polypeptide containing 39 amino acids. The active component of the molecule is the initial segment of 23 amino acids. The hormone is secreted in irregular bursts throughout the day, but the most active secretion occurs in the early morning, causing the diurnal secretion of cortisol. Cortisol secretion increases within minutes of an elevation in plasma ACTH levels. ACTH binds to an adrenal plasma membrane receptor and activates adenylate cyclase, which in turn raises tissue cyclic adenosine monophosphate (cAMP) levels. The cAMP activates critical protein kinases, which effect the phosphorylation of proteins that increase steroidogenesis.

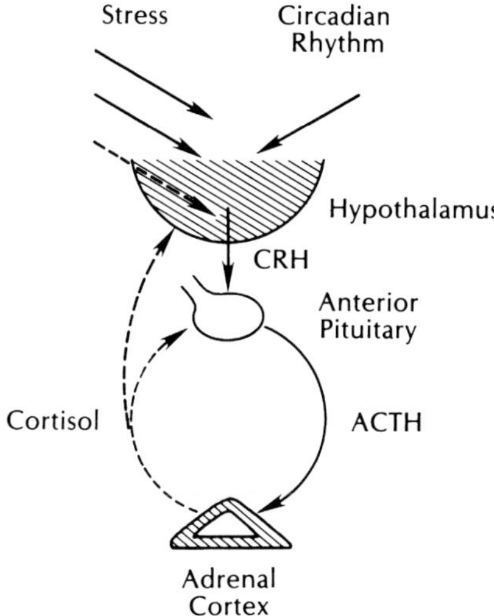

FIGURE 13.6. Hypothalamic pituitary adrenal axis including the long- and short-loop feedback circuits.

The secretion of ACTH is controlled primarily by corticotropin-releasing factor (CRF), a protein with 41 amino acid residues, which is synthesized in the median eminence of the hypothalamus and travels to the pituitary by means of the portal-hypophyseal vessels (Fig. 13.6). Arginine vasopressin from the hypothalamus and several nonhypothalamic factors such as lymphokines (60) also can cause ACTH release (82). The peripheral plasma level of CRF in normal human subjects is 0.4 to 6.0 pmol/L (58). CRF secretion is regulated by four main factors: circadian rhythm, glucocorticoid feedback, ACTH feedback, and stress. Stress increases the secretion of CRF and ACTH, whereas there is a negative feedback relationship between plasma glucocorticoid levels and ACTH secretion. This inhibition of ACTH secretion is probably mediated at both the hypothalamus and the pituitary.

Three clinically relevant points related to ACTH secretion are as follows: (a) Some neoplasms secrete ACTH-like substances that can stimulate the adrenal gland to release glucocorticoids and thus cause Cushing's syndrome. (b) After treatment with large doses of exogenous glucocorticoids, not only is the adrenal gland unresponsive, but the hypothalamic-pituitary axis may be unable to secrete normal quantities of ACTH. (c) ACTH is not required for aldosterone synthesis and secretion, and therefore a patient with hypopituitarism does not require mineralocorticoid replacement.

Actions of Glucocorticoids

Glucocorticoids are essential for life. An adrenalectomized person will die even if provided with mineralocorticoids. Adrenal steroids and, indeed, all steroid hormones easily cross the cell membrane to bind with cytoplasmic receptor proteins that are present in target tissues. The steroid may be metabolized within the cell to a more or less active form. The steroid–receptor complex migrates to the cell nucleus, where it attaches to a specific group of genes. This causes the production of new ribonucleic acid, which in turn effects the synthesis of proteins that serve as structural building blocks of enzymes that regulate cellular function in various tissues.

Glucocorticoids are so named because they have major effects on carbohydrate metabolism, including the promotion of liver glycogen deposits and gluconeogenesis. In the starving patient, they allow survival by enhancing proteolysis, preventing death from hypoglycemia. They also have an antiinsulin effect. Thus they are diabetogenic, causing hyperglycemia during stress or when present in pharmacologic quantities.

Glucocorticoids have many permissive actions in that they facilitate processes that they do not initiate. Several additional effects of glucocorticoids are listed in Table 13.1 along with their clinical implications.

Actions of Adrenal Androgens and Estrogens

The mechanism of action of the major adrenal androgens DHEA, DHEAS, and androstenedione is similar to that described for the glucocorticoids. These compounds are weak androgens that have little effect in physiologic quantities. In disease states, however, they may virilize a female fetus (adrenogenital syndrome) (see Chapter 57), causing

TABLE 13.1. EFFECTS AND IMPLICATIONS OF GLUCOCORTICOIDS

Effect	Clinical Implications
Enhance skeletal and cardiac muscle contraction	Absence results in weakness
Cause protein catabolism	Excess results in wastage and weakness
Inhibit bone formation	Excess decreases bone mass
Inhibit collagen synthesis	Excess causes thin skin and fragile capillaries
Increase vascular contractility and decrease permeability	Absence makes it difficult to maintain blood pressure
Have antiinflammatory activity	Exogenous steroid useful in treating inflammatory diseases
Have antiimmune system activity	Exogenous steroids useful in treating transplantation and various immune diseases
Maintain normal glomerular filtration	Absence reduces glomerular filtration

pseudohermaphroditism, and virilize either prepubertal children or adult females with Cushing's syndrome. The effects of excess adrenal androgens are not clinically evident in the adult male, which delays the diagnosis of Cushing's syndrome in some men. Excess adrenal estrogens may cause breast enlargement in children and men.

Regulation of Glomerulosa Function

The primary regulator of aldosterone secretion is the renin-angiotensin system. Renin is an enzyme synthesized in the juxtaglomerular apparatus of the nephron. When released into the circulation, renin cleaves renin substrate, a globulin secreted from the liver, releasing the decapeptide angiotensin I. Angiotensin I is hydrolyzed to angiotensin II, an octapeptide, by converting enzyme, which is found primarily in the lung. Angiotensin II is a potent stimulator of aldosterone secretion. It is rapidly destroyed in the plasma by angiotensinases.

Renin secretion is regulated by a complex intrarenal mechanism (see Chapter 23). Decreased perfusion pressure in the renal artery and decreased chloride absorption at the macula densa cause increased renin release and thus ultimately increased circulating levels of aldosterone. Angiotensin II and aldosterone can inhibit renin secretion through short- and long-loop feedback systems, respectively. Catecholamines may increase renin release, but dopamine inhibits aldosterone secretion in sodium-depleted individuals. ACTH increases the sensitivity of the zona glomerulosa to angiotensin II and stimulates aldosterone secretion, but the latter effect is not long lasting. Potassium also causes an increase in aldosterone secretion. Thus aldosterone secretion is increased in the following clinical settings: (a) stress, (b) hemorrhage, (c) sodium depletion, (d) dehydration, (e) hyperkalemia, (f) congestive heart failure, (g) hepatic cirrhosis, (h) nephrotic syndrome, (i) estrogen administration, and (j) renal artery stenosis.

Effects of Mineralocorticoids

Mineralocorticoids are steroid hormones that effect ion transport in the epithelial cells of the kidney, gastrointestinal tract, sweat glands, and salivary glands, causing sodium absorption and loss of potassium. The target tissue specificity appears to be enzyme and not receptor mediated. Indeed, mineralocorticoid receptors are rather similar to glucocorticoid receptors and are saturated by glucocorticoids in most tissues because of the tenfold higher concentration of circulating glucocorticoids. The physiologic action of aldosterone is due to aldosterone synthetase and 11-β-hydroxysteroid dehydrogenase in target tissues, which metabolizes glucocorticoids into receptor-inactive 11-keto congeners. The C-11 hydroxyl group in aldosterone is protected from this target tissue enzyme by its aldehyde at C-18 (30).

TABLE 13.2. RELATIVE ACTIVITIES OF GLUCOCORTICOID AND MINERALOCORTICOID

Steroid	Glucocorticoid Activity	Mineralocorticoid Activity
Cortisol	1.0	1.0
Corticosterone	0.3	15.0
Aldosterone	0.3	3,000.0
Deoxycorticosterone	0.2	100.0
Cortisone	0.7	1.0
Prednisolone	4.0	0.8
9-α Fluorocortisol	10.0	125.0
Dexamethasone	25.0	0

The mechanism of action is to increase production of an uncharacterized protein. Because protein synthesis requires time, the effect of mineralocorticoids is not seen until 1 or 2 hours after the tissue is exposed to the steroid. The most important physiologic effects of these compounds are to increase reabsorption of sodium and secretion of potassium and hydrogen ions in the distal tubule of the kidney. Mineralocorticoids do not cause excessive potassium excretion in sodium-depleted subjects. This fact is clinically important because sodium-depleted patients with hyperaldosteronism do not demonstrate a significant kaluresis. Excess aldosterone causes weight gain, increased blood pressure, hypokalemia, and mild metabolic alkalosis as a result of the physiologic effects described earlier. However, normal subjects "escape" the effects of excessive mineralocorticoids after approximately 14 days, and eventually blood volume returns to baseline levels. The mechanisms of the escape phenomenon, which has been studied intensely for years, remain uncertain. It appears that the rise in blood pressure may produce a pressure natriuresis, and also the arterial natriuretic factor may play a role. Mineralocorticoid deficiency results in sodium loss, and if uncorrected, death from hypovolemic shock. The naturally occurring mineralocorticoids are, in order of potency, aldosterone, deoxycorticosterone, 18-hydroxy-deoxycorticosterone, corticosterone, and cortisol. Table 13.2 lists the active mineralocorticoid and glucocorticoid activity of several naturally occurring and synthetic steroids.

Adrenal Medulla

The adrenal medulla secretes catecholamines into the circulation. The primary compound secreted by the medulla is epinephrine. Small quantities of norepinephrine and trace amounts of dopamine also are released from the gland. The adrenal medulla usually, but not invariably, acts in concert with the rest of the sympathetic nervous system. The hormones from the medulla are not essential for life.

Synthesis and Metabolism of Catecholamines

Catecholamines are synthesized from tyrosine in the adrenal medulla. The pathways of catecholamine synthesis are illustrated in Fig. 13.7. In approximately 15% of the granules in the normal medulla, the last step in biosynthesis is the conversion of dopamine to norepinephrine (NE), accounting for the secretion of NE by the normal adrenal and by tumors of the gland. Most of the granules contain phenylethanolamine-*N*-methyltransferase, which converts NE to epinephrine (E), the major hormone of the adrenal medulla. In contrast, sympathetic nerves and other extraadrenal chromaffin tissue do not contain phenylethanolamine-*N*-methyltransferase and thus do not secrete E. This point is clinically useful in attempts to localize a catecholamine-secreting tumor.

NE and E have short half-lives in plasma, ranging from 1 to 3 minutes. They are degraded by two principal enzymes, catechol-*O*-methyl transferase and monoamine oxidase. Figure 13.8 illustrates the major metabolic pathways for circulating catecholamines. Catechol-*O*-methyl transferase converts NE and E, respectively, to normetanephrine (NMN) and metanephrine (MN). Determination of NMN or MN produces vanillylmandelic acid (VMA), a major metabolic product of catecholamine degradation. Less than 5% of the circulating NE and E are secreted intact in the urine. In a normal individual, NE from sympathetic nerve terminals makes up most of the intact urinary catecholamines, whereas E composes 20% of the total. The vast majority of the catecholamines are secreted in the urine as NMN, MN, VMA, and other metabolites shown in Fig. 13.6. Measurement of these various products is important in the diagnosis of pheochromocytoma.

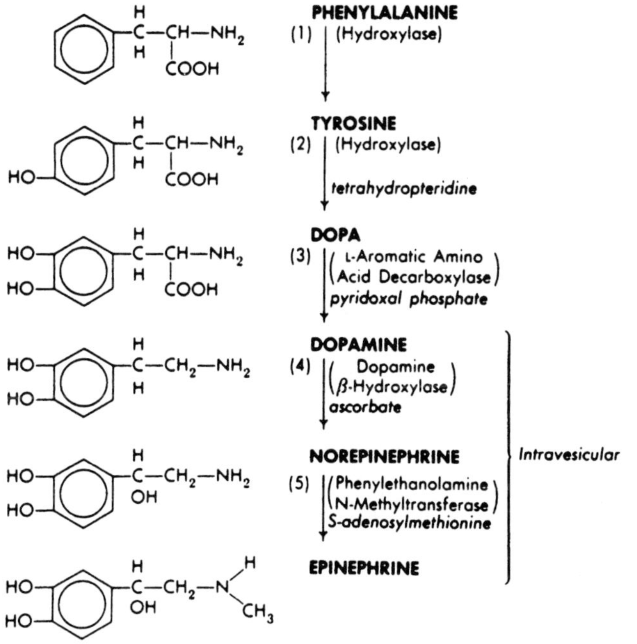

PHENYLALANINE
(1) (Hydroxylase)
TYROSINE
(2) (Hydroxylase) tetrahydropteridine
DOPA
(3) (L-Aromatic Amino Acid Decarboxylase) pyridoxal phosphate
DOPAMINE
(4) (Dopamine β-Hydroxylase) ascorbate
NOREPINEPHRINE — Intravesicular
(5) (Phenylethanolamine N-Methyltransferase) S-adenosylmethionine
EPINEPHRINE

FIGURE 13.7. Biochemical pathways for the synthesis of norepinephrine and epinephrine.

Regulation of Adrenal Medullary Catecholamine Synthesis and Secretion

Stimulation of the sympathetic nervous system during stress caused by stimuli such as fear, pain, or hemorrhage results in increased secretion of catecholamines from the adrenal medulla. Hypoglycemia is also a potent stimulator of adrenal catecholamine secretion. In most situations, the ratio of NE to E remains stable, although exceptions do occur. The basal plasma levels of E are 25 to 50 pg/mL. A total of approximately 150 mg is secreted daily. NE release at sympathetic nerve endings may spill over into the intracellular fluid or be retaken up by the tissues. The plasma level of NE is determined by a balance between the amount released into the circulation and the quantities metabolized and retaken up by the tissues.

Actions of Catecholamines

E and NE are potent hormones that activate α_1-, α_2-, β_1-, and β_2-plasma membrane receptors. E primarily stimulates β-receptors but also has some effect on α-receptors, particularly when the plasma levels of the hormone are high. Conversely, NE primarily affects α-receptors. Because these catecholamines can have α and β action, the effects of intravenously administered hormones vary quantitatively and qualitatively with the dose.

For example, at low dosages E causes vasodilation (a β-effect), which may result in hypotension, whereas at higher dosages there is a net increase in vascular resistance, causing hypertension with a larger increment in systolic than diastolic pressure, resulting in an increased pulse pressure. Both compounds have a positive inotropic effect on the heart and therefore increase cardiac output. Intravenously administered E causes tachycardia, whereas NE results in bradycardia because of the vagal reflex response to the increase in blood pressure.

Catecholamines help restore plasma glucose during exercise or stress by stimulating glycogenolysis in the liver, inhibiting insulin secretion, and increasing glucagon secretion. They also facilitate the reuse of lactate by exercising muscle and increase the release of free fatty acids into the circulation.

Excessive concentrations of catecholamines from exogenous sources or endogenous secretion in patients with pheochromocytoma may cause symptoms relating to the

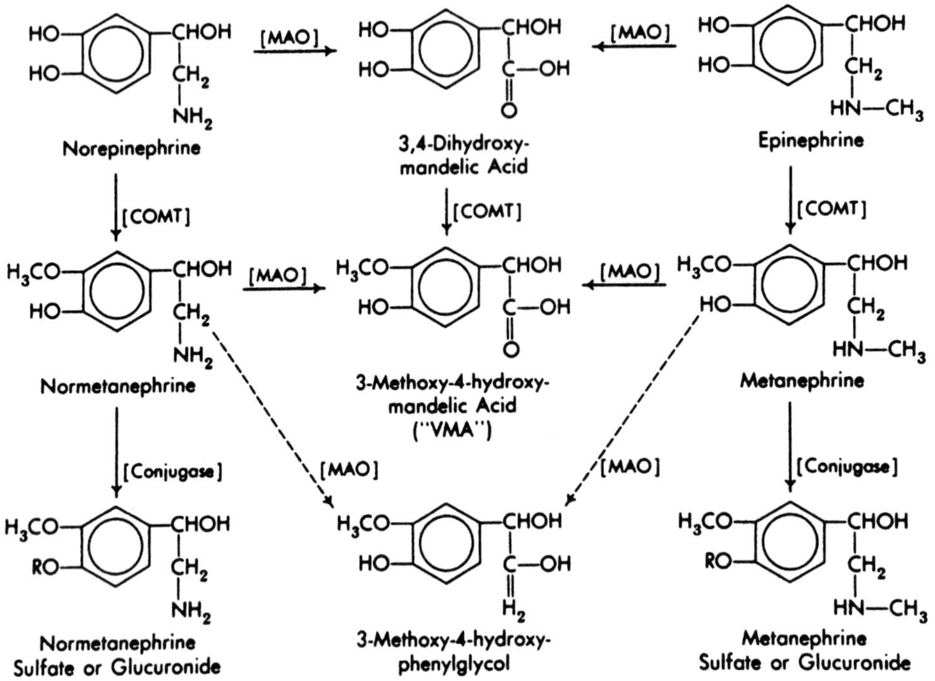

FIGURE 13.8. Metabolic pathways for the degradation of norepinephrine and epinephrine. The urinary metabolites are important in diagnostic evaluation of patients with suspected pheochromocytomas.

previously described effects (see Pheochromocytomas). The symptoms in patients with pheochromocytoma are caused by E and NE. NE elevates the blood pressure and thus may cause headaches.

CUSHING'S SYNDROME

Introduction

Cushing's syndrome is a complex of symptoms and signs caused by excess circulating glucocorticoids. The term is used to describe all patients with the clinical syndrome regardless of the cause. It is important to understand that Cushing's *disease* refers to the form of Cushing's *syndrome* caused by pituitary hypersecretion of ACTH. The most common cause of Cushing's syndrome is exogenously administered glucocorticoids. Twenty-five percent of endogenous Cushing's syndrome is caused by primary adrenal disease (i.e., adenoma or carcinomas). Seventy-five percent of the endogenous disease is excessive ACTH secretion, usually from the pituitary gland but occasionally from an ectopic source. Most patients with pituitary hypersecretion of ACTH (Cushing's disease) have microadenomas, although they may not be obvious during surgery. It is easier to understand the evaluation and treatment of patients with Cushing's syndrome if one keeps in mind that the *first* task of the clinician is to determine whether the patient has Cushing's syndrome. The *second* goal is to determine the cause of the syndrome, and the *final* assignment is to formulate a treatment plan.

Symptoms and Signs

Cushing's syndrome occurs in men, women, and children of all races but is most commonly diagnosed in women between the ages of 20 and 60 years. It is usually characterized by plethoric "moon" facies and central or "buffalo" obesity in the nuchal, truncal, and girdle areas (Fig. 13.9A and B). Protuberance of superclavicular fat pads is the cardinal physical finding that distinguishes Cushing's syndrome from obesity. Serial photographs of the patient are helpful in making the diagnosis because these pictures always document a shift in fat distribution, even if the patient is not obese. The protein wasting secondary to excess glucocorticoids causes easy bruising and thin skin, which results in pink or purple striae. Muscle wasting may cause severe weakness. The weakness is generally proximal and can be observed by asking the patient to do deep knee bends. Emotional symptoms and headaches are common. Adrenal androgens often cause hirsutism in women and prepubertal boys. Oligomenorrhea in women and acne also are common symptoms related to adrenal androgens. Fifteen percent of the patients have urinary stones caused by hypercalciuria. The full-fledged syndrome is easy to recognize, but the differential diagnosis may be difficult, particularly in men and also in women with hirsutism unrelated to Cushing's syndrome. The most prevalent symptoms and signs of the syndrome are listed in Table 13.3.

Common physical findings in patients with Cushing's syndrome are hypertension and edema secondary to the mineralocorticoid activity of the adrenal steroids and, as mentioned previously, plethoric moon facies, central obesity, striae, acne, and hirsutism.

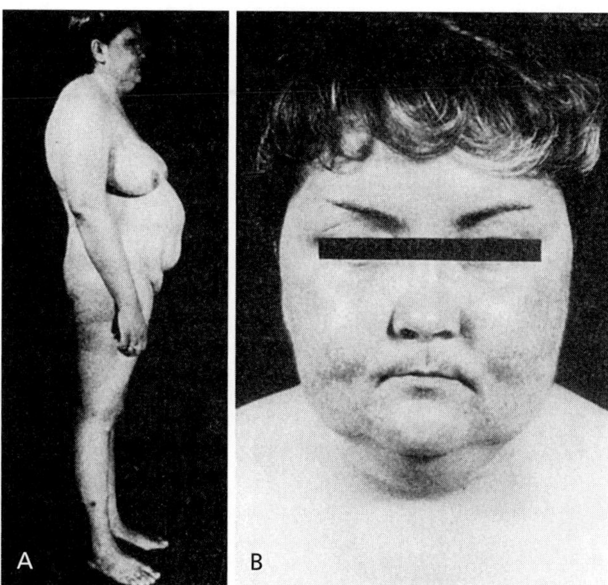

FIGURE 13.9. Typical appearance of a patient with Cushing's syndrome. **A:** Central obesity striae, buffalo hump, and moon facies. **B:** Protuberance of the subclavicular fat pads, hirsutism, facial pigmentation, and the fact that one cannot see the ears, which is typical of patients with Cushing's syndrome. There are also acne fold lesions on the skin.

TABLE 13.3. SYMPTOMS AND SIGNS OF CUSHING'S SYNDROME IN ORDER OF FREQUENCY

Symptoms	Signs
Central obesity	Central obesity
Hirsutism	Hypertension
Oligomenorrhea	Hirsutism
Purple striae	Purple striae
Plethoric facies	Plethoric facies
Easy bruisability	Acne
Personality change	Edema
Acne	Muscle weakness
Edema	
Muscle weakness	
Poor wound healing	
Backache	
Polyuria	
Polydipsia	
Impotence	
Growth arrest (children)	

Differential Diagnosis

Cushing's syndrome is caused by the actions of glucocorticoids. Therefore anything that causes excess circulating levels of these hormones can evoke the syndrome. The most common cause is iatrogenic administration of glucocorticoids. Pituitary Cushing's syndrome or Cushing's disease accounts for the majority of the noniatrogenic cases. Approximately 95% of the patients with pituitary Cushing's syndrome have detectable pituitary tumors.

Evidence is mounting that the primary problem in these patients is hypersecretion of ACTH independently or CRF secretion (82). Ectopic secretion of ACTH or CRF (16) from tumors also can cause the syndrome. Finally, primary adrenal adenomas or carcinomas may secrete enough hormone to produce the syndrome. Adrenal tumors tend to be autonomous in their secretion of glucocorticoids, a characteristic that assists in the differential diagnosis of Cushing's syndrome. Most of these tumors are unilateral, but bilateral tumors do occur. Most children with Cushing's syndrome have adrenal neoplasms.

In patients younger than 15 years of age, adrenal carcinoma is the most common cause of Cushing's syndrome. Because most patients with adrenal cortical carcinoma have endocrine symptoms or a mass in the retroperitoneum, the syndrome is rarely suspected because of distant metastasis, although pulmonary and liver metastases are not uncommon and skeletal, brain, pleura, and mediastinal metastases do occur (45). Patients with ectopic or pituitary ACTH-dependent Cushing's syndrome may have hyperpigmentation. Galactorrhea occurs occasionally and only in individuals with pituitary hypersecretion of ACTH. Patients with adrenal carcinoma are characterized by hirsutism and virilism resulting from androgenic adrenal steroids, and individuals with ectopic ACTH tend to have severe manifestations of the syndrome attributable to the high levels of ACTH. The presence of a decreased serum potassium level in patients with this finding is highly suggestive of ectopic ACTH secretion, and the diagnosis should be pursued even if there is also suspicion of a pituitary cause.

The diagnosis of Cushing's syndrome is most frequently entertained when a physician is consulted by an overweight woman concerned about hirsutism. Most of these patients have excessive secretion of androgens from the ovary (50) rather than hyperadrenocorticism. Late-onset adrenal hyperplasia, however, has been reported in 24 of 400 women with hirsutism (54).

Laboratory Diagnosis of Cushing's Syndrome

There are two basic steps in the laboratory evaluation of individuals with suspected Cushing's syndrome: first, determining whether they have the syndrome, and second, identifying the cause.

Many tests have been recommended for diagnosis of Cushing's syndrome. We prefer to screen patients with a determination of the free cortisol in a 24-hour urine specimen. In our laboratory, the normal value is lower than 80 mg per 24 hours. Values vary with age and from laboratory to laboratory. Following are examples of such results (29).

A normal finding rules out Cushing's syndrome unless the clinical level of suspicion is high. If the urinary free cortisol is elevated, we then do a low-dose dexamethasone test. Dexamethasone is a biologically active glucocorticoid that suppresses the secretion of ACTH and thus endogenous adrenal glucocorticoids but does not affect the measurement of the endogenous hormones in the serum and their metabolism in the urine. The patient is given dexamethasone 0.5 mg orally every 6 hours four times daily. At 9 A.M. after the last 3 A.M. dosage, a blood sample is obtained. The normal individual will have a suppressed serum cortisol level of less than 2 to 5 mg/dL. Twenty-four-hour urine levels of free cortisol also should be depressed to less than 20 mg/L on the second and third days. Porter-Silber 17-OH corticoids and ketogenic steroids in the urine should be less than 2.0 and 5.0 mg/g of creatinine, respectively. The best criterion to use for the dexamethasone test is the value of 17-OH corticoids per gram of creatinine. The creatinine corrects for surface area. If the serum and urinary values are normal, the patient does not have Cushing's syndrome; if the values are elevated, Cushing's syndrome is likely. There are exceptions, however, including endogenous depression and alcoholic pseudo-Cushing's syndrome.

In other institutions the morning and afternoon serum cortisol levels and overnight dexamethasone test are used to make the diagnosis of Cushing's syndrome. In the normal individual, there is a diurnal rhythm in serum cortisol concentration, with a peak of 8 to 25 mg/dL at 6 to 9 A.M. and a nadir of less than 7 to 10 mg/dL in the afternoon (Fig. 13.10). Therefore the test is done by drawing blood samples at 8 A.M. and 4 P.M. Normal persons should conform to the stated values and display at least a 50% decrease between morning and afternoon determinations. This diurnal rhythm is not present in young patients (Fig. 13.10). Patients with Cushing's syndrome usually have elevated values, particularly in the afternoon, and also do not exhibit the normal diurnal rhythm. The overnight dexamethasone suppression test is done by giving the patient 1.0 mg of dexamethasone at 11 P.M. and obtaining a blood sample the next morning at 8 A.M. The normal individual will have a suppressed serum cortisol level less than 5.0 mg/dL, whereas the patient with Cushing's syndrome will have a serum cortisol level greater than 5.0 mg/dL (usually greater than 20 mg/dL).

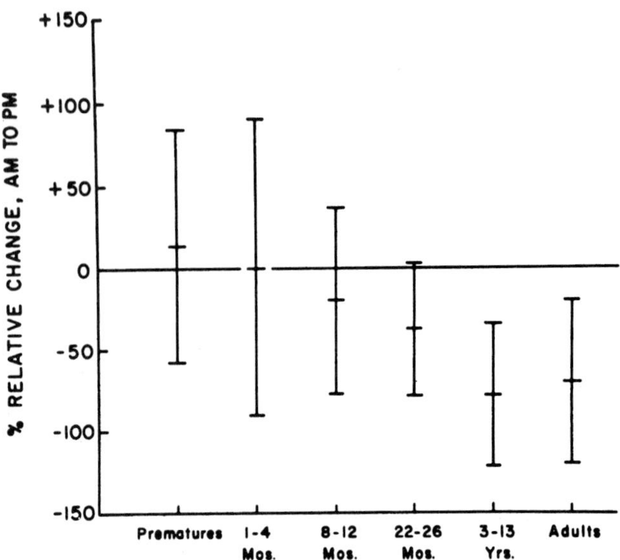

FIGURE 13.10. Diurnal rhythm in serum cortisol levels and its variation with age.

Laboratory Determinations of the Cause of Cushing's Syndrome

Many tests are available to facilitate the differential diagnosis of Cushing's syndrome. None of these tests is always correct, and the diagnosis can be difficult. Disagreement among test results is the rule rather than the exception. The diagnosis can be confused by the fact that pituitary Cushing's syndrome can cause autonomous adrenal hyperfunction when adrenal hyperplasia develops into a discrete adenoma (41). Among the many tests available, we prefer three: plasma ACTH, high-dose dexamethasone suppression, and the metyrapone test. The normal plasma ACTH level in an adult is 10 to 80 pg/mL in the morning and at least 50% in the evening (5,72). The morning plasma ACTH is suppressed to undetectable levels in patients with adrenal adenomas or carcinomas. In patients with ectopic secretion of ACTH, the value is elevated (200 to 1000 pg/mL), and in patients with Cushing's disease, it is normal or high (40 to 100 pg/mL) but elevated inappropriately for the level of cortisol. The high-dose dexamethasone test is done in the same manner as the low-dose test described earlier, except that each dose of the drug is 2.0 mg. Patients with ectopic ACTH secretion or adrenal tumors do not suppress, but those with Cushing's disease do.

Metyrapone inhibits the enzyme 11-β-hydroxylase, thus preventing 11-β-hydroxylation during steroidogenesis (Fig. 13.4). This eliminates the production of cortisol, which in turn increases the secretion of ACTH (because the negative feedback has been removed) and the secretion of adrenal steroids such as 11-deoxycortisol. In patients with ectopic ACTH secretion or adrenal tumors, metyrapone has no effect. Patients with Cushing's disease have an exaggerated response. There is a potential danger that metyrapone will cause adrenal insufficiency and adrenal crisis.

The administration of corticotropin-releasing hormone to patients with Cushing's syndrome caused by adrenocortical tumor usually results in little change in ACTH levels, whereas patients with pituitary microadenomas usually have an exaggerated ACTH response. Nonetheless, because of large individual variations, corticotropin-releasing hormone testing is not recommended for routine use in the differential diagnosis of Cushing's syndrome (82). Oldfield and associates measured the levels of adrenocorticotropin in the peripheral blood and the plasma from both of the inferior petrosal sinuses in 281 patients with Cushing's syndrome. They found that an inferior petrosal sinus adrenocorticotropin level of twice the plasma concentration identified Cushing's disease in 205 of 215 patients (sensitivity 95%) with no false-positive results (specificity 100%). After CRF administration a measured ratio of greater than 3.0:1 was 100% accurate with no false-positive or false-negative results (68).

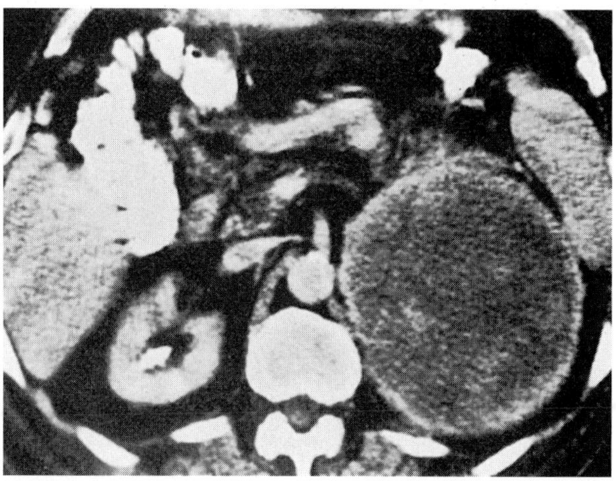

FIGURE 13.11. Computed tomography (CT) scan of a patient with a large adrenal hematoma. CT scans of patients with tumors causing Cushing's syndrome might be quite similar in configuration, although the intratumor density would vary.

Localization of Adrenal Causes of Cushing's Syndrome

The techniques currently used to localize adrenal tumors are listed in Table 13.4. Intravenous pyelography, arteriography, and adrenal vein venography are no longer recommended for localizing adrenal lesions in patients with Cushing's syndrome.

Most tumors of the adrenal that cause Cushing's syndrome are larger than 2 cm and therefore are easily visualized with CT or magnetic resonance imaging (MRI) (Figs. 13.11 and 13.12) (1,75). The adrenal gland on the affected side in patients with renal agenesis or inferior ectopy is a paraspinal disk-shaped organ that has a linear appearance on CT scan (49). Unilateral Cushing's adenomas are associated with contralateral adrenal atrophy. Adrenal hyperplasia is associated with diffuse thickening, occasionally with bilateral cortical nodularity in 10% to 20%. Adrenal carcinomas are usually larger in size (greater than 6 cm), irregular, with evidence of necrosis, calcification, or local invasion. Upon MRI, adenomas are generally isointense as compared with the liver on T_2-weighted images, whereas carcinomas are hyperintense and inhomogeneous. An intravenous pyelography, especially with tomography, also may reveal an adrenal mass, although it is less sensitive. Adrenal tumors typically displace the upper pole of the kidney laterally (Fig. 13.13), changing the axis of the kidney and the collecting system. They rarely displace the kidney caudally without shifting the axis. Sonography can be a useful screening technique, particularly for large tumors, and is useful in determining whether a retroperitoneal mass extends from or into the kidney or is separated from the kidney and/or the liver. If it is unclear whether a retroperitoneal mass is of adrenal or renal origin, arteriography may be useful because it is often pathognomonic of renal cell carcinoma and also may be useful in planning surgery. However, we do not routinely perform arteriograms in patients with suspected adrenal or renal tumors.

Venography with catheterization of the adrenal veins is an extremely precise technique for diagnosing and localizing endocrinologically active adrenal tumors. However, it is difficult to catheterize the adrenal veins, particularly on the right, and even in experienced hands this method may fail. Also there is danger of damaging the adrenal gland if undue pressure is exerted in the adrenal vein. Adrenal masses also can be identified with scintillation scanning techniques using NP-59 (Fig. 13.14). We have found this technique useful in the evaluation of patients with Conn's syndrome.

TABLE 13.4. LOCALIZATION TEST FOR CUSHING'S SYNDROME

Computed tomography or magnetic resonance imaging
Scintiscan: 6-β-iodomethyl norcholesterol (NP-59)
Ultrasonography

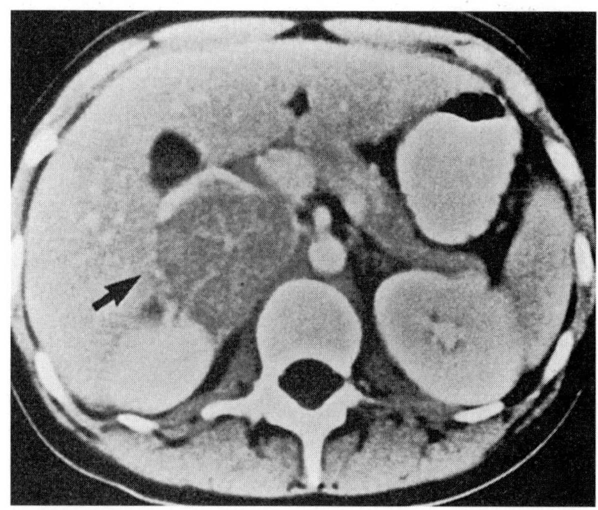

FIGURE 13.12. Computed tomography scan of a patient with pheochromocytoma *(arrow)*.

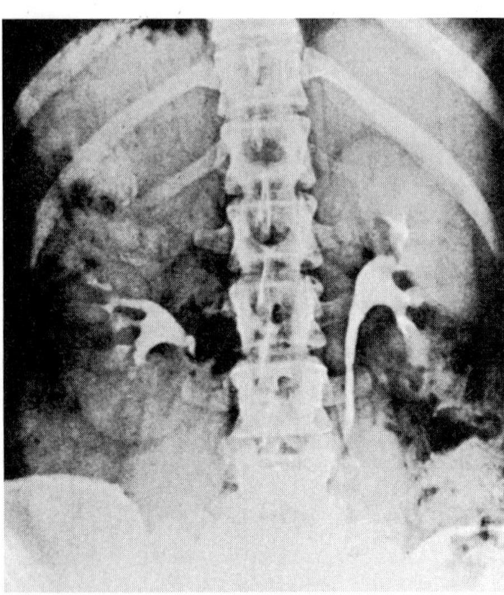

FIGURE 13.13. Intravenous pyelography of a patient with an adrenal mass. Note that the renal axis and the axis of the collecting system are deviated with the upper pole pushed outward. This is quite typical of an adrenal tumor. The tumors of the adrenal usually push the upper pole outward rather than pushing the kidney down.

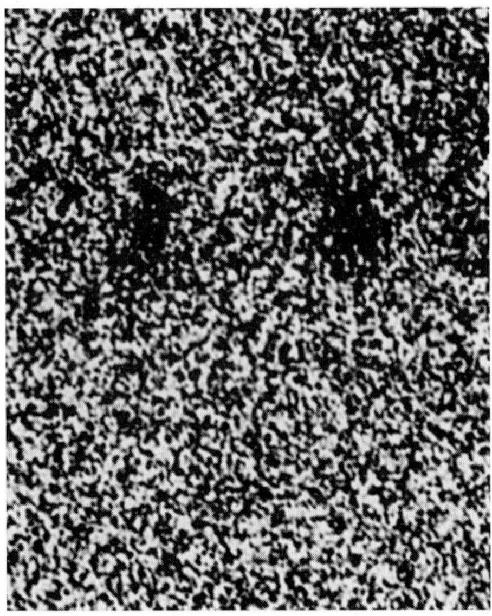

FIGURE 13.14. IP-59 scintillation scan of a patient with bilateral adrenal hyperplasia. Note that both adrenal glands are seen on this scan and are of approximately equal density. If the patient had an adrenal adenoma, the side with the adenoma would be highlighted, whereas the other side would not be visualized.

CUSHING'S DISEASE

Transsphenoidal hypophysectomy, pituitary irradiation, bilateral adrenalectomy, and medical therapy are all used to treat Cushing's disease. The treatment of choice in most centers is transsphenoidal removal of the microadenoma (10,59,81). The current success rate is between 85% and 95%. This treatment is less morbid than bilateral adrenalectomy and avoids the complication of Nelson's syndrome. Pituitary irradiation (cobalt-60) with 4,000 to 5,000 rad has a reasonable success rate in children, approximately 80%, but only approximately a 20% cure rate in adults. Pituitary irradiation with a cyclotron (proton beam) may have a higher cure rate in adults, but this technique is available in only a few locations in the United States. We reserve bilateral adrenalectomy for patients who have failed pituitary surgery. Bilateral adrenalectomy may be complicated in 10% to 20% of cases by rapid postoperative growth of pituitary tumors and hyperpigmentation (Nelson's syndrome). Preoperative pituitary irradiation decreases the incidence of Nelson's syndrome.

Medical treatment with cyproheptadine 6 mg orally four times daily has been reported to cause remission in 60% to 65% of patients with Cushing's disease after 6 to 8 weeks. Mitotane, o,p-DDD, 6.0 g per day, or aminoglutethimide has also been used to treat patients with Cushing's disease, but because of significant side effects, we do not recommend these compounds except for inoperable cases. We prefer metyrapone 1.0 g per day. This drug has a short half-life and must be given every 4 hours. It is monitored by following serum and not urinary cortisol. Hypertension may result from accumulation of deoxycorticosterone. This can be treated with spironolactone. In general, in Cushing's disease medical therapy is used only when indicated to prepare patients for surgical treatment. The major use of medical treatment is in palliation of patients with Cushing's syndrome as a result of malignancies.

Adrenal Tumors

The distinction between a benign adenoma and a malignant adrenal cortical neoplasm is important because of the difference in long-term patient survival. Ultimately, the only method certain to establish the difference is pathologic analysis (86). Nonetheless, a reasonable assessment of the malignant potential can be made using clinical, biochemical, and radiographic information. A recent review of 40 patients (27 adenomas, 13 carcinomas) with ACTH-independent Cushing's syndrome was undertaken at our institution with the primary aim of establishing criteria for the preoperative delineation of adrenal adenomas from carcinomas (22).

The two demographic features that distinguished adenomas from carcinomas were age and tumor size. As compared with carcinoma patients, adenoma patients were significantly younger (39.6 versus 51.5 years) and their tumors were significantly smaller (3.3 versus 8.6 cm). Women constituted the majority of patients in both groups, and left-sided tumors accounted for 70% of cases in both groups. No specific physical finding differentiated adenomas from carcinomas.

All patients had elevated 24-hour urinary free cortisol values and low-normal ACTH levels. No specific biochemical abnormality identified either adenoma or carcinoma patients. Nevertheless, urinary free cortisol, 17-ketosteroid (17-KS), dehydroepiandrosterone sulfate (DHEAS-S), and lactate dehydrogenase (LDH) levels tended to be higher in carcinoma patients. A pure biochemical syndrome of glucocorticoid excess without elevation of 17-KS, DHEA-S, testosterone, or aldosterone was present in 68% of adenoma patients as opposed to only 8% of carcinoma patients.

Some groups have noted the presence of virilization/ hirsutism as an important clinical clue suggesting the presence of carcinoma (69). This is based on the premise that carcinomas are less effective than adenomas at converting steroid precursors to glucocorticoids. In our recent review, this was not a discriminating feature (22). Whereas most carcinoma patients presented with a mixed endocrine syndrome (92%), adenoma patients commonly had virilization (93%), and 32% presented with a mixed endocrine syndrome as determined by biochemical analysis. There were a few noteworthy observations. Of the adenoma patients in whom DHEA-S was measured, 44% had subnormal values, and in the two patients with elevated levels the values were only mildly raised. In contrast, only one carcinoma patient had a subnormal level of DHEA-S, and 50% of the carcinoma patients had elevations that exceeded four times the normal value. Overall, the magnitude of the biochemical abnormalities were more severe for the carcinoma patients. These findings support the notion that adenomas in general are more efficient than carcinomas at converting steroid precursors to glucocorticoids; however, significant tumor-to-tumor variability remains. Although steadfast rules do not exist with regard to the preoperative hormonal profile capable of predicting the presence of adenoma versus that of carcinoma, it is likely that patients with ACTH-independent CS, normal 17-KS levels, and subnormal DHEA-S values have an adenoma, whereas those with greatly elevated 17-KS and DHEA-S levels have a carcinoma. Although steroid profiling may not dramatically enhance the management of patients with a small adrenal mass that is likely to be an adenoma, it is important for patients with suspected carcinoma because the steroid values can be helpful in the follow-up of these patients, serving as markers of recurrent disease.

The treatment of Cushing's syndrome secondary to adrenal tumors is surgical removal unless the tumor is unresectable. Preoperative preparation requires specific measures to correct metabolic abnormalities caused by Cushing's syndrome. These patients are prepared for surgery by treatment with metyrapone (250 to 500 mg orally every 4 hours) while awake. To the extent that these drugs reverse Cushing's syndrome, they decrease the operative morbidity and the mortality. Malignant adrenal tumors causing Cushing's syndrome in the adult do not have a good prognosis. The Cleveland Clinic series revealed a 44% 5-year survival in patients with localized disease who made up 49% of 82 patients, and a 13% and 6% 5-year survival in patients with regional and metastatic disease (9). In the M.D. Anderson series, 13 of 18 patients (72%) had recurrent disease (78). Of the 13, 8 patients had local recurrence. The prognosis is better in children.

Bilateral adrenalectomy is indicated for patients with Cushing's disease refractory to hypophysectomy. Postoperatively, these patients require replacement glucocorticoids and mineralocorticoids indefinitely. We usually give hydrocortisone sodium succinate (Solu-Cortef) 100 mg intravenously every 8 hours for the first few days and taper to an oral dose of 25 to 37.5 mg of cortisone acetate and 0.1 mg of fluorocortisone acetate (Florinef) daily.

PRIMARY HYPERALDOSTERONISM

Deming and Luetscher (24) described a sodium-retaining substance in the urine in 1950. Three years later Simpson and associates chemically identified the compound as the 18-aldehyde of corticosterone, aldosterone. Within a year, aldosterone had been synthesized and, remarkably, Conn (19) described the clinical syndrome of primary hyperaldosteronism, or Conn's syndrome. Never before in the history of medicine had an important clinical advance followed so closely on the heels of a basic scientific discovery.

Conn's syndrome is defined as the adrenal hypersecretion of aldosterone in a hypertensive, nonedematous patient. The exact incidence of the disease is not known, but it accounts for approximately 1% of hypertensive patients. It should be pointed out that 1% of 35 million hypertensive patients in the United States is 350,000 people. Women outnumber men approximately 2.5 to 1, and 75% of the patients are between 30 and 50 years of age. Primary hyperaldosteronism should be suspected in any hypertensive patient with hypokalemia. The patients typically have hypertension, muscle weakness, polyuria, hypokalemia, and mild metabolic alkalosis. Table 13.5 gives the incidence of the common symptoms of primary hyperaldosteronism reported in Conn's original description of 103 cases.

In recent years, the diagnosis of Conn's syndrome has been confirmed in many individuals with no obvious symptoms of hypokalemia. There are rare patients with primary

TABLE 13.5. SYMPTOMS OF CONN'S SYNDROME

Symptom	%
Muscle weakness	73%
Polyuria (nocturia)	72%
Headache	51%
Polydipsia	46%
Paresthesia	24%
No symptoms	6%

hyperaldosteronism who do not have unprovoked hypokalemia.

The headaches are caused by the hypertension, whereas the muscle weakness, polyuria, and paresthesias relate to the effect of hypokalemia on skeletal muscle, the renal concentrating mechanism, and peripheral nerves, respectively.

The major physical finding in patients with primary hyperaldosteronism is hypertension without edema. Mild retinopathy may be present. Routine laboratory evaluation reveals (a) a persistently dilute urine with a pH of 6.5 or higher, (b) a plasma potassium level below 3.5 to 4.0 mEq/L with the patient off all diuretic medication, and (c) mild metabolic alkalosis (elevated serum bicarbonate radical). The serum sodium concentration may be slightly elevated, and mild proteinuria is often present. The electrocardiogram often reveals premature ventricular contractions, depression of the ST segments, T waves, and the presence of U waves. When the diagnosis of primary hyperaldosteronism is entertained, three questions must be sequentially answered: (a) Does the patient have primary hyperaldosteronism? (b) If so, what is the cause? (c) If the disease is the result of an adenoma, what is the location of the tumor?

Does the Patient Have Primary Hyperaldosteronism?

By far the most common cause of hypertension and hypokalemia is essential hypertension treated with diuretics. Also, hypertension, hypokalemia, and hypersecretion of aldosterone are more often caused by secondary hyperaldosteronism than by primary hyperaldosteronism. Any stimulus that compromises renal blood flow may increase renin secretion and thus cause secondary hyperaldosteronism. Common clinical situations that evoke secondary hyperaldosteronism are listed in Table 13.6.

Rare causes of secondary hyperaldosteronism include renin-secreting renal tumors and Bartter's syndrome. Bartter's syndrome is characterized by elevations in plasma renin and aldosterone, hypokalemia, and hyperplasia of the juxtaglomerular cells in the kidney.

It is not always easy to determine whether a patient has primary hyperaldosteronism. Many different approaches to diagnosis have been recommended. One of the most difficult problems facing the clinician is which patients should be screened for primary hyperaldosteronism. Certainly, individuals with spontaneous hypokalemia (less than 4.0 mEq/L) and inappropriate kaluresis (greater than 3.0 mEq per day) may have primary hyperaldosteronism. To make the diagnosis we first perform a saline suppression test. With the patient in the supine position a serum sample is obtained for aldosterone, saline is infused at 500 mL per hour for 4 hours, and then another serum sample is drawn. A normal individual will suppress serum aldosterone to less than 10 ng/dL, whereas in patients with primary hyperaldosteronism, the serum aldosterone after saline infusion will be greater than 10 ng/dL. In addition, patients with the disease will have an increased plasma concentration and urinary secretion of aldosterone after potassium repletion to more than 3.5 mEq/L (12).

The captopril test is advocated by many investigators, but we find it less precise than the approach just outlined. The test is done by obtaining serum before and 2 hours after administration of 25 mg of captopril. In secondary hyperaldosteronism, the serum renin rises after the captopril, whereas in primary hyperaldosteronism it does not. Also, the aldosterone-to-renin ratio decreases in secondary hyperaldosteronism but not in primary.

TABLE 13.6. CAUSES OF SECONDARY HYPERALDOSTERONISM

Shock	Cardiac failure
Dehydration	Hepatic cirrhosis
Renal artery stenosis	Pregnancy

What Is the Cause of Primary Hyperaldosteronism?

Primary hyperaldosteronism may be caused by an adrenal tumor (usually a unilateral adenoma), adrenal hyperplasia ("idiopathic"), deoxycorticosterone acetate-suppressible adrenal hyperplasia (indeterminate hyperplasia), or glucocorticoid-remediable family hyperplasia. The last two forms of the disease occur in adolescents and children, respectively, and are rare. Approximately two-thirds of patients with primary hyperaldosteronism have adrenal adenomas. The major differential diagnosis is between adenoma and hyperplasia. We make the diagnosis of adenoma if (a) there is an anomalous decrease in plasma aldosterone during ambulation, (b) the blood pressure is normalized on spironolactone (400 mg/L for 6 weeks), (c) the serum aldosterone-stimulating factor is *not* elevated (16), and (d) CT or MRI scanning shows a discrete adrenal mass. Biglieri and associates (7) also have noted that the plasma 18-hydrocorticosterone level after overnight recumbency is much higher (greater than 100 ng/dL) in patients with an adenoma than in individuals with hyperplasia. Despite these tests, the differential diagnosis may be difficult. Once the diagnosis of adenoma is made, we attempt to localize the tumor.

Where Is the Tumor?

Methods used to localize adrenal adenomas have included intravenous pyelography, aortography, phlebography, adrenal vein catheterization, radionuclide scan, CT, and nuclear resonance imaging. The NP-59 scan is a useful noninvasive technique. The patient is prepared for 3 days with Lugol's solution (5 drops twice daily) and oral dexamethasone (0.5 mg every 6 hours). The Lugol's solution is continued for 2 weeks. Imaging is done after the 3-day preparation and again in 4 more days. CT scanning often identifies an adenoma (85), but false-negative results may occur because these adenomas are typically rather small. When CT scanning is used, thin-section CT techniques with section thicknesses of 1.5 to 3 mm should be used (37). The accuracy of CT scanning alone in patients with low-renin hyperaldosteronism has been estimated at 73% to 90% (90). This imprecision is due to the fact that CT scans may miss adenomas smaller than 1 cm. Ironically, with the increased sensitivity of CT scans, an additional, perhaps even prevalent, source of inaccuracy is the fact that modern CT scans overdiagnose adenomas because they find small nonfunctioning masses and confuse unilateral macronodular hyperplasia with adenomas (25).

MRI with and without gadolinium administration also can identify an adenoma-causing primary aldosteronism with the same efficacy as CT scanning. Adrenal vein catheterization with sampling and analysis of the effluent is perhaps the most precise way to localize a tumor, but, as pointed out in the discussion of Cushing's syndrome, it is technically difficult (33).

Treatment

The preferred management of primary hyperaldosteronism secondary to adrenal hyperplasia is medical treatment with spironolactone, which inhibits the action of aldosterone on the distal renal tubule. Reduction of plasma volume by diuretic therapy is an important aspect of treating hypertension in these patients. Administration of 200 mg of spironolactone per day (50 mg four times daily) normalizes serum potassium with relatively little effect on the pressure. The addition of hydrochlorothiazide (HCTZ) 50 mg per day (25 mg twice daily) rapidly reduces blood pressure while maintaining serum potassium concentrations within the normal range. Painful gynecomastia is a distressing side effect of spironolactone. Occasionally, agents that interfere with renal tubular ion transport, such as triamterene or amiloride, are also incorporated into a pharmacologic treatment program. Bilateral adrenalectomy has no place in the management of primary aldosteronism because complete adrenal insufficiency may be more difficult to treat than hypertension from aldosteronism.

The treatment of choice for an aldosterone-producing adrenal cortical adenoma is surgical adrenalectomy, which carries minimal morbidity and provides definitive therapy in most cases. Blumfeld and colleagues (8) demonstrated in 1994 that 35% of patients with a unilateral adenoma had normal blood pressure postoperatively without any concurrent antihypertensive medications. In an additional 56% of patients with residual hypertension postoperatively, addition of an antihypertensive agent decreased their blood pressure below 140/90 mm Hg. Thus more than 90% of patients with an adenoma had cure or significant improvement of hypertension following surgical excision. Medical therapy with spironolactone may be indicated for poor surgical risk patients with an adenoma. Occasionally, an adrenal gland removed for a suspected adenoma is found to contain one or more hyperplastic nodules. Although the results of adrenalectomy for hyperplasia are less satisfactory, some patients experience improvement of hypertension postoperatively (56). This therapeutic response is not completely understood and may result from a simple reduction in the amount of adrenal tissue.

Patients with primary hyperaldosteronism from an adrenal adenoma have a significant potassium deficit, which must be corrected preoperatively because hypokalemia increases the risk of cardiac arrhythmias during anesthesia. Supplemental oral potassium alone is not sufficient to overcome the kaluresis experienced by these patients. Preoperative treatment with spironolactone is also necessary both to correct hypokalemia and to facilitate blood pressure control. Some patients with a unilateral adenoma develop contralateral mineralocorticoid suppression, which may become manifest postoperatively as clinical hyperaldosteronism. This problem may also be prevented by preoperative spironolactone therapy because this allows reactivation of the renin-angiotensin-aldosterone system.

Because aldosterone-producing adenomas are invariably small and benign, laparoscopic adrenalectomy has now become the preferred surgical approach. Following adrenalectomy in such cases, there is usually a moderate urinary diuresis of sodium and retention of potassium. This requires appropriate volume replacement and close monitoring of serum electrolyte levels for the first week postoperatively. In some cases, hyponatremia and hyperkalemia develop in the immediate postoperative period secondary to suppression of the contralateral zona glomerulosa, with a resulting aldosterone deficiency. This phenomenon will necessitate mineralocorticoid replacement until the remaining adrenal gland recovers. In general, patients experience a rapid and uneventful postoperative recovery from adrenalectomy for hyperaldosteronism. Hypertension may take several weeks to resolve completely; however, ultimately 80% of patients are cured (56).

ADRENAL INSUFFICIENCY

Adrenal insufficiency was described in 1855 by Thomas Addison—thus the eponym *Addison's disease.* Addison's disease is a rare entity, usually secondary to tuberculosis or autoimmune adrenocortical atrophy. Other causes include amyloidosis, histoplasmosis, blastomycosis, and metastatic carcinoma. Iatrogenic adrenal insufficiency secondary to high-dose adrenal steroid therapy or surgical adrenalectomy is more common. Urologists should be aware that ketocona-

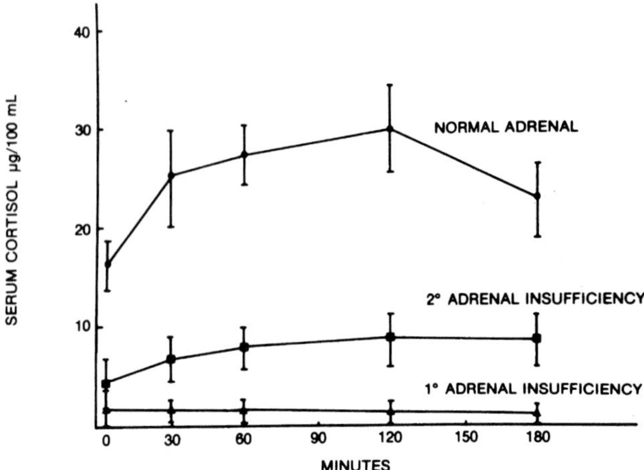

FIGURE 13.15. Serum cortisol response and response to adrenocorticotropin hormone infusion in normal persons and in patients with primary and secondary adrenal insufficiency.

zole therapy for prostatic cancer may cause reversible adrenal insufficiency (83).

The symptoms of adrenal insufficiency include muscular weakness, fatigability, weight loss, hyperpigmentation, anorexia, nausea, vomiting, and diarrhea. Cardiac tamponade is a rare, often fatal complication of adrenal insufficiency. Hypotension is the cardinal sign. Hyponatremia and hyperkalemia are common. Plasma cortisol levels are low, as are levels of the various urinary metabolites of the endogenous adrenal steroids. The diagnosis can be confirmed by finding an elevated level of serum ACTH and a lack of significant response in serum cortisol after administration of ACTH (Fig. 13.15). Corticotropin-releasing hormone levels have been reported to be either elevated or normal in patients with Addison's disease (82).

The initial treatment is 100 mg of hydrocortisone every 8 hours. All patients maintained on adrenal steroid therapy should receive this dose for several days after any surgical procedure. The dose is tapered to a maintenance dose of 30 mg per day, given as 20 mg in the morning and 10 mg in the evening, to mimic the physiologic diurnal variations in serum levels. In patients with adrenal insufficiency secondary to pituitary disease, it is usually not necessary to provide mineralocorticoid replacement. In patients with no functioning adrenal tissue, fluorocortisol 0.05 to 1.0 mg per day will provide adequate mineralocorticoid replacement. The adequacy of the replacement therapy can be determined by monitoring blood pressure, serum electrolytes, renal function, and plasma ACTH and renin activity.

PHEOCHROMOCYTOMAS

Pheochromocytomas are fascinating tumors that secrete catecholamines that cause a variety of symptoms, usually including hypertension. Most pheochromocytomas secrete NE and E. Occasional tumors release only NE, and rare lesions secrete dopa, dopamine, serotonin, somatostatin, ACTH, or E. The tumors are composed of chromaffin cells and may arise anywhere in the body where chromaffin tissue derived from primitive neuroectoderm is located. Approximately 95% of the tumors are located in the adrenal gland, but pheochromocytomas have been found in the bladder, Zuckerkandl's organ, and anywhere in the body that sympathetic nervous tissue is located. Three percent of pheochromocytomas are extraabdominal. Although only 0.1% to 0.2% of hypertensive patients have a pheochromocytoma, they should always be screened because the tumors are curable in 90% of the patients, and untreated pheochromocytomas frequently cause fatal complications such as cardiac arrhythmias, congestive heart failure, myocardial infarct, cerebral vascular accidents, and hemorrhage.

Pheochromocytomas may be familial. Patients with familial pheochromocytomas often have multiple tumors. These Sturge-Weber syndrome cases also are often associated with one of the variants of the multiple endocrine neoplasia syndrome, the most common of which is type 2A, characterized by carcinoma of the thyroid, hyperparathyroidism, and pheochromocytoma. DNA-polymorphism analysis facilitates identification of individuals at risk for this syndrome (80). Pheochromocytoma is also linked with von Recklinghausen's disease (café-au-lait spots) and von Hippel–Lindau disease (angiomatosis of the retina and hemangioblastoma of the cerebellum). Patients with von Hippel–Lindau disease also may have neurologic symptoms including seizures and mental retardation. Neumann and associates (64) reported that 19 of 82 (23%) unselected patients with pheochromocytoma were carriers of von Hippel–Lindau disease or had multiple endocrine neoplasia type 2. They recommended that all patients with pheochromocytoma should be screened for these abnormalities to reduce morbidity in the patients and their families.

Patients with a pheochromocytoma usually present with hypertension, although 15% to 20% are normotensive, and rare patients are hypotensive. Approximately 50% of the hypertensive patients have sustained elevations in blood pressure, and the remainder have characteristic paroxysmal hypertension. Hypertensive patients with sweating, tachycardia, and headaches have more than a 90% chance of having a pheochromocytoma, whereas individuals with none of these characteristics have less than a 1% incidence of pheochromocytomas (70). The common symptoms and signs are listed in Table 13.7.

Patients, even those with sustained hypertension, often experience paroxysmal symptoms that may occur dramatically and suddenly. The frequency of these attacks is rather variable, and the duration is usually less than an hour. The attacks may be precipitated by emotional, physical, or pharmacologic stimuli. Neurocutaneous lesions, progressive diabetes associated with hypertension, and unexplained

TABLE 13.7. SYMPTOMS AND SIGNS OF PHEOCHROMOCYTOMA

	Frequency (%)
Symptom	
Headache	80–85
Weakness	75–80
Diaphoresis	65–70
Palpitations	60–65
Orthostatic hypotension	50–60
Nausea and vomiting	35–60
Nervousness	35–40
Constipation	30–35
Sign	
Hypertension	80–85
Retinopathy	50–70
Decreased body weight	40–70
Fasting hyperglycemia	40–50

Adapted from Atuk NO. Pheochromocytomas: diagnosis, localization, and treatment. *Hosp Pract* 1983;18:187.

intraoperative hypertension all should suggest the presence of pheochromocytoma.

The hypertension is caused by the release of catecholamines from the tumor *and* increased sympathetic neural tone. Bravo and associates (13) have shown that clonidine, a drug that decreases sympathetic tone, reduces blood pressure and heart rate in patients with pheochromocytoma without affecting plasma catecholamines or renin concentrations. Tumors that produce only NE are associated with fewer symptoms than those that release NE and E. The latter compound has a more pronounced affect on β-receptors, causing symptoms such as diaphoresis and palpitations.

Laboratory Evaluation

The diagnosis of pheochromocytoma is made by documenting elevated levels of catecholamines in the blood or urine. The assays are rather precise, but false-positive results can occur secondary to drugs, stress, and other diseases that increase the concentrations of catecholamines (Table 13.8). Modest elevations in hematocrit levels are common as a result of a decreased plasma volume secondary to vasoconstriction.

TABLE 13.8. SOME CAUSES OF INCREASED CATECHOLAMINES

Drugs	Diseases
Methyldopa	Guillain-Barré syndrome
Theophylline	Neuroblastoma
Ephedrine	Porphyria
Levodopa	Brain tumor
Tricyclic antidepressants	Carcinoid syndrome
Clonidine (withdrawal)	Intrahepatic cholelithiasis

Patients can be screened for pheochromocytoma by analysis of a 24-hour urine sample for combined MN (normal 0.2 to 1.3 mg per 24 hours) and VMA. Normal values are shown in Table 13.9. Urinary MN is the best single test. Urinary free catecholamines also can be useful; Duncan and associates (26) have shown that 24-hour urinary NE had a 100% sensitivity and a 98% specificity in a large group of hypertensive patients. An advantage of measuring urinary free catecholamines is that if E is present and NE is absent, the tumor is extremely likely to be located in an adrenal gland. These tests in combination are more than 95% accurate. The pattern most typical of malignant pheochromocytomas is elevated dopamine secretion, often with comparably high NE levels and low E secretions. This is because malignant pheochromocytomas often are deficient in dopamine β-hydroxylase and phenylethanolamine N-methyltransferase.

Some authorities have recommended screening patients with an assay of plasma catecholamines. Bravo and Gifford (11) from The Cleveland Clinic have had excellent results with the plasma assay. The blood test also must be carefully done, with a supine and relaxed patient, and the laboratory must be experienced with the assay. In patients with equivocal values of plasma catecholamines, provocative testing may be necessary. Plasma catecholamines greater than 2,000 pg/mL are diagnostic of pheochromocytoma. If the catecholamine levels are between 1,000 and 2,000 pg/mL, clonidine suppression test (11) is performed. The principle behind this test is that in essential (neurogenic) hypertension, activation of the sympathetic nervous system results in an increase in plasma catecholamine. However, in patients with a pheochromocytoma, the increased catecholamines are due to the tumor itself, bypassing normal storage and release mechanisms. Therefore clonidine will not suppress catecholamine release in patients with a pheochromocytoma but will suppress catecholamine release in patients with essential (neurogenically mediated) hypertension. Following a 0.3-mg oral dose of clonidine, a 50% reduction in

TABLE 13.9. NORMAL VALUES FOR CATECHOLAMINES IN URINE[a]

	Adult (μg)	Infant and Child (Range μg/kg)
NE	80	0.4–1.6
E	25	0.02–1.6
VMA	8	83 ± 26
NMN	450	4.9–20.8
MN	300	3.1–15.6

[a]Catecholamine values for 24-hour urine collection.
E, epinephrine; MN, metanephrine; NE, norepinephrine; NMN, normetanephrine; VMA, vanilylmandelic acid.

plasma catecholamines and a catecholamine level less than 500 pg/mL is diagnostic of essential hypertension. However, postclonidine catecholamine levels greater than 500 pg/mL are indicative of pheochromocytoma. If resting plasma catecholamine levels are less than 1,000 pg/mL, a glucagon stimulation test is employed. Glucagon 2 mg is administered intravenously. One to three minutes later, a threefold increase in plasma catecholamine (greater than 2,000 pg/mL) is diagnostic of pheochromocytoma.

Localization of Pheochromocytomas

Once the diagnosis of pheochromocytoma has been made, it is necessary to localize the tumor for surgical planning. CT or MRI of the abdomen and pelvis are the best initial examinations (Fig. 13.12). These are performed because 97% of all tumors, including extraabdominal tumors, are located below the diaphragm. CT is widely available, is cost-effective, and can resolve masses as small as 1 cm. MRI is an alternative that requires no radiation exposure or intravenous contrast; however, it is more expensive. MRI has superior tissue characterization and, unlike benign adrenal adenomas, pheochromocytomas exhibit a high signal intensity on T_2-weighted images (37). MRI also avoids metallic clip artifact, which may be present on CT. Iodine-131-meta-iodobenzylguanidine scintigraphy is also an accurate method for anatomically and functionally characterizing pheochromocytomas (77,79) (Fig. 13.16). Its main advantage is the ability to image the whole body so that occult extraadrenal or metastatic disease may be identified. Its expense, limited availability, and diminished sensitivity restrict its utility. At present, it is a complementary study to CT or MRI in patients in whom there is a high suspicion of extraadrenal or metastatic disease.

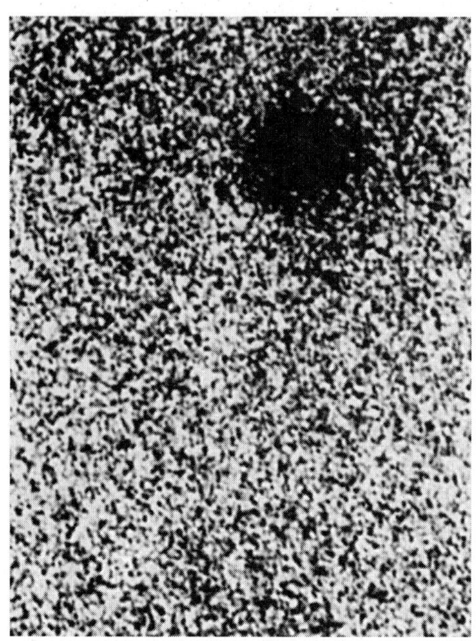

FIGURE 13.16. MIBG scan of a pheochromocytoma.

Treatment

The treatment of pheochromocytoma is surgical removal unless the operation is contraindicated. In the latter situations, medical therapy is indicated. In 10% of patients who have malignant pheochromocytomas, treatment should be governed by the basic principles of cancer management. The diagnosis is not frequently made preoperatively and may be difficult to confirm histologically. Tumors that invade adjacent structures or metastasize are considered malignant. Both α- and β-adrenergic blocking agents and α-methyl-L-tyrosine (metyrosine, which blocks synthesis of NE by inhibiting tyrosine hydroxylase) all can be used to alleviate symptoms in patients with inoperable malignant pheochromocytomas.

The goal of perioperative medical management of the pheochromocytoma patient is to minimize cardiovascular morbidity. Preoperative α-blockade is indicated for 2 to 3 weeks to control the blood pressure and to facilitate intravascular volume expansion. Oral phenoxybenzamine is widely used, although some groups prefer a shorter-acting agent such as prazosin. Calcium channel blockers (verapamil SR, nifedipine XL) also are used. Advantages of calcium channel blockers include normalization of blood pressure without any of the side effects of chronic α-blockade. There is no orthostatic or "overshoot" hypotension. Furthermore, calcium channel blockers may prevent catecholamine-induced vasospasm and myocarditis. At The Cleveland Clinic, calcium channel blockers are the drug of choice for preoperative preparation of patients with pheochromocytoma. If additional control of hypertension is necessary, we add selective α_1-blockade with prazosin. β-Blockade is indicated to treat cardiac arrhythmias or tachycardias, but only in patients with complete α-blockade. Propranolol should be avoided in patients with a history of bronchospastic disease because it causes bronchospasm. If a β-blocker is indicated, low-dose metoprolol is more appropriate.

The other important aspect of preoperative preparation is volume repletion. Most patients with a pheochromocytoma are volume depleted due to catecholamine-induced vascular constriction. Whereas transfusion of whole blood was routine before 1985, it is now more appropriate to hydrate these patients aggressively with a combination of colloid and normal saline the night before surgery. Some groups also use adjunctive preoperative salt loading with a high-salt diet. These measures are integral to preventing hypotension following surgical removal of the tumor.

The surgical approach to pheochromocytoma is based on the size and anatomic location of the tumor. Large pheochromocytomas are removed through an anterior transperitoneal or a thoracoabdominal incision. With the availability of improved localization techniques, it is no longer necessary to explore the abdomen routinely in patients with pheochromocytoma. Therefore, in select patients with a small adrenal tumor and no evidence of extraadrenal disease or multiple tumors, a unilateral extraperitoneal surgical approach may be used (21,46). Laparoscopic adrenalectomy is also currently being performed in some of these cases. Intensive intraoperative hemodynamic monitoring and the availability of rapidly acting vasoactive agents are essential to managing hypertension related to manipulation of the tumor. The anesthetic agent of choice is enflurane, which does not stimulate catecholamine secretion or increase catecholamine-induced cardiac variability. Intraoperatively, one may be faced with hypertensive crises before and during tumor removal, and hypotension following removal of tumor. To manage the hypertensive crisis, phentolamine or sodium nitroprusside may be employed. Bolus diffusion of esmolol, a β-blocker, is especially helpful if phentolamine or sodium nitroprusside affords insufficient control. For hypotension, norepinephrine (4 to 8 mg in 500 mL normal saline) can be used judiciously.

After the tumor is removed, significant hypotension may occur as a result of arterial and venous dilation secondary to catecholamine withdrawal. This situation can be compounded by prior α-blockade or inadequate volume repletion. The primary treatment of choice is volume replacement with crystalloid; pressors should be administered only when volume expansion does not correct the hypotension. Hypoglycemia is another complication that can occur postoperatively and may manifest as hypotension resistant to volume repletion or vasopressors. The blood glucose level should routinely be checked in the postoperative period, and if hypoglycemia is identified, appropriate replacement therapy should be administered.

After removal of a pheochromocytoma, the blood pressure response depends on whether the patient's hypertension was sustained or paroxysmal. Only 75% of patients with sustained hypertension remain normotensive after surgery, whereas 95% of patients with paroxysmal hypertension remain normotensive. The presence of concomitant essential hypertension is the most common reason for treatment failure; however, the possibility of undiagnosed multicentric disease should be aggressively evaluated and ruled out. Long-term follow-up of all patients is important because recurrent or metastatic disease may develop many years postoperatively. Annual measurement of the blood pressure and plasma or urinary catecholamine levels should be used to follow these patients.

We recently reviewed the experience with surgical management, complications, and treatment outcome of histologically confirmed pheochromocytoma in 113 patients at The Cleveland Clinic (84). There were no surgical mortalities. Average length of stay in the intensive care unit was 1.2 days. There were only six major cardiovascular complications all of which occurred in patients who received preoperative medications, including five with α-blockade. Patients receiving no preoperative α-blockade required an average of 956 mL less in total intraoperative fluids, which approached statistical significance, and 479 mL less fluids on postoperative day 1, which was statistically significant. These findings suggest that preoperative α-adrenergic blockage is not essential in pheochromocytoma patients. In our experience, calcium channel blockers were just as effective and safer when used as the primary mode of antihypertensive therapy. These data also affirm that surgery for pheochromocytoma is safe in the modern era.

Malignant pheochromocytomas are difficult to diagnose histologically and often are resected incompletely because of metastases in the lung, liver, bone, or brain. There is no good chemotherapy. Streptozocin has limited antitumor activity. Treatment with cyclophosphamide, vincristine, and dacarbazine has resulted in some response (3). The metabolic effects of residual malignant pheochromocytoma can be ameliorated with phenoxybenzamine, propranolol, or α-methyl-L-tyrosine.

INCIDENTAL ADRENAL MASSES

The incidental adrenal mass is a diagnostic and management dilemma created by the widespread availability of CT scanning (20). Such an "adrenaloma" or "incidentaloma" is a serendipitous finding in 0.3% to 5% of patients undergoing abdominal CT scanning. Most of these tumors (70% to 94%) are benign and biochemically inert (8, 63). However, a small minority may be biochemically active or malignant. In this group, the most common abnormality is a Cushing's or pre-Cushing's syndrome in 0% to 18% of patients. Interestingly, in patients with a known extraadrenal malignancy, the autopsy incidence of adrenal metastases ranges from 8% to 38%.

Evaluation of an incidental adrenal mass should be limited and focused. A detailed history and physical examination, stool for occult blood, and a chest radiograph are mandatory. To look for occult malignancy, a mammogram may be performed in the female. Biochemical workup includes serum potassium, and 24-hour urine estimation for catecholamines, metanephrines, and urinary free cortisol. If there is any concern, a low-dose dexamethasone suppression may be performed. In hypertensive patients, a paired serum aldosterone level and an upright PRA should be obtained.

CT characteristics of adrenal masses that suggest malignancy include an irregular ill-defined margin, internal heterogeneity, and larger size. However, significant overlap and inconsistencies in these criteria have limited the diagnostic accuracy of CT scanning in the individual patient. In general, it is accurate to say that 90% of adrenal cortical carcinomas are larger than 6 cm in diameter, with adenomas rarely obtaining such large sizes (4,32,71,42).

However, size criteria per se, are weak and inconsistent discriminators between a benign and malignant adrenal nodule. In Korobkin's (53) analysis of 135 adrenal masses, adenomas were smaller than nonadenomas (2.4 cm versus 4.5 cm); however, the authors emphasized that the considerable overlap between the two groups precluded identification of a highly specific threshold value. Kloos and colleagues (51) mentioned three patients with a 3- to 5-cm, biochemically inert adrenal mass, who were initially advised against an operation at an outside institution. Upon referral to the author's center 3 to 7 years later, these patients were found to have obviously progressed adrenal cortical carcinomas. Linos and Stylopoulos (57) reported three patients who were "incidentally found to have an adrenal cancer measuring 2.6 to 2.9 cm on CT." An important factor to be considered when discussing adrenal mass size is the reported 20% to 40% CT scan underestimation of adrenal size when compared with their actual size on histopathology examination. CT densitometry has a higher sensitivity-to-specificity ratio. Using a threshold of 10 Hounsfield units, the sensitivity and specificity were 73% and 96%, respectively, for differentiating adenomas from nonadenomas (53).

Although, typically, MRI has been used to differentiate benign from malignant adrenal masses, one must be aware that an overlap of 20% to 30% exists. Compared with the liver or spleen, adenomas are usually isotense on T_1-weighted images and slightly hypertense or isotense on T_2-weighted images. Basically, adenomas change little in intensity from T_1- to T_2-weighted studies. In contrast, adrenal cancer is hypointense compared with liver-spleen on T_1-weighted and hyperintense on T_2-weighted images. Thus a mean signal intensity ratio between the adrenal mass and spleen of less than 0.8 indicates benign adenoma. However, hyperintensivity on MRI is not specific to adrenal carcinoma and can be seen with adrenal metastases, hemorrhage, neural tumors, or other retroperitoneal masses. More recently, chemical-shift MRI imaging was shown to detect a relative loss of signal intensity in 95% of adrenal adenomas compared with 0% of nonadenomas (62). It appears that future diagnostic algorithms may combine the accuracy of chemical-shift MRI and unenhanced CT densitometry for accurate nonoperative differentiation between adrenal adenomas and nonadenomas.

This critical decision when faced with an incidental adrenal mass is whether to perform surgical excision or continue with observation. Surgical excision is indicated for hormonally active masses, tumors 5 cm or larger, tumors with suspicious characteristics on CT or MRI, and masses that are documented to enlarge over time. Observation and periodic (every 6 to 12 months) radiographic follow-up are recommended for those who do not fall into one of the above categories.

Recently, several investigators have reported that a significant minority of patients with incidentally discovered adrenal masses have preclinical or subclinical functioning tumors with no clinical evidence of endocrinologic function, but they demonstrated autonomous cortisol production. Removal of these tumors results in improvement in hypertension, obesity, or diabetes in many of the patients (52,73).

The adrenal is also an extremely common site of metastatic lesions because of its intense vascular supply (6 to 7 mL/g per minute). In fact, adrenal metastatic lesions are more common than primary adrenal cancer. In the presence of a known extraadrenal malignancy, the chance that an adrenal mass is cancerous is approximately 8% to 38% (51). Fine-needle aspiration should be performed if a metastatic etiology is suspected. This can enable diagnosis of a metastatic adrenal lesion but is of limited value in delineating an adrenal adenoma from an adrenal cortical carcinoma (15). Surgical removal of the adrenal gland is indicated only if the adrenal represented the solitary site of metastatic disease.

ADRENOCORTICAL CARCINOMA

Adrenocortical carcinoma is an uncommon disease, with only 80 to 130 cases per year in the United States (14). Approximately 50% of the tumors are endocrinologically functional. Cushing's syndrome, virilization, and feminization occur in 20%, 9%, and 3% of these patients, respectively, and primary hyperaldosteronism is present in less than 4% (39). Less than 30% of the tumors are localized to the adrenal gland at presentation. Surgical excision or debulking is the treatment of choice. Radiotherapy and chemotherapy have been disappointing, although approximately half of the patients will respond to mitotane for 10 to 12 months (61). Mean survival for localized disease is 5.0 years and for more extensive lesions is 2.3 years (9,18).

OPERATIVE APPROACHES TO THE ADRENAL GLANDS

A wide spectrum of adrenal pathology may warrant surgical intervention. A variety of operative approaches are available for adrenal surgery. The optimal technique must be individualized according to the adrenal pathology, the patient's body habitus and surgical history, and the familiarity of the surgeon with each operative approach.

Posterior Approach

The posterior surgical approach to the adrenal gland was first described more than 50 years ago (89) and continues to find useful application in selected patients undergoing adrenalectomy. The advantages of this approach are that it is extraperitoneal and that adrenalectomy can be done with minimal disturbance of adjacent viscera. Anatomically, a posterior incision represents the most direct approach to the adrenal gland. Because no major muscles are transected, patient discomfort is generally minimal and early ambulation is possible. If indicated, both adrenal glands can be exposed simultaneously through bilateral posterior incisions.

The major disadvantage of the posterior approach is the relatively small operative field, which restricts visualization and exposure of the great vessels. Therefore this approach should not be used to remove large adrenal lesions where wide exposure and early avascular control are necessary. This approach is also contraindicated in patients with a potentially malignant process, in whom an exploratory laparotomy must be done. Based on these limitations, the primary indication for posterior adrenalectomy is in patients with bilateral hyperplasia from Cushing's disease who have failed transsphenoidal hypophysectomy. This approach has also been used in the past to treat small benign adrenal lesions such as adrenal cortical adenomas causing hyperaldosteronism or Cushing's syndrome, and small adrenal pheochromocytomas; these small benign unilateral tumors are now being treated by laparoscopic adrenalectomy at many centers.

The posterior anatomic relation of the adrenal glands is illustrated in Fig. 13.17. The pleural reflection extends below most of the eleventh rib and a variable portion of the medial aspect of the twelfth rib. The right adrenal gland lies more superiorly in the retroperitoneum than its counterpart on the left side. The left adrenal gland can usually be adequately approached posteriorly through the bed of the twelfth rib. The optimal incision for exposing the right adrenal gland is generally through the bed of the rib. In most cases, the location of the adrenal gland in relation to the ribs is known from preoperative imaging studies.

The patient is placed in the prone position on a laminectomy frame, which provides flexion at the hips and allows gentle dorsal curvature of the spine from the midthoracic to the lower lumbar levels. An oblique incision is made over the eleventh rib or twelfth rib and extended laterally almost to the midaxillary line (Fig. 13.18). The incision is developed to expose the entire length of the rib and the sacrospinalis muscle medially. The rib is resected subperiosteally, including as much of its medial aspect as possible to optimize exposure of the adrenal gland; such exposure also is facilitated by medial retraction of the sacrospinalis muscle. In operating through a twelfth rib incision, the diaphragm and pleura can readily be mobilized and retracted superiorly. However, in operating through an eleventh rib incision, attempting to mobilize the pleura superiorly may be tedious and can lead to one or more inadvertent pleural entries. In such cases, simply opening the pleural and diaphragmatic layers of the thoracic cavity in line with the incision can be done safely and provides excellent direct exposure of the adrenal gland (66,67). After the retroperitoneal space is entered, Gerota's fascia is incised

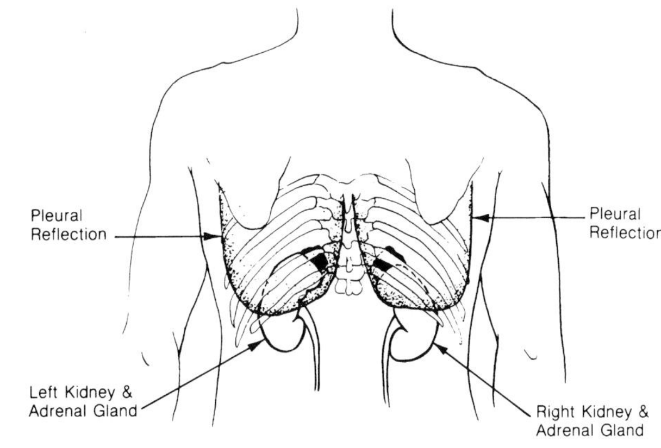

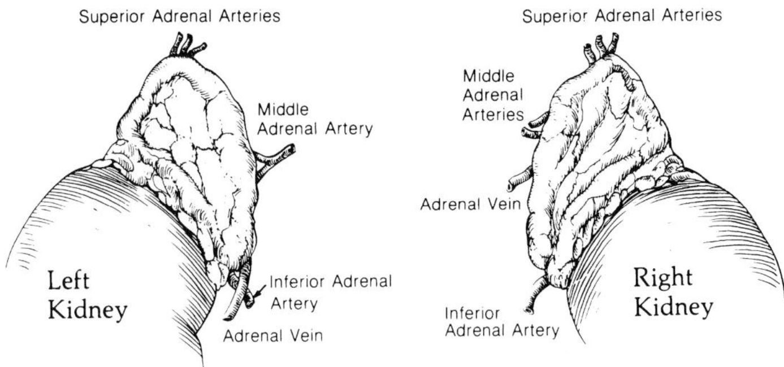

FIGURE 13.17. Sketch illustrating the posterior anatomic relations of the adrenal glands. (From Novic AC. Adrenal surgery. In: Novick AC, ed. *Stewart's operative urology,* 2nd ed. Baltimore: Williams & Wilkins, 1989, with permission.)

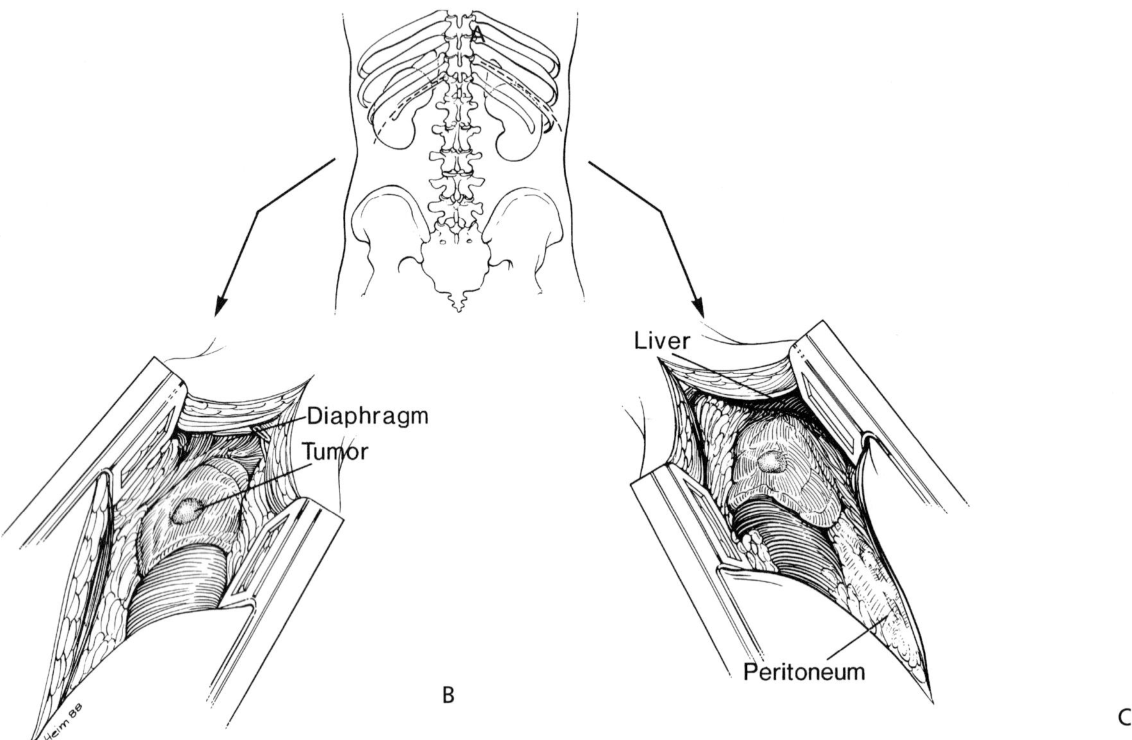

FIGURE 13.18. Sketch illustrating the posterior approach for adrenal surgery **(A)**, through the eleventh rib on the right side **(C)** and through the twelfth rib on the left side **(B)**. (From Novick AC. Surgery for primary hyperaldosteronism. *Urol Clin North Am* 1989;16:535, with permission.)

and the posterior surface of the kidney and adrenal gland is exposed.

On the left side (Fig. 13.19), the attachment between the upper pole of the kidney and the inferior aspect of the adrenal gland is kept intact, so that gentle downward traction on the kidney can be done to enhance exposure. The apical vascular ligament is identified and transected between silver clips to deliver the gland more extensively into the operative field. The lateral borders of the gland are then freed, and the gland is retracted medially to expose its anterior surface. Care must be taken not to injure the pancreas, which lies just beneath the adrenal gland through this approach. The left adrenal vein is exposed as it courses downward just medial and anterior to the upper pole of the kidney to enter the left renal vein. The left adrenal vein is then ligated with 2-0 silk and divided. The upper stump of the vein can be left long and used as a handle for additional lateral traction on the gland. The inferior adrenal artery also is secured at this stage as it courses upward from the proximal aspect of the renal artery. Through use of lateral and upward traction, the left adrenalectomy is completed by securing and dividing the middle adrenal arteries as they course inward medially from the aorta.

On the right side (Fig. 13.20), the kidney is retracted downward, and the liver is gently retracted upward to facilitate exposure of the adrenal gland. In some cases, the apex of the adrenal gland is adherent to the liver and must be carefully dissected free. The dissection is continued cephalad, and the apical vascular ligament is divided between silver clips. The lateral and inferior aspects of the gland are easily mobilized, and the dissection is carried around to expose the anterior surface medially to the level of the inferior vena cava. The gland is then returned to its normal anatomic position to expose the remaining inferior and medial vascular attachments. Gentle lateral traction on the gland is applied to facilitate identification, ligation, and division of the right adrenal vein. The remaining arterial supply is divided between silver clips to complete the removal of the right adrenal gland.

When adrenalectomy is completed, if a transthoracic incision has been used, the diaphragm is reapproximated with interrupted 2-0 silk mattress sutures. Airtight closure of the pleura is achieved using 3-0 silk or chromic sutures with the lung under positive-pressure expansion. Chest tube drainage is generally not necessary unless there has been difficulty in reapproximating the pleura. No surgical drains are used. A chest film is obtained several hours postoperatively in the recovery room to verify that the lung is fully expanded. Incisional discomfort with this approach is mild, and ambulation is generally possible on the day after surgery.

Flank Approach

The extraperitoneal flank approach is an alternative to the posterior approach for removal of relatively small benign unilateral tumors. The flank approach has the advantage of relative simplicity and familiarity to the urologic surgeon. Also, in particularly obese patients, exposure of the adrenal gland through a posterior incision may be compromised; in such cases, the use of a generous extraperitoneal flank incision is preferable for performing adrenalectomy.

When an extraperitoneal flank adrenalectomy is performed, either the twelfth or the eleventh rib is resected to allow entrance to the retroperitoneal space. Alternatively, the retroperitoneum can be entered through an incision in the tenth or eleventh intercostal space. A classic subcostal flank incision is not recommended because of the difficulty in obtaining adequate superior exposure of the adrenal gland.

On the right side (Fig. 13.21), the colon and duodenum are reflected medially, and the liver is reflected upward to expose the kidney and adrenal gland. The kidney with its attached adrenal gland is retracted downward. The anterior, posterior, and apical aspects are mobilized by blunt dissection from the undersurface of the liver posteriorly and from the duodenum and hepatic flexure of the colon anteriorly. The apical attachments of the gland are then divided between silver clips. With the gland retracted laterally, small arterial branches entering the medial aspect of the gland are identified as they course beneath the vena cava. Branches of the inferior adrenal artery coursing upward from the proximal right renal artery are similarly identified. After these

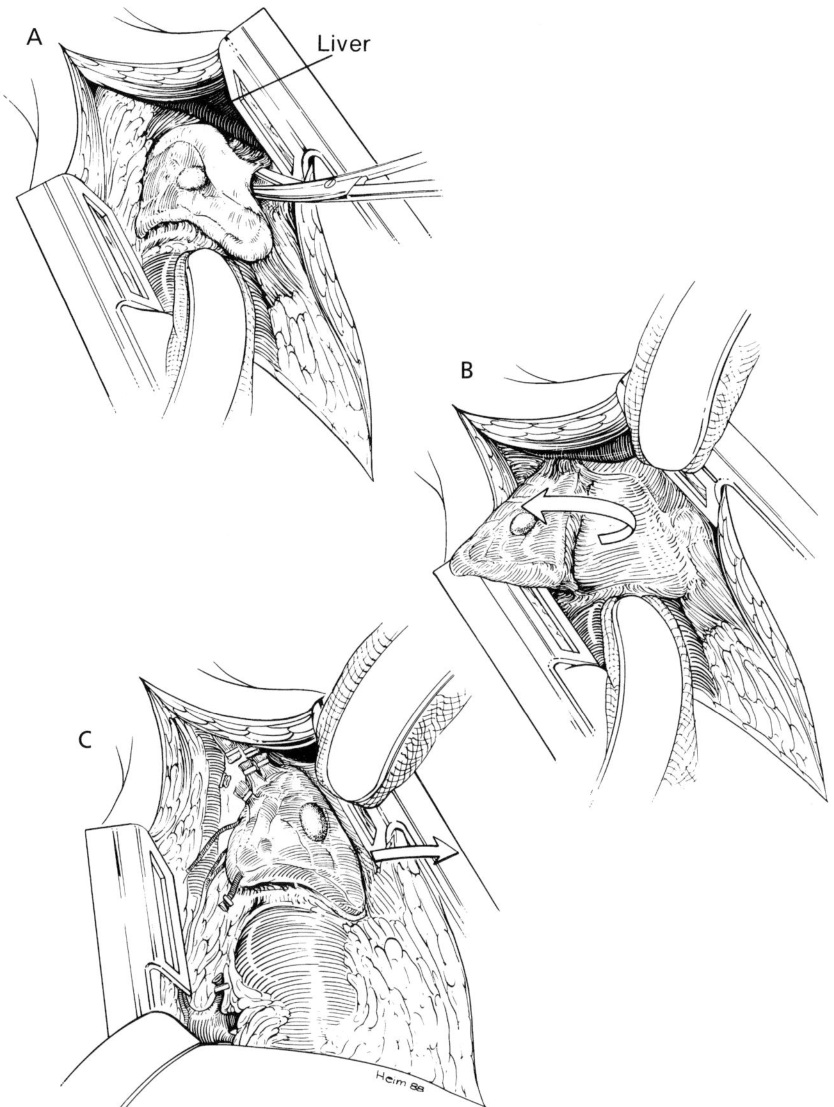

FIGURE 13.19. A–C: The technique of left adrenalectomy through a posterior incision. (From Novick AC. Surgery for primary hyperaldosteronism. *Urol Clin North Am* 1989;16: 535, with permission.)

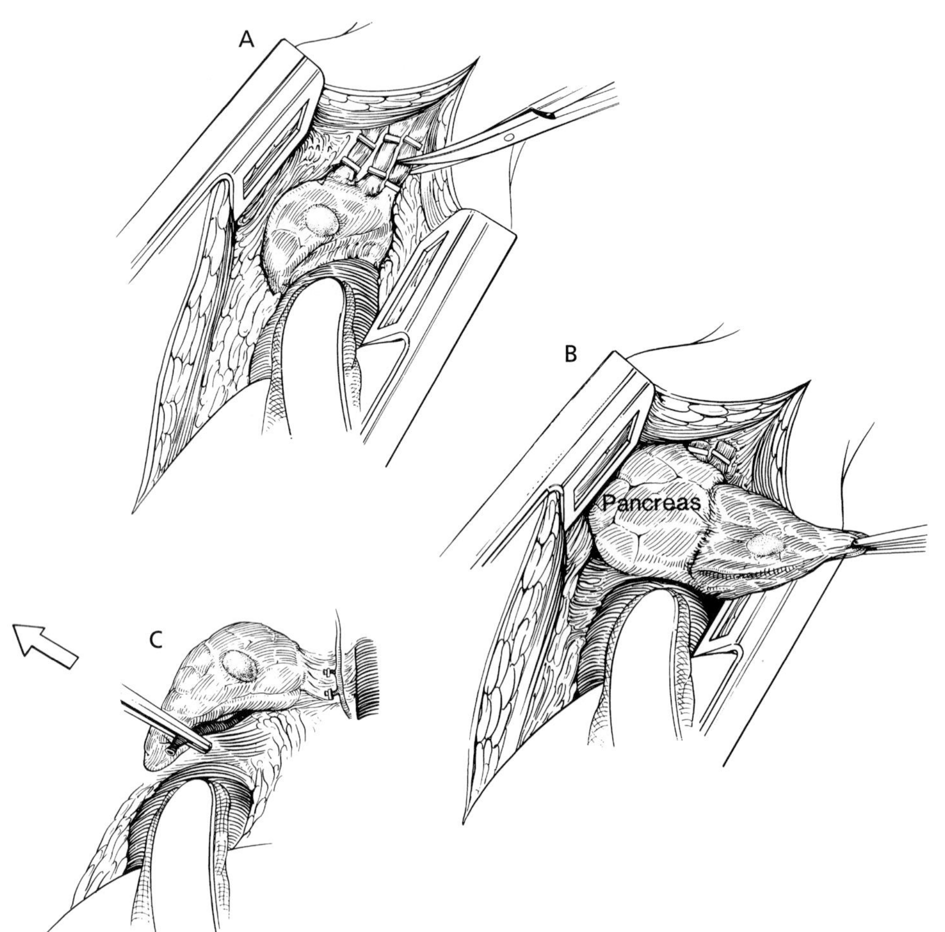

FIGURE 13.20. A–C: The technique of right adrenalectomy through a posterior incision. (From Novick AC. Surgery for primary hyperaldosteronism. *Urol Clin North Am* 1989;16:535, with permission.)

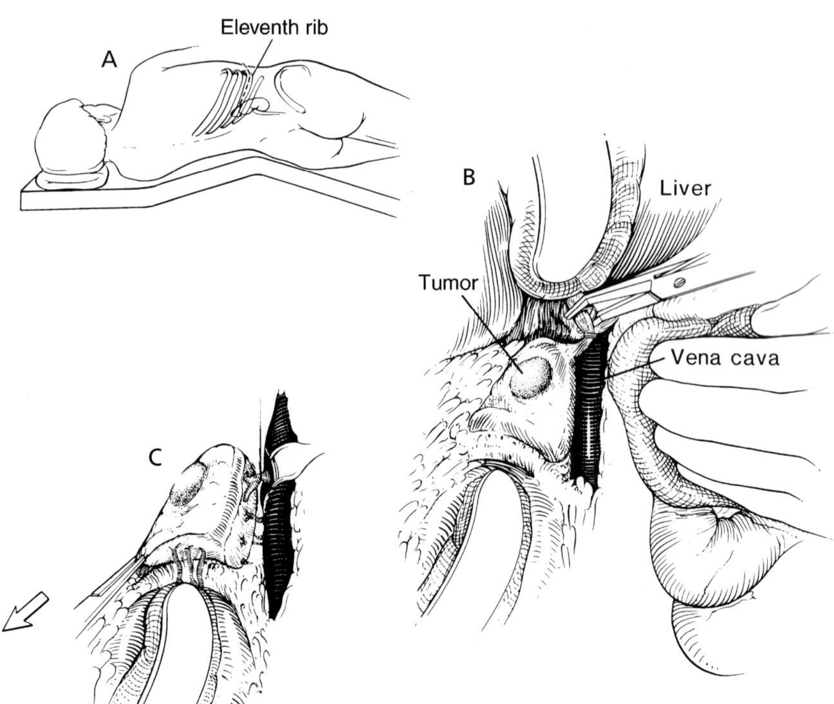

FIGURE 13.21. A–C: The technique of right adrenalectomy through an eleventh rib flank incision. (From Novick AC. Surgery for primary hyperaldosteronism. *Urol Clin North Am* 1989;16:535, with permission.)

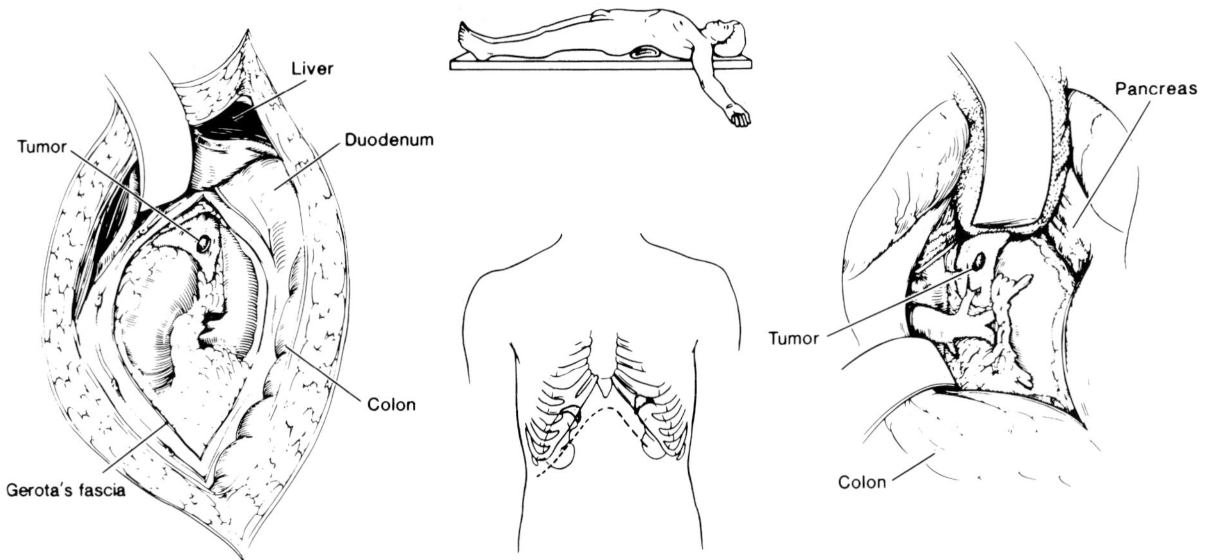

FIGURE 13.22. Anterior transabdominal approach to the adrenal glands. (From Guz B, Straffon R, Novick AC. Operative approaches to the adrenal gland. *Urol Clin North Am* 1989;16:527, with permission.)

vessels have been secured and transected, the right adrenal veinis located, secured, and divided. Residual apical vascular branches are then similarly secured and transected to complete the adrenalectomy.

Anterior Transabdominal Approach

The anterior transabdominal approach is indicated for adrenal lesions that are either large or potentially malignant. These include suspected or proven adrenal cortical carcinomas, large adrenal cortical adenomas, and large adrenal pheochromocytomas. In these cases, wide exposure is necessary, which cannot be achieved to the same extent through an extraperitoneal incision. With potentially malignant adrenal masses, intraabdominal inspection of other organs for metastatic disease is required. An anterior approach is also mandatory for adrenal malignancies that involve the inferior vena cava (74). The optimal anterior approach is through a bilateral subcostal or chevron incision, which provides much better exposure of the superior and lateral aspects of the adrenal gland than a midline incision. A unilateral extended subcostal incision can be used if the patient is thin and only one adrenal gland needs to be exposed. A vertical midline incision is used only if an extraadrenal pheochromocytoma is suspected in the retroperitoneum along the great vessels or in the pelvis.

The main advantage of the transabdominal approach is that it provides excellent exposure of both adrenal glands, the vascular pedicles, the abdominal organs, and the retroperitoneum. Its principal disadvantage is that the peritoneal cavity is entered. It is not the most direct avenue to the adrenal glands, and in an obese patient, exposure may be more difficult. Postoperative morbidity is higher than with extraperitoneal approaches because of an increased incidence of ileus, atelectasis, and incisional discomfort.

The patient is placed with a rolled sheet beneath the lumbar spine, and a unilateral extended subcostal or bilateral subcostal incision is made to enter the peritoneal cavity (Fig. 13.22). On the right side, the posterior peritoneum lateral to the ascending colon is incised, the colon and the duodenum are reflected medially, and the liver is retracted superiorly to expose the kidney and adrenal gland. The kidney is gently retracted downward to bring the anterior surface of the right adrenal gland into view. In most cases, it is necessary to release the upper margin of the gland from the liver with sharp dissection to obtain complete exposure. In cases of pheochromocytoma, it is important to secure the adrenal vein as soon as possible to interrupt catecholamine release from the tumor into the systemic circulation. If the vein lies far cephalad, as it often does, division of the arterial supply medially and inferiorly may be necessary before the vein can be exposed satisfactorily and safely. Surgical exposure is facilitated by medial retraction of the inferior vena cava. In cases of suspected malignancy, it is also best to isolate the medial blood supply first and to carry out the lateral dissection later. For tumors confined to the adrenal gland, after the blood supply has been secured, the remaining lateral and inferior attachments of the gland are mobilized and divided to complete the adrenalectomy.

On the left side, the adrenal gland is exposed by incising the posterior peritoneum lateral to the descending colon and dividing the ileorenal ligament with medial retraction of the colon and superior retraction of the spleen. The left adrenal vein is identified at its entry into the left renal vein and is then ligated and divided. The inferior adrenal artery also is secured and divided at this time. The adrenal gland is mobilized posteriorly and laterally by blunt dissection. The gland is then retracted downward to expose the superior vascular attachments, which are secured and divided. The gland is then retracted laterally to expose the remaining medial arterial blood supply, which is secured and divided. Residual attachments of the gland to the upper pole of the kidney are divided into sharp dissection to complete the adrenalectomy.

In some cases, an adrenal malignancy may invade the upper pole of the kidney. In this event, radical en bloc removal of both the kidney and adrenal gland within Gerota's fascia is the indicated procedure (Fig. 13.23). The main renal artery and vein are secured and divided in sequence, as in a radical nephrectomy; the ureter also is secured and divided. A plane is then developed posteriorly along the psoas muscle, bluntly mobilizing both the kidney and adrenal mass from behind and laterally. With downward and lateral retraction on the kidney, the medial blood supply to the tumor mass can be better identified. This exposure is facilitated by medial retraction of the vena cava. The medial adrenal arteries are secured and transected. On the right side, as the dissection proceeds upward, the adrenal vein also is identified, secured, and divided. This vein is large and friable, often lies higher than the surgeon expects, and must be carefully dissected free from surrounding structures to prevent avulsion from the vena cava. Should such an avulsion occur, the caval entry is immediately secured with Allis clamps and the defect is oversewn with a continuous 5-0 arterial suture. After the blood supply is secured, the dissection is carried upward and laterally to completely remove the tumor mass and kidney en bloc within Gerota's fascia. A regional lymphadenectomy is then performed from the level of the inferior mesenteric artery to the crus of the diaphragm. Splanchnic nerves and celiac ganglia may be sacrificed if adjacent nodes appear involved by neoplasm.

Thoracoabdominal Approach

The thoracoabdominal approach to the adrenal gland is desirable for very large tumors that cannot be removed safely through an anterior transabdominal incision. It can be particularly advantageous for large right-sided adrenal masses, where the overlying liver and vena cava can limit exposure. There is less indication for this incision on the left side because the spleen and pancreas usually can be elevated away from the adrenal without difficulty. The thoracoabdominal incision provides excellent exposure of the suprarenal area (17,75); however, exposure of the contralateral adrenal is more difficult than with the anterior approach. Additional operative time is required to open and close a thoracoabdominal incision. Because the thoracic cavity is entered and the diaphragm divided, potential pulmonary morbidity is greater. For these reasons, the thoracoabdominal approach is reserved for patients in whom exposure beyond that provided by an anterior subcostal incision is considered important for complete and safe tumor removal.

The patient is placed in a semioblique position with a rolled sheet inserted longitudinally between the flank and hemithorax (Fig. 13.24). The incision is begun in the eighth or ninth intercostal space near the angle of the rib and is carried medially across the umbilicus. The intercostal muscles are divided to reveal the pleura and diaphragm; the diaphragm is divided circumferentially. On the right side, the hepatic flexure of the colon and duodenum are reflected medially and the liver is retracted upward to expose the adrenal tumor. On the left side, the descending colon is reflected medially with superior retraction of the pancreas

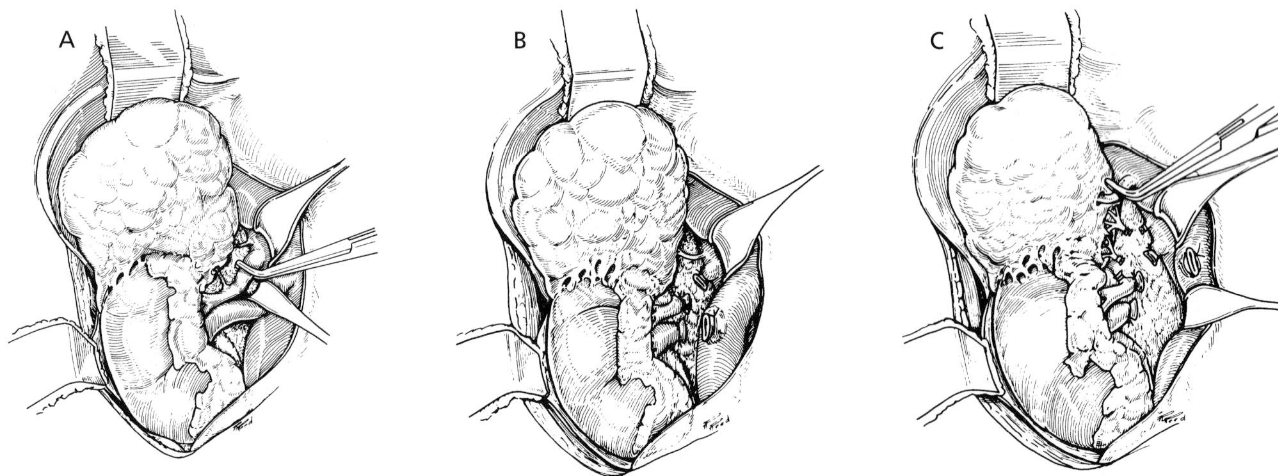

FIGURE 13.23. A–C: Technique of radical nephroadrenalectomy on the right side. (From Novic AC: Adrenal surgery. In Novick AC, ed. *Stewart's operative urology,* 2nd ed. Baltimore, Williams & Wilkins, 1989, with permission.)

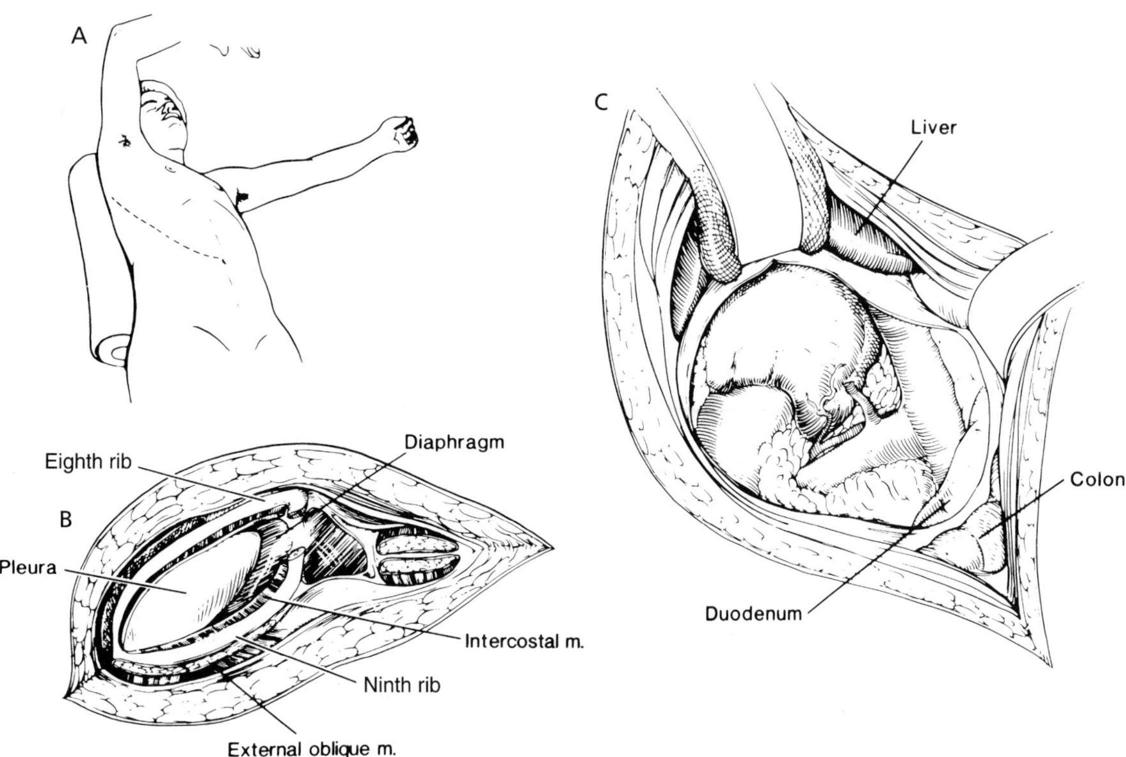

FIGURE 13.24. A–C: Thoracoabdominal approach to the adrenal gland. (From Guz B, Straffon R, Novick AC. Operative approaches to the adrenal gland. *Urol Clin North Am* 1989;16:527, with permission.)

and spleen to expose the adrenal gland. The details of adrenalectomy or nephroadrenalectomy are the same as those described for the anterior transabdominal surgical approach.

Laparoscopic Adrenalectomy

Laparoscopic adrenalectomy was initially described by Gagner and colleagues in 1992. Since then, the rapid advances in minimally invasive surgery have led to laparoscopy becoming the technique of choice for many surgical adrenal disorders. Advantages of the laparoscopic approach include a shorter hospital stay, less postoperative pain, decreased patient morbidity, more rapid patient recovery, and a superior cosmetic result.

Several studies have confirmed the safety and efficacy of laparoscopic adrenalectomy for benign adrenal disorders such as (a) primary aldosteronism (36,38,88), (b) Cushing's disease or Cushing's syndrome due to an adrenal adenoma (27,38,55), or (c) other benign lesions such as a cyst or myelolipoma. Other indications have included small nonfunctioning adrenal masses with radiographic features suspicious for malignancy, small solitary adrenal metastases, and small adrenal pheochromocytomas (28,47). Laparoscopic adrenalectomy is currently contraindicated in large pheochromocytoma or clinical overt adrenal cortical carcinomas. As an extension of the latter, any radiographic evidence of local tumor invasion, venous extension, or lymphadenopathy would definitely contraindicate a laparoscopic approach.

Laparoscopic adrenalectomy can be performed by either a transperitoneal or lateral retroperitoneal approach. In a recent prospective, but as yet unpublished study, Gill compared these two approaches and found no advantage for the extraperitoneal approach in this setting. Most centers currently employ the transperitoneal approach for laparoscopic adrenalectomy. The availability of 2-mm instrumentation and camera technology has led to the emergence of needlescopic surgery. Data from our group (36) have shown that needlescopic adrenalectomy is feasible and does offer some advantages over conventional laparoscopic adrenalectomy. A description of the technique of needlescopic adrenalectomy follows.

The patient is secured in the flank (lateral decubitus) position with the table flexed and the kidney bridge elevated. With the use of the closed (puncture) technique, a needlescopic (2 mm) port, with *in situ* Veress needle introducer, is inserted into the abdomen just below the costal margin in the anterior axillary line (for a right adrenalectomy) or at the lateral border of the rectus muscle (for a left adrenalectomy). Proper intraperitoneal placement of the tip of the Veress needle is evaluated by the routine saline suction-injection-suction technique. Carbon dioxide pneumoperitoneum is established (15 mm Hg). The 2-mm port assembly is advanced an additional 2 cm into the abdomen, and the Veress needle introducer is removed. A 1.9-mm needlescopic inserted through the 2-mm port visually confirms safe intraperitoneal access. Under needlescopic guidance, a 10/12-mm trocar sheath is placed into the peritoneal cavity at the superior crease of the umbilicus. The needlescope is removed and a 10-mm, 45-degree laparoscope is inserted through the umbilical port. Two additional secondary trocars, whose location varies depending on the side of the adrenalectomy, are inserted under visualization of the 10-mm laparoscope: (a) for a right adrenalectomy, a 2-mm port is located lateral to the xiphoid at the costal margin and a 5 mm port at the lateral border of the rectus muscle, 2 cm below the costal margin; (b) for a left adrenalectomy, a 2-mm port is located at the midaxillary line and a 5-mm port is located at the midclavicular line, both at the costal margin.

Right Needlescopic Adrenalectomy

The surgeon works through the lateral 2-mm port and the 5-mm port, whereas the assistant works through the medial 2-mm port (Fig. 13.25). The procedure is initiated under visualization by the 10-mm, 45-degree laparoscope placed through the umbilical port. The assistant retracts the liver cephalad with a 2-mm grasper placed through the medial 2-mm port; extreme care must be taken to avoid injury to the gall bladder and liver during this maneuver. With the use of 5-mm scissors, introduced through the 5-mm trocar, the triangular ligament of the liver is incised; this allows more secure cephalad retraction of the liver by the 2-mm grasper. The posterior parietal peritoneum is incised parallel to, and 1 cm below, the inferior edge of the liver. Located between the liver and the hepatic flexure of the colon, this horizontal peritoneal incision extends from the paracolic gutter laterally up to the inferior vena cava medially. With the use of a 2-mm grasper, inserted through the lateral 2-mm port, the incised edges of the peritoneum are retracted, and the adrenal gland is identified in the retroperitoneum.

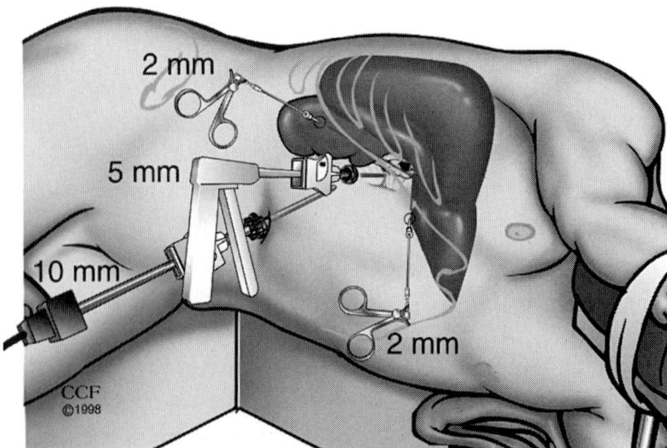

FIGURE 13.25. Needlescopic right adrenalectomy: port placement. Note that the 10-mm, 45-degree laparoscope is placed at the umbilicus. (From Gill IS, Soble JJ, Sung GT, et al. Needlescopic adrenalectomy—the initial series: comparison with conventional laparoscopic adrenalectomy. *Urology* 1998;52:180, with permission.)

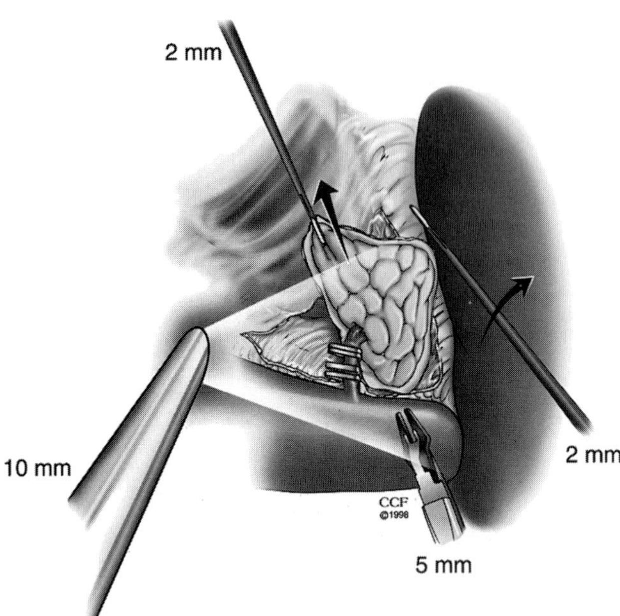

FIGURE 13.26. Needlescopic right adrenalectomy: dissection between the adrenal gland and the inferior vena cava brings the main adrenal vein into view. Care must be taken while retracting the liver cephalad with the 2-mm instrument. The main adrenal vein is clip-ligated by a 5-mm clip-applier inserted through the 5-mm subcostal port. Note that visualization is provided by the 10-mm, 45-degree laparoscope placed at the umbilicus. (From Gill IS, Soble JJ, Sung GT, et al. Needlescopic adrenalectomy—the initial series: comparison with conventional laparoscopic adrenalectomy. *Urology* 1998;52:180, with permission.)

Dissection is performed between the medial border of the adrenal gland and the inferior vena cava. This step is facilitated by lateral retraction of the adrenal gland and surrounding adipose tissue by the 2-mm grasper placed through the lateral 2-mm port (Fig. 13.26). Dissection along the right lateral edge of the inferior vena cava brings the main right adrenal vein into view. A 5-mm clip-applier, introduced through the 5-mm port, is used to secure the adrenal vein, which is then divided (Fig. 13.26). At this point in the dissection, the psoas muscle can be visualized through the laterally retracted adrenal gland and the inferior vena cava, signifying the posterior extent of the dissection.

Dissection proceeds along the superomedial border of the adrenal gland, where adrenal branches from the inferior phrenic vessels are clip-ligated and divided. After the superior edge of the adrenal gland is completely freed, the adrenal gland is retracted anteromedially, placing its inframedially and inferior attachments on gentle retraction. With the use of a combination of hook-blade electrocautery and the 5-mm clip-applier, small adrenal branches from the renal artery and vein are secured, and the adrenal gland is mobilized meticulously from the superior aspect of the renal hilum. The avascular plane between the upper pole of the kidney and the adrenal is developed, thus mobilizing the inferior edge of the adrenal gland. The tail of the adrenal gland is freed, completely excising the specimen.

The 10-mm laparoscope is now removed, and the needlescope is introduced through the medial 2-mm port. A plastic bag is inserted through the umbilical port, and under needlescopic visualization, the specimen is entrapped and extracted intact from the umbilicus. After confirming hemostasis, fascial closure of the umbilical port is performed and all ports are removed under needlescopic visualization. The umbilical incision and the 5-mm port-site incision are closed with subcuticular sutures. Each 2-mm port-site puncture hole is closed with a single Steri-Strip.

Left Needlescopic Adrenalectomy

The surgeon works through the medial 2-mm port and the 5-mm port, whereas the assistant works through the lateral 2-mm port. The main differences in a left adrenalectomy include mobilization and medial retraction of the splenic flexure and descending colon, cephalad retraction of the spleen, and control of the left main adrenal vein. Although virtually no colonic mobilization is required during a right adrenalectomy, performance of a left adrenalectomy requires incision of the line of Toldt and formal mobilization of the splenic flexure and part of the descending colon. The splenocolic, splenorenal, and splenophrenic ligaments are incised to completely mobilize the spleen in a medial and cephalad direction. Occasionally, for a larger adrenal mass, the tail of the pancreas must be mobilized off the anterior surface of the adrenal gland.

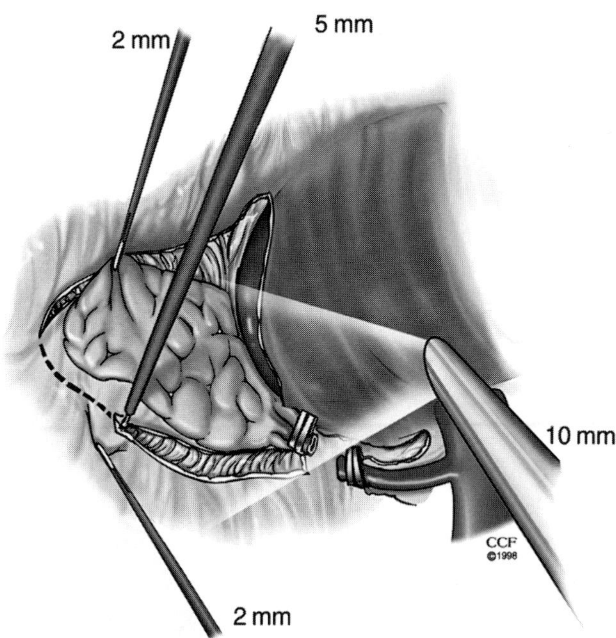

FIGURE 13.28. Needlescopic left adrenalectomy: clip-ligation of the main adrenal vein with 5-mm clip appliers. (From Gill IS, Soble JJ, Sung GT, et al. Needlescopic adrenalectomy—the initial series: comparison with conventional laparoscopic adrenalectomy. *Urology* 1998;52:180, with permission.)

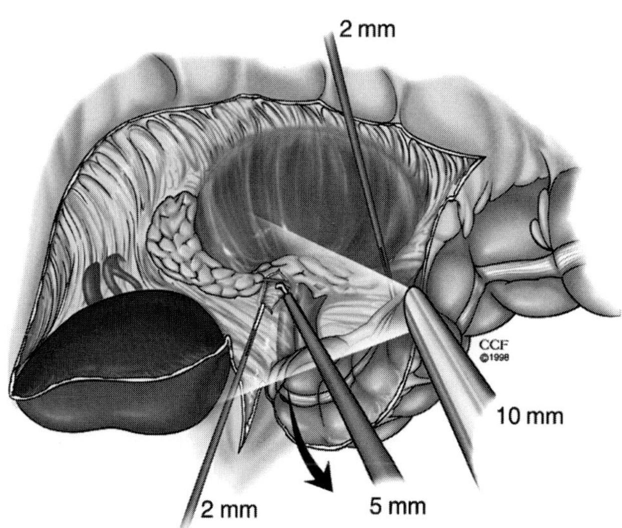

FIGURE 13.27. Needlescopic left adrenalectomy: identification of the left main adrenal vein. Note the T-incision along the line of Toldt. If adequate mobilization of the spleen is performed initially, the spleen stays retracted away from the operative site by gravity alone. Care must be taken while retracting the spleen and colon with 2-mm instruments. (From Gill IS, Soble JJ, Sung GT, et al. Needlescopic adrenalectomy—the initial series: comparison with conventional laparoscopic adrenalectomy. *Urology* 1998;52:180, with permission.)

Dissection along the superior border of the left renal vein identifies the left main renal vein (Fig. 13.27). Clip-ligation of the main adrenal vein is performed with 5-mm clip-appliers (Fig. 13.28). Many aortic branches to the adrenal vein are clip-occluded and divided to free the adrenal gland.

During needlescopic adrenalectomy, visualization is provided by the 10-mm 45-degree laparoscope placed through an umbilical 10/12-mm trocar. From a cosmetic standpoint, the umbilicus is the optimal location to "hide" the mandatory 2- to 3-cm skin incision ultimately required for intact extraction of the excised adrenal gland. Our experience has shown that the diminished trauma of access by the needlescopic technique results in diminished port-site pain, and a superior cosmetic result (Fig. 13.29) (36). Currently, at our center, the needlescopic approach is the technique of choice when performing transperitoneal endoscopic adrenalectomy, except in patients with marked obesity or large adrenal tumors. In the latter settings, a conventional laparoscopic technique is employed with four 10/12-mm trocar sheets placed along the costal margin. The primary port is placed by the closed (Veress needle) technique, and the three secondary ports are inserted under laparoscopic guidance. The technique of laparoscopic adrenalectomy is otherwise similar to the needlescopic technique.

Recent studies also have shown that needlescopic adrenalectomy is less expensive than the open approach (43) and can be performed on an outpatient basis in select patients (34).

In a recent retrospective study, the results of laparoscopic/needlescopic adrenalectomy were compared with those of open adrenalectomy in 210 patients at The Cleveland Clinic Foundation (35). Laparoscopic/needlescopic adrenalectomy was performed in 110 patients from March 1996 through November 1998. Open adrenalectomy was performed in 100 patients from May 1987 through March 1996. Detailed data are outlined in Table 13.10. There was no significant difference in operative time and the mean specimen weight was similar in the two groups. The laparoscopic/needlescopic approach was clearly advantageous with respect to less blood loss, reduced narcotic analgesic requirements, earlier postoperative oral intake, and a reduced hospital stay. Currently, needlescopic adrenalectomy is currently being performed as an outpatient procedure in many patients (34). Additional recent data from our group have demonstrated that needlescopic adrenalectomy has a reduced overall cost compared with open adrenalectomy (43). Based on data such as these, laparoscopic/needlescopic adrenalectomy is emerging as the standard of care for many patients with surgical adrenal disease.

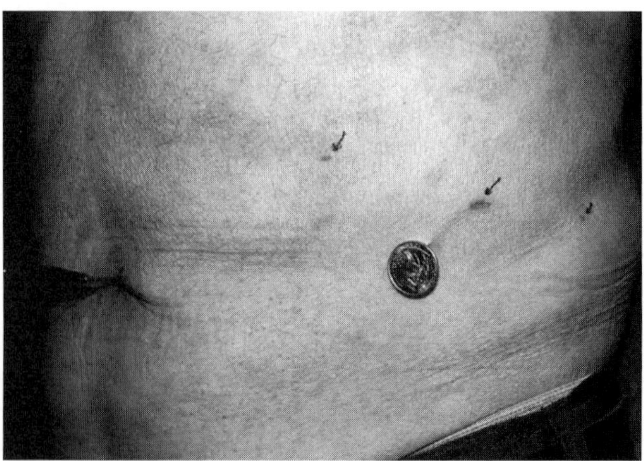

FIGURE 13.29. Patient photograph 2 weeks after needlescopic left adrenalectomy. The port-site skin incisions *(arrows)* are barely visible. (From Gill IS, Soble JJ, Sung GT, et al. Needlescopic adrenalectomy—the initial series: comparison with conventional laparoscopic adrenalectomy. *Urology* 1998;52:180, with permission.)

TABLE 13.10. CLEVELAND CLINIC EXPERIENCE WITH LAPAROSCOPIC VERSUS OPEN SURGICAL ADRENALECTOMY

	Laparoscopic[a] (n = 110)	Open[a] (n = 100)	
Specimen weight (g)	29	28.6	
Surgical time (min)	188	218	
Blood loss (mL)	125	563	p = .0001
Narcotics (mg)	38	471	p = .0001
Oral intake (days)	1.0	3.2	p = .0001
Hospital stay (days)	1.9	7.6	p = .0001

[a]Mean values.
From Gill IS, Schweizer D, Nelson D, et al. Laparoscopic vs open adrenalectomy: Cleveland Clinic experience with 210 cases. *J Urol* 1999; 161:21.

REFERENCES

1. Adams JE, Johnson RJ, Richards D, et al. Computed tomography in adrenal disease. *Clin Radiol* 1983;34:39.
2. Atuk NO. Pheochromocytomas: diagnosis, localization, and treatment. *Hosp Pract* 1983;18:187.
3. Averbuch SD, Steakley CS, Young RC, et al. Malignant pheochromocytoma-effective treatment with a combination of cyclophosphamide, vincristine and dacarbazine. *Ann Intern Med* 1988;109:267.
4. Belldegrun A, Hussain S, Seltzer SE. Incidentally discovered mass of the adrenal gland. *Surg Gynecol Obstet* 1986;163:203.
5. Besser GM. ACTH and MSH assays and their clinical application. *Clin Endocrinol* 1973;2:175.
6. Bethune JE. *The adrenal cortex, a Scope monograph.* Kalamazoo, MI: Upjohn Co., 1974.
7. Biglieri EG, Schambelan M. The significance of elevated levels of plasma 18-hydroxycorticosterone in patients with primary aldosteronism. *J Clin Endocrinol Metab* 1979;49:87.
8. Blumfeld JD, Schulssel Y, Sealey JE, et al. Diagnosis and treatment of primary hyperaldosteronism. *Ann Intern Med* 1994; 121:877.
9. Bodie B, Novick AC, Pontes JE. The Cleveland Clinic experience with adrenal cortical carcinoma. *J Urol* 1989;141:257.
10. Boggan JE, Tyrrell JB, Wilson CB. Transsphenoidal microsurgical management of Cushing's disease: report of 100 cases. *J Neurosurg* 1983;59:195.
11. Bravo EL, Gifford RW Jr. Current concepts: pheochromocytoma: diagnosis, localization, and management. *N Engl J Med* 1984;311:1298.
12. Bravo EL, Tarazi RC, Dustan HP, et al. The changing spectrum of primary aldosteronism. *Am J Med* 1983;74:641.
13. Bravo EL, Tarazi RC, Fetnat M, et al. Blood pressure regulation in pheochromocytoma. *Hypertension* 1982;4[Suppl II]:193.
14. Brennan M. Cancer of the endocrine system. In: Devita V, Hellman S, Rosenberg S, eds. *Cancer: principles and practice of oncology,* 2nd ed, Philadelphia: Lippincott, 1985:198.
15. Candel AG, Gattuso P, Reyes CV, et al. Fine-needle aspiration biopsy of adrenal masses in patients with extra-adrenal malignancy. *Surgery* 1993;114:1132.

16. Carey RM, Sen S, Solan IM, et al. Idiopathic hyperaldosteronism: a possible role of aldosterone-stimulating factor. *N Engl J Med* 1984;311:94.
17. Chute R, Soutter L, Kerr WS. The value of the thoracoabdominal incision in the removal of kidney tumors. *N Engl J Med* 1949;241:951.
18. Cohn K, Gottesman L, Brennan M. Adrenocortical carcinoma. *Surgery* 1986;100:1170.
19. Conn JW, Knopf RF, Nesbit RM. Clinical characteristics of primary aldosteronism from an analysis of 145 cases. *Am J Surg* 1964;107:159.
20. Copeland PM. The incidentally discovered adrenal mass. *Ann Surg* 1984;199:116.
21. Cullen ML, Staren ED, Straus AK, et al. Pheochromocytoma: operative strategy. *Surgery* 1985;98:927.
22. Daitch JA, Goldfarb DA, Novick AC. Cleveland Clinic experience with adrenal Cushing's syndrome. *J Urol* 1997;158:2051.
23. Davies CJ, Joplin GF, Welbourn RB. Surgical management of the ectopic ACTH syndrome. *Ann Surg* 1982;196:246.
24. Deming QB, Leutscher AJ Jr. Bioassay of desoxycorticosterone-like material in urine. *Proc Soc Exp Biol* 1950;73:171.
25. Doppman JL, Gill I Jr, Miller DL, et al. Distinction between hyperaldosteronism due to bilateral hyperplasia and unilateral aldosteronoma: reliability of CT. *Radiology* 1992;18:677.
26. Duncan MW, Compton P, Lazarus L, et al. Measurement of norepinephrine and 3,4 dihydroxyphenylglycol in urine and plasma for the diagnosis of pheochromocytoma. *N Engl J Med* 1988;319:136.
27. Fernandez-Cruz L, Saenz A, Benarroch G, et al. Laparoscopic unilateral and bilateral adrenalectomy for Cushing's syndrome: transperitoneal and retroperitoneal approaches. *Ann Surg* 1996; 224:727.
28. Fernandez-Cruz L, Taura P, Saenz A, et al. Laparoscopic approach to pheochromocytoma: hemodynamic changes and catecholamine secretion. *World J Sur* 1996;20:762.
29. Franks RC. Urinary 17-hydroxycorticosteroid and cortisol excretion in childhood. *J Clin Endocrinol Metab* 1973;36:702.
30. Funder JW. Mineralocorticoid, glucocorticoids, receptors and response elements. *Science* 1993;259:1132.
31. Gagner M, Lacroix A, Bolte E. Laparoscopic adrenalectomy in Cushing's syndrome and pheochromocytoma [Letter]. *N Engl J Med* 1992;327:1033.
32. Geelhoed GW, Druy EM. Management of adrenal "incidentaloma." *Surgery* 1982;92:866.
33. Geisinger MA, Zelch MG, Bravo EL, et al. Primary hyperaldosteronism: comparison of CT, adrenal venography and venous sampling. *AJR Am J Roentgenol* 1983;141:299.
34. Gill IS, Hobart MG, Schweizer D, et al. Outpatient adrenalectomy. *J Urol* 2000;163:717.
35. Gill IS, Schweizer D, Nelson D, et al. Laparoscopic vs open adrenalectomy: Cleveland Clinic experience with 210 cases. *J Urol* 1999;161:21.
36. Gill IS, Soble JJ, Sung GT, et al. Needlescopic adrenalectomy—the initial series: comparison with conventional adrenalectomy. *Urology* 1998;52:180.
37. Glazer GM, Francis IR, Quint LE. Imaging of the adrenal glands. *Invest Radiol* 1988;23:3.
38. Go H, Takeda M, Imai T, et al. Laparoscopic adrenalectomy for Cushing's syndrome: comparison with primary aldosteronism. *Surgery* 1995;117:11.
39. Gruhn JG, Could VE. The adrenal glands. In: Kissane JM, ed. *Anderson's pathology,* ed 9, St. Louis: Mosby, 1990:1580.
40. Guz B, Straffon R, Novick AC. Operative approaches to the adrenal gland. *Urol Clin North Am* 1989;16:527.
41. Hermus AR, Pieters GF, Smals AG. Transition from pituitary dependent to adrenal dependent Cushing's syndrome. *N Engl J Med* 1988;318:966.
42. Herra MF, Grant CS, Van Heerden JA, et al. Incidentally discovered adrenal tumors: an institutional perspective. *Surgery* 1991;110:1014.
43. Hobart MG, Gill IS, Schweizer D, et al. Financial analysis of needlescopic versus open adrenalectomy. *J Urol* 1999;162:1264.
44. Reference deleted in proofs.
45. Hutter AM. Adrenal cortical carcinoma: clinical features of 138 patients. *Am J Med* 1966;41:572.
46. Irvin GL, Fishman LM, Sher JA. Pheochromocytoma: lateral versus anterior operative approach. *Am Surg* 1989;209:774.
47. Janetschek G, Finkenstedt G, Gasser R, et al. Laparoscopic surgery for pheochromocytoma: adrenalectomy, partial resection, excision of paragangliomas. *J Urol* 1998;160:330.
48. Junqueira LC, Carneiro J. Adrenal islets of Langerhans, thyroid, parathyroids, and pineal body. In: *Basic histology,* ed 4, Los Altos, CA: Lange Medical Publishers, 1984:428.
49. Kenney PJ, Robbins GL, Ellis DA, et al. Adrenal glands in patients with congenital renal anomalies: CT appearance. *Radiology* 1985;155:181.
50. Kirschner MA, Zucker IR, Jespersen D. Idiopathic hirsutism—an ovarian abnormality. *N Engl J Med* 1976;294:637.
51. Kloos RT, Korobkin M, Thompson NW, et al. Incidentally discovered adrenal masses. In: Arnold A, ed. *Endocrine neoplasms.* Boston: Kluwer Academic Publishers, 1997:63.
52. Kobayashi S, Seki T, Nonomura K, et al. Clinical experience of incidentally discovered adrenal tumor with particular reference to cortical function. *J Urol* 1993;150:8.
53. Korobkin M, Brodeur FJ, Yutzy GG, et al. Differentiation of adrenal adenomas from nonadenomas using CT attenuation values. *AJR Am J Roentgenol* 1996;166:531.
54. Kuttenn F, Couillin P, Girard F, et al. Late-onset adrenal hyperplasia in hirsutism. *N Engl J Med* 1985;313:224.
55. Lanzi R, Montorsi F, Losa M, et al. Laparoscopic bilateral adrenalectomy for persistent Cushing's disease after transsphenoidal surgery. *Surgery* 1998;123:144.
56. Lim RC, Nakayama DK, Biglieri EG, et al. Primary aldosteronism: changing concepts in diagnosis and management. *Am J Surg* 1986;152:116.
57. Linos DA, Stylopoulos N. How accurate is computed tomography in predicting the real size of adrenal tumors? A retrospective study. *Arch Surg* 1997;132:740.
58. Linton EA, McLean C, Kruseman CAN. Direct measurement of human plasma corticotropin-releasing hormone by "two-site" immunoradiometric assay. *J Clin Endocrinol Metab* 1987;64: 1047.
59. Ludecke DK, Niedworok G. Results of microsurgery in Cushing's disease and effect on hypertension. *Cardiology* 1985;72:91.
60. Lumpkin MD. The regulation of ACTH secretion by IL-1. *Science* 1987;238:452.
61. Luton JP, Cerdas S, Billaud L, et al. Clinical features of adrenocortical carcinoma, prognostic factors, and the effect of mitotane therapy. *N Engl J Med* 1990;3221:1195.
62. Mayo-Smith WW, Lee MJ, McNicholas MM, et al. Characterization of adrenal masses (<5 cm) by use of chemical shift MR imaging. Observer performance vs quantitative measures. *AJR Am J Roentgenol* 1995;165:91.
63. Muller SC, Schreyer T, Rumpelt HJ. Myelolipoma of the adrenal gland. *Urol Int* 1985;40:132.

64. Neumann HPH, Berger DP, Sigmund G, et al. Pheochromocytoma, multiple endocrine neoplasia type 2, and von Hippel-Lindau disease. *N Engl J Med* 1993;329:1531.
65. Neville AM, O'Hare MJ. Aspects of structure, function, and pathology. In: James VAT, ed. *The adrenal gland,* New York: Raven Press, 1979.
66. Novick AC. Operations upon the adrenal gland. In Novick AC, Streem SB, Pontes JE, eds. *Stewart's operative urology,* Baltimore, Williams & Wilkins, 1989:65–95.
67. Novick AC. Adrenal surgery. In: Novick AC, ed. *Stewart's operative urology,* 2nd ed, Baltimore: Williams & Wilkins, 1989.
68. Oldfield EH, Doppman JL, Nieman LK, et al. Petrosal sinus sampling with and without corticotropin-releasing hormone for the differential diagnosis of Cushing's syndrome. *N Engl J Med* 1991;325:897.
69. Orth DN. Cushing's syndrome. *N Engl J Med* 1995;332:791.
70. Plouin PF, Degoulet P, Tugaye A, et al. Le depistage du pheochromocytoma: chez quels hypertendus? Etude semiologique chez 2585 hypertendus don't 11 ayant un pheochromocytome. *Nouv Presse Med* 1981;10:869.
71. Prinz RA, Brooks MH, Churchill R, et al. Incidental asymptomatic adrenal masses detected by computed tomographic scanning: is operation required? *JAMA* 1982;248:701.
72. Ratcliffe JG, Knight RA, Besser GM, et al. Tumor and plasma ACTH concentration in patients with and without the ectopic ACTH syndrome. *Clin Endocrinol* 1972;1:27.
73. Reincke M, Nieke J, Krestin G, et al. Preclinical Cushing's syndrome in adrenal "incidentalomas": comparison with adrenal Cushing's syndrome. *J Clin Endocrinol Metab* 1992;75:826.
74. Ritchey ML, Kinard R, Novick DE. Adrenal tumors: involvement of the inferior vena cava. *J Urol* 1987;138:1134.
75. Scott HW Jr, Abumrad NN, Orth DN. Tumors of the adrenal cortex and Cushing's syndrome. *Ann Surg* 1985;201:586.
76. Seddon JM, Baranetsky N, Boxel PJV. Adrenal "incidentalomas." Need for surgery. *Urology* 1985;25:1.
77. Shapiro B, Sisson JC, Eyre P, et al. ^{131}I-MIBG-new agent in diagnosis and treatment of pheochromocytoma. *Cardiology* 1985;72(1):137.
78. Shirkhoda A. Computed tomography after adrenalectomy in adrenal cortical carcinoma. *Urol Radiol* 1985;7:132.
79. Sisson JC, Frager MS, Valk TW, et al. Scintigraphic localization of pheochromocytoma. *N Engl J Med* 1981;305:12.
80. Sobol H, Naroo SA, Nakamura Y. Screening for multiple endocrine neoplasia type 2a with DNA-polymorphism analysis. *N Engl J Med* 1989;301:996.
81. Styne DM, Grumbach MM, Kaplan SL, et al. Treatment of Cushing's disease in childhood and adolescence by transsphenoidal microadenomectomy. *N Engl J Med* 1984;310:889.
82. Taylor AL, Fishman LM. Corticotropin-releasing hormone. *N Engl J Med* 1988;319:213.
83. Tucker WS, Snell BB, Island DP, et al. Reversible adrenal insufficiency induced by ketoconazole. *JAMA* 1985;253:2413.
84. Ulchaker JC, Goldfarb DA, Bravo EL, et al. Successful outcomes in pheochromocytoma surgery in the modern era. *J Urol* 1999; 161:764.
85. Vetter H, Fischer M, Galanski M, et al: Primary aldosteronism: diagnosis and noninvasive lateralization procedures. *Cardiology* 1985;71:57.
86. Weiss LM. Comparative histologic study of 43 metastasizing and nonmetastasizing adrenocortical tumors. *Am J Surg Pathol* 1984; 8:163.
87. Wilson JD, Foster DW. *Williams textbook of endocrinology,* ed 7, Philadelphia: WB Saunders, 1985.
88. Winfield HN, Hamilton BD, Bravo EL, et al. Laparoscopic adrenalectomy: the preferred choice? A comparison to open adrenalectomy. *J Urol* 1998;160:325.
89. Young HH. A technique for simultaneous exposure and operation on the adrenals. *Surg Gynecol Obstet* 1936;54:179.
90. Young WF Jr, Hogan MJ, Klee GG, et al. Primary aldosteronism: diagnosis and treatment. *Mayo Clin Proc* 1990;65:96.

14

THE KIDNEY

W. SCOTT McDOUGAL

RENAL ANATOMY

The renal parenchyma is divided into an outer cortical zone and an inner medullary area. The medulla is subdivided into inner and outer portions, the former containing the 4 to 12 renal papillae. Each papilla is surrounded by transitional cell epithelium, the complex referred to as a *calyx.* It drains into an infundibulum, and the infundibula join one to another and then to the renal pelvis. A detailed knowledge of the calyceal anatomy is important, because endoscopic location of lesions within the kidney requires the ability to identify, on the two-dimensional roentgenogram, the location of the calyx in which the lesion is present and to correlate it with the gross anatomy of the kidney when visualizing the infundibula from the renal pelvis. The calyces located in the upper and lower poles often are compound and project directly to their respective poles. The remainder are arranged into an anterior and posterior row (Fig. 14.1). The anterior row of calyces forms an angle 70 degrees to the frontal plane; these are the calyces visualized laterally on an anteroposterior (AP) view of an intravenous (IV) urogram. The posterior calyces form a 20-degree angle with the frontal plane and are those visualized medially on the urogram (Fig. 14.2).

Segments of the cortex and medulla are served by end arteries, that is, arteries that do not anastomose with other arteries and therefore have little potential for the development of collateral vessels. The segments of the kidneys are the two polar, the anterosuperior, the anteroinferior, and the posterior (Fig. 14.3). The first main branch off the renal artery serving the renal parenchyma supplies the posterior segment. Thus location of this artery allows for identification of the subsegmental anatomy of the kidney. It allows identification of the avascular plane, adjacent to

W.S. McDougal: Department of Urology, Harvard Medical School; Massachusetts General Hospital, Boston, MA 02111.

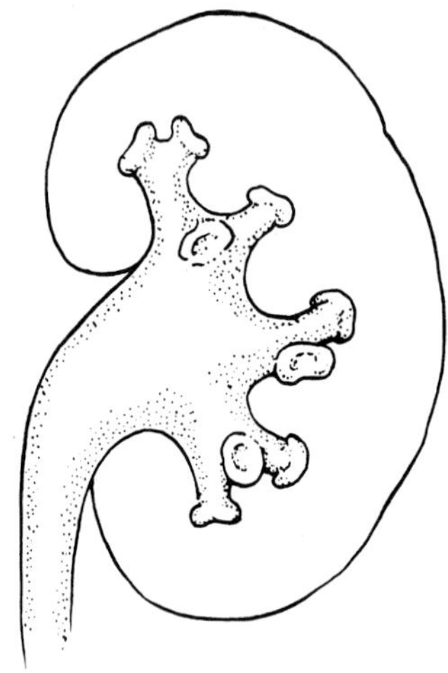

FIGURE 14.1. Calyceal anatomy. The polar calyces project to their respective poles while the middle calyces form an anterior and posterior row.

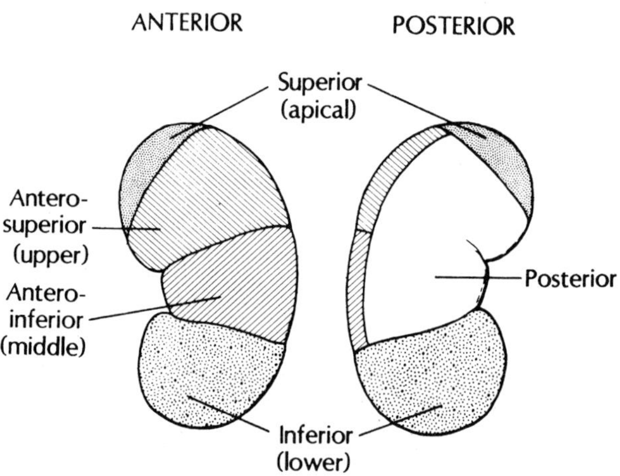

FIGURE 14.3. Segmental anatomy of the kidney. There are five segments: superior, inferior, posterior, anterosuperior, and anteroinferior.

Brödel's line between the anterior and posterior segments, along which the kidney may be split and calyces entered through the parenchyma without violation of the blood supply to segments of the parenchyma (Fig. 14.2). The arteries branch from the main renal artery into, successively, the interlobar; arcuate; interlobular; and afferent, glomerular, and efferent arterioles. The efferent arterioles supply the proximal tubule from the glomerulus in the cortex from which it arose, and supply the proximal tubule and Henle's loop when it arises from a juxtamedullary glomerulus. The venous drainage follows the arterial supply; however, unlike the arteries, veins intercommunicate between the segments.

There are two types of lymphatic networks in the kidney: a superficial system that drains the capsule and a deeper system that drains from the hilum (5). Lymphatic vessels in the kidney follow the arterial vessels from interlobular arteries proximally. The exact course of the lymphatic vessels distal to the interlobular arteries is not known. It has been suggested that the medulla contains few if any lymphatic vessels, whereas the cortex may be drained by regional areas from lymphatic vessels that actually do not penetrate deeply into the parenchyma (59). The renal capsule is supplied richly by lymphatic vessels. Capsule lymphatic vessels and parenchyma lymphatic vessels drain to the renal hilum and from there to the great vessel closest to the respective kidney.

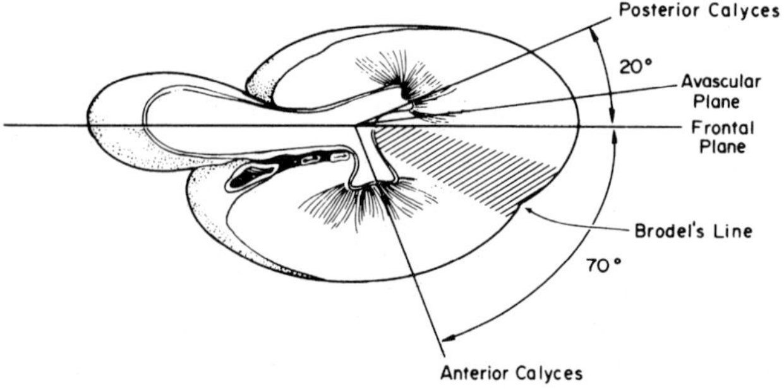

FIGURE 14.2. Location of anterior and posterior calyces. Notice that the anterior calyces form a 70-degree angle with the frontal plane and the posterior calyces a 20-degree angle with that plane. The avascular plane adjacent to Brödel's line, through which the calyces may be entered without violating segmental vasculature, is depicted.

The kidneys are supplied by sympathetic nerves from T4 to L4, which course to the celiac, superior, and inferior mesenteric and aorticorenal ganglia. The postganglionic fibers course to the renal hilum and then to the renal parenchyma. Once in the renal parenchyma, they travel with the vessels, eventually making contact with the juxtaglomerular apparatus and the basement membranes of the proximal and distal tubule cells. Innervation of the glomerulus is controversial. Stimulation of these nerves causes vasoconstriction and a short-term reduction in renal blood flow (RBF). Denervation of the kidney results in an increase in electrolyte excretion primarily caused by a diminished proximal tubule fractional reabsorption.

The hilum of the kidney contains the renal vessels, renal nerves, lymphatic vessels, lymph node tissue, and renal pelvis. The renal capsule extends to the renal sinus and incorporates it into the kidney proper.

There are two types of nephrons: cortical nephrons with short Henle's loops and juxtamedullary nephrons with long Henle's loops (Fig. 14.4). There are approximately 2 million nephrons per kidney, seven-eighths of which are cortical and one-eighth juxtamedullary. The arterial supply to the cortical nephrons differs from that of the juxtamedullary nephrons. In the former, the efferent arteriole courses along the proximal tubule belonging to the glomerulus from

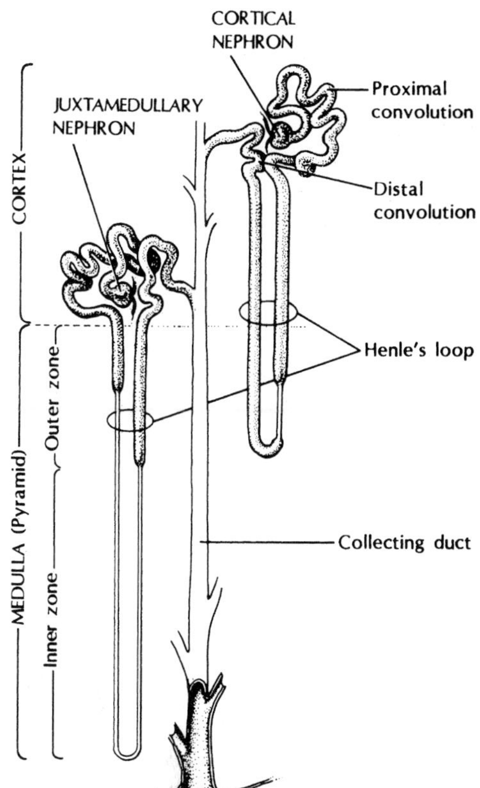

FIGURE 14.4. The renal parenchyma is divided into cortex and medulla and contains two types of nephrons: cortical and juxtamedullary.

which it came. This allows that arteriole to reabsorb filtrate that it left behind in the glomerulus. Because these nephrons have short Henle's loops, they play a lesser role in maximum urinary concentration than do the juxtamedullary nephrons with long Henle's loops. The efferent arterioles from the juxtamedullary nephrons course not only along the proximal tubule from the respective glomerulus but also dive deep into the medulla, coursing along their respective Henle's loops. The vessels that follow Henle's loops are called *vasa recta.*

The components of the nephron include the glomerulus, the proximal tubule, Henle's loop, the distal tubule, and the collecting duct. The glomerulus consists of an afferent arteriole, capillary and efferent arterioles, a juxtaglomerular apparatus, and Bowman's space and capsule (Fig. 14.5). The afferent arteriole, and to a lesser extent the efferent arteriole, are in intimate contact with the first portion of the distal tubule belonging to that glomerulus. This association is called the *juxtaglomerular apparatus* and consists of two parts: the macula densa, or the dark cells of the distal tubule, and the juxtaglomerular cells, or the endothelial cells of the afferent and efferent arterioles that contain renin granules. It has been postulated that this structure is responsible for the regulation of sodium conservation through the stimulation of aldosterone production and that it acts as a feedback mechanism for the intrarenal regulation of each nephron's blood flow and therefore glomerular filtration rate (GFR) (see the following discussion).

The glomerular capillary network is the area through which plasma is filtered. The capillaries contain an endothelium, which lies on a basement membrane. On the other side of the basement membrane is Bowman's space. It is on this side of the basement membrane that the epithelial cells, or foot processes (podocytes), are found (Fig. 14.6A). Finally, mesangial cells that support the structures of the glomerulus are found within the glomerular tuft. These cells may play a role in causing arteriole constriction and in providing support for the aforementioned structures. Bowman's space empties into the convoluted proximal tubule. The cells of this portion of the nephron have a dense brush border on the luminal side (Fig. 14.6B) and are attached to each other by impermeable tight junctions. At the end of the proximal tubule, the nephron dives toward the medulla, where it attaches to the thin limb of Henle's loop. This portion of the proximal tubule is called the *pars recta.* Its brush border is less dense, and this area perhaps is less active in filtrate reabsorption than the other portion of the proximal tubule. The thin limb of Henle's loop descends and then turns back on itself and ascends toward its respective glomerulus. As it ascends, it changes to the thick limb of Henle's loop, which has notably different permeability and transport characteristics than the thin limb. The thick limb joins the first portion of the distal tubule whose cells are called the *macula densa*—a component of the juxtaglomerular apparatus. The distal convoluted tubule joins with many others to enter a collecting duct. The collecting duct traverses the parenchyma to the renal papilla (59).

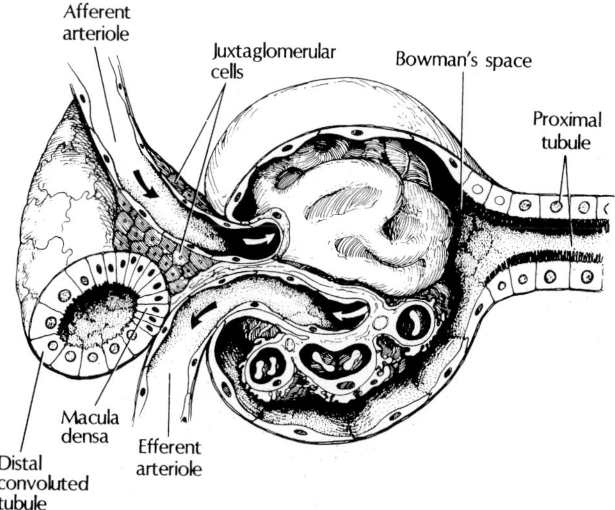

FIGURE 14.5. Glomerulus and juxtaglomerular apparatus.

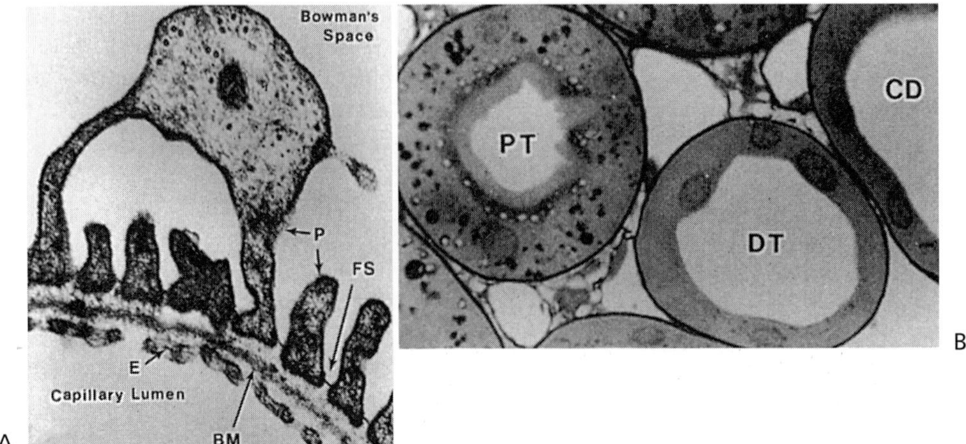

FIGURE 14.6. **A:** Electron photomicrograph of the glomerulus. BM, basement membrane; E, endothelial cell; FS, filtration slit; P, podocyte. **B:** Light photomicrograph of renal tubules. CD, collecting duct; DT, distal tubule; PT, proximal tubule (notice dense brush border). Notice the dense staining basement membrane surrounding each tubule.

RENAL PHYSIOLOGY

Glomerular Filtration

Plasma, water, and nonprotein crystalloids are separated from blood cells and protein within the glomerulus by a process called *ultrafiltration* (43). Nonchanged molecules with a molecular radius less than 20 Å are freely filtered (60). The forces involved in ultrafiltration are the hydrostatic pressure within the glomerular capillary, the permeability of the glomerular membrane called *hydraulic permeability,* the oncotic pressure of the plasma, and the hydrostatic pressure in Bowman's space. The hydrostatic pressure in the glomerular capillary remains relatively constant throughout its length, whereas the oncotic pressure rises along the course of the capillary as filtrate leaves. The net filtration pressure is the hydrostatic pressure minus the oncotic pressure minus the pressure in Bowman's space. Net filtration is determined by this pressure and the hydraulic permeability of the glomerular membrane. As blood courses along the length of the capillary, the net ultrafiltration pressure declines because oncotic pressure rises as a result of the increased protein concentration as fluid is removed from the capillary lumen (Fig. 14.7). This serves to keep the amount of filtrate constant despite capillary length and thus prevents loss of excessive fluid into Bowman's space. The permeability of the membrane is a function of the permeability of its component parts: the endothelium, the basement membrane, and the epithelial cells (podocytes or foot processes). The basement membrane and filtration slits account for 98% of the resistance, with the endothelium accounting for only 2% of the resistance (18). The podocytes are separated by filtration slits that contain pores having dimensions of 40 to 140 Å. Negatively charged glycoproteins are attached to the surfaces of the endothelial cells, basement membrane, and podocytes. Thus the membrane acts as a barrier by discriminating according to both the molecule's size and its electric charge (an electrostatic barrier).

The glomerular mesangium and renal vasculature are sensitive to a number of endogenous hormones. Angiotensin II, norepinephrine, the leukotrienes, platelet activating factor, adenosine triphosphate (ATP), endothelin, vasopressin, serotonin, and epidermal growth factor all may cause vasoconstriction.

The measurement of the quantity of plasma filtered by the glomeruli can be determined by a clearance technique. A clearance is defined as the volume of plasma from which the kidney removes a substance per unit of time. To measure the amount of fluid arriving in Bowman's space or the GFR, a substance is chosen that is freely filtered at the glomerulus

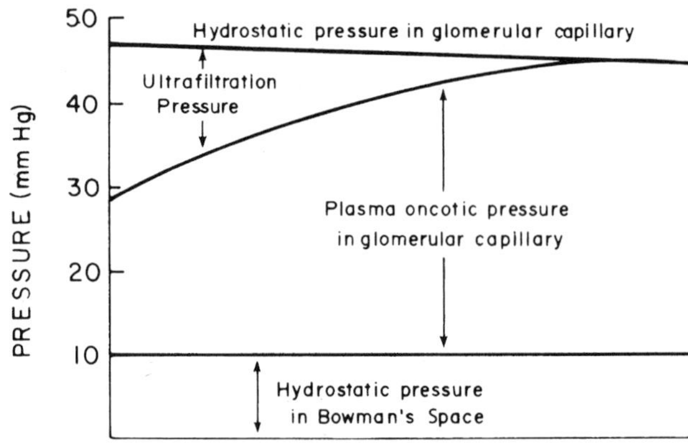

FIGURE 14.7. Forces of glomerular ultrafiltration. As fluid traverses the capillary and as some is filtered into Bowman's space, oncotic pressure within the capillary increases until it completely counteracts the hydrostatic pressure gradient. This limits the amount of fluid filtered into the proximal tubule.

but is neither secreted nor reabsorbed by the tubule. Inulin, a starchlike polymer of fructose with a molecular weight of approximately 5,000, is such a substance, the standard against which other substances used to measure GFR are compared. Inulin clearance is independent of serum concentration and urine flow. The clearance is calculated from the following formula:

$$\frac{UV}{P}$$

where *U* is the urine concentration, *V* is the urine volume per unit of time, and *P* is the plasma concentration.

The amount of filtrate removed from the plasma remains relatively constant as a result of the forces previously described. The fraction of fluid in the glomerular capillary bed entering Bowman's space is called the *filtration fraction* and is approximately 20%; that is, 20% of the plasma arriving in the glomerulus leaves as filtrate into Bowman's space.

Tubule Reabsorption

Reabsorption by the tubule epithelium of substances essential to normal body function, such as water, sugars, amino acids, and electrolytes, is critical for homeostasis. Reabsorption of a substance may be determined by comparing its clearance with that of inulin: if the clearance of the filtered substance is less than that of inulin, it must be reabsorbed. Many substances that are reabsorbed are actively transported, thus having the potential to saturate the carrier mechanism, at which time a transport maximum (T_m) is achieved. T_m is the maximum amount of substance that can be actively transported when all carriers are saturated. Glucose, other sugars, sulfate, amino acids, phosphate, uric acid, and albumin have a T_m. The transport of a number of compounds can be facilitated by sodium transport. Glucose, uric acid, amino acids, and phosphate movement are enhanced in the presence of sodium, a process called *cotransport.*

Not all substances are reabsorbed by an active process. Passive reabsorption accounts for urea movement across the tubule. This type of transport is strongly affected by urine flow. At low flow rates, reabsorption of urea is increased, and at high flow rates urea is flushed from the tubule, thereby lessening its absorption. The flow of urea after filtration is not unidirectional. In certain portions of the tubule, urea is reabsorbed and in others it is secreted. Potassium and weak acids and bases (including drugs) also are secreted and reabsorbed in different portions of the nephron. The process is called *bidirectional transport.*

Tubule Secretion

Substances secreted are usually either weak acids or weak bases; they are foreign to the body and are either not metabolized or are metabolized slowly or incompletely. Secretion is confirmed when a filtered substance's clearance exceeds that of the inulin clearance. Examples of substances secreted include drugs (e.g., diuretics, antibiotics, salicylates), *para*-aminohippuric acid (PAH), and thiamine.

Renal Hemodynamics

Approximately 20% to 25% of the cardiac output flows to the kidneys, more than 90% of which perfuses the cortical region. Even though the medullary region gets only a small fraction of the total RBF, in absolute amounts it is perfused with approximately the same amount of blood as is resting muscle. The blood flow is sensitive to hemorrhage, the cortex being primarily affected. Antidiuretic hormone (ADH), the prostaglandins, renin, and sympathetic nerve stimulation affect RBF. ADH causes vasoconstriction and therefore prevents washout of osmotically active particles from the medulla. Prostaglandins are both vasodilatory and vasoconstrictive. Their vasodilatory action exerts a protective role in diseases causing vasoconstriction (20). Thromboxane, a potent prostaglandin vasoconstrictor, may play a role in altering RBF during obstructive uropathy (49). Others are not convinced that it alters renal hemodynamics. Renin, through the release of angiotensin, also causes vasoconstriction, and its release may be stimulated by an alteration of distal tubule sodium concentration, sympathetic nerve stimulation, and changes in intrarenal blood pressure. Angiotensin II exerts constrictive effects on both afferent and efferent arterioles, with an increased effect on the efferent arteriole. The subtype angiotensin II-2 receptor has been shown to have vasodilatory effects in selected circumstances. Angiotensin receptors also are located on mesangial cells, resulting in changes in glomerular surface area (12).

The renin-angiotensin system has been implicated in distribution of RBF; in regulation of GFR through its effects on afferent and efferent arterioles, on filtration coefficient, and on mesangial contraction; in sodium reabsorption by proximal and distal tubules; in renal concentrating mechanism; in potentiation of renal sympathetic activity; in interaction with prostaglandins; and as a renal growth factor (33). Stimulation of the sympathetic nerves supplying the kidney, through their innervation of the arterioles, causes vasoconstriction by stimulating contraction of endothelial muscle cells.

Finally, endothelin and endothelin-derived relaxing factor play a role in vasoconstriction and relaxation of the renal microcirculation. Under most conditions RBF remains relatively constant by a phenomenon known as *autoregulation.* Over a range of systolic blood pressures from 80 to 180 mm Hg, RBF and GFR remain constant. It has been suggested that the renin-angiotensin system, prostaglandins, the catecholamines, kinins, leukotrienes, ATP, serotonin, epidermal growth factor, platelet activating factor, and other substances regulate RBF by altering vascular resistance in the afferent and efferent arterioles by a complex set of interactions. Through this combined effect, intraglomerular hydrostatic pressure is maintained relatively constant over wide variations in systemic pressure.

RBF usually is measured by a clearance technique (see the following). PAH is used, because it is filtered and secreted by the kidney. Thus the amount of plasma that delivers the amount of PAH found in the urine per unit of time is the amount of plasma that passed through the kidney, or the *renal plasma flow* (RPF). The calculation is simple. However, from a practical point of view its determination is difficult, because both the renal vein and renal artery concentrations must be known to calculate the amount of plasma delivered to the kidney because the arteriovenous difference is the amount removed in one pass. The renal artery concentration is easily determined from a peripheral venous sample; however, an invasive technique must be used whereby a catheter is passed to sample the renal vein directly. This difficulty can be obviated if the renal vein concentration approaches zero. If the PAH concentration is kept low enough in the systemic circulation, essentially all PAH entering the renal artery is cleared in one pass. Thus the calculation simplifies to a clearance as follows: UV/P of PAH. Because approximately 10% of the arterial concentration remains in the renal vein at low systemic PAH concentrations and because this may vary by as much as 20% under differing experimental conditions, the calculation of RPF determined without actual measurement of renal venous concentration is termed *effective renal plasma flow* to indicate that it is not actual RPF but rather an approximation thereof, because renal vein concentration is assumed to be zero, which actually may not be the case. If the renal vein concentration were known, then actual RPF could be calculated by the clearance technique previously described. RBF may be calculated by dividing the plasma flow by the following quantity: (1 – hematocrit).

Sodium and Water Balance

Sodium is actively transported from the luminal contents to the interstitium. The bulk of energy expended by the kidney is involved in this active process. In the proximal tubule, approximately 60% to 70% of the filtered sodium and fluid is reabsorbed. Because water follows sodium passively and because the proximal tubule is freely permeable to water, the fluid in this portion of the tubule is reabsorbed isosmotically. A constant fraction of the filtered sodium is reabsorbed in the proximal tubule (i.e., glomerulotubular balance), normally approximately 70% despite variations in the GFR.

Glomerulotubular balance appears to be brought about by two processes. The first involves changes in filtration fraction, perhaps brought about by nervous or humoral factors. The second involves the process of cotransport. Because sodium reabsorption is linked to the reabsorption of various substances that are almost completely reabsorbed by the proximal tubule (e.g., glucose), when increases in the filtered load of the substance occur, an increase in sodium reabsorption is stimulated and vice versa.

In the thin limb of Henle's loop, water moves according to its concentration gradient. Thus in the proximal portion, water moves out, whereas in the distal portion it moves back in. Sodium follows passively. In the thick ascending limb, sodium and chloride are actively pumped from the lumen; however, this portion is impermeable to water, and thus the fluid becomes hypotonic. In the distal tubule, sodium is actively removed under the influence of aldosterone. Water moves according to the movement of sodium and its concentration gradient. In the collecting duct, sodium is reabsorbed, and water movement (collecting duct permeability to water) is influenced by the concentration of ADH.

Mechanisms responsible for sodium balance may be classified into three groups. The first factor responsible for sodium homeostasis is GFR, which alters sodium reabsorption through the mechanism of glomerular tubule balance. Occasionally, glomerular tubular balance may be disrupted under circumstances of excessive sodium loads.

The second group of factors include angiotensin and aldosterone. Angiotensin II exerts potent effects on sodium and bicarbonate transport in the proximal tubule (12). Aldosterone is released either as a direct action of hyperkalemia or angiotensin II on the adrenal gland or as a result of the release of renin or adrenocorticotropic hormone (ACTH) (23). Renin is released from the juxtaglomerular cells as either a consequence of a low afferent arteriolar pressure (secondary to hypotension) or decreased distal tubule sodium concentration. Stimulation of the sympathetic nervous system, various prostaglandins, and calcium channel blockers also stimulate renin production. Angiotensin II, vasopressin, endothelin, and adenosine inhibit renin release. Renin is produced in an inactive form and is activated by a serum proteinase. Activated renin acts on a protein substrate to cleave a decapeptide, angiotensin I. Angiotensin I is converted by a converting enzyme to a vasoactive octapeptide, angiotensin II (Fig. 14.8). Angiotensin II results in vasoconstriction and stimulation of the adrenal gland to release aldosterone (33).

Factors in the third group are nervous and/or humoral influences, which alter sodium transport. They are not well-defined; however, their effects are known. For example, volume expansion with sodium results in natriuresis that is caused by a decreased fractional reabsorption in the proximal tubule from 70% to 40% and a decreased sodium reabsorption in the distal tubule. This is not dependent on factors in either group one or two. A substance that may be responsible for some of these effects is *atrial natriuretic factor,* a 28–amino acid polypeptide that has been identified in the atrium. The 28–amino acid residue is the circulating form that is derived from a 126-residue precursor—the principal storage form. It has potent diuretic, natriuretic, and vasorelaxant properties. It also inhibits the release of ADH. The atria are the only established source of atrial

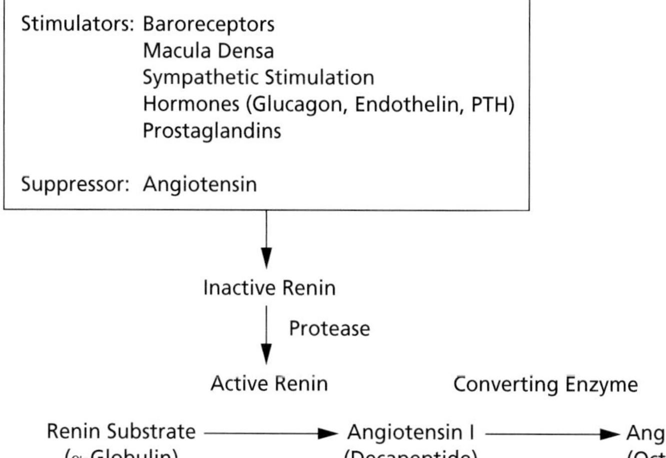

FIGURE 14.8. The renin-angiotensin system. PTH, parathyroid hormone.

natriuretic factor. Its release is stimulated by stretch of the atrium, volume expansion, sodium concentration, osmolality, and certain vasopressor agents (69). Finally, prostaglandins play a minor role in the modulation of sodium and water excretion. Prostaglandins synthesized in the renal medulla act locally to enhance water and sodium excretion by (a) increasing RBF, (b) inhibiting sodium transport from the thick ascending limb of Henle's loop, (c) antagonizing the action of vasopressin on the collecting duct, and (d) inhibiting urea and sodium reabsorption from the collecting duct (19).

Concentration and Dilution

The ascending limb of Henle's loop is impermeable to water, and because sodium and chloride are actively reabsorbed, electrolyte transport occurs without water following. This establishes a hyperosmotic medullary interstitium, which is the primary determinant of the kidney's ability to concentrate. Henle's loop acts as a countercurrent multiplier increasing the concentration of solutes, whereas the vasa recta coursing along with Henle's loop preserve medullary tonicity by serving as countercurrent exchangers. This is particularly important, because plasma flow to the medulla is approximately ten times greater than tubule fluid flow. This unique relationship preserves medullary tonicity and thus concentration capabilities.

Urea recycling helps maintain osmolality in the medulla, both in the medullary interstitium and the tubule lumen. Urea concentration in Henle's loop increases as water leaves. Under the influence of ADH, urea reabsorption in the collecting duct is facilitated as water is reabsorbed. This maintains a high medullary tonicity. Thus during antidiuresis, urea provides 40% of the medullary osmotically active particles, whereas in diuretic states urea constitutes only 10% of the medullary solutes.

ADH adjusts the amount of water that is reabsorbed from the late distal tubule and collecting ducts. ADH increases tubule permeability, thus allowing water to travel according to its concentration gradient. In the collecting duct, where medullary tonicity is high, water is reabsorbed. ADH also causes vasoconstriction of the vasa recta, preventing the removal of solute from the medulla, thereby maintaining a high medullary tonicity. Prostaglandins also may play a role in this regulation by opposing the action of ADH. ADH is released as a result of stimuli from volume receptors or osmoreceptors. Osmoreceptors located in the hypothalamus, when exposed to increased osmolality, stimulate the posterior pituitary to release ADH. Similarly, volume receptors located in the left atrium or pulmonary veins also result in the release of ADH.

Acid–Base Balance

The daily production of 40 to 70 mmol of inorganic and organic acids (i.e., the fixed acids) and 13,000 mmol of carbon dioxide (CO_2), which momentarily generates hydrogen (the volatile acid), requires elimination by the body. This acid load requires buffering so that major pH shifts do not occur locally. The buffers include hemoglobin, protein, inorganic phosphate, organic phosphate, and bicarbonate. Organic phosphate is the major intracellular buffer, whereas the main extracellular buffer is the carbonic acid bicarbonate system. The latter is particularly effective, because the concentration of one component of the pair, CO_2 can be altered rapidly by the lungs.

Perhaps one of the most effective initial methods of buffering the volatile acid load is the reaction hydrogen has with hemoglobin. Oxygenated hemoglobin is more acidic than nonoxygenated hemoglobin. Thus when hemoglobin gives up its oxygen, it can take up a great deal of hydrogen without any overall change in local pH. CO_2 arising from metabolism is hydrated to carbonic acid and dissociates into hydrogen and bicarbonate. The hydrogen is taken up by hemoglobin, and the CO_2 travels to the lungs as bicarbonate. The reverse reaction occurs in the lungs where hydrogen is given up, CO_2 is eliminated, and hemoglobin is oxygenated. Fixed acids initially are buffered by bicarbonate, phosphate, and proteins, thus lessening their effect on systemic pH. In the process of buffering, fixed acids consume bicarbonate. The volatile acid is excreted by the lungs and the fixed acids by the kidney, thus restoring buffer capacity.

The kidney reclaims bicarbonate by two mechanisms. Filtered bicarbonate is reclaimed in the proximal tubule, where 80% to 90% of that which is filtered is reabsorbed. This process occurs by (a) the secretion of hydrogen ion by the proximal tubule cell, (b) the combination of the hydrogen with filtered bicarbonate to form carbonic acid, (c) the dehydration of carbonic acid to CO_2 and water within the tubule lumen, (d) the diffusion of CO_2 into the proximal tubule cell, (e) the formation of carbonic acid, and (f) the removal of hydrogen to be secreted into the lumen thereby, in effect, reabsorbing bicarbonate. Filtered bicarbonate is reclaimed in this manner; however, bicarbonate consumed in the process of buffering fixed acid is restored and the hydrogen eliminated by hydrogen secretion in the cortical collecting tubule. The hydrogen arises from carbonic acid and thus results in bicarbonate generation within the tubule cell. The bicarbonate stores are thus replenished. The hydrogen ion secreted in the cortical collecting tubule by the Na-H antiport is fixed to phosphate, creatinine, and urate. These act as buffers and are excreted as weak acids. Hydrogen excreted in this manner is called *titratable acid* and, as such, lowers urinary pH. Because an intraluminal hydrogen concentration cannot exceed a concentration difference of more than 1,000 : 1, any amount excreted in excess of this back-diffuses into serum. The kidney is therefore incapable of lowering urinary pH values to less than a pH of 4.4. This mechanism limits the amount of hydrogen ion capable of being secreted. Fortunately, the ammonium system allows for further elimination of hydrogen ion without the need to lower urinary pH.

Ammonia is generated from glutamine in the proximal tubule. Ammonia diffuses across the membrane into the tubule lumen, flows to the distal tubule/cortical collecting duct, and combines with a hydrogen ion to form ammonium. Ammonium may be secreted by a number of transporters, NH4/H exchange being one. The quantitative role of this mechanism is not firmly established. Ammonium is trapped and combines with an available anion—usually chloride, sulfate, or phosphate—to form a neutral salt. The neutral salts do not influence pH and are excreted as such. Distal hydrogen secretion is promoted by increasing the severity of the acidosis, the presence of aldosterone, depletion of potassium, and increased delivery of sodium to the distal nephron. Factors that alter bicarbonate reabsorption in the proximal tubule include the serum concentrations of CO_2, potassium, chloride, phosphate, calcium, and parathormone, and the volume status of the patient. Increased bicarbonate reabsorption occurs with elevated CO_2, decreased potassium, diminished chloride, and elevated phosphate and decreased volume. Increased parathormone, hyperkalemia, and reduced CO_2 decrease bicarbonate reabsorption.

The final regulation of urinary acid excretion occurs in the collecting duct. Collecting duct acid–base balance is regulated by systemic acid–base states, potassium balance, sodium reabsorption, mineralocorticoids, and other peptide hormones (27).

Potassium

Only approximately 10% to 20% of the filtered load of potassium is excreted. It is reabsorbed in the proximal tubule and also may be reabsorbed in the distal tubule and collecting duct under certain experimental conditions. It is secreted in the distal tubule, and it is by this mechanism that most potassium is excreted in the urine. The rate of secretion is influenced by the presence of mineralocorticoids, urine flow, acid–base balance, and sodium intake. Mineralocorticoids stimulate the secretion of potassium, mainly in the cortical collecting duct. Their presence results in sodium reabsorption, but there is not a 1 : 1 ratio of sodium for potassium. Alkalosis results in increased potassium secretion, whereas acidosis results in hydrogen secretion at the expense of potassium secretion. Potassium and hydrogen ion transport are linked in some manner explaining this phenomenon. An increased flow rate keeps the concentration gradient high between tubule cell and lumen and therefore promotes secretion. Sodium, by increasing flow rates in the distal tubule or by its effect on the sodium-potassium cellular exchange pump, also increases potassium secretion.

Calcium

The bulk of filtered calcium is reabsorbed in the proximal tubule. However, the remainder is reabsorbed in the thick ascending limb of Henle's loop and the distal tubule. Its reabsorption depends on phosphate, magnesium, and parathormone. Hypophosphatemia decreases calcium reabsorption as does an increase in magnesium concentration. Parathormone increases calcium reabsorption and reduces phosphate reabsorption. Parathormone also stimulates the kidney to produce 1,25-dihydroxyvitamin D_3, which increases gut absorption and bone reabsorption for calcium. Magnesium, calcium, and sodium may share some of the same carriers, because if there is an excess of one, others tend to be excreted; that is, the common pump is saturated by the ion in excess.

Magnesium

Magnesium is reabsorbed in the proximal tubule, thick ascending limb, and distal tubule. Increased sodium, calcium, and mineralocorticoid reduce reabsorption. Osmotic agents, renal vasodilation, glucose, and hyperthyroidism increase excretion (68).

DETERMINATION OF RENAL FUNCTION

Because of the complexity and wide range of functions the kidney performs, the assessment of renal function requires measurement of individual processes occurring in various portions of the nephron. It is not practical to measure each one; therefore, selected functions are determined and, unless otherwise indicated, it is assumed that these reflect the general function of the entire kidney. For convenience these studies are divided into five groups: (a) glomerular filtration, (b) RBF, (c) tubule electrolyte transport, (d) concentration and dilution, and (e) protein conservation.

Glomerular Filtration Rate

GFR is the amount of filtrate arriving in the proximal tubule per unit of time. It assesses the normalcy of RBF, glomerular integrity, and proximal tubule pressure. Its measurement is based on the concept of a clearance (see the following equation). The ideal substance for this measurement is freely filtered at the glomerulus and is not metabolized, secreted, or reabsorbed by the tubule. The material used to perform the clearance must be maintained at a constant concentration in the serum. For inulin this requires maintaining a constant IV infusion, because the substance is not endogenous to the body. Once a constant serum level is obtained, the amount of inulin excreted in the urine is measured per unit time (urine concentration, *U*, multiplied by the volume, *V*, of urine excreted: $U \times V$). To find the amount of serum from which this amount of inulin was extracted, the product is divided by the serum concentration, *P*. Thus $U \times V/P$ gives the amount of serum completely cleared of the substance per unit time or the GFR.

A normal GFR (measured by inulin clearance) for a young adult is 130 mL per minute for males and 120 mL per minute for females per 1.73 m^2 of body surface area. Exercise lowers GFR, whereas pregnancy may increase it by as much as 50%. Hydration, either extreme overhydration or dehydration, also may affect filtration rate. In children older than the age of 1 year, when the GFR is corrected to 1.73 m^2 of body surface area, it is the same amount as for adults. In children younger than the age of 1 year, it is less—only approximately 50% of the corrected adult value in the neonatal period. Similarly, the GFR falls with age, until by the age of 60 years it is only 60% to 80% of the young adult value.

Several formulas have been developed to assess GFR from the measurement of serum creatinine alone without the need for a urine collection (30). Perhaps the most widely used formula is the following:

$$\frac{(140 - \text{age}) \times \text{Body weight (kg)}}{72 \times \text{Cr}_s}$$

where Cr_s is the serum creatinine concentration.

This gives the GFR for males; for females the value is multiplied by 0.85. This formula is useful for calculating GFR when the need to adjust drug doses arises. It is reasonably accurate when the GFR exceeds 40 mL per minute. This formula is inaccurate in patients with spinal cord injury (muscle wasting), in those with bowel interpositions in the urinary tract, and in those in whom one of the interfering substances is present (see previous discussion). It must be remembered that serum creatinine concentrations vary with muscle mass (more muscular individuals have a higher serum creatinine level), daily protein consumption, and metabolic state of the patient (13,52). Alterations in serum creatinine are a less accurate method of determining renal function.

Because of the inaccuracies of creatinine, other substances and methods have been developed in an attempt to measure GFR accurately without the difficulties encountered with the inulin clearance. Vitamin B_{12}, edetate (EDTA), sodium iothalamate, and sodium diatrizoate have been shown to have clearance rates similar to inulin. However, they appear to have no advantages over endogenous creatinine clearances except in selected circumstances.

Radiopharmaceuticals have enjoyed popularity as a less cumbersome method of determining renal function. The radiopharmaceutical technetium, labeled *pentetic acid* [diethylenetriaminepentaacetic acid (DTPA)], is used for GFR measurements, and iodohippurate sodium ^{131}I (Hippuran) is used for RBF determination. Two methods are commonly used to determine GFR and RBF. The GFR or RBF can be calculated from an empiric formula that requires knowledge of the amount of isotope taken up by the kidneys over a 6-minute period (25). The second method involves injecting the isotope and withdrawing serial blood samples over several hours. The amount of isotope is determined in the blood samples, and a disappearance curve is plotted. GFR or RBF is calculated from the half-life of the disappearance curve (10). In patients with relatively normal renal function who are in good health, these methods correlate well with inulin clearances. However, they are inaccurate in patients with significant edema or ascites, in those with intestine interposed in the urinary tract, and in patients with poor renal function.

Renal Blood Flow

The kidneys receive approximately 20% of the cardiac output. Measurement of RBF allows an assessment of the vascular integrity of the kidney and, to a lesser extent, the viability of the renal parenchyma. A clearance technique or isotope washout method is usually employed. Clinically, the clearance method is most convenient, because it requires no special instrumentation and is based on the Fick principle. The amount excreted in the urine (urine concentration, *U*, multiplied by urine volume, *V*) divided by the renal artery minus the renal vein concentration difference gives the amount of plasma required to deliver the substance. Because it is from renal plasma that the substance is extracted, RPF is determined as follows:

$$\text{RPF} = \text{UV/A} - \text{RV}$$

where *U* is urine concentration; *V*, urine volume per unit time; *A*, renal artery concentration; and *RV*, renal vein concentration. Because the determination of renal vein concentration is cumbersome, a substance that is completely extracted in one pass is chosen so that renal vein concentration is zero. Thus the calculation simplifies to UV/P. Because no known substance is extracted completely in one pass, the measurement is called *effective RPF*. PAH, iodopyracet (Diodrast), and Hippuran, when administered at low-dose levels, are removed almost completely and are the agents employed to measure RPF. The renal extraction is approximately 90%; thus there is approximately a 10% error rate. Moreover, not all blood to the kidney is exposed to functioning tubules and glomeruli, so this technique may be significantly inaccurate in disease. Normal values are 600 to 700 mL per minute per 1.73 m^2. RBF may be calculated from RPF by the following equation:

$$\text{RBF} = \text{RPF}/(1 - \text{Hct})$$

where *Hct* is the patient's hematocrit level.

Washout methods involve injecting a bolus of isotope (xenon or krypton) in the renal artery and then measuring the speed with which the isotope leaves renal parenchyma by recording the rate at which radioactivity diminishes over the kidney by conventional scanning techniques. The concentration of isotope in the kidney as a function of time is plotted. The equation that describes the disappearance curve is of the fourth order or greater. By stripping the curve, that is, generating the equation for the curve, RBF to various segments (cortex and medulla) may be determined (58).

Finally, the disappearance of isotopically labeled Hippuran from the blood or timed accumulation by the kidney may be used as a gross estimate of RBF (see previous discussion).

Tubule Electrolyte Transport

Integrity of transport processes can be determined by assessing the transport of various electrolytes. This is important in certain disease entities, such as renal tubular acidosis (RTA) in which there is a defect in hydrogen ion secretion. That defect may be brought to light by stressing the kidney's hydrogen ion transport process. Other defects, such as distal tubule ammonium dysfunction, as occurs in certain patients who form uric acid stones, and salt-losing nephropathy, may be assessed similarly.

Sodium extraction rate may be used as a crude index of proximal and distal tubule function. The normal kidney under conditions of severe salt restriction should be able to excrete less than 0.1% of the filtered load of sodium in a urine concentration of less than 1 mEq/L.

Distal tubule function may be assessed by the administration of a mineralocorticoid and observation of a decrease in urine sodium concentration and a rise in urine potassium concentration. Distal tubule hydrogen secretion also may be assessed by administering hydrochloric acid, ammonium chloride, or one of the cationic amino acids (lysine, arginine, or histidine) and observing a decrease in the urine pH to less than 5 and/or a lack of ammonia generation.

Concentration and Dilution

Alterations in concentration and dilution indicate distal tubule and collecting duct dysfunction. Many entities affect these functions (Table 14.3), most often pyelonephritis and urinary obstruction. The normal kidney can dilute to an osmolality of 40 mOsm/kg and concentrate to 1,200 mOsm/kg. Concentrating ability is determined by either water deprivation or the administration of vasopressin. Diluting ability is determined by having the patient drink 1 L of water over a short time. The patient will excrete more than half the volume over 3 hours with a urine osmolality of 80 mOsm/kg or less.

DETERMINATION OF RENAL FUNCTION IN THE PRESENCE OF INTESTINAL SEGMENTS

The assessment of renal function in patients in whom a segment of intestine is interposed in the urinary tract requires modifying the techniques normally employed to determine renal function in the intact collecting system. This is necessary because the intestine, which is used as a conduit, functions as a vehicle of urine transport and as an absorptive and secretory surface. Thus urine may be modified considerably after transversing intestine, making it difficult to determine whether the measured substance has been altered by bowel absorption or secretion. Many of the substances used to assess renal glomerular function or RBF are absorbed by the intestinal segment. Urea is perhaps the most permeable, but creatinine, inulin, and PAH also are significantly absorbed (36). Their absorption depends on their concentration and the amount of time they remain in contact with the intestine, which is a function of the surface area to which they are exposed and the urine flow rate.

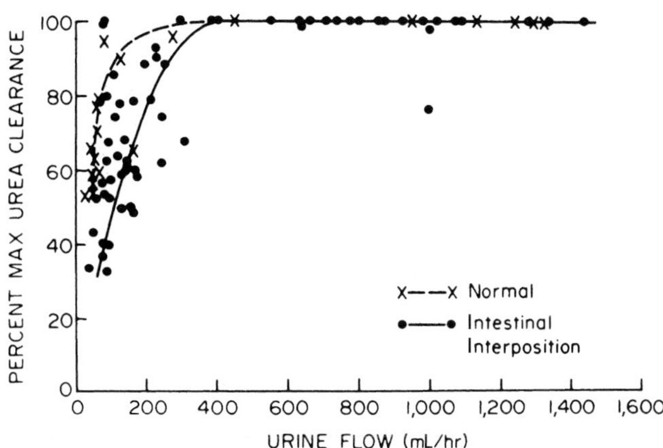

FIGURE 14.9. Flow dependency of urea clearance in patients with normal urinary tracts compared with those with ileal and colon interpositions.

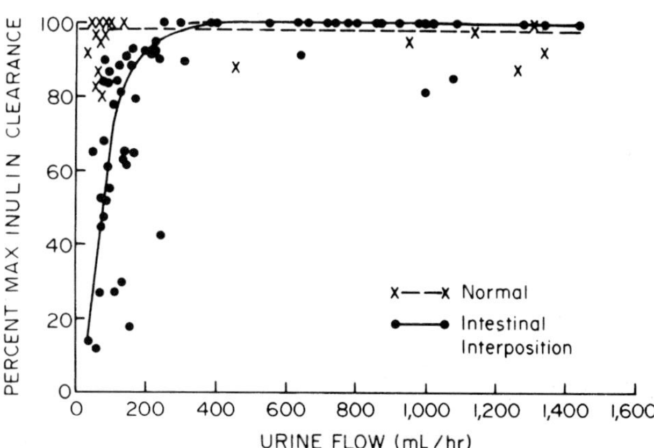

FIGURE 14.11. Flow dependency of inulin clearance in patients with normal urinary tracts compared with those with ileal and colon interpositions.

Figures 14.9 through 14.11 illustrate the dependency of urine flow rate on absorption of urea, creatinine, and inulin in patients with ileal and colon conduits. For clarity, the figures compare the percentage of maximum clearance achieved as a function of flow rate in normal collecting systems and ileal and colon interpositions. The illustrations demonstrate that when urine flow rates exceed 250 mL per hour, intestinal absorption for creatinine and inulin is negligible, and at these flow rates the substances more closely measure the true GFR and RPF (PAH shows a similar flow dependency). These curves were derived from a group of patients with ileal conduits, colon conduits, and intact urinary tracts. Because renal function varied from poor to normal, the patients were compared by factoring each measured clearance by the maximum clearance obtained for that patient. At high flow rates, patients with stomal stenosis tend to diminish their clearance, indicating that at these flows the intestine serves as a functional obstruction (45).

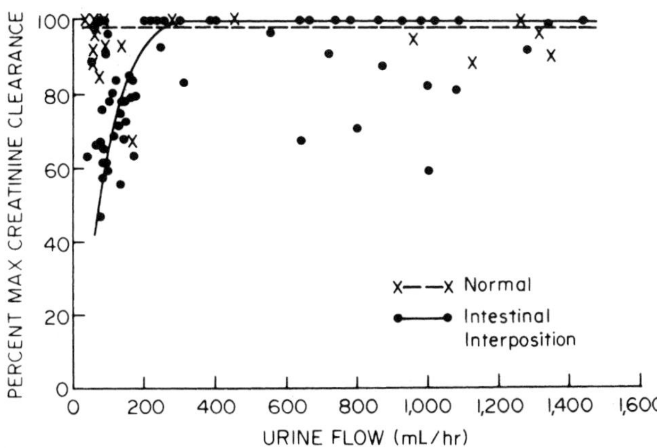

FIGURE 14.10. Flow dependency of creatinine clearance in patients with normal urinary tracts compared with those with ileal and colon interpositions.

Measurement of Glomerular Filtration Rate

Because clearance is flow dependent, it is necessary to establish a diuresis in patients with ileal and colonic segments at urine flows between 300 and 700 mL per hour. These flows may be achieved by fluid administration alone. Rarely, a diuretic such as furosemide also may be required. The urine is collected over 1 hour. The volume is measured, and the substance used for the clearance is measured in the serum and urine. Creatinine is perfectly adequate in these patients, provided the serum does not contain excessive ketoacids, cephalosporins, cimetidine, trimethoprim-sulfamethoxazole, or propranolol (51). Because diuretic creatinine clearance parallels diuretic inulin clearance, the former is the clinically expedient method of determining the GFR. Creatinine clearance measured in this manner is approximately 20% less than inulin clearance at GFRs that exceed 20 mL per minute. If the GFR is less than 20 mL per minute, the creatinine clearance may overestimate the inulin clearance as a result of secretion by the renal tubule. At low GFRs (i.e., less than 10 mL per minute), the error rate may be as great as 50% (Fig. 14.12).

Renal isotope determination of GFRs in these patients is not useful, because there is little correlation between GFRs obtained by this method and those obtained by inulin clearance. This is true at all levels of renal function (45).

Because the bowel absorbs, secretes, and metabolizes creatinine, the calculation of the GFR from serum creatinine, age, weight, and gender by empiric formulas is totally unreliable and not useful in these patients (45).

Renal Blood Flow

PAH clearance obtained when urine flows range between 300 and 700 mL per hour accurately reflects effective RPF.

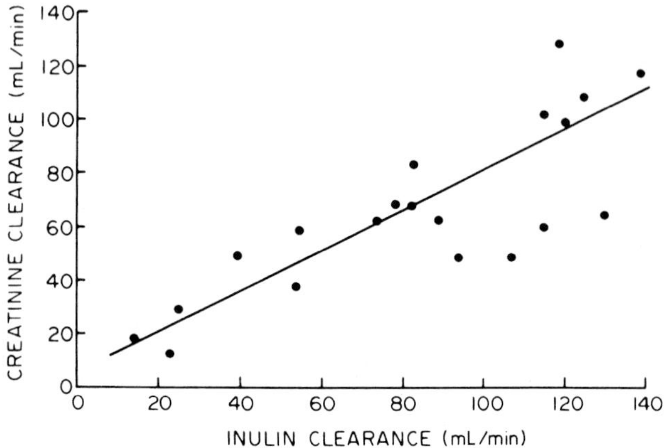

FIGURE 14.12. Diuretic inulin and creatinine clearances in patients with normal urinary tracts compared with those with ileal and colon interpositions. Notice the excellent correlation and that creatinine clearance is consistently 20% less than inulin clearance.

Isotope scans are not accurate in determining RBF in these patients.

Tubule Function

The determination of tubule function by the measurement of sodium excretion and hydrogen ion secretion under conditions of sodium deprivation or hydrogen loading (see previous discussion) cannot be accurately performed in these patients. Although some qualitative indication of the way electrolytes are handled can be obtained, the maximum capabilities of the kidneys with respect to electrolyte transport cannot be determined when urine is analyzed after it has traversed an intestinal segment.

Concentration and Dilution

Because the bowel cannot concentrate much more than 50 mOsm/kg greater than serum, urine traversing an intestinal segment, if more concentrated than serum, is diluted. Thus in patients with ileal and colon conduits, maximum urinary concentration usually does not exceed 400 mOsm/kg. The determination of maximum urinary concentrating ability of the kidney cannot be performed accurately in patients with intestinal segments (45). Although the kidney's ability to dilute can be assessed with the techniques described previously, maximum dilutional capabilities cannot be determined because of absorption by the intestine. Therefore statements about distal tubule and collecting duct function based on maximum concentrating ability in patients with colon or ileal segments are meaningless.

It is clear that patients who have colon or ileal conduits, those with intestine interposed in the urinary tract, and those in whom intestine is used as a urinary reservoir require special manipulations to measure renal function. GFR and RPF can be accurately assessed if, while they are being measured, urine flows range between 300 and 700 mL per hour. They must be measured by classic clearance techniques, not by either isotopic scans or empiric calculation from serum creatinine. Tubule function is most difficult to assess in these patients, and at present there is no good way of determining the kidney's maximum capacity for conserving sodium, excreting hydrogen, or reabsorbing water.

ACUTE RENAL FAILURE

Acute renal failure (ARF) in surgical patients has numerous causes (Table 14.1). Whatever the primary cause, it is associated with significant morbidity and mortality and presents as a progressive rise in blood urea nitrogen (BUN) and creatinine levels, often with a decrease in urine output. ARF is said to be oliguric when the urine output is less than 400 mL per 24 hours and nonoliguric when the urine output exceeds this amount. The initial therapy and prognosis for ARF are determined not only by examining the serum chemistries and state of fluid balance but also depend on the expeditious assignment of patients to one of the three subdivisions of this disease: prerenal, intrarenal, or postrenal. Therefore it is necessary to begin diagnostic procedures

TABLE 14.1. CAUSES OF ACUTE RENAL FAILURE

- Prerenal failure
  - Excessive nitrogen load
  - Myocardial pump failure
  - Hypovolemia
- Intrarenal failure
  - Occlusion of renal arteries or renal veins
  - Arteriolar damage
    - Malignant hypertension
    - Polyarteritis
    - Hypersensitivity angiitis
  - Disseminated intravascular coagulation
  - Glomerulonephritis
    - Lupus erythematosus
    - Poststreptococcal glomerulonephritis
  - Parenchymal damage
    - Acute interstitial nephritis
    - Acute pyelonephritis
    - Papillary necrosis
      - Diabetes mellitus
      - Nephrosclerosis
      - Sickle cell anemia
      - Analgesic medications
    - Cortical necrosis
    - End-stage renal disease
  - Hepatorenal syndrome
  - Hepatic artery ligation
  - Vasomotor nephropathy
    - Shock
    - Sepsis
    - Transfusion reactions
    - Crush injury
  - Tubule toxins
    - Drugs
    - Myoglobin
    - Poisons
- Postrenal failure
  - Obstruction of the collecting system
    - Tumors
    - Calculi
    - Infection and inflammatory lesions
    - Fibrosis
    - Blood clots
    - Renal papillae
    - Increased intraabdominal pressure
    - Retroperitoneal hemorrhage
  - Osmolality, mOsm/L
- Occasional hyaline
  - Occasional hyaline P cast
- Tubule epithelial casts
  - Variable, initially low

that will determine the type of ARF simultaneously with therapy directed at correcting fluid imbalance and electrolyte abnormalities.

Immediate Management of Acute Renal Failure

A careful history and physical examination often will suggest the type of ARF; however, the immediate management of this disease is dictated by the extent of serum chemical aberrations and fluid imbalance. Thus initial steps are directed at defining these abnormalities. An electrocardiogram (ECG), serum electrolytes, and urine for microscopic and chemical analysis are obtained. If the serum potassium is elevated, the ECG changes will indicate the rapidity with which the hyperkalemia must be corrected and will serve not only as a baseline against which the success of therapy may be measured but also as an immediate approximation of potassium concentration during the patient's course. Hyperkalemia results in progressive peaking of the T wave, prolongation of the QRS complex, and at high concentrations, absence of the P wave. When the serum potassium is greater than 7 mEq/L or when prominent alterations of the ECG occur (particularly when the P wave is absent), immediate reduction in serum potassium is accomplished by infusing hypertonic sodium bicarbonate and/or administration of insulin and glucose in a ratio of 1 unit per 5 g. Calcium is administered intravenously to stabilize myocardial conductivity. Acidosis and hyperkalemia may be partially corrected by giving bicarbonate, which results in a shift of potassium into the cell with preservation of electroneutrality by concomitant movement of hydrogen ion out of the cell. If some renal function is preserved, potassium secretion is increased in the distal tubule, because bicarbonate reduces the amount of hydrogen ion competing for the common hydrogen-potassium secretory mechanism, thus allowing it increased access to potassium. Glucose and insulin result in movement of potassium into the cell, either by binding it during glucose transport or during glycolytic phosphorylation. These mechanisms result in a transitory decrease in serum potassium, because it moves out of the cell in the former when acidosis recurs and in the latter when substrate has been metabolized. Therefore it is important to lower the total body serum potassium by simultaneously employing an ion exchange resin, such as polystyrene sulfonate (Kayexalate), 10 to 20 g orally or 50 g by enema, both given with sorbitol, or by peritoneal dialysis or hemodialysis. Usually 2 to 3 hours are required before ion exchange resins show an effect or before dialysis can be instituted. Most commonly, alkalization, ion exchange resins, and occasionally, dialysis are all that are required, with glucose and insulin being reserved only for those cases in which hyperkalemia is immediately life-threatening. The state of fluid balance is determined by analysis of intake and output, weight, venous or left atrial filling pressure, physical examination, and history. Inappropriate intake for the amount of output usually accounts for the imbalance; however, therapeutic maneuvers used to treat electrolyte abnormalities also may be contributory. Kayexalate, by exchanging sodium for potassium and sodium bicarbonate, can cause an excessive sodium load and fluid retention. When either overhydration or hypernatremia becomes an urgent problem, dialysis is most effective in correcting the disorder. Usually time is not of the essence, and sodium and fluid restriction will suffice. Low venous or pulmonary wedge pressure, clinical signs of dehydration, a history of blood loss, and hypotension indicate volume depletion and are treated by appropriate fluid replacement.

During the short-term treatment of hyperkalemia and fluid imbalance, an attempt should be made to define the type of ARF involved. A careful history and physical examination often can be diagnostic. The aseptic and atraumatic passage of a Foley catheter is helpful from both a diagnostic and, occasionally, a therapeutic point of view. If the patient is capable of voiding spontaneously and the residual is less than 30 mL, the catheter is withdrawn. If the diagnosis remains unclear after these simple maneuvers, a more sophisticated workup is in order and will include chemical analysis of the urine and serum for sodium, potassium, urea, creatinine, and osmolality; central venous or right atrial pressure determinations; and ultrasonograms of the kidneys. IV pyelography is rarely indicated. The degree of renal deterioration is usually of such an extent that visualization does not occur. Indeed, the contrast material may cause further deterioration of the severely compromised kidney; therefore indiscriminate use of contrast material is to be condemned. If the diagnosis is still in doubt, retrograde or antegrade pyelography or sonography is indicated. The characteristics and therapy for each type of ARF are described in detail in the following sections.

Prerenal Failure

Prerenal failure occurs when there is an excessive nitrogen load or reduced blood supply to the kidney. The former may result from increased muscle catabolism, blood breakdown within the gastrointestinal tract, or excessive protein alimentation. The latter appears in the presence of volume depletion, congestive heart failure, valvular heart disease, or any disease that causes myocardial pump failure.

Pathophysiology

In prerenal oliguria RBF is reduced. When the blood flow is reduced to a level such that the afferent arteriolar pressure falls below 60 mm Hg, reduced filtration pressure results in a decrease in the amount of filtrate delivered to the proximal tubule; glomerulotubular balance is disrupted; and sodium, water, and urea are reabsorbed in increased amounts. A BUN-to-creatinine ratio of greater than 10:1 occurs because creatinine, when filtered, is not reabsorbed by the tubule, whereas urea is reabsorbed in increased amounts. The proportional excretion of BUN and creatinine, which occurs in health, is disrupted and the urea recirculates, thus resulting in the abnormally high BUN-to-creatinine ratio.

Diagnosis

Diagnostic indications of prerenal failure include a serum BUN-to-creatinine ratio that is greater than 10:1, and a central venous pressure (CVP) and right arterial pressure in volume depletion that are low, provided coexisting myocardial disease is not present. The small volume of urine excreted is highly concentrated with a low sodium content (less than 15 mEq/L). The urine urea concentration divided by the plasma urea concentration (U ÷ P urea) is greater than 20:1, and the U/P osmolality is greater than 1.5. The fractional excretion of sodium or the ratio of U/P sodium to U/P creatinine (U/P_{Na}-to-U/P_{Cr}) is less than 1%. The urine sediment may reveal hyaline casts but generally will be free of casts and red and white blood cells (Table 14.2).

Treatment

The treatment of prerenal oliguria is directed at the primary disease: (a) correction of the lesion that has caused the increased nitrogen load, (b) improvement of the failing myocardium, or (c) volume repletion.

Intrarenal Failure

Acute intrarenal failure may follow an ischemic or a nephrotoxic injury or interstitial or glomerular nephritis. Examples of ischemic injury include sepsis, hemorrhagic shock, aortic cross clamping, and surgical or obstetric misadventures; causes of nephrotoxic injury include drugs (aminoglycosides), crush injuries (myoglobin), and diagnostic agents (IV contrast), whereas the etiology of interstitial nephritis often includes drugs. One-half to two-thirds of the patients will be oliguric, whereas the remainder will have urine outputs exceeding 400 mL per 24 hours. Patients who present with nonoliguric ARF have higher sodium concentrations, greater fractional sodium excretions, shorter hospital stays, and a lower mortality and require fewer dialyses than do those who present with oliguria. Indeed, oliguric renal failure has a mortality of 50% to 70%, whereas mortality is approximately 25% in nonoliguric patients. The importance of the sodium excretion rate is emphasized by the finding that less frequently fatal, nonoliguric renal failure patients have higher sodium excretion rates than oliguric patients. Moreover, in the oliguric ARF patient, a persistent urine sodium concentration less than 40 mEq/L is associated with only a 37% survival, whereas those with a urinary concentration greater than 40 mEq/L have a survival rate of 56% (3). It has been suggested that a low fractional excretion for sodium indicates that the cause of the injury

TABLE 14.2. DIFFERENTIAL DIAGNOSIS OF PRERENAL, INTRARENAL, AND POSTRENAL FAILURE

Measurement	Normal	Prerenal	Intrarenal	Postrenal
Blood				
CVP, cm water	5–8	Low to normal	Normal to elevated	Normal to elevated
BUN-to-creatinine ratio	10:1	>10:1	10:1	10:1+
Urine				
Sodium, mEq/L	15–40	<15	>40	>40
Potassium, mEq/L	15–40	Variable	Variable	Variable
Osmolality, mOsm/L	400–600	>450	<300	<300
Volume, mL	800–1200	Low	Variable	Variable, initially low
Urine-to-blood ratio				
Urea	20:1	>20:1	<10:1	<5:1
Osmolality	1.5–2.0	>1.5:1	<1.2:1	<1.0:1
Creatinine	20:1	>40:1	<20:1	<20:1
Fractional sodium excretion, %	Variable	<1.0	>1.0	>1.0
Urine—microscopic analysis	0–1 RBC	Occasional hyaline P cast	Tubule epithelial casts	RBCs and WBCs
	0–1 WBC		RBCs, free heme, or myoglobin	Malignant cells
	Occasional hyaline P cast No cellular casts			Crystals

BUN, blood urea nitrogen; CVP, central venous pressure; RBC, red blood cell; WBC, white blood cell.

involves tubular obstruction or alterations in renal hemodynamics rather than direct tubular nephrotoxicity (16). The recovery also somewhat depends on the cause of the ARF. Approximately 80% of patients with acute cortical necrosis and 66% of those with thrombotic thrombocytopenic purpura or the hemolytic uremic syndrome do not recover renal function adequate to support life. This is in contrast to patients with acute tubular necrosis and acute interstitial nephritis in whom 62% recover normal renal function. Thirty-one percent show a partial recovery, and only 6% have no recovery whatsoever (7). Another indication of recoverability is correlated with the length of time anuria occurs and the degree to which the kidney takes up nuclide on a renal scan. In one study, infants who remained anuric for at least 4 days after the acute insult and revealed no uptake of radionuclide on scan invariably died of their ARF, whereas infants with ischemic ARF who were nonoliguric and whose kidneys took up the nuclide had a more favorable prognosis (14).

Pathophysiology

A great deal of clinical and experimental data have been accumulated trying to define a pathophysiology for ARF. Unfortunately, most of the information comes from experimental animals, and correlation with the clinical situation often is contrived. A number of proposed mechanisms can be grouped into three areas: (a) vasomotor, increased nephron permeability, tubule obstruction, and decreased ultrafiltration (29); (b) injury to the cell resulting in necrosis or apoptosis; and (c) production of inflammatory mediators that cause injury often introduced by activated neutrophil infiltrations. Because the initiating events are multiple and varied, it is likely that in each case the ARF has been caused by a combination of some of these factors. It is important to understand each of the mechanisms because therapy of established ARF is based on these hypotheses.

The vasomotor theory proposes that there is not only a decrease in total RBF but also a redistribution of intrarenal blood flow. Xenon washout and microsphere injection studies have demonstrated a shift of blood flow away from the cortical nephrons toward the juxtamedullary nephrons (62). Some have suggested that this shift may be protective. Although under normal circumstances the whole kidney receives a blood flow resulting in oxygen delivery that far exceeds demand, the blood flow to the medulla is much less than to the cortex, resulting in limited oxygen reserves. It has been suggested that the medulla is most susceptible to ischemic injury and that the shift in blood flow to the medulla is an attempt to protect this segment (2). The renin-angiotensin system may play a role in the RBF shift. Moreover, prostaglandins also may be contributory. If the initial injury causes an increased release of renin, cortical afferent and efferent arteriolar constriction would result in reduction of cortical blood flow. Because stimulation of the autonomic nervous system releases renin, its role in the cause is unclear, but it may partially explain the occurrence of ARF in patients whose aortas have been cross-clamped. Further evidence for the importance of renin is demonstrated by depleting it in experimental models by either long-term salt loading or antirenin antibodies. A renin-depleted animal has not only a greater chance of recovery but also a more rapid return of function. Moreover, in many patients, renin activity is elevated early in the course of ARF (63). Unfortunately, specific antagonists of renin or angiotensin do not alter the course of these patients once the ARF is established.

Additional evidence for the significance of hormonal regulation of intrarenal blood flow during ARF comes from reports of indomethacin-induced ARF. Indomethacin blocks the synthesis of prostaglandins. PGE_2, a vasodilating prostaglandin, appears to play a significant role in maintaining RBF in the face of pathologic forces that tend to compromise it. Thus in the proper setting, eliminating PGE_2 results in the development or exacerbation of ARF (67). In addition to angiotensin II and prostaglandins, adenosine, increased cytosolic calcium, oxygen-free radicals, and endothelin have been implicated. Although renal vasoconstriction and low RBF may play key roles in the early stages of intrinsic renal failure, later spontaneous increases in RBF often occur without a concomitant increase in the GFR.

The hypothesis of increased tubule permeability proposes that although filtration pressure may or may not be reduced when the filtrate arrives in the proximal tubule, it leaks out, resulting in an effective reduction in filtration. Conflicting data supporting this theory have been reported. Some investigators have demonstrated leakage of labeled inulin and mannitol from the tubule. Moreover, the dye, lissamine green, has been observed to leak out of the tubule. However, others using micropuncture techniques have failed to show increased permeability in split-drop experiments.

Tubule blockade may play a major role in ARF after surgery. Myoglobin can precipitate in the tubule and cause mechanical blockage of the tubule lumen. In models of renal artery cross-clamping, up to 90% of the proximal tubules have been found to be occluded by swollen cells and desquamated proximal tubule microvilli; however, other experimental models that simulate medical causes of ARF are less convincing.

A decrease in ultrafiltration probably plays a major role in many causes of ARF. Numerous studies have demonstrated alterations in the glomerular basement membrane and supporting structures. These alterations result in a decrease in the membrane permeability by as much as 60%. This, coupled with decreased blood flow, results in a lessened hydrostatic pressure gradient and a marked decrease in the delivery of filtrate to the proximal tubule. Perhaps the changes that occur in glomerular membrane properties may explain the dissociation between RBF and GFR, because a decreased glomerular capillary permeability would continue to cause a decreased GFR even with increased RBF (38).

The aforementioned theories fail to explain all aspects of ARF and, indeed, seem not to explain some circumstances of injury. Following severe injuries, cellular necrosis and the initiation of apoptosis occur—the latter resulting in progressive loss of renal tubule cells (31).

Finally, a variety of inflammatory mediators, including tumor necrosis factor, interleukin-1, interleukin 8, and macrophage chemoattractant protein, are produced by the injured kidney. Some of these may be provided by activated neutrophils, which infiltrate the interstitium of the injured kidney.

Diagnosis

The diagnosis of intrarenal failure is based on historic, chemical, and radiologic determinations. The BUN-to-creatinine ratio is 10:1, and the CVP or left arterial filling pressure is normal or elevated. The urinary sodium concentration exceeds 40 mEq/L with a variable potassium secretion—usually less than 20 mEq/L. The U/P osmolality is less than 1.2 and the U/P urea is less than 10. The fractional sodium excretion exceeds 1%. Tubule epithelial cells and tubule epithelial cell casts may be observed in the urine (Table 14.2). A radioimmunoassay of tubule antigens has been developed that successfully diagnoses 80% of patients with acute tubule necrosis (71). This test has not gained popularity because the diagnosis of intrarenal failure may be made with this degree of accuracy by conventional techniques.

Ultrasonography or roentgenographic studies of the abdomen without the administration of pyelographic contrast should be used in an effort to determine whether the acute problem is superimposed on prior renal disease. Preexisting renal disease may be demonstrated by unilateral or bilateral small kidneys indicative of a vascular or infectious cause. An enlarged renal outline may imply either acute renal vein thrombosis or an infiltrative lesion, such as myeloma or lymphoma, or postrenal failure when it is associated with dilated calyces. Radionuclide renal scans or magnetic resonance arteriography occasionally are helpful in cases of bilateral renal artery thrombosis and may suggest that therapy is needed.

The BUN rises between 10 and 20 mg/dL per day, whereas creatinine increases 0.5 to 1.0 mg/dL per day. Plasma potassium increases 0.5 mEq/L per day, and because 50 to 100 mEq of fixed acid is retained, the plasma bicarbonate decreases by 1 to 2 mEq/L per day. In the posttraumatic state, the hypercatabolic response may result in a more rapid rise in the BUN, potassium, and fixed-acid accumulation. A crush injury involving muscle necrosis and myoglobin nephropathy can result in rises in serum creatinine up to 2 mg/dL per day and rapid increases in serum potassium and uric acid. Hypocalcemia often is noted and may have significant cardiac consequences, particularly if the serum potassium is elevated.

Treatment

Careful fluid balance, the judicious use of ion-exchange resins, dialysis, and administration of a potent diuretic when oliguria occurs are the hallmarks of therapy (66). The use of furosemide in the treatment of acute oliguric intrarenal failure is controversial. Several studies have failed to demonstrate more rapid recovery, improved GFR, or reduction in the number of dialyses required, except when cardiac decompensation is present (11). On the other hand, converting oliguria to nonoliguria makes subsequent fluid management less cumbersome. If furosemide is given, a dose of 80 mg is tried; if unsuccessful, it is doubled. One of three responses occurs:

1. Oliguria persists. The patients are treated with replacement of net water requirements (insensible loss – water of metabolism = 10 to 15 mL/kg per 24 hours). If a return in urine output does not occur within 21 days, the chance of recovery of renal function is poor.
2. A diuresis ensues, GFR increases, and an immediate reversal in the rise of BUN and creatinine occurs. It is important to rehydrate the patient in this setting, because this response suggests prerenal oliguria. These patients recover, often obtaining normal renal function.
3. A diuresis occurs, GFR remains low, and BUN and creatinine continue to rise. These patients are treated with replacement of net water loss (10 mL/kg per 24 hours) plus urine output and gastrointestinal and tube losses.

Large sodium losses occur during this phase and require replacement. Potassium losses are small, although rarely they may be excessive and require replacement. Appropriate serum potassium concentrations are maintained by restriction of potassium and the use of ion exchange resins and dialysis.

Mannitol has been found to be useful in patients with ARF resulting from crush injury, but has not been shown to be particularly helpful in other types of renal injury.

Low-dosage dopamine (1 to 2 μg/kg per minute) has not altered the course of ARF; however, some evidence indicates that it is helpful in the hepatorenal syndrome and in preventing ARF if used during the early prodromal period (65). The administration of dopamine to these patients results in a significant increase in the diuresis and natriuresis and, when combined with furosemide, may improve renal function in at least some patients with ARF. Experimental evidence shows a synergistic protective effect with the combination of dopamine and furosemide in several models of ARF. Dopamine causes marked vasodilation of both afferent and efferent arterioles (26). Mannitol has been helpful in preventing ARF (if given before interrupting renal artery flow) and in lessening the toxic effects of myoglobin. No study to date that has been properly performed has shown dopamine to be of any benefit in reducing morbidity or mortality.

β-Blockers have produced variable results, and angiotensin and renin inhibitors have not proved useful. Alkalizing agents, by solubilizing organic acids (drugs) when they are causative, and diuresis, by diluting toxic substances (cisplatin and myoglobin), are helpful prophylactically. Finally, if given early in the course of the disease, calcium channel blockers may be helpful by reducing intracellular calcium in tubule cells that have suffered an ischemic injury and are deprived of ATP.

Atrial natriuretic peptide has been shown to convert some patients from oliguric renal failure to nonoliguric renal failure, but generally has not been found to be helpful in reducing mortality. Insulin-like growth factor has been shown to prevent the decline in GFR in patients with ARF in selected circumstances but also has not been helpful in changing morbidity or mortality.

Perhaps the one drug regimen that all agree is most helpful, particularly in severely malnourished surgical patients, is nutritional support. Hyperalimentation with essential L-amino acids has improved recovery and reduced the number of dialyses required (22).

Dialysis plays an important role in the management of these patients. If the BUN is greater than 100 mg/dL and the creatinine exceeds 12 mg/dL, dialysis is mandatory. Evidence suggests that if the BUN is kept below 70 mg/dL, the incidence of sepsis is reduced from 88% to 63%, bleeding from 60% to 36%, and mortality from 80% to 36% (15). Others have shown consistently that mortality is lowered, extrarenal complications are less frequent, and the clinical course is better in any type of ARF when dialysis is employed before the clinical signs of uremia occur, emphasizing the need to evaluate each patient rather than basing dialysis on some arbitrary number. Dialysis may be accomplished either peritoneally or hemically.

Recent evidence indicates that in the critically ill patient, dialysis under certain circumstances may in fact prolong ARF. This is particularly apparent in unstable patients who become hypotensive when placed on dialysis. In addition, the dialysis membrane may activate the inflammatory cascades, further compromising the recovery of the injured kidney.

Plasma exchange may be useful in treating patients whose renal failure is the result of nondialyzable substances, such as dextran. Slow continuous ultrafiltration with a filter placed between two limbs of a Scribner shunt has been useful in selected critically ill patients. Its advantages include hemodynamic stability, ability to remove large fluid volumes (thus making treatment modalities such as IV nutrition feasible), and no requirement for systemic anticoagulation. It has many disadvantages, among them electrolyte abnormalities, bleeding, clotting of the shunt filter, excessive drug removal, azotemia, hypotension, and bacteremia (57,64).

Mortality in this group is high; however, between 25% and 70% of patients surviving an acute tubule injury eventually recover sufficient renal function to support life without dialysis. Of those recovering, 20% to 40% will have a reduced GFR for 1 year or longer. Abnormalities of tubule function, including renal glucosuria and decreased concentrating ability, may persist indefinitely.

The most frequent cause of death is infection (61). It causes 36% of the deaths and is usually pulmonary in origin. The next most common cause of death is gastrointestinal hemorrhage. Delayed wound healing, poor generation of granulation tissue, anorexia, anemia, and bleeding abnormalities caused by platelet malfunction contribute to the high level of morbidity in this disease. Indeed, even mild ARF significantly affects morbidity, even in the absence of significant comorbid disease (41).

Because of the high mortality of ARF, perhaps the most effective treatment is prophylaxis. Adequate hydration and selective use of dopamine, mannitol, furosemide, and alkalization in patients undergoing surgery who are known to have a high risk for the development of postoperative ARF should lessen the incidence of the disease. Risk factors that carry with them an increased incidence of postoperative ARF include advanced age, cardiac or hepatic failure, sepsis, jaundice, rhabdomyolysis, and massive blood transfusions.

Myoglobin Nephrotoxicity

Rhabdomyolysis has been reported to be the cause of ARF in approximately 5% of all patients with acute renal insufficiency. The prognosis for recovery is excellent, provided rhabdomyolysis is recognized promptly and therapy is begun immediately. There are traumatic and nontraumatic causes of rhabdomyolysis (37). The former include crush injuries, electric burns, arterial occlusion, and surgery. Nontraumatic causes include increased muscle exertion, inflammatory muscle diseases, infection, toxic drugs, and metabolic abnormalities (particularly hypokalemia). In urologic patients, prolonged, exaggerated lithotomy position has been associated with rhabdomyolysis and ARF (24).

After the precipitating event the patient becomes acutely ill with fever, weakness, and pain. The urine is brownish and is dipstick-positive for heme. Because the molecular weight of myoglobin is much lower than that of hemoglobin, it is cleared rapidly from the serum. Thus a spun blood sample will reveal a clear serum in contradistinction to hemolysis, where the serum will be red as a result of retained hemoglobin. A high serum creatinine phosphokinase level establishes the diagnosis. Serum potassium and phosphate often are elevated, and hyperuricemia may be severe. The mechanism of ARF is unclear, but it probably is caused by a combination of events including low flow, prolonged contact of the tubule lumen with myoglobin, and high uric acid concentration. Therapy is directed at establishing a diuresis with either a loop diuretic or by volume expansion, with saline solution combined with either mannitol or a loop diuretic. The diuresis dilutes the toxic myoglobin, removes it from the kidney, reduces the serum uric acid concentration, and modestly alkalizes the urine. Alkalization is advisable initially, because an acid medium promotes myoglobin dissociation into ferroprotoporphyrin and globin. The former is toxic (21).

Radiocontrast-induced Acute Renal Failure

The incidence of reduced renal function resulting from radiocontrast material has been reported to be as high as 12%. The incidence of contrast nephropathy in patients with normal renal function is lower than 2% after angiography and approximately 1.5% after IV urography. In contrast, among patients with diabetes and coexisting renal insufficiency, more than half develop substantial renal damage after IV urography (6). The occurrence of clinically significant ARF in the general population is exceedingly low; it is most commonly found after angiography or IV urography in patients with significant risk factors for the development of the disease. Almost all patients who develop clinically significant ARF have either previously existing renal disease with compromised renal function or diabetes with moderate renal impairment. However, adult-onset diabetic patients with normal renal function do not appear to be at increased risk for development of ARF. Patients with juvenile-onset diabetes are more likely to develop renal insufficiency even though they do not demonstrate significant renal impairment before the injection of contrast medium. Other factors that have been less well correlated with the development of renal insufficiency after the injection of radiocontrast include advanced age, dehydration, multiple contrast exposure within 24 hours, hyperuricemia, proteinuria, hypoalbuminemia, multiple myeloma, and impaired hepatic function. Dehydration per se does not appear to be a specific risk factor unless the patient has preexisting renal disease. Conversely, in patients with prior renal disease, establishing a diuresis after the injection of contrast medium appears to lessen the incidence of renal deterioration. In patients with multiple myeloma, there is no compelling evidence of any increased risk for contrast-induced renal failure unless there is preexisting renal insufficiency. However, contrast-induced renal failure in patients with multiple myeloma often has catastrophic implications because it is irreversible.

In summary, existing renal insufficiency is the single most important predisposing factor. Moreover, diabetes does not increase the risk of contrast-induced renal failure if renal function is normal and the patient is well hydrated and does not have juvenile-onset diabetes. When radiocontrast-induced renal failure does occur, 75% of patients are oliguric for the first 24 hours after contrast exposure. Prolonged oliguria results in only partial return of renal function. The serum creatinine generally peaks by the seventh postinsult day, and renal function returns to normal in 75% of the cases. Dialysis rarely is required, and almost all patients have an adequate return of function and do not require long-term dialysis (50). The pathogenesis of the disorder has been hypothesized to be the result of direct tubule toxicity, to renal ischemia caused by alterations in blood flow with shunting of blood from cortex to medulla, and to intratubular obstruction. Because contrast agents are uricosuric, tubule obstruction by crystals of uric acid has been proposed as the pathogenic mechanism. Finally, immunologic factors have been proposed, but the evidence is not compelling. It appears that the renal toxicity after contrast exposure is probably the result of direct tubule toxicity and renal ischemia (6).

Postrenal Failure

The causes of postrenal failure are divided into lower and upper urinary tract obstruction. The lower urinary tract is evaluated in the preliminary treatment, as previously indicated, by the passage of the Foley catheter. Obstruction of the upper urinary tract may be the result of ureteral calculi, blood clots, sloughed papillae, ureterovesical or ureteropelvic junction obstruction, ureteral tumors, ureteral stricture, extrinsic compression by retroperitoneal tumors, hemorrhage, fibrosis, tumor, or an inflammatory lesion. Recently, increased intraabdominal pressure has been reported as a cause of postrenal failure.

Pathophysiology

In the patient with postrenal failure, RBF is markedly reduced with a reduction in GFR to 10% of normal or less, causing a decline in filtration with decreased delivery of filtrate to the proximal tubule (47). This may be mediated through the renin-angiotensin system (46) and/or the prostaglandin system. Elevated concentrations of renin, the vasodilator PGE_2, and the vasoconstrictor thromboxane A_2 have been reported in obstructive uropathy (49). The significance of the prostaglandins in the pathophysiology of obstructive uropathy has been questioned recently. Specific inhibitors of thromboxane synthesis have failed to show any major effect on renal hemodynamics (42). Moreover, inhibition of prostaglandin synthesis during the obstructive phase has little influence on return of renal function, whereas inhibition of renin during this phase results in a major improvement in the return of renal function (44). Interstitial infiltration by lymphocytes and activated neutrophils result in cytokine release, which may explain some of the pathologic events. Moreover, apoptosis in the distal tubule and cortical collecting duct are initiated in animals with uretal obstruction. Even though complete obstruction does occur, GFR does not cease but remains modest, and the fluid that is filtered is reabsorbed by the renal tubules, the peripelvic lymphatic vessels and veins, and the perirenal tissues when the urine extravasates around the fornices of the calyx. With the increased hydrostatic pressure within the ureter, destruction of tubule tight junctions occurs, causing increased tubule permeability (46). Permeability is increased throughout the entire nephron, proximal tubule, loop, distal tubule, and collecting duct; there is a reduction in the net sodium and water reabsorption with net addition of sodium by the collecting duct. Increased potassium secretion by the distal tubule occurs in the postobstructed phase, and during recovery, concentrating ability remains impaired for days (47). Although reduced, RBF persists and removes solute from the medulla. Thus after the relief of such obstructions, there is often an excessive volume output with large sodium losses and inability of the kidney to concentrate and excrete an acid load. The loss of medullary tonicity and the rapidity with which it is built up determines the degree and length of time urinary concentration is impaired. Rarely, concentrating ability may take as long as 6 to 9 months to return to normal. Should obstruction occur in the presence of infection or protein depletion and exist for prolonged periods, parenchymal destruction occurs. Under these circumstances complete return of renal function does not occur. The longest report of complete obstruction with the return of renal function to support life is 90 days.

Diagnosis

The diagnosis of upper tract obstruction is established by retrograde pyelography or occasionally by percutaneous puncture and antegrade pyelography. However, it should be remembered that indiscriminate manipulation of the urinary tract must be avoided, because sepsis, the most common cause of death in patients with intrarenal failure, all too often is a consequence of genitourinary manipulation. After lower urinary tract obstruction has been ruled out by the introduction of a Foley catheter, complete anuria demands retrograde or antegrade pyelography. In addition to obstruction, total anuria may be the result of bilateral renal artery thrombosis, aortic vascular catastrophes, acute glomerulonephritis, or cortical necrosis, and it may be present during the first 12 to 24 hours of acute tubular injury.

Abdominal roentgenograms, computed tomography scans, and renal ultrasonograms are useful. The diagnosis may be suggested by the presence of calcification in the course of the ureters; osteoblastic lesions of the bones implying carcinoma of the prostate, which may have invaded the bladder; or large pelves on ultrasonography, implying obstruction. Rarely, the ultrasonogram will show a nondilated system even in the presence of bilateral obstruction (56). Therefore if one's index of suspicion is high, retrograde or antegrade pyelography should be performed even though the ultrasonogram does not show hydronephrosis.

These patients are well hydrated; have normal or slightly elevated CVP; have a BUN-to-creatinine ratio of 10 : 1 or greater; and a urine microscopic examination may reveal red blood cells, white blood cells, crystals, or malignant cells. Urine sodium concentration is greater than 40 mEq/L, and potassium concentration is variable, usually ranging between 20 and 40 mEq/L. The renal concentrating ability is severely impaired, which is reflected by a U/P urea of less than 5 and a U/P osmolality of less than 1.0. The fractional sodium excretion is in excess of 1%.

Treatment

Therapy is directed at the site of obstruction, requiring a urethral catheter, a suprapubic cystotomy, a nephrostomy, a cutaneous ureterostomy, or indwelling ureteral catheters; double-J stents may be left temporarily until the metabolic status of the patient is stable enough to permit the appropriate surgical procedure. During the postobstructed period, large quantities of urine are excreted with a low osmolality and a high sodium concentration (50 to 70 mEq/L). These defects are unresponsive to ADH and mineral corticoid administration. Volume and sodium should be replaced as lost. D_5½NS is usually the appropriate infusion. Potassium losses are therapeutic initially, but if prolonged and excessive, replacement of potassium may be necessary later. Sodium and potassium conservation return to normal within 48 to 72 hours; however, the concentrating defect may persist for 7 to 12 days, making dehydration a potential danger should fluid be inappropriately restricted. Most of these patients, if they respond with a diuresis, will go on to recovery of renal function. If oliguria persists, the obstruction has caused destruction of parenchyma, and such patients are managed as described for intrarenal ARF.

Postrenal Polyuria

Postrenal polyuria occurs during partial chronic urinary obstruction or after the release of complete bilateral ureteral occlusion (postobstructive diuresis), provided that significant parenchymal damage has not occurred. As described previously, basic defects involve a washout of the medullary concentration gradient and increased tubule permeability. Such patients lose excessive volumes of fluid that generally contain 40 to 80 mEq/L of sodium and variable concentrations of potassium. They are incapable of both concentrating and acidifying their urine. Because there is no medullary osmotic gradient, ADH is ineffective. The management of these patients is as previously described and involves careful intake and output records, daily weights, frequent serum osmolalities, and careful physical examination to determine the presence of dehydration or edema.

TABLE 14.3. DIFFERENTIAL DIAGNOSIS OF POLYURIA

- Postrenal polyuria
  - Obstruction
- Intrarenal polyuria
  - Anatomic disruption
    - Sickle cell anemia
    - Pyelonephritis
    - Amyloidosis
    - Nephrocalcinosis
  - Metabolic abnormalities of ADH–collecting duct interaction
    - Hypercalcemia
    - Hypokalemia
    - Renal tubular acidosis
  - Functional abnormalities
    - Nephrogenic diabetes insipidus
    - Medullary washout
- Prerenal polyuria
  - Lack of ADH
    - Suppressed expanded extracellular fluid
    - Diabetes insipidus
    - Trauma
  - Diuretic agents (other than doxycycline or neuromuscular agents)

ADH, antidiuretic hormone.

Intrarenal Polyuria

Intrarenal polyuria results from an intrinsic impairment of the renal concentrating mechanism. It may be caused by anatomic disruption from disease, metabolic aberrations affecting the ADH–collecting duct interaction, or functional renal derangements (Table 14.3). A reduction in renal medullary tonicity may be caused by anatomic disruptions such as those found in sickle cell anemia. In such patients, portions of the renal medulla are infarcted as a result of low oxygen tonicity and sickling of the erythrocytes. Other diseases, such as medullary cystic disease, pyelonephritis, nephrocalcinosis, and amyloidosis, may similarly disrupt the medulla. Metabolic aberrations of the ADH–collecting duct interaction include hypercalcemia, prolonged hypokalemia, and RTA. These disorders are not uncommon in postsurgical and posttrauma patients.

Hypercalcemia initially interferes with the action of ADH on the collecting duct epithelium, and if it is corrected early, reversal of the concentrating defect is immediate. Prolonged hypercalcemia with calcium deposition in the thick ascending limb of Henle's loop, the distal tubule, and the collecting duct may result in permanent loss of renal concentrating ability. Prolonged hypokalemia may exert its effect by inhibition of the generation of adenyl cyclase, cyclic adenosine monophosphate (cAMP), or protein kinase and their interaction between ADH and the collecting duct. Restoration of the appropriate potassium level corrects the concentrating disorder. RTA also may cause a lack of concentrating ability. Because RTA often results in low serum potassium concentrations, it may be hypokalemia, not the RTA as such, that is responsible for the concentrating defect. In any event, restoration of normal serum acid–base and electrolyte balance corrects the problem, provided nephrocalcinosis has not complicated the disease.

Finally, other causes of polyuria include functional derangements, such as nephrogenic diabetes insipidus in which the collecting duct appears to be insensitive to circulating levels of ADH, and lack of medullary tonicity from persistent excessive urine output. The management of intrarenal polyuric states involves daily monitoring of body weight and serum osmolality and fluid replacement, volume for volume. Specific metabolic disorders, such as hypercalcemia, hypokalemia, and systemic acidosis, are corrected. Anatomic abnormalities, such as sickle cell disease, pyelonephritis, polycystic disease, myeloma, amyloidosis, and polyarteritis, are not amenable to any specific treatment with respect to polyuria, and therefore these patients are best treated in a supportive manner. Exogenous ADH is not effective in these disorders unless they have a metabolic cause and then only when the abnormality has been corrected.

Prerenal Polyuria

Prerenal polyuria is caused by insufficient ADH or by exogenous or endogenous diuretic agents. The intrinsic ability of the concentrating mechanism to function is maintained; however, if the polyuria is prolonged, it may result in washout of the medullary osmotic gradient, in which case an intrinsic renal defect would be superimposed on a prerenal defect (17). Insufficient ADH activity may result from suppression of ADH release in the pituitary, either as a normal consequence of volume overload or as a consequence of iatrogenic-induced reduction in serum osmolality. The common causes in volume expansion include over-administration of IV fluids, compulsive water drinking, and pathologic stimulation of the thirst center. Dilution of plasma osmolality occurs when sodium loss exceeds that replaced or when water is replaced in an electrolyte-poor fluid. Absence of or insufficient ADH production occurs in cerebral trauma and diabetes insipidus, which may be an inherited or acquired abnormality. Because the intrinsic concentrating mechanism is unaffected in these states, it is of paramount importance to determine the primary cause. If a lack of ADH is responsible, administration of this hormone is therapeutic. However, if volume abnormalities have caused this disorder, their correction will be curative.

Prolonged, persistent diuresis can cause dilation of the collecting system. After the prolonged diuresis, IV urography may reveal bilateral hydronephrosis. This hydronephrosis occurs on the basis of excessive diuresis and not on the basis of any mechanical obstruction. Because diuresis results in an increase in intraureteral pressure as bladder filling occurs, it is easy to understand why ureteral dilation occurs (see Physiology in Chapter 24).

CHRONIC RENAL FAILURE

Chronic renal failure occurs most commonly as a result of glomerulonephritis caused by immunopathogenic mechanisms; diabetes, infection, toxins, obstruction, congenital disorders, and hereditary nephropathies account for the majority of the remaining causes. The loss of renal function is usually insidious, not manifesting itself until late in the disease. The initial symptoms that herald a significant lack of renal function are protean and include fatigue, lassitude, and weakness. As the renal function continues to deteriorate, the patient may complain of a metallic taste, anorexia, nausea, vomiting, abdominal pain, hiccups, and diarrhea. With progression, there is an inability to concentrate, somnolence, twitching, bone pain, pericarditis, and hypertension (and its sequelae). All organ systems are affected at various stages in the disease. The detrimental effects of renal failure can be ameliorated by proper recognition and anticipation of the various complications with appropriate prophylactic therapy instituted before the abnormalities become clinically manifest.

Pathophysiology

As renal function decreases, those nephrons that continue to function increase in size, as do their respective glomeruli. This concept was originally suggested by Bricker and coworkers (9) and is known as the *intact nephron hypothesis.* Although this hypothesis has been questioned, because micropuncture data suggest a heterogeneity of tubule function in disease, it appears that within the constraints of biologic variability, the intact nephron hypothesis has the most evidence to support it and thus best explains the observed deterioration of renal function in chronic renal failure. GFR and RPF decrease, and functional mass decreases in parallel, whereas each individual nephron that continues to function increases its single-nephron filtration rate. Because fewer nephrons are functioning and those that are have increased their activity, if solute excretion is to be maintained, the fractional excretions for the respective solutes must increase. Sodium homeostasis is maintained until late in the disease by the mechanism of increasing single-nephron fractional excretion from less than 1% in health to 10% to 20% in disease. Late in the disease sodium excretion becomes fixed, and the nephron is incapable of varying its fractional excretion according to the needs of the patient, thus resulting in a salt-losing nephropathy. Salt restriction in such patients will result in substantial hyponatremia. This occurs late in the disease process. Similarly, water conservation and excretion are maintained until the GFR falls below 20 mL per minute, at which time the kidney is incapable of compensating for varying water loads or significant water deprivation. The kidney retains a remarkable ability to excrete potassium until late in the process. The increased flow rate obtained by the remaining functional nephrons facilitates potassium secretion. Acidosis, which is associated with increasing renal failure, also promotes potassium secretion. Mild hyperkalemia occurs when the GFR falls below 10 mL per minute. Significant hyperkalemia is uncommon until oliguria supervenes with a urine output less than 500 mL per 24 hours.

Acid–base balance is reasonably well maintained until the GFR falls below 20 mL per minute, then acid–base imbalance is a result of the failure of the distal tubule to maintain ammonia excretion (39). Even in advanced renal failure, not much alkali is excreted. Bicarbonate reabsorption is strongly influenced by the extracellular volume so that late in the disease, when the kidney is not capable of responding to fluid loads, excessive fluid intake often results in bicarbonate wasting.

The determination of renal function using creatinine presents certain difficulties in patients with chronic renal failure. Serum creatinine levels may be deceptively low because of increased metabolism by the gut and decreased muscle mass as a result of muscle wasting from the uremia. When the GFR is less than 15 mL per minute, the creatinine clearance will overestimate the true GFR (inulin clearance) as a result of tubule secretion of creatinine, often by as much as 50% to 100%.

Unfortunately, some aspects of renal function are maintained at the expense of others. Phosphate homeostasis is an excellent example of this "trade-off" phenomenon. As the need to excrete phosphate continues with decreased renal function, the intact nephrons are not capable of increasing their fractional excretion for phosphate. Serum phosphate rises, which results in a fall in serum calcium and the subsequent release of parathormone. Parathormone acts on tubules to increase phosphate excretion, thereby returning serum phosphate to normal levels. The other effect of parathormone on bone reabsorption also occurs, resulting in bone destruction. Bone destruction is the price, or trade-off, paid for maintaining a normal level of serum phosphate.

The increased filtration that each nephron must maintain appears to be responsible for its ultimate demise. It has been shown experimentally that increasing single-nephron GFR results in stripping off the glomerular endothelial cells, thus destroying the charge barrier that prevents deposition of circulating proteins in the glomerular basement membrane (55). The circulating serum proteins are then deposited and accumulate in the mesangium, resulting in the histologic appearance of glomerulosclerosis. Thus an initial insult that reduces renal mass, such as segmental injuries caused by obstruction, reflux, or dysplasia, may have occurred in the distant past, with renal failure occurring slowly over the ensuing years as a result of an increased workload of the remaining functional nephrons, with protein deposition causing their ultimate failure. In chronic renal failure patients in the Christchurch series, 12% of cases were the result of reflux nephropathy, few of which had been infected. These patients began dialysis at approximately 18 years of age, suggesting that the initial insult caused progressive renal deterioration as each remaining nephron was required to do more work (4).

The fact that protein is detrimental to renal function was suggested many years ago (1) and led to the development of the protein-restricted "renal failure diet." When patients eat this diet, many of the symptoms of uremia are alleviated or reduced. Administration of essential amino acids and their keto analogs have been successful in slowing the rise in BUN; however, the substances are not generally palatable. More recently it has been suggested that dietary protein may cause renal failure in patients who have sustained a renal insult (8). Thus dietary protein restriction may not only alleviate symptoms of uremia in patients with severely compromised renal function but may also prevent the progression of the disease in patients who have a modest decrease in renal function of insufficient degree to manifest signs or symptoms. Protein induces an acute increase in GFR through renal vasodilation and glomerular hyperperfusion. The elevated intracapillary pressures and transcapillary flux of ultrafiltrate eventually disrupt the integrity of the glomerular capillary membrane. Proteinuria ensues, and the increased flux of proteins exacerbates the glomerular capillary injury and causes progressive accumulation of mesangial deposits—the forerunner of focal glomerulosclerosis. Others have suggested that it may not be protein per se that causes the renal injury but rather the high phosphate intake from the protein. The phosphorus-induced renal injury is mediated through calcium-phosphate deposition in the kidney as a result of an increased filtered load of phosphate per nephron (28). Several prospective studies have shown that dietary restrictions of protein lessen the progression of renal deterioration in certain subgroups of patients, particularly those with advanced disease (54). Other studies have shown a nonsignificant slowing in the progression (34). In children, a multiinstitutional study has failed to show any effect of low-protein diets on slowing the progression of chronic renal failure (70). Proper control of blood pressure has been found to be one of the most important methods of slowing the progression of chronic renal failure.

Complications

Chronic renal failure is a systemic disease and, as such, affects every organ system in the body. The more common complications most relevant to the urologist include bladder and renal and/or perirenal infections, acquired renal cystic disease and renal carcinoma, infertility, impotence, and gynecomastia.

Renal, Perirenal, and Bladder Infections

Urinary tract infection is an important cause of morbidity and mortality in chronic renal failure and has been reported to be responsible for up to 20% of all deaths in patients with end-stage renal disease (ESRD) (35,48). As many as 10% of patients receiving hemodialysis have had, at any one time, a bacteremia secondary to an infection (53). Pyocystis, pyonephrosis, perinephric abscesses, and infected polycystic kidneys are not uncommon (40). The frequent absence of leukocytosis and fever coupled with a low index of suspicion (because a poorly functioning urinary tract is often dismissed) results in a delayed or missed diagnosis. A history of stone disease, congenital abnormalities of the collecting system, and pus from the urethra, coupled with urethral catheterization, renal ultrasonography, or computed tomography usually will lead to the diagnosis.

Acquired Renal Cystic Disease and Renal Cell Carcinoma

Patients on chronic dialysis for extended periods of time have a high propensity to develop cysts in their native kidneys. The incidence has been reported to vary between 35% and 80%. There is also a 100-fold increased risk of developing renal cell cancer in these cysts when compared with the general population (32). The acquired cysts make detection of renal cell cancers difficult. Patients who require periodic follow-up with ultrasound include those who have hematuria, flank pain, or other symptoms or signs that indicate a change in the kidneys.

Infertility

Both men and women who have ESRD are infertile. Even dialysis does not seem to restore their fertility. Serum hormone studies reveal an elevated level of luteinizing hormone and follicle-stimulating hormone and a depressed level of testosterone in the male patients. It appears that the failure occurs at the level of the testes.

Impotence

Gonadotropins are elevated, prolactin is elevated, and testosterone is depressed. Some patients respond to dialysis and others respond to androgen supplementation. A trial of bromocriptine to inhibit the elevated prolactin has been used with success in some patients, but the side effects of the drug usually prevent patients from continuing therapy.

Gynecomastia

Gynecomastia is not unusual, particularly early in dialysis. There is no satisfactory treatment; however, certain drugs aggravate the situation and should be discontinued if possible. The drugs include digitalis preparations, methyldopa (Aldomet), and spironolactone (Aldactone).

Gastrointestinal Tract

Mucosal ulcerations, ascites, pancreatitis, pruritus, and peptic ulceration are not uncommon. However, the symptoms of anorexia, nausea, vomiting, diarrhea, uremic breath, and metallic taste are more common.

Cardiovascular Disorders

Hypertension occurs in more than 80% of patients with ESRD. Three-quarters of these patients are hypertensive because of volume overload. The patient must be overloaded by at least 5% of body weight for hypertension to occur. This can be completely corrected by dialysis and the selected use of potent diuretics. The other 25% of uremic hypertensive patients are volume independent. These patients are labile when dialyzed and often require potent antihypertensives for blood pressure control. Even so, some patients ultimately require nephrectomy for control of their hypertension. Congestive heart failure is not infrequent in these patients. Uremic pericarditis continues to be a frequent complication, even with dialysis. These patients often present with fever, chest pain, leukocytosis, and sometimes, a pericardial friction rub. Often they will respond to dialysis alone, but indomethacin or corticosteroid administration may be necessary. Rarely, cardiac tamponade occurs, signaled by an enlarging cardiac silhouette on chest x-ray films, an elevated venous pressure, and hypotension. Surgical drainage is the treatment of choice. Echocardiography has been used with great success to follow the size of pericardial effusions.

Neuromuscular System

Peripheral neuropathy is usually sensory, with patients complaining of burning sensation in the feet and legs, particularly at night. Its incidence has decreased with the advent of early dialysis. Left untreated, the neuropathy will progress to loss of sensation, muscle atrophy, and motor nerve involvement. Therapy consists of dialysis and replacement of nutritional deficits. Renal transplantation reverses the disorder. Central nervous system disorders include loss of attention, short memory, and disturbed sleep. Without treatment, agitation, seizures, and psychotic behavior with eventual coma supervene. Aluminum intoxication has been implicated, but its role remains controversial.

Hematologic Disorders

The major cause of anemia in uremic patients is the lack of bone marrow production. Other contributing factors include gastrointestinal bleeding; vitamin deficiency states, particularly folate, pyridoxine, and iron; and hemolysis. Therapy consists of dialysis, replacement of nutritional deficits, minimization of blood loss, and occasionally, the use of androgens. The recent introduction of recombinant erythropoietin has markedly changed the management of anemia of renal failure. Most patients can maintain a hematocrit level of approximately 35% if given erythropoietin. These patients report an improvement in their sense of well-being. Transfusion should be reserved for situations in which active bleeding occurs or in cases in which the anemia is severe and unresponsive to erythropoietin, that is, the hematocrit is less than 14%. These patients also have a bleeding diathesis, because platelet function appears to be disturbed. It is a qualitative rather than a quantitative defect. This abnormality will reverse with dialysis alone.

Skeletal System

Osteomalacia and hyperparathyroidism often are seen together in uremia. Renal osteodystrophy includes osteitis fibrosa cystica, osteoporosis, osteomalacia, and osteosclerosis. Hyperparathyroidism results in subperiosteal resorption of bone and, rarely, brown tumor formation. Growth retardation in children and deforming skeletal rickets also occur. Chronic acidosis leads to the osteopenia and depression of skeletal growth in children. The osteomalacia may be a result of aluminum intoxication. The complications are fractures, aseptic necrosis of the hips, bone pain, and deformities. Treatment involves correction of serum phosphorus, usually with antacids that do not contain aluminum, and the administration of calcium supplements and dihydroxyvitamin D_3. (Care must be taken not to give calcium or vitamin D until the serum phosphorus is normal, because metastatic calcification will occur and damage many organs.) Parathyroidectomy is indicated if roentgenographic changes of hyperparathyroidism or metastatic calcification occur.

Arthropathy or joint pain is usually secondary to gout when there is hyperuricemia or to pseudogout when serum uric acid is relatively normal but serum calcium and phosphorus are both high. Both disorders respond to correction of the met abolic disturbances.

Metabolic Disturbances

Metabolic acidosis occurs late in the disease. Hypercalcemia occasionally occurs, usually as a result of secondary hyperparathyroidism or excessive calcium or vitamin D supplementation. Hyperuricemia is extremely common and generally is not associated with gout. Hypermagnesemia is common in patients who are not receiving dialysis. This can be significantly aggravated by compounds that contain magnesium (e.g., antacids). It is important not to give drugs that contain magnesium to patients with ESRD, because these patients are prone to magnesium intoxication.

Treatment

Currently, treatment of ESRD involves four basic approaches. Early in the disease dietary manipulation with the use of selected drugs to maintain serum electrolytes is all that is necessary. As the GFR falls below 10 mL per minute, either peritoneal dialysis or hemodialysis generally will be required. Renal transplantation is the ultimate therapy for the disorder.

Drug Administration

The kidneys are the major route of drug metabolism and secretion. Renal failure necessitates altered handling of most drugs and giving them in the usual dosages to uremic patients will lead to elevated blood levels, toxic symptoms, and perhaps even death. Antibiotics, sedatives,

TABLE 14.4. DRUGS TO AVOID IN UREMIC PATIENTS

Antimicrobials	Antihypertensives
Methenamine mandelate	Methyldopa
Nalidixic acid	Guanethidine
Nitrofurantoin	Reserpine
Tetracyclines (other than doxycycline or minocycline)	Diuretics
Neomycin	Acetazolamide
	Mercurials
Analgesics—narcotics	Triamterene
Salicylates	Spironolactone
Acetaminophen	Thiazides
Phenacetin	Arthritis—gout
Phenazopyridine	Gold salts
Meperidine	Probenecid
Morphine	Phenylbutazone
Sedatives—tranquilizers	Antineoplastics
Barbiturates	Nitrosourea
Glutethimide	Cisplatin
Lithium	Neuromuscular agents
Ethchlorvynol	Gallamine
Methaqualone	Pancuronium
Phenothiazines	Succinylcholine
Antacids—laxatives	Antiarrhythmics
With magnesium	Bretylium
With phosphate	Others
Mineral oil	Terbutaline
	Acetohexamide
	Chlorpropamide

TABLE 14.5. DRUGS REQUIRING MAJOR DOSAGE REVISION IN UREMIC PATIENTS

Antimicrobials	Cardiac glycosides
Aminoglycosides[a]	Digoxin
Cephalosporins[a]	Digitoxin
Penicillins[a]	Arthritis—gout
Polymyxins	Allopurinol
Vancomycin	Antineoplastics
Flucytosine[a]	Bleomycin
Trimethoprim-sulfamethoxazole	Cyclophosphamide[a]
Amantadine	Methotrexate
Analgesics—narcotics	Mithramycin
Salicylates[a]	Neuromuscular agents
Meperidine	Neostigmine
Morphine	Miscellaneous
Antiarrhythmics	Insulin
Procainamide[a]	Cimetidine[a]
Quinidine[a]	Clofibrate
N-acetylprocainamide[a]	Methimazole
Antihypertensives	Niacin
Clonidine	Propylthiouracil
Diazoxide[a]	
Nitroprusside[a]	

[a]Dialyzed significantly.

narcotics, and cardiovascular drugs often must be adjusted to an appropriate dosage level. Certain drugs should be totally avoided in uremic patients (Table 14.4). Drugs that commonly require altered dosage schedules are listed in Table 14.5.

REFERENCES

1. Addis T. *Glomerular nephritis: diagnosis and treatment.* New York: Macmillan, 1948:222.
2. Agmon Y, Buczis M. Acute renal failure: a multifactorial syndrome. *Contrib Nephrol* 1993;102:23.
3. Baek S, Makabali G. Clinical determinants of survival from postoperative renal failure. *Surg Gynecol Obstet* 1975;140:685.
4. Bailey RR, Lynn KL. End-stage reflux nephropathy. *Contrib Nephrol* 1984;39:102.
5. Bell RD, Keyl MJ, Shrader FR, et al. Renal lymphatics: the internal distribution. *Nephron* 1968;5:454.
6. Berkseth RO, Kjellstrand CM. Radiologic contrast-induced nephropathy. *Med Clin North Am* 1984;68:351.
7. Bonomini V, Stefoni S, Vangelista A. Long-term patient and renal prognosis in acute renal failure. *Nephron* 1984;36:169.
8. Brenner BM, Meyer TW, Hostetter TH. Dietary protein intake and the progressive nature of renal disease: the role of hemodynamically mediated injury in the pathogenesis of progressive glomerulosclerosis in aging, renal ablation and intrinsic renal disease. *N Engl J Med* 1982;307:652.
9. Bricker NS, Morris PAD, Kime JW Jr. The pathologic physiology of chronic Bright's disease: an exploration of the intact nephron hypothesis. *Am J Med* 1960;28:77.
10. Britton KE, Maisey MN. Renal radionuclide studies. In: Maisey MN, Britton KE, Gilday DL, eds. *Clinical nuclear medicine.* London: Chapman & Hill, 1983:99.
11. Brown CB, Ogg CS, Cameron JS. High-dose furosemide in acute renal failure: a controlled trial. *Clin Nephrol* 1981;15:90.
12. Burns KD, Homma T, Harris RC. The intrarenal renin-angiotensin system. *Semin Nephrol* 1993;13:13.
13. Caregaro L, Menon F, Angel P, et al. Limitations of serum creatinine level and creatinine clearance as filtration markers in cirrhosis. *Arch Intern Med* 1994;154:201.
14. Chevalier RL, Campbell F, Brenbridge AN. Prognostic factors in neonatal acute renal failure. *Pediatrics* 1984;74:265.
15. Conger JP. A controlled evaluation of prophylactic dialysis in post-traumatic case renal failure. *J Trauma* 1975;15:1056.
16. Corwin HL, Schreiber MJ, Fang LST. Low fractional excretion of sodium: occurrence with hemoglobinuric- and myoglobinuric-induced acute renal failure. *Arch Intern Med* 1984;144:981.
17. DeWardener HE, Herxheimer AW. The effect of a high water intake in the kidney's ability to concentrate the urine in man. *J Physiol (Lond)* 1957;139:42.
18. Drumond MC, Dean WM. Structural determinants of glomerular hydraulic permeability. *Am J Physiol* 1994;266:F1.
19. Dunn MJ. Renal prostaglandins. In: Dunn MJ, ed. *Renal endocrinology.* Baltimore: Williams & Wilkins, 1983.
20. Dunn MJ, Zambraski EJ. Renal effects of drugs that inhibit prostaglandin synthesis. *Kidney Int* 1980;18:609.
21. Eneas JF, Schoenfeld PY, Humphreys MH. The effect of infusion of mannitol-sodium bicarbonate on the clinical course of myoglobinuria. *Arch Intern Med* 1979;139:801.
22. Freund H, Atarmain S, Fischer J. Comparative study of parenteral nutrition in renal failure using essential and nonessential amino acid containing solutions. *Surg Gynecol Obstet* 1980; 151:652.

23. Funder JW. Aldosterone action. *Ann Rev Physiol* 1993;55:115.
24. Gabrielli A, Caruso L. Postoperative acute renal failure secondary to rhabdomyolysis from exaggerated lithotomy position. *J Clin Anesthesia* 1999;11:257.
25. Gates GF. Glomerular filtration rate: estimation from fractional renal accumulation of ^{99m}Tc-DPTA (stannous). *AJR Am J Roentgenol* 1982;138:565.
26. Graziani G, Cantaluppi A, Casati S, et al. Dopamine and furosemide in oliguric acute renal failure. *Nephron* 1984;37:39.
27. Hamm LL, Hering-Smith KS. Acid–base transport in the collecting duct. *Semin Nephrol* 1993;13:246.
28. Haut LL, Alfrey AC, Guggenheim S, et al. Renal toxicity of phosphate in rats. *Kidney Int* 1980;17:722.
29. Hermreck AS. The pathophysiology of acute renal failure. *Am J Surg* 1982;144:605.
30. Hull JH, Hals LJ, Koch GG, et al. Influence of range of renal functions and liver disease in predictability of creatinine clearance. *Clin Pharmacol Ther* 1981;29:516.
31. Humes HD, Liu S. Cellular and molecular basis of renal repair in acute renal failure. *J Lab Clin Med* 1994;124:749-754.
32. Ishikawa I, Saito Y, Shikura N, et al. Ten year prospective study on the development of renal cell carcinoma in dialysis patients. *Am J Kidney Dis* 1990;16:452.
33. Johnston CI, Fabris B, Jandeleit K. Intrarenal renin-angiotensin system in renal physiology and pathophysiology. *Kidney Int* 1993;44[Suppl 42]:S59.
34. Jovanovic DB, Djukanovic L. Analysis of factors influencing chronic renal failure progression. *Ren Fail* 1999;21:177-87.
35. Keane WF, Shapiro FL, Raij L. Incidence and type of infections occurring in 445 chronic hemodialysis patients. *Trans Am Soc Artif Intern Organs* 1977;23:41.
36. Koch ML, McDougal WS. Determination of renal function following urinary diversion through intestinal segments. *J Urol* 1985;133:517.
37. Koffler A, Friedler R, Massry S. Acute renal failure due to nontraumatic rhabdomyolysis. *Arch Intern Med* 1976;85:23.
38. Kon V, Ishikawa I. Physiology of acute renal failure. *J Pediatr* 1984;105:351.
39. Kurtzman NA. Chronic renal failure: metabolic and clinical consequences. *Hosp Pract* 1982;7:114.
40. Lees JA, Falk RM, Stone WJ, et al. Pyocystis, pyonephrosis, and perinephric abscess in end-stage renal disease. *J Urol* 1985; 134:716.
41. Levy EM, Viscol CM, Horwitz RI. The effect of acute renal failure on mortality—a cohort analysis. *JAMA* 1996;275:1489.
42. Loo MH, Marion DN, Vaughn ED. Failure of thromboxane inhibition to improve renal blood flow in dogs with complete unilateral ureteral obstruction. *Abstr Am Urol Assoc* 1985;63:129.
43. Maddox DA, Brenner BM. Glomerular ultrafiltrates. In: Brenner BM, ed. *Breamer & Restor's the kidney*. Philadelphia: WB Saunders, 2000:329.
44. McDougal WS. Pharmacologic preservation of renal mass and function in obstructive uropathy. *J Urol* 1982;128:418.
45. McDougal WS, Koch MO. Accurate determination of renal function in patients with ileal and colon interpositions in the urinary tract. *J Urol* 1986;135:1175.
46. McDougal WS, Rhodes RS, Persky L. A histochemical and morphologic study of postobstructive diuresis in the rat. *Invest Urol* 1976;14:169.
47. McDougal WS, Wright FS. Defect in proximal and distal sodium transport in post-obstructive diuresis. *Kidney Int* 1972; 2:304.
48. Montgomerie JZ, Kalmanson GM, Guze LB. Renal failure and infection. *Medicine* 1968;47:1.
49. Morrison AR, Nishikawa K, Needleman P. Unmasking of thromboxane A_2 synthesis by ureteral obstruction in the rabbit kidney. *Nature* 1977;267:259.
50. Mudge G. Nephrotoxicity of urographic radiocontrast drugs. *Kidney Int* 1980;19:540.
51. Muther RS. Drug interference with renal function tests. *Am J Kidney Dis* 1983;3:118.
52. Nanji AA, Campbell DJ. Falsely-elevated serum creatinine values in diabetic ketoacidosis-clinical implications. *Clin Biochem* 1981; 14:91.
53. Nsouli KA, Lazarus JM, Shoenbaum SC, et al. Bacteremic infection in hemodialysis. *Arch Intern Med* 1979;139:1255.
54. Oldrizzi L, Rugin C, Maschio G. Diet and chronic renal failure. *Contrib Nephrol* 1993;102:37.
55. Olson JL, Hostetter TH, Rennke HG, et al. Altered glomerular permeability and progressive sclerosis following ablation of renal mass. *Kidney Int* 1982;22:112.
56. Rascoff JH, Golden RA, Spinowitz BS, et al. Nondilated obstructive nephropathy. *Arch Intern Med* 1983;143:696.
57. Ronco C. Continuous renal replacement therapy for the treatment of acute renal failure in intensive care patients. *Clin Nephrol* 1993;40:187.
58. Rosen SM, Hollenberg NK, Dealy JB, et al. Measurement of the distribution of blood flow in the human kidney using the intra-arterial injection of ^{133}Xe: relationship to function in the normal and transplanted kidney. *Clin Sci* 1968;34:287.
59. Rouiller C, Muller AF. *The kidney*, vol. 1. New York: Academic Press, 1969.
60. Scandling JD, Myers BD. Glomerular size-selectivity and microalbuminuria in early diabetic glomerular disease. *Kidney Int* 1992;41:840.
61. Schrier RW. Acute renal failure. *Kidney Int* 1979;15:205.
62. Siegel NJ, Gunstream SK, Handler RI, et al. Renal function and cortical blood flow during the recovery phase of acute renal failure. *Kidney Int* 1977;12:199.
63. Stein JH, Lifschitz MD, Barnes LD. Current concepts in the pathophysiology of acute renal failure. *Am J Physiol* 1978;234: F171.
64. Synhaivsky A, Kurtz SB, Wochos DN, et al. Acute renal failure treated by slow-continuous ultrafiltration. *Mayo Clin Proc* 1983; 58:729.
65. Tiller DJ, Mudge GH. Pharmacologic agents used in the management of acute renal failure. *Kidney Int* 1980;18:700.
66. Topley N, Lameire N, Jörres A, et al, eds. Treatment of acute renal failure. *Kidney Int* 1998;54(6):1817.
67. Torres VE, Strong CG, Romero JC, et al. Indomethacin enhancement of glycerol-induced acute renal failure in rabbits. *Kidney Int* 1975;7:170.
68. Valtin H. *Renal function*. Boston: Little, Brown, 1983.
69. Volpe M. The physiologic role of atrial natriuretic factor. *Cardioscience* 1992;3:217.
70. Wingen AM, Fabian-Bach C, Schaefer F, et al. Randomised multicenter study of a low-protein diet on the progression of chronic renal failure in children. *Lancet* 1997;349:1117.
71. Zager R, Rubin N, Ebert T, et al. Rapid radioimmunoassay for diagnosing acute tubular necrosis. *Nephron* 1980;26:7.

Adult and Pediatric Urology, 4/e, edited by Jay Y. Gillenwater, John T. Grayhack, Stuart S. Howards, and Michael E. Mitchell.

15

ALTERNATIVE MEDICAL THERAPIES FOR UROLOGIC DISEASES

CHARLES E. MYERS, JR.

DIETARY SUPPLEMENT HEALTH AND EDUCATION ACT OF 1994

The past few years have witnessed a dramatic increase in the use of herbal products as well as other methods associated with alternative and complementary medicine. This has led to considerable attention on the part of the media, including a cover story in *Time* magazine. Estimates of the amount spent on supplements yearly generally are in excess of one billion dollars per year. Recent reports document that supplement use is common among prostate cancer patients. Unfortunately, these studies also show that patients often do not share this information with their physicians. During my initial visit with patients, I often find that patients spend more on supplements than they do on prescription medications.

What has fueled this shift toward herbal and nutritional supplements? Many patients view herbal products as offering a gentler, more natural form of therapy with fewer side effects. Although this may be true for some supplements, such as valerian, the side effects of many herbal products simply have not been publicized adequately. There is no question that it is much more convenient and pleasant to visit the local health food store than to make an appointment to see a physician, get a prescription, and have it filled. For many patients, this is then followed by a battle to have the cost reimbursed by an insurance company. The use of herbal products also puts the patient in control of his or her treatment.

As the American public turned their attention to natural healing products, the political and legal environment also began to change. One key event was the passage by Congress of a major new law governing the marketing and sale of these products. This law, called the *Dietary Supplement Health and Education Act of 1994,* severely restricted the ability of the U.S. Food and Drug Administration (FDA) to regulate supplements (9). This act represents the result of a struggle, dating back to the early 1960s, between the FDA and forces seeking to provide Americans with less restricted access to supplements. In this process, the FDA has managed to assemble a consistent pattern of failure in the courts and in Congress.

Two elements characterized the FDA strategy. Their stance was that supplements were either unapproved drugs or they were unapproved food additives. If they were drugs, then they had to pass the same review processes that a drug would. If they were to be used as a food additive, they had to pass through the strict review process that a new food additive would pass through. The supplement industry argued that it could not afford to take either path because of the limited profit potential involved. After all, at the end they would not have the exclusivity our system guarantees a new prescription drug.

The FDA sought to restrict the distribution of information on supplements in the form of books, articles, or pamphlets. In this effort, they attacked balanced and scien-

C.E. Myers, Jr.: Professor of Medicine and Urology, University of Virginia School of Medicine, Charlottesville, VA 22908.

tifically sound as well as distorted and misleading material. The stance was that in any case these represented a marketing effort for unapproved food additives or drugs. In one case, the FDA objected to health food stores selling an herbal product and books on that same product. In the process, they managed to gain the opposition of free speech advocates, further complicating their political and legal difficulties.

The passage of the Dietary Supplement Health and Education Act of 1994 represented a clear repudiation of the FDA position. It is worthwhile to directly quote some of the text of this Act so that you can get a sense of the will of Congress.

> Despite a voluminous scientific record indicating the potential health benefits of dietary supplements, the Food and Drug Administration has pursued a heavy-handed enforcement agenda against dietary supplements for over 30 years. The agency's approach has forced the Congress to intervene on two previous occasions, and yet again with the adoption of S.784.

Key aspects of the Act represent a clear statement of differing philosophy than the philosophy that dominated the FDA and much of establishment medicine.

- "There is a link between the ingestion of certain nutrients or dietary supplements and the prevention of chronic diseases such as cancer, heart disease, and osteoporosis."
- "Healthful diets may mitigate the need for expensive medical procedures, such as coronary bypass surgery or angioplasty."
- "Preventive health measures, including education, good nutrition, and appropriate use of safe nutritional supplements will limit the incidence of chronic diseases, and reduce long-term health expenditures."
- "There is a growing need for emphasis on the dissemination of information linking nutrition and long-term health."
- "Consumers should be empowered to make choices about preventative health care programs based on data from scientific studies on health benefits related to particular dietary supplements."
- "Studies indicate that consumers are placing increasing reliance on the use of nontraditional health care providers to avoid the excessive costs of traditional medical services and to obtain more holistic considerations of their needs."
- "Dietary supplements are safe within a broad range of intake, and safety problems with supplements are relatively rare."
- "Legislative action that protects the right of access of consumers to safe dietary supplements is necessary in order to promote wellness."

This Act countered FDA strategy in several ways. First, they declared dietary supplements were foods, not drugs. Instead, they created a new category of food by specifically defining dietary supplements to include dietary ingredients such as vitamins, minerals, herbs or other botanicals, amino acids, or other dietary supplements. A dietary supplement must be intended for ingestion, such as a tablet, capsule, powder, soft gel, gelcap, or liquid form. The Act also specifically states that customers can be provided with publications on supplements in connection with the sale of the dietary supplements. These publications must not be false or misleading, not promote a specific brand of supplement, and provide a balanced view of the available scientific literature. In the store, it must be physically separated from the supplement.

The Act allowed supplements to carry claims that they help preserve general well-being. In addition, they can claim that they help preserve the structure or function of parts of the body. However, they cannot state that the supplements are effective treatment of any disease, because this would be a drug claim. This section of the Act has been the subject of continual discussion and litigation between the FDA and representatives of the supplement industry. In retrospect, this aspect of the Act was not well thought out and was probably not enforceable.

The case of lovastatin is a good example of some of the difficulties involved in distinguishing a drug from a supplement. Lovastatin is an FDA-approved drug for the treatment of elevated cholesterol, marketed by Merck as Mevacor. However, lovastatin also can be found in a range of natural products such as oyster mushrooms and a form of red yeast used in China to season rice, and ingestion of these natural products will lower cholesterol levels. Extract of red yeast is now being marketed to people concerned about heart disease and information about its lovastatin content is widely available. As far as I can determine, there is no reason why, milligram for milligram, lovastatin in this red yeast extract is not as active as that in Mevacor. Yet, red yeast extract must be marketed as a supplement with an obscure structure-function claim about preserving the structure and function of the heart, whereas Mevacor is marketed specifically for its ability to lower cholesterol: once in the body, they act identically.

The end result of this Act has been mixed. There is no doubt that Americans now have much greater access to nutritional or herbal supplements. However, these supplements range radically in their value. Among these supplements are therapeutic agents with a strong scientific basis and proven clinical value. Most of these lack FDA approval because no company has been willing to take them through the expensive process the FDA mandates. In contrast, other herbal products have no scientific basis and no sound clinical trial documentation of efficacy, and even pose a health risk.

The Act specifically empowers the FDA to oversee quality control of supplements and they are given the power to remove unsafe supplements from the market. In practice, this process has not worked very well. The plain fact is that the quality of supplements on the market is variable. Studies have shown that supplements from some manufacturers can contain 25% or less of the active ingredient than stated on the label. It also appears that supplements on the market are not adequately monitored for hazardous contaminants.

It would appear that there is a great need for increased regulatory supervision of the supplement industry. It would be best if Americans were ensured of the potency and safety of the supplements they purchase. While we wait for these changes, there are some promising trends. Several major pharmaceutical firms have purchased supplement companies and this promises improvement in quality control and standardization. In addition, several major supplement manufacturers are funding clinical trials that specifically document the value of their herbal extracts.

STRESS

Time and again, patients relate how their prostate cancer appeared to develop following a period of stress. They then commonly ask if the stress was responsible for the fact that they now had cancer. Evidence from laboratory experiments do suggest that the stress hormones, epinephrine, norepinephrine, and cortisol, may play a role in the progression of prostate cancer. Patients often turn to alternative or complementary medicine for tools effective in the management of stress.

Problems with the Stress Response

It is important to realize that this stress response is very much designed to handle acute problems. When humans or other mammals are subjected to chronic stress, the continuous elevation of cortisol and catecholamines delays healing; suppresses the immune system; and contributes to high blood pressure, heart disease, and diabetes. Other diseases, such as duodenal ulcers, ulcerative colitis, rheumatoid arthritis, and psoriasis, also worsen during periods of stress. In essence, we are best designed by nature for a life where acute stress is followed by periods of peace and security.

Much of modern thinking about the biology of stress is based on the work of the Canadian scientist, Hans Selye (87). Through elegant laboratory experimentation and astute observation of human behavior, Selye developed a theoretic basis for analyzing the impact of stress that is still useful more than half a century after he first articulated these ideas. He pointed out that there were two distinct types of stress: distress and eustress. Distress would be loss of a job, death of a loved one, threat of debt, or similar events. Eustress would be the excitement associated with skiing down a mountain, reading an exciting novel, watching a football game, a new love, or other consuming passion. Although chronic distress obviously is not good, too much eustress also is a problem. Indeed, blood levels of catecholamines and cortisol elevate in response to both distress and eustress. The conclusion of this line of thinking is that it is important to keep a balance between periods of distress and eustress and periods of peace and quiet.

TABLE 15.1. SIGNS OF STRESS

▪ Forgetfulness	▪ Irritability
▪ Insomnia	▪ Substance abuse
▪ Altered eating habits	

How can you judge the stress in a patient's life? I have found the stress scale developed by Miller and Rahe to be particularly useful (72). A sense of perspective is necessary in interpreting the results of this test. People differ in how well they tolerate stress. One person may become sick from stress-related illness even though his or her total score on this test may be relatively low. Others tolerate and even prefer a relatively high level of stress. In fact, some people appear to be addicted to catecholamines and only feel fully alive when they are under a high level of stress.

What are some of the symptoms that might tell you when your patients are under too much stress (Table 15.1)? They may find it difficult to concentrate or experience forgetfulness. They may awaken in the middle of the night with their minds churning over unresolved problems from the previous day. They may find that they have lost their appetite or suddenly find themselves overeating. They may become impatient or intolerant of others. They may find themselves losing their temper over minor issues. Their blood pressure may suddenly become higher or other stress-related diseases may worsen. It is important for you to become attuned to how your patients respond to stress and to develop a sense for when you need to advise them of the need to decrease life's stress. I think that having them take the Miller and Rahe stress test will help you recognize when stress has become too much.

Epinephrine and Prostate Biology

The prostate gland is well supplied with sympathetic nerves. Activation of these sympathetic nerves plays a central role in ejaculation: without their activity, men experience a dry ejaculation. Obviously, this involves a sudden surge in sympathetic nerve activity. What about catecholamines from the adrenal medulla? Experiments in dogs indicate that ejaculation is fostered by a sudden increase in catecholamine release from the adrenal medulla plus action by the prostatic sympathetic nerves (Table 15.2).

What about chronic activation of the prostatic sympathetic nerves? Lee and his colleagues from Northwestern University in Chicago showed that if one cuts the sympathetic nerves to the prostate gland, it shrinks (70,71,98). If one cuts the sympathetic nerves to one side of the prostate

TABLE 15.2. CATECHOLAMINES AND THE PROSTATE

▪ Important for ejaculation ▪ Enhances response to testosterone and epidermal growth factor by normal and malignant prostatic epithelial cells	▪ Blockade of α_1-adrenoreceptors leads to apoptosis of prostatic epithelial cells and associated stroma

gland, that side will shrink. It appears that activity of the sympathetic nerves act in conjunction with testosterone to allow the prostate gland to reach its mature size.

These findings suggest that catecholamines stimulate the growth and/or survival of prostate cells. Direct evidence of this comes largely from the work of Kyprianou from the University of Maryland (22,60). When catecholamines interact with cells, they act through proteins found on the surface of these cells. These proteins, called *adrenoreceptors,* bind to the catecholamines and trigger the cell's response. A wide range of different adrenoreceptors are found in tissues throughout the body. Drug companies have made use of this fact to develop drugs that block the action of only one adrenoreceptor type at a time. Examples of this are the drugs Hytrin, Cardura, and Flomax. These drugs are selective for α_1-adrenoreceptors. Activation of the α_1-adrenoreceptors in the bladder and urethra blocks the flow of urine out of the bladder. Hytrin, Cardura, and Flomax block these α_1-adrenoreceptors, causing relaxation of the muscles in the urethra and bladder, making it easier for men to urinate.

These same α_1-adrenoreceptors also are found on the cells that line the ducts of the prostate gland and the fibroblasts that make up the support network for the gland. Kyprianou and others have shown that the α_1-adrenoreceptor–blocking drugs cause prostate lining cells and the fibroblasts to die. The same appears to be true, at least in the laboratory, for human prostate cancer cells.

How do catecholamines foster the growth and survival of human prostate cancer cells? The best insight into this issue comes from research done by Weber at the University of Virginia. All growth signals coming from cell surface receptors do so by activating an enzyme called *mitogen-activated protein* (MAP) kinase. Epidermal growth factor is one of the most important growth and survival factors for human prostate cancer cells. This growth factor acts by binding to a protein on the surface of these cells that is called the *epidermal growth factor receptor.* The resulting growth signal causes activation of MAP kinase, resulting in increased cancer cell growth. Catecholamines dramatically increase the ability of epidermal growth factor to activate MAP kinase (21).

Stress also has been shown to impair the function of the immune system. The function of natural killer cells appears to be consistently decreased following stress. This may be important for cancer patients because natural killer cells have the capacity to kill cancer cells. Natural killer cells have adrenoreceptors on their surface, and activation of these receptors by norepinephrine or epinephrine blocks the effectiveness of these immune cells. The adrenoreceptor in this case is a β-receptor rather than the α-receptor involved in prostate biology. In the laboratory and in tissue culture, drugs that block the β_2-receptor protect natural killer cells during periods of stress.

In summary, stress causes an increase in the release of epinephrine and norepinephrine from sympathetic nerve endings and from the adrenal medulla. These catecholamines stimulate the response of prostate cells, normal or malignant, to epidermal growth factor and testosterone. In addition, these catecholamines suppress the function of the immune system. If these factors are biologically important, it would be predicted that prostate cancer cells would spread preferentially to the adrenal gland. This is indeed the case. Recent detailed autopsy studies performed in men showed that the adrenal gland is the fourth most common site involved in metastatic prostate cancer (15).

Medical Approaches to Stress Reduction

The benzodiazepines are the most widely prescribed anxiety-relieving drugs. This drug class includes diazepam (Valium), chlordiazepoxide hydrochloride (Librium), and alprazolam (Xanax). The latter is now commonly used to relieve anxiety in cancer patients. There are several problems with the benzodiazepines. The most disturbing issue is that these drugs can be addicting (66). They also can impair coordination, leading to falls, accidents, and motor vehicle crashes. In addition, people treated chronically with these drugs can be troubled by loss of intellectual function. Both loss of coordination and impaired intellectual function are markedly increased if alcohol consumption follows ingestion of these drugs.

Buspirone and antidepressants, such as venlafaxine hydrochloride (Effexor), appear to circumvent many of these problems. Effexor may worsen high blood pressure, and in this situation, sertraline hydrochloride (Zoloft) has been found to be of value. These drugs are much less likely to impair coordination or intellectual function. In addition, they are safer to take in conjunction with recreational use of alcohol. Finally, their use is much less likely to result in addiction. However, as a note of caution, buspirone and the serotonin-reuptake inhibitor class of antidepressants can elevate circulating prolactin levels. Because prolactin promotes the growth and survival of prostatic epithelial cells, it is theoretically possible that these antianxiety drugs might adversely affect the outcome of treatment for prostate cancer.

A number of herbal products are reported to reduce stress. Valerian root is probably the best documented of these (31,59). Valerian is mildly sedating, has no addiction potential, and seems quite safe. Its major limitation is that it appears to be less effective than Effexor or buspirone in lessening anxiety.

Drug-free Stress Reduction

Most communities of any size have programs where patients are taught stress reduction techniques. Often, these are associated with progressive community hospitals or other community-based health care delivery organizations. For many patients, these programs are of great value.

Most of these stress reduction programs are based on what is called the *relaxation response* (Table 15.3). During this response, pulse rate and blood pressure drop, the flow of blood to the hands and feet improves, and brain wave frequency slows (8,18,52). This occurs when a person places himself or herself in a quiet, pleasant environment and focuses his or her attention on something neutral and nonthreatening, such as a single candle flame or fish in an aquarium.

Many men are reluctant to engage in these techniques. Some of them are associated with religious or political connotations with which they may not agree. A relatively simple approach will give your patient a sense of what is involved.

First, find a comfortable chair in a quiet, pleasant place. After the patient has relaxed, take his blood pressure.

Have him pick some short word or syllable that he will repeat over and over again. In Hindu meditation, they use the word *om,* but the patient can just as easily use the word one, five, six, or ten. The key is that it should either have no emotional connotation or a pleasant one.

Next, have the patient close his eyes and repeat the chosen word or syllable. While he does this, have him purge his thoughts of any other concern. He also should try to ignore his surroundings and focus on the rhythm of the repeating word. He should continue this for 20 minutes. At the end of this period, his pulse and blood pressure should be remeasured; nearly always both will have declined significantly.

Patients should approach this with the idea that they are learning a new skill, like playing tennis or golf. They should expect that their comfort and skill will improve with practice. It is a common experience for people to think their initial attempts at meditation are failures. Even when they think they have not done well, it is very likely that engaging in this relaxation response will have had considerable impact on their stress level. If the patient plans to use the relaxation response optimally, he should plan to set aside 20 minutes at least once and, preferably, twice per day.

TABLE 15.3. RELAXATION RESPONSE

- Easy to elicit
- Decrease in pulse rate
- Decrease in blood pressure
- Increase in blood flow to hands and feet
- Decrease in blood catecholamine levels

Will the relaxation response alter the progression of prostate cancer? There have been no clinical trials testing this idea. What we can say is that the relaxation response will lead to a decrease in blood epinephrine levels and a decrease in the activity of the sympathetic nervous system. As we have seen, there is a scientific basis for the hypothesis that blood epinephrine concentration and activation of the sympathetic nervous system might increase the growth of prostate cancer cells. At the very least, this technique may lessen the impact of stress on your patient's health and anxiety level.

ANTIOXIDANTS

Antioxidants represent one of the most common supplement classes ingested by prostate cancer patients. Widely used examples include vitamin C; vitamin E; selenium; and plant polyphenols, such as those from green tea, grape seed, and pine bark. A growing body of scientific and clinical work supports the use of these compounds by patients with cancer and other diseases.

Antioxidant Defense Network

Many biochemical reactions essential for life carry with them the threat of oxidative damage to the tissues of the body. For example, the process by which mitochondria produce the adenosine triphosphate (ATP) that drives your muscles and other tissues creates side products such as hydrogen peroxide that can damage tissues by oxidation. Exposure to sunlight can enhance oxidative damage to skin cells. Chemicals that naturally occur in food can cause oxidative damage. We are able to safely eat these foods only because our bodies do such a great job defending us against oxidative damage; fava beans can cause severe injury if consumed by people who lack the normal defenses against oxidative damage.

It is now known that the body has a comprehensive antioxidant defense network in which each component part has a role to play (25,44). What are the components of this antioxidant defense network?

One group of enzymes function to destroy or detoxify common oxidants. For example, hydrogen peroxide is one oxidant commonly formed as a byproduct as the tissues in the body perform their daily tasks. Several enzymes are capable of detoxifying hydrogen peroxide. The enzyme catalase binds two hydrogen peroxide molecules together to form oxygen and water. A second family of enzymes, called *glutathione peroxidases,* reduces hydrogen peroxide to water. Most of the known glutathione peroxidases require selenium.

A second group of components are vitamins that act as antioxidants. Vitamins C and E are prominent members of this group. Vitamin C is soluble in water and acts as an antioxidant in the water phase of the cell. Vitamin E is soluble in body fat and other lipids, but not in water. For this reason, vitamin E acts as an antioxidant for body lipids.

A third group of components is the dietary antioxidants. It is now apparent that most vegetables and grains contain antioxidants. Tomatoes contain the red pigment, lycopene. Green tea contains antioxidant polyphenols. Onions and garlic have large amounts of sulfur-containing chemicals that are strong antioxidants. Fruits such as blueberries, strawberries, and raspberries are another rich source of antioxidants. It now appears that these plant antioxidants act to bolster the effectiveness of other members of the antioxidant network.

The final component of the antioxidant defense network is a group of proteins that sequester iron and copper. This is important because free iron and copper can stimulate the conversion of peroxides into free radicals that rapidly react with and destroy normal tissues. Under normal conditions, this system is so effective that free iron and copper do not exist in body fluids or tissues. When sequestration of iron fails, it causes hemochromatosis and hemosiderosis. When sequestration of copper fails, it causes Wilson's disease.

When all four components of the antioxidant defense network are functioning optimally, the body can effectively handle attack by a wide range of oxidants without sustaining serious injury. Oxidative damage can include injury to DNA, the genetic material in a cell. This genetic damage can foster the development of cancer or promote the progression of cancer from a slow-growing local problem to one that grows and spreads rapidly. Thus a fully functioning antioxidant network can lower the risk that cancer will develop. However, this network operates so that various components overlap in their function, so that a deficiency in one component can be compensated by the others. For example, a low level of vitamin E may not be of great consequence if selenium, vitamin C, and dietary antioxidants are present at optimal levels. This is an important point to keep in mind when reading the results of clinical trials: any antioxidant can appear to have no impact if the subjects are taking in large amounts of other antioxidants and/or are not exposed to significant oxidant stress. Conversely, if the people in the trial are all subject to some oxidative stress, antioxidants may prove more effective than they would in normal subjects. For example, cigarette smoking subjects the body to increased oxidative stress and smokers may have a greater need for antioxidants than nonsmokers. This will prove important when we discuss some of the clinical trials involving antioxidants and prostate cancer.

Oxidants and the Development of Prostate Cancer

Why should antioxidants alter the risk of dying from prostate cancer? Wilding and his colleagues from the University of Wisconsin have published a series of papers that provide a possible answer to this question (83,84). They have shown that prostate cancer cells exposed to testosterone produce hydrogen peroxide and other oxidants. This led them to propose that testosterone exposure results in the production of oxidants that cause genetic damage. Genetic damage can play a role in the progression as well as the genesis of cancer. The implication of this line of research is that strengthening the antioxidant network may lessen the risk of developing prostate cancer. It may also slow the progression of this disease from a slow-growing cancer limited to the prostate gland to one that has spread throughout the body and become resistant to all therapies. Several antioxidants may alter the natural history of prostate cancer.

Selenium

Over the past few years, our knowledge about selenium and its effects on living organisms has increased dramatically. A search of the National Library of Medicine's online database, PubMed, shows more than 1,000 scientific articles published on selenium since January 1998.

One major factor behind this surge in interest about the health effects of selenium has been Clark and colleague's 1996 publication of a large, randomized, controlled clinical trial that demonstrated a marked reduction in cancer deaths associated with increased selenium intake (23,24). This trial was initiated in 1983 as a randomized controlled trial testing the impact of supplementation with 200 μg of selenium-yeast per day on the risk of skin cancer. This clinical trial enrolled 1,300 individuals residing in the Mid-Atlantic Coastal Plain from Virginia to South Carolina, an area long known to have low soil and water selenium levels. After 10 years, the overall cancer death rate was 50% lower in the subjects taking selenium as compared with the control group (Table 15.4). The cancers responsible for this difference were carcinomas of the prostate, colon, and lung: prostate cancer deaths were decreased by 64%, colon cancer by 40%, and lung cancer by 30%. The four major causes of cancer death are those of the lung, prostate, colon, and breast. Thus selenium dramatically reduced the death rate of

TABLE 15.4. SELENIUM

- Deficiency exists where high rainfall and acid soils are present
- 200 μg of selenium per day reduces prostate cancer deaths by 60%–70%
- The 200-μg dose is recognized as safe and costs $0.10 per day
- Markedly enhances cytotoxic T-cell activity in cancer patients

three of the four most common causes of cancer death in the United States. Furthermore, no cases of selenium toxicity were reported among the people in this trial who took selenium supplements for years.

Selenium and Prostate Cancer

Since the publication of Clark's paper, there has been one major study designed to test the validity of his findings. In his paper, Clark reported on the correlation between serum selenium levels and the risk of prostate cancer. One criticism of this approach is that serum selenium levels are just a "snap shot" of selenium levels at one point in time, whereas the development of prostate cancer takes many years and is more likely to be influenced by the average selenium level during that time period. Hair and nails are formed at the rate of approximately 1 mm per day, and thus hair or nail clippings are a better estimate of average selenium level. Giovannucci, from the Harvard School of Public Health, examined the selenium content of nail clippings from approximately 34,000 men and found that the risk of developing metastatic prostate cancer decreased as the selenium content of the nail clippings increased (103). When Giovannucci compared the men with the highest and lowest nail selenium content, he found a 65% reduction in the risk of metastatic prostate cancer.

What is the next step in this line of investigation? The National Cancer Institute (NCI) has just funded a large, randomized, controlled trial in which men will be randomized between control, vitamin E, selenium, and vitamin E plus selenium. Colteman, from the University of Texas, San Antonio, is the lead investigator on this clinical trial.

Selenium and the Immune System

A number of studies suggest adequate selenium levels are necessary for proper function of the immune system. The most convincing study is a randomized, controlled clinical trial in patients with head and neck cancer (56). Most patients with this cancer exhibit depression of the immune system. Cytotoxic T cells and natural killer cells are the most important parts of the immune system in terms of resistance to cancer. Natural killer cell function usually is profoundly depressed in head and neck cancer patients. Cytotoxic T-cell number and function also are commonly suppressed. Patients in this study all had untreated squamous carcinoma of the head and neck and were randomized to placebo or selenium at a dosage of 200 µg per day for 8 weeks. This trial was double blind, which means that neither the patients nor the doctors knew who was receiving placebo or selenium until the study was completed.

Plasma selenium levels were measured at the start and during the trial to ensure patients took the selenium as directed. During the 8 weeks, 88.3% of the patients took the assigned selenium dose. At the start of the trial, the average selenium levels in the two groups were 91.3 and 94.4 µg/L of blood plasma. After 8 weeks of selenium supplementation, the average selenium level increased from 91.3 to 105.3 µg/L.

Despite this minor increase in plasma selenium, there were major changes in the immune system. In the patients on placebo, cytotoxic T cells killed only 7% of the tumor cells. After 8 weeks of selenium supplementation, the T cells were able to kill 78% of the tumor cell targets. This is a rather remarkable shift given the short duration of treatment and small increase in selenium levels. To place these findings in perspective, in the Clark study, prolonged administration of the same dose of selenium, 200 µg per day, eventually increased the selenium levels to close to 200 µg/L, rather than the 105.3 µg/L after 8 weeks reported in this paper on head and neck cancer.

Other lines of evidence show the importance of the antioxidant defense network and selenium in protecting the immune system. HIV-1, the virus that causes AIDS, kills because it destroys T cells that are important in the immune response. HIV-1 increases oxidant stress in the T cells at the same time as it appears to weaken key elements of the antioxidant defense system. Selenium plays a major role in the ability of glutathione to act as an antioxidant. A selenium-containing protein, glutathione peroxidase, uses glutathione to convert hydrogen peroxide to water. Without selenium, glutathione peroxidase is unable to accomplish this task. Given this background, the fact that children and adults infected with HIV-1 live much longer if their selenium levels are adequate is not surprising (10,17).

In addition, one additional study examined restoration of normal immune function in the elderly by selenium combined with other nutrients. This study by Girodon, from the Scientific and Technical Institute for Foods and Nutrition, Conservatiore National des Arts et Metiers, Paris, involved a group of institutionalized elderly patients (40). It showed that 20 mg of zinc and 100 µg of selenium significantly increased antibody response to influenza vaccine and decreased the risk of upper respiratory infection.

Selenium and Viral Infections

In addition to its effects on the immune system, selenium can have a direct effect on the progress of viral infections (12). This is best studied in a virus called *coxsackie B.* Although not a household name, coxsackie B infections are common, and this virus can cause serious, life-threatening illness. Coxsackie virus infections typically start in the gastrointestinal (GI) tract, where they can cause nausea, vomiting, and diarrhea. From there, the virus can enter the blood stream and spread throughout the body. This virus can attack the nervous system, causing a disease that results in paralysis similar to that caused by polio. Coxsackie virus can enter muscles, where it can cause severe muscle damage and pain. For example, it can infect the muscles of the rib cage that are used to breathe and make it very painful to take a deep breath. When this virus enters the heart muscle, the damage can be sufficient to require a heart transplant. In fact, coxsackie B virus infections are one of the leading reasons for heart transplant.

The link between selenium and coxsackie B virus starts in China. In the Keshan province of China, soil and water contain little selenium. Residents of this area can have daily intakes of selenium of less than 20 µg per day, compared with 200 µg per day in Clark's trial. Residents of Keshan can develop a form of fatal heart failure called *Keshan's disease.* However, this disease does not occur in residents of this area who manage to receive more than 20 µg of selenium per day. Subsequent studies showed that a disease similar to Keshan disease can be found in several parts of China, all of which are selenium deficient. In addition to being limited to geographic regions low in selenium, Keshan disease only appeared during certain seasons of the year: summer in Southern China and winter in Northern China. Seasonal patterns like this are characteristic of disease of infectious origin. This led the Chinese to isolate viruses from the hearts of people who had succumbed to Keshan's disease. Coxsackie B virus emerged as a common isolate. The Chinese scientists then showed that coxsackie B virus would infect mice and cause heart damage. Furthermore, the damage was much worse in mice on a low selenium diet compared with those on a high selenium diet.

This phenomenon was subsequently investigated by Beck from the University of North Carolina, Chapel Hill (12). Several strains of coxsackie B virus that are able to infect mice are available. These strains differ in the severity of the infection they cause in the mice, ranging from those causing mild disease to those that cause serious illness. Beck showed that the viral strains causing serious illness did much less damage to mice on high selenium diets compared with those on low selenium diets. Of even greater interest, when a viral strain that normally caused mild disease was allowed to infect a selenium-deficient mouse, the virus was permanently altered into a virus that would cause severe disease. Beck then showed that this change in viral virulence induced by selenium was always associated with the same genetic changes. In other words, passage of a mild virus in a selenium-deficient animal caused changes in the genetics of the virus, rendering it much more dangerous. This is currently the best explanation for why severe selenium deficiency can result in potentially fatal heart damage.

Vitamin E deficiency also worsens the impact of coxsackie B virus infection on the heart. In addition, when a mild form of the virus infects vitamin E–deficient mice, it becomes more virulent, just as it did in selenium-deficient mice. Again, the evidence shows that the antiviral activity is not specific for selenium, but reflects the fact that an optimally functioning antioxidant network suppresses the progression of coxsackie B virus.

Selenium and Heavy Metals

Metals such as arsenic, lead, mercury, cadmium, and thallium are all poisonous. Furthermore, industrial uses of these metals have led to large-scale environmental contamination. One of these metals, cadmium, has been specifically implicated as a cause of prostate cancer. Selenium alters the toxicity of heavy metal ions in several ways (99,105). It is important to note that selenium can bind these metal ions into complexes not soluble in water. To a certain extent, selenium can bind to these metal ions in the GI tract, diminishing the absorption of both selenium and the toxic metals. Once selenium has been absorbed, it can form complexes with these metal ions, lessening or delaying the toxicity of these metal ions. One of the side benefits of taking selenium supplements to decrease the risk of prostate cancer or to slow its progression is protection from the toxicity of these metal ions.

TABLE 15.5. DOSAGE FORMS OF SELENIUM

▪ Selenium-yeast	▪ Selenomethionine
▪ Sodium selenate	▪ Selenocysteine
▪ Sodium selenite	▪ Selenodiglutathione

Selenium Dose

A daily selenium dose of 400 µg per day is now recognized as the maximum safe daily dose. This number may be increased as studies currently in progress are completed. In Clark's study, a dose of 200 µg of selenium-yeast was ingested for years without a single reported side effect, but with a major impact on cancer deaths. A number of additional studies, both short and long term, document the safety and effectiveness of this dose of selenium.

Forms of Selenium

Commercially available selenium supplements come in a wide range of chemical forms (Table 15.5). The most widely available form is as selenium-yeast, and 200 µg per day costs about 10 cents. This is also the form used in Clark's study.

Unfortunately, some individuals are allergic to selenium-yeast. Selenomethionine also is widely available and appears safe. However, selenomethionine is not directly used by any of the selenium-requiring proteins in the body. Instead, it gets randomly taken up by all proteins in the body. After these proteins are broken down, the selenium gets recycled into biologically useful forms. Thus although it eventually acts to reverse selenium deficiency, it would not offer the rapid reversal most cancer patients might desire.

Sodium selenate and selenite are available and are rapidly reduced in the body to selenide. The latter is rapidly incorporated into the key selenoproteins in the body. The only disadvantage of these selenium salts is that their absorption from the GI tract is not consistent.

Selenocysteine is the form of selenium that is directly incorporated into the key selenoproteins in the body. Selenocysteine is commercially available and also is present in preparations such as selenoglutathione or selenodiglutathione.

Vitamin E

Vitamin E is soluble in lipids, but not in water. As a result, it largely acts to prevent oxidative damage to the lipids in a cell. In laboratory studies, vitamin E has been shown to act in concert with antioxidants present in the cytosol, such as vitamin C, glutathione, and selenium.

The first evidence that vitamin E might alter the progression of prostate cancer came as an unexpected result of a clinical trial designed to test the role of this vitamin in the prevention of lung cancer in smokers. In this trial, approximately 23,000 male cigarette smokers were randomized to placebo, beta-carotene, vitamin E, or beta-carotene plus vitamin E (48). At the point where men had been on the trial for 5 to 8 years, death rates from prostate cancer were 40% less in the men taking vitamin E alone compared with placebo. In contrast, the men taking beta-carotene experienced a 30% increase in mortality from this malignancy. The group taking beta-carotene plus vitamin E were not significantly different from the control group.

Vitamin E is not a single chemical substance, but a name given to a family of fat-soluble antioxidants (Table 15.6). These compounds differ in their content in foods as well as their ability to act as antioxidants. Although alpha-tocopherol is widely available and the form most commonly is used in laboratory and clinical studies, it is not the most active antioxidant. Recently, the work of two groups suggests that alpha-tocopherol may also not be the most active against cancer cells, including those of the prostate.

Moyad and Pienta, from the University of Michigan, have recently reported that gamma-tocopherol is more active against prostate cancer cells than is the alpha form of this vitamin (74). In contrast, other groups have found gamma-tocopherol no more active than alpha-tocopherol as an anticancer agent (42,53,69). Instead, they have found the most active tocopherol is the delta form. In addition, tocotrienols are considerably more active than the corresponding tocopherols, and the most active preparation currently available commercially is concentrated palm oil tocotrienols. Finally, vitamin E succinate appears to exert anticancer activity equal to or greater than any of the naturally occurring tocopherols or tocotrienols.

There is now evidence that vitamin E kills prostate cancer cells by a unique mechanism. All cells in the body have the capacity to commit "suicide." This suicide can be triggered by several means. One means of accomplishing this is by activating certain proteins, called *death receptors,* on the surface of cells. These death receptor proteins are designed so that when they are activated, the cell bearing them rapidly destroys itself. One of the most common of these proteins is called *Fas.* When vitamin E–like chemicals kill prostate cancer cells, Fas rapidly appears on the surface of the prostate cancer cells and appears to undergo activation, leading to cell death. These findings suggest that vitamin E does more than prevent genetic damage caused by oxidants released as a result of testosterone exposure. In fact, it may well be that vitamin E–like molecules actually may be orally active chemotherapeutic agents with low toxicity. This concept has led at least one group to chemically synthesize analogs of vitamin E with the hope of increasing the anticancer activity of this family of compounds.

TABLE 15.6. VARIOUS TOCOPHEROL AND TOCOTRIENOLS

Alpha-tocopherol	Alpha-tocotrienol
Beta-tocopherol	Beta-tocotrienol
Gamma-tocopherol	Gamma-tocotrienol
Delta-tocopherol	Delta-tocotrienol

Plant Monophenols and Polyphenols

Plant phenols are one of the most potent groups of antioxidants. They can occur as monophenols or as clusters of monophenols, called *polyphenols.* Polyphenols are found in a wide range of plant products that have health benefits.

Green Tea

Green tea intake has been associated with a decreased risk of cancers of the prostate, colon, pancreas, skin, and other organs (2,62,93). It seems that green tea prevents the damage caused by a large number of cancer-causing chemicals and even excessive sun exposure.

It appears that green tea cannot only prevent cancer, but is able to stop the growth of or even kill human cancer cells. This ability was documented in human breast, lung, colon, pancreatic, and prostate cancers in tissue culture and in animal models. Growth arrest occurs at the G2/M interface, a portion of the cell cycle where tumor cells are most sensitive to radiation therapy. This is also the same portion of the cell cycle in which paclitaxel (Taxol) and docetaxel (Taxotere) act to block the cell cycle.

The major polyphenols from green tea are epigallocatechin-3-gallate (EGCG), epigallocatechin, and epicatechin-3 gallate. Together, these make up 30% to 40% of the solids extracted from green tea leaves during brewing. The contents of green tea have been examined carefully to determine the chemical in the tea responsible for the anticancer activity. The growing consensus is that most of the useful activity is caused by the polyphenol, EGCG. This compound caused the rapid shrinkage of human prostate cancers growing in mouse xenograft models. It should be pointed out that there is no known mechanism by which an antioxidant can cause cancer cells to stop growing or cause rapid shrinkage of a tumor mass. For this reason, it is likely that EGCG exerts its anticancer activity by a mechanism independent of its antioxidant activity.

EGCG and other green tea polyphenols are sensitive to light and air; they are most stable at a pH of less than 5.5 and when the tea is brewed at 180°F or less.

The amount of EGCG found in green tea appears to be effective as a cancer prevention agent. The amount needed to stop the growth of cancer cells or to cause the cancer to shrink rapidly in mice is much larger—projecting from the animal experiments, a dose equivalent to 10 or more cups per day would be necessary. Human clinical trials have progressed to phase 1, where a dose of green tea extract of 1,000 mg per day (equivalent to 10 to 12 cups per day) was well tolerated. At present, there are no published phase II or III clinical trials.

Proanthocyanidins

Proanthocyanidins are a large group of polyphenols that are widely marketed by the health food industry. Proanthocyanidins are very effective antioxidants, exceeding vitamins E and C in this regard. The proanthocyanidins are made up of the monophenols, catechin and procyandin, strung together like beads on a chain. There are a wide range of specific proanthocyanidins, each with a specific sequence of catechin and procyandins. When these compounds enter the stomach, the stomach acid breaks these chains into fragments composed of one individual catechin and procyandin units, each of which can act as a potent antioxidant. Some of the plant sources of proanthocyanidins can be found in Table 15.7 (45).

The two richest sources of proanthocyanidins are cocoa and apples. Apples can vary widely in proanthocyanidin content: Red Delicious and Granny Smith have more than twice the concentration of McIntosh and Golden Delicious. Even McIntosh and Golden Delicious look impressive compared with other plant sources of proanthocyanidin. For comparison, red wine and cranberries have only one-third the concentration of these compounds as is found in Golden Delicious and less than one-sixth that found in cocoa.

Total proanthocyanidin content is not the whole story because some of these compounds have unique activities not related to their activity as antioxidants, which is likely based on specific combinations of catechin and procyandin units. For example, cranberries have a proanthocyanidin that blocks the ability of bacteria to adhere to the bladder lining, making cranberry juice a valuable adjunct in the treatment of bladder infections (33).

Cocoa. Chocolate is made by combining cocoa butter with cocoa liquor. Cocoa powder is dried cocoa liquor. Alone or mixed with water, cocoa powder is dark brown, tastes quite bitter, and is marketed as cooking cocoa. Chocolate made only with cocoa powder, cocoa butter, and emulsifying agents is also dark and bitter and is marketed as cooking or baking chocolate. Sweet, dark chocolate that is free of milk or milk fat is marketed with up to 70% cocoa powder and can be quite tasty. It should be mentioned that the cocoa powder content sometimes is listed as "cocoa mass," not cocoa powder. The antioxidant content of cocoa is very high and helps prevent chocolate from spoiling, making it very stable during prolonged storage.

After ingestion of chocolate rich in cocoa powder, the proanthocyanadins in the chocolate will break down, releasing epicatechins in large amounts. Within 2 hours of consuming 80 g of chocolate, blood levels of epicatechin increase by 1,200% (97). It takes approximately 6 hours for blood levels of this antioxidant to return to baseline. This sudden increase in epicatechin is so effective that it causes a 40% decline in oxidative damage to the fats in the blood.

This information about cocoa is relatively new and the full biologic impact of cocoa has not been fully investigated. In terms of total polyphenols and even epicatechins, cocoa is much richer than green tea. However, green tea has very specific epicatechins, such as EGCG, that act not only as antioxidants, but also act to kill cancer cells, including prostate cancer cells. In addition, extensive epidemiologic studies show a decrease in prostate cancer risk in men who chronically ingest green tea. Similar information is not available for cocoa powder.

TABLE 15.7. SOURCES RICH IN PROANTHOCYANADINS

▪ Cocoa	▪ Cranberries
▪ Apples	▪ Red wine
▪ Grape seed	▪ Grape skins
▪ French Maritime Pine Bark (pycnogenol)	▪ Blueberries

Grape Seed Extract. Grape seed extract is another rich, natural source of proanthocyanadins that is widely available and on which a number of papers have been published (85,89). The proanthocyanadins from grape seed extract have been shown to kill head and neck cancer cells without damaging normal cells. It also blocks the development of cancer in rodent skin exposed to chemical carcinogens. It will protect vitamin E in cells exposed to strong oxidants.

In animal models, grape seed extract exhibits potential beneficial effects that do not directly relate to the development or progression of cancer. When the blood supply to the heart is blocked temporarily and then restored, there is an intense wave of oxidative damage to the heart, called *reperfusion injury*. In animals subjected to this, administration of grape seed extract significantly lessens the damage. Finally, again in animals, application of grape seed extract to the skin was reported to increase hair growth by 230%.

Unfortunately, there are no useful clinical trials testing this preparation in humans. This is particularly striking in view of its widespread commercial availability and its popularity among cancer patients.

Pycnogenol. Pycnogenol, a proanthocyanidin preparation, is an extract obtained from the bark of the French Maritime Pine and is widely available (50,65,78,95). As with grape seed extract, a number of interesting papers have been published on this preparation. In laboratory experiments, pycnogenol protected the cells that line blood vessels from oxidative damage. In animal experiments, it reduced blood pressure by inhibiting angiotensin-converting enzyme. In aged mice, administration over 2 months increased the number of B and T cells, key members of the immune system. It also increased growth of bone marrow stem cells in tissue culture.

Like grape seed extract, the absence of useful clinical trials is striking in view of pycnogenol's wide commercial availability and popularity with patients.

Cranberries. For *Escherichia coli* to successfully attack the bladder, it must be able to attach to the wall of the bladder so that it can avoid being flushed out with the passage of urine. The bacteria does this through the use of fimbria. Cranberries contain a proanthocyanadin that blocks the ability of *E. coli's* fimbria to attach to surfaces (3,33). Even more interesting, prolonged contact with cranberry proanthocyanadin changes the *E. coli* so that it loses the capacity to make fimbria.

There is currently a controversy regarding whether the consumption of cranberries, their juice, or their extract plays a role in the management of urinary tract infections. One comprehensive review of the literature has concluded that the evidence is too weak to support its use (55). Others support the opposite, concluding that cranberries do have a role to play in the treatment of urinary tract infections. The most impressive study was published in the *Journal of the American Medical Association* (JAMA) (6). In this study, women with urinary tract infections were randomized to receive 300 mL of cranberry juice a day or placebo. Those taking cranberry juice had a significant improvement in their recovery from the infection. Conversely, there is little evidence that cranberry juice intake prevents urinary tract infection and it did not help children with recurrent bladder infections (86).

The cranberry is a member of the *Vaccinum* genus, which also includes the blueberry, bilberry, and lignonberry. One paper examined the ability of proanthocyanadins from various members of this genus to block the action of chemicals that cause cancer. In laboratory tests, low-bush blueberry, cranberry, and lignonberry all showed significant activity (13). Blueberry extracts also have been shown to reverse the loss of coordination and the ability to solve maze problems in aged rodents. Unfortunately, there is no evidence that cranberries or other members of this genus prevent cancer or improve mental function in humans.

DIETARY FAT AND PROSTATE CANCER

Enormous controversies exist regarding the link between diet and the risk of metastatic prostate cancer. The situation is so contentious that one can almost pick studies to support any conclusion he or she might favor. There are a number of reasons for this situation. Most studies use crude tools, such as requiring people to remember what they ate in the past or measuring the disappearance of certain foodstuffs from the economy of various countries. The determination of prostate cancer incidence also is difficult because different cultures vary in their willingness to accurately report prostate cancer as a cause of death. Given these problems, only the most robust associations between diet and prostate cancer will be reliable. One of these is the association between a diet rich in animal products, especially red meat, and prostate cancer, suggesting a strong link between a component of meat and the risk of prostate cancer.

Of course, not all studies of prostate cancer and diet are of equal quality. The best type of study would be a clinical trial in which patients were randomly assigned to diets high or low in specific fats. Trials that fit this description are currently in progress. Until they are complete, we have to fall back to our next best option. In this author's opinion, the best studies on diet and prostate cancer are those published by the investigators at the Harvard School of Public Health (34,38). These investigators conducted two trials, one involving physicians and a second involving other health care professionals. In both studies, information on diet was conducted prospectively and did not depend on people accurately recalling the composition of their diet in the distant past. The information from the two studies indicates that dietary fat did not influence the risk of localized prostate cancer, but did increase the risk of metastatic prostate cancer. When specific foods were examined, red meat, dairy fat, egg yolks, and creamy salad dressings emerged as significant risk factors.

Potential Dangers of Omega-3 Fatty Acids

One finding reported by Gann and associates (34) has elicited considerable controversy. These investigators reported that dietary intake of alpha-linolenic acid (ALA) was associated with a dramatic increase in the risk of developing metastatic prostate cancer. ALA is the major plant omega-3 fatty acid and increased intake of this lipid is thought to confer many health benefits. Extensive literature shows the ability of ALA and other omega-3 fatty acids to lower cholesterol, moderate high blood pressure, and suppress inflammation associated with rheumatoid arthritis and other diseases. Many dietitians and other health care professionals recommend that patients increase their intake of ALA to ensure a sufficient intake of omega-3 fatty acid. This fatty acid is present in large amounts in flax seed oil, where it comprises 50% of the total fatty acids present. Canola and soy bean oil are also rich in ALA. However, in addition to the Gann paper, a number of studies on the impact of ALA on prostate cancer have shown either no benefit or an adverse impact (4,27,41,47). These clinical studies have been matched with laboratory research that also shows increased growth of prostate cancer cells exposed to ALA. For this reason, it probably is not prudent for prostate cancer patients to take dietary supplements rich in ALA, such as flax seed oil or essential fatty acid mixtures.

ALA is not the only omega-3 fatty acid. Two others, eicosapentaenoic acid (EPA) and docosahexaenoic acid (DHA), are found in the fat of ocean fish, such as wild salmon or haddock. Fish do not make EPA or DHA, but obtain it from the algae that they ingest. For this reason, the fat in farm-raised salmon will reflect the fact that they have been fed corn or soy meal rather than algae and may not differ significantly from cattle or pigs fed a similar diet. Oil obtained from wild fish appears to have all of the same health benefits of ALA but is not associated with an increased risk of prostate cancer. In fact, several studies suggest a decreased risk of prostate cancer in men who eat several servings of fish a week (77). For more than a century, industrialized countries have made the oceans the garbage dumps of last resort. A large amount of literature can be found on the toxic chemicals that concentrate in the flesh and oils of fish living in the ocean. These range from toxic heavy metals such as mercury, to chemicals such as dioxin. For this reason, fish or fish oil may not be the best source for EPA and DHA.

Fortunately, DHA that is free of ALA and from a source that is not likely to be contaminated by heavy metals or toxic chemicals can now be purchased. Algae that produce DHA are now grown commercially, and the DHA is extracted and sold as 100- or 200-mg capsules. This preparation appears to represent the best source for omega-3 fatty acids (49, 57,91).

Animal Fat

Although dietary intake of red meat and animal fat consistently have been associated with increased risk of metastatic prostate cancer, the specific components of meat and animal fat responsible for this increased risk remain controversial.

One fatty acid, arachidonic acid, is present in much greater concentration in animal products. Vegans typically have arachidonic acid levels that are 10% to 30% of those found in meat eaters (81). This fatty acid is known to have a dramatic impact on the behavior of cancer cells, including cancer of the prostate. Arachidonic acid has been shown to enhance prostate cancer growth, to stimulate its spread, and to facilitate its ability to form new blood vessels. In addition, arachidonic acid products have been shown to kill cells of the immune system involved in the control of cancer.

Although a diet rich in meat can supply large amounts of arachidonic acid, most mammals can also produce their own. The "essential" fatty acid, linoleic acid, can be converted to arachidonic acid. Linoleic acid commonly is present in large amounts in many plant oils. In most animals used in diet experiments, such as rats and mice, this conversion is so efficient that a diet rich in plant oils will support high levels of arachidonic acid. This is not the case for humans, who are much less efficient in converting linoleic acid to arachidonic acid.

Dietary arachidonic acid does not cause any acute side effects. The typical American ingests approximately 100 mg of arachidonic acid each day. In clinical studies, people have tolerated five to ten times this amount for close to 2 months with no problems of any kind. It is only at doses of 7,000 mg a day that acute side effects have been seen in humans. The serious problems appear to develop only after chronic ingestion and in the context of preexisting disease, such as cancer (75).

Some investigators have argued that a diet rich in meat, and thus arachidonic acid, should not be of concern because humans evolved eating a diet rich in wild animal meat (67). Because humans survived hundreds of thousands of years on this diet, it is suggested that we must be well adapted to it. Although this idea is attractive superficially, the average life span of humans in primitive societies was typically less than 40 years. The diseases linked to high intake of animal fat, such as heart disease and cancer, are not common before the age of 50 years, long after the majority of people in primitive cultures would have died. Modern civilization has created an artificial situation, effectively doubling the life span of humans, thereby exposing us to diseases we are evolutionarily ill equipped to handle.

Arachidonic Acid and Prostate Cancer Biology

There is evidence that arachidonic acid is able to stimulate directly the growth of some cancer cells. This does not appear to be the case for prostate cancer cells. Arachidonic acid must be converted to one of several metabolites, called *eicosanoids.* For example, aspirin is able to relieve pain because it blocks the conversion of arachidonic acid to an eicosanoid, prostaglandin E_2 (PGE_2), which causes pain. Table 15.8 shows the major eicosanoids that can be made from arachidonic acid. Of these, 5-hydroxyeicosatetaraenoic acid (5-HETE), 12-HETE, and PGE_2 are known to be made by prostate cancer cells and to play a role in the growth and spread of this disease.

In men older than 50, lymphocytes are common throughout the normal prostate tissue. In radical prostatectomy specimens, it will be found that lymphocytes are

TABLE 15.8. SOME MAJOR EICOSANOIDS FORMED FROM ARACHIDONIC ACID

Products of cyclooxygenase Prostaglandin E_2 and thromboxane A_2	Products of 12-Lipoxygenase 12-HETE and 5,12-HETE
Products of 5-Lipoxygenase 5-HETE and Leukotrienes	Products of 15-Lipoxygenase 15-HETE and 5,15-HETE

uncommon in prostate cancers of Gleason grades of 7 or higher. Arachidonic acid can be converted to a chemical PGE_2. Human prostate cancer cells have long been known to produce PGE_2 from arachidonic acid. In radical prostatectomy specimens, the cancer produced ten times as much PGE_2 as the surrounding normal prostate tissue (20). PGE_2 is toxic to both natural killer cells and cytotoxic T cells and is one potential mechanism by which prostate cancer evades the immune system.

Arachidonic acid also markedly stimulates the ability of human prostate cancer cells to move and invade. This process requires the conversion of arachidonic acid to a substance called *12-HETE.* Inhibitors of 12-HETE formation are remarkably effective at arresting the movement of human prostate cancer cells (64).

Honn, from Wayne State Medical School in Detroit, has shown that conversion of arachidonic acid to 12-HETE by prostate cancer cells stimulates angiogenesis required for the growth of human prostate cancer (76). Honn and his colleagues first showed that simply adding 12-HETE to prostate cancer cells did not increase the growth rate of these cells. They then inserted additional copies of the gene controlling 12-HETE formation into these human prostate cancer cells. The original cancer cells and those engineered to make large amounts of 12-HETE were injected into mice. The cancers making increased amounts of 12-HETE grew much more rapidly and exhibit increased vascularity, suggesting increased angiogenesis.

In a separate study, Honn and colleagues examined radical prostatectomy specimens to see which cancers had the capacity to make 12-HETE and which did not (35). They found that patients with tumors able to make 12-HETE were much more likely to develop metastatic prostate cancer after radical prostatectomy. These findings are consistent with the capacity of 12-HETE to stimulate cancer cell invasiveness and angiogenesis in laboratory models.

Beginning in the mid-1980s, a series of investigators reported that the addition of arachidonic acid stimulated the growth of prostate cancer cells. None of these investigators was able to determine how arachidonic acid managed to increase the growth of these cancer cells. In a series of papers, it was confirmed that arachidonic acid stimulated the growth of both hormone-sensitive and hormone-independent human prostate cancer cells. It could then be shown that a specific metabolite of arachidonic acid, 5-HETE, was responsible for the growth stimulus provided by arachidonic acid. Furthermore, 5-HETE also acted as a potent survival factor for human prostate cancer cells (36,37).

The pathway by which arachidonic acid is converted to 5-HETE plays a major role in other diseases, including asthma, rheumatoid arthritis, and psoriasis. On the other hand, this pathway does not seem to be necessary for the health of humans or other mammals. Genetic engineering has been used to produce mice that make no 5-HETE. These mice bear offspring that are normal and that mature into normal adults. Therefore a drug that blocks the formation of 5-HETE might be effective against prostate cancer and have few side effects. In fact, several of the herbal products widely used to treat prostatic diseases, such as saw palmetto, block eicosanoid formation, including 5-HETE, in prostate cells (Table 15.9).

TABLE 15.9. HERBAL PRODUCTS THAT BLOCK EICOSANOID FORMATION

▪ Saw palmetto	▪ Cernilton
▪ Pygeum africanum	▪ Boswellia
▪ Stinging nettle	

In summary, prostate cancer cells are known to metabolize arachidonic acid to eicosanoid products that stimulate the survival, growth, and invasiveness of these cancer cells (Table 15.10). Other arachidonic acid metabolites suppress immune function and facilitate tumor angiogenesis. Considered together, these findings provide a rationale for why a diet rich in animal fat might speed the progression of human prostate cancer. As presented in the following sections, a range of herbal products traditionally used to treat prostatic diseases are now known to inhibit the formation of PGE_2, 5-HETE, and various leukotrienes.

Conjugated Linoleic Acid

Conjugated linoleic acid (CLA) recently has appeared on the market as a nutritional supplement, and this was accompanied by a report of significant activity against human prostate cancer in a mouse xenograft model (19). As a result, this supplement is now widely used by prostate cancer patients.

When animals with a rumen, such as cows, goats, or sheep, are fed grass and not grain, they make a special fatty acid called *conjugated linoleic acid.* CLA is incorporated into the meat as well as the milk made by grass-fed animals. It reduces the amount of body fat in the animals and lessens the amount of fat in the milk they produce. This is one reason grain-fed beef has a higher fat content than animals raised on the range.

Originally, CLA was discovered as a component in diary fat that blocked the ability of chemical carcinogens to cause cancer. The benefits of this compound were quickly shown

TABLE 15.10. ARACHIDONIC ACID AND PROSTATE BIOLOGY

▪ Stimulates growth and survival	▪ Contributes to immunosuppression
▪ Increases invasiveness	
▪ Increases angiogenesis	

to extend to other diseases in animal models (79). In animal models of diabetes mellitus, CLA was shown to make insulin's action more effective and reduced triglycerides. CLA acts to reduce inflammation in a manner similar to drugs such as aspirin or ibuprofen by blocking the conversion of arachidonic acid into PGE_2.

The initial observations that CLA would reduce the number of cancers in animals exposed to cancer-causing chemicals have been duplicated and appear to be quite impressive (51). In tissue culture, CLA slows or arrests the growth of a wide range of cancers, including human malignant melanoma, colorectal, breast, prostate, and lung cancer cell lines. The activity of CLA against breast cancer has been extended to experiments in mouse models of breast cancer. In these models, CLA slows or arrests the growth of the breast cancer masses. When these CLA-treated cancers are examined under the microscope, CLA is seen to cause an increase in apoptosis (a form of suicide), as well as slowing the rate at which the cancer cells duplicate.

There is currently only one paper on the activity of CLA against human prostate cancer (19). Cesano and colleagues used the most aggressive human prostate cancer cell line available, DU145. When DU145 is implanted in a mouse, it grows and spreads rapidly, killing the mouse in a short period of time. This cell line is hormone independent and is resistant to most cancer drugs. In fact, very few men have prostate cancers even remotely as aggressive as DU145. In this experiment, animals were given a food mixture that contained 1% CLA by weight. In the control mice, the cancer grew and spread rapidly to other tissues. In the mice on CLA, the cancer grew normally for a few weeks, gradually slowed and then stopped. After a few additional weeks, the cancers in approximately 30% of the CLA-fed mice began to turn black and fell off. In the control mice, the cancer had spread to the lungs in 80% of the mice, compared with only 10% in the CLA-fed mice. This dose of CLA caused no side effects in the mouse.

What mechanism best explains all of these effects? In one important study, the growth of human prostate cancers in a mouse model was markedly enhanced by feeding the mice corn oil, a fat rich in linoleic acid. CLA very effectively prevents the conversion of linoleic acid to arachidonic acid and can be expected to block the ability of arachidonic acid to foster the growth and spread of prostate cancer cells (7).

CLA has functions other than just blocking the conversion of linoleic acid to arachidonic acid. A group of proteins called *peroxisome proliferator–activated receptors* (PPAR) mediate the action of a group of cholesterol-lowering drugs, the most common of which is clofibrate. In addition to the ability to lower cholesterol, these drugs cause fat to accumulate in the liver and can lower the blood sugar. CLA has been shown to activate potently all three PPAR receptors (α, β, and γ) (68,73). *In vivo,* CLA exhibits many of the effects one would anticipate from a PPAR agonist: improved glucose tolerance, lowered blood lipids, and increased liver lipids.

The interaction of CLA with the PPARs may play a role in the antitumor activity of these compounds. PPAR-γ agonists, such as troglitazone, have shown activity against human prostate cancer *in vitro* and *in vivo* (58). A clinical trial of troglitazone in men with prostate cancer showed slowing or arrest of tumor growth in a significant number of patients. However, no PPAR agonists have been reported to cause tumor necrosis such as that seen in the CLA-treated mice bearing DU145. For these reasons, it is suspected that the ability of CLA to block the growth and spread of prostate cancer cells may result from a combination of its ability to block synthesis of arachidonic acid and its ability to activate PPARs.

Despite these promising results, there are a number of problems with the widespread use of CLA by prostate cancer patients. First, all commercially available CLA preparations are complex mixtures of closely related isomers that differ in their biology and, presumably, their therapeutic effects. For example, one of the isomers appears to be the most active in altering the synthesis of milk fat; no one has identified the isomers most active against prostate cancer. It would be best to have a CLA preparation with a defined isomer composition, preferably limited to those with documented anticancer activity.

Second, no clinical trials have tested the effectiveness of any CLA preparation against cancer. In the mouse studies, the anticancer activity is apparent only after more than 1 month of continuous administration. The action of many drugs is ten times faster in mice than in humans, therefore an effect exhibited in mice after 1 month might take 10 months to be seen in humans. Based on this information, the most promising test of this compound would be in patients who could afford to wait close to a year for its therapeutic impact. On the other hand, humans and mice may differ in some way that allows CLA to act much more rapidly in humans. Without human studies, it is difficult to know if CLA is of benefit to patients with prostate cancer or even in which clinical situation this product will be of greatest value.

Saw Palmetto

Saw palmetto is a compound derived from the fruit extract of the American Dwarf palm tree that is native to the Atlantic Coastal Plain from North Carolina south through Northern Florida. The common herbal preparation of saw palmetto represents the extracted lipids and sterols.

All clinical trials testing saw palmetto in the treatment of benign prostatic hyperplasia (BPH) were reviewed in *JAMA* in 1998 (101). After critically evaluating the quality of the clinical trials and the consistency of the results, the authors concluded that saw palmetto was an effective treatment for BPH. This conclusion has been confirmed in two subsequent extensive literature reviews (14,100). Proscar currently is approved by the FDA as a treatment for BPH and for male-pattern hair loss. In the clinical trials comparing finasteride (Proscar) with saw palmetto as treatment for BPH, finasteride was found to be less successful than saw palmetto.

One problem with these reviews is that they do not take into account the varying potency and quality of commercially available saw palmetto products. There are many different ways to extract these lipids and sterols, yielding products with differences in their biologic effects. In addition, the different brands and preparations are available with varying amount of extract per capsule. Consumer Labs, Inc., has tested 27 of the products on the market and found that only 17 contain an adequate amount of the specific fatty acids and sterols needed to produce a therapeutic effect. A list of the manufacturers that passed this test is available at their website, www.consumerlabs.com.

The only sure way of knowing whether a given saw palmetto extract is active is for the manufacturer to sponsor clinical trials that document its activity. Clinical trials are expensive and most herbal product companies have been reluctant to participate in such stringent tests of the value of their products. The economic justification was that the consumer did not demand this investment and the cost of such trials eroded the profitability of their business. A few companies have been foresighted enough to take part in clinical testing of their herbal extracts. In those few situations, we have solid evidence of the value of an herbal product as well as sound information about the effective dose and possible side effects.

The biochemical basis for the activity of saw palmetto against benign enlargement of the prostate almost certainly includes inhibition of the formation of dihydrotestosterone (DHT) within the prostate gland. Interestingly, although saw palmetto inhibits formation of DHT in the prostate gland, it does not inhibit formation in many other tissues and may not alter blood levels of this hormone (11,28). However, Proscar is effective at reducing prostatic DHT levels but is relatively ineffective in relieving the symptoms of BPH. The action of testosterone and DHT on the prostate gland is markedly stimulated by the hormone, prolactin. Saw palmetto is reported to block the response of prostate cells to prolactin (Table 15.11) (94).

Saw palmetto also has been reported to inhibit the enzyme 5-lipoxygenase, which converts arachidonic acid to the eicosanoid 5-HETE. This eicosanoid is known to stimulate the growth of prostate cells (80). Other products of 5-lipoxygenase, the leukotrienes, are potent mediators of inflammation.

TABLE 15.11. SAW PALMETTO

- Decreases synthesis of dihydrotestosterone in the prostate gland
- Decreases responsiveness to prolactin
- Decreases formation of 5-HETE and leukotrienes

In BPH, the increased size of the gland can arise from an increase in the number of cells lining the prostate ducts as well as an increase in the number of stromal cells in the space between the ducts. With this background, it is interesting to note that saw palmetto has been shown to cause the death of both the stromal cells and the cells lining the prostate ducts (82,92). This has been followed by one study showing that saw palmetto was able to slow the growth of prostate cancer cells and, at high enough concentrations, even kill these cancer cells. To date, there are no clinical trials testing saw palmetto in the treatment of prostate cancer, so it is difficult to know whether this observation is clinically relevant.

In summary, specific saw palmetto extracts appear to have useful activity in the treatment of BPH. This product appears to alter prostate biology through a number of mechanisms, some of which might also be relevant to the treatment of prostatitis and prostate cancer. Unfortunately, clinical trial documentation of the activity of saw palmetto extract is inadequate in the case of prostatitis and completely lacking in the case of prostate cancer.

Black Cohosh Root

The alcoholic extract of black cohosh root is widely used by women in Europe, and now in the United States, as a treatment for menopausal symptoms (46,63,96). Virtually all of the clinical studies have been performed with one preparation, Remifemin, which was originally developed in Europe and is now marketed in the United States. Many men with prostate cancer on hormonal therapy are using Remifemin or other black cohosh root preparations as treatment for their hot flashes and other symptoms of male menopause. In addition, some physicians caring for prostate cancer patients have been recommending it to their patients.

Black cohosh was one of the medicinal plants widely used by various Native Americans. It was also one of the first native herbal products adapted by early European settlers. Interestingly, the most common use for this herbal product by Native Americans and early European settlers appeared to be as a treatment for rheumatism. There is no convincing evidence that the Native Americans used it for menopausal symptoms. The use of black cohosh for this latter problem became widespread during the 1800s in both America and Europe. Its use in America subsided by 1900, but continued in Europe, especially in Germany. At present, virtually all significant clinical and laboratory investigations on black cohosh have been performed by European investigators.

Numerous clinical trials, including randomized controlled trials, have compared black cohosh root, almost always using Remifemin, with placebo and a variety of estrogen preparations commonly used as hormone replacement therapy for women. It is now well documented that this herbal preparation effectively reduces hot flashes in women. Remifemin also appears to be effective in countering the depression, insomnia, and other psychiatric complications of female menopause. This black cohosh extract appears to prevent bone loss in animals after surgical removal of the ovaries, raising the possibility that it might also ameliorate the development of osteoporosis. This possibility has yet to be tested in humans. Remifemin also appears to act on the female genitalia, where it has been reported to cause estrogen-like effects on the vaginal mucosa.

The production of estrogen by the ovaries is stimulated by luteinizing hormone (LH). When the brain senses that sufficient estrogen is present, it decreases the production of LH, shutting down the production of additional estrogen (32). During menopause in women, LH production increases because the brain senses the absence of estrogen. The magnitude of this LH rise has been reported to correlate with the severity of menopausal symptoms. A majority of the studies indicate that a dose of Remifemin sufficient to reverse menopausal symptoms also blocks the release of LH.

As with most herbal preparations, Remifemin is composed of a mixture of different chemicals. Fractions have been identified that can bind to the estrogen receptor and appear to mimic the actions of estrogen. Another fraction can block LH release even though it has no estrogenic activity. These results suggest that it would be possible to prepare black cohosh extracts that selectively suppress the response of the brain to menopausal symptoms, such as hot flashes, depression, and insomnia, that lack any activity at the estrogen receptor.

The side effects of Remifemin appear to be mild. The most common side effect is transient gastric distress, which is seen in approximately 7% of women. In fact, it seems to be as well or better tolerated than the commonly used estrogenic medications. In particular, it appears to be much less likely to cause uterine bleeding. In standard test systems, it also does not cause mutations or stimulate the development of cancers. This is important because naturally occurring estrogens are known to promote the development of cancers of the breast and uterus.

In women with breast cancers that contain the estrogen receptor, there is concern that use of estrogen-based drugs might enhance the growth of the cancer. One of the concerns about soy phytoestrogens is that, at low concentrations, they enhance the growth of the estrogen-responsive human prostate cancer cell line, MCF-7 (30). It is only at higher concentrations that soy phytoestrogens retard the growth of this and other breast cancer cell lines. In contrast, several studies now show that Remifemin retards the growth of MCF-7 in tissue culture at all of the concentrations tested. This has led several commentators to suggest that this herbal product might be safe for postmenopausal women with breast cancer. However, it is dangerous to use such tissue culture data as proof of safety. The only valid study would be to directly test the impact of Remifemin in women with estrogen receptor–positive breast cancer. This testing has not been performed, and the author therefore hesitates to recommend Remifemin to women with established breast cancer or women at high risk for breast cancer because of family history.

How efficacious is the use of Remifemin and other black cohosh extracts in men? No clinical trials in which Remifemin or other black cohosh extracts were administered to men could be found. Black cohosh definitely should not be recommend to men who are not on hormonal therapy. The concern is that it might suppress LH production and this might lead to testicular atrophy. In men already on hormonal therapy, the estrogenic activity of this supplement may cause breast enlargement and other estrogen-dependent side effects. No information could be found about the impact of Remifemin and other black cohosh preparations on prostate cancer growth and spread, and it is impossible to predict its impact on this disease. Its use in men is questionable at best until there is a better understanding of its impact on the physiology of the human male and its effects on prostate cancer.

Lycopene

It has long been known that intake of fruits, vegetables, and grains are associated with a decrease in the risk of many cancers, but the specific components of these foods responsible for this reduced risk remain a matter of controversy. Lycopene is a member of a broad group of plant pigments, called *carotenoids,* that includes beta-carotene (orange color of carrots) and lutein (yellow color in many vegetables). Carotenoids, especially beta-carotene, have long been thought to play an important role in cancer prevention (93). Lycopene is the red pigment found in tomatoes, pink grapefruit, watermelon, and apricots and is related to beta-carotene and other carotinoids in structure (1). Evidence strongly indicates that intake of tomato products and lycopene offer protection against cancers of the stomach, lung, and prostate. Lycopene also appears to reduce the risk of cancers of the oral cavity, esophagus, breast, pancreas, cervix, and colon. What is more interesting is that none of the 72 studies reviewed in preparation of this chapter report a link between lycopene and an increase in the risk of any cancer. Furthermore, there are no reports of toxicity, regardless of dose.

In a recent review, Giovannucci discussed study after study in which the intake of lycopene, but not other carotenoids such as beta-carotene, correlates with protection from cancer (39). This is consistent with a recent randomized, controlled trial that found that supplemental beta-carotene actually increased the risk of death from prostate cancer. This is an important point, because many dietitians and alternative health practitioners are still recommending beta-carotene to men with prostate cancer. It is important to stress that there is no evidence to support this practice.

Lycopene is well absorbed from cooked tomato products such as tomato sauce or tomato paste, but not from fresh tomatoes. In addition, lycopene absorption is enhanced by the addition of oil (61). The traditional practice around the Mediterranean of consuming cooked tomato products in combination with olive oil appears to have a strong rationale.

Why should lycopene reduce the risk of cancer? Carotenoids can act as antioxidants and as precursors to Vitamin A. Among the common carotenoids, lycopene is the most effective antioxidant and this property may be important given the activity of vitamin E and selenium against this cancer.

Several observations instill confidence in the importance of lycopene. First, the studies that report a reduced risk of cancer associated with lycopene involved the United States, Italy, the Netherlands, Spain, Sweden, Australia, Iran, China, and Japan, indicating the protective effect persists despite widely different dietary patterns, lifestyles, and ethnic background. Second, the protective effect extends to a wide range of human cancers, each of which has its own unique biology and is caused by different mechanisms. Third, in every country and with every cancer examined, lycopene intake never correlated with a significant increase in the risk of cancer.

What is lacking? Final proof of lycopene's importance will require a randomized, controlled clinical trial in which large numbers of people take a placebo or a defined amount of lycopene over a prolonged time period and the impact on cancer frequency and cancer deaths is measured. Because tomato products often are used in prepared foods in ways that are not obvious, this study will be difficult to conduct.

PC-SPES

PC-SPES is a combination of seven Chinese medicinal herbs with the addition of one North American herb, saw palmetto. This herbal product appeared a few years ago and is widely used by patients as a treatment for prostate cancer. The story of this herbal product illustrates the positive and negative aspects of the current regulatory environment with regard to supplements. This product did not proceed through the standard process by which prescription drugs are approved by the FDA. Shortly after this product was introduced, many in the medical field became aware that, in some patients, this product induced a significant decrease in tumor size. Physicians initially had no information about appropriate dosing, side effects, and antitumor activity of this preparation. Physicians specializing in prostate cancer have gathered experience with the use of this herbal product, largely because patients decided to try it on their own.

Reports about PC-SPES began to appear in medical literature. One noteworthy article by DiPaola and co-workers, of the Robert Wood Johnson School of Medicine, New Brunswick, New Jersey, appeared in the New England Journal of Medicine (29). The article showed that this preparation has estrogenic activity, but is distinct from known estrogenic drugs such as diethylstilbestrol (DES) and estradiol. They also found that PC-SPES caused a significant drop in blood levels of the male sex hormone, testosterone. It caused a greater than 50% drop in prostate-specific antigen (PSA) in 6 of 8 patients. The findings reported by DiPaola and co-workers suggest that the activity of PC-SPES in these patients represents a "hormonal" response equivalent to that caused by conventional estrogenic substances such as DES and estradiol.

A phase II clinical trial designed to establish the true effectiveness of PC-SPES was recently reported by Small of the University of California at San Francisco (90). In this study, essentially all of the patients who had not yet received hormonal treatment responded, consistent with the ability of PC-SPES to mimic the action of DES. Of even greater interest, almost half of the patients with hormone-refractory prostate cancer also responded. This response rate in hormone-refractory prostate cancer compares well with the most active cytotoxic chemotherapy regimens. Other groups also have documented the activity of this herbal preparation against human prostate cancer (26).

PC-SPES is not without significant side effects (Table 15.12). Virtually all men treated with this herbal product develop breast tenderness and gynecomastia. In addition, most men experience a loss in sex drive. GI toxicity in the form of diarrhea also can be a problem. Leg cramps are common and usually associated with a low serum magnesium level. Of greater concern, men with preexisting hypertension find its management more difficult. Shortly after the introduction of PC-SPES, a number of men were reported to develop thrombophlebitis and pulmonary embolism. For this reason, it became common practice to place patients on warfarin as prophylaxis against blood clots. However, in the large phase II trial conducted by Small, blood clots were no more common than one would anticipate from that normally seen in men with prostate cancer.

Soy and Genistein

It has long been known that the risk of prostate cancer is low in populations where soy consumption is common. Soy contains isoflavones, such as genistein, that are thought to account for the health benefits of this legume. These compounds are alternatively referred to by their specific chemical name, such as genistein; as isoflavones; or as phytoestrogens. The latter term arises from the fact that these isoflavones mimic some of the biologic effects of the female sex hormone, estrogen.

TABLE 15.12. SIDE EFFECTS OF PC-SPES

- Gynecomastia and gynecodynia
- Loss of sex drive
- Diarrhea
- Hypertension
- Thrombophlebitis

In the laboratory, genistein has well-documented activity against prostate cancer (5,16,88,102,104). High concentrations of genistein and other soy isoflavones cause the death of prostate cancer cells. At somewhat lower concentrations, these isoflavones arrest the growth of prostate cancer and block tumor cell invasiveness. In addition, there are now several studies in which soy products or isolated soy isoflavones have been demonstrated to slow the growth of human prostate cancer cells in mouse xenograft models.

The mechanism by which soy isoflavones might slow the growth and/or spread of prostate cancer remains unclear. Genistein, at concentrations obtainable in humans, can block the action of both the epidermal growth factor and *Her-2/neu* receptors. This means that genistein can theoretically block one of the major mechanisms by which prostate cancer cells become hormone-refractory. Although these isoflavones act as estrogenic compounds in laboratory assays, men on soy-rich diets have only minor alterations in sex hormone levels. Finally, soy isoflavones appear to block tumor angiogenesis in laboratory models.

There is also considerable controversy about the best soy product to use to obtain high blood levels of genistein and other soy isoflavones. Genistein is absorbed much more effectively from fermented soy products such as miso, natto, and tempeh than it is from soy beans, tofu, or soy milk. In addition, soy phytoestrogen or genistein tablets or capsules currently on the market would easily permit the ingestion of several grams of soy isoflavones per day. An additional complication is that blood levels of genistein may underestimate the levels in the prostate. When genistein levels are measured in prostatic fluid, the concentration is five to ten times higher than in the blood.

Clinical use of soy isoflavones in the treatment or prevention of prostate cancer is made questionable by several problems. Although quite a few epidemiology studies show a correlation between high soy intake and a reduced risk of prostate cancer, a randomized, controlled clinical trial showing that these soy products prolong the life of men with this disease is still lacking (43,54). Clinical trials that show that soy products arrest or slow the growth of prostate cancer are even lacking. The dose and schedule for the administration of soy isoflavones most likely to affect human prostate cancer is not known. On the other hand, many health benefits appear to be associated with the use of soy protein as a substitute for animal proteins. The FDA recently has allowed firms marketing soy protein to claim that these products have a favorable impact on the course of coronary heart disease.

SUMMARY

The Dietary Supplement Health and Education Act of 1994 guarantees Americans ready access to herbal products. Although selected herbal products have impressive therapeutic activity in tissue culture and animal models, with few exceptions, clinical trial documentation of activity is less than impressive. In fact, the common pattern is for initially promising laboratory findings to lead to widespread commercial availability without any intervening clinical investigation. An additional problem of great concern is that the commercially available herbal products vary widely in their quality.

REFERENCES

1. Agarwal S, Rao AV. Tomato lycopene and its role in human health and chronic diseases. *CMAJ* 2000;163(6):739.
2. Ahmad N, Feyes DK, Nieminen AL, et al. Green tea constituent epigallocatechin-3-gallate and induction of apoptosis and cell cycle arrest in human carcinoma cells. *J Natl Cancer Inst* 1997;89(24):1881.
3. Ahuja S, Kaack B, Roberts J. Loss of fimbrial adhesion with the addition of *Vaccinum macrocarpon* to the growth medium of P-fimbriated *Escherichia coli. J Urol* 1998;159(2):559.
4. Andersson SO, Wolk A, Bergstrom R, et al. Energy, nutrient intake and prostate cancer risk: a population-based case-control study in Sweden. *Int J Cancer* 1996;68(6):716.
5. Aronson WJ, Tymchuk CN, Elashoff RM, et al. Decreased growth of human prostate LNCaP tumors in SCID mice fed a low- fat, soy protein diet with isoflavones. *Nutr Cancer* 1999; 35(2):130.
6. Avorn J, Monane M, Gurwitz JH, et al. Reduction of bacteriuria and pyuria after ingestion of cranberry juice [Comments]. *JAMA* 1994;271(10):751.
7. Banni S, Angioni E, Casu V, et al. Decrease in linoleic acid metabolites as a potential mechanism in cancer risk reduction by conjugated linoleic acid. *Carcinogenesis* 1999;20(6): 1019.
8. Barnes VA, Treiber FA, Turner JR, et al. Acute effects of transcendental meditation on hemodynamic functioning in middle-aged adults. *Psychosom Med* 1999;61(4):525.
9. Bass IS, Young AL. *Dietary supplement health and education act: a legislative history and analysis.* Washington, DC: The Food and Drug Law Institute, 1996.
10. Baum MK, Shor-Posner G. Micronutrient status in relationship to mortality in HIV-1 disease. *Nutr Rev* 1998;56(1 Pt 2):S135.
11. Bayne CW, Ross M, Donnelly F, et al. The selectivity and specificity of the actions of the lipido-sterolic extract of *Serenoa repens* (Permixon) on the prostate. *J Urol* 2000;164 (3 Pt 1):876.
12. Beck MA. Nutritionally induced oxidative stress: effect on viral disease [Review]. *Am J Clin Nutr* 2000;71[6 Suppl]:1676S.
13. Bomser J, Madhavi DL, Singletary K, et al. In vitro anticancer activity of fruit extracts from *Vaccinum* species. *Planta Med* 1996;62(3):212.
14. Boyle P, Robertson C, Lowe F, et al. Meta-analysis of clinical trials of Permixon in the treatment of symptomatic benign prostatic hyperplasia. *Urology* 2000;55(4):533.
15. Bubendorf L, Schopfer A, Wagner U, et al. Metastatic patterns of prostate cancer: an autopsy study of 1,589 patients. *Hum Pathol* 2000;31(5):578.
16. Bylund A, Zhang JX, Bergh A, et al. Rye bran and soy protein delay growth and increase apoptosis of human LNCaP prostate adenocarcinoma in nude mice. *Prostate* 2000;42(4):304.

17. Campa A, Shor-Posner G, Indacochea F, et al. Mortality risk in selenium-deficient HIV-positive children. *J Acquir Immune Defic Syndr Hum Retrovirol* 1999;20(5):508.
18. Castillo-Richmond A, Schneider RH, Alexander CN, et al. Effects of stress reduction on carotid atherosclerosis in hypertensive African Americans. *Stroke* 2000;31(3):568.
19. Cesano A, Visonneau S, Scimeca JA, et al. Opposite effects of linoleic acid and conjugated linoleic acid on human prostatic cancer in SCID mice. *Anticancer Res* 1998;18(3A):1429.
20. Chaudry AA, Wahle KW, McClinton S, et al. Arachidonic acid metabolism in benign and malignant prostatic tissue in vitro: effects of fatty acids and cyclooxygenase inhibitors. *Int J Cancer* 1994;57(2):176.
21. Chen T, Cho RW, Stork PJ, et al. Elevation of cyclic adenosine 3',5'-monophosphate potentiates activation of mitogen-activated protein kinase by growth factors in LNCaP prostate cancer cells. *Cancer Res* 1999;59(1):213.
22. Chon JK, Borkowski A, Partin AW, et al. Alpha 1-adrenoceptor antagonists terazosin and doxazosin induce prostate apoptosis without affecting cell proliferation in patients with benign prostatic hyperplasia. *J Urol* 1999;161(6):2002.
23. Clark LC, Dalkin B, Krongrad A, et al. Decreased incidence of prostate cancer with selenium supplementation: results of a double-blind cancer prevention trial. *Br J Urol* 1998; 81(5):730.
24. Clark LC, Combs GF Jr, Turnbull BW, et al. Effects of selenium supplementation for cancer prevention in patients with carcinoma of the skin. A randomized controlled trial. Nutritional Prevention of Cancer Study Group [Comments]. [Published erratum appears in JAMA 1997;277(19):1520.] *JAMA* 1996;276(24):1957.
25. Clinton S. The dietary antioxidant network and prostate carcinoma. *Cancer* 1999;86:1629.
26. de la Taille A, Buttyan R, Hayek O, et al. Herbal therapy PC-SPES: in vitro effects and evaluation of its efficacy in 69 patients with prostate cancer. *J Urol* 2000;164(4):1229.
27. De Stefani E, Deneo-Pellegrini H, Boffetta P, et al. Alpha-linolenic acid and risk of prostate cancer: a case-control study in Uruguay. *Cancer Epidemiol Biomarkers Prev* 2000;9(3):335.
28. Di Silverio F, Monti S, Sciarra A, et al. Effects of long-term treatment with *Serenoa repens* (Permixon) on the concentrations and regional distribution of androgens and epidermal growth factor in benign prostatic hyperplasia. *Prostate* 1998; 37(2):77.
29. DiPaola RS, Zhang H, Lambert GH, et al. Clinical and biologic activity of an estrogenic herbal combination (PC- SPES) in prostate cancer [Comments]. *N Engl J Med* 1998;339 (12):785.
30. Dixon-Shanies D, Shaikh N. Growth inhibition of human breast cancer cells by herbs and phytoestrogens. *Oncol Rep* 1999;6(6):1383.
31. Donath F, Quispe S, Diefenbach K, et al. Critical evaluation of the effect of valerian extract on sleep structure and sleep quality. *Pharmacopsychiatry* 2000;33(2):47.
32. Duker EM, Kopanski L, Jarry H, et al. Effects of extracts from *Cimicifuga racemosa* on gonadotropin release in menopausal women and ovariectomized rats. *Planta Med* 1991;57(5):420.
33. Foo LY, Lu Y, Howell AB, et al. The structure of cranberry proanthocyanidins which inhibit adherence of uropathogenic P-fimbriated Escherichia coli in vitro. *Phytochemistry* 2000; 54(2):173.
34. Gann PH, Hennekens CH, Sacks FM, et al. Prospective study of plasma fatty acids and risk of prostate cancer [Comments]. [Published erratum appears in *J Natl Cancer Inst* 1994;86(9): 728.] *J Natl Cancer Inst* 1994;86(4):281.
35. Gao X, Porter AT, Honn KV. Involvement of the multiple tumor suppressor genes and 12-lipoxygenase in human prostate cancer. Therapeutic implications. *Adv Exp Med Biol* 1997; 407:41.
36. Ghosh J, Myers CE. Arachidonic acid stimulates prostate cancer cell growth: critical role of 5-lipoxygenase. *Biochem Biophys Res Commun* 1997;235(2):418.
37. Ghosh J, Myers CE. Inhibition of arachidonate 5-lipoxygenase triggers massive apoptosis in human prostate cancer cells. *Proc Natl Acad Sci USA* 1998;95(22):13182.
38. Giovannucci E, Rimm EB, Colditz GA, et al. A prospective study of dietary fat and risk of prostate cancer [Comments]. *J Natl Cancer Inst* 1993;85(19):1571.
39. Giovannucci E. Tomatoes, tomato-based products, lycopene, and cancer: review of the epidemiologic literature [Comments]. *J Natl Cancer Inst* 1999;91(4):317.
40. Girodon F, Galan P, Monget AL, et al. Impact of trace elements and vitamin supplementation on immunity and infections in institutionalized elderly patients: a randomized controlled trial. MIN. VIT. AOX. geriatric network. *Arch Intern Med* 1999;159(7):748.
41. Godley PA, Campbell MK, Gallagher P, et al. Biomarkers of essential fatty acid consumption and risk of prostatic carcinoma [Comments]. *Cancer Epidemiol Biomarkers Prev* 1996; 5(11):889.
42. Gunawardena K, Murray DK, Meikle AW. Vitamin E and other antioxidants inhibit human prostate cancer cells through apoptosis. *Prostate* 2000;44(4):287.
43. Habito RC, Montalto J, Leslie E, et al. Effects of replacing meat with soyabean in the diet on sex hormone concentrations in healthy adult males. *Br J Nutr* 2000;84(4):557.
44. Halliwell B. Antioxidant defense mechanisms: from the beginning to the end (of the beginning). *Free Radic Res* 1999; 31(4):261.
45. Hammerstone JF, Lazarus SA, Schmitz HH. Procyanidin content and variation in some commonly consumed foods. *J Nutr* 2000;130(8):2086S.
46. Hardy ML. Herbs of special interest to women [Review]. *J Am Pharm Assoc (Wash)* 2000;40(2):234.
47. Harvei S, Bjerve KS, Tretli S, et al. Prediagnostic level of fatty acids in serum phospholipids: omega-3 and omega-6 fatty acids and the risk of prostate cancer. *Int J Cancer* 1997;71(4):545.
48. Heinonen OP, Albanes D, Virtamo J, et al. Prostate cancer and supplementation with alpha-tocopherol and beta-carotene: incidence and mortality in a controlled trial [Comments]. *J Natl Cancer Inst* 1998;90(6):440.
49. Horrocks LA, Yeo YK. Health benefits of docosahexaenoic acid (DHA) [Comments]. *Pharmacol Res* 1999;40(3):211.
50. Huynh HT, Teel RW. Selective induction of apoptosis in human mammary cancer cells (MCF-7) by pycnogenol. *Anticancer Res* 2000;20(4):2417.
51. Ip MM, Masso-Welch PA, Shoemaker SF, et al. Conjugated linoleic acid inhibits proliferation and induces apoptosis of normal rat mammary epithelial cells in primary culture. *Exp Cell Res* 1999;250(1):22.
52. Irvin JH, Domar AD, Clark C, et al. The effects of relaxation response training on menopausal symptoms. *J Psychosom Obstet Gynaecol* 1996;17(4):202.
53. Israel K, Yu W, Sanders BG, et al. Vitamin E succinate induces apoptosis in human prostate cancer cells: role for Fas in vitamin E succinate-triggered apoptosis. *Nutr Cancer* 2000;36(1):90.
54. Jacobsen BK, Knutsen SF, Fraser GE. Does high soy milk intake reduce prostate cancer incidence? The Adventist Health Study (United States) [Comments]. *Cancer Causes Control* 1998;9(6):553.

55. Jepson RG, Mihaljevic L, Craig J. Cranberries for treating urinary tract infections [Review]. *Cochrane Database Syst Rev* 2000;(2):CD001322.
56. Kiremidjian-Schumacher L, Roy M, Glickman R, et al. Selenium and immunocompetence in patients with head and neck cancer. *Biol Trace Elem Res* 2000;73(2):97.
57. Kremer JM. ω-3 fatty acid supplements in rheumatoid arthritis. *Am J Clin Nutr* 2000;71[1 Suppl]:349S.
58. Kubota T, Koshizuka K, Williamson EA, et al. Ligand for peroxisome proliferator-activated receptor gamma (troglitazone) has potent antitumor effect against human prostate cancer both in vitro and in vivo. *Cancer Res* 1998;58(15):3344.
59. Kuhlmann J, Berger W, Podzuweit H, et al. The influence of valerian treatment on "reaction time, alertness and concentration" in volunteers. *Pharmacopsychiatry* 1999;32(6):235.
60. Kyprianou N, Benning CM. Suppression of human prostate cancer cell growth by alpha1-adrenoceptor antagonists doxazosin and terazosin via induction of apoptosis. *Cancer Res* 2000;60(16):4550.
61. Lee A, Thurnham DI, Chopra M. Consumption of tomato products with olive oil but not sunflower oil increases the antioxidant activity of plasma. *Free Radic Biol Med* 2000; 29(10):1051.
62. Liao S, Umekita Y, Guo J, et al. Growth inhibition and regression of human prostate and breast tumors in athymic mice by tea epigallocatechin gallate. *Cancer Lett* 1995;96(2):239.
63. Liske E. Therapeutic efficacy and safety of *Cimicifuga racemosa* for gynecologic disorders. *Adv Ther* 1998;15(1):45.
64. Liu B, Maher RJ, Hannun YA, et al. 12(S)-HETE enhancement of prostate tumor cell invasion: selective role of PKC alpha. *J Natl Cancer Inst* 1994;86(15):1145.
65. Liu FJ, Zhang YX, Lau BH. Pycnogenol enhances immune and haemopoietic functions in senescence-accelerated mice. *Cell Mol Life Sci* 1998;54(10):1168.
66. Longo LP, Johnson B. Addiction: Part I. Benzodiazepines—side effects, abuse risk and alternatives. *Am Fam Physician* 2000;61(7):2121.
67. Mann N. Dietary lean red meat and human evolution. *Eur J Nutr* 2000;39(2):71.
68. McCarty MF. Activation of PPAR-gamma may mediate a portion of the anticancer activity of conjugated linoleic acid. *Med Hypotheses* 2000;55(3):187.
69. McIntyre BS, Briski KP, Gapor A, et al. Antiproliferative and apoptotic effects of tocopherols and tocotrienols on preneoplastic and neoplastic mouse mammary epithelial cells. *Proc Soc Exp Biol Med* 2000;224(4):292.
70. McVary KT, Razzaq A, Lee C, et al. Growth of the rat prostate gland is facilitated by the autonomic nervous system. *Biol Reprod* 1994;51(1):99.
71. McVary KT, McKenna KE, Lee C. Prostate innervation. *Prostate Suppl* 1998;8:2.
72. Miller MS, Rahe RH. Life changes scaling for the 1990s. *J Psychosom Res* 1997;43:279.
73. Moya-Camarena SY, Van den Heuvel JP, Belury MA. Conjugated linoleic acid activates peroxisome proliferator-activated receptor alpha and beta subtypes but does not induce hepatic peroxisome proliferation in Sprague-Dawley rats. *Biochim Biophys Acta* 1999;1436(3):331.
74. Moyad MA, Brumfield SK, Pienta KJ. Vitamin E, alpha- and gamma-tocopherol, and prostate cancer. *Semin Urol Oncol* 1999;17(2):85.
75. Nelson GJ, Kelley DS, Emken EA, et al. A human dietary arachidonic acid supplementation study conducted in a metabolic research unit: rationale and design. *Lipids* 1997;32(4):415.
76. Nie D, Hillman GG, Geddes T, et al. Platelet-type 12-lipoxygenase in a human prostate carcinoma stimulates angiogenesis and tumor growth. *Cancer Res* 1998;58(18):4047.
77. Norrish AE, Skeaff CM, Arribas GL, et al. Prostate cancer risk and consumption of fish oils: a dietary biomarker-based case-control study. *Br J Cancer* 1999;81(7):1238.
78. Packer L, Rimbach G, Virgili F. Antioxidant activity and biologic properties of a procyanidin-rich extract from pine (Pinus maritima) bark, pycnogenol. *Free Radic Biol Med* 1999; 27(5-6):704.
79. Park Y, Albright KJ, Storkson JM, et al. Changes in body composition in mice during feeding and withdrawal of conjugated linoleic acid. *Lipids* 1999;34(3):243.
80. Paubert-Braquet M, Mencia Huerta JM, Cousse H, et al. Effect of the lipidic lipidosterolic extract of *Serenoa repens* (Permixon) on the ionophore A23187-stimulated production of leukotriene B4 (LTB4) from human polymorphonuclear neutrophils. *Prostaglandins Leukot Essent Fatty Acids* 1997;57(3):299.
81. Phinney SD, Odin RS, Johnson SB, et al. Reduced arachidonate in serum phospholipids and cholesteryl esters associated with vegetarian diets in humans. *Am J Clin Nutr* 1990; 51(3):385.
82. Ravenna L, Di Silverio F, Russo MA, et al. Effects of the lipidosterolic extract of *Serenoa repens* (Permixon) on human prostatic cell lines. *Prostate* 1996;29(4):219.
83. Ripple GH, Wilding G. Drug development in prostate cancer. *Semin Oncol* 1999;26(2):217.
84. Ripple MO, Henry WF, Rago RP, et al. Prooxidant-antioxidant shift induced by androgen treatment of human prostate carcinoma cells [Comments]. *J Natl Cancer Inst* 1997;89(1):40.
85. Sato M, Maulik G, Ray PS, et al. Cardioprotective effects of grape seed proanthocyanidin against ischemic reperfusion injury. *J Mol Cell Cardiol* 1999;31(6):1289.
86. Schlager TA, Anderson S, Trudell J, et al. Effect of cranberry juice on bacteriuria in children with neurogenic bladder receiving intermittent catheterization [Comments]. *J Pediatr* 1999; 135(6):698.
87. Selye H. Syndrome produced by diverse noxious agents. *Nature* 1936;138:32.
88. Shen JC, Klein RD, Wei Q, et al. Low-dose genistein induces cyclin-dependent kinase inhibitors and G(1) cell-cycle arrest in human prostate cancer cells. *Mol Carcinog* 2000;29(2):92.
89. Shirataki Y, Kawase M, Saito S, et al. Selective cytotoxic activity of grape peel and seed extracts against oral tumor cell lines. *Anticancer Res* 2000;20(1A):423.
90. Small EJ, Frohlich MW, Bok R, et al. Prospective trial of the herbal supplement PC-SPES in patients with progressive prostate cancer. *J Clin Oncol* 2000;18(21):3595.
91. Stordy BJ. Dark adaptation, motor skills, docosahexaenoic acid, and dyslexia. *Am J Clin Nutr* 2000;71[1 Suppl]:323S.
92. Vacherot F, Azzouz M, Gil-Diez-De-Medina S, et al. Induction of apoptosis and inhibition of cell proliferation by the lipidosterolic extract of *Serenoa repens* (LSESr, Permixon(R)) in benign prostatic hyperplasia. *Prostate* 2000;45(3):259.
93. Valcic S, Timmermann BN, Alberts BS, et al. Inhibitory effect of six green tea catechins and caffeine on the growth of four selected human tumor cell lines. *Anticancer Drugs* 1996; 7(4):461.
94. Van Coppenolle F, Le Bourhis X, Carpentier F, et al. Pharmacological effects of the lipidosterolic extract of *Serenoa repens* (Permixon) on rat prostate hyperplasia induced by hyperprolactinemia: comparison with finasteride. *Prostate* 2000;43(1):49.

95. Virgili F, Kim D, Packer L. Procyanidins extracted from pine bark protect alpha-tocopherol in ECV 304 endothelial cells challenged by activated RAW 264.7 macrophages: role of nitric oxide and peroxynitrite. *FEBS Lett* 1998;431(3):315.
96. Wade C, Kronenberg F, Kelly A, et al. Hormone-modulating herbs: implications for women's health. *J Am Med Womens Assoc* 1999;54(4):181.
97. Wang JF, Schramm DD, Holt RR, et al. A dose-response effect from chocolate consumption on plasma epicatechin and oxidative damage. *J Nutr* 2000;130[8S Suppl]:2115S.
98. Wang JM, McKenna KE, McVary KT, et al. Requirement of innervation for maintenance of structural and functional integrity in the rat prostate. *Biol Reprod* 1991;44(6):1171.
99. Whanger PD. Selenium in the treatment of heavy metal poisoning and chemical carcinogenesis. *J Trace Elem Electrolytes Health Dis* 1992;6:209.
100. Wilt T, Ishani A, Stark G, et al. Serenoa repens for benign prostatic hyperplasia [Review]. *Cochrane Database Syst Rev* 2000;(2):CD001423.
101. Wilt TJ, Ishani A, Stark G, et al. Saw palmetto extracts for treatment of benign prostatic hyperplasia: a systematic review [Comments]. [Published erratum appears in *JAMA* 1999;281 (6):515.] *JAMA* 1998;280(18):1604.
102. Yang Z, Liu S, Chen X, et al. Induction of apoptotic cell death and in vivo growth inhibition of human cancer cells by a saturated branched-chain fatty acid, 13-methyltetradecanoic acid. *Cancer Res* 2000;60(3):505.
103. Yoshizawa K, Willett WC, Morris SJ, et al. Study of prediagnostic selenium level in toenails and the risk of advanced prostate cancer [Comments]. *J Natl Cancer Inst* 1998;90(16): 1219.
104. Zhou JR, Gugger ET, Tanaka T, et al. Soybean phytochemicals inhibit the growth of transplantable human prostate carcinoma and tumor angiogenesis in mice. *J Nutr* 1999;129(9):1628.
105. Zikic RV, Stajn AS, Ognjanovic BI, et al. The effect of cadmium and selenium on the antioxidant enzyme activities in rat heart. *J Environ Pathol Toxicol Oncol* 1998;17 (3–4):259.

16

RENAL TUMORS

CHAD W.M. RITENOUR
ROBERT O. NORTHWAY
FRAY F. MARSHALL

Much of what is known today about renal tumors revolves around data from just the past century. Advances in both pathologic diagnosis and surgical technique have been steady since the first known nephrectomy approximately 140 years ago. Unfortunately, at this time, there is still no highly effective therapy, apart from surgery, for most malignant renal tumors. Nonetheless, continued research in this arena has yielded some important discoveries, and this challenge persists for future generations. As more is learned about the cellular characteristics, and specifically the molecular nature of these tumors, researchers will further target surgical and medical approaches to improve the prognosis of patients with advanced disease.

CLASSIFICATION

Although less common than benign renal cysts, solid tumors of the kidney are most often malignant in nature. The majority of these are adenocarcinomas, commonly called *renal cell carcinomas (RCCs).* However, numerous other lesions have been described in the kidney, and these have been found in all aspects of renal and perirenal tissue including epithelial tissue, vascular structures, neurogenic tissue, and mesenchymal derivatives. Childhood renal tumors [predominantly Wilms' tumor (nephroblastoma)], from embryonic tissue also are seen and are discussed elsewhere in this text.

Over the past decades, investigators have proposed several classification schemes for renal masses, although not one has been universally accepted as being both simple and comprehensive. Stratification has been based on tissue origin, behavior (malignant, benign, or inflammatory), and radiographic appearance. Histopathologic diagnosis, as related to molecular genetics, also has been examined in attempts to find common links between different tumors as well as to locate potential prognostic markers at the gene level (283).

With the advent of new molecular genetic data, specific morphologic and cytogenetic characteristics of the most common renal neoplasms, epithelial tumors, were recently integrated into a standard classification system. In 1997, at a consensus conference (the Diagnosis and Prognosis of Renal Cell Carcinoma) held by the World Health Organization (WHO) in combination with the Union Internationale Contre le Cancer (UICC) and the American Joint Committee of Cancer (AJCC), old categorization systems were modernized. An appreciation for the histologic diversity led investigators to reclassify on the basis of morphology and yet remain consistent with known genetic facts. The descriptive terms applied had historic reference, reflected salient morphologic features, and were unambiguous. The contemporary classification of adult renal epithelial neoplasia was generated as listed in Table 16.1 (239). Regardless of the classification scheme, the clinician must be aware of the behavioral characteristics of the mass once a diagnosis is made.

C.W.M. Ritenour, R.O. Northway, and F.F. Marshall: Department of Urology, Emory University, Atlanta, GA 30322.

TABLE 16.1. CLASSIFICATION OF RENAL EPITHELIAL TUMORS

Benign Neoplasms	Malignant Neoplasms
Papillary adenoma	Conventional (clear cell) renal carcinoma
Renal oncocytoma	Papillary renal carcinoma
Metanephric adenoma	Chromophobe renal carcinoma Collecting duct carcinoma Renal cell carcinoma, unclassified

From Störkel S, Eble J, Adlakha K, et al. Classification of renal cell carcinoma. Workgroup No. 1. *Cancer* 1997;80(5):987, with permission.

BENIGN EPITHELIAL TUMORS

Papillary Adenoma

Several previous classifications of renal epithelial tumors have included adenoma as a distinct pathologic entity. However, significant controversy exists over the differentiation of adenomas from adenocarcinomas by histologic criteria (88). Distinction is important because adenomas generally are regarded as benign lesions, which do not progress to metastasis, whereas adenocarcinomas have known metastatic potential.

Asymptomatic papillary adenomas are the most common renal epithelial neoplasm. They are exclusive to the renal cortex and have been identified in 4% to 37% of autopsy specimens (88). Based on ultrastructural studies, papillary adenomas originate from a distal tubular cell (71). In addition, associated chromosomal changes (including trisomy 7, trisomy 17, and loss of the Y chromosome) similar to those seen with papillary RCC have been identified (125). Increased frequency of papillary adenomas has been found with smoking (279), end-stage renal disease with hemodialysis (107), and arteriosclerotic renal vascular disease (21).

On gross examination, papillary adenomas appear as very small yellow to pale gray spots in the renal cortex. Recently, Grignon and Eble (88) proposed a constellation of three histologic features to assist in identifying these lesions. First, the cellular architecture must be tubular, papillary, or tubulopapillary in character. Second, the diameter of the tumor should measure less than or equal to 5 mm. Although certain slightly larger lesions may be adenomas, the chance of malignancy is greater with increased sizes. Third, the cells should not histologically resemble clear cell, chromophobe, or collecting duct RCCs. If these criteria are satisfied, the diagnosis of papillary adenoma can be made with greater confidence.

Renal Oncocytoma

Renal oncocytomas are distinct pathologic lesions associated with benign clinical courses. Although earlier reports suggest metastatic potential of certain oncocytomas, these reports now are thought to have represented cases of chromophobe RCC, a similar but histologically different tumor not recognized at that time. Because chromophobe RCCs are known to metastasize, the distinction between oncocytomas and these carcinomas currently is important for therapeutic decisions and follow-up.

Oncocytoma and chromophobe RCC have many overlapping morphologic, histochemical, and ultrastructural features. Both are thought to arise from cells of the distal nephron (73,285). Some specific nuclear parameters such as binucleation or multinucleation or staining with an antimitochondrial antibody (113-1) can be valuable in distinguishing between the two tumors (252,253). Characteristically, the cytoplasm of oncocytoma cells is uniformly eosinophilic and granular, whereas that of chromophobe RCC is more variable. Both tumors exhibit chromosomal loss on chromosomes Y and 1, but recent research with oncocytomas has revealed a unique recurring chromosomal translocation about 11q13, in proximity to the BCL1 locus, that may serve as a marker for improved classification (167,224).

Oncocytomas are thought to account for 3% to 7% of solid renal tumors (136). They are approximately two times more common in males than in females. Most often, they are discovered as incidental findings on radiographic studies performed for other reasons. Occasionally, oncocytomas present with flank pain, hematuria, or an abdominal mass, but they usually are asymptomatic. The median age of patients at presentation is in the seventh decade, which is slightly older than for RCC.

On gross appearance, oncocytomas (Fig. 16.1) are a tan-brown color and are well circumscribed from surrounding renal parenchyma. Often, a central scar highlights the neoplasm. Necrosis and hemorrhage are not prominent. Although most oncocytomas are unilateral, approximately 4% to 6% are bilateral (46). Histologically, the cells show regular granular cytoplasm due to numerous mitochondria and uniform nuclei with few mitoses. Cases of oncocytosis with innumerable oncocytic nodules throughout the kidney and associated with one dominant tumor have been reported (254). Coexistence of oncocytoma with RCC also has been described in up to 10% of cases (46).

Radiographic studies rarely are diagnostic for oncocytoma because it often appears as any other solid renal tumor. Occasionally, a central scar is visualized on ultrasound studies or computed tomography (CT) scans, but this is nonspecific. Although angiography is now rarely performed for these tumors, a characteristic "spoke-wheel" appearance has been used to describe oncocytoma (273).

Due to lack of a pathognomonic radiographic sign, the diagnosis of oncocytoma rarely is made without an operation. The potential presence of concurrent malignant tumors within oncocytoma makes diagnosis by percutaneous needle biopsy risky. Partial nephrectomy with an adequate margin is the surgical therapy of choice for small tumors, but large or multifocal tumors may require radical nephrectomy for complete excision.

Metanephric Adenoma

Metanephric adenoma is a recently recognized benign epithelial tumor. In a report of 50 cases, investigators concluded that it occurs most commonly in the fifth to sixth decades, with a 2 : 1 female predilection (44). Some of these tumors present with symptoms of polycythemia, flank pain, mass, or hematuria; however, approximately half are incidental findings on radiographic studies.

Metanephric adenomas characteristically range in size from 3 to 6 cm, with occasional reports of larger tumors (44). The tumors are well circumscribed with a gray, tan, or yellow color and occasional foci of hemorrhage and necrosis (115). Cysts may also be present. Calcifications, represented histologically by Psammoma bodies, are common. Cells are tightly packed and uniform with prominent nuclei and scant cytoplasm (88). Mitoses are rare or absent. Adherence to these histologic criteria will avoid having other, more common renal lesions misdiagnosed as metanephric adenomas (182).

Differentiation of metanephric adenomas from other renal tumors by ultrasound or CT scans is difficult (60). Although no known case has recurred following removal of the tumor, synchronous RCC has been found in several isolated specimens (45). Therefore all solid lesions of the kidney should be treated as malignant unless proven otherwise with tissue diagnosis.

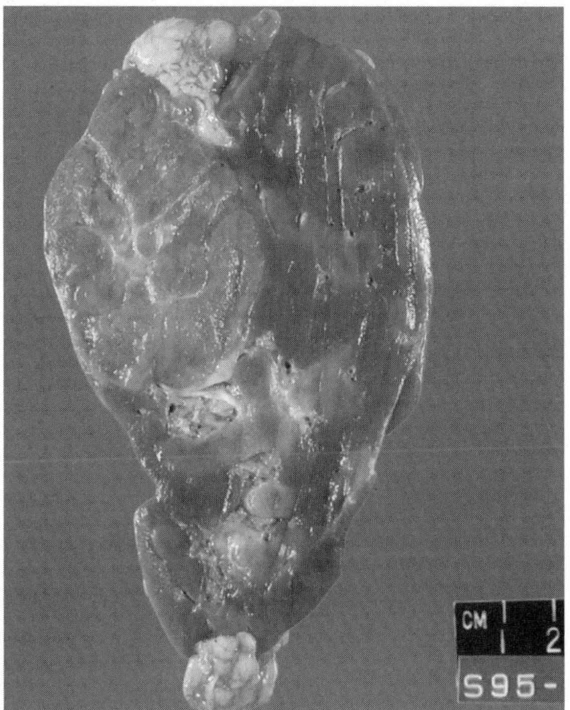

FIGURE 16.1. Oncocytoma with characteristic central scar and demarcation from surrounding renal tissue.

A variant of metanephric adenoma has been termed *metanephric adenofibroma.* In one of the first descriptions, Hennigar and Beckwith (98) reported several tumor cases with an epithelial component identical to metanephric adenoma along with a spindle cell component similar to congenital mesoblastic nephroma. (They originally termed this new tumor a *nephrogenic adenofibroma,* but given its similarity to metanephric adenoma, the name was later modified to metanephric adenofibroma.) The combination of both histologic components is necessary for the diagnosis of metanephric adenofibroma, but careful sampling may be necessary to avoid missing small epithelial nodules (214). Patients with metanephric adenofibroma have ranged in age from 3.5 to 36 years, younger than most patients with metanephric adenomas, and appear to have a benign course.

MALIGNANT EPITHELIAL TUMORS

Renal Cell Carcinoma

Epidemiology

Malignant tumors of the kidney are estimated to represent approximately 2.5% of all new cancer cases in the United States each year. Statistical analysis showed that, for the year 2000, approximately 31,000 new cases and 12,000 deaths would occur (87). Most of these diagnoses are related to malignant renal epithelial tumors, or RCCs, which comprise approximately 85% of all renal neoplasms (161). Males show more than twice the incidence of females in studies of RCCs, with most patients presenting in the seventh and eighth decades of life. The highest rates occur in North America and Europe, especially Scandinavia (161).

Over the past several decades, both the incidence of diagnosis and numbers of related deaths for RCC have risen in the United States and other countries (34). This parallels higher numbers of incidentally discovered tumors found during radiographic screening studies performed for the diagnosis and management of other disorders. Routine ultrasonography, CT, and magnetic resonance imaging (MRI) now discover increased numbers of small lesions in the absence of symptoms (113,251). However, most epidemiologists do not believe that these incidental tumors fully explain the rising incidence of renal cancer (34).

Aside from the rise in small, early-stage kidney tumors, there has also been a smaller percentage increase in the number of higher-stage lesions found (33). This expanding discovery mirrors the overall rising mortality rates that have been observed in recent years. In the United States, these changes are most evident in the African American population, which shows greater increases in both incidence and

TABLE 16.2. SELECTED RISK FACTORS ASSOCIATED WITH RENAL CELL CARCINOMA

Cigarette smoking	Occupational exposures (e.g., asbestos, petroleum, cadmium, lead)
Hypertension	Genetic predisposition (e.g., von Hippel–Lindau disease)
Elevated body weight	
Medications (e.g., diuretics)	
Acquired renal cystic disease	

mortality for RCC when compared with Caucasians (34). The reasons for this racial difference are unclear.

Etiology

Based on information from case-control, genetic, and cohort studies, several risk factors have been associated with the development of RCC (Table 16.2). Most studies with sufficient sample size demonstrate a positive correlation between RCC and smoking cigarettes, which has been associated with up to a 35% increase in risk (282). The data suggest a dose-response relationship, with relative risk increasing with the numbers of cigarettes smoked, as well as a significant reduction in risk associated with cessation. Obesity also has shown positive associations with RCC (33). Greater risk exists for women with elevated weight than for their male counterparts, and the risk appears proportionate to the severity of obesity (161). With its increasing prevalence in the United States, obesity may contribute to the rising incidence of RCC.

Several epidemiologic studies link hypertension to elevated risks for RCC, with up to a threefold increase in risk reported (33). Diuretics, which often are used in the medical treatment of hypertension, have been particularly implicated (89,213). Acquired cystic disease, found in renal failure patients on hemodialysis, has been associated with higher rates of RCC (110,111). Occupational exposure to asbestos, petroleum, cadmium, and lead also has been reported to produce increased levels of risk (33).

Although relatively rare, familial cases of RCC have been linked to genetic causes. von Hippel–Lindau (VHL) disease, an autosomal-dominant genetic disorder, has long been associated with the development of RCC. The condition is characterized by hemangioblastomas of the retina and the central nervous system, especially the cerebellum, as well as cysts of the kidneys, liver, and pancreas. Pheochromocytomas also have been linked to the syndrome (69). Renal tumors in these patients tend to be small, multifocal, and bilateral.

Pathology and Molecular Genetics

Although collectively termed RCCs, malignant renal epithelial neoplasms are now subdivided under the new classification system, based on prominent morphologic features (239). However, in the past, pathologists long debated the varied histologic appearance of RCC. Of particular note, in the nineteenth century, Grawitz and others advanced the idea that these tumors were derived from malignant transformation of adrenal rest cells within the kidney. This belief led to later use of the term *hypernephroma,* first used to symbolize origin from cells above the kidney but now recognized as a misnomer to describe these tumors (116). Today, investigators know RCCs originate from renal tubular cells.

Although early study was limited to gross structural or numeric chromosomal alteration, investigators later discovered that discrete and specific loss of gene product from somatic cells could be linked to the origination and evolution of certain cancers (Table 16.3). Such thorough cytogenetic analysis of both sporadic and familial forms of RCC helped localize areas of suspect genetic alteration. In a particular major breakthrough, Seizinger and colleagues initially mapped the VHL gene to the short arm (3p25) of chromosome 3 (211).

In one study, researchers noted VHL gene mutations in 57% of patients with sporadic RCC and confirmed its potential involvement with tumorigenesis of that entity (79). Further research has demonstrated that multiple mechanisms of VHL gene mutation, including methylation, deletion, insertion, transition, and transversion, are responsible for the phenotypic variability of the syndrome (79,99). Meanwhile, others have chosen to focus on the inhibitory function of the VHL gene. Current theory proposes that the VHL protein plays a role in tumor suppression by modulating a transcription elongation complex, elongin or SIII, and negatively regulating the accumulation of vascular endothelial growth factor (VEGF) (109,219).

Concurrent with the ongoing research of the VHL protein, there were multiple reports of chromosomal deletions in the same region (3p) with sporadic forms of RCC. Since the late 1980s, the loss of loci on the short arm of chromosome 3 has been the predominant mutation linked to clear cell carcinoma (Fig. 16.2), the most common subtype of RCC (67,284). Increasing focus on a cohort of sporadic tumors identified 86% of cytogenically examined specimens as having a detectable anomaly distal to band 3p11.2-p13 (124). Allelic loss of 3p now is thought to be an early event

TABLE 16.3. LOCATION OF POTENTIAL CHROMOSOMAL CHANGES IN RENAL CELL CARCINOMA

Tumor	Affected Chromosomes
Conventional (clear cell) RCC	3p, 17
Papillary RCC	3q, 7, 12, 16, 17, 20, Y
Chromophobe RCC	1, 2, 6, 10, 13, 17, 21
Collecting duct carcinoma	1q, 6p, 8p, 13q, 21q

RCC, renal cell carcinoma.

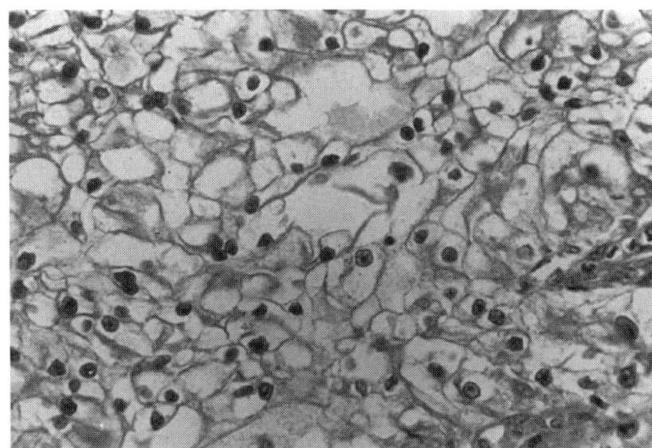

FIGURE 16.2. Histologic appearance of conventional (clear cell) renal cell carcinoma.

in the pathogenesis of clear cell carcinoma, whereas others now consider additional allelic losses on chromosome 17 to be associated with the advanced disease.

Among 60 nonpapillary RCCs studied at Memorial Sloan-Kettering Cancer Center, a significant correlation associating the deletion of chromosome 17p with tumor grade, pathologic stage, and nodal metastasis has been seen (188). Whether deletions of 3p occur in all renal cell cancers is under scrutiny, and many other chromosomal aberrations have been identified. Research to date shows that 3p genomic changes are conspicuously absent from the papillary variant of RCC and therefore reinforces the linkage between genes and representative histology.

Representing 10% to 15% of all renal cell cancers, the papillary carcinoma variant can be inheritable, multifocal, and bilateral, but generally suggests a more favorable prognosis. Long differentiated through immunohistochemistry, papillary RCC has distinct cytogenetic character, associated with loss of the Y chromosome along with trisomies of chromosomes 3q, 7, 12, 16, 17, and 20 (239). Recent research on those affected by hereditary papillary renal carcinoma implicates mutations, activating the MET protooncogene, to chromosome 7q31.1-34 (210). Investigators continue to propose that mutations in the MET protooncogene render the cells more susceptible to errors in chromosomal replication resulting in nonrandom duplication, a proliferative advantage, and the frequent occurrence of trisomy (286).

Chromophobe RCC accounts for approximately 5% of malignant renal epithelial tumors (239). Histologically, they are composed of two distinct cell types, those with granular eosinophilic cytoplasm and those with pale cytoplasm. Ultrastructural analysis shows numerous cytoplasmic microvesicles, and characteristic cytoplasm staining with Hale's colloidal iron is typical (42). Microscopic similarities exist between chromophobe RCC and oncocytoma, although distinctive nuclear features, including wrinkled "raisinoid" nuclei with frequent binucleation and perinuclear clearing are helpful in distinguishing between the two (253). A clinical analysis of patients with chromophobe carcinoma shows that the majority of tumors appear to be localized to the kidney at the time of diagnosis, but clinical behavior seems to be similar to respective stages of clear cell carcinoma (42). Large tumors and those with synchronous papillary carcinoma may be particularly prone to metastasis (192). DNA aneuploidy, especially hypodiploidy, is seen in the majority of cases with noted monosomy of different chromosomes (1,6,10,13,17,21,184) (239).

Collecting duct carcinomas represent a rare group of renal neoplasms. Unlike clear cell carcinoma, they arise from the distal portion of the nephron, commonly strike in a young population, and carry an unusually poor prognosis. Application of the aforementioned chromosomal inspection has discovered a frequent loss of heterozygosity at chromosome regions on 1q, 6p, 8p, 13q, and 21q (184). High density mapping of arm 1q in 13 collecting duct tumors shows an area of minimal deletion around the area located at 1q32.1-32.2 in 69% of the examined specimens (238). Considering these data together gives credence to the idea of a potentially unique set of molecular events in tumorigenesis, different from that of clear cell carcinoma.

RCC, unclassified, is a category reserved for malignant epithelial tumors that do not conform to any of the other subtypes. Of the total group of RCCs, they comprise approximately 4% to 5% (239). Specifically, composites of recognized subtypes, tumors with mucin production, and tumors with extensive sarcomatoid changes without recognizable epithelial elements are examples of this classification.

Pathologic grading of tumor cells has been shown to have prognostic value in cases of RCC (233). Several grading systems exist, although most pathologists rely on nuclear grading for renal lesions. The Fuhrman nuclear grading system is the most widely used in North America, and several studies confirm its relevance for prognosis (82). Nonetheless, all grading is subjective, and problems with standardization are recognized (154).

Clinical Presentation

Significant variability exists in the clinical presentation of RCC. However, a significant number of lesions are not discovered until reaching an advanced stage because small tumors isolated to the kidney are often asymptomatic. Aside from local symptoms produced by the tumor itself, a variety of systemic manifestations have been described. Therefore the clinician must be familiar with some of the extrarenal manifestations and must harbor a high suspicion for diagnosis. Although a classic triad of symptoms (pain, hematuria, and flank mass) has been associated with RCC, all three symptoms rarely are present together (150). Single symptoms occur much more frequently. Hematuria often is listed as the most common symptom, occurring in up to 60% of patients (161). Nonspecific symptoms such as fever, malaise, weight loss, and night sweats are also common.

TABLE 16.4. PARANEOPLASTIC SYNDROMES ASSOCIATED WITH RENAL CELL CARCINOMA

Erythrocytosis	Acute hepatic dysfunction
Anemia	Amyloidosis
Hypercalcemia	Thrombocytosis
Hypertension	

Occasionally, a varicocele from compression or obstruction of the testicular vein is found.

Few other disease entities possess such a propensity for paraneoplastic syndromes as RCC (Table 16.4). Erythrocytosis, anemia, hypercalcemia, hypertension, acute hepatic dysfunction, and amyloidosis all have been associated with renal cancer (150) and sometimes have been the hallmark features at presentation. Questions remain regarding which signals, substances, or cytokines initiate the manifesting signs and whether these are markers for prognosis or recurrence.

Several blood and serologic markers have been evaluated, and many have potential utility. Serum ferritin levels have been shown to be significantly elevated and higher than controls when looking at patients with RCC. In this group of patients, a statistically significant increase with advancing stage exists (57). Erythropoietin also can be elevated, presenting in as many as 63% of patients (242). More routine laboratory studies, including hematocrit and platelet levels, can likewise prove credible in regards to prognosis. In a series of stage IV tumors, patients with a normal platelet count had a mean increased survival of 59 months over those with thrombocytosis (platelet count more than 400,000) when controlling for pathologic stage, nuclear grade, and cell type (245). Others point to anemia and serum iron as useful tumor markers for initial evaluation and in follow-up (281). Anemia is the most common hematologic abnormality associated with RCC. Characteristically normocytic, normochromic anemia of chronic disease has been implicated. Following tumor resection, the anemia has usually resolved and some have shown that disease progression coincided with recurrent anemia (86,281).

Hypercalcemia has been associated with RCC and, like anemia, often resolves after removal of the primary tumor. Some elevation in serum calcium will be seen in 10% of patients. Experience shows that recurrent hypercalcemia can be an early sign of undetected skeletal metastasis or herald secondary sites that secrete an inciting humoral factor. Although parathyroid hormone–related protein (PTHrP) has been linked to the syndrome of humoral hypercalcemia of malignancy and has been detected in more than 95% of RCC, no significant correlation was identified when observing intensity of immunostaining of PTHrP and serum calcium levels (84).

Hypertension has been identified in many patients with RCC. A patient may be hypertensive as a consequence of hypercalcemia, but other factors such as polycythemia, arteriovenous fistulae, ureteral obstruction, or renin secretion may be responsible. Sufrin and colleagues noted that the elevated levels of renin were associated with high-stage renal tumors and hypertension (241). In fact, renin secretion is a known characteristic of RCC (103) but lacks specificity, because renin production has been reported with other cancers as well (55).

Acute elevation of liver enzymes (Stauffer's syndrome) has been described with certain cases of RCC (236). The majority of these cases show no evidence of hepatic metastasis from the tumor (19). Moreover, the enzymes often return to normal levels following removal of the renal lesion. Failure of liver function to return to normal has been significantly correlated with decreased survival (66). Recent work has shown that elevated liver enzymes, as well as other paraneoplastic syndromes, may be related to increased systemic levels of interleukin-6 (15,268).

Radiographic Diagnosis

The revolutionary improvements in radiographic diagnosis have radically changed the preoperative, intraoperative, and follow-up investigation of renal lesions. Standard historic, radiographic evaluation consisted of a chest x-ray film, intravenous (IV) pyelography, renal angiography, and possibly, bone scintigraphy. However, radiologists increasingly discover renal lesions incidentally through the newer modalities of ultrasonography, CT, or MRI while pursuing other suspected diagnoses. Although some may consider the plain film dated, one must recognize that 10% of RCCs will contain calcium and be detectable on abdominal plain films (112). Besides abdominal films, a chest radiograph has significant use and is a cost-effective tool for follow-up examination.

Intravenous Pyelography

Although there have been recent shifts away from excretory urography toward new imaging modalities, the intravenous pyelogram (IVP) remains a standard evaluation of the upper tracts for hematuria. On this study, renal masses may produce changes in the nephrogram and/or distortion of the collecting system. Occasionally, calcifications are present and also may be suggestive of a mass (133). The main limitation of IVP is its low sensitivity for small lesions compared with other studies (270). In addition, poor technique may lead to missed lesions altogether.

Angiography

Currently, angiography rarely is used in the initial diagnosis of renal masses, which historically show marked hypervascularity on angiogram. This study has been replaced almost completely by less invasive modalities such as CT and MRI. Nonetheless, angiography still proves useful for surgical planning in certain cases of partial nephrectomy.

Ultrasound

Recent reviews show that in as many as two-thirds of patients with localized RCC, lesions are found fortuitously on ultrasound examination (4). Moreover, incidentally detected tumors are of a lower stage than the comparative symptomatic lesions and result in improved survival (122,187). Noninvasive and cost-effective, ultrasound has inherent advantages. Echogenic criteria are well described and categorized to differentiate simple lesions from complex lesions with malignant potential. The sensitivity of sonography exceeds that of IVP in detecting small renal lesions, but both fall short of CT in relation to lesions less than 2 cm (270). Although descriptive, echogenic features unreliably determine histology. Recent attempted modifications, such as digitization with measuring of the grayscale (221) and Doppler vascularity determinations (119), have provided little absolute data on differing histology.

Real-time dynamic imaging capability does allow for intraoperative sonographic assessment of deep parenchymal lesions (i.e., difficult to palpate), tumor extension into adjacent structures, and pathology with uncertain preoperative staging (185). With the expanding role of nephron-sparing surgery and partial nephrectomy, intraoperative ultrasonography helps determine the boundaries of resection, multicentricity, venous extension, and associated cysts that may not be appreciated with visual inspection or preoperative radiographic evaluation (28,146).

Transabdominal ultrasound has been used to assess the inferior vena cava (IVC) for tumor extension in those undergoing radical nephrectomy. Recently, intraoperative ultrasound has been used to help clarify preoperative findings at the time of surgery (96,138). Newer ultrasound studies including color-flow Doppler and transesophageal echocardiography (TEE) also have proved valuable for diagnosis. Even when a tumor extends beyond the proximal cava or renal vein, TEE facilitates the identification of tumor thrombus migration and air embolization, allowing for immediate intraoperative intervention (220). Color-flow Doppler has been used for cases of equivocal CT scans and has shown excellent accuracy for caval tumor (91,121, 220,256).

An occasional diagnostic dilemma involves the identity of a renal cystic lesion by ultrasound. Bosniak developed a classification system for standardizing such lesions and identifying those with higher risk for malignancy (18). In a review comparing Bosniak classification with confirmed pathologic diagnosis, Seigel and colleagues found the incidence of malignancy with Bosniak I, II, III, and IV lesions to be 0%, 13%, 45%, and 90%, respectively (218a). One limitation of the Bosniak classification, which has been extended to cysts found by CT, is its subjectivity.

Computed Tomography

CT has distinct advantages over ultrasound and other modalities. Physicians can rapidly measure cyst densities, gain relational perspective between organs, and provide tumor staging with improving accuracy. New generation, multiphasic helical scanners enable greater detection of lesions, particularly small renal tumors, and foster a more thorough understanding of the capability. In contrast to conventional CT, helical scanning eliminates respiratory misregistration, and rapid acquisition allows for comparison of identical levels obtained before and after contrast. This is helpful in assessments of tumor extension into the renal vein (274). For maximum sensitivity, research shows that the differentiation of attenuation between a lesion and normal renal parenchyma is greatest during the nephrogenic phase, just before excretion of contrast into the collecting system, and not during the corticomedullary phase (39,246). Helical CT technology permits the production of detailed, high-quality three-dimensional (3D) reconstruction in a format remarkably similar to actual parenchymal, vascular, and adjacent structural anatomy. In one study, preoperative staging with 3D helical CT accurately depicted the pathologic character in 95 of 97 tumors; almost all of the renal arteries (96%) and renal veins (93%) were detected (40). Using these data obtained preoperatively readily simulates the surgical perspective and has proven a useful adjunct in nephron-sparing surgery (228,229).

For such reasons, CT has become the preferred method for staging of RCC (Fig. 16.3). Although the patient must ingest oral contrast and receive IV contrast, the procedure has less inherent risk than angiography and provides the surgeon with superior information (201). With CT, one can better define the regional extension of the mass through the renal capsule or into adjacent organs, such as the liver or

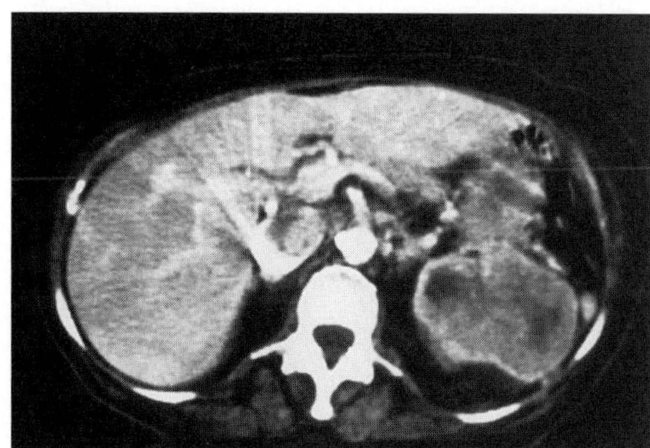

FIGURE 16.3. Axial view of computed tomography scan demonstrating large left renal mass. Also note contrast-filling defect in vena cava from associated tumor thrombus.

colon, and detect lymph node and distant visceral metastatic disease. Regarding venous involvement, Lang first reported the efficacy of CT scanning in evaluating extension into the renal vein and vena cava in comparison with angiography and sonography (131). CT has been criticized for its inability to identify the true cephalad extension of tumor thrombus, especially in the intrahepatic vena cava, but the advent of 3D reconstruction has added benefit in the detection of small accessory renal arteries and unusual venous branches (Fig. 16.4). Some suggest comparable vascular anatomic detail and even superior accuracy in relation to arteriography (40). Such data will only further reduce the indications for angiography in the evaluation of renal lesions.

Magnetic Resonance Imaging

Currently, physicians use MRI in situations in which the patient has preexisting medical conditions such as renal insufficiency or a serious contrast allergy that preclude the administration of contrast material. MRI historically has held an advantage to CT in evaluating renal lesions because it depends less on technique and the first modality capable of multiplanar imagery. RCC appears heterogeneous on T_1-weighted images and then typically becomes hyperintense when compared with normal parenchyma on T_2-weighted images. Spin-echo sequences are used to assess venous involvement.

In particular, MRI has been extremely useful in assessing vascular invasion (Fig. 16.5) by RCC (80). Specifically, MRI is noted for its accuracy in assessing superior extent of tumor thrombus (240). It also delineates the tumor within the cava even when there is total caval occlusion. The modern addition of gradient-recalled echo (GRE) sequences enhances the detail, reducing flow and respiratory motion artifact, and facilitates precise localization and more confident detection of thrombus. In a 1992 study, caval thrombus was identified correctly in 13 of 13 (100%), renal vein thrombus in 23 of 26 (88%), and right atrial thrombus in 4 of 5 (80%) patients (200). In general, MRI remains the preferred study for caval assessment.

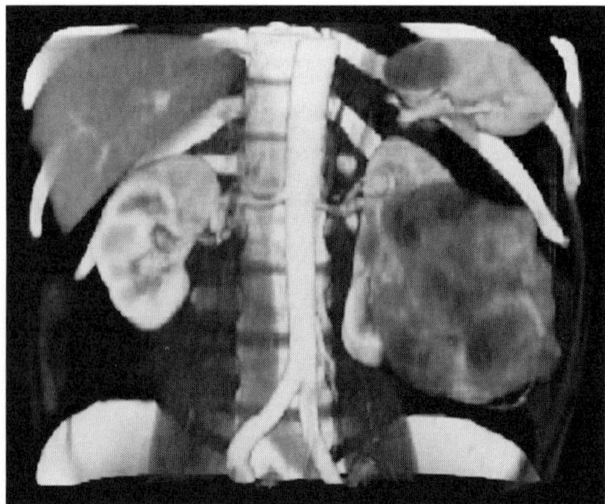

FIGURE 16.4. Three-dimensional computed tomography reconstruction view demonstrating excellent anatomic detail of left renal mass.

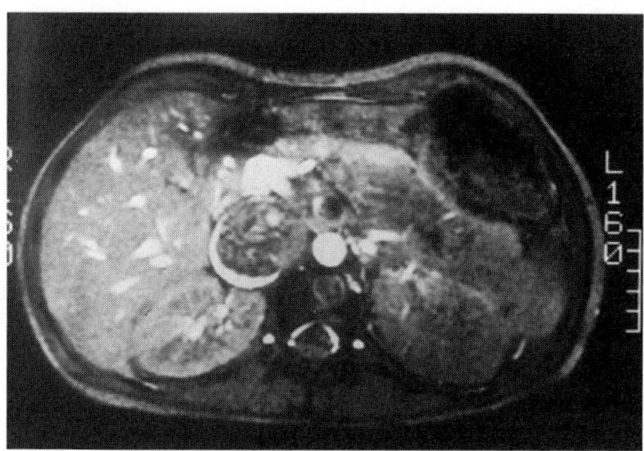

FIGURE 16.5. Axial magnetic resonance imaging view showing left renal mass with caval extension and surrounding contrast material.

Relatively long test time, high cost, obese body habitus that prohibits entry into the scanner, and ferro-magnetic prostheses or subcutaneous metallic foreign bodies are the current obstacles to MRI. Technology is advancing rapidly with open scanners and improving technical software. Much like CT angiography, researchers are using three-dimensional dual-phase MRI with gadolinium in the preoperative staging of renal carcinoma. Of the 18 patients enrolled in a prospective study, 30 of 31 (97%) surgically confirmed renal arteries were detected on preoperative scanning (35).

Positron Emission Tomography

Positron emission tomography (PET), like MRI, is another emerging noninvasive technology with potential applications to staging and detecting tumor recurrence. PET uses select endogenous substances with positron-emitting radioisotopes that accumulate in known sites of biologic activity. The most common radiotracer, 18-fluoro-2-deoxyglucose (FDG), resembles endogenous glucose and readily accumulates in the brain and myocardial tissue due to tissue demand. The renal tubules are unable to reabsorb FDG following filtration, and tracer detection consequently is prominent in the kidneys and bladder as well. In addition to these areas of resultant high uptake, malignant tumor foci generally possess a high rate of glycolysis and can be isolated on whole body imaging.

In one of the few studies that applied FDG PET scanning to RCC, Bachor and colleagues found that FDG PET detected 20 of 26 histologically confirmed renal tumors. Six cases failed to note the tumor focus, and three benign lesions were deemed falsely positive for malignancy (8). These data suggest some limitations with the modality. However, 10 of 10 patients with known progressive RCC in another study had their active metastasis identified with PET, whereas conventional modalities noted only an increasing lesion in 7 of the 10 (102).

FDG allows for detection of small malignant nodes not meeting the pathologic size criteria of CT scanning. Moreover, PET also may prove superior to CT or MRI in situations where postsurgical anatomy or artifactual distortion due to surgical clips decrease the sensitivity and specificity of those examinations (264). Technical considerations such as bowel preparation, IV bolus hydration, bladder irrigation, furosemide washout, procedural length, and cost limit PET to select clinical and investigational situations.

Staging

Staging, like histologic classification, has undergone several modifications to better characterize renal tumors and to establish some prognostic information. In the 1960s, Robson (194) improved the earlier work of Flocks and Kadesky (66a), and his system formed the basis of staging in the following several decades (Fig. 16.6). However, this arrangement suffered prognostically by grouping tumors with renal vein involvement alone, with vena cava involvement, or with lymph node involvement all within the third stage. As a result, this classification basically has been replaced by the tumor, node, and metastasis (TNM) system proposed by the International Union Against Cancer in the 1990s (10).

In 1997, the TNM system was further revised, as listed in Table 16.5 (230). Analysis of the first classification of tumor stages revealed little difference in survival between T_1 and T_2 lesions when the distinction was tumor size reaching 2.5 cm (90,250). Therefore the discriminating size between T_1 and T_2 lesions was changed to 7.0 cm in the tumor's greatest dimension. Analysis of this change shows that the new system permits better stratification of cases according to survival, thereby increasing its clinical use (112,157).

Therapy

The only consistently successful therapy for RCC to date has been surgical treatment for local, locally advanced, and minimally metastatic disease. Nonetheless, case reports of spontaneous tumor regression suggest that the malignancy may be susceptible to immune attack. This consideration, combined with new insights into molecular biology, has spawned significant research into potential immunotherapy for renal tumors. Unfortunately, although some regression has been seen in selected cases, complete response rates remain low. Likewise, both chemotherapy and radiotherapy demonstrate little success in treating this relatively resistant tumor. As the human genetic code is unraveled, clues into

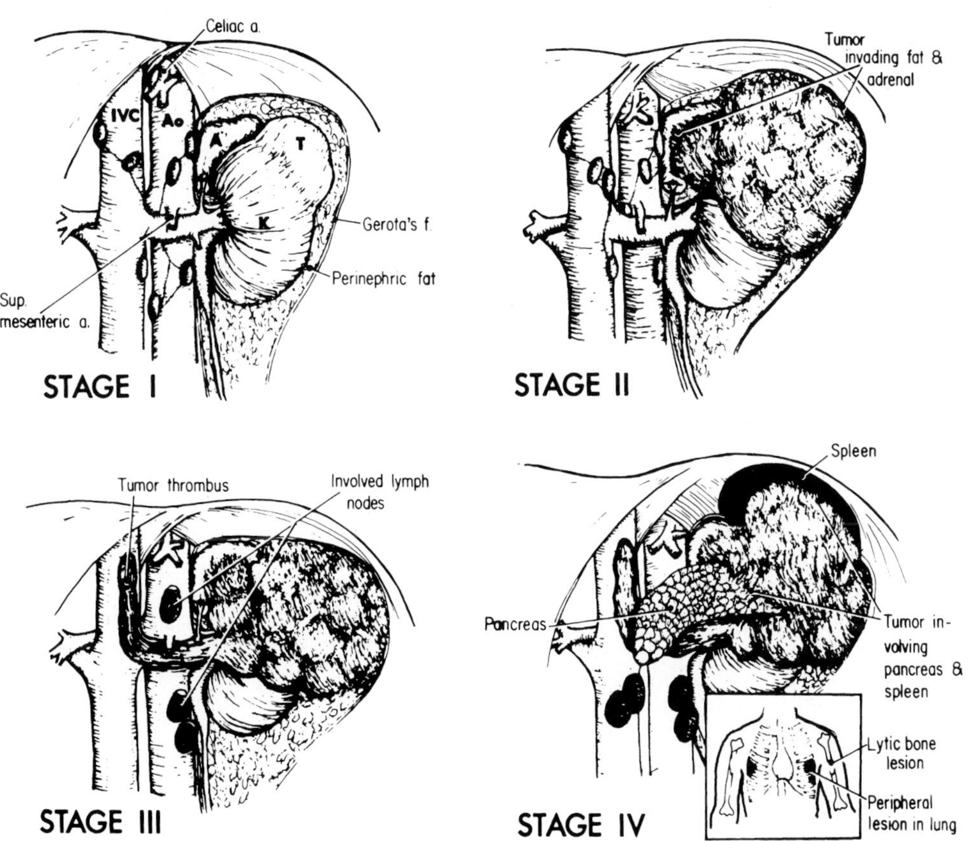

FIGURE 16.6. Robson staging classification of renal cell carcinoma.

TABLE 16.5. TUMOR NODE METASTASIS CLASSIFICATION FOR RENAL CELL CARCINOMA (1997)

T—Primary Tumor

T_X Primary tumor cannot be assessed
T_1 Tumor is ≤7.0 in greatest dimension and limited to kidney
T_2 Tumor is >7.0 cm in greatest dimension and limited to kidney
T_3 Tumor extends into major veins or invades adrenal gland or perinephric tissues but not beyond Gerota's fascia
T_{3a} Tumor invades adrenal gland or perinephric tissues but not beyond Gerota's fascia
T_{3b} Tumor grossly extends into renal vein or vena cava below diaphragm
T_{3c} Tumor grossly extends into vena cava above diaphragm
T_4 Tumor extends beyond Gerota's fascia

N—Regional Lymph Nodes

N_X Regional lymph nodes cannot be assessed
N_0 No regional lymph node metastasis
N_1 Metastasis in a single regional lymph node
N_2 Metastasis in more than one regional lymph node

M—Distant Metastasis

M_X Distant metastasis cannot be assessed
M_0 No distant metastasis
M_1 Distant metastasis

From Sobin L, Wittekind C. *International Union Against Cancer (UICC): TNM classification of malignant tumors,* 5th ed. Philadelphia: Lippincott-Raven, 1997:180, with permission.

the genetic abnormalities of patients with RCC will provide directions for new research that may yield new forms of treatment.

Radical Nephrectomy

The traditional gold standard therapy for patients with localized RCC and a normal contralateral kidney is the radical nephrectomy. This includes removal of the tumor-containing kidney and perirenal tissue within Gerota's fascia (Fig. 16.7). Theoretically, this encompasses the ipsilateral adrenal gland, although the issue of concomitant adrenalectomy often is debated. The question of whether to remove the lymph nodes draining the kidney at the time of nephrectomy is also controversial.

In 1869, the first elective nephrectomy was reportedly performed by Gustav Simon to treat a refractory ureterovaginal fistula (158). Removal of the tumorous kidney followed and the method was further developed in the twentieth century. Simple nephrectomy alone for cancer has fallen out of favor and currently is not recommended.

In 1963, Robson described a classic series in which he reported a 66% 10-year survival rate following radical nephrectomy for RCC (195). He attributed this excellent survival rate to early ligation of the renal pedicle and broader removal of the kidney with surrounding tissue, including perinephric fat and lymph nodes, from the crus of the diaphragm to the bifurcation of the aorta. Despite the small number of patients in this particular series, Robson continued to accrue patients for further reports (194) and can be credited with popularizing the concept of radical nephrectomy.

The kidney can be approached through several different incisions because of its location in the retroperitoneum. The urologic surgeon should be familiar with these different approaches and consequently tailor the operation to the individual patient while considering size of the tumor, location of the tumor within the kidney, and body habitus of the patient. Sometimes, the pleural and/or peritoneal cavities are entered as part of the nephrectomy procedure; often, neither of these spaces are violated. The choice of incision depends on the individual surgeon and hospital center, but currently, the most often used approach is the extraperitoneal flank incision. However, all approaches have two basic requirements: early ligation of the renal pedicle and adequate margins of tumor resection.

For the flank incision, the patient is placed in the lateral position with the operating table in the flexed position and the kidney rest elevated. The surgeon usually makes the incision over the eleventh or twelfth rib, and occasionally removes part of the rib to facilitate exposure. The goal is to stay in the extraperitoneal space and to avoid the potential complications of entering the peritoneum. Disadvantages include relatively more postoperative pain from incision of the flank muscles and the risk of pneumothorax from inadvertent entrance into the pleural cavity. Nonetheless, the flank approach provides excellent access to the renal fossa and is especially useful for small, localized tumors.

The transperitoneal approach has been used since the time of early nephrectomies. At that time, there were

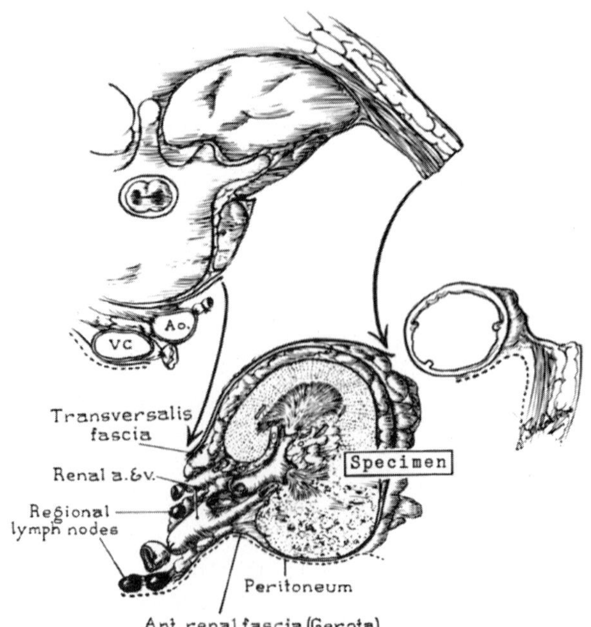

FIGURE 16.7. Radical nephrectomy specimen. Ao, aorta; VC, vena cava. (From Marshall FF. Radical nephrectomy: flank approaches. In: Marshall FF, ed. *Textbook of operative urology.* Philadelphia: WB Saunders, 1996:249, with permission.)

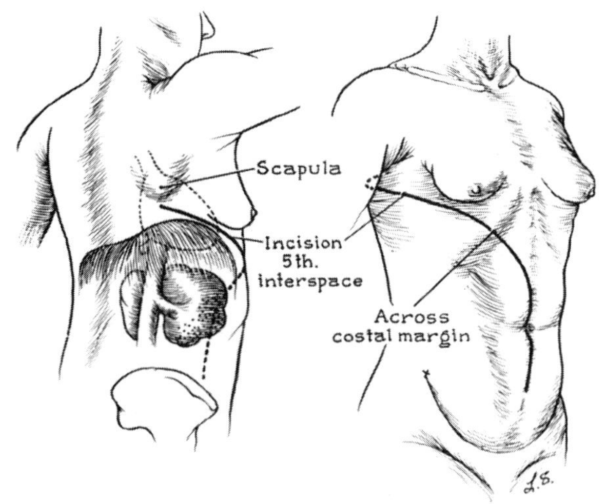

FIGURE 16.8. Thoracoabdominal incision. (From Marshall FF, Reitz BA. Radical nephrectomy with excision of vena caval tumor thrombus. In: Marshall FF, ed. *Textbook of operative urology.* Philadelphia: WB Saunders, 1996:265, with permission.)

significant complications of postoperative, often fatal, infections of the peritoneal space; however, these are rare with modern antibiotics. Today, the midline upper abdominal incision and the chevron incision are the most commonly used transperitoneal approaches. Advantages of these include easy identification of the renal pedicles and the ability to examine the abdominal organs. Moreover, the chevron incision permits much easier access to larger tumors. Disadvantages include poor exposure of the upper lateral quadrants with the midline incision and potential for ileus and intestinal adhesions.

The thoracoabdominal incision (Fig. 16.8), popularized by Chute, provides excellent exposure of upper pole tumors but involves entering the pleural space and, usually, the peritoneal cavity (37). With this approach, there is excellent exposure of the vena cava, so many surgeons prefer it for accessing tumors with caval thrombus. Entry into the chest cavity also allows for removal of any concomitant metastatic lung lesions, if necessary. A chest tube is required postoperatively.

Few surgeons use the subcostal incision for radical nephrectomy. Although this incision avoids the risk of unintentional entry into the pleural space, it generally provides relatively poor exposure of the kidney if the approach is kept extraperitoneal. Nonetheless, the benefit of examination of abdominal organs is possible if the incision is carried transperitoneally.

Lymphadenectomy

It has been established that RCC spreads through lymphatic routes. Studies have reported an approximate 20% to 25% average incidence of positive retroperitoneal lymph nodes when the nodes are sampled at the time of surgery (234). In 1935, Parker reported on the lymphatic drainage of the kidney. Based on his work, there are noted differences between lymphatics of the left and right kidneys (177). The left kidney most often drains to paraaortic nodes in the lumbar region, whereas the right kidney drains primarily to the interaortocaval and paracaval nodes (Fig. 16.9). These patterns have important implications when performing lymphadenectomy of nodes draining the kidney (147). One must also consider that anomalous vasculature and retroperitoneal processes, such as large tumors, ureteral obstruction, and caval extension, can alter these diagrammed routes.

In 1963, Robson suggested that extended lymphadenectomy at the time of surgery would be beneficial in terms of survival (195). Since that time, several others have advocated the removal of nodes found in the drainage pattern of the kidney as a means of preventing tumor spread. How-

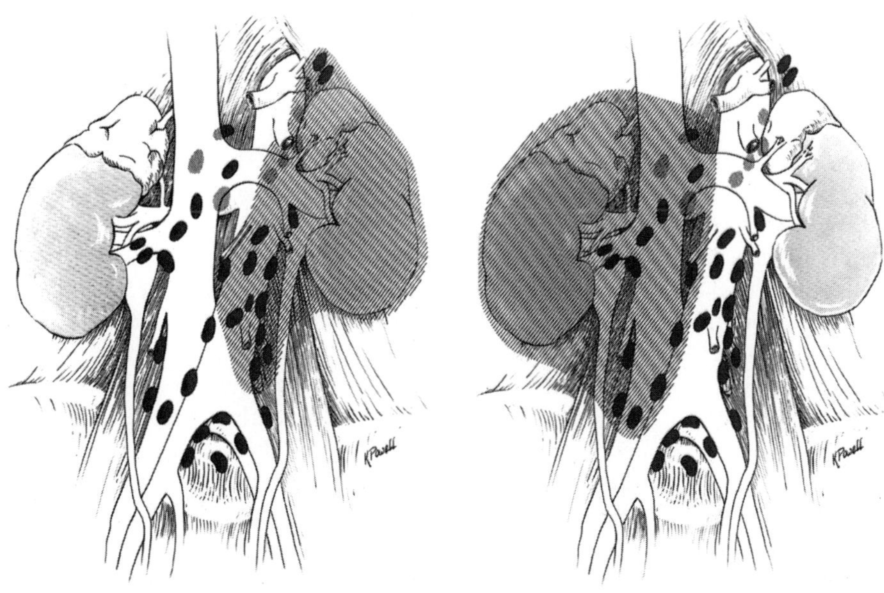

FIGURE 16.9. Lymphatic drainage patterns of the kidneys. (From Marshall FF, Powell K. Lymphadenectomy for renal cell carcinoma: anatomical and therapeutic considerations. *J Urol* 1982;128: 677, with permission.)

ever, the question of whether to remove nodes at the time of nephrectomy remains a controversial issue (181). In essence, all debate focuses on whether the benefits of the added procedure outweigh its risks. Currently, little data exist on patients prospectively randomized to receive nephrectomy with lymphadenectomy versus nephrectomy alone. Preliminary data from a randomized trial sponsored by the European Organization for Research on Treatment of Cancer (EORTC) showed little difference in disease progression between the aforementioned two groups (16,17).

Both proponents and opponents of lymphadenectomy make significant points. Those favoring lymphadenectomy in combination with nephrectomy argue that removal of nodes for pathologic examination will assist with true staging of the tumor and therefore may have prognostic implications. In addition, removing nodes may prove curative by excising metastatic spread along with the primary tumor and consequently improving survival rates. Those against lymphadenectomy argue that distant, often blood-borne metastases, for which lymph node excision provides no therapeutic benefit, occur commonly in advanced RCC (114). Moreover, considering the frequently aberrant distribution of lymph nodes draining the kidney, the removal of retroperitoneal nodes does not guarantee complete removal of lymphatic metastases. Studies that report increased survival with lymphadenectomy are limited by cohort size, lack of standardization, and retrospective analysis (234).

The extent of dissection when performing lymphadenectomy varies between individual surgeons. Limited regional dissection of the hilar nodes will have a much higher false-negative rate than will an extended retroperitoneal dissection. Until a prospective, randomized study with strict protocol regarding extent of node dissection is completed, the role of lymphadenectomy in RCC will be questioned.

Adrenalectomy

Available series report that the incidence of ipsilateral adrenal gland involvement in RCC ranges from 3.2% to 5.7% (202,206,212,257,266). Acknowledging this potential for adrenal involvement, Robson initially described ipsilateral adrenalectomy as part of the radical nephrectomy procedure (195). Recently, however, there has been considerable debate over the necessity of removing the adrenal gland at the time of nephrectomy (212,257,266). Reported benefits of avoiding adrenalectomy include lowered risk for adrenal insufficiency, preservation of adrenal tissue should the contralateral adrenal gland develop metastasis, decreased operative time, and decreased morbidity. Others point to studies showing that patients with adrenal involvement have a higher likelihood of positive lymph nodes or distant metastasis and therefore question the utility of excising the adrenal gland (202,212).

Research shows upper pole tumor location, left-sided tumors, and large tumors as risk factors for adrenal involvement in cases of RCC (202). Renal vein thrombosis also has been described as a risk factor (258). Most surgeons believe that extensive upper pole tumors, which have the propensity to spread to the ipsilateral adrenal gland by local extension, require adrenalectomy as part of the surgical procedure. However, tumors in the midpole and lower pole of the kidney also have shown adrenal gland metastasis, albeit in a much lower percentage; these tumors are thought to spread by hematogenous routes. Adrenalectomy also has been recommended when the adrenal gland contains a single metastatic lesion (212).

CT shows excellent sensitivity for adrenal lesions, and several investigators advocate its use to determine the need for adrenalectomy (75,193,206). Series report the negative predictive value of CT scans to be as high as 100% for adrenal abnormalities (257). Therefore a normal adrenal gland by CT scan makes the possibility of adrenal metastasis quite low. When abnormalities are detected, not all prove to be metastatic lesions because large tumors can cause displacement or poor visualization of the adrenal gland.

Overall, most studies report the yield of routine ipsilateral adrenalectomy at the time of nephrectomy to be quite low. As a result, many surgeons will avoid the adrenal gland in cases of small renal tumors not involving the upper pole. Certainly, those patients with risk factors for adrenal involvement can be identified preoperatively with radiographic studies, acknowledging that some with microscopic disease may be missed by this method. However, careful follow-up on these patients should identify the development of any other new lesions.

Nephron-sparing Surgery

In 1950, Vermooten was one of the first to suggest the idea of removing only part of a kidney affected by tumor (263). Nonetheless, the standard therapy for renal tumors soon thereafter became radical nephrectomy (145). Nephron-sparing surgery was later revisited, primarily for patients with marginal renal function, bilateral tumors, or a solitary kidney. Long-term studies of nephron-sparing surgery and outcomes now exhibit results comparable with radical nephrectomy in terms of tumor recurrence and survival. As a result, many urologists now advocate the use of partial nephrectomy for patients with a normal contralateral kidney. Overall, nephron-sparing renal surgery now has an increasingly expanded role in the management of even the most difficult localized renal tumors.

Enucleation. Simple enucleation involves separating the pseudocapsule of a tumor from surrounding normal renal parenchyma and coring out the neoplastic tissue from the remainder of the kidney. The advantages of enucleation are its simplicity and minimal disturbance of the kidney, whereas its main disadvantage is the risk of leaving behind residual tumor. Approximately 20 years ago, two small series reported the success of enucleation with regards to renal tumors (30,85). Later investigation also showed enucleation

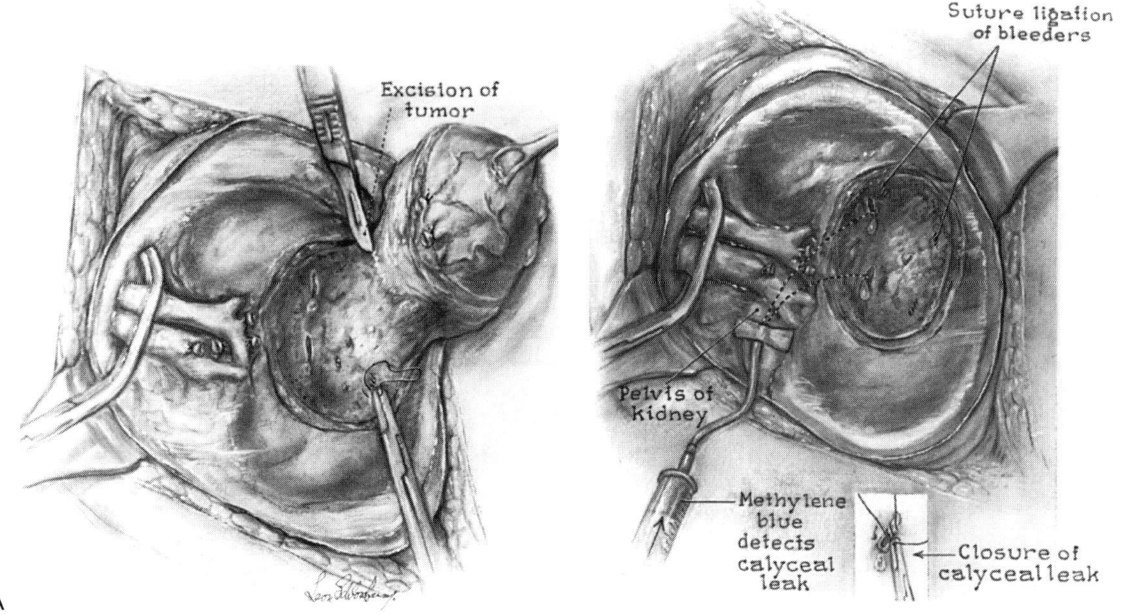

FIGURE 16.10. Technique of partial nephrectomy. **A:** Excision of the renal tumor after occlusion of the main renal vasculature. Vessels are ligated as encountered at the tumor base. **B:** Dye is injected into the collecting system to check for urinary leaks, which are then repaired. (From Marshall FF. Partial nephrectomy. In: Marshall FF, ed. *Textbook of operative urology.* Philadelphia: WB Saunders, 1996:274, with permission.)

feasible and successful in certain cases of well-circumscribed tumors (149,169). However, CT scans cannot always predict which tumors would be good candidates for enucleation. At this time, most surgeons do not recommend enucleation as a primary treatment for the majority of tumors but rather suggest partial nephrectomy. Nonetheless, in cases of VHL syndrome, where salvage of as much functional parenchyma as possible is preferable, enucleation remains an acceptable procedure.

Partial Nephrectomy. Standard partial nephrectomy differs from enucleation in that a normal rim of renal parenchyma is excised around the tumor specimen. While preserving renal tissue, partial nephrectomy also risks leaving tumor behind and therefore has risk of local recurrence. Studies report such recurrence to occur in approximately 4% to 8% of cases and attribute most instances to undetected multifocal tumors. Nonetheless, partial nephrectomy has proven to have disease-specific and overall survival rates comparable with radical nephrectomy.

The indications for partial nephrectomy have broadened over the years. Previous contraindications such as centrally located tumors (31) and tumors associated with normal contralateral kidneys (100) no longer prohibit consideration of nephron-sparing surgery. However, concerns regarding increased numbers of local recurrences with larger-sized tumors have led several investigators to suggest specific size limitations for the procedure. No consensus exists, but recent recommendations suggest elective partial nephrectomy only for tumors smaller than 2.5 cm (156) or tumors 4.0 cm or smaller (92).

The technique of partial nephrectomy (Fig. 16.10) most often involves the flank approach. Gerota's fascia and the overlying perinephric tissue are resected along with the tumor (186). In most instances, the renal vasculature is temporarily clamped to prevent significant bleeding during removal of the tumor. This requires cooling the kidney with ice slush to lessen chances of ischemic damage. Preoperative knowledge of the renal vasculature supplying the tumor allows for better surgical planning. Although this previously has been accomplished with angiography, newer, less invasive methods, such as 3D helical CT angiography, also are effective (228).

Long-term follow-up of partial nephrectomy patients yields excellent survival rates. In a recent review of 485 patients at the Cleveland Clinic, overall and cancer-specific 5-year survival rates were 81% and 92%, respectively (92). Others also have shown excellent long-term tumor control with partial nephrectomy (261), and higher disease-free rates have been reported in patients with a normal contralateral kidney (100). Adequate selection of both individual patients and tumors appears to be the key to successful outcomes.

Cryotherapy. Cryosurgical ablation of renal tumors has received attention over the past few years as an *in situ* form of nephron-sparing surgery. The benefits of freezing tumors in other organs including liver, prostate, cervix, and skin have been described. Several small series have reported minimal complications with excellent local tumor control (14,197). Currently, no sufficient long-term data are available to compare cryosurgery with other modalities.

Cryotherapy may be performed through an open incision or laparoscopically. Typically, there are two phases, freezing and thawing, that cause cellular disruption and tissue ablation (197). In an examination of acute histologic changes of renal tissue after cryoablation, investigators reported extensive coagulative necrosis and hemorrhage beyond the boundaries of the tumor (56). Negative tumor margins apparently are obtained, but long-term pathologic changes are unknown.

High-intensity Focused Ultrasound. Another attempt at nephron-sparing therapy for RCC includes high-intensity focused ultrasound (HIFU). HIFU involves ultrasound waves generated extracorporeally and then focused to a point inside the body, where they induce thermonecrosis of the tissue. Initial studies report HIFU therapy to be safe and efficacious (1,120), yet further investigation regarding long-term results of this new modality is needed for the future.

Laparoscopic Surgery

With the rapid development of minimally invasive surgery, urologists increasingly are using laparoscopy for the treatment of malignant renal tumors. The utility of the laparoscopic approach has been well documented (27,118,153, 191), and the addition of hand-assisted techniques also further broadens its appeal, adding dexterity and tactile sensation (278). Retroperitoneoscopy, without violation of the peritoneal cavity, also has been described (76). Initial concerns about tumor implantation at trochar sites and recurrence in the renal fossa have not proven to be significant complications. In a multicenter review of 157 patients with a mean follow-up period of 19.3 months, no patient developed tumor implantation or recurrence in the fossa (27).

Inferior Vena Cava Extension

Studies of RCC show that vena caval extension occurs in approximately 4% to 10% of cases, with a strong male predominance (38,80,135,148,152). All levels of caval tumor thrombus, from the renal vein ostia to the right atrium of the heart, occur. Because there is no adequate medical regimen, surgery offers the only cure for caval extension of tumor. The difficulty of the surgical approach is related to the degree of cephalad extension by the tumor thrombus, and intracaval neoplastic extension may even necessitate cardiopulmonary bypass for a safe and complete excision.

A thorough preoperative history to evaluate intercurrent health problems is mandatory for all surgical candidates. Anesthesia, and sometimes medical, consultations are needed to optimize conditions and prepare patients for often long procedures with intense hemodynamic shifts. Particular attention should be applied to cardiovascular status, especially when cardiopulmonary bypass is considered. Patients with IVC invasion may also have unique presentations. Although rare, symptoms can include massive lower extremity edema from IVC occlusion, ascites from Budd-Chiari syndrome, severe congestive heart failure, intestinal malabsorption, varicocele, or engorgement of the abdominal wall veins. Embolization of a portion of the tumor thrombus also may produce signs consistent with pulmonary embolus.

A full radiographic evaluation of patients with RCC and vascular extension is required before any operative intervention. The purpose of this is twofold: to discover any metastatic disease and to establish the true cephalad extension of the intracaval tumor. This evaluation can be accomplished by a variety of studies including venacavography, ultrasound, CT, and MRI. Venacavography involves the direct injection of contrast dye into the vena cava. Intravascular tumor can be visualized as filling defects in the contrast-filled cava (Fig. 16.11). However, cavography sometimes requires both antegrade (femoral) and retrograde (basilic) injections to fully delineate tumor extent (Fig. 16.12) (80). Cavography has the obvious disadvantage of exposing remaining normal renal parenchyma to a potentially nephrotoxic contrast load. Because of its invasive nature, there is also a risk of dislodging intravascular tumor.

Approximately one-third of patients with IVC extension have at least one metastatic lesion (227). Multiple studies have shown that survival rates are poor with radical surgery in the setting of vascular extension and metastatic disease (243,244). Therefore a complete workup for metastatic disease is important before surgical intervention. Radiologic tests, including bone scans, play a valuable role in this setting. Routine serum chemistries and liver function tests also may provide clues to possible disease outside the kidney. Thorough knowledge of preoperative lesions will allow much better follow-up in the postoperative course.

Surgical approach in cases of renal neoplasms extending into the vena cava is dictated by the superior extent of the intracaval or intracardiac tumor. Involvement of intrahepatic and suprahepatic caval levels can create numerous potential technical problems, thereby lengthening operative time. When sections of vena cava must be resected, reconstruction to allow for adequate venous drainage poses new challenges. Furthermore, extension into the right atrium exposes one to the additional potential complications of cardiac surgery and cardiopulmonary bypass.

Exposure of the neoplastic kidney and associated tumor thrombus can be achieved through several operative approaches. Most cases of RCC with IVC involvement occur on the right side, but tumors in the left kidney require bilateral dissection. Regardless of laterality, full exposure is necessary to ensure complete resection of both tumor and

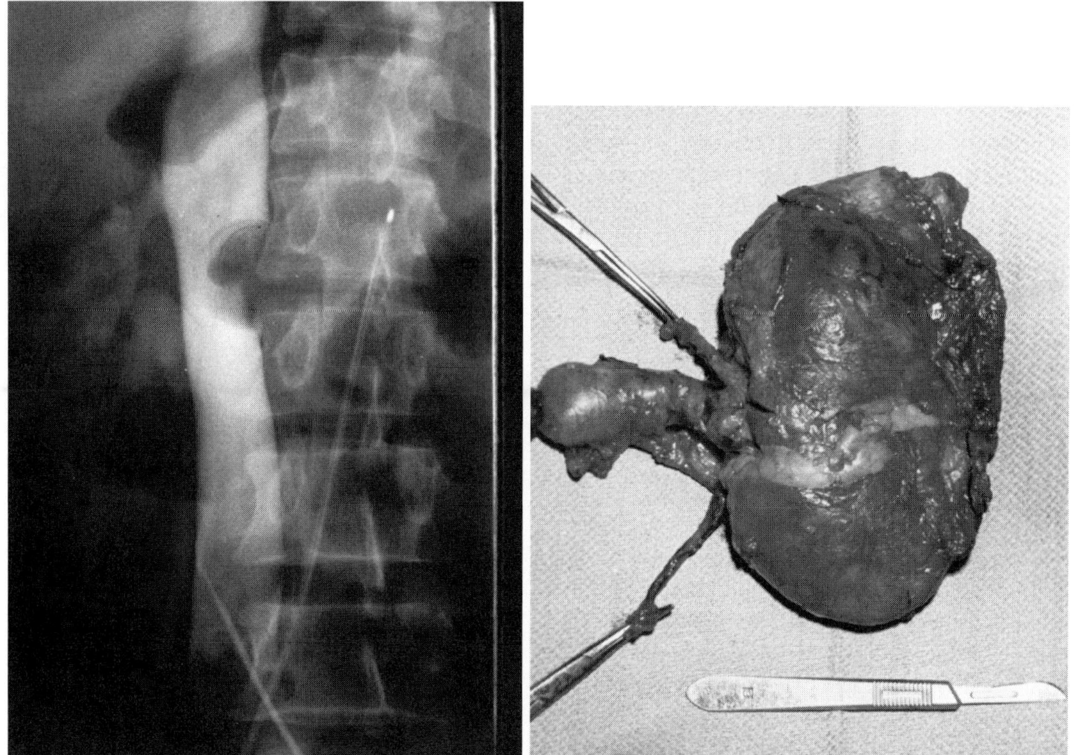

FIGURE 16.11. A: Venacavography demonstrates filling defect, suggesting extension of known left renal mass. **B:** Gross nephrectomy specimen in the same patient demonstrating distended renal vein from tumor thrombus.

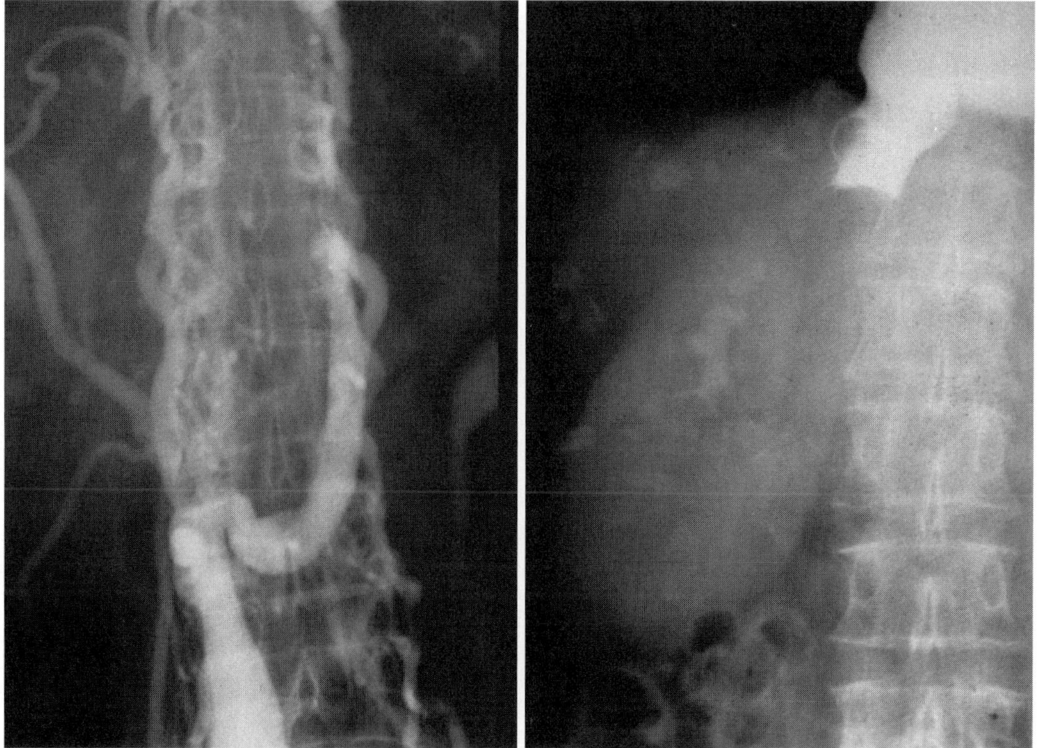

FIGURE 16.12. A: Antegrade venacavography with cutoff of contrast flow in the middle interior vena cava. **B:** Retrograde venacavography in the same patient demonstrating superior extent of tumor thrombus.

thrombus. The thoracoabdominal incision provides excellent exposure for renal tumors but more limited access to the aortic arch for cardiopulmonary bypass. The midline abdominal incision with extended sternotomy also allows for excellent visualization and has the added benefit of more direct access to the heart for cardiopulmonary bypass and hypothermia. However, this approach requires entry into the peritoneal cavity and therefore displacement of the bowel. The chevron incision with extended sternotomy may prove superior for exposure of large tumors in large patients. The most important goal of surgery for renal cell tumors with IVC extension is complete resection, including full removal of caval tumor and resection of any involved caval wall, if possible, because this has tremendous prognostic implications.

Following tumor excision, the vena cava can be reconstructed to allow for venous return from other structures including the contralateral kidney. Reconstitution of venous drainage after tumor removal depends on the extent of the cavotomy incision. Several studies report that at least 50% of the original IVC lumen diameter must be maintained with caval reconstruction to prevent blood thrombus formation and caval occlusion (151). Occasionally, synthetic graft material is used to construct new portions of the IVC (173,174), but harvested native pericardium for this purpose also has been described (151). In some situations, segmental cavectomy with ligation of proximal and distal ends has been used with satisfactory results (265).

Reconstruction of drainage for the contralateral kidney depends on the side of the lesion. For right-sided tumors, the left renal vein can be ligated, if necessary, because there is good collateral blood flow for venous drainage of the left kidney. Anatomic studies have shown this collateral flow to mainly depend on the left ascending lumbar vein, which receives a branch from the left renal vein and then joins the hemiazygous venous system to drain into the superior vena cava (38). The right ascending lumbar vein bypasses the right renal vein and therefore no collateral drainage for the right kidney exists. Because of this finding, the IVC must be reconstructed for left-sided tumors to allow venous return from the right renal unit.

Caval tumor extending into the retrohepatic and suprahepatic IVC requires extensive dissection (148). Significant bleeding can be encountered in posterior mobilization of the liver, particularly the caudate lobe. Some surgeons use division of the caudate lobe veins to allow for improved exposure of the vena cava and associated thrombus (Fig. 16.13). Even resection of the caudate lobe has been described (172).

Perioperative morbidity and mortality have been well described with surgery involving tumor in the inferior vena cava. Pulmonary embolization of tumor thrombus is a well-recognized complication that sometimes can be avoided by preoperative or intraoperative placement of a vena caval (e.g., Greenfield) filter (20,68). However, a filter can complicate surgery and pose additional risks such as IVC occlusion or renal vein compromise (20). Operative blood loss can be massive, and significant hemorrhage can produce hemodynamic and cardiac effects. Coagulopathy can sometimes occur with prolonged cardiopulmonary bypass. If adequate venous drainage is not ensured for the contralateral kidney, renal failure can ensue.

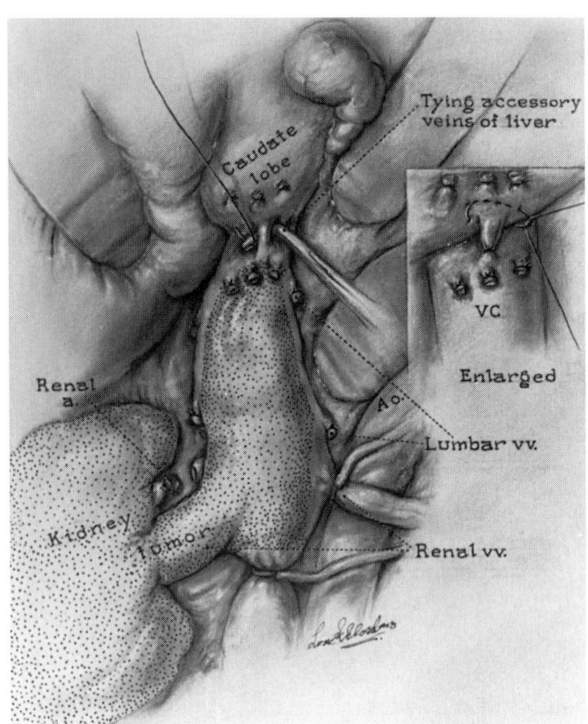

FIGURE 16.13. Removal of vena cava tumor thrombus often requires division of the veins from the caudate lobe of the liver. Ao, aorta VC, vena cava.

A variety of studies have examined characteristics of RCCs with tumor thrombi to assess prognostic factors both preoperatively and postoperatively from pathologic diagnosis. However, many of these studies contradict others examining the same factors. Therefore several questions have not been completely answered, and confusion still exists. There is almost complete agreement that incomplete resection of tumor thrombus portends a much worse prognosis than total removal.

Whether tumor extension into the vena cava alone affects prognosis has been examined in several studies. In a retrospective analysis of 71 cases (median survival, 81 months), isolated caval extension offered little prognostic impact (32). However, a later European study reported a significant survival advantage for patients with tumors confined to the kidney versus those with venous extension (137). Most would agree that survival is affected more by associated tumor factors than venous extension alone. Microscopic invasion of the vein wall by tumor cells has been reported as the single most relevant prognostic factor in one study, which showed a 45% chance of disease progression within 1 year of nephrectomy in this group of patients (262). A significant improvement in survival also was noted for patients with freely mobile tumor as compared with invading tumor (69% versus 26% 5-year survival, respectively). Of particular note, resection of the involved caval wall was associated with improved survival (97). Nonetheless, in one series of 26 patients, there was no survival difference between those patients with venous wall involvement and those without (137). Most studies have shown that the cranial extent of tumor thrombus alone has no bearing on prognosis in terms of survival (77,97,127, 137). However, several studies report that higher-extending thrombi are associated with significantly decreased survival rates (159,232).

Spread to regional lymph nodes has repeatedly been shown to be a poor prognostic indicator for RCC (12,127). A significant decrease in life expectancy was found in this subgroup when compared with a full cohort of patients with tumors invading the vena cava (13 versus 32 months median survival; $p < .001$) (127). Investigators showed that 5-year survival in a group of 37 patients with IVC tumor extension was 0% for the subset with lymph node metastases (versus 33.6% overall). Multiple studies have also confirmed that the preoperative or intraoperative demonstration of distant metastatic disease combined with caval extension leads to a poor prognosis, even with radical nephrectomy (32,127, 244). Such patients have much lower long-term survival rates, usually less than 15%, when compared with those without metastases (135,159,226,244).

For patients with caval thrombi from RCC, 5-year survival rates have ranged from approximately 30% to 60% following surgery, as in Table 16.6 (166). Again, these rates depend on the aforementioned factors. The presence of lymph node or distant metastases is associated with much shorter long-term survival, whereas the superior anatomic extent of the thrombus often does not appear to be as important. Excellent long-term survival has been achieved with complete surgical removal, so the preoperative evaluation to select suitable surgical candidates will have the greatest impact on survival rates.

TABLE 16.6. FIVE-YEAR SURVIVAL RATES IN STUDIES OF RENAL CELL CARCINOMA WITH CAVAL EXTENSION

Investigator (Year)	No. of Patients	Percentage of Patients Alive at 5 Years
Pritchett, et al. (1986)	25	28
Libertino, et al. (1987)	44	44
Hatcher, et al. (1991)	44	42
Swierzewski, et al. (1994)	100	54
Glazer and Novick (1996)	18	57
Nesbitt, et al. (1997)	37	34
Babu, et al. (1998)	15	55

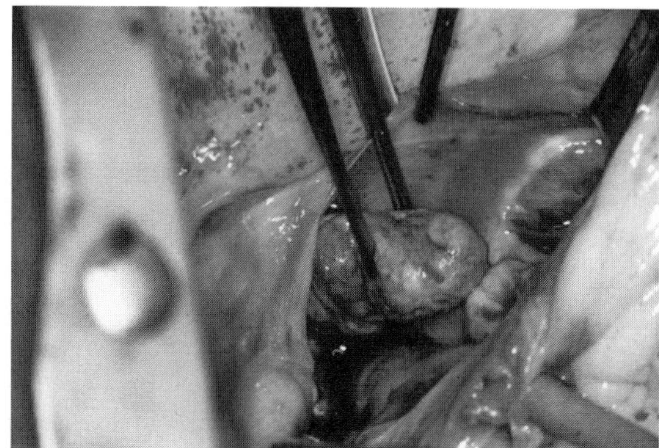

FIGURE 16.14. Removal of atrial tumor thrombus in the bloodless field allowed by cardiopulmonary bypass. Note the close vicinity of the tricuspid valve.

Cardiopulmonary Bypass and Hypothermia. The use of cardiopulmonary bypass and hypothermia has revolutionized surgery for IVC tumor thrombus extending into the right atrium. Bypass allows for an essentially bloodless field, which greatly assists in accessing and viewing pieces of caval and atrial tumor (Fig. 16.14). Moreover, this helps decrease the risk of tumor embolization during surgical manipulation (275). To date, use of cardiopulmonary bypass has not been shown to decrease survival in cases of renal tumors, but it does allow for full resection of the tumor. Perioperative mortality appears to be related to myocardial dysfunction, whereas short-term survival depends on lymph node and distant metastases (53). Length of bypass and arrest time also impacts survival. The surgeon places cannulas in the aorta and right atrium to allow for shunting of blood through the bypass machine. Systemic heparinization is used to prevent thrombosis. Once bypass has started, a cardioplegic solution is applied to the heart. To avoid subsequent permanent effects, optimal time for bypass is less than 45 minutes (148). Recently, a technique of minimally invasive (small incision) bypass has been described (64).

Metastatic Renal Cell Carcinoma

Years of intervention have done little to improve survival in patients with metastatic RCC. Regardless of the therapy used, results have been disappointing, and the search for effective treatment regimens remains a challenge for urologists and oncologists alike. Nonetheless, failure has fortunately bred an ever-expanding list of potential therapies, including chemotherapy and a multitude of immunomodulating options. Few sites in the body are safe from potential metastatic deposits with RCC; however, the most common sites are the lungs, bones, lymph nodes, adrenal glands, and brain (203). At autopsy of patients with RCC, no significant difference in metastatic locations was seen in patients who had undergone previous nephrectomy versus those who had not had surgery (204).

Radiotherapy

RCC has been characteristically regarded as a radioresistant tumor. In the past, several studies have addressed the issue of adjunctive radiotherapy in the treatment of metastatic disease, but none have documented significantly increased survival in that group of patients. Today, radiotherapy most often is used for palliative treatment of symptomatic tumors or metastatic lesions (51,123). Several investigators have used brachytherapy for this purpose (129).

Specifically, radiation has proven effective under circumstances of osseous or brain metastasis by rendering palliation, possibly preventing progression, and improving quality of life. Stereotactically guided high-precision irradiation selectively destroys small intracranial lesions and preserves surrounding brain tissue (11,160). Externally applied radiation alleviates bone pain in up to 77% of treated sites (94). Future applications linking radiation and immunotherapy are under investigation. In an effort to improve tumor targeting, novel phase I trials are investigating both the accumulation and the therapeutic potential of radiolabeled (I-131) monoclonal antibodies (G250) in metastatic RCC (52,237). Early results are encouraging, but much research still is needed to prove efficacy.

Chemotherapy

Standard historic chemotherapeutic regimens have failed to impact disease progression, and ultimately survival, in the majority of patients. An extensive review of more than 83 published trials from 1983 to 1993 showed a 6% response rate in 4,093 adequately treated patients with advanced RCC. The most efficacious agents were continuously infused 5-fluorouracil and floxuridine, with remissions in 10% and 12%, respectively. Circadian infusion, meant to optimize drug metabolism, modestly improved the remission rate to 15% of the patients treated with floxuridine (280). A recent review confirms that chemotherapy options for treatment are limited and suggests use in advanced cases only (3).

Scientists attribute, in part, the unyielding multidrug resistance of RCC to a plasma membrane glycoprotein (P-glycoprotein) that promotes the efflux of therapeutic agent away from the targeted cell. Overexpression of P-glycoprotein has been shown in 80% of tumors, which is much higher than in normal proximal tubular cells (81). Several medications, including cyclosporine (196), tamoxifen (205), and calcium channel blockers (176), have been used in attempts to block the multidrug resistant activity and to enhance the effect of chemotherapeutic agents, but no additive responses beyond that of chemotherapy alone are documented.

Immunotherapy

Because of RCC's resistance to chemotherapy and radiotherapy, alternative approaches have been sought. Physicians long ago suspected an integral role for the immune system in cases of spontaneous regression, and immunotherapy has gathered increased consideration for systemic treatment of metastatic tumors. The first recorded case of spontaneous regression (from the Mayo Clinic in 1928) postulated that antibodies produced by the body were responsible for either rendering the tumor cells inert or destroying them (26). Admittedly rare, almost 100 cases of spontaneous regression exist in the literature (58), and 2 recent reports document partial, transient regression in 5% to 7% of patients with pulmonary nodules without the impact of therapy (144,175). Additional supportive data include modern immunohistochemical analysis demonstrating infiltration of T lymphocytes and macrophages (63) as well as observed clinical responses to infused cytokines, interferons, and interleukins. Approaches applying biologic response modifiers (cytokines), vaccination, and gene therapy are under current study.

Interferons. Since its initial discovery in the 1950s, the family of homologous proteins known as *interferons* has expanded in both number and function. Interferons act on the cellular level, binding to a surface receptor and transducing important regulatory signals. The exact mechanism of antitumor activity is unknown, but research has shown interferons to impart, via signal transduction, potent antiviral, antiproliferative, and immunomodulatory function *in vivo* (106). Specifically, leukocytes produce interferon-α(IFN-α), which subsequently enhances natural killer cell function and induces major histocompatibility complex antigen expression.

Within the family of interferons, many individual proteins have been studied (126). Results from a well-constructed, randomized trial proved no difference, relative to placebo, in outcome of patients treated with interferon-γ (IFN-γ)-1b for metastatic RCC (78). IFN-α also has been thoroughly tested as a single agent, and promising initial data with this agent prompt further consideration of IFN-α as a therapeutic approach in patients with metastatic disease. An average of 3 to 4 months may transpire before the occurrence of an objective response from the initiation of therapy, but multiple studies show a reproducible response rate of 10% to 20% (24,61,163,260) and a complete response rate ranging as high as 5% (24). The patients most likely to respond are those who have undergone prior nephrectomy with good performance status, have a long disease-free interval, and have lung-predominant metastatic disease (143,208). Nonetheless, the duration of response rarely exceeds 2 years, with a mean time ranging from 5 to

15 months (276), and randomized trials have shown only a modest increase, 2 to 7 months, in survival time (231). In attempts to apply reports of *in vitro* synergy, randomized trials combining IFN-α with vinblastine failed to show improved survival over using interferon as the sole therapy and showed exacerbation of the subsequent interferon side effects, including leukopenia, nausea, vomiting, and neurotoxicity (165).

Interleukins. Another of the biologic response modifiers, interleukin-2 (IL-2), was approved on the basis of safety and efficacy for the treatment of RCC by the U.S. Food and Drug Administration in 1992. Interleukins indirectly affect tumorigenesis by enhancing the proliferation and function of T lymphocytes, and clinical studies for renal tumors suggest an approximate 15% to 19% objective response rate with IV bolus administration (25, 74,199). Moreover, the complete response rate registers as high as 9.3% and is durable. More than 75% of the complete responders remain disease free for 3 years, and some in excess of 10 years without evidence of recurrent RCC. Treatment favors those with good performance status, absence of prior immunotherapy, total dose administered, and maximal rebound lymphocytosis after cessation of IL-2 (199).

Toxicity of interleukins can be severe. Many patients suffer with relatively minor symptoms of fever, chills, nausea, vomiting, diarrhea, and general malaise, but high-dose IL-2 treatment also can spur significant hypotension, fluid retention, acute respiratory distress, confusion, and renal failure as a physiologic consequence of the resultant cytokine cascade (178). Intensive monitoring and, frequently, aggressive support that includes maintenance of blood pressure with volume and pharmacologic vasopressors is required with bolus infusion. Even though side effects generally subside with discontinuation of therapy, treatment-related mortality ranges as high as 4% yearly with early experience (74). More recent analysis from the National Cancer Institute accounting for all 1,241 individuals treated with high-dose bolus IL-2 reveals an overall mortality rate of 0.7% with no treatment-related deaths in the last consecutive 680 patients (199).

Attempts have been made to optimize results and diminish the significant and sometimes life-threatening side effects of IL-2. Modifying dosage may diminish the toxicity without changing efficacy in regards to partial or complete tumor regression (22,235). However, the data currently are inconclusive. An ongoing randomized trial specifically addressing the issue reports preliminary results showing the high-dose IV bolus regimen to be the most effective (162). Adding complementary products such as lymphokine-activated killer cells (132,198), tumor-infiltrating lymphocytes (23,62), or IFN-α (164) currently does not produce statistically significant improvement in regards to overall survival over IL-2 alone.

Gene Therapy

Another novel approach, gene therapy, has garnered much attention, and clinical trials of therapeutic gene transfer in the treatment of urologic cancer are underway. Fundamentally, all gene therapy is a procedure of molecular surgery, because physicians sterilely introduce therapeutic DNA into diseased cells by way of a vector. Successful chromosomal integration allows for replication with the remainder of the treated cell's genes. Through the introduction of normal or modified genetic code, the process of carcinogenesis may be reversed or prevented.

Two entirely different gene therapy strategies can be defined. The first is corrective gene therapy, which involves the replacement or inactivation of defective genetic material with genes that prevent, slow, or reverse the events that encompass tumorigenesis. Significant insight into the molecular mechanisms of carcinogenesis is emerging, and potential mutational targets such as the VHL gene are being identified. In fact, introduction of a normal chromosome 3p has been shown to modulate tumor growth rate in an RCC cell line *in vitro* as long as 10 years ago (218). Nonetheless, several impressive limitations, including targeting, efficacy, and efficiency of vector transfer, exist currently with respect to corrective therapy. The second strategy includes treatment with recombinant DNA that selectively enhances killing of malignant cells, directly or indirectly. This cytoreductive gene therapy is further along than corrective gene therapy in terms of clinical application. More than 80 clinical protocols have been approved worldwide (223).

Previous research involving multiple cytokine genes shows that granulocyte-macrophage colony-stimulating factor (GM-CSF) gene–transduced vaccines incite the most vigorous, durable, and specific tumor immunity (5,54). Additional study has found preliminary evidence that GM-CSF genetically transduced, irradiated tumor vaccines induce potent T-cell–mediated antitumor activity without toxicity (222). The action of GM-CSF after gene transfer involves local spread of the cytokine at high concentrations, triggering antigen-presenting cell ingress and activation. This paracrine physiology more closely mimics the natural biology of cytokine action compared with the systemic IV administration of recombinant cytokines. Similar to other immunotherapies, treatment parameters such as mode of delivery, the ideal concentration of stimulatory cytokine, and minimum number of tumor cells for antigen presentation have yet to be determined. The nascent frontier of gene therapy will continue to grow, along with the other novel immunologic approaches under study such as tumor-specific vaccination (105) and monoclonal antibody treatments (52).

Surgical Resection

The role of surgical resection in the setting of metastatic disease has been questioned (209). Specifically, with the development of improved immunotherapy regimens, the benefits of adjuvant nephrectomy and/or resection of metastatic lesions have been addressed (248,267,277). Nephrectomy also has been performed for the palliation of severe symptoms, such as pain or hematuria. In addition, reasonable 5-year survival rates have been seen in cases of solitary metastatic lesions that have undergone metastasectomy. In all cases, the risks of surgical therapy must be weighed against the potential benefits of removing the malignant lesion. The lack of randomized studies in this area makes this a difficult comparison.

Controversy exists regarding whether to perform adjuvant cytoreductive surgery with immunotherapy and also regarding appropriate timing for the operation. Critics of surgery point to a meager rate of spontaneous regression (1% to 4.4%) with frequent recurrence (144), increased morbidity and operative mortality (13), and deferred subsequent cytokine therapy in some cases (190). On the other hand, proponents believe that excision of the primary tumor serves as an adjunct to systemic immunotherapy for purposes of tissue procurement and elimination of a suspected immunomodulator. Recently, adjuvant surgery for immunotherapy in metastatic RCC has been reported to have beneficial results in terms of survival, although studies are not conclusive (65). Previously, however, it was suggested that nephrectomy alone did not improve survival rates in patients with metastatic disease (47) or, at best, affected outcome in certain favorable patients only (83,168).

Patients with known metastatic disease who present with significant symptoms, including those from pain, hematuria, or paraneoplastic syndromes, may benefit from palliative surgery. Although occasional reports of spontaneous regression of metastatic lesions following nephrectomy have surfaced, palliative surgery has not been shown to have significant effects on overall survival. Nonetheless, palliation of symptoms may improve quality of life. Again, the risks of surgical intervention must be weighed against potential benefits of improved symptoms. A less invasive method of palliation for certain patients involves angioinfarction, in which blood flow to the kidney is blocked by use of an embolic material placed in the renal vasculature. Although theoretically appealing, angioinfarction conveys little prognostic benefit.

The percentage of RCC patients who present with a single detectable metastatic lesion ranges from approximately 1% to 3%, according to available studies (155,170,255). Evidence suggests that aggressive surgical therapy may have beneficial results in this select group of patients. The prototype metastatic lesion responding to surgical therapy is the pulmonary nodule. Moreover, improved survival has been associated with normal performance status, and a disease progression–free interval of more than 24 months from time of nephrectomy (142). Other types of metastatic lesions, including those to the central nervous system (179) and bone, also have shown effective long-term results.

The Future: Molecular Prognostic Markers

Recent evaluation reaffirmed the statistic significance of pathologic staging and nuclear grade in relation to survival (258). On a macroscopic level, metastasis can be qualified and generally portends a poor prognosis. However, the prognosis for patients with locally confined RCC is known to be variable. With ever finer focus, scientists are identifying morphologic character, proteins, antigens, and other prognostic markers that aid in both diagnosis and characterization of a particular lesion. Less specific prognostic signs and symptoms such as weight loss, anemia, hypercalcemia, and elevated liver function tests are giving way to clinicopathologic features discovered through application of immunohistochemistry, flow cytometry, polymerase chain reaction technology, and nucleic acid analysis. Already proven techniques have been expanded to generate better outcome data. For instance, distortion of nuclear shape has a long history in the histologic evaluation of tumors, but by using modern digital technology and mathematic equations for nuclear roundness and ellipticity, investigators found significantly improved prognostication (29).

Modern markers of proliferation such as Ki-67, silver-staining nucleolar organizer regions (AgNOR), and proliferating-cell nuclear antigen (PCNA) are present in cycling cells and therefore have potential utility in estimating the biologic aggressiveness of a given tumor. Several studies have identified the Ki-67 antigen and PCNA to be significant prognostic parameters in regards to survival and tumor recurrence, comparing favorably or even superior to grade and pathologic stage (48,101,249). In contrast to nuclear grading, the evaluation of positive staging is not only less subjective, but also reproducible and simple. In addition, AgNOR, Ki-67, and PCNA all have been shown to be independent predictors of survival and of greater prognostic value than histologic grade in multivariate analysis (48,93). Another measure of abnormal proliferation can be ascertained through detection of aneuploidy. Determinations of ploidy by flow cytometry are proving less reliable however, and in studies of locally confined tumors, conclusions regarding in its relationship to grade, stage, and prognosis are mixed (249).

Along with high proliferative indices, RCC has other inherent qualities ripe for prognostic analysis. Metastasis involves a complex series of events and depends on the cancer's ability to break from the primary location and implant in another area of the body. Two elements believed to be essential in this process are cell adhesion molecules and angiogenesis factors. Cadherins are a large family of transmembrane proteins responsible for mediating cell-to-cell adhesion, and when expression decreases, their inherent ability to modulate and preserve epithelial integrity diminishes. Lack of E-cadherin expression correlates with aggressiveness in several tumors, but only 20% of RCCs express the glycoprotein (117). E-cadherin appears to be localized to Bowman's capsule and other tubular segments rather than to the proximal tubular epithelium. Such evidence brings to question whether E-cadherin plays an integral role in renal cell carcinogenesis.

As a result, more recent focus has shifted to cadherin-6. Shimazui showed this cadherin to be the major one in the proximal renal tubules and RCC itself. Investigating this relationship as related to prognosis, Shimazui's group found that aberrant expression of cadherin-6 connoted poor survival (216,217). These data have been reproduced in a series wherein the majority of renal cell cancers with histology-associated poor prognosis (e.g., high-grade clear cell cancers) showed aberrant expression. The tumors with a historically good prognosis (e.g., low-grade clear cell carcinomas and papillary cancers) exhibited normal cadherin-6 expression (180).

In a similar fashion, the degree of angiogenesis has been shown to correlate with the development of metastases in several cancers including melanoma (225), prostate (271), breast (272), and non–small-cell lung carcinoma (140). In one study, when investigating the relationship to malignant renal epithelial tumors, an immunohistochemical marker of angiogenesis, microvessel density, exhibited no correlation to clinical stage, pathologic stage, or tumor grade (141). However, another investigation showed that higher microvessel density was associated with longer patient survival in clear cell carcinoma; this relationship is contrary to that reported with other types of malignancies (49). RCC is a vascular tumor, but its direct relationship to angiogenesis has yet to be completely determined.

Proteins responsible for apoptosis, such as p53, have been extensively studied in many cancer models, including RCC. The p53 protein binds DNA and is believed to regulate transcription, acting as a "checkpoint" to induce cell cycle arrest (128). When mutated, this tumor suppressor gene inactivates the normal function of DNA damage surveillance. Aneuploid cells originate, carcinogenesis occurs, and tumor progression can ensue (104). Mutant p53 proteins have a prolonged half-life, and with accumulation are detectable with immunohistochemical analysis (130). Yet controversy exists in regards to the frequency of the mutation in RCC (ranging from 4% to 40% of specimens tested) and consequently, its resultant prognostic power. Uhlman found an 87% 10-year, disease-specific survival rate for patients with nonstaining Robson stage I tumors versus a 62% survival with p53 positive-staining tumors ($p < .01$). Moreover, p53 positivity was an independent predictor of survival, whereas tumor grade was not (259). More recently, others have demonstrated a significant correlation between p53 and nuclear grading and PCNA expression, and these researchers claim p53 to be an independent predictor of survival. Nonetheless, they also recognize the infrequency of staining and believe it to be a useful adjunct to the standard criteria of stage and grade (215). The clinical significance of p53 and other apoptotic markers has yet to be completely elucidated.

MISCELLANEOUS RENAL TUMORS

Renal Angiomyolipoma

Renal angiomyolipomas (Fig. 16.15) are generally benign tumors of the kidney that are named based on their three characteristic histologic components: blood vessels, smooth muscle, and mature adipocytes. Their extensive vascularity is associated with a significant propensity for hemorrhage, which can produce clinical symptoms. However, angiomyolipomas often may grow to large sizes before diagnosis. They can occur as a solitary lesion, in multiple sites within one kidney, or in both kidneys. Rare cases of malignant degeneration have been described (36,59,139), as well as coexistence with RCC (95).

Angiomyolipomas also are commonly associated with tuberous sclerosis, an inherited syndrome characterized by mental retardation, epilepsy, adenoma sebaceum, and hamartomas of multiple organs including retina, heart, bone, lung, and kidney (108). A significant number of patients with tuberous sclerosis will develop renal angiomyolipomas; therefore careful screening is required. In this group of patients, the tumors tend to occur at a younger age and to be multifocal and bilateral (238).

The size of the tumor appears to significantly affect its symptomatology. Steiner and associates (238) reported that tumors smaller than 4 cm produced no symptoms in their series of patients. However, tumors larger than 4 cm commonly produce symptoms (171,238). Flank pain is the most prevalent symptom at presentation, occurring in up to 70% of symptomatic patients (9). A palpable mass and hematuria, usually microscopic, also are seen. More rare presentations include hypertension and anemia. Rupture of the tumor with subsequent retroperitoneal hemorrhage also may produce significant hypotension, which can progress to hemorrhagic shock.

Often, radiographic imaging alone confirms the diagnosis of angiomyolipoma. The numerous fat–nonfat interfaces

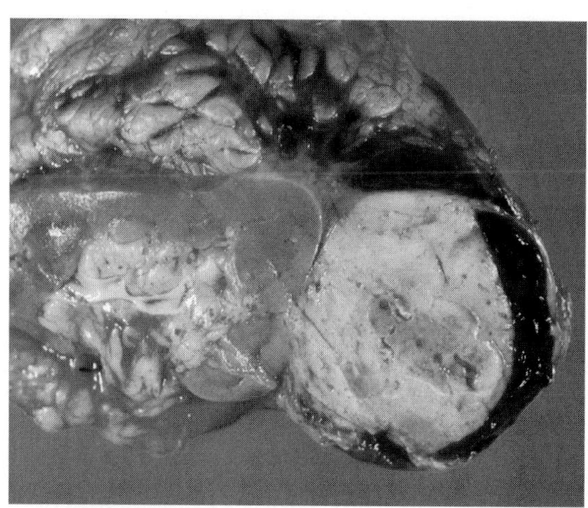

FIGURE 16.15. Gross view of angiomyolipoma.

with sonography produce an intensely echogenic lesion. Quantifying these echoes with computer assistance may aid in differentiation of angiomyolipomas from other renal tumors (221). CT scans can detect fat densities (−70 to −30 Hounsfield units) within the tumor, and the presence of fat is essentially pathognomonic for angiomyolipoma. The characteristic high signal intensity of fat on T_1-weighted images of MRI scans also can assist in the diagnosis. If fat cannot be detected in the lesion using radiographic studies, the tumor should be treated as malignant until a pathologic diagnosis confirms angiomyolipoma. Percutaneous needle sampling of the tumor for tissue analysis has been described (207).

The management of angiomyolipomas varies based on the individual patient. Once a diagnosis is made, the size of the tumor and the presence of symptoms determine the future course. The goal for therapy is renal preservation, when possible. Small, asymptomatic tumors may be followed with yearly ultrasounds, with no treatment necessary unless tumors become large or symptomatic. Tumors larger than 4 cm that are asymptomatic or mildly symptomatic also may be followed, but investigators recommend semiannual radiographic monitoring (171,238). Patients with extremely large tumors or those with severe symptoms should undergo therapy before the development of retroperitoneal hemorrhage. Embolization of angiomyolipomas often has been successful in control of bleeding and also can be therapeutic (171). Tumors that are poorly suited for angioinfarction or those with questionable diagnosis require surgical exploration for treatment. Nephron-sparing surgery with preservation of normal parenchyma is the preferred approach, when possible. Tumors that replace the entire kidney, multifocal lesions, and those with uncontrollable hemorrhage necessitate total nephrectomy.

Renal Medullary Carcinoma

Renal medullary carcinoma is a tumor found in patients with SC trait or hemoglobin sickle cell disease. It has been described mainly in African American adolescents and young adults, with a male predominance (6,41,43,45,70). This highly aggressive tumor quickly progresses to metastatic disease. Mean survival after diagnosis averages approximately 3 months (6,45), with only rare reports of survival past 1 year (41,183). Multiple failed chemotherapy regimens demonstrate the chemoresistance of this tumor (6,183).

Patients most often present with gross hematuria; therefore this symptom in a patient with sickle cell trait should prompt an appropriate workup (269). The tumor is concentrated in the medulla of the kidney, but satellite nodules in the renal cortex and renal sinus are often noted (45). Infiltrative growth is common (43), and venous and lymphatic invasion usually is present (45). Abnormalities on chromosome 3 and monosomy 11 have been identified in some patients (6). On radiographic studies of the kidney, contrast enhancement and echotexture are consistently heterogeneous (43). Hypovascularity also has been noted on renal angiogram (43,70).

TABLE 16.7. OTHER RENAL TUMORS

Fibroma	Lymphangioma
Fibrosarcoma	Lymphoma
Fibrous histiocytoma	Mesoblastic nephroma
Hemangioma	Metastatic tumors
Hemangiopericytoma	Myxoma
Juxtaglomerular cell tumor	Neurogenic tumors
Leiomyoma	Osteogenic sarcomas
Leiomyosarcoma	Renomedullary interstitial cell tumors
Lipoma	Rhabdomyosarcomas
Liposarcoma	

Other Tumors

Aside from the more common tumors discussed previously, numerous other lesions have been described as occurring within the kidney (Table 16.7). In general, these are exceedingly rare tumors; many are derived from mesenchymal elements and are benign in nature (247). Metastatic deposits from other primary malignancies also are seen. Often, no symptoms are present and discovery of the lesion occurs as an incidental or autopsy finding.

REFERENCES

1. Adams J, Moore R, Anderson J, et al. High-intensity focused ultrasound ablation of rabbit kidney tumors. *J Endourol* 1996;10(1):71.
2. Reference deleted in proofs.
3. Amato R. Chemotherapy for renal cell carcinoma. *Semin Oncol* 2000;27(2):177.
4. Amendola M, Bree R, Pollack H, et al. Small renal cell carcinoma: resolving a diagnostic dilemma. *Radiology* 1988;166:637.
5. Asher A, Mule J, Kasid A, et al. Murine tumor cells transduced with the gene for tumor necrosis factor-alpha. *J Immunol* 1990;146:3327.
6. Avery R, Harris J, Davis C Jr, et al. Renal medullary carcinoma: clinical and therapeutic aspects of a newly described tumor. *Cancer* 1996;78(1):128.
7. Babu SC, Mianoni T, Shah PM, et al. Malignant renal tumor with extension to the inferior vena cava. *Am J Surg* 1998;176(2):137.
8. Bachor R, Kotzerke J, Gottfried H, et al. Positron emission tomography in diagnosis of renal cell carcinoma. *Urologe A* 1996;35:146.
9. Bardot S, Montie J. Renal angiomyolipoma: current concepts of diagnosis and management. *AUA Update Series* 1992;11:306.
10. Beahrs O, ed. American Joint Committee on Cancer: manual for staging cancer, 4th ed. Philadelphia: J.B. Lippincott, 1992:201.

11. Becker G, Duffner F, Kortman R, et al. Radiosurgery for the treatment of brain metastasis in renal cell carcinoma. *Anticancer Res* 1999;19(2c):1611.
12. Belis J, Kandzari S. Five-year survival following excision of renal cell carcinoma extending into the inferior vena cava. *Urology* 1990;35(3):228.
13. Bennett R, Lerner S, Taub H, et al. Cytoreductive surgery for stage IV renal cell carcinoma. *J Urol* 1995;154:32.
14. Bishoff J, Chen R, Lee B, et al. Laparoscopic renal cryoablation: acute and long-term clinical, radiographic, and pathologic effects in an animal model and application in a clinical trial. *J Endourol* 1999;13:233.
15. Blay JY, Rossi JF, Wijdenes J, et al. Role of interleukin-6 in the paraneoplastic inflammatory syndrome associated with renal-cell carcinoma. *Int J Cancer* 1997;72(3):424.
16. Blom JH, van Poppel H, Marechal JM, et al. Radical nephrectomy with and without lymph node dissection: preliminary results of the EORTC randomized phase III protocol 30881. EORTC Genitourinary Group. *Eur Urol* 1999;36(6):570.
17. Blom JHM, Schroeder FH, Sylvester R, et al. European Organization for Research on Treatment of Cancer Genitourinary Group. The therapeutic value of lymphadenectomy in conjunction with radical nephrectomy in non-metastatic renal cancer—results of an EORTC phase III study [Abstract]. *J Urol* 1992; 147:422a.
18. Bosniak MA. The current radiological approach to renal cysts. *Radiology* 1986;158(1):1.
19. Boxer R, Waisman J, Lieber M, et al. Non-metastatic hepatic dysfunction associated with renal carcinoma. *J Urol* 1978; 119:468.
20. Brenner D, Brenner C, Scott J, et al. Suprarenal Greenfield filter placement to prevent pulmonary embolus in patients with vena caval tumor thrombi. *J Urol* 1992;147:19.
21. Budin R, McDonnell P. Renal cell neoplasms: their relationship to arteriolonephrosclerosis. *Arch Pathol Lab Med* 1984; 108:138.
22. Bukowski R, Goodman P, Crawford D, et al. Phase II trial of high dose intermittent interleukin-2 in metastatic renal cell carcinoma: a southwest oncology group study. *J Clin Oncol* 1990;82(2):143.
23. Bukowski R, Sharfman W, Murthy S, et al. Clinical results and characterization of tumor-infiltrating lymphocytes with or without recombinant interleukin-2 in human metastatic renal cell carcinoma. *Cancer Res* 1991;51:4199.
24. Bukowski R. Immunotherapy in renal cell carcinoma. *Oncology* 1999;801:810.
25. Bukowski R. Natural history and therapy of metastatic renal cell carcinoma: role of interleukin-2. *Cancer* 1997;80:1198.
26. Bumpus H. The apparent disappearance of pulmonary metastasis is a case of hypernephroma following nephrectomy. *J Urol* 1928;20:185.
27. Cadeddu J, Ono Y, Clayman R, et al. Laparoscopic nephrectomy for renal cell cancer: evaluation of efficacy and safety: a multicenter experience. *Urology* 1998;52:773.
28. Campbell S, Fichtner J, Novick A, et al. Intraoperative evaluation of renal cell carcinoma: a prospective study of the role of ultrasonography and histopathological frozen sections. *J Urol* 1996;155:1191.
29. Carducci M, Piantadosi S, Pound C, et al. Nuclear morphometry adds significant prognostic information to stage and grade for renal cell carcinoma. *Urology* 1999;53:44.
30. Carini M, Selli C, Minaro GB, et al. Conservative surgery for renal cell carcinoma. *Eur Urol* 1981;7:19.
31. Chan D, Marshall F. Partial nephrectomy for centrally located tumors. *Urology* 1999;54(6):1088.
32. Cherrie R, Goldman D, Lindner A, et al. Prognostic implications of vena caval extension of renal cell carcinoma. *J Urol* 1982;128(5):910.
33. Chow W, Devesa S, Fraumeni J Jr. Epidemiology of renal cell carcinoma. In: Vogelzang N, Scardino P, Shipley W, et al, eds. *Comprehensive textbook of genitourinary oncology,* 2nd ed. Philadelphia: Lippincott Williams & Wilkins, 2000:101.
34. Chow W, Devesa S, Warren J, et al. Kidney cancer incidence trends in the United States. *JAMA* 1999;281:1628.
35. Choyke P, Walther M, Wagner J, et al. Renal cancer: preoperative evaluation with dual-phase three-dimensional MR angiography. *Radiology* 1997;205:767.
36. Christiano A, Yang X, Gerber G. Malignant transformation of renal angiomyolipoma. *J Urol* 1999;161(6):1900.
37. Chute R, Soutter L, Kerr WS Jr. The value of the thoracoabdominal incision in the removal of kidney tumors. *N Engl J Med* 1949;241:951.
38. Clayman R, Gonzalez R, Fraley E. Renal cell cancer invading the inferior vena cava: clinical review and anatomical approach. *J Urol* 1980;123:157.
39. Cohan R, Sherman L, Korobkin M, et al. Renal masses: assessment of corticomedullary-phase and nephrogenic-phase CT scans. *Radiology* 1995;196:445.
40. Coll D, Uzzo R, Herts B, et al. 3-dimensional volume rendered computerized tomography for preoperative evaluation and intraoperative treatment of patients undergoing nephron-sparing surgery. *J Urol* 1999;161:1097.
41. Coogan C, McKiel C Jr, Flanagan M, et al. Renal medullary carcinoma in patients with sickle cell trait. *Urology* 1998;51: 1049.
42. Crotty T, Farrow G, Lieber M. Chromophobe cell renal carcinoma: clinicopathological features of 50 cases. *J Urol* 1995; 154(3):964.
43. Davidson A, Choyke P, Hartman D, et al. Renal medullary carcinoma associated with sickle cell trait: radiologic findings. *Radiology* 1995;195(1):83.
44. Davis C Jr, Barton J, Sesterhenn I, et al. Metanephric adenoma: clinicopathological study of fifty patients. *Am J Surg Pathol* 1995;19(10):1101.
45. Davis C Jr, Mostofi F, Sesterhenn I. Renal medullary carcinoma. The seventh sickle cell nephropathy. *Am J Surg Pathol* 1995;19(1):1.
46. Dechet C, Bostwick D, Blute M, et al. Renal oncocytoma: multifocality, bilateralism, metachronous tumor development and coexistent renal cell carcinoma. *J Urol* 1999;162(1):40.
47. DeKernion J, Ramming K, Smith R. The natural history of metastatic renal cell carcinoma: a computer analysis. *J Urol* 1978;120(2):148.
48. Delahunt B, Bethwaite P, Nacey J, et al. Proliferating cell nuclear antigen (PCNA) expression as a prognostic indicator for renal cell carcinoma: comparison with tumor grade, mitotic index and silver staining nucleolar organizer region numbers. *J Pathol* 1993;170:471.
49. Delahunt B, Bethwaite PB, Thornton A. Prognostic significance of microscopic vascularity for clear cell renal cell carcinoma. *Br J Urol* 1997;80(3):401.
50. Reference deleted in proofs.
51. DiBiase S, Valicenti R, Schultz D, et al. Palliative irradiation for focally symptomatic metastatic renal cell carcinoma: support for dose escalation based on biological model. *J Urol* 1997;158(3):746.
52. Divgi C, Bander N, Scott A, et al. Phase I/II radioimmunotherapy trial with iodine-131-labeled monoclonal antibody G250 in metastatic renal cell carcinoma. *Clin Cancer Res* 1998; 4:2729.

53. Donatelli F, Pocar M, Triggiani M, et al. Surgery of cavo-atrial renal carcinoma employing circulatory arrest: immediate and mid-term results [Abstract]. *Cardiovasc Surg* 1998;6:166.
54. Dranoff G, Jaffee E, Lazenby A, et al. Vaccination with irradiated tumor cells engineered to secrete murine GM-CSF stimulates potent, specific and long lasting tumor immunity. *Proc Natl Acad Sci USA* 1993;90:3539.
55. Eddy R, Sanchez S. Renin-secreting renal neoplasm and hypertension with hypokalemia. *Ann Intern Med* 1971;75:725.
56. Edmunds T Jr, Shulsinger D, Durand D, et al. Acute histologic changes in human renal tumors after cryoablation. *J Endourol* 2000;14:139.
57. Esen A, Ozen H, Ayhan A, et al. Serum ferritin: a tumor marker for renal cell carcinoma. *J Urol* 1991;145:1134.
58. Fairlamb D. Spontaneous regression of metastases of renal cancer. *Cancer* 1981;47:2102.
59. Ferry J, Malt R, Young R. Renal angiomyolipoma with sarcomatous transformation and pulmonary metastases. *Am J Surg Pathol* 1991;15(11):1083.
60. Fielding J, Visweswaran A, Silverman S, et al. CT and ultrasound features of metanephric adenoma in adults with pathologic correlation. *J Comput Assist Tomogr* 1999;23(3):441.
61. Figlin R, deKernion J, Mukamel E, et al. Recombinant interferon alpha 2a in metastatic renal cell carcinoma: assessment of antitumor activity and anti-interferon antibody formation. *J Clin Oncol* 1988;6:1604.
62. Figlin R, Pierce W, Kaboo R, et al. Treatment of metastatic renal cell carcinoma with nephrectomy, interleukin-2 and cytokine-primed or CD8(+) selected tumor-infiltrating lymphocytes from primary tumor. *J Urol* 1997;158:740.
63. Finke J, Tubbs R, Connelly B, et al. Tumor infiltrating lymphocytes in patients with renal cell carcinoma. *Ann NY Acad Sci* 1987;532:387.
64. Fitzgerald J, Tripathy U, Svensson L, et al. Radical nephrectomy with vena caval thrombectomy using a minimal access approach for cardiopulmonary bypass. *J Urol* 1998;159:1292.
65. Flanigan R, Blumenstein S, Bearman S, et al. Cytoreduction nephrectomy in metastatic renal cancer: the results of Southwestern Oncology Group trial 8949 [Abstract 685]. *J Urol* 2000;163(4):156.
66. Fletcher M, Packham D, Pryor J, et al. Hepatic dysfunction in renal cell carcinoma. *Br J Urol* 1981;53:533.
66a. Flocks RH, Kadesky MC. Malignant neoplasms of the kidney: an analysis of 353 patients followed 5 years or more. *J Urol* 1958;79:196.
67. Foster K, Crossey P, Cairns P, et al. Molecular genetic investigation of sporadic renal cell carcinoma: analysis of allele loss on chromosomes 3p,5q,11p,17 and 22. *Br J Cancer* 1994;69:230.
68. Friedell M, Sujka S, Welch J, et al. Massive pulmonary embolus after surgery for renal cell carcinoma extending into the inferior vena cava: a case report. *Am Surg* 1997;63(6):516.
69. Friedrich CA. Von Hippel-Lindau syndrome. A pleomorphic condition. *Cancer* 1999;86[11 Suppl]:2478.
70. Friedrichs P, Lassen P, Canby E, et al. Renal medullary carcinoma and sickle cell trait. *J Urol* 1997;157(4):1349.
71. Fromowitz PB, Bard RH. Clinical implications of pathologic subtypes in renal cell carcinoma. *Semin Urol* 1990;8:31.
72. Frydenberg M, Gunderson L, Hahn G, et al. Preoperative external beam radiotherapy followed by cytoreductive surgery and intraoperative radiotherapy for locally advanced primary or recurrent renal malignancies. *J Urol* 1994;152(1):14.
73. Fukushima T, Nagashima Y, Nakatani Y, et al. Chromophobe renal cell carcinoma: a report of two cases. *Pathol Int* 1994; 44(5):401.
74. Fyfe G, Fisher R, Rosenberg S, et al. Results of treatment of 255 patients with metastatic renal cell carcinoma who received high dose recombinant interleukin-2 therapy. *J Clin Oncol* 1995;13:688.
75. Gill I, McClennan B, Kerbl K, et al. Adrenal involvement from renal cell carcinoma: predictive value of computerized tomography. *J Urol* 1994;152(4):1082.
76. Gill I, Rassweiler J. Retroperitoneoscopic renal surgery: OM approach. *Urology* 1999;54(4):734.
77. Glazer A, Novick A. Long-term followup after surgical treatment for renal cell carcinoma extending into the right atrium. *J Urol* 1996;155:448.
78. Gleave M, Elhilali M, Frodet Y, et al. Interferon gamma-1b compared with placebo in metastatic renal cell carcinoma. *N Engl J Med* 1998;338:1265.
79. Gnarra J, Tory K, Weng Y, et al. Mutations of the VHL tumor suppressor gene in renal carcinoma. *Nature Genetics* 1994;7:85.3
80. Goldfarb D, Novick A, Bretan L, et al. Magnetic resonance imaging for assessment of vena caval tumor thrombi: a comparative study with venacavography and computerized tomography scanning. *J Urol* 1990;144:1100.
81. Goldstein L, Galski H, Fojo A, et al. Expression of a multidrug resistance gene in human cancers. *J Natl Cancer Inst* 1989;81:116.
82. Goldstein NS. The current state of renal cell carcinoma grading. *Cancer* 1997;80(5):977.
83. Golimbu M, Al-Askari S, Tessler A, et al. Aggressive treatment of metastatic renal cancer. *J Urol* 1986;136:805.
84. Gotoh A, Kitazawa S, Mizuno Y, et al. Common expression of parathyroid hormone–related protein and no correlation of calcium level in renal cell carcinoma. *Cancer* 1993;71(9):2803.
85. Graham SD Jr, Glenn JF. Enucleative surgery for renal malignancy. *J Urol* 1979:122:546.
86. Greenberg PL, Creger WP. The anemia of chronic disorders due to renal cell carcinoma: ferrokinetic and morphologic documentation of its surgical correction. *Am J Med Sci* 1971; 261:265.
87. Greenlee R, Murray T, Bolden S, et al. Cancer statistics, 2000. *CA Cancer J Clin* 2000;50:7.
88. Grignon D, Eble J. Papillary and metanephric adenomas of the kidney. *Semin Diag Pathol* 1998;15(1):41.
89. Grossman E, Messerli FH, Glodbourt U. Does diuretic therapy increase the risk of renal cell carcinoma? *Am J Cardiol* 1999; 83(7):1090.
90. Guinan P, Saffrin R, Studhldreher D, et al. Renal cell carcinoma: comparison of the TNM and Robson stage groupings. *J Surg Oncol* 1995;59:186.
91. Habboub H, Abu-Yousef M, Williams R, et al. Accuracy of color Doppler sonography in assessing venous thrombus extension in renal cell carcinoma. *AJR Am J Roentgenol* 1997; 168:267.
92. Hafez K, Fergany A, Novick A. Nephron sparing surgery for localized renal cell carcinoma: impact of tumor size on patient survival, tumor recurrence and TNM staging. *J Urol* 1999;162: 1930.
93. Haitel A, Weiner H, Migschitz B, et al. Proliferating cell nuclear antigen and MIB-1. An alternative to classic prognostic indicators in renal cell carcinomas? *Am J Clin Path* 1997; 107:229.
94. Halperin EC, Harisiadis L. The role of radiation therapy in the management of metastatic renal cell carcinoma. *Cancer* 1983; 51:614.
95. Hardman J, McNicholas T, Kirknam N, et al. Recurrent renal angiomyolipoma associated with renal carcinoma in a patient with tuberous sclerosis. *Br J Urol* 1993;72:983.

96. Harris D, Wang Y, Ruckle H, et al. Intraoperative ultrasound: determination of the presence and extent of vena caval tumor thrombus. *Urology* 1994;44:189.
97. Hatcher P, Anderson E, Paulson D, et al. Surgical management and prognosis of renal cell carcinoma invading the vena cava. *J Urol* 1991;145:20.
98. Hennigar R, Beckwith J. Nephrogenic adenofibroma: a novel kidney tumor of young people. *Am J Surg Pathol* 1992;16(4)325.
99. Herman J, Latif F, Weng Y, et al. Silencing of the VHL tumor-suppressor gene by DNA methylation in renal cell carcinoma. *Proc Natl Acad Sci USA* 1994;91:9700.
100. Herr H. Partial nephrectomy for unilateral renal cell carcinoma and a normal contralateral kidney: 10-year followup. *J Urol* 1999;161:33.
101. Hofmockel G, Tsatalpas P, Muller H, et al. Significance of conventional and new prognostic factors for locally confined renal cell carcinoma. *Cancer* 1995;76(2):296.
102. Hoh C, Seltzer M, Franklin J, et al. Positron emission tomography in urological oncology. *J Urol* 1998;159:347.
103. Hollifield J, Page D, Smith C, et al. Renin-secreting clear cell carcinoma of the kidney. *Arch Intern Med* 1975;135:1989.
104. Hollstein M, Sidransky D, Vogelstein B, et al. p53 mutations in human cancers. *Science* 1991;253:49.
105. Holti L, Rieser C, Papesh C, et al. Cellular and humoral immune responses in patients with metastatic renal cell carcinoma after vaccination with antigen pulsed dendritic cells. *J Urol* 1999;161:777.
106. Horoszewicz J, Murphy G. An assessment of the current use of human interferons in therapy of urological cancers. *J Urol* 1989;142:1173.
107. Hughson M. Renal neoplasia and acquired cystic kidney disease in patients receiving long-term dialysis. *Arch Pathol Lab Med* 1986;110:592.
108. Hyman M, Whittemore V. National Institutes of Health Consensus Conference: tuberous sclerosis complex. *Arch Neurol* 2000;57(5):662.
109. Illiopoulos O, Kaelin W. The molecular basis of von Hippel-Lindau disease. *Mol Med* 1997;3(5):289.
110. Ishikawa I, Kovacs G. High incidence of papillary renal cell tumours in patients on chronic haemodialysis. *Histopathology* 1993;22:135.
111. Ishikawa I. Renal cell carcinoma in chronic hemodialysis patients—a 1990 questionnaire study in Japan. *Kidney Int* 1993;41:S167.
112. Javidan J, Stricker H, Tamboli P, et al. Prognostic significance of the 1997 TNM classification of renal cell carcinoma. *J Urol* 1999;162:1277.
113. Jayson M, Sanders H. Increased incidence of serendipitously discovered renal cell carcinoma. *Urology* 1998;51:203.
114. Johnson JA, Hellsten S. Lymphatogenous spread of renal cell carcinoma: an autopsy study. *J Urol* 1997;157(2):450.
115. Jones E, Pins M, Dickersin G, et al. Metanephric adenoma of the kidney: a clinicopathological, immunohistochemical, flow cytometric, cytogenic, and electron microscopic study of seven cases. *Am J Surg Pathol* 1995;19(6):615.
116. Judd E, Hand J. Hypernephroma. *J Urol* 1929;22:10.
117. Katagiri A, Wantanabe R, Tomita Y. E-cadherin expression in renal cell cancer and its significance in metastasis and survival. *Br J Urol* 1995;71:376.
118. Kerbl K, Clayman R, McDougall E, et al. Transperitoneal nephrectomy for benign disease of the kidney: a comparison of laparoscopic and open surgical techniques. *Urology* 1994; 43:607.
119. Kier R, Taylor K, Feyock A, et al. Renal masses: characterization with Doppler US. *Radiology* 1990;176:703.
120. Koehrmann K, Michel M, Fruhauf J, et al. High intensity focused ultrasound for noninvasive tissue ablation in the kidney, prostate, and uterus [Abstract]. *J Urol* 2000;163(4) [Suppl]:J56.
121. Koide Y, Mizoguchi T, Ishii K, et al. Intraoperative management for removal of tumor thrombus in the inferior vena cava of the right atrium with multiplane transesophageal echocardiography. *J Card Surg* 1998;39:641.
122. Konnak J, Grossman H. Renal cell carcinoma as an incidental finding. *J Urol* 1985;134:1094.
123. Kortman R, Becker G, Classen J, et al. Future strategies in external radiation therapy of renal cell carcinoma. *Anticancer Res* 1999;19:1601.
124. Kovacs G, Erlandsson R, Boldog F, et al. Consistent chromosome 3p deletion and loss of heterozygosity in renal cell carcinoma. *Proc Natl Acad Sci USA* 1988;85:1571.
125. Kovacs G. Molecular differential pathology of renal cell tumours. *Histopathology* 1993;22:1.
126. Krown S. Interferon treatment of renal cell carcinoma: current status and future prospects. *Cancer* 1987;59:647.
127. Kuczyk M, Bokemeyer C, Kohn G, et al. Prognostic relevance of intracaval neoplastic extension for patients with renal cell cancer. *Br J Urol* 1997;80(1):18.
128. Kuerbitz S, Plunkett B, Walsh W, et al. Wild-type p53 is a cell cycle checkpoint determinant following irradiation. *Proc Natl Acad Sci USA* 1992;89:7491.
129. Kwiatkowski J, Schmidt B, Merkle P, et al. Perioperative brachytherapy as an additional therapeutic option in patients with renal cell carcinoma, either inoperable or after completed percutaneous radiotherapy. *Anticancer Res* 1999;19:1597.
130. Lane D, Benchimol S. p53 oncogene or anti-oncogene? *Genes Dev* 1990;4:1.
131. Lang E. Comparison of dynamic and conventional computed tomography, angiography and ultrasonography in the staging of renal cell carcinoma. *Cancer* 1984;54(10):2205.
132. Law T, Motzer R, Mazumdar M, et al. Phase III randomized trial of interleukin-2 with or without lymphokine-activated killer cells in the treatment of patients with advanced renal cell carcinoma. *Cancer* 1995;76:824.
133. Leder R, Walther P. Radiologic imaging of renal cell carcinoma: its role in diagnosis, staging, and management. In: Vogelzang NJ, Scardino PT, Shipley WU, et al, eds. *Comprehensive textbook of genitourinary oncology,* 2nd ed. Philadelphia: Lippincott Williams & Wilkins, 2000:143.
134. Levy DA, Slaton JW, Swanson DA, et al. Stage specific guidelines for surveillance after radical nephrectomy for local renal cell carcinoma. *J Urol* 1998:159(4):1163.
135. Libertino J, Zinman L, Watkins E Jr. Long-term results of resection of renal cell cancer with extension into inferior vena cava. *J Urol* 1987;137:21.
136. Lieber MM. Renal oncocytoma. *Urol Clin North Am* 1993; 20(2):355.
137. Ljungberg B, Stenling R, Osterdahl B, et al. Vein invasion in renal cell carcinoma: impact on metastatic behavior and survival. *J Urol* 1995;154:1681.
138. Long J, Choyke P, Shawker T, et al. Intraoperative ultrasound in the evaluation of tumor involvement of the inferior vena cava. *J Urol* 1993;150:13.
139. Lowe B, Brewer J, Houghton D, et al. Malignant transformation of angiomyolipoma. *J Urol* 1992;147:1356.
140. Macchiarini P, Fontanini G, Hardin M, et al. Relation of neovascularization to metastasis of non-small cell lung cancer. *Lancet* 1992;340:145.

141. MacLennan G, Bostwick D. Microvessel density in renal cell carcinoma: lack of prognostic significance. *Urology* 1995; 46(1):27.
142. Maldazys JD, deKernion JB. Prognostic factors in metastatic renal carcinoma. *J Urol* 1986;136(2):376.
143. Mani S, Tood M, Katz K, et al. Prognostic factors for survival in patients with metastatic renal cancer treated with biologic response modifiers. *J Urol* 1995;154:35.
144. Marcus S, Choyke P, Reiter R, et al. Regression of metastatic renal cell carcinoma after cytoreductive nephrectomy. *J Urol* 1993;150:463.
145. Marsh CL, Lange PH. Rationale for total nephrectomy for suspected renal cell carcinoma. *Semin Urol Oncol* 1995; 13(4):273.
146. Marshall F, Holdford S, Hamper U. Intraoperative sonography of renal tumors. *J Urol* 1992;148:1393.
147. Marshall F, Powell K. Lymphadenectomy for renal cell carcinoma: anatomical and therapeutic considerations. *J Urol* 1982; 128:677.
148. Marshall F, Reitz B. Technique for removal of renal cell carcinoma with suprahepatic vena caval tumor thrombus. *Urol Clin North Am* 1986;13:551.
149. Marshall F, Taxy J, Fishman E, et al. The feasibility of surgical enucleation for renal cell carcinoma. *J Urol* 1986;135:231.
150. Marshall F, Walsh P. Extrarenal manifestations of renal cell carcinoma. *J Urol* 1977;117:439.
151. Marshall F. Supradiaphragmatic renal cell carcinoma tumor thrombus: indications for vena caval reconstruction with pericardium. *J Urol* 1985;133:266.
152. Marshall V, Middleton R, Holswade G, et al. Surgery for renal cell carcinoma in the vena cava. *J Urol* 1970;103:414.
153. McDougall E, Clayman R, Elashry O. Laparoscopic radical nephrectomy for renal tumor: the Washington University experience. *J Urol* 1996;155:1180.
154. Medeiros LJ, Jones EC, Aizawa S, et al. Grading of renal cell carcinoma. Workgroup No. 2. *Cancer* 1997;80(5):990.
155. Middleton RG. Surgery for metastatic renal cell carcinoma. *J Urol* 1967;97:973.
156. Miller J, Fischer C, Freese R, et al. Nephron-sparing surgery for renal cell carcinoma—is tumor size a suitable parameter for indication? *Urology* 1999;54(6):988.
157. Moch H, Gasser T, Amin MB, et al. Prognostic study of the recently recommended histologic classification and revised TNM staging system of renal cell carcinoma: a Swiss experience with 588 tumors. *Cancer* 2000;89(3):604.
158. Moll F, Rathert P. The surgeon and his intention: Gustav Simon (1824–1876), his first planned nephrectomy and further contributions to urology. *World J Urol* 1999;17(3):162.
159. Montie J, el Ammar R, Pontes J, et al. Renal cell carcinoma with inferior vena cava tumor thrombi. *Surg Gynecol Obstet* 1991;173:107.
160. Mori Y, Kondzioka D, Flickinger J, et al. Stereotactic radiosurgery for brain metastasis from renal cell carcinoma. *Cancer* 1999;83(2):344.
161. Motzer R, Bander N, Nanus D. Renal-cell carcinoma. *N Engl J Med* 1996;335(12):865.
162. Mulders P, Figlin R, deKernion J, et al. Renal cell carcinoma: recent progress and future directions. *Cancer Res* 1997;57:5189.
163. Muss H, Constanzi J, Leavitt R, et al. Recombinant alfa interferon in renal cell carcinoma: a randomized trial of two routes of administration. *J Clin Oncol* 1987;5(2):286.
164. Negrier S, Escudier B, Lasset C, et al. Recombinant human interleukin-2, recombinant human interferon alfa-2a, or both in metastatic renal-cell carcinoma. *N Engl J Med* 1998;338: 1272.
165. Neidhart J, Anderson S, Harris J, et al. Vinblastine fails to improve response of renal cancer to interferon alfa-n1: high response rate in patients with pulmonary metastases. *J Clin Oncol* 1991;9(5):832.
166. Nesbitt J, Soltero E, Dinney C, et al. Surgical management of renal cell carcinoma with inferior vena cava tumor thrombi. *Ann Thorac Surg* 1997;63(6):1592.
167. Neuhaus C, Dijkhuizen T, van de Berg E, et al. Involvement of the chromosomal region 11q13 in renal oncocytoma: case report and literature review. *Cancer Genet Cytogenet* 1997;94:95.
168. Neves R, Zincke H, Taylor W. Metastatic renal cell cancer and radical nephrectomy: identification of prognostic factors and patient survival. *J Urol* 1988;139:1173.
169. Novick A, Zincke H, Neves R, et al. Surgical enucleation for renal cell carcinoma. *J Urol* 1986;135:235.
170. O'dea MJ, Zincke H, Utz DC, et al. The treatment of renal cell carcinoma with solitary metastasis. *J Urol* 1978;120(5):540.
171. Oesterling J, Fishman E, Goldman S, et al. The management of renal angiomyolipoma. *J Urol* 1986;135:1121.
172. Ohwada S, Satoh Y, Nakamura S, et al. Left-sided approach to renal cell carcinoma tumor thrombus extending into suprahepatic inferior vena cava by resection of the left caudate lobe. *Angiology* 1997;48(7):629.
173. Okada Y, Kumada K, Havuchi T, et al. Total replacement of the suprarenal inferior vena cava with an expanded polytetrafluoroethylene tube graft in 2 patients with tumor thrombi from renal cell carcinoma. *J Urol* 1989;141:111.
174. Okada Y, Kumada K, Terachi T, et al. Long-term followup of patients with tumor thrombi from renal cell carcinoma and total replacement of the inferior vena cava using an expanded polytetrafluoroethylene tubular graft. *J Urol* 1996;155:444.
175. Oliver R, Mehta A, Barnett M. A phase II study of surveillance in patients with metastatic renal cell carcinoma and assessment of response of such patients to therapy on progression. *Mol Biother* 1998;1:13.
176. Overmayer B, Fox K, Tomaszewski J, et al. A phase II trial of R-verapamil and infusional vinblastine (Velban) in advanced renal cell carcinoma (RCC). *Proc Am Soc Clin Oncol* 1993;12: 251(792A).
177. Parker A. Studies on the main posterior lymph channels of the abdomen and their connections with the lymphatics of the genitourinary system. *Am J Anat* 1935;56:409.
178. Parkinson D, Sznol M. High-dose interleukin-2 in the therapy of metastatic renal cell carcinoma. *Semin Oncol* 1995;22(1):61.
179. Patchell R, Tibbs P, Walsh J, et al. A randomized trial of surgery in the treatment of single metastases to the brain. *N Engl J Med* 1990;332:494.
180. Paul R, Ewing C, Robinson J, et al. Cadherin-6, a cell adhesion molecule specifically expressed in the proximal renal tubule and renal cell carcinoma. *Cancer Res* 1997;57:2741.
181. Phillips E, Messing E. Role of lymphadenectomy in the treatment of renal cell carcinoma. *Urology* 1993;41(1):9.
182. Pins MR, Jones EC, Martul EV, et al. Metanephric adenoma-like tumors of the kidney: report of 3 malignancies with emphasis on discriminating features. *Arch Pathol Lab Med* 1999; 123(5):415.
183. Pirich L, Chou P, Walterhouse D. Prolonged survival of a patient with sickle cell trait and metastatic renal medullary carcinoma. *J Pediatr Hematol Oncol* 1999;21(1):67.
184. Polascik TJ, Cairns P, Epstein JI. Distal nephron renal tumors: microsatellite allelotype. *Cancer Res* 1996;56:1892.
185. Polascik T, Meng M, Epstein J, et al. Intraoperative sonography for the evaluation and management of renal tumors: experience with 100 patients. *J Urol* 1995;154:1676.

186. Polascik T, Pound C, Meng M, et al. Partial nephrectomy: technique, complications, and pathological findings. *J Urol* 1995;154:1312.
187. Porena M, Vespasiani G, Rosi P, et al. Incidentally detected renal cell carcinoma: role of ultrasonography. *J Clin Ultrasound* 1992;20:395.
188. Presti JC, Reuter VE, Cordon-Cardo C, et al. Allelic deletions in renal tumors: histopathological correlations. *Cancer Res* 1993;53(23):5780.
189. Pritchett TR, Lieskovsky G, Skinner DG. Extension of renal cell carcinoma into the vena cava: clinical review and surgical approach. *J Urol* 1986;135(3):460.
190. Rackley R, Novick A, Klein E, et al. The impact of adjuvant nephrectomy on multimodality treatment of metastatic renal cell carcinoma. *J Urol* 1994;152:1399.
191. Rassweiler J, Fornara P, Weber M, et al. Laparoscopic nephrectomy: the experience of the laparoscopy working group of the German Urologic Association. *J Urol* 1998;160:18.
192. Renshaw A, Henske E, Loughlin K, et al. Aggressive variants of chromophobe renal cell carcinoma. *Cancer* 1996;78(8):1756.
193. Robey E, Schellhammer P. The adrenal gland and renal cell carcinoma: is ipsilateral adrenalectomy a necessary component of radical nephrectomy? *J Urol* 1986;135(3):453.
194. Robson C, Churchill B, Anderson W. The results of radical nephrectomy for renal cell carcinoma. *J Urol* 1969;101:297.
195. Robson C. Radical nephrectomy for renal cell carcinoma. *J Urol* 1963;89:37.
196. Rodenburg C, Nooter K, Herweijer H, et al. Phase II study of combining vinblastine and cyclosporin-A to circumvent multidrug resistance in renal cell cancer. *Ann Oncol* 1991;2:305.
197. Rodriguez R, Chan D, Bishoff J, et al. Renal ablative cryosurgery in selected patients with peripheral renal masses. *Urology* 2000;55:25.
198. Rosenberg S, Lotze M, Muul L, et al. A progress report on the treatment of 157 patients with advanced cancer using lymphokine-activated killer cells and interleukin-2 or high-dose interleukin-2 alone. *N Engl J Med* 1987;316:889.
199. Rosenberg S, Yang J, White D, et al. Durability of complete responses in patients with metastatic cancer treated with high-dose interleukin-2. Identification of the antigens mediating response. *Ann Surg* 1998;228(3):307.
200. Roubidoux M, Dunnick N, Sostman H, et al. Renal cell carcinoma: detection of venous extension with gradient-echo MR imaging. *Radiology* 1992;182:269.
201. Roy C, Tuchmann C, Saussine C, et al. Is there still a role for angiography in the management of renal lesions? *Eur Radiol* 1999;9(2):329.
202. Sagalowsky A, Kadesky K, Ewalt D, et al. Factors influencing adrenal metastasis in renal cell carcinoma. *J Urol* 1994;151(5):1181.
203. Saitoh H, Hida M, Nakamura K, et al. Metastatic processes and a potential indication of treatment for metastatic lesions of renal adenocarcinoma. *J Urol* 1982;128(5):916.
204. Saitoh H, Nakayama M, Nakamura K, et al. Distant metastasis of renal adenocarcinoma in nephrectomized cases. *J Urol* 1982;127(6):1092.
205. Samuels B, Hollis D, Rosner G, et al. Modulation of vinblastine resistance in metastatic renal cell carcinoma with cyclosporin A or tamoxifen: a cancer and leukemia group B study. *Clin Cancer Res* 1997;3:1977.
206. Sandock D, Seftel A, Resnick M. Adrenal metastases from renal cell carcinoma: role of ipsilateral adrenalectomy and definition of stage. *Urology* 1997;49(1):28.
207. Sant G, Ayers D, Bankoff M, et al. Fine needle aspiration biopsy in the diagnosis of renal angiomyolipoma. *J Urol* 1990;143:999.
208. Sarna G, Figlin R, deKernion J. Interferon I renal cell carcinoma: the UCLA experience. *Cancer* 1987;59:610.
209. Sawczuk S, Pollard J. Renal cell carcinoma: should radical nephrectomy be performed in the presence of metastatic disease? *Curr Opin Urol* 1999;9:399.
210. Schmidt, L, Duh F, Chen F, et al. Germline and somatic mutations in the tyrosine kinase domain of the MET protooncogene in papillary renal carcinomas. *Nat Genet* 1997;16:68.
211. Seizinger B, Rouleau G, Ozelius L, et al. Von Hippel-Lindau disease maps to the region of chromosome 3 associated with renal cell carcinoma. *Nature* 1988;332:268.
212. Shalev M, Cipolla B, Guille F, et al. Is ipsilateral adrenalectomy a necessary component of radical nephrectomy? *J Urol* 1995;153(5):1415.
213. Shapiro JA, Williams MA, Weiss NS, et al. Hypertension, antihypertensive medication use, and risk of renal cell carcinoma. *Am J Epidemiol* 1999;149(6):521.
214. Shek T, Luk I, Peh W, et al. Metanephric adenofibroma: report of a case and review of the literature. *Am J Surg Pathol* 1999;23(6):727.
215. Shiina H, Igawa M, Urakami S, et al. Clinical significance of immunohistochemically detectable p53 protein in renal cell carcinoma. *Eur Urol* 1997;31:73.
216. Shimazui T, Giroldi L, Bringuier P, et al. Complex cadherin expression in renal cell carcinoma. *Cancer Res* 1996;56:3234.
217. Shimazui T, Oosterwijk E, Akaka H, et al. Expression of cadherin-6 as a novel diagnostic tool to predict prognosis of patients with E-cadherin-absent renal cell carcinoma. *Clin Cancer Res* 1998;4:2419.
218. Shimizu M, Yokota J, Mori N, et al. Introduction of normal chromosome 3p modulates the tumorigenicity of human renal cell carcinoma cell line YCR. *Oncogene* 1990;5:185.
218a. Siegel CL, McFarland EG, Brink JA, et al. CT of cystic renal masses: analysis of diagnostic performance and intraobserver variation. *AJR Am J Roentgenol* 1997;169(3):813.
219. Siemester G, Weindel K, Mohrs K, et al. Revision of deregulated expression of vascular endothelial growth factor in human renal cell carcinoma cells by von Hippel-Lindau tumor suppressor protein. *Cancer Res* 1996;56:2299.
220. Sigman D, Hasnain J, Del Pizzo J, et al. Real-time transesophageal echocardiography for intraoperative surveillance of patients with renal cell carcinoma and vena caval extension undergoing radical nephrectomy. *J Urol* 1999;161:36.
221. Sim J, Seo C, Kim S, et al. Differentiation of small hyperechoic renal cell carcinoma from angiomyolipoma: computer-aided tissue echo quantification. *J Ultrasound Med* 1999;18:261.
222. Simons J, Jaffe E, Weber C, et al. Bioactivity of autologous irradiated renal cell carcinoma vaccines generated by ex vivo granulocyte-macrophage colony-stimulating factor gene transfer. *Cancer Res* 1997;57:1537.
223. Simons J, Marshall F. The future of gene therapy in the treatment of urologic malignancies. *Urol Clin North Am* 1998;25(1):23.
224. Sinke R, Dijkhuizen T, Janssen B, et al. Fine mapping of the human renal oncocytoma-associated translocation (5;11)(q35;q13) breakpoint. *Cancer Genet Cytogenet* 1997;94:95.
225. Sirvastava A, Laidler P, Davies R, et al. The prognostic significance of tumor vascularity in intermediate-thickness (0.76–4.0 mm thick) skin melanoma. *Am J Pathol* 1988;133:419.
226. Skinner D, Prichett T, Lieskovsky G, et al. Vena caval involvement by renal cell carcinoma. Surgical resection provides meaningful long-term survival. *Ann Surg* 1989;210(3):387.

227. Slaton J, Balbay M, Levy D, et al. Nephrectomy and vena caval thrombectomy in patients with metastatic renal cell carcinoma. *Urology* 1997;50:673.
228. Smith P, Marshall F, Corl F, et al. Planning nephron-sparing renal surgery using 3D helical CT angiography. *J Comput Assist Tomogr* 1999;23(5):649.
229. Smith P, Marshall F, Fishman E. Spiral computed tomography evaluation of the kidneys: state of the art. *Urology* 1998;15:3.
230. Sobin L, Wittekind C. *International Union Against Cancer (UICC): TNM classification of malignant tumours,* 5th ed. Philadelphia: Lippincott-Raven, 1997.
231. Solchok J, Motzer R. Management of renal cell carcinoma. *Oncology* 2000;14(1):29.
232. Sosa R, Muecke E, Vaughn E, et al. Renal cell carcinoma extending into the inferior vena cava: the prognostic significance of the level of vena cava involvement. *J Urol* 1984;132(6):1097.
233. Srigley JR, Hutter RVP, Gelb AB, et al. Current prognostic factors—renal cell carcinoma. Workgroup No. 4. *Cancer* 1997; 80(5):994.
234. Srougi M. Lymph node dissection in the treatment of renal cell carcinoma. In: Vogelzang N, Scardino P, Shipley W, et al, eds. *Comprehensive textbook of genitourinary oncology,* 2nd ed. Philadelphia: Lippincott Williams & Wilkins, 2000:201.
235. Stadler W, Vogelzang N. Low-dose interleukin-2 in the treatment of metastatic renal-cell carcinoma. *Semin Oncol* 1995; 22(1):67.
236. Stauffer M: Nephrogenic hepatosplenomegaly [Abstract]. *Gastroenterology* 1961;40:694.
237. Steffens M, Boerman O, de Mulder P, et al. Phase I radioimmunotherapy of metastatic renal cell carcinoma with 131I-labeled chimeric monoclonal antibody G250. *Clin Cancer Res* 1999;5(10s):3268s.
238. Steiner M, Goldman S, Fishman E, et al. The natural history of renal angiomyolipoma. *J Urol* 1993;150:1782.
239. Störkel S, Eble J, Adlakha K, et al. Classification of renal cell carcinoma. Workgroup No. 1. *Cancer* 1997;80:987.
240. Straton C, Libertino J, Larson C. Is magnetic resonance imaging alone accurate enough in staging renal cell carcinoma? *Urology* 1992;40:351.
241. Sufrin G, Chasa S, Golio A, et al. Paraneoplastic and serologic syndromes of renal adenocarcinoma. *Semin Urol* 1989;7:158.
242. Sufrin G, Mirand EA, Moore RH. Hormones in renal cancer. *J Urol* 1977;117:433.
243. Suggs W, Smith R III, Dodson T, et al. Renal cell carcinoma with inferior vena cava involvement. *J Vasc Surg* 1991;14:413.
244. Swierzewski D, Swierzewski M, Libertino J. Radical nephrectomy in patients with renal cell carcinoma with venous, vena caval, and atrial extension. *Am J Surg* 1994;169:205.
245. Symbas N, Townsend M, El-Galley R, et al. Poor prognosis associated with thrombocytosis in patients with renal cell carcinoma. *BJU Int* 2000;86(3):203.
246. Szolar D, Kammerhuber F, Altziebler S, et al. Multiphasic helical CT of the kidney: increased conspicuity for detection and characterization of small (<3 cm) renal masses. *Radiology* 1997;202:211.
247. Tamboli P, Ro JY, Amin MB, et al. Benign tumors and tumor-like lesions of the adult kidney. Part II: Benign mesenchymal and mixed neoplasms, and tumor-like lesions. *Adv Anat Pathol* 2000;7(1):47.
248. Tanguay S, Swanson D, Putman J Jr. Renal cell carcinoma metastatic to the lung: potential benefit in the combination of biological therapy and surgery. *J Urol* 1996;156:1586.
249. Tannapfel A, Hahn H, Katalinic A, et al. Prognostic value of ploidy and proliferation markers in renal cell carcinoma. *Cancer* 1996;77(1):164.
250. Targonski P, Frank W, Stuhldreher D, et al. Value of tumor size in predicting survival from renal cell carcinoma among tumors, nodes, metastasis stage I and stage II patients. *J Urol* 1994;152:1389.
251. Thompson I, Peek M. Improvement in survival of patients with renal cell carcinoma—the role of the serendipitously detected tumor. *J Urol* 1988;140:487.
252. Tickoo S, Amin M, Linden M, et al. Antimitochondrial antibody (113-1) in the differential diagnosis of granular renal cell tumors. *Am J Pathol* 1997;21(8):922.
253. Tickoo S, Amin M. Discriminant nuclear features of renal oncocytoma and chromophobe renal cell carcinoma. Analysis of their potential utility in the differential diagnosis. *Anat Pathol* 1998;110:782.
254. Tickoo S, Reuter V, Amin M, et al. Renal oncocytosis: a morphologic study of fourteen cases. *Am J Surg Pathol* 1999; 23(9):1094.
255. Tolia BM, Whitmore WF Jr. Solitary metastasis from renal cell carcinoma. *J Urol* 1975;114(6):836.
256. Trieger B, Humphrey L, Peterson Jr C, et al. Transesophageal echocardiography in renal cell carcinoma: an accurate diagnostic technique for intracaval neoplastic extension. *J Urol* 1991; 145:1138.
257. Tsui K, Shvarts O, Barbaric Z, et al. Is adrenalectomy a necessary component of radical nephrectomy? UCLA experience with 511 radical nephrectomies. *J Urol* 2000;163(2):437.
258. Tsui K, Shvarts O, Smith R, et al. Prognostic indicators for renal cell carcinomas: a multivariate analysis of 643 patients using the revised 1997 TNM stage criteria. *J Urol* 2000;163(4): 1090.
259. Uhlman D, Nguyen P, Manivel C, et al. Association of immunohistochemical staining for p53 with metastatic progression and poor survival in patients with renal cell carcinoma. *J Natl Cancer Inst* 1994;86(19):1470.
260. Umeda T, Nijima T. Phase II study of alpha interferon on renal cell carcinoma. *Cancer* 1986;58:1231.
261. Van Poppel H, Bamelis B, Oyen R, et al. Partial nephrectomy for renal cell carcinoma can achieve long-term tumor control. *J Urol* 1998;160:674.
262. Van Poppel H, Vandendriessche H, Boel K, et al. Microscopic vascular invasion is the most relevant prognosticator after radical nephrectomy for clinical nonmetastatic renal cell carcinoma. *J Urol* 1997;158:45.
263. Vermooten V. Indications for conservative surgery in certain renal tumors: a study based on the growth pattern of the clear cell carcinoma. *J Urol* 1950;64:200.
264. Vesselle H, Miraldi F. FDG PET of the retroperitoneum: normal anatomy, variants, pathologic conditions and strategies to avoid diagnostic pitfalls. *Radiographics* 1998;18:805.
265. Vicente Prados E, Tallada Bunuel M, Pastor J, et al. Renal adenocarcinoma with vena cava invasion: current status of its diagnosis and treatment using total segmentary cavectomy [Abstract]. *Arch Esp Urol* 1998;51(1):35.
266. Von Knobloch R, Seseke F, Riedmiller H, et al. Radical nephrectomy for renal cell carcinoma: is adrenalectomy necessary? *Eur Urol* 1999;36(4):303.
267. Walther M, Alexander R, Weiss G, et al. Cytoreductive surgery prior to interleukin-2-based therapy in patients with metastatic renal cell carcinoma. *Urology* 1993;42:250.
268. Walther MM, Johnson B, Culley D, et al. Serum interleukin-6 levels in metastatic renal cell carcinoma before treatment with interleukin-2 correlates with paraneoplastic syndromes but not patient survival. *J Urol* 1998;159:718.

269. Warren K, Gidvani-Diaz V, Duval-Arnould B. Renal medullary carcinoma in an adolescent with sickle cell trait. *Pediatrics* 1999;103:490.
270. Warshauer D, McCarthy S, Street L, et al. Detection of renal masses: sensitivities and specificities of excretory urography/linear tomography, US and CT. *Radiology* 1988;169:363.
271. Weidner N, Carroll P, Flax J, et al. Tumor angiogenesis correlates with metastasis in invasive prostate carcinoma. *Am J Pathol* 1993;143:401.
272. Weidner N, Semple J, Welch W, et al. Tumor angiogenesis and metastasis—correlation in invasive breast carcinoma. *N Engl J Med* 1991;324:1.
273. Weiner SN, Bernstein RG. Renal oncocytoma angiographic features of two cases. *Radiology* 1977;125(3):633.
274. Welch T, LeRoy A. Helical and electron beam CT scanning in the evaluation of renal vein involvement in patients with renal cell carcinoma. *J Comput Assist Tomogr* 1997;21:467.
275. Welz A, Schmeller N, Schmitz C, et al. Resection of hypernephromas with vena caval or right atrial tumor extension using extracorporeal circulation and deep hypothermic circulatory arrest: a multidisciplinary approach. *Eur J Cardiothorac Surg* 1997;12(1):127.
276. Wirth M. Immunotherapy for metastatic renal cell carcinoma. *Urol Clin North Am* 1993;20:283.
277. Wolf J, Aronson F, Small E, et al. Nephrectomy for metastatic renal cell carcinoma: a component of systematic treatment regions. *J Surg Oncol* 1994;55:7.
278. Wolf J, Moon T, Nakada S. Hand assisted laparoscopic nephrectomy: comparison to standard laparoscopic nephrectomy. *J Urol* 1998;160:22.
279. Xipell J. The incidence of benign renal nodules (a clinicopathologic study). *J Urol* 1971;106:503.
280. Yagoda A, Abi-Rached B, Petrylak D. Chemotherapy for advanced renal cell carcinoma: 1983–1993. *Semin Oncol* 1995; 22(1):42.
281. Yu C, Chen K, Chen M, et al. Serum iron as a tumor marker in renal cell carcinoma. *Eur Urol* 1991;19:54.
282. Yuan J, Castelao J, Gago-Dominguez M, et al. Tobacco use in relation to renal cell carcinoma. *Cancer Epidemiol Biomarkers Prev* 1998;7:429.
283. Zambrano N, Lubensky I, Merino M, et al. Histopathology and molecular genetics of renal tumors toward unification of a classification system. *J Urol* 1999;162(4):1246.
284. Zbar B, Brauch H, Talmadge C, et al. Loss of alleles of loci on the short arm of chromosome 3 in renal cell carcinoma. *Nature* 1987;372:721.
285. Zerban H, Nogueira E, Riedasch G, et al. Renal oncocytoma: origin from the collecting duct. *Virchows Arch* 1987;52(5):375.
286. Zhuang Z, Park W, Pack S, et al. Trisomy 7-harboring nonrandom duplication of the mutant MET allele in hereditary papillary renal carcinomas. *Nat Genet* 1997;16:68.

Adult and Pediatric Urology, 4/e, edited by Jay Y. Gillenwater, John T. Grayhack, Stuart S. Howards, and Michael E. Mitchell.
Lippincott Williams & Wilkins, Philadelphia © 2002

17

UROTHELIAL CARCINOMA OF THE UPPER URINARY TRACT

MEIDEE GOH
JAMES E. MONTIE
J. STUART WOLF, JR.

EPIDEMIOLOGY AND ETIOLOGY

Incidence

Urothelial (transitional cell) carcinoma of the upper urinary tract is an uncommon disease, accounting for 4.5% to 9% of all renal tumors and 5% to 6% of all urothelial tumors (27,43,108,159,160). Renal pelvis urothelial tumors are two to four times more common than ureteral urothelial tumors (89,100,104,117). Upper urinary tract tumors rarely occur before age 40 years and have a peak incidence in the sixth and seventh decades of life, with a mean age at diagnosis of 65 years (7,54). Upper tract urothelial cancers are two to four times more common in men than in women and two times more common in Caucasians than in African Americans (7).

M. Goh, J.E. Montie, and J.S. Wolf, Jr.: Department of Urology, University of Michigan, Ann Arbor, MI 48109.

Risk Factors

Association with Balkan Nephropathy

In regions of Bulgaria, Greece, Romania, and Yugoslavia, the presence of an endemic form of nephropathy (termed *Balkan nephropathy*) has been associated with a high frequency of renal pelvic and ureteral tumors. Balkan nephropathy is a degenerative interstitial disease resulting in renal failure in its late stages. The upper tract tumors associated with this nephropathy tend to be low grade and slow growing, which encourages conservative management in these cases. Interestingly, there is no increase in the incidence of bladder urothelial cancer (118). These urothelial tumors occur bilaterally in 10% of these patients and account for 40% of all renal cancers in these geographic regions (125).

Occupational Risk Factors

Workers in the chemical, petrochemical, and plastics industries have been shown to be four times more likely to develop renal pelvic and ureteral cancers compared with the population at large. In addition, workers who are exposed to coal, coke, asphalt, tar, and aniline dyes experience a similar increase in risk (122).

Smoking

Cigarette smoking is a major risk factor for urothelial cancer of the upper urinary tract, as well as the bladder. In a study by Jensen and colleagues (64), 56% of upper tract cancers in eastern Denmark were thought to be caused by cigarette smoking. The associated risk increased with lifetime amount of tobacco use and degree of inhalation. This study suggested that the association of tobacco use with upper tract urothelial cancer was even stronger than with bladder urothelial cancer. The addition of other types of tobacco increased the relative risk from 2.6 to 3.8. McLaughlin and associates (92) calculated that of upper tract urothelial tumors in three areas of the United States, 7 of 10 in men and 4 of 10 in women were attributable to smoking. Cigarette smoking appears to be the most significant acquired risk factor for upper tract urothelial cancer.

Analgesic Use

A number of case reports and epidemiologic studies have linked heavy use of analgesic mixtures with urothelial carcinoma of the renal pelvis. In particular, phenacetin, an aromatic amide with *N*-hydroxylated amines, has been linked in one study to 22% of patients with renal pelvis cancer and 11% of those with ureteral cancers (148). Other studies have been supportive of this association (91,99). The phenacetin metabolite *N*-hydroxyphenacetin, a potent liver carcinogen, may be responsible for the increased risk. The latency period can be as long as 25 years (45).

Prolonged use of nonsteroidal antiinflammatory drugs has been associated with the development of interstitial nephritis. This nephropathy is characterized by capillarosclerosis, a thickening of the basement membrane around the subepithelial capillaries, which is pathognomonic for analgesic abuse. Palvio and associates (114) noted capillarosclerosis in 15% of cases of upper tract urothelial cancer. Combination analgesics result in an even greater frequency of nephropathy, possibly as a result of synergy between aspirin, phenacetin, and other nonsteroidal agents. In a study by Jensen and associates (65), the relative risk for upper tract urothelial cancer attributed to analgesic abuse was greater for women than for men (4.2 versus 2.4).

Coffee Drinking and Artificial Sweeteners

There has been controversy over the association of upper tract urothelial cancer with coffee drinking or the use of saccharin. Although some have noted a slightly increased risk with the former (132), others have not (99). The preponderance of evidence suggests that saccharin is not associated with urothelial tumors (63,99).

Infectious Agents

Although there has been some evidence that human papillomavirus (HPV) may predispose to the development of bladder urothelial cancer, studies of HPV in upper tract urothelial cancer have not provided confirmation of a similar relationship (6,21,38,161). Chronic bacterial infections of the upper urinary tract have been linked to the development of squamous cell carcinoma, but the association with urothelial cancer is uncertain.

Cyclophosphamide

Cyclophosphamide is an alkylating chemotherapeutic agent widely used to treat lymphomas, leukemia, and other solid tumors. In addition, it has been used in the management of patients with autoimmune disorders such as rheumatoid arthritis, lupus erythematosus, and polyarteritis nodosa. One product of cyclophosphamide metabolism, acrolein, is toxic to the urothelium and thought to be responsible for injury to the mucosa. Cyclophosphamide exposure has been associated with an increased risk of both bladder and upper tract urothelial cancer (18,156).

Heredity

There have been several reported cases of familial urothelial carcinoma of the upper urinary tract. In particular, increased risk has been suggested among families with hereditary nonpolyposis colon cancer (47,84). Increased risk of urothelial carcinoma of the upper urinary tract has been associated with Muir-Torre syndrome, which is a rare autosomal-dominant disorder characterized by sebaceous tumors and at least one visceral malignancy (i.e., colon cancer) (48,73). There has been the suggestion of overlap with hereditary nonpolyposis colon cancer.

Chromosomal Abnormalities

Chromosomal abnormalities have been described in upper tract urothelial cancers. Reports describe gain of chromosome 7, complete or partial loss of chromosome 9, partial loss of chromosome 10, and partial loss of chromosome 21 (11,35,134,155). Some studies suggest that the changes seen are similar to those for bladder urothelial cancer.

Through mapping studies and examination of recurrent bladder tumors, there has been a suggestion that multifocal urothelial tumors arise from a monoclonal origin (83,144, 157). In a molecular study of three patients, Sidransky and colleagues (144) showed that inactivation of the same X chromosome occurred in multiple tumor samples. A similar clonal pattern was also seen in the allelic loss of chromosome 9q, a loss that is thought to occur early in tumorigenesis (151). Similarly, Van der Poel and colleagues (157) demonstrated that the same p53 mutation was present in multiple urothelial tumors present in one patient. While allelic loss of chromosome 9 is thought to be an early event, loss of chromosome 17p, containing the site for p53, is thought to be late event (52).

The chronology of genetic alterations in urothelial tumors might shed light on their development. Takahashi and colleagues (151) found that low-grade papillary urothelial tumors rarely acquire additional genetic alterations; genetic divergence and heterotopic spread appear to occur after alterations in chromosome 9. Their findings suggest that most multifocal low-grade superficial urothelial tumors are genetically stable and that alterations in chromosome 9 may be an early event in tumorigenesis.

Location and Distribution

Urothelial carcinoma is two to four times as common in the renal pelvis as in the ureter (89,100,104,117). In the ureter, lesions are more common in the distal portion (40). Zungri and colleagues (168) found that among patients with upper tract tumors, 78% had tumors in the distal ureter and 27% in the proximal ureter.

Upper tract urothelial carcinomas occur in a bilateral and synchronous fashion in 1.5% to 2%; 6% to 8% develop as bilateral metachronous lesions (103,160). Upper tract tumors occur in 2% to 4% of patients with previous bladder cancer. The mean interval between the diagnosis of bladder cancer and upper tract disease varies from 17 to 170 months (109). Carcinoma *in situ* (CIS) of the bladder increases the likelihood of upper tract urothelial cancer in patients with bladder cancer from 13.4% to 21%. The median time from diagnosis of bladder tumor to occurrence of upper tract tumor ranges from 62 to 88 months (25,95,138). Despite successful bacille Calmette-Guérin (BCG) treatment of CIS in the bladder, these individuals have a lifelong risk for developing upper tract tumors and thus should have continued evaluation of the upper tracts in addition to the bladder.

The risk of developing bladder tumors following the diagnosis of upper tract urothelial cancer is significantly higher. This incidence has been estimated at 20% to 48% (40,58,68,76,101,102,129). Although, as noted, some of these bladder tumors are found before or at the time of diagnosis of the upper tract tumor, most occur after the diagnosis of upper tract disease. In a series of 69 patients reported by Mukamel and colleagues (102), most of these bladder tumors occurred within the first year following nephroureterectomy, although late occurrences are noted as well (93). There has been some controversy as to the impact that the diagnosis of a bladder tumor has on survival of patients with upper tract urothelial cancer. In the two series compiled by Krogh and colleagues (76) and Charbit and associates (23), the additional diagnosis of a bladder tumor did not affect survival. However, the two series collected by Reitelman and colleagues (129) and Mukamel and associates (102) suggest that the additional diagnosis of a bladder tumor decreases survival significantly.

The higher rate of metachronous as compared with synchronous bladder tumors following the diagnosis of an upper tract tumor has led to speculation about the method by which urothelial carcinoma is disseminated in the urinary tract. These phenomena suggest that many of the tumors that recur do so as a result of direct seeding downstream or from longer exposure of the causative agent in the bladder.

Some investigators have pursued urothelial mapping as a method of determining the causal link between urothelial cancers in the bladder and the upper tract. Several studies indicate that there are widespread abnormalities in the urothelium of the renal pelvis and ureter in patients with upper tract urothelial carcinoma (68,82,85). Thus the entire urothelium is at risk for the precancerous and cancerous event. Furthermore, there appears to be a correlation between the grade of tumor seen and the degree of disturbance seen in the surrounding epithelium. McCarron and colleagues (90) evaluated 30 consecutive nephroureterectomy specimens and found that in most high-grade neoplasms, the remote urothelium expressed marked atypia or carcinoma. Conversely, the low-grade neoplasms were accompanied by the presence of only varying degrees of simple hyperplasia of the surrounding urothelium. These findings suggest that conservative approaches will be less effective in the setting of high-grade neoplasm because urothelium remains at risk. The incidence of subsequent ipsilateral upper tract urothelial cancer lesions has been reported to range from 14% to 30%, and the incidence of ipsilateral ureteral stump recurrence has been shown to range from 19% to 48% (76,89,150,164).

Others have theorized that tumors in the upper urinary tract occur as a consequence of seeding that occurs as a result of vesicoureteral reflux (164). This suggestion is supported by the findings reported by Babaian and Johnson (7) that 73% of ureteral cancers were in the distal ureter, 24% in the midureter, and 3% in the proximal ureter.

PATHOLOGY

Of upper tract collecting system tumors, 90% are urothelial carcinomas. These may occur as single or multifocal lesions. Grading for these lesions is similar to that for bladder cancer and is based on the worst grade seen. The current World Health Organization/International Society for Urological Pathology (WHO/ISUP) consensus classification of urothelial (transitional cell) lesions was developed in 1998 out of a need to have a universally accepted classification system (Table 17.1) (34,131). The term *urothelial* is preferred over the term *transitional cell.* Although investigators had all

TABLE 17.1. THE 1998 WHO/ISUP CONSENSUS CLASSIFICATION OF UROTHELIAL (TRANSITIONAL CELL) NEOPLASMS

Flat lesions with atypia
- Reactive (inflammatory) atypia
- Atypia of unknown significance
- Dysplasia (low-grade intraurothelial neoplasia)
- Carcinoma *in situ* (high-grade intraurothelial neoplasia)

Papillary neoplasms
- Papilloma
- Inverted papilloma
- Papillary neoplasm of low malignant potential
- Papillary carcinoma, low grade
- Papillary carcinoma, high grade (option to add comment regarding presence of anaplasia)

Adapted from Reuter VR, Epstein JI, Amin MB, et al. A newly illustrated synopsis of the World Health Organization/International Society of Urological Pathology (WHO/ISUP) consensus classification of urothelial (transitional-cell) neoplasms of the urinary bladder. *J Urol Pathol* 1999;11:1.

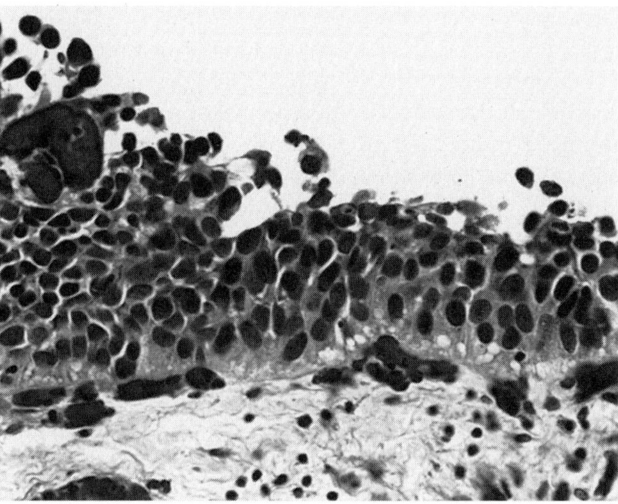

FIGURE 17.1. Urothelial carcinoma *in situ* with pleomorphic cells and hyperchromatic nuclei replacing the full thickness of the urothelium (×200 magnification). (Photo courtesy of Dr. Nader H. Bassily.)

agreed that grade was an important predictor of outcome, the use of multiple systems of grading had resulted in a lack of reproducibility. The goal of the WHO/ISUP 1998 classification was to define a classification continuum from normal tissue to invasive neoplasms (Table 17.1) (34,131). Comparison of this 1998 consensus grading system and previous three- and four-tiered grading system is shown in Table 17.2.

Carcinoma *In Situ* (High-grade Intraurothelial Neoplasia)

CIS (Fig. 17.1) has been characterized as a precursor lesion to invasive cancer. Cells with large, irregular hyperchromatic nuclei that compose a portion of or the entire urothelium define this high-grade lesion. Mitotic activity is commonly seen in the middle to upper urothelium. This designation encompasses lesions that used to be described as severe dysplasia or marked atypia.

TABLE 17.2. HISTOLOGIC GRADING CATEGORIES FOR PAPILLARY UROTHELIAL TUMORS

WHO 1998	WHO 1973	Murphy	Bergkvist
Papilloma	Papilloma	Papilloma	Papilloma
Papillary neoplasm of low malignant potential	Grade 1	Papilloma	Grade 1
Low-grade papillary carcinoma	Grade 2	Low-grade	Grade 2
High-grade papillary carcinoma	Grade 3	High-grade	Grade 3
			Grade 4

Adapted from Grignon DJ. Neoplasms of the urinary bladder. In: Bostwick DG, Eble JN, eds. *Urologic surgical pathology.* St. Louis: Mosby, 1997:246.

Papillary Urothelial Neoplasms

Papilloma is a discrete papillary growth with a central fibrovascular core. The surface of the papilloma is covered by urothelium of normal thickness and cytology. Although they do not have the ability to invade or metastasize, papillomas do have a tendency to recur. This propensity for recurrence has been associated with subsequent development of carcinoma (17,34,131).

Papillary urothelial neoplasm of low malignant potential is the designation for a lesion in which there is an orderly polar arrangement of cells within papillae. The papillae exhibit minimal architectural abnormalities and minimal nuclear atypia. However, the nuclei are significantly enlarged or the urothelium has more layers than normal. Mitotic figures are infrequent. These lesions pose little risk for invasion or metastases.

Low-grade papillary urothelial carcinomas (Fig. 17.2) represent the next step in the continuum of urothelial change. Although the orderly appearance of the cell layers is preserved, there is now variation in the architectural or cytologic features. Despite the presence of cellular atypia, mitotic figures remain rare (34,131).

High-grade papillary urothelial carcinomas (Fig. 17.3) demonstrate disordered appearance even at low magnification. Both the architecture and cytologic features are involved. Marked to moderate cellular pleomorphism, clumped nuclear chromatin, prominent nucleoli, and mitotic figures all can be present. The pathologist may also add

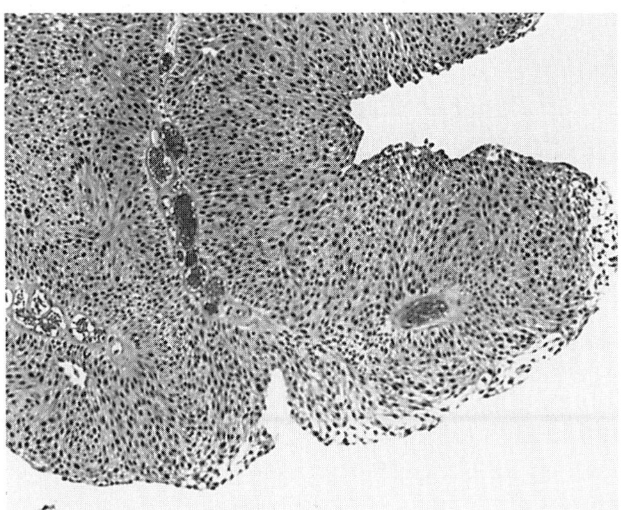

FIGURE 17.2. Low-grade papillary urothelial carcinoma with exophytic papillary fronds covered by thick urothelium. Note the mild nuclear atypia, intact basement membrane, and preservation of normal architecture (×40 magnification). (Photo courtesy of Dr. Nader H. Bassily.)

an additional comment on the degree of anaplasia during grading (34,131).

NATURAL HISTORY

Patterns of Spread

Urothelial carcinoma of the upper urinary tract can spread by (a) direct extensions through the wall of the collecting system into the renal parenchyma or surrounding structures, (b) lymphatic invasion, or (c) more rarely, vascular invasion.

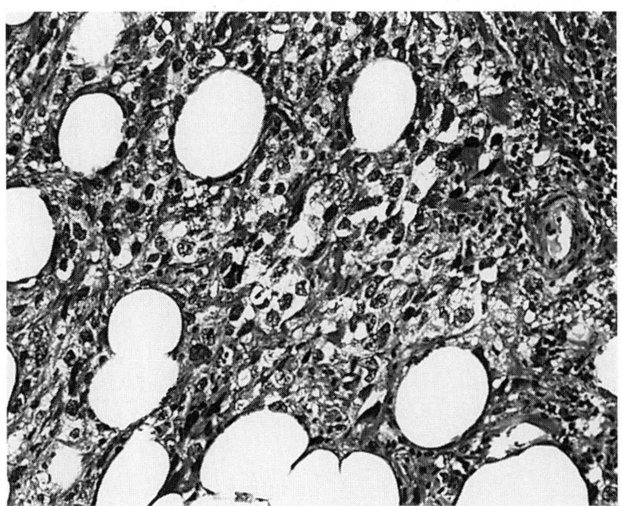

FIGURE 17.3. Invasive high-grade urothelial carcinoma growing in large solid sheet into periureteral fibrofatty tissue. Note the pleomorphic nuclei and disorganized pattern of growth (×200 magnification). (Photo courtesy of Dr. Nader H. Bassily.)

The paraaortic, paracaval, and pelvic lymph nodes are the most common sites for lymphatic invasion. Venous extension into the renal vein and the vena cava has been reported and is associated with poor prognosis (53,66,130). The most common metastatic sites for urothelial cancer of the upper tract are lung (31%), bone (22%), and liver (9%) (58).

Mucosal Spread

Global field changes present in the urothelium at the time of resection of the primary urothelial upper tract lesions may predispose the remainder of the upper tract to recurrence. Mahadevia and colleagues (85) demonstrated with urothelial mapping of nephroureterectomy specimens that widespread abnormalities of the entire urothelium are present concomitantly with the diagnosis of upper tract urothelial cancer. McCarron and colleagues (90) confirmed this finding. This group also demonstrated that the degree of urothelial disturbance parallels the grade of the principal lesion. The widespread nature of urothelial abnormalities may provide a plausible explanation for the high incidence (20% to 64%) of recurrent urothelial carcinoma in ureteral stumps (67,150).

Others have suggested that urothelial upper tract cancers are seeded from bladder tumors when malignant cells are washed into the upper tract through an incompetent ureteral orifice (113). Studies have suggested that patients with bladder cancer and vesicoureteral reflux are 16 to 22 times more likely to develop upper tract urothelial cancer than are bladder cancer patients without concomitant reflux (5,29).

TUMOR STAGE

Stage, along with grade, is an important prognostic indicator for upper tract urothelial carcinomas. Depth of tumor invasion is inversely correlated with survival. In a study of 103 subjects, patients with tumors of the renal pelvis or ureter without invasion beyond the midpoint of the muscularis experienced a 72% 5-year survival rate. Patients with tumors that had extended more deeply (Fig. 17.4) had a 5-year survival rate of only 32% (16).

Renal pelvic and ureteral carcinomas are staged according to an assessment of the degree of tumor infiltration, nodal involvement, and presence of metastatic disease. The American Joint Committee on Cancer (AJCC) system (Tables 17.3 and 17.4) uses combinations of tumor, node, metastasis (TNM) categories to form stage groupings.

SIGNS AND SYMPTOMS

Gross hematuria is the most common symptom of urothelial carcinoma of the upper urinary tract, present in 70% to

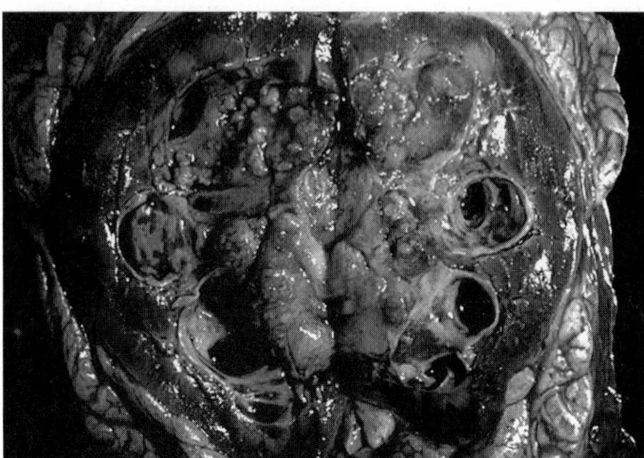

FIGURE 17.4. Gross specimen of stage T_3 urothelial carcinoma of the renal pelvis (extensive tumor, with focal invasion into peripelvic fat).

90% of patients. Flank pain may be present in 8% to 50% of patients and occurs as a result of ureteral obstruction by blood clots or tumor. Constitutional symptoms, such as weight loss, anorexia, and bone pain, are rarely present unless there is metastatic disease. A flank mass due to hydronephrosis or the actual tumor mass is noted in up to 10% to 20% of patients (39).

TABLE 17.3. TUMOR, NODE, METASTASIS (TNM) STAGING FOR TUMORS OF THE RENAL PELVIS AND URETER

T	**Primary tumor**
T_X	Primary tumor cannot be assessed
T_0	No evidence of primary tumor
T_{is}	Carcinoma *in situ*
T_a	Papillary noninvasive carcinoma
T_1	Tumor invades subepithelial connective tissue
T_2	Tumor invades muscularis
T_3	Tumor invades beyond muscularis into periureteric or peripelvic fat or renal parenchyma but not adjacent organs
T_4	Tumor invades adjacent organs or through the kidney into perinephric fat
N	**Regional lymph nodes**
N_X	Regional lymph nodes cannot be assessed
N_0	No regional lymph node metastasis
N_1	Metastasis in a single lymph node, ≤2 cm in greatest dimension
N_2	Metastasis in a single lymph node, >2 cm but <5 cm in greatest dimension; or multiple lymph nodes, none >5 cm in greatest dimension
N_3	Metastasis in a lymph node(s) >5 cm in greatest dimension
M	**Distant metastasis**
M_X	Presence of distant metastasis cannot be assessed
M_0	No regional lymph node metastasis
M_1	Distant metastasis

Adapted from Fleming ID, Cooper JS, Henson DE, et al, eds. *AJCC cancer staging manual,* 5th ed. Philadelphia: Lippincott-Raven, 1998.

DIAGNOSIS

Excretory Urography

Upper urinary tract collecting system tumors may produce an intraluminal filling defect, unilateral nonvisualization of the collecting system, or hydronephrosis (4,10,162) on either excretory urography (IVP) or retrograde pyelography. The differential diagnosis primarily includes nonopaque calculi, blood clots, sloughed renal papillae, and fungus balls. Other considerations include fibroepithelial polyp (56), air bubble, granuloma, renal tuberculosis, and leiomyoma.

Although 50% to 75% of patients may exhibit a filling defect (Fig. 17.5), 10% to 30% of patients diagnosed with upper tract urothelial tumors demonstrate obstruction or nonvisualization of the collecting system, which limits the usefulness of excretory urography. Further evaluation of a nonvisualized collecting system usually requires retrograde pyelography.

Retrograde Pyelography

Retrograde pyelography allows for excellent visualization of the collecting system and provides opportunity for direct collection of specimens for cytology. A bulb- or cone-tipped ureteral catheter is inserted through the ureteral orifice, and contrast is injected to visualize the collecting system under fluoroscopy. The contrast medium should be diluted to one-third or one-half its original concentration before use, which will allow better visualization of subtle filling defects. Care is taken to fill and view the entire renal pelvis and collecting system. Filling of the collecting system is performed with fluoroscopic monitoring in order to prevent overfilling, which may result in rupture of the renal fornices. Occasionally, dilation of the ureter distal to the ureteral tumor is noted, creating a "goblet" appearance. In this dilated region, a catheter passed distal to the tumor may form a coil; this radiologic appearance is called Bergman's sign (12).

When urine is being collected from the upper tracts for cytology, it is important to consider that the hyperosmotic contrast material injected for the retrograde pyelography may affect the interpretation of the cytology. Thus, once the ureteral catheter has been inserted, it might be advisable to first collect urine and saline barbotage for cytology before injection of contrast material.

Antegrade Pyelography

Puncture of the renal pelvis for either an antegrade study or a needle biopsy is not recommended. Although fine-needle

TABLE 17.4. STAGING OF URETERAL AND RENAL PELVIC TUMORS

Description	Stage	Tumor	Nodes	Metastases
Confined to the mucosa	Stage 0a	T_a	N_0	M_0
Carcinoma *in situ*	Stage 0is	T_{is}	N_0	M_0
Invasion into the lamina propria	Stage I	T_1	N_0	M_0
Invasion into the muscularis	Stage II	T_2	N_0	M_0
Extension through the muscularis into fat or renal parenchyma	Stage III	T_3	N_0	M_0
Spread to adjacent organs	Stage IV	T_4	N_0	M_0
Lymph node metastasis	Stage IV	Any T	N_1 to N_3	M_0
Distant metastasis	Stage IV	Any T	Any N	M_1

Adapted from Fleming ID, Cooper JS, Henson DE, et al, eds. *AJCC cancer staging manual,* 5th ed. Philadelphia: Lippincott-Raven, 1998.

biopsy has been reported as a diagnostic technique for renal pelvis filling defects (107,135), seeding of the tumor along the needle tract has also been reported (145). Alternatives for evaluation of a nonvisualized collecting system, such as retrograde pyelography, ureteroscopy with or without biopsy, or computed tomography (CT) scanning, generally should be used first unless there are specific contraindications.

Computed Tomography

CT can be useful in differentiating between a radiolucent uric acid stone and an upper tract urothelial cancer as the source of the filling defect seen during IVP, as well as for staging of upper tract urothelial cancer. Following intravenous injection of contrast material, pelvic or ureteral urothelial tumors typically have an average radiodensity of between 60 and 80 Hounsfield units (HU). In contrast, uric acid stones have much higher radiodensity, usually greater than 200 HU. Other causes of filling defects have less distinctive radiodensities: papillary necrosis at 20 to 40 HU and blood clot at 40 to 80 HU (94). In a review of 343 published cases, 43% to 77% clinicopathologic correlation between upper tract urothelial cancer and CT scan imaging was accomplished, with 7% to 31% overstaging and 13% to 36% understaging (19,22,94,121). Some of the understaging occurred due to small tumor volume. The most common findings were hydronephrosis in the case of ureteral tumors and filling defects in the case of renal pelvis tumors.

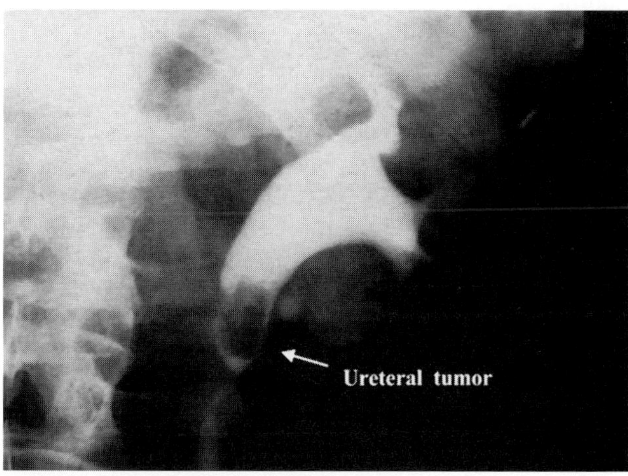

FIGURE 17.5. Intravenous urogram demonstrating a filling defect indicating a proximal ureteral tumor.

Renal parenchymal invasion (Fig. 17.6) can be seen on CT as an alteration in renal contour. The invasive renal urothelial cancer appears as a centrally located mass that distorts the renal contour. Poorly defined margins of the tumor, obliteration of renal sinus fat, and obliteration or entrapment of the collecting system all may be signs of renal parenchymal involvement (37). The specificity of these finding ranges from 75% to 97%, and the sensitivity ranges from 64% to 78% (19,22,94,121).

In the case of ureteral tumors, determination of extension is less accurate, with a sensitivity of 67% and a specificity of 77% (94). Lymph node enlargement as a determinant of lymph node metastases has a sensitivity of 47% to 87.5% and a specificity of 94% to 100% (19,22,94,121).

CT urography is an evolving technique that attempts to duplicate and then improve on intravenous urography, taking advantage of the resolution and volumetric data acquisition of CT (149). The protocol varies from institution to institution, but generally it involves imaging during several phases of contrast excretion with three-dimensional reconstruction of images using a variety of algorithms. Although there are no large series yet describing the results of this new technique, it is likely that it will play an increasingly important role as an alternative to intravenous urography. Yet to be determined is the sensitivity of this technique for subtle tissue-density filling defects.

Ultrasonography

Surface ultrasonography provides a noninvasive method for evaluating the upper tracts that does not depend on the adequacy of renal function. In a series collected over a 9-year period (50), ultrasound identified the presence of hypo-

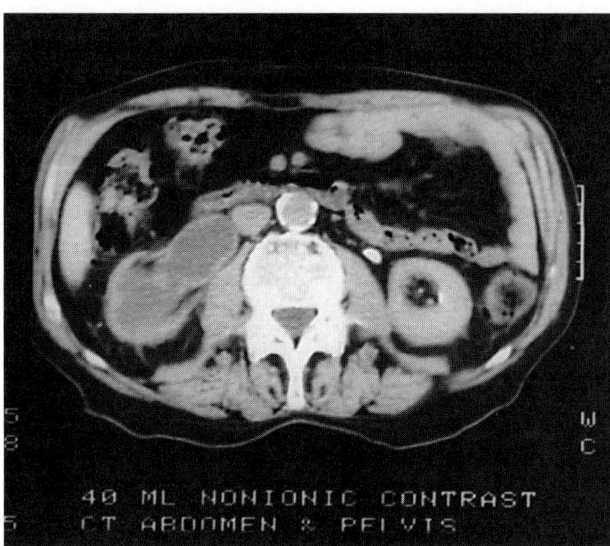

FIGURE 17.6. Computed tomography scan demonstrating a centrally located tumor with distortion of the renal contour.

echoic intraluminal tissue in 16 patients with ureteral tumors. All 10 IVPs and all 3 retrograde pyelograms performed in these patients were abnormal, but only 7 of 11 CT scans clearly demonstrated the tumor. The utility of ultrasonography may be limited if hydronephrosis is absent, or by large body habitus or interference from overlying bowel gas. Information regarding the depth of invasion is unavailable with this technique, and ultrasonography is extremely operator dependent.

To provide more useful information with ultrasonographic imaging, some investigators have employed endoluminal ultrasonography. A 12.5- or 20-MHz transducer is housed within a 6.2-Fr ureteral catheter that is passed in a retrograde fashion up the ureter under fluoroscopic guidance. Liu and colleagues (81) suggest that use of endoluminal ultrasonography can provide information regarding the size and location of the lesion, as well as some estimation of the depth of penetration. In addition to diagnosis of other nonneoplastic causes of filling defects (i.e., stones, air bubbles, and blood clots), this technique may allow for the determination of the location of adjacent vessels before endoscopic resection. The technique has not been widely accepted, however, because it requires an invasive procedure, and as such, it is usually performed at the time of the intended definitive procedure. In this setting, the ultimate utility of the information is uncertain.

Cystoscopy

Cystoscopic examination of the bladder is necessary to rule out the coexistence of a bladder urothelial cancer. As noted, patients with upper tract urothelial cancers are at 20% to 48% risk of having a bladder tumor, either synchronous or metachronous (40,58,68,76,101,102,129).

Cytopathology

Upper urinary tract urothelial cancers can be diagnosed by the examination of voided urine cytology. As with urine cytology in the bladder, the accuracy of diagnosis depends on the grade of the tumor. Accuracy of voided urine cytology ranges from 23% to 92% (30). Improvement in diagnostic accuracy (77% to 92%) can be achieved by obtaining the urine sample through ureteral catheterization. It is worth noting that in a study of retrograde catheterization for urine cytology done following transurethral resection of bladder tumors, 25% of patients with low-grade urothelial neoplasms and 32% of patients with high-grade urothelial neoplasms in the bladder had positive upper tract urinary cytology (133). All of these patients had negative IVP or retrograde pyelography. This suggests that the results from upper tract sampling in the face of concurrent bladder urothelial cancer should be viewed with caution.

The best yields of cytology occur when samples are obtained by saline barbotage of the ureter following catheterization: 87% sensitivity and 100% specificity have been reported with this technique (78). The saline barbotage may improve the accuracy by providing a shearing force to loosen cells from the urothelial lining. Minimo and associates (97) report that the addition of computed DNA measurements and assays for p53 expression can enhance the accuracy of material submitted for cytology in terms of correlation with final histologic grade.

Brush Biopsy

Brush biopsies of the upper urinary tract lesions are performed by passing a fine brush mounted on the end of a guidewire passed through a ureteral catheter into the collecting system up to the level of the filling defect (44). Under fluoroscopic guidance, the brush is gently moved back and forth over the filling defect. Confirmation of the location of the filling defect is obtained fluoroscopically with the injection of dilute contrast. The brush is then removed and the sample is sent for cytologic examination. In one study by Gill and colleagues (42), both sensitivity and accuracy approached 100%. In other series, accuracy has ranged from 78% to 92% (15,165). Accuracy was greater if the cytologic specimens were read as either positive or negative for tumor, rather than requiring accurate grading of the tumor.

Although complications are rare, hematuria and occasionally some flank pain can occur following the brush biopsy of the upper urinary tract. The hematuria is often self-limiting, although severe hemorrhage and perforation of the ureter have been reported (15). There is some concern that denuding the urothelium as a result of the brush biopsy may provide an area for tumor implantation; however, in one retrospective study of 45 patients, there was no evidence of this (143).

Ureteroscopy

Flexible ureteroscopy was first reported in 1964 by Marshall (86), who passed a 9-Fr fiberscope into the ureter to visualize an impacted ureteral calculus. Since then, improvements in miniaturization, light-carrying capacity, fiber optics, and two-way active deflection have made flexible ureteroscopy an important part of the diagnostic armamentarium for upper tract urothelial cancer. Initially, Bagley and colleagues (9) had reported a 79% success rate in visualization of the whole intrarenal collecting system. However, with improvements in the equipment, one group was able to report in 1997 a 100% success rate (32). Ureteroscopy is an excellent modality to assist in the diagnosis of upper tract urothelial cancer when a filling defect of tissue density has been confirmed radiographically, but cytology is not positive for tumor. It is also useful for the evaluation of upper tract tumors to assist in treatment planning and, as described in a later section, the resection of selected tumors.

Use of flexible cup biopsy forceps or basket through the flexible ureteroscope has improved diagnostic accuracy for upper tract tumors. In the study by Keeley and colleagues (71) of 51 cases of upper tract urothelial cancer, 94% of the cases were diagnosed based on cytologic material collected. Grading of the ureteroscopic specimens was achieved in 82% of all cases (88% of diagnostic ones). The authors attributed their success to their sampling technique: ureteroscopic examination followed by aspiration, saline wash, biopsy of the lesions, and then another saline wash following the biopsy. In another study of 45 upper tract urothelial carcinomas, 40 (89%) were definitively diagnosed with ureteroscopic biopsy, and of these, the ureteroscopic biopsy grade matched the surgical pathology grade in 78% (49).

The possibility of pyelovenous or pyelolymphatic migration of malignant cells during ureteroscopy has raised some concerns. In one case report, tumor cells were noted in the submucosal lymphatic and vascular spaces when ureteropyeloscopy was performed immediately before nephroureterectomy (80). The authors suggested that the high-pressure irrigation required during ureteropyeloscopy played a role in forcing tumor cells into these spaces. A more recent study of 96 patients evaluating the long-term consequences of diagnostic ureteroscopy for upper tract urothelial carcinoma was unable to find any adverse effect on overall or disease-specific survival (55). Attempts to make definitive diagnoses of tumor stage with endoscopic biopsies of the upper tract collecting system risk perforation. Fortunately, deep biopsies are not required because in most cases the grade of the upper tract urothelial tumor is an adequate surrogate for stage, at least for the purposes of planning treatment (70,71).

Ureteral perforation following ureteroscopy has been reported with an incidence of 0% to 4.6% (1,13,46,51). Long-term complications of ureteroscopy, most notably ureteral strictures, have an incidence of 0.5% to 1.4% (1,13,46,51). It is important to note that the lower rates cited for ureteral perforations and strictures have come from more recent series using smaller-diameter (6.9- to 7.5-Fr) flexible ureteroscopes (46,51,154). With these instruments, formal dilation of the intramural ureter is not usually required and ureteral trauma is minimal. These small-diameter ureteroscopes make possible direct visual confirmation and sampling of almost any upper tract urothelial cancer, which should provide for more exact identification and assessment of lesions than was previously available with only radiography and ureteral catheterization.

TREATMENT

Prognosis

Tumor grade and stage are important determinants of long-term outcome in upper tract urothelial cancer. Low-grade and low-stage upper tract urothelial tumors have a good outcome regardless of whether a conservative or more radical surgical approach is taken. Patients with intermediate grade or multifocal disease ultimately have a better outcome with radical surgery. Unfortunately, patients with high-stage and high-grade disease often do poorly regardless of the approach.

In one study, patients with grade 1 tumors had a 100% 5-year survival rate, those with grade 2/4 had an 80% 5-year survival rate, and those with grade 3/4 had a 60% 5-year survival rate (33). Both patients with grade 4/4 cancer succumbed to their disease. In another report, 27% of patients with grade 2 and 73% of patients with grade 3 disease died of their disease (107). In contrast, Mufti and colleagues (101) found survival to be greater than 90% for patients with superficial well-differentiated tumors regardless of whether they were treated with nephroureterectomy or more conservative methods.

Some have found multiplicity of the tumors to be a negative prognostic indicator. In Mazeman's 1976 review (89), patients with multiple tumors in the upper urinary tract experienced a decreased 5-year survival rate (20% versus 37% in individuals with single tumors).

DNA ploidy has been evaluated as an independent prognostic indicator. DNA ploidy relies on flow cytometric measurement of DNA content. Al-Abadi and Nagel (3) were able to find a correlation between DNA ploidy and tumor grade or stage. Although they did not find ploidy to be an independent predictor of prognosis, they did demonstrate that patients with aneuploid tumors did poorly. The poor response of aneuploid tumors was confirmed by Badalament and colleagues (8). In their series, patients with aneuploid tumors had a median disease-free survival of 19 months, and those with diploid tumors had a median disease-free survival of 59 months.

In an attempt to create a uniform management protocol for patients with upper tract urothelial cancer, the National Comprehensive Cancer Network guideline was created (136). Listed in the guideline are treatment algorithms using the latest information available on treatment outcomes. The guidelines incorporate the grade and stage in the management protocols.

Nephroureterectomy

Nephroureterectomy continues to be the preferred treatment for most upper tract urothelial carcinomas. The technique involves a simple nephrectomy and ipsilateral ureterectomy with the removal of a 2-cm cuff of urinary bladder. This procedure may be performed through a single midline incision or through two separate incisions such as a flank incision and a Pfannenstiel or lower midline incision to remove the distal ureter. Others have described endoscopic resection or mobilization of the intramural ureter followed by open en bloc resection of both the kidney and the ureter.

Johansson and Wahlqvist (67) advocate a transabdominal radical nephrectomy with adrenalectomy, in addition to a complete ureterectomy with bladder cuff. The 5-year survival rate of patients who had undergone the radical procedure was 84%, versus 51% for patients who had undergone more conventional resection. This difference was most marked in the high-stage patients (74% versus 37% 5-year survival). For small tumors, a simple nephrectomy with ureterectomy is probably sufficient, but in doubtful cases, or in the presence of a large tumor at high risk for invasion into the renal parenchyma, the inclusion of perinephric tissue as for radical nephrectomy (with or without adrenal gland, depending on tumor extent) is prudent. Komatsu and colleagues (75) also suggest that lymphadenectomy may provide some therapeutic benefit in selected patients. They found two long-term survivors whose nodes were located close to the original tumor. Other authors have not found a survival advantage to lymphadenectomy, reporting the likelihood of cancer death with uninvolved lymph nodes to be essentially the same as for those who had not undergone lymphadenectomy (23).

More recently, there has been the emergence of laparoscopic nephroureterectomy. This technique has been performed using both a transperitoneal and a retroperitoneal approach (41,90,127). Although requiring more specialized surgical skill and (usually) greater operative time, laparoscopic nephroureterectomy appears beneficial to the patient in terms of reduced blood loss, decreased postoperative narcotic use, and more rapid resumption of daily activities. In a series by Shalhav and colleagues (140), the disease-specific survival was identical for both laparoscopic nephroureterectomy and open nephroureterectomy (77%). Keeley and Tolley (72) reported similar success in 18 cases, in which only one patient with pT3 ureteral tumor developed a bladder and retroperitoneal recurrence.

Although laparoscopic nephroureterectomy appears to be a promising new minimally invasive technique, the technical demands and needs for specialized instrumentation make its widespread use unlikely at present. In addition, recent reports (2,111) of port site metastasis of urothelial carcinoma occurring following laparoscopic nephrectomy are worrisome, although in one of these cases (111) the urothelial carcinoma was unsuspected and the entrapment sac was torn during removal. Not only does urothelial carcinoma appear to have a propensity for wound seeding, but also intact specimen removal is desirable because the pathologic stage may have therapeutic implications. As such, when laparoscopic nephroureterectomy is performed for urothelial carcinoma, an incision large enough for extraction of the intact kidney is recommended. The addition of hand assistance to the laparoscopic technique, which allows the use of one hand within the operative field while maintaining pneumoperitoneum, takes advantage of this incision throughout the procedure rather than just at its conclusion. Hand assistance probably shortens operative time and appears to maintain the reduced morbidity of the laparoscopic procedure (163).

Renal-sparing Surgery

In the case of a pelvic tumor, a heminephrectomy or partial excision of the renal pelvis can be performed to remove the neoplasm with preservation of the kidney. Distal ureteral lesions can be managed by simple segmental resection and reimplantation; segmental resection of upper ureteral and midureteral tumors may require ileal interposition or autotransplantation. Conservative management may be indicated for patients with a solitary kidney, bilateral disease, or renal insufficiency. In patients with a functioning, disease-free, contralateral kidney, the indications for renal-sparing management (except for distal ureteral lesions) are less certain. The results of conservative management vary with the grade, stage, and multifocality of the neoplasm.

Open Surgical Approach

Localized surgical resection has been advocated for low-grade, low-stage distal ureteral tumors. Zungri and colleagues (168) demonstrated that survival for pTa disease was 100% regardless of whether the patient underwent more conservative or more radical surgery. In one series, Babaian and Johnson (7) reviewed the records of 44 patients with primary ureteral tumors and found that all of those with low-grade noninvasive disease confined to the distal third of their ureter were disease free following ureterectomy at the time of last follow-up. Segmental resection for low-grade and low-stage ureteral tumors produces results similar to that for nephroureterectomy. Zoretic and Gonzales (167) found that following nephroureterectomy, the 5-year survival rate was 50%. In contrast, the 5-year survival rate following segmental resection for low-grade and low-stage lesions was 71.4%, with ureteral recurrence rate of 6%. Similarly, Mufti and colleagues (101) reported 100% survival for low-grade disease treated with conservative resection.

In the middle and upper ureter, there has been less success with local resection—partially due to the technical difficulties resulting from insufficient remaining ureteral length to allow for reimplantation. Ileal interposition and autotransplantation with direct pyelovesical anastomosis have been described in these situations. In one series of 50 patients who had tumors too proximal to allow for complete resection of the distal portion of ureter, the investigators reported a recurrence rate of 50% at 3 years (89). Similar results have been noted by Strong and Pearse (150), who found a 30% recurrence rate in the portion of the ureter distal to the tumor in patients treated with local resection.

Local resection of the renal pelvic or calyceal tumors has usually been associated with a less favorable outcome. During open surgical local resection of renal pelvic tumors, the luminal surface of the tumor being removed cannot be isolated as it can be for ureteral resection, and thus there is increased risk of tumor spillage into the surgical field. Open surgical resection of urothelial tumors in a renal calyx may require removal of renal parenchyma as well. Visualization of the calyces is limited, and multifocal disease that is not suspected radiographically might easily be overlooked. Open surgical resection of multifocal renal pelvic and calyceal tumors is technically difficult.

Mazeman (89) and Zincke and Neves (166) have reported recurrence rates as high as 45% to 65% following local resection of the renal pelvic tumors; the actual recurrence rates were dependent on grade. This is worrisome because Charbit and associates (23) noted that as many as 33% of patients had multifocal disease that was not recognized until histopathologic examination was complete, and that when recurrences occurred, 66% of these patients experienced an increase in grade or stage, or both. Mills and Vaughan (96) reported worse prognoses for invasive lesions in their series of 53 cases: patients with submucosal infiltration had an 80% 5-year survival rate, and those with periureteral fat invasion had only a 33% 5-year survival rate.

Findings suggest that the greater the length of the ureter remaining, the greater the chance for recurrence. Many investigators report that partial removal of the ureter results in a high ureteral stump recurrence rate. Recurrence rates range from 20% to as high as 58% (74,106,150) and may occur from 1 to 45 years after resection (102). Mazeman (89) showed that following subtotal nephroureterectomy, nephrectomy and partial ureterectomy, and simple nephrectomy, patients had recurrence rates of 24%, 32%, and 48%, respectively.

All these results taken together would suggest that elective open surgical renal-sparing management of upper tract urothelial cancers should be limited to distal ureteral tumors, or low-grade and low-stage lesions in the middle and upper ureter. Other tumors, such as those in the renal pelvis or higher-grade upper ureteral and midureteral cancers, are ideally treated with nephroureterectomy in the setting of a contralateral upper tract that is functioning and disease free. When open surgical renal-sparing management is chosen for such tumors because renal sparing is imperative (i.e., solitary kidney, bilateral disease, and renal insufficiency), it is technically difficult and carries a substantial risk of recurrence.

Endoscopic Approach

The first series describing ureteroscopic treatment of upper tract collecting system tumors involved the use of 12- to 13-Fr rigid ureteral resectoscopes. Size and rigidity limited the usefulness of these endoscopes. Endoscopic treatment for upper urinary tract disease has been simplified considerably by the development of small-diameter semirigid and flexible ureteroscopes. These have allowed clear visualization of tumors throughout the collecting system (Fig. 17.7). In addition, the application of the neodymium:yttrium-aluminum-garnet (Nd:YAG) laser and the holmium:yttrium-aluminum-garnet (Ho:YAG) laser through small-diameter fibers has made the endoscopic treatment of larger tumors more feasible.

Simple fulguration with electrocautery can be used to treat small lesions or the base of a lesion following resection of the bulk of the tumor. However, fulguration of large portions of ureter may risk stricture formation. The depth of penetration (5 to 6 mm) of the Nd:YAG laser allows coagulation of full-thickness urothelium, but tissue ablation

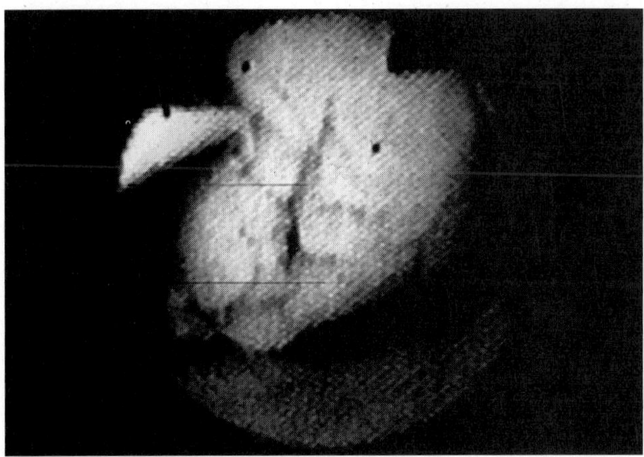

FIGURE 17.7. Endoscopic view of upper tract papillary urothelial carcinoma.

is not optimal with this laser. The Ho:YAG laser produces more ablation than coagulation of tissue, although the process is slow through the small fibers that can be passed through ureteroscopes. Combinations of Nd:YAG and Ho:YAG lasers have been used, taking advantage of the coagulative power of the Nd:YAG laser and the ablative power of the Ho:YAG laser (153).

In one retrospective review of 92 patients treated ureteroscopically, 76% of patients with grade 1 and 2 disease were able to become tumor free (70). Tumor size (larger than 1.5 cm), greater tumor grade, and multifocality predicted poor outcome. Similar favorable outcomes in the endoscopic treatment of low-grade upper tract urothelial cancer were reported by Martinez-Pineiro and colleagues (87). They reported that patients with grade 1 disease had a much lower recurrence rate than patients with grade 2 disease, 27% and 40%, respectively.

Controversy surrounds whether location of the tumor may play a role in treatment outcomes. Ureteral cancers have a lower recurrence rate than renal pelvic tumors. Blute and colleagues (14) reported a 63% failure rate for patients with renal pelvic tumors. One possible explanation to account for this difference is the greater accessibility of the ureter for endoscopic treatment than the renal pelvis. In contrast, Martinez-Pineiro and colleagues (87) reported a higher failure rate for ureteral tumors (36.6% versus 10% for renal pelvic tumors). Tawfiek and Bagley (153) reported that local recurrence rate was essentially the same for renal pelvic tumors (33%) and ureteral tumors (31.2%).

Complications resulting from endourologic management include formation of ureteral strictures and ureteral perforation. The risk of stricture disease following ureteroscopic treatment may be related to need for dilation at the ureterovesical junction and the extent of cautery and ablation required for treatment of the lesion. The use of small-diameter flexible ureteroscopes has reduced the need for formal dilation of the intramural ureter. Although initial reports described stricture rates as high as 25% (137), more recent series have reported more modest rates of 5% to 13% (33,70,87).

Ureteral perforations occur as a result of deep resection and can be managed conservatively with stent placement. Elliot and colleagues (33) report successfully treating two cases of ureteral perforation during endoscopic resection with double-J stent placement. In addition, the theoretic risk of dissemination of malignant cells into the retroperitoneal space has been raised. A case report of extravasation and propagation of tumor cells beyond the collecting system and into the parenchyma following ureteroscopic examination supports this fear (80).

Percutaneous management, another alternative for the renal-sparing management of upper tract urothelial cancer, is more suited for large tumors in the intrarenal collecting system or proximal ureter (Fig. 17.8). Once percutaneous access has been obtained, the tract is dilated to allow placement of a sheath, through which an endoscope with resection loop or biopsy forceps can be used to remove the tumor. Ablation and fulguration with a flexible electrode, rollerball electrode, or laser (Nd:YAG or Ho:YAG) following biopsy of the tumor(s) is useful when disease is extensive or difficult to access (105,110).

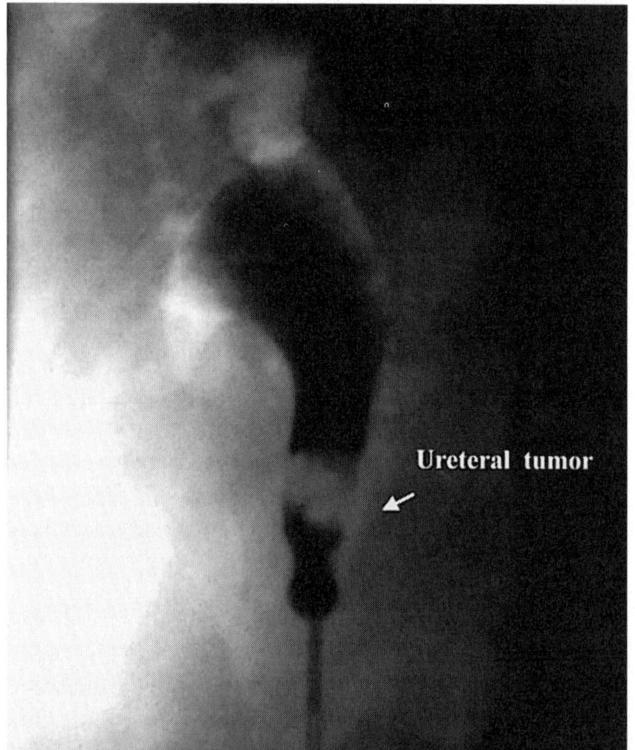

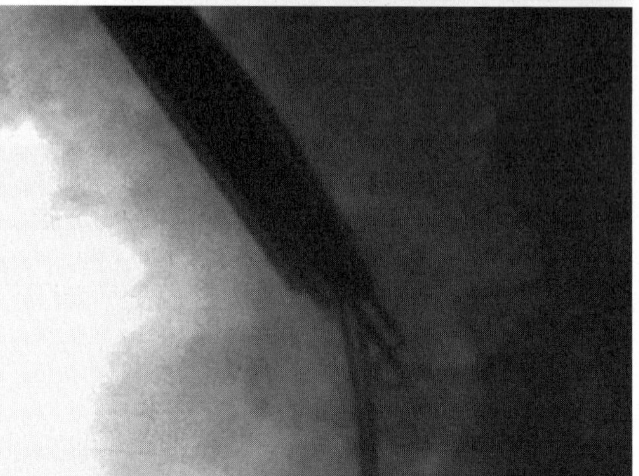

FIGURE 17.8. Percutaneous resection of large proximal ureteral tumor. **A:** Fluoroscopic view of lesion. **B:** Resectoscope in place for resection.

Similar to results obtained for ureteroscopic treatment, percutaneous resection or ablation of urothelial cancer has been most successful for low-grade and low-stage disease. In a series of 61 patients followed for a mean duration of four years, investigators reported 95% overall disease-specific survival: 100% for pTa lesions and 80% for T_1 lesions (61). Recurrence rates correlate with grade and stage of disease (24,62,77,116). Jarrett and colleagues (62) reported an 18% recurrence rate for grade 1 disease and a 50% recurrence rate for grade 3 disease. They strongly advocated second- and third-look procedures performed approximately 1 week apart to ensure that complete resection had occurred. Similarly, Clark and colleagues (24) reported a 28% recurrence rate for patients with grade 1 or 2 disease and 50% recurrence for grade 3 disease. Patel and colleagues (116) found a 12.5% recurrence rate for T_a disease and 50% for T_{2b} disease. Other reported recurrence rates range from 11% to 45% (61,120). Orihuela and Smith (110) found lower recurrence rates if second-look nephroscopy was performed, if Nd:YAG laser had been used for ablation, and if BCG had been instilled following resection.

Most complications of percutaneous management of upper tract urothelial cancer are similar to those for percutaneous management of stone disease. The most common complications are bleeding and extravasation. In addition to the cancer-specific risk of forcing cells into the systemic circulation as a result of pyelovenous or pyelolymphatic backflow (as in ureteroscopy), a unique concern associated with percutaneous treatment is the risk of tumor cells seeding the nephrostomy tube tract. Reports of seeding of the nephrostomy tract are numerous (24,36,57,139,141). One group advocates iridium wire brachytherapy within the nephrostomy tube tract to prevent recurrences (116). With this technique, this group did not experience seeding in their series of 28 patients. Others suggest the use of single-stage percutaneous access, tract dilation, and tumor resection as methods to reduce the seeding risk (119). Additional suggestions to prevent pyelovenous or pyelolymphatic backflow include keeping the irrigation fluid bag less than 40 cm above the level of the kidney and making sure that there is a loose fit between the working sheath and the nephroscope. Some investigators have gone as far as to suggest use of sterile water as the working irrigant to take advantage of its cytolytic properties; however, this practice may be associated with dilutional hyponatremia. The long-term effect of percutaneous treatment on renal function is not known. Jarrett and colleagues (62) reported two cases of chronic renal insufficiency that developed following percutaneous treatment.

Adjuvant Therapy

Topical Agents

As in the case of superficial bladder cancer, many investigators have explored the use of topical therapy with BCG, mitomycin C, and thiotepa. Drug delivery into the collecting system has occurred in a variety of manners: retrograde installation using ureteral catheters, direct installation through a percutaneous nephrostomy tube, or resection of the ureteral orifice inducing reflux into the collecting system (56,126,142). Although these reports suggest some benefit from these agents, there have not been any randomized trials to unequivocally demonstrate survival benefit due to the rarity of their application for upper tract urothelial tumors.

Herr (56) described creation of a pyelovesicostomy to allow reflux of BCG into the collecting system. The patient remained tumor free at 13 months of follow-up. Orihuela and Smith (110) reported on six patients who received six weekly courses of BCG via nephrostomy tube following percutaneous resection. The BCG was well tolerated and no incidence of sepsis was reported. Although they had a small number of patients, they found a lower recurrence rate with the use of BCG (16.6% versus 80% without BCG). Patel and Fuchs (115) showed that BCG could be instilled in a retrograde fashion via a transvesical single-J ureteral stent. At 1 year of follow-up, 15 of 17 renal units treated were preserved. In addition, there has been report of reflux of BCG through a ureteroileal anastomosis used as a method to keep one patient recurrence free at 1 year of follow-up (126). The direct routes of administration offer more assured contact of BCG with the upper tract tissue.

Several investigators have reported use of mitomycin C. Smith and colleagues (146) reported the treatment of superficial papillary urothelial carcinoma in the distal ureter with mitomycin C. Despite leaving the primary lesions unresected, both patients became tumor free and remained so after more than 2 years of follow-up. Eastham and Huffman (31) reported on the delivery of mitomycin C via percutaneous nephrostomy tube (continuous infusion of 40 mg in 1,000 mL of saline infused continuously at 50 mL hour) or ureteral catheter (5 mg in 20 mL of saline instilled and held for 30 minutes). Five of their seven patients were disease free 1 to 12 months following treatment.

De Kock and Breytenbach (28) reported the use of six weekly courses of topical thiotepa via retrograde ureteral catheter following local excision of a renal pelvis tumor in a solitary kidney. The patient required two 6-week courses to become disease free and subsequently developed thrombocytopenia. Although there was no recurrence of her renal pelvic tumor, with 6.5 years of follow-up, the thrombocytopenia points out a potential risk of thiotepa. One unusual report of intraureteral use of thiotepa involves the use of a subcutaneously placed Ommaya reservoir in the treatment of bilateral primary urothelial carcinoma of the ureter (123). The patient received four courses of thiotepa injected through the reservoir and continued to receive maintenance treatment via a retrograde ureteral catheter following removal of the reservoir. At 8.5 years following his initial treatment, the patient remained recurrence free.

In the absence of comparative studies between BCG, mitomycin, and thiotepa for topical upper tract therapy, at our institution we prefer percutaneous administration of mitomycin for treatment of residual upper tract urothelial neoplasms or prophylaxis following resection of high-grade disease, in patients who have imperative indications for renal sparing. Our protocol involves six weekly instillations of 30 mg of mitomycin in 60 mL of saline, instilled through a nephrostomy tube continuously for 2 hours at 30 mL hour. The nephrostomy tube is clamped between treatments, minimizing the inconvenience for the patient. Ureteroscopic reevaluation is performed 6 weeks after the last instillation, with repeat endoscopic fulguration or repeat topical therapy (possibly with BCG) in case of disease persistence, and removal of the nephrostomy tube if there is no evidence of disease.

Radiation Therapy

In an attempt to reduce local and regional failure rate, some investigators have explored the use of adjuvant radiotherapy. Cozad and colleagues (26) reported that adjuvant radiation decreased the 5-year local recurrence rate from 25% to 10%. This improvement in local control was also noted by Brookland and Richter (20), who noted an 11% local recurrence rate in patients with high-risk (stage III or grade 3) disease treated with radiation and a 45% local recurrence rate in patients who had not received adjuvant treatment. Although local control was possible, there was no improvement in the recurrence of distant metastasis and in overall survival. Maulard-Durdux and colleagues (88) reported that despite an improvement in local control, metastatic dissemination still occurred in 54% of patients. Ozahin and colleagues (112) also demonstrated this lack of improvement in overall survival in their review of 138 patients.

Chemotherapy

As in the treatment of advanced bladder urothelial cancer, cisplatinum-based chemotherapeutic regimens such as methotrexate, vinblastine, adriamycin, and cisplatinum (MVAC) have been used in both a neoadjuvant and an adjuvant setting (60,79,152). The effectiveness of cisplatinum-based chemotherapy regimens has been similar to that for bladder urothelial cancer. Lerner and colleagues (79), in a study of 28 patients with high-grade and advanced urothelial carcinoma of the upper tract, found a 54% overall response rate [18% complete response (CR) and 36% partial response (PR)] to platinum-based chemotherapy. However, 89% of these patients eventually succumbed to their disease. They suggested that their outcome might have been better if their patients had been able to tolerate a full course of treatment. Owing to renal insufficiency following their nephroureterectomy, all of these patients had required dose reduction. Similarly, Igawa and colleagues (59) found a 52.9% overall response rate for treatment of advanced renal pelvic and urothelial tumors. Although they were able to achieve durable CR, mean time to recurrence for patients with partial response was only 6.4 months.

More recently, investigators have reported success rates similar to that for MVAC using a combination of paclitaxel and carboplatin. Redman and colleagues (128) reported a 51.5% overall response rate (19% CR and 30.6% PR) in phase II trial. Similar results were also seen in a study of 32 patients at the University of Vienna, with a response rate of 71.9% (31.3% CR and 40.6% PR) (124). The toxicities associated with this combination, including myalgias, arthralgias, alopecia, and neutropenia, occur less often than with MVAC (124,128). Despite promising results, the mean time to progression after CR was reported at 7 months and after PR was only 5.9 months (124).

Others have reported additional success with a combination of gemcitabine and cisplatin. Gemcitabine, a cytosine analog, was shown to be active as a single-agent therapy in urothelial cancer (147). In combination with cisplatin, gemcitabine results in an overall response rate ranging from 41% to 52% (69,98,158). Toxicity associated with this combination was mainly hematologic. Median time to progression ranged from 5.5 months to 7.2 months, and median survival ranged from 12.5 to 14.3 months (69, 98,158).

Although these new combinations present new therapeutic options in the management of advanced urothelial cancer, the long-term outlook for these patients remains poor.

REFERENCES

1. Abdel-Razzak OM, Bagley DH. Clinical experience with flexible ureteroscopy. *J Urol* 1992;148(6):1788.
2. Ahmed I, Shaikh NA, Kapadia CR. Track recurrence of renal pelvic transitional cell carcinoma after laparoscopic nephrectomy. *Br J Urol* 1998;81(2):319.
3. Al-Abadi H, Nagel R. Transitional cell carcinoma of the renal pelvis and ureter: prognostic relevance of nuclear deoxyribonucleic acid ploidy studied by cytometry: an 8-year survival time study. *J Urol* 1992;148(1):31.
4. Almgard LE, Freedman D, Ljungqvist A. Carcinoma of the ureter with special reference to malignancy grading and prognosis. *Scand J Urol Nephrol* 1973;7(2):165.
5. Amar AD, Das S. Upper urinary tract transitional cell carcinoma in patients with bladder carcinoma and associated vesicoureteral reflux. *J Urol* 1985;133(3):468.
6. Anwar K, Naiki H, Nakukuki K, et al. High frequency of human papilloma virus infection in carcinoma of the urinary bladder. *Cancer* 1992;70(7):1967.
7. Babaian RJ, Johnson DE. Primary carcinoma of the ureter. *J Urol* 1980;123(3):357.
8. Badalament RA, O'Toole RV, Kenworthy P, et al. Prognostic factors in patients with primary transitional cell cancer of the upper urinary tract. *J Urol* 1990;144(4):859.
9. Bagley DH, Huffman JL, Lyon ES. Flexible ureteropyeloscopy: diagnosis and treatment of the upper urinary tract. *J Urol* 1987;138(2):280.
10. Batata MA, Whitmore WF Jr, Hilaris BS. Primary carcinoma of the ureter: a prognostic study. *Cancer* 1975;35(6):1626.

11. Berger CS, Sandbergt AA, Todd IA, et al. Chromosomes in kidney, ureter, and bladder cancer. *Cancer Genet Cytogenet* 1986;23(1):1.
12. Bergman H, Friedenberg RM, Sayegh V. New roentgenologic signs of carcinoma of the ureter. *AJR Am J Roentgenol* 1961; 86:707.
13. Blute ML, Segura JW, Patterson DE. Ureteroscopy. *J Urol* 1988;139(3):510.
14. Blute ML, Segura JW, Patterson DE, et al. Impact of endourology on diagnosis and management of upper urinary tract urothelial cancer. *J Urol* 1989;141(6):1298.
15. Blute RD, Gittes RR, Gittes RF. Renal brush biopsy: survey of the indications, techniques and results. *J Urol* 1981; 126(2):146.
16. Booth CM, Camaeron KM, Pugh RCB. Urothelial carcinoma of the kidney and ureter. *Br J Urol* 1980;52(6):430.
17. Bostwick DG, Ramnani D, Cheng L. Diagnosis and grading of bladder cancer and associated lesions. *Urol Clin North Am* 1999;26(3):493.
18. Brenner DW, Schellhammer PE. Upper tract urothelial malignancy after cyclophosphamide therapy: a case report and literature review. *J Urol* 1987;137(6):1226.
19. Bretheau D, Lechevallier E, Uzan E, et al. Value of radiologic examinations in the diagnosis and staging of upper urinary tract tumors. *Prog Urol* 1994;4(6):966.
20. Brookland RK, Richter MP. The post operative irradiation of transitional cell carcinoma of the renal pelvis and ureter. *J Urol* 1985;133(6):952.
21. Bryant P, Davies P, Wilson D. Detection of human papilloma virus DNA in cancer of the urinary bladder by *in situ* hybridization. *Br J Urol* 1991;68(1):53.
22. Buckley JA, Urban BA, Soyer P, et al. Transitional cell carcinoma of the renal pelvis: a retrospective look at CT staging with pathologic correlation. *Radiology* 1996;201(1):194.
23. Charbit L, Gendreau MC, Mee S, et al. Tumors of the upper urinary tract: 10 years of experience. *J Urol* 1991;146(5):1243.
24. Clark PE, Streem SB, Geisinger MA. 13-year experience with percutaneous management of upper tract transitional cell carcinoma. *J Urol* 1999;161(3):772.
25. Cookson MS, Herr HW, Zhang Z, et al. The treated natural history of high risk superficial bladder cancer: 15 year outcome. *J Urol* 1997;158(1):62.
26. Cozad SC, Smalley SR, Austenfeld M, et al. Transitional cell carcinoma of the renal pelvis or ureter: patterns of failure. *Urology* 1995;46(6):796.
27. Cummings KB. Nephroureterectomy: rationale in the management of transitional cell carcinoma of the upper urinary tract. *Urol Clin North Am* 1980;7(3):569.
28. De Kock MLS, Breytenbach IH. Local excision and topical thiotepa in the treatment of transitional cell carcinoma of the renal pelvis: a case report. *J Urol* 1985;135(3):566.
29. De Torres Mateos JA, Banus Gassol JM, Palou Redorta J, et al. Vesicorenal reflux and upper urinary tract transitional cell carcinoma after transurethral resection of recurrent superficial bladder carcinoma. *J Urol* 1987;138(1):49.
30. Dodd LG, Johnson WW, Roberstson CN, et al. Endoscopic brush cytology of the upper urinary tract. Evaluation of its efficacy and potential limitations in diagnosis. *Acta Cytologica* 1997;41(2):377.
31. Eastham JA, Huffman JL. Technique of mitomycin C installation in the treatment of upper urinary tract urothelial tumors. *J Urol* 1993;150(2 Pt 1):324.
32. Elashry OM, Elbahnasy AM, Ganesh SR, et al. Flexible ureteroscopy: Washington University experience with the 9.3 F and 7.5 F flexible ureteroscopes. *J Urol* 1997;157(6):2074.
33. Elliott DS, Blute ML, Patterson DE, et al. Long term follow-up of endoscopically treated upper urinary tract transitional cell carcinoma. *Urology* 1996;47(6):819.
34. Epstein JJ, Amin MB, Reuter VR, et al. The World Health Organization International Society of Urological Pathology consensus classification of urothelial (transitional cell) neoplasms of the urinary bladder. Bladder consensus conference committee. *Am J Surg Pathol* 1998;22(12):1435.
35. Fadl-Elmula I, Gorunova L, Mandahl N, et al. Cytogenetic analysis of upper urinary tract transitional cell carcinomas. *Cancer Genet Cytogenet* 1999;115(2):123.
36. Fuglsig S, Krarup T. Percutaneous nephroscopic resection of renal pelvic tumors. *Scand J Urol Nephrol* 1995;172[Suppl]:15.
37. Fukuya T, Honda H, Nakata H, et al. Computed tomographic findings of invasive transitional cell carcinoma of the kidney. *Radiat Med* 1994;12(1):6.
38. Furihata M, Inoue K, Ohtsuki Y, et al. High-risk human papilloma virus infection and overexpression of p53 protein as prognostic indicators of transitional cell carcinoma of the urinary bladder. *Cancer Res* 1993;53(20):4823.
39. Geerdsen J. Tumours of the renal pelvis and ureter. Symptomatology, diagnosis, treatment and prognosis. *Scand J Urol Nephrol* 1979;13(3):287.
40. Ghazi M, Morales P, Al-Askari S. Primary carcinoma of the ureter. *Urology* 1979;14(1):18.
41. Gill IS, Munch LC, Lucas BA, et al. Initial experience with retroperitoneoscopic nephroureterectomy: use of a double balloon technique. *Urology* 1995;46(5):747.
42. Gill WB, Lu CT, Thomsen S. Retrograde brushing: a new technique for obtaining histologic and cytologic material from ureteral, renal pelvic and renal calyceal lesions. *J Urol* 1973; 109(4):573.
43. Gittes RF. Management of transitional cell carcinoma of the upper tract: case for conservative local excision. *Urol Clin North Am* 1980;7(3):559.
44. Gittes RF. Retrograde brushing and nephroscopy in the diagnosis of upper tract urothelial cancer. *Urol Clin North Am* 1984;11(4):617.
45. Goyer R. Environmentally related diseases of the urinary tract. *Med Clin North Am* 1990;74(2):377.
46. Grasso M, Bagley D. Small diameter, actively deflectable, flexible ureteropyeloscopy. *J Urol* 1999;160(5):1648.
47. Greenland JE, Weston PM, Wallace DM. Familial transitional cell carcinoma and the Lynch syndrome II. *Br J Urol* 1993; 72(2):177.
48. Grignon DJ, Shum DT, Bruckschwaiger O. Transitional cell carcinoma in the Muir-Torre syndrome. *J Urol* 1987; 138(2):406.
49. Guarnizo E, Pavlovich CP, Seiba M, et al. Ureteroscopic biopsy of upper tract urothelial carcinoma: improved diagnostic accuracy and histopathological considerations using a multi-biopsy approach. *J Urol* 2000;163(1):52.
50. Hadas-Halpern I, Farkas A, Patlas M, et al. Sonographic diagnosis of ureteral tumors. *J Ultrasound Med* 1999;18(9):639.
51. Harmon WJ, Sershon PD, Blute ML, et al. Ureteroscopy: current practice and long-term complications. *J Urol* 1997; 157(1):28.
52. Harris AL, Neal DE. Bladder cancer—field versus clonal origin. *N Engl J Med* 1992;326(11):759.
53. Hartman DS, Pyatt RS, Dailey E. Transitional cell carcinoma of the kidney with invasion into the renal vein. *Urol Radiol* 1983;5(2):83.
54. Hawtrey CE. Fifty-two cases of primary ureteral carcinoma: a clinical-pathologic study. *J Urol* 1971;105(2):188.

55. Hendin BN, Streem SB, Levin HS, et al. Impact of diagnostic ureteroscopy on long-term survival in patients with upper tract transitional cell carcinoma. *J Urol* 1999;161(3):783.
56. Herr HW. Durable response of a carcinoma *in situ* of the renal pelvis to topical bacillus Calmette-Guérin. *J Urol* 1985; 134(3):531.
57. Huang A, Low RK, Whie RD. Nephrostomy tract tumor seeding following percutaneous manipulation of a ureteral carcinoma. *J Urol* 1995;153(3 Pt 2):1041.
58. Huben RP, Mounzer AM, Murphy GP. Tumor grade and stage as prognostic variables in upper tract urothelial tumors. *Cancer* 1988;62(9):2016.
59. Igawa M, Ueki T, Ueda M, et al. MVAC (methotrexate, vinblastine, adriamycin and cisplatinum) in chemotherapy in advanced renal pelvic and ureteral carcinoma. *Jpn J Cancer Chemother* 1989;16(8 Pt 1):2577.
60. Igawa M, Urakami S, Shiina H, et al. Limitations of ureteroscopy in the diagnosis of invasive upper tract urothelial cancer. *Urol Int* 1996;56(1):13.
61. Jabbour ME, Desgrandchamps F, Cazin S, et al. Percutaneous management of grade II upper urinary tract transitional cell carcinoma: the long-term outcome. *J Urol* 2000;163(4):1105.
62. Jarrett TW, Sweetser PM, Weiss GH, et al. Percutaneous management of transitional cell carcinoma of the renal collecting system: 9 year experience. *J Urol* 1995;154(5):1629.
63. Jensen OM, Kamby C. Intra-uterine exposure to saccharin and risk of bladder cancer in man. *Int J Cancer* 1983;29(5):507.
64. Jensen OM, Knudsen JB, McLaughlin JK, et al. The Copenhagen case-control study of renal pelvis and ureter cancer: role of smoking and occupational exposures. *Int J Cancer* 1988; 41(4):557.
65. Jensen OM, Knudsen JB, Tomasson H, et al. The Copenhagen case-control study of renal pelvis and ureter cancer: role of analgesics. *Int J Cancer* 1989;44(6):965.
66. Jitsukawa S, Nakamura K, Nakayama M, et al. Transitional cell carcinoma of the kidney extending into renal vein and inferior vena cava. *Urology* 1985;25(3):310.
67. Johansson S, Wahlqvist L. A prognostic study of urothelial renal pelvic tumors: comparison between the prognosis of patients treated with intrafascial nephrectomy and perifascial nephrectomy. *Cancer* 1979;43(6):2525.
68. Kakizoe T, Fujita J, Murase T, et al. Transitional cell carcinoma of the bladder in patients with renal pelvic and ureteral cancer. *J Urol* 1980;124(1):17.
69. Kaufman D, Raghavan D, Carducci M, et al. Phase II trial of gemcitabine plus cisplatin in patients with metastatic urothelial cancer. *J Clin Oncol* 2000;18(9):1921.
70. Keeley FX, Bibbo M, Bagley DH. Ureteroscopic treatment and surveillance of upper urinary tract transitional cell carcinoma. *J Urol* 1997;157(5):1560.
71. Keeley FX, Kulp DA, Bibbo M, et al. Diagnostic accuracy of ureteroscopic biopsy in upper tract transitional cell carcinoma. *J Urol* 1997;157(1):33.
72. Keeley FX, Tolley DA. Laparoscopic nephroureterectomy: making management of upper-tract transitional cell carcinoma entirely minimally invasive. *J Endourol* 1998;12(2):139.
73. Kiemeney LALM, Schoenberg M. Familial transitional cell carcinoma. *J Urol* 1996;156(3):867.
74. Kimball FN, Ferris HW. Papillomatous tumor of the renal pelvis associated with similar tumors of the ureter and bladder. *J Urol* 1934;31:257.
75. Komatsu H, Tanabe N, Kubodera S, et al. The role of lymphadenectomy in the treatment of transitional cell carcinoma of the upper urinary tract. *J Urol* 1997;157(5):1622.
76. Krogh J, Kvist E, Rye B. Transitional cell carcinoma of the upper urinary tract. Prognostic variables in upper tract urothelial tumors. *Br J Urol* 1988;67(1):32.
77. Lee BR, Jabbour ME, Marshall FF, et al. 13-year survival comparison of percutaneous and open nephroureterectomy approaches for management of transitional cell carcinoma of the renal collecting system: equivalent outcomes. *J Endourol* 1999; 13(4):289.
78. Leistenschneider W, Nagel R. Lavage cytology of the renal pelvis and ureter with special reference to tumors. *J Urol* 1980;124(5):597.
79. Lerner SE, Blute ML, Richardson RL, et al. Platinum based chemotherapy for advanced transitional cell cancer of the upper urinary tract. *Mayo Clin Proc* 1996;71(10):945.
80. Lim DJ, Shattuck MC, Cook WA. Pyelovenous lymphatic migration of transitional cell carcinoma following flexible ureterorenoscopy. *J Urol* 1993;49:109.
81. Liu J, Bagley DH, Conlin MJ, et al. Endoluminal sonographic evaluation of ureteral and renal pelvic neoplasms. *J Ultrasound Med* 1997;16(8):515.
82. Lomax-Smith JD, Seymour AE. Neoplasia in analgesic nephropathy. A urothelial field change. *Am J Surg Pathol* 1980; 4(6):565.
83. Lunec J, Challen C, Wright C, et al. c-erbB-2 amplification and identical p53 mutations in concomitant transitional carcinomas of renal pelvis and urinary bladder. *Lancet* 1992;339:439.
84. Lynch H, Ens JA, Lynch JF. The Lynch syndrome II and urological malignancies. *J Urol* 1990;143(1):24.
85. Mahadevia PA, Karwa GL, Koss LG. Mapping of urothelium in carcinomas of the renal pelvis and ureter. A report of nine cases. *Cancer* 1983;51(5):890.
86. Marshall VF. Fiber optics in urology. *J Urol* 1964;91:110.
87. Martinez-Pineiro JA, Garcia MJ, Martinez-Pineiro L. Endourological treatment of urothelial carcinomas: analysis of a series of 59 tumors. *J Urol* 1996;156(2 Pt 1):377.
88. Maulard-Durdux C, Dufour B, Chrétien HY, et al. Postoperative radiation therapy in 26 patients with invasive transitional cell carcinoma of the upper urinary tract: no impact on survival? *J Urol* 1996;155(1):115.
89. Mazeman E. Tumors of the upper urinary tract calyces, renal pelvis and ureter. *Eur Urol* 1976;2(3):120.
90. McCarron JP Jr, Chasko SB, Gray GF Jr. Systematic mapping of nephroureterectomy specimens removed for urothelial cancer: pathological findings and clinical correlations. *J Urol* 1982; 128(2):243.
91. McCredie M, Stewart JH, Ford JM, et al. Phenacetin-containing analgesics and cancer of the bladder or renal pelvis in women. *Br J Urol* 1983;55(2):220.
92. McLaughlin JK, Silverman DT, Hsing AW, et al. Cigarette smoking and cancers of the renal pelvis and ureter. *Cancer Res* 1992;52(2):254.
93. Melamed MR, Reuter VE. Pathology and staging of urothelial tumors of the kidney and ureter. *Urol Clinic North Am* 1993; 20(2):333.
94. Millán-Rodriguez F, Palou J, de la Torre-Holguera P, et al. Conventional CT signs in staging of transitional cell tumors of the upper urinary tract. *Eur Urol* 1999;35(4):318.
95. Miller EB, Eure GR, Schellhammer PF. Upper tract transitional cell carcinoma following treatment for superficial bladder cancer with BCG. *Urology* 1993;42(1):26.
96. Mills C, Vaughan ED. Carcinoma of the ureter: natural history, management and 5-year survival. *J Urol* 1983;129(2):275.
97. Minimo C, Tawfiek ER, Bagley DH, et al. Grading of upper tract transitional cell carcinoma by computed DNA content and p53 expression. *Urology* 1997;50(6):869.

98. Moore MJ, Winquist EW, Murray N, et al. Gemcitabine plus cisplatin, an active regimen in advanced urothelial cancer: a phase II trial of the National Cancer Institute of Canada Clinical Trials Group. *J Clin Oncol* 1999;17(9):2876.
99. Morrison AS. Advances in the etiology of urothelial cancer. *Urol Clin North Am* 1984;11(4):557.
100. Morrison AS. Epidemiology and environmental factors in urologic cancer. *Cancer* 1987;60[3 Suppl]:632.
101. Mufti GR, Gove JR, Badenock DF, et al. Transitional cell carcinoma of the renal pelvis and ureter. *Br J Urol* 1989; 63(2):135.
102. Mukamel E, Simon D, Edelman A, et al. Metachronous bladder tumors in patients with upper urinary tract transitional cell carcinomas. *J Surg Oncol* 1994;57(3):187.
103. Mullen JB, Kovacs K. Primary carcinoma of the ureteral stump: a case report and review of the literature. *J Urol* 1980; 123(1):113.
104. Murphy DM, Zinke H, Furlow WL. Primary grade 1 transitional cell carcinoma of the renal pelvis and ureter. *J Urol* 1980;123(5):629.
105. Nakada SY, Clayman RV. Percutaneous electrovaporization of upper tract transitional cell carcinoma in patients with functionally solitary kidneys. *Urology* 1995;46(5):751.
106. Newman DM, Allen LE, Wishard WN Jr, et al. Transitional cell carcinoma of the upper urinary tract. *J Urol* 1967; 98(3):322.
107. Nguyen GK, Schumann GB. Needle aspiration cytology of low grade transitional cell carcinoma of the renal pelvis. *Diagn Cytopathol* 1997;16(5):437.
108. Nocks BN, Heney NM, Dally JJ, et al. Transitional cell carcinoma of the renal pelvis. *Urology* 1982;19(5):472.
109. Oldbring J, Glifberg I, Mikulowski P, et al. Carcinoma of the renal pelvis and ureter following bladder carcinoma: frequency, risk factors and clinicopathological findings. *J Urol* 1989;141(6):1311.
110. Orihuela E, Smith AD. Percutaneous treatment of transitional cell carcinoma of the upper urinary tract. *Urol Clin North Am* 1988;15(3):425.
111. Otani M, Shinichiro I, Tsuji Y. Port site metastasis after laparoscopic nephrectomy: unsuspected transitional cell carcinoma within a tuberculous atrophic kidney. *J Urol* 1999; 162(2):486.
112. Ozahin M, Zouhair A, Villa S, et al. Prognostic factors in urothelial renal pelvis and ureter tumours: a multicenter rare cancer network study. *Eur J Cancer* 1999;35(5):738.
113. Palou J, Farina LA, Villavicencio H, et al. Upper tract urothelial tumor after transurethral resection for bladder tumor. *Eur Urol* 1992;21(2):110.
114. Palvio DH, Andersen JC, Falk E. Transitional cell tumors of the renal pelvis and ureter associated with capillarosclerosis indicating analgesic abuse. *Cancer* 59(5):972.
115. Patel A, Fuchs GJ. New techniques for the administration of topical adjuvant therapy after endoscopic ablation of upper urinary tract transitional cell carcinoma. *J Urol* 1998;159(1):71.
116. Patel A, Soonawalla P, Shepherd SF, et al. Long-term outcome after percutaneous treatment of transitional cell carcinoma of the renal pelvis. *J Urol* 1996;155(3):868.
117. Petkovic SD. Conservation of the kidney in operations for tumors of the renal pelvis and calcyes: a report of 26 cases. *Br J Urol* 1972;44(1):1.
118. Petkovic SD. Epidemiology and treatment of renal pelvic and ureteral tumors. *J Urol* 1975;114(6):858.
119. Pettersson S, Brynger H, Johansson S, et al. Extracorporeal surgery and autotransplantation for carcinoma of the pelvis and ureter. *Scand J Urol Nephrol* 1979;13(1):89.
120. Plancke HRF, Strijbos EM, Delaere KPJ. Percutaneous endoscopic treatment of urothelial tumours of the renal pelvis. *Br J Urol* 1995;75(6):736.
121. Planz B, George R, Adam G, et al. Computed tomography for detection and staging of transitional cell carcinoma of the upper urinary tract. *Eur Urol* 1995;27(2):146.
122. Poole-Wilson DS. Occupational tumors of the renal pelvis and ureter arising in the dye-making industry. *Proc R Soc Med* 1969;62(1):93.
123. Powder JR, Mosberg WH, Pierpont RZ, et al. Bilateral primary carcinoma of the ureter: topical intraureteral thiotepa. *J Urol* 1984;132(2):349.
124. Pycha A, Grbovic M, Posch B, et al. Paclitaxel and carboplatinum in patients with metastatic transitional cell cancer of the urinary tract. *Urology* 1999;53(3):510.
125. Radovanovic Z, Krajinovic S, Jankovic S, et al. Family history of cancer among cases of upper urothelial tumors in a Balkan nephropathy area. *J Cancer Res Clin Oncol* 1985;110(2):181.
126. Ramsey JC, Soloway MS. Instillation of bacillus Calmette-Guérin into the renal pelvis of a solitary kidney for treatment of transitional cell carcinoma. *J Urol* 1990;143(6):1220.
127. Rassweiler JJ, Henkel TO, Potempa DM, et al. The technique of transperitoneal laparoscopic nephrectomy, adrenalectomy, and nephroureterectomy. *Eur Urol* 1993;23(4):425.
128. Redman BG, Smith DC, Flaherty L, et al. Phase II trial of paclitaxel and carboplatinum in the treatment of advanced urothelial carcinoma. *J Clin Oncol* 1998;16(5):1844.
129. Reitelman C, Sawczuk IS, Olsson CA, et al. Prognostic variables in patients with transitional cell carcinoma of the renal pelvis and proximal ureter. *J Urol* 1987;138(5):1144.
130. Renart WA, Rudin LJ, Casarella WJ. Renal vein thrombosis in carcinoma of the renal pelvis. *AJR Am J Roentgenol* 1972; 114:735.
131. Reuter VR, Epstein JI, Amin MB, et al. A newly illustrated synopsis of the World Health Organization/International Society of Urological Pathology (WHO/ISUP) consensus classification of urothelial (transitional-cell) neoplasms of the urinary bladder. *J Urol Pathol* 1999;11:1.
132. Ross RK, Paganini-Hill A, Landolph J, et al. Analgesics, cigarette smoking, and other risk factors for cancer of the renal pelvis and ureter. *Cancer Res* 1989;49(4):1045.
133. Sadek S, Soloway MS, Hook S, et al. The value of upper tract cytology after transurethral resection of bladder tumor in patients with bladder transitional cell cancer. *J Urol* 1999; 161(1):77.
134. Sandberg AA, Berger CA, Haddad FS, et al. Chromosome change in transitional cell carcinoma of the ureter. *Cancer Genet Cytogenet* 1986;19(3–4):335.
135. Santamaria M, Jauregui I, Urtasun F, et al. Fine needle aspiration biopsy of urothelial carcinoma of the renal pelvis. *Acta Cytologica* 1995;39(3):443.
136. Scher H, Bahnson R, Cohen S, et al. NCCN urothelial cancer practice guidelines. National Comprehensive Cancer Network. *Oncology* 1998;12(7A):225.
137. Schmeller NT, Hofstetter AG. Laser treatment of ureteral tumors. *J Urol* 1989;141(4):840.
138. Schwalb DM, Herr HW, Sogani PC, et al. Upper tract disease following intravesical BCG for superficial bladder cancer: five year followup. *J Urol* 1992;147(2):273A.
139. Sengupta S, Harewood L. Transitional cell carcinoma growing along an indwelling nephrostomy tube tract. *Br J Urol* 1998; 82(4):591.
140. Shalhav AL, Dunn MD, Portis AJ, et al. Laparoscopic nephroureterectomy for upper tract transitional cell cancer: the Washington University experience. *J Urol* 2000;163(4):1100.

141. Sharma NK, Nicol A, Powell CS. Tract infiltration following percutaneous resection of renal pelvic transitional cell carcinoma. *Br J Urol* 1994;73(5):597.
142. Sharpe JR, Duffy G, Chin JL. Intrarenal bacillus Calmette-Guérin therapy for upper urinary tract carcinoma *in situ. J Urol* 1993;149(3):457.
143. Sheline M, Amedola MA, Pollack HM, et al. Fluoroscopically guided retrograde brush biopsy of transitional cell carcinoma of the upper urinary tract: results in 45 patients. *AJR Am J Roentgenol* 1989;153(2):313.
144. Sidransky D, Frost P, Von Eschenbach A, et al. Clonal origin of bladder cancer. *N Engl J Med* 1992;326(11):737.
145. Slywotzky C, Maya M. Needle tract seeding of transitional cell cancer following fine-needle aspiration of a renal mass. *Abdom Imaging* 1994;19(2):174.
146. Smith AY, Vitale PJ, Lowe BA, et al. Treatment of superficial papillary transitional cell carcinoma of the ureter by vesicoureteral reflux of mitomycin C. *J Urol* 1987;138(5):1231.
147. Stadler WM, Kuzel T, Roth B, et al. Phase II study of single-agent gemcitabine in previously untreated patients with metastatic urothelial cancer. *J Clin Oncol* 1997;15(11):3394.
148. Steffens J, Nagel R. Tumours of the renal pelvis and ureter: observations in 170 patients. *Br J Urol* 1988;61(4):277.
149. Stenzl A, Frank R, Eder R, et al. Three-dimensional computerized tomography and virtual reality endoscopy of the reconstructed lower urinary tract. *J Urol* 1998;159(3):741.
150. Strong DW, Pearse HD. Recurrent urothelial tumors following surgery for transitional cell carcinoma of the upper urinary tract. *Cancer* 1976;38(5):2173.
151. Takahashi T, Habuchi T, Kakehi Y, et al. Clonal and chronological genetic analysis of multifocal cancers of the bladder and upper urinary tract. *Cancer Res* 1998;58(24):5835.
152. Tannock I, Gospodarowicz M, Connolly J, et al. M-VAC (methotrexate, vinblastine, doxorubicin and cisplatinum) chemotherapy for transitional cell carcinoma: the Princess Margaret Hospital experience. *J Urol* 1989;142(2 Pt 1):289.
153. Tawfiek ER, Bagley DH. Upper tract transitional cell carcinoma. *Urology* 1997;50(3):321.
154. Tawfiek ER, Bagley DH. Management of upper urinary tract calculi with ureteroscopic techniques. *Urology* 1999;53(1):25.
155. Tsai YC, Nichols PW, Hiti AL, et al. Allelic losses of chromosomes 9, 11, and 17 in human bladder cancer. *Cancer Res* 1990;50(1):44.
156. Tuttle TM, Williams GM, Marshall FF. Evidence for cyclophosphamide-induced transitional cell carcinoma in a renal transplant patient. *J Urol* 1988;140(5):1009.
157. Van der Poel HG, Hessels D, Van Leenders GJLH, et al. Multifocal transitional cell cancer and p53 mutation analysis. *J Urol* 1998;160(1):124.
158. von der Maase H, Andersen L, Crino L, et al. Weekly gemcitabine and cisplatinum combination therapy in patients with transitional cell carcinoma of the urothelium: a phase II clinical trial. *Ann Oncol* 1999;10(12):1461.
159. Wagle DG, Moore RH, Murphy GP. Primary carcinoma of the renal pelvis. *Cancer* 1974;33(6):1642.
160. Wallace DMA, Wallace DM, Whitfield HN, et al. The late results of conservative surgery for upper tract urothelial carcinomas. *Br J Urol* 1981;53(6):537.
161. Wang J, Tseng H, Lin S, et al. Transitional cell and uncommon urothelial carcinoma of the renal pelvis/ureter and bladder: low incidence of human papilloma virus. *Chin Med J* 1997; 59(3):151.
162. Williams CB, Mitchell JP. Carcinoma of the ureter: a review of 54 cases. *Br J Urol* 1973;45(4):377.
163. Wolf JS Jr, Moon TD, Nakada SY. Hand assisted laparoscopic nephrectomy: comparison to standard laparoscopic nephrectomy. *J Urol* 1998;160(1):22.
164. Yousem DM, Gatewood OM, Goldman SM, et al. Synchronous and metachronous transitional cell carcinoma of the urinary tract: prevalence, incidence, and radiographic detection. *Radiology* 1988;167(3):613.
165. Zaman SS, Sack MJ, Ramchandani P, et al. Cytopathology of retrograde renal pelvis brush specimens: an analysis of 40 cases with emphasis on collecting duct carcinoma and low-intermediate grade transitional cell carcinoma. *Diagn Cytopathol* 1996;15(4):312.
166. Zincke H, Neves RJ. Feasibility of conservative surgery for transitional cell cancer of the upper urinary tract. *Urol Clin North Am* 1984;11(4):717.
167. Zoretic S, Gonzales J. Primary carcinoma of the ureters. *Urology* 1983;21(4):354.
168. Zungri E, Chechile G, Algaba F, et al. Treatment of transitional cell carcinoma of the ureter: is the controversy justified? *Eur Urol* 1990;17(4):276.

18

ADULT LAPAROSCOPIC UROLOGY

JAIME LANDMAN
ELSPETH M. McDOUGALL
INDIBER S. GILL
RALPH V. CLAYMAN

HISTORY OF LAPAROSCOPY

Urologists have recently embraced laparoscopic surgery as another extension of their endourologic skills. Initially, this would appear to be a new era in urologic surgery. However, careful evaluation illustrates the extent to which we are the products of our past. The curiosity and adventurous thinking of past clinicians established a groundwork on which innovative modern surgeons have developed the potential of many basic concepts of laparoscopy. The first documented attempt to visualize a living human internal organ was by Philipp Bozzini in Frankfurt in 1806 (Table 18.1). He inspected the urethra with a double-lumen cannula; one lumen transmitted light from a candle and the other was for visualization (40). In 1877, Max Nitze in Germany first utilized a lens system for cystoscopy (147). This enabled him to view a magnified image of the urethra and bladder. Nitze, in collaboration with Joseph Leiter, refined his instrument to produce a practical endoscope, which consisted of a metal catheter with light provided from heated platinum wire loops sheathed in a goose quill and cooled by a continuous flow of water (147). Thomas Edison's invention of the incandescent light bulb in the United States in 1880 generated a new era of endoscopes (21).

The birth of laparoscopy can be attributed to Georg Kelling, a surgeon of Dresden, Germany. In 1901, he described "coelioscopy," a technique in which he filled the abdomen of a living dog with air and inserted a Nitze cystoscope to inspect the viscera. In the same year, D.O. Ott, a Russian gynecologist, published his "ventroscopic" technique in which he used a head mirror as a light source and inserted a speculum through a small abdominal or cul-de-sac incision to view the abdominal viscera (318).

J. Landman: Department of Surgery, Division of Urology, Washington University Medical Center, Barnes-Jewish Hospital, St. Louis, MO 63110.

E.M. McDougall: Department of Urologic Surgery, Vanderbilt University Medical Center, Nashville, TN 37232.

I.S. Gill: Section of Laparoscopic and Minimally Invasive Surgery, Cleveland Clinic Urological Institute, Cleveland Clinic Foundation, Cleveland, OH 44195.

R.V. Clayman: Division of Minimally Invasive Surgery, Department of Surgery and Radiology, Washington University, Barnes-Jewish Hospital, St. Louis, MO 63110.

TABLE 18.1. HIGHLIGHTS IN THE HISTORY OF LAPAROSCOPIC SURGERY

1806	Bozzini uses a tube and a candle as a light source ("Lichtleiter") to visualize the human urethra.
1877	Nitze creates the prototype for the modern cystoscope.
1880	Edison invents the incandescent bulb.
1901	Kelling inserts a cystoscope into the inflated abdomen of a dog and describes "celioscopy."
1910	Jacobaeus performs laparoscopy in patients with ascites.
1929	Kalk introduces the foroblique (35-degree) lens and advocates a separate pneumoperitoneum needle and "dual trocar" technique.
1938	Veress develops a special needle to induce pneumothoraces to treat TB.
1952	Forrestier, Gladu, and Valmiere develop an endoscope with a proximal light source and a quartz rod system to transmit the light to the distal end of the scope.
1970s	Semm develops an automated insufflation device that monitors gas flow and intraabdominal pressure, and numerous instruments still used in modern laparoscopy.
1976	Cortesi uses the laparoscope for the first time in urology to localize a cryptorchid testis.
1987	Mouret performs the first laparoscopic cholecystectomy in a human.
1988	Mouret is denounced at Lycee Chirurgical de Francais.
1988	Dubois and Perissat in Europe and Reddick in the United States popularize laparoscopic cholecystectomy.
1989	Mouret is reinstated and given the Croix de Chirque, the highest honor of Lycee Chirurgical.
1990	Clayman and associates perform the first laparoscopic nephrectomy.

Further work by H.C. Jacobaeus in Stockholm, Sweden, involved insertion of a trocar to create pneumoperitoneum in humans, and then insertion of a cystoscope to inspect the peritoneal or pleural space. In 1910, he reported on a series of patients in whom "laparoscopy" was performed, and he commented on cirrhotic changes in the liver, metastatic cancer, and tuberculous peritonitis (189). Bertram Bernheim, in 1911, performed the first diagnostic laparoscopy in the United States when he used a proctoscope and an ordinary light to examine the abdominal cavity (26). Subsequent to the pioneering work of these laparoscopists, new instruments and techniques were developed. Nordentoft used the Trendelenburg position to more easily view the pelvis of a cadaver (157). The sharp pyramidal-pointed trocar was developed by Orndoff in 1920 to facilitate trocar insertion (147).

The introduction of the oblique-viewing (35-degree) lens system by a German, H. Kalk, in 1929 allowed laparoscopy to become widely accepted as a diagnostic tool (205). Kalk also advocated the use of the pneumoperitoneum needle and the dual trocar to allow simultaneous visualization of and passage of instruments into the abdomen. He reported on more than 100 cases of laparoscopy using this technique and published the first color atlas of laparoscopy in 1935 (445). Ruddock, in the United States in 1934, performed peritoneoscopy with a device having integrated biopsy forceps (361). In 1938, Janos Veress of Hungary developed a special needle for inducing pneumothoraces to treat pre-antibiotic-era tuberculosis (429). This needle had a spring-loaded central blunt tip that protected the lung from injury after the needle passed through the pleura and currently is often used for the creation of pneumoperitoneum.

A major advance in the technology of laparoscopy occurred in France in 1952 when Forrestier, Gladu, and Valmiere used a quartz rod to efficiently transmit a proximal light source to the distal end of the endoscope (15). At the same time, in England, Hopkins and Kapany introduced early fiberoptic technology to endoscopy (157). These developments resulted in a wider acceptance of laparoscopy, particularly for gynecologic diagnostic purposes.

The concept of monitoring intraabdominal pressure during pneumoperitoneum was promoted initially by Raoul Palmer of Paris, as early as 1947 (320). Professor Kurt Semm of Kiel, Germany, a gynecologist and engineer, developed an automatic insufflation device to monitor intraabdominal pressure and gas flow (147). He was one of the innovative researchers and clinicians in the field of laparoscopy. Many of the instruments and techniques devised by Semm are still used today, including thermocoagulation during laparoscopic procedures, hooked scissors, tissue morcellators, the endoloop suture applicator, an irrigation and aspiration device, techniques for intracorporeal and extracorporeal knot tying, needle-holders, clip-appliers, atraumatic forceps, microscissors, and the "pelvic trainer," designed to teach surgeons laparoscopic techniques (378). Semm expanded the indications for laparoscopy by advocating laparoscopic lysis of adhesions, bowel suturing, tumor biopsy, and incidental appendectomy.

The first case report of laparoscopy in the urologic literature appeared in 1976 when Cortesi and associates (66) used the laparoscope to successfully localize bilateral abdominal testicles in a cryptorchid adult patient. However, surgeons were generally slow to recognize laparoscopy as a valuable diagnostic tool, considering it to be a "blind" procedure, providing incomplete examination of the abdominal cavity. Laparoscopy lost further ground when computed tomography (CT) was developed for clinical use and ultrasonographically directed biopsies became generally available. Despite this turn of events, many pioneering surgeons continued to enthusiastically popularize laparoscopy as a valuable diagnostic and therapeutic modality with significant clinical benefits (135,136,159,180,320).

Therapeutic laparoscopy necessarily lagged behind diagnostic laparoscopy (137). Frimdberg, in Europe in 1978, performed laparoscopic cholecystectomy in pigs (105). In 1987, Philippe Mouret in Lyon, France, performed the first laparoscopic cholecystectomy in a human (328). Interestingly, Mouret was denounced the following year at the Lycee Chirurgical de Francais for performing what was considered a surgical procedure with unwarranted risk for the patient. However, during 1988, Dubois and Perissat in Europe and Reddick in the United States popularized laparoscopic cholecystectomy (86,328,352). Within a matter of months, it became apparent that this minimally invasive approach to the gallbladder was going to revolutionize the practice of general surgery. Laparoscopic cholecystectomy has since become the standard of therapy for routine gallbladder removal. In 1989, Mouret not only was vindicated by reinstatement, but was awarded the Croix de Chirurgue, the highest honor of the Lycee Chirurgical.

Presently, laparoscopic surgery has pervaded not only gynecology and general surgery, but also thoracic surgery. The gynecologic procedures commonly performed are myriad: hysterectomy, ovariectomy, tubal ligation, and, more recently, tubal reconstruction. In general surgery, the three most commonly performed open procedures are all now in the realm of laparoscopy: herniorrhaphy, cholecystectomy, and appendectomy. In addition, other procedures are becoming more commonplace: adhesiolysis, bowel resection, choledocholithotomy, posterior truncal vagotomy, anterior seromyotomy, and Nissen fundoplication (71,81,208,330, 377). With regard to thoracic surgery, the laparoscope has also made inroads in the treatment of emphysematous blebs and reflex sympathetic dystrophy and is also being used to perform lung biopsy and to drain loculated empyema. Similarly in cardiac surgery, single-vessel coronary artery bypass is now just beginning to be performed laparoscopically; the entire procedure is done in the closed chest on a beating heart.

The use of laparoscopic surgery in urology paralleled, to a large extent, the aforementioned developments in general surgery. Although Cortesi reported the first urologic laparoscopy to localize cryptorchid testes in adults in 1976, the initial pediatric laparoscopic localization of an undescended testicle was reported by Silber in 1980 (390). Since then, more than 350 laparoscopic procedures to identify an undescended testicle have been reported in the literature (260). The laparoscopic approach is more rapid, less morbid, and of equal accuracy compared with open surgical exploration for an undescended testicle. Over the past 15 years, laparoscopy has supplanted open surgical approaches to the localization of undescended testicles, management of intersex disorders, and the biopsy of pelvic gonadal organs.

However, it was not until the late 1980s, with the advent of interest in pelvic lymph node dissection, that laparoscopy made its entry into mainstream urology. Gynecologists were the first to advocate laparoscopic lymphadenectomy for staging of pelvic cancers (353). The first staging laparoscopic pelvic lymphadenectomy for prostate cancer was attempted by Hald in 1980. However, he found the extraperitoneal approach to be limited and unsatisfactory (150). It was the clinical work of Schuessler and Vancaillie in 1989 that demonstrated the feasibility of completing the staging of patients who had carcinoma of the prostate with the minimally invasive technique of transperitoneal, laparoscopic obturator node dissection (375). The reports of this work initiated a new era in urologic surgery, and soon laparoscopy was applied to a variety of urologic procedures previously approachable only by a flank or an abdominal incision.

The development of a surgical entrapment sack and a high-speed, 10-mm electrical tissue morcellator was integral to the concept of removing large, solid tissue specimens via a laparoscopic approach. In 1990, Clayman and colleagues (62) used this technology to perform the first laparoscopic nephrectomy. Since that time, unique laparoscopic techniques have been used in several medical centers to accomplish a variety of other urologic procedures, including nephroureterectomy, bladder neck suspension, pelvic lymphocelectomy, ureterolysis, and adrenalectomy (5,6,209, 215,255,407). Anecdotal reports have included cystectomy, renal cyst decortication, renal exploration, partial nephrectomy, ureteroureterostomy, nephropexy, prostatectomy, and ileal conduit formation (225,265,300,301,322,372, 426,441). Many recent applications of laparoscopy to urologic surgery have demonstrated the feasibility of these techniques to complete the intended diagnostic or therapeutic objective and provide the patient with a more comfortable and shorter recuperative period compared with more traditional open surgery. Continued laboratory and clinical research will expand the field of laparoscopic urologic surgery for both therapeutic and reconstructive techniques.

GENERAL LAPAROSCOPIC TECHNIQUE

Laparoscopy has been applied recently to myriad surgical procedures for the urologic patient. Despite this increasing diversity, there exists a set of basic concepts and principles associated with laparoscopic techniques in general.

Access with Gas

The basic principle of laparoscopy is to maximally distend the potential space of the peritoneal cavity, facilitate visualization of the viscera, and insert various instruments to complete the surgical procedure. Various gases have been used to create the working environment of the pneumoperitoneum, including filtered room air, nitrous oxide, carbon dioxide, argon, and helium.

Types of Insufflants

Nitrous oxide will support combustion if present in a high concentration (98). Therefore this gas is not acceptable as an insufflant for modern laparoscopy because of the increased use of laser and electrocautery techniques in most surgical laparoscopic procedures. Indeed, nitrous oxide should not even be used as an anesthetic during any therapeutic laparoscopic procedures. It has been shown that during extended laparoscopic surgery, nitrous oxide may diffuse from the bowel into the peritoneal cavity in concentrations that could support combustion of bowel gas (298). There has been a report of a case of colonic explosion during colonic diathermy in a patient with rectal cancer (9). Thus it is advisable to avoid the use of nitrous oxide even as an anesthetic agent during long laparoscopic procedures.

Carbon dioxide is readily available in most operating rooms and is relatively inexpensive; thus it has become the most commonly used insufflant. Carbon dioxide absorption into the blood during laparoscopic surgery may lead to respiratory acidosis, increased ventilation requirements, and potentially serious cardiovascular compromise. In the clinical setting, the increased CO_2 load is not a problem if the patient is managed with controlled ventilation. As a result, most patients undergoing laparoscopic urologic procedures are managed with cuffed endotracheal general anesthesia and controlled ventilation. Mullet and colleagues (290) showed that CO_2 diffusion into the body, as measured by end-tidal CO_2, increases gradually and then plateaus approximately 10 minutes after insufflation; this observation is not influenced by the duration of intraperitoneal insufflation. During extraperitoneal pelvioscopy, CO_2 diffusion into the body is more marked and does not tend to plateau with the duration of insufflation. The anesthetic records of 62 patients undergoing laparoscopic renal surgery at Washington University were evaluated for hourly estimates of CO_2 expiration (V_{CO_2}) during the preinsufflation period and the first 4 hours of insufflation (446). V_{CO_2} increased with time, although the increase over the previous interval was less pronounced every hour after the first. Most of the increase occurred during the first 2 hours of insufflation. Multifactorial analysis revealed that the extraperitoneal, as compared with the transperitoneal, approach and the presence of subcutaneous emphysema were strongly and independently associated with a greater increase in V_{CO_2}. Pneumothorax and pneumomediastinum were significantly more common during extraperitoneal (37%) than transperitoneal (3%) laparoscopy. There were five postoperative cardiopulmonary complications, none of which was related to hypercapnia. Thus CO_2 absorption during laparoscopic renal surgery, which is greater than occurs during pelvic laparoscopy, was highest in patients approached through an extraperitoneal route and in those with subcutaneous emphysema. Nonetheless, with aggressive intraoperative mechanical ventilation, no sequelae of hypercapnia were noted in this series. Also, it must be noted that if one uses a cuffed Hasson cannula, the risk of hypercarbia with the retroperitoneal approaches appears to be eliminated. This type of cannula seals the port site, thereby effectively eliminating subcutaneous emphysema and the associated problems of hypercarbia (303).

Helium is biologically and chemically inert and therefore has been proposed as an alternative insufflating agent. Leighton and colleagues (234), in animal studies, showed that helium insufflated intraperitoneally did not cause hypercarbia, aciduria, or pulmonary hypertension when using the same insufflation conditions as for CO_2. These results support the concept that the transperitoneal absorption of CO_2, not increased dead space, is responsible for the respiratory acidosis observed during pneumoperitoneum.

Argon is an inexpensive inert gas that also has been used for intraabdominal insufflation. Animal studies at Washington University School of Medicine demonstrated that an argon pneumoperitoneum of 20-mm Hg pressure had the same hemodynamic and renal effects as 20 mm Hg of CO_2 (271). Argon is not absorbed as easily as CO_2; thus the degree of respiratory acidosis is less when using this agent as an insufflant. However, any of the inert gases, which are slow to reabsorb, may result in prolonged duration of subcutaneous emphysema that may occur during laparoscopy and also put the patient at a higher risk for problems should a gas embolus develop. There has been one report in the literature of an argon gas embolism during laparoscopic cholecystectomy when an argon beam coagulator was used for hemostasis of the liver bed (249). Gas embolism can occur whenever a large amount of any gas is administered directly into the vascular system; however, the poor solubility of the inert gases compared with CO_2 exacerbates the potential problems due to a gas embolism.

Method of Introduction

The pneumoperitoneum can be established using either a closed or an open technique. The Veress needle is used to penetrate the abdominal wall and deliver CO_2 gas into the abdomen for the closed technique of insufflation. This 14-gauge needle may be 12 or 15 cm in length and is either disposable or nondisposable. The 15-cm needle is useful in the very obese patient to facilitate successful access to the peritoneal cavity. The reusable needle is made entirely of metal and tends to be heavier than the disposable needle, which has a plastic hub; the needle point may become dull with repeated use and therefore must be sharpened regularly. Also, the reusable needle must be disassembled and all the parts cleaned after each use.

The Veress needle consists of an outer 14-gauge sheath with a sharp beveled tip and an inner spring-loaded, blunt tip. The blunt tip retracts back inside the outer sheath on meeting resistance of the fascia or peritoneum. This presents the sharp beveled tip to the fascia and peritoneum, allowing penetration (Fig. 18.1A). The inner blunt tip springs forward immediately on entry into the abdominal cavity and release of resistance (Fig. 18.1B). The hub of the Veress needle may have an indicator to show when the inner blunt tip is retracted or presented. The hub also has a Luer-Lok connector for attaching the aspirating-irrigating syringe of

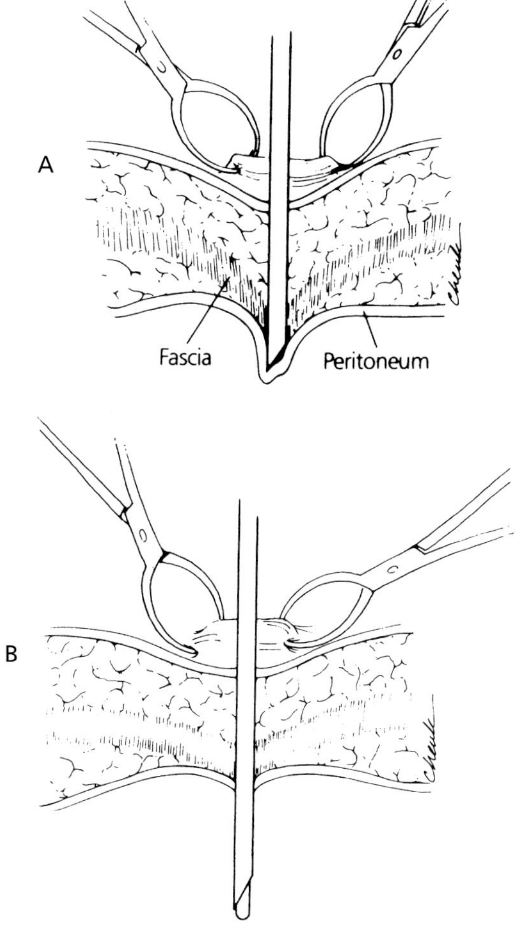

FIGURE 18.1. A: The Veress needle has a spring-loaded, blunt-tip obturator that is pushed back inside the sheath to expose the sharp tip of the sheath during penetration of the fascia and peritoneum. **B:** Immediately upon passing through the fascia and peritoneum, the inner blunt tip springs forward to protect the intraabdominal structures from the sharp needle tip. (Reprinted from Clayman RV, McDougall EM, eds. *Laparoscopic urology.* St. Louis: Quality Medical Publishing, 1993, with permission.)

saline and the CO_2 insufflating tubing. There may be a stopcock on this side arm to interrupt the flow of CO_2 into the abdomen.

The Veress needle is most commonly inserted at the umbilicus because the peritoneum is closer to the skin at this point on the abdominal wall (Fig. 18.2). The properitoneal layer of fatty tissue, which lies between the linea alba and the peritoneum, is thinnest at the level of the umbilicus. The extremely obese or very thin patient may require special consideration during Veress needle and initial port insertion. Hurd and associates (181) studied the relationship of the umbilicus to the aortic bifurcation using magnetic resonance imaging (MRI) and CT. They assessed the effect obesity has on this relationship. In nonobese patients weighing less than 160 pounds (73 kg), the umbilicus is a mean distance of 0.4 cm caudal to the aortic bifurcation, with a skin-to-peritoneum distance of 2 cm. In obese patients weighing between 160 and 200 pounds (73 and 91 kg), the umbilicus is 2.4 cm caudal to the aortic bifurcation, with a skin-to-peritoneum distance of 2 cm. In obese patients weighing more than 200 pounds (91 kg), the umbilicus is located 2.9 cm caudal to the bifurcation of the aorta, with a skin-to-peritoneum median distance of 12 cm. The authors concluded that Veress needle insertion in the nonobese patient should be at a 45-degree angle from the horizontal (Fig. 18.3) to reduce the risk of major abdominal vascular

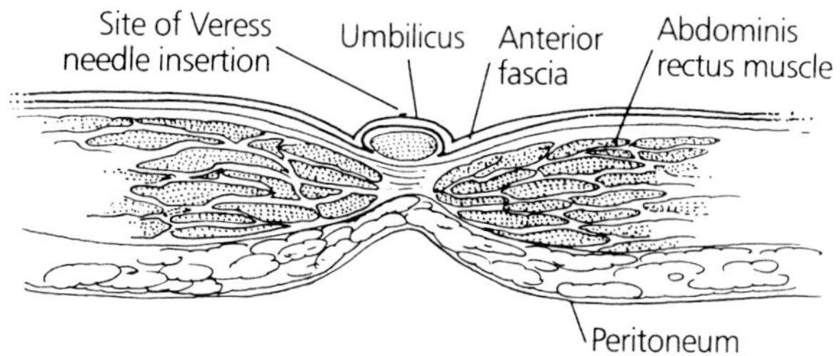

FIGURE 18.2. The properitoneal layer of fatty tissues is thinnest at the umbilicus, providing this site with the shortest distance between the skin and peritoneum. (Reprinted from Clayman RV, McDougall EM, eds. *Laparoscopic urology.* St. Louis: Quality Medical Publishing, 1993, with permission.)

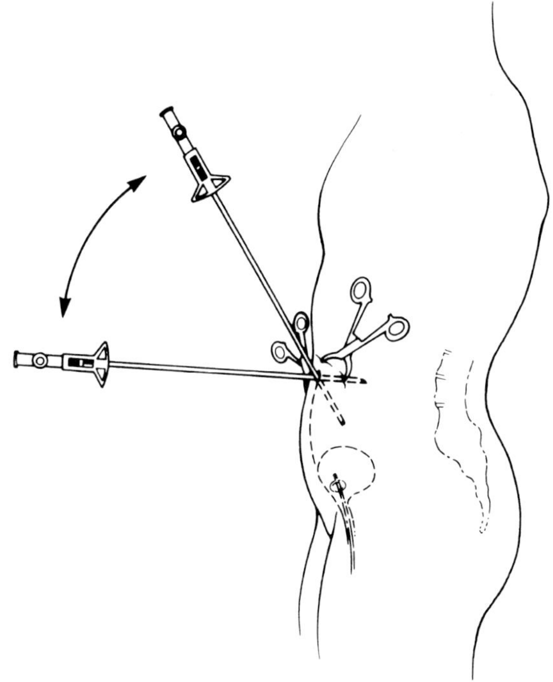

FIGURE 18.3. In the nonobese patient, the Veress needle should be inserted at a 45-degree angle from the horizontal to minimize the risk of injury to the retroperitoneal great vessels. In the obese patient, the increased fatty tissue space between the skin and the peritoneum dictates a Veress needle insertion at a 90-degree angle to the umbilicus to achieve intraperitoneal placement of the needle tip. (Reprinted from Clayman RV, McDougall EM, eds. *Laparoscopic urology.* St. Louis: Quality Medical Publishing, 1993, with permission.)

injury and properitoneal placement (182). Because of the increased distance to the peritoneum in the obese patient and the caudal displacement of the umbilicus in relationship to the aortic bifurcation, the Veress needle should be inserted at a 90-degree angle from horizontal to achieve intraperitoneal placement. In patients who have had previous abdominal surgery, alternative sites may be used for the Veress needle insertion to avoid adhesions.

A small skin incision is made with a no. 12 hook blade at the supraumbilical or infraumbilical crease. A sharp towel clip is placed on the skin edges, on either side of the incision, to stabilize the skin during needle insertion. The Veress needle is held like a dart in the dominant hand and passed into the wound. As the needle passes through the anterior abdominal fascia and then the peritoneum, resistance will be felt and also observed due to movement at the spring-loaded hub. A click may be heard as the blunt trocar springs forward into the peritoneal cavity.

The intraabdominal positioning of the Veress needle is confirmed by performing four test maneuvers. First, a 10-mL syringe with 5 mL of saline is attached to the hub of the needle. The syringe is aspirated to determine that no blood or bowel contents enter the barrel of the syringe. Second, the saline is injected through the needle; it should inject easily without any resistance. In the third step, the syringe is used to reaspirate the needle. With a true intraabdominal positioning of the needle, there should be no return of fluid into the syringe. As the syringe is removed from the needle, the small amount of saline remaining in the hub should flow easily into the abdomen. The final test is to advance the needle 1 to 2 cm into the abdomen; neither the tip indicator nor the hub should show any indication of encountering resistance. Only after all of these tests confirm satisfactory intraperitoneal positioning of the Veress needle should CO_2 insufflation begin.

The sterile insufflation tubing, which has been connected to the insufflator, is placed on the Luer-Lok of the Veress needle hub as the needle is held steady by the surgeon. CO_2 insufflation is commenced with a flow rate of 2 L minute or less, and the intraabdominal pressure limit is set at 10 mm Hg. The initial intraabdominal pressure should be less than 10 mm Hg. If the intraabdominal pressure is greater than 10 mm Hg, the needle should be rotated or withdrawn slightly. If the pressure remains high, the insufflation should be terminated and the Veress needle removed and reinserted; alternatively, an open technique for establishing the pneumoperitoneum can be used. The intraabdominal pressure usually remains less than or equal to 10 mm Hg until 500 to 1,000 mL of CO_2 have been insufflated. After 500 mL of gas is instilled into the peritoneal cavity, the abdomen will be slightly and symmetrically distended and tympanic on percussion. The insufflation flow rate can then be maximized and the desired pressure limit set for the primary trocar insertion.

Retroperitoneal Veress needle insufflation can also be performed in those patients in whom a retroperitoneoscopic approach is planned. The procedure is commenced by inserting a Veress needle through either the inferior posterior lumbar triangle (Petit's) in the posterior axillary line just above the iliac crest or the superior posterior lumbar triangle, just posterior to the tip of the twelfth rib. The retroperitoneum is inflated with approximately 2 to 3 L of CO_2, and then a 10- or 12-mm port is inserted at this site. Visualization of the retroperitoneal space with the laparoscope and blunt dissection with this instrument creates a small space within the retroperitoneum that will allow introduction of the dilating balloon catheter.

The dilating balloon catheter is created by cutting the middle finger off of a size 8 Triflex sterile latex surgeon's glove (Baxter Health Care Corp., Valencia, California). The finger of the glove is placed over the tip of a 16-Fr red rubber catheter and secured in place with two 0-silk ligatures so that the openings in the tip of the catheter lie within the finger of the glove. The balloon catheter is back-loaded through a 30-Fr Amplatz sheath until the balloon is retracted just inside the sheath. The assembled unit is inserted through the 10- or 12-mm primary trocar until the tip of the Amplatz sheath lies just at the port opening. The balloon catheter is advanced through the Amplatz sheath 3 to 4 cm into the perirenal space (outside Gerota's fascia), and then the balloon is filled with 1 L of normal saline. This provides an adequate working space and minimizes the risk of balloon rupture from overdistention. The fluid is aspirated from the balloon catheter, which is then withdrawn into the Amplatz sheath, and the balloon and Amplatz sheath are removed from the port. The pneumoperitoneum is established to a pressure of 10 to 15 mm Hg and the laparoscope is inserted.

For the neophyte laparoscopic surgeon, the open technique for obtaining a pneumoperitoneum is recommended. Indeed, some surgeons advocate this approach in all patients undergoing laparoscopic surgery to minimize the risk of vascular, bowel, or omental injury (204). One study has shown that the open technique for placement of the primary port, including establishment of the pneumoperitoneum, is faster, safer, and more cost-effective compared with the closed technique (16). However, this study used the closed technique in the initial 150 patients, changing to the open technique for the subsequent 150 patients (41). It is important to realize that complications can occur, albeit rarely, with the open technique for pneumoperitoneum (363).

The open technique should be used whenever intraperitoneal positioning of the Veress needle cannot be confirmed with confidence. Similarly, patients with multiple previous surgical procedures on the abdomen may have significant adhesions, obviating blind access to the peritoneal cavity.

The open technique of accessing the abdominal cavity involves a small (2- to 3-cm) laparotomy for insertion of a blunt-tip, Hasson cannula. The skin incision is usually made at or just below the umbilicus, unless there are preexisting abdominal scars, in which case a point lateral to the abdominus rectus muscle, farthest from the incisions, is

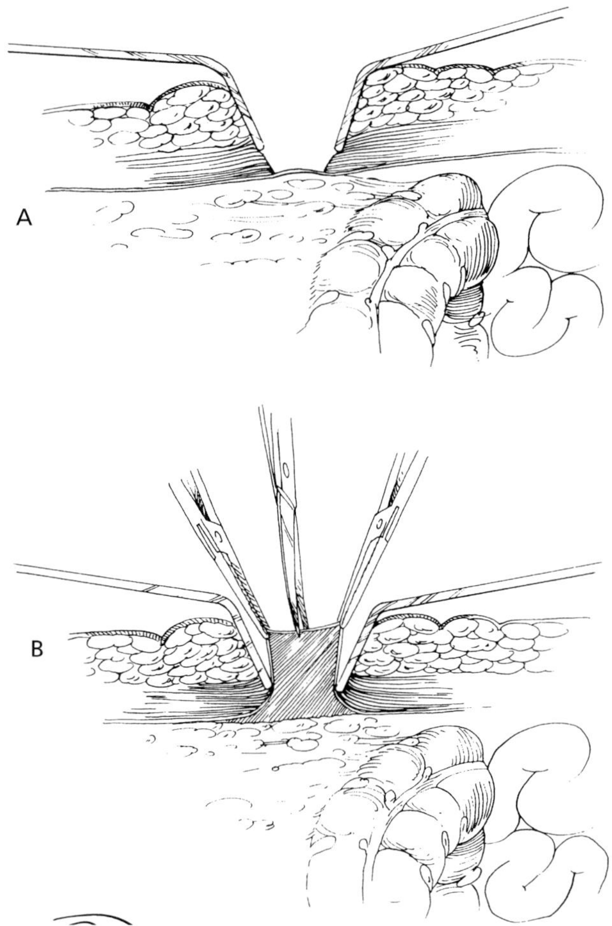

FIGURE 18.4. A: The open technique of port placement requires incision of the skin and fascia to accommodate the planned port and exposure of the peritoneum by bluntly retracting the peritoneal fat. **B:** The peritoneum is grasped and elevated by two small hemostats, and scissors incise the peritoneum to admit the surgeon's finger and then the blunt-tip port. (Reprinted from Clayman RV, McDougall EM, eds. *Laparoscopic urology.* St. Louis: Quality Medical Publishing, 1993, with permission.)

used. Through a transverse incision, the subcutaneous tissue is dissected and the anterior abdominal fascia is exposed and incised (2 cm) (Fig. 18.4A). The properitoneal fat is then bluntly swept off the peritoneum. The peritoneum is grasped, using small hemostats, and elevated (Fig. 18.4B). Scissors are used to incise the peritoneum to admit the surgeon's index finger. Satisfactory entry into the abdominal cavity is confirmed by digital palpation or visual inspection. A 0 Vicryl or silk suture is placed on either side of the fascial incision.

The Hasson-type cannula used in the open approach consists of three components: a cone-shaped sleeve, a metal sheath with a trumpet valve to which two struts are affixed for tying the suture, and a blunt-tipped obturator. The metal sheath can be moved up and down through the cone-shaped sleeve to allow proper positioning before tightly affixing the sleeve to the sheath.

The blunt tip of the obturator within the Hasson cannula is inserted through the peritoneal incision, and the cone-shaped sleeve is slid down snugly against the fascia (Fig. 18.5). The two fascial sutures are secured to the struts on the sheath of the cannula, after the sleeve is secured to the sheath with the set screw. The fascial sutures fix the cannula in place. Sterile insufflation tubing is connected to the cannula and the blunt-tipped obturator is removed. The CO_2 insufflator is set at a high flow rate and the intraabdominal pressure is raised to 15 mm Hg. This port may now receive the laparoscope.

An open insertion can also be performed for retroperitoneoscopy. The Hasson cannula is usually placed at the superior posterior lumbar triangle. A 1.5-cm skin incision is made to accommodate the appropriate size of Hasson cannula chosen. A Kelly forceps is used to spread the subcutaneous fatty tissue and expose the fascia overlying the musculature. A 1.5-cm incision is made through the fascia with a no. 12 hook blade. The Kelly forceps are then used to spread the muscle layers into the retroperitoneal space. Next, blunt finger dissection can be performed confirming the retroperitoneal positioning of this incision; the surface of the psoas

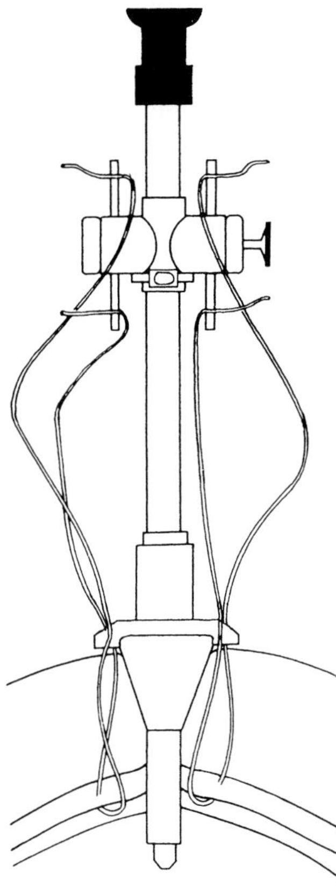

FIGURE 18.5. The blunt tip of the Hasson cannula is inserted through the peritoneotomy, and the cone-shaped sleeve is slid down snugly against the fascia. Two preplaced fascial sutures are secured to the struts on the sheath to hold the port in place. (Reprinted from Clayman RV, McDougall EM, eds. *Laparoscopic urology.* St. Louis: Quality Medical Publishing, 1993, with permission.)

muscle should be easily palpated with the tip of the surgeon's finger. The balloon catheter, back-loaded through a 30-Fr Amplatz sheath, can then be delivered directly into the retroperitoneal space. The Amplatz sheath is withdrawn, leaving the balloon catheter in position. The balloon is filled with 1 L of normal saline creating the retroperitoneal working space. The balloon is aspirated of the fluid and withdrawn. Alternatively, extensive blunt finger dissection of the retroperitoneal space can be performed in smaller patients in lieu of using the balloon.

The Hasson cannula is now positioned. Stay sutures placed on the fascia are used to secure the Hasson cannula in place. Alternatively, a Hasson with a balloon retention mechanism and an outer soft foam cuff device (Origin Medsystems, Inc., Menlo Park, California) can be used; with this device, no sutures need to be placed and the chances of subcutaneous emphysema appear to be decreased. The pneumoretroperitoneum is established to a pressure of 10 to 15 mm Hg.

Insufflator

The insufflator allows the laparoscopist to create and maintain the pneumoperitoneum. It consists of a valve mechanism, which can be adjusted and monitored, to allow the flow of pressurized gas from the tank into the patient's abdomen. The insufflator unit should consist of gauges that will (a) indicate the rate of flow (liters per minute) of CO_2 from the insufflator; (b) constantly display, on an analog or digital gauge, abdominal pressure (millimeters of mercury); and (c) indicate the total volume of CO_2 (in liters) that has been instilled into the abdomen. A separate indicator measures the line pressure of the gas tank, providing the surgeon with information regarding the amount of CO_2 remaining in the gas tank. The CO_2 is transported from the insufflator to the patient by flexible, inert tubing. The tubing may have an incorporated filter and a Luer-Lok fitting end to snugly attach to the Luer-Lok of the Veress needle or the side arm of one of the laparoscopic ports.

The CO_2 flow rate is adjustable to between 0 and 10 L per minute. A low flow rate of 1 to 2 L per minute is generally used at commencement of the insufflation process. After satisfactory instillation of 500 to 1,000 mL of CO_2, the flow rate is increased to a medium or high flow rate (6 to 10 L per minute) for the duration of the procedure. The insufflator should be placed just below the surgeon's monitor so that a continuous display of intraabdominal pressure is clearly visible to the surgeon throughout the operative procedure.

The insufflator can be preset for a specific intraabdominal pressure so that the flow of CO_2 gas will cease automatically if the preset pressure is exceeded and an alarm will sound to draw attention to the elevated pneumoperitoneum pressure. Intraabdominal pressures greater than 15 mm Hg are associated with decreased venous return due to vena caval compression, impaired ventilation as a result of pressure on the diaphragm, increased risk of CO_2 absorption causing systemic acidosis, and decreased urine output (269). For adult laparoscopic procedures, the intraabdominal pressure set point should be 10 to 15 mm Hg.

The insufflator should be tested for satisfactory functioning before each laparoscopic procedure. An additional reserve of CO_2 should always be available in the operating room.

Clinical studies at Washington University have shown that the volume of CO_2 insufflated and the insufflation pressure of the pneumoperitoneum during laparoscopy are directly related. However, this volume and pressure relationship is completely independent of patient weight, height, and body mass index (a measure of obesity) (267). Increasing the intraabdominal pressure from 15 to 30 mm Hg increases the volume of CO_2 insufflated by 50%. However, in animal studies, when the pneumoperitoneum pressure is compared with the estimated actual intraabdominal volume, the intraabdominal volume increases by only 5% to 6% when the intraabdominal pressure is increased from 15 to 30 mm Hg. These results suggest that increasing the pneumoperitoneum to 30 mm Hg does not significantly increase the actual intraabdominal volume, but the increased pressure may effect greater compression of the intraperitoneal viscera and put the peritoneum under more tension. Therefore increasing the intraabdominal pressure to 25 to 30 mm Hg for the primary port placement may facilitate this step of laparoscopy and minimize potential complications. Clinical studies at Washington University have shown that elevating the pneumoperitoneum pressure to 30 mm Hg for the primary port placement has no deleterious effect on the heart rate, blood pressure, cardiac output, or end-tidal CO_2 (284). Following placement of the initial port, which usually takes less than 10 minutes, the pneumoperitoneum is reduced to 15 mm Hg or less for the duration of the procedure.

Access Without Gas

Increased intraabdominal pressure is associated with significant changes in systemic vascular resistance, blood pressure, and cardiac return (207,235). Insufflation of gas into the peritoneal cavity results in an increase in intraabdominal pressure and vena caval compression with subsequent reduction in venous return to the heart. Insufflation to pneumoperitoneum pressures of 15 to 20 mm Hg is generally well tolerated; however, increases greater than 20 mm Hg often decrease cardiac output and arterial blood pressure.

The Trendelenburg position causes the weight of the abdominal contents to rest on the diaphragm. Insufflation of the abdomen exerts an additional force against the diaphragm. Together these factors restrict lung expansion and decrease pulmonary compliance, resulting in ventilation-perfusion mismatching (376). Absorption of insufflated CO_2 into the vascular system combined with the ventilation-perfusion mismatching leads to significant hypercarbia during laparoscopic procedures (287). General anesthesia with controlled ventilation and close monitoring is able to minimize these effects (8).

Intraperitoneal pressures of 10 mm Hg or greater are associated with decreased renal vein flow and a concomitant decrease in urine output (269). Release of the pneumoperitoneum does result in a return of the renal vein flow and the urine output to preinsufflation values when the prolonged pneumoperitoneum has been at 10-mm Hg pressure. However, after prolonged pneumoperitoneum pressure of 15 or 20 mm Hg, the renal vein flow does not return to preinsufflation levels for up to 2 hours after desufflation.

Alterations in renal vein flow and urine output are seen also with insufflation of CO_2 into the retroperitoneum at a pressure of 20 mm Hg. Animal studies have demonstrated a significant increase in the end-tidal CO_2 following retroperitoneal insufflation. Accordingly, an increased ventilation rate was required to maintain the end-tidal CO_2 between 30 and 40 mm Hg. At necropsy in these study animals, diffuse bilateral distribution of gas throughout the retroperitoneum was noted, although the insufflation was performed through one port on one side of the retroperitoneum.

Wakizaka and colleagues (430) studied the effects of CO_2 insufflation during laparoscopic cholecystectomy on arterial blood gas analysis and urine output. Both the increase in $Pa{CO_2}$ and the decrease in pH was larger in the group of patients undergoing laparoscopy at an intraabdominal pressure of 15 cm H_2O, as compared with patients operated at an intraabdominal pressure of 10 mm Hg. At a pneumoperitoneum of 15 cm H_2O, the increase in $Pa{CO_2}$ was significantly higher if the operative time was more than 60 minutes, compared with patients with an operative time less than 60 minutes. This change in $Pa{CO_2}$ with respect to the operative time was not noted when the intraabdominal pressure was maintained at 10 cm H_2O. Also, obese patients (obesity index greater than 120) developed significantly higher levels of $Pa{CO_2}$ during CO_2 insufflation, compared with patients who were not obese.

In an attempt to avoid these complications of pneumoperitoneum, the Laparolift device (Origin Medsystems, Inc., Menlo Park, California) has been developed (299). The abdomen is accessed in a manner similar to the open technique. After the skin, fascia, and peritoneum are incised, a double-bladed lift device is inserted through the peritoneotomy with the blades closed. Once the blades are within the peritoneal cavity and resting against the undersurface of the anterior abdominal wall, they are opened to their maximum angle of 45 degrees. A hydraulic L-arm is secured to the operating table edge and directed over the patient. After endoscopically the positioning of the device's blunt blades are satisfactorily confirmed under the anterior abdominal wall, the lift device is connected to the hydraulic arm. The hydraulic arm then can be raised mechanically to apply between 0 and 15 kg of force on the abdominal wall. Animal studies at Washington University on the effect of pneumoperitoneum on renal function included evaluation of the Laparolift (269). As expected, unlike with a CO_2 pneumoperitoneum, the Laparolift did not have an associated increase in end-tidal CO_2 levels during its use. There was no associated decrease in urine output when applying the Laparolift at forces of 5, 10, or 15 kg. These devices have been used successfully to perform laparoscopic cholecystectomy and pelvic procedures (17,160). However, they are somewhat limiting during procedures, such as laparoscopic nephrectomy, in which the laparoscope and instruments are moved to different port sites during the operative procedure. The hydraulic arm positioned over the patient may limit easy access to some of the ports.

Other mechanical devices have been developed to elevate the anterior abdominal wall, thus creating an intraabdominal space for performing laparoscopic procedures. One of the original concepts used for elevating the abdominal wall was described by Kitano and colleagues (221a). After first obtaining a standard CO_2 pneumoperitoneum, they used a U-shaped trocar to traverse the peritoneal cavity and travel around the falciform ligament; the trocar then was lifted by a winch and framework located above the patient's anterior chest wall. Other groups have used long surgical wires placed in the subcutaneous tissue of the abdomen, or large-caliber suture material passed through the abdominal wall, to winch the abdominal wall anteriorly for exposure (17,160,293). The limited current clinical application of these devices suggests that they may be less than ideal for most laparoscopic surgical procedures.

Transperitoneal Approach: Pneumoperitoneum

Placement of the Primary Port

In the open technique, the primary port (Hasson cannula) is placed first, followed by establishment of the pneumoperitoneum. In the closed technique, the primary port is inserted after establishing an adequate pneumoperitoneum with the Veress needle. The pneumoperitoneum may be established between 15- and 30-mm Hg pressure before insertion of the port (267).

Before the Veress needle is removed, the skin incision is extended to accommodate the size of the planned port (usually 10 or 12 mm). The incision should approximate the diameter of the port as closely as possible to reduce gas leakage around the port during the procedure.

Trocars are available in a vast array of sizes and types and may be reusable or disposable. Trocars consist of two components: a sharp-pointed, removable obturator to facilitate insertion through the abdominal fascia and peritoneum, and an outer sheath through which the obturator passes. The sheath contains a valve or diaphragm through which instruments may be passed without any loss of the CO_2 pneumoperitoneum. A side-arm stopcock on the port allows connection of the insufflating tubing. Laparoscopic trocars have a safety shield that retracts during insertion of the trocar through the fascia and peritoneum to allow exposure of the sharp pyramidal tip of the obturator. When the port tip enters the gas-filled peritoneal cavity, resistance from the fascial and peritoneal tissue is released and the spring-loaded shield moves forward and locks in place to cover the sharp tip of the obturator and reduce the risk of injury to the underlying viscera.

Corson and colleagues (65) studied the force required to insert nondisposable and disposable ports during a pneumoperitoneum of 11.57 mm Hg. Nondisposable trocars required twice the force used to pass through the anterior abdominal wall as compared with disposable trocars. In the animal laboratory, McDougall and colleagues (267) assessed the force required to insert four different types of 10-mm disposable trocars at 15- and 30-mm Hg pneumoperitoneum pressure. There was no significant difference in the force necessary for the insertion of each of the ports at 15- versus 30-mm Hg pressure. Also, there was no significant difference in force of insertion between the two trocar systems with a safety shield versus the nonshielded trocar. A trocar that used an electrocautery cutting current wire at the tip of the blunt obturator did require significantly less force by 1 to 2 kg during insertion when compared with the other three ports at both 15- and 30-mm Hg pressure. Therefore, after placement of the first port at an intraabdominal pressure of 30 mm Hg, it is reasonable to reduce the pneumoperitoneum to 15 mm Hg for all subsequent port placements.

In preparation for primary port placement, the patient is positioned slightly head-down, and the intraabdominal pressure may be increased transiently to 20 to 30 mm Hg. Following an adequate incision at the supraumbilical or infraumbilical crease, the subcutaneous tissues are spread with Kelly forceps in a cephalocaudal direction. This helps push small blood vessels from the path of insertion of the port and allows the incision to assume a more rounded configuration. The abdominal wall may be stabilized by grasping and raising it, beneath the umbilicus, in the surgeon's nondominant hand. Alternatively, a sharp towel clip may be placed just at the skin edge on either side of the incision; one towel clip is held and stabilized by the assistant, and the other is held by the surgeon's nondominant hand.

The surgeon holds the fully assembled trocar in the palm of the dominant hand with the hub of the trocar secured against the thenar eminence. The middle finger is extended along the shaft of the trocar to act as a brake and prevent too sudden or deep an advancement into the abdomen during insertion.

The trocar is inserted with a steady downward pressure and a twisting motion as the fascia is traversed. The pressure must be constant and maintained to prevent disengagement of the obturator from the sheath. If disengagement occurs, a click will be audible, which signifies that the safety shield has locked into position over the sharp obturator tip and further attempts to pass the trocar through the fascia will be futile. The trocar must then be removed and reset before proceeding with insertion.

Immediately upon entering the gas-filled abdominal cavity, the click of the secured safety shield will be heard, and the hissing of CO_2 gas escaping from the open side arm will confirm this position. The side arm is closed, the port is gently advanced 2 cm deeper into the peritoneal cavity, and the obturator is removed. The CO_2 insufflation tubing is connected to the side arm, which is then opened, and insufflation is commenced at a maximum flow rate with the maximum intraabdominal pressure set at between 10 and 15 mm Hg.

A nondisposable trocar may be used as a primary port, although it does not have the safety shield mechanism for the sharp pyramidal tip. Surgeons using nondisposable trocars may prefer to use the open technique for primary port placement to reduce the risk of intraabdominal injuries possibly associated with an unshielded trocar passed blindly into the peritoneal cavity. The Endotip port (Storz Endoscopy, Inc.) is a unique nondisposable trocar. It has a blunt leading tip and a screw configuration along the body of the cannula. This port is screwed through the abdominal wall until the hiss of CO_2 gas from the open sidearm confirms positioning in the abdominal cavity. The port minimizes trauma to the abdominal wall and reduces the risk of intraabdominal injury by providing a blunt leading tip.

Abdominal Inspection

Light Source

An efficient light source will optimize depth perception and image detail during laparoscopic surgery. Laparoscopic light sources are high intensity and use a xenon, mercury, or halogen vapor bulb with an output of 250 to 300 W. There should always be a reserve light bulb available in the operating room.

The intensity of the light output is manually adjustable. Some light-source units have an automatic light-level adjustment that varies according to the level of light reaching the camera; however, they should also have a manual control. Light is transmitted from the light source of the laparoscope by a flexible fiberoptic cable. These cables are light-source and laparoscope specific. It is essential that all the connections fit correctly and snugly to ensure no loss of light transmission to the surgical field. These cables are sterilized before each use and must be handled with care to avoid breakage of the individual fiberoptic fibers of the light cord. The integrity of the light cord can be reviewed before each procedure by connecting the cable to the light source and observing for an even emission of light from the end of the cable; dark areas indicate broken fibers.

Camera

The camera system comprises the camera and a video monitor. The camera locks onto the eyepiece of the endoscope and magnifies the laparoscopic image to provide excellent visualization of fine anatomic details. The camera transmits the optical information from the laparoscope via a cable to the camera box. The camera box electronically reconstructs the image and transmits it to the video monitor where the optical information is displayed for viewing by all operating room personnel. Currently, most laparoscopic cameras are sterilized by soaking or by gas before each use, thereby precluding use of any plastic sterile camera wraps.

Recently, innovative digital technology has been put to use in endoscopic imaging equipment. Image enhancement is a digital-subtraction image processing system that works between the camera and the video monitor; the digital-subtraction process results in contrast enhancement, detail enhancement, edge enhancement, and edge correction of the endoscopic video images in real time. This allows the viewer to accentuate structures that are obscure or otherwise poorly visible to the naked eye. The increased detail recognition improves the potential video diagnostic capabilities and facilitates monitoring of technical operative procedures such as endoscopic suturing and dissection of fine structures.

Depth perception is the product of human binocular vision. Because the pupils of human eyes are separated by approximately 5 cm, each of the eyes sees an object from a slightly different perspective. The optic nerves relay the separate left and right views from the eyes to the brain. The two images are merged by the brain into a single, three-dimensional (3D) image that provides more information than either view separately. Developments in endoscopic video systems have attempted to replicate human binocular vision (367). These video systems consist of a camera system that acquires two separate endoscopic images; a signal processor that digitizes, accelerates, and synchronizes the two video signals; and a video display that alternately displays the two images at a rate of 120 frames per second so that the eyes and brain assemble the two images as if they were coincident. The resultant brain image is a single, three-dimensional image, as in normal binocular vision. The advantages of a 3D video system include restoration of depth perception to aid in definition of the relationship of anatomic structures, easier instrument placement and manipulation, and enhancement of the image, which facilitates more precise intracorporeal tasks such as suturing and knot tying. Some preliminary studies suggest that 3D video has the potential to make minimal-access surgery easier, quicker, less prone to error, and more applicable to advanced procedures (274,282). Work continues with these prototype 3D video systems to improve and refine this technology. At present, these systems are more expensive than the existing one-chip 2D video system and three-chip 2D video system. However, these costs may equalize in time.

The camera should be oriented so that the monitor image is in a "true," upright position, which is the same as would be seen through an open abdominal incision. This is particularly important when using the 30-degree laparoscope. With this instrument, the camera must be held at all times in the true, upright position; the laparoscope can then be rotated through 360 degrees to provide visualization around and over intraabdominal structures, as well as up to the anterior abdominal wall. When a 0-degree laparoscope is used, the camera should be positioned in the true, upright position; then the laparoscope eyepiece can be locked onto the camera because rotation of the 0-degree endoscope will not change the straight-ahead field of vision as long as the camera is maintained in its true orientation.

Insertion of a cold or room temperature laparoscope into the warmer abdominal cavity may produce fogging of the lens and blurring of the monitor image. Accordingly, it is helpful to keep the laparoscope immersed in hot saline until insertion into the abdomen. Wiping the end of the lens with an antifog solution or povidone-iodine solution may also reduce condensation forming on the instrument. The insufflation of the cold CO_2 gas through the laparoscope port may also produce cooling and subsequent fogging of the laparoscope during the procedure. Therefore, following insertion of the second port, it is helpful to transfer the CO_2 insufflation tubing to the side arm of this port. It is important to maintain a watertight seal between the camera and the endoscope. Moisture collecting on the eyepiece or camera will produce blurring of the image and require disconnection of the two pieces and careful wiping to completely dry these surfaces before reconnection.

Video monitors are available from a variety of manufacturers in 13- or 19-inch sizes. The larger monitors provide a larger picture but poorer image resolution. Most monitors with higher resolution capabilities of 1,125 lines of resolution must be used with a camera system capable of providing the appropriate input.

Abdominal Inspection

The initial critical function of the first port inserted into the abdomen is to facilitate insertion of a 10-mm laparoscope to perform a complete inspection of the abdomen. The endoscope must be fully prepared for use before establishment of the pneumoperitoneum. The preparation of the endoscope involves several steps. The camera is locked onto the eyepiece of a 0- or 30-degree laparoscope. The 30-degree laparoscope allows more versatility in visualizing around or over intraabdominal structures, but this endoscope requires a conscientious camera operator to maintain proper orientation because the camera must remain true and stable while the shaft of the endoscope is rotated to take full advantage of the 30-degree angulation of the lens. The light cable is connected to the light post of the laparoscope and the intensity of the light is turned up to the maximum setting. The laparoscope is then directed toward a white gauze pad and the image on the monitor is focused sharply on the monitor screen. While still focused on the white gauze pad, the camera "white balance" button is pressed until the indicator shows that white balancing has been completed. This ensures a naturally colored monitor image. As a final step it is helpful to prewarm the endoscope with warm saline and wipe the tip of the endoscope with an antifogging solution to reduce fogging of the endoscope on introduction into the warm abdominal cavity.

For primary ports of 10 mm or greater in size, a 10.5-mm reducer must be applied to the sheath before insertion of the laparoscope. These reducers may be detachable, or attached and flip on and off the sheath. With the sheath appropriately reduced, the 10-mm laparoscope is introduced into the abdominal cavity. The bowel immediately below the port should be examined for any evidence of bleeding or injury that may have occurred during the primary port placement. Blood dripping from the port may suggest a through-and-through bowel injury or abdominal wall vessel injury, which is better delineated after the second port has been placed, facilitating transfer of the laparoscope and examination of the primary port site. Blood dripping along the port may obscure the lens and make visualization difficult until the endoscope can be moved to an alternative port and the bleeding vessel controlled with electrocautery or a transcutaneous hemostatic suture.

With the laparoscope positioned satisfactorily in the peritoneal cavity, the surgeon proceeds with a systematic examination of the entire abdomen. The laparoscope is first directed caudally toward the pelvis, where the midline posterior wall of the bladder can be seen with the broad urachus (i.e., median umbilical ligament) extending up toward the umbilicus (Fig. 18.6). On either side of the bladder, the medial umbilical ligaments are usually quite prominent as they travel just lateral to the bladder; they also are umbilically directed. In very obese patients, the medial umbilical ligament may be difficult to identify. Lateral to the medial umbilical ligaments are the internal inguinal rings on either side of the pelvis. Extending from the internal inguinal ring, the vas deferens (male; Fig. 18.6A) or the round ligament (female; Fig. 18.6B) can be identified, passing medially to cross the free edge of the medial umbilical ligament before descending deeper into the pelvis. Also exiting from the internal inguinal ring are the gonadal vessels as they course cephalad just under the peritoneal membrane in the retroperitoneum. In female patients the midline uterus and laterally positioned ovaries are visualized. The laterally lying colon will also be visualized, and on the right side the cecum and appendix are apparent. There are often adhesions from the descending colon to the lateral pelvic wall. Coursing along the anterior abdominal wall are the inferior epigastric vessels, just medial to the internal inguinal ring and lateral to the medial umbilical ligament. These structures are more easily visualized using the 30-degree laparoscope.

The laparoscope is then rotated to a cephalad orientation to view the upper abdomen. The liver, gallbladder, stomach, and spleen are examined. The omentum and small bowel should be assessed for any possible injury during Veress needle insertion or port placement. Also, there is usually an adhesion present from the splenic flexure of the colon to the abdominal sidewall.

Placement of Additional Trocars

After the abdominal examination has been completed, attention is directed to placement of additional ports to facilitate performance of the planned surgical procedure. The exact pattern of the port arrangement will depend on the type of procedure to be performed and the surgeon's preference. It is advisable to use a 10-mm trocar for the second port placement, allowing transfer of the 10-mm, 30-degree laparoscope for visualization of the primary port. This size endoscope is mandatory if omental, bowel, or abdominal wall vascular injury during primary port placement is suspected. Also, if one is planning to use any of the GIA-type laparoscopic staplers, a 12-mm port is necessary.

Secondary ports are positioned such that they are not too close to each other; if placed too close together, they will limit maneuverability because the sheaths interfere with each other on the abdominal surface, and the movement of instruments within the ports causes them to strike against one another and impede access to the surgical site (Fig. 18.7A).

Pressure on the abdominal wall at the planned secondary port site and simultaneous laparoscopic visualization assist in determining the exact port site in relationship to the surgical field; the 30-degree laparoscope is most useful for this procedure. After selection of the port site, the room lights are dimmed and the area of the abdominal wall is transilluminated with the laparoscope inside the abdomen. The tip of the laparoscope is moved upward until it is just underneath the abdominal wall. Large superficial abdominal wall blood vessels can be identified and avoided using this technique. Trocars should not be placed through the abdominus rectus muscle. The inferior epigastric vessels can be visualized with the laparoscope; they are positioned just lateral to the medial umbilical ligament and caudal and medial to the internal inguinal ring. The 30-degree endoscope is useful for this maneuver to facilitate the secondary port placement immediately medial or lateral to the inferior epigastric vessels.

A transverse skin incision is made with the no. 12 hooked blade to precisely accommodate the size of the chosen port. Pressing the port, without the obturator, against the skin to

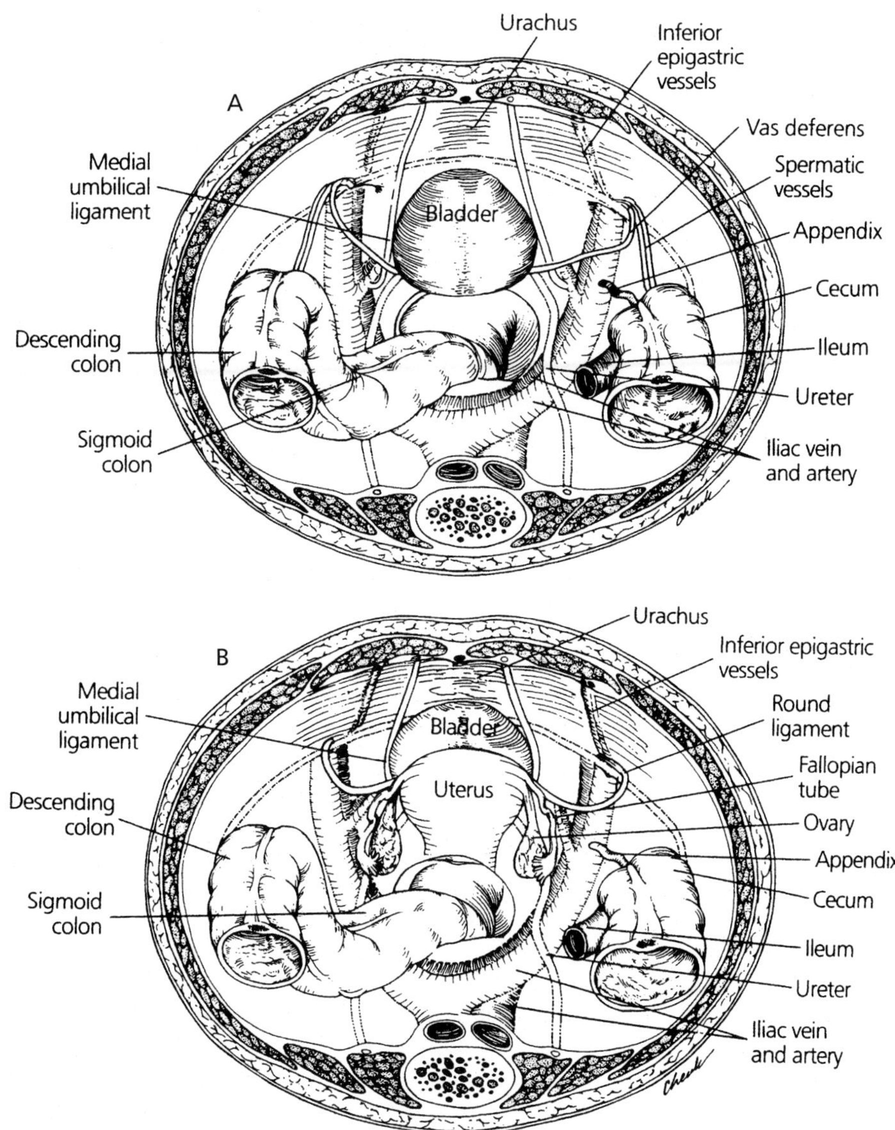

FIGURE 18.6. **A:** Laparoscopic examination of the male pelvis will include identification of the midline urachus and bladder, medial umbilical ligaments on either side of the bladder, bilateral internal inguinal rings, and spermatic vessels. The vas deferens may be seen just beneath the peritoneum, passing medially from the internal ring and crossing the medial umbilical ligament. **B:** Laparoscopic examination of the female pelvis will include identification of the midline urachus, bladder and uterus, medial umbilical ligaments on either side of the bladder, bilateral internal inguinal rings, and ovaries and fallopian tubes. The round ligament passes from the internal inguinal ring medially to cross the medial umbilical ligament. (Reprinted from Clayman RV, McDougall EM, eds. *Laparoscopic urology.* St. Louis: Quality Medical Publishing, 1993, with permission.)

leave an imprint of the port circumference assists in determining the correct length of the skin incision. All secondary ports should be directed through the fascia and peritoneum in a direct line with the planned surgical site. If this principle is followed during port placement, the sheaths will naturally point toward the surgical fields. This minimizes the amount of torque applied to the port site during manipulation of the instruments and reduces tearing of the peritoneum, which may cause CO_2 leakage. It also improves the surgeon's limited tactile sensation during intraabdominal handling of the tissues with the instruments. Using continuous laparoscopic monitoring, the secondary port is advanced through the fascia and peritoneum with a constant pressure and a slow, twisting action. The tip of the obturator will be seen laparoscopically to enter the abdominal cavity, and the safety shield will snap forward over the sharp obturator tip. Insertion of the port is continued until the shaft of the sheath is seen to protrude 1 to 2 cm inside the peritoneum.

The resistance of the abdominal wall may not allow the obturator to pass through the fascia and peritoneum without placing the sharp obturator tip dangerously close to the underlying viscera. To counteract this situation, sharp towel clips may be placed on the skin edges of the port site to elevate the abdominal wall away from the viscera. Also, after the sharp obturator point has passed through the fascia and peritoneum, the port can be redirected toward the laparoscopic lens for the remainder of the sheath insertion, thereby directing the sharp obturator point way from the viscera.

It is important to secure the port to the insertion site so that it does not become dislodged during instrument ma-

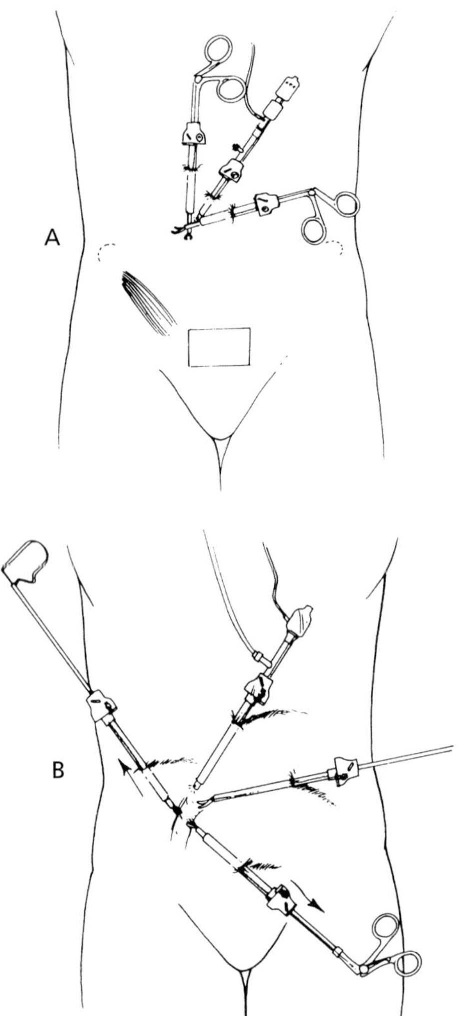

FIGURE 18.7. A: Ports placed too close together will limit the movement of the sheaths on the abdominal surface and cause the instruments to strike against one another and obstruct access to the surgical site. **B:** Optimal port placement allows the assistant to grasp tissue opposite the surgeon's grasper, thus creating traction and countertraction. The surgeon may then use a cutting device to incise the intervening exposed tissue. (Reprinted from Clayman RV, McDougall EM, eds. *Laparoscopic urology.* St. Louis: Quality Medical Publishing, 1993, with permission.)

nipulation. Some ports consist of a self-retaining device, including (a) a Malecot flange system that will open on removal of the obturator or by opening a lever on the upper sheath; (b) inflation of a balloon at the distal end of the port sheath by injecting air through a side port; (c) a plastic retentive sleeve that is screwed down, over the sheath, through the fascia and peritoneum 1 to 2 cm, and tightened onto the shaft of the port; or (d) an integral screw edge on the outside of the port cannula. When using any of the retentive sleeves, it is essential to *never* use a plastic retentive sleeve in combination with a metal sheath because this can create a problem with electrosurgical capacitive coupling and subsequent bowel injury. Alternatively, the port may be sutured to the skin with a no. 2 Prolene suture; this technique has the advantage of allowing the port to be advanced farther into the abdomen, yet it cannot be inadvertently removed from the abdomen.

The first crucial function of the second inserted port is to facilitate examination and confirmation of accurate positioning of the primary port. Immediately following the securing of the second port, the laparoscope is transferred to the second port and the primary port is examined. This will ensure that no bowel or omental injury has occurred and that the port site has satisfactory hemostasis. The sheath of the initial port is then positioned so that 2 cm extends inside the abdominal cavity; a retentive device or suture may be used to secure this port in this position.

The laparoscope is then returned to the umbilical port position, and the remaining secondary ports for the surgical procedure are inserted. It is important to place these other ports to facilitate traction and countertraction of tissues held in grasping forceps by the surgeon and assistant, respectively. The surgeon's electrocautery scissors should enter the abdomen from the same side and in a similar trajectory to the laparoscope to allow the surgeon to work with a "true" monitor image and manipulate or cut the tissue held between the two grasping forceps (Fig. 18.7B).

Instrumentation

The selection of laparoscopic equipment has increased exponentially over the past 4 to 5 years, reflecting how much laparoscopic surgery relies on the associated technology. Many of the instruments are available as disposable or nondisposable products. The nondisposable instruments have the advantage of representing a single monetary expenditure for the hospital, but the disadvantage of becoming dull or less efficient with repeated use. The disposable instruments are more expensive, which is of increasing concern in our present era of health care cost awareness. Until recently, disposable instruments have provided more versatility and specific functions than the more traditional nondisposable instruments. Presently, some instruments are being developed as "reposable" units: They have components (e.g., the blades of the scissors or jaws of a forceps) that can be discarded or replaced and that are mounted on a nondisposable shaft; this combination makes their use less expensive than classic disposable units while providing the surgeon with optimal instrumentation for each procedure.

Laparoscopy remains limited by the loss of 3D and wide-field vision perspective and the reduction of tactile sensation. Many features of the instrumentation of laparoscopy attempt to accommodate or compensate for these limitations. It is important for the laparoscopist to be familiar with the equipment used in each laparoscopic case and to determine which additional instruments will better facilitate the performance of a specific planned procedure.

The intention of this review is not to provide an exhaustive list of available laparoscopic equipment, but rather to discuss the basic principles of the laparoscopic instrumentation available to surgeons and some of the more recent adaptations that may be useful in specific circumstances.

Grasping Instruments

Many grasping instruments are available for laparoscopy. These instruments vary in size from 3 to 12 mm and may be reusable or disposable. Grasping forceps are insulated, allowing them to be used for cauterization of the tissue they are grasping. The opening mechanism of grasping forceps may be single action, where only one jaw moves when the instrument is opened, or double action, with opening movement of both jaws. The double-action grasping forceps are usually preferable because they more closely approximate those used during open surgical dissection.

Grasping forceps may be locking or nonlocking. Two mechanisms have been developed to produce locking of the grasping forceps: the spring-loaded locking handle and the ratchet-style locking handle. The spring-loaded grasping forceps remains securely locked closed until the handle, which fits in the surgeon's hand, is firmly squeezed to open the jaws and release the held tissue. The ratchet-style locking grasper has a bar-type finger-activated ratchet that locks the jaws in the closed position with varying degrees of tension on the tissue. The jaws will not open until the ratchet lock is released.

The main difference between grasping forceps is the tip design. Grasping-forceps tips may be classified as traumatic or atraumatic. Atraumatic graspers have serrated grasping surfaces for gentle manipulation of tissues. The tip shape is variable and includes blunt, pointed (e.g., dolphin), straight (e.g., duck bill), curved, and right-angled. Traumatic graspers are designed to hold fibrous tissues securely and tightly and usually are toothed or clawed. The jaws of these instruments tend to be broader and longer. These instruments also include Allis, Babcock, and bowel clamps and may have tip-rotating and articulating functions to better access the operative site.

Cutting Instruments

Tissues can be transected using laparoscopic scissors, scalpels, electrosurgical probes, laser fibers [neodymium: yttrium-aluminum-garnet (Nd:YAG) or potassium titanyl phosphate (KTP)], or high-speed ultrasonic instruments. Endoscopic scissors may be reusable or disposable and are available in a variety of shapes. Scissor blades may be straight or curved for dissection. Serrated tips are useful for cutting fascia, and a hooked tip facilitates transection of sutures. The scissors may be insulated to facilitate simultaneous electrocoagulation and transection of tissues. The ability to rotate or angulate the tips of the scissors, by turning a finger control knob, allows easier access to a variety of surgical sites. Scissors with angulating blades are useful for adhesiolysis between the bowel or omentum and the anterior abdominal wall. Curved electrosurgical scissors with rotating tip provide for excellent access to most surgical sites, rapid dissection of tissues, transection of tissues with mechanical (i.e., cold) cutting when near delicate structures such as the bowel, and electrical currents for incision and coagulation of tissues.

Laparoscopic scalpel blades are also available. These were initially developed for incising the common bile duct and have had limited applicability to laparoscopic urology. Recently, they have been used for incision of the urethra during a laparoscopic radical prostatectomy. Great care should be used when inserting, manipulating, or removing these instruments to avoid inadvertent intraabdominal injuries.

Electrosurgical currents may be applied to insulated instruments with needle-point, flat-spatula, or right-angled hook tips. A thin metal tip provides the greatest current density and the most efficient cutting. A needle electrode (i.e., Corson needle) creates a very fine incision of the peritoneum or tissues. A right-angle or hooked tip can be manipulated under tissues and used to draw the tissues away from underlying structures before electrical activation and incision of the tissue. The most common setting for cutting and coagulation currents on electrosurgical instruments is 25 to 50 W; the lowest setting necessary to achieve effective coagulation is recommended. It is imperative that the insulation material on the shaft of the instrument be completely intact to prevent inadvertent sparking of current between instruments or to adjacent tissues. Also, the entire active tip of the electrosurgical instrument should be visualized laparoscopically while being used, to avoid injury to adjacent structures (438). As previously noted, metal trocar sheaths should not be used in conjunction with plastic retention sleeves when electrocautery is being used. The plastic sleeve acts as an insulator and may allow electric charge to build up in the metal sheath. Inadvertent contact between the bowel and the metal sheath could result in a bowel injury or perforation.

The most effective electrocoagulation of small blood vessels is achieved by using an insulated grasper to grasp the tissue and oppose the walls of the vessel. Directly applying an electric current to the grasping forceps, or touching the tips of the forceps with an activated electrosurgical instrument in the coagulation mode, will coagulate the coapted vessel. Last, many electrosurgical instruments are combined with an aspirator-irrigator. This facilitates suctioning of the smoke generated during fulguration and cutting of tissues.

Monopolar electrosurgical instruments are most commonly used and require a remote ground so that the electric current applied to the tissues passes through the patient's body to the ground pad. Bipolar laparoscopic electrosurgical instruments are available. They incorporate both the live and ground contacts in the tip of the instrument; no ground pad is used and the electric current passes only between the two contacts. Less energy is required for bipolar electrocautery, as compared with monopolar; thus inadvertent injury to surrounding structures is reduced.

Laser probes, including KTP (532 nm) and Nd:YAG (1,064 nm), also may be used for cutting and fulgurating tissues. The KTP laser facilitates noncontact cutting and noncontact fulguration. The Nd:YAG laser provides contact cutting and noncontact fulguration. A 600-micron fiber is usually passed through an aspirator-irrigator instrument for stabilization. Wavelength-specific protective eyeglasses must be worn by all operating room personnel whenever laser energy is being used. In addition, a special filter is necessary on the camera to prevent disturbance of the image during laser firing.

A recent development in tissue cutting and hemostasis is the harmonic knife. This instrument uses high-frequency ultrasound to create rapid vibration of the tip of the instrument. Using different frequencies and the edge or flat portion of the spatula tip, the surgeon can selectively cut or coagulate tissues.

Retractors

Retractors often are required to expose a surgical site by retracting liver, spleen, or bowel, or to facilitate dissection by retracting the kidney to place the hilar vessels on slight stretch. Although many retractors have been developed, the simplest remains a blunt-tip grasping forceps in either a 5- or 10-mm size, depending on the available port site. These instruments can be used to elevate the liver or spleen or medially retract the bowel. Instruments specifically designed to be retractors possess a feature that, when opened, increases the surface area against which they are placed. This allows dispersion of the force of retraction over a larger surface of the retracted structure, thereby reducing the risk of visceral injury. Also, better visualization results because a large amount of tissue can be retracted. Retractors include 5- and 10-mm instruments.

Fan retractors consist of three or four blunt-tip blades that can be opened after intraabdominal positioning. A variation of the fan retractor consists of two blades with an interposing V-hinge joint. When the V hinge is opened, the outer blades spread apart, creating a broad retracting surface. This retractor can be opened to the desired width and locked into position. Recently, the fan retractor has been modified by the addition of an inflatable balloon around the blades of the fan. After positioning the instrument into the abdominal cavity, the blades are opened. A syringe is attached to a side-arm connector, and the balloon covering the blades is inflated with 10 to 20 mL of air. This provides a larger surface area for retraction and thus better distributes the pressure applied to the tissues, potentially causing less ischemia and less chance of organ injury. Vein retractors are available in 5- or 10-mm diameter and consist of a broad, bluntly curved tip for gentle retraction of vascular structures. In addition, 14-gauge needle hook retractors are available; these are inserted separately into the abdomen, and the small hook end is advanced and secured on the peritoneal edge or tissue for retraction. A major advantage of this retractor is that it does not have to be passed through any of the ports.

There are several options for the surgeon to create his or her own retraction devices in the operating room. For example, a 24-inch length of umbilical tape, suture material, or vessel loop may be placed around the ureter or blood vessel for retraction purposes. The needle-pointed grasper of the Carter-Thomason device (see Exiting the Abdomen) can be used, through a small stab wound on the flank, to deliver and retrieve the ends of the tape, suture, or loop. A mosquito clamp on the abdominal wall side maintains tension on the retraction around the ureter or vessel, without using a port site for this purpose.

Sewing Instruments

Laparoscopic suturing and knot tying are two of the most challenging skills for the laparoscopic surgeon to acquire. Recent technologic developments have helped simplify some aspects of these techniques.

Laparoscopic ports used during suturing may vary from 5 to 12 mm in diameter. It is important to plan the surgical procedure and determine the most appropriate port size for each location according to the anticipated need for needle introducers, clip-appliers, or stapling devices. Reducer caps allow working instruments of smaller diameter (3.5 to 10.5 mm) to be used through larger laparoscopic ports (5 to 12 mm) without loss of the pneumoperitoneum. These reducers may be an integral part of the port or may be readily affixed to the top of the laparoscopic cannula.

Laparoscopic 5-mm needle-holders are used to grasp and manipulate needles during suturing of tissues. These devices may be single or double action. The single-action needle-holder has one fixed jaw and one moveable jaw, which is opened by squeezing the spring-loaded handle of the instrument. The double-action needle-holder more closely simulates the traditional needle-holder in that both jaws open when the ring handles are spread apart. The jaws may be serrated to provide a more secure grip on the needle. The hinge mechanism of the jaws should be flush with the shaft of the instrument when closed to facilitate intracorporeal knot tying; this design allows formed loops of suture to slide off the shaft easily without getting caught in the hinge mechanism.

Tissue graspers are usually 5 mm in diameter and should be atraumatic to facilitate grasping of the tissue to be sewn, to grasp the suture material without tearing it, and to assist in proper positioning of the needle within the needle-holder. It is helpful to have a locking feature on this instrument to facilitate these functions.

The suture introducer is helpful to allow introduction of the needle and suture without entanglement on the flap valve system of the port. The needle-holder securing the needle and suture within the introducer are moved as a unit through the designated port, and the needle-holder and suture with needle are advanced into the abdomen. Alternatively, if one is working through a 12-mm port, the suture can be grasped just behind the needle by the needle-holder; the flap valve is then inactivated and the entire assembly is passed through the port.

Knot-pushers facilitate delivery of extracorporeally tied knots into the abdomen; they may be independent or an integral part of the suture material. The independent knot-pusher is used to slide (Clarke-Reich) or to slide and cinch (Gazayerli) the knot into place. The integral knot-pusher is attached to a preformed knotted loop in the suture. After the loop is passed over the tissues to be secured, the plastic knot-pusher is snapped free of its terminal plastic base and used to deliver and secure the preformed knot within the abdomen.

The most significant advancement in laparoscopic suturing technology is the development of the EndoStitch device (U.S. Surgical Corporation, Norwalk, Connecticut). This device consists of a double-sided needle (9 mm, straight) with the suture attached to the midshaft of the needle, a built-in needle-holder on both jaws of the instrument, and a toggle mechanism that allows the needle to be transferred from one jaw of the needle-holder to the other. With the loading unit provided, the needle with the attached suture is loaded into the laparoscopic needle-holder. The needle's position is fixed on the needle-holder, eliminating the need for repositioning the needle. Closing the handles passes the needle through the tissue. A switch of the toggle lever secures the needle in the opposite jaw of the needle-holder, thereby completing passage of the suture when the handles are relaxed and allowing the jaws of the EndoStitch to separate (Fig. 18.8). This instrumentation has greatly facilitated reconstructive laparoscopic urologic procedures such as the pyeloplasty (4).

Performing an intracorporeal knot is one of the more challenging skills for a laparoscopist to acquire. The vast array of techniques that have been described attests to the confusion and frustration that can be associated with learning this skill (256). Mechanical aids developed to facilitate or replace traditional surgical knots include, respectively, a polydioxanone (Vicryl) suture clip to secure a suture and metal clips or staples for occluding blood vessels, excising tissue, and reapproximating tissue edges (241).

The Lapra-Ty suture clip-applier (Ethicon EndoSurgery Inc., Cincinnati, Ohio) is a reusable device, and the Lapra-Ty (polydioxanone) suture clip is available in packets of six clips. The clips are individually loaded into the clip-applier and then positioned on a single strand of 0 Vicryl, 3-0 Vicryl, or 4-0 Vicryl. Tightly squeezing the handle of the clip-applier locks the suture clip onto the suture to act as a knot. Tensile-strength studies in the laboratory have shown that these suture clips, acutely, are as secure as a hand-tied surgeon's knot using the same suture

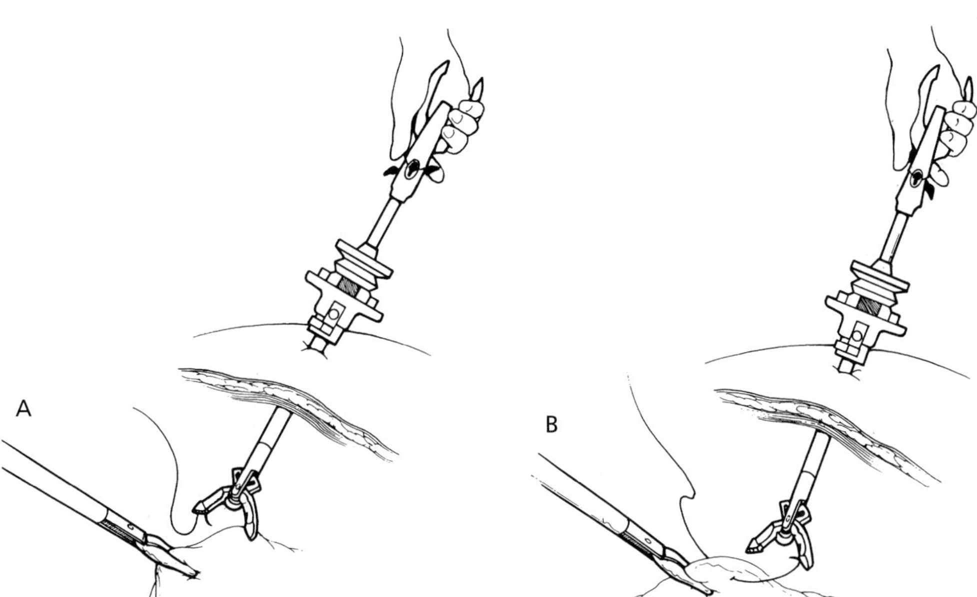

FIGURE 18.8. A: Automatic suturing device from U.S. Surgical Corp., Norwalk, Connecticut. The needle has a point on either end, and the suture is attached at midshaft. **B:** Either side of the jaws of the instrument alternately functions as the "needle-driver" to allow rapid back-and-forth passage of the needle, thereby providing the surgeon with a running suture. The same mechanism can be used to complete intracorporeal knotting of the ends of the suture.

materials. These suture clips may be used to secure the ends of the suture material when performing interrupted or running suture techniques laparoscopically. Used in conjunction with the EndoStitch device, these clips have further simplified reconstructive laparoscopy.

Laparoscopic clipping instruments are available in two forms: (a) occlusive for occluding blood vessels and (b) tacking for approximating tissue edges or securing various foreign materials (e.g., cadaveric fascia, mesh) to tissues. Occlusive clips come in lengths of 6, 9, and 11 mm. The applier is passed into the abdomen via a 10-mm port. The clip-applier may be either a single-load reusable type or a multiload, disposable type, which comes with 15 to 30 clips already loaded in the applier; the latter device, especially if it comes with a semiautomatic feed system, is capable of firing clips in rapid succession. The tips of the clip are approximated by the jaws of the clip-applier before closure of the body of the clip, thereby allowing the surgeon to slide a clip up or down along a given vessel before securing it in place (Fig. 18.9). The 9-mm clips are as secure as a hand-tied surgeon's knot of 0 silk on the renal artery when pressure tested (216). The tacking clips close in either a rectangular or B configuration, and the applier is passed into the abdomen via an 11-mm port (Fig. 18.10). All clip-appliers have a rotating shaft, and some allow angulation of the working end, to help align the tip of the clip-applier with the structure to be clipped or tacked.

Laparoscopic stapling devices are available only as disposable instruments and have rotating and articulating capabilities at the working end. Staple sizes range from 2.5 to 4.8 mm; smaller staples are used to occlude vascular structures, whereas larger staples are used to secure bulkier tissues. The length of each row of staples is 3 or 6 cm, and each cartridge delivers six separate rows of staples. As the staples are pushed into the tissues and closed, a knife simultaneously cuts the tissue between the third and fourth staple lines.

Developments in laparoscopic staplers (occlusive and reconstructive) have been most impressive. Indeed, bowel anastomoses can be readily performed laparoscopically using the same staple technology that was developed for open surgery. This technology has only begun to be transferred to urologic reconstructive surgery because of concerns over the potential of stone formation on the titanium staples that would be continuously exposed to urine within the reconstructed collecting system. However, in the bladder, titanium staples have apparently been well tolerated, and to date, there are no reports of stone formation on the staples used to secure a cuff of bladder during a nephroureterectomy (214,215).

Further advances in the realm of staple and clip technology will likely revolve around the development of extremely small absorbable clips. Already, absorbable clips have been developed for use in creating a right colon pouch for urinary

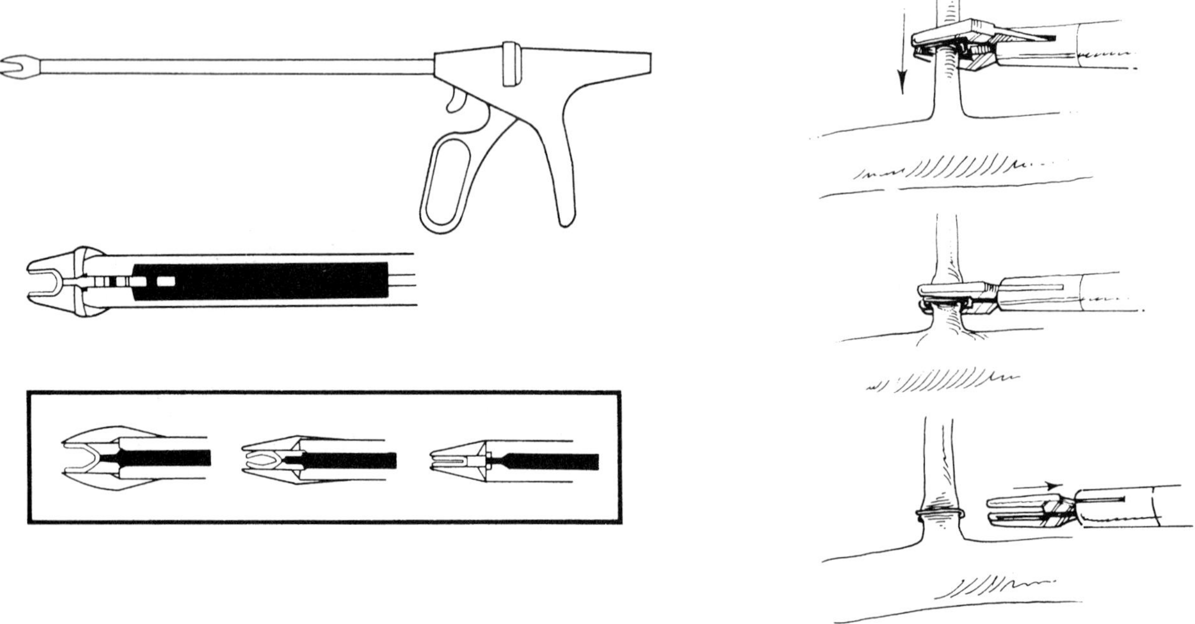

FIGURE 18.9. The clip-applier contains preloaded occlusive clips. After the jaws of a clip are placed around the suture to be clipped, the handle of the instrument is squeezed half-closed. This approximates the tips of the clip, which can be moved along the structure for precise placement. The handle is then fully closed, which securely closes the body of the clip on the structure. (Reprinted from Clayman RV, McDougall EM, eds. *Laparoscopic urology.* St. Louis: Quality Medical Publishing, 1993, with permission.)

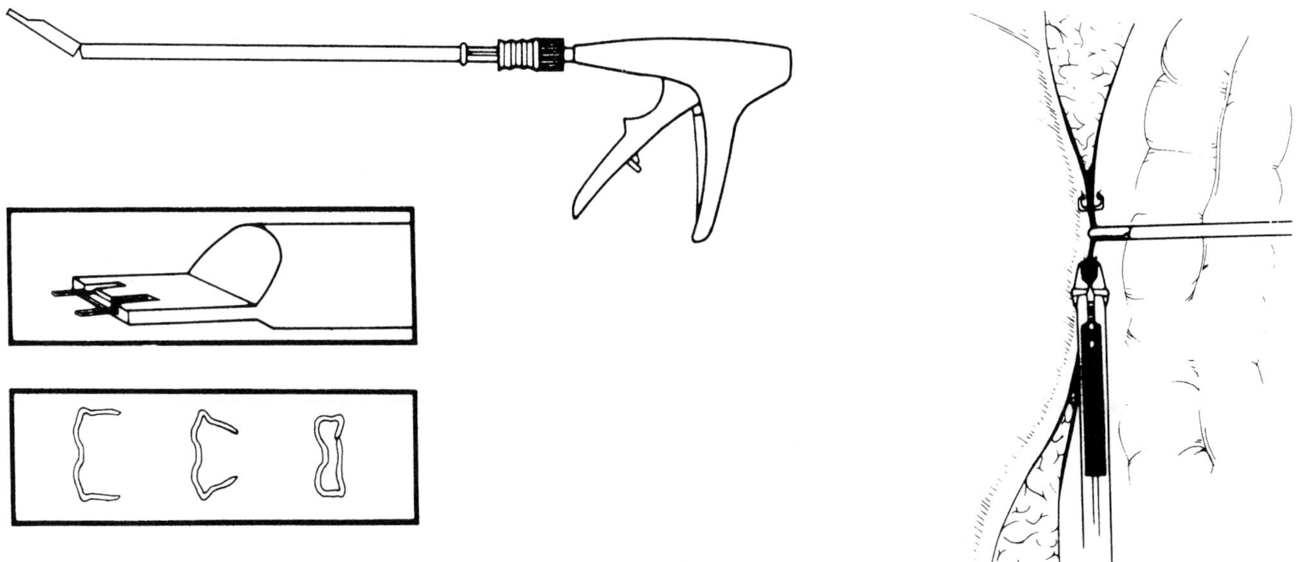

FIGURE 18.10. The tacking clips close in a rectangular or B configuration and are used to reapproximate tissue edges such as peritoneum to peritoneum or Marlex mesh to peritoneum. (Reprinted from Clayman RV, McDougall EM, eds. *Laparoscopic urology.* St. Louis: Quality Medical Publishing, 1993, with permission.)

diversion (138,312). Presently, these staples are too large to be used for the delicate reconstruction of the ureter or renal pelvis.

The recent development of fibrin glue is further expanding the range of reconstructive laparoscopic urology. The first clinically effective use of tissue glue was in 1972 by Matras and colleagues (249a), who used a fibrin glue to join peripheral nerves. At present, there are two commercially available preparations: Tisseel and Beriplast (120). These systems consist of fibrinogen (70 to 100 mg/mL) in one part of a dual syringe, and a second solution in the opposite chamber of the syringe. The second solution contains thrombin, factor XIII, fibronectin, and ionized calcium with or without aprotinin, an antifibrinolytic agent. In theory, the fibrinogen determines the strength of the glue while the amount of thrombin directly determines the speed of reaction, which may vary from 5 seconds to several minutes. Aprotinin prolongs the presence of the glue at the anastomotic site for 2 to 4 weeks. The glue used in combination with cellulose has been used to perform hand-assisted laparoscopic partial nephrectomy for tumor (194). This technique provides excellent hemostasis of the transected renal parenchyma. The glue has also been used experimentally to aid in the creation of anastomoses, such as tubal reconstruction, vasovasostomy, or ureteroureterostomy (117,237,271,306).

Miscellaneous

Other instruments and devices are available that facilitate specific laparoscopic functions. The organ entrapment sack is made of either a durable double layer of impermeable nylon and plastic or a single layer of thick-walled plastic. The sacks vary in size from 2 by 5 inches to 10 by 8 inches. The sack is tightly rolled over an introducing device and inserted through a 10-mm port. Within the abdomen the sack is unrolled, and the neck of the sack is triangulated open with traumatic grasping forceps placed on the three equidistant tabs on the sack edge or by a metallic band that causes the mouth of the sack to spring open when inserted into the abdomen. The surgical specimen is deposited into the sack, the neck of the sack is closed, and the neck of the entire sack is pulled out by its drawstring through a 12-mm port site. If just the neck of the sack is delivered, the tissue is fragmented and removed from the sack using forceps; a 10-mm, high-speed electric tissue morcellator [note that this morcellator can only be used with a LapSac (Cook Urological Inc., Spencer, Indiana)]; or a jaw-system mechanical morcellator. The morcellation process is monitored laparoscopically to ensure that sack perforation or incorporation of bowel or omentum into a fold of the sack does not occur. Landman and colleagues (229) recently reported their evaluation of the various tissue morcellators in the animal model. They determined that all three presently available morcellators were feasible for renal morcellation. The Steiner morcellator (Karl Storz Inc., Culver City, California) resulted in more rapid morcellation, larger morcellation products, and comparable safety in their experimental model.

Aspiration devices are necessary during laparoscopy, and combined aspiration-irrigation devices are preferable. The aspirating channel may be attached directly to an operating room vacuum and collection system. The aspirator consists of a 5- or 10-mm metal tube and trumpet valve. The irrigating channel is controlled with a one-way stopcock or trumpet valve. The irrigant must be pressurized to 250 to 700 mm Hg to allow adequate flushing of tissues and blood clots. The irrigation fluid most commonly used is saline and heparin (5,000 U/L); a broad-spectrum antibiotic (e.g., 500 mg of cephalosporin per liter) may be added to the irrigant. It is important for the aspirating tip of the instrument to have sideholes, in addition to the endhole, to maximize the suction ability of the instrument.

The development of laparoscopic ultrasound probes allows sonographic examination of tissues and Doppler detection of blood vessels during the surgical procedure. This may be useful in directing wedge resection of small renal lesions, identifying the testicular artery during laparoscopic varix ligation, or identifying the renal artery during a laparoscopic nephrectomy. The laparoscopic ultrasound probe is now articulating, which is helpful in performing intraoperative renal ultrasonography, especially during laparoscopic cryotherapy of renal lesions.

An argon beam coagulator may be used with 5- or 10-mm probes. This device uses argon gas (at a flow rate of 4 L per minute) to clear blood and fluid from the surgical field and deliver electrical current to a bleeding surface, thereby electrofulgurating the tissue. The surface temperature of the fulgurated tissue remains below 100°F, limiting the depth of injury to 1 to 2 mm (versus 5 mm, with standard electrocautery). This may be particularly helpful during wedge resection of the kidney or for a partial nephrectomy.

Another device, which recently completed clinical trials, is the pneumodissector. This instrument applies brief blasts of CO_2 gas at a pressure of 50 psi to facilitate dissection of connective tissues. Animal studies have confirmed that the pneumodissector will not cause laceration of the liver, kidney, aorta, or vena cava, even at a maximum pressure of 100 psi (63). After sharp incision of the peritoneum, the pneumodissector effectively assists in dissection of the fatty tissues and exposure of the renal hilar vessels. It has been shown, in clinical evaluation, to be a safe and efficacious technique for rapid blunt tissue dissection (327).

There has been recent interest in hand-assisted laparoscopy (HAL) as a method for inexperienced laparoscopists to acquire the skills necessary for performing laparoscopic renal surgery. It also has particular relevance to procedures that require an incision to remove the surgical specimen intact, such as laparoscopic nephroureterectomy for upper tract transitional cell carcinoma or live donor nephrectomy (212,295,393). It may also facilitate the successful performance of laparoscopic partial nephrectomy (2).

For placement of a hand-assist device, it is necessary to first obtain a Veress needle pneumoperitoneum and placement of a primary port in the midclavicular line. Under laparoscopic visualization, a skin, fascial, and peritoneal incision, of 6 to 8 cm in length, is performed at the midline. For a right-hand–dominant surgeon, this incision is made overlying and just above the umbilicus for left renal surgery, and overlying and just below the umbilicus for right renal surgery. Various HAL devices are available, but essentially they all provide an airtight seal of the abdominal wall and allow the surgeon to insert the nondominant hand, through a plastic sleeve, into the abdominal cavity to assist with tissue dissection and retraction while maintaining the pneumoperitoneum. The presently available devices include Pneumosleeve (Dexterity Inc., Blue Bell, Pennsylvania), Intromit (Applied Medical Resources, Laguna Hills, California), and Hand Port (Smith-Nephew, Worcester, Massachusetts).

Exiting the Abdomen

At the conclusion of the laparoscopic procedure, it is essential to exit the abdomen in an organized and systematic manner to minimize the risk of complications. Intraabdominal pressure should be reduced to 5 mm Hg because this will allow any venotomy previously tamponaded by the 15 mm Hg pneumoperitoneum to be recognized. The surgical sites and all the port sites should be examined closely for hemostasis. The abdominal cavity should be scanned from the pelvic region to the upper quadrants to rule out any injury to abdominal viscera.

After satisfactory examination of the abdomen, the 10-mm laparoscope is removed and replaced by a 5-mm laparoscope through one of the secondary 5-mm ports. The primary 10-mm (or larger) port is removed from the abdomen under laparoscopic visualization. The assistant places a finger over the port site to maintain the pneumoperitoneum. If hemostasis of the port site remains satisfactory, the fascia is closed using a figure-of-eight of 0 absorbable suture under continuous laparoscopic observation. A small S-curved or Sinn retractor is used to retract the skin and expose the fascia. The fascia is grasped with a Kocher clamp or toothed forceps. The suture is passed through the fascia, and laparoscopic visualization ensures that the bowel or omentum is not incorporated into the stitches. This procedure of port removal and fascial closure is repeated for all the remaining ports larger than 5 mm.

Identifying the fascia for placement of a figure-of-eight suture is often difficult, especially in an obese patient. Several companies have developed devices to simplify this final step in the laparoscopic procedure. The device that we have found consistently to be the most useful and least expensive is the Carter-Thomason closure device (47) (Fig. 18.11). This device consists of two parts: a metal cone with two through-and-through oblique channels drilled in it and a needle-tip 2-mm grasping forceps. The two channels in the cone part of the device serve to direct the sharp, needle-pointed suture-grasper through the fascia and peritoneum; this is always performed under laparoscopic visualiza-

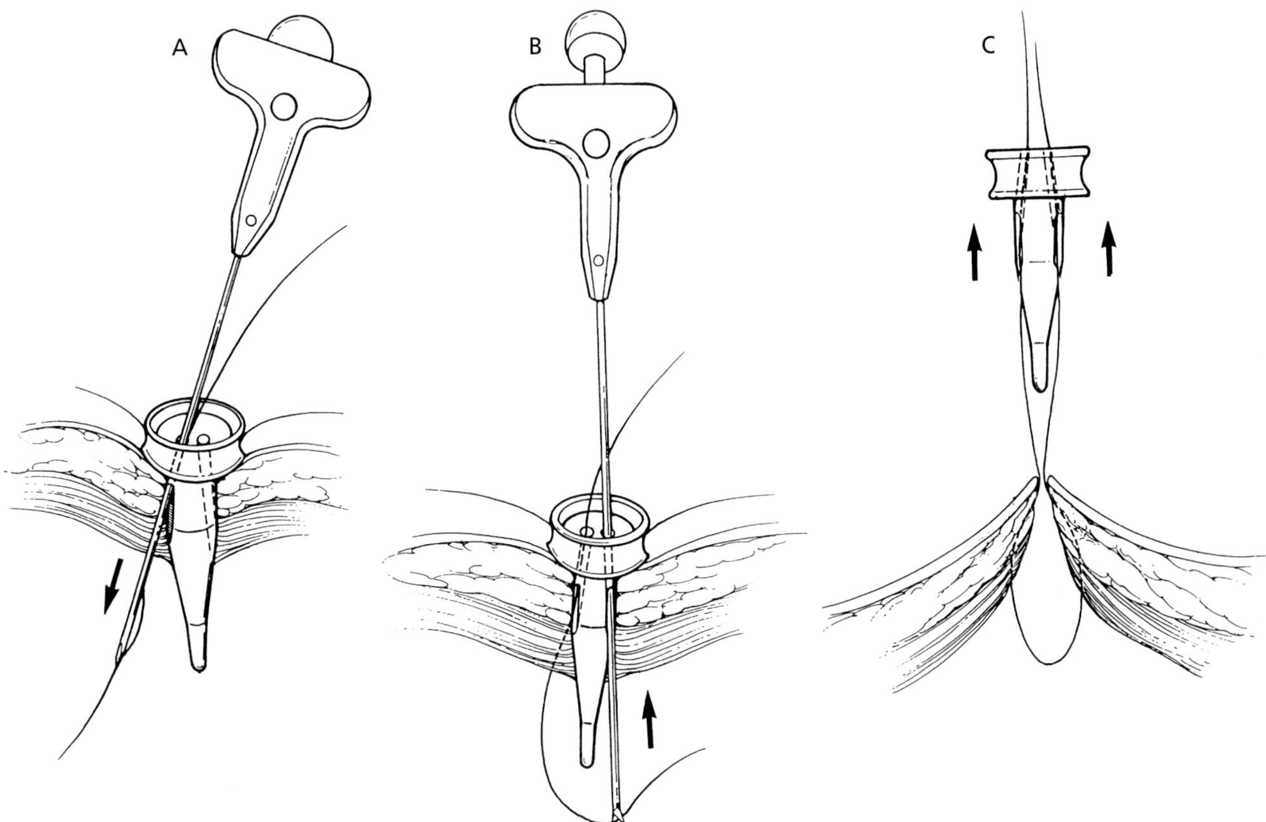

FIGURE 18.11 **A:** The Carter-Thomason laparoscopic wound closure device is inserted into the port site after removing the port. The suture end secured in the needle-pointed grasper is inserted through the channel, directing it through the fascia and peritoneum. **B:** The needle-pointed grasper is inserted through the second channel, is passed through the fascia and peritoneum opposite the initial suture insertion, and grasps the intraabdominal end of the suture. **C:** The two ends of the suture are tied down to complete the closure of the fascia and peritoneum.

tion. The suture chosen for closure should be a minimum of 12 inches in length. One end of the suture is grasped by the sharp, needle-pointed grasper. After removal of the port, the metal cone piece is placed into the port site; its tip is visualized by the laparoscope. The needle-point grasper is then inserted through one of the channels of the cone. Passage of the instrument through the fascia and peritoneum is monitored laparoscopically to avoid any intraperitoneal injury. When positioned well into the abdomen, the jaws of the needle-point grasper are opened to drop the suture. The jaws are then closed and the instrument is withdrawn from the working channel. The needle-pointed grasper is then inserted through the second channel, which directs the instrument through the fascia and peritoneum, 180 degrees from its initial insertion, on the opposite side of the peritoneotomy. After the needle-pointed grasper is positioned within the abdomen, the grasping jaws are used to secure the intraabdominal end of the suture and draw it out through the working channel. A 5-mm locking grasper can be used through another port to facilitate removal of the suture from the needle-grasper and for positioning the suture so that it can be easily grasped by the needle grasper on its second pass. The two ends of the suture should now lie on the abdominal wall, having passed through both sides of the fascia and peritoneum. The metal cone device is withdrawn from the port site and off the suture, which is tied down snugly to close the port site.

After all of the sheaths larger than 5 mm have been removed and the fascia closed, all but the laparoscope-bearing 5-mm sheath are pulled from the abdomen under laparoscopic visualization. Fascial sutures are not necessary at these port sites if no bleeding is present from the sites; the only exception is in the child, in which case even the 5-mm ports require a fascial suture. If any bleeding is noted from a 5-mm port site, either electrocoagulation of the site or placement of a 0 absorbable suture is necessary.

The last sheath to be removed is the 5-mm sheath through which the 5-mm laparoscope has been passed. The pneumoperitoneum is maintained by having the assistant occlude the 5-mm port sites with a finger. The laparoscope is backed out until the tip is just protruding from the end of the port sheath. The last sheath and laparoscope are then slowly backed out of the abdomen as a unit. As the 5-mm laparoscope is withdrawn, the site of the peritoneotomy and fasciotomy are examined to rule out bleeding. If bleeding is noted, the site may be coagulated through the sheath, or if this fails, one of the other 5-mm port sites should be replaced. The bleeding port site may then be sutured with a 0 absorbable suture.

The CO_2 is allowed to escape from the 5-mm port sites. The skin incisions of the port sites larger than 5 mm are closed in a subcuticular fashion using a 4-0 absorbable suture. The skin incisions of all the port sites are closed and secured with sterile adhesive strips. This method of exiting the abdomen should obviate bowel or omentum becoming entrapped by the fascial sutures and eliminate herniation through any of the port sites.

Retroperitoneal Approach

Following balloon dilation or blunt-finger dissection access to the retroperitoneum, a Hasson-type cannula or 10- to 12-mm trocar is inserted. The 10-mm, 30-degree laparoscope is inserted and the retroperitoneal space is inspected. On initial examination, the psoas muscle and genitofemoral nerve should be clearly seen. Gerota's fascia and the ureter are typically visible, although this may be difficult in the obese patient or in those patients with any degree of scarring or fibrosis in the retroperitoneal space. A small amount of venous blood overlying the tissues is normal, but there should be no active bleeding.

Insertion of additional working ports is performed under endoscopic guidance. A 10- or 12-mm port is placed at the inferior lumbar triangle; a 5-mm port is placed at the level of the twelfth rib on the anterior axillary or midclavicular line; and a 5-mm port is placed at the level of the twelfth rib on the posterior line. The placement of the ports should form a T shape.

When a retroperitoneal approach is used, only minimal dissection in the area of the ureter is needed to completely expose this structure. Likewise, pulsations from the renal artery are often visible early in the case as the surgeon moves the endoscope up along the medial border of the psoas muscle. Instrumentation for the laparoscopic retroperitoneoscopic procedure is similar to that for the transperitoneal approach.

As with the peritoneal approach to renal surgery, it is important to systematically exit the retroperitoneal space. Following completion of the surgical procedure, the CO_2 pressure in the retroperitoneum is reduced to 5 mm Hg and the operative and port sites are examined to ensure adequate hemostasis. With the retroperitoneal approach, the port sites do not require a fascial suture closure because there is minimal risk of hernia formation. Therefore the ports are removed under direct visualization. The port sites are irrigated with saline and the skin is closed with a subcuticular 4-0 nonabsorbable suture.

Physiology of CO_2 Insufflation

Cardiopulmonary Function

There are two very nonphysiologic situations that occur during laparoscopy. The first is insufflation of the abdominal cavity with gas, usually CO_2, and the second is the elevation of intraabdominal pressure. Studies comparing the effect of insufflants on hemodynamic and respiratory function indicate that the type of gas used does not significantly affect cardiac output.

However, CO_2 gas may increase the central venous pressure and the mean arterial pressure (MAP). Likewise, argon gas can markedly increase cardiac afterload by elevating arterial pressures and systemic vascular resistance, even more so than CO_2 gas. In addition, CO_2 has been demonstrated to have a negative effect on respiratory function, whereas argon and helium do not appear to have these limitations. Thus it appears that the best alternative to CO_2 as an insufflant is helium because of the limited effect on hemodynamic function and essentially no effect on respiratory function (203). Wolf and colleagues (447) reported that conversion to helium insufflation was able to successfully reverse a significant respiratory acidosis caused by a CO_2 pneumoperitoneum in a patient with severe chronic obstructive pulmonary disease during a laparoscopic radical nephrectomy.

Aside from the choice of gas used for insufflation, the increased intraabdominal pressure itself can lead to unfavorable hemodynamic changes, which are essentially pressure dependent. Cardiovascular, pulmonary, and renal effects of elevated intraabdominal pressure have been extensively studied in the laboratory and clinical setting.

An elevated intraabdominal pressure has been shown to increase atrial filling pressures, increase systemic vascular resistance, decrease venous return, decrease cardiac output, and reduce stroke volume (70,223,269). Peak inspiratory pressures have been shown to increase in conjunction with the elevated abdominal pressure. These effects are pressure dependent, usually not becoming evident until pressures reach 14 to 15 mm Hg (269,439). In animal studies concerning the effects of laparoscopic surgery on hemodynamic responses, it has been shown that the changes are minimal when intraabdominal insufflation is performed in healthy, well-hydrated, and hyperventilated animals (173). Similarly, for healthy patients in the clinical setting, these hemodynamic changes do not appear to have any significant adverse effect (132,284). Clinically, the respiratory effect of the elevated intraabdominal pressure is monitored using pulse oximetry and capnography. The pulse oximeter saturation should be maintained at greater than 93% and the end-tidal CO_2 should be maintained between 35 and 45 mm Hg, which usually ensures that the $Pa{CO_2}$ is less than 50 mm Hg. Increasing respiratory rate and tidal volume can usually control these levels satisfactorily. Even in the face of moderate pulmonary disease, despite an elevation of the

$Paco_2$ and respiratory acidosis, the impairment of pulmonary function usually causes no significant negative hemodynamic effect (85). However, in laboratory studies on septic animals, although laparoscopy could be performed, the hemodynamic compromise in the form of acidosis with cardiodepression was more apparent. Therefore the clinical application of laparoscopy in the septic patient should be approached with caution (141).

Renal Function

It is well recognized that a prolonged period of increased intraabdominal pressure is associated with decreased urine output, even to the point of anuria (269). This continues to be the most marked intraoperative renal effect observed from the pneumoperitoneum, and it is pressure dependent. In a human study, the use of a lower intraabdominal pressure (4 mm Hg), plus the aid of a retraction device, for performing the laparoscopic cholecystectomy led to no significant changes in urine output, effective renal plasma flow, or glomerular filtration rate (GFR) as opposed to the transient renal dysfunction that was noted with an intraabdominal pressure of 12 mm Hg (280). Although this transient renal dysfunction has been well documented, various mechanisms have been described to explain these changes: choice of insufflant, decreased cardiac output, ureteral obstruction, renal vein compression, renal parenchymal compression, and systemic hormonal effects (156,221). The choice of insufflant does not appear to have a direct affect on renal function (269). In animal studies comparing CO_2 to argon gas for pneumoperitoneum, no change in urine output was noted for intraabdominal pressures less than 15 mm Hg. For intraabdominal pressures of 15 mm Hg or greater, a similar impairment in urine output and GFR was seen for both types of gas.

The body of evidence also eliminates a decrease in cardiac output as a direct etiologic factor responsible for the renal dysfunction (221). Although cardiac output has been reported to decrease to as much as 37% of normal at 40 mm Hg, normalizing cardiac output with plasma expanders failed to improve the diminished renal blood flow and GFR (156).

In addition, ureteral obstruction resulting from extrinsic compression does not appear to play a role in oliguria (269). Placement of ureteral stents during pneumoperitoneum does not improve urine output. Likewise, intraoperative urograms in animals with decreased urine output during pneumoperitoneum confirm the absence of ureteral obstruction (221).

In contrast, changes in renal vein flow do appear to be linked to the oliguria associated with the pneumoperitoneum. To determine the etiology of oliguria, Kirsch and colleagues (221) subjected rats to intraabdominal pressures of 5 and 10 mm Hg. Urine output did not diminish until the pressure reached 10 mm Hg. At that level of pneumoperitoneum, vena caval blood flow decreased 92% and aortic blood flow decreased 46%, leading to the conclusion that the renal effect was due to renal vascular insufficiency from central venous compression. Similarly, McDougall and colleagues (269), using a porcine model, demonstrated a significant decrease in renal vein flow concomitant with a drop in urine output, but only at a pressure of 15 mm Hg or greater. Interestingly, renal vein flow and creatinine clearance remained diminished even after 2 hours of desufflation, although no long-term effects were noted (269). Subsequent animal studies, using MRI to provide a noninvasive evaluation of renal vessel blood flow and parenchymal perfusion, also demonstrated reduced cardiac output, reduced flow velocity in the renal vessels, decreased renal parenchymal perfusion, and a concomitant reduction in urine output. The changes seen in renal perfusion were similar in the cortex and medulla of the kidneys; these findings confirmed that a shunting phenomenon was *not* occurring in the renal parenchymal during the time of the elevated pneumoperitoneum pressure (258).

Although the renal vein compression hypothesis is supported to some extent by the foregoing studies, the most likely mechanism for oliguria during laparoscopy appears to be direct renal parenchymal compression, similar to that seen with a Page kidney. Razvi and associates (351) placed a pressure cuff around canine kidneys subjecting them to pressures of 15 mm Hg. This resulted in a decreased urine output of 63% in the treated kidney along with decreased GFR and reduced effective renal blood flow. As other investigators have observed, even after 2 hours of desufflation, renal blow flow did not return to baseline levels. The control kidney showed no significant changes in urine output or GFR.

From a hormonal standpoint, it is of note that aldosterone has been reported to be elevated during the oliguric period in the animal model, which correlates with the decreased urinary sodium and increased urinary potassium observed (56). It also supports the Page kidney effect as a significant component of the intraoperative oliguria observed during the pneumoperitoneum.

In healthy patients, this acute renal dysfunction appears to completely resolve postoperatively following desufflation; however, there is concern that in patients with preexisting renal disease, these transient changes may become clinically significant. To address this, Cisek and colleagues (59), in an animal model, performed renal reductive surgery to mimic chronic renal insufficiency. After being exposed to intraabdominal pressures of 20 mm Hg for 6 hours, simulating a complex laparoscopic procedure, a dramatic drop in urine output (80%), GFR (63%), and renal blood flow (20%) was noted, which did not return to baseline after 90 minutes of desufflation postprocedure. An increase in the urinary *N*-acetyl-β-D-glucosaminidase (NAG) was observed, as was acute renal failure despite hydration and central venous pressure monitoring (59). However, at 1 week following the insufflation tests, the GFR returned to the baseline, chronic renal failure level, indicating that no long-term effect on the renal function from the acute insufflation was identified, even in the face of preexisting renal insufficiency.

The observed blood flow changes have suggested the possibility of renal tubular damage secondary to ischemia, as a cause of the oliguria associated with pneumoperitoneum. NAG is present in renal tubular cells and is released into the urine in response to tubular cell injury. Micali and colleagues (277) measured preoperative and postoperative NAG levels in 31 patients undergoing laparoscopic surgery compared with 28 patients undergoing conventional open surgery. No differences in NAG were noted between the preoperative and postoperative levels in either of the groups or between the groups. They demonstrated that pneumoperitoneum was not associated with the change in the urinary concentration of NAG. Similarly, there was no correlation between urinary NAG levels and the total operative time. This observation suggests that significant ischemic renal injury is not associated with laparoscopic-related oliguria. This biochemical finding has been confirmed histologically in animal models. In a rat study, after a 5-hour pneumoperitoneum at a pressure of 15 mm Hg, acutely and chronically, no significant histologic differences could be identified when compared with control rat kidneys (232). McDougall and colleagues (269), in the porcine model, also confirmed a lack of histologic abnormality in kidneys rendered oliguric at pressures of 15 mm Hg.

Elevated intraabdominal pressures may also act via stimulation of a variety of systemic hormones, which contribute to the hemodynamic and renal effects. Independent of the type of gas used, excessive intraabdominal pressures (20 mm Hg or greater) are responsible for increasing serum catecholamines (279). Likewise, endothelin, a potent vasoconstrictor, has also been shown to increase in response to renal vein compression and during pneumoperitoneum in animal models. In fact, compression of a unilateral renal vein leads to a decrease in GFR and urine output in both kidneys and is associated with elevated renal vein endothelin concentrations, thus implicating it as a contributing factor to the oliguria observed during long laparoscopic cases (151). In other animal studies, the administration of a vasopressin antagonist improved renal function when compared with control animals, suggesting that the endogenous release of arginine vasopressin also contributes to the oliguria seen with increased abdominal pressures (84).

Methods to improve urine output during pneumoperitoneum, which have included the use of ureteral stents, fluid hydration, and intravenous dopamine infusion, have been unsuccessful in changing urine output. However, altering the temperature of the insufflated CO_2 has been found to partially counteract the hemodynamic and renal effects of increased intraabdominal pressure. A comparison of the use of warm (37°C) versus room temperature CO_2 during prolonged (greater than 90 minutes) laparoscopic surgery demonstrated a higher core temperature, urine output, and cardiac index with warm insufflation, suggesting that local vasodilation in the compressed kidney may restore enough blood flow to maintain GFR and urine output (14).

In conclusion, oliguria is a recognized component of the physiologic effect of increased intraabdominal or retroperitoneal pressure. The etiology is multifactorial, emanating from vascular and parenchymal compression and associated with systemic hormonal effects. Ureteral obstruction does not play a significant role. These changes are pressure dependent and are usually not apparent until pressures reach 15 mm Hg or greater. Likewise, this effect is not associated with any histologic pathology or evidence of renal tubular damage. Following the release of the pneumoperitoneum or pneumoretroperitoneum, the renal function and urine output return to normal with no long-term sequelae, even in patients with preexisting renal disease. It is important for the entire operative team to have an understanding of the physiologic effects of CO_2 insufflation. This will allow appropriate intraoperative monitoring and management and minimize intraoperative and postoperative complications.

Pneumoretroperitoneum

For the most part, gas insufflation into the retroperitoneal or extraperitoneal space has been associated with greater CO_2 absorption and hypercarbia as compared with intraperitoneal insufflation, especially in the presence of subcutaneous emphysema (133,269,448). This, however, is not entirely without controversy. Other animal and human studies have demonstrated the opposite results. In a canine model, Wolf and colleagues (446) noted a higher increase in $Paco_2$ and a greater drop in serum pH in the intraperitoneal insufflation group compared with the extraperitoneal insufflation group. Conversely, risk of thoracic dissection of gas was greater during extraperitoneal insufflation than during intraperitoneal insufflation. Wright and colleagues (453), in a human study, noted a more rapid increase in the $Paco_2$ in the transperitoneal group than the extraperitoneal group, although no significant difference in the overall magnitude of the rise was demonstrated. Nonetheless, regardless of the method of laparoscopy, appropriate ventilatory management, with hyperventilation, usually avoids any adverse sequelae of hypercarbia.

The renal and hemodynamic effects of pneumoretroperitoneum are similar to those seen with a pneumoperitoneum. A unilateral pneumoretroperitoneum leads to elevated systolic and diastolic aortic pressures, although the effect is less than that seen with the pneumoperitoneum (55). In contrast, at 15-mm Hg pressure, the decrease in renal vein flow is similar to that seen with the pneumoperitoneum (269). An elevated retroperitoneal pressure also leads to oliguria, and when maintained for 2 hours, it leads to a gradual decrease in the contralateral kidney perfusion and a concomitant increase in the intraabdominal pressure (55). Likewise, this reduction in urine output is reversible after desufflation and leads to no identifiable pathologic renal abnormalities (269).

SPECIFIC LAPAROSCOPIC PROCEDURES

Laparoscopic access was initially applied within urologic surgery only for diagnostic purposes. Slowly, with advances in technology and skill, the indications for laparoscopic access have evolved such that diagnostic, ablative, and even complex reconstructive procedures are presently performed laparoscopically at academic centers throughout the world. The subsequent section is a comprehensive listing and description of the current state of the art of laparoscopic procedures in urology. The procedures have been stratified into diagnostic, ablative, and reconstructive designations and have been further subdivided into operations for either benign or malignant disease processes. For each procedure, a systematic review of the literature describing the indications, technique(s), efficacy, efficiency, equanimity, and economy is provided.

Benign Disease: Diagnostic Procedures

Renal Biopsy

Renal biopsy is often indispensable in the diagnostic evaluation of various kidney diseases. Since its original description by Iversen and Brun (188), the percutaneous approach has been the preferred procedure for sampling renal tissue for almost half a century. Percutaneous renal biopsy is indicated for patients with occult acute renal failure, nephrotic syndrome in an adult without signs of systemic disease, significant proteinuria, hematuria after urologic studies indicate no specific upper or lower tract causes, or systemic disease with suspected renal involvement (114, 417). Valuable diagnostic and prognostic information can be obtained and treatment tailored to the patient based on biopsy results.

As a result of the efficacy and minimally invasive nature of percutaneous biopsy, biopsy under vision is reserved for patients for whom percutaneous biopsy is either unsuccessful or contraindicated. Percutaneous renal biopsy is sometimes difficult or impossible because of anatomic constraints such as mobility of the kidney, morbid obesity, positioning of the kidney high under the rib cage, spinal deformity, or the presence of impenetrable scar tissue or other organs around the kidney (e.g., a retrorenal colon). Absolute and relative contraindications for percutaneous renal biopsy vary among nephrologists. Reasons for referral for a renal biopsy under direct vision include failure of previous percutaneous biopsy attempts, inadequate tissue sample with the percutaneous biopsy, an uncooperative patient, marked obesity, a solitary functioning kidney, patients of the Jehovah's Witness faith, presence of renal artery aneurysm, calcific arteriosclerosis, or a coagulopathy (30,161,228,371).

Laparoscopic renal biopsy was initially described via a transperitoneal approach (396). Currently, however, the procedure is most commonly performed in a retroperitoneal fashion with the patient in the flank position under general anesthesia. Via a two-port approach, a pneumoretroperitoneum is obtained and the retroperitoneum is dissected bluntly. Renal biopsy is typically obtained with a single stroke of a laparoscopic cup forceps. Hemostasis of the biopsy site is then achieved with electrocautery or argon beam coagulation. The procedure has been described with mean operating room times ranging from 35 (115) to 90 minutes (131).

Diagnostic yield using this technique for laparoscopic renal biopsy has been high. Gaur and colleagues (115) described adequate tissue for diagnosis in 17 of 17 consecutive renal biopsies. Subsequently, other series have recorded 100% diagnostic yield in an additional combined total of 40 patients using either single or multiple biopsies under laparoscopic vision (53,131). These results are better than the reported diagnostic yield with percutaneous biopsy, which ranges from 80% to 95% (30,36,80,206,291).

Complications from laparoscopic renal biopsy have usually been minimal and self-limiting. Gaur and colleagues (115) reported 2 complications in 17 consecutive renal biopsies (12%). One patient required extension of a laparoscopic port site for hemostasis. The other patient had macroscopic hematuria, which resolved spontaneously after 2 days; this patient did not require a blood transfusion (116). In a series of 32 consecutive patients, Gimenez and co-workers (131) reported two complications (6%). An anticoagulated patient experienced postoperative pain, and evaluation revealed a perinephric hematoma. The hematoma resolved without intervention and the patient did not require transfusion. A single postoperative death was reported in this series. In this case, a female patient who underwent an uncomplicated biopsy and was found to have lupus nephritis was treated with high-dose steroids and experienced a perforated gastric ulcer. She was a Jehovah's Witness and refused blood transfusions, which ultimately resulted in her death. In a review of renal biopsy in eight morbidly obese patients, Chen and colleagues (53) reported no complications.

The overall frequency of complications after percutaneous needle biopsy of the kidney has been reported as 5% to 10% (114). In a comparison of percutaneous and open renal biopsies, Bolton and Vaughan (30) describe a 12% (20 of 171) complication rate for percutaneous biopsy and an 11% (11 of 100) complication rate for open renal biopsy. The severity of complications was similar, and transfusion requirements were equal at 3% for both the percutaneous and open renal biopsy group.

Convalescence from laparoscopic renal biopsy is rapid. Although Gimenez and colleagues (131) reported a mean hospital stay of 1.7 days (range 0 to 7 days), others have performed the procedure on an outpatient basis (53). Return to activity has been reported to be less than 2 weeks (116,131). Postoperative analgesic requirements are minimal, ranging from no parenteral medications (131) to an average of 3 mg of morphine (range of 0 to 8 mg) (53). Cost data on laparoscopic renal biopsy have not been published.

Evaluation of the Acute Abdomen: Posttraumatic and Postoperative

Exploratory laparotomy offers the greatest accuracy in the diagnosis of intraabdominal injury, but it is associated with significant morbidity. Laparoscopy may provide diagnostic capabilities equivalent to that of open exploration with less morbidity. Initial reports from the general surgery and gynecologic literature demonstrated the utility of laparoscopy in the diagnosis of the acute abdomen associated with trauma.

Laparoscopy was introduced as an alternative diagnostic modality for the evaluation of patients with abdominal injuries associated with trauma in the late 1970s (24,118). Since these reports, the diagnostic and therapeutic potentials of laparoscopy for the acute abdomen have expanded. Cuesta and colleagues (69) prospectively evaluated 65 patients with laparoscopic evaluation of their acute abdomen (excluding free-air and bowel obstruction) and were able to avoid exploratory laparotomy in 80%. In addition, these patients received smaller, more limited incisions for appropriate open surgical management of any laparoscopically defined problems. In a similar study, Chung and co-workers (58) prospectively evaluated 55 patients with an acute abdomen. They determined the accuracy of laparoscopic diagnosis to be the same as exploratory laparotomy. They managed 62% of patients laparoscopically, and these patients required significantly shorter hospitalization than matched controls treated by open operations. Morbidity was not increased by laparoscopy in patients who required conversion to open operation. The additional cost of the laparoscopic approach was not quantitated.

The urologic community is only beginning to explore the potential applications of laparoscopy in the setting of the acute abdomen. Bauer and colleagues (20) described the successful application of laparoscopic diagnosis and treatment of the acute abdomen in the urologic postoperative setting in three patients. In the first two patients, the laparoscopy revealed misplacement and malfunction of a suprapubic cystotomy tube and a gastrostomy tube, respectively. In the third patient, a large postoperative urinoma was managed by laparoscopic drainage and placement of a retroperitoneal drain and a suprapubic cystotomy tube.

Benign Disease: Ablative

Pelvis: Lymphocelectomy

The development of a lymphocele after surgical dissection was first documented by Mori in 1955 (286). The reported incidence of lymphoceles after pelvic lymphadenectomy for prostate cancer and renal transplant has ranged from 0.5% to 10% and 1% to 15%, respectively (304,310).

Small asymptomatic lymphoceles do not require treatment and may be followed with serial ultrasound evaluations. Spontaneous regression has been well documented, although absorption may take several months. Symptomatic or infected lymphoceles require intervention. Lymphoceles are most frequently symptomatic due to pressure exerted on one or more adjacent structures: the external iliac vein (edema of the lower extremity or venous thrombosis), lymphatics (lower extremity lymphedema), bladder (voiding symptoms), allograft ureter (renal dysfunction and obstruction of the collecting system), and anterior abdominal wall (pain and swelling).

The management of lymphoceles has evolved over the past two decades. Sterile lymphoceles have traditionally been managed by open transperitoneal marsupialization with or without omentoplasty. In 1983, Aronowitz and Kaplan (13) reported the first percutaneous drainage of a postoperative pelvic lymphocele. Lymphocele resolution was noted 3 weeks after insertion of a 9-Fr silastic pigtail catheter. More recently, the addition of sclerosing agents to percutaneous drainage has become increasingly popular. Tetracycline was initially used (270,387). Subsequently, successful management of lymphoceles with povidone-iodine has been described (38,130,413). In 1991, the first laparoscopic lymphocelectomy was performed by McCullough and colleagues (255).

Laparoscopic lymphocelectomy is accomplished via the transabdominal approach, and usually is performed with three trocar sites. After inspection of the abdominal cavity, the bluish-gray bulge of the lymphocele is identified in the pelvis (Fig. 18.12). If the lymphocele is readily identified, needle aspiration may be performed to further confirm the diagnosis. If the lymphocele is not readily apparent, decreasing the pressure of the pneumoperitoneum to 5 mm Hg may allow the lymphocele to appear more prominent. Alternatively, laparoscopic sonographic guidance can be used to identify the lymphocele. Failing this, transabdominal standard sonographic guidance can be used to allow for percutaneous puncture of the lymphocele, which can then be expanded with indigo carmine–stained saline. Occasionally, the location of the bladder relative to the lymphocele may be unclear. If this is the case, the bladder can be distended through the Foley catheter to help identify it relative to the lymphocele; the bladder should then be drained with an indwelling catheter.

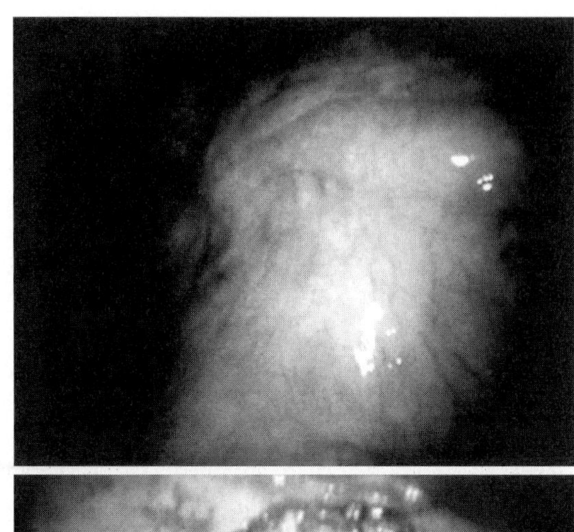
A

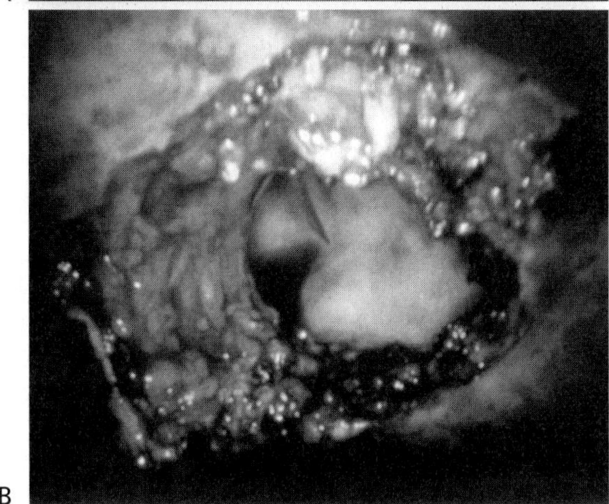
B

FIGURE 18.12. **A:** Laparoscopic inspection revealing the bluish-gray bulge of the lymphocele in the pelvis. **B:** Unroofed lymphocele with percutaneously placed needle visible within. See also Color Figure 18.12.

After confirmation of the lymphocele, using electrocautery scissors a 3- to 4-cm window is excised from the most translucent, thinnest portion of the lymphocele wall. Meticulous hemostasis about the edges of the peritoneal defect is obtained. The laparoscope is advanced into the lymphocele cavity, and intracystic loculations are disrupted by circular motions of the laparoscope. Complete decompression of the lymphocele can be further confirmed with intraoperative transabdominal or laparoscopic ultrasonography. If readily available, a pedicle of omentum may be advanced into the lymphocele cavity and anchored to the cut edge of the lymphocele with titanium clips.

Gill and co-workers (124) compared laparoscopic and open internal marsupialization of pelvic lymphoceles. This retrospective review compared three populations: 12 patients who underwent laparoscopic lymphocelectomy, 13 patients who had open surgery between 1990 and 1993, and 13 patients who had open surgery between 1980 and 1989. Baseline demographics were comparable among these three nonrandomized groups.

No patient managed laparoscopically experienced recurrence of a lymphocele. In contrast, 7 of the 26 patients (27%) managed with open surgery had recurrent lymphoceles. Although laparoscopic management required a longer operative time (177 versus 155 minutes), the patients who were managed laparoscopically had decreased blood loss (23 versus 68 mL), earlier resumption of oral food intake (0.9 versus 2.3 days), and an abbreviated convalescence (2.2 versus 5.6 weeks) (124).

Several other authors have addressed the issue of post–renal transplant lymphoceles and laparoscopic management. Bischof and colleagues (27) reported on 919 kidney transplants that were complicated by 63 (6.8%) symptomatic lymphoceles. Thirty-five of the 63 patients were drained percutaneously, with 47 aspirations (without associated sclerotherapy); 20 lymphoceles were drained by open surgery; and eight lymphoceles were drained laparoscopically. In both surgical groups, six patients each had previously been treated with percutaneous drainage, but reaccumulation of lymph fluid prompted more definitive management. The patients who underwent primary percutaneous drainage experienced local infection in 8 of 47 (17%) cases. One of these patients required open surgery after developing an abscess. Fourteen of 47 (30%) patients had recurrence. There was a single complication in the open surgery population: recurrence of a lymphocele that required a second open procedure. There were no complications and no recurrences in the population undergoing laparoscopic lymphocelectomy. Operative times were not reported. Similar excellent efficacy for laparoscopic lymphocelectomy has been reported by Melvin and co-workers (272) and by Shaver and colleagues (382), with eight and seven patients treated, respectively, without any recurrences.

However, not all reports have demonstrated superior efficacy with laparoscopic drainage. In a series reporting 59 lymphoceles associated with renal transplants, Gruessner and colleagues (142) reported recurrence rates of 48% (13 of 27), 22% (5 of 23), and 33% (3 of 9) for percutaneous, open, and laparoscopic drainage of lymphoceles, respectively. Patients drained laparoscopically had a shorter mean hospital stay than the patients treated with open surgery (3 versus 7 days). Operative time was not reported. Hospital costs for patients undergoing successful laparoscopic drainage were $8,300; for patients with primary open drainage, the costs were $15,680. In 36% (5 of 14), however, there was conversion from laparoscopic to open technique. Hospital cost for this population was $18,550. The only complication reported by the authors was intraoperative bleeding from the right inferior epigastric artery caused by a 5-mm trocar. The injury was repaired without conversion to open surgery (142). On the basis of this series, the authors concluded that posttransplant lymphoceles located lateroposterior and lateroinferior to the renal allograft were technically difficult to access, and may be better managed by open drainage.

Laparoscopic lymphocelectomy has clearly become a viable option for the management of lymphoceles after both renal transplant and pelvic lymphadenectomy. In cases of multiloculated and recurrent lymphoceles, the laparoscopic lymphocelectomy is the procedure of choice, offering patients excellent efficacy, low morbidity, and an expeditious and more comfortable convalescence. Although limited data are available, it appears that laparoscopic management of lymphoceles may have the additional benefit of reduced overall cost.

Pelvis: Varicocelectomy

Normally manifesting in the adolescent period, varicoceles are found in 15% of the male population (369); however, they are described in up to 40% of men seeking treatment for infertility (64). Most men with varicoceles are asymptomatic, but in some cases, patients may have testicular pain or signs of testicular atrophy (140).

Before 1990, clinically significant varicoceles were treated with either surgical ligation or a percutaneous approach using an occlusive transvenous technique under fluoroscopic guidance (414). Surgical ligation of the spermatic veins has been accomplished by an inguinal (187), retroperitoneal (321), or subinguinal approach (248). The laparoscopic varicocelectomy was first described by Sanchez de Badajoz and co-workers (364) and subsequently was developed in the United States by Winfield and Donovan (440).

Laparoscopically, the varicocele is typically managed via a transperitoneal approach. The ipsilateral internal spermatic vessels are identified and the peritoneum is incised laterally. A T-shaped incision is made by incising toward the iliac vessels. Having gained access to the retroperitoneum, the packet of testicular vessels is dissected from the psoas muscle. Testicular traction may be intermittently applied to aid in the identification of the spermatic cord. Dissection of the testicular veins from the testicular artery is then performed. Identification of the testicular artery is aided by intraoperative laparoscopic Doppler sonography or the topical application of 1% lidocaine or papaverine to the spermatic cord. Spermatic veins are isolated, interrupted with clips, and transected. In contrast, other authors have greatly simplified the laparoscopic varicocelectomy by proceeding to secure and divide both the testicular veins and the testicular artery. Interestingly, the positive impact on fertility has been similar with either approach.

Several studies have compared the results of the different modalities for management of varicoceles. Trials comparing the results of sclerotherapy, open varicocelectomy, and laparoscopic varicocelectomy are presented in Table 18.2. Abdulmaaboud and colleagues (3) retrospectively compared 301 patients with 417 varicoceles undergoing treatment with open surgery (131 cases), percutaneous retrograde sclerotherapy (163 cases), or laparoscopic varicocelectomy (123 cases). All three modalities were equally efficacious with regard to recurrence rate and improvement in semen parameters postoperatively. Specifically, the recurrence rates with open, percutaneous sclerotherapy, and laparoscopic treatment were 10.5%, 11.2%, and 9.1%, respectively. Comparison of semen parameters before and after treatment showed significant and equal increases in density and motility, as well as a significant reduction in abnormal forms in all groups. There was no significant difference in pregnancy rates with open surgery, sclerotherapy, and laparoscopy (37%, 41%, and 39%, respectively) (3).

However, the efficacy of percutaneous sclerotherapy is often overestimated; in the Adulmaaboud and colleagues (3) series, 26% of patients failed attempted percutaneous sclerotherapy due to technical difficulties. Problems resulting in failure of percutaneous management included perforation of the spermatic vein (4.3%), abnormal anatomy (10.4%), or spasm of the spermatic vein with failed catheterization (11.6%). If technical failures are included, the efficacy of percutaneous sclerotherapy decreases to 66%. This reported technical failure rate is consistent with most contemporary reports. In addition, although the overall success rate with left-sided varicoceles was 83%, the success rate with right-sided varicoceles was only 51% (3). Minor complications were associated with sclerotherapy; these included a groin hematoma, three femoral artery punctures, and minor contrast media reactions in seven patients. There were no operative complications reported in patients undergoing open or laparoscopic varicocele repair.

Sclerotherapy was carried out as an outpatient procedure performed under local anesthesia. Open surgery used a retroperitoneal approach and was performed with regional anesthesia in most cases, and laparoscopy was done under general anesthesia. Operative time for open surgery was significantly shorter than either sclerotherapy or laparoscopy. Open surgery required an average of only 22 minutes compared with 59 minutes and 35 minutes for management by sclerotherapy and laparoscopy, respectively. Patients undergoing sclerotherapy typically returned to normal activity within 1 day, significantly faster than the other management modalities. The open group experienced a significantly longer convalescence (8 days) than the laparoscopic group (3 days). Although not quantitated, the cost of sclerotherapy was reported to be one-fifth to one-fourth the cost of open surgery, and the cost of laparoscopy was approximately double that of open surgery (3).

In another large series, the relative merits of open and laparoscopic varicocele repair were prospectively evaluated by Mandressi and co-workers (247). Comparison of 120 patients managed by open surgery using Palomo's retroperitoneal technique with 160 patients who underwent laparoscopic repair revealed equal efficacy regarding both recurrence and improvement in semen parameters. Recurrence

TABLE 18.2. VARICOCELECTOMY—COMPARATIVE TRIALS

Source	Indications	Technique	No.	Complications		OR Time (min)	Analgesics	Length of Stay	Full Recovery (days)	Cost	Failure Rate	Follow-up Period	Pregnancy Rate
				Minor	Major								
Abdulmaaboud et al. (3)	Infertility/pain	Open retroper	131	7.60%	None	22	NA	Outpatient	8	1X	11.20%	13 months	36.6%
		Sclerotherapy	163	6.70%	None	59	NA	Outpatient	1	0.2X	36.90%	12 months	41.4%
		Lap transper	123	4.90%	None	35	NA	Outpatient	3	2X	9.10%	12.5 months	39.1%
Winfield and Donovan (440)	Infertility	Lap transper	15	NA	NA	82.3	13.7 tab Tylenol No. 3	Outpatient	4.9	NA	0%	NA	NA
		Lap transper lift	7	NA	NA	170	22.5 tab Tylenol No. 3	Outpatient	6.6	NA	0%	NA	NA
		Open subinguinal	19	NA	NA	35.6	10.9 tab Tylenol No. 3	Outpatient	5.1	NA	0%	NA	NA
Mandressi et al. (247)	Infertility/pain	Open retroper	120	0.60%	None	21	26% required	3.2 days	11	$1,128	6.70%	NA	NA
		Lap transper	160	7.50%	None	32.1	6% required	2.1 days	5	$1,810	3.10%	NA	NA
Nickel et al. (305)	Infertility	Open subinguinal	27	NA	NA	38.8	9.2 tab Tylenol No. 3	Outpatient	4.2	NA	NA	NA	NA
		Open retroper	28	NA	NA	44.1	7.5 tab Tylenol No. 3	Outpatient	3.4	NA	NA	NA	NA
		Lap transper	14	NA	NA	118	8.4 tab Tylenol No. 3	Outpatient	3.4	NA	NA	NA	NA
Totals—laparoscopic			**319**	**6.40%**	**None**	**42.4 min**			**4.06**	**$1,810**	**5.70%**		
Totals—open			**325**	**4.20%**	**None**	**25.4 min**			**8.2**	**$1,128**	**9%**		
Totals—sclerotherapy			**163**	**6.70%**	**None**	**25.4 min**			**1**	**NA**	**36.90%**		

Note: "X" in the Cost column means that the author's institution does not permit publication of cost. Open surgery was therefore assigned an arbitrary value (X), and the other values are arbitrary.
All columns list mean values.
Lap, laparoscopic; NA, not available; retroper, retroperitoneal; transper, transperitoneal.

rates of 6.7% (8 of 120) and 3.1% (5 of 160) were reported for the open and laparoscopic groups, respectively. Both populations manifested significant and equal improvement in postoperative semen parameters, including volume, sperm count, motility, and morphology. Pregnancy rates were not reported.

The mean total operative time for the laparoscopic group was 32 minutes, which was significantly longer than the open population, which had a mean operative time of 21 minutes. There were no intraoperative complications in either group. Minor postoperative complications occurred in 0.6% and 7.5% of the laparoscopic and open surgery groups, respectively. The only complication in the laparoscopic group was a case of shoulder pain that resolved spontaneously over 3 days. In the surgical group, two hydroceles (1.6%) and seven wound infections (5.8%) were recorded. The number of patients requiring postoperative analgesia was significantly higher in the surgical group. Only 6% of patients in the laparoscopic group required pain medications, whereas 26% of patients managed by open surgical venous ligation required pain medicines (247).

Hospital stay was significantly shorter for patients undergoing laparoscopic versus open varicocelectomy (2.1 days versus 3.2 days, respectively). On average, patients treated laparoscopically returned to normal preoperative activity within 5 days, whereas the patients treated surgically required 11 days. Overall costs were significantly more expensive for the laparoscopic than for the open procedure: $1,810 versus $1,130.

In contrast to a retroperitoneal open approach (i.e., Palomo technique), the subinguinal repair of a varicocele is thought to be less invasive and potentially less morbid. In this regard, Hirsch and colleagues (168) prospectively reported a comparison of open subinguinal and laparoscopic varicocele repair. Seventeen patients undergoing laparoscopic varicocele repair were compared with nineteen patients managed with the open subinguinal approach. Recurrence rates and changes in semen parameters were not reported. Average operating time was significantly longer for the laparoscopic group than for the open group (82 versus 36 minutes).

There were two reported complications in the open group: a minor wound infection and a subcutaneous hematoma. Both resolved promptly with conservative management. In the group treated laparoscopically, two patients failed laparoscopic management due to technical difficulties. In addition, two of the remaining 15 laparoscopically managed patients experienced complications that required overnight admission. One patient was observed after repair of laparoscopic trocar injury to the inferior epigastric vein. A second patient experienced nausea necessitating overnight observation (168).

All subinguinal cases were performed under local anesthesia with sedation; the laparoscopic group received general anesthesia. Postoperative analgesic requirements and convalescence were not significantly different for either management modality (168). Cost analysis was not performed in this study.

Nickel and colleagues (305) compared results of inguinal and subinguinal bilateral varicocele repairs with a published series of laparoscopic bilateral varicocele repairs. Twenty-seven patients underwent bilateral subinguinal repairs, and 28 patients underwent bilateral inguinal repairs. Results were compared with 14 patients undergoing laparoscopic bilateral varicocele repairs. Mean operative times for subinguinal, inguinal, and laparoscopic repairs were 39, 44, and 118 minutes, respectively. Pain medication was reported in number of pills of Tylenol with Codeine No. 3. Mean number of pills for subinguinal, inguinal, and laparoscopic bilateral repairs were 9.2, 7.5, and 8.4 pills, respectively. Mean time for return to work for the three groups was 4.2, 3.4, and 3.4 days, respectively. No advantage was noted for the laparoscopic approach.

To date, there does not exist a prospective, randomized trial comparing the efficacy of different modalities for varicocele repair regarding improvement in semen parameters or pregnancy rate. It seems clear, however, that percutaneous sclerotherapy provides an inexpensive, least invasive, and cost-effective first-line solution to the problem of a left varicocele. For those patients who do not respond to sclerotherapy, the next most reasonable option would appear to be a subinguinal open approach. Laparoscopic varicocelectomy, although feasible and safe, remains more costly and less efficient than either of the other two approaches; its use should be reserved for the rare patients in whom the percutaneous or subinguinal approach fails or when another laparoscopic procedure is to be accomplished concomitantly. Although only limited data are available, it appears that even when bilateral varicocele repair is required, laparoscopy should still not be the first line of therapy; indeed, in these patients, the subinguinal approach requires less operative time and results in equal postoperative discomfort and an equally expeditious convalescence.

Retroperitoneum: Adrenalectomy

Laparoscopic adrenalectomy was introduced by Gagner and colleagues (110) in 1992. Subsequent advances in minimally invasive surgery have allowed laparoscopy to become the technique of choice for management of the majority of surgical diseases of the adrenal gland. Indications for adrenalectomy include aldosteronoma, pheochromocytoma, adrenal cysts, adrenal myelolipoma, Cushing's disease, and Cushing's adenoma.

Although initially described as a transperitoneal approach, laparoscopic adrenalectomy can currently be performed using either a transperitoneal or retroperitoneal technique. The transperitoneal approach is performed with the patient in the flank position. Typically, for a right adrenal lesion, after achieving a pneumoperitoneum and placing four subcostal ports, a transverse incision is made in the posterior parietal peritoneum (i.e., hepatic posterior coronary ligament) parallel to and just below the inferior edge of the liver. The incision extends from the line of Toldt, laterally, to the inferior vena cava, medially. Dissection begins between the medial border of the adrenal gland and the lateral border of the vena cava (Fig. 18.13); Gerota's fascia is incised and the main adrenal vein is identified and secured with three clips. The adrenal vein is then divided, leaving two clips on the caval side. Superiorly, the gland is dissected free from the diaphragm, where the diminutive inferior phrenic tributaries to the adrenal are encountered and secured with electrocautery. Next, the inferior portion of the dissection is completed, staying well away from the renal hilum. Last, the gland is freed laterally, following which it is placed in a laparoscopic sack and removed. For much of the periadrenal dissection through the perirenal fat, the harmonic scalpel can be helpful.

Left transperitoneal adrenalectomy requires mobilization of the spleen and the splenic flexure of the descending colon; dissection of the latter also allows safe medial displacement of the tail of the pancreas. An incision in the peritoneum is made along the line of Toldt extending from the diaphragm caudal, past the splenic flexure of the descending colon; in doing this, any connections between the spleen and diaphragm are released (i.e., splenophrenic ligaments). A counterincision is then made perpendicular to the line of Toldt at the inferior border of the spleen; with this T-shaped incision, the splenic flexure of the colon is mobilized as the lienocolic ligament is secured and divided. Next, the kidney is further separated from the spleen by incising the lienorenal ligament. Occasionally, for a large adrenal mass, the tail of the pancreas must be identified and mobilized off the anterior surface of the adrenal gland.

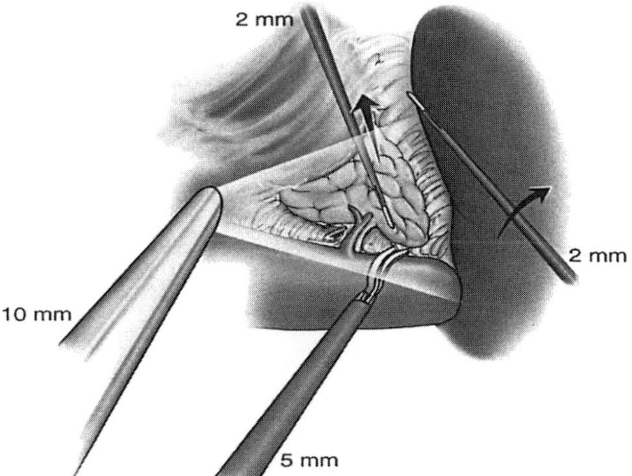

FIGURE 18.13. After incision of Gerota's fascia, the main adrenal vein is identified. (Reprinted from Spencer JR, O'Conor VJ Jr. Comparison of procedures for stress urinary incontinence. *AUA Update Series* 1987;18:259, with permission.)

At this time, the left renal vein may or may not be visible; if it is not, it may be necessary to trace the gonadal vein upward to identify its juncture with the left renal vein. In doing this, the anterior part of Gerota's fascia is incised. Dissection of the anterior and superior portions of the left renal vein allows identification of the left adrenal vein; it is secured with four vascular clips and divided. The medial dissection is then performed with any of the diminutive aortic branches to the adrenal gland being electrocoagulated. The gland is then freed laterally from the medial surface of the kidney. The specimen is placed into a laparoscopic entrapment sack for extraction.

Access for retroperitoneal laparoscopic adrenalectomy is gained via a 2-cm muscle-splitting incision in the midaxillary line just caudal to the tip of the twelfth rib. Balloon or blunt dilation is used to create a working space, and insufflation to 12 mm Hg is performed. A second trocar is placed on the vertebral side of the first trocar. The peritoneum is mobilized medially, allowing for placement of a third trocar on the medial side of the first trocar. Gerota's fascia is opened, exposing the adrenal gland. At times, a laparoscopic ultrasound unit is helpful to demarcate the location of the adrenal gland, especially in patients with Cushing's disease. The gland is dissected circumferentially. The adrenal vein is clipped and divided during the final phase of the dissection. The specimen is then placed in an entrapment sack and removed.

Although a prospective study comparing the merits of laparoscopic and open adrenalectomy has not been performed, a number of authors have retrospectively compared these modalities. Trials comparing the results of open and laparoscopic adrenalectomies are presented in Table 18.3. In the following few paragraphs, studies have been selected in which transperitoneal open and laparoscopic, retroperitoneal open and laparoscopic, and transperitoneal laparoscopic versus open retroperitoneal approaches have been compared. In each comparison, the advantages of laparoscopy are apparent.

Guazzoni and co-workers (143) compared 20 transperitoneal laparoscopic and 20 open (both transperitoneal and retroperitoneal) adrenalectomies in the management of benign hyperfunctioning adrenal tumors. There were no conversions to open procedures. There was no significant difference in operative times noted, with laparoscopic and open adrenalectomies requiring 2.8 and 2.4 hours for completion, respectively (143). Estimated blood loss was significantly lower in the laparoscopic population at 100 versus 450 mL. Complications were encountered significantly more frequently in the open group (two patients experienced pneumothorax, two patients experienced wound infections, three patients required transfusion, two patients experienced postoperative ileus, and two patients had postoperative fevers greater than 38°C). In the laparoscopic group there was only one complication, a port site wound infection (143). Postoperatively, the patients

TABLE 18.3. ADRENALECTOMY—COMPARATIVE TRIALS

Source	Indications	Technique	Number	Complications: Minor	Complications: Major	EBL (mL)	OR Time (hr)	Analgesics	Hospital Stay	Full Recovery	Cost
Aldrighetti et al. (7)	Incidental	Open	12	2/12 (17%)	2/12 (17%)	NA	2.9	3 days	7.9 days	NA	NA
		Lap/transper	8	2/8 (25%)	0	NA	2.5	1.7 days	3.5 days	NA	NA
Bonjer et al. (31)	<7 cm	Open	30	8/30 (27%)	0	125	1	3.0 days	7.0 days	NA	NA
		Lap/retroper	42	3/42 (7%)	0	20	1.5	1.0 days	4.0 days	NA	NA
Brunt et al. (37)	All benign lesions, <8 cm	Open/transper	25	16/25 (64%)	3/25 (12%)	408	2.4	142 mg morphine	8.7 days	NA	$16,972
		Open/retroper	17	9/17 (53%)	0	366	2.3	54 mg morphine	6.2 days	NA	$12,266
		Lap/transper	24	4/24 (16.7%)	0	104	3.1	15.9 mg morphine	3.2 days	10.6 days	$13,184
Guazzoni et al. (143)	Benign hyperfunctioning	Open	20	7/20 (35%)	4/20 (20%)	450	2.4	320 mg ketoprofen	9 days	16 days	NA
		Lap/transper	20	0	1/20 (5%)	100	2.8	175 mg ketoprofen	3.4 days	9.7 days	NA
Jacobs et al. (190)	All benign lesions	Open	19	6/19 (32%)	0	263	2.5	NA	5.1 days	NA	$13,720
		Lap/transper	19	1/19 (5%)	0	109	2.7	NA	2.3 days	NA	$10,929
Linos et al. (240)	All lesions (<6 cm)	Open/transper	86	1/86 (1.2%)	4/86 (4.7%)	NA	2.6	3.4 days	8.0 days	NA	$2,724
		Open/retroper	61	5/61 (8.2%)	0	NA	1.8	2.3 days	4.5 days	NA	together
		Lap/transper	18	0	0	NA	1.9	1.1 days	2.3 days	NA	$2,920
MacGillivray et al. (246)	All lesions	Open	12	2/12 (16.7%)	3/12 (25%)	NA	2.8	NA	7.9 days	11.6 days	NA
		Lap/transper	14	3/14 (21.4%)	0	NA	4.3	NA	3.0 days	7.6 days	NA
Naito et al. (294)	<4 cm	Open	11	1/11 (9%)	0	150	2.8	11/11 (100%) needed	9.0 days	NA	NA
		Lap/transper	6	1/6 (16.7%)	1/6 (16.7%)	200	3.8	1/6 (16.7%) needed	9.0 days	NA	NA
Printz (341)	<10 cm	Open/transper	11	NA	NA	391	2.9	1002 mg meperidine	6.4 days	NA	NA
		Open/retroper	13	NA	NA	288	2.3	801 mg meperidine	5.5 days	NA	NA
		Lap/transper	10	NA	NA	228 (ant. only)	3.5	93 mg meperidine	2.1 days	NA	NA
Shen et al. (384)	Hyperaldosteronism	Open	38	2/38 (5.3%)	2/38 (5.3%)	NA	NA	NA	NA	NA	NA
		Lap	42	0	0	NA	NA	NA	NA	NA	NA
Staren et al. (397)	All lesions	Open	20	NA	NA	NA	3	NA	6.1 days	NA	NA
		Lap/both	21	NA	NA	NA	3.4	NA	2.2 days	NA	NA
Thompson et al. (415)	All lesions	Open/retroper	50	5/50 (10%)	0	NA	2.8	48 mg morphine	5.7 days	7.0 wk	$6,000
		Lap/transper	54	17/54 (32%)	0	NA	2.1	28 mg morphine	3.1 days	3.8 wk	$7,000
Winfield et al. (444)	<6 cm and nonmalignant	Open	17	3/17 (17.6%)	0	266	2.3	28.8 mg morphine	6.2 days	6.5 wk	NA
		Lap/transper	20	9/20 (45%)	2/20 (10%)	183	3.7	14.8 mg morphine	2.7 days	3.1 wk	NA
Yoshimura et al. (457)	All lesions	Open	25	2/25 (8%)	0	345	2.2	3.4 doses	18.0 days	NA	NA
		Lap/both	28	8/28 (28.6%)	0	370	6.2	2.7 doses	12.0 days	NA	NA
Totals											
Laparoscopic			326	16%	1.40%	94 mL	3 hr		3.5 days	18.3 days	$8,301
Open			467	16%	4.20%	303 mL	2.4 hr		6.0 days	37.2 days	$6,152

All columns list mean values.
Both, transperitoneal and retroperitoneal approaches combined; EBL, estimated blood loss; lap, laparoscopic; NA, not available; retroper, retroperitoneal; transper, transperitoneal.

treated laparoscopically experienced significantly less pain: 175 mg of ketoprofen compared with 320 mg of ketoprofen. Length of hospital stay and convalescence were also significantly shorter for patients treated laparoscopically: 3.4 days versus 9 days and 9.7 days versus 16 days, respectively (143).

Thompson and colleagues (415) retrospectively compared 50 patients managed with open retroperitoneal adrenalectomy to 54 patients managed by transperitoneal laparoscopic technique. Seven patients in this series required conversion to open adrenalectomy. However, experience significantly affected the conversion rate; the conversion rate of 12% in the first 11 patients was reduced to 4.5% in the last 43 patients. Operative times were 40 minutes less for patients managed via the open approach: 2.1 versus 2.8 hours. Complications in the laparoscopic group occurred in 10% versus 18% in the open group. Most interestingly, these authors also sought to document the incidence of late complications. Late complications in the open group occurred in 54% of patients, including chronic pain at the wound site, severe laxity of the abdominal wall musculature, and bothersome flank numbness. In contrast, no late complications occurred in patients managed laparoscopically. The laparoscopic approach tended to be more expensive than the open approach: $7,000 versus $6,000.

Adrenal tumors less than 7 cm in diameter managed with either open retroperitoneal or laparoscopic retroperitoneal technique were retrospectively compared by Bonjer and colleagues (32). Forty-two laparoscopic adrenalectomies were compared with thirty open procedures. Two laparoscopic adrenalectomies required conversion to open surgery. Complications were significantly less in the laparoscopic population, 7% versus 27% (32). Mean operative times were 30 minutes longer for the laparoscopic group (1.5 versus 1.0 hours). However, the laparoscopic group experienced significantly less discomfort, requiring an average of only 1 day as opposed to 3 days of pain medication. Hospital stay for the laparoscopic group was also significantly shorter: 4 days versus 7 days (32).

Whereas most authors have sought to compare open to laparoscopic techniques, Takada and associates (410) compared the two types of laparoscopic approaches to each other: transperitoneal (27 cases) versus retroperitoneal (11 cases). In four cases (36%), laparoscopic retroperitoneal exploration was converted to transperitoneal adrenalectomy because of difficulty during the retroperitoneal exploration in three cases and secondary to a pancreatic injury in one case. In contrast, with the transperitoneal approach, there were no conversions. Mean operative time for retroperitoneal adrenalectomy was 4.1 hours, which was not significantly longer than the 3.9 hours required for transperitoneal laparoscopic adrenalectomy (410). Similarly, there was no difference in time to oral intake and time to ambulation. However, the complications and length of stay associated with each technique were not reported.

Overall, the laparoscopic transperitoneal approach is preferred by some authors for left adrenalectomy and the retroperitoneal approach is preferred for the right adrenal due to the posterior insertion of the right adrenal vein into the inferior vena cava. Also, some authors prefer a transperitoneal approach in cases of Cushing's syndrome due to the large amount of fatty tissue surrounding the adrenal gland that can greatly impede a retroperitoneal dissection.

Of all the indications for adrenalectomy, none is more challenging than pheochromocytoma given its potential to cause a hypertensive crisis and volume-related problems. A drawback to the laparoscopic approach is that it precludes thorough exploration of the para-aortic region and the contralateral adrenal gland. However, scintigraphy with ^{131}I-meta-iodobenzylguanidine, CT scanning, and MRI of the abdomen are capable of localizing pheochromocytomas very precisely, thereby, in many centers, precluding the need for additional surgical exploration. Bonjer and co-workers (32) reported successful laparoscopic management of eight pheochromocytomas. In this series, intraoperative systolic blood pressure did not exceed 180 mm Hg, heart rate remained below 140 beats per minute, and cardiac arrhythmias were not encountered. Similarly, Gagner and co-workers (109) reported on 17 patients who had 23 pheochromocytomas; 6 patients had bilateral tumors. All cases were completed laparoscopically. Unilateral adrenalectomy required an average of 3.8 hours and bilateral cases required 6.3 hours for completion. Hypertensive crises with systolic blood pressures greater than 200 mm Hg or diastolic pressure greater than 100 mm Hg occurred in nine patients, and all were well controlled pharmacologically. Hypotension, defined as systolic blood pressure less than 80 mm Hg, occurred at induction or after venous clamping in three bilateral and six unilateral cases and was corrected with volume expansion or pressor agents (109). These findings are consistent with recent recommendations from The Cleveland Clinic demonstrating good blood pressure control in patients with pheochromocytomas with hydration and calcium channel blockers, thus obviating the use of α-blockers for a prolonged period preoperatively (424). Only 4 of 17 patients (24%) required continued antihypertensive medications postoperatively. Complications were noted in 6% of patients.

When all of the series are reviewed it becomes apparent that the laparoscopic approach, whether retroperitoneal or transperitoneal, provides the following benefits: less blood loss, less need for analgesics, shorter hospital stay, and more rapid convalescence. When comparing the laparoscopic transperitoneal and retroperitoneal approaches for adrenalectomy, no significant differences have been reported. In sum, at this time, the laparoscopic adrenalectomy, like cholecystectomy, has largely supplanted open surgery for adrenal disease.

Retroperitoneum: Renal Cyst Decortication—Simple Peripheral Cyst

Simple renal cysts are common incidental findings. They occur in at least 24% of all individuals older than 40 years of age and in 50% of individuals older than 50 years of age who are evaluated with abdominal CT scans performed for nonurologic indications (230). Simple cysts only rarely are discovered due to clinical manifestations. However, flank pain, abdominal pain, hematuria, recurrent infection, hypertension, and obstructive uropathy alone or in combination are the most common reasons that simple cysts require intervention (10).

Historically, open decortication was the treatment modality of choice for a symptomatic renal cyst. Although highly efficacious for eliminating cysts, one-third of patients undergoing open surgical management experienced perioperative complications, including wound infections, urinary retention, atelectasis, pneumonia, and venous thrombosis (227). Open surgical management is also associated with significant postoperative pain from the flank or abdominal wound and a postoperative convalescence of 1 month or more.

The advent of minimally invasive urologic technologies engendered less invasive techniques for the management of renal cysts. Alternative techniques for ablation of renal cysts include percutaneous cyst aspiration with sclerosis, retrograde endoscopic cyst incision with marsupialization, and percutaneous resection with fulguration (172,178,210). The least invasive of these options is cyst aspiration with sclerosis. This is an easily performed procedure done with local anesthesia on an outpatient basis with a low morbidity rate. Sclerosis of the cyst can be performed with a number of agents: bismuth phosphate, isophendylate, ethanol, and autologous blood. Reports of aspiration and sclerosis have demonstrated varying degrees of success.

Holmberg and Hietala (172), using sclerotherapy with bismuth phosphate, reported elimination of 10% of cysts and decrease in the size of another 36% at 3 years follow-up among 54 cysts. Complications included eight (15%) patients with postprocedure pain, two patients (4%) with perirenal hematomas not requiring transfusion, and five patients (9%) with fever for 1or 2 days (172). Liatsikos and colleagues (239) reported a series of 24 patients with large symptomatic renal cysts. Treatment consisted of aspiration under ultrasound guidance and sclerosis with alcohol and tetracycline. Two patients experienced mild pain with alcohol injection, but the procedure was successfully completed. One patient reported severe pain with tetracycline injection necessitating termination of the procedure. This patient underwent surgical unroofing of the cyst 3 weeks later. With a mean follow-up period of 20 months, all patients remained asymptomatic. Follow-up ultrasound evaluations revealed resolution in 11 of 24 (46%) and small residual cyst cavities in 12 of 24 (50%). There were no complications in this series.

Aspiration and sclerosis should be the primary form of intervention for symptomatic renal cysts. It should be noted, however, that cyst puncture cytology has been shown to be only 80% to 85% sensitive in diagnosing renal malignancy (359,416); however, in the face of a Bosniak 1–type cyst with the aspiration of clear fluid and a negative cytology, the cyst is invariably benign.

Laparoscopic renal cyst ablation has been described using both transperitoneal and retroperitoneal approaches; it has been used as both a primary and secondary modality for cyst therapy, but as previously stated, it should be most commonly used only when percutaneous aspiration and sclerosis fails in the treatment of a documented, symptomatic benign cyst. The transperitoneal approach is performed with the patient in the lateral decubitus position. If the cyst is in close proximity to the renal collecting system, a ureteral catheter may be placed before laparoscopy to facilitate identification of the ureter and renal pelvis. Typically the procedure can be performed with three trocar sites: umbilical, below the costal margin in the midclavicular line, and infraumbilical in the midclavicular line. The line of Toldt is incised and the colon reflected medially to expose the kidney. The cyst is typically readily identified as a bulge in Gerota's fascia. The fascia and perirenal fat are dissected off of the cyst. The outer cyst wall is then excised and sent for histopathology. The cyst base is then carefully inspected; any mural nodule or lesion is biopsied at this time and sent for frozen section. If the cyst is peripheral and not in close contact with the collecting system, the argon beam coagulator can then be used to fulgurate the base of the cyst.

The laparoscopic retroperitoneal approach is performed with the patient in the lateral decubitus position. Access just behind the tip of the twelfth rib is performed with either balloon dilation or digital dissection of the retroperitoneal space. Two additional trocars are placed: one anterior and slightly superior and one inferior and slightly posterior to the original access site. Incision of Gerota's fascia and blunt dissection of the perirenal fat are performed to expose the cyst. As with the transperitoneal approach, a segment of the cyst wall is excised and the base of the cyst is treated in the same manner.

Jahnsen and Solhaug (191) first described laparoscopic management of the symptomatic renal cyst. Rubenstein and colleagues (359) subsequently reported a series of ten patients with symptomatic renal cysts that were managed laparoscopically. Six patients had simple cysts, two patients had polycystic renal disease, and there was a single case each of a peripelvic cyst and multiple simple cysts. The indication for surgery in all ten patients was chronic pain; six patients had undergone prior needle aspiration of their cyst. Two patients, both of whom had undergone a negative preoperative aspiration, were discovered to have renal malignancies at the time of surgery, and both underwent radical nephrectomy. The eight remaining patients were all asymptomatic without radiographic evidence of cyst recurrence at a mean follow-up of 10 months. Operative times ranged from 50 minutes to 4 hours (mean of 2 hours, 27 minutes), including one patient who underwent radical nephrectomy under the same anesthesia. There were no intraoperative complications and only two postoperative complications. Six patients did not require any postoperative parenteral narcotics. Median postoperative parenteral narcotic requirement was two tablets. Seven patients were discharged from the hospital on postoperative day 1, and overall mean hospital stay was 2.2 days. The mean interval to resumption of normal activity was 9 days. There were no long-term complications at a mean follow-up of 10 months (359).

Rassweiler and colleagues (347) reported experience with retroperitoneal management of 50 renal cysts. This report incorporated patients with septated or suspicious cysts, large simple cysts after failure of percutaneous aspiration and sclerotherapy, multiple renal cysts with deterioration of renal function, and simple hilar cysts that obstructed the collecting system. Operative time ranged from 30 to 130 minutes (mean of 80 minutes), and average hospital stay was 5.4 days. Mean opiate dose was 1.2 doses per patient. There were two (4%) complications, including one retroperitoneal hematoma requiring transfusion (347).

All of these studies suffer from the same problem: lack of long-term (i.e., longer than 1 year) objective follow-up and a uniform patient population. In this regard, because follow-up data are largely unavailable, no valid statements can be made regarding the need to fulgurate the base of the cyst, whether a transperitoneal or retroperitoneal approach is preferable, or whether it is necessary to place fat or omentum into the cyst cavity to prevent a recurrence.

Simple cysts are common and rarely have clinical manifestations. Although laparoscopic simple cyst decortication is feasible, safe, and effective, this type of intervention is rarely required. Initial management of symptomatic cysts should include aspiration and sclerosis for two reasons. First, this will largely preclude the unwelcome "surprise" of a renal cell cancer. Second, many simple cysts will respond well to sclerotherapy, thereby avoiding a more invasive, albeit laparoscopic procedure. As such, laparoscopic simple cyst decortication should be reserved for those patients who continue to suffer symptoms when percutaneous sclerotherapy fails.

Retroperitoneum: Simple Nephrectomy

Gustav Simon from the Medical School of Heidelberg University performed the first successful open nephrectomy in 1869. Despite technical modifications, this open surgical procedure remained essentially unchanged until the first laparoscopic total nephrectomy was performed by Clayman and colleagues in 1990 (61). The indications for simple laparoscopic nephrectomy parallel those of open nephrectomy and include any benign renal pathology resulting in sepsis, bleeding, pain, compression of surrounding structures, or hypertension that is difficult to control medically. Certain conditions, such as xanthogranulomatous pyelonephritis (XGP) or nephrectomy in patients with autosomal-dominant polycystic kidney disease (ADPKD), require special consideration (see sections on XGP and ADPKD).

Laparoscopic simple nephrectomy has been performed using either a transperitoneal or retroperitoneal technique (144). The transperitoneal procedure is performed in the lateral decubitus position. Twelve-millimeter trocars are placed at the umbilicus, in the midclavicular line under the costal margin, and 3 cm inferior to the umbilicus in the midclavicular line. Two additional 5-mm trocars are placed in the anterior axillary line at the tip of the twelfth rib and at the level of the umbilicus. Recent modifications have included elimination of one or both of the 5-mm trocars and reduction of one of the 12-mm trocars to 5 mm. At times, on the right side, an additional 5-mm trocar is placed just beneath the xiphoid process to aid in retraction of the liver during the hilar dissection.

Using monopolar electrosurgical scissors, the surgeon incises the line of Toldt from the hepatic or splenic flexure caudal across the iliac vessels until the ureter is identified. The ureter is dissected from surrounding tissues up to the level of the kidney. Gerota's fascia is entered and the dissection is continued on the renal capsule until the entire kidney has been freed from the perirenal fat (Fig. 18.14). The kidney can be retracted laterally and the renal hilum exposed. The renal vessels are carefully dissected. The renal artery is clipped five times and cut between the second and third clips (leaving two clips on the side of the specimen). Attention is then turned to the renal vein; it is secured with an Endo-GIA vascular stapler. The ureter is secured with four clips and divided; the kidney is then freed from any remaining retroperitoneal attachments. The specimen is then placed in an endoscopic sack and either morcellated with forceps or, after enlarging one of the port sites, the specimen can be removed intact.

Access for retroperitoneal simple nephrectomy is gained by a 2-cm incision just posterior to the tip of the twelfth rib. After balloon or blunt digital dissection of the retroperitoneum around Gerota's fascia, a Hasson cannula is placed. Three additional trocars are placed: a 5-mm posterior trocar, located at the angle of the twelfth rib and the erector spinae muscle; a 5- or 12-mm trocar in the midaxillary line, 2 cm cephalad to the iliac crest; and a 5-mm trocar subcostal in the anterior axillary line, thereby describing a T configuration for the four ports. Attention is first directed to the renal hilum, and the renal artery and vein are sequentially controlled with clip ligation and the vascular Endo-GIA stapler, respectively. Gerota's fascia is incised and the kidney is dissected from the perirenal fat. The ureter is dissected

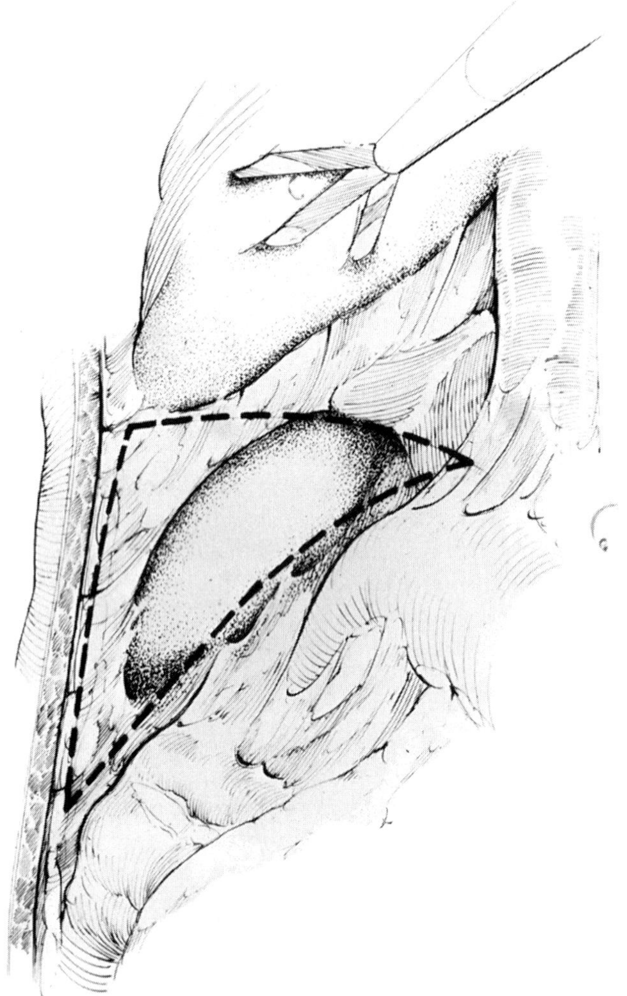

FIGURE 18.14. Dissection template for simple laparoscopic right transperitoneal nephrectomy.

from the surrounding tissues, clipped, and cut. The specimen may then be entrapped and morcellated.

Results of trials comparing open and laparoscopic simple nephrectomy are presented in Table 18.4. Parra and coworkers (323) compared 12 patients undergoing laparoscopic transperitoneal nephrectomy for benign renal disease with 13 patients managed with a traditional flank incision. All laparoscopic procedures were performed via a transperitoneal approach. One patient in the laparoscopic group required conversion to open surgery after injury to a lower pole artery with minimal blood loss. A second patient in the laparoscopic group experienced a bowel injury that was repaired laparoscopically. Both patients had had previous open abdominal surgery. There were no intraoperative complications in the open group. Mean specimen weights were similar: 169 g in the open group and 157 g in the laparoscopic group. Operative times for the open and laparoscopic procedures were similar (157 minutes and 145 minutes, respectively). Mean blood loss in the open population was twice that of the group treated laparoscopically: 141 versus 295 mL.

All parameters of convalescence favored laparoscopic simple nephrectomy. Patients in the open group had eight times the morphine equivalents for pain relief: 130 versus 14 mg. Mean hospital stay was 8 days for open simple nephrectomy and 3.5 days when the procedure was performed laparoscopically. Similarly, return to full activity was more expeditious in the laparoscopic group (16 versus 32 days, respectively). Postoperative complications included a wound infection and a urinary tract infection in the open group. No postoperative complications were reported in the patients treated with laparoscopic simple nephrectomy.

Rassweiler and co-workers (346) reported results comparing the open and the transperitoneal laparoscopic approaches and the retroperitoneal laparoscopic approach for simple laparoscopic nephrectomy. Results from 18 transperitoneal and 17 retroperitoneal laparoscopic simple nephrectomies were compared with the results of 19 open simple nephrectomies. Two conversions to an open procedure were required in the transperitoneal group, and one conversion was required in the retroperitoneal group. Mean operative times for laparoscopic transperitoneal and retroperitoneal nephrectomies were similar, and significantly longer than times required for open simple nephrectomy: 207 minutes, 211 minutes, and 117 minutes, respectively. Transfusion rates were lowest in the retroperitoneal group: 5.9% versus 17% in the laparoscopic transperitoneal patients and 16% in the open group (346).

All parameters of convalescence favored the laparoscopic approaches. Mean time for analgesia requirement for the transperitoneal and retroperitoneal laparoscopic groups was 2 days and 1 day, respectively, significantly shorter than the 4 days of analgesic administration that patients undergoing open simple nephrectomy required. Hospital stay reflected a similar pattern with transperitoneal and retroperitoneal simple nephrectomy requiring mean hospital stays of 6.6 and 6.3 days, respectively, versus 10 days in the open group. Time to complete recuperation was again similar for transperitoneal and retroperitoneal simple nephrectomy (24 and 21 days, respectively); both results were significantly shorter than the mean 40 days of recuperation time for open simple nephrectomy (346).

Overall complication rates were similar for the three approaches. Complication rates for transperitoneal, retroperitoneal, and open simple nephrectomy were 39%, 29%, and 26%, respectively. In the transperitoneal laparoscopic group, three patients experienced bleeding during dissection; one patient required conversion to open surgery. The other two were well controlled and did not require blood transfusion. There was also a bowel injury that was managed by conversion to open surgery. In addition, there were two cases of subcutaneous emphysema and a subcutaneous abscess, both of which resolved with conservative management. In the retroperitoneal laparoscopic group, there was

TABLE 18.4. SIMPLE NEPHRECTOMY—COMPARATIVE TRIALS

Source	Indications	Technique	Number	Minor Complications	Major Complications	Extraction	OR Time	EBL (mL)	Analgesia	Length of Stay	Full Recovery	Cost
Kerbl et al. (218)	All benign	Lap-transper	20	15%	15%	Morcellated	355 min	200	54 mg morphine	3.7 days	1.8 mo	NA
		Open-retroper	23	None	None	Intact	165 min	332	23 mg morphine	7.4 days	9.85 mo	NA
Parra et al. (323)	All benign	Lap-transper	12	17%	None	8% morcellate	145 min	141	14 mg morphine	3.5 days	16 days	NA
		Open-retroper	13	15%	None	Intact	56.6 min	295	29 mg morphine	8.0 days	32.3 days	NA
Rassweiler et al. (346)	All benign	Lap-transper	18	22%	17%	Intact	06.5 min	NA	2 days	6.6 days	24 days	NA
		Lap-retroper	17	12%	18%	Intact	11.2 min	NA	1 day	6.3 days	21 days	NA
		Open-retroper	19	16%	11%	Intact	117 min	NA	4 days	0.1 day	40 days	NA
Totals												
Laparoscopic			**67**	**17%**	**14%**		**241 min**	**179**		**5.1 days**	**30.8 days**	
Open			**55**	**9%**	**4%**		**146 min**	**319**		**8.5 days**	**145 days**	

All columns list mean values.
EBL, estimated blood loss; Lap, laparoscopic; NA, not available; retroper, retroperitoneal; transper, transperitoneal.

also a conversion to open surgery as a result of intraoperative bleeding. One patient also required subsequent reexploration for a pancreatic fistula. As in the transperitoneal group, there was a single case of subcutaneous emphysema and a subcutaneous abscess, both of which resolved with conservative management. In the open population, two cases of intraoperative bleeding were reported that required blood transfusion. There was also a case of intercostal neuralgia that was managed with pain medications, a retroperitoneal hematoma that was successfully observed, and an incisional hernia that required surgical repair (346).

Eraky and colleagues (99) reported the largest experience with laparoscopic simple nephrectomy. In their report, 106 laparoscopic transperitoneal simple nephrectomies were performed for chronic pain ($n = 73$), recurrent urinary tract infection ($n = 28$), or hypertension ($n = 5$). All kidneys were entrapped in a LapSac and underwent manual morcellation with a blunt scissors and surgical clamps. Ninety-seven (92%) nephrectomies were successfully completed laparoscopically. Conversion was necessitated to overcome failure of entrapment in one patient, because of uncontrollable bleeding in three cases, and because of severe perirenal adhesions in five patients. Mean operative time was 186 minutes. When stratified by experience, however, the mean operative times were 217 minutes and 154 minutes, respectively, for the first 53 and second 53 cases. Twenty-four (23%) patients experienced minor complications consisting of low-grade fevers (less than 38°C) and small asymptomatic hematomas. Four (3.8%) patients developed trocar site hernias. There were four (3.8%) major complications. These included a pulmonary embolism requiring anticoagulation, renal vein bleeding requiring reexploration, a colonic perforation requiring colostomy construction, and an infected hematoma that was drained percutaneously. Three of the four (75%) major complications and 17 of the 26 (65%) minor complications occurred in the first 53 cases. The mean hospital stay was 2.9 days, and mean follow-up period for the series was 14 months (range of 6 to 22 months). Analgesic requirements were not reported.

Laparoscopic simple nephrectomy accomplishes the objectives of its traditional open counterpart without exposing patients to additional risks or complications. The procedure offers the advantages of decreased pain, more rapid short- and long-term convalescence, and improved cosmesis.

Prospective, randomized comparison of the transperitoneal and retroperitoneal approaches for simple nephrectomy has not been performed; therefore there are no data demonstrating the superiority of either approach.

Retroperitoneum: Nephroureterectomy (Simple)

Laparoscopic simple nephroureterectomy was initially described in 1992 (92). Indications for simple nephroureterectomy include various benign diseases with concomitant renal and ureteral pathology that result in a kidney with poor renal function. Such clinical scenarios include vesicoureteral reflux in a single or duplicated system with recurrent episodes of pyelonephritis or pyoureteronephrosis.

Laparoscopic nephroureterectomy has been described using either a transperitoneal or retroperitoneal technique. The procedure is performed in the lateral decubitus position. In the transperitoneal approach the initial trocar is placed 2 cm superior and medial to the anterior superior iliac spine. Next, under endoscopic control three additional trocars are placed: just below the costal margin in the midclavicular line, several centimeters lateral and a few centimeters superior to the umbilicus, and in the midline approximately 2 to 3 cm above the pubis. A 5-mm trocar is placed in the midaxillary line subcostal. For operations on the right side, it is sometimes helpful to insert another 5-mm trocar subcostally near the xiphoid process to aid in retraction of the inferior border of the liver during the hilar dissection.

Using monopolar electrosurgical scissors, the surgeon incises the line of Toldt from the hepatic or splenic flexure caudal across the iliac vessels. The ureter is identified at the point where it crosses the iliac vessels. The ureter is dissected from surrounding tissues up to the level of the kidney. The renal hilum is exposed and the renal vessels carefully dissected. The renal artery is clipped five times and cut between the second and third clips (leaving only two clips on the side of the specimen). Attention is then turned to the renal vein, which is secured with an Endo-GIA vascular stapler. Gerota's fascia is incised and the kidney is dissected from the surrounding perirenal tissues. The ureter is then mobilized further caudally into the pelvis. In these patients it is sufficient to take the ureter at a point just below the iliac vessels, rather than attempting to secure a cuff of bladder; the ureter is divided between two pairs of clips. The specimen is then placed in an entrapment sack and morcellated; thereby completing the procedure without the need to enlarge any port site beyond its original 12-mm size.

Doehn and co-workers (83) described results with nephroureterectomy performed for benign disease. Sixteen patients who underwent transperitoneal laparoscopic nephroureterectomy were retrospectively compared with fifteen patients who underwent open retroperitoneal nephroureterectomy. All procedures were successfully accomplished laparoscopically. Operative time between the two groups was statistically similar: 100 minutes for the laparoscopic approach and 124 minutes for the open approach. Estimated blood loss for patients managed laparoscopically was significantly less (mean of 140 mL) than for open nephroureterectomy (470 mL) (83). Four (25%) minor complications were reported in the laparoscopic population. Three patients had a postoperative fever that was presumed to be from urinary tract infection. All three resolved within 2 to 5 days with antibiotic administration. One patient had back and shoulder pain for 3 days, which resolved with analgesics. There were three (20%) complications in the open population.

One patient had a pneumonia that resolved after 8 days of antibiotic treatment, and a second patient was successfully managed with antibiotics for a urinary tract infection. There was a single wound dehiscence that was managed conservatively on an outpatient basis (83). Oral intake in the laparoscopic population (11 hours) resumed significantly more quickly than in the open population (39 hours). Mean hospital stay was significantly shorter for patients managed laparoscopically: 6 versus 12.7 days. Similarly, patients in the laparoscopic group required significantly less analgesics in the form of morphine sulfate equivalents: 12 versus 40 mg. Patients undergoing laparoscopic simple nephroureterectomy returned to full activity almost twice as fast as patients undergoing open nephroureterectomy: 21 versus 39 days (83).

Prabhakaran and Lingaraj (339) reported on four pediatric patients who underwent simple nephroureterectomy for dysplastic kidneys. All four procedures were accomplished laparoscopically with a mean operative time of 176 minutes. Blood loss was minimal, and no intraoperative complications were noted. All patients resumed regular feeding on the first postoperative day, and mean hospital stay was less than 3 days (339). Similarly, Seibold and co-workers (379) reported on three children, 6 to 15 months of age, who underwent nephroureterectomy for nonfunctioning multicystic dysplastic kidneys and for reflux nephropathy. A single complication was documented: an incarcerated hernia through one of the 5-mm trocar sites.

Data regarding nephroureterectomy performed for benign disease are limited. However, these small series support the contention that laparoscopic simple nephroureterectomy is feasible, safe, efficacious, and accompanied by a rapid convalescence.

Benign Disease: Ablative—On the Horizon

Peripelvic Renal Cyst Decortication

Most peripelvic cysts are asymptomatic. However, they can occasionally enlarge and obstruct portions of the urinary collecting system. These cysts may rarely require surgical management.

One of the earliest reports of laparoscopic treatment of a peripelvic cyst was by Rubenstein and colleagues (359). They reported laparoscopic management of a symptomatic peripelvic cyst that was obstructing the upper pole renal collecting system (359). After transabdominal exposure, the cyst was unroofed, and a polytetrafluoroethylene wick was anchored within the cyst to maintain patency. Although the patient remained asymptomatic, a small cystic persistence (2 cm) was noted on follow-up at 10 months.

Hoenig and co-workers (169) reported on four patients with peripelvic cysts who were managed laparoscopically. Mean operative time was 338 minutes, and mean estimated blood loss was 90 mL. One intraoperative complication occurred: an injury to the renal pelvis that was sutured laparoscopically. Mean narcotic requirement was 385 mg of meperidine hydrochloride. Patients were discharged from the hospital at a mean of 2.8 days postoperatively and returned to normal activity at a mean of 3.3 weeks. Pain resolved in all four patients postoperatively but recurred 2 months after the procedure in the one patient who had been managed via a retroperitoneal approach. CT revealed recurrence of the peripelvic cyst, and the patient underwent open cyst marsupialization. With a mean follow-up of 13.5 months, the remaining three patients remained pain free. However, one of the three patients had radiographic evidence of a 2-cm, asymptomatic reaccumulation (169).

Laparoscopic management of peripelvic cysts is feasible and efficacious. The procedure is more technically challenging than management of simple peripheral renal cysts because of the proximity of the renal vessels and urinary collecting system. To date, only a few cases have been reported, and no long-term results are available.

Cystectomy

Laparoscopic simple cystectomy was first described by Parra and co-workers (322) in 1992. The procedure was performed in a 27-year-old female paraplegic with severe incontinence and urinary tract infections. She was initially managed with an ileocolonic reservoir with a continent stoma, but she subsequently developed multiple infections with purulent bladder drainage despite conservative management. A transperitoneal simple cystectomy was performed. Endo-GIA vascular staplers were used to ligate and divide the vascular pedicles and urethra and to separate the bladder from the vagina that was left intact. Operative time was 130 minutes, and estimated blood loss was 115 mL. The specimen weighed 22 g. Two 50-mg injections of meperidine hydrochloride and four tablets of acetaminophen with codeine were required for pain control. The patient was discharged home on postoperative day 5. Subsequently, Parra and co-workers (324) described a second laparoscopic simple cystectomy in a male paraplegic in 1995. The prostate was left *in situ.*

Laparoscopic cystectomy has been described in case reports and small series. Until further refinements of techniques and technology are available, the procedure remains investigational. Specifically, although the cystectomy itself seems to be rather straightforward, it is the bladder reconstruction or substitution that remains the key challenge to making laparoscopic simple cystectomy a viable clinical alternative.

Seminal Vesiculectomy

Isolated pathologic conditions of the seminal vesicles are uncommon. The advent of transrectal ultrasonography, CT, and MRI has made the discovery of isolated benign lesions of the seminal vesicles more frequent. The decision to surgically manage seminal vesicle cysts depends on the degree of symptoms experienced by the patient. Surgical treatment is challenging due to the deep pelvic location of the seminal vesicles.

The initial report on a laparoscopic approach to the seminal vesicles was produced by Kavoussi and colleagues (211) in 1993. They reported their technique for bilateral seminal vesicle mobilization as part of radical perineal prostatectomy for carcinoma of the prostate. A 12-mm trocar is placed infraumbilically, and two 10-mm trocars are placed at the level of the umbilicus just lateral to the rectus muscles. Two additional 10-mm trocars are placed in each lower quadrant. A transverse incision is made through the anterior peritoneum overlying the rectovesical pouch. The ampullae and vasa deferentia are identified and dissected from surrounding tissue. Each ampulla is then separately isolated, clipped, and transected. The dissection is kept close to the seminal vesicles and prostate to avoid injury to the ureter, the rectum, or the adjacent neurovascular bundle of the prostate. Working medially to laterally, the surface of the seminal vesicle is defined by blunt dissection, and the artery to each seminal vesicle is isolated, ligated with clips, and divided. Gentle medial traction of the seminal vesicles allows for further lateral dissection, thereby freeing the seminal vesicle down to its base.

Successful seminal vesicle mobilization was performed in 15 of 16 (95%) patients. The solitary failure had extensive tumor involving the seminal vesicles. Mean operative time was not reported, but a range of 1 to 2.5 hours was described. Blood loss was minimal, and no short-term complications were reported. Long-term follow-up was not provided.

Carmignani and co-workers (46) reported laparoscopic unilateral seminal vesiculectomy in a symptomatic 19-year-old male patient. The patient complained of lower urinary tract symptoms and pain with ejaculation. Transrectal ultrasound demonstrated cystic dilation of the right seminal vesicle, and needle aspiration demonstrated immotile spermatozoa. Transabdominal laparoscopic cyst excision was performed. Total operative time was 180 minutes, and the patient was discharged home on the second postoperative day. There were no intraoperative or postoperative complications. At 6-month follow-up, the patient was asymptomatic and transrectal ultrasonography revealed a normal left and absent right seminal vesicles.

Ikari and colleagues (183) reported laparoscopic seminal vesiculectomy in two patients. The first case was a 24-year-old man complaining of left pelvic pain. Ultrasound and CT revealed a large left seminal vesicle cyst. A transperitoneal laparoscopic seminal vesiculectomy was performed. Operative time was 90 minutes, and the patient was discharged on the second postoperative day. There were no complications, and transrectal ultrasound 120 days postoperatively was remarkable only for absence of the left seminal vesicle. The second case presented was of a 10-month-old child with recurrent Gram-negative urinary tract infections. Ultrasonography revealed a 5-cm retrovesical cystic tumor. This was confirmed with MRI. Laparoscopic seminal vesiculectomy was performed in 120 minutes, and the patient was discharged on postoperative day 2. With 4-year follow-up, the child was asymptomatic and had not had recurrence of urinary tract infections (183).

Bilateral seminal vesicle mobilization to facilitate perineal prostatectomy is safe and feasible. However, due to the additional surgical time required for this portion of the procedure and given the now rare indications for a pelvic lymph node dissection, this approach is rarely used. In contrast, isolated pathology of the seminal vesicles, although unusual, is well resolved by a laparoscopic approach.

Partial Adrenalectomy

Partial adrenalectomy was first described by Janetschek and co-workers (193,198) for management of bilateral aldosterone-producing adenomas. Criteria for partial adrenalectomy continue to be defined; however, complete absence of adrenal function necessitates glucocorticoid and mineralocorticoid replacement therapy. This form of medical management is associated with a decreased quality of life (412). Accordingly, the preservation of any functioning adrenal tissue is preferable from the patient's standpoint.

For aldosterone-producing adenomas, Nekada and co-workers (297) demonstrated superior physiologic responses in patients undergoing open enucleation compared with open adrenalectomy. There were no cases of recurrent hyperaldosteronism in either group. Reported indications for partial adrenalectomy have included small functioning masses, renal masses with bilateral adrenal metastases, and syndromes associated with bilateral adrenal pathology.

Advances in the technology and quality of intraoperative ultrasonography have made laparoscopic partial adrenalectomy feasible (164,184,289). Presently available flexible 10-mm probes now afford the laparoscopic surgeon the ability to determine tumor characteristics and borders. Ultrasound can establish the presence of tumor, demonstrate that large tumors are without signs of malignancy, determine the degree of infiltration of the adrenal gland and surrounding structures, and help locate the adrenal vasculature (164). These criteria can be used to determine whether small adenomas are technically resectable via partial adrenalectomy. If a tumor is peripheral and the remnant after resection with an adequate margin is expected to be greater than 50% of the gland, partial adrenalectomy is feasible.

Janetschek and colleagues (194) reported results of four patients managed with six partial adrenalectomies (two bilateral). Laparoscopic partial adrenalectomies were performed in patients with inherited syndromes associated with von Hippel–Lindau disease or the multiple endocrine neoplasia (MEN) 2b syndrome. Operative data specific for partial adrenalectomy were not separated from other laparoscopic adrenalectomies in this series. However, 2 of 6 (33%) patients undergoing partial adrenalectomy experienced complications. One patient experienced intraoperative bleeding that did not require transfusion, postoperative pneumonia, and lymphatic ascites in the postoperative period. Another patient developed a trocar site hernia. Patients undergoing partial adrenalectomy were able to return to full activity in 22 days and had complete recovery in a mean of 8 weeks.

Sasagawa and co-workers (366a) reported results of 15 laparoscopic retroperitoneal partial adrenalectomies for benign adrenal tumors. Adrenal transection was accomplished successfully in all cases using an endoscopic stapling device. Mean operative time was 162 minutes, and mean estimated blood loss was 12 mL. A single (7%) complication was reported; a pneumothorax was created due to intraoperative injury to the crus of the diaphragm. Postoperative parameters were not reported.

Most recently, Walther and colleagues (432) reported partial adrenalectomies performed on three patients with Von Hippel–Lindau disease. Mean operative time was 324 minutes, with an estimated blood loss of 100 mL. Postoperatively, the patients required a mean of 22 mg of morphine sulfate, and no patient required hormonal replacement. In two cases, partial adrenalectomy was unilateral, and in the last case bilateral partial adrenalectomy was performed. Mean hospital stay was 4 days, and patients returned to full activity in 12 days. No intraoperative or postoperative complications were reported. There was no evidence of tumor recurrence with follow-up of 3 years, 5 months, and 3 weeks reported for the three patients.

Laparoscopic partial adrenalectomy is feasible and, in properly selected patients, has demonstrated efficacy in controlling functioning adrenal tumors. Patients with bilateral adrenal disease may benefit from this management strategy because the morbidity and decreased quality of life associated with exogenous steroid replacement is thereby precluded.

Partial Nephrectomy and Wedge Excision

Partial nephrectomy is used therapeutically for various benign renal abnormalities. These maladies include vascular lesions, trauma, segmental obstruction or infection, and renal stone disease localized to either pole. Winfield and colleagues (441) performed the first laparoscopic partial nephrectomy for benign disease in 1992. The procedure was performed using a technique developed by McDougall and co-workers in a porcine model (265). In these animal studies, successful partial nephrectomies were performed using a plastic cable as a renal tourniquet and electrosurgical scissors for renal transection. Hemostasis was achieved with argon beam coagulation.

Numerous technologies have been studied for use in laparoscopic partial nephrectomy due to the suboptimal clinical results and technical difficulty of the procedure. Elashry and colleagues (97) compared the use of an electrosurgical snare and ultrasound dissection in a porcine model. Gill and co-workers (122) reported the first successful retroperitoneal laparoscopic partial nephrectomy in 1994. The procedure was performed using a double-loop sling used to secure the kidney and achieve circumferential hemostatic compression. Despite determined efforts, a safe, effective, and reproducible technique for a purely laparoscopic partial nephrectomy remains elusive.

Several series describe laparoscopic nephron-sparing surgery. Winfield and co-workers (443) described four successful laparoscopic partial nephrectomies in six attempts. All cases were performed without control of the renal vasculature using a 5-mm electrosurgical blade for parenchymal transection and argon beam coagulation for hemostasis. No attempts at closure of the collecting system were made. Two of their six attempts resulted in conversion to open surgery due to an inadequate specimen in one case and to hemorrhage in another patient.

In comparing their experience to open partial nephrectomy, although the blood loss was less in the laparoscopic group (525 versus 708 mL) and the analgesic requirements were lower (52 versus 118 mg of morphine sulfate equivalents), there were many drawbacks to the laparoscopic procedure. Mean operative time for the laparoscopic procedure (6.1 hours) was 2 hours longer than for the open procedures and the hospital stay was no different. Minor complications occurred in two of the laparoscopic patients (a residual stone and an obstructed drain). However, of note, full convalescence was 6 weeks shorter in the laparoscopic group (443).

McDougall and colleagues (266) described results from nephron-sparing surgery in 12 patients. This series included nine attempted polar partial nephrectomies, three of which required conversion to open surgery (i.e., dense fibrosis, hemorrhage, and inability to properly judge the point of incision). Of the nine polar nephrectomy patients, two had masses suspicious for malignancy, four had symptomatic calyceal dilation with or without stone disease, two had upper pole atrophy associated with a duplicated collecting system, and one patient had a nonfunctioning upper pole. Renal vessels were not controlled in any case, and parenchymal transection was performed with electrosurgical scissors in five cases, an electrosurgical snare in three cases, and an Endo-GIA stapling device in one case. Exposed parenchyma was then fulgurated with the argon beam coagulator. Intracorporeal suturing was used to close defects in the collecting system. Mean operative time for the successful partial nephrectomies was 6.5 hours, and mean estimated blood loss was 217 mL. A mean of 52 mg of morphine sulfate equivalent was required for postoperative pain management. Mean hospital stay was 5.3 days, and mean time to complete convalescence was 4.2 weeks. There were three (50%) postoperative complications: nephrocutaneous fistula requiring placement of a percutaneous nephrostomy, retroperitoneal urinoma requiring drainage, and a 48-hour ileus (266).

Hoznek and colleagues (176) recently described a series of 13 patients who underwent a laparoscopic retroperitoneal approach to nephron-sparing surgery for benign disease. A complete partial nephrectomy was performed in only three cases, and in the other situations, a wedge-type excision was done (176). Surgery was performed for benign conditions in six (hydrocalyx with overlying atrophy in five and upper pole atrophy in one), equivocal solid masses in four, and indeterminate renal cysts in three patients. Intraoperative ultrasound was used to assess intrarenal anatomy in cases of borderline cysts and solid masses. Transection was performed with a rotating-tip electrosurgical scissors or a harmonic scalpel. In five patients, an atraumatic vascular clamp was placed on the renal vessels before transection. The transected raw parenchymal surface was covered with oxidized regenerated cellulose mesh impregnated with gelatin resorcinol formaldehyde glue (176). All procedures were successfully accomplished laparoscopically. Average operating time was 1.9 hours, and average intraoperative blood loss was 72 mL. There were only two postoperative complications, both urinomas. Mean hospital stay was 6.1 days. Analgesic requirements and time to full recovery were not reported.

Laparoscopic partial nephrectomy for benign disease in the adult is technically difficult and, even in the hands of experienced urologic laparoscopists, results in high conversion rates and significant complications. In contrast, reported results with wedge resection of benign renal lesions have been superior to those for partial nephrectomy. Many wedge resections are completed successfully with minimal bleeding and rapid postoperative convalescence.

Cyst Decortication in Autosomal-dominant Polycystic Kidney Disease

Autosomal-dominant polycystic kidney disease (ADPKD) is characterized by bilateral, multiple, nonfunctioning, and noncommunicating renal cysts. Typically, symptoms appear in the third and fourth decades of life and include hypertension, hematuria, and abdominal pain. Although the disease has protean manifestations, the most common presentation is abdominal pain; hypertension, pyelonephritis, hematuria, and palpable abdominal masses also are common. End-stage renal disease is the major late sequela of ADPKD and occurs in approximately 40% of patients.

It is widely believed that the progressive renal dysfunction seen in ADPKD patients is due to compression and distortion of adjacent noncystic renal parenchyma by the expanding cysts. However, cyst decortication has not been shown to result in improved renal function. As such, surgical treatment is indicated only for pain control after failure of medical management.

Minimally invasive methods have been used to treat these patients. Ultrasound- or fluoroscopically guided percutaneous cyst aspiration has been performed to drain a few large symptomatic renal cysts (23,112). However, this therapy has resulted in durable pain relief at 1.5 years in only 33% of patients (23). Likewise, percutaneous endourologic techniques have been used to treat one or several larger cysts; pain relief has usually been only transient. Better results have been obtained with open surgical extensive cyst decortication, but this is a major and often morbid procedure. However, Bennett and co-workers (23) reported that 81% of ADPKD patients treated with open decortication were still benefited at 1.5 years with regard to decreased discomfort.

Morgan and Rader (285) performed the first laparoscopic cyst decortication for a complex renal cyst in 1991. Subsequently, Barry and Lowe (18a) reported laparoscopic cyst marsupialization in patients with ADPKD. More recently, Brown and co-workers (35) reported results with 13 consecutive laparoscopic cyst decortications for patients with symptomatic ADPKD. Of the 13 patients, 6 (46%) had undergone prior cyst aspiration with or without attempted sclerosis. The procedure was technically successful in 12 of 13 (92%) patients. Estimated blood loss was less than 150 mL, and mean operative time was 2.7 hours. No intraoperative or postoperative complications were reported. Of 13 patients, 11 (85%) experienced immediate relief of symptoms. In two patients, a less than complete decortication of all large cysts was done; both failed to benefit. However, 3 of the 11 successful patients had recurrent pain at 7, 11, and 16 months postoperatively. The remaining eight (62%) had good pain relief (80% to 100%) with follow-up of 12 to 28 months.

Lifson and colleagues (238) reported results of cyst decortication in eight patients with ADPKD. All procedures were successfully accomplished laparoscopically. Mean estimated blood loss was 116 mL, and mean operative time was 137 minutes. There was one postoperative complication, a self-limited retroperitoneal hemorrhage that was managed with a 2-unit blood transfusion. Mean hospital stay was 2.3 days. During early follow-up, all patients had significant pain relief. A second procedure was performed in three patients with recurrent pain; it was successful in two of these patients. Overall, 71% were pain free at 6 months, and 57% were pain free at 2 years (238). Although this report did not include follow-up data on hypertension or renal function, an earlier report on these patients recorded late deterioration of renal function as manifested by progression of serum creatinine in 2 of 6 (33%) patients. Because there was no control group, it is unknown what effect the laparoscopic procedure had on the natural history of this patient population.

Laparoscopic cyst decortication for ADPKD is efficacious in resolving pain. Most patients experience resolution of pain postoperatively, and approximately 60% have satisfactory pain control for up to 2 years. However, the effects of laparoscopic cyst decortication on renal function and hypertension remain undefined. Longer follow-up (i.e., 3 to 5 years) is necessary to delineate the long-term efficacy of the procedure for pain control and to carefully track the impact of this surgery on hypertension and renal function.

Donor Nephrectomy

Renal transplantation is the treatment of choice for end-stage renal failure. Live-donor renal transplantation offers advantages to the recipient when compared with cadaveric kidney transplantation. One-year patient and graft survivals for live-donor kidney transplants are 97% and 91%, respectively. In contrast, 1-year recipients of cadaveric renal transplants have patient and graft survivals of 93% and 81%, respectively (425). The incidence of delayed function and need for posttransplant dialysis are decreased with a live-donor kidney.

Despite the aforementioned advantages of live-donor transplantation, there has been reluctance on the part of prospective donors. In large part, this appears to be due to the anticipated 7- to 10-day hospital stay, 6-week convalescence period, significant postoperative pain, and large flank incision characteristic of open donor nephrectomy (77). The prolonged convalescence can lead to financial hardship, strains on the family unit, and job insecurity.

In 1994, the endourology group at Washington University reported the feasibility of laparoscopic donor nephrectomy in a porcine model. They described a series of laparoscopic donor nephrectomies with successful renal extraction associated with mean renal artery and vein length equivalent to open donor nephrectomy (121). Subsequently, in 1995, Ratner and colleagues (349) reported the first clinical laparoscopic donor nephrectomy. In this case, the allograft produced urine immediately, and the recipient's creatinine normalized by postoperative day 2. The donor experienced minimal postoperative pain and was discharged home on the first postoperative day. He returned to work as a welder 2 weeks after surgery.

Laparoscopic donor nephrectomy is performed with the patient in the lateral decubitus position; in most cases, the left kidney is selected. Trocar placement is similar to that described for laparoscopic radical nephrectomy. During the procedure, it is important to keep the patient volume expanded because vigorous hydration and low insufflation pressure combine to help maintain urine output (242). The administration of parenteral diuretics (12.5 g of mannitol and 40 mg of furosemide) is also beneficial.

The descending colon and splenic flexure are mobilized and reflected medially by incising the line of Toldt and dissecting the colon off of Gerota's fascia. Diaphragmatic attachments to the spleen are divided, allowing it to fall medially. Gerota's fascia is incised, and attention is directed to the renal hilum. The renal vein is freed from its adventitial attachments, and the gonadal, adrenal, and any associated lumbar veins are identified, clipped, and divided. The renal artery, usually behind the vein, is then identified and freed from surrounding tissue. Maximum length of the renal artery is achieved by dissecting it to its proximal origin at the aorta. The renal artery may be bathed with a topical solution of papaverine to prevent vasospasm. At this point, the patient is given mannitol and furosemide intravenously. Attention is turned to the ureteral dissection. The ureter is broadly dissected to the level of the iliac vessels, and it is taken en bloc along with the gonadal vein via an Endo-GIA stapler. The remaining attachments to the kidney are then divided.

An extraction incision is then made, leaving the underlying peritoneum intact to maintain insufflation. Right upper quadrant, midline, and Pfannenstiel incisions have been described; the last is cosmetically preferable. The incision should be generous enough for atraumatic extraction of the kidney. Before the surgeon divides the vascular pedicle, 3,000 units of heparin sulfate is administered intravenously. The Endo-GIA vascular stapler is then used to sequentially divide the renal artery and renal vein. An endoscopic extraction sack is then used to entrap the kidney, the peritoneum is opened, and the specimen is delivered. The incision should be lengthened as necessary to ensure atraumatic extraction. After injection of protamine sulfate to reverse the effects of the heparin, the fascia is closed and the pneumoperitoneum reestablished. The renal bed is inspected for bleeding. After adequate hemostasis is confirmed, all incision sites are closed.

Hand-assist techniques for laparoscopic donor nephrectomy have also been described. Access is achieved via the umbilicus, where a 12-mm trocar is placed. A second 12-mm trocar is placed in the midaxillary line midway between the iliac crest and the costal margin. The hand-assist device is placed in the midline above the umbilicus, and an incision equal in length in centimeters to the surgeon's glove size is created. The use of the surgeon's hand facilitates the procedure because it allows for manual blunt dissection, rapid renal exposure, and hand delivery of the kidney.

Philosophe and colleagues (331) from the University of Maryland have reported the largest single-center experience with laparoscopic donor nephrectomy. The records of 193 patients undergoing laparoscopic donor nephrectomy were compared with results from 168 open donor nephrectomies performed at the same institution before the advent of the laparoscopic technique. Mean warm ischemia times for laparoscopic donor nephrectomy was 158 seconds (307). Immunosuppression regimens were similar for both groups. Mean follow-up for the laparoscopic population was 10.7 months, and follow-up for the open population was 41.5 months. Donor characteristics were similar between the two groups.

The 2-year graft survival rates for laparoscopic and open donor nephrectomy were similar at 98% and 96%, respectively. The 2-year patient survival rate was also similar, with laparoscopic and open donor nephrectomies resulting in survivals of 98% and 97%, respectively. Graft function, as assessed by serum creatinine levels at 3 months and 1 year, were similar between the two groups. Specifically, 3-month serum creatinine values for laparoscopic and open donor nephrectomies were both 1.6 mg/dL. At 1 year the serum creatinine values were 1.6 and 1.7 mg/dL, respectively. Philosophe and co-workers (331) reported delayed graft function to be similar for laparoscopic and open donor nephrectomy (6.2% and 5.1%, respectively).

Philosophe and colleagues (331) specifically addressed the incidence of ureteral complications, which had been reported as being as high as 11% in the initial series versus only 3% for the open donor nephrectomy group. There were 15 (7.7%) operations for ureteral complications in the laparoscopic group, compared with only 1 (0.6%) from kidneys procured using the open technique. Modifications to the laparoscopic surgical technique were made in October 1997 to try to decrease the rate of ureteral complications. Specifically, an Endo-GIA stapler was used to divide the ureter and a broad expanse of periureteral fat distally to include more periureteral tissue. Since the modification, the authors have had only a single ureteral complication in 62 consecutive patients; the complication was managed with a ureteral stent (331).

Data on complications were reported in an earlier article comparing laparoscopic and open donors from the University of Maryland (307). In the open population, there were two (2%) cases of delayed graft function due to acute tubular necrosis (ATN), three (3%) cases of early acute rejection, one (1%) ureteral complication, and two (2%) cases of sepsis resulting in allograft dysfunction. In the laparoscopic donor nephrectomy group, there were ten (7.6%) cases of ATN, three (2.3%) cases of early acute rejection, six (4.5%) cases of ureteral complications, two (1.5%) cases of pyelonephritis, one (0.8%) case of hemorrhage, one (0.8%) lymphocele, and two (1.5%) complications reported as "no records."

Ratner and co-workers (350) described the Johns Hopkins University School of Medicine experience. Donors undergoing laparoscopic donor nephrectomy had significantly less intraoperative blood loss: 266 versus 393 mL. Postoperative analgesic requirements were significantly decreased in the laparoscopic group: 40 versus 124 mg of morphine equivalents. Similarly, oral intake was resumed more quickly in the laparoscopic group (0.8 versus 2.6 days). Hospital stay in the group of laparoscopic donors was 3.0 days versus 5.7 days required in the open population. Return to work was significantly faster in the laparoscopic population: 4 versus 6.4 weeks (350).

Results of 110 recipients of laparoscopically procured kidneys were compared with 48 patients receiving kidneys from open donors (350). Recipient serum creatinine in the laparoscopic group was significantly higher on postoperative days 2 and 3, but by day 4 there was no significant difference. There was no significant difference in creatinine clearance at 24 months: 75 versus 63 mL per minute. In addition, there was no significant difference in patient or graft survival, need for dialysis, or incidence or severity of rejection episodes. Recipients' complications were not significantly different when laparoscopic and open groups were compared. Ureteral complications occurred in ten (9.1%) of laparoscopically procured kidneys, compared with three (6.3%) of kidneys retrieved via the open approach. Vascular thrombosis occurred in three (2.7%) and two (4.2%) of laparoscopically procured and open donor kidneys, respectively.

Odland and colleagues (311) retrospectively compared 30 laparoscopic donor nephrectomies with 30 open donor nephrectomies. Of 30 procedures, 10 (87%) were successfully completed laparoscopically. The laparoscopic group had significantly longer operative times than the open group: 183 versus 148 minutes, respectively. Estimated blood loss and transfusion requirements were not significantly different between the two populations. Three laparoscopic donors (12%) required reexploration, two for bleeding and one for retrieval of a foreign body. All three explorations were successfully accomplished laparoscopically. No patient in the open donor nephrectomy group required reexploration. Persistent wound problems were significantly more common among open donors. Of patients in the open group, 55% experienced chronic wound problems, compared with 11% of laparoscopic donors.

Kidneys in the laparoscopic donor nephrectomy group had a significantly longer warm ischemia time when compared with the open donors (5.8 versus 1.7 minutes). There was no significant difference in serum creatinine at 2 weeks or 6 months. Similarly, there was no significant difference in delayed graft function between laparoscopic and open donor nephrectomy (12% and 3%, respectively). Acute graft rejection rates at 6 months were also similar between the laparoscopic and open donor groups: 27% and 37%, respectively. Graft survival rates for laparoscopic and open donor groups were 96% and 90%, respectively (311).

Total hospital costs were slightly higher for the laparoscopic than the open donor population: $11,123 versus $9,335, respectively. The shorter hospital stay associated with the laparoscopic approach was negated by the higher intraoperative costs for laparoscopy; mean operative procedure costs for the laparoscopic and open groups were $7,218 and $5,583, respectively.

Slakey and co-workers (393) reported results comparing 10 laparoscopic donor nephrectomies to 12 laparoscopic donor nephrectomies performed using the hand-assist device. When the hand-assist device was used, mean operative times were significantly reduced: 2.0 versus 3.1 hours with the pure laparoscopic technique. Similarly, warm ischemia times were significantly reduced with the hand-assist technique: 1.2 versus 3.9 minutes. Only one patient required parenteral narcotics after leaving the recovery room, and all patients tolerated a regular diet when fully awake. There was a single complication in the series. One patient in the standard laparoscopy group experienced a deep venous thrombosis that was successfully managed with anticoagulation. All recipient kidneys functioned immediately, and all grafts had normal function with follow-up of 1 to 12 months (393). Comparative data on length of stay and convalescence were not presented.

Laparoscopic donor nephrectomy is clearly feasible and has removed some of the disincentives to live-donor kidneys. The operation provides donors the benefits characteristic of the laparoscopic approach to renal surgery in general, including decreased pain and more rapid recovery. Given these results, it is not surprising that Ratner and colleagues (350) have noted a greater than 100% increase in live donor transplants at their institution since the inception of the laparoscopic donor nephrectomy program. Although there is a "learning curve" that each surgeon must traverse, it would appear that the laparoscopic approach to donor nephrectomy has proven itself; in the larger series, the technique has equaled or surpassed the high standards achieved by open donor surgery for donor safety and graft function and survival. It appears that hand-assisted laparoscopic donor nephrectomy may help flatten the learning curve while improving the efficiency, without impairing the equanimity, of the laparoscopic approach.

Nephrectomy for Xanthogranulomatous Pyelonephritis

XGP is an atypical form of chronic renal infection characterized by destruction of the renal parenchyma and its replacement by masses of lipid-laden macrophages. XGP is usually associated with nephrolithiasis, obstructive uropathy, and an ongoing urinary tract infection. The treatment of choice is nephrectomy, which is challenging given the extent of the disease and the not uncommon involvement of the renal hilum and contiguous structures by the ongoing inflammatory process. Few authors have examined the role of laparoscopy in the setting of XGP.

Keeley and Tolley (213) described two cases of simple nephrectomy for XGP in a series of 100 nephrectomies. One of the two cases required conversion to open surgery. In the same year, Merrot and co-workers (275) reported a 13-year-old girl with XGP managed via a retroperitoneal laparoscopic approach. The procedure was successfully completed in 150 minutes, and the patient was discharged on postoperative day 4 without complication. Cadeddu and colleagues (43) reported results on three laparoscopic nephrectomies performed for XGP. Two cases (67%) required conversion to open surgery due to extensive perinephric scarring. No intraoperative or postoperative complications were reported (43).

Bercowsky and co-workers (25) compared the results of five patients who underwent laparoscopic nephrectomy for XGP with four patients managed with the open technique. Of note, in only 5 of the 9 patients (56%) was the diagnosis of XGP suspected preoperatively. Two cases were performed via the retroperitoneal approach. Laparoscopic nephrectomy was successful in 4 of 5 (80%) patients managed laparoscopically. Conversion to open surgery was necessary in one patient. In all patients, the dissection was considered very difficult because it was challenging to define lines of cleavage between the retroperitoneal structures and to dissect the renal hilum. Mean operative time was 6 hours in the laparoscopic group and 2.5 hours in the open population. Estimated blood loss was less in the laparoscopic group than in the open nephrectomy group: 260 versus 438 mL. Unlike most reports in which laparoscopy is compared with open surgery, among these patients, analgesic requirements and hospital stay were similar; however, time to normal activity (4.6 versus 9.3 weeks) and complete recovery (13.6 versus 16 weeks) were more rapid in the laparoscopic nephrectomy group (25). Complications occurred in three patients (60%) in the laparoscopic group: ileus in two patients and multiple complications in another patient (5-unit blood transfusion, retroperitoneal hematoma, pulmonary embolus, and a retroperitoneal abscess). No complications were reported in the open group.

Although simple nephrectomy for XGP is feasible, it is technically very challenging. The laparoscopic approach has been associated with a high conversion rate and has an increased risk of postoperative complications. In addition, the short-term benefits characteristic of laparoscopy are not as pronounced as in other laparoscopic procedures. As such, at most centers, a preoperative diagnosis of XGP remains a relative to absolute contraindication for laparoscopic nephrectomy.

Nephrectomy for Autosomal-dominant Polycystic Kidney Disease

The laparoscopic approach to these giant kidneys has only recently been described. These patients, despite being on dialysis or having undergone a successful renal transplant, continue to have symptoms and signs of their markedly enlarged kidneys: flank and abdominal pain, shortness of breath, gastrointestinal problems (early satiety, constipation), and renal-related hypertension.

Laparoscopic nephrectomy in these patients was initially reported by Elashry and colleagues (95) in 1996 at Washington University; this was performed in two patients with renal failure. The case time was 4.5 hours with a 3.5-day hospital stay. Patients returned to their baseline activity in 2 weeks. More recently, Dunn and colleagues (89) have updated the Washington University experience with nine ADPKD patients undergoing 11 nephrectomies for pain. In this group, the average operating time was 6.3 hours with an average hospital stay of 3 days. Six significant complications occurred: blood transfusion, a vena cavotomy repaired laparoscopically, splenic cyanosis, pulmonary embolism, clotted arteriovenous fistula, and brachial plexus injury. Incisional hernias occurred in 2 of the 3 patients who underwent open intact removal. Patients returned to their baseline activities in 5 weeks. Relief of pain was achieved in all patients. In three patients, hypertension improved or resolved, whereas in three other patients, hypertension worsened postoperatively.

In these patients, the use of hand-assist laparoscopy would appear to offer a favorable compromise between a pure laparoscopic approach and intact removal. The hand-assist approach allows for rapid mobilization of these giant kidneys and provides a workable incision through which the cysts can be decompressed as the specimen is removed. In addition, because of the increased efficiency of hand-assisted laparoscopy, bilateral nephrectomy becomes a more feasible undertaking in these patients.

Benign Disease: Reconstructive

Pelvis: Bladder Neck Suspension

Stress urinary incontinence is the involuntary loss of urine from the urethra resulting from an increase in intraabdominal pressure and in the absence of a detrusor contraction. In 1996, the Agency for Health Care Policy and Research estimated that approximately 14 million Americans suffer from urinary incontinence, at an estimated annual cost of $46 billion (102). Factors involved in the normal continence mechanism in the female include an intrinsic coapting ability of the proximal urethra, a critical functional and anatomic urethral length, the ability of the pelvic floor to increase urethral pressure at the time of stress, and the proper anatomic location of the sphincter mechanism (398).

Multiple surgical procedures have been developed to suspend or support the bladder neck and thereby correct female stress incontinence. These include anterior colporrhaphy, anterior cystourethropexy, endoscopic needle suspensions, and sling procedures. Laparoscopic bladder neck suspension was first described as a transperitoneal approach by Vancaillie and Schuessler in 1991 (427).

At present, laparoscopic bladder neck suspension is usually performed in an extraperitoneal retropubic fashion. A 2-cm incision is created in the upper one-third of the distance between the symphysis pubis and the umbilicus. A dilating balloon is placed in the retropubic space and inflated with 1 L of saline. A laparoscopic trocar is placed and insufflation performed. Two additional trocars are placed just lateral to the lateral border of the rectus abdominus muscle. For a right-handed surgeon, one trocar is placed on the right side just opposite the initial trocar placement, and the other trocar is placed on the left side, several centimeters above the pubic ramus. Using intracorporeal suturing technique, sutures are placed on either side of the bladder neck, and are then passed through the midline cartilaginous notch of the posterior symphysis [modified Marshall-Marchetti-Krantz (MMK)] (Fig. 18.15A), through Cooper's ligament bilaterally (modified Burch) (Fig. 18.15B), or through the ileal pectinate line (modified

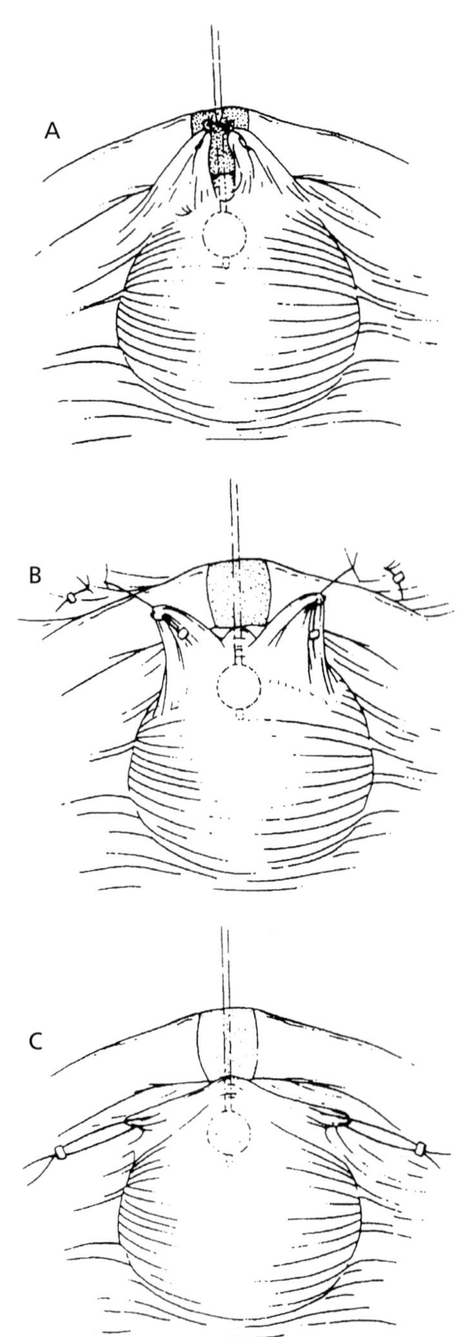

FIGURE 18.15. Laparoscopic bladder neck suspension. **A:** Modified Marshall-Marchetti-Krantz: Sutures are placed on either side of the bladder neck and are then passed through the midline cartilaginous notch of the posterior symphysis. **B:** Modified Burch: Sutures are passed through Cooper's ligament bilaterally. **C:** Modified Richardson: Sutures are passed through the ileal pectinate line.

Richardson) (Fig. 18.15C). Sutures are tightened down to gently elevate the bladder neck and proximal urethra behind the pubic symphysis; the sutures are secured with an anchoring device (e.g., Lapra-Ty clip) or by intracorporeal or extracorporeal knotting techniques. A Foley catheter is placed in the bladder for 24 hours.

Albala and co-workers (6) reported results of 22 bladder neck suspensions using transperitoneal MMK (n = 22) or Burch (n = 10) procedures. Twenty-nine (91%) procedures were successfully accomplished laparoscopically. Two conversions resulted from inability to place sutures, and one conversion was the result of bladder injury during dissection of the space of Retzius. All three of these patients were discharged on the third postoperative day without further complication. Mean operative times for the Burch and MMK procedures were 105 and 65 minutes, respectively. Estimated blood loss and analgesic requirements were not reported. Twenty-eight patients (88%) were discharged in less than 18 hours postoperatively. Nineteen (59%) patients were discharged home without a Foley catheter, and thirteen (41%) had catheters placed for 3 days. In the MMK group, all patients were cured of their incontinence more than 1 year after surgery. With a mean follow-up of only 7 months, all patients in the Burch group were also cured of their incontinence. Postoperative complications included urinary retention in two patients (6%) requiring cystotomy tube placement.

Ou and co-workers (319) reported results of 40 women with stress incontinence treated with a modified laparoscopic Birch procedure. A transperitoneal approach was used, and Proline hernia mesh was stapled to both the periurethral tissues and Cooper's ligament, thereby obviating intracorporeal suturing. Operative times and estimated blood loss were not reported. All 40 procedures were successfully accomplished laparoscopically. Average length of hospital stay was 1.2 days, and average duration of catheterization was less than 24 hours. Minor complications were reported in 6 of 40 (15%) patients: hematuria, low-grade fevers, urinary retention, and urinary tract infection. All complications were self-limiting and were successfully managed without intervention or transfusion. With a mean follow-up of 16 months, all patients had resolution or improvement of incontinence. Specific details regarding postoperative leakage of urine were not reported (319).

Although there was an initial rush toward performing laparoscopic bladder neck suspension, the success of the procedure began to unravel when it was reexamined in the light of longer follow-up (73). In this regard, Su and co-workers (403) reported a prospective comparison of laparoscopic and open bladder neck suspension. Forty-six women were randomized to extraperitoneal laparoscopic bladder neck suspension, and forty-six women were randomized to the open procedure. Operative times were not significantly different for laparoscopic and open procedures (66.5 and 72.8 minutes, respectively). However, mean estimated blood loss was significantly decreased in the laparoscopic population (53 versus 134 mL, respectively). Bladder drainage was significantly longer in the open group compared with the patients managed laparoscopically (6.8 versus 3.9 days, respectively). Analgesic requirements were not reported. With a minimum of 1 year of follow-up, postoperative urodynamic evaluation revealed both groups to have a significant and similar increase in leak point pressure. However, the continence rate was significantly better in the patient population managed with the open technique (96%) than with the laparoscopic technique (80%). In the laparoscopic group, there was a complication rate of 11%: two patients experienced outflow obstruction, two patients experienced *de novo* detrusor instability, and one patient developed a urinary tract infection. In the open group, there was a 17% complication rate: two patients with outflow obstruction, two patients with hematuria, three patients with detrusor instability, and one patient who developed a urinary tract infection.

Subsequent studies with even longer follow-up have shown further erosion of the success of laparoscopic bladder neck suspension. Specifically, McDougall and colleagues (268) compared results of 58 patients undergoing laparoscopic extraperitoneal bladder neck suspension with results of 42 patients managed by transvaginal Raz bladder neck suspension. Mean follow-up was the longest of any reports on this procedure: 45 months in the laparoscopy group and 59 months in the transvaginal group. Of 58 patients, 50 (86%) were available for follow-up in the laparoscopy group, and 29 of 42 (69%) of the transvaginal group were available for follow-up. Operative time was significantly longer in the population managed laparoscopically: 1.7 hours versus 45 minutes. Estimated blood loss was similar between patients managed with laparoscopic and vaginal technique (84 and 74 mL, respectively). Mean days of postoperative catheterization was 0.9 days for the laparoscopic bladder neck suspension group and 13.2 days for patients managed transvaginally.

Using the strict definition of absolutely no stress incontinence, 30% of patients in the laparoscopy group were completely dry and another 20% had occasional stress incontinence requiring no pads. This was not quite as sanguine an outcome as in the transvaginal group, among whom 34% were completely dry and 28% had occasional stress incontinence requiring no pads. In the remainder of the laparoscopy group, 46% of patients were using one to two pads daily and 4% required more than two pads per day. Of the 19 remaining patients in the transvaginal group, 31% were using one to two pads daily and 7% required more than two pads per day. Fourteen (28%) and eleven (38%) patients in the laparoscopy and transvaginal groups, respectively, experienced postoperative urge incontinence.

With any reconstructive procedure, it is important to determine that point in time when the "success" of the procedure becomes durable. For bladder neck suspension, it would appear that follow-up of less than 2 years is not sufficient. Indeed, in a review of the literature, Spencer and

O'Conor (395) established that failures occurred anywhere between 6 months and 23 years after surgery. They concluded that accurate determination of the efficacy of continence surgery should be established only after 5 years of follow-up. Although laparoscopic bladder neck suspension offers women with incontinence the advantages of minimally invasive surgery, the sparse long-term follow-up data to date suggest that the procedure, as it presently exists, probably does not offer women reasonable long-term continence. In addition, because recent information has shown that a significant population of women with type I and type II incontinence will also manifest some degree of intrinsic sphincter deficiency, many incontinence surgeons currently favor sling procedures that are efficacious in the management of both forms of stress urinary incontinence and have withstood the 5-year test of time (49).

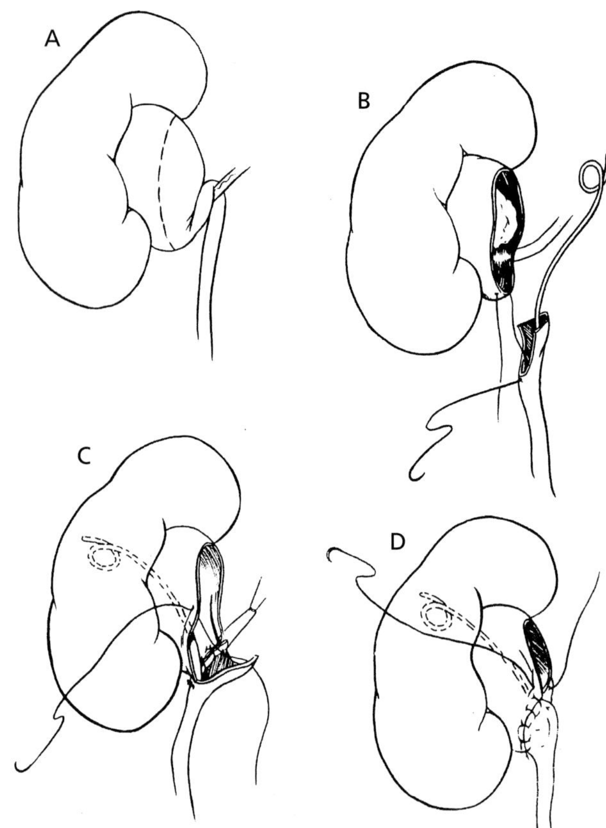

FIGURE 18.16. Laparoscopic dismembered pyeloplasty. **A:** Circumferential incision transecting the renal pelvis above the ureteropelvic junction (UPJ). **B:** The proximal ureter is spatulated through the level of the UPJ laterally. **C, D:** The anastomosis is then completed using intracorporeal suturing with 4-0 absorbable suture.

Retroperitoneum: Pyeloplasty

Open pyeloplasty is the gold standard for correction of ureteropelvic junction (UPJ) obstruction in both pediatric and adult populations. Success rates following open pyeloplasty in contemporary series exceed 90%. However, because of the postoperative morbidity associated with open surgery, including significant pain and a prolonged convalescence period from the flank incision, several alternative, less invasive techniques to manage UPJ obstruction have been developed. Endoscopic or fluoroscopic retrograde and endoscopic percutaneous antegrade management strategies are both efficacious and decrease the convalescence period compared with open pyeloplasty; however, these techniques are associated with a lower success rate.

Laparoscopic pyeloplasty was first reported by Schuessler and co-workers in 1993 (372). The transperitoneal laparoscopic procedure attempts to duplicate the high success rate associated with open surgery while affording patients the advantages of minimally invasive management strategies.

Laparoscopic pyeloplasty can be performed in almost all patients with UPJ obstruction. Patients with a secondarily obstructed UPJ who have failed retrograde or antegrade percutaneous endopyelotomy are especially good candidates for this approach. The presence of ipsilateral renal calculi does not preclude laparoscopic pyeloplasty because flexible or rigid endoscopes can be used to access the renal collecting system during the laparoscopic procedure. Similarly, the laparoscopic approach is effective when there is a complex vascular arrangement around the renal pelvis. Only the presence of a small intrarenal pelvis is currently a contraindication to the procedure.

The procedure is performed via a transperitoneal approach using three or four trocars. After reflection of the colon, the ipsilateral ureter and renal pelvis are identified and fully mobilized. Dissection of an extensive length of ureter is avoided to prevent devascularization of this structure. If a crossing lower pole renal artery is present, it is preserved; all other vessels and peri-UPJ fibrotic tissue are divided. Next, a circumferential incision is made transecting the renal pelvis above the UPJ (Fig. 18.16A). The proximal ureter is spatulated through the level of the UPJ laterally (Fig. 18.16B). If anterior crossing vessels are present, the ureter and renal pelvis are transposed anterior to the vessels before performing the anastomosis. If the renal pelvis is markedly enlarged, pelvic reduction is performed. This is done using laparoscopic scissors and suturing techniques. The anastomosis is then completed using intracorporeal suturing with 4-0 absorbable suture (Fig. 18.16C and D). Suturing can be performed using a free needle and suture or with the assistance of a suturing device (e.g., EndoStitch, U.S. Surgical Inc., Norwalk, Connecticut). The anastomosis can be done either with interrupted or running sutures, depending on the surgeon's preference. An indwelling ureteral stent is placed along with a retroperitoneal drain; the stent is removed 2 to 3 weeks later, and the drain is usually removed before the patient's discharge from the hospital.

Initially, Schuessler and colleagues (372) reported results of four primary and one secondary UPJ obstruction managed with laparoscopic dismembered pyeloplasty. All procedures were accomplished laparoscopically. Operative time ranged from 3 to 7 hours. Estimated blood loss was not reported. Mean hospital stay was 3 days, and all patients returned to normal activity within 1 week. No complications were reported. The procedure was immediately successful in 4 of the 5 cases; one patient, after removal of the stent, reported flank pain and was found to have a stricture distal to the UPJ. The patient underwent balloon dilation and was pain free with a patent ureter after 9 months of follow-up. All other patients remained symptom free and without radiologic signs of obstruction with follow-up ranging from 9 to 17 months (372).

Brooks and colleagues (34) retrospectively compared antegrade endopyelotomy, Acucise endopyelotomy, and laparoscopic pyeloplasty in the management of adult patients with a UPJ obstruction. There were 15 patients evaluated in each group. Mean operative times for antegrade endopyelotomy, Acucise endopyelotomy, laparoscopic pyeloplasty, and open pyeloplasty were 2.5 hours, 46 minutes, 6 hours, and 3.8 hours, respectively. Mean postoperative analgesic requirements for the different procedures varied widely. Analgesic requirements for antegrade endopyelotomy, Acucise endopyelotomy, laparoscopic pyeloplasty, and open pyeloplasty were 18, 1.2, 19, and 190 mg of morphine sulfate equivalents, respectively. Similarly, there was a wide variation in the mean hospital stay. Hospital stays for antegrade endopyelotomy, Acucise endopyelotomy, laparoscopic pyeloplasty, and open pyeloplasty were 3, 0.2, 3.1, and 7.3 days, respectively. A similar pattern was noted with time for full recovery: 4.7 weeks, 1 week, 2.3 weeks, and 10.3 weeks, respectively. Of 13 patients undergoing antegrade endopyelotomy, 3 (23%) required transfusion, as did 2 of 9 (22%) patients undergoing Acucise endopyelotomy. No patient in the laparoscopic pyeloplasty or open pyeloplasty groups required blood transfusion.

Complications were comparable among the four groups. One patient each from the antegrade and Acucise endopyelotomy groups experienced obstruction of their stents necessitating replacement. Two patients in the laparoscopic pyeloplasty group and one patient in the open pyeloplasty group experienced transient obstruction after stent removal. All three patients responded favorably to repeat stent placement. Other complications included a bulbar urethral stricture in the antegrade endopyelotomy group and a midureteral stricture in the laparoscopic pyeloplasty group. There was a single case of urosepsis related to a postoperative antegrade nephrostogram in the open pyeloplasty group (34). All 15 pyeloplasties in both the open and laparoscopic groups had successful outcomes. Success for the two incisional techniques, antegrade and Acucise endopyelotomy, were 77% and 78%, respectively.

Bauer and colleagues (19) retrospectively compared complications and outcomes of 42 patients undergoing laparoscopic pyeloplasty with 35 patients who underwent open pyeloplasty. All laparoscopic procedures were successfully accomplished. Operative time and hospital stay were not reported. There were five (12%) complications in the laparoscopy group: two cases of obstruction after stent removal requiring an additional month of stenting, one intraoperative colon injury that was repaired, one case of thrombophlebitis, and one case of pneumonia. In the open population, there were four (11%) complications: three cases of obstruction after stent removal necessitating stent or nephrostomy tube placement for more than 2 months and one patient with postoperative hemorrhage requiring transfusion.

There were no significant differences between preoperative and postoperative pain and activity scores between the procedures. Specifically, in the laparoscopic group, with a mean follow-up of 22 months, 62% of patients were pain free, 29% of patients had significant improvement in their pain, and 9% of patients experienced minimal or no change in symptoms. In the open surgery group, with a mean follow-up of 58 months, 60% of patients were pain free, 31% of patients reported improvement in their pain, and 3% of patients percent experienced minimal or no change. Objective success was based on the most recent radiographic follow-up (sonogram, intravenous pyelogram, or renal scan). Of the 42 patients in the laparoscopic group, with a mean follow-up of 15 months, 1 (2%) had a failure that was noted within 24 hours of stent removal. In the open group, two patients (6%) had postoperative obstruction with a mean follow-up of 30 months (19).

Laparoscopic pyeloplasty in the adult is a feasible but technically demanding procedure. In adults, the procedure matches the efficacy of open pyeloplasty while offering the benefits of a less invasive approach. However, laparoscopic pyeloplasty remains more morbid than the percutaneous or retrograde approaches to endopyelotomy. As such, although it is generally accepted as an excellent salvage procedure, its use as front-line therapy currently remains controversial.

Retroperitoneum: Nephropexy

Perhaps no urologic procedure has had as checkered a history as the surgical treatment of the patient with a ptotic kidney. Early in the twentieth century, renal ptosis was blamed for myriad symptoms and surgical therapy was applied to a large patient population who, despite fixation of their ptotic kidney, failed to benefit symptomatically (149). As such, nephropexy rightfully fell into disfavor. However, as with many controversial operations, the truth lies somewhere in the middle, and many urologists have come to realize that there is a certain, albeit small, number of patients whose lower quadrant abdominal discomfort is due to renal ptosis. This select group is almost invariably thin and female with the problem occurring almost uniformly on the right side. Classically, their pain is relieved with lying down, and it is common for their right kidney, when in its ptotic position, to be readily palpable in the right lower quadrant. Lying and standing urograms and renal scans are helpful in the diagnosis; the latter may show evidence of decreased blood flow and reduced clearance when the kidney is ptotic. Myriad open procedures have been described to "pex" the kidney high in the retroperitoneum. Hence, it was only a natural progression of laparoscopic renal surgery that led Urban and colleagues (426) to report the first successful laparoscopic nephropexy in 1993.

Laparoscopic transperitoneal nephropexy is initiated by mobilization of the colon to expose Gerota's fascia. Gerota's fascia is then incised and the kidney is dissected along its anterior, posterior, and lateral aspects. Blunt dissection is performed to expose the fascia over the psoas muscle. The patient is then placed in a steep Trendelenburg position, and the kidney is fixed in place, high in the retroperitoneum. The kidney is anchored with four to five nonabsorbable interrupted intracorporeal sutures, placed between the lateral border of the kidney and the psoas or quadratus lumborum muscles (Fig. 18.17). In some cases, a second suture line is run between the anterior surface of the kidney and the upper edge of the incised posterior coronary hepatic ligament (94).

Hubner and co-workers (177) described results of ten women treated for symptomatic nephroptosis who were managed with laparoscopic nephropexy. All ten patients had two nuclear renal scans that demonstrated a change in renal perfusion with alterations in posture. Operative time averaged 2.7 hours; there were no intraoperative complications. Patients required a mean of 10 mg of morphine sulfate for adequate pain control. Postoperatively, all patients underwent intravenous pyelography, which demonstrated no renal descent. With follow-up ranging from 6 to 42 weeks, all patients reported resolution of their symptoms.

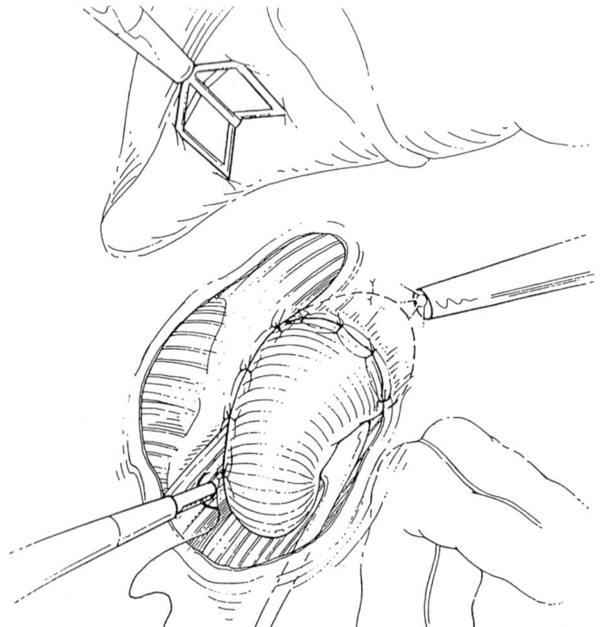

FIGURE 18.17. Laparoscopic nephropexy. Nonabsorbable interrupted intracorporeal sutures are placed between the lateral border of the kidney and the psoas and quadratus lumborum muscles.

Fornara and colleagues (106) compared results of 23 laparoscopic nephropexies with a historical control group of 12 patients who underwent open nephropexy. The laparoscopic group consisted of 1 man and 22 women, and all 12 patients in the open group were female. Of 23 patients, 22 (96%) in the laparoscopic group manifested pathology on the right side. In the laparoscopic group, pain scales were administered preoperatively and at follow-up. All laparoscopic procedures were successfully accomplished with a mean operative time of 61 minutes. Open nephropexies required a mean operative time of 49 minutes. Estimated blood loss was not reported. There were no intraoperative complications in either group.

Postoperative analgesic requirements were 15 and 38 mg of morphine equivalents for laparoscopic and open nephropexy, respectively. Mean hospital stay was 3.7 days in the laparoscopic group and 16 days in the patients managed with open surgery. Time to return to work was not available in the open group, but patients in the laparoscopic group returned to work in a mean time of 19 days. In the laparoscopic group, there were three (13%) minor complications: a urinary tract infection that resolved with antibiotic therapy and two retroperitoneal hematomas that were managed with observation only. In the open group, there was a single (8%) complication: a perirenal hematoma that required transfusion of 2 U of packed RBCs. Of the 21 patients in the laparoscopic group available for follow-up evaluation, all reported significant improvement in pain scores and none required regular analgesics for pain control. Three patients (25%) managed with open surgery had pain similar to what was experienced preoperatively (106).

McDougall and colleagues (257) reported long-term results of 14 women who had undergone laparoscopic nephropexy. The procedure was successfully accomplished in all 14 patients. Operative time was 4.1 hours, with an estimated blood loss of less than 50 mL in every case. The patients resumed oral intake in a mean time of 16.5 hours, and mean hospital stay was 2.6 days. Patients required an average of 37 mg of morphine sulfate for pain control in the postoperative period. There were no intraoperative complications, and there was a single postoperative complication. This patient experienced nausea and vomiting, which required a 5-day hospitalization for intravenous hydration. The symptoms resolved without intervention. Patients returned to their usual activities after a 6-week convalescence.

With a mean follow-up of 3.3 years, the patients experienced an average improvement of 80% on pain scales. Overall, 21% were considered cured, 71% were improved, and 7% failed. The one patient (7%) reported as a failure still had more than 50% improvement in pain. All patients experienced radiographic resolution of nephroptosis; no patient manifested descent of the kidney of more than one vertebral body. Renal function as evaluated by serum creatinine was stable or improved in all patients (257).

Patients with symptomatic nephroptosis have excellent results with nephropexy. Laparoscopic nephropexy is feasible and effective in pain control in properly selected patients. Patients undergoing laparoscopic nephropexy have less postoperative discomfort and a more rapid convalescence than their open surgical counterparts.

Retroperitoneum: Ureterolithotomy and Pyelolithotomy

Until the 1980s, most upper ureteric and renal pelvic calculi that required treatment were managed by open surgery. With the development of extracorporeal shock wave lithotripsy (ESWL), ureteroscopy, percutaneous renal surgery, and improved endourologic instrumentation, the need for open ureterolithotomy and pyelolithotomy has become minimal. Despite the rare indication for open stone surgery, several authors have taken even these few cases and proceeded to perform the necessary stone removal using laparoscopic techniques. The first laparoscopic ureterolithotomy and pyelolithotomy were performed via a retroperitoneal approach by Wickham (437) in 1979 and Gaur and colleagues (115) in 1992, respectively.

Laparoscopic ureterolithotomy has been described via the transperitoneal and retroperitoneal approaches. When done via the transperitoneal approach, the procedure is accomplished with a three-trocar technique. The primary trocar is typically placed infraumbilically in the midline, and two additional trocars are positioned in the midclavicular line, based on the location of the stone (i.e., one above and one below the stone's location). After mobilization of the colon, the ureter is identified and the stone located visually. The ureter is incised and the stone is extracted. The ureter is then closed with interrupted sutures, and a drain is left in the retroperitoneum.

Access for retroperitoneal laparoscopic ureterolithotomy is gained via an incision at the tip of the twelfth rib. The retroperitoneal space is created and two additional trocars are placed, usually one posterior to the initial trocar and a second directly inferior to the initial trocar and two fingerbreadths above the iliac crest. Additional trocar placement is dependent on stone location. The ureter is identified and the stone located visually. After incision of the ureter and stone extraction, one of several paths may be taken: (a) the ureter is closed with intracorporeal sutures, a stent is placed, and a drain is left in the retroperitoneum; (b) the ureter is not closed, but a stent is placed and a drain is left in the retroperitoneum; or (c) the ureter is not closed, a stent is not placed, but a drain is left in the retroperitoneum. Although laparoscopic suturing remains a challenging task, formal closure and stenting of the ureter along with placement of a retroperitoneal drain appears to be the surest way to preclude urinoma or other complications.

Transperitoneal pyelolithotomy is usually performed using three trocars. One trocar is placed at the umbilicus and the other two are placed in the midclavicular line (one subcostal and the other in the lower quadrant). The colon is reflected medially and the renal pelvis identified by following the proximal ureter in a cephalad direction. The renal pelvis is dissected from surrounding structures. A transverse pyelotomy is then made above the ureteropelvic junction. Renal stones are visualized and extracted by passing a flexible cystoscope through a 10- or 12-mm midclavicular cannula. Grasping forceps or a stone basket is used to extract calculi through the trocar. Stones too large to pass through a 10-mm trocar may be placed in a sack and extracted at the termination of the procedure. The pyelotomy is closed with a watertight running or interrupted 3 or 4-0 absorbable suture. A suction drain is left in the retroperitoneum, and an indwelling stent is left in the ureter.

Harewood and co-workers (155) reported results of nine ureterolithotomies. Patients all had large, longstanding, impacted, or obstructing calculi located in the upper or middle ureter. In six patients, a transperitoneal approach was used, and in three cases, the approach was retroperitoneal. The retroperitoneal approach was successful in one patient but required conversion to a transperitoneal approach in the other two patients. In all nine patients, the stones were successfully extracted with the laparoscopic approach. Ureterotomy incisions were closed after indwelling stent placements with two or three interrupted 3-0 chromic catgut sutures to achieve a watertight closure. These sutures were placed using an Ethicon semiautomatic suturing device (Johnson and Johnson Medical, Cincinnati, Ohio). Mean operative time was 158 minutes. Significant drainage occurred in the first five patients; this lasted from 1 to 3 days. Mean hospital stay was 5.2 days. Mean analgesic requirement was 27 mg of morphine sulfate. No intraoperative or postoperative complications were reported.

Turk and colleagues (422) reported results of 21 patients undergoing laparoscopic ureterolithotomy. The transperitoneal approach was used in 20 patients, and the retroperitoneal approach was applied in a single case. The procedure was successfully accomplished in 19 of 21 (90%) cases. Mean operative time was 90 minutes. In two patients, safe location of the calculus by laparoscopy was not possible and open surgery was performed. After indwelling ureteral stent placement, the ureterotomies were closed with running 4-0 PDS suture. Postoperative analgesic requirements were not specified. Patients were discharged between 2 and 7 days after surgery. In two patients, the ureteral stent was left in position for more than 4 weeks due to extravasation on radiographic evaluation. No other intraoperative or postoperative complications were reported.

Gaur and co-workers (115) reported results of eight attempted laparoscopic pyelolithotomies performed via a retroperitoneal approach. The procedure could not be performed in three (38%) patients. Two procedures were converted to open surgery because retroperitoneal access could not be adequately gained. In a third case, conversion to open surgery was necessitated by a tear in the peritoneum. Average operative time was 2 hours. Estimated blood loss was less than 250 mL in all cases. No attempt was made to close the pyelolithotomy incisions, and no indwelling stents were left in position. Average hospital stay was not stated. Drains were removed as outpatients within 7 to 15 days. Analgesic requirements were reported as minimal.

Micali and colleagues (276) presented results of 17 patients undergoing laparoscopic management of renal and ureteral calculi. Eleven patients were treated for renal calculi, and the remaining six patients had ureteral calculi. All procedures were performed using a transperitoneal approach. For renal stones a transverse pyelotomy was created, and stones were extracted using a flexible cystoscope. In 9 of 11 patients with renal calculi, a concomitant laparoscopic pyeloplasty was performed. A suction drain was placed in all 11 patients. A longitudinal ureterotomy was used in all ureteral cases. After stone extraction, ureterotomies were closed with one or two interrupted 4-0 absorbable sutures. Three (50%) patients undergoing ureterolithotomy had a suction drain placed.

Laparoscopic stone removal was successful in 15 (88%) cases. In one case, an investigational camera resulted in disorientation of the surgical team, requiring conversion to open surgery to locate the ureter. The second conversion resulted from inability to fragment a large stone that could not be removed intact. An incision was required to pass a lithotrite to crush the stone. Mean operative time including ancillary procedures was 4.9 hours. Mean estimated blood loss was 133 mL, and no patient required blood transfusion. Patients required 26 mg of morphine sulfate for pain control and had a mean hospital stay of 4.5 days. Return to full activity required 3 weeks. With a mean follow-up of 13.7 months, all patients were asymptomatic and stone free without obstruction on intravenous urography. There were three (18%) postoperative complications. One patient had a prolonged ileus and another patient experienced a *Clostridium difficile* infection, requiring hospital stays of 5 and 15 days, respectively. One patient experienced fever and abdominal pain 2 weeks after distal ureterolithotomy, and a retroperitoneal urinoma was identified and drained percutaneously. This patient did not have a drain placed after ureterolithotomy.

Laparoscopic ureterolithotomy and pyelolithotomy are feasible procedures. However, present-day technology, including ESWL, ureteroscopy, and percutaneous access techniques, offers patients a less invasive alternative for stone management. In general, laparoscopic management should be considered only when these modalities are unavailable or have been tried and failed or the patient is undergoing a concomitant laparoscopic procedure (e.g., pyeloplasty).

Retroperitoneum: Ureterolysis

Extrinsic compression and obstruction of the ureters is relatively uncommon and is often associated with significant patient discomfort and functional renal loss. Retroperitoneal fibrosis (RPF) and ovarian pathology are among the most common benign conditions associated with extrinsic obstruction of the ureter. Although ureterolysis for RPF is highly efficacious, it is associated with significant morbidity and occasional mortality. Laparoscopic ureterolysis has been described as a minimally invasive alternative to the open procedure. Laparoscopic ureterolysis was introduced by Kavoussi and co-workers (209) in 1992; Puppo and colleagues (343) subsequently reported the first bilateral procedure in 1994.

The technique is usually a four-port transperitoneal approach. In all cases, an external ureteral stent is placed immediately before the laparoscopy. After incising the line of Toldt and reflecting the colon, the surgeon circumferentially dissects the unaffected portions of the ureter proximal and distal to the fibrosis. Following this, the affected ureter is dissected out of the thick fibrotic tissue, being careful to remove it from the layers of periureteral fibrotic tissue without entering the ureteral lumen. Once freed, the ureter is brought into the peritoneal cavity, and the line of Toldt is then reestablished posterior to the ureter, using intracorporeal suturing or placement of apposing clips. An omental wrap of the ureter is usually not performed. At the end of the procedure, the external stent is exchanged for an internal ureteral stent; the ureteral stent is left in place for 4 to 6 weeks.

Elashry and colleagues (96) compared six patients undergoing unilateral laparoscopic ureterolysis for extrinsic ureteral obstruction with seven patients undergoing open unilateral ureterolysis for similar pathologic conditions. Laparoscopic unilateral ureterolysis was successfully accomplished in all six patients. Mean operative times for laparoscopic and open ureterolysis were similar (255 versus 232 minutes); however, in the open group, an omental wrap of the ureter was usually performed in addition to the ureterolysis. Estimated blood loss was decreased with the laparoscopic approach: 140 versus 373 mL. Hospital stay was shortened in the laparoscopic group: 2.8 versus 10.5 days. Similarly, return to full activity was expedited by the laparoscopic approach: 2.1 versus 7 weeks. There were no major or minor complications in the laparoscopically managed group. In the open group, there was one (14%) intraoperative complication and four (57%) postoperative complications. Intraoperatively, a ureter was avulsed during ureterolysis, requiring psoas hitch reimplantation. In addition, among the open surgery patients, two patients (29%) required postoperative blood transfusions, one patient (14%)

had a 6-day ileus, and one patient (14%) experienced wound cellulitis that resolved with intravenous antibiotic treatment. All patients in both groups were symptomatically improved or cured, and all had evidence of radiologic resolution of obstruction on follow-up evaluations (96).

Nezhat and colleagues (302) described laparoscopic ureterolysis in 28 women with severe urinary tract endometriosis. Twenty-one women in this series had partial or complete obstruction of the ureter. After ureteral catheter placement, the affected ureter was dissected free from surrounding tissues with hydrodissection and the CO_2 laser. Any evidence of ureteral endometriosis or fibrosis was vaporized using the laser. When the ureteral lumen was grossly entered, closure was performed with intracorporeal suturing. Pinpoint entries were not repaired. If the lumen was completely occluded and catheter placement was impossible, the affected segment was excised and primary laparoscopic anastomosis performed.

Seventeen women had extrinsic ureteral compression causing partial obstruction and four had full-thickness complete obstruction. Of the four with full-thickness involvement, three underwent primary repair and one was treated with ureteroneocystostomy. Mean postoperative hospital stay was 1.8 days. A single postoperative complication was reported. On postoperative day 1, a woman developed a pleural effusion requiring thoracocentesis and aspiration. On follow-up evaluation, 20 of 21 (95%) patients had patent ureters and functional kidneys. One woman (5%), who presented with unilateral complete ureteral obstruction, had a patent ureter postoperatively but only 10% to 20% function on the affected side; unfortunately, there was no preoperative functional evaluation in this patient (302).

Laparoscopic ureterolysis is feasible and effective. Benefits include rapid convalescence and minimal morbidity. Of interest is the success of laparoscopic ureterolysis as a singular procedure, devoid of using an omental wrap; elimination of this step from the ureterolysis procedure may well account for the reasonable operating room time and the markedly lower morbidity of the laparoscopic approach.

Abdominal: Peritoneal Dialysis Catheter Placement and Repair

Peritoneal dialysis (PD) was described by Ganter in 1923 (111). Despite offering several advantages over hemodialysis, complications related to the peritoneal catheter such as exit site infection, tunnel infection, incorrect positioning of the catheter within the abdomen, peritonitis, pericatheter hernia, pain, or mechanical dysfunction with related fluid drainage remain troublesome. Complications have limited catheter survival to only 51% to 60% at 18 months and 22% to 50% at 36 months (152,355).

The most common approach to PD catheter placement is the open surgical approach. Other methods for PD catheter placement, using guidewire techniques, have also been described. However, these methods have not gained widespread acceptance because of concerns over possible visceral injury.

Kimmelstiel and colleagues (220) first reported laparoscopic placement of peritoneal dialysis catheters in 1993. At present, the laparoscopic technique for PD catheter placement employs a 1.5-cm infraumbilical incision. After inspection of the abdomen for adhesions or other anatomic abnormalities that could hinder catheter flow, a second trocar is inserted in a lower paramedian position. The PD catheter is then positioned with its tip in the pouch of Douglas. After fascial closure, a subcutaneous tunnel is created for the PD catheter entry port. Intraabdominal position of the catheter is confirmed with a sterile saline flush before termination of the procedure.

Crabtree and Fishman (68) reported results of 29 patients undergoing laparoscopic PD catheter placement. All catheters were placed via two paramedian trocars placed at the level of the umbilicus. Twenty-nine attempted catheter placements were described with a single (3.4%) failure due to injury of an inferior epigastric artery. Operative times and estimated blood loss were not provided. Median follow-up was 4.4 months. Two patients experienced intraperitoneal bleeding that required transfusion in the postoperative period. All catheters were functional at the time of the report. Ten (36%) patients experienced delayed complications: six exit site infections, one exit site/tunnel tract infection, one case of peritonitis, one catheter leak, and one episode of outflow obstruction requiring laparoscopic manipulation for repair.

Wright and colleagues (454) performed a randomized prospective trial comparing 21 laparoscopic and 25 open PD catheter placements. Laparoscopic placement was accompanied by creation of a 2.5- to 3.0-cm lower midline incision for catheter placement. Complications were divided into an early group (occurring within 6 weeks of surgery) and a late group (occurring after 6 weeks). Four laparoscopic procedures required conversion to an open approach due to technical, nonhemorrhagic problems (i.e., unable to establish a pneumoperitoneum and obesity). Open surgery was faster than the laparoscopic approach: 14 versus 22 minutes. Estimated blood loss was not reported. There was no significant difference in the early or late complication rates between the laparoscopic and open groups: 48% versus 29% early problems and 48% versus 63% late complications. These problems, both early and late, were almost invariably due to exit site infections or peritonitis. The duration of hospital stay, pain scores, and analgesic requirements were not significantly different between the two groups. However, the laparoscopic group tended to have lower pain scores after the initial six postoperative hours. In sum, these authors found no significant benefit to the laparoscopic approach.

In contrast, Gadallah and co-workers (107) compared complications of 72 open surgical placements with 76 peritoneoscopic PD catheter placements in a prospective randomized fashion. Peritoneal dialysis catheters were placed via a single 2-cm paramedian incision after laparoscopic visualization of the abdominal contents. Convalescence parameters and surgical data were not reported. Complications were considered early if they occurred within 2 weeks of PD catheter placement and late if they occurred more than 2 weeks after catheter placement. Early complications, commonly peritonitis or leakage, were significantly more common in the open group: 33% versus 13%. There was no significant difference in the frequency of late complications between open and peritoneoscopic approaches: 61% versus 58%, respectively. These complications included infection, catheter malfunction, and hernias (107).

Laparoscopic salvage of malfunctioning PD catheters has also been described. Amerling and co-workers (11) reported results of 25 patients with 28 episodes of PD catheter obstruction undergoing laparoscopic salvage procedures. In 23 (92%) cases, the catheter was successfully restored to function. In two cases, adhesions were so dense that the distal end of the catheter could not be identified. Obstruction was secondary to omental entrapment in 18 cases and to local adhesion formation in 10 cases. Operative time ranged from 40 to 120 minutes. When performed on low-risk patients, many could be discharged on the same day as the laparoscopic procedure. Only oral analgesics were required postoperatively.

Subsequently, the salvaged catheters remained patent for a mean of 9.2 months (range = 0 to 36 months). Overall, the procedural complication rate was 39%: catheter occlusion (one case), peritonitis (four cases), subcutaneous leakage (four cases), and trocar site hernia (two cases). The latter two problems were largely rectified with the routine use of a trocar site closure device (11).

Laparoscopic peritoneal dialysis catheter placement is a feasible procedure. A two-trocar site approach for access, placement, and manipulation of the PD catheter provides satisfactory results without the need for any incision larger than the port itself (i.e., 10 to 12 mm); likewise, fascial closure of all port sites is recommended to prevent subsequent leakage. The laparoscopically implanted PD catheters tend to have fewer early complications, perhaps because of better positioning and use of a smaller incision; however, the overall benefits of the laparoscopic approach appear to be minimal, and the operative time is longer. In contrast, salvage of nonfunctioning PD catheters is a feasible and perhaps more beneficial application of laparoscopy among these patients.

Benign Disease: Reconstructive—On the Horizon

Sling Procedure

Pubovaginal sling, artificial sphincter placement, and periurethral injection therapies are the treatment options for intrinsic sphincter deficiency (type III) stress urinary incontinence. The pubovaginal sling has also become the primary modality for repair of type I and type II stress incontinence. The technique for performing a pubovaginal sling has been described for either a transvaginal or transabdominal approach. In an attempt to minimize postoperative pain and convalescence, the laparoscopic approach has been applied to the procedure.

Kreder and Winfield (226) described the initial laparoscopic sling placement for stress urinary incontinence via an extraperitoneal approach. Fascia lata was harvested from the patient's thigh in the usual fashion. Five trocar sites were placed in the lower abdomen, and a plane was created between the bladder neck and the vagina. The fascial sling was passed through the defect at the bladder neck and anchored to the rectus fascia 0.5 cm above the pubis with nonabsorbable sutures passed through two of the previously placed trocar sites. Two cases were described, one of which had to be converted to open due to an inadvertent urethrotomy. The successful laparoscopic case had an operative time of 6.5 hours with an estimated blood loss of less than 100 mL. The patient required 16 mg of intramuscular morphine postoperatively. Sluggish return of bowel function resulted in a 5-day hospital stay. At 3-week follow-up, the patient was doing well with a normal voiding cystourethrogram, and the catheter was removed. At 4-month follow-up, the patient was continent.

A laparoscopic pubovaginal sling procedures is technically feasible. However, with the evolution of a transvaginal approach in conjunction with synthetic or allograft materials for sling construction, the open procedure has become minimally invasive. Indeed, most of these patients are now treated on an outpatient basis. As such, it is unlikely there will be any advantage to patients in the application of laparoscopic technology for this purpose.

Sacral-colposuspension

Vaginal wall prolapse has been managed by abdominal sacral colpopexy or transvaginal sacrospinous ligament vaginal vault suspension. In an attempt to apply minimally invasive technology to vaginal wall prolapse, laparoscopic sacral-colposuspension has been described.

The procedure, as described by Ostrzenski (317), is performed via an extraperitoneal approach. The retropubic space is entered bilaterally between the urachus and the medial umbilical folds, and the space of Retzius is opened until the obturator foramen is visualized bilaterally. The vagina is digitally elevated to its normal position, and using 0-polydioxanone suture, the surgeon anchors it to the surrounding pelvic structures. Posteriorly, the vaginal apex is suspended to the deep layer of the uterosacral ligaments. The posterolateral vaginal cuff is suspended to the cardinal ligaments. Anteriorly, the vaginal vault is suspended to the pubocervical fascia. Finally, the pubocervical fascia and the anterolateral vaginal sulci are suspended to the fascia of the obturator internus muscle and tendinous arch bilaterally. The peritoneum is closed after vaginal suspension has been accomplished.

Ostrzenski (317) reported the use of this technique in 27 patients with iatrogenic total vaginal prolapse after hysterectomy. The initial 17 patients underwent the procedure without suspension of the pubocervical fascia to the obturator internus and tendinous arches. The procedure was subsequently modified and the two groups compared. All procedures were successfully accomplished laparoscopically, and estimated blood loss was minimal. Mean operative time was 3.6 hours. Twenty-four (89%) patients were discharged on the day of surgery, with the remaining three (11%) discharged on postoperative day 1. No intraoperative complications were described. Two patients (7%) experienced postoperative urinary tract infections.

Of the initial 16 patients, 1 (6%) experienced complete vaginal prolapse within 6 months of the procedure. Eleven patients (69%) had no significant laxity of the vaginal apex or walls. Four patients (25%) displayed some degree of vaginal cuff descent postoperatively. After modification of the procedure, an additional 11 patients were evaluated. No patient experienced prolapse of the vaginal apex over a 42-month follow-up period. Ten patients (91%) displayed no laxity of the vaginal apex or walls. One patient (9%) demonstrated moderate vaginal wall descent.

There are limited data on laparoscopic sacral-colposuspension. However, the procedure appears to be safe and feasible. Preliminary results are promising, and patients may benefit from a more rapid convalescence with decreased pain. Data comparing open and laparoscopic techniques are required before a more definitive conclusion can be drawn.

Mitrofanoff Procedure

Clean intermittent catheterization is the preferred management option for the patient with a neurogenic bladder. When the urethra cannot be used, cutaneous appendicovesicostomy, as described by Mitrofanoff (283), offers a reliable alternative. The Mitrofanoff principle entails the use of a supple conduit, typically the appendix, brought to the skin as a catheterizable stoma with an antireflux connection to the urinary reservoir. Laparoscopic urinary diversion using the Mitrofanoff principle was initially described by Strand and colleagues (402).

Hedican and colleagues (162) reported their experience with a laparoscopic assisted Mitrofanoff procedure in eight patients ages 7 to 26 years. The laparoscopic technique was used to mobilize the cecum and harvest a gastric segment, thereby eliminating the need for an upper abdominal incision. The vermiform appendix was mobilized and a stapler fired across the base to isolate this segment. A laparoscopic suture was placed through the appendix to allow withdrawal through a trocar site. The remainder of the reconstruction was performed through a Pfannenstiel incision. The time for the laparoscopic portion of the procedures was not reported, and analgesic requirements were not quantitated. Median hospital stay was 8 days. One (12.5%) complication was reported: a patient required open reexploration for small bowel obstruction caused by a knuckle of ileum trapped between crossed mesenteries.

Lorenzo and co-workers (245) compared results of four open Mitrofanoff procedures with four laparoscopic Mitrofanoff procedures performed with the same basic technique in patients ages 17 to 58 years. Using four access trocars, the physician isolated the vermiform appendix with the vascular pedicle. Using a linear laparoscopic stapler, the physician transected the appendiceal base with a 3-mm cuff of cecum. The distal appendix was cut, and a direct anastomosis to the bladder was accomplished with four to six interrupted 4-0 Vicryl sutures. The proximal appendix, with the attached 3-mm cecal segment, was used to create the skin stoma. A 10-Fr Foley catheter was placed through the lumen of the appendicular lumen, and a skin stoma was created at the umbilicus. A Penrose drain was left in position.

All four procedures were successfully accomplished laparoscopically with a mean operative time of 2.45 hours versus 1.55 hours for the open procedures. Mean estimated blood loss was 200 mL in both groups. Mean hospital stay for the open and laparoscopic procedures was 5 and 3 days, respectively. The postoperative narcotic requirements of patients managed laparoscopically were reported to be significantly less than the requirements of patients managed with open surgery. The mean recovery time for the open procedure was 4 weeks; after the laparoscopic procedure it was 1.5 weeks. Postoperative laboratory tests demonstrated that all patients had sterile urine, and there was no laboratory or radiographic evidence of upper tract deterioration with a mean follow-up of 19.5 months (245). All eight patients remain continent both subjectively and by urodynamic assessment.

Laparoscopic urinary diversion applying the Mitrofanoff principle is feasible. Limited data are available; however, the procedure seems to afford patients the benefits of minimally invasive surgery while resulting in reliable urinary continence.

Ileal Conduit

Since its introduction by Bricker (33) in the 1950s, the ileal conduit has become a staple in the urologist's armamentarium. Indications for ileal conduit construction include the need for urinary diversion due to a diseased or otherwise nonfunctional bladder. Several groups have reported laparoscopic ileal conduit construction.

Kozminski and Partamian (225) described the first laparoscopic assisted ileal conduit. Bilateral ureteral dissection was performed. Bowel transection was performed by pulling the ileum through one of the trocar sites. A small mesenteric window was made at the edge of the bowel wall and a GIA stapler was used to transect the bowel. After the ileal segment had been isolated, the free ends of the remaining transected bowel were pulled through a trocar site using previously placed suture tags. An extracorporeal antimesenteric side-to-side anastomosis was then performed using GIA and TA-55 staplers. The mesenteric window was then closed with Endoclips. Both ureters were anastomosed to the ileal loop in an end-to-side fashion. Each ureter was brought through a trocar site with the ileal conduit, and a standard hand-sewn anastomosis was performed on the abdominal wall. Operative time was 6.3 hours. The patient required no narcotic medications after the first 12 postoperative hours. He was started on a diet on postoperative day 5 and discharged home on postoperative day 7. He was able to resume normal activity 10 days after surgery. The patient had not experienced any complications at follow-up 3 months later (225).

Vara-Thorbeck and Sanchez-de-Bandajoz (428) reported laparoscopic assisted ileal conduit construction for a high-risk elderly patient with bladder cancer. The patient had a solitary kidney and known invasive bladder cancer with several episodes of urinary retention secondary to blood clots. Distal ureteral dissection was performed unilaterally. Sufficient ureteral length was dissected to allow an extracorporeal ureteroileal anastomosis to be performed. A 15-cm segment of ileum was isolated and bowel continuity reestablished with a side-to-side sutured anastomosis. A single-J stent was placed in the ureter before implantation in the ileal segment through an extended trocar site 4 cm in length. Operative time was 4 hours, and intestinal motility was noted on the first postoperative day. With a 4-month follow-up, the patient was symptom free and receiving radiation therapy.

Potter and colleagues (338) reported long-term follow-up of an ileal conduit constructed in 1995 with a completely intracorporeal technique. The ileal conduit was constructed in a 28-year-old man with a neurogenic bladder. The ileal segment was isolated with laparoscopic staplers, and ureteral anastomoses were performed using a "dunk" technique. After placement of 1 cm of distal ureter into the ileal conduit, four anchoring adventitial sutures were placed in the ureter. During 5 years of follow-up, the patient had no urinary tract infections and the skin stoma remained patent and viable. Intravenous urography performed 1, 2, 3, and 5 years after creation of the conduit revealed prompt, symmetric renal function and preservation of renal parenchyma without evidence of obstruction of the urinary tract. Retrograde contrast studies of the ileal conduit revealed no evidence of reflux, and the patient's serum creatinine remained stable at 0.8 mg/dL.

Laparoscopic assisted ileal conduit construction has been described and is feasible. The procedure is time-consuming, and the benefits of the laparoscopically assisted ileal conduit have not been clearly demonstrated due to the few number of procedures and the variations in technique. Comparison with traditional open techniques is lacking, and long-term follow-up data are just beginning to emerge, albeit in only a handful of patients.

Enteric Bladder Augmentation

Open enteroplasty is the most commonly used technique for augmentation of bladder capacity. Anastomosis of a well-vascularized patch of detubularized bowel can significantly and durably increase the storage capacity of the urinary bladder. Several investigators have described laparoscopic enterocystoplasty with different segments of the gastrointestinal tract.

Docimo and colleagues (82) described gastrocystoplasty in a young female patient with a neurogenic bladder. The patient had a small poorly compliant bladder with a capacity of 150 mL. Stomach was chosen as the source for augmentation because the authors believed it would be more technically straightforward. Using blunt and sharp dissection, the surgeon dissected the anterior bladder wall free of surrounding structures to the level of the urethra. Attention was turned to the stomach, where the greater omentum was divided distal to the gastroepiploic arcade and the transverse mesocolon was displaced posteriorly. The right gastroepiploic pedicle was dissected free of the right side of the greater curvature of the stomach to the level of the pylorus. After division of the omentum, a gastric wedge, 20 cm in length, was removed using five firings of a laparoscopic stapler. An EndoStitch suturing device was used to oversew the stomach. An EndoStitch device with 3-0 Vicryl suture was used to run the edges of the anastomosis of the gastric segment to the bladder. A 24-Fr Malecot suprapubic tube and a 20-Fr Foley urethral catheter were left to drain the bladder. The patient also underwent a needle bladder neck suspension. Total operative time was 10 hours, 55 minutes. The patient received a transfusion of 2 units of packed RBCs despite an estimated blood loss of 250 mL. Postoperatively, the patient received 247 mg of morphine via her patient-controlled analgesia device. Because of a transient urine leak, she was not discharged until postoperative day 13. Urodynamic evaluation 3 months after surgery revealed a bladder capacity of 315 mL. She remained dry on intermittent catheterization.

Gill and colleagues (127) reported results of laparoscopic assisted enterocystoplasty in three patients with reduced bladder capacity. Augmentation was performed with ileum in the first case and sigmoid colon in the second. The third patient underwent augmentation with cecum and right colon, and the terminal ileum was refashioned to create a continent conduit, which was brought out at the umbilicus as a catheterizable stoma. After selection of the appropriate bowel segment, 15 cm of bowel was delivered outside the abdomen via a 2-cm extension of the umbilical trocar site. Using open surgical techniques, each bowel segment with its mesenteric pedicle was isolated, bowel continuity reestablished, and the mesenteric window closed (Fig. 18.18A).

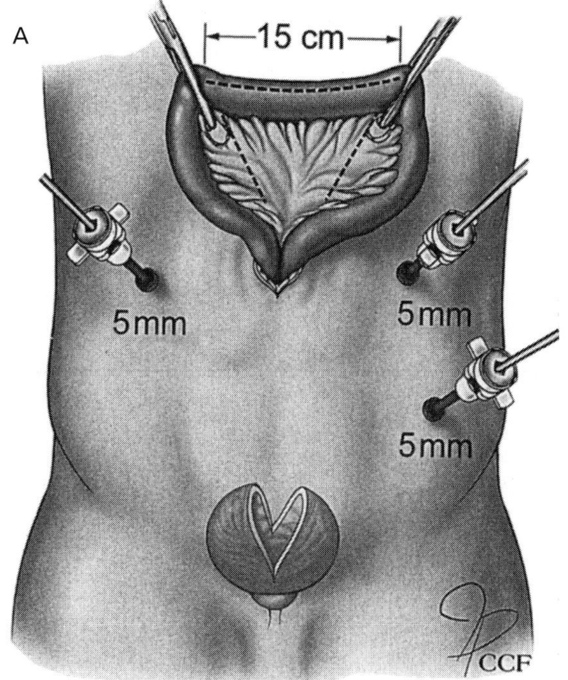

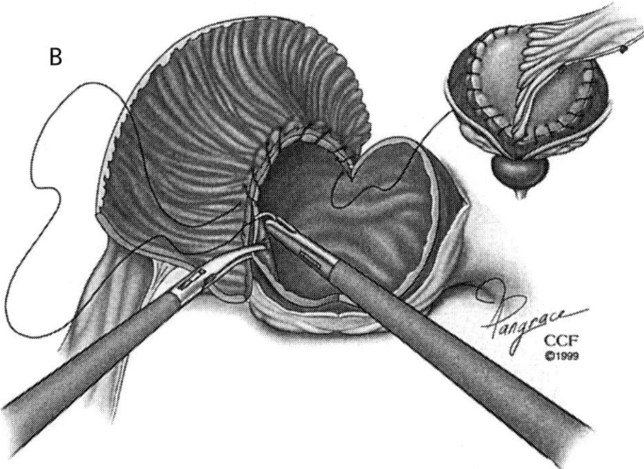

FIGURE 18.18. Laparoscopic bladder augmentation. **A:** Ileal segment is isolated and bowel continuity reestablished using open technique. **B:** After detubularization, the isolated ileal segment is anastomosed to the bladder with intracorporeal suturing.

After detubularization, the bowel segments were anastomosed to the bladder with intracorporeal suturing (Fig. 18.18B). In the third patient, the terminal ileum was narrowed, the ileocecal junction was imbricated, and the ileum was brought out the umbilicus as a catheterizable stoma. Mean operative time was 6.8 hours. Mean estimated blood loss was 150 mL. The only intraoperative complication was a rectus sheath hematoma, which was controlled laparoscopically. Postoperative Jackson-Pratt drainage was minimal in all three cases, and drains were removed on postoperative days 3, 5, and 4, respectively. The first patient developed an ileus that delayed his discharge until postoperative day 7. The subsequent two patients were discharged on postoperative days 4 and 5. Analgesic requirements were 44, 55, and 229 mg of morphine. Follow-up bladder capacities and long-term patient outcomes were not reported.

Pure laparoscopic and laparoscopic assisted procedures for enterocystoplasty are feasible; however, in only one case has long-term data been provided as to the efficacy of the procedure. Further experience and eventual comparison with traditional open techniques are needed. At present, this laparoscopic approach remains under study.

Bladder Autoaugmentation

A consistent feature of the urologic approach to bladder augmentation has been the application of components of the alimentary tract as a vascularized source of graft material. Aside from the morbidity of harvesting the graft material, the use of bowel for urologic reconstruction is associated with significant late sequelae, including segment-specific metabolic disturbances arising from chronic contact with urine, pouch rupture, urolithiasis, and, rarely, carcinogenesis. Autoaugmentation (vesicomyotomy or vesicomyomectomy) represents an alternative approach to increasing the capacity of the urinary bladder while avoiding the incorporation of foreign epithelium. This technique entails the incision or excision of the detrusor layer of the bladder to create a large wide-mouthed diverticulum of urothelium. First described by Couvelaire and Agrandir (67) in 1955, the technique has undergone a significant evolution with variable results.

The technique of laparoscopic autoaugmentation was first described by Ehrlich and Gershman (91). Briefly, a transperitoneal pneumoperitoneum is established to 10 mm Hg. Four trocars are placed: umbilical, two midclavicular trocars on either side midway between the iliac crest and umbilicus, and a right lower quadrant trocar just lateral to the rectus sheath and inferior to the midclavicular right-sided trocar. The bladder is distended via a urethral catheter. Using curved laparoscopic scissors and low-power cutting current, the posterior wall of the bladder is incised until the urothelium is visualized. Using graspers, the surgeon teases the bladder muscle laterally, exposing additional amounts of urothelium. Any bleeding detrusor muscle is carefully coagulated with special care to avoid coagulation of the urothelium. The incision is extended posteriorly to the cul-de-sac and superiorly to the anterior fusion of the peritoneum and bladder. The bladder muscle is teased laterally for approximately one-third of the circumference of the bladder. A drain is left in the space of Retzius. The bladder is drained with a urethral catheter; a cystogram is performed 5 to 7 days postoperatively, and if there is no extravasation, the bladder catheter is removed.

In Ehrlich and Gershman's initial case report (91), an 8-year-old boy with a nonneurogenic neurogenic bladder underwent a 1.2-hour laparoscopic autoaugmentation. The patient was discharged in less than 24 hours, and the drain was removed on postoperative day 2. On postoperative day 8, the patient's urethral catheter malfunctioned, resulting in a small bladder perforation that was treated with a percutaneous cystotomy tube. Voiding cystourethrogram at 2 weeks demonstrated no extravasation. One year postoperatively, the patient's persistent daytime and nighttime incontinence had markedly improved, with only minor leakage with strenuous athletic activity.

McDougall and colleagues (264) also reported their initial experience, albeit with an extraperitoneal laparoscopic autoaugmentation, in a 26-year-old woman with a traumatic spinal cord injury. Urodynamic evaluation revealed poor compliance, a decreased leak point pressure, and a bladder capacity of 85 mL. An extraperitoneal laparoscopic seromyotomy autoaugmentation was performed using a 3-Fr right-angle Greenwald electrode. The bilateral detrusor flaps were sutured to Cooper's ligament bilaterally with 1-0 polyglactin suture. Operative time was 6.5 hours, and estimated blood loss was 75 mL. The patient was discharged on postoperative day 2 with bladder drainage in place. Bladder drainage was continued for 1 month, at which time a cystogram revealed no extravasation. At 6-month follow-up, the patient had a normal cystogram, good compliance, a bladder capacity of 285 mL, and improved leak point pressure. The patient had daytime and nighttime continence, and she was catheter-free voiding by Valsalva with a residual of 30 mL.

Subsequently, Poppas and co-workers (337) reported two cases of laparoscopic seromyotomy autoaugmentation that were performed with KTP laser assistance. Two children with myelodysplasia and high-pressure neurogenic bladders unresponsive to conservative management underwent laparoscopic autoaugmentation. The detrusorotomy was performed with the KTP laser. A right-angle backstop device was used for the final portions of the detrusorotomy after initial access to the urothelium had been achieved. There were no reported complications. Initial results were promising, with improvement in symptoms, decreased peak detrusor pressures, and increased bladder capacity in both cases. However, at 5 months, both cases failed and went on enterocystoplasty.

Autoaugmentation is an attractive, minimally invasive method for the treatment of the contracted, high-pressure bladder. Although the technique is amenable to a laparoscopic approach, there is little experience and inconsistent results. Further detailed studies in the laboratory and clinical arena are needed to determine the appropriate application and best technique for autoaugmentation surgery.

Ureteroureterostomy

The need for ureteral reconstruction is usually due to an intrinsic stricture (e.g., trauma, infection, stone impaction) or extrinsic compression (e.g., endometriosis, retrocaval ureter). Whereas the former can often be managed by endoscopic techniques, the latter usually requires a formal ureteroureterostomy for therapy. Several authors have described laparoscopic ureteroureterostomy in the management of ureteral pathology.

Nezhat and colleagues (301) reported the use of laparoscopic ureteroureterostomy for the management of ureteral obstruction secondary to endometriosis. Using laparoscopic techniques, the surgeon excised the diseased segment of the ureter and performed a ureteroureterostomy using four evenly spaced full-thickness 4-0 PDS sutures. The sutures were tied intracorporeally. Operative time was 117 minutes, with an estimated blood loss of less than 100 mL. The patient was discharged on postoperative day 1. Two months postoperatively, the ureteral stent was removed and intravenous urography revealed a patent ureter. Twenty-one months postoperatively, the patient was asymptomatic with a normal ultrasound evaluation of the kidney.

Laparoscopic ureteroureterostomy for retrocaval ureter was initially described by Ishitoya and colleagues (186) and later by Matsuda and co-workers (250) in 1996. Polascik and Chen (332) also reported ureteroureterostomy in the management of an obstructed retrocaval ureter. Using three trocars, the surgeon identified and mobilized the affected portion of the ureter. The ureter was divided at the most visible portion of the dilated proximal segment. The distal segment was spatulated for approximately 2 cm. The ureter was repositioned to lie anterior to the vena cava, and a previously placed stent was advanced into the renal pelvis. Anastomosis was performed using several interrupted 4-0 polyglactin sutures with an EndoStitch device. A double-J stent was left in position at the end of the procedure. Operative time was 3.75 hours. The patient was discharged on postoperative day 2. Analgesics were not required after the first day, and the patient resumed full activity on postoperative day 4. Retrograde ureteropyelogram performed 4 months after surgery revealed a patent ureter (332).

Laparoscopic ureteroureterostomy is feasible and has demonstrated good results in the few reported cases. The procedure is technically demanding, but future advances in laparoscopic tissue apposition may result in simplification. In a porcine model, Maxwell and co-workers (251) reported successful laparoscopic ureteroureterostomy using vascular closure staple (VCS) clips to perform the anastomosis. Operative times to perform the ureteroureterostomy were reduced from 39.7 and 39.5 minutes with hand suturing and EndoStitch suturing, respectively, to 22 minutes using the VCS clips. The procedure resulted in patent ureters without stones or encrustation at subsequent evaluation 12 weeks later.

Calyceal Diverticulum

Most calyceal diverticula remain asymptomatic. The incidence of calculi within calyceal diverticula varies from 10%

to 50% (278). Options for management of these stones, when they become symptomatic, have included percutaneous extraction, ureteroscopic lithotripsy, and ESWL.

Gluckman and colleagues (134) reported the initial procedure of laparoscopic treatment of a stone-bearing, calyceal diverticulum. Subsequently, Ruckle and Segura (360) reported transperitoneal laparoscopic management of a stone-filled calyceal diverticulum. Later, Chen and colleagues (52) reported using a retroperitoneal approach for unroofing a calyceal diverticulum filled with milk of calcium.

Harewood and co-workers (154) described a series of three patients with calyceal diverticula that were managed by an extraperitoneal laparoscopic approach. All three patients had diverticula associated with calculi. All three cases were successfully completed laparoscopically with a mean operative time of 127 minutes. Blood loss was minimal in the first two patients, but hemorrhage was troublesome in the third patient, necessitating a transfusion of 3 units of packed RBCs. All calculi were eliminated, but there was a small recurrence of one (33%) of the diverticula. Patients received an average of six doses of meperidine and were discharged in 4 days. One patient experienced drainage from one of the trocar sites for 2 months that resolved without intervention. There were no other complications reported.

Hoznek and co-workers (175) reported results of retroperitoneal laparoscopic management of three patients with symptomatic calyceal diverticula. All procedures were successfully accomplished with a mean operative time of 80 minutes and minimal blood loss. The calyceal diverticular cavities were filled with surgical mesh impregnated with gelatin resorcinol formaldehyde glue. Average hospital stay was 6.7 days with patients requiring analgesics only during the first postoperative day. There were no complications reported. At 6 months, follow-up CT scan revealed no calculi or recurrence of the diverticula.

Laparoscopic calyceal diverticulectomy is a feasible procedure. However, for the most part, a laparoscopic approach is only considered first-line therapy by some endourologists for a large, anterior calyceal diverticulum, because all others can be expeditiously managed by percutaneous or ureteroscopic techniques.

Bladder Diverticulum

A urinary bladder diverticulum creates a separate, poorly contractile chamber and can lead to complications such as recurrent urinary tract infection, stone formation, ureteral obstruction, vesicoureteral reflux, and rarely, transitional cell carcinoma. Das (72) first described laparoscopic bladder diverticulectomy in 1992. Subsequently, there have been several reports regarding laparoscopic management of bladder diverticula.

Jarrett and colleagues (200) detailed their laparoscopic management of a large bladder diverticulum. After cystoscopic placement of a balloon catheter into the diverticulum, a transperitoneal approach was used to access the bladder. The peritoneum was reflected laterally and the diverticulum excised. The bladder was closed in a single layer with intracorporeal suturing expedited with Lapra-Ty clips. A cystotomy tube was left in position for bladder drainage, and Jackson-Pratt drains were left in position for drainage. Operative time was 6.5 hours. The retroperitoneal drain was removed on postoperative day 1. The patient was discharged on postoperative day 3. Analgesic requirement included 4 mg of morphine and 225 mg of intramuscular meperidine. On postoperative day 9, the patient had a cystogram that demonstrated no leakage and the Foley catheter was removed.

Iselin and co-workers (185) compared two laparoscopic urinary bladder diverticulectomies with four open cases. Patients in both groups underwent transurethral resection of the prostate followed by either laparoscopic or open urinary bladder diverticulectomy. Both laparoscopic diverticulectomies were performed successfully. Mean operative times for laparoscopic and open procedures were 4.2 and 1.7 hours, respectively. All cases had successful resolution of the bladder diverticula on follow-up. One complication occurred in the laparoscopy group: a pelvic hematoma was associated with a drop in hematocrit. The hematoma was observed and no blood transfusion was required. There were no significant complications in the open group. Hospital stay was 4.5 days in the laparoscopy group and 10.8 days in the open group. Mean time to full recovery was 2.5 weeks in the laparoscopic group and 8.7 weeks in the open population. The mean combined intraoperative and postoperative cost for the laparoscopic group was $9,800 versus $5,700 for the open group.

Laparoscopic bladder diverticulectomy is feasible, and the limited data available demonstrate that patients who undergo laparoscopic treatment of a bladder diverticulum have less pain and a more expeditious convalescence. Hospital costs are a major deterrent; however, the financial impact of the markedly shortened convalescence should also be considered.

Malignant Disease: Diagnostic

Pelvic Lymph Node Dissection

The staging of a malignancy is of paramount importance before treatment. No noninvasive imaging modality or technique has proven adequate for determining lymph node status. Accordingly, surgical pelvic lymphadenectomy has been accepted as the most precise method to assess nodal disease in the setting of prostate, penile, urethral, and cervical cancers. Laparoscopic pelvic lymph node dissection (LPLND) was first described by Schuessler and colleagues (375) in 1991. It was this procedure, more than any other, that introduced laparoscopy into mainstream adult urology. Since then, LPLND has been evaluated as a less invasive alternative to the traditional open pelvic lymph node dissection at many centers.

Prostate cancer is the most common noncutaneous malignancy in men. The status of pelvic lymph nodes has a major impact on treatment and long-term prognosis in men with clinically localized prostate cancer. Clinical parameters including digital rectal examination, serum prostate-specific antigen (PSA) level, and Gleason's score can be used in conjunction with statistical tables to exclude the need for pelvic node sampling in patients with favorable characteristics (158,326). As such, the question arises as to which patients should be candidates for a lymph node dissection. We believe this is based on the potential therapy should the lymph node dissection reveal no metastatic disease. Specifically, when the risk of lymph node involvement is greater than 5% to 10%, staging pelvic lymphadenectomy is indicated if the treatment plan is for either perineal prostatectomy or radiation therapy. In contrast, among patients who are candidates for a radical retropubic prostatectomy, the threshold for performing LPLND is higher. These individuals should have upward of a 40% risk of nodal disease before proceeding with an LPLND because in this case, a positive LPLND will merely spare the patient a lower midline incision rather than avoiding needless extirpative perineal surgical or radiation therapy. Using these guidelines, fewer than 10% of patients with clinically localized prostate cancer are candidates for LPLND.

Transperitoneal LPLND is performed with the patient in the Trendelenburg position and rotated laterally. Peritoneal access and laparoscope insertion are through an incision at the umbilicus. Two additional trocars are placed bilaterally, lateral to the rectus abdominus muscle and approximately 2 cm inferior to the umbilicus. A fourth trocar is inserted in the midline above the symphysis pubis, thereby completing the "diamond" array of trocar placement. An incision is created in the parietal peritoneum just lateral to the medial umbilical ligament. The vas deferens is isolated and divided between clips or is electrocoagulated and cut. (In this regard, it is essential that each patient be told that following this procedure he will be infertile.) The external iliac artery is identified and dissected along its medial aspect; the external iliac vein is then identified and dissected anterior and medial along its length. The pubic ramus is identified medial to the external iliac vein and is dissected toward the midline. Next, the obturator space is carefully dissected, and the obturator nerve is identified and gently teased out of the nodal packet. The obturator vein can be divided if necessary, but the obturator artery should be preserved. The dissection is continued cephalad to the level of the bifurcation of the common iliac artery. All tissue bounded by the medial edge of the external iliac artery laterally, the pubis caudally, the obturator nerve and obturator vessels posteriorly, and the bifurcation of the common iliac artery cranially are removed. In those patients in whom there is a high suspicion for nodal disease, the dissection is "extended" by removing any nodal tissue along the common iliac artery up to the point where the ureter crosses the common iliac vessels; in addition, the nodal tissue in the presciatic (i.e., deep to the obturator nerve), presacral (i.e., medial to the hypogastric artery), and lateral/posterior to the upper portion of the external iliac artery areas may also be included in the dissection.

Another laparoscopic approach to LPLND, albeit less widely used, is extraperitoneal. This is performed by creating a 2-cm incision in the midline just below the umbilicus. After digital dissection, a balloon is used to expand the extraperitoneal space to 700 to 1,000 mL. Next, the balloon is deflated and removed; a Hasson-type trocar is placed into this incision. Three additional trocars are placed, in the same configuration as described for a transperitoneal pelvic lymph node dissection. The dissection proceeds laterally along the external iliac vein. Laparoscopic clips are used to control any lymphatics or venous branches visualized, in particular the inferior epigastric vein. All nodal tissue is taken from within the boundaries previously described.

Results of trials comparing open and laparoscopic LPLND are presented in Table 18.5. Schuessler and colleagues (373) reported results of 147 consecutive patients with localized carcinoma of the prostate undergoing LPLND. Initially, the laparoscopic procedure was performed in a limited manner; however, the final 86 patients underwent an extended LPLND (hypogastric, external iliac, and obturator lymph node dissection). Mean operative time was 2.5 hours, and mean estimated blood loss was 100 mL. Mean postoperative hospital stay was 2 days. Only 20% of patients required analgesics at the time of discharge from the hospital, and 85% of patients returned to full activity within 2 weeks after surgery. The overall complication rate was 31%. The reoperation rate among all 147 patients was 7% (11 of 147). Of 11 patients, 7 were reexplored laparoscopically. Reexploration was performed in five patients (3%) for hemorrhage, one patient (0.6%) for a bowel laceration, one patient (0.6%) for a ureteral injury, and four patients (3%) for lymphoceles. The mean number of lymph nodes removed was the highest in any series: 45 (range of 13 to 86); the overall positive nodal involvement rate was 23%.

Stone and co-workers (400) reported results of 130 LPLNDs performed for T_{1a} to T_{2a} carcinoma of the prostate. All LPLNDs were successfully performed laparoscopically. A median of five nodes per side was removed. Operative parameters were not reported. Five (3.8%) patients experienced major complications: two patients required transfusion of 1 unit of blood for injuries to an inferior epigastric vessel and an obturator vessel, respectively, one (0.7%) patient experienced a cerebrovascular accident, one (0.7%) patient experienced a bladder injury, and one (0.7%) patient required rehospitalization for intravenous antibiotics to treat an infected pelvic hematoma.

In a subsequent report, Stone and colleagues (401) compared standard, "limited" LPLND to extended LPLND for

TABLE 18.5. PELVIC LYMPH NODE DISSECTION—COMPARATIVE TRIALS

Source	Indications	Technique	Number	Minor Complication	Major Complications	OR Time	Estimated Blood Loss	Analgesia	Length of Stay	Full Recovery	Number of Nodes Taken	Cost
Parra et al. (322)	PreRRP	Lap-transper	12	None	None	3.1 hr	100 mL	NA	NA	NA	10.7	NA
		Open-retroper	12	NA	NA	NA	NA	NA	NA	NA	11	NA
Kerbl et al. (217)	PreCAPTx	Lap-transper	30	13.3%	16.6%	3.3 hr	100 mL	1.6 mg morphine	1.7 days	10.8 days	NA	NA
		Open-retroper	16	None	None	1.7 hr	12.5 mL	47 mg morphine	5.4 days	65.5 days	NA	NA
Troxel and Winfield (419)	PreCAPTx	Lap-transper	11	NA	NA	3.9 hr	NA	NA	1.6 days	7 days	NA	$10,068
		Open-retroper	50	NA	NA	2.7 hr	NA	NA	4.5 days	17 days	NA	$8,723
Perrotti et al. (329)	PreCAPTx	Lap-transper	20	None	25%	3.2 hr	NA	4.5 mg morphine	1.2 days	NA	NA	$4,245
		Open-retroper	7	NA	NA	1.5 hr	NA	NA	7 days	NA	NA	$4,262
		Minilap-retrope	13	None	15%	1.5 hr	NA	3.7 mg morphine	1.3 days	NA	NA	$2,516
Herrell et al. (165)	PreCAPTx	Lap-transper	19	None	None	3.5 hr	NA	NA	1.6 days	NA	8.5	NA
		Open-retroper	38	16%	5%	1.9 hr	NA	NA	5.6 days	NA	9.2	NA
		Minilap-retrope	11	None	None	1.7 hr	NA	NA	2.2 days	NA	8.8	NA
Totals												
Laparoscopic			**92**	**4.90%**	**12.30%**	**3.4 hr**	**100 mL**	**2.8 mg morphine**	**1.5 days**	**9.8 days**	**9.4**	**$6,311**
Open			**123**	**11.30%**	**3.50%**	**2.2 hr**	**215 mL**	**47 mg morphine**	**5.7 days**	**28.8 days**	**9.6**	**$8,175**
Minilaparotomy			**24**	**None**	**8.10%**	**1.6 hr**	**NA**	**3.7 mg morphine**	**1.7 days**	**NA**	**8.8**	**$2,516**

All columns list mean values.
Lap, laparoscopic; NA, not available; retroper, retroperitoneal; RRP, radical retropubic prostatectomy; transper, transperitoneal.

detection of carcinoma of the prostate. Thirty-nine patients underwent an extended LPLND that included obturator, hypogastric, common, and external iliac nodes. These results were compared with patients undergoing LPLND that included only the obturator and hypogastric lymph nodes. A mean of 9.3 nodes was removed during modified LPLND, compared with 18 nodes removed during extended LPLND. Extended dissection was positive in the extended area in only one patient (2.6%). Even when patients were stratified into high-risk groups based on PSA greater than 20 ng/mL, Gleason score 7 or higher, or stage T_{2b} or T_{3a}, patients in the extended LPLND group did not have a significantly higher node positivity rates: 30% and 26.4% ($p = .8$), 27% and 19% ($p = .4$), and 25% and 15% ($p = .17$), respectively. Of note, the extended LPLND was associated with a significant increase in complications: 14 of 25 patients (36%) undergoing the extended dissection had complications, compared with only 3 of 147 patients (2%) in the standard group. Complications in the extended group included 11 (28%) cases of scrotal or penile edema, 4 (10%) cases of lower extremity edema, and 2 (5%) cases each of obturator nerve palsies, pelvic abscesses, and urinary retention (401).

Kerbl and colleagues (217) compared 30 patients undergoing a standard limited LPLND with 16 patients undergoing open pelvic lymph node dissection during the same period. All laparoscopic procedures were successfully completed. Mean operative time was significantly longer for the laparoscopic group: 3.3 hours compared with 1.7 hours for the open group. However, postoperative analgesic requirement was markedly less in patients undergoing LPLND: 1.6 mg of morphine sulfate equivalents versus 47 mg in the open group. Major and minor complications occurred in 13% and 17% of patients in the laparoscopic group, respectively. No complications were reported in the open group. A learning curve was noted in the laparoscopic group, with all major complications occurring in the first 12 patients. Major complications included a bladder perforation, a pelvic hematoma, a pelvic collection requiring drainage, and a delayed bowel fistula. Minor complications included subcutaneous emphysema in one patient, two instances of scrotal swelling, a scrotal hematoma, and one case of urinary retention. Hospital stay was 1.7 days in the laparoscopic group and 5.4 days in the open group. Similarly, return to full activity was expedited with the laparoscopic technique: 11 versus 66 days. Cost evaluation was also performed (217). Unilateral and bilateral LPLNDs cost $7,700 and $10,300, respectively. Open pelvic lymph node dissection was more cost-effective, with unilateral and bilateral procedures costing $6,600 and $8,200, respectively.

In 1994, Troxel and Winfield (419) performed a financial analysis comparing open and laparoscopic pelvic lymph node dissection. The total overall cost from hospital admission to discharge was $1,350 more for the laparoscopic approach. The same authors later performed a financial analysis comparing LPLND and open pelvic lymph node dissection during two separate time periods to evaluate the effect of the learning curve on overall cost (420). Cost analysis was performed comparing 50 men undergoing LPLND between 1990 and 1992 with 55 men undergoing LPLND between 1993 and 1994. Despite a decrease in preoperative and postoperative expenses (112% and 31%, respectively) in the laparoscopic group, the overall cost of the laparoscopic procedure remained unchanged because of increased operating room costs. Indeed, despite operative time decreasing by a mean of 19 minutes, the cost of surgical supplies increased $910 (104%), resulting in an increased overall absolute cost.

Ferzli and co-workers (104) compared 18 patients undergoing transperitoneal LPLND with 18 patients undergoing extraperitoneal LPLND in a nonrandomized, retrospective fashion. All prostate cancer patients received LPLND before brachytherapy or radical perineal prostatectomy. All laparoscopic procedures were successfully completed; one extraperitoneal procedure required open conversion due to dense adhesions from prior surgery. Mean operative time was similar between the two groups: 2.25 hours for transperitoneal laparoscopic LPLND versus 2.5 hours for the extraperitoneal LPLND. The mean number of lymph nodes removed was eight for both groups. Average length of stay was 3.2 days for the transperitoneal group and 2.7 days for the extraperitoneal LPLND group. The authors reported an increased complication rate in the transperitoneal laparoscopic group: 28% versus 0% in the extraperitoneal group. Complications included two patients (11%) requiring transfusions, one (5.5%) omental hernia, one (5.5%) prolonged postoperative ileus, and one (5.5%) infected lymphocele requiring percutaneous drainage. In the extraperitoneal population, there were no postoperative complications. However, one extraperitoneal procedure required conversion to open surgery and another procedure was converted to a transperitoneal laparoscopic approach when the peritoneum was entered during the dissection. Analgesic requirements and return to full activity were not reported (104).

Several groups have compared LPLND with mini-laparotomy incisions. Among these studies, two stand out. Both clearly favor the mini-laparotomy while also corroborating the benefits of LPLND as well as mini-laparotomy over a standard open surgical approach. Perrotti and co-workers (329) reported results comparing a standard open lower midline incision, a 6-cm mini-laparotomy incision, and LPLND. In their series, 7 patients underwent open lymphadenectomy, 13 patients underwent mini-laparotomy, and 20 patients underwent LPLND. Mean operative times for open and mini-laparotomy procedures were both 90 minutes. Mean operative time for LPLND was 190 minutes. Postoperative hospital stay for open, mini-laparotomy, and LPLND were 7, 1.3, and 1.2, respectively. Analgesic requirements were not reported for patients who underwent open pelvic lymph node dissection. However, patients in the mini-laparotomy and LPLND groups required a mean of 3.7 and 4.5 mg of morphine sulfate equivalents, respectively.

One (5%) patient in the LPLND group required conversion to open surgery for control of hemorrhage. In addition, one (5%) patient in the LPLND group experienced mild left lower extremity discomfort that resolved without intervention, one (5%) patient experienced self-limited abdominal discomfort and bloating 1 week postoperatively, and two (10%) patients experienced scrotal swelling for 4 days postoperatively. In the mini-laparotomy group, no intraoperative complications occurred and only two postoperative complications were seen: one (8%) patient complained of vague abdominal pain, and one (8%) patient experienced a small area of skin separation at the wound site. Complications for the open group were not reported. Operative costs for both mini-laparotomy and open lymphadenectomy were $1,311, compared with $2,100 for LPLND. Total costs for open lymphadenectomy, mini-laparotomy, and LPLND were $4,300, $2,500, and $4,200, respectively (329).

Herrell and colleagues (165) similarly compared three techniques for pelvic lymphadenectomy. In their series, 38 patients underwent open lymphadenectomy, 11 patients underwent mini-laparotomy, and 19 patients underwent LPLND. The mean number of lymph nodes removed for open, mini-laparotomy, and LPLND were 9.2, 8.8, and 8.5, respectively. LPLND required significantly more operative time (3.5 hours) than either open lymphadenectomy (1.9 hours) or mini-laparotomy (1.7 hours). Hospital stay was significantly longer for open lymphadenectomy: 5.6 days compared with 2.2 days for the mini-laparotomy group and 1.6 days for the LPLND group. No complications occurred in either the mini-laparotomy or LPLND groups. In the open lymphadenectomy group, there were several complications (22%): three (8%) cases of ileus, two (5%) patients with urinary retention, and one (3%) case each of a lymphocele, a deep venous thrombosis, and a pelvic abscess.

One major criticism of LPLND has been the concern that this approach may result in seeding of cancer cells in patients with positive lymph nodes. Problems of this sort have been noted in patients with ovarian and other gynecologic cancers, but usually these cases were complicated by malignant ascites or direct violation of the tumor's borders during the dissection. Nonetheless, because of this hypothetical problem, Cadeddu and colleagues (44) evaluated the effect of LPLND on the natural history of carcinoma of the prostate in 52 men with node-positive LPLND. There were three (5.8%) deaths from prostate cancer at 3.0, 3.5, and 4.0 years, respectively, after LPLND; however, at a mean follow-up of 3.1 years, none of the patients developed trocar site tumor implantation. Adjuvant radiation therapy was administered in 12 (23%) men. Of 45 men treated with androgen ablation, 19 (42%) demonstrated biochemical progression during the study period. Among these men with node-positive prostate cancer, the 5-year actuarial biochemical progression-free rate was 45%, similar to the results with open surgery. As such, LPLND appears to neither alter the natural history of stage D_1 carcinoma of the prostate nor lead to trocar site implantation.

LPLND is feasible and is an adequate staging modality for carcinoma of the prostate. When performed by experienced laparoscopic surgeons, LPLND offers patients the comfort, low morbidity, and rapid convalescence characteristic of most laparoscopic procedures. However, it must be stressed that in skilled hands mini-laparotomy provides patients an equally comfortable and expeditious convalescence at less cost. The choice of which less invasive modality to use for pelvic lymph node sampling is dependent on the experience of the individual surgeon; however, it is equally clear that either method remains far superior to a standard open surgical node dissection.

Retroperitoneal Lymph Node Dissection

Patients with nonseminomatous germ cell tumors are at risk for retroperitoneal lymph node involvement. Although noninvasive staging techniques are somewhat accurate, 20% to 25% of patients with clinical stage I disease are understaged when only clinical nonsurgical staging modalities are used. Laparoscopic retroperitoneal lymph node dissection (LRPLND) was originally reported by Hulbert and Fraley in 1992 (179) and has subsequently been performed in patients with stage I disease after orchiectomy and, rarely, in patients with stage IIb disease after chemotherapy.

Gerber and co-workers (119) reported results of 20 laparoscopic retroperitoneal lymph node dissections performed in men with stage I nonseminomatous germ cell tumors. A modified unilateral retroperitoneal lymphadenectomy was performed in all patients. Anatomic boundaries for the dissection included the renal hilum superiorly, ureter laterally, medial aspect of the vena cava or aorta medially (right and left dissection, respectively) (i.e., the interaortocaval lymph nodes), and level of the origin of the inferior mesenteric artery inferiorly; the dissection was extended to the bifurcation of the common iliac vessels on the ipsilateral side, and the stump of the spermatic cord was excised. The retrocaval and retroaortic nodes were not removed.

Of 20 cases, 18 (90%) were successfully completed laparoscopically. In two cases, conversion to an open procedure was necessitated because of bleeding from gonadal vessels. One of these two cases required transfusion. Two additional patients required blood transfusion in the postoperative period [total transfusions = three (15%) patients]. Median operative time was 6 hours, and median estimated blood loss was 250 mL. A median of 14.5 nodes were removed per patient, with 3 of 18 (17%) manifesting disease in the lymph nodes. Most patients required intramuscular or intravenous narcotics for less than 1 day. Hospital stay was 3 days, and patients returned to full activity in 2 weeks.

Complications occurred in 6 of 20 patients (30%), including the 2 patients (10%) requiring conversion to open surgery. Other complications included two additional patients (10%) requiring transfusion in the postoperative period, one patient (5%) with myonecrosis that resolved with observation, and one patient (5%) with lymphocele. Of the 15 patients who successfully underwent retroperitoneal lymph node dissection and had no evidence of disease, none manifested retroperitoneal disease recurrence with a mean follow-up of 10 months. Of 15 patients, 1 (7%) presented with a lung nodule 4 months after retroperitoneal lymphadenectomy. CT scan demonstrated no evidence of retroperitoneal disease, and the patient received chemotherapy. There was no evidence of disease 9 months later. All 20 patients (100%) reported normal antegrade ejaculation.

Rassweiler and colleagues (348) reported results of 26 retroperitoneal lymph node dissections. Seventeen patients were managed for stage I disease, and the remaining nine patients underwent retroperitoneal lymph node dissection for stage II disease after chemotherapy. The procedure was successfully completed in 16 of 17 stage I patients (94%); however, it was successfully completed in only 2 of 9 stage II patients (22%). The stage I conversion resulted from bleeding that could not be controlled laparoscopically. Stage II conversions were all the result of difficult dissection attributed to the desmoplastic reaction associated with the disease process and chemotherapy. Mean operative time for stage I and stage II patients was 4.9 and 5.9 hours, respectively. Estimated blood loss was not reported. There were four (24%) postoperative complications in the stage I group. These consisted of a patient with a retroperitoneal hematoma who subsequently developed ureteral stenosis. This patient required ureterolysis 8 weeks later. Another patient developed a pulmonary embolism that was successfully managed with anticoagulation. In addition, there was a single case of retrograde ejaculation. There was one (11%) postoperative complication in the stage II group, a lymphocele. Patients managed for stage I disease had a mean follow-up of 27 months. No patient manifested a regional relapse, but two patients had pulmonary metastases that were treated successfully with three cycles of chemotherapy. Histopathology in all nine cases of stage II cases revealed necrotic material only, and no patient had evidence of disease with a median follow-up of 29 months.

Janetschek and co-workers (196) have done the most extensive work in the area of LRPLND. They reported results of 105 patients undergoing laparoscopic retroperitoneal lymphadenectomy either for stage I nonseminomatous germ cell tumors after radical orchiectomy or stage IIb nonseminomatous germ cell tumors after chemotherapy. The procedure was successfully accomplished laparoscopically in 103 of 105 (98%) patients. Two (2%) patients required conversion to an open procedure because of bleeding. Mean operative time was 6.3 hours; however, the authors reported a "long and steep learning curve." Operative time for the first 14 patients was 8 hours; this progressively decreased such that operative time for patients 45 through 64 was reduced to 3.7 hours. Minor postoperative complications were not quantitated but included a small asymptomatic lymphocele, transient lower extremity edema, and transient chylous ascites. Chylous ascites was noted in 21% of patients undergoing retroperitoneal lymph node dissection after chemotherapy. In all patients, the ascites improved with conservative measures, including low-fat diet or medium-chain triglyceride diet. No major complications were reported. Of the 64 patients managed for stage I tumors, 47 (73%) were negative for malignant disease. With a mean follow-up period of 25 months, one patient (1.5%) developed a retroperitoneal recurrence outside the surgical field. Retrospective review of this patient's specimen revealed that a positive lymph node had been missed on the original pathologic evaluation. In contrast, among the patients who received chemotherapy, LRPLND yielded necrotic tissue in 61% of cases and mature teratoma in 37%; active tumor was found in only one patient (2%). With a mean follow-up of 27 months, no recurrences were reported.

In a subsequent report, Janetschek and co-workers (197) expanded their series of retroperitoneal node dissection for stage I nonseminomatous testicular cancer to 73 patients. The operative time continued to decrease; the last 13 patients had a mean operative time of 3.6 hours. Mean estimated blood loss in this group was 156 mL, including one of the two conversions with an estimated blood loss of 2,600 mL. Postoperatively, antegrade ejaculation was normal in all patients. There were no major complications, and a single (1.5%) minor complication was reported. One patient experienced transient irritation of the genitofemoral nerve. Only patients with a minimum follow-up of 6 months were reported; as such, the mean follow-up for this group was 43.3 months. There was only one recurrence, as previously described.

In 1996, Janetschek and co-workers (195) reported comparison between open retroperitoneal lymph node dissection and an earlier portion of their series. This report included the initial 29 patients treated for stage I nonseminomatous testicular tumors. To demonstrate the effects of the learning curve, data for the laparoscopic group were stratified into two groups. Group 1 represented the first 14 cases, and group 2 represented the latest 15 cases. Mean operative times for the open population, group 1, and group 2 were 4.2, 8, and 5.1 hours, respectively. Mean decrease in hemoglobin for the open group, group 1, and group 2 was 2.5, 3.6, and 1.8 g/dL, respectively. Patients managed laparoscopically had a significantly shorter hospital stay. Mean hospital stay for open, group 1, and group 2 patients was 10.6, 5.5, and 4.0 days, respectively. Analgesic requirements and time to full recovery were not reported.

Cost analysis revealed significantly higher operative costs in the laparoscopic group ($3,200 versus $2,500). In contrast, the cost for hospital stay was less for the laparoscopic group. Overall, in Austria, laparoscopic retroperitoneal lymph node dissection was more cost-effective than open surgery ($4,000 versus $4,150). These calculations did not include cost of patient convalescence, which would have only added to the cost-saving benefits of the laparoscopic approach.

Laparoscopic retroperitoneal lymph node dissection is technically challenging but feasible, especially for staging of stage I nonseminomatous disease; for stage II postchemotherapy patients, a sanguine experience has been reported from only one center (197). The procedure offers these often very young patients the benefits of a minimally invasive approach, while accomplishing the goals of open retroperitoneal lymphadenectomy of effective lymphadenectomy and preservation of the sympathetic nerves responsible for ejaculation.

Malignant Disease: Ablative

Adrenalectomy

Laparoscopic adrenalectomy for malignant disease is highly controversial. Early reports have included removal of solitary adrenal metastases and smaller primary adrenocortical carcinomas. With small differences, the technique for laparoscopic adrenalectomy for malignant disease is essentially the same as previously described for benign adrenal pathology. However, in these cases, the dissection is more en bloc to include all of the periadrenal fatty tissue. On the right side, the borders of the dissection are the renal vein inferiorly, the line of Toldt and upper pole of kidney laterally, and the posterior coronary hepatic ligament superiorly. On the left side, the borders include the kidney laterally, the renal vein inferiorly, and the area of the lienorenal ligament superiorly. Gerota's fascia over the upper border of the adrenal is removed en bloc with the specimen.

Suzuki and co-workers (408) reported results of two patients who underwent laparoscopic adrenalectomy for malignant disease. The first patient underwent a transperitoneal laparoscopic adrenalectomy for what was thought to be a 5-cm cortisol-producing adenoma; however, the final pathology revealed an adrenocortical carcinoma. Despite removal of the tumor as an en bloc specimen, the patient presented with local recurrence and abdominal dissemination 19 months after surgery. The patient died 3 years after the initial procedure. In the second case, a patient with a 5.5-cm adrenal metastasis from poorly differentiated adenocarcinoma of the lung underwent a retroperitoneal laparoscopic adrenalectomy. The procedure required conversion to open surgery because of severe adhesions between the kidney and the adrenal tumor. The patient died of multiple metastases from lung cancer 8 months after surgery.

Elashry and colleagues (93) reported on two patients who underwent laparoscopic adrenalectomy for a solitary metachronous contralateral adrenal metastasis from renal cell carcinoma. The first patient presented 5 years after laparoscopic radical nephrectomy for T_2 disease; a 4-cm adrenal mass was detected during routine postoperative radiologic studies. The patient underwent an uncomplicated laparoscopic adrenalectomy. Operative time was 2.5 hours, with an estimated blood loss of 50 mL. Pathology of the specimen revealed metastatic clear cell renal cell carcinoma. The patient was without evidence of disease at 11-month follow-up. The second patient also presented 5 years after laparoscopic radical nephrectomy for T_2 disease; a 5-cm adrenal mass was detected during routine postoperative radiologic studies. CT-guided biopsy revealed malignant cells, and the patient underwent an uncomplicated adrenalectomy. Operative time was 4.3 hours and estimated blood loss was 75 mL. At 16-month follow-up, the patient remained free of disease. Both patients returned to full activity in 2 weeks.

Bendinelli and colleagues (22) reported results of six patients who underwent laparoscopic adrenalectomy for suspected solitary non–small cell carcinomas of the lung. The tumors ranged from 2.8 to 4.7 cm in diameter. In all cases, laparoscopic adrenalectomy was successfully performed without complication. There were no postoperative complications, and patients were discharged on postoperative day 2 or 3. Histology revealed metastatic disease in four cases and adrenal cortical adenoma in the remaining two patients. With a mean follow-up of 13.5 months, two patients were disease free. The remaining two patients with malignant disease died of other causes (myocardial infarct and trauma).

Because of the rarity of primary or resectable secondary adrenal cancer, to date, there are only a handful of reports of laparoscopic adrenalectomy for malignancy. The procedure is feasible and appears to be as effective as open surgery, but further evaluation is required before the long-term efficacy of laparoscopic adrenalectomy for malignant disease can be determined.

Radical Nephrectomy

Radical nephrectomy is the definitive surgical treatment for localized renal cell carcinoma as described by Robson and colleagues (354) in 1969. The procedure includes en bloc resection of the kidney and enveloping Gerota's fascia, along with the ipsilateral adrenal gland, proximal half of the ureter, and renal hilar lymph nodes. An important part of radical nephrectomy is early ligation of the renal artery followed by ligation of the renal vein. Recently, total nephrectomy rather than radical nephrectomy has been recommended for renal tumors occupying the middle or lower portions of the kidney, thereby sparing the ipsilateral adrenal gland (380,421).

Laparoscopic nephrectomy, as originally described by Clayman and co-workers (60) in 1991, was initially applied to a tumor-bearing kidney (i.e., oncocytoma) and was a total nephrectomy in that the adrenal gland was spared. Initial application of the laparoscopic technique for radical nephrectomy, by the same urologists, was controversial. However, its role in the management of renal malignancies has evolved over the past decade, and the laparoscopic approach is presently accepted as a management strategy for selected renal masses.

Recommended size limitations for laparoscopic management of renal masses has been quite variable. Most series report results for localized tumors that are 7 cm in greatest diameter. However, recently, Walther and co-workers (433) reported a series of laparoscopic cytoreductive radical nephrectomies for renal masses up to 15 cm in greatest diameter, and in an early series, the Washington University group (262) reported successful removal of a stage T_{3b} lesion involving the renal vein. With experience, all renal tumors, short of those involving the inferior vena cava or larger than 15 cm, are currently considered at major centers for laparoscopic removal.

The surgical technique for laparoscopic radical nephrectomy was originally described via a transperitoneal approach. The transperitoneal procedure is performed with the patient in the lateral decubitus position. Three 12-mm trocars are placed: at the umbilicus, in the midclavicular line under the costal margin, and in the midclavicular line 3 cm inferior to the umbilicus. Two additional 5-mm trocars are placed: in the anterior axillary line off the tip of the twelfth rib and in the anterior axillary line at the level of the umbilicus. At times, on the right side, an additional 5-mm trocar is placed in the midline, just beneath the xiphoid, to aid in retraction of the liver, during the hilar dissection.

Templates for laparoscopic right- and left-sided radical nephrectomy are presented in Fig. 18.19. Monopolar electrosurgical scissors are used to incise the line of Toldt from the hepatic or splenic flexure caudal to the iliac vessels and cephalad to the diaphragm. On the right side, this incision is continued cephalad to include division of the triangular ligament of the liver, whereas on the left side, the splenic attachments to the diaphragm are divided. Further dissection in the retroperitoneum on the right side takes the shape of a trapezoid: (a) the colon is dissected from the inferior surface of the kidney and the duodenum is dissected medially (i.e., Kocher maneuver) to reveal the surface of the inferior vena cava; (b) the posterior coronary hepatic ligament is incised from the line of Toldt, laterally, to the inferior vena cava, medially; and (c) the inferior vena cava is dissected from above the adrenal gland to the level of the insertion of the gonadal vein, and the gonadal vein is secured with two pairs of clips and divided. At this point, the hilar dissection can be accomplished by clipping and dividing the renal artery followed by stapling of the renal vein. The adrenal vein is then dissected, clipped, and divided. The ureter can then be dissected and divided, and the entire specimen can be moved onto the surface of the liver pending entrapment and morcellation or direct extraction by extension of one of the port sites or manually via a previously placed hand-assist device.

On the left side, the dissection takes on the shape of an inverted cone: (a) the line of Toldt and splenophrenic attachments are divided; (b) the colon is dissected from the inferior surface of the kidney and Gerota's fascia and moved medially; and (c) the "opening" of the cone (defined as the splenocolic ligament) is divided anteriorly, and the splenorenal ligament, in the same plane, is divided posteriorly. The gonadal vein is then followed to its insertion into the renal vein where it is clipped and divided along with the ascending lumbar vein; the adrenal vein superiorly is likewise dissected, clipped, and divided. In this regard, the gonadal vein is the key to the entire subsequent dissection of the left renal hilum; tracing this vein cephalad reliably and safely leads the surgeon to the left renal vein. The renal artery is then dissected and divided followed by stapling and division of the renal vein. The ureter is then dissected, clipped, and divided. The entire specimen can be moved onto the surface of the spleen pending entrapment and morcellation or direct extraction by extension of one of the port sites or manually, through a previously placed hand-assist device.

Laparoscopic radical nephrectomy may also be performed via a retroperitoneal approach. Access to the retroperitoneum is gained with the Hasson technique through a 2-cm skin incision at the tip of the twelfth rib. After balloon or blunt dissection of the retroperitoneum outside Gerota's fascia, a second trocar (12 mm) is placed at the angle of the twelfth rib and the erector spinae muscle. Next, a third trocar (5 mm) is placed subcostally in the anterior axillary line and a fourth trocar (12 mm) is placed in the midaxillary line just cephalad to the iliac crest. Dissection is initiated around the renal hilum, with sequential control of the renal artery and vein with clip ligation and Endo-GIA stapling, respectively. Circumferential mobilization of the kidney within Gerota's fascia is performed. The adrenal gland may be spared depending on the size and location of the renal mass. The ureter is transected between clips. Next, off of one of the lower port sites, the incision may be extended horizontally to 8 to 10 cm, and the entire specimen retrieved intact; alternatively, an entrapment sack can be placed and the specimen can be secured in the sack. The latter approach often requires opening of the peritoneal cavity to provide sufficient space to maneuver the sack and the specimen. The specimen is then morcellated or removed intact depending on surgeon preference.

In an effort to simplify the technical aspects of laparoscopic surgery, hand-assisted techniques have been developed. This technique requires making a 7- to 8-cm transperitoneal incision over which one of a variety of wound-occlusive devices is affixed; the surgeon's hand and

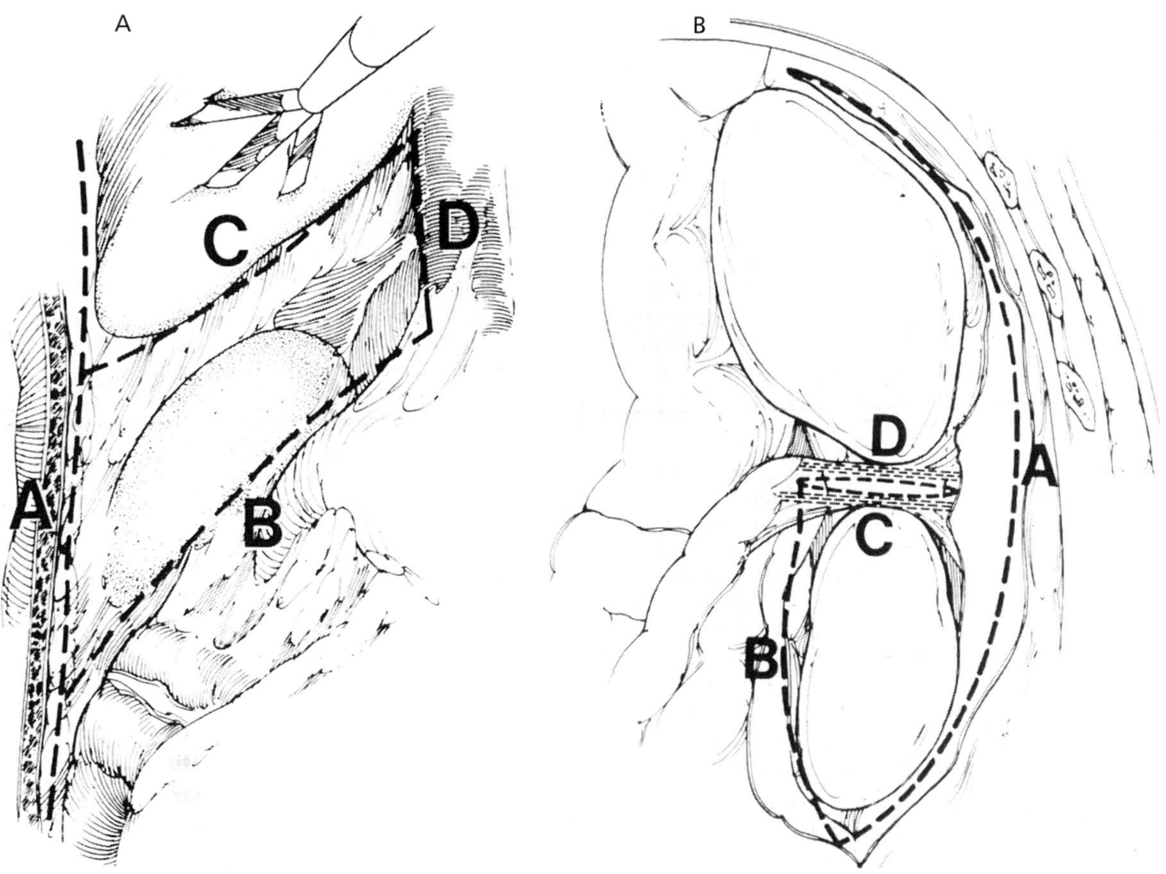

FIGURE 18.19. A: Trapezoid template for right-sided radical nephrectomy. *A,* The line of Toldt is incised from the hepatic flexure caudal to the iliac vessels and cephalad to the diaphragm. The incision is continued cephalad to include division of the triangular ligament of the liver. *B,* Reflection of colon and duodenum. *C,* Incision of posterior coronary hepatic ligament. *D,* Incision overlying the inferior vena cava from above the adrenal vein down to the insertion of the gonadal vein. **B:** Inverted cone template for left-sided radical nephrectomy. *A,* Incision of line of Toldt and medial through any splenophrenic attachments. *B,* Mobilization of the descending colonic mesentery off of Gerota's fascia. *C,* Incision of splenocolic ligament. *D,* Incision of splenorenal ligament.

forearm are inserted through the secured "airtight" device into the peritoneal cavity while maintaining a pneumoperitoneum. Wolf and co-workers (449) detailed their technique for hand-assisted laparoscopic nephrectomy. Peritoneal access is gained via a 12-mm incision at the lateral border of the rectus muscle inferior to the umbilicus. A second 12-mm trocar is placed in the midclavicular line 2 cm beneath the costal margin. An upper midline incision is made above the umbilicus with its length in centimeters equaling the surgeon's glove size. One of the commercially available occlusion devices is then applied to the incision, allowing the surgeon's hand to be inserted into the peritoneal cavity. For a right-sided nephrectomy, the surgeon's left arm is placed through the hand-assist incision; for a left-sided nephrectomy, the surgeon's right arm is placed in the incision. The laparoscopic instruments are placed in the subcostal trocar site. Alternatively, the hand-assist device may be placed periumbilically; a 12-mm port is then placed in the midline, midway between the xiphoid and umbilicus, and a second 12-mm port is placed in the midclavicular line, subcostal. The laparoscopic instruments are again passed via the subcostal port.

With the hand-assist approach, radical nephrectomy proceeds as previously described. Tissues are picked up with the surgeon's hand and managed using routine laparoscopic techniques. The renal hilum may be identified by palpation, and retroperitoneal dissection of the kidney is greatly facilitated by blunt finger dissection. For suture ties, a "one-handed" knot can be created by using the intraperitoneal hand and grasping the free end of the suture with a laparoscopic instrument. At the termination of the case, the specimen is extracted via the hand-assist incision.

Results of trials comparing open and laparoscopic radical nephrectomy are presented in Table 18.6. To date, three large series have appeared in the literature, among which two directly compared laparoscopic and open radical or total nephrectomy techniques. In the largest published series, Barrett and co-workers (18) reported results from 72 attempted laparoscopic nephrectomies. Tumor size ranged from 1 to 9 cm (mean of 4.5 cm). The transabdominal approach and specimen morcellation were used in all patients. Eight patients underwent concomitant procedures, including six cholecystectomies, a tubal ligation, and a bowel resection.

Of the 72 patients, 6 (8%) required conversion to open radical nephrectomy. The six conversions were the result of unrecognized tumor-associated venous thrombus, large parasitic veins servicing a large renal tumor, adhesions to the spleen, scarring of the renal hilum from prior infection, hilar bleeding, and a case of sudden hypoxia and suspected gas embolus. Sixty-six patients underwent successful laparoscopic nephrectomy with morcellation. Mean operative time was 2.9 hours, including the eight concomitant nonrenal laparoscopic procedures. There was a single (1.4%) intraoperative mortality. In this case, the patient suddenly became hypoxemic during the morcellation of the entrapped specimen; immediate open exploration failed to reveal a source of hemorrhage or other life-threatening surgical problem. Resuscitation attempts failed. At autopsy, extensive miliary lung disease was identified; the precise cause of death could not be determined. A gas embolus was suspected, but never proven.

Two patients (3%) required blood transfusion. Three patients (4%) experienced bowel complications, including one trocar site hernia. The hernia occurred at the extraction site in a patient who had undergone concomitant bowel resection. There was a single case each of a wound infection and transient unstable angina. Hospital stay for the 66 patients undergoing successful laparoscopic radical nephrectomy was 4.4 days. Fifty-seven patients had the diagnosis of a renal malignancy. With a mean follow-up of 21 months, there were no port site recurrences, no intraabdominal or retroperitoneal recurrences, and no evidence of metastatic disease. Analgesic requirements and time to full convalescence were not reported (18). Longer follow-up by this group has revealed one patient who developed a port site recurrence along with distant metastatic disease; of note, the port site recurrence was not at the site through which the tumor was morcellated. This occurred in a patient with a T_2 lesion with sarcomatous elements. This is the first and, to date, only report of seeding following radical nephrectomy (17a).

Dunn and colleagues (88) described the Washington University experience with radical nephrectomy. Clinical data on 60 consecutive patients undergoing laparoscopic radical nephrectomy for renal tumors 10 cm in diameter or smaller were compared with 33 open radical nephrectomies performed for tumors 10 cm in diameter or smaller. The majority of the specimens were morcellated. Two patients (3%) in the laparoscopic group required conversion to open surgery: one received 2 units of packed red blood cells because of intraoperative bleeding, which at the time of open conversion was found to be due to back-bleeding from the 1,100-g specimen, and the other patient had an injury to the superior mesenteric artery requiring repair. The overall transfusion rate was 12%. In the open group, the overall transfusion rate was 15%. Mean estimated blood loss was significantly less for laparoscopic nephrectomy: 172 versus 451 mL. Operative time was significantly longer for patients managed with the laparoscopic technique: 5.5 versus 2.8 hours. There were fewer major and minor complications in the laparoscopic group than in the open group: 3% versus 9% and 34% versus 45%, respectively.

Major differences in recovery were noted. Patients managed laparoscopically required significantly less analgesics for adequate pain control: 28 versus 78 mg of morphine sulfate equivalents. Resumption of oral intake was significantly faster in the laparoscopic group: 18 versus 59 hours. Hospital stay was also significantly reduced with the laparoscopic technique: 3.4 versus 5.2 days. Full recovery was expedited by the laparoscopic approach: 8 versus 29 weeks. The average follow-up in the laparoscopic group was 25 months (range of 3 to 73 months) among 44 patients with documented localized renal cell cancer; 91% were disease free. Among the three patients who failed therapy, two patients developed metastatic disease in the liver, lung, bone, or a paracaval node. Both patients subsequently died: one 52 months postoperatively, presumably due to metastatic disease, and the other 2 years later from aspiration pneumonia. A local recurrence occurred in the third patient; this patient developed recurrent disease in the ipsilateral ureteral stump, which was subsequently excised at open surgery. In the open group, the average follow-up was 28 months; 90% remained disease free, similar to the laparoscopic group.

A cost evaluation was also performed. Mean total operating room cost for laparoscopic radical nephrectomy was $6,300. Operating room cost for open radical nephrectomy was $4,400. The large discrepancy in operating room expenditures was not offset by the decreased hospital stay, such that overall cost for the laparoscopic procedure was $15,800; the open procedure required $13,700.

Ono and co-workers (314) reported results of 60 laparoscopic radical nephrectomies performed for renal masses less than 5 cm in diameter; the majority of specimens were morcellated. These results were compared with a contemporary series of 40 open radical nephrectomies. Forty-five patients (75%) underwent transperitoneal radical nephrectomy, and the remaining fifteen patients (25%) were managed via the retroperitoneal approach. Only one patient (2%) required conversion to an open procedure; this was prompted by uncontrollable bleeding from a left renal artery. Mean operative time for laparoscopic radical ne-

TABLE 18.6. LAPAROSCOPIC RADICAL NEPHRECTOMY—COMPARATIVE TRIALS

Source	Indications	Technique	Number	Minor Complications	Major Complications	Extraction	OR Time	EBL (mL)	Analgesia	Length of Stay	Full Recovery	Follow-up	Recurrence	Cost
Dunn et al. (88)	<10-cm masses	Lap-both	61	34.40%	3.30%	65% morcellated	5.5 hr	172	28 mg morphine	3.4 days	3.6 wk	25 mo	8%	$15,816
		Open-NA	33	45%	9%	Intact	2.8 hr	451	78.3 mg morphine	5.2 days	8.1 wk	27.5 mo	9%	$13,672
Ono et al. (313)	<5-cm masses	Lap-both	60	8.30%	5%	57% morcellated	5.2 hr	255	30 mg pentazocine	NA	3.3 wk	24 mo	3.40%	NA
		Open-NA	40	2.50%	5%	Intact	3.3 hr	512	68 mg pentazocine	NA	8.1 wk	28.5 mo	2.50%	NA
Abbou et al. (1)	<9-cm masses	Lap-retroper	29	0%	6.90%	Intact	2.4 hr	100	1.8 mg morphine	4.8 days	NA	15 mo	3.40%	NA
		Open-NA	29	10%	17.20%	Intact	2.0 hr	285	2.3 mg morphine	9.7 days	NA	13 mo	3.40%	NA
Walther et al. (433)	Cytoreductive	Lap-transper	11	9%	9%	55% morcellated	7.5 hr	1409	283 mg morphine	7.3 days	NA	NA	NA	NA
		Open-NA	19	0%	18%	Intact	4.2 hr	1000	442 mg morphine	8.2 days	NA	NA	NA	NA
Totals														
Laparoscopic			**161**	**16.70%**	**5.00%**		**5 hr**	**274.5 mL**		**4.2 days**	**3.5 wk**	**22.4 mo**	**6.10%**	
Open			**121**	**15.50%**	**11.10%**		**3 hr**	**517.6 mL**		**7.5 days**	**8.1 wk**	**23.8 mo**	**4.90%**	

All columns list mean values.
Both, transperitoneal and retroperitoneal approaches combined; EBL, estimated blood loss; lap, laparoscopic; NA, not available; retroper, retroperitoneal; transper, transperitoneal.

phrectomies was significantly longer than open surgery: 5.2 versus 3.3 hours. Mean estimated blood loss, however, was significantly decreased in the laparoscopic population: 255 versus 513 mL. Patients undergoing laparoscopic radical nephrectomy required significantly less pain medication: 31 versus 68 mg of pentazocine. Hospital stay was not reported; however, mean time to full convalescence was significantly shorter in patients undergoing laparoscopic management: 3 versus 8 weeks (314). There was no significant difference in the complication rate between open and laparoscopic radical nephrectomy. Two patients (3%) in the laparoscopic group required intraoperative blood transfusions. There were five intraoperative complications, including the injury to the left renal artery. Other complications included a splenic injury, an adrenal injury, and bleeding from a periureteral artery. In addition, a duodenal injury was recognized on postoperative day 1; the patient was successfully managed by open duodenojejunostomy. In the postoperative period, there were two cases of paralytic ileus that resolved with conservative management and a pulmonary thrombosis that was managed by anticoagulation. There were only two intraoperative complications in the open population: an injury to the renal vein and a splenic injury. Postoperative complications in this population included a single case of paralytic ileus that resolved with conservative management. Three patients (8%) required blood transfusions.

All 60 patients in the laparoscopic group were alive with a median follow-up of 24 months. Of the 60 patients, 58 had no evidence of recurrence, metastatic disease, or trocar site seeding. The calculated 5-year survival was 95%. One patient had lung metastases discovered 3 months postoperatively by chest CT scan. The other patient had a right iliac bone metastasis, which was discovered 19 months postoperatively by CT scan and bone scintigraphy. Both patients were treated with α-interferon and were alive at the time of publication. Of the 40 patients managed by open radical nephrectomy, 39 (97.5%) were alive without evidence of metastasis or recurrence. There was no statistically significant difference in the calculated disease-free rates between the two techniques. One patient had both lung and bone metastases discovered 5 months postoperatively; α-interferon therapy was administered. The patient died of progressive disease after 11 months (314).

With regard to the retroperitoneal approach, Abbou and co-workers (1) reviewed 29 patients who underwent retroperitoneal laparoscopic radical nephrectomy and 29 patients who underwent open radical nephrectomy. A single laparoscopic procedure (3%) required conversion after a vascular staple was dislodged from the renal artery during specimen extraction. Mean operative time for the laparoscopic group was 2.5 hours, significantly longer than the 2 hours required for open radical nephrectomy. Mean hospital stay for patients managed laparoscopically was 4.8 days, significantly less than the 9.7-day hospital stay reported in patients undergoing open radical nephrectomy. There were two intraoperative complications in the laparoscopic group. The patient requiring conversion to open surgery was managed with transfusion of 2 units of packed red blood cells intraoperatively. Another patient experienced a colonic injury that was managed with a temporary colostomy. In the open population, eight complications (24%) in seven patients were reported: two cases of pneumonia, two cerebrovascular accidents, a case of phlebitis, a pulmonary embolus, a colonic injury, and an eventration. With a mean follow-up of 15 months, there was a single case of local recurrence and hepatic metastasis in the patient requiring conversion from laparoscopic to open technique. This patient had a 9-cm tumor with final pathology revealing a pT3b grade 2 renal cell carcinoma confined within the surgical specimen. The recurrence was noted 9 months postoperatively (1).

Ono and colleagues (314) compared transperitoneal and retroperitoneal laparoscopic techniques. Thirty-four transperitoneal laparoscopic nephrectomies with morcellation of the specimen were compared with 15 retroperitoneal laparoscopic radical nephrectomies. All but one transperitoneal (97%) and all (100%) retroperitoneal procedures were completed successfully using laparoscopic techniques. Mean operative times for the retroperitoneal and transperitoneal approaches were similar (4.9 and 5.1 hours, respectively). Estimated blood loss was also similar for the retroperitoneal and transperitoneal approaches (276 and 176 mL, respectively). Both procedures required the same amount of postoperative analgesia (29 mg of pentazocine), and the complication rate was similar.

With regard to the hand-assist approach, Wolf and colleagues (450) compared standard laparoscopic nephrectomy (8 cases) with laparoscopic nephrectomy performed with the hand-assist device (13 cases). The series consisted of 15 simple nephrectomies, 4 radical nephrectomies, and 2 nephroureterectomies. Mean operative times for hand-assist and standard laparoscopic nephrectomies were 4 and 5.4 hours, respectively (p = .04). Estimated blood loss for hand-assist and standard laparoscopic nephrectomies was 211 and 340 mL, respectively. There was no significant difference in hospital stay with hand-assist and standard laparoscopic nephrectomy patients: 3.1 and 3.0 days, respectively. Hand-assist patients required 57 mg of morphine sulfate in the postoperative period compared with 48 mg for the standard laparoscopic population (p >.5). The hand-assist patients returned to normal activity in 14 days, compared with 10 days for standard laparoscopic nephrectomy (p >.1). There was a single (8%) major complication in the hand-assist group, and there were three (38%) major complications in the standard laparoscopy group.

The most important aspect of laparoscopic total or radical nephrectomy for renal cell cancer has to do with the long-term efficacy of the procedure. In this regard, Cadeddu and colleagues (42) reported results of a multicenter study encompassing 157 patients undergoing laparoscopic radical nephrectomy for pathologically proven renal cell carcinoma. Six patients (3.8%) required conversion to an open approach as a result of difficult dissection or hemorrhage. There were 16 (9.6%) perioperative complications in 15 patients and one intraoperative death. Mean follow-up was 19.2 months. There were no trocar site recurrences, and 151 patients (96%) had no evidence of disease recurrence at last follow-up. Four patients had progressive disease but were alive at the time of publication. All four patients had stage T_2 disease at the time of surgery. Three of four recurrences were at distant sites. One patient had a local recurrence in the ureteral stump 8 months postoperatively, as described in the Dunn series.

Another possible indication for laparoscopic nephrectomy has recently been examined by Walther and coworkers (433): cytoreductive surgery in patients with metastatic renal cell carcinoma before initiation of interleukin (IL)-2 immunotherapy. Patients with tumor thrombus, massive retroperitoneal lymphadenopathy, or liver invasion were excluded. Laparoscopically managed patients were stratified into two groups depending on whether the specimen was morcellated or removed intact. Results were compared with a contemporary group of open radical nephrectomies in similar patients. Open procedures were performed through a chevron incision extending from the midaxillary line of the ipsilateral side to the anterior axillary line of the contralateral side. After surgery, patients were randomized to treatment with either high- or low-dose IL-2.

Of the 11 patients, 3 (27%) in the laparoscopic groups were electively converted to open surgery because of tedious dissection. Transfusion requirements tended to be higher in the laparoscopic intact extraction group: 3.1 units (open group), 2.3 units (laparoscopic morcellated), and 5.2 units (laparoscopic intact extraction); of note, the estimated blood loss was greater in the laparoscopic intact extraction group (3,600 mL versus 1,300 to 1,600 mL in the other two groups). Patients in both laparoscopic groups had significantly longer operative times than patients undergoing open radical nephrectomy: 8.5 hours (laparoscopic morcellated) and 6.4 hours (laparoscopic intact) versus 4.2 hours for open removal. Postoperative complications occurred in four patients. In the laparoscopic group, a port site hernia and pressure necrosis of the skin occurred. In the open population, there was a pulmonary embolus and a small bowel obstruction. There was no significant difference in complications among the three groups.

Patients undergoing laparoscopic management of their tumors with morcellation were discharged from the hospital sooner (6.3 days) than patients undergoing open nephrectomy (8.2 days). Of note, patients with laparoscopic intact removal had a hospital stay similar to the open nephrectomy group: 9.2 days. Patients undergoing laparoscopic management with tumor morcellation had significantly less narcotic requirements (243 mg of morphine sulfate equivalents) than the laparoscopic intact removal group (332 mg of morphine sulfate equivalents) or the open surgery group (442 mg of morphine sulfate equivalents). Most important, the laparoscopic approach reduced time to treatment by almost 1 month; mean time to treatment with IL-2 for the open nephrectomy, laparoscopic intact, and laparoscopic morcellated groups was 11, 8, and 6 weeks, respectively. Time to full convalescence was not reported.

Overall, results comparing open and laparoscopic radical nephrectomy, by either a transperitoneal or retroperitoneal approach, are remarkably consistent. Patients treated laparoscopically undergo a procedure that respects the oncologic principles required for optimal management, while experiencing the benefits of a minimally invasive procedure. Specifically, patients managed by laparoscopic radical nephrectomy have significantly less pain, shorter hospital stays, and more rapid return to full activity when compared with patients undergoing an open procedure. These benefits are not associated with an increase in either intraoperative or postoperative morbidity. Tumor-free survival appears to be similar, in the short run (i.e., 2 years), between patients managed by open and laparoscopic approaches; 5- and 10-year data are needed. The expeditious convalescence associated with laparoscopic radical nephrectomy may be of value in patients with higher-stage malignancies. In this select group of patients, after a laparoscopic nephrectomy, adjuvant treatment can be initiated earlier.

Radical Nephroureterectomy

Laparoscopic radical nephroureterectomy for the treatment of upper tract transitional cell cancer was introduced by Clayman and colleagues in 1991 (62,261). Laparoscopic radical nephroureterectomy has been performed via both transabdominal and retroperitoneal techniques. Several techniques have been described for the management of the distal ureteral segment: transurethral resection ("pluck"), unroofing and stapled ureteral resection, intussusception, and needlescopic transvesical dissection. The usual recommendation for this procedure has been to proceed with any transurethral manipulation of the ureteral orifice and tunnel initially and then continue with the laparoscopic portion of the nephroureterectomy. However, because of concerns about possible local seeding of tumor cells, Clayman and colleagues (381) have recommended proceeding with the laparoscopic part of the procedure first, reserving any unroofing of the ureteral orifice and tunnel to the end of the procedure, thereby precluding any spillage of tumor cell–laden urine into the retroperitoneum.

Transurethral ureteral resection ("pluck" ureterectomy) is performed cystoscopically with the patient in a dorsal lithotomy position. The ureteral orifice, tunnel, and ureterovesical junction (UVJ) are transurethrally resected out to the perivesical fat. The ureter is thereby released from the bladder. Hemostasis is obtained and a urethral catheter is placed. If done early in the procedure, as soon as the laparoscopic portion of the procedure is initiated, the ureter should be isolated and clipped to prevent further leakage of urine into the retroperitoneum. After laparoscopic dissection of the kidney, the surgeon can "pluck" the ureter cephalad, thereby precluding any pelvic dissection of the ureter. The major drawback of this approach is concern about leakage of malignant cell–laden urine into the retroperitoneum until the ureter is laparoscopically occluded. Instances of seeding after an open "pluck" procedure have been reported by several urologists (12,167,201).

Ureteral unroofing and stapling is performed with the patient in the dorsal lithotomy position. A guidewire is placed in the ureter, and a 7-Fr ureteral dilating balloon (5-mm diameter, 10-cm length) is inserted over the guidewire. An Orandi electrosurgical knife is used to unroof the intramural ureter at the 12 o'clock position. The dilating balloon is then removed, and a 7-Fr 11.5-mm occlusion balloon catheter is inserted, inflated in the renal pelvis, and snugged down at the ureteropelvic junction. A roller electrode is used to fulgurate the cut edges and interior of the opened ureteral tunnel. Later in the procedure, after the kidney has been completely dissected laparoscopically, the ureter is dissected caudally until the detrusor muscle fibers at the UVJ are identified. The retrograde 7-Fr occlusion balloon is deflated and removed. An Endo-GIA stapler is applied to the cuff of bladder at the UVJ, thereby simultaneously incising and securing the bladder cuff and the UVJ specimen. For this portion of the procedure, an angulating Endo-GIA stapler is most helpful because it allows a more direct approach to the UVJ, thereby securing an ample cuff of bladder. If there is concern about the contralateral ureteral orifice or tunnel, this portion of the procedure can be monitored intravesically by having the assistant pass a flexible cystoscope while the bladder cuff is being secured.

Application of a needlescopic technique for management of the distal ureter was described by Gill and colleagues in 1999 (128). The patient first undergoes cystoscopy to rule out a concomitant bladder tumor and to ensure adequate bladder capacity. Diminished bladder capacity (less than 200 mL) increases the technical difficulty due to limited working space. Cystoscopy is performed with the patient in a 30-degree Trendelenburg position. Two needlescopic trocars (2 mm) are inserted suprapubically into the bladder under cystoscopic vision. A 2-mm Endoloop is inserted through the needlescopic trocar. A 6-Fr ureteral catheter is passed through the loop and into the affected ureter with the assistance of a guidewire. A 24-Fr continuous-flow resectoscope is then passed into the bladder alongside the ureteral catheter. A Collings' knife is used to electrosurgically score the urothelium circumferentially around the intramural ureter such that a 2- to 3-cm cuff is outlined. With use of a 2-mm grasper, the ureteral orifice and hemitrigone are retracted anteriorly and a full-thickness incision is made with the Collings' knife. In this manner, approximately 3 to 4 cm of ureter may be dissected free from surrounding tissues. The previously placed Endoloop is then positioned over the ureter and closed tightly, occluding the lumen as the ureteral catheter is withdrawn. The tail of the Endoloop is then cut with 2-mm laparoscopic scissors. The bladder edges about the excised ureter are then coagulated. All instruments are removed from the bladder and a Foley catheter is left indwelling. The laparoscopic nephrectomy is then performed, and the ureter is pulled up with the specimen via a 7- to 10-cm incision (128).

The intussusception technique is only used when the patient has transitional cell cancer of the renal pelvis; it cannot be used in patients with ureteral transitional cell cancer. In this approach, the ureterectomy is done after the laparoscopic nephrectomy portion of the procedure. A stone basket is passed retrograde up to the middle ureter. The ureter is occluded just proximal to the stone basket and incised, thereby allowing the stone basket to exit the ureterotomy site. The ureter is then incised vertically for a distance of 1 to 2 cm, to create two or three flaps; the stone basket is opened and the flaps of ureter are passed through the wires of the basket. The basket is then closed and pulled caudal while the surgeon holds the sidewalls of the middle ureter stationary; this results in the ureter intussuscepting. The surgeon then releases the sidewalls as they too become intussuscepted; the ureter is thus pulled through the ureterovesical junction and into or out the urethra, in males and females, respectively. The surgeon can then either continue to pull the ureter out, thereby avulsing it at the level of the trigone, or introduce a resectoscope to release the ureter at the ureteral tunnel (76).

Laparoscopic nephroureterectomy has been performed using either a transperitoneal or retroperitoneal technique; the former is more commonly described. The trocar placement is identical to that for a radical nephrectomy, except that for the transperitoneal approach an additional 12-mm trocar is placed in the midline 2 to 3 cm above the symphysis pubis for passage of the Endo-GIA stapler to secure the bladder cuff. For a hand-assist approach, placement of the hand-assist device is in the lower midline so the surgeon's hand can be used to facilitate both the nephrectomy and ureterectomy portions of the procedure.

The nephrectomy portion, whether performed by a transperitoneal or a retroperitoneal route, is identical to that for a total nephrectomy. For the ureterectomy portion, if a pluck or needlescopic dissection was used, the ureter is simply pulled cephalad out of the pelvis; alternatively, if a ureteral unroofing approach is selected, the ureter is mobilized caudally into the pelvis, as described, and secured with the Endo-GIA stapler. The specimen is entrapped in an entrapment sack and removed intact.

Recently, Shalhav and colleagues (381) reported on 25 patients at Washington University who underwent transperitoneal laparoscopic nephroureterectomy; these patients were retrospectively evaluated, and the results were compared with those of 17 patients who underwent open nephroureterectomy during a similar time period. Operative time was significantly longer for patients treated laparoscopically: 7.7 versus 3.9 hours. However, estimated blood loss was significantly less in the laparoscopic group: 199 versus 441 mL. All measures of patient comfort and convalescence favored the laparoscopic group. These patients resumed oral intake in a mean time of 1 day, compared with 4.8 days for the open group. The laparoscopic group averaged 37 mg of morphine sulfate equivalents versus 144 mg of morphine sulfate equivalents for pain relief in the open group. Hospital stay was also significantly shorter for patients undergoing laparoscopic nephroureterectomy: 3.6 versus 9.6 days. Resumption of full activity was facilitated by the laparoscopic approach: 2.8 versus 10 weeks. Major and minor complications occurred in 8% (postoperative bleeding, adult respiratory distress syndrome) and 40% of the laparoscopic group, respectively, and in 29% (e.g., pneumonia, myocardial infarction, acute renal failure) and 29% of the open group, respectively. There was one death in the laparoscopic group and none in the open group. At a mean follow-up of 2 years and 3.6 years for the laparoscopic and open groups, respectively, the bladder recurrence rate of transitional cell cancer was 23% and 54%, respectively. Of note, at 2 years in the open group, the bladder recurrence rate was similar to that in the laparoscopic group. Cancer-specific survival in the two groups was 77%, albeit with longer follow-up in the open cohort.

Of concern in the laparoscopic group was the identification of two retroperitoneal recurrences in the pelvis; this occurred despite neither patient having had any identifiable gross extravasation of urine at the time of the procedure. Because of these two cases, the authors have changed their protocol such that the integrity of the bladder and the ipsilateral ureter and kidney are absolutely maintained throughout the procedure. Accordingly, transurethral unroofing of the ureter is now done at the end of the procedure, following dissection, entrapment, and removal of the entire specimen (i.e., kidney, ureter down to the ureterovesical junction, and periureteral cuff of bladder). At that time, using the resectoscope equipped with an Orandi knife, the ipsilateral ureteral orifice and tunnel are unroofed until the staple line is visualized; then the roller electrode is used to electrocoagulate the interior of the opened ureteral tunnel from the level of the incised orifice out to the staple line.

Recently, there has been increasing experience with the hand-assist approach to laparoscopic nephroureterectomy. The largest series to date is from Stifelman and associates (399), who presented 22 cases of hand-assisted laparoscopic nephroureterectomy for upper tract transitional cell cancer. The average operative time was 4.5 hours, with an estimated blood loss of 180 mL. Of note, there were no intraoperative complications. Mean narcotic requirements were 55 mg of morphine sulfate equivalents; the average hospital stay was 4.1 days with a convalescence of 2.7 weeks. At 13-month follow-up, bladder recurrences were noted in 18% and metastatic disease had developed in 9%. Compared with a pure laparoscopic nephroureterectomy, this approach markedly decreases the operative time with only a slight increase in the amount of pain medications required and a minimal increase in hospital stay. Data on the cost-effectiveness of the hand-assisted nephroureterectomy have yet to be compiled.

Laparoscopic radical nephroureterectomy is a viable option for the management of upper tract transitional cell carcinoma. The procedure respects the oncologic principles of the open procedure and does not appear to increase morbidity. Of note, the characteristic advantages of laparoscopy, including decreased pain and expedited convalescence, are particularly evident. The hand-assist approach appears to greatly facilitate laparoscopic nephroureterectomy while providing nearly similar benefits. However, concerns over retroperitoneal recurrence have discouraged the more widespread use of this approach. More long-term data are needed to realistically address these misgivings. Likewise, data are needed with regard to the best way of managing the distal ureter to minimize the risk of an extravesical recurrence. To this end, meticulous follow-up with pelvic CT scans is essential among these patients.

Malignant Disease: Ablative—On the Horizon

Partial Nephrectomy and Renal Wedge Excision for Renal Tumors

Recently, several papers have revealed the excellent survival achievable with partial nephrectomy or, to a lesser extent, wedge excision among patients with small renal tumors (4 cm or smaller). The technical success rates and long-term patient survival with nephron-sparing surgery have been shown to equal results with radical or total nephrectomy for the management of stage I renal malignancies (103,148,259,309,442). Laparoscopically, renal wedge excision is technically much easier to accomplish than a formal partial nephrectomy. As such, it is not surprising that the initial experience with laparoscopic wedge excision was reported in 1993, but the initial successful laparoscopic partial nephrectomy for renal cancer was not reported until 1997 (97,263).

In general, only lesions of 2 cm or smaller that are predominantly exophytic are candidates for laparoscopic wedge excision. The basic method is to use a transperitoneal approach for anterior lesions and a retroperitoneal approach for posterior lesions. After renal mobilization, the lesion is identified either endoscopically or with an intracorporeal ultrasonographic probe. For the latter purpose, a flexible ultrasonic probe is most useful. Dissection around the lesion proceeds down to the renal capsule, being careful to keep the perinephric fat over the lesion undisturbed. If the fat overlying the tumor is displaced, it should be sent as a separate specimen for staging purposes.

After the lesion is well delineated, excision of the lesion with a margin of normal tissue is performed. Ultrasonic hook, ultrasonic shears, monopolar scissors, bipolar instruments, and other modalities have all been used for the wedge excision. To date, no transection modality has provided consistently reliable hemostasis. In this regard, a 5-mm argon beam coagulator is extremely useful to control small and medium-sized vessels and to stop parenchymal bleeding. Other hemostatic techniques include application of fibrin glue, gelatin formaldehyde resorcinol glue, bovine collagen, Surgicel (oxidized regenerated cellulose, Johnson and Johnson, Somerville, New Jersey), and Gelfoam (absorbable gelatin sponge, Pharmacia and Upjohn Co., Kalamazoo, Michigan). If the collecting system has not been violated, no drain is left.

Several techniques for laparoscopic partial nephrectomy have been described; however, these have largely been limited to single or several case reports. In general, these lesions are in the 2- to 4-cm size range. The approach is similar to the wedge excision with regard to locating the affected area of the kidney. No indwelling stent is placed. To try to prevent hemorrhage, a variety of devices have been employed: cable tie, double loop sling, and Endoloop suture occlusion (380a). More recently, hand-assist techniques have enabled the surgeon to use hand compression, thereby facilitating the transection of the affected area. The incision through the parenchyma is accomplished with any of the aforementioned modalities used for the wedge excision. Clayman and colleagues (97) have attempted to do this with an electrosurgical snare; however, their sanguine animal experience did not transfer into the clinical realm. Once the affected area is excised, the underlying incised parenchyma and collecting system can be most easily closed using a combination of fibrin glue and a hemostatic fabric. Alternatively, the collecting system can be sutured closed and parenchymal hemostasis can be obtained using a combination of the argon beam coagulator and the application of bovine collagen. By giving the patient an intravenous dose of furosemide (Lasix) and indigo carmine, the surgeon can make a final check to rule out any urine leak. A drain is left in the retroperitoneum.

McDougall and colleagues (266) reported results of nine partial nephrectomies and three wedge resections. The partial nephrectomies were for benign disease and have been previously reviewed. All three wedge resections were for small renal masses and were successfully completed laparoscopically. Mean operative time for these three cases was 3.5 hours. Mean estimated blood loss was 92 mL. Patients had a mean hospital stay of 2.7 days and required an average of 21 mg of morphine sulfate for pain control. Mean time for complete convalescence was 4 weeks, and there were no intraoperative or postoperative complications. Pathology revealed a renal cell carcinoma, an oncocytoma, and an old infarction. At 46 months, there was no recurrence of tumor in the one kidney with renal cell cancer (266).

Janetschek and co-workers (194) reported results of seven patients undergoing laparoscopic wedge resection for renal tumors up to 2 cm in diameter. Final pathology revealed five lesions to be renal cell carcinoma; the remaining two were multilocular cysts. All procedures were successfully completed laparoscopically. Mean operative time was 3.7 hours, and mean estimated blood loss was 311 mL. There was a single intraoperative complication: high abdominal pressures from the argon beam coagulator resulted in pneumothorax that resolved without the need to place a chest tube. No patient required analgesia after the second postoperative day. Mean hospital stay was 4.6 days, and patients returned to full activity between 7 and 21 days postoperatively. Long-term follow-up data were not available.

The initial laparoscopic partial nephrectomy for a renal cell cancer was reported in 1997 by Elashry and colleagues (97). This initial case required 5 hours; an electrosurgical snare was used to incise the renal parenchyma. The snare failed to provide satisfactory hemostasis; the argon beam coagulator proved effective in this regard. The collecting system was closed using intracorporeal suturing. The procedure was complicated by a urinoma requiring percutaneous nephrostomy tube drainage; the patient was in the hospital for 5 days. Total analgesic requirement consisted of 60 mg of ketorolac. Long-term follow-up was not available in this case report.

Wolf and colleagues (451) reported results of ten laparoscopic nephron-sparing procedures performed in nine patients; eight of these procedures were completed using hand assistance. They compared their results with 11 open procedures. Of 11 tumors, 8 (73%) were malignant. There was no significant difference in operative time between the laparoscopic and open approaches (3.3 versus 2.7 hours). Estimated blood loss for the laparoscopic and open groups was 460 and 210 mL, respectively. This included a laparoscopic wedge resection complicated by a 1,860-mL blood loss. There were three complications in each group. Laparoscopic complications included a patient requiring a transfusion of 4 units of packed red blood cells and transient urinary retention in two patients. Complications in the open group included two transfusions of 4 units of packed red blood cells and an arteriovenous fistula requiring embolization. Patients managed laparoscopically required less analgesic medications (40 versus 105 mg of morphine sulfate equivalents). Hospital stay was 2.0 days for the laparoscopic group and 3.5 days for the open group. Return to normal activity was also more expeditious in the laparoscopic group (8 versus 23 weeks). Long-term follow-up data were not available.

Division of the laparoscopic procedures into polar nephrectomy, wedge resection, and enucleation revealed that the operative time and estimated blood loss are higher with a

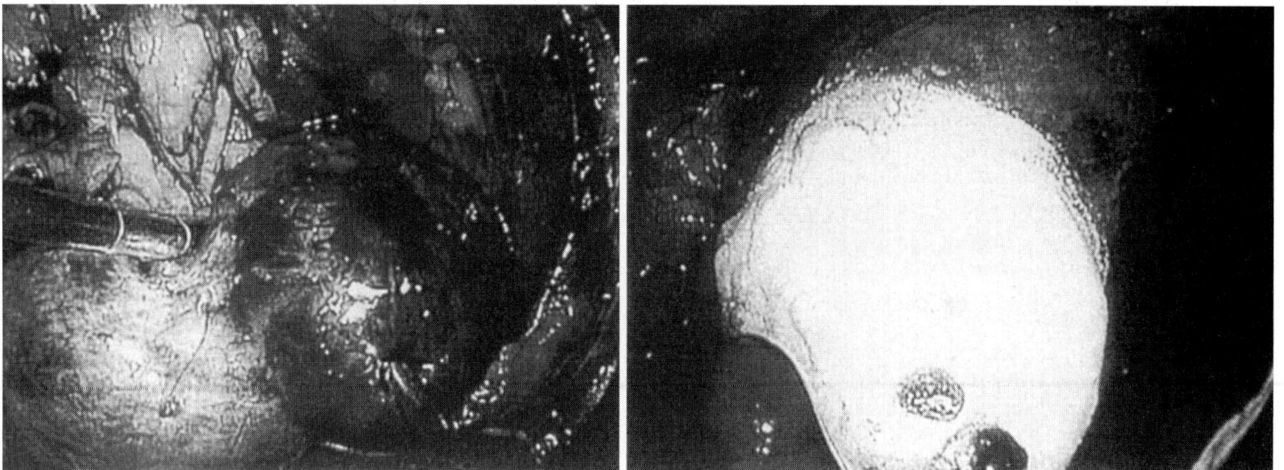

FIGURE 18.20. Renal cryotherapy. **A:** Mobilized kidney with cryoprobe inserted in renal mass. **B:** Ice ball engulfing renal mass. (Reprinted from Elsevier Science, with permission.)

partial nephrectomy (445a). The operative times for laparoscopic partial nephrectomies, wedge resections, and enucleations were 4.2, 3.3, and 2.4 hours, respectively. Estimated blood loss for uncomplicated laparoscopic partial nephrectomy, wedge resection, and enucleation was 550, 300, and 300 mL, respectively. Mean length of stay for all three procedures was similar at 2 days.

Results for laparoscopic partial nephrectomy and laparoscopic wedge resection are frequently difficult to distinguish in the literature. Both procedures, although technically challenging with present technology, are feasible. Laparoscopic wedge resection has been described with results demonstrating the procedure to be effective, in the short run, and safe. Laparoscopic partial nephrectomy remains challenging, with the optimal technique yet to be developed. Both procedures suffer from a lack of cases and an absence of any long-term follow-up data.

Renal Cryoablation for Renal Tumors

The management of small renal masses continues to evolve with the progression from open radical nephrectomy, to open partial nephrectomy, to laparoscopic nephrectomy, and most recently to laparoscopic nephron-sparing surgery. Presently, the next step in minimally invasive therapy is just beginning to be explored: needle ablative therapy. Recently, cryotherapy has been used in the clinical management of small renal masses (Fig. 18.20). The ability of intraoperative laparoscopic ultrasound probes to accurately monitor the progression of the resulting ice ball has further stimulated interest in this modality. Other renal ablative modalities just beginning to be explored in the laboratory include wet and dry radiofrequency, photon irradiation, thermal rods, ethanol gel, and microwave therapy (Fig. 18.21).

Zegal and co-workers (458) performed cryotherapy in six patients with renal masses less than 4 cm in greatest diameter. The kidneys were accessed via open laparotomy incisions, and one to three cryoprobes were inserted into the renal masses under ultrasonographic guidance. Two cycles of cryoablation were applied to each tumor with a 1.5- to 2.0-cm ice ball margin created around each mass. All patients were successfully treated. During a follow-up period of 3 to 22 months, all patients were followed with CT scan, MRI, or both. There was no evidence of tumor recurrence during this relatively brief follow-up period.

Bishoff and co-workers (28) reported results of eight patients with T_1 renal tumors managed with laparoscopic-guided cryosurgical ablation. Mean tumor size was 2 cm. A transperitoneal laparoscopic approach was used to access anterior or medial tumors, and a retroperitoneal approach

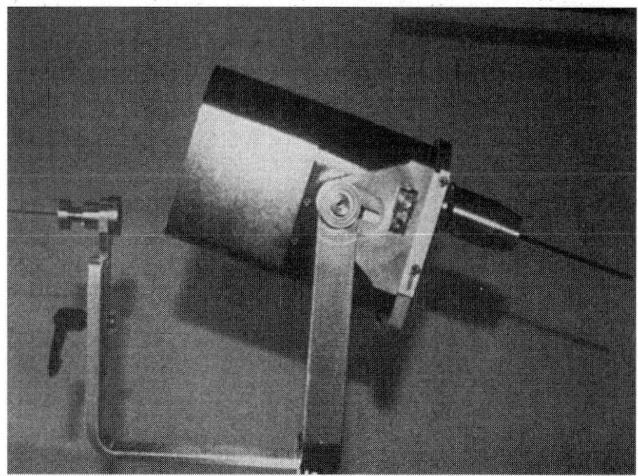

FIGURE 18.21. Photo beam irradiation source. (Reprinted from Mary Ann Liebert Co., with permission.)

was used to access posterior and lateral tumors. A cryoprobe, 4.8 mm in diameter, was used for tumor ablation, and a double freeze cycle of 5 minutes with a single thaw cycle of 15 minutes was applied. Renal biopsies at the time of surgery revealed renal cell carcinoma in six patients and were indeterminate in two patients. There were no intraoperative or postoperative complications reported. Mean operative time was 3.7 hours, and the mean estimated blood loss was 87 mL. Hospital stay was 3 days. With a mean follow-up of 7.7 months, no patient had radiographic evidence of tumor recurrence.

Gill and colleagues (126) reported laparoscopic cryoablation of 11 exophytic renal tumors ranging in size from 1.5 to 3.0 cm. A 4.8-mm conical-tipped cryoprobe was used (Fig. 18.20A). All procedures were successfully completed via a retroperitoneal approach. Laparoscopic ultrasound guidance was used for probe placement and to monitor the ice ball (Fig. 18.20B). Mean surgical time was 2.4 hours, and estimated blood loss was 75 mL. Hemostasis was achieved using the argon beam coagulator and Surgicel (oxidized regenerated cellulose, Johnson and Johnson, Somerville, New Jersey). Mean postoperative analgesic requirements consisted of 21 mg of morphine sulfate equivalents. Nine of ten patients were discharged within 23 hours. One patient tolerated the procedure well but required an 8-day hospital stay for stabilization of his cardiac status and systemic anticoagulation therapy. Intraoperatively, there was a single complication (a small liver laceration that was coagulated). Postoperatively, the only complication was a perirenal hematoma. Mean follow-up was 5.5 months and consisted of CT scan and MRI radiologic evaluation. All lesions continued to decrease in size during the follow-up period. Three patients underwent follow-up CT-guided biopsy of the cryoablation site. There was no evidence of tumor on any of the three biopsies.

Follow-up data from The Cleveland Clinic series was subsequently presented by Levin and co-workers (236) in a patient group now expanded to 22 patients. Needle biopsies were performed in all patients 3 and 6 months after cryotherapy. No patient had recurrent disease on these biopsies. However, one patient with a negative biopsy at 6 months had a local recurrence at 12 months; laparoscopic radical nephrectomy was performed and revealed a 1.3-cm focus of renal cell carcinoma.

Laparoscopic cryoablation of small renal masses (less than 3 cm) under ultrasonic guidance is feasible. In small series of highly selected patients, the procedure has so far been safe and resulted in a rapid convalescence. However, follow-up has been relatively brief, and one case of oncologic failure has already been reported at less than 2 years postprocedure. Accordingly, at this point in time, renal cryosurgery for small renal masses remains a largely investigational technique pending further long-term (i.e., 3- to 5-year) follow-up.

The next decade will be of great interest as each of the forms of needle ablative therapy comes under clinical investigation. By the year 2010, effective needle ablative therapy may well become the norm for renal lesions in the 1- to 4-cm size range. With advances in this arena, nephron-sparing surgery, as we currently know it, may well begin to fade from the scene.

Radical Prostatectomy

Radical prostatectomy was performed for the first time by Proust (342) in 1901 via a transperineal incision. Developments in this form of surgery occurred slowly; indeed, it took more than 40 years before Millin (281) proposed a retropubic approach. Likewise, it took almost another 40 years for another major change to occur in this operation; in 1983, Walsh and co-workers (431) modified the retropubic approach to make it "nerve-sparing," thereby preserving potency.

Laparoscopic transperitoneal radical prostatectomy was introduced by Schuessler and colleagues (374) in 1997. The technique has been subsequently modified and its application greatly expanded by Guillonneau and Vallancien (145). Recently, an extraperitoneal approach to laparoscopic radical prostatectomy has also been described by Savad and Ferzli (368).

Guillonneau and Vallancien (146) reported results of 120 consecutive patients undergoing laparoscopic transperitoneal radical prostatectomy. Mean operative time was 4.0 hours. The authors used a five-port array. The prostatectomy was done in the following order: infravesical mobilization of the seminal vesicles and division of the vasa, anterior dissection of the bladder, entry into the endopelvic fascia, suture ligation of the dorsal venous complex, incision of the bladder neck, take-down of the pedicles with bipolar electrosurgical coagulation, urethral dissection and incision, take-down of the rectourethralis, and entrapment of the specimen. The urethrovesical anastomosis was completed using completely intracorporeal sutures; six to eight individual sutures were placed and tied. When patients were stratified by thirds, operative times for the first, second, and third groups were 4.8, 4.1, and 3.9 hours, respectively. Mean estimated blood loss for all patients was 402 mL. When stratified by sequential experience, estimated blood loss was 534, 517, and 277 mL for the three groups, respectively. Conversion to an open procedure occurred in 7 (5.8%) patients, all of whom were among the initial 80 patients. Conversion resulted from bleeding in three cases and from difficult dissection in four cases. Twelve patients (10%) required transfusion; however, the transfusion rates decreased with experience: 15%, 12.5%, and 2.5% for the first, second, and third group of 40 cases, respectively.

There were three (2.5%) intraoperative complications: an epigastric vessel injury that was repaired laparoscopically, an obturator nerve palsy that resolved with conservative management, and a rectal injury that was repaired laparoscopically. Postoperative complications included two patients (1.7%) with a 5-day ileus and nine patients (7.5%) with leakage from the urethrovesical anastomosis. In seven of these nine patients, the leakage resolved spontaneously by postoperative day 5 with suction drainage alone. In one case, percutaneous aspiration of a urinoma was required, and one patient required anastomotic repair that was performed laparoscopically. One patient required open exploration for bleeding from an injured epigastric artery that was not appreciated intraoperatively. In addition, 14 patients (10%) experienced urinary tract infections, and three patients (1.5%) had transient urinary retention. Morphine sulfate was requested by only 9% of patients by postoperative day 1 and by only 2% of patients by postoperative day 2.

Definitive histologic examination revealed prostatic intraepithelial neoplasia in 2 patients (1.7%), stage pT2a disease in 37 patients (30.8%), pT2b in 68 patients (56.7%), stage pT3a in 7 patients (5.8%), and stage pT3b in 6 patients (5%). The overall positive surgical margin rate was 15%. With a mean follow-up of only 2.2 months, PSA levels were 0.1 ng/mL or less in 95% of the 94 patients studied. No instances of port site seeding were noted.

Mean postoperative catheterization time was 6.6 days. Catheterization times for the first, second, and third groups of patients were 7.9, 7.3, and 5.7 days, respectively. The 120 patients had a mean functional follow-up of 1.7 months. Eighty-five patients (71%) were completely continent (no pads), with 58% of patients regaining continence within 30 days. No patient had experienced a postoperative bladder neck contraction. Of the 60 patients with at least 6 months of follow-up, the continence rate was 73%.

Preservation of the neurovascular bundles was routinely performed only in the final 40 patients. Twenty of these patients (50%) were potent and sexually active before surgery. In 9 of these 20 (45%), spontaneous erections were reported postoperatively; however, only one patient (5%) reported rigidity sufficient for sexual intercourse. Of interest, the authors noted that the overall cost of laparoscopic radical prostatectomy in France was $1,237 less than that for an open retropubic radical prostatectomy (146).

The work of Abbou and co-workers (2) has been contemporaneous with that of Guillonneau and Vallancien (145,146). Laparoscopic transperitoneal radical prostatectomy was performed in 43 men. The approach was similar to that described by Guillonneau and Vallancien except that running sutures were used to effect the urethrovesical anastomosis. The median operative time for the first ten patients was 7 hours (n = 5) without lymphadenectomy and 8.6 hours (n = 50) with lymphadenectomy. After the first ten patients, the operative time for laparoscopic radical prostatectomy dropped to 4.3 hours in 21 patients without lymphadenectomy and 5.1 hours in patients with lymphadenectomy. Estimated blood loss was not reported.

Complications included two (4.7%) cases of prolonged lymphatic drainage, one (2.3%) rectal injury managed with open suture repair and colonic diversion, and four (9.3%) vesicoureteral anastomotic leakages that were managed by open surgery in three cases and laparoscopically in one case. One month after surgery, 36 patients (84%) were continent. Of the remaining seven patients (16%), five had only minor and occasional leakage during extreme stress; this population did not require use of pads. The remaining two patients wore only one pad daily for minor stress incontinence. With a mean follow-up of 6.3 months, all 43 patients had a serum PSA of less than 0.1 mg/dL. Positive surgical margins were identified in 12 (28%) specimens.

Laparoscopic radical prostatectomy is feasible. Subsequent modifications have made the procedure more expeditious, and initial results for both cancer control and patient morbidity are promising. At present, the procedure remains technically challenging as demonstrated by lengthy learning curves even in the hands of experienced laparoscopic surgeons. Long-term comparative data with open radical retropubic prostatectomy and with open perineal prostatectomy are needed to determine the role of the laparoscopic approach.

Radical Cystectomy

The first laparoscopic radical cystectomy and urinary diversion was reported by Sanchez de Badajoz and colleagues (365) in 1993. Denewer and co-workers (78) subsequently reported a series of ten patients who underwent laparoscopic radical cystectomy and continent pouch construction performed through a limited incision. Seven of the ten patients (70%) had received radiation therapy 1 to 4 months before laparoscopic cystectomy. Bilateral pelvic lymphadenectomy was performed. The rectovesicle pouch was sharply entered, and dissection of Denonvilliers' fascia was performed to mobilize the posterior portion of the bladder. Both bladder pedicles were secured with the laparoscopic stapler. A stapler or electrosurgical scissors dissection was used to separate the urethra at the pelvic floor. An 8-cm subumbilical midline incision was then used to create a sigmoid pouch with an intussusception antireflux valve. Individual ureteral anastomoses were also performed in an open fashion via the same 8-cm incision. In this series, the mean operative time was 160 minutes for cystectomy, and an additional 55 minutes was required for pouch construction. Mean intraoperative blood transfusion rate was 2.2 units of packed red blood cells per patient. Hospital stay was 10 to 13 days. A single intraoperative complication was reported: the external iliac artery was divided in one patient. The vessel was successfully repaired during the open portion of the procedure. Postoperative complications occurred in four patients (40%). These included a case of urinary leakage that resolved without any need for stenting or reoperation, a deep venous thrombosis, and a pelvic collection that required percutaneous drainage. One patient died postoperatively; this individual developed postoperative hemorrhage. Reexploration was followed by disseminated intravascular coagulation, multisystem organ failure, and death (78).

Puppo and associates (344) reported results of five laparoscopically assisted transvaginal radical cystectomies in women with invasive bladder cancer. A bilateral cutaneous ureterostomy was performed in the first case. In the remaining four cases, an ileal conduit was accomplished through a mini-laparotomy at the stoma site. The specimen was removed transvaginally in four cases. In one case, vaginal atrophy necessitated removal through a midline laparotomy.

All procedures were successfully accomplished laparoscopically. Mean operative time was 7.1 hours, and although estimated blood loss was not reported, three patients (60%) required transfusion (mean of 3 units of packed red blood cells). Analgesic requirements were not reported. Hospital stay was 10.6 days. No major complications occurred intraoperatively. Two patients had significant lymphatic drainage for 1 week that resolved without intervention. All patients were reported to be alive with a mean follow-up of 10.8 months, but their disease status was not reported.

Gill and co-workers (123) reported results of two laparoscopic radical cystoprostatectomies with ileal conduits performed for invasive transitional cell carcinoma. In both cases, for the first time, the cystoprostatectomies and ileal conduits were constructed completely intracorporeally. Mean operative time was 11 hours, and mean estimated blood loss was 1,100 mL. Both patients resumed ambulation on postoperative day 2. Oral intake was resumed on postoperative day 4, and the patients were discharged on postoperative day 6. The two patients required 108 and 17 mg of morphine sulfate equivalents for analgesia, respectively. No intraoperative or postoperative complications were reported. Time to full convalescence was not reported. Long-term follow-up data were not available.

Laparoscopic cystectomy and diversion appears to be feasible. However, its application has been limited to very few institutions, and to date, there have been no large series and no direct comparisons with open cystectomy and diversion. Follow-up is too brief to comment on the long-term efficacy of this approach or to address concerns regarding possible seeding.

NEWER TECHNOLOGY

As the era of industrialization wanes, the age of computer-based information technology has become ascendant. Medical application of these advanced technologies will lead to major diagnostic and therapeutic advances. In this section, the impact of these newer technologies on laparoscopic surgery is presented. In this regard, the following areas are addressed: needle ablative therapy for renal tumor ablation, robotics, virtual reality as applied to laparoscopy, improvements in optics, newer laparoscopic tissue approximation techniques, and newer tissue dissection techniques.

Needle-invasive Ablation of Renal Tissue

Nephron-sparing surgery for renal tumors has become an established practice in select patients with a compromised global nephron mass and in patients with small tumors (less than 4 cm) (308). Within the past decade, minimally invasive techniques have been increasingly implemented for renal surgery. In keeping with these trends, various alternative energy sources for tumor ablation have also been developed. In urology, the majority of alternative treatments for solid organ tumors were originally investigated for treatment of benign and cancerous pathologies of the prostate. These treatments have now been adapted for renal surgery as well. The anatomic location and laparoscopic accessibility of the kidneys, as well as advances in imaging, have permitted accurate localization and ablation of renal tumors using these newer techniques. The various alternative energy sources described herein include cryoablation, radiofrequency ablation, microwave thermotherapy, high-intensity focused ultrasound (HIFU), and interstitial photon radiation energy.

Cryoablation

Uchida and colleagues (423) pioneered clinical renal cryoablation in 1995, using the percutaneous technique. Delworth and colleagues (76a) first reported open renal cryoablation, and Gill and colleagues (125) published the initial experience with laparoscopic renal cryoablation in 1996. At present, cryoablation is the most widely investigated and clinically used energy source for renal tumor ablation.

During renal cryoablation, tissue destruction is achieved by alternate cycles of freezing and thawing (108). Alternate freeze–thaw cycles are responsible for cell injury as a result of progressive metabolic failure secondary to extracellular and intracellular ice formation. As tissue temperatures approach the freezing zone, extracellular fluid is transformed into ice. Increased extracellular osmotic pressure relative to the intracellular compartment results, which draws water out of the cells. The ensuing increased intracellular solute concentration is detrimental to cell survival (254). Subsequently, intracellular ice formation occurs as a result of extension of extracellular ice directly, or as a result of continued rapid tissue cooling. The incorporation of minute blood vessels within the growing ice ball results in regional vascular occlusion that further accentuates tissue destruction. Profound tissue hypothermia inhibits tissue metabolism, adversely affecting cellular repair and survival following the cryotherapy insult.

During the thaw cycle, the osmotic effect is reversed. Extracellular ice melts, causing hypotonicity and thereby shifting water into the intact cells, causing cell swelling and disruption of cellular membranes. Thawing causes vasodilation and increased vascular permeability, tissue congestion, and edema. Platelet aggregation and microthrombi formation occur as a result of endothelial damage. Several small blood vessels are occluded following the thaw cycle. The microcirculatory failure and vascular stasis that result from cryoablation further augment the cytocidal effect of intracellular freezing. The resultant tissue anoxia is the basis of delayed cryoinjury. Repetition of the freeze–thaw cycle further potentiates tissue destruction (292). Sindelar and colleagues (392) proposed that an enhanced host cryoimmunologic response to the cryoablated tissue may be an additional mechanism of tissue destruction.

At the advancing edge of the ice ball, a 1- to 2-mm transition zone separates the zone of lethal destruction from the nontargeted normal renal parenchyma (296). This zone typically demonstrates a less pronounced and variable degree of cellular destruction.

Early to intermediate changes occurring a few weeks after cryosurgery include coagulative necrosis, which reduces the tubular cell remnants into proteinaceous aggregates, and variable amounts of chronic inflammation (273). The tubular basement membrane and collagenous network remain intact and form the framework for the subsequent deposition of fibrin. Late changes, occurring 3 months after surgery, include tissue destruction and autoabsorption within the lethal zone. Fibrin is laid down as part of the reparative process.

Chosy and colleagues (57) studied the lethal temperature required for renal cell destruction in the porcine model. Using thermosensors, a temperature of −19.4°C was found to be necessary for uniform cell death. This lethal temperature was achieved up to 3.1 mm inside the edge of the ice ball. Temperatures achieved at the tip of the cryoprobe are typically in the range of −140° to −180°C. Clinically, to ensure complete tumor destruction the freeze zone is extended approximately 1 cm beyond the edge of the tumor. To maximize the cold effect on tissues, concurrent renal artery clamping during the procedure has been suggested as a possible method for prevention of temperature conduction (the heat sink effect). However, Campbell and colleagues (45) demonstrated no significant advantage associated with this maneuver in the porcine model.

It is critical at all times to ensure that the ice ball is not in contact with any surrounding organ structure. Porcine studies have demonstrated deleterious effects such as small bowel obstruction and pelviureteral obstruction due to inadvertent injury caused by direct contact of these structures with the ice ball (45,125). However, Sung and colleagues (406) have recently demonstrated spontaneous watertight urothelial regeneration following intentional cryoinjury to the renal collecting system, thereby potentially paving the way for the cryotreatment of more centrally located tumors.

Percutaneous interventional MRI-guided cryoablation in 17 patients was recently reported by Shingleton and colleagues (386). The technique represents a less invasive form of renal cryoablation than the laparoscopic technique. Cryoprobes as small as 1.8 mm can be used. Short-term follow-up appeared promising.

Radiofrequency Interstitial Tumor Ablation

The role of hyperthermia in tumor destruction was noted initially by Busch (39) as early as 1866, in a patient with a sarcoma. Radiofrequency waves are low-frequency electromagnetic waves (frequency ranging from 0.5 to 1.0 MHz) that have the potential to alter the molecular kinetics of the tissues that they traverse. Radiofrequency waves cause ionic and molecular agitation, which results in a rise in kinetic energy. The resulting heat is the basis for thermotherapy (404). These low-frequency electromagnetic waves have greater tissue penetration than microwaves.

Clinical utility of radiofrequency ablation was established for the destruction of accessory cardiac conduction pathways responsible for arrhythmias (366). Radiofrequency ablation has also been employed for the treatment of hepatocellular cancer and osteoid osteomas and for performing neurotomy (75,244,357). In urology, transurethral needle ablation (TUNA) and transperineal radiofrequency interstitial tumor ablation (RITA) have been used for the treatment of benign prostatic hyperplasia and cancer of the prostate, respectively. Zlotta and colleagues (460) initially described RITA of a renal tumor in 1997. Their study included renal tumor radioablation before ipsilateral radical nephrectomy.

The size of the radiolesion depends on the length of the probe, the duration of contact, and the power used. Electrodes may be monopolar or bipolar. RITA induces vaporization and tissue charring in the immediate vicinity of the electrode tip. As a result, tissue impedance rises, thus limiting the size of the radiolesion. To overcome this problem, saline-infused RITA has recently been described using a probe through which hypertonic saline can also be infused (333). Radiofrequency waves spread along the interstitial saline infusion, minimizing tissue charring, thus resulting in larger radiolesions in an extremely short period of time; indeed, with this approach, tissue impedance is reduced by upward of 66% at 1 minute. Hoey and colleagues (170) demonstrated lesions ranging from 2.5 to 22.8 cm^3 (mean of 8.5 cm^3) using this technique, compared with lesions of only 0.06 to 0.93 cm^3 (mean of 0.34 cm^3) when using the dry radiofrequency probe. Polascik and colleagues (333) produced lesions involving 25% to 50% of the rabbit kidney (i.e., up to 2- by 1.3- by 1-cm lesions) with a 30- to

45-second treatment with "wet" RITA at 50 W. Clinical trials using wet RITA for the treatment of renal tumors are yet awaited.

Microwave Thermotherapy

Microwaves are electromagnetic waves with high frequencies, ranging from 300 to 3,000 MHz. In 1979, Tabuse (409) initially reported using microwaves for tissue during hepatic surgery. Its initial application as a method of thermotherapy was described by Yerushalmi and colleagues (455) in 1982 for the treatment of prostate cancer. Transrectal and transurethral heat applicators have been described for treatment of patients with prostate cancer and benign prostatic hyperplasia, respectively.

Laparoscopic microwave thermotherapy has been described for the experimental destruction of rabbit VX-2 renal tumors (219). The needle electrode was 1 mm in diameter and 8 mm in length with a 5-mm coaxial cable. Microwaves (2,450 MHz) were generated at a maximum output of 110 W. Coagulative necrosis was achieved over a 5- to 6-mm radius around the probe. During microwave thermotherapy, temperatures of 84° ± 3.3°C were achieved at a distance of 5 mm from the electrode, and temperatures of 55° ± 1.6°C were achieved at a distance of 10 mm from the electrode. The procedure is rapid, with desired effects being seen within 30 seconds. An advantage of the coagulative effect of microwaves is that tissue hemostasis is achieved simultaneously. However, lesions of a limited size are produced, which may necessitate the placement of multiple probes. Furthermore, a considerable amount of steam may be generated during treatment, which may interfere with laparoscopic visualization. Clinical trials using microwave therapy for the treatment of renal tumors are pending.

High-intensity Focused Ultrasound

Several studies have investigated the effects of HIFU for treatment of prostate cancer. Tissue temperatures of 85°C and lesions 18 mm in size have been reported within a few seconds of initiating treatment. HIFU is performed with a 1- to 2.25-MHz ultrasound transducer. Low-intensity exposure (less than 500 W/cm^2) for longer than 1 second is typically associated with thermal coagulative damage of the targeted tissue, whereas higher-intensity exposure (greater than 3,000 W/cm^2) causes tissue cavitation resulting in punched-out lesions (87). Cavitation is induced by conversion of tissue water into vapor. The vapor bubbles absorb energy from the ultrasound waves and grow larger. Once the bubbles reach their resonance they collapse, releasing high pressure and temperature, which induces tissue destruction. Pressure and temperature as high as 28,000 bars and 10,000 K, respectively, may be generated. Ultrasound waves of intermediate intensities tend to produce changes, which include cavitation surrounded by an area of coagulative necrosis. However, the ultrasound waves must be accurately focused on targeted tissues. Misfiring or inaccurate focusing may result in destruction of nontargeted neighboring tissues.

Chapelon and colleagues (51) studied the effects of HIFU on renal tissues of rats and dogs. Subsequent human trials resulted in incomplete tumor destruction and production of superficial burns (436). Although studies to determine the true efficacy and safety of this developmental treatment modality are yet necessary, it has the potential to be a completely noninvasive ablative modality for destruction of renal tumors.

Interstitial Photon Radiation

The role of interstitial photon therapy for stereotactic ablation of brain tumors is well established. Radiosurgery has also been used for the treatment of brain metastasis from metastatic renal cell cancer. Chan and colleagues (50) studied the feasibility of using intracavitary photon radiation for renal ablation in dogs. A 3.2-mm-diameter probe was inserted into the renal parenchyma, and local radiation of 15 Gy was delivered. An average lesion of 2.5 cm was produced. The animals maintained normal renal function over a 6-month survival period. The exposed tissues demonstrated changes suggestive of coagulative necrosis with a sharply demarcated rim, signifying unaffected surrounding renal parenchyma.

Compared with the high intensity and high energy of external beam radiation and the low intensity and low energy of brachytherapy, interstitial radiation is associated with high intensity and low energy. Hence, it does not produce the excessive tissue destruction seen with external beam radiation, nor does it require the prolonged treatment time necessary with brachytherapy. Furthermore, interstitial photon radiation may be delivered percutaneously. The potential of this form of treatment has not yet been explored at the level of clinical urology.

Robotics

Advances in robotics in the fields of industrial and aerospace-related technology have led to the simultaneous growth of medical robotics (153). A robot is a programmable automated task performance system controlled by microprocessors. Telerobotic devices synergistically integrate machine and real-time remote human interactions via electronic interfaces. Surgical procedures performed in such a manner are referred to as telepresence robotic surgery.

Robotic surgery has triggered advances in microsurgery (including vascular surgery) and laparoscopy. For totally robotic procedures, the surgeon is seated at a control station from where the robotic arms can be telemanipulated (one arm holds the laparoscope, and two arms hold laparoscopic instruments) using two robotic ergonomically designed handles. A dedicated computer and coaxial cables link the two systems. For laparoscopic procedures, the robotic arms operate specially designed laparoscopic instruments that are inserted through standard laparoscopic ports.

AESOP (Automated Endoscope System for Optimal Positioning, Computer Motion, Goleta, California) is an example of a single robotic arm for control of the laparoscope (362) (Fig. 18.22). It was the first robotic system approved by the U.S. Food and Drug Administration (FDA) for laparoscopic intervention. The system obeys the surgeon's voice based on a preprogrammed voice card and voice recognition software. A safety feature incorporated into the AESOP arm is a mechanism that automatically releases the laparoscope from its clasp when any pressure in excess of 5 pounds is applied. A technical drawback of the current system is the inability to control telescopic zoom and angular rotation of forward-oblique laparoscopes.

The Green Telemanipulator Surgical System (SRI International, Menlo Park, California) was originally designed as a remote operational system that could perform surgical tasks in the battlefield (139). The system consisted of robotic arms with four degrees of freedom. The da Vinci Surgical System (Intuitive Surgical, Inc., Mountain View, California) is a sophisticated robotic system developed from the Green prototype with 3D image capability (385). A feature unique to this system is the Endo-wrist technology of the robotic arms. The arms have six degrees of freedom of motion, and a seventh degree of motion is provided by distally located computer-enhanced joints designed to further accentuate surgical dexterity. The ARTEMIS (Advanced Robotic Telemanipulator for Minimally Invasive Surgery) and the Zeus Microsurgical Robotic System (Computer Motion, Goleta, California) are other robotic systems designed for minimally invasive surgery. The Zeus system may be used in conjunction with the AESOP laparoscopic manipulator and consists of robotic arms with six degrees of freedom. Newer robotic systems have been designed to provide force and tactile feedback to the operator. Currently, however, these haptic interfaces are still largely developmental.

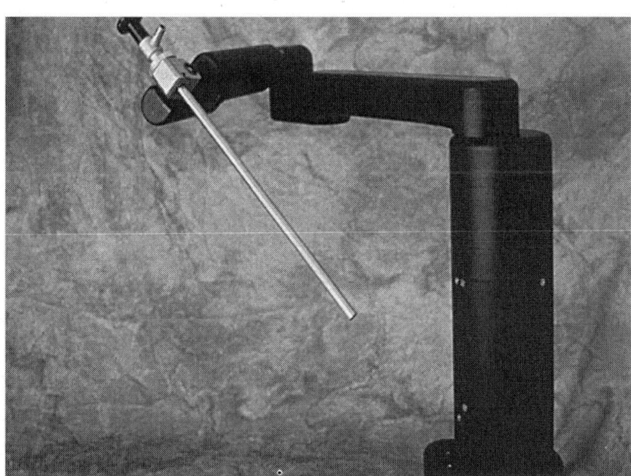

FIGURE 18.22. AESOP robotic arm.

Initially, clinical applications in urology included transurethral resection of the prostate and prostatic biopsy (74,358). Kavoussi and colleagues, in a comparison between human versus AESOP robotic laparoscopic control (eight laparoscopic pelvic lymphadenectomies and three laparoscopic Burch colposuspensions), concluded that the robotic system was more effective and accurate than human laparoscopic control (209a). In another study, Partin and colleagues (325) successfully performed 82% of 17 cases using one or two AESOP robotic arms with a single surgeon. Human intervention was warranted in the event of any intraoperative complications such as significant hemorrhage. At The Cleveland Clinic, experimental robotic-assisted laparoscopic pyeloplasty (405) and the initial study on completely robotic laparoscopic nephrectomy and adrenalectomy in the porcine model have been performed.

The Future of Robotics

During laparoscopy, a fulcrum is created on the shaft of the instrument at the site of entry into the body (the trocar). As a result, the surgeon's movements are inverted before being transmitted to the distal instrument tip. To eliminate this inversion, the Human Interface Technology Laboratory at the University of Washington is developing an immersive robotic interface (315). This futuristic system proposes to give the surgeon the perspective of being shrunk and immersed into the patient's body for direct control of the distal tips of the laparoscopic instruments. This would involve the use of robotics and virtual reality images and would eliminate the inversion effect produced during routine laparoscopy. Furthermore, this may improve precision while shortening the learning curve associated with laparoscopy. Current robotic surgery is based on a "master-slave" interaction in a telerobotic manner. The rapid developments in information technology and neural networks may well pave the way for completely automated robotic surgery performed independently. Using computer algorithms and artificial intelligence with sensory inputs from the environment, future robotic systems may be able to perform complex preprogrammed tasks without the need for any interference from the human "master."

Remote Robotic Surgery

Advanced telecommunication technology has incredibly hastened the speed of data transfer over the past few years. Using high-bandwidth telecommunications, a surgeon can remotely control a surgical procedure being performed transcontinentally. Lee and colleagues (231) at Johns Hopkins University in Baltimore reported telementoring of a laparoscopic adrenalectomy performed in Innsbruck, Austria, 5,083 miles away, and telementoring of a laparoscopic varicocelectomy in Bangkok, Thailand, 10,880 miles away, in 1998. With further development of telecommunications and optics for data transfer, long-distance remote robotic surgery may become part of standard clinical teaching and practice.

Virtual Reality

Similar to flight simulators, which are designed to train pilots, virtual reality systems are being developed as a potential method for surgical training. Virtual reality systems seek to simulate real-patient situations by means of a series of synthetic computer-generated animations. Besides its potential use to train surgical residents, it will also enable more experienced surgeons to rehearse steps of a procedure before the actual operation. By entering patient-specific sophisticated imaging data into the simulator, a surgeon will be navigated through the area of interest. Such "enhanced" reality systems seek to augment reality with patient-specific images.

A laparoscopic virtual reality simulator comprises a manikin in which the laparoscopic instruments are manipulated. The surgeon wears a head-mounted display or alternatively uses a 3D video monitor. The system is equipped with a stereolaparoscope and auditory and haptic feedback (174). In addition, head, hand, and instrument-tracking technology is incorporated (435). A series of computer-generated images are relayed, consisting of representations of various anatomically correct cartoons. The images respond to movements of the surgeon by producing tissue deformation effects, bleeding, and other real-life physical situations (54). A state-of-the-art graphics computer with texture mapping capabilities is essential to generate these images. Alternatively, instead of the use of a manikin, systems are being developed that incorporate the use of a "dataglove." The MIST-VR (Minimally Invasive Surgery Trainer—Virtual Reality) is an example of a developmental virtual reality system for laparoscopic training (171).

Optics

Image clarity and optimal visualization are key to the success of any laparoscopic procedure. Analog images are being replaced by higher-resolution digital images. Charge-coupled devices (CCDs) form the core of all digital and electronic cameras. A CCD chip is a light-sensitive solid-state silicon chip containing a series of pixels. Pixels are electronic sensors that discharge an electric charge when struck by light. When a photon strikes the CCD, an electrical potential is generated, creating a digital image. These images can be relayed, printed, or stored for future reference in computers or using optic computer disks. Current laparoscopic cameras may contain one to three CCD chips with 25,000 to 50,000 pixels. Higher-resolution triple-chip cameras function in a manner such that each chip is dedicated to one of the three primary colors: red, green, and blue (RGB). Images are transmitted employing RGB video channels. Advances in digital technology have enabled the production of cameras with several megapixels of image resolution. When clinically available for laparoscopic applications, these cameras will provide unparalleled visualization and definition.

In its present design, the laparoscopic camera is typically mounted to the proximal end of the laparoscope. An air interface exists between the laparoscope and the camera, which hampers image quality. Eliminating this air interface by directly mounting the CCD on the distal tip of the laparoscope would provide for clearer images.

Newer high-definition television monitors provide better sharpness and definition of displayed images. These monitors display up to 1,125 lines of resolution compared with 525 lines of resolution displayed by the ordinary television monitor. High-definition head-mounted displays incorporating liquid crystal on silicon microdisplays are available (OptiVu, Optimize, Los Gatos, California). Video images archived in the digital format are permanent, are easily retrievable, and can be stored on desktop computers that can be used for multimedia presentations. Digital video disc (DVD) technology with improved Moving Pictures Expert Group (MPEG-2)–quality images has resulted in crisp image storage and playback. Desktop and notebook computers with DVD cards and optimal memory capacity can store and display these high-quality movie images. Video imaging is a rapidly advancing field. Currently, MPEG-4 through MPEG-7 image qualities are being developed. In the years to come, these images will provide far superior resolution than current technology.

Stereoscopic Laparoscopy

Standard current laparoscopy involves 2D image technology. A disadvantage is the lack of depth perception. With increased operator experience, laparoscopic procedures are becoming more technically complex, necessitating superior visualization. Stereoscopic images have the potential to provide precise high-quality images with depth perception.

To produce 3D images, a video system must convey differing offset images to each eye. Stereoscopic images are obtained by using a stereolaparoscope, which consists of a laparoscope with two optical lenses. The laparoscope is equipped with a stereo camera containing two CCD chips. The surgeon wears a head-mounted device (HMD) with a liquid crystal display and active shutter glasses. Images are alternately cycled at 120 Hz to each eye (282). The right eye exclusively views the right image and the left eye the left image. While an image is provided to one eye, the shutter covers the opposite eye. Images cycled at less than 120 Hz cause perceptible flickering. Currently available

HMDs are rather heavy and somewhat uncomfortable when worn for prolonged periods. Alternatively, a 3D monitor with lenticular lenses in front of the screen or passive-polarized glasses may be used. The left eye image is selectively displayed to the left eye and the right eye image to the right eye.

Widespread use of 3D technology in its current form has not gained popularity. In its current form, stereoscopic laparoscopy does not yet provide optimal depth perception. Moreover, trained laparoscopic surgeons attain a sense of depth perception over time, and hence may not feel the need for this expensive technology (166). Learned 3D vision is akin to watching 2D television or movies and yet being able to perceive depth efficiently. Nevertheless, advances in the field of optics such as the use of high-definition video displays with improved clarity and improvements in stereoscopic technology may render stereoscopic laparoscopy more useful.

Optics for Ergonomic Comfort

Laparoscopic surgery involves peering into a television monitor positioned straight ahead on a vertical rack for hours at end. Thus the surgeon's line of vision is away from the actual operative field. This dissociation of the surgeon's vision from the line of work may be associated with significant physical strain. This problem can be rectified by using an image projector and a sterile screen, which can be intraoperatively manipulated by the surgeon to provide a direct line of view of the surgical field at the patient's skin level, thereby eliminating the need to look up at the television monitor during the procedure (ViewSite, Karl Storz Inc., Culver City, California; and Inside View, LSI Solutions, Rochester, New York). The advent of flat screen technology will similarly enable the surgeon to view the laparoscopic field comfortably.

Techniques for Laparoscopic Tissue Approximation

Fibrin Glue

Fibrin glue is produced by mixing appropriate quantities of fibrinogen with thrombin. The latter cleaves fibrinogen into fibrin monomers, which crosslink with one another to produce a sealant (388). The initial use of fibrin glue was directed toward achieving tissue hemostasis. Currently, it is employed for tissue approximation as well. The ability to obtain fibrinogen concentrates in the 1970s led to the high-level production of fibrin glue; however, the risk of transmission of blood-borne viral diseases such as hepatitis and HIV led the FDA to withhold its use (120). Recently, autologous fibrin glue has been prepared using cryocentrifugation, cryofiltration, and ethanol precipitation methods, making it safer for commercial use (456). In addition, with recombinant DNA technology large quantities of safe blood products are becoming available.

Fibrin glue is commercially available in a double-barreled syringe containing fibrinogen and aprotinin in one barrel and thrombin admixed with calcium chloride in the other barrel. The fibrinogen content determines the strength of the glue, and the thrombin content determines the rate at which glue stabilizes. The addition of aprotinin protects against rapid resorption of the glue. Fibrin glue has been used for several reconstructive procedures, such as vasovasostomies, and for sealing splenic injuries (391,418). In laparoscopic urologic surgery it has been used to perform pyeloplasties and ureteral reanastomosis. McKay and colleagues (271) demonstrated the feasibility of performing laparoscopic ureteral reanastomosis with fibrin glue in pigs. Compared with the animals that underwent open ureteral reanastomosis, animals treated with fibrin glue had more pronounced inflammation and fibrosis. In another porcine animal study conducted by Wolf and colleagues (452), ureteral repair with fibrin glue was associated with better flow characteristics and histology than laparoscopic suturing. Eden and colleagues (90) reported the clinical use of fibrin glue for laparoscopic dismembered pyeloplasty.

Cyanoacrylate Glue

Cyanoacrylate glue, or superglue as it is known, is a heavy-duty adhesive. It has powerful hemostatic and adhesive qualities. It rapidly polymerizes on contact with any ionic medium, including blood or saline. Indeed, polymerization can be so rapid that iophendylate or glacial acid may need to be added to slow the reaction (48). It has been clinically used as a hemostatic agent in interventional radiology and as a skin sealant. Experimentally, it has been associated with some degree of fibroblast and human tendon cell cytotoxicity, and it has also been associated with a marked inflammatory response and fibrosis (100,202). Cyanoacrylate is nonabsorbable, and its effect on mucosal approximation must be studied in detail before its utilization for tissue approximation in urology.

Laser Welding

The use of lasers in urology for tissue ablation and for hemostasis is well established. The initial successful laser weld for achieving vascular anastomosis was performed by Jain and colleagues (192). The concept was derived from the use of electrocautery for closure of venotomies, described by Sigel and Acevido (389). The basis of tissue welding is the photothermic effect of lasers on tissue proteins. At approximately 60°C, collagen fibrils tend to uncoil and then crosslink (370). The ideal tissue-welding laser should have optimal tissue penetration and should be associated with a strong weld while limiting the thermal damage and lateral spread of heat. Advances in the field of laser welding include the use of laser solders, thermal feedback, and chromophore enhancement. In 1988, Poppas and colleagues (336) developed tissue solders for improving the strength of the weld and for limiting the lateral spread of heat by acting as a heat sink. The protein solder is effectively incorporated into the weld, thereby strengthening the tissue approximation (434). Albumin in concentrations of 40% to 50% is the most commonly used solder. The endpoint of laser welding may be determined by studying the color of the lased tissue. This is a rather inaccurate method that can lead to overheating of the tissues. The use of infrared thermal sensors (222) and chromophore enhancement with substances such as indocyanate and fluorescein may provide more accurate real-time thermal feedback and thereby prevent tissue damage. Nd:YAG lasers with a penetration of 3 to 5 mm and KTP lasers that penetrate up to 1 mm have been used for tissue approximation (335). Also, the use of the 1.9-μm diode laser for gastrocystoplasty in the canine model has been associated with good results; Bleustein and colleagues (29) demonstrated better results and less thermal damage with the use of the diode than Nd:YAG. The tensile strengths achieved with the diode lasers were comparable with that attained during tissue suturing (29). Laser welding appears to be an impressive and effective way of achieving sutureless tissue approximation.

Alternative Tissue Dissection Techniques

Alternative energy sources for laparoscopic tissue dissection include the use of ultrasound energy, pneumodissection, and hydrodissection. The harmonic scalpel (UltraCision) is driven by ultrasound vibrations. The power box is attached to forceps or a blade and vibrates at 55,500 cycles per second. The rapid vibration is associated with release of thermal energy, which facilitates simultaneous tissue coagulation. However, there is minimal risk of lateral spread of tissue coagulation (233).

Gardner and colleagues (113) reported the feasibility of high-pressure CO_2 for laparoscopic tissue dissection. Pneumodissection at 50 psi could be safely performed in the porcine model with a 5-mm pneumodissector. Short bursts of high-pressure CO_2 were used as a blunt dissector. The use of higher pressures (greater than 60 psi) was associated with splenic trauma when the pneumodissector was fired directly on the spleen. The same group presented their experience with the use of this technique in 20 patients (327). Acid–base imbalances were documented, although they were not statistically significantly different from the level of hypercarbia noted in patients undergoing a CO_2 pneumoperitoneum without use of pneumodissection. In their studies, gas embolism did not occur in either the animal or clinical cases.

Another tissue dissection technique involves the use of water under pressure. Hydro-jet dissection was employed to perform laparoscopic partial nephrectomy in the porcine model by Shekarriz and colleagues (383). An ultracoherent stream of normal saline, with a pressure of up to 30 atm, was used for dissection of the renal parenchyma during a partial nephrectomy. An average of 195 mL of saline was used per case. The saline stream effectively cut through the parenchymal tissue, preserving the intrarenal vasculature and collecting system.

Microlaparoscopic and Needlescopic Instruments

Instruments of smaller caliber than regular laparoscopic instruments have been developed to further decrease the morbidity and improve the cosmetic result associated with laparoscopic procedures. Needlescopic instruments are introduced through 2-mm (i.e., 14-gauge) trocars. A minute skin puncture results that needs no more than a single Steri-Strip for closure (129).

However, currently available mini-laparoscopic instruments are inferior in performance to larger 5-mm instruments. A 2-mm laparoscope does not provide the image clarity seen with a 10-mm laparoscope. Moreover, 2-mm clip applicators are not available and adequate suctioning cannot be performed. A judicious combination of conventional laparoscopic and mini-laparoscopic instruments is currently the best use of this technology. Significant advantages such as decreased pain and better cosmesis are noted when the 2-mm access is substituted for 5- or 10-mm ports. With further technologic development and improvement of instruments, it is possible that reconstructive procedures will be performed entirely via 2-mm ports.

CONCLUSION

With the incorporation of newer technologies, laparoscopic procedures of greater technical difficulty will be addressed in the future. More complex reconstructions and challenging ablations will be performed laparoscopically, with increasing confidence. Progressive technologic development is directed toward achieving increased efficiency, precision, and cost-effectiveness.

Computers in the 1950s were room-sized machines and had the storage capability equivalent to a few silicon chips of today's computers. Newer machines and instruments are smaller and yet vastly more powerful. We are presently in a transition from bulk technology to molecular technology. The future will witness progress in the fields of artificial intelligence and nanotechnology. A nanometer is one-billionth of a meter, and nanotechnology is the anticipated technology involving the use of molecular-sized devices. It has been envisaged that these micromachines will be able to perform a range of diagnostic and therapeutic procedures intracorporeally. When injected into the circulation, they will be able to find their way in a preprogrammed manner into the area of interest and intelligently execute the task for which they were programmed. Molecular-scale surgery and cell repair machines involving nanorobotics may be possible in the future. In the years to come, the role of the master surgeon may well be reduced to that of today's house officer: to just "put in a line."

REFERENCES

1. Abbou CC, Cicco A, Gasman D, et al. Retroperitoneal laparoscopic versus open radical nephrectomy. *J Urol* 1999;161: 1776.
2. Abbou CC, Salomon L, Hoznek A, et al. Laparoscopic radical prostatectomy: preliminary results. *Urology* 2000;55:630.
3. Abdulmaaboud MR, Shokeir AA, Farage Y, et al. Treatment of varicocele: a comparative study of conventional open surgery, percutaneous retrograde sclerotherapy, and laparoscopy. *Urology* 1998;52:294.
4. Adams JB, Schulam PG, Moore RG, et al. New laparoscopic suturing device: initial clinical experience. *Urology* 1995; 46:242.
5. Albala DM, Schuessler WW, Vancaillie TG. Laparoscopic bladder neck suspension. *J Endourol* 1992;6:137.
6. Albala DM, Schuessler WW, Vancaillie TG. Laparoscopic bladder neck suspension for the treatment of stress incontinence. *Semin Urol* 1992;10:222.
7. Aldrighetti L, Giacomelli M, Calori G, et al. Impact of minimally invasive surgery on adrenalectomy for incidental tumors: comparison with laparoscopic technique. *Int Surg* 1997; 82:160.
8. Alexander GD, Noe FE, Brown EM. Anesthesia for pelvic laparoscopy. *Anesth Analg* 1969;48:14.
9. Altmore DF, Memeo V. Explosion during diathermy colotomy. Report of a case. *Dis Colon Rectum* 1993;36:291.
10. Amar AD, Das S. Surgical management of benign renal cysts causing obstruction of the renal pelvis. *Urology* 1984;24:429.
11. Amerling R, Vande Maele D, Spivak H, et al. Laparoscopic salvage of malfunctioning peritoneal catheters. *Surg Endosc* 1997;11:249.
12. Arango O, Bielsa O, Carles J, et al. Massive tumor implantation in the endoscopic resected area in modified nephroureterectomy. *J Urol* 1997;157:1893.
13. Aronowitz J, Kaplan AL. The management of pelvic lymphocele by the use of a percutaneous indwelling catheter inserted with ultrasound guidance. *Gynecol Oncol* 1983;16:292.
14. Backlund M, Kellolumpu I, Scheinin T, et al. Effect of temperature of insufflated CO_2 during and after prolonged laparoscopic surgery. *Surg Endosc* 1998;12:1126.
15. Balin H, Wan LS, Israel SL. Recent advances in pelvic endoscopy. *Obstet Gynecol* 1966;27:30.
16. Ballem RV, Rudomanski J. Techniques of pneumoperitoneum. *Surg Laparosc Endosc* 1993;3:42.
17. Banting S, Shimi S, Velpen GV, et al. Abdominal wall lift: low pressure pneumoperitoneum in laparoscopic surgery. *Surg Endosc* 1993;7:57.

17a. Barrett DH, personal communication, 1997.

18. Barrett PH, Fentie DD, Taranger LA. Laparoscopic radical nephrectomy with morcellation for renal cell carcinoma: the Saskatoon experience. *Urology* 1998;52:23.

18a. Barry JM, Lowe BA. Laparoscopic marsupialization of renal cysts in a patient with painful adult polycystic kidneys. Presented at the annual meeting of the Western Section American Urological Association. Maui, HI Oct 25–30, 1992.

19. Bauer JJ, Bishoff JT, Moore RG, et al. Laparoscopic versus open pyeloplasty: assessment of objective and subjective outcome. *J Urol* 1999;162:692.
20. Bauer JJ, Schulam PG, Kaufman HS, et al. Laparoscopy of the acute abdomen in the postoperative urologic patient. *Urology* 1998;51:917.
21. Belt AE, Charnock DA. The history of the cystoscope. In: Cabot H, ed. *Modern urology.* Philadelphia: Lea & Febiger, 1936.
22. Bendinelli C, Lucchi M, Buccianti P, et al. Adrenal masses in non–small cell lung carcinoma patients: is there any role for laparoscopic procedures? *J Laparoendoscop Adv Surg Tech* 1998; 3:119.
23. Bennett WM, Elzinga L, Golper TA, et al. Reduction of cyst volume for symptomatic management of autosomal dominant polycystic kidney disease. *J Urol* 1987;137:620.
24. Berci G, Dunkelman D, Nucgek SL, et al. Emergency minilaparoscopy in abdominal trauma: an update. *Am J Surg* 1983; 143:261.
25. Bercowsky E, Shalhav AL, Portis A, et al. Is the laparoscopic approach justified in patients with xanthogranulomatous pyelonephritis? *Urology* 1999;54:437.
26. Bernheim BM. Organoscopy: cystoscopy of the abdominal cavity. *Ann Surg* 1911;53:764.
27. Bischof G, Rockenschaub S, Berlakovich G, et al. Management of lymphoceles after kidney transplantation. *Transpl Int* 1998; 11:227.
28. Bishoff JT, Chen RB, Lee BR, et al. Laparoscopic renal cryoablation: acute and long-term clinical, radiographic, and pathologic effects in an animal model and application in a clinical trial. *J Endourol* 1999;13:233.
29. Bleustein CB, Cuomo B, Mingin GC, et al. Laser-assisted demucosalized gastrocystoplasty with autoaugmentation in a canine model. *Urology* 2000;55:437.
30. Bolton WK, Vaughan ED Jr. A comparative study of open surgical and percutaneous renal biopsies. *J Urol* 1977;142:696.
31. Bonjer HJ, Lange JF, Kazemier G, et al. Comparison of three techniques for adrenalectomy. *Br J Surg* 1997;84:679.
32. Bonjer HJ, van der Harst E, Steyerberg EW, et al. Retroperitoneal adrenalectomy: open or endoscopic. *World J Surg* 1998;22: 1246.
33. Bricker EM. Bladder substitution after pelvic evisceration. *Surg Clin North Am* 1950;30:1511.
34. Brooks JD, Kavoussi LR, Preminger GM, et al. Comparison of open and endourologic approaches to the obstructed ureteropelvic junction. *Urology* 1995;46:791.
35. Brown JA, Torres BE, King BF, et al. Laparoscopic marsupialization of symptomatic polycystic kidney disease. *J Urol* 1996; 156:22.
36. Brun C, Raaschou F. Kidney biopsies. *Am J Med* 1958;24:676.
37. Brunt LM, Doherty GM, Norton JA, et al. Laparoscopic adrenalectomy compared to open adrenalectomy for benign adrenal neoplasms. *J Am Coll Surg* 1996;183:1.
38. Burgos J, Teruel JL, Mayayo T, et al. Diagnosis and management of lymphoceles after renal transplantation. *J Urol* 1983; 61:289.
39. Busch W. Uber den Einfluss welchen eftigere Erysipeln zu Weilen auf Organ: Neubildungen Ausuben. *Verhandl Naturn Preuss Rhein Westpmal* 1866;23:28.
40. Bush RB, Leonhardt H, Bush IM, et al. Dr. Bozzini's Lichtleiter. A translation of his original article (1806). *Urology* 1974; 3:119.
41. Byron JW et al. A randomized comparison of Veress needle and direct trocar insertion for laparoscopy. *Gynecol Obstet* 1993; 177:259.

42. Cadeddu JA, Ono Y, Clayman RV, et al. Laparoscopic nephrectomy for renal cell cancer. Evaluation of efficacy and safety: a multicenter experience. *Urology* 1998;52:773.
43. Cadeddu JA, Chan DY, Hedican SP, et al. Retroperitoneal access for transperitoneal laparoscopy in patients at high risk for intra-abdominal scarring. *J Endourol* 1999;13:567.
44. Cadeddu JA, Elashry OM, Snyder O, et al. Effect of laparoscopic pelvic lymph node dissection on the natural history of D_1 (T_{1-3}, N_{1-3}, M_0) prostate cancer. *Urology* 1997;50:391.
45. Campbell SC, Krishnamurthy V, Chow G, et al. Renal cryosurgery: experimental evaluation of treatment parameters. *Urology* 1998;52:29.
46. Carmignani G, Gallucci M, Puppo P, et al. Video laparoscopic excision of a seminal vesicle cyst associated with ipsilateral renal agenesis. *J Urol* 1995;153:437.
47. Carter JE. A new technique of fascial closure for laparoscopic incisions. *J Laparoendosc Surg* 1994;4:143.
48. Cekirge S, Oguzkurt L, Saatçi I, et al. Embolization of a high-output postnephrectomy aortocaval fistula with Gianturco coils and cyanoacrylate. *Cardiovasc Intervent Radiol* 1996; 19:56.
49. Chaikin DC, Rosenthal J, Blaivas JG. Pubovaginal fascial sling for all types of stress urinary incontinence: long-term analysis. *J Urol* 1998;160:1312.
50. Chan DY, Koniaris L, Magee C, et al. Feasibility of ablating normal renal parenchyma by interstitial photon radiation energy: study in a canine model. *J Endourol* 2000;14:111.
51. Chapelon JY, Margonari J, Theillère Y, et al. Effects of high-energy focused ultrasound on kidney tissue in the rat and the dog. *Eur Urol* 1992;22:147.
52. Chen RN, Kavoussi LR, Moore RG. Milk of calcium within a calyceal diverticulum. *Urology* 1997;49:620.
53. Chen RN, Moore RG, Micali S, et al. Retroperitoneoscopic renal biopsy in extremely obese patients. *Urology* 1997;50:195.
54. Chinnock C. Virtual reality in surgery and medicine. *AHA Hospital Technology Series* 1994;13:1.
55. Chiu AW, Chang LS, Birkett DH, et al. The impact of pneumoperitoneum, pneumoretroperitoneum, and gasless laparoscopy on systemic and renal hemodynamics. *J Am Coll Surg* 1995;181:395.
56. Chiu AW, Chang LS, Birkett DH, et al. Changes in urinary output and electrolytes during gaseous and gasless laparoscopy. *Urol Res* 1996;24:361.
57. Chosy SG, Nicety So, Lee FT, et al. Thermosensor-monitored renal cryosurgery in swine: predictors of tissue necrosis. *J Urol* 1996;157:250.
58. Chung RS, Diaz JJ, Chari V. Efficacy of routine laparoscopy for the acute abdomen. *Surg Endosc* 1998;12:219.
59. Cisek LJ, Gobet RM, Peters CA. Pneumoperitoneum produced reversible renal dysfunction in animals with normal and chronically reduced renal function. *J Endourol* 1998;12:95.
60. Clayman RV, Kavoussi LR, Soper NJ, et al. Laparoscopic nephrectomy. *N Engl J Med* 1991;324:1370.
61. Clayman RV, Kavoussi LR, Soper NJ, et al. Laparoscopic nephrectomy: initial case report. *J Urol* 1991;146:278.
62. Clayman RV, Kavoussi LR, Figenshau RS, et al. Laparoscopic nephroureterectomy: initial case report. *J Laparoendosc Surg* 1991;1:343.
63. Clayman RV, McDougall EM, Gardner SM, et al. Laparoscopic pneumodissection: a unique means of tissue dissection. *J Urol* 1994;151:498A(abst 1082).
64. Cockett ATK, Takihara H, Cosentino MJ. The varicocele. *Fertil Steril* 1970;21:606.
65. Corson, SL, Butzer FR, Gocial B, et al. Measurement of the force necessary for laparoscopic trocar entry. *J Reprod Med* 1989;34:282.
66. Cortesi N, Ferrari P, Zambarda E, et al. Diagnosis of bilateral abdominal cryptorchidism by laparoscopy. *Endoscopy* 1976;8:33.
67. Couvelaire R, Agrandir A. La vessie. In: *Chirurgie de la vesie.* Paris: Masson, 1955.
68. Crabtree JH, Fishman A. Videolaparoscopic implantation of long-term peritoneal dialysis catheters. *Surg Endosc* 1999; 13:186.
69. Cuesta MA, Eijsbouts QA, Gordijn RV, et al. Diagnostic laparoscopy in patients with an acute abdomen of uncertain etiology. *Surg Endosc* 1998;12:915.
70. Cullen DJ, Coyle JP, Teplick R, et al. Cardiovascular, pulmonary and renal effect of massively increased intraabdominal pressure in critically ill patients. *Crit Care Med* 1989;17:118.
71. Dallemagne B, Weerts JM, Jehales C, et al. Laparoscopic Nissen fundoplication: preliminary report. *Surg Laprosc Endosc* 1991;1(3):138.
72. Das S. Laparoscopic removal of bladder diverticulum. *J Urol* 1992;148:1837.
73. Das S, Palmer JK. Laparoscopic colposuspension. *J Urol* 1995; 154:1119.
74. Davies BL, Hibberd RD, Coptcoat MJ, et al. A surgeon robot prostatectomy: a laboratory evaluation. *J Med Eng Technol* 1989;13:273.
75. De Berg JC, Pattynama PMT, Obermaun WRI, et al. Percutaneous computed-tomography-guided thermocoagulation for osteoid osteomas. *Lancet* 1995;346:350.
76. Dell'Adami G, Breda G. Transurethral or endoscopic ureterectomy. *Eur Urol* 1976;2:156.
76a. Delworth MG, Pisters LL, Fornage BD, et al. Cryotherapy for renal cell carcinoma and angiomyolipoma. *J Urol* 1996; 155:252.
77. Demarco T, Amin M, Harty JI. Living donor nephrectomy: factors influencing morbidity. *J Urol* 1982;127:1082.
78. Denewer A, Kotb S, Hussein O, et al. Laparoscopic assisted cystectomy and lymphadenectomy for bladder cancer: initial experience. *World J Surg* 1999;23:608.
79. Reference deleted in proofs.
80. Diaz-Buxo JA, Donadio JV. Complications of percutaneous renal biopsy: an analysis of 1,000 consecutive biopsies. *Clin Nephrol* 1975;4:223.
81. Dion YM, Morin J. Laparoscopic inguinal herniorrhaphy. *Can J Surg* 1992;35:209.
82. Docimo SG, Moore RG, Adams J, et al. Laparoscopic bladder augmentation using stomach. *Urology* 1995;46:565.
83. Doehn C, Fornara P, Fricke L, et al. Comparison of laparoscopic and open nephroureterectomy for benign disease. *J Urol* 1998;159:732.
84. Dolgar B, Kitano S, Yoshida T, et al. Vasopressin antagonist improves renal function in a rat model. *J Surg Res* 1998; 79:109.
85. Dorsam J, Bucuras CV, Mieck U, et al. The effects of CO_2 pneumoperitoneum in pigs with impaired pulmonary function. *J Endourol* 1997;11:185.
86. Dubois F, Icard P, Berthelot G, et al. Coelioscopic cholecystomy. Preliminary report of 36 cases. *Ann Surg* 1990;211:60.
87. Dunn F, Fry FJ. Ultrasonic threshold dosages for the mammalian central nervous system. *IEEE Engin Med Biol* 1971; 18:253.
88. Dunn MD, Portis AJ, Shelhav AL, et al. Laparoscopic versus open radical nephrectomy: a 9-year experience. *J Urol* 2000; 164(4):1153.

89. Dunn MD, Portis AJ, Elbahnassy AM, et al. Laparoscopic nephrectomy in patients with end-stage renal disease and adult polycystic kidney disease. *Am J Kidney Dis* 2000;35:720.
90. Eden CG, Sultana SR, Murray KHA, et al. Extraperitoneal laparoscopic dismembered fibrin-glued pyeloplasty: medium-term results. *Br J Urol* 1997;80:382.
91. Ehrlich RM, Gershman A. Laparoscopic seromyotomy (auto-augmentation) for non-neurogenic neurogenic bladder in a child: initial case report. *Urology* 1993;42:175.
92. Ehrlich RM, Gershman A, Mee Sharon, et al. Laparoscopic nephrectomy in a child: expanding horizons for laparoscopy in pediatric urology. *J Endourol* 1992;6:463.
93. Elashry OM, Clayman RV, Soble JJ, et al. Laparoscopic adrenalectomy for solitary metachronous contralateral adrenal metastasis from renal cell carcinoma. *J Urol* 1997;157:1217.
94. Elashry OM, Nekada SY, McDougall EM, et al. Laparoscoic nephropexy: Washington University experience. *J Urol* 1995; 154:1655.
95. Elashry OM, Nakada SY, Wolf JS, et al. Laparoscopy for adult polycystic kidney disease: a promising alternative. *Am J Kidney Dis* 1996;27:224.
96. Elashry OM, Nakada SY, Wolf JS, et al. Ureterolysis for extrinsic ureteral obstruction: a comparison of laparoscopic and open surgical techniques. *J Urol* 1996;156:1403.
97. Elashry OM, Wolf JS, Rayala HJ, et al. Recent advances in laparoscopic partial nephrectomy: comparative study of electrosurgical snare electrode and ultrasound dissection. *J Endourol* 1997;11:15.
98. El-Kady AA, Abd-El-Razek M. Intraperitoneal explosion during female sterilization by laparoscopic electrocoagulation: a case report. *Int J Gynaecol Obstet* 1976;14:487.
99. Eraky I, El-Kappany HA, Ghoneim MA. Laparoscopic nephrectomy: Mansoura experience with 106 cases. *Br J Urol* 1995;75:271.
100. Evans CE, Lees GC, Trail IA. Cytotoxicity of cyanoacrylate adhesives to cultured tendon cells. *J Hand Surg* 1999; 24:658.
101. Reference deleted in proofs.
102. Fantl JA, Newman DK, Colling J, et al. *Urinary incontinence in adults: acute and chronic management.* Clinical practice guideline. No. 2, 1996 update. Rockville, Md: US Department of Health and Human Services. Public Health Service, Agency for Health Care Policy and Research.
103. Fergany AF, Hafez KS, Novick AC. Long-term results of nephron sparing surgery for localized renal cell carcinoma: 10 year followup. *J Urol* 2000;163:442.
104. Ferzli G, Raboy A, Kleinerman D, et al. Extraperitoneal endoscopic pelvic lymph node dissection vs. laparoscopic lymph node dissection in the staging of prostatic and bladder carcinoma. *J Laparoendoscop Surg* 1992;2:219.
105. Filipi CJ, Fitzgibbons RJ, Salerno G. Historical review: diagnostic laparoscopy to laparoscopic cholecystectomy and beyond. In: Zucker KA, ed. *Surgical laparoscopy.* St. Louis: Quality Medical Publishing, 1991.
106. Fornara P, Doehn C, Jocham D. Laparoscopic nephropexy: 3 year experience. *J Urol* 1997;158:1679.
107. Gadallah MF, Pervez A, El-Shahawy MA, et al. Peritoneoscopic versus surgical placement of peritoneal dialysis catheters: a prospective randomized study on outcome. *Am J Kidney Dis* 1999;33:118.
108. Gage AA, Baust JJ. Mechanisms of tissue injury in cryosurgery. *Cryobiology* 1998;37:171.
109. Gagner M, Breton G, Pharand D, et al. Is laparoscopic adrenalectomy indicated for pheochromocytomas? *Surgery* 1996;120: 1076.
110. Gagner M, Jacroix A, Bolte E. Laparoscopic adrenalectomy in Cushing's syndrome and pheochromocytoma [Letter]. *N Engl J Med* 1992;327:1033.
111. Ganter G. Uber die besitigening giftiger stroffe ans dem blut durch dialyse. *Munch Med Wochenschr* 1923;70:1478.
112. Garcia M, Bru C, Campistol JM, et al. Effect of reduction of cytsic volume by percutaneous cystic puncture on the renal function in polycystic kidney disease. *Nephron* 1990; 56:459.
113. Gardner SM, Clayman RV, McDougall EM, et al. Laparoscopic pneumodissection: unique means of tissue dissection. *J Urol* 1995;154:591.
114. Gault MH, Muehrcke RC. Renal biopsy: current views and controversy. *Nephron* 1983;4:1.
115. Gaur DD, Agarwal DK, Khochikar MV, et al. Laparoscopic renal biopsy via a retroperitoneal approach. *J Urol* 1994; 151:925.
116. Gaur DD, Agarwal DK, Purohit KC, et al. Retroperitoneal laparoscopic pyelolithotomy. *J Urol* 1994;151:927.
117. Gauwerkiy JFH, Klose R. An experimental model for pelviscopic tubal anastomoses. *Hum Reprod* 1990;5:439.
118. Gazzaniga AB, Stanton WW, Barlett RH. Laparoscopy in the diagnosis of blunt and penetrating injuries to the abdomen. *Am J Surg* 1976;131:315.
119. Gerber GS, Bissada NK, Hulbert JC, et al. Laparoscopic retropertioneal lymphadenectomy: multi-institutional analysis. *J Urol* 1994;152:1188.
120. Gibble JW, Ness PM. Fibrin glue: the perfect operative sealant? *Transfusion* 1990;30:741.
121. Gill IS, Carbone JM, Clayman RV, et al. Laparoscopic live-donor nephrectomy. *J Endourol* 1994;8:143.
122. Gill IS, Delworth MG, Much LC. Laparoscopic retroperitoneal partial nephrectomy. *J Urol* 1994;152:1539.
123. Gill IS, Fergany A, Klein E, et al. Laparoscopic radical cystoprostatectomy with ileal conduit performed completely intracorporeally: the initial 2 cases. *Urology* 2000;56:26.
124. Gill IS, Hodge EE, Munch LC, et al. Transperitoneal marsupialization of lymphoceles: a comparison of laparoscopic and open techniques. *J Urol* 1995;153:706.
125. Gill IS, Matamoros A, Heffron TG, et al. Laparoscopic renal cryoablation. *J Urol* 1997;157:210.
126. Gill IS, Novick AC, Soble JJ, et al. Laparoscopic renal cryoablation: initial clinical series. *Urology* 1998;52:543.
127. Gill IS, Rackley RR, Meraney AM, et al. Laparoscopic enterocystoplasty. *Urology* 2000;55:178.
128. Gill IS, Soble JJ, Miller SD, Sung GT. A novel technique for management of the en bloc bladder cuff and distal ureter during laparoscopic nephroureterectomy. *J Urol* 1999; 161:430.
129. Gill IS, Soble JJ, Sung GT, et al. Needlescopic adrenalectomy—the initial series: comparison with conventional laparoscopic adrenalectomy. *Urology* 1998;52:180.
130. Gilliland JD, Spies JB, Brown S, et al. Lymphoceles: percutaneous treatment with povidone-iodine sclerosis. *Radiology* 1989; 171:227.
131. Gimenez LF, Micali S, Chen RN, et al. Laparoscopic renal biopsy. *Kidney Int* 1998;54:525.
132. Girardis M, Broi UD, Antonutto G, Pasetto A. The effect of laparoscopic cholecystectomy on cardiovascular function and pulmonary gas exchange. *Anesth Analg* 1996;83:134.

133. Glascock JM, Winfield HN, Lund GO, et al. CO_2 hemostasis during transperitoneal or extraperitoneal laparoscopic pelvic lymphadenectomy: a real time intraoperative comparison. *J Endourol* 1996;10:319.
134. Gluckman GR, Stoller M, Irby P. Laparoscopic pyelocaliceal diverticula ablation. *J Endourol* 1993;4:315.
135. Gomel V. Laparoscopy. *Can Med Assoc J* 1974;111:167.
136. Gomel V. Laparoscopy in general surgery. *Am J Surg* 1976; 131:319.
137. Gomel V. Operative laparoscopy: time for acceptance. *Fertil Steril* 1989;52:1.
138. Grainger DA, Meyer WR, De Cherney AH, et al. Laparoscopic clips: evaluation of absorbable and titanium with regard to hemostasis and tissue reactivity. *J Reprod Med* 1991; 36:493.
139. Green PS, Hi JW, Jensen JF, et al. Telepresence surgery. *IEEE Eng Med Biol* 1995;14:324.
140. Greenberg SM, Lipshultz LI, Wein AJ. Experience with 425 subfertile patients. *J Urol* 1978;119:507.
141. Greif WM, Forse RA. Hemodynamic effects of the laparoscopic pneumoperitoneum during sepsis in the porcine endotoxic shock model. *Ann Surg* 1998;227:474.
142. Gruessner RWG, Fasola C, Benedetti E, et al. Laparoscopic drainage of lymphoceles after kidney transplantation: indications and limitations. *Surgery* 1995;117:288.
143. Guazzoni G, Montorsi F, Bocciardi A, et al. Transperitoneal laparoscopic versus open adrenalectomy for benign hyperfunctioning adrenal tumors: a comparative study. *J Urol* 1995; 153:1597.
144. Guillonneau B, Ballanger P, Lugagne PM, et al. Laparoscopic versus lumboscopic nephrectomy. *Eur Urol* 1996;29:288.
145. Guillonneau B, Vallancien G. Laparoscopic radical prostatectomy: initial experience and preliminary assessment after 65 operations. *Prostate* 1999;39:71.
146. Guillonneau B, Vallancien G. Laparoscopic radical prostatectomy: the Montsouris experience. *J Urol* 2000;163:418.
147. Gunning JE. The history of laparoscopy. *J Reprod Med* 1974; 12:222.
148. Hafez KS, Fergany AF, Novick AC. Nephron sparing surgery for localized renal cell carcinoma: impact of tumor size on patient survival, tumor recurrence and TNM staging. *J Urol* 1999;162:1930.
149. Hahn E. Die Operative Behandlung der beweglicken niere durch fixation. *Zbl Chir* 1881;8:449.
150. Hald T, Rasmussen F. Extraperitoneal pelvioscopy: a new aid in staging of lower urinary tract tumors. A preliminary report. *J Urol* 1980;124:245.
151. Hamilton BD, Chow GK, Inman SR, et al. Increased intraabdominal pressure during pneumoperitoneum stimulates endothelin release in a canine model. *J Endourol* 1998;12:193.
152. Handt AE, Ash SR. Longevity of Tenckoff catheters placed by the VITEC peritoneoscopic technique. *Perspect Perit Dial* 1984;2:30.
153. Hannaford B, Trujillo J, Sinanan M, et al. Computerized endoscopic surgical grasper. In: *Proceedings of Medicine Meets Virtual Reality.* San Diego: 1998.
154. Harewood LM, Agarwal D, Lindsay S, et al. Extraperitoneal laparoscopic caliceal diverticulectomy. *J Endourol* 1996; 10:425.
155. Harewood LM, Webb DR, Pope AJ. Laparoscopic ureterolithotomy: the results of an initial series, and evaluation of its role in the mangement of ureteric calculi. *Br J Urol* 1994; 74:170.
156. Harman RK, Kron IL, McLachlan HD, et al. Elevated intraabdominal pressure and renal function. *Ann Surg* 1982; 196:594.
157. Harrison RM. The development of modern endoscopy. *J Med Primatol* 1976;5:73.
158. Harrison SH, Seale-Hawkins C, Schun CW, et al. Correlation between side of palpable tumor and side of pelvic node metastasis in clinically localized prostate cancer. *Cancer* 1992;69:750.
159. Hasson HM. Open laparoscopy: a report of 150 cases. *J Reprod Med* 1974;12:234.
160. Hayakawa H, Nimura Y, Kamiya J, et al. Laparoscopic cholecystectomy using retraction of the falciform ligament. *Surg Laparosc Endosc* 1991;1:26(abst).
161. Healey DE, Newman RC, Cohen MS, et al. Laparoscopically assisted percutaneous renal biopsy. *J Urol* 1993;150:1218.
162. Hedican SP, Schulam PG, Docimo SG. Laparoscopic assisted reconstructive surgery. *J Urol* 1999;161:267.
163. Reference deleted in proofs.
164. Heniford BT, Iannitti DA, Hale J, et al. The role of intraoperative ultrasonography during laparoscopic adrenalectomy. *Surgery* 1997;122:1068.
165. Herrell SD, Trachtenberg J, Theodorescu D. Staging pelvic lymphadenectomy for localized carcinoma of the prostate: a comparison of 3 surgical techniques. *J Urol* 1997;157:1337.
166. Herron DM, Lantis JC II, Maykel J, et al. The 3-D monitor and head-mounted display. A quantitative evaluation of advanced laparoscopic viewing technologies. *Surg Endosc* 1999; 13:751.
167. Hetherington JW, Ewing R, Philip NH. Modified nephroureterectomy: a risk of tumor implantation. *Br J Urol* 1986; 58:368.
168. Hirsch IH, Abdel-meguid TA, Gomella LG. Postsurgical outcomes assessment following varicocele ligation: laparoscopic versus subinguinal approach. *J Urol* 1998;51:810.
169. Hoenig DM, McDougal EM, Shalhav AL, et al. Laparoscopic ablation of peripelvic renal cysts. *J Urol* 1997;158:1345.
170. Hoey MF, Mulier PM, Leveillee RJ, et al. Transurethral prostate ablation with saline electrode allows controlled production of larger lesions than conventional methods. *J Endourol* 1997; 11:279.
171. Hoffman H. Developing network compatible instructional resources for UCSD core curriculum. In: *Proceedings of Medicine Meets Virtual Reality.* San Diego: 1992.
172. Holmberg G, Hietala SO. Treatment of simple renal cysts by percutaneous puncture and instillation of bismuth-phosphate. *Scand J Urol Nephrol* 1989;23:207.
173. Horvath KD, Whelan RL, Lier B, et al. The effects of elevated intraabdominal pressure, hypercarbia, and positioning on hemodynamic responses to laparoscopic colectomy in pigs. *Surg Endosc* 1998;12:107.
174. Howe RD, Peine WJ, Kotarinis DA. Remote palpation technology for surgical applications. *IEEE Eng Med Biol* 1995; 14:318.
175. Hoznek A, Herard A, Ogiez N, et al. Symptomatic caliceal diverticula treated with extraperitoneal laparoscopic marsupialization, fulguration and gelatin resorcinol formaldehyde glue. *J Urol* 1998;160:352.
176. Hoznek A, Salomon L, Antiphon P, et al. Partial nephrectomy with retroperitoneal laparoscopy. *J Urol* 1999;162:1922.
177. Hubner WA, Schramek P, Pfluger H. Laparoscopic nephropexy. *J Urol* 1994;152:1184.

178. Hulbert JC, Hunter D, Young AT, et al. Percutaneous intrarenal marsupialization of a perirenal cystic collection—endocystolysis. *J Urol* 1988;139:1039.
179. Hulbert JC, Fraley EE. Laparoscopic retroperitoneal lymphadenectomy: new approach to pathologic staging of clinical stage I germ cell tumors of the testis. *J Endourol* 1992;6:123.
180. Hulka JF, Mercer JP, Fishburne JI, et al. Spring clip sterilization: one year follow-up of 1079 cases. *Am J Obstet Gynecol* 1976;125:1039.
181. Hurd WH, Bude RO, Delancey JO, et al. Abdominal wall characterization by magnetic resonance imaging and computed tomography. The effect of obesity on laparoscopic approach. *J Reprod Med* 1991;36:473.
182. Hurd WW, Bude RO, DeLancey JO, et al. The relationship of the umbilicus to the aortic bifurification: implications for laparoscopic techniques. *Obstet Gynecol* 1992;80:48.
183. Ikari O, Castilho LN, Lucena R, et al. Laparoscopic excision of seminal vesicle cysts. *J Urol* 1999;162:498.
184. Imai T, Tanaka Y, Kikumori M, et al. Laparoscopic partial adrenalectomy. *Surg Endosc* 1999;13:343.
185. Iselin CE, Winfield HN, Rohner S, et al. Sequential laparoscopic bladder diverticulectomy and transurethral resection of the prostate. *J Endourol* 1996;10:545.
186. Ishitoya S, Okubo K, Arai Y. Laparoscopic ureterolysis for retrocaval ureter. *Br J Urol* 1996;77:155.
187. Ivanisovich O, Gregorini H. A new operation for the cure of the varicocele. *Semana Med* 1918;61:17.
188. Iversen P, Brun C. Aspiration biopsy of the kidney. *Am J Med* 1951;11:324.
189. Jacobaeus Von VC. Ueber die moglichkeit die zystoscopie bei untersuchung seroser hohlungen anzyuwenden. *Munch Med Wochenschr* 1910;57:2090.
190. Jacobs JK, Goldstein RE, Geer RJ. Laparoscopic adrenalectomy: a new standard of care. *Ann Surg* 1997;225:495.
191. Jahnsen JU, Solhaug JH. Extirpation of benign renal cysts with laparoscopic technique. *Tidsskr Nor Laegenforen* 1992;112:3552.
192. Jain KK, Gorisch W. Repair of small blood vessels with the Nd:YAG laser. A preliminary study. *Surgery* 1979;85:684.
193. Janetschek G, Altarac S, Finkenstedt G, et al. Technique and results of laparoscopic adrenalectomy. *Eur Urol* 1996;30:475.
194. Janetschek G, Daffner P, Peschel R, et al. Laparoscopic nephron sparing surgery for small renal cell carcinoma. *J Urol* 1998;159:1152.
195. Janetschek G, Hobisch A, Holt L, et al. Retroperitoneal lymphadenectomy for clinical stage I nonseminomatous testicular tumor: Laparoscopic versus open surgery and impact of learning curve. *J Urol* 1996;156:89.
196. Janetschek G, Hobisch A, Peschel R, et al. Laparoscopic retroperitoneal lymph node dissection. *Urology* 2000;55:136.
197. Janetschek G, Hobisch A, Peschel R, et al. Laparoscopic retroperitoneal lymph node dissection for clinical stage I nonseminomatous testicular carcinoma: long-term outcome. *J Urol* 2000;163:1793.
198. Janetschek G, Lhotta K, Gasser R, et al. Adrenal-sparing laparoscopic surgery for aldosterone producing adenoma. *J Endourol* 1997;11:145.
199. Reference deleted in proofs.
200. Jarrett TW, Pardalidis NP, Sweetser P, et al. Laparoscopic transperitoneal bladder diverticulectomy: surgical technique. *J Laparoendosc Surg* 1995;5:105.
201. Jones DR, Moisey CU. A cautionary tale of the modified "pluck" nephroureterectomy. *Br J Urol* 1993;71:486.
202. Juan GM, Kawamura S, Yasui N, et al. Histological changes in the rat common carotid artery following simultaneous topical application of cotton sheet and cyanoacrylate glue. *Neurol Med Chir (Tokyo)* 1999;39:908.
203. Junghans T, Bohm B, Grundel K, et al. Effects of pneumoperitoneum with CO_2, argon or helium on hemodynamic and respiratory function. *Arch Surg* 1997;132:272.
204. Kaali SG, Barad DH. Incidence of bowel injury due to dense adhesions at the site of direct trocar insertion. *J Reprod Med* 1992;37:617.
205. Kalk H. Erfahrungen mit der laparoskopicie (zugleich mit beschreiburg eines neuen instrumentes). *Z Klin Med* 1929;111:303.
206. Kark RM, Muehrcke RC, Pollack VE, et al. An analysis of five hundred percutaneous renal biopsies. *AMA Arch Int Med* 1958;101:439.
207. Kashtan J, Green JF, Parsons EQ, et al. Hemodynamic effects of increased abdominal pressure. *J Surg Res* 1981;30: 249.
208. Katkhouda N, Mouiel J. A new technique of surgical treatment of chronic duodenal ulcer without laparotomy by videocoelioscopy. *Am J Surg* 1991;161:361.
209. Kavoussi LR, Clayman RV, Brunt LM, et al. Laparoscopic ureterolysis. *J Urol* 1992;147:426.

209a. Kavoussi LR, Moore RG, John B. et al. Comparison of robotic versus human laparoscopic camera control. *J Urol* 1995;154:2134.

210. Kavoussi LR, Clayman RV, Mikkelsen DJ, et al. Ureteronephroscopic marsupialization of obstructing peripelvic renal cyst. *J Urol* 1991;146:411.
211. Kavoussi LR, Schuessler WW, Vancaillie TG, et al. Laparoscopic approach to the seminal vesicles. *J Urol* 1993;150:417.
212. Keeley FX, Sharma NK, Tolley DA. Hand-assisted laparoscopic nephroureterectomy. *BJU Int* 1999;83:504.
213. Keeley FX, Tolley DA. A review of our first 100 cases of laparoscopic nephrectomy: defining risk factors for complications. *Br J Urol* 1998;82:615.
214. Kerbl K, Chandhoke PS, Clayman RV, et al. Ligation of the renal pedicle during laparoscopic nephrectomy: a comparison of staples, clips, and sutures. *J Laparoendosc Surg* 1993;3:9.
215. Kerbl K, Chandhoke PS, McDougall EM, et al. Laparoscopic stapled bladder closure: laboratory and clinical experience. *J Urol* 1993;149:1437.
216. Kerbl K, Clayman RV, McDougall EM, Urban DA, et al. Laparoscopic nephroureterectomy: evaluation of first clinical series. *Eur Urol* 1993;23:431.
217. Kerbl K, Clayman RV, Petros JA, et al. Staging pelvic lymphadenectomy for prostate cancer: a comparison of laparoscopic and open techniques. *J Urol* 1993;150:396.
218. Kerbl K, Figenshau RS, Clayman RV, et al. Retroperitoneal laparoscopic nephrectomy: laboratory and clinical experience. *J Endourol* 1993;7:23.
219. Kigure T, Harada T, Yuri Y, et al. Laparoscopic microwave thermotherapy on small renal tumors: experimental studies using implanted VX-2 tumors in rabbits. *Eur Urol* 1996;30:377.
220. Kimmelsteil FM, Miller RE, Molinelli BM, et al. Laparoscopic management of peritoneal dialysis catheters. *Surg Gynecol Obstet* 1993;176:565.
221. Kirsch AJ, Hensle TW, Chang DT. Renal effects of CO_2 insufflation: oliguria and acute renal dysfunction in a rat model. *Urology* 1994;43:453.

221a. Kitano S, Tomikawa M, Iso Y, et al. A safe and simple method to maintain a clear field of vision during laparoscopic cholecystectomy. *Surg Endosc* 1992;6:197.

222. Klioze SD, Poppas DP, Rooke CT, et al. Development and initial application of a real time thermal control system for laser tissue welding. *J Urol* 1994;152:744.

223. Knauer CM, Lowe HM. Hemodynamics in cirrhotic patient during paracentesis. *N Engl J Med* 1967;276:491.
224. Reference deleted in proofs.
225. Kozminski M, Partamian KO. Case report of laparoscopic ileal loop conduit. *J Endourol* 1992;6:147.
226. Kreder KJ, Winfield HN. Laparoscopic urethral sling for treatment of intrinsic sphincter deficiency. *J Endourol* 1996; 10:255.
227. Kropp KA, Grahyack JT, Wendel RM, et al. Morbidity and mortality of renal exploration for cysts. *Surg Gynecol Obstet* 1967;125:803.
228. Krueger RP. Renal biopsy. In: Glenn JF, ed. *Urologic surgery.* Philadelphia: Lippincott, 1983.
229. Landman J, Collyer WC, Olweny EO, et al. Laparoscopic renal ablation—new techniques in morcellation. *J Urol* 2000; 163:361.
230. Laucks SP, McLachlan MSF. Aging and simple cysts of the kidney. *Br J Radiol* 1981;54:12.
231. Lee BR, Bishoff JT, Janetschek G, et al. A novel method of surgical instruction: international telementoring. *World J Urol* 1998;16:367.
232. Lee BR, Cadeddu JA, Molmar-Nadasdy G, et al. Chronic effect of pneumoperitoneum on renal histology. *J Endourol* 1999;13:279.
233. Lee SJ, Park KH. Ultrasonic energy in endoscopic surgery. *Yonsei Med J* 1999;40:545.
234. Leighton TA, Liu SY, Bongard FS. Comparative cardiopulmonary effects of carbon dioxide versus helium pneumoperitoneum. *Surgery* 1993;113:527.
235. Lenz RJ, Thomas TA, Wilkins DG. Cardiovascular changes during laparoscopy. Studies of stroke volume and cardiac output using impedance cardiography. *Anesthesia* 1976;31:4.
236. Levin HS, Meraney AM, Novick AC, et al. Needle biopsy histology of renal tumors 3–6 months after laparoscopic renal cryoablation. *J Urol* 2000;163[4 Suppl]:153.
237. Levinson KA, Swanson DA, Johnson DE, et al. Fibrin glue for partial nephrectomy. *Urology* 1991;38:314.
238. Lifson BJ, Teichman JMH, Hulbert JC. Role and long-term results of laparoscopic decortication in solitary cystic and autosomal dominant polycystic kidney disease. *J Urol* 1998; 159:702.
239. Liatsikos EN, Siablis D, Karnabatidis D, et al. Percutaneous treatment of large symptomatic renal cysts. *J Endourol* 2000; 14:257.
240. Linos DA, Stylopoulos N, Boukis M, et al. Anterior, posterior, or laparoscopic approach for the management of adrenal diseases? *Am J Surg* 1997;173:120.
241. Lipsky H, Wuernschimmel E. Laparoscopic lithotomy for ureteral stones. *J Min Inv Ther* 1993;2:19.
242. London E, Neuhaus A, Ho H, et al. Beneficial effect of volume expansion on the altered renal hemodynamics of prolonged pneumoperitoneum [A85]. In: *American Society of Transplant Surgeons book of abstracts.* Chicago: 1998.
243. Reference deleted in proofs.
244. Lord SM, Barnsley L, Wallis BJ, et al. Percutaneous radiofrequency neurotomy for chronic cervical zygapophyseal-joint pain. *N Engl J Med* 1996;335:1721.
245. Lorenzo JL, Castillo A, Serrano EA, et al. Urodynamically based modification of Mitrofanoff procedure. *J Endourol* 1999; 11:77.
246. MacGillivray DC, Shichman SJ, Ferrer FA, et al. A comparison of open vs. laparoscopic adrenalectomy. *Surg Endosc* 1996; 10:987.
247. Mandressi A, Buizza C, Antonelli D, et al. Is laparoscopy a worthy method to treat varicocele? Comparison between 160 cases of two-port laparoscopic and 120 cases of open inguinal spermatic vein ligation. *J Endourol* 1996;5:435.
248. Marmer JL, DeBenedictis TJ, Praiss D. The management of varicoceles by microdissection of the spermatic cord at the external inguinal ring. *Fertil Steril* 1985;43:583.
249. Mastragelopulos N, Sarkar MR, Kaissling C, et al. Argon gas embolism in laparoscopic cholecystectomy with the argon beam coagulator. *Chirurg* 1992;63:1053.
249a. Matras H, Dinges HP, Lassmann H, Mamoli B. Suture-free interfasicular nerve transplantation in animal experiments. *Wein Med Wochenschr* 1972;122:517.
250. Matsuda T, Yasumoto R, Tsujino T. Laparoscopic treatment of a retrocaval ureter. *Eur Urol* 1996;29:115.
251. Maxwell KL, McDougall EM, Elbahnasy AM, et al. Laparoscopic ureteroureterostomy using vascular closure staples in a porcine model. *J Endourol* 1998;12:131.
252. Reference deleted in proofs.
253. Reference deleted in proofs.
254. Mazur P. The role of intracellular freezing in the death of cells cooled at supraoptimal rates. *Cryobiology* 1977;14:251.
255. McCullough CS, Soper NJ, Clayman RV, et al. Laparoscopic drainage of a posttransplant lymphocele. *Transplantation* 1991; 51:725.
256. McDougall EM. Laparoscopic knot tying. In: Clayman RV, McDougall EM, eds. *Laparoscopic urology.* St. Louis: Quality Medical Publishing, 1993.
257. McDougall EM, Afane JS, Dunn MD, et al. Laparoscopic nephropexy: long-term follow-up—Washington University experience. *J Endourol* 2000;14:247.
258. McDougall EM, Bennett HF, Monk TG, et al. Functional MR imaging of the porcine kidney: physiologic changes of the prolonged pneumoperitoneum. *J Soc Laparoendosc Surg* 1997;1:29.
259. McDougall EM, Clayman RV, Anderson K. Laparoscopic wedge resection of a renal tumor: initial experience. *J Laparosc Endosc Surg* 1993;42:201.
260. McDougall EM, Clayman RV, Anderson KR, et al. Laparoscopic gonadectomy in the case of testicular feminization. *Urology* 1993;42:201.
261. McDougall EM, Clayman RV, Elashry OM. Laparoscopic nephroureterectomy for upper tract transitional cell cancer: the Washington University experience. *J Urol* 1995;154:975.
262. McDougall EM, Clayman RV, Elashry OM. Laparoscopic radical nephrectomy for renal tumor: the Washington University experience. *J Urol* 1996;155:1180.
263. McDougall EM, Clayman RV, Fadden PT. Retroperitoneoscopy: the Washington University Medical School experience. *Urology* 1994;43:446.
264. McDougall EM, Clayman RV, Figenshau RS, et al. Laparoscopic retropubic auto-augmentation of the bladder. *J Urol* 1995;153:123.
265. McDougall EM, Clayman RV, Paramjit S, et al. Laparoscopic partial nephrectomy in the pig model. *J Urol* 1993;149: 1633.
266. McDougall EM, Elbahnasy AM, Clayman RV. Laparoscopic wedge resection and partial nephrectomy—the Washington University experience. *J Soc Laparoendosc Surg* 1998;2:15.

267. McDougall EM, Figenshau RS, Clayman RV, et al. Laparoscopic pneumoperitoneum: impact of body habitus. *J Laparoendosc Surg* 1994;4:385.
268. McDougall EM, Heidorn CA, Portis AJ, et al. Laparoscopic bladder neck suspension fails the test of time. *J Urol* 1999;162: 2078.
269. McDougall EM, Monk TG, Wolf JS, et al. The effect of prolonged pneumoperitoneum on renal function in an animal model. *J Am Coll Surg* 1996;182: 317.
270. McDowell GC, Babaian RJ, Johnson DE. Management of symptomatic lymphocele via percutaneous drainage and sclerotherapy with tetracycline. *Urology* 1991;37:237.
271. McKay TC, Albala DM, Gehrin BE, et al. Laparoscopic ureteral reanastomosis using fibrin glue. *J Urol* 1994;152: 1637.
272. Melvin WS, Bumgardner GL, Davies EA, et al. The laparoscopic management of post-transplant lymphocele. *Surg Endosc* 1997;11:245.
273. Meraney AM, Gill IS, Sung GT, et al. Histology of renal tumors 3–6 months post-cryoablation. J Endourol 1999; 13[Suppl 1]:A13.
274. Merritt JO, Cole RE, Ikehara C. A rapid-sequential-positioning task for evaluating motion parallax and stereoscopic 3-D cues in teleoperator displays. In: *IEEE conference proceedings,* 91CH3067-6. New York, New Hampshire: 1991.
275. Merrot T, Ordorica-Flores R, Steyeart H, et al. Is diffuse xanthogranulomatous pyelonephritis a contraindication to retroperitoneoscopic nephrectomy? *Surg Laparosc Endosc* 1998; 8:366.
276. Micali S, Moore RG, Averch TD, et al. The role of laparoscopy in the treatment of renal and ureteral calculi. *J Urol* 1997;157:463.
277. Micali S, Silver RI, Kaufman HS, et al. Measurement of urinary and *N*-acetyl-beta-D-glucosaminidase to assess renal ischemia during laparoscopic operations. *Surg Endosc* 1999;13:503.
278. Middleton AW, Pfister RC. Stone-containing pyelocalyceal diverticulum: embryogenic, anatomic, radiologic and clinical characteristics. *J Urol* 1974;111:2.
279. Mikami O, Fujise K, Matsumoto S, et al. High intraabdominal pressure increases plasma catecholamine concentrations during pneumoperitoneum for laparoscopic procedures. *Arch Surg* 1998;133:3.
280. Miki Y, Iwase K, Kmiike W, et al. Laparoscopic cholecystectomy and time course changes in renal function: the effect of the retraction method on renal function. *Surg Endosc* 1997; 11:838.
281. Millin T. Retropubic prostatectomy: a new extravesical technique. *Lancet* 1945;4:473.
282. Mitchell TN, Robertson J, Nagy AG, et al. Three-dimensional endoscopic imaging for minimal access surgery. *J R Coll Surg Edinb* 1993;38:285.
283. Mitrofanoff P. Cystostomic continente trans-appendiculane dans le traitement des vesse neurologiques. *Chir Pediatr* 1980; 21:297.
284. Monk TG, Despotis GJ, Hoghe CW, et al. Hemodynamic and echocardiographic alterations during laparoscopic surgery. *Anesthesiology* 1993;79:A54.
285. Morgan C, Rader D. Laparoscopic unroofing of a renal cyst. *J Urol* 1992;148:1835.
286. Mori N. Clinical and experimental studies on so-called lymphocyst which develop after radical hysterectomy in cancer of the uterine cervix. *J Jpn Soc Obstet Gynecol* 1955;2:178.
287. Motew M, Ivankovich AD, Bieniarz J, et al. Cardiovascular effects and acid-base and blood gas changes during laparoscopy. *Am J Obstet Gynecol* 1973;115:1002.
288. Reference deleted in proofs.
289. Mugiya S, Suzuki K, Kazuhiro S, et al. Unilateral laparoscopic adrenalectomy followed by contralateral retroperitoneal partial adrenalectomy in a patient with multiple endocrine neoplasia type 2a. *J Endourol* 1999;13:99.
290. Mullet CE, Viale JP, Sagnard PE, et al. Pulmonary CO_2 elimination during surgical procedures using intra- or extraperitoneal CO_2 insufflation. *Anesth Analg* 1993;76:622.
291. Muth RG. The safety of percutaneous renal biopsy: an analysis of 500 consecutive cases. *J Urol* 1965;94:1.
292. Myers RS, Hammond WG, Ketcham AS. Cryosurgery of experimental tumors. *J Cryosurg* 1969;2:225.
293. Nagai H, Inabo T, Kamiya S, et al. A new method of laparoscopic cholecystectomy: an abdominal wall lifting technique without pneumoperitoneum. *Surg Laparosc Endosc* 1991; 1:26(abst).
294. Naito S, Uozumi J, Ichimiya H, et al. Laparoscopic adrenalectomy comparison with open adrenalectomy. *Eur Urol* 1994; 26:253.
295. Nakada SY. Hand-assisted laparoscopic nephrectomy. *J Endourol* 1999;13:9.
296. Nakada SY, Lee FT Jr, Warner T, et al. Laparoscopic cryosurgery of the kidney in the porcine model: an acute histological study. *Urology* 1998;51:161.
297. Nekada T, Kubota Y, Sasagawa I, et al. Therapeutic outcome of primary aldosteronism: adrenalectomy versus enucleation of aldosterone producing adenoma. *J Urol* 1995;153:1775.
298. Neuman GG, Sidebotharn G, Negoianu E, et al. Laparoscopy explosion hazards with nitrous oxide. *Anesthesiology* 1993; 78:875.
299. Newman L, Luke JP, Ruben DM, et al. Laparoscopic herniorrhaphy without pneumoperitoneum. *Surg Laparosc Endosc* 1993;3:213.
300. Nezhat C, Nezhat F, Green B, et al. Laparoscopic ureteroureterostomy. *J Endourol* 1992;6:143.
301. Nezhat C, Nezhat F, Green B. Laparoscopic treatment of obstructed ureter due to endometriosis by resection and ureteroureterostomy: a case report. *J Urol* 1992;148:865.
302. Nezhat C, Nezhat F, Nezhat CH, et al. Urinary tract endometriosis treated by laparoscopy. *Fertil Steril* 1996;66:920.
303. Ng CS, Gill IS, Sung GT, et al. Retroperitoneoscopic surgery is not associated with increased cabon dioxide absorption. *J Urol* 1999;162:1268.
304. Nicholson ML, Veitch PS. Treatment of lymphocele associated with renal transplant. *Br J Urol* 1990;65:240.
305. Nickel KG, Hollander MB, Lipschultz LI. Treatment of bilateral varicoceles—postoperative morbidity data for open surgical versus laparoscopic techniques. *J Urol* 1993;149:389A.
306. Niederberger C, Ross LS, Mackenzie B Jr, et al. Vasovasostomy in rabbits using fibrin adhesive prepared from a single human source. *J Urol* 1993;149:183.
307. Nogueira JM, Cangro CB, Fink JC, et al. A comparison of recipient renal outcomes with laparoscopic versus open live donor nephrectomy. *Transplantation* 1999;6:722.
308. Novick AC. Partial nephrectomy for renal cell carcinoma. *Urol Clin North Am* 1987;14:419.
309. Novick AC, Streem S, Montie JE, et al. Conservative surgery for renal cell carcinoma: a single-center experience with 100 patients. *J Urol* 1989;141:835.
310. Novicki DE, and Ferrigni RG. Non-malignant processes of the lymphatic system of clinical importance to the urologist. *AUA Update Series* 1987;Vol. VI.lesson 22.

311. Odland MD, Ney AL, Jacobs DM, et al. Initial experience with laparoscopic live donor nephrectomy. *Surgery* 1999;126:603.
312. Olsson CA, Kirsch AJ, Whang MIS. Rapid construction of right colon pouch. *Current Surgical Techniques in Urology* 1993;6:1.
313. Ono Y, Katoh N, Kinukawa T, et al. Laparoscopic radical nephrectomy: the Nagoya experience. *J Urol* 1997;158:719.
314. Ono Y, Kinukawa T, Hattori R, et al. Laparoscopic radical nephrectomy for renal cell carcinoma: a five-year experience. *Urology* 1999;53:280.
315. Oppenheimer P, Weghorst S, MacFarlane M, et al. Immersive surgical robotic interfaces. In: Westwood JD et al, eds. *Medicine meets virtual reality.* IOS Press, 1999.
316. Reference deleted in proofs.
317. Ostrzenski A. Laparoscopic colposuspension for total vaginal prolapse. *Int J Gynecol Obstet* 1996;55:147.
318. Ott DO. Ventroscopic illumination of the abdominal cavity in pregnancy. *Akush Zhenskikh Boleznei* 1901;15:7.
319. Ou C, Presthus J, Beadle E. Laparoscopic bladder neck suspension using hernia mesh and surgical staples. *J Laparoendoscop Surg* 1993;3:563.
320. Palmer R. Instrumentation et technique de la coelioscopie gynecologique. *Gynecol Obstet (Paris)* 1947;46:420.
321. Palomo A. Radical cure of varicocle by a new technique: preliminary report. *J Urol* 1949;61:604.
322. Parra RO, Andrus CH, Jones JP, et al. Laparoscopic cystectomy: initial report on a new treatment for the retained bladder. *J Urol* 1992;148:1140.
323. Parra RO, Perez MG, Boullier JA, et al. Comparison between standard flank versus laparoscopic nephrectomy for benign renal disease. *J Urol* 1995;153:1171.
324. Parra RO, Worischeck JH, Hagood PG. Laparoscopic simple cystectomy in a man. *Surg Laparosc Endosc* 1995;5:161.
325. Partin AW, Adams JB, Moore RG, et al. Complete robot-assisted laparoscopic urologic surgery: a preliminary report. *J Am Coll Surg* 1995;181:552.
326. Partin AW, Yoo J, Carter HB, et al. The use of prostate specific antigen, clinical stage, and Gleason score to predict the pathological stage in men with localized prostate cancer. *J Urol* 1993;150:110.
327. Pearle MS, Nakada SY, McDougall EM, et al. Laparoscopic pneumodissection: results in initial 20 patients. *J Am Coll Surg* 1997;184:579.
328. Perissat J, Vitale CC. Laparoscopic cholecystectomy: gateway to the future. *Am J Surg* 1991;161:408.
329. Perrotti M, Gentle DL, Barada JH, et al. Mini-laparotomy pelvic lymph node dissection minimizes morbidity, hospitalization and cost of pelvic lymph node dissection. *J Urol* 1996; 155:986.
330. Petelin JB. Laparoscopic approach to common duct pathology. *Surg Laparosc Endosc* 1991;1:33.
331. Philosophe B, Kuo PC, Schweitzer EJ, et al. Laparoscopic versus open donor nephrectomy. *Transplantation* 1999;68:497.
332. Polascik TJ, Chen RN. Laparoscopic ureteroureterostomy for retrocaval ureter. *J Urol* 1998;16:121.
333. Polascik TJ, Hamper U, Lee BR, et al. Ablation of renal tumors in a rabbit model with interstitial saline-augmented radiofrequency energy: preliminary report of a new technology. *Urology* 1999;53:465.
334. Reference deleted in proofs.
335. Poppas DP, Schlossberg SM. Laser tissue welding in urologic surgery. *Urology* 1994;43:143.
336. Poppas D, Schlossberg S, Richmond I, et al. Laser welding in urethral surgery: improved results with a protein solder. *J Urol* 1988;139:415.
337. Poppas DP, Uzzo RG, Britanisky RG, et al. Laparoscopic laser assisted auto-augmentation of the pediatric neurogenic bladder: early experience with urodynamic follow-up. *J Urol* 1996;155: 1057.
338. Potter SR, Charambura TC, Adams JB, et al. Laparoscopic ileal conduit: five-year follow-up. *Urology* 2000;56:22.
339. Prabhakaran K, Lingaraj K. Laparoscopic nephroureterectomy in children. *J Pediatr Surg* 1999;34:556.
340. Reference deleted in proofs.
341. Printz RA. A comparison of laparoscopic and open adrenalectomies. *Arch Surg* 1995;130:489.
342. Proust R. Technique de la prostatectomie perineale. *Assoc Franc Urol* 1901;5:361.
343. Puppo P, Carmignani G, Gallucci M, et al. Bilateral laparoscopic ureterolysis. *Eur Urol* 1994;25:82.
344. Puppo P, Perachino M, Ricciotti G, et al. Laparoscopically assisted transvaginal radical cystectomy. *Eur Urol* 1995;27:80.
345. Reference deleted in proofs.
346. Rassweiler JJ, Frede T, Henkel TO, et al. Nephrectomy: a comparative study between the transperitoneal and retroperitoneal laparoscopic versus the open approach. *Eur Urol* 1998; 33:489.
347. Rassweiler JJ, Seemann O, Frede T, et al. Retroperitoneoscopy: experience with 200 cases. *J Urol* 1998;169:1265.
348. Rassweiler JJ, Seemann O, Henkel TO, et al. Laparoscopic retroperitoneal lymph node dissection for nonseminomatous germ cell tumors: indications and limitations. *J Urol* 1996;156: 1108.
349. Ratner LE, Ciseck LJ, Moore RG, et al. Laparoscopic live donor nephectomy. *Transplantation* 1995;60:1047.
350. Ratner LE, Montgomery RA, Kavoussi LR. Laparoscopic live donor nephrectomy: the four year Johns Hopkins University experience. *Nephrol Dial Transplant* 1999;14:2090.
351. Razvi HA, Fields D, Vargas JC, et al. Oliguria during laparoscopic surgery: evidence for direct renal parenchymal compression as an etiologic factor. *J Endourol* 1996;10:1.
352. Reddick EJ, Olsen DO. Laparoscopic laser cholecystectomy. A comparison with mini-lap cholecystectomy. *Surg Endosc* 1989; 3:131.
353. Reich H, McGlynn F, Wilkie W. Laparoscopic management of stage I ovarian cancer. A case report. *J Reprod Med* 1990; 35:601.
354. Robson CJ, Churchill BM, Anderson W. The results of radical nephrectomy for renal cell carcinoma. *J Urol* 1969;101:297.
355. Rodriguez-Carmona A, Garcia-Falcon T, Perez-Fontan M, et al. Survival on chronic peritoneal dialysis: have results improved in the 1990's? *Perit Dial Int* 1996;16:s410.
356. Reference deleted in proofs.
357. Rossi S, Stasi M, Buscarini E, et al. Percutaneous radiofrequency interstitial thermal ablation in the treatment of small hepatocellular carcinoma. *Cancer J Sci Am* 1995;1:73.
358. Rovetta A, Sala R, Wen Z, et al. Sensorization of a surgeon robot for prostate biopsy operation. In: *Proceedings of the First International Symposium on Medical Robotics and Computer Assisted Surgery.* Pittsburgh: 1994.

359. Rubenstein SC, Hulbert JC, Pharand D, et al. Laparoscopic ablation of symptomatic renal cysts. *J Urol* 1993;150:1103.
360. Ruckle HC, Segura JW. Laparoscopic treatement of a stone-filled caliceal diverticulum: a definitive, minimally invasive therapeutic option. *J Urol* 1994;151:122.
361. Ruddock JC. Peritoneoscopy in surgery. *Gynecol Obstet* 1937; 65:523.
362. Sackier JM, Wang Y. Robotically assisted laparoscopic surgery. *Surg Endosc* 1994;8:63.
363. Sadeghi-Mejad H, Kavoussi LR, Peters CA. Bowel injury in open technique laparoscopic cannula placement. *Urology* 1994; 43:559.
364. Sanchez de Badajoz E, Diaz Ramirez F, Marin Marin J. Endoscopic treatment of varicocele. *Arch Esp Urol* 1988; 41:15.
365. Sanchez de Badajoz E, Perales G, Reche Rosado JL. Laparoscopic radical cystectomy and ileal conduit. *Arch Esp Urol* 1993;46:621.
366. Saoudi N. Evolving modes of energy delivery for catheter ablation of accessory pathways. *Circulation* 1992;85:1208.
366a. Sasagawa I, Suzuki H, Izumi T, et al. Posterior retroperitoneoscopic partial adrenalectomy using ultrasonic scapel for aldosterone-producing adenoma. *J Endourol* 2000;14:573.
367. Satava RM. 3-D vision technology applied to advanced minimally invasive surgery systems. *Surg Endosc* 1993;7:429.
368. Savad P, Ferzli G. The extraperitoneal approach and its utility. *Surg Endosc* 1999;13:1168.
369. Saypol DC. Varicocele. *J Androl* 1981;41:5.
370. Scherr DS, Poppas DP. Laser tissue welding. *Urol Clin North Am* 1998;25:123.
371. Schow DA, Vinson RK, Morrisseau PM. Percutaneous renal biopsy of the solitary kidney: a contraindication? *J Urol* 1992; 147:1235.
372. Schuessler WW, Grune MT, Tecuanhuey LV, et al. Laparoscopic dismembered pyeloplasty. *J Urol* 1993;150;1795.
373. Schuessler WW, Pharand D, Vancaillie TG. Laparoscopic standard pelvic node dissection for carcinoma of the prostate: is it accurate? *J Urol* 1993;150:898.
374. Schuessler WW, Schulam PG, Clayman RV, et al. Laparoscopic radical prostatectomy: initial short-term experience. *Urology* 1997;50:854.
375. Schuessler WW, Vancaillie TG, Reich H, et al. Transperitoneal endosurgical lymphadenectomy in patients with localized prostate cancer. *J Urol* 1991;145:988.
376. Scott DB. Some effects of peritoneal insufflation of carbon dioxide during anesthesia for laparoscopy. *Anesthesia* 1970; 25:590.
377. Semm K. Endoscopic appendectomy. *Endoscopy* 1983;15:59.
378. Semm K. *Operative manual for endoscopic abdominal surgery.* Chicago: Year Book Medical, 1987:175, 181, 184, 216.
379. Seibold J, Janetschek G, Bartsch G. Laparoscopic surgery in pediatric urology. *Eur Urol* 1996;30:394.
380. Shalev M, Cipolla B, Guille F, et al. Is ipsilateral adrenalectomy a necessary component of radical nephrectomy? *J Urol* 1995; 153:1415.
380a. Shalhav A, Cadeddu J. Personal communication, 1999.
381. Shalhav AL, Dunn MD, Portis AJ, et al. Laparoscopic nephroureterectomy for upper tract transitional cell cancer: the Washington University experience. *J Urol* 2000;163:1100.
382. Shaver TR, Swanson SJ, Fernandez-Bueno C, et al. The optimal treatment of lymphoceles following renal transplantation. *Transpl Int* 1993;6:108.
383. Shekarriz H, Shekkariz B, Upadhyay J, et al. Hydro-jet assisted laparoscopic partial nephrectomy: initial experience in porcine model. *J Urol* 2000;163:1005.
384. Shen WT, Lim RC, Siperstein AE, et al. Laparoscopic vs open adrenalectomy for the treatment of primary hyperaldosteronism. *Arch Surg* 1999;134:628.
385. Shennib H, Bastawisy A, Mcloughlin J, et al. Robotic computer-assisted telemanipulation enhances coronary artery bypass. *J Thorac Cardiovasc Surg* 1999;117:310.
386. Shingleton WB, Sewell P. Renal tumor cryoablation utilizing interventional magnetic resonance imaging (IMRI). *J Urol* 2000;163:155.
387. Shokeir AA, el-Diasty TA, Ghoneim MA. Percutaneous treatment of lymphoceles in renal transplant recipients. *J Endourol* 1993;7:481.
388. Sierra DH. Fibrin sealant adhesion systems: a review of their chemistry, material properties and clinical applications. *J Biomaterials Applications* 1993;7:309.
389. Sigel B, Acevedo F. Vein anastomosis by electrocoaptive union. *Surg Forum* 1962;13:291.
390. Silber SJ, Cohen R. Laparoscopy for cryptorchidisms. *J Urol* 1980;124:928.
391. Silverstein JI, Mellinger BC. Fibrin glue vassal anastomosis compared to conventional suture vasovasostomy in the rat. *J Urol* 1991;145:988.
392. Sindelar WF, Javadpour N, Bagley DH. Histological and ultrastructural changes in rat kidney after cryosurgery. *J Surg Oncol* 1981;18:363.
393. Slakey DP, Wood JC, Hender D, et al. Laparoscopic live donor nephrectomy: advantages of the hand-assisted method. *Transplantation* 1999;68:581.
394. Reference deleted in proofs.
395. Spencer JR, O'Conor VJ Jr. Comparison of procedures for stress urinary incontinence. *AUA Update Series* 1987;6(28):1.
396. Squadrito JF, Coletta AV. Laparoscopic renal exploration and biopsy. *J Laparosc Surg* 1991;1:235.
397. Staren ED, Printz RA. Adrenalectomy in the era of laparoscopy. *Surgery* 1996;120:706.
398. Staskin DR, Zimmern PE, Hadley HR, et al. The pathophysiology of stress incontinence. *Urol Clin North Am* 1985; 12:271.
399. Stifelman MD, Sosa RE, Andrade A, et al. Hand assisted laparoscopic nephroureterectomy for the treatment of transitional cell carcinoma of the upper urinary tract. *Urology* 2000; 56(5):741.
400. Stone NN, Stock RG, Unger P. Indications for seminal vesical biopsy and laparoscopic pelvic lymph node dissection in men with localized carcinoma of the prostate. *J Urol* 1995; 154:1392.
401. Stone NN, Stock RG, Unger P. Laparoscopic pelvic lymph node dissection for prostate cancer: comparison of the extended and modified techniques. *J Urol* 1997;158:1891.
402. Strand WT, McDougall EM, Leach FS, et al. Laparoscopic creation of a catheterizable cutaneous ureterovesicostomy. *Urology* 1997;49:272.
403. Su T, Wang K, Hsu C, et al. Prospective comparison of laparoscopic and traditional colposuspension in the treatment of genuine stress incontincence. *Acta Obstet Gynecol Scand* 1997;76:576.
404. Sulman A, Aschoff AJ, Martinez M, et al. Perfusion modulated MRI guided radiofrequency (RF) interstitial thermal ablation of the kidney in a porcine model. *J Urol* 2000;163:213.
405. Sung GT, Gill IS, Hsu TH. Robotic-assisted laparoscopic pyeloplasty: a pilot study. *Urology* 1999;53:1099.

406. Sung GT, Gill IS, Hsu THS, et al. Effect of intentional cryoinjury to the renal collecting system. *J Endourol* 2000; 13[Suppl 1]:A14.
407. Suzuki K, Kageyama S, Ueda D, et al. Laparoscopic adrenalectomy: clinical experience with 12 cases. *J Urol* 1993;150: 1099.
408. Suzuki K, Ushiyama T, Mugiya S, et al. Hazards of laparoscopic adrenalectomy in patients with adrenal malignancy. *J Urol* 1997;158:2227.
409. Tabuse K. A new operative procedure of hepatic surgery using a microwave tissue coagulator. *Arch Jpn Chir* 1979;48:160.
410. Takada M, Go H, Watanabe R, et al. Retroperitoneal laparoscopic adrenalectomy for functioning adrenal tumors: comparison with conventional transperitoneal laparoscopic adrenalectomy. *J Urol* 1997;157:19.
411. Reference deleted in proofs.
412. Telenuis-Berg M, Ponder MA, Berg B, et al. Quality of life after bilateral adrenalectomy in MEN 2. *Henry Ford Hosp Med J* 1989;37:160.
413. Teruel JL, Escobar ME, Quereda C, et al. A simple and safe method for management of lymphoceles after renal transplantation. *J Urol* 1983;130:1058.
414. Thomas AJ Jr, Geisinger MA. Current management of varicoceles. *Urol Clin North Am* 1990;17:893.
415. Thompson GB, Grant CS, van Heerden JA, et al. Laparoscopic versus open posterior adrenalectomy: a case-control study of 100 patients. *Surgery* 1997;122:1132.
416. Tikkakoski T et al. Ultrasound guided aspiration cytology of renal expansions. *Roentgenblatter* 1990;43:502.
417. Tisher CC. Indications for and interpretation of renal biopsy. In Schrier RW, Gottshalk CW, eds. *Diseases of the kidney*. Atlee Brown, 1988.
418. Tricarico A, Tartaglia A, Taddeo F, et al. Videolaparoscopic treatment of spleen injuries. Report of two cases. *Surg Endosc* 1994;8:910.
419. Troxel SA, Winfield HN. Comparative financial analysis of laparoscopic versus open pelvic lymph node dissection for men with cancer of the prostate. *J Urol* 1994;152:675.
420. Troxel SA, Winfield HN. Comparative financial analysis of laparoscopic pelvic lymph node dissection performed in 1990–1992 v 1993–1994. *J Endourol* 1996;10:353.
421. Tsui K, Shvarts O, Barbaric Z, et al. Is adrenalectomy a necessary component of radical nephrectomy? UCLA experience with 511 radical nephrectomies. *J Urol* 2000;163:437.
422. Turk I, Deger S, Roigas J, et al. Laparoscopic ureterolithotomy. *Tech Urol* 1998;4:29.
423. Uchida M, Imaide Y, Sugimoto K, et al. Percutaneous cryosurgery for renal tumors. *Br J Urol* 1995;75:132.
424. Ulchaker JC, Goldfarb DA, Bravo EL, et al. Successful outcomes in pheochromocytoma surgery in the modern era. *J Urol* 1999;161:764.
425. UNOS and the Division of Transplantation, Bureau of Health Resources and Services Administration. *Annual report of the US Scientific Registry of Transplant Recipients and Organ Procurement and Transplantation Network—transplant data: 1988–1994.* Rockville, Md: US Department of Health and Human Services, 1995.
426. Urban DA, Clayman RV, Kerbl K, et al. Laparoscopic nephropexy for symptomatic nephroptosis: initial case report. *J Endourol* 1993;7:27.
427. Vancaillie TG, Schuessler W. Laparoscopic bladder neck suspension. *J Laparoendoscop Surg* 1991;1:169.
428. Vara-Thorbeck C, Sanchez-de-Bandajoz E. Laparoscopic ileal-loop conduit. *Surg Endosc* 1994;8:114.
429. Veress J. Neues Instrument zur Ausfuhrung von brusto der Bachpunktionen und Pneumothoraxbehandlung. *Deutsch Med Wochenschr* 1938;64:1480.
430. Wakizaka Y, Sano S, Koike Y, et al. Changes of arterial CO_2, $PaCO_2$ and urine output by carbon dioxide insufflation of the peritoneal cavity during laparoscopic cholecystectomy. *Nippon Geka Gakkai Zasshi* 1994;95:336.
431. Walsh PC, Lepor H, Eggleston JC. Radical prostatectomy with preservation of sexual function: anatomical and pathological considerations. *Prostate* 1983;4:473.
432. Walther MM, Herring J, Choyke PL, et al. Laparoscopic partial adrenalectomy in patients with hereditary forms of pheochromocytoma. *J Urol* 2000;164:14.
433. Walther MM, Lyne JC, Libutti SK, et al. Laparoscopic cytoreductive nephrectomy as preparation for administration of systemic interleukin-2 in the treatment of metastatic renal cell carcinoma: a pilot study. *Urology* 1999;53:496.
434. Wang S, Grubbs P, Basu S, et al. Effect of blood bonding on bursting strength of laser-assisted microvascular anastomosis. *Microsurgery* 1988;9:10.
435. Wang YF, Uecker DR, Wang Y. A new framework for vision-enabled and robotically assisted minimally invasive surgery. *Comput Med Imag Graph* 1998;22:429.
436. Watkin NA, Morris SB, Rivens IH, et al. High-intensity focused ultrasound ablation of the kidney in a large animal model. *J Endourol* 1997;11:191.
437. Wickham JEA. The surgical treatment of renal lithiasis. In: *Urinary calculous disease.* New York: Churchill Livingstone, 1979.
438. Willson PD, McAnena OJ, Peters EE. A fatal complication of diathermy in laparoscopic surgery. *J Min Inv Ther* 1994;3:19.
439. Windberger U, Siegel H, Woisetchlager R, et al. Hemodynamic changes during prolonged laparoscopic surgery. *Eur Surg Res* 1994;26:1.
440. Winfield HN, Donovan JF. Laparoscopic varicocelectomy. *Semin Urol* 1992;10:152.
441. Winfield HN, Donovan JF, Godet AS, et al. Human laparoscopic partial nephrectomy, case report. *J Min Inv Ther* 1992; 1[Suppl]:66.
442. Winfield HN, Donovan JF, Godet AS, et al. Laparoscopic partial nephrectomy: initial case report for benign diease. *J Endourol* 1993;7:521.
443. Winfield NH, Donovan JF, Lund GO, et al. Laparoscopic partial nephrectomy: initial experience and comparison to the open surgical approach. *J Urol* 1995;153:1409.
444. Winfield HN, Hamilton BD, Bravo EL, et al. Laparoscopic adrenalectomy: the preferred choice? A comparison to open adrenalectomy. *J Urol* 1998;160:325.
445. Wittman I. *Peritoneoscopy.* Budapest: Publishing House of the Hungarian Academy of Sciences, 1966:3–5.
445a. Wolf JS Jr. Personal communication, 1999.
446. Wolf JS Jr, Carrier S, Stoller ML. Intraperitoneal vs. extraperitoneal insufflation of carbon dioxide gas as for laparoscopy. *J Endourol* 1995;9:63.
447. Wolf JS Jr, Clayman RV, McDougall EM, et al. Carbon dioxide and helium insufflation during laparoscopic radical nephrectomy in a patient with severe pulmonary disease. *J Urol* 1996;155:2021.
448. Wolf JS Jr, Monk TG, McDougall EM, et al. The extraperitoneal approach and subcutaneous emphysema are associated with greater absorption of CO_2 during laparoscopic renal surgery. *J Urol* 1995;154:959.

449. Wolf JS Jr, Moon TD, Nakada SY. Hand-assisted laparoscopic nephrectomy: technical considerations. *Tech Urol* 1997; 3:123.
450. Wolf JS Jr, Moon TD, Nakada SY. Hand-assist laparoscopic nephrectomy: comparison to standard laparoscopic nephrectomy. *J Urol* 1998;160:22.
451. Wolf JS Jr, Seifman BD, Montie JE. Nephron sparing surgery for suspected malignancy: open surgery compared to laparoscopy with selective use of hand assistance. *J Urol* 2000;163: 1659.
452. Wolf SJ Jr, Soble JJ, Nakada SY, et al. Comparison of fibrin glue, laser weld and mechanical suturing device for the laparoscopic closure of ureterotomy in a porcine model. *J Urol* 1997;157:1487.
453. Wright DM, Serpell MG, Baxter JN, et al. Effect of extraperitoneal CO_2 insufflation on intraoperative blood gas and hemodynamic changes. *Surg Endosc* 1995;9:1169.
454. Wright MJ, Bel'eed K, Johnson BF, et al. Randomized prospective comparison of laparoscopic and open peritoneal dialysis catheter insertion. *Perit Dial Int* 1999;19:372.
455. Yerushalmi A, Servadio C, Leib Z, et al. Local hyperthermia for treatment of carcinoma of the prostate: a preliminary report. *Prostate* 1982;6:623.
456. Yoshida H, Hirozane K, Kamiya A. Comparative study of autologous fibrin glues prepared by cryo-centrifugation, cryofiltration, and ethanol precipitation methods. *Biol Pharm Bull* 1999;22:1222.
457. Yoshimura K, Yoshioka T, Miyake O, et al. Comparison of clinical outcomes of laparoscopic and conventional open adrenalectomy. *J Endourol* 1998;12:555.
458. Zegal HG, Holland GA, Jennings SB, et al. Intraoperative ultrasonographically guided cryoablation of renal masses: initial experience. *J Ultrasound Med* 1998;17:571.
459. Reference deleted in proofs.
460. Zlotta AR, Djavan B, Matos C, et al. Percutaneous transperineal radiofrequency ablation of prostate tumor: safety, feasibility and pathological effects on human prostate cancer. *Br J Urol* 1998;81:265.

19

ENDOUROLOGY OF THE UPPER URINARY TRACT: NONCALCULOUS APPLICATIONS

ELSPETH M. McDOUGALL
RALPH V. CLAYMAN
R. SHERBURNE FIGENSHAU

Although initially limited to calculous disease, today the span of endourology encompasses almost all types of maladies affecting the upper urinary tract. This is due to significant advances in the endoscopic and auxiliary instrumentation available to the urologic surgeon. Presently, rigid working endoscopes have become as small as 6 Fr, and their flexible counterparts are only 7.5 Fr. Despite the small size of these endoscopes, a working channel of 3 Fr or larger is available for the passage of myriad instruments, ranging from biopsy forceps to electrosurgical and laser probes.

As a result of these developments, diagnostic and therapeutic procedures, previously possible only through a large incision, now can be performed effectively endoscopically. From a diagnostic standpoint, a minimally invasive approach has been most beneficial in the upper urinary tract in the areas of lateralizing hematuria, filling defects, renal masses, and obstruction. Likewise, the therapeutic approach to many upper urinary tract disease entities has progressed from an open to an endourologic treatment. In the ureter, endourologic approaches have been used for treating strictures, transitional cell cancer, and ureterovesical fistulae. In the kidney, a minimally invasive approach has been used to deal with ureteropelvic junction (UPJ) and infundibular obstruction, calyceal diverticula, and transitional cell cancer. In addition, benign renal masses, including cysts and abscesses, have been treated successfully endourologically. Most recently, these same techniques have been used to resolve similar problems affecting a renal transplant. In these patients, both stricture and fistula problems have been managed successfully endoscopically. The endourologic approach also has been applied to perirenal processes, such as abscesses, urinomas, and lymphoceles.

R.V. Clayman and R.S. Figenshau: Department of Surgery (Urology) and Radiology, Washington University, Barnes-Jewish Hospital, St. Louis, MO 63110.

E.M. McDougall: Department of Urologic Surgery, Vanderbilt University Medical Center, Nashville, TN 37232.

DIAGNOSTIC RENAL AND URETERAL APPLICATIONS

Lateralizing Hematuria

In the diagnosis of lateralizing hematuria, an endourologic approach has become the final and definitive step in the diagnostic regimen (200). Among patients with macroscopic hematuria, the laboratory evaluation usually includes urine for cytology, urinalysis to rule out proteinuria associated with medical renal disease, coagulation studies, and when appropriate, a sickle cell preparation.

Aside from these basic studies, much has been written about examination of the morphology of the red blood cells in the urine in order to differentiate bleeding attributable to a glomerular problem (i.e., dysmorphic red blood cells) from bleeding caused by an anatomic lesion (i.e., normal-shaped red blood cells). Using interference microscopy, Tomita and associates (358) have identified five different red blood cell shapes indicative of a glomerular or nonglomerular (i.e., anatomic) site of bleeding. In patients with 15% glomerular red blood cells, the sensitivity and specificity of the test for glomerular bleeding was 90% and 98%, respectively. The accuracy of this study is further enhanced if the urine has a pH of less than 6.4 or is highly concentrated (osmolality greater than 400 mOsm/kg H_2O); likewise, identification of one subtype of the glomerular red blood cells (a doughnut cell) further increased the certainty of glomerular bleeding (196). Other reports have been less encouraging, with a sensitivity and specificity of 73% and 60%, respectively; however, these values were substantially improved when obvious causes of hematuria, such as urinary tract infection or urolithiasis, were eliminated from the data pool. Accordingly, in the patient with no obvious cause for lateralizing hematuria (i.e., negative radiologic studies), the appearance of deformed red blood cells on phase contrast microscopy or on a Coulter counter can be more than 90% accurate in diagnosing the presence of a glomerular, nonsurgical problem (4,270,311).

Also of interest are recent reports on detailed protein analysis of the urine among patients with hematuria of undetermined etiology. A nonglomerular source of hematuria is associated with an increase in high-molecular-weight proteins. Specifically, when the urine albumin exceeds 100 mg/L, the measurement of α_2-macroglobulin in the second voided morning specimen is recommended; if it is also elevated (i.e., α_2-macroglobulin-to-albumin ratio greater than 2.0×10^{-2}), a nonglomerular, postrenal site of bleeding is likely (127).

After the aforementioned studies, the next tests are usually radiologic and endoscopic: an intravenous urogram and cystoscopy. The intravenous urogram should clearly show the examiner all of the calyces and the entire length of the ureter; this might require additional radiographs and repositioning the patient to fill the entire ureter. Failure to image all of the calyces or the entire ureter necessitates completion of a retrograde ureterogram. If intravenous urography (IVU) fails to reveal an obvious cause for the hematuria (i.e., no filling defects, stones, or apparent renal masses) and cystoscopy reveals blood emanating from the right or left ureteral orifice, the next procedure is usually a computed tomogram or ultrasound (US) examination to rule out an occult renal mass that might have been missed on the IVU (227). If this study is unremarkable, there is some support for proceeding to a renal arteriogram to rule out an arteriovenous malformation or other large vascular anomaly; if discovered, the vascular abnormality can be embolized during the same angiographic session (Fig. 19.1).

When radiographic studies have failed to identify an obvious cause for lateralizing hematuria, it is necessary to proceed with ureteroscopic evaluation of the ipsilateral urinary tract. The role of percutaneous nephroscopy in these patients is limited; indeed, this approach would be considered only in the rare event that ureteroscopic examination was not possible (e.g., patient with a cross-trigonal reimplantation) or was unsatisfactory (i.e., inability to closely examine the lower-pole calyces in the face of an otherwise negative examination).

Technique

Diagnostic ureteroscopy is performed routinely under intravenous sedation, thereby eliminating the more morbid effects and prolonged recovery time incurred by general or spinal anesthesia (368). The patient's urine culture must be sterile. In examining the upper urinary tract in a patient with lateralizing hematuria, it is essential that the examiner visualize each area of the ureter and renal collecting system *before it is traumatized by a guidewire or other blindly passed instrument.* Accordingly, the procedure is begun by examining the distal ureter with a short, rigid, less than 7-Fr ureteroscope. This endoscope is introduced directly into the affected ureteral orifice and slowly advanced up the distal ureter, being certain to visualize the full circumference of the ureteral lumen. The irrigant pressure is kept at or below 40 cm H_2O. At this point, no guidewire has been passed into the ureter. (In rare cases, it may be necessary to extend a 2- to 3-cm length of guidewire from the end of the ureteroscope to help open the ureteral orifice and to serve as a guide for the passage of the ureteroscope. However, this is done under direct endoscopic, not fluoroscopic, monitoring. Again, the goal is to see each area of the ureter before it is manipulated.)

The rigid endoscope is passed as far up the ureter as possible. However, if passage of the endoscope becomes difficult, a guidewire is introduced. The guidewire is passed only to the most proximal point of ureteroscopic examination. Under fluoroscopic control, the rigid ureteroscope is withdrawn; during this time, the examiner's eyes should be focused on the tip of the guidewire to make certain that while withdrawing the ureteroscope the guidewire is not inadvertently advanced up the ureter. A less than 10-Fr, or

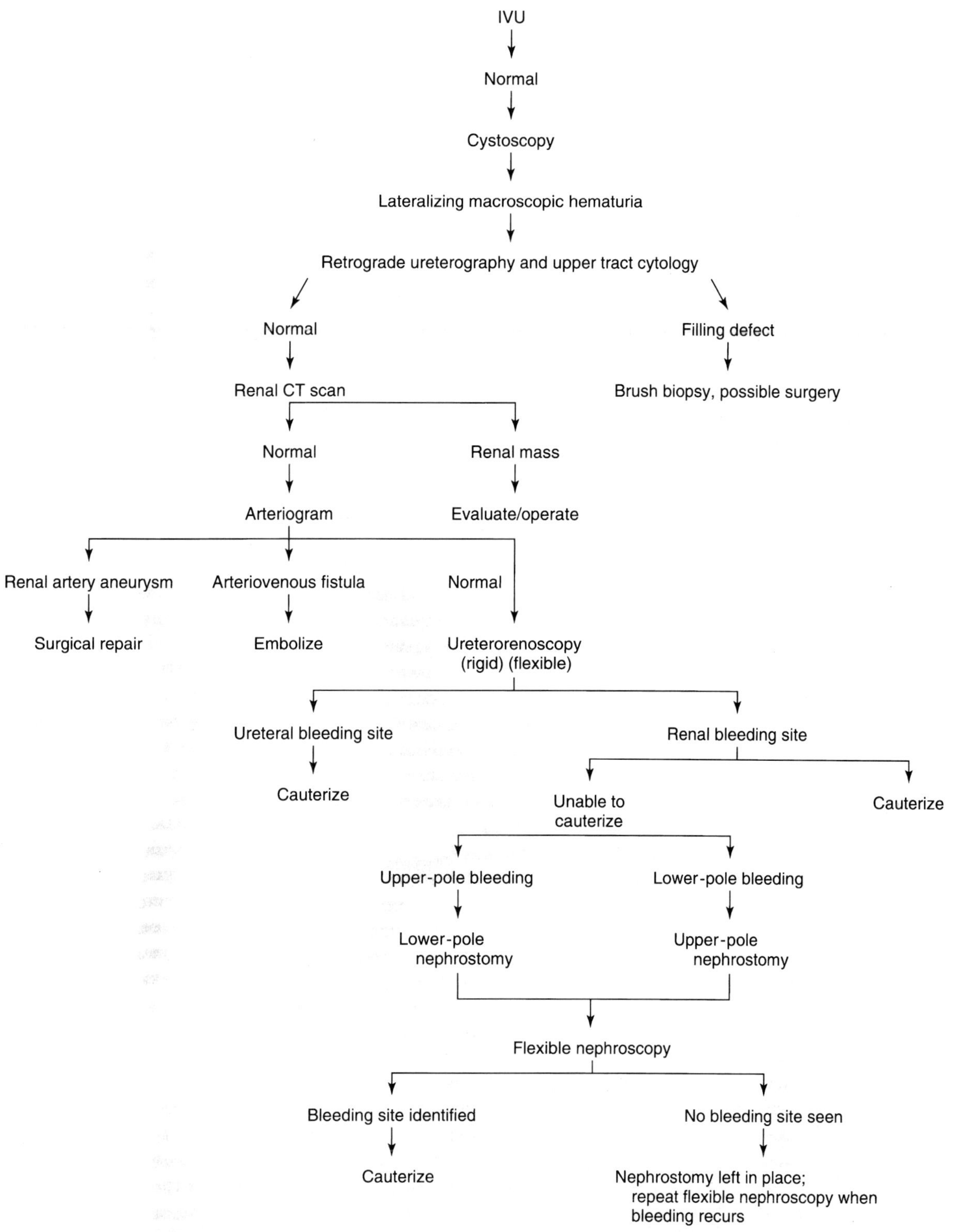

FIGURE 19.1. Lateralizing essential hematuria: evaluation. CT, computed tomography; IVU, intravenous urography. (From McMurtry JM, Clayman RV, Perminger GM. Endourologic diagnosis and treatment of essential hematuria. *J Endourol* 1987;1:145, with permission.)

preferably less than 8-Fr, flexible ureteroscope is introduced over the solitary guidewire; the flexible ureteroscope is passed up to the point where the rigid ureteroscopic evaluation of the ureter ended (121). The guidewire is removed and the proximal portion of the ureter is examined carefully with the flexible ureteroscope up to the ureteropelvic junction.

Now the previously obtained IVU is examined carefully and each calyx is numbered. The endoscopist then proceeds to examine the renal pelvis, upper-pole calyces, middle calyces, and lower-pole calyces in sequence (Fig. 19.2A to C). Adhering to this sequence precludes the creation of iatrogenic lesions (i.e., bruising) along the os of the upper-pole infundibulum during flexion of the endoscope into the lower pole. As each calyx is entered, a small amount of dilute contrast is injected through the endoscope to determine the exact location of the endoscope; the assigned number of the entered calyx is then checked off. It is important to use minimum pressure on the irrigant flow during the ureterorenoscopic procedure (less than 40 mm Hg). Also, aspirating the upper collecting system through the flexible ureteroscope will reduce the volume of fluid and pressure within the upper collecting system and may help identify an area of venous bleeding. Any obvious lesion, such as a hemangioma, is treated directly with either neodymium:yttrium-aluminum-garnet (Nd:YAG) laser or electrocautery (via a 2-Fr electrode) (Fig. 19.2D); similarly, if a small tumor is noted, it is biopsied and then fulgurated.

After completely examining the collecting system, a guidewire is passed through the ureteroscope, and the ureteroscope is withdrawn. A 5- to 7-Fr indwelling ureteral stent is then placed, and the bladder is drained. The patient usually can be discharged on the same day (376). The stent is removed 3 days later in the office. Oral antibiotic coverage is given preoperatively and for 4 days after the procedure.

Results

Successful examination of the entire collecting system with the previously described approach is high. Bagley (12) noted that with a small (8.5-Fr), flexible ureteroscope, equipped with both primary and secondary deflection, the intrarenal collecting system could be examined satisfactorily in 92% of patients. The most difficult area to examine was invariably the lower-pole calyces.

Among patients coming to ureteroscopy for lateralizing hematuria of undetermined origin, approximately 50% are found to have a discrete vascular lesion that can be fulgurated. These vascular lesions (i.e., hemangioma or arteriovenous malformation) appear to be equally distributed throughout the kidney. Coagulation of the lesion results in an immediate successful outcome in more than 90% of patients; however, follow-up data at only 7 months reveals rebleeding in 12% of "successfully" treated individuals. This is not overly surprising given the finding that 12% of renal hemangiomas are multiple, thus implying that although the hemangioma that was bleeding may have been treated at the initial ureteroscopic session, a smaller, nonbleeding lesion may have been missed only to bleed at a later date (181). Nakada and colleagues (259) reported an average 58-month follow-up in 17 patients undergoing flexible ureteroscopy and intrarenal ureteroscopic therapy for lateralizing essential hematuria. Among 11 patients with a discrete lesion, only 18% subsequently rebled; however, for patients in whom no pathology or multiple bleeding sites were noted, the recurrence of hematuria was high (83%) (Table 19.1).

In 5% to 10% of patients, despite a completely negative cytology and unremarkable radiologic evaluation, a renal calculus or small, upper tract transitional cell cancer will be detected. This usually can be treated at the same time as the diagnostic ureteroscopy, using ureteroscopic lithotripsy or electrical or laser lithotripsy, respectively (12,13,189,210, 259,353) (Table 19.1).

In the remaining patients, multiple, putative sites of bleeding are noted; in these patients, the success rate of *in situ* endoscopic electrocoagulation is less effective. As an alternative, intrarenal instillation or systemic therapy may be attempted. Bahnson (17) reported instilling 10 mL of

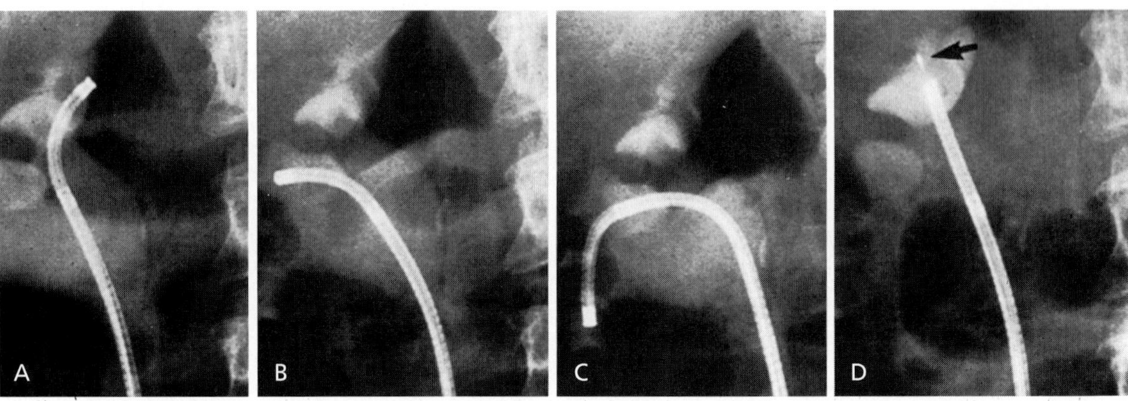

FIGURE 19.2. A–C: Flexible uteroscope examining collecting system of adult female patient with essential hematuria. **D:** Vascular lesion was identified and fulgurated with a 3-Fr electrosurgery probe *(arrow)*.

TABLE 19.1. ESSENTIAL HEMATURIA: DIAGNOSIS AND TREATMENT

			Unilateral Diagnosis								
Authors	No. of Patients	Method of Nephrostomy	Ureteroscopy	Discrete Vascular Abnormality	Diffuse Vascular Abnormality	Stone	Tumor	No Diagnosis	Treatment	Rebleeding	Average Mean Follow-up Range (mo)
Gittes and Varady (115)	12	Operative (12)	None	5	7	0	0	0	Nephrectomy (1) Partial nephrectomy (11)	None	—
Patterson et al. (285)	4	Percutaneous (3)	Rigid (4)	1	3	0	0	0	Fulguration (4) Nephroscope (3) Ureteroscope (1)	None	5 (2–10)
McMurtry et al. (241)	8	Percutaneous (7)	Right (2) Flexible (1)	4	3	1	0	0	Fulguration (8) Nephroscope (7) Ureteroscope (1)	25% (4–6 mo)	6 (2–41)
Kavoussi et al. (181)	8	None	Flexible (6)	Not specified		0	0	0	Fulguration (6) Ureteroscope (6)	12% (7 mo)	11 (7–18)
Bagley and Allen (13)	32	None	Flexible (30)	14	9	1	1	5	Fulguration (16) Nephroureterectomy (1) Stone removal (1)	Discrete: 8% (1 of 12) Diffuse: 100% (4 of 4)	—
Kumon et al. (210)	12	None	Flexible (12)	9	1	0	0	2	Fulguration (9)	None	10.3 (6–21)
Nakada et al. (259)	17	None	Flexible (17)	10	2	1	1	3	Fulguration (11)	Discrete: 18% (2 of 11) Diffuse: 83% (5 of 6)	58 (24–103)
Tawfiek and Bagley (353)	23	None	Flexible (23)	11	2	2	3	5	Nephroureterectomy (1) Fulguration (16) Stone removal (1)	Discrete: 0 Diffuse: 20% (1 of 5)	8 (4–18)
Summary	**116**			**47%**	**23%**	**4%**	**4%**	**13%**		**Discrete: 12%** **Diffuse: 40%**	

1% silver nitrate into the renal pelvis via a retrograde ureteral catheter in three patients with lateralizing hematuria caused by sickle cell hemoglobinopathy; in all three patients, the bleeding ceased after one or two instillations. During an average follow-up of 13 months, no rebleeding was reported. Likewise, Stefanini and associates (342) noted that oral epsilon aminocaproic acid at a daily dose of 150 mg/kg divided into four 6-hour intervals, given for up to 3 weeks, appeared to control hematuria in the short term in four patients with upper tract hematuria caused by tumor or trauma.

Renal Mass

An endoscopic approach to a renal mass is rarely necessary. Modern imaging modalities, including US, computed tomography (CT), and magnetic resonance imaging (MRI), largely have supplanted the need to obtain a confirmatory tissue diagnosis.

All renal masses can be separated into three broad categories: cystic, solid, and indeterminant. The vast majority of renal masses are simple cysts. Renal US can definitively diagnose a renal cyst provided the lesion fulfills the diagnostic criteria of being anechoic at high and low gain and has a strong posterior wall. Similarly, CT criteria for a cyst are likewise reliable: a thin-walled lesion with a homogenous interior of low density [i.e., 0 Hounsfield units (HU)] is invariably a simple renal cyst (Fig. 19.3). If these criteria are not met, the lesion is considered indeterminant and further diagnostic studies are indicated.

For solid, noncystic lesions, the CT or MRI study is essential. One advantage of MRI is in the patient with renal insufficiency or a contrast allergy; in these patients the gadolinium-enhanced scan is of particular value (204,325). For the diagnosis of a solid lesion, the key point is to determine whether there is any fat within the lesion. If fat is found within the lesion, an angiomyolipoma is probably present; a solid lesion without any fat is more likely a renal cell cancer. The former, if smaller than 3.5 to 4 cm and asymptomatic, can be followed, whereas the diagnosis of a renal cell cancer leads to surgical ablation (269,363) (Fig. 19.4).

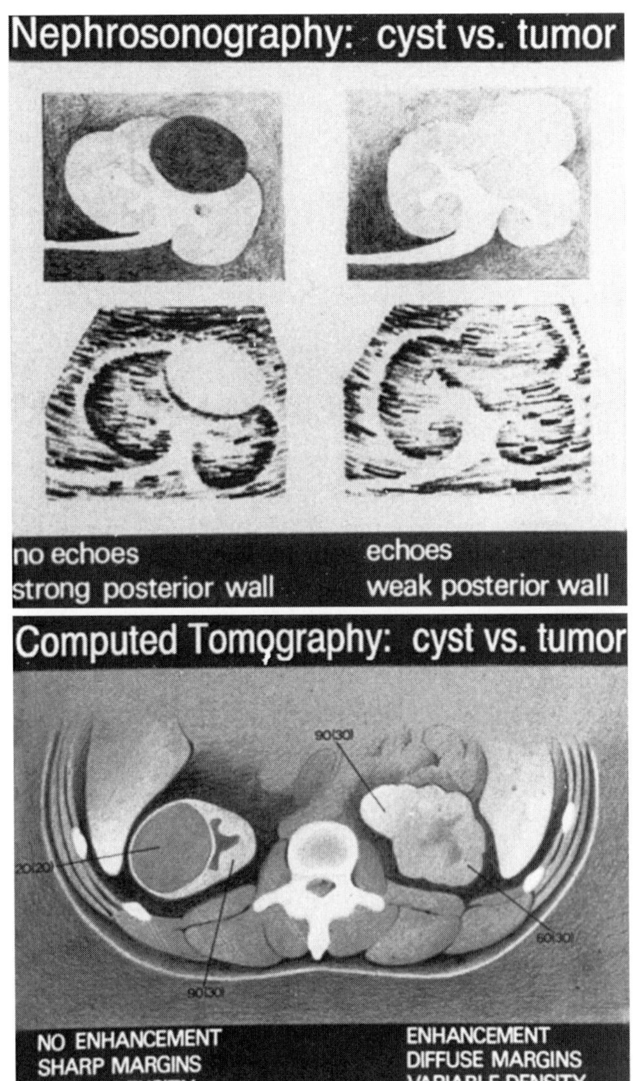

FIGURE 19.3. A: Characteristics of cystic *(left side)* and solid tumorous *(right side)* renal mass as each would appear on a renal ultrasound study. **B:** Characteristics of a cystic *(left side)* and tumor-bearing *(right side)* kidney as each would appear on a computed tomogram study. Numbers refer to Hounsfield units with and without *(in parentheses)* intravenous contrast administration.

Technique

Only in the case of an indeterminant lesion or a solid lesion in a patient with a known cancer (i.e., differential diagnosis of primary renal cancer versus a metastatic lesion) does it behoove the urologist to seek a more definitive diagnosis. In this regard, a US- or CT-guided puncture or biopsy of the lesion is indicated. If the contents are fluid, cytology, culture, and electrolytes can be obtained on the specimen; however, if the lesion has a solid component, an aspiration or needle biopsy can be obtained.

Needle biopsy of a renal lesion may be done either percutaneously or via a transrenal approach. The percutaneous approach to renal biopsy is by far the better-known procedure, having been used since 1950. The Vim Silverman needle and Tru-Cut needle have been the mainstays of percutaneous renal biopsy; however, recent advances in biopsy guns have provided the physician with much smaller 18-gauge, spring-loaded systems, which can be accurately guided to the lesion under US or CT imaging.

Leal (219) has described a transurethral, transrenal approach to renal biopsy. Using a torque control guidewire and 5- and 8-Fr catheters, the calyx closest to the parenchymal mass is accessed. The guidewire is pushed into the mass and the 8-Fr catheter is then advanced into the mass. The guidewire and 5-Fr catheters are removed, and aspiration is applied to the end of the 8-Fr catheter during fluoroscopic imaging. The 8-Fr catheter is then removed and the plug of tissue is flushed out and sent for histologic evaluation; an indwelling ureteral stent is placed.

If all of these methods fail to yield a definitive diagnosis, a retroperitoneal laparoscopic or open approach may be necessary, at which time both a diagnostic biopsy and definitive therapy can be accomplished (Fig. 19.4) (53).

Results

Overall, the vast majority of incidentally discovered renal masses are cysts. A simple renal cyst is identified during abdominal CT in 25% to 33% of patients more than 50 years of age. In contrast, Tosaka and colleagues (359) noted

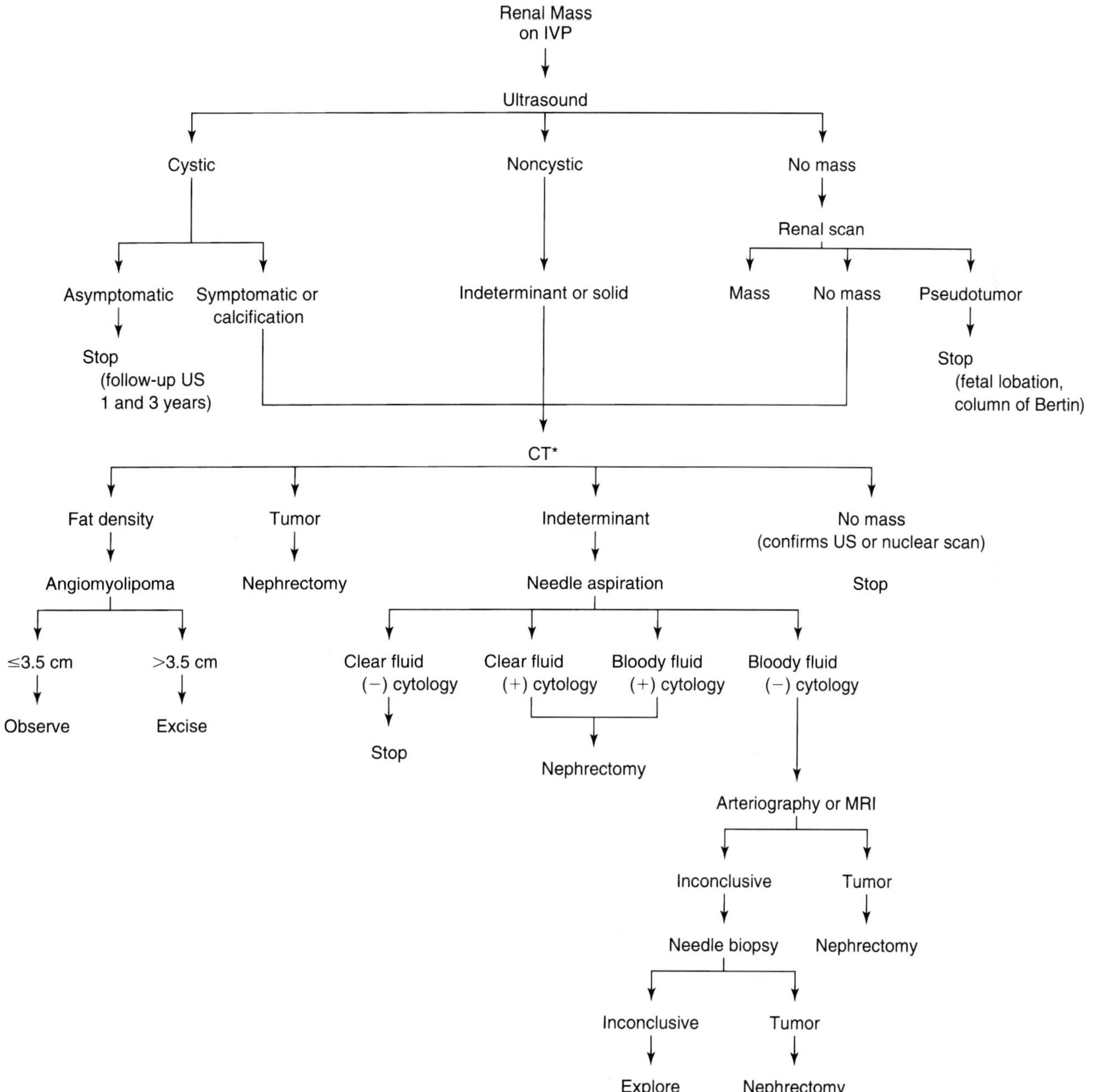

FIGURE 19.4. Diagnosis of renal cell cancer. CT, computed tomography; IVP, intravenous pyelogram; MRI, magnetic resonance imaging; US, ultrasound. (*If contrast allergy or renal insufficiency, substitute MRI for CT scan.)

that among 46,000 adults undergoing US screening for renal masses, a mass was noted in only 1%. Among these masses, two-thirds proved to be a normal renal variant; cystic lesions (23%) greatly outnumbered renal cancers (5.4%). However, when the patient has a renal mass in association with macroscopic hematuria, flank pain, or a palpable flank mass, the chance of a renal cell cancer being present exceeds 50% (53). Other renal masses, specifically angiomyolipoma, renal pelvic tumors, and other benign lesions, are all relatively uncommon, accounting for approximately 5% of all renal masses among asymptomatic patients (359,363).

Complications from percutaneous renal biopsy with the larger 14-gauge needles occurred in 2% to 11% of patients; however, most of these problems were of a minor nature. The nephrectomy rate from renal biopsy is 0.06%, with a mortality rate of 0.08%. However, the advent of 18-gauge biopsy needles has resulted in the apparent elimination of major complications such as death or nephrectomies in some series; minor complications occur in only 5% (predominantly symptomatic perirenal hematoma or hematuria). The improved safety margin of this approach now has made it feasible to pursue a percutaneous biopsy even in the case of a solitary kidney (79,81,320).

Concerns about possible postbiopsy seeding of the needle tract are not sufficient to alter the course from percutaneous biopsy to renal exploration. Reported cases of seeding of the needle tract are few and are usually associated with unusual circumstances, such as multiple biopsies of a lesion over time, the use of large needles, or other extenuating circumstances (112,222,369).

Although the intrarenal biopsy method is of interest, it has been used successfully in only three patients, according to Leal's original report. Subsequent information has yet to be published. There is no information regarding complications from this approach. Overall, it remains significantly more invasive than currently available percutaneous biopsy techniques and thus would be of greatest value in those few patients in whom a percutaneous approach was unsuccessful or not feasible (e.g., massive obesity).

Diagnosis of Filling Defects Within the Upper Urinary Tract

As with the evaluation of a renal mass, the workup of the patient with a filling defect in the upper urinary tract should proceed in an orderly fashion from less invasive to more invasive studies. The patient's prior history and a fresh urinalysis with urine cytology and urine culture can help steer the clinician toward the correct diagnosis from the outset (Fig. 19.5). As such, patients with a history of stone disease or transitional cell cancer of the bladder are immediately suspect for similar upper tract conditions. Likewise, individuals with a history of diabetes, recurrent upper tract infections, analgesic abuse, or sickle cell disease may have papillary necrosis or an associated blood clot. Patients with a history of inflammatory bowel disease are at risk for developing a filling defect because of the presence of air in the collecting system from a ureteroenteric fistula. In addition, a long-term history of *Escherichia coli* urinary tract infection can be associated with malakoplakia or, in the diabetic patient, with emphysematous pyelonephritis. Pneumaturia may similarly indicate a fistulous bowel communication with the upper or, more commonly, lower urinary tract.

A complete urinalysis, performed by the urologist, is essential (Fig. 19.5). If the urine pH is above 6.5, the likelihood of a uric acid stone becomes remote. The presence of a significant amount of hematuria may indicate that the filling defect is secondary to a blood clot. A urine sample sent for cytology can be helpful if it is positive for malignant cells; however, the accuracy of this test is highly dependent on the skill of the cytologist. In one report, a false-positive cytology was noted in 17% of patients, and false-negative cytologies ranged from 10% to 80%, depending on the grade of the tumor (16,71,242,310,322). The urine culture also is helpful; the presence of fungi may indicate a fungal ball, whereas the presence of mixed aerobic and anaerobic bacteria would indicate a ureteroenteric fistula.

The next step in the diagnostic evaluation of a filling defect discovered on intravenous urography is either US or CT (Fig. 19.5) (301). US is safe, is relatively inexpensive, and has the ability to clearly show a larger stone because of its characteristic acoustic shadowing; however, the resolution of US is not as reliable as CT scanning (74). In Bagley's series, US evaluation of 14 patients with an upper tract filling defect failed to image 5 of 6 tumors and 4 of 4 stones. In contrast, CT imaged 57% of the stones (4 of 7) and 36% (5 of 14) of the transitional cell tumors (16).

When a stone is definitively identified, urinary alkalinization, high fluid intake, and if hyperuricemia is present, the use of a xanthine oxidase inhibitor are indicated (74). This should result in dissolution of the presumably uric acid stone within weeks to months. If, on subsequent radiographic studies, the stone persists unchanged in size, extracorporeal shock wave lithotripsy (ESWL) can be undertaken. Failing ESWL, a ureteroscopic or percutaneous approach is the next step.

When despite these studies the lesion remains indeterminant, retrograde ureterography and ureteroscopy are the next steps (Fig. 19.6). Even in the face of a positive cytology, given the 17% false-positive cytology rate in Bagley's series, a strong case can still be made for proceeding with diagnostic ureteroscopy and biopsy (16).

Technique

In the past decade, the diameter of the rigid ureteroscope has decreased rapidly from 12.5 Fr to only 6 to 7 Fr; these diminutive endoscopes still contain working channels in the 3- to 4-Fr range. Their small size enables the urologist to

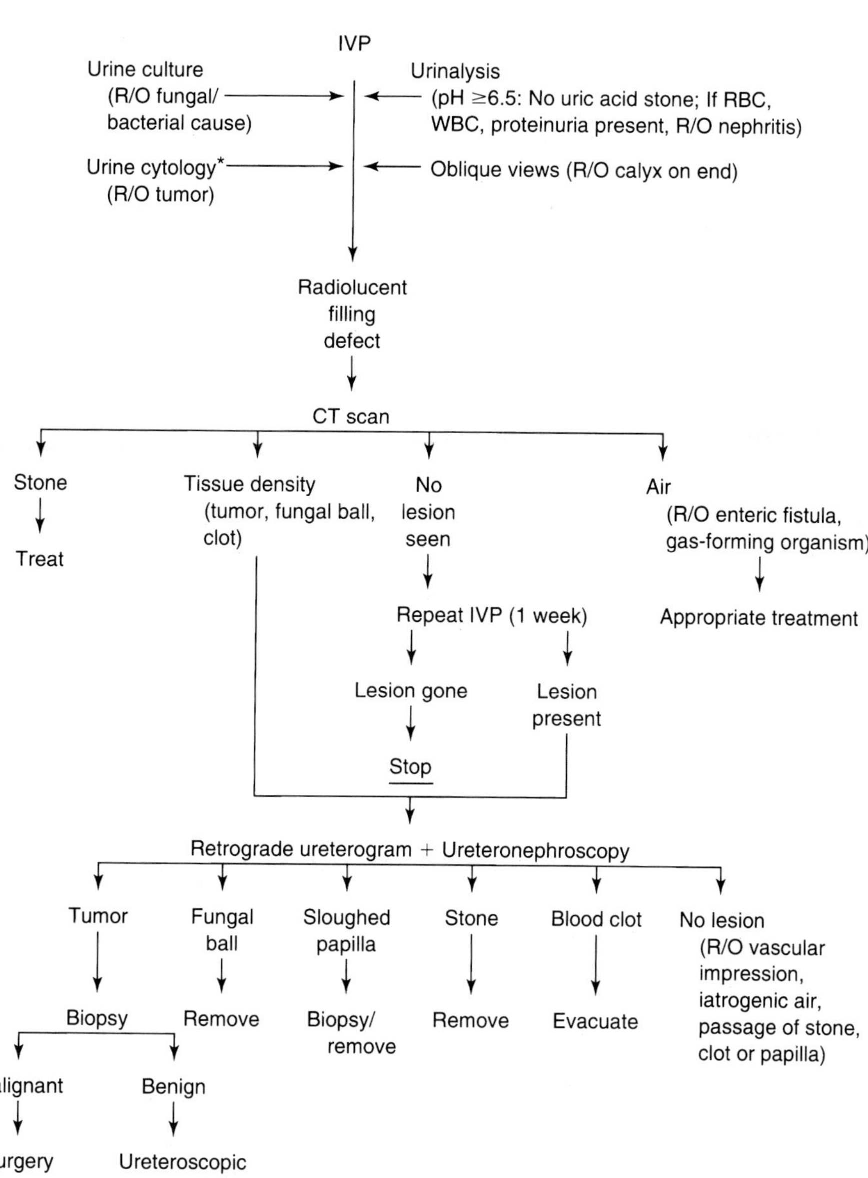

FIGURE 19.5. Radiolucent filling defect in the upper urinary tract: evaluation. CT, computed tomography; IVP, intravenous pyelogram; RBC, red blood cell; R/O, rule out; WBC, white blood cell. (*With a positive urine cytology, sterile urine, and a soft-tissue filling defect, a surgical procedure—that is, ureteroscopic confirmation versus surgical ablation—for suspected transitional cell carcinoma is reasonable.) (Modified from Resnick MI. Radiolucent filling defects. In: Resnick ME et al, eds. *Decision making in urology.* St Louis: Mosby, 1985:18, with permission.)

perform ureteroscopy without the need to dilate the distal ureter. However, although these semirigid endoscopes can usually traverse the entire length of the ureter in the female, manipulation over the iliac vessels in the male may be difficult. As such, for upper ureteral lesions in the male or for lesions located in the renal collecting system, flexible ureteroscopy is necessary.

Like their rigid counterpart, the flexible endoscopes have undergone a significant decrease in size over the last 10 years, from 13 to 7.5 Fr. The latter endoscope still has a 3.6-Fr channel; thus it can usually be passed up the ureter without ureteral dilation and yet allows the urologist the ability to use a full range of instruments, including biopsy forceps, electrosurgical probes, and laser fibers. In addition, these endoscopes have an actively deflectable tip mobility of 170 degrees and passive secondary deflection, thereby facilitating their introduction into the lower-pole calyces (121). Also of interest are reports of even more diminutive, 2-Fr diagnostic passive flexible videoureteronephroscopes that can be passed through a 6-Fr guide tube to provide both vision and a 3-Fr working channel (380). However, experience with these endoscopes is limited.

Unlike in the case of lateralizing essential hematuria, the patient with a filling defect in the collecting system provides the endoscopist with an identifiable target. The endoscopist can approach the site of interest directly; however, in patients with suspected transitional cell cancer or stone, a systematic examination of the entire collecting system is still indicated to rule out other sites of stone or tumor growth. The normal saline irrigating fluid is kept at 75 mm Hg or less to prevent pyelovenous or pyelosinous backflow. Only when the biopsy forceps or a stone basket is in the endoscope's channel is the irrigant pressure increased to maintain flow (i.e., 150 mm Hg). As soon as the instrument is withdrawn, the irrigant pressure is lowered to 75 mm Hg.

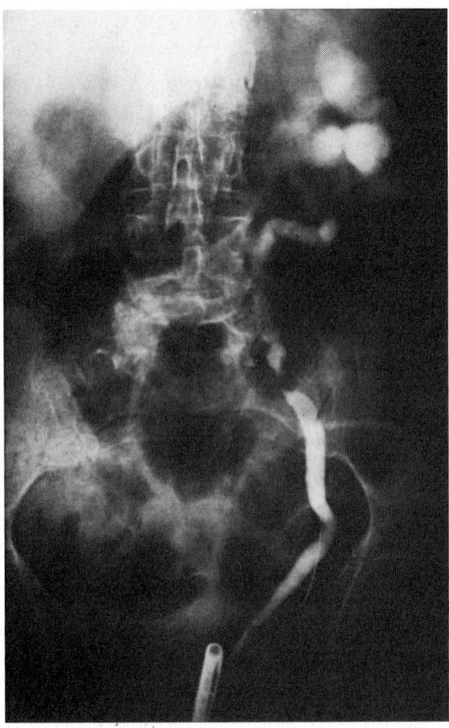

FIGURE 19.6. Retrograde uterogram reveals a midureteral filling defect with associated obstruction. The patient had macroscopic hematuria. Subsequent uteroscopy and biopsy established the diagnosis of a high-grade transitional cell cancer of the ureter.

After the ureter and renal collecting system are fully examined, the lesion can be addressed directly. If it is a stone, intracorporeal lithotripsy with a holmium : yttrium-aluminum-garnet (Ho : YAG) laser or a 1.9-Fr electrohydraulic lithotripsy probe through the flexible ureteroscope, or laser, electrohydraulic, ultrasonic, or pneumatic lithotripsy via the rigid ureteroscope, can be accomplished. If a cystic lesion is found, a biopsy can be obtained and the lesion unroofed and fulgurated (Fig. 19.7). If a tumor is discovered and a flexible ureteroscope is being used, the ureteroscope can be removed and an 8-Fr catheter and 10-Fr sheath can be introduced into the ureter. After withdrawing the 8-Fr catheter, a second guidewire is placed in the upper urinary tract. The 10-Fr sheath can then be replaced with a ureteral access sheath. This is passed over one of the guidewires, the dilator is removed, and the 12- or 14-Fr sheath is left in place. As such, when the ureteroscope is withdrawn during the biopsy process, the sheath maintains access to the ureter so the ureteroscope can be returned easily to the site of the lesion. If a rigid ureteroscope is being used, an access sheath is usually not placed.

When a suspected transitional cell tumor is viewed ureteroscopically, cytology samples are obtained immediately before any biopsies and just after the biopsy procedure via a saline irrigation directly in front of the lesion (186). Next, at least four to five biopsies are obtained. To do this, a 3-Fr biopsy forceps or a diminutive stone basket is passed. In the former instance, the opened biopsy jaws are advanced deep into the lesion; the jaws are then closed and withdrawn from the lesion by pulling the entire endoscope caudal (Fig. 19.8). Thus a larger piece of tissue may be obtained than if the closed biopsy forceps were pulled into the working channel, thereby shearing off the specimen. Alternatively, a stone basket may be opened at the site of the lesion and

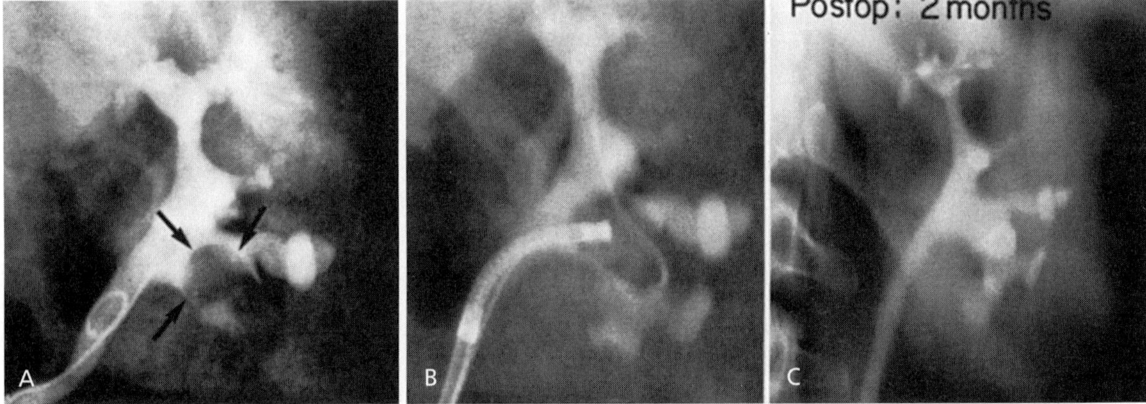

FIGURE 19.7. A: Filling defect *(arrows)* previously identified on an intravenous urogram is clearly delineated on this retrograde ureterogram. A guidewire has been passed up the ureter in preparation for introduction of the flexible ureteroscope. **B:** Via the flexible ureteroscope, a biopsy of the lesion was taken. It was found to be a benign cyst; accordingly, an electrosurgical probe was passed through the ureteroscope and the interior of the cyst was fulgurated. **C:** Two months later a follow-up intravenous urogram reveals no recurrence of the cyst.

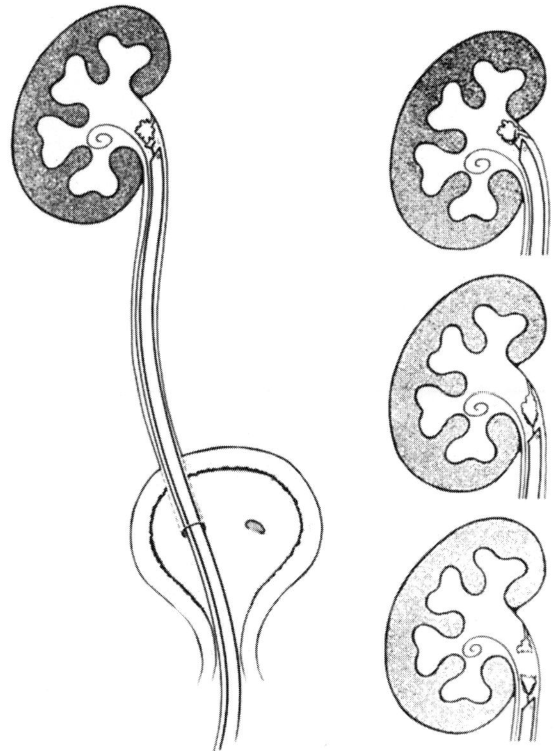

FIGURE 19.8. A 3-Fr biopsy forceps has been passed through the flexible ureteroscope in preparation for biopsying a papillary tumor. Once the jaws have been secured on the tumor, the entire endoscope with the biopsy forceps extended is pulled out of the ureter and urethra, thereby removing a large piece of the tumor. Note that a safety guidewire remains in the ureter. If the forceps is pulled into the endoscope, pieces of the tumor may be sheared off, thereby rendering the specimen too small for diagnostic purposes. Alternatively, a stone basket can be used to trap and avulse the tumor, thereby providing a large specimen for histologic analysis. (From Clayman RV, Kavousi LR. Endosurgical techniques for noncalculous disease. In: Walsh PC et al, eds. *Campbell's urology,* ed 6. Philadelphia: Saunders, 1992:2254, with permission.)

twirled into the lesion, thus entrapping a large amount of tissue; as the basket is twisted amidst the papillary fronds, tissue is detached and trapped on the wires of the basket. The partially closed basket and endoscope are then withdrawn as a unit, again to preclude shearing tissue from the basket. In Bagley's experience, the use of a biopsy forceps or stone basket produced equivalent results with regard to obtaining a definitive diagnosis, 68% to 76% (186).

Two of the biopsies can be sent for cytologic analysis, and the remaining biopsies are sent for routine histologic analysis. It is also helpful to have the pathologist come to the operating room so that the pathologist can appreciate the intact appearance of the lesion; this can be invaluable during the pathologist's subsequent histologic assessment of the diminutive biopsy specimens.

Following the procedure, an indwelling ureteral stent usually is placed; the stent is removed in the office 3 days later. Most of these procedures are completed on an outpatient basis under intravenous sedation. Antibiotic coverage may be given immediately before the procedure and continued orally for 4 days after the procedure.

With regard to antegrade nephroscopy via a percutaneous tract, this is a less desirable means for accessing the upper urinary tract, especially in the patient with a suspected transitional cell cancer. It is far more invasive and morbid than ureteroscopy and does not provide any more information than a ureteroscopic examination (282). As such, antegrade nephroscopy would be used only in the rare instance in which an upper tract lesion could not be visualized adequately, biopsied, or treated through the ureteroscope. In this regard, the nephrostomy tract is positioned as far from the lesion as possible while still remaining on a fairly direct line with the lesion. Accordingly, if the lesion is in the ureter, an upper-pole or middle-posterior-calyceal approach is chosen; however, if the lesion is in the kidney, a remote calyx is selected as long as the surgeon will still be provided with a sufficiently direct route to the tumor such that rigid endoscopic equipment can be used. In addition, concerns over seeding the nephrostomy tract from an unsuspected transitional cell cancer remain a valid albeit unlikely consideration. There has been only one report of such an occurrence (147).

Results

For the most part, the actively deflectable ureteroscopes are preferred to their passive cousins because they allow reliable access to most lesions and permit the examiner to perform a more complete examination of the entire collecting system. Endoscopes smaller than 7.5 Fr have been used usually for diagnostic purposes; these diminutive passive endoscopes are as small as 2 Fr. However, considerably more skill and patience are necessary. Nonetheless, Yoshida and colleagues (380) were able to obtain diagnostic information in 87% of their patients using a 2-Fr passive endoscope, positioned through a 6-Fr guide tube.

Among patients coming to ureteroscopy, a transitional cell cancer is diagnosed in 16% to 40%, and a stone is noted in 18% to 44% (121,181,295). The other common finding is that of a vascular impression or essentially normal urothelium in 16% to 24% (16,181). Less common diagnoses are blood clot, papillary necrosis, fibroepithelial polyp, inverted papilloma, intrarenal cyst, pyelitis cystica, "eccentric" papilla, fungal ball, submucosal hemorrhage, air, and malakoplakia (Table 19.2). In addition, on rare occasions, a renal cell cancer may produce a filling defect in the collecting system without a significant accompanying mass effect in the renal parenchyma (123).

Obstruction of the Upper Urinary Tract

In evaluating the patient with upper urinary tract obstruction, the urologist needs to determine both the functional significance and the cause of the obstruction.

TABLE 19.2. RADIOLUCENT FILLING DEFECTS IN THE UPPER URINARY TRACT: DIFFERENTIAL DIAGNOSIS

	Diagnosis
Common Entities	
Tumor	Transitional cell carcinoma
Urolithiasis	Uric acid calculi
Blood clot	Trauma/tumor
Air	Iatrogenic (retrograde ureterogram)
Infection/ inflammation	Papillary necrosis Fungal ball
Uncommon Causes	
Tumors	Leukemic infiltrate Angiomyolipoma Multiple myeloma Lymphoma Wilms' tumors Renal cell carcinoma Cysts Fibroepithelial polyp Squamous cell carcinoma Adenocarcinoma Leukoplakia Amyloid Sarcoma Connective-tissue tumors Metastatic tumors
Urolithiasis	Matrix Xanthine Indinavir
Blood clot	Coagulopathy Nephritis Anticoagulants
Air	Enteric fistula Gas-forming organism
Congenital	Vessel crossing Ectopic papilla End-on-calyx
Vascular	Renal artery aneurysm Vascular impression (vessel crossing renal pelvis/upper pole infundibulum, lower pole vessel, ovarian vein) Arteriovenous fistula
Infection/ inflammation	Pyelitis cystica Ureteritis cystica Tuberculosis Malacoplakia Helminths Fistula
Foreign body	Iatrogenic

From Clayman RV, Lange PH, Fraley EE. Transitional cell cancer of the upper urinary tract. In: Javadpour N, ed. *Principles and management of urologic cancer,* ed 2. Baltimore: Williams & Wilkins, 1983, with permission.

The diagnosis of functional obstruction is of primary importance because this, along with the patient's symptoms, helps determine whether the obstruction requires therapeutic intervention. In general, abnormal dilation of the upper urinary tract is initially diagnosed by renal US or intravenous urography. However, the presence of dilation does not mean that there is obstruction (e.g., congenital megacalycosis). Likewise, the presence of dilation may occur in the face of either functionally insignificant narrowing or longstanding obstruction to which the kidney has accommodated, such that the renal pelvis pressure is low and the threat to renal function is nil. Radiographic studies, such as retrograde ureterography or antegrade nephrostogram, provide only anatomic, not functional, information.

As such, once hydronephrosis is noted, the next and most important step is to determine if there is any functional impact. Today, urologists have three studies available to define the significance of narrowing in the upper urinary tract: duplex Doppler renal US, Lasix washout renal nuclear scan, and the antegrade pressure-flow study (i.e., Whitaker test). Of these, the simplest study is duplex Doppler renal US. In this study, an external Doppler US probe is used to determine peak systolic and end-diastolic velocity over the renal interlobar and arcuate arteries. The *resistive index* (RI) is defined as peak systolic velocity minus end-diastolic velocity, divided by the peak systolic velocity. In the face of functionally significant obstruction, the peak systolic velocity is blunted, and thus the RI rises. In general, a RI above 0.75 and a difference in resistive indices of 0.10 or more between the two kidneys is believed to be consistent with functionally significant obstruction. Values between 0.70 and 0.75 with a differential that is greater than 0.05 are equivocal (i.e., gray zone) (275,303,354). In these indeterminate cases, the administration of a diuretic followed by repeat determination of the resistive indices may help classify more accurately the nature of the obstruction (275). Resistive indexes less than 0.70 with a differential of less than 0.05 are normal. Using these parameters, Gilbert and co-workers (113) noted that the results with duplex Doppler renal US were similar to diuretic renography. Similarly, Rodgers and associates (303) noted that among 20 adults with acute renal colic caused by a ureteric calculus, the RI was elevated in 93%. However, other investigators have shown that renal RI measurements may not be valuable in detecting acute urinary tract obstruction. Older and colleagues (272) demonstrated, in 54 patients evaluated by renal RI, that although the mean RIs of the obstructed and nonobstructed patients were statistically different, the wide overlap of the values for each group precluded clinical usefulness for the individual patient. The sensitivity of RI was only 42%, with 11 false-negative results; specificity of RI for obstruction was 79%.

Diuresis renography is the major study used to determine the presence or absence of functionally significant obstruction; however, the test must be administered properly and a standard protocol must be followed in order to obtain meaningful data. Significant variables include the state of renal function, degree of patient hydration, fullness of the bladder at the time of the study, the amount of diuretic given, the type of radiopharmaceutical used, and the point in the examination when the diuretic is administered (235). In the adult, the diuresis renogram is accomplished using intravenous ^{131}I Hippuran (*o*-iodohippurate), ^{123}I Hippuran, or technetium-99m diethylenetriamine pentaacetic acid (DTPA). Renal imaging is done at 2, 5, 10, 15, and 20 minutes after giving the radionuclide with the patient in a supine position. At the 20-minute point, if it appears that the adult kidney may be obstructed, furosemide (40 mg) is given intravenously. In the normal unobstructed, two-kidney situation, half of the radionuclide tracer should drain from the kidney within 12 minutes. If it takes longer than 20 minutes, the kidney is considered obstructed (Fig. 19.9); results between 12 and 20 minutes are considered to be in a gray zone, and the test is deemed inconclusive. The presence of medical renal disease, renal artery disease, or massive hydronephrosis may blunt the response of the kidney to furosemide or alter the dilution of the excreted radionuclide, thereby resulting in a false-positive study; this occurs in 9% to 30% of diuretic scans. On the other hand, a false-negative diuretic scan is rare; hence, if a normal curve is obtained, the system is probably not obstructed. An equivocal result or suspicion of a false-positive result should lead to performance of a Whitaker perfusion test (vide infra) (231,277,278,349).

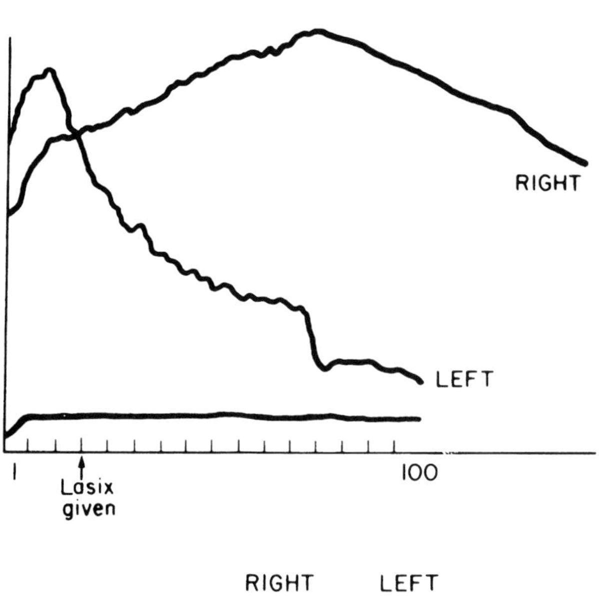

FIGURE 19.9. Lasix washout renogram performed in a patient with an obstructed right kidney. The right kidney shows an abnormal rising curve even before the Lasix is administered. On administration of the Lasix, the normal left kidney clears half of the radionuclide tracer in 6 minutes; however, the obstructed right kidney does not clear half of the tracer until 48 minutes, thus indicating its obstructed status. (From Clayman RV, Kavousi LR. Endosurgical techniques for noncalculous disease. In: Walsh PC et al, eds. *Campbell's urology,* ed 6. Philadelphia: Saunders, 1992:2269, with permission.)

In an effort to obtain more accurate information from diuresis renography, work by the Society for Fetal Urology and the Pediatric Nuclear Medicine Club of the Society of Nuclear Medicine has resulted in development of a standardized regimen for diuresis renography in children; as yet, a similar protocol is not available for adults (58). In the pediatric regimen, the bladder is catheterized; the patient receives intravenous hydration for at least 15 minutes before the study (15 mL/kg per 30 minutes); urine output response to the diuretic is measured; and the diuretic dose is standardized at 1 mg/kg of furosemide. The preferred radionuclide is 99m-technetium mercuroacetylglycylglycylglycine (^{99m}Tc MAG3) because it is rapidly cleared by the kidney and is primarily excreted by the tubules. The percent function of the affected kidney is determined; a half-life is calculated; and a clearance curve is generated. The curves can be divided into one of four groups: normal, obstructed, hypotonic pelvis, and equivocal (277). In general, a normal study would include renal function of 50% plus or minus 10% and a half-life of 10 minutes or less. If the half-life is 10 to 20 minutes, this is considered equivocal for obstruction, and a half-life greater than 20 minutes is compatible with significant obstruction (278,349).

In addition, other investigators have used the data accrued during diuretic renography to calculate a variety of other indicators that at times are useful in uncovering obstruction when the diuresis renogram is otherwise equivocal. These calculations include the normalized renal slope ratio, renal output efficiency, and calculations designed to relate renal volume to the rate of emptying of the collecting system (34,38,382). These other determinations are used to neutralize the two major causes of false-positive renal scans: compromised renal function and a dilated, phlegmatic renal pelvis. With use of these additional calculations, specificity could be increased from 85% to the 94% to 98% range using the normalized renal slope ratio, and accuracy rates of 94% were attained in patients with compromised renal function using the renal output efficiency formula. In another effort to overcome potential problems caused by a dilated system, Rossleigh and co-workers (305) have advocated obtaining an additional view after standard diuresis renography; this view is obtained after the child ambulates for 5 minutes or after the infant has been held upright for 10 to 15 minutes. In examining 12 children suspected of recurrent obstruction after a pyeloplasty; 64% of the postoperative patients who appeared to be obstructed on routine diuresis renography were not obstructed on the gravity-assisted drainage views. However, the gravity-assisted view was helpful in only 1 of 12 patients with suspected obstruction before a surgical procedure; for these children, routine diuresis renography was satisfactory. Upsdell and associates (361) have described giving furosemide 15 minutes before administering the radionuclide (the F-15 renogram); this results in a marked diuresis at the inception of the study. The authors found that this method of performing the renogram resulted in fewer equivocal results.

The Whitaker test is the most invasive means of determining the presence or absence of functionally significant obstruction in the upper urinary tract (374) (Fig. 19.10). This test is done in the interventional radiology area under fluoroscopic control with the patient in a prone position. Usually a 20- or 22-gauge nephrostomy needle or an 8-Fr catheter is percutaneously passed into the collecting system. A Foley catheter is placed in the bladder. Using a three-way stopcock, dilute contrast is infused through the nephrostomy tube until the collecting system is fully distended. Then the flow is increased to 10 mL per minute; pressure readings of the renal pelvis and the bladder are taken at 5-minute intervals until a steady state is reached. If the pressure differential between the renal pelvis and the bladder remains less than 15 cm H_2O, the test is negative for obstruction; if the differential pressure exceeds 22 cm H_2O, the test is considered positive. Differential pressures between 15 and 22 cm H_2O are in the gray zone. For patients with an indeterminate reading, the flow rate can be increased to 15 mL per minute; the differential pressure, once a steady state is reached, should not exceed 18 cm H_2O (262).

In contradistinction to the diuretic renogram, the most common problem with the Whitaker test is that of a false-negative study. This occurs because of inadequate filling of a large floppy renal pelvis, extravasation during the study, recording "final" pressures before a steady state has been reached, and renal intravasation caused by pyelovenous, pyelosinus, or pyelolymphatic backflow. Also, in some patients the UPJ obstruction is of an intermittent nature depending on the patient's position and the amount of urine output at a given point in time. As such, the obstruction actually may be relieved when the patient is lying prone; thus it may be necessary to repeat the Whitaker study with these patients in either a supine or sitting position.

The overall reliability of the Whitaker test is high. Laboratory studies by Ryan and colleagues (306) have confirmed the accuracy of the Whitaker test in detecting

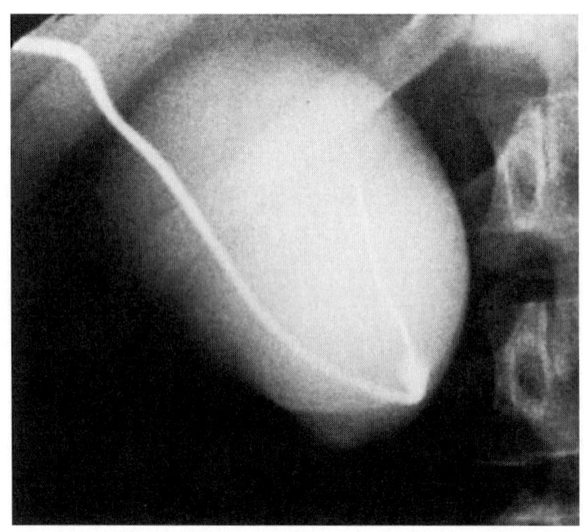
A

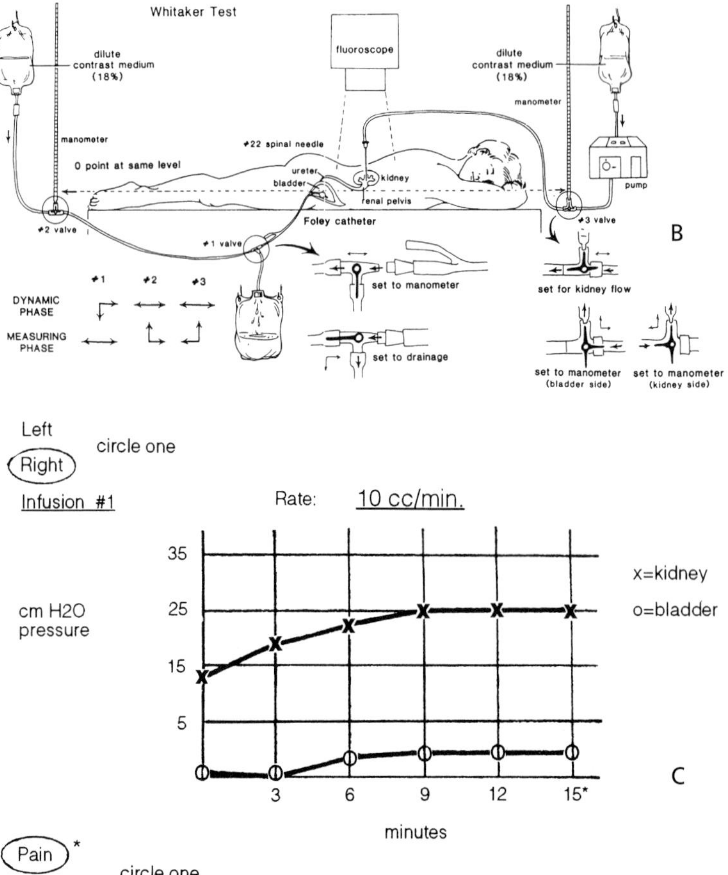

FIGURE 19.10. A: An antegrade nephrostogram reveals a hydronephrotic right kidney secondary to ureteropelvic junction obstruction. **B:** The setup for the Whitaker test consists of a pump to deliver fluid through the nephrostomy cannula, a pressure manometer connected to the nephrostomy cannula, a bladder catheter, and a pressure manometer connected to the bladder catheter. **C:** The values from the Whitaker test are plotted on a graph. In this patient, the pressure differential between the bladder and the kidney is 23 cm; the test indicates that there is a functionally significant obstruction at the ureteropelvic junction. (From Clayman RV, Kavousi LR. Endosurgical techniques for noncalculous disease. In: Walsh PC et al, eds. *Campbell's urology,* ed 6. Philadelphia: Saunders, 1992:2270, with permission.)

functional obstruction in a canine model. Clinically, Bouchot and co-workers (32) reviewed their findings with Whitaker tests and diuretic renograms in 47 children. They noted that the overall accuracy of the Whitaker test was 90.5% among children with hydronephrosis. However, the Whitaker and diuretic renogram studies were *not* in agreement in 43% of the cases. Again, most of the problems were due to false-positive or equivocal renogram curves. Similarly, O'Reilly (277) and Krueger and associates (206) independently noted that in 9% to 30% of cases in which the diuretic renogram was positive, the Whitaker test was negative for obstruction. However, in the same series, the Whitaker test was inaccurate in 15% of patients largely because of a false-negative result. Overall, the most diagnostically reliable situation occurs when both the diuresis renogram and the Whitaker test are positive; this occurs in only 40% to 60% of cases overall.

THERAPEUTIC URETERAL APPLICATIONS

Ureteral Strictures

With respect to ureteral strictures, from an endourologic standpoint, the ureter can be divided into three areas: proximal, middle, and distal. When discussing stricture disease, the proximal and distal portions of the ureter are quite short: the proximal ureter is primarily the few centimeters of the ureter just below the UPJ, and the distal ureter stretches from the ureteral orifice to just above the ureterovesical junction. The middle ureter includes the ureter beginning just below the iliac vessels, crossing the bony pelvis, and the majority of the ureter lying in the soft tissues of the retroperitoneum. The predominant cause of a ureteral stricture is iatrogenic (i.e., ureteroscopy, gynecologic surgery, or ureteral surgery). The distal ureter is most commonly the site of stricture disease.

Endoscopic ureteral dilation was described initially in 1891 by Pawlick, when he used ureteral bougies cystoscopically to dilate strictures secondary to tuberculosis (249). In 1907, Nitze designed a catheter with a terminal inflatable balloon to dilate and occlude the ureter (264). In 1926, Dourmashkin (77,78) dilated the ureter with a series of rubber bags attached to hollow bougies. He regularly dilated ureters up to 20 Fr and, on occasion, up to 30, 46, and 54 Fr, enabling a stone expulsion rate of 68% in his patients. In 1978, Gruntzig (126) reported percutaneous transluminal coronary angioplasty using a dilating catheter with a 3.0- to 3.8-mm balloon at the tip; these balloons were later used to dilate ureteral strictures. The concomitant development of the 9- and 11-Fr ureteroscope by Perez-Castro and Martinez-Pineiro (289) led to a renewed interest by urologists in the endourologic treatment of ureteral strictures. With improved optical capabilities and smaller endourologic instrumentation came the advent of diagnostic biopsy and therapeutic incision of endoscopic ureteral strictures.

Technique

Catheter Dilation

Catheter dilation is performed over a guidewire with multiple tapered, ureteral dilators passed under fluoroscopic control. The 0.035-inch, floppy-tip guidewire is passed into the upper collecting system under fluoroscopic control. The 5-Fr angiographic catheter is passed over the floppy-tip guidewire to secure access to the upper collecting system, and the guidewire is exchanged for an Amplatz superstiff guidewire. The 5-Fr catheter is removed. The ureteral dilators are sequentially passed over the guidewires, progressing from a 5-Fr up to a 14-Fr dilator. Following the dilation, a 7- or 8-Fr ureteral stent is placed for 4 to 6 weeks (378). However, serial, rather than single, ureteral dilations may be necessary for stricture resolution.

Balloon Dilation

Since the introduction of transluminal balloon dilation by Gruntzig in 1978 (126), this concept has been accepted widely by urologic surgeons as a technique to dilate the ureteral orifice and intramural ureter before ureteroscopy. Balloon dilation also has been used in the management of stricture disease.

The technique of balloon dilation of the ureter involves four steps to complete the procedure: (a) access to the upper urinary tract, (b) placement of the dilating balloon catheter, (c) activation of the dilating balloon, and (d) placement of a ureteral stent. Fluoroscopy is essential to each of these steps to ensure appropriate positioning and activation of the dilating balloon catheter.

The patient is positioned in the lithotomy position, usually under general or regional (e.g., spinal or epidural) anesthesia. Cystoscopy is performed and a 0.035-inch Bentson guidewire is introduced into the ureteral orifice. Using fluoroscopic guidance, the surgeon advances the guidewire along the course of the ureter, past the stricture, and positions it with the floppy tip coiled in the renal pelvis.

When the Bentson guidewire will not traverse past the stricture, a Terumo guidewire may be used. The lubricated, hydrophilic polymer coating of this guidewire greatly facilitates its passage through the narrowest ureteral stricture. It is essential to keep the surface of this guidewire constantly moistened with water or saline to achieve the maximum reduction of surface friction. However, because of its slippery nature, once positioned in the upper collecting system this guidewire can fall out easily. Therefore, once this guidewire has been passed, a 5-Fr angiographic catheter is passed over it. The Terumo guidewire is exchanged for a 0.035-inch Bentson or a 0.035-inch Amplatz superstiff guidewire. The 5-Fr angiographic catheter is then removed, leaving the stiffer guidewire in position in the upper collecting system.

Ureteral dilating balloon catheters are available in a wide variety of sizes (5 to 12 mm) and balloon lengths (2 to

8 cm). For dilating ureteral strictures, an 8-mm-diameter, 4-cm-long balloon is usually used; the balloon should be rated to withstand pressures of greater than 10 atm. The dilating balloon exerts a radially distributed force perpendicular to the ureteral mucosa and is designed to be inflated with fluid. A pressure gauge is placed between the syringe and the balloon; the recommended pressure limit of the balloon should not be exceeded, or else the balloon may rupture within the ureter and cause significant ureteral damage.

The dilating balloon catheter is passed over the guidewire into the ureter under fluoroscopic monitoring. Proximal and distal metal markers on the balloon catheter indicate radiographically the borders of the balloon and allow it to be positioned accurately; the balloon should straddle the "contrast"-outlined stricture. Using a handheld pressure-generating syringe (e.g., LeVeen) with an incorporated pressure gauge, the clinician inflates the balloon with a 50:50 mixture of contrast medium and saline solution under fluoroscopic monitoring. The balloon is initially inflated up to 1 atm of pressure, following which it is inflated at a rate of 1 mL of contrast mixture per minute under fluoroscopic control until the waist in the balloon at the site of the stricture disappears. If the pressure rating of the balloon is reached and the waist is still present, an endoincision (vide infra) will be necessary. Once the waist disappears, the inflated balloon is maintained in position for 2 to 5 minutes before it is deflated; the balloon is then reinflated. If the stricture has truly been torn, the balloon should now fill out at a low pressure. In contrast, if the balloon fails to fill out at low pressure, the stricture has not been treated adequately and an endoincision (vide infra) will be necessary. Following deflation of the balloon, the catheter is removed from the ureter leaving the guidewire in position. An indwelling ureteral stent (either a 7- or 8-Fr or a 7-/14-Fr stent) is then placed fluoroscopically over the guidewire. The ureteral stent is maintained for 4 to 6 weeks.

Clayman and colleagues (50) studied the effects of rapid and slow balloon dilation of the distal ureter to 8 mm (24 Fr) in the pig model. They showed that dilating the ureter to 8 mm (24 Fr) was safe. Slow dilation, over a 10-minute period, produced less residual inflammation 6 weeks following dilation compared with the rapid-dilation (less than 10 seconds) group. However, both groups had similar epithelial denudation, inflammation, and submucosal hemorrhage immediately following the dilation. Selmy and colleagues (324) studied the effect of balloon dilation of the ureter on upper tract dynamics and ureteral wall morphology in the pig model. They found that 1 week after ureteral dilation there was circumferential edema in the lamina propria and thinning of the muscularis propria; this correlated with obstructive urodynamic changes and grade 2 reflux in one-third of the animals. Over a 6-week period, there was gradual resolution of the pathologic inflammatory changes, disappearance of the obstructive changes, and return to radiographically normal ureters. Their observations favor a 6-week stinting period.

Endoincision

The development of the smaller rigid ureteroscope (6.9 Fr), the smaller flexible ureteroscope (7.5 Fr), and accompanying ancillary instruments for use with these endoscopes has made visualization and manipulation of the ureter and upper urinary tract an easier and safer procedure. Cutting modalities for incision of a ureteral stricture include the cold knife, electrosurgical probes, and the Ho:YAG laser.

Strictures in the proximal ureter are incised using a technique similar to an antegrade endopyelotomy. A percutaneous nephrostomy tract is established such that there is a straight-line access to the UPJ region and ureter. The straight posterior or posterolateral incision in the ureteral stricture is full thickness until retroperitoneal fat is seen. The caudal extent of the incision should be 1 cm beyond the area of the stricture. The cephalic portion of the ureteral incision should be into the renal pelvis. Following the incision, an indwelling 7- or 8-Fr double pigtail or 7-/14-Fr endopyelotomy stent is placed in an antegrade fashion. A small 14-Fr nephrostomy tube and Foley catheter also are inserted postoperatively. A nephrostogram is performed 36 to 48 hours postoperatively.

When there is no evidence of extravasation at the site of the ureteral incision, the nephrostomy tube and Foley catheter may be removed. The ureteral stent is usually maintained for 4 to 6 weeks (88,183,318).

The middle ureteral stricture is the most difficult to manage endosurgically. Middle ureteral strictures may be approached in an antegrade or a retrograde fashion. The antegrade approach is identical to an antegrade endopyelotomy except that the cephalad extent of the incision travels 1 cm into normal ureter rather than entering the UPJ. The retrograde approach is similar to a retrograde endopyelotomy except that the proximal limb of the incision remains in the confines of the middle ureter, and in some cases, the short rigid ureteroscope with or without an insulated sheath may be used. In the retrograde approach, after securing a guidewire across the stricture and into the upper collecting system, the intramural ureter is balloon dilated to 15 Fr. This allows introduction of the 12-Fr ureteroscope, through which a cold knife may be passed. Alternatively, ureteral dilation may be omitted and the rigid 6.9-Fr or flexible 7.5-Fr ureteroscope may be introduced, through which a 3-Fr or smaller electrosurgical device or 200-micron holmium laser probe may be passed to perform the incision (Fig. 19.11). The stricture is incised posterolaterally if it lies above the iliac vessels, anterior if it overlies the iliac vessels, and anteromedially if it lies just below the iliac vessels; the full-thickness incision through the stricture is extended 1 cm above and 1 cm below the stricture region into normal-caliber ureter.

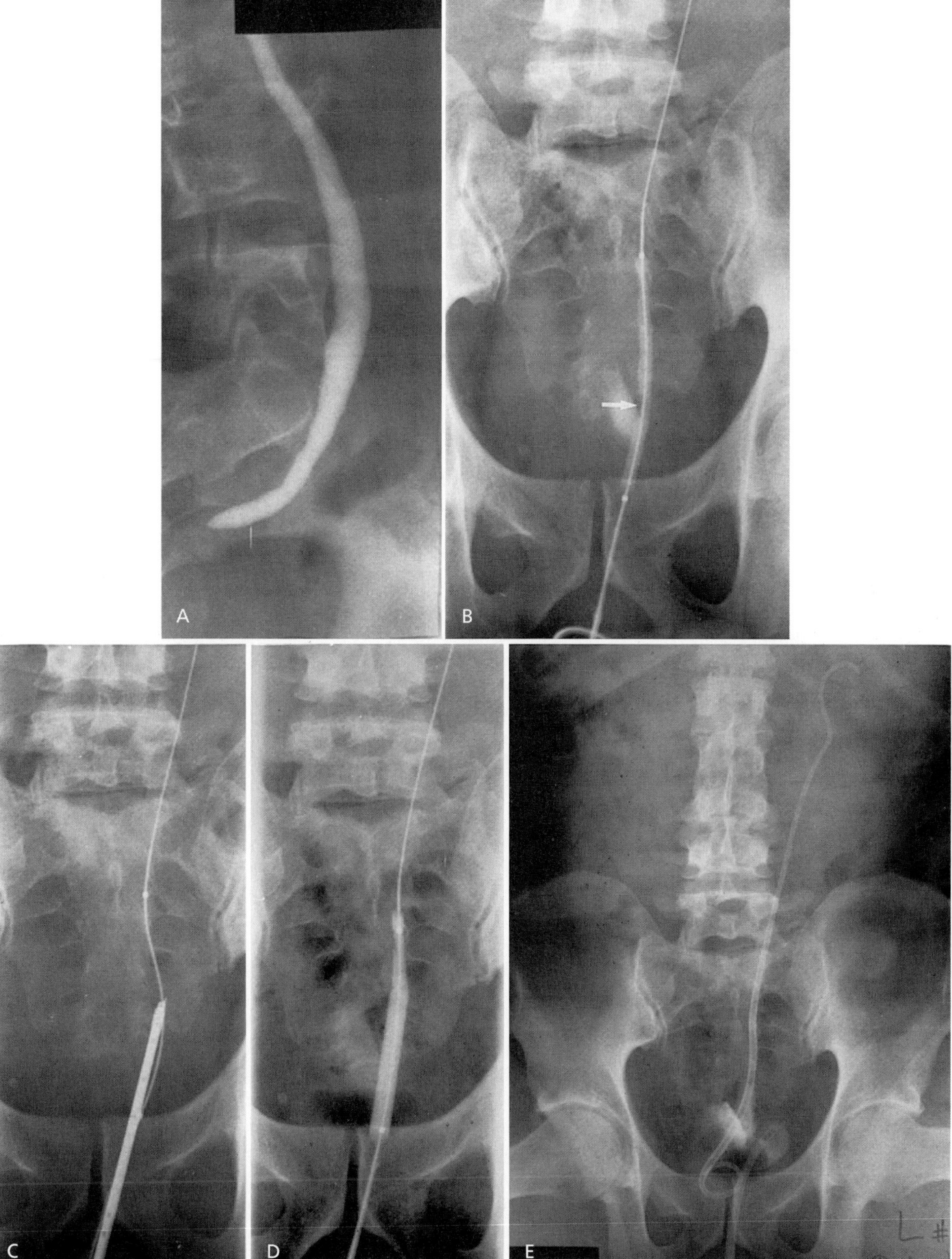

FIGURE 19.11. A: A benign, left ureteral stricture with hydroureter on intravenous pyelography. **B:** A guidewire has been passed retrograde into the upper collecting system. The ureteral dilating balloon catheter is filled to 1 atm pressure, and persistent waisting *(arrow)* of the balloon corresponds to the area of stricture. **C:** With the deflated dilating balloon catheter still in position, the short, rigid ureteroscope is inserted to the level of the stricture. A 3-Fr, right-angle electrosurgical probe is used to incise the stricture full thickness, extending the incision 1 cm above and 1 cm below the strictured region. **D:** Following incision of the stricture, inflation of the ureteral dilating balloon to 1 atm pressure demonstrates resolution of the area of waisting, confirming adequate incision of the stricture. **E:** A 7-/14-Fr double pigtail ureteral stent is positioned in the upper collecting system with the 14-Fr portion traversing the region of the ureteral incision.

In male patients, with a middle ureteral stricture above the iliac vessels, a 7.5-Fr flexible ureteroscope is recommended. A nonconducting Terumo guidewire is passed across the stricture, followed by passage of an 8-Fr dilator and 10-Fr sheath. The 8-Fr dilator is removed, and a side-arm adaptor is placed on the 10-Fr sheath; a retrograde ureterogram is performed to delineate the stricture, following which a second guidewire is passed by the ureter and into the renal pelvis. The 10-Fr sheath is removed. One guidewire is fixed to the drapes with a clamp, thereby becoming the safety guidewire. The flexible ureteroscope is passed over the second (i.e., working) guidewire. Once the ureteroscope is delivered to the ureter, the working guidewire is removed.

If the flexible ureteroscope buckles at the ureteral orifice or does not pass easily up the ureter to the site of the stricture, the flexible ureteroscope is exchanged for a ureteral access sheath. Once the 14-Fr end of the sheath is delivered well into the distal ureter, the 12-Fr dilator is removed. The flexible ureteroscope is then passed over the working guidewire through the 14-Fr sheath and into the ureter. The safety guidewire remains in place alongside the access sheath.

The flexible ureteroscope necessitates the use of a 2- or 3-Fr electrosurgical or less than 400-micron laser Ho:YAG probe. Periureteral damage from use of electrosurgical devices with a greater than 400-micron tip is similar to a cold-knife incision (75). Using visual orientation in combination with fluoroscopy in two planes, a full-thickness incision is made posterolaterally in the ureter above the iliac crossing, anteriorly in the ureter overlying the iliac vessels, or anteromedially in the ureter below the iliac vessels. Retroperitoneal or periureteral fat should be exposed by the endoincision, which extends 1 cm proximal and 1 cm distal to the ureteral stricture. After the stricture incision is completed, an indwelling ureteral stent (a 7- or 8-Fr double pigtail stent or a 7-/14-Fr endopyelotomy stent) is placed. When the 7-/14-Fr stent is used, it should be positioned such that the 14-Fr portion traverses the region of the ureteral incision. A Foley catheter is used to drain the bladder postoperatively. A cystogram 36 to 48 hours postoperatively usually confirms cessation of extravasation at the region of the ureteral incision, which permits removal of the urethral catheter. If extravasation is still present, the patient is discharged from the hospital with the urethral catheter still in place. An outpatient cystogram and catheter removal can be done 1 week later provided that a postoperative urine culture is sterile.

The distal ureteral stricture is usually at the ureteral orifice, the intramural tunnel, or just at or slightly above the ureterovesical junction. These strictures are incised such that the lower limb of the incision extends through the ureteral orifice (61). The retrograde approach is used most commonly for distal strictures. Cystoscopically, a guidewire is manipulated past the region of the stenosis and positioned fluoroscopically in the upper collecting system. An 8-mm, 4-cm-long ureteral dilating balloon catheter is passed over the guidewire after the cystoscope has been removed. Fluoroscopically, the balloon is positioned in the distal ureter such that the metal, lower radiopaque markers on the balloon lie just caudal to the ureteral orifice in the bladder. The balloon is inflated with a 50:50 mixture of contrast solution and saline stained with indigo carmine to a low pressure (i.e., 1 atm). The site of the stricture thus should be well outlined (i.e., a visible waist should appear in the balloon at the stricture site). A standard Iglesius resectoscope sheath is then inserted into the bladder. The proper positioning of the balloon catheter in the intramural ureter is confirmed visually. A right-angle, Orandi or Collins, electrocautery knife attachment is placed through the resectoscope sheath. Using 50 W pure cut, the surgeon begins the incision at the 12 o'clock position of the ureteral orifice and extends it cephalad through the ureteral orifice, ureteral tunnel, and for a distance of 1 cm cephalad to the area of stricturing. Following completion of an adequate incision, the 8-mm balloon should inflate fully at less than 1 atm of pressure. The dilating balloon is then deflated and removed. An indwelling 7- or 8-Fr double pigtail stent or a 7-/14-Fr endopyelotomy stent is placed over the guidewire; when the latter is used, the 14-Fr portion of the stent traverses the distal ureter. A Foley urethral catheter is used to drain the bladder. A cystogram 36 to 48 hours postoperatively is performed to confirm the resolution of any extravasation, following which the urethral catheter may be removed. The indwelling stent is removed on an outpatient basis 4 to 6 weeks following the stricture incision.

The Acucise cutting balloon device also has been used in the management of proximal and distal ureteral strictures (40) (Fig. 19.12). This technique involves placement of a nonconducting Terumo guidewire past the stricture and into the upper collecting system. The balloon catheter is positioned across the strictured region of the ureter under fluoroscopic control. In the proximal ureter above the iliac vessels, the cutting wire is oriented posterolateral, whereas below the iliac vessels the balloon cutting wire is directed anteromedially to avoid the branches of the internal iliac artery and vein, which are lateral to the ureter. *Strictures lying directly over the iliac vessels should not be approached with the cutting balloon device.* This type of ureteral stricture is better approached using direct ureteroscopic visualization and an electrosurgical probe because the surgeon can more accurately confirm visually the precise anterior location of the planned incision.

After positioning the cutting balloon catheter in the appropriate orientation, using two-plane fluoroscopy, the surgeon inflates the balloon with 2 mL of a 50:50 contrast solution and saline mixture while simultaneously activating the cutting wire with 75 to 100 W of pure cut electrical current. Inflation of the balloon carries the activated wire through the tissues. This portion of the procedure should take less than 3 seconds. The balloon is left inflated for 10 minutes, and then it is deflated and pulled retrograde. By

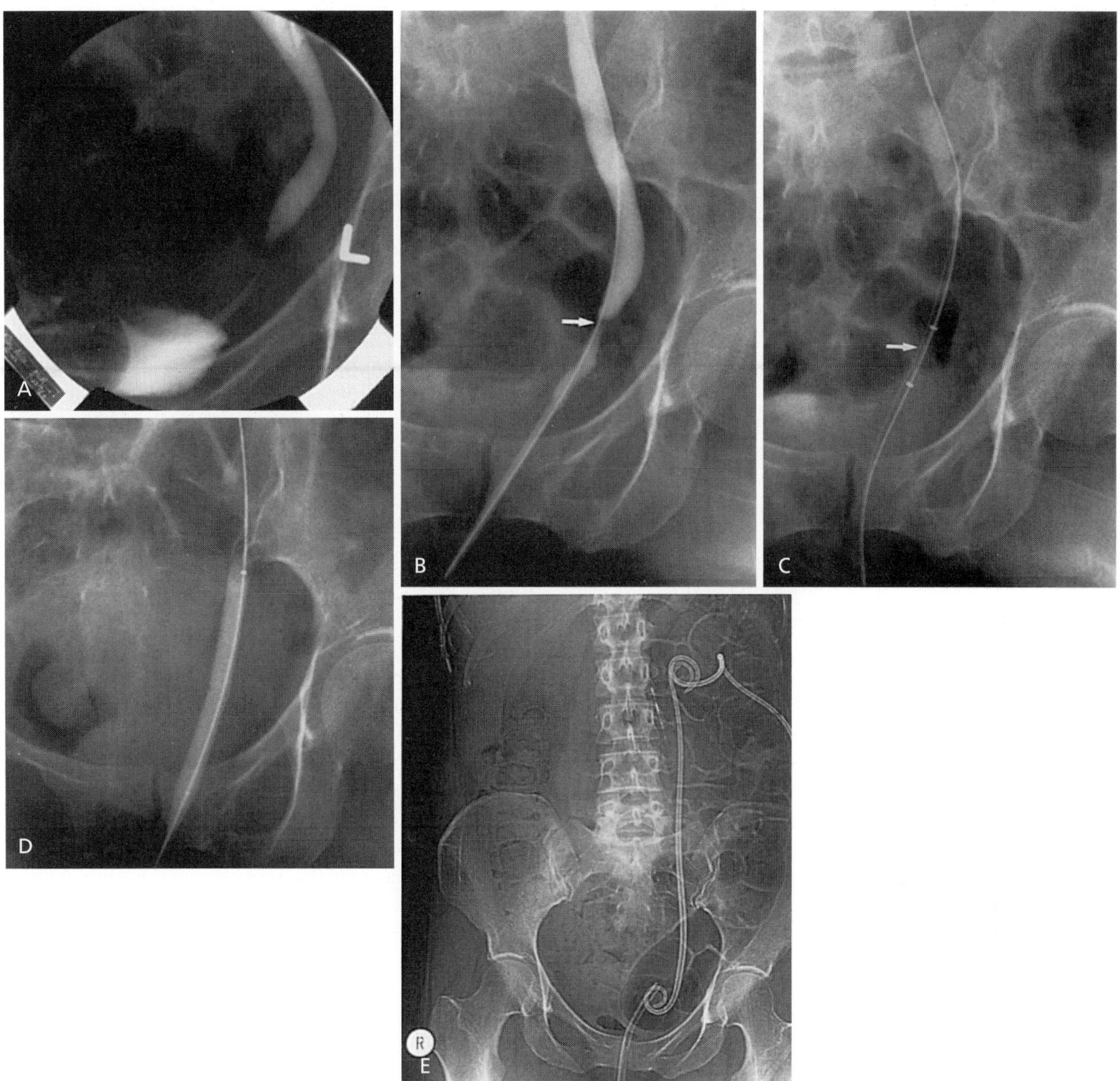

FIGURE 19.12. **A:** Distal left ureteral stricture with hydroureter on nephrostogram evaluation. **B:** Flexible cystoscopy is performed, and a 0.035-inch Terumo guidewire is passed through the strictured region *(arrow)* of the ureter in the upper collecting system. **C:** The cutting balloon catheter is passed over the guidewire and positioned with the cutting wire *(arrow)* oriented medially and traversing the region of the ureteral stricture. The radiopaque markers outline the exposed cutting wire, which is presented to the tissues as the balloon is inflated at a low pressure. **D:** Following incision of the stricture, a ureteral dilating balloon catheter inflated to 1 atm pressure confirms no residual waisting at the level of the stricture. **E:** A 7-/14-Fr double pigtail ureteral stent is positioned in the upper collecting system with the 14-Fr segment traversing the region of the ureteral stricture. The nephrostomy tube (placed preoperatively) and the Foley catheter are removed 24 to 48 hours postoperatively when a cystogram or nephrostogram indicates no residual extravasation at the site of the ureteral incision.

affixing a side-arm adaptor over the guidewire and onto the cutting balloon catheter, a retrograde ureterogram can be obtained. This study should confirm extravasation from the site of the incision. The cutting balloon catheter is then removed. A 5-Fr angiographic catheter is passed over the Terumo guidewire into the upper collecting system. The Terumo guidewire is exchanged for a 0.035-inch Amplatz superstiff guidewire, and the 5-Fr catheter is removed. An indwelling ureteral stent (a 7- or 8-Fr double pigtail stent or a 7-/14-Fr endopyelotomy stent) is passed over the guidewire and positioned fluoroscopically in the upper collecting system. The 7-/14-Fr endopyelotomy stent is positioned such that the 14-Fr portion of the stent traverses the region of the ureteral incision.

The more challenging problem, associated with ureteral stricture disease, occurs when the retrograde ureterogram reveals complete ureteral obstruction. A percutaneous nephrostomy tract is established. With the patient lying prone, the extent of the stricture can then be estimated through a combined antegrade nephrostogram and retrograde ureterogram. The latter is secured after using prone flexible cystoscopy to place the retrograde catheter; in some cases, the flexible ureteroscope can also be passed with the patient prone so a "cut-to-the-light" procedure can be done. A short (less than 1 cm) occlusion may be approached endosurgically. Bagley (11) has reported successful recanalization of complete ureteral obstructions up to 5 cm in length. However, in general, ureteral occlusions longer than 2 cm are better managed with an open surgical procedure.

The site of complete ureteral occlusion may be accessed antegrade by developing the percutaneous nephrostomy tract and passing a flexible nephroscope or short rigid ureteroscope down to the obstruction. Concomitantly, a flexible ureteroscope may be passed in a retrograde fashion to the distal end of the occlusion. If the ureteral stricture is short, the light from the retrograde endoscope may be identified and the tips of the two endoscopes may be aligned using fluoroscopy in an anteroposterior and then oblique projection. With a rigid ureteroscope passed antegrade, a direct incision using a cold knife may be performed onto the tip of the retrograde endoscope. Also, the surgeon can be guided by the light coming from the retrograde endoscope. In this case, the light through the antegrade endoscope is turned off. If the two endoscopes are properly aligned, a bright pink light should be seen through the stricture. As the incision is made toward the light, the light should become more white in appearance until the tip of the retrograde endoscope is clearly visualized. A 260-cm exchange guidewire is then passed through the retrograde instrument and retrieved by the antegrade endoscope. After establishing a guidewire across the stricture, the surgeon can complete the incision through full thickness of the scar and balloon dilation to 8 mm can be used to confirm the adequacy of the incision before placing a ureteral stent. When a flexible endoscope has been passed antegrade, an electrosurgical probe is used to incise the stricture. Alternatively, a stylet guidewire (e.g., rocket wire with a sharp tip from a Lawson retrograde nephrostomy kit) may be passed through the retrograde endoscope to create an indentation on the scarred ureteral tissue and to guide the incision by the antegrade instrument under direct visualization. Alternatively, this sharp wire can be passed, under fluoroscopic control, through the lower end of the stricture and retrieved proximally; the stricture can then be balloon dilated.

Following incision of the stricture, a long-acting steroid (e.g., triamcinolone 40 mg/mL) may be injected into the bed of the incised stricture (243). A 3-Fr Greenwald injecting needle catheter is passed via the rigid or flexible ureteroscope, and 3 to 5 mL of triamcinolone (40 mg/mL) is injected into any dense scar tissue bordering the ureteral incision. A pressure syringe (e.g., LeVeen) is helpful to inject the medication into this area.

Among patients with a particularly long stricture (i.e., longer than 2 cm), a rarely used alternative to open surgical repair is the placement of a free urothelial graft (49,243). With use of a 28-Fr Iglesius resectoscope equipped with an Orandi knife, a 2- to 4-cm-long piece of urothelium from the bladder is incised and carefully lifted off of the dome or base of the bladder. The donor site is cauterized with a roller electrode. The graft is meticulously defatted, following which the thin urothelial surface of the graft is sutured, facing inward, onto a 7-Fr ureteral stent using 5-0 chromic suture. Via a 14-Fr ureteral access sheath, the stent is fluoroscopically positioned in place so the graft-bearing portion of the stent traverses the area of the incised stricture; as the 14-Fr sheath is pulled retrograde, the stent-bearing graft is kept in place with a metal tip stent pusher. A urethral catheter is left in place and the patient is kept on bed rest for 48 hours. The urethral catheter is removed on postoperative day 7; the stent is removed after 6 weeks.

For totally occlusive strictures of the distal ureter, a percutaneous nephrostomy is placed. Through this site, a guidewire and ureteral dilating balloon catheter may be positioned into the distal ureter to the level of the obstruction. The balloon of the catheter should be constructed such that it is *flush* with the tip of the catheter. The balloon is inflated with a 50:50 mixture of contrast medium and saline solution stained with indigo carmine until a pressure of 1 atm is reached. An Iglesius resectoscope sheath is inserted into the bladder; after fluoroscopically aligning the tip of the Orandi electrosurgical knife over the balloon in two planes, an incision is made through the intervening tissue directly onto the inflated balloon. The balloon is thereby uncovered as the overlying sclerotic bladder and ureteral tissues are incised. A 260-cm exchange guidewire is passed through the balloon catheter and retrieved through the bladder. This through-and-through guidewire is then used to place a 7-Fr or 7-/14-Fr indwelling ureteral stent.

A Foley urethral catheter is inserted into the bladder to complete the procedure. A cystogram, 36 to 48 hours postoperatively, usually shows no evidence of extravasation, and the urethral catheter is removed. If extravasation per-

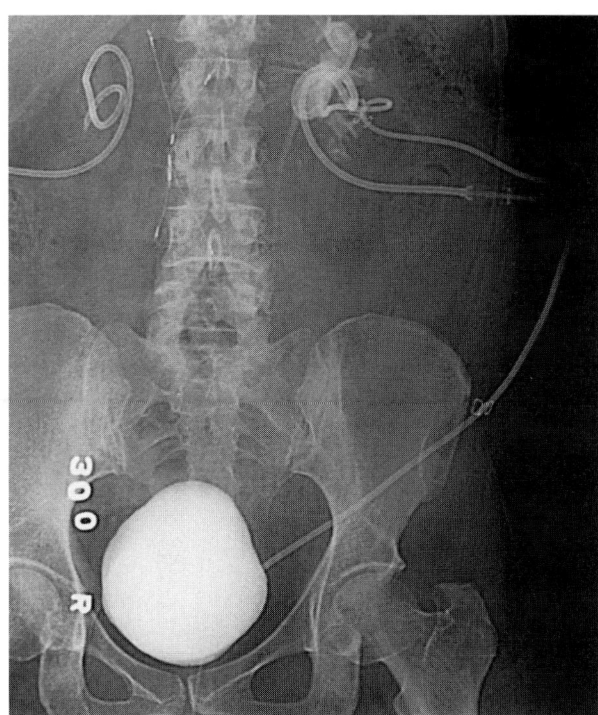

FIGURE 19.13. A left, subcutaneous nephrovesical stent has been placed in this 32-year-old woman with complete obstruction of both distal ureters secondary to metastatic breast carcinoma.

sists, the catheter is maintained for another 7 days before repeating the cystogram. The indwelling stent is removed on an outpatient basis 4 to 6 weeks postoperatively.

Recently, Nissenkorn and Gdor (263) reported their experience with a nephrovesical stent for management of complete ureteral obstruction secondary to metastatic prostate or invasive bladder cancer (Fig. 19.13). The proximal end of a specially designed 7-Fr double pigtail stent is inserted into the renal pelvis via a percutaneous nephrostomy puncture. A subcutaneous tunnel is created from the flank to the suprapubic region, down which the distal end of the stent is passed. The stent is passed into the bladder through a suprapubic bladder puncture. This stent is changed every 4 months over a guidewire, using a small flank incision to access the subcutaneous nephrovesical stent.

Results

When evaluating the literature with regard to the management of ureteral stricture disease, it is important to review the cause of the stricture. Ureteral strictures secondary to radiation therapy or resulting from extraluminal metastatic malignancies, causing periureteral compression, respond poorly to endoureterotomy (216). In contrast, patients with a concomitant ureteral stone and an apparent ureteral stricture usually have resolution of the stricture following removal of the stone and alleviation of the inflammatory response to the stone; incising these strictures may falsely inflate the endoureterectomy success rate.

The development of high-pressure arterial balloon-dilating catheters allowed this technology to be applied to ureteral stricture disease. Several investigators have reported favorable results with balloon dilation of ureteral strictures. Success rates range from 48% to 88%, with an overall average of 55% in 271 patients (19,24,41,170,193,203, 216,261,268) (Table 19.3). However, there appears to be limited consensus among the reports of balloon dilation on the optimal balloon size and technique to perform the procedure. In the literature, the dilating balloon size varies from 4 to 10 mm and the duration of balloon inflation ranges from 30 seconds to 10 minutes for anywhere from one to several inflation cycles. Also, there is no agreement on the size of stents or duration of stinting following balloon dilation; stent sizes range from 6 to 16 Fr, and stent duration ranges from 2 days to 12 weeks. In many of the reports, the success of the procedure is assessed on the basis of subjective relief of the patients' pain or symptoms. When objective studies are provided, they are often not more than 6 months after the procedure. These criteria are unreliable and could inaccurately inflate the success rate reported by 15% or more.

Endoureterotomy, either endosurgical or fluoroscopic (i.e., cutting balloon), for middle and distal ureteral stricture disease appears to have good clinical results with success rates ranging from 66% to 88%. The overall success rate for 156 patients undergoing endoureterotomy is 78%, which appears to be better than the overall success rate of 67% noted for balloon dilation (Table 19.3). However, there is no apparent consensus on the ideal cutting modality used for the endoureterotomy. Cold-knife incision of the ureteral stricture appears to be as efficacious as electrosurgery and Ho:YAG laser in performing endoureterotomy (40,293, 318,335). Figenshau and colleagues (95) investigated the acute tissue changes occurring in the pig ureter following balloon dilation (5 mm), cutting balloon, and endoscopic incision with a cold knife, Nd:YAG laser, or electrocautery as endosurgical management of ureteral strictures. This study used small 250- and 660-micron electrocautery probes. There was no significant difference in the degree of tissue injury among the various cutting modalities used except for the larger 660-micron electrosurgical probe. Unlike a ureteral incision balloon, dilation resulted in injury to the lamina propria but did not appear to split the muscularis and adventitial layers.

The optimal stent size and duration of stenting remain undetermined. Animal studies have shown that for middle ureteral stricture, the larger size stent (i.e., 14 Fr) provides similar results to a 7-Fr stent (247). Similarly, Kerbl and co-workers (187) could find no difference in the healing of ureteral strictures regardless of whether a 1-, 3-, or 6-week period of stenting was selected.

Although balloon dilation and endoureterotomy for ureteral strictures have impressive success rates, these do not

TABLE 19.3. MANAGEMENT OF URETERAL STRICTURES

Authors	No. of Patients	Balloon Size	Method of Incision	Stent Size (Fr)	Stent Duration (wk)	Overall Success Rate (%)	Average Follow-up (mo)
Balloon Dilation							
Banner and Pollack (19)	44	4 mm		7–10	4 days–12 wk	48	—
Chang et al. (41)	11	5–8 mm		8–16	4–8	88	10
Johnson et al. (170)	13	4–10 mm		5–16	2 days–mo	69	3–21
Lang and Glorioso (216)	127	4–6 mm		7–10	3–6	50	—
O'Brien et al. (268)	20	4–6 mm		—	—	60	17
Beckman et al. (23)	17	4–8 mm		7–10	4–8	82	15
Kramolowsky et al. (203)	20	5–10 mm		6–12	6	64	—
Netto et al. (261)	19	4–6 mm		8.5	2–8	53	—
Osther et al. (276)	37	10 mm		7	4–6	90	29
Total	**308**	**4–10 mm**		**6–11**	—	**67%**	—
Endoureterotomy							
Eshghi et al. (88)	40		Cold knife	6–10	4–6	88	—
Schneider et al. (318)	12		Cold knife	14	3–6	71	15
Chandhoke et al. (40)	8		Electrosurgical cutting balloon	7/14[a]	4	75	4
Cohen et al. (56)	6		Electrosurgical cutting balloon	7/14[a]	4–6	66	29
Preminger et al. (293)	40		Electrosurgical cutting balloon	7–7/14[a]	4–6	71	9
Wolf et al. (379)	38		Electrosurgical probe or cutting balloon	7–7/14[a]	4–6	82	28
Singal et al (335)	12		Holmium laser and balloon dilation	6/12	4–6	75	11
Total	**156**			**6–14**	**3–7**	**78%**	**4–29**
Surgical Repair							
Smith (338)	36		Surgical repair			97	
Kramolowsky et al. (203)	11		Surgical repair	5–7	2.5	91	21

[a]Endopyelotomy stent.

duplicate the very high 91% to 97% success rate achieved with open surgical repair of ureteral strictures (203,261). There may be several reasons for the discrepancies noted in these comparisons. The success of any treatment modality may depend on the length of the ureteral stricture, the cause of the stenosis, and the location of the stricture; until now, strictures of similar nature have not been studied in an effort to cull from the general category of ureteral stricture those strictures that would best respond to an endourologic approach.

Several investigators have noted that long ureteral strictures tend to be associated with poorer success rates despite the use of balloon dilation or endoincision. Beckmann and colleagues (24) noted that in 25 patients with strictures shorter than 2 cm, balloon dilation was successful in 84%. Conversely, among eight patients with strictures longer than 2 cm, dilation succeeded in only 50%. Chang and colleagues (41) and Netto and colleagues (261) separately concluded that strictures longer than 1 cm rarely responded well to balloon dilation. The same observation has been noted in the literature on the use of incision of ureteral strictures. Meretyk and colleagues (243) found that the best results following endoureterotomy were in those patients with strictures less than 2 cm. Schneider and colleagues (318) reported that the longest stricture they treated by cold-knife incision was 2.5 cm in length, and this patient reobstructed 24 hours after removal of the ureteral stent. Therefore it would appear appropriate to apply endosurgical management to only patients with strictures less than 2 cm in length.

The cause of the ureteral stricture also has a significant impact on the success of the endosurgical treatment results. The most common cause (23%) of ureteral stricture in the Meretyk series was postoperative fibrosis following open pelvic surgery or a ureteroscopic procedure (243). These relatively nonischemic strictures respond better to endosurgical treatments than do poorly vascularized strictures (19,41,216,243,318). Other causes of ureteral stricture include intrinsic inflammatory processes, such as schistosomiasis, tuberculosis, or radiation injury (82,170,193,261,299, 328). The ischemic stricture associated with radiation responds poorly to endoureterotomy.

Extrinsic processes resulting in ureteral stricturing include retroperitoneal fibrosis, endometriosis, and retroperitoneal malignancies (170,243,261). Those processes causing extrinsic compression of the ureter do not respond to balloon dilation or incision of the ureter. As such, ureteral strictures secondary to retroperitoneal fibrosis are more appropriately managed by releasing the ureter from the retroperitoneal fibrosis and transposing it into an intraabdominal position or treating the underlying disease process.

Likewise, for ureteral strictures associated with a malignancy, a nephrovesical stent or endoluminal metal stent (i.e., Wallstent) or a permanent nephrostomy tube is indicated (62,226,263,286). Lopez-Martinez and colleagues (226) have used the nephrovesical stent in eight patients with metastatic prostate cancer. The average duration of stent patency was 19 months (range of 1 to 48 months). Five patients reobstructed because of recurrent tumor, and in two patients additional stents were telescopically placed. Three patients died of metastatic cancer with the stent *in situ.* Six patients at risk at 12 months had patent stents compared with 3 of 5 at 24 months, 2 of 2 at 36 months, and 1 of 1 at 48 months. Nissenkorn and Gdor (263) have used the nephrostomy-diverting stent in eight patients with metastatic prostate and invasive bladder cancer. With a mean follow-up of 5.5 months, the stents functioned well and eliminated the percutaneous nephrostomy during the terminal stages of the patients' disease.

The anatomic location of the ureteral stricture also has been cited as a factor affecting the success of endoureterotomy. Smith (338) showed that in a series of 28 patients with ureteral stricture disease, all 4 patients with a middle ureteral stricture failed balloon dilation. Similarly, Meretyk and colleagues (243) noted a 25% success rate for endourologic incision of middle ureteral strictures compared with an 80% success rate for distal ureteral strictures. Likewise, proximal ureteral strictures, specifically secondary UPJ obstruction, respond well (i.e., 80%) to an endoincision. As such, marsupializing one limb of the stricture into the bladder or renal pelvis appears to provide a better success rate than strictures in the middle ureter, which by definition remain bound by normal ureter above and below the treatment region.

Contrary to earlier reports, it now appears that the duration of a ureteral stricture before treatment has no significant effect on the success rate of the therapy. When the factors of stricture length, location, and cause are controlled, the duration of the stricture does not alter the ultimate outcome. Successful endosurgical therapy has been reported in strictures ranging from 8 weeks' to 18 months' duration (261).

Clearly, the success of endosurgical treatment depends to some extent on the previously described characteristics of the stricture: cause, length, and location. Unfortunately, rarely do study reports subdivide the patient groups according to their stricture characteristics. This factor, when combined with the inconsistencies of the technique of balloon dilation or endoincision and the variability in posttreatment stent size and stent duration, results in a significant amount of clinical confusion such that cumulative data on the endosurgical management of ureteral stricture can only be judged in the broadest anecdotal manner.

Meretyk and colleagues (243) have described the use of long-acting steroid injection and free urothelial grafts in the stricture region to improve the results of endoincision of ureteral strictures. Triamcinolone injection appears to be clinically beneficial in patients undergoing incision of urethral and bladder neck contractures (65,92). One of the actions of triamcinolone is to block collagen formation. In three patients with recurrent stricture after endoscopic ureterotomy, Schmeller and colleagues (315) demonstrated that histologically the area of the ureterotomy consisted of collagen-rich connective tissue with few fibroblasts and a scarcity of smooth muscle fibers. Therefore the application of triamcinolone into the incised bed of the ureteral stricture may inhibit collagen formation and improve the success of endoureterotomy. Wolf and colleagues (379) demonstrated that a nonischemic etiology, more recent etiology (less than 24 months), shorter stricture (1 cm), use of a 12-Fr or larger stent, and injection of triamcinolone into the bed of the stricture were associated with better outcomes for ureteral strictures treated endosurgically.

Experimental results with free tissue grafts (i.e., tunica vaginalis) to repair the ureter have been inconsistent and complicated by hydronephrosis and graft sloughing (102, 204,146). However, a free graft of bladder urothelium has worked well for urethral stricture disease (139) and could possibly be of value for ureteral replacement (124). In Urban's series, six patients underwent a free urothelial graft for ureteral strictures between 1.5 and 8 cm. Mean follow-up at 30 months revealed a patency rate of 83% (362). Presently, this time-consuming approach may be a reasonable procedure in high-risk surgical patients with strictures longer than 2 cm.

Several investigators have evaluated absorbable biocompatible materials as substitutes in the urinary tract (321). However, these have been unsatisfactory because of urine leakage, shrinkage of the repair site, and stone formation. Improvement in cell-culture techniques have enabled some investigators to create a monolayer of urothelial cells on synthetic graft materials before implantation (179). These studies are encouraging for improved cellular lining, prolonged patency, and selective permeability of the graft, but follow-up is limited and clinical trials have yet to be instituted. Cussenot and colleagues (62) reported on the use of a flexible, expandable, tantalum wire stent in the management of four patients with ureteral stricture disease. All of the patients had complicated pathology, including periureteral malignancy and several failed endourologic balloon dilation attempts. Radiographic and endourologic follow-up showed mucosal hyperplasia of varying intensity in all four patients and recurrent obstruction in three (75%). This hyperplastic reaction to metal stent implantation also has been observed in the human urethra. In contrast, Pauer and Lugmayr (286) used a self-expanding, stainless steel alloy, 7-mm stent (Wallstent) to treat ureteral obstruction secondary to a metastatic retroperitoneal tumor in 12 patients; an indwelling double-J stent was used during the first 4 weeks of Wallstent placement. Hyperplasia and edema of the urothelium was observed in all cases during the initial 4 weeks of stent placement; however, the hyperplasia appeared to resolve after the initial 4 weeks. However, during an average follow-up of 27 weeks, 87% of the stents remained open. Two patients developed encrustation of the stent after 30 weeks.

In conclusion, endourologic management of ureteral strictures has not acquired the same degree of acceptance as endourologic management of UPJ obstruction. Overall, the endosurgical management of distal and upper ureteral strictures less than 2 cm and not associated with radiation or other ischemic injury is highly successful and results in minimal morbidity. Also, failure to establish patency does not preclude a subsequent open reconstructive repair. Strictures longer than 2 cm and those associated with radiation or ischemic injury or a middle ureteral location may be managed more appropriately by open reconstruction because of the high failure rate associated with this group of patients treated endosurgically. Further clinical studies are necessary to determine the long-term feasibility and success of adjuvant therapy, such as triamcinolone injection and free urothelial grafting.

Ureteroenteric Strictures

Ureteroenteric strictures are a late complication of urinary diversion. There is no predilection to the type of urinary diversion and the rate of development of stenosis at the ureteroenteric anastomosis, which ranges from 4% to 8% (128,316). The mechanism of stenosis is usually idiopathic. Compression of the ureter by recurrent tumor or inflammation secondary to radiation therapy is a rare cause of late stricture formation. The patient with ureteroenteric stenosis may have flank pain, urinary tract infection, sepsis, or fever. However, these strictures often may be asymptomatic, thereby leading to permanent renal damage. For this reason, it is important to follow urinary diversion patients annually with routine evaluation of the upper urinary tract to obviate silent, slowly developing, renal obstruction.

The standard therapy for a ureteroenteric anastomotic stricture is usually exploratory laparotomy and revision of the ureteroenteric anastomosis with reimplantation of the viable ureter into the conduit. The development of percutaneous nephrostomy drainage and external ureteral stents initially provided a therapeutic alternative to the surgical approach, especially in patients with recurrent malignant disease (304,339). However, chronic nephrostomy tubes and ureteral stents are associated with considerable morbidity and must be exchanged at regular intervals to minimize the risk of obstruction (253,371). As such, in patients without recurrent cancer, this approach is only of a temporizing value. In 1979, Smith and colleagues (339) reported endoscopic dilation of ureteroileal strictures with Teflon dilators and insertion of a Gibbons ureteral stent. Subsequently, in 1988, Kramolowsky and colleagues (202) treated nine patients with ten ureterointestinal strictures with either balloon dilation or an endoureterotomy, followed by stent removal.

Technique

It is important to completely assess the patient with regard to the etiology of the ureteral anastomotic stricture and the location and extent of the stenosis before embarking on the endosurgical manipulation. As such, a CT scan and renal scan are helpful. If the stricture is complete or secondary to recurrent malignancy, the objective of endourologic therapy is to establish a retrograde external ureteral catheter, which may be changed on an outpatient basis every 12 to 16 weeks. If the stricture is totally occluding the ureter, a nephrostomy tube can be placed for a 4- to 6-week period. If, despite optimal drainage, the function of the affected kidney remains below the 15% level, nephrectomy may be the next best step provided the contralateral kidney is normal. Likewise, if the patient has evidence of urosepsis, a nephrostomy tube should be placed immediately.

For benign, partial ureteroenteric anastomotic obstruction of a well-functioning kidney, the goal is to reestablish a permanent, nonstinted, patent ureteral conduit. A percutaneous nephrostomy is placed. An antegrade ureterogram is performed in combination with a loopogram to determine the extent of the stenosis. The ureteroenteric stricture may be approached from an antegrade or a retrograde access or from a combined antegrade and retrograde approach.

The antegrade approach is commonly used for balloon dilation of the stricture. The patient is placed in a flank position, with the affected side superior. Both the stoma and flank are prepared and draped. Percutaneous access is easily established because the kidney is commonly hydronephrotic. After the percutaneous nephrostomy has been established, a guidewire is manipulated antegrade through the dilated UPJ and down the ureter. If the guidewire does not easily pass through the region of stenosis, a 5-Fr angiographic catheter is placed over the guidewire. The guidewire is exchanged for a Terumo guidewire, which because of its lubricity can usually pass through even the tightest stricture. The 5-Fr angiographic catheter is then advanced over the Terumo guidewire across the stenosis and into the conduit loop. The Terumo guidewire is then exchanged for a 260-cm exchange guidewire. A flexible cystoscope is passed into the conduit through the stoma, and grasping forceps are used to retrieve the end of the exchange wire from the stoma. The 5-Fr angiographic catheter is removed. An 8-mm, 4-cm-long, 7-Fr ureteral dilating balloon catheter is passed over the through-and-through guidewire under fluoroscopic control until it straddles the stricture. The balloon of the catheter should be rated to a minimum of 15 atm of pressure. A pressure syringe (i.e., LeVeen type) with an in-line pressure gauge is attached to the balloon inflation port and used to slowly inflate the balloon with a 50:50 contrast and saline mixture. The inflation is continued until the waist in the balloon at the level of the stricture disappears. The balloon is left inflated for 1 minute and deflated. This cycle of inflation followed by deflation may be repeated once or twice.

Following completion of the balloon dilation, the dilating catheter is removed. A 10- to 16-Fr nephroureteral stent is then placed antegrade, or preferably a single pigtail 12-Fr biliary urinary drainage catheter can be placed retrograde. The latter has sideholes only in the stent coil, which resides in the renal pelvis; the butt end of the tube exits the conduit stoma. A 2-0 Prolene suture is used to secure the shaft of the stent to the peristomal skin. The patient's urine collection device is passed over the end of the stent and secured in the usual manner to the peristomal skin. If a retrograde stent is placed, an 8- or 10-Fr nephrostomy tube also is positioned. On postoperative day 2 or 3, a nephrostogram may be performed, and if the collecting system is intact, the nephrostomy tube is removed. The nephrostent or retrograde ureteral stent is removed 4 to 8 weeks postoperatively.

Retrograde balloon dilation of ureteroenteric strictures also may be performed. However, this may be more difficult than an antegrade approach. Flexible cystoscopy of the conduit is performed through the stoma. If a nephrostomy tube is in place, indigo carmine–stained saline can be instilled to help identify the narrowed ureteroenteric anastomosis. Via the cystoscope, a Terumo guidewire is inserted into the ureter and advanced under direct endoscopic and fluoroscopic control. Once coiled in the renal pelvis, a 5-Fr angiographic catheter is passed over the guidewire through the strictured region and into the upper collecting system. The Terumo guidewire is exchanged for a 0.035-inch Amplatz superstiff guidewire, and the 5-Fr angiographic catheter and the cystoscope are removed. An 8-mm, 4-cm-long, 7-Fr ureteral dilating balloon catheter is passed over the guidewire until the balloon straddles the region of the stricture fluoroscopically. The same technique of balloon dilation and retrograde stent placement described for the antegrade approach is used for the retrograde approach (i.e., sideholes only in the renal pelvic coil of the stent). An indwelling ureteral stent should not be used because it may become occluded with mucus. This scenario may result in obstruction and fatal urosepsis (371). The stent is removed 4 to 8 weeks postoperatively under fluoroscopic guidance; a retrograde ureterogram is obtained.

Endoincision of a ureteroenteric stricture carries with it the risk of an inadvertent enterotomy or significant hemorrhage. Therefore these patients should receive a complete mechanical and antibiotic bowel preparation preoperatively. If the bowel is appropriately prepared, an enterotomy may be managed conservatively with an external ureteral stent and an elemental diet. In the situation of significant bleeding, an open procedure may be necessary; if the patient is stable, revision of the ureteroenteric anastomosis may be performed at the same time. In general, a left ureteral stricture that extends more than 1 cm above the ureteroenteric anastomosis site is a contraindication to an endoincision.

The endoscopic incision of the ureteroenteric stricture also may be approached in an antegrade or a retrograde fashion. In either case, the patient is placed in the flank position with the affected side superior, and both the stoma and posterior flank are prepared and draped.

To perform an antegrade endoincision of a ureteroenteric stricture, an 18-Fr nephrostomy tract should be established in a middle or upper posterior calyx to provide straight-line access to the affected distal ureter. The flexible 7.5- or 9.4-Fr ureteroscope, or 15-Fr nephroscope, is inserted through the nephrostomy tract into the renal pelvis, and under direct visualization the endoscope is delivered to the stricture. A 0.035-inch Terumo guidewire is visually passed through the stricture and into the conduit. A flexible cystoscope is passed via the conduit stoma and is used to retrieve the end of the Terumo guidewire. The flexible ureteroscope or nephroscope is removed, and a 5-Fr angiographic catheter is passed fluoroscopically over the Terumo guidewire until the tip is through the conduit. The Terumo guidewire is exchanged through the 5-Fr angiographic catheter for a 0.035-inch, 260-cm exchange guidewire. The 5-Fr angiographic catheter is removed. A 6- or 8-mm, 7-Fr ureteral dilating balloon catheter is passed retrograde over the guidewire until the balloon straddles the stricture. The balloon is inflated with dilute radiographic contrast solution stained with indigo carmine, using a pressure syringe (i.e., LeVeen type) with an in-line pressure gauge, to 1 atm. With the balloon inflated, the flexible endoscope is introduced antegrade, and a 2- or 3-Fr straight-tip or right-angle electrosurgery probe is passed through the endoscope. A right-angle electrosurgery probe allows for highly accurate stricture incision. An incision is made in the ureter alongside the balloon using 50 to 100 W of pure cut energy. The incision is extended distally until the conduit is entered; the cut is made through the full thickness of the ureter until retroperitoneal fat can be seen. The ureteral dilating balloon should now expand to its full size; if the balloon was punctured during the incision, it is removed and replaced with a 10-mm nephrostomy dilating balloon. Visually and fluoroscopically, the balloon is positioned across the region of the incision. If the incision in the stricture is successful, the balloon should fully inflate at 1 to 2 atm without any evidence of a waist. If the scar tissue of the incised ureteral stricture appears to be particularly dense and no fat is seen, 3 to 5 mL of triamcinolone (40 mg/mL) may be injected into the bed of the incised stricture using a 3-Fr Greenwald needle mounted on a flexible shaft. A LeVeen pressure syringe is used to perform the injection into the dense scar tissue.

The balloon catheter and flexible endoscope are removed. A 12-Fr retrograde single pigtail catheter with sideholes only in the pigtail is inserted retrograde into the upper collecting system; the butt end of the catheter exits the stoma. A 14-Fr nephrostomy tube is inserted into the renal pelvis. A nephrostogram is performed on postoperative day 1 or 2, and if the collecting system is intact, the nephrostomy tube is removed. The external ureteral stent is maintained for 4 to 8 weeks postoperatively.

Retrograde endoincision is performed under direct vision with the Sachs urethrotome, 12-Fr, short, rigid therapeutic ureteroscope, or 15-Fr flexible cystoscope. The endoscope is inserted alongside the guidewire. An 8-mm ureteral dilating balloon catheter is passed retrograde, until the balloon straddles the area of the stricture. The balloon is inflated with 50 : 50 contrast material and saline in a pressure syringe (LeVeen type) with an in-line pressure gauge, to 1 atm pressure to delineate the stricture fluoroscopically. The balloon is then deflated and the area of the stricture is incised using a cold knife through the rigid ureteroscope. Alternatively, the balloon may be left inflated, and a 2- or 3-Fr straight-tip or right-angle Greenwald electrode may be used through the ureteroscope or flexible cystoscope to incise the ureter alongside the balloon. The incision should be extended through the full thickness of the ureter; ideally, periureteral fat should be seen. The incision is extended cephalad until the dilated normal ureter is identified. The ureteroscope is withdrawn and the 8-mm balloon is reinflated to confirm that the ureter is widely patent. A 12-Fr single pigtail ureteral catheter is passed retrograde as previously described. If on postoperative day 2 a nephrostogram shows no evidence of extravasation, the 8-Fr nephrostomy tube is removed. The retrograde catheter is removed 4 to 8 weeks postoperatively.

If the ureteroenteric obstruction is complete, a combined antegrade and retrograde approach is necessary. In the combined approach, the rigid endoscope is passed through the conduit, and the flexible ureteroscope or flexible nephroscope is passed through the developed nephrostomy tract. When the tips of the two endoscopes are fluoroscopically close (less than 1 cm), the light from the antegrade endoscope is turned off. The endoscopist then seeks the light coming from the rigid retrograde endoscope lying within the conduit, which will appear as a bright pink light transilluminating the intervening tissue. The C-arm fluoroscope is used in two planes of projection to further confirm the close alignment of the tips of the two endoscopes. At this point a cut-to-the-light procedure can be performed as previously described for treatment of the completely obstructing ureteral stricture (253). Alternatively, the light of the antegrade endoscope can be sought via the retrograde endoscope; a retrograde incision is then made (Fig. 19.14).

Once a guidewire has been established across the area of the stricture, the incision can be extended using an antegrade or retrograde technique to complete the endoincision. This incision should be performed slowly under direct endoscopic control to avoid inadvertent injury to an underlying artery or segment of bowel.

If the bowel is entered, a 10-Fr ureteral pigtail catheter is placed across the area of incision and into the renal pelvis. The fistula will usually close spontaneously over several weeks with the patient on an elemental diet (244). If an artery is incised, there will be immediate hemorrhage; a 10-mm balloon catheter or a Kaye catheter can be passed over the through-and-through guidewire to straddle the region of the incision, and the balloon is inflated to tamponade the bleeding site. The balloon can usually be deflated 2 days later. If bleeding recurs, the balloon is reinflated, and

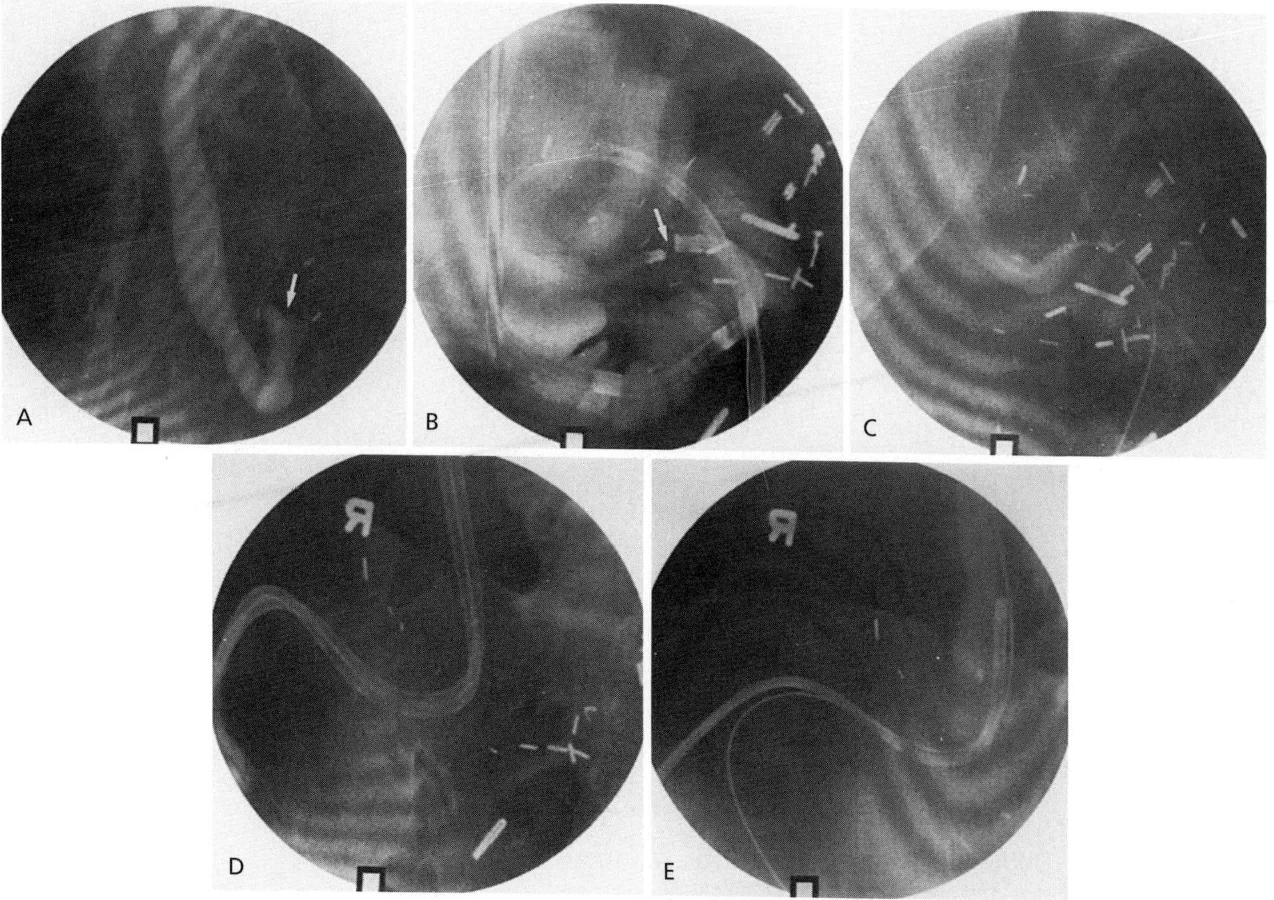

FIGURE 19.14. **A:** Right uteroenteric stricture *(arrow)* with moderate hydroureteronephrosis on antegrade nephrostogram. **B:** A flexible uteroscope has been passed antegrade to the level of the stricture. A flexible cystoscope is passed retrograde through the ileoconduit to the stricture. A cut-to-the-light technique is used by passing an electrosurgical cutting device through the cystoscope to incise the intervening stricture *(arrow)*. **C:** After incising the stricture, a guidewire is passed antegrade and retrieved by the cystoscope to establish a through-and-through guidewire across the region of the stricture. **D:** A stent is then placed. In this case, two 7-Fr single pigtail catheters have been placed across the region of the incised stricture. Note: there are no sideholes in the shaft of the stents; the drainage holes are only in the pigtail portion. **E:** At the time of stent removal, ureteroscopy is performed through the ileal conduit to confirm patency of the incised stricture.

angiography followed by selective embolization or an open surgical repair is performed. If there is no bleeding, the balloon is exchanged for a 12-Fr single pigtail retrograde external ureteral catheter.

Results

The reported experience with ureterointestinal strictures is even more limited than that of UPJ and ureteral strictures. The largest single-center series used balloon dilation to treat 37 ureteroenteric anastomotic strictures in 29 patients (329). Most of these patients had undergone cystectomy and diversion for bladder or uterine/cervical carcinoma and had received adjuvant radiation therapy before cystectomy. All but three patients underwent diversion to an isolated segment of terminal ileum; in the remainder, a colon conduit was created. All of the ureteroenteric strictures were dilated in an antegrade fashion using a 4- to 10-mm dilating balloon catheter. The goal of the dilation was to eliminate the waist in the balloon at the area of the stricture; this required between one and three inflations at the same procedure. The balloon was left inflated for 1 to 2 minutes. Most of the ureters were stinted with an 8.3- or 10-Fr stent, although six ureters had stents ranging in size from 14 to 24 Fr. The stents were placed retrograde following the dilation and were maintained for 1 to 6 weeks. In short-term follow-up, only 30% of the cases were considered to be clinical successes. At 1 year of follow-up, only 6 of 37 strictures (16%) were patent. Half of the successful cases subsequently required repeat dilation and stent placement to maintain ureteral patency; these late restenoses occurred between 14 and 73 months following the initial dilation.

TABLE 19.4. ENDOUROLOGIC MANAGEMENT OF URETEROINTESTINAL ANASTOMOTIC STRICTURE

Authors	No. of Patients	Balloon Size	Method of Incision	Stent Size (Fr)	Stent Duration (wk)	Overall Success Rate (%)	Average Follow-up (mo)	Complications
Balloon Dilation								
Chang et al. (41)	8	5–8 mm		8–16	4–6	50	20	0
Johnson et al. (170)		4–10 mm		5–16	2 days–mo	43	3–21	0
O'Brien et al. (268)	6	4–6 mm		—	—	17	12	—
Shapiro et al. (329)	37	4–10 mm		8–24	1–6	16	12	1 urosepsis
Beckman et al. (23)	5	4–8 mm		7–10	4–8	60	22	0
Aliabdi et al. (6)	3	6–8 mm		—	6	67	12	0
Total	**66**	**4–10 mm**		**5–24 Fr**	**1–8 wk**	**29%**	**14 mo**	**2%**
Endoincision		**Approach**						
Meretyk et al. (244)	19	Antegrade	2–5 Fr electrosurgery probe	18–20	3–6	57	29	1 ureteroenteric fistula
Cornud et al. (59)	9	Antegrade	7 Fr sphincterotome	18	8	67	8	1 urinoma
Ahmadzadeh (5)	5	Antegrade	3 Fr needle electrode	7	4	60	14	1 peritoneal urine leak 1 fever
Germinale et al. (109)	9	Antegrade and Retrograde	Balloon dilation and electrode (2) or cold knife (2)	10	8	45	12	0
Chandhoke et al. (40)	3	Antegrade	Electrosurgical cutting balloon	14	4	33	4	1 ureteroarterial fistula
Wolf et al. (379)	30	—	Electrosurgical probe or cutting balloon	7–16 Fr	4–6	50	23	1 blood transfusion, 1 sepsis 3 febrile UTI, 1 lacerated iliac artery
Singal et al. (335)	9	—	Holmium laser and balloon dilation	6/12	4–6	75	11	0
Lin et al. (224)	9	—	Electrosurgical cutting balloon	10	6	30	24	0
Total	**74**	—	—	**10–20 Fr**	**3–8 wk**	**52%**	**16 mo**	**10%**
Surgical Repair								
Kramlowsky et al. (202)	7 (9 strictures)	—	—	7–8 F	—	89	33 mo	1 peritoneal urine leak 1 conduit enterotomy 1 bowel resection caused by enterotomies

UTI, urinary tract infection.

These investigators were unable to identify distinguishing or predictive factors for success of balloon dilation of the ureterointestinal anastomotic strictures.

Several other investigators have reported on balloon dilation of ureterointestinal anastomotic strictures (6,24,41, 170,268) (Table 19.4). There does not appear to be any consensus as to the size of dilating balloon to use, the size of the ureteral stent to place following the dilation, or the duration of stent placement. In these other series, the success rates for balloon dilation of ureterointestinal strictures range from 16% to 67%. Among all series, the overall average success rate was 29% at an average follow-up of 14 months. Of note, the highest success rate of 67% occurred among pediatric patients with a conduit and a benign etiology of the stricture (6). Many of these reports had short-term follow-up (less than 12 months) of their patients, and as Shapiro and colleagues (329) have demonstrated, longer follow-up significantly decreases the initially favorable results (Table 19.4).

The experience with endosurgical incision of the ureterointestinal anastomotic stricture also is limited. This procedure may be performed in an antegrade or a retrograde fashion, although most investigators have used the antegrade technique (5,40,59,109,224,335,379).

The largest single-center study was reported by Wolf and colleagues (379) and consisted of 30 ureterointestinal anastomotic strictures in 25 patients. Most of the patients (26 of 30) had an ileal conduit for transitional cell carcinoma or cervical carcinoma. Of 30 strictures, 16 occurred less than 24 months and 13 occurred more than 24 months from the time of the diversion procedure. A variety of approaches to the endoureterotomy were taken, including antegrade, retrograde, and combined antegrade and retrograde. The success rates of endoureterotomy for ureteroenteric strictures at 1, 2, and 3 years were 72%, 51%, and 32%, respectively. There was an improved outcome for right rather than left strictures (68% versus 17% 3-year success rates, respectively) and for strictures treated less than 24 months after the etiologic insult (37% 3-year success rate compared with 27% for those treated longer than 24 months after the insult). Stricture length, diameter, and previous treatment did not alter the results. Those strictures that were amenable to treatment in a purely retrograde fashion, as opposed to those requiring an antegrade or combined approach, tended to have a better outcome (75% and 18% 3-year success rates, respectively). More favorable results were also noted with the use of 12-Fr or larger stents (38% compared with 0% 3-year success rate when using smaller stents) and stinting longer than 4 weeks (35% compared with 26% 3-year success when stinting 4 weeks or less). The use of triamcinolone did not appear to affect the results. One of the patients in this series had a major postoperative complication. During incision with the cutting balloon device, a left ureteral–left iliac artery fistula was created. The bleeding was controlled with a high-pressure, 10-mm tamponade balloon catheter in the ureter. Angiography confirmed the presence and location of the fistula. Open surgical management was required. Overall, use of the cutting balloon for ureterointestinal strictures is advisable only if the stricture is at the ureteroenteric site and if initial attempts at an endoscopic incision have been unsuccessful.

Additional reports in the literature have shown an overall success rate of 52% for endoincision of the ureterointestinal anastomotic stricture (Table 19.4). A variety of cutting modalities have been used, including electrosurgical, cold knives of various sizes and configurations, and Ho:YAG laser (5,59,109,335,379). Following the endoincision, all patients have been stinted (10 to 20 Fr) for 3 to 8 weeks postoperatively. Kramolowsky and colleagues (202) compared their nine patients who underwent open surgical revision of a ureteroenteric stricture with their six patients who underwent endoscopic incision and balloon dilation of a ureterointestinal stricture. The ureter was patent with no ureteral stent in 89% of the patients treated with open surgical revision at 33 months and in 71% of patients undergoing the endoscopic incision at 18 months. Although the endoscopic procedure was less successful than the open surgical revision, it was associated with a significantly shorter hospitalization, decreased blood loss, reduced patient discomfort, and decreased cost compared with the open surgical procedure. Although the standard open surgical revision of a ureteroenteric anastomotic stricture is usually successful, it can be difficult to perform because of surrounding scar tissue or previous radiation therapy, making intraoperative and postoperative morbidity significant. Postoperative complications can occur in 30% of the open-surgery patients, and these problems often necessitate reoperation (202). Many patients with ureterointestinal strictures are poor surgical candidates because of age, longstanding urosepsis, or renal insufficiency. As such, the endoscopic incision of the ureterointestinal stricture provides a less invasive, less morbid approach that is successful in alleviating the problem in as many as 75% of otherwise surgical candidates (335).

In patients with known metastatic disease, the endoscopic approach allows placement of an external stent for drainage purposes. This may facilitate optimization of the patient's renal function before chemotherapy. All stents used in a ureterointestinal unit should have side drainage holes present only in the portion of the stent in the renal pelvis and at the end where the stent exits the stoma. No holes should be placed along the catheter where it traverses the conduit to preclude mucous obstruction and possible fatal urosepsis (371). Stents should be changed every 3 to 4 months as an outpatient procedure under fluoroscopic control.

Transitional Cell Cancer of the Ureter

Primary transitional cell carcinoma of the ureter (TCCU) represents only 2% of all urothelial malignancies seen in the urinary tract. Patients most commonly have hematuria, flank pain, or urinary frequency and dysuria, although lower abdominal mass, fever, or weight loss may be the presenting complaint. Batata and colleagues (20) demonstrated that 65% of ureteral cancer patients have cancer in other parts of the urinary tract concurrent with or before or after a diagnosis of ureteral cancer. The most common malignancy of the ureter is transitional cell carcinoma (93%); rarely, squamous cell carcinoma (5%) or mucoid adenocarcinoma (2%) may occur in the ureter. Most ureteral tumors occur in the distal ureter (65%), followed by the middle (17%) and upper (12%) ureter; the entire ureteral length is affected by malignancy in 7% of ureteral tumor patients (8).

Several investigators have evaluated prognostic factors in carcinoma of the ureter (30,140). As with transitional cell carcinoma of other areas of the urinary tract, ureteral transitional cell carcinoma has an excellent (greater than 90% survival rate at 5-year follow-up) prognosis if it is well differentiated and confined to the mucosa. Eighty-two percent of patients without muscle-invasive tumor survive 5 years. However, dissemination of the carcinoma into regional lymph nodes or beyond results in a 10% patient survival 5 years from the time of diagnosis. Local extension of the tumor into the periureteral tissues also has a poor prognosis, with only 29% of patients surviving 5 years (20,234).

The accuracy of clinical diagnosis of TCCU becomes crucial in predicting the patient's prognosis and determining the most appropriate therapy. Batata and colleagues (20) showed that 72% of ureteral tumors could be diagnosed reliably radiographically by intravenous pyelography (19%), retrograde urography, or ureteral catheterization (53%). However, that leaves more than one-fourth of the patients with indeterminate radiographic studies. Neither urine cytology nor flow cytometry is consistently reliable in diagnosing transitional cell carcinoma of the upper urinary tract. Although high-grade tumors often have an associated abnormal cytology, negative urine cytology is seen in as many as 10% of patients with high-grade lesions and in up to 60% of patients with low-grade lesions (310). Flow cytometry measures cellular DNA and RNA content. A false-negative flow cytometry may be seen in 66% of superficial papillomas and in 8% of invasive cancers (242). Blute and colleagues (31a) showed that imaging studies and cytology together correctly diagnosed a ureteral tumor in only 52% of 21 patients who eventually were found to have a ureteral malignancy.

In 1929, Young (381) performed the first recorded ureteroscopic examination when he inserted a pediatric endoscope into a dilated ureter and passed it up to the level of the renal pelvis in a child with posterior urethral valves. Fifty years later, Lyon and colleagues (229) reported on their experience with endoscopy of the distal ureter using pediatric instruments. Subsequently, Perez-Castro and Martinez-Pineiro (289) created the first custom-built ureteroscope; they described their experience in ureteroscopy, including initial examination of the ureter to the level of the renal pelvis in both men and women.

First-generation rigid ureteroscopes were developed with the goal of visualizing the distal ureter and generally measured 20 cm long with a diameter of 13 to 14.5 Fr. As indications were extended into the middle ureter, proximal ureter, and renal pelvis, working lengths increased and endoscope diameters decreased. Presently, rigid ureteroscopes are available in 6.9 Fr with working lengths up to 40 cm; these diminutive endoscopes also incorporate single (4 to 5 Fr) or dual (2.3 and 3.4 Fr) working channels to allow simultaneous passage of instruments and effective irrigation. Subsequently, flexible ureteroscopes with active deflection up to 180 degrees and a diameter of 7.5 Fr have been developed. The working channel size in these endoscopes is smaller (3.6 Fr) than in their rigid counterparts, hence the irrigant must be pressurized when using diagnostic or therapeutic instruments.

Presently, the indications for diagnostic ureteroscopy include radiographic filling defects or obstruction, unilateral malignant urinary cytology, or macroscopic, essential lateralizing hematuria (149). The indications for ureteroscopic treatment of upper tract tumors are less well defined.

Technique

Ureteroscopy is an adjuvant procedure in the diagnostic evaluation of the patient. Therefore all patients should have preprocedural evaluations, including a thorough history, physical examination, and radiographic evaluation. The urethra and bladder must be examined carefully with the cystoscope to eliminate the possibility of a lower tract tumor. If this is present, it should be resected and the surgical site allowed to heal completely before manipulation of the upper urinary tract to reduce the potential risk of tumor seeding and implantation (341).

The technique for ureteroscopy in patients with suspected upper tract TCCU involves no use of an initial ureteral guidewire to avoid inadvertent injury to the collecting system (259). The procedure is initiated by passing a small-caliber (6.9-Fr), short, rigid ureteroscope to study the distal ureter and rule out any pathologic condition. Through the ureteroscope, a guidewire is advanced to the uppermost point to which the 6.9-Fr ureteroscope was advanced, and the short rigid ureteroscope is removed. A small-caliber, actively deflectable flexible ureteroscope is passed over the guidewire and into the ureter under fluoroscopic guidance, being careful not to push the guidewire any higher in the ureter. If upper tract biopsies are anticipated, it is helpful to place a ureteral access sheath to the level of the ureter visualized with the rigid ureteroscope. This facilitates subsequent placement of the flexible ureteroscope, through the distal ureter, into the upper collecting system. In addition, following biopsy of a lesion, the ureteroscope can be removed without having to pull the biopsy device through the endoscope, which may shear off the tissue of the specimen within the scope. Multiple biopsies can be performed because the flexible ureteroscope can be easily reintroduced into the collecting system through the access sheath. Once the flexible ureteroscope is positioned at the upper level of the already examined ureter, the guidewire is removed. With the availability of smaller-caliber ureteroscopes, dilation of the distal ureter usually is not necessary.

Proximal ureteroscopy is performed, followed by examination of the renal pelvis. Systematic evaluation of the upper-, middle-, and lower-pole calices, in that order, is performed. This procedure prevents confusion due to contusion of the mouth of the upper-pole infundibulum caused by passive deflection of the shaft of the endoscope against this area during inspection of the lower-pole calices. Nonionic contrast medium is injected under fluoroscopic guidance to verify endoscopic entry into all calices of the renal collecting system. If a lesion is identified, its location is marked on the fluoroscope screen. After complete inspection of the collecting system, the lesion is addressed. The lesion is then biopsied by passing a 3-Fr biopsy forceps or a 3-Fr basket through the ureteroscope. The latter is twirled into the lesion and then closed; as it is withdrawn, the entrapped papillary fronds are detached from the tumor.

Brush biopsy catheters for the flexible ureteroscope are also available and may be of value if the biopsy material is not adequate. It is helpful to place a ureteral access sheath to facilitate passage of the flexible ureteroscope and removal of the biopsy specimen. After removal of the biopsied material, a 2- or 3-Fr electrosurgical probe or a 200- to 400-micron

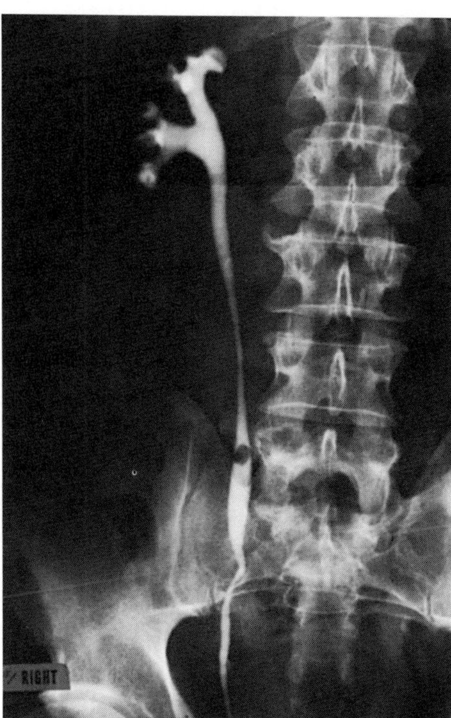

FIGURE 19.15. This midureteral filling defect is a low-grade transitional cell cancer. The diagnosis and therapy both were completed using the ureteroscope. Follow-up over 2 years revealed no recurrence.

Nd:YAG laser probe (20 W) may be used to fulgurate the area; alternatively, if a large 12.5-Fr, rigid ureteroscope is being used, a resectoscope loop can be used to resect the tumor down to ureteral muscle (Fig. 19.15) (99). Last, the flexible endoscope is advanced into the renal pelvis, and the collecting system is systematically examined for any additional occult tumors. The aspirate and biopsy specimens should be sent immediately to the cytopathology laboratory, where they are evaluated by smear and cytospin. When any tissue fragments are visible in the specimen, a cell block is prepared.

Following resection of the primary tumor, a withdrawal retrograde ureterogram should be performed to assess extravasation. The ureteroscope is removed, and an indwelling ureteral stent is inserted over the safety guidewire; a urethral catheter is also placed. If there is no extravasation, the urethral catheter is removed on the first postoperative morning. The ureteral catheter is removed 3 to 5 days later as an outpatient. In the event of extravasation, the urethral catheter is maintained for 2 or 3 days, at which time a cystogram is performed. When the extravasation has resolved, the urethral catheter may be removed. The ureteral stent is left in place for 4 to 6 weeks.

Results

Grasso and Bagley (121) used the small-diameter, actively deflectable, flexible ureteroscope to investigate 584 patients suspected to have urothelial malignancies. They were able to successfully complete the ureteropyeloscopy in 94% of the patients. Ureteral dilation was required in only 12% of procedures. Lower-pole access required secondary or passive deflection in 60% of procedures. Keeley and colleagues (185) performed diagnostic ureterorenoscopy in 92 consecutive patients with upper tract transitional cell carcinoma. Fifty-one open surgical procedures were subsequently performed, including distal ureterectomy in four and nephroureterectomy in forty-seven. Cytologic evaluation was positive for malignancy in 48 of 51 cases (94%). Grading of ureteroscopic specimens was possible in 42 cases (82%) (Table 19.5). Transitional cell carcinoma grade on ureteroscopy accurately predicted tumor grade and stage in the surgical specimens. There was no significant perioperative morbidity.

The success of intravesical agents in the treatment of superficial transitional cell carcinoma of the bladder has motivated some investigators to apply these agents in the management of upper urinary tract tumors (83,185,233). Among these reports a variety of topical chemotherapeutic agents have been used, including bacille Calmette-Guérin (BCG), mitomycin C, thiotepa, and interferon-α_2. There has been no standardization to determine which patients receive this adjuvant therapy, although it tends to be given to patients judged to be at high risk for recurrence. The therapy is usually administered via a ureteral catheter, after retrograde pyelography has confirmed no extravasation and

TABLE 19.5. ENDOSCOPIC MANAGEMENT OF PRIMARY URETERAL TRANSITIONAL CELL CARCINOMA

Authors	No. of Patients	Treatment	Adjuvant Therapy	Local Recurrance Rate (%)	Metastasis	Average Follow-up (mo)
Huffman et al. (153)	17	3 segmental ureterectomy 14 ureteroscopic excision	0 0	33 36	0 0	15 16
Eastham and Huffman (83)	4	4 ureteroscopic excision	Mitomycin C 5 mg in 20 mL saline × 30 min	25	0	8
Elliott et al. (86)	23	8 ureteroscopy/Nd:YAG 13 ureteroscopy/electrocautery 2 PCN/Nd:YAG	0 0 0	39	9	58
Martinez-Pineiro et al. (233)	22	14 ureteroscopy/Nd:YAG 6 ureteroscopy/electroresect 2 ureteroscopy/electrocautery	BCG/mitomycin/VAC, 5-FU not specified who received what treatment	57 0 0	Not specified	30
Keeley et al. (185)	18	Ureteroscopy/Nd:YAG/Ho:YAG	Mitomycin 40 mg/3 doses via ureteral catheter	28	Not specified	35
Grasso et al. (122)	8	7 ureteroscopy/Nd:YAG 1 ureteroscopy resection	0 0	63	0	18
Total	**92**			**47**		**28**

good flow around the ureteral catheter. Keeley and colleagues (185) administered 40 mg of mitomycin C in three divided doses in the immediate postoperative period in 15 patients with no attributable toxicity. Seven patients received intravesical BCG with a ureteral stent in place; again with no significant toxicity. However, no attempt was made to randomize the patients; therefore little can be determined regarding the efficacy of either treatment.

A low-grade, low-stage ureteral tumor may be associated with urothelial dysplasia and carcinoma *in situ* in other areas of the ureter in 50% and 9% to 13% of cases, respectively (140). Bloom and associates (30) reported ureteral stump tumors in 4 of 10 patients (40%) with primary ureteral carcinoma who underwent nephrectomy and partial ureterectomy. Strong and colleagues (346) had 5 of 13 patients (40%) with ureteral stump recurrences following segmental ureterectomy or incomplete nephroureterectomy for primary ureteral carcinoma. Therefore, when management other than radical surgical excision is chosen for a patient with transitional cell carcinoma of the ureter, ongoing surveillance of the entire urinary tract is mandatory. In most situations, this should follow the same regimen that is used among bladder cancer patients. Specifically, ureteroscopic examination of the ureter should be performed every 3 months for 1 year, then every 6 months for 1 year, and then on an annual basis. Although intravenous or retrograde urography and cytology may be substituted for the endoscopic evaluation, these studies may be less accurate in detecting early, diminutive, low-grade recurrences.

Kerbl and Clayman (188) described a method of transurethrally unroofing the ureteral orifice in two patients undergoing endoscopic management of upper tract transitional cell carcinoma. At presentation, neither patient had a history of bladder tumor. By creating a widely patent ureteral orifice, the clinician could perform flexible ureteroscopy (10 Fr) in the office without the need for dilation of the intramural ureter, without oral or parenteral analgesics, and without postureteroscopy stent placement. The entire length of the ureter and all of the calyces could be completely examined in this manner. These two patients have been followed for over 5 years. One patient has had a small, recurrent, superficial, papillary lesion in the renal pelvis treated with electrosurgical fulguration 4 years after the initial procedure; pathologic evaluation was not performed on this lesion. The other patient has had three small upper tract recurrences. Both patients have had grade I to II pathologic stage A bladder tumors during the 5 years of follow-up and have received intravesical BCG or interferon therapy following transurethral resection of the bladder tumor.

Incision of the intramural ureter creates low-grade asymptomatic reflux. Guthman and colleagues (133) have shown that sterile reflux in the adult does not impair renal function or result in increased urinary tract infections. The primary concern is whether reflux will result in more frequent upper tract recurrences in these patients because of seeding from the lower tract. Some investigators have shown that among patients with recurrent bladder tumors and reflux, the incidence of upper tract tumors may be as high as 20% (7,254). Long-term, clinical follow-up will be necessary to study this hypothetical concern.

A significant concern with regard to endoscopic management of patients with transitional cell carcinoma of the ureter is the potential for tumor implantation or tumor seeding. Soloway and Masters (341) have shown in an animal model that disruption of the urothelial cell layer by cauterization increased implantation of transitional cell tumors by fourfold. During balloon dilation of the distal ureter and passage of the ureteroscope, abrasion of the urothelium may occur. Kulp and Bagley (208) reported on 13 patients, all of whom underwent ureteropyeloscopy with biopsy and treatment one to four times before nephroureterectomy for TCC of the renal pelvis. Only one patient had vascular-lymphatic extension, and because of the tumor growth characteristics, extension was suspected before endoscopy. This patient had no intravascular-lymphatic free cells or clumps of cells noted on the final pathologic specimen. There were no local recurrences in the follow-up of the remaining patients, at 3 months to 6 years (average of 34 months).

Ureteral perforation and subsequent retroperitoneal tumor implantation are a concern during ureteroscopy for TCCU. Perforation is more likely to occur with electrosurgical resection of the ureteral lesion than with excisional biopsy and Nd:YAG laser fulguration of the tumor base. However, to date in none of the reports of ureteroscopic management of primary ureteral transitional cell carcinoma has there been a case of retroperitoneal seeding documented during clinical follow-up up to 21 months (83,86,122,151, 187,233).

Nephroureterectomy or distal ureterectomy remains the treatment of choice in most patients with TCCU. For patients with a solitary kidney, renal insufficiency, or medical illnesses rendering them poor candidates for an open surgical procedure, endoscopic modalities for treatment of upper tract transitional cell carcinoma are reasonable alternatives for management. However, the overall long-term (i.e., longer than 5 years) efficacy of these endoscopic modalities remains unproven. Continued long-term follow-up of patients with ureteral transitional cell carcinoma managed with ureteroscopic excision and fulguration is essential to delineate the effectiveness and long-term complications and cost of this minimally invasive procedure.

Benign Ureteral Fistulae

The ureter may be damaged easily during abdominal or pelvic surgery because of its proximity to the peritoneum. Gynecologic operations are the primary cause of iatrogenic ureteral injury. The incidence of these lesions ranges from 0.5% to 1% for common pelvic operations and up to 10% for radical pelvic surgery (80). Ureteroscopy also can result in ureteral injury. In addition, ureteral fistulae to the peritoneal space, retroperitoneum, adjacent viscera, or skin may result from other benign (i.e., regional enteritis) disease. Perforation, resection, or ligation of the ureter leads to extravasation of urine, formation of a urinoma, and late development of ureterocutaneous or ureterovaginal fistulae. Many ureteric injuries are identified at the time of the surgical procedure and managed with repair or stinting without significant sequelae to the patient. Ureteric injuries that are not recognized intraoperatively or in the early postoperative period are complicated by periureteric fibrosis or epithelialization of the fistulous tract.

Technique

The approach to urinary fistulae is based on the principle that the urine must be diverted from the site of the extravasation. The placement of a percutaneous nephrostomy tube effectively diverts the urine away from the fistula; in addition, an indwelling ureteral stent, with sideholes only in the intrapelvic and intravesical pigtail, is positioned across the fistulous tract.

The stent may be passed antegrade or retrograde. The antegrade approach is performed more easily because of the dilation of the upper collecting system. If a guidewire cannot be manipulated across the ureter, a flexible ureteroscope can be passed antegrade, and the ureter can be cannulated under direct vision. Likewise, if a retrograde approach is chosen, ureteroscopy may be helpful to cannulate the ureter. Ureteroscopy is also helpful if the obstruction and fistula formation are the result of a prior surgical procedure. In this case, retrograde rigid ureteroscopy is advisable because any visualized obstructing suture can be incised with a ureterotome before placing a stent (198).

Results

Early diagnosis and treatment are key to the successful management of ureteral injuries. Endourologic techniques have a higher success rate when instituted as soon as possible following the ureteral injury (198). Successful endourologic treatment reduces the patient's hospitalization, incidence of complications, and postoperative discomfort. Placement of the ureteral stent seems to decrease stricture formation at the site of injury (212). Chang and colleagues (41) reported 12 patients with ureteral fistulae treated with percutaneous nephrostomy and 8- to 12-Fr ureteral stents. The stent was left in place for 4 to 6 weeks. In 10 of 12 patients (83%), the ureteral fistula healed without stricture formation or further intervention. One patient required continued stinting for recurrence of a pelvic malignancy. One patient had a persistent ureterovaginal fistula and required a psoas hitch and ureteral reimplantation. At the time of surgery, the ureter was noted to be angulated as a result of cicatrization and a chronic urinoma.

Malignant Ureteral Fistulae

The most difficult ureterovaginal or vesicovaginal fistulae to manage are those associated with incurable pelvic cancer. These patients often have been treated with radiation therapy, are terminally ill, and are not suitable candidates for open urinary diversion.

Technique

Nephrostomy tube drainage is usually instituted in these patients; although the drainage of urine is diminished, it is rarely stopped by this modality alone. Usually the ureter must be occluded to truly stop the leakage of urine. This can be accomplished with either of two antegrade approaches: electrocoagulation of the urothelium of the lower ureter or fluoroscopic placement of obstructing material in the distal ureter. Ureteral coagulation is performed through a flexible nephroscope introduced via the nephrostomy tract. Beginning approximately 6 to 7 cm below the ureteropelvic junction, the urothelium is circumferentially electrocoagulated using a 3- or 5-Fr round-tip or ball electrode. The procedure is continued until 4 to 5 cm of proximal ureter has been treated; the nephrostomy tube is then replaced. Alternatively, under fluoroscopic control, an antegrade angiographic catheter can be delivered to the fistulous site. A large sponge of Gelfoam (38 inches thick, 34 inches long, 14 inches wide) is instilled through the catheter; Gianturco coils also may be delivered to the fistulous site. These materials are superior to instillation of cyanoacrylate or placement of a detachable balloon for closing the ureter (129).

Results

Gunther and colleagues (130) first attempted to perform transrenal ureteral occlusion with the tissue adhesive butyl-2-cyanoacrylate. However, long-term follow-up showed that this substance softened in urine and was expelled by ureteral peristalsis. Subsequently, they adopted a detachable balloon filled with low-viscosity silicone rubber and released in the distal ureter (129). An advantage to the occlusion balloon is that the ureter is not irreparably destroyed should ureteral surgery or diversion become necessary at a later date. In their clinical report, five patients with urinary fistulae secondary to pelvic cancer and two patients with severe painful pollakisüria underwent ureteral occlusion with a detachable balloon (129). In all patients, urinary flow via the ureter ceased by ureteral balloon occlusion and combined nephrostomy drainage. Follow-up ranged from 1 month to 6 months. No complications occurred.

Kinn and associates (194) combined the insertion of nylon plugs with injection of polidocanol for ureteral occlusion in 15 patients with vesicovaginal fistulae. Urine leakage ceased in 73% of patients; however, the plug did migrate to the renal pelvis in six patients and was associated with pyelonephritis in one patient. More recently, a high success rate has been attained using Gianturco coils in combination with gelatin sponge material to occlude the ureter (103).

Reddy and colleagues (300) described the technique of percutaneous ureteral fulguration for occlusion of the ureter combined with nephrostomy drainage in three patients with urinary tract fistulae secondary to pelvic cancers. In their report, three patients were treated with percutaneous ureteral fulguration and nephrostomy tube drainage for lower urinary tract fistulae secondary to advanced pelvic malignancy. All patients were completely dry at the fistula site 4 to 10 days following the ureteral fulguration. Follow-up ranged from 1 to 21 months with stable renal function and no complications.

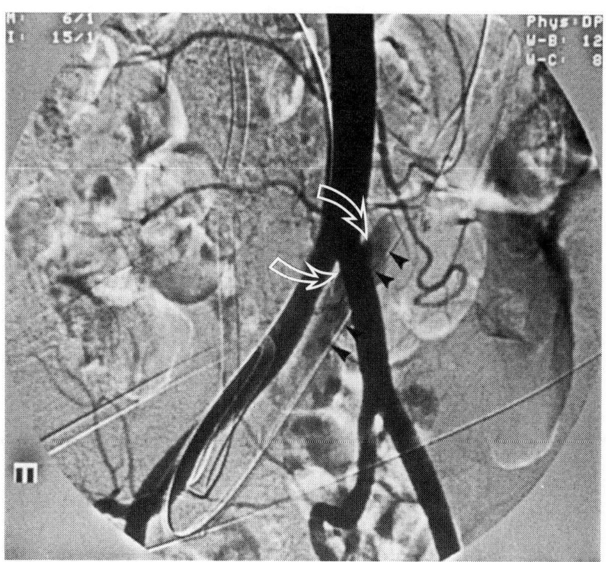

FIGURE 19.16. An arterial-ureteral *(curved arrows)* fistula is demonstrated on this flush aortogram. The arrowheads outline the ureter. This fistula developed 3 days following an endoureterotomy for a left ureteroenteric anastomotic stricture. This patient underwent an uneventful open repair of the left common iliac artery.

Arterial Ureteral Fistulae

Arterioureteral fistulae are rare, with less than 40 cases reported in the literature (72). The primary clinical presentation is massive hematuria, which may result in shock and cardiovascular arrest. In many cases the hematuria did not become apparent until the time of ureteral stent removal. In a review of the literature, Dervanian and colleagues (72) found that 57.5% of the arterioureteral fistulae reported in the literature were associated with prolonged (average of 5.6 months) ureteral catheterization. They hypothesized that the stent may result in ischemia of the ureter as it crosses the iliac vessels, thereby resulting in localized necrosis of the ureteral and arterial walls. Other factors that may contribute to arterioureteral fistula formation include primary iliac artery disease (e.g., mycotic infection, aneurysm), prior iliac artery surgery (e.g., endarterectomy, prosthetic graft), pelvic neoplasm, radiation fibrosis, postsurgical ischemia of the ureter, and endoureterotomy. Patients with known common iliac artery disease are poor candidates for chronic indwelling ureteral stents. In these patients, a permanent nephrostomy or a nephrovesical stent is a safer alternative.

Technique

Among patients with a chronic indwelling ureteral stent, it is advisable to remove the stent over a guidewire. This ensures the urologist's control over the upper urinary tract. The immediate treatment of sudden onset of hematuria after stent removal is to pass a 5- or 8-mm ureteral dilating balloon catheter over the guidewire until the balloon straddles the area of the common iliac vessels. On inflation, the fistulous tract is effectively occluded, thereby allowing time to stabilize the patient with intravenous fluids.

Treatment of the arterioureteral fistula is by embolization and bypass or by direct surgical repair. These fistulae are amenable to embolization. However, careful coordination between the interventional radiologist and vascular surgeon is essential to avoid lower limb ischemia. The advantage of this approach is that a femoral-femoral bypass can be performed, thereby obviating a major transabdominal procedure. The direct surgical procedure involves management of the blood vessel by ligation and bypass, direct suture repair, or patch repair. The urinary tract involvement may be managed with nephroureterectomy, cutaneous ureterostomy, ureteral resection and anastomosis, or ureteral ligation followed by percutaneous nephrostomy. The choice of surgical procedure depends on the local tissue conditions and the patient's overall medical status. However, the least invasive therapy is to embolize the common iliac vessel, proceed with a femoral-to-femoral bypass, and place a percutaneous nephrostomy tube.

Results

If an arterioureteral fistula is suspected, arteriograms and retrograde pyelograms should be performed (Fig. 19.16). Of the 33 cases in Dervanian's report, direct visualization of the arterioureteral fistula by retrograde pyelograms occurred in 27% and by arteriography in 23% of the patients studied. The common iliac artery was most often involved (55%); other vessels involved were the internal iliac artery (9%), external iliac artery (6%), inferior mesenteric artery (3%), and iliac patch angioplasty or anastomosis site (30%). The right ureter was involved in 58% of the cases and the left ureter in 42% of cases. The mortality rate of arteriovenous fistulae is approximately 15%. Knowledge of this rare problem and its efficient management are essential for all urologists.

THERAPEUTIC RENAL APPLICATIONS

There are four areas in which endourology has a significant effect on the handling of noncalculous renal disease: obstruction, transitional cell cancer, cysts, and infection (e.g., abscess, fungal bezoar). In each of these areas, retrograde ureteroscopic and antegrade nephroscopic techniques are used. In this section, each of these four areas is reviewed from the standpoint of technique and results. Endourologic techniques as they apply to the transplant kidney are also reviewed.

Renal Obstruction

There are two types of stricture disease that affect the kidney: UPJ obstruction and calyceal abnormalities. In the latter category are the calyceal diverticulum and hydrocalyx.

Ureteropelvic Junction

Historical Aspects

Precedence in the surgical treatment of UPJ obstruction belongs to Friedrich Trendelenburg, who in 1886 performed the first recorded reconstructive procedure on the ureteropelvic junction. Unfortunately, the death of his patient probably tempered enthusiasm for this approach; it was not until 5 years later that Ernest Kuster accomplished a dismembered pyeloplasty unaccompanied by surgical mortality (257). Other innovative open surgical approaches to repairing the obstructed UPJ soon followed: renal pelvis plication, Y-V flap advancement, straight flap insertion, and spiral flap repair.

In the early 1900s, faced with what appeared to be an inoperable situation, Joachim Albarran performed the first endopyelotomy when he incised an upper tract stricture and left a catheter in place. Surprisingly, the incised-but-not-reconstructed ureter healed and remained patent; Albarran termed this fortuitous occurrence a *ureterotome externe* when he first reported it in 1909. Subsequently, during a visit to Europe, Keyes learned of the technique and brought it back to the United States in 1915. However, it was not until the 1940s that David M. Davis, in the twilight of his career in urology, rediscovered Albarran's work. Between 1943 and 1948, Davis developed the technique of "intubated ureteroplasty." He reported an 89% subjective and a 60% objective success rate at 1- to 2-year follow-up (67,68).

Much interest resulted from Davis' reports, and during the ensuing decade many laboratory studies were undertaken in an effort to better understand how the intubated ureterotomy worked. From these studies it became apparent that the urothelium covered the ureteral incision, usually within 5 days. Ureteral muscle appeared to regenerate and grow around the incised ureter between 6 and 12 weeks; contracture appeared to play less of a role with regard to the development of an intact circumferential muscle layer. In addition, peristalsis was noted to return across the area of the incision within 6 weeks (135,136,230, 274,372). Despite these revelations, by the late 1960s intubated ureterotomy had become a rarely performed procedure, having been superseded by the more successful and aesthetically more pleasing plastic reconstructive procedures of the renal pelvis, specifically the Anderson Hynes dismembered pyeloplasty.

The 1970s brought an explosion in interest in percutaneous nephrostomy; in the late 1970s, this new method for minimally invasive access to the kidney rapidly replaced open nephrostomy first, and later, open urolithiasis surgery. It was in this environment that in 1983, Mr. J.E.A. Wickham developed the concept for performing a percutaneous intubated ureterotomy by incising the UPJ from inside out (i.e., "pyelolysis"). Wickham, working with Miller, Whitfield, and Ramsey, used a cold-knife urethrotome to incise the ureteropelvic junction. Via a preplaced nephrostomy tract, the kidney was traversed, and the UPJ was incised until periureteric fat could be seen. A nephrostomy tube was placed at the end of the procedure; an indwelling stent was maintained across the incised UPJ for 4 weeks. The reported success rate was 64% (287,298).

Subsequently, A.D. Smith brought Mr. Wickham's pyelolysis to the United States; he renamed the procedure *endopyelotomy.* Using a cold-knife endoscopic technique with a newly developed hook blade, Smith, Badlani, Karlin, and associates achieved success rates of 87.5% in patients with both primary and secondary UPJ obstruction (10,176, 250). In their series, a 14-Fr tapered external nephrostent was left indwelling for 6 weeks. By 1993, they had expanded their series to 189 patients; overall success rate was 86% at 6 to 96 months' follow-up regardless of a primary or secondary type of UPJ obstruction (251).

The approach and method of UPJ incision are variable. The approach may be either antegrade by endoscopic means or retrograde by endoscopic, fluoroscopic, or combined means. Nonetheless, the classic antegrade percutaneous approach is still a very popular method for performing an endopyelotomy (Fig. 19.17). Via an upper pole or middle posterior calyx nephrostomy tract, the UPJ is visualized directly and incised with a cold knife until periureteric fat is seen clearly.

Variations of the antegrade method include using a retrograde inflated balloon to invaginate the UPJ into the renal pelvis, using a wire-guided ureterotome blade, and a transpelvic approach. In the invagination method, the balloon is inflated just beneath the UPJ, provided the ureter has a low insertion into the renal pelvis. The inflated balloon is then pushed cephalad so that the UPJ is carried into the renal pelvis itself; as such, when the tissue overlying the balloon is incised, a double length of tissue is cut because the UPJ has been folded into the renal pelvis. This method should preclude any inadvertent incision of a crossing vessel and speeds the overall completion of the procedure (106,107). Alternatively, a wire-guided cutting instrument can be passed antegrade over the guidewire and through the

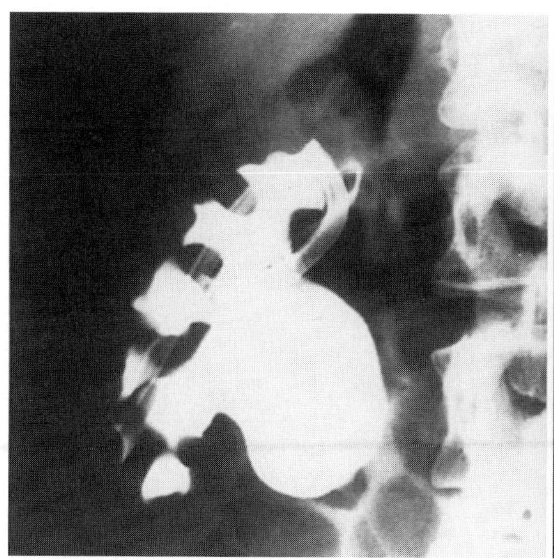

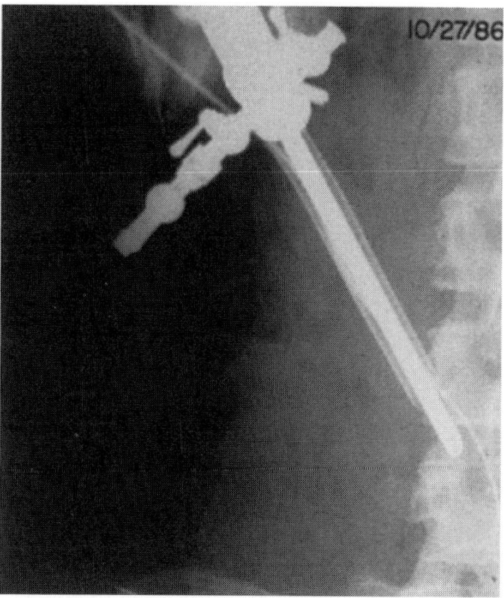

FIGURE 19.17. A: An antegrade nephrostogram reveals marked ureteropelvic junction obstruction. **B:** A cold-knife urethrotome has been introduced via the nephrostomy tract. A guidewire traverses the ureteropelvic junction. An incision in the ureteropelvic junction (UPJ) was then made along the lateral border of the UPJ.

narrowed UPJ, thereby incising it. This technique has been used successfully by both Korth and Schneider (201,318). Another technique is the transpelvic approach in which the renal pelvis is purposely incised along its lateral or posterolateral surface and the urethrotome is passed *outside* of the pelvis. The UPJ is then incised from the outside inward (273).

The retrograde approach varies from a purely fluoroscopic to an endoscopic technique. In 1987, Beckman and Roth (22) reported passing a retrograde angioplasty-type balloon to dilate the obstructed UPJ. Since then there have been few reports of a similar approach (Table 19.6). In general, an 8- to 10-mm dilating balloon catheter rated to 10 to 15 atm of pressure is passed retrograde until it straddles the obstructed UPJ. The balloon is then inflated until the obstruction disappears; the inflated balloon is left in place for a variable period of time (usually 1 minute). In some cases, the balloon is then deflated and reinflated for two more 60-second cycles.

At about the same time that Beckman and Roth described their retrograde fluoroscopic technique, Inglis and Tolley (160) reported a retrograde ureteroscopic approach to performing an endopyelotomy. In their approach, the rigid ureteroscope was passed up to the site of the UPJ obstruction, and the ureter was then incised with an electrosurgical probe until periureteric fat could be seen. Subsequently, several other urologists reported on a similar approach using electrocautery or a cold knife to make the incision (Fig. 19.18) (47). To facilitate delivery of the rigid or flexible ureteroscope, Thomas suggested stinting the ureter for 1 week before the planned endopyelotomy (356).

A third variation on the retrograde approach was reported by Clayman and colleagues (52) in 1992. In this fluoroscopic technique, a 13-Fr electrosurgical wire-bearing, 8-mm balloon catheter is advanced over a guidewire until the balloon straddles the UPJ (Fig. 19.19). For primary UPJ obstruction before insertion over the guidewire, the balloon catheter is rotated until the electrosurgical wire faces laterally. The catheter is advanced halfway up the ureter, at which point a side-arm adaptor is placed on the throughput channel of the catheter. A retrograde ureterogram with dilute contrast is obtained, thereby defining the UPJ area. Next, the catheter is advanced across the UPJ; the electrosurgical wire should remain in a lateral orientation. The position of the electrosurgical wire is carefully checked with fluoroscopy (Fig. 19.20A,B). At this point, 0.5 mL of dilute contrast is placed in the balloon to define its position and to raise the electrosurgical wire slightly off of the catheter's shaft. Then the electrosurgical wire is simultaneously activated at 75 W of pure cutting current while the balloon is completely inflated to its full 2 mL volume (Fig. 19.20C). The inflated balloon is left in place for 10 minutes, and then it is deflated. There should be prompt extravasation from the incision site (Fig. 19.20D). If this is not the case, the cutting device can be activated one more time. If extravasation still is not appreciable, the cutting balloon catheter is deflated, pulled back to the midureter, and a retrograde ureterogram is repeated. If there is still no extravasation, the cutting balloon catheter is removed and a flexible ureteroscope can be passed to the site; if no incision in the ureter is seen, a cut can be made with a 2-Fr electrosurgical probe or a 360-micron Ho:YAG laser fiber passed through the flexible ureteroscope.

After the UPJ is opened, an external or internal stent varying in size from 8 to 14 Fr is placed. The stent duration is usually 4 to 6 weeks. A follow-up intravenous pyelogram

TABLE 19.6. ENDOPYELOTOMY: RETROGRADE BALLOON AND ANTEGRADE TECHNIQUE

Authors	No. of Patients	Approach	Method of Incision	Stent Size (Fr)	Stent Duration (wk)	Overall Success Rate (%)	Success Rate (%) 1° UPJ	Success Rate (%) 2° UPJ	Hospital Stay (days)	Average Follow-up (range) (mo)	Secondary Pyeloplasty (%)	Secondary Nephrectomy (%)
Balloon Series												
Beckman et al. (23)	11	Antegrade or retrograde	6 to 10-mm balloon	8–10	4–8	73	86	50	—	10 (2–22)	—	—
Webber et al.	76	Retrograde	10-mm balloon	10	6–8	67	—	—	—	(8–120)	3	11
Oakley et al. (267)	20	Retrograde (15) Antegrade (5)	10-mm balloon	6	6	67	72	33	4	22 (6–30)	—	15
Total	**80**		**10-mm balloon**	**6–10**	**4–8**	**73**	**81**	**46**	**4.2**	**17**	—	—
Antegrade Endopyelotomy												
Van Cangh et al. (365)	102	Antegrade	Cold-cut knife	10–12	6	73	—	—	6.7	60 (12–120)	11	0
Kletscher et al. (197)	50	Antegrade	Cold-cut knife	7–14	6	88	90	82	3–8	12 (4–74)	14	0
Brooks et al. (35)	13	Antegrade	Cold knife	7 or 14	4–6	77	—	—	3	20 (4–53)	2	0
Korth et al. (201)	286	Antegrade	Cold knife	Primestent PCN/EP	3–6	73	80	67	—	20 (6–120)	—	—
Gallucci and Alpi (100)	46	Antegrade	Cold knife	5 or 6	3	80	—	—	4	— (12–60)	4	—
Khan et al. (189)	220	Antegrade	Cold knife	8–12 PCN/EP	6	86.7	—	—	5.2	—	5	3
Danuser et al. (66)	80	Antegrade	Cold knife	8/14 or 7/12 PCN/EP	6	89	—	—	6	26 (1.5–72)	11	1
Shalhav et al. (326)	83	Antegrade	Electrosurgical	7 or 7/14	4–6	83	89	77	4	32	—	—
Total	**880**			**5–7/14**	**3–6**	**81**	**86**	**75**	**4.7**	**28**	—	—

UPJ, ureteropelvic junction.

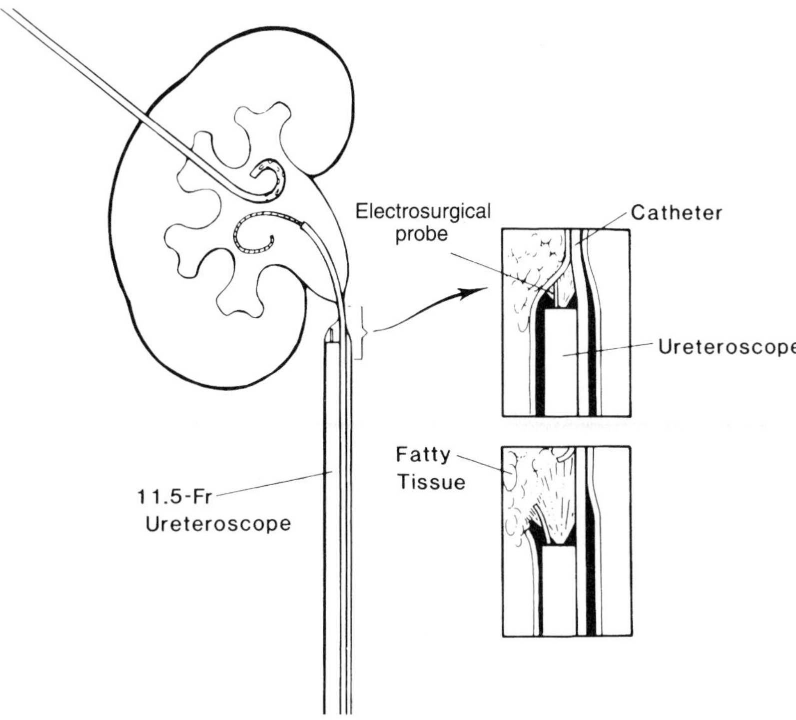

FIGURE 19.18. The 11.5-Fr long, rigid ureteroscope has been passed through the ureter; an electrosurgical probe tip can be seen protruding from the tip of the ureteroscope. The tip of the ureteroscope is covered with a nonconductive material. A nephrostomy rube remains from a preoperative Whitaker test. A safety guidewire and a 5-Fr nonconductive catheter have been placed up the ureter. The *inset* shows a close-up of the actual incision in the lateral aspect of the UPJ; the incision is continued until the full thickness of the ureteral wall has been cut and periureteral fat can be seen clearly. (From Clayman RV, Kavousi LR. Endosurgical techniques for noncalculous disease. In: Walsh PC et al, eds. *Campbell's urology,* ed 6. Philadelphia: Saunders, 1992:2277, with permission.)

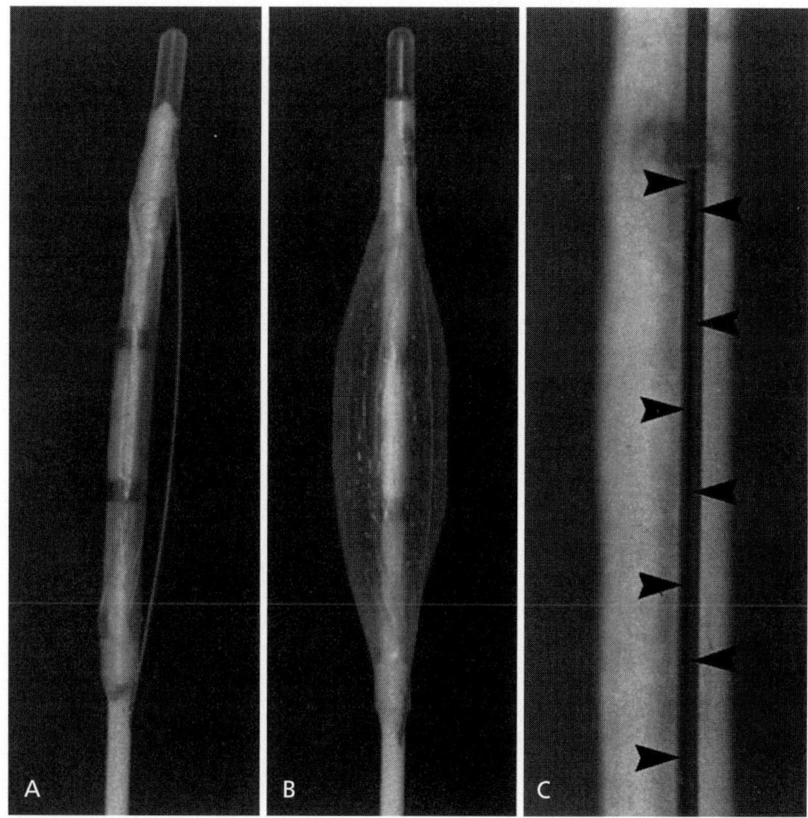

FIGURE 19.19. A: A cutting balloon (i.e., Acucise) is shown in its uninflated state. The cutting wire is clearly seen overlying the balloon. **B:** With the balloon inflated, the cutting wire is stretched over the balloon. **C:** A close-up of the cutting wire shows that the actual cutting surface of the wire *(arrowheads)* is only 150 microns in width but 2.8 cm in length.

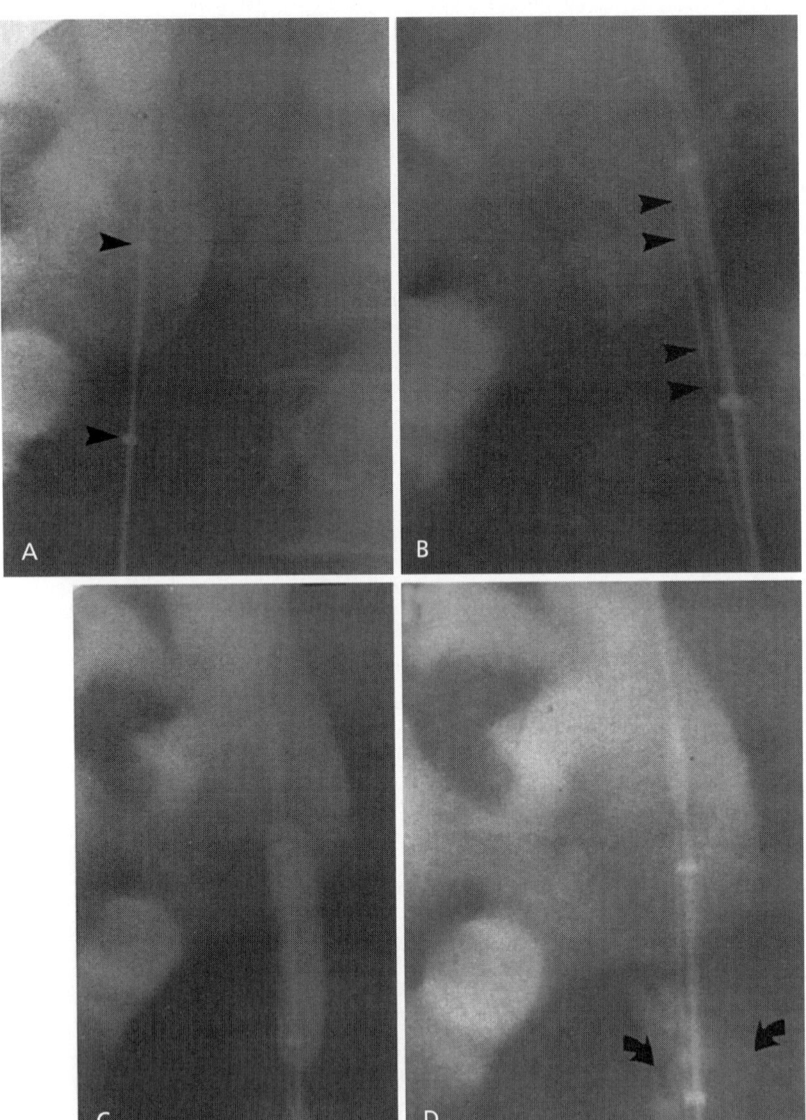

FIGURE 19.20. A: The cutting balloon has been passed up over the guidewire until the cutting wire straddles the ureteropelvic junction (UPJ) area. Note that the cutting wire lies between the two radiopaque markers *(arrowheads).* The cutting wire cannot be seen in this projection. **B:** The catheter has been turned so that the cutting wire is facing laterally *(arrowheads)* along the UPJ area. **C:** The cutting wire has been activated and the balloon has been fully inflated. **D:** As the balloon is deflated, extravasation of contrast *(arrows)* can be seen. Following this, the balloon is removed and an indwelling ureteral stent is placed along with a bladder catheter.

(IVP) or Lasix washout renogram is obtained 1 to 2 weeks after stent removal and again at 3 months, 6 months, 1 year, and then annually for 5 years.

Results

The results of endopyelotomy, regardless of approach or method of incision, have been highly satisfactory. Although not quite equal to open pyeloplasty, the overall success rate has been high enough that, when combined with the minimal morbidity and short hospital stay associated with the procedure, endopyelotomy has become the preferred method of many urologists for treating adult UPJ obstruction.

The largest endopyelotomy experience to date is with an antegrade approach using a cold knife to incise the UPJ. Motola and colleagues (251) reported the initial large series of patients. Among 212 patients treated by antegrade endopyelotomy over an 8-year period between 1983 and 1991, the overall success rate was 89%. For patients followed 6 months or more, the success rate hardly changed: 86%. In addition, primary UPJ and secondary UPJ obstruction fared equally well (85% versus 86% success rate). Other urologists have independently reported success rates of 73% to 89% in series ranging from 13 to 286 patients (33,35,63,66,189,197,201,326,364). Overall, results for primary and secondary UPJ obstruction were comparable (Table 19.6).

In Motola and colleagues' (251) large series, operative time averaged 90 minutes with a hospital stay of 6.2 days. When compared with open pyeloplasty at their institution, they noted that endopyelotomy resulted in a shorter hospital stay (6.2 versus 10 days) and less operative time (90 minutes versus 106 minutes). Also, convalescence was much quicker in the endopyelotomy groups: 20 days versus 42 days. Brooks and colleagues (35) compared open and endourologic approaches with UPJ obstruction in 45 patients. Successful relief of obstruction was achieved in 100% of patients undergoing open and laparoscopic dismembered pyeloplasty, 78% undergoing Acucise endopyelotomy, and 77% undergoing antegrade percutaneous endopyelotomy. The Acucise endopyelotomy resulted in shorter convalescence (1 week) than the antegrade endopyelotomy (4.7 weeks), laparoscopic pyeloplasty (2.3 weeks), or open pyeloplasty (10.3 weeks). Complication rates were similar among all the groups.

Gupta and colleagues (132) reviewed 401 percutaneous endopyelotomy procedures performed over a 12-year period. Eighty-five percent of the failures occurred within 6 months of the endopyelotomy; although 2% failed as late as 5 years following the endopyelotomy. They noted that patients with high-grade hydronephrosis and poor initial renal function were much less likely to have a successful endopyelotomy than those with moderate hydronephrosis or good renal function. Other investigators have demonstrated similar results. The success rate for endopyelotomy in patients with UPJ obstruction caused by high insertion is similar to that reported for endopyelotomy in patients without high insertion (43,326).

Complications from endopyelotomy have been relatively few. Bleeding requiring transfusion has been noted in only 1% of patients in Smith's antegrade endopyelotomy series; however, others have noted significant hemorrhage in 8% to 9% of their cases (207,245). Cassis and co-workers (37) noted an overall major complication rate of 11%. Other serious complications have included ureteral avulsion, ureteral necrosis, and arteriovenous fistula formation (232,251, 347). Urinoma, hematoma, and urinary tract infection also have been reported, albeit rarely.

For retrograde ureteroscopic endopyelotomy, success rates similar to antegrade endopyelotomy have been reported (Table 19.7) (44). An overall success rate of 80% was published by Meretyk and colleagues (245); however, in their series, there was a 16% incidence of intraoperative hemorrhage and a 20% incidence of distal ureteral strictures postoperatively. This resulted in their abandoning the retrograde endoscopic approach in favor of the antegrade technique. However, Thomas and colleagues (356) reported excellent results and low morbidity with a ureteroscopic approach, providing the ureter was stinted for 1 week before ureteroscopic endopyelotomy. In their series the success rate was 87%; one patient (2.5%) required urgent nephrectomy for acute bleeding. Of note, notwithstanding the early experience of Meretyk and associates (245), other urologists have reported an 82% to 90% success rate with the electrosurgical or Ho:YAG laser cutting modality (352,356). Interestingly, in two out of the three reports a dilating balloon is used following the incision at the UPJ to dilate the area. The overall experience with this approach remains small.

The retrograde, fluoroscopic approach to performing an endopyelotomy is the simplest method yet developed (Tables 19.6 and 19.7). However, experience with either balloon dilation to 30 Fr or a balloon incision is less than with the antegrade approach. Although originally described by Kadir and colleagues (173) in 1982 in a patient with a secondary UPJ obstruction, balloon dilation of the UPJ did not undergo any significant testing until 1989, when Beckman and colleagues (23) and O'Flynn and colleagues (271) independently reported on its use in a series of 11 and 31 patients, respectively. After balloon dilation to 18 to 30 Fr, a 7- to 10-Fr stent was left indwelling for 4 to 8 weeks. Overall success rates of 68% to 73% were recorded at follow-up of 10 months. Of note, the procedure appeared to work better for primary (86% success rate) than for secondary (50% success rate) UPJ obstruction (23,173,271). Subsequently, McClinton and colleagues (236) expanded O'Flynn and colleagues' (271) original series and reported on 76 patients treated with endoballoon rupture of the UPJ using a 30-Fr balloon; follow-up of 8 months to 10 years revealed an overall success rate of 67%, with a re-treatment rate of 28%. With a single treatment, only 42% of patients had a durable successful outcome. Recent reports of balloon dilation of UPJ obstruction have used a 10-mm balloon catheter with reported success rates averaging 73%. Success with primary UPJ appears to be better than for secondary obstruction (Table 19.6). However, in a recent long-term follow-up, McClinton noted a durable response rate of only 52%.

Reports on the outcome of the endopyelotomy using a retrograde fluoroscopically guided cutting balloon are now available. In long-term follow-up of the Washington University series, at an average of 33 months' follow-up, the cure rate was 81% on diuretic renal scan evaluation (258). In this same group of patients, subjective analysis done with analog pain scales demonstrated that 61% had a favorable response with 36% totally free of pain and 25% markedly improved. Preminger and colleagues (293) reported a multi-institutional clinical trial, with the cutting balloon catheter, in 66 patients with UPJ obstruction. With a mean follow-up of 7.8 months, the patency rate was 77% for the endopyelotomy, with 72% of the primary and 100% of the secondary UPJ obstructions remaining patent. Postoperative hemorrhage was the most significant complication, occurring in 3% of the patients, and controlled in both cases by embolization. Brooks and associates (35) compared the retrograde balloon incision to a standard antegrade endopyelotomy and to a laparoscopic pyeloplasty. The success rate for the antegrade and retrograde endopyelotomies was similar (77% to 78%) at 20 to 24 months' follow-up; however, the hospital stay (0.2 versus 3.0 days), analgesic use (1.2 versus 18 mg of morphine sulfate), and operative time (46 versus 145 minutes) were all less for the retrograde balloon

TABLE 19.7. RETROGRADE ENDOPYELOTOMY AND OPEN PYELOPLASTY

Authors	No. of Patients	Approach	Method of Incision	Stent Size (Fr)	Stent Duration (wk)	Overall Success Rate (%)	Success Rate (%)		Hospital Stay (days)	Average Follow-up (range) (mo)	Secondary Pyelo-plasty (%)	Secondary Nephrectomy (%)
							1° UPJ	2° UPJ				
Ureterscopic Series												
Thomas et al. (356)	39	Retrograde	Electrocautery and 8-mm balloon	7/14	6–8	90	—	—	1.2	16 (7–37)	—	8
Tawfiek et al. (352)	32	Retrograde	Electrosurgical or Ho:YAG laser	6–7/14	6–10	87.5	87.5	87.5	—	18 (5–49)	3	16
Gerber & Kim (107a)	22	Retrograde	Electrosurgical or Ho:YAG laser + 7-mm balloon	7–7/14	6–7	82	—	—	<1	21 (4–61)	5	—
Total	**93**			**6–7/14**	**6–10**	**87**	—	—	—	**16**	—	—
Acucise												
Brooks et al. (35)	9	Retrograde	Acucise	7 or 14	4–6	78	—	—	0.2	24 (15–32)	2	—
Nadler et al. (258)	28	Retrograde	Acucise	7 or 7/14	4–6	81	78	100	1.6	33 (24–43)	4	4
Faeber et al. (90)	32	Retrograde	Acucise	7/14	6–8	87.5	—	—	1.8	14 (3–28)	12.5	—
Preminger et al. (293)	66	Retrograde	Acucise	7–7/14	6	77	72	100	—	7.8 (1–17.9)	—	—
Shalhav et al. (326)	66	Retrograde	Acucise	7 or 7/14	4–6	77	71	83	2.2	20	—	—
Lechevallier et al. (220)	36	Retrograde	Acucise	9	4–12	75	74	77	3	24 (6–42)	11	—
Total	**237**			**7–7/14**	**4–12**	**79**	**74**	**90**	**1.8**	**17**	—	—
Open Pyeloplasty												
Scardino and Scardino (313)	2,481	Open	Open pyeloplasty	—	—	88	—	—	—	8–10	2	3
Brooks et al. (35)	11	Open	Open pyeloplasty	—	—	100	—	—	7.3	26 (9–44)	—	—
Total	**2,492**			—	—	**94**	—	—	—	—	—	—

UPJ, ureteropelvic junction.

incision. However, as with all of the retrograde approaches, there is no single series with more than 75 patients, and the number of published reports is limited.

Endopyelotomy: Unsettled Issues on Indication

In an effort to maximize the success rate of endopyelotomy, numerous investigations have been made into patient selection, procedural modifications, and the fate of endopyelotomy failures. Each of these areas is of vital importance because the answers to these questions may enable the urologist to preselect patients in whom endopyelotomy will have the best chance of working while providing the surgeon with the best instrumentation and appropriate guidelines necessary to maximize the chances of a favorable outcome. In addition, knowledge concerning the fate of endopyelotomy failures is essential so that urologists can provide their patients with accurate information on which to decide between an endourologic versus open procedure.

With regard to patient selection, concerns have been voiced regarding the use of endopyelotomy in the following seven circumstances: concomitant presence of renal calculi, children, the elderly, a high ureteral insertion, poor renal function, massive hydronephrosis, and a crossing renal vessel. First, it is important that the diagnosis of a UPJ be made in the absence of renal calculi. Szewcyzk and colleagues (348) have shown that patients with renal pelvic stones may appear to have a UPJ obstruction on preliminary testing. However, following percutaneous removal of these calculi, the associated edema in the area of the UPJ region resolves, indicating that the apparent UPJ obstruction was of a secondary, transient nature. Obviously, performing an endopyelotomy in this patient group or having a large number of these types of patients in an endopyelotomy series may result in an inflated success rate (348).

Pediatric endopyelotomy has been performed sparingly. In 1987, Towbin and co-workers (360) reported on the results of endopyelotomy for primary UPJ obstruction in three children, 11 to 18 years of age; the procedure was successful in two out of the three cases. Lingeman and colleagues (225) reported on seven children undergoing endopyelotomy for primary UPJ obstruction; in their series, a successful outcome occurred in 100% of children followed for an average of 13 months. More recently, Figenshau and colleagues (94) expanded Kavoussi and colleagues' (184) earlier report on pediatric endopyelotomy to 17 children ranging in age from 3 months to 17 years old. Endopyelotomy was performed for primary (eight cases) and secondary (nine cases) UPJ obstruction; at a mean follow-up of 25 months, the success rate in the primary group was only 62%, whereas the success rate in the secondary UPJ group was 100%. In two patients with a secondary UPJ obstruction, an additional percutaneous procedure was required to obtain a successful end result. All failures were found within the first year of follow-up. Schenkman and Tarry (312) compared 8 children undergoing endopyelotomy with a contemporary group of 20 children having an open pyeloplasty for UPJ obstruction. The endopyelotomy success rate at 1.5 years of follow-up was 88%. The open pyeloplasty success rate was 93%. The hospital stay was similar for the two groups (2.5 days versus 3.4 days for the endopyelotomy and open pyeloplasty, respectively). The operative time was longer for the endopyelotomy than for the pyeloplasty (220 versus 132 minutes, respectively), and this resulted in a higher average hospital cost for the endopyelotomy group ($8,474 versus $5,931, respectively).

At the other end of the age spectrum, endopyelotomy for primary and secondary UPJ obstruction in the geriatric population has proven quite successful. Horgan and colleagues (145) reviewed 18 patients ranging in age from 66 to 83 years; the success rate in these patients mimicked the success rate in the overall adult population: 88% for either primary or secondary UPJ obstruction. There were no intraoperative complications, and the average hospital stay was 6.3 days; these results were also identical to the hospital stay for their younger adult endopyelotomy patients.

Of ongoing concern to all urologists performing endopyelotomy is that the success rate is only 72% to 88%. In an effort to better identify ideal candidates for endopyelotomy, the following factors have been studied: high insertion, poor renal function, hydronephrosis, and the presence of a crossing vessel. Several investigators have determined that high insertion of the ureter has no adverse effect on outcome (43,327,364). In contrast, it was the opinion of Meretyk and associates (245) that poor renal function (i.e., less than 20%) augured a poor outcome; indeed, for these patients a nephrectomy was recommended. Gupta and colleagues (132) have similarly shown that patients with poor renal function were less likely to have a successful endopyelotomy (54% success rate if renal function is less than 25% versus 92% success rate if renal function is greater than 40%). With regard to hydronephrosis, Van Cangh and colleagues (365), Glinz and colleagues (117), and Gupta and colleagues (132) have each independently noted that massive hydronephrosis bodes ill. In Gupta and colleagues' (132) series, fully 89% of the failed endopyelotomies were among patients with severe or massive hydronephrosis. Similarly, Van Cangh and colleagues (365) noted a 76% success rate in patients with minimal hydronephrosis versus a 66% success rate in patients with grade 3 to 4 hydronephrosis. Glinz and colleagues (117) noted that among patients undergoing a successful endopyelotomy, the average volume of the renal pelvis was less than 60 mL.

The one area that has stimulated the greatest amount of debate regarding patient selection for endopyelotomy has been the issue of the crossing vessel (343). Cassis and associates (37) had first voiced concern about the potential importance of diagnosing the presence of a crossing vessel preoperatively; for this purpose the IVP was inadequate, and only an angiogram provided the necessary information.

However, the seminal work on the impact of a crossing vessel on the outcome of an endopyelotomy was performed by Van Cangh and colleagues (365). They obtained preoperative angiograms in patients before endopyelotomy. The presence of a crossing vessel with either mild (grade 1 to 2) or severe (grade 3 to 4) hydronephrosis resulted in success rates of only 50% and 39%, respectively; whereas absence of a crossing vessel was associated with a successful outcome in 95% of patients with mild hydronephrosis and 77% of patients with moderate to severe hydronephrosis. In this series, the crossing vessel was the single most important prognostic factor (365). Including all series of open surgery, angiography, endoluminal US, and spiral CT, the incidence of crossing vessels in patients with UPJ obstruction averages 50% (33% to 79%) (131).

In the quest to diagnose a crossing vessel, the advent of two minimally invasive studies has been most timely. Today, endoluminal US and spiral CT provide the urologist with the ability to closely examine the UPJ area before proceeding with a given therapy (15,138). Endoluminal US involves the retrograde passage of a 7.2-Fr catheter over a 0.025-inch guidewire (Fig. 19.21). The tip of the catheter contains a 12.5- or 20-MHz US unit. The catheter is set up to scan 10 degrees from the perpendicular, providing a 360-degree cross section with a 1.5-cm radius. By slowly pulling the catheter through the UPJ area, the examiner can clearly identify any vein or artery crossing the UPJ and measure its size. Drawbacks to the technique, however, include the cost of the catheter (several hundred dollars), the invasive nature of the test, and the learning curve for the observer, which includes recognition of vessels, categorizing them as arteries or veins, and determining the anterior or posterior direction of vessel passage.

Nonetheless, using this method Tawfiek and colleagues (352) reported on 37 successful examinations in 27 patients with a primary UPJ obstruction and in 10 patients with a secondary UPJ obstruction. Crossing vessels were seen in 53%; the vessels crossed the UPJ anteriorly (16%), posteriorly (6%), anteromedially (9%), anterolaterally (19%), and anteriorly and posteriorly (3%); none were noted directly lateral (Fig. 19.22). This variation in vessel distribution is similar to that observed by Sampaio and Favorito (309) in their postmortem study of the normal UPJ, in which they noted 65% of patients had a crossing vessel at the UPJ; however, no vessels crossed the lateral surface. In Tawfiek and Bagley's report (352), the information gleaned from the endoluminal US study helped determine the site of endopyelotomy incision in 16 patients and changed the planned therapy in 5 patients.

Spiral (helical) CT differs from the standard tomography the way a bread slicer differs from a potato peeler (138) (Fig. 19.23). In the former situation, only sections of the area of interest can be studied; although these sections can be made quite thin, an accurate reconstruction of the area is difficult. In the latter situation, a dynamic ongoing record of the entire area of interest is made; this continuous radiographic recording then can be reconfigured to provide the observer with views of the area from every conceivable angle. To accomplish this, during CT scanning the x-ray source undergoes rotation in a spiral pattern while the patient is moved through the CT scanner. With this arrangement, an entire scan of the area of interest usually can be done with a single breath hold (i.e., less than 25 seconds). Both the total amount of radiation exposure and the amount of image noise are reduced compared with conventional CT technology. With this technique, overlapping images at intervals as small as 1 mm can be obtained. The ability to detect small vessels around the UPJ is further improved by giving a bolus of intravenous contrast just before scanning. As such, vessels as small as 2 mm in size that cross the UPJ area can be detected. In addition, by reconstructing the renal pelvis, an accurate measurement of its size can be obtained, further enabling the surgeon to better determine the suitability of a given patient for endopyelotomy. Quillin and colleagues (296) imaged 24 consecutive patients, with symptomatic UPJ obstruction, with dual-phase, contrast-enhanced heli-

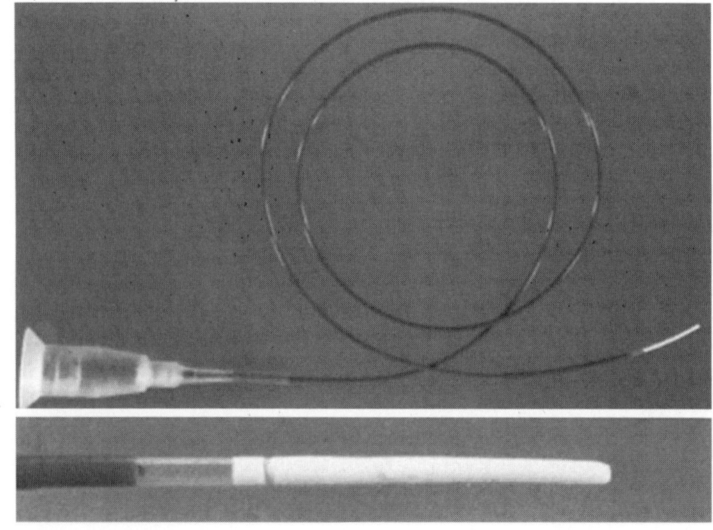

FIGURE 19.21. A: An endoluminal ultrasound catheter for intraluminal ultrasonography. The 7.2-Fr catheter passes over a 0.025-inch guidewire. **B:** The tip of the endoluminal ultrasound unit contains either a 12.5- or 20-MHz ultrasound unit capable of providing 360-degree scans of the ureter with a radius of 1.5 cm.

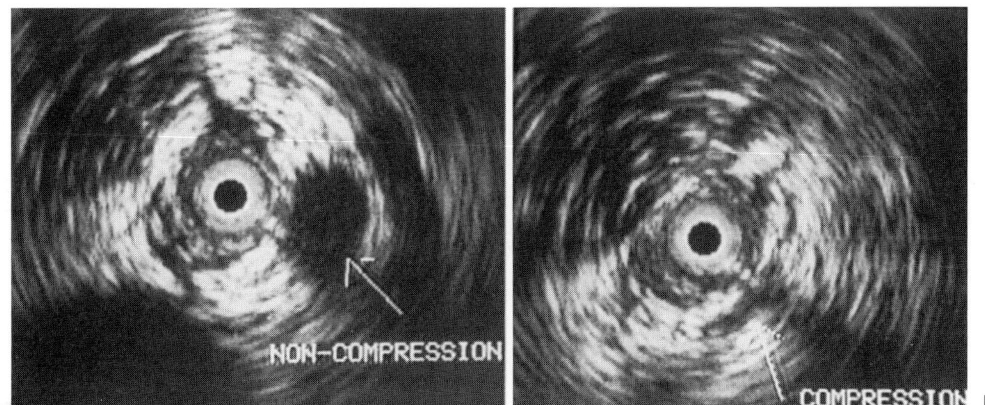

FIGURE 19.22. A: An endoluminal ultrasound study performed at the level of the ureteropelvic junction (UPJ) reveals a large vessel crossing the UPJ directly posterior *(arrow).* Noncompression refers to the conditions at the time of scanning: no manual pressure was put over the kidney area. **B:** By pressing down on the flank directly overlying the area of the scanning, the crossing vessel *(arrow)* can be compressed, thereby indicating its probably venous nature.

cal CT. Eleven (46%) of the patients collectively had 11 anterior and three posterior vessels (2 mm or greater in diameter) crossing the UPJ on helical CT. Laparoscopy and open surgery findings were in agreement with the helical CT angiogram for five of five patients in this study. Uncomplicated endopyelotomy was performed for 11 patients in whom no significant vessels were seen posterior or posterolateral to the UPJ.

Armed with endoluminal US and spiral CT, several investigators are seeking to corroborate Van Cangh and colleagues' (365) findings because many questions remain unanswered. Specifically, it remains puzzling that despite the presence of a crossing vessel, even in Van Cangh and colleagues' (365) series the endopyelotomy was still successful in approximately 50% of patients depending on the degree of hydronephrosis. Nakada and colleagues (260) demonstrated in 16 patients, who had undergone successful cutting balloon endopyelotomy for UPJ obstruction, with greater than 2-year follow-up, that six (38%) had anterior or posterior crossing vessels based on CT angiography. Could it be that only some and not other vessel configurations are directly responsible for the UPJ obstruction? Perhaps only an anterior crossing vessel causes problems or perhaps a crossing artery is of greater concern than a crossing vein. The next question arises that if a crossing vessel is found, what should be the next step: open pyeloplasty, laparoscopic pyeloplasty, laparoscopic exploration and incision of the vessel if it is not a major renal arterial branch, or laparoscopic exploration and incision of the vessel combined with endopyelotomy? Further clinical evaluation will be necessary to determine the significance and implication of the crossing vessel associated with UPJ obstruction. Ideally, appropriate laboratory and clinical studies will allow the urologist in the future to confidently select patients for endopyelotomy knowing that the procedure will then be as successful as its open surgical counterpart. In all respects, this continues to be the goal of each endourologic procedure: to offer the patient a minimally invasive approach of efficacy equal to, but with morbidity less than, a standard open surgical procedure.

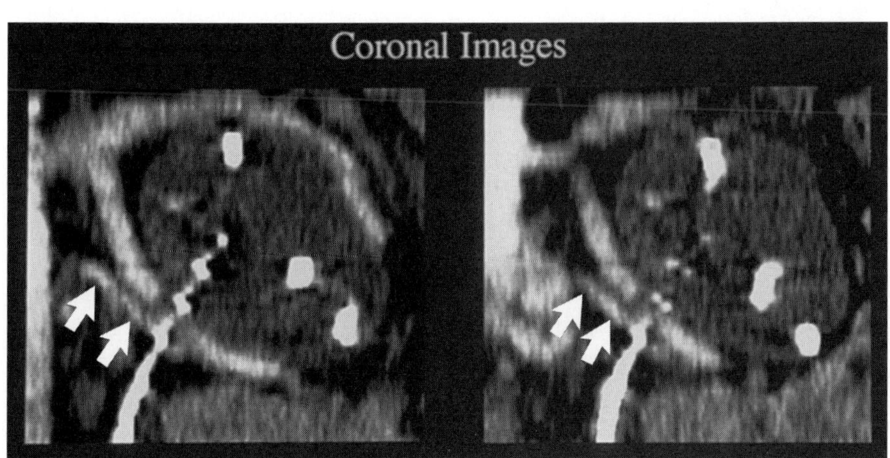

FIGURE 19.23. In this spiral computed tomography scan of a 34-year-old male patient with a UPJ obstruction, the coronal reconstruction reveals a vessel *(arrows)* crossing the UPJ posteriorly. The density of the vessel suggests that it is probably an artery.

Endopyelotomy: Unsettled Technical Issues

To what extent differences in the technical aspects of performing an endopyelotomy affect the ultimate success rate remains unknown. Controversy continues in several areas: the method of incision, the size of the indwelling stent placed after the endopyelotomy, and the period of time that the stent is left indwelling. From an incisional standpoint, although a cold-knife urethrotome continues as the preeminent method for opening the ureteropelvic junction, a variety of apparently equally efficacious methods have been described. Hulbert and colleagues (155) and Meretyk and colleagues (245) have independently reported on using a minute electrosurgical probe for making the incision; similarly, Chandhoke and colleagues (40) have reported on using an electrosurgical cutting balloon, whereas O'Flynn and colleagues (271) have written about using a 10-mm dilating balloon presumably to split the UPJ along its weakest point, and Tawfiek and Bagley (353), Gerber and Alsikafi (107b), and Renner and others (300a) have individually reported using the Ho:YAG laser to incise the UPJ stricture. As noted, the results with any of these techniques appear to be remarkably similar. Studies examining electrosurgical incisions have shown that when the cutting surface of the probe is less than or equal to 400 microns, the resulting incision and peripheral damage are indistinguishable from the incision achieved with a cold knife. However, probes that have a 1-mm or larger tip cause significantly more damage and should be avoided (75). With balloon disruption of the UPJ area, laboratory studies have shown that although the balloon splits the ureteral mucosa and muscularis, the adventitia usually remains intact, thereby precluding any significant retroperitoneal extravasation. The balloon at times splits the ureter along a single plane; however, the site of the split and the overall length of the tear are highly variable (288). With regard to other endoscopic cutting modalities, such as bipolar electrosurgical probes or special laser fibers (e.g., side-firing fiber with a KTP laser), data are unavailable.

Controversy continues over the size of the stent to leave indwelling after an endopyelotomy. For years, the notion has been that the stent serves as a mold around which the ureter heals. This philosophy was strongly endorsed in Davis's classic writings; based on his clinical experience, Davis recommended that as large a stent as possible should be placed following an intubated ureterotomy (68). As such, many urologists have advocated leaving a 14-Fr stent in place, in the hope that the healed UPJ will then assume the same size as a normal UPJ. These large stents have a dual taper so that the portion traversing the incised UPJ is 14 Fr, while the portion in the bladder is only 7 to 8 Fr. Both an external nephrostent and internal double pigtail design have been used. However, laboratory studies have challenged Davis's notion. Moon and colleagues (247) could show no difference in ureteral healing in a pig model after a cutting-balloon endoureterotomy whether a 7- or 14-Fr stent was used. Similarly, there have been a few clinical reports suggesting that the stent, rather than a mold, is actually serving as a *scaffold* along which the orderly growth of the urothelium and subsequent ingrowth of the ureteral musculature is guided, a concept attributed to Hinman (274). In several series, indwelling stents of 8 to 10 Fr have been placed; the outcomes have been highly favorable, with success rates of 83% to 88% reported (44,197,236). If stent size is ultimately shown not to affect the outcome of an endopyelotomy, the need to prestint the ureter before a retrograde endopyelotomy would be decreased, and the ease and safety of postendopyelotomy stent placement and removal would be facilitated.

Research has challenged the 6-week stent practice. Animal studies by Kerbl and colleagues (187) revealed that in a pig ureteral stricture model, stinting for 1 week with a 7-Fr stent provided results as good as stinting for 3 or 6 weeks. In the 1-week group, the results for endoureterotomy of longer strictures were statistically significantly better than in either the 3- or 6-week groups. Clinically, Kuenkel and Korth (207) noted in their series of 143 endopyelotomies that a stent for 3 weeks produced superior results to leaving a stent for 6 weeks. Abdel-Hakim (1) has noted that as short a stinting period as 4 days was successful in five patients, each of whom was stinted with a 7-Fr external ureteric catheter. However, maximum follow-up in this series was only 6 months. Kumar and colleagues (209) demonstrated that 2 weeks of stent placement were as effective as 4 weeks in the successful outcome of antegrade endopyelotomy. Obviously, in this regard we again have much to learn; prospective, randomized clinical studies of patients with similar types of UPJ obstruction are sorely needed to answer this and other questions regarding stinting after endopyelotomy.

Endopyelotomy: Fate of Failed Procedures

One last question regarding endopyelotomy is of paramount importance. Specifically, is the patient in whom an endopyelotomy fails placed at a disadvantage for subsequent surgical salvage? Certainly, if this is the case, one would be most hesitant to proceed with a minimally invasive procedure in which a failure rate as high as 30% could be expected. Kavoussi and colleagues (180) and Motola, Smith, and colleagues (252) have independently written on the fate of the failed endopyelotomy patient. Both reports noted that although salvage open pyeloplasty is at times a bit more difficult to perform than a primary pyeloplasty, the overall success rate was excellent. Among 15 patients in Motola and colleagues' (252) series and 5 patients in Kavoussi and colleagues' (180) report, all underwent a successful salvage dismembered pyeloplasty. Follow-up at 1 to 7 years revealed that all 20 patients had a successful outcome. Of note, in the Kavoussi and colleagues (180) series, one patient underwent a nephrectomy because of decreased renal function, whereas in the Smith series there were no subsequent nephrectomies.

Calyceal Diverticulum and Hydrocalyx

The calyceal diverticulum and the hydrocalyx are two entities related by the narrowness of their communication with the collecting system. Whereas in the former, there is no associated functioning renal tissue, in the latter, the relief of obstruction can have a potentially positive effect on renal function. As such, the endosurgical approach to these two conditions is quite different.

Calyceal diverticula are noted on 0.45% of intravenous urograms. Most commonly these outpouchings are unilateral and emanate from a minor calyx and are more of anatomic than clinical interest. Only one-third become symptomatic because of the development of urolithiasis, pain, hematuria, or recurrent infection (357).

Far more rare than calyceal diverticula is the hydrocalyx. This is usually an acquired condition caused by infection (e.g., tuberculosis, urolithiasis, prior intrarenal surgery). A congenital isolated hydrocalyx may be either developmental or associated with extrinsic compression from a crossing segmental renal vessel; the latter has been described most commonly in the upper pole of the kidney (Fraley's syndrome) (89,97). At times, the distinction between a hydrocalyx and a calyceal diverticulum only can be made during nephroscopy; the absence or presence of a papilla differentiates between a diverticulum and a hydrocalyx, respectively.

Calyceal Diverticulum: Technique

For the few calyceal diverticula requiring surgical therapy, the standard approach has been to excise or marsupialize the diverticulum; the neck of the diverticulum is then closed with a suture. For a very large diverticulum, partial nephrectomy is performed. However, beginning in the late 1980s these lesions began to be managed successfully endourologically by percutaneous and ureteroscopic methods. There have also been a few case reports of successful laparoscopic treatment of a calyceal diverticulum (118).

When approached percutaneously, the diverticulum should be entered directly; the renal pelvis or normal part of the collecting system is not initially entered (Fig. 19.24) (158). Once inside the diverticulum, any stones are removed. Next, the opening of the diverticulum into the collecting system is identified and cannulated with a guidewire; the guidewire is then covered with a 5-Fr angiographic catheter. With use of a roller electrode, the entire inner surface of the diverticulum, except the neck of the diverticulum, is electrocoagulated. Following this, the neck of the diverticulum is enlarged by multiple electrosurgical (less than 400-micron tip) endoscopically guided, shallow (less than 2 mm in depth) incisions, balloon dilation to 12 to 24 Fr, and/or dilation with coaxial dilators to 26 to 28 Fr. Next, a nephrostomy tube is placed such that it traverses the diverticulum and terminates in the renal pelvis. This tube is usually removed 2 to 7 days later (48,157,171,211).

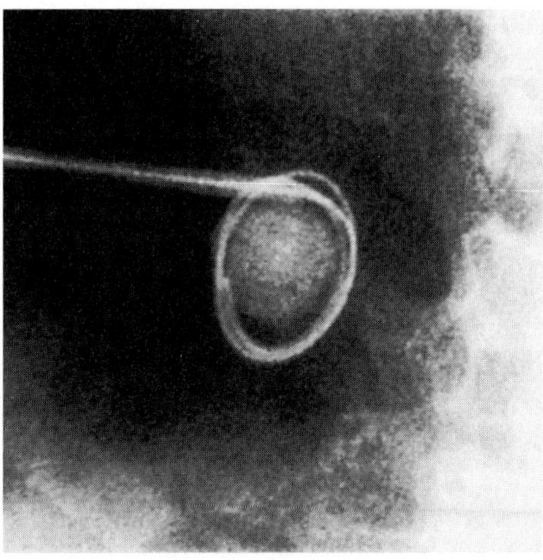

FIGURE 19.24. Direct percutaneous puncture of a stone-containing calyceal diverticulum. The wire has been coiled several times within the diverticulum to enable the urologist to dilate the tract over the stiff part of the guidewire. (From Hulbert JC, Reddy PK, Hunter DW, et al. Percutaneous techniques for the management of caliceal diverticula containing calculi. *J Urol* 1986;135:225, with permission.)

There are two alternatives to percutaneously cannulating and incising the neck of the diverticulum. In both situations, the neck of the diverticulum is not sought. In one technique, the entire inner surface of the diverticulum, including the presumably unidentified diverticular neck, is electrocoagulated under endoscopic control; a tube is left in the diverticulum for 2 to 3 days and then removed. The true collecting system of the kidney is never entered (323). In the other approach, a transdiverticular puncture into the collecting system is made; the interior of the diverticulum is either electrocoagulated as previously described or left intact. The neoinfundibulum is either dilated (12 to 18 Fr for 2 minutes), thereby creating a new drainage path, or is allowed to heal closed. In the former situation, an 8- to 10-Fr nephrostent is placed, whereas in the latter circumstance, the tip of the tube is placed only into the diverticulum. In Lang's (214) series, the stent was left in place for 4 weeks, following which it was exchanged for an indwelling stent of unspecified size and duration (27).

When approached ureteroscopically, the neck of the diverticulum is first identified, following which a safety guidewire may be passed into the diverticulum or into the renal pelvis. The lens of the ureteroscope is removed so that a 4-mm dilating balloon catheter can be passed over the guidewire through the sheath of the ureteroscope; the balloon is passed retrograde until it straddles the neck of the diverticulum. The balloon is then inflated, thereby dilating the neck of the diverticulum; the balloon is then deflated and removed. The ureteroscope's lens is replaced and the ureteroscope is advanced into the diverticulum. Alternatively, flexible ureteroscopy can be done and a nonconducting guidewire can be passed into the diverticulum. Next, a 2- or 3-Fr electrosurgical probe can be used to incise the neck of the diverticulum; several radial incisions (less than 2 mm) are made, and the ureteroscope is advanced into the diverticulum (Fig. 19.25). The calculus is then fragmented with laser or electrohydraulic energy, and the walls of the diverticulum can be treated with either electrocautery or Nd:YAG energy. An indwelling ureteral stent is placed in the collecting system; the stent does not transverse the diverticulum. Alternatively, following dilation of the neck of the diverticulum, the calculi may be treated by shock wave lithotripsy; however, in this case the diverticulum will probably remain intact (98,157,246).

Another approach to treating the stone-bearing calyceal diverticulum is extracorporeal shock wave lithotripsy. Although this results in successful fragmentation of the stone in the majority of patients, in most cases, the stone fails to pass; however, many patients do become at least transiently asymptomatic. Of note, the diverticulum remains unaltered; hence, the potential for recurrent stone disease in the diverticulum remains a real risk. According to Streem and Yost (345), the ideal diverticulum for a primary ESWL approach is one in which the neck of the diverticulum is visibly patent on the pretreatment radiographs and the stone burden is less than 1.5 cm.

Hydrocalyx: Technique

In contrast to the calyceal diverticulum, the traditional approach to treating a hydrocalyx has been open partial nephrectomy or transposition of an obstructing vessel. Minimally invasive approaches to this problem have included both ureteroscopic and percutaneous therapy; however, the more common endourologic approach has been via a percutaneous route (165). With the endourologic approach, the goal is twofold: to open the narrowed infundibulum and to preserve the functioning calyceal tissue. A direct percutaneous approach into the hydrocalyx may be attempted. In this case, the technique is identical to that described for treating a calyceal diverticulum except that after incising or dilating the neck of the infundibulum (12- to 18-Fr balloon or 20- to 24-Fr Amplatz dilators), the walls of the hydrocalyx are not disturbed in an effort to preserve the function of the now unobstructed calyx (25).

In incising an infundibulum, it is important to limit the depth of any incision to only 2 mm in order not to injure any of the larger vessels that may surround the infundibulum (48). Anatomically, the vessels surrounding an infundibulum are most prevalent along its anterior and posterior surfaces; the superior and inferior surfaces of the infundibulum are less vascular. Based on anatomic studies, Sampaio (308) recommended that the initial incision should be on the superior surface of the infundibulum; if need be, a counterincision can be made along the inferior surface. These surfaces in a middle calyx would be akin to the medial and lateral surfaces of an upper- or lower-pole calyx; in these cases, a lateral incision has been recommended (159). Again, anterior and posterior incisions should be avoided because they may result in significant hemorrhage.

Overall, the least invasive yet most effective form of therapy for a symptomatic, stone-containing calyceal diverticulum is a direct percutaneous approach with stone removal and obliteration of the walls of the diverticulum. Using this approach, up to 100% of patients can be rendered asymptomatic; more than 90% of patients become stone free; and in two-thirds or more of cases, the calyceal diverticulum is obliterated, thereby precluding recurrent urolithiasis or infection (Table 19.8) (89,154,171,318). In these cases, either cannulation and dilation of the true neck of the diverticulum or electrocoagulation of the entire diverticulum is recommended. In contrast, balloon dilation of a newly created drainage path from the diverticulum into the collecting system results in diverticular obliteration in only 20% of cases; however, in 70% of cases, the neoin-

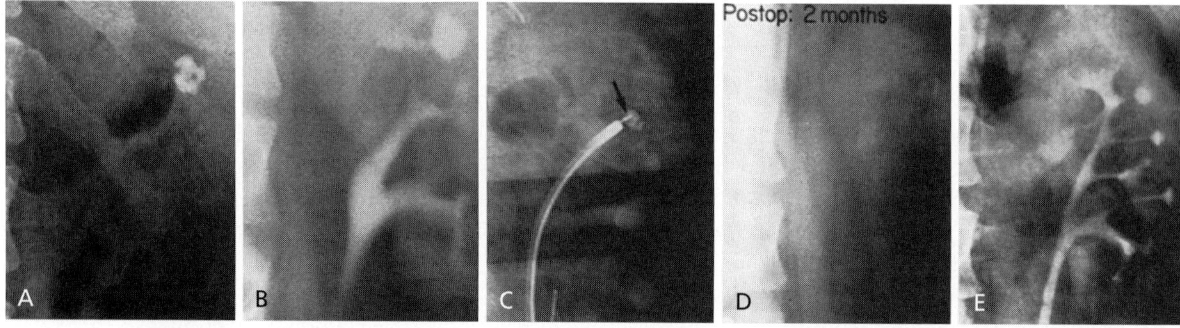

FIGURE 19.25. A: A plain abdominal radiograph reveals multiple calculi lying in the kidney just above the eleventh rib. **B:** An intravenous urogram reveals that the stones are lying in an upper pole calyceal diverticulum. **C:** The flexible ureteroscope has been advanced retrograde, and the neck of the calyceal diverticulum has been identified. With a 3-Fr electrosurgical probe, the neck of the diverticulum is incised, following which the stones are fragmented using laser lithotripsy. **D:** At 2 months after the operation, a plain abdominal radiograph reveals only a few stone flecks in the area of the diverticulum. **E:** The intravenous urogram at 2 months after the procedure reveals that the diverticulum has decreased markedly in size.

TABLE 19.8. CALYCEAL DIVERTICULA: PERCUTANEOUS APPROACH

Authors	No. of Patients	Technique	Symptom Free (%)	Stone Free[a] (%)	Diverticulum Obliterated	Average Follow-up (range) (mo)	Catheter Duration
Hulbert et al. (154)	12	Antegrade PCN (neck dilated)	NS	100[b]	100	9 (3–15)	2 wk
Eshghi et al. (89)	14[c]	Antegrade PCN (cold knife)	NS	100	86	NS	3 days–2 wk
Jones et al. (171)	14	PCN	100	96	100[b]	35 (16–60)	—
Lang (214)	10	PCN	NS	NS	20[d]	≤7 yr	—
Lagha et al. (218)	18	PCN ± fulguration (neck dilated to 26–28 Fr)	—	100	72	1–3	2 days

[a]Stone status of diverticulum.
[b]Electrocoagulate walls of diverticulum.
[c]Did not differentiate between calyceal diverticulum or hydrocalyx.
[d]In 60% the calyceal diverticulum had a patent neck after dilation.
NS, not specified.

fundibulum remains patent, thereby draining the calyceal diverticulum (214).

The other endourologic methods for approaching this disease entity are less effective. With regard to ESWL, its success rate is highly variable dependent on how selective the physician has been (Table 19.9). In patients with a small stone burden (i.e., less than 1.5 cm) and with a patent diverticular neck on radiographic studies, Streem and Yost (345) achieved an 86% rate of asymptomatic or less symptomatic patients and a 58% stone-free rate; at follow-up 2 years later, 8% of these preselected patients had re-formed a stone in the treated calyceal diverticulum. Also, they noted that of nine patients treated in this manner who also had infection, recurrent infection occurred in 67%. Other urologists, using no selective criteria, have reported post-ESWL symptom-free rates of only 36% and stone-free rates of only 0% to 20% (101,171, 294). A purely ureteroscopic approach was effective in only two of six patients treated by Mikkelsen and colleagues (246). In sum, percutaneous calyceal diverticulectomy with removal of the calculus and obliteration of the walls of the diverticulum remains the most definitive and long-lasting less invasive method of treating the symptomatic calyceal diverticulum. Other less morbid procedures are often less effective.

Unlike with calyceal diverticula, there is scant experience in treating infundibular stenosis endourologically. Schneider and co-workers (317) reported on six patients

TABLE 19.9. CALYCEAL DIVERTICULA: EXTRACORPOREAL SHOCK WAVE LITHOTRIPSY (ESWL)

Authors	No. of Patients	Technique	Symptom Free (%)	Stone Free[a] (%)	Diverticulum Obliterated	Average Follow-up (range) (mo)	Catheter Duration
Garcia et al. (101)	13	ESWL	37	0	NS	NA	
Jones et al. (171)	26	ESWL	36[b]	12	NS	35 (16–60)	
Psihramis and Dretlee (294)	10	ESWL	70	20	NS	5.9	
Streem and Yost (345)	19[d]	ESWL	86[e]	58	NS	24	
Fuchs and David (98)	15[f]	URS and ESWL	87	73	7[g]	7.4	3 wk

[a]Stone status of diverticulum.
[b]Thirty-nine percent required PCN salvage because of symptoms.
[c]All stones <1.5 cm.
[d]All diverticula with radiographically patent neck.
[e]Includes symptom free and improved.
[f]Twelve were truly calyceal diverticula.
[g]Twenty percent more had decrease in size of diverticulum.
NS, not specified; NA, not applicable.

with a hydrocalyx among whom a cold-knife incision was successful in 66%; the catheter was left indwelling for 3 to 6 weeks. The length of follow-up was not stated. Similarly, Lang (214) reported a 67% success rate in six patients with a hydrocalyx, treated by percutaneous infundibuloplasty (i.e., balloon dilation) who were followed for 2 to 7 years. In his series, the infundibulum was dilated with a 12- to 18-Fr balloon, which was left inflated for 2 minutes. Following this, an 8- to 10-Fr nephrostent was placed; the external stent was left in place for 4 weeks, after which it was exchanged for an internalized stent of unspecified size and duration. Hwang and Park (159) reported an 80% success rate with cold-knife infundibulotomy among 10 patients with tuberculous infundibular strictures followed for longer than 1 year after their percutaneous procedure.

Transitional Cell Cancer of the Renal Pelvis

Transitional cell cancer rarely affects the upper urinary tract: 94% of all transitional cell tumors occur in the bladder, whereas only 5% are found in the renal pelvis and 1% in the ureter (51,375). Traditionally, the therapy for all upper tract tumors has been an open surgical ablative approach. For the kidney and upper ureter, this has entailed a nephroureterectomy with excision of a cuff of bladder, whereas for the distal ureteral tumor, distal ureterectomy and ureteral reimplantation usually has been sufficient. The feasibility of an endosurgical approach to these tumors was championed by Gittes (114), who in 1980 questioned why low-stage, low-grade tumors of the ureter and renal pelvis could not be treated by local excision just as it is common practice for similar types of lesions affecting the bladder. For many years, the stumbling block to this approach remained one of access. However, with the advent of percutaneous and ureteroscopic techniques in the 1980s, this minimally invasive hypothesis could be examined more directly (383,384).

A major area of contention with regard to the endosurgical therapy of upper tract TCC is the appropriate indications for such therapy. On the one hand, some urologists believe this to be "heroic" therapy and thus would limit its application to individuals with a solitary kidney, with renal insufficiency, or who are a high surgical risk. On the other hand, other urologists believe equally as strongly that for low-grade, low-stage disease, an endosurgical excision should be offered to all patients as a simpler, less morbid, renal-sparing form of therapy. This controversy continues to grow because advances in endoscopic equipment and in electrosurgical and laser technology have greatly facilitated the ability of the urologist to access and treat superficial lesions anywhere in the upper urinary tract. As such, today an endosurgical approach would technically be feasible in approximately 40% to 50% of all patients (i.e., patients with low-grade and low clinical stage disease) with upper tract transitional cell cancer (375).

Technique

When approaching transitional cell cancer of the renal pelvis (TCCP), the ureteroscope may be most effectively used if the lesion is small (i.e., less than 1 cm). In males, except for the distal ureter, a flexible ureteroscope is commonly used, and the tumor, after excisional biopsy, is usually treated with electrocautery, the Nd:YAG laser, or Ho:YAG laser (314) (Fig. 19.26). In females, a rigid ureteroscope usually can be used to reach the renal pelvis and the upper-pole calyx, whereas a flexible ureteroscope is needed to approach lesions in the middle or lower calyces (14).

In all ureteroscopic cases, a nonconducting guidewire (i.e., Terumo or guidewire) is passed into the kidney to serve as a safety guidewire. This safety guidewire remains in place throughout the procedure and is used at the end of the procedure for the passage of an indwelling ureteral stent.

In procedures involving the upper ureter and renal pelvis, the distal ureter is dilated with a 4-mm balloon if a 9.4-Fr flexible ureteroscope is to be used or with an 8- to 10-Fr fascial dilator set if a 7.5-Fr flexible ureteroscope is available. If the patient previously has undergone diagnostic ureteroscopy and an indwelling stent was placed, the ureter usually will have dilated passively around the stent, precluding the need for active, acute dilation. Also in this situation, the surgeon is benefited by knowing the diagnosis such that the goal at the second session is therapy alone. If a preoperative diagnosis has not been obtained, the urologist will have to biopsy the lesion and then proceed with definitive therapy. In this circumstance, there is usually bleeding from the biopsy site, and subsequent therapy may be compromised because of impaired visibility. If this occurs, it is prudent to stop the procedure, place an indwelling stent, and plan to return on another day to therapeutically address the tumor.

If, during the procedure, the flexible ureteroscope cannot be easily advanced to the tumor site, the procedure should end. In the upper ureter, the ureteral wall is much thinner than in the distal ureter and it can be perforated easily. As such, it is not recommended to use a 4-mm balloon to dilate the upper ureter because ureteral perforation and possible retroperitoneal seeding may occur. In this case, it is far more prudent to place an indwelling ureteral stent and return in a few days to 1 week to perform the ureteroscopy. As previously noted, with an indwelling ureteral stent in place, the ureter will dilate passively, thereby facilitating subsequent ureteroscopy.

Throughout the ureteroscopic procedure, the irrigant pressure is kept below 100 mm Hg in order to preclude hypothetical renal backflow of any tumor cells. The only time the pressure on the irrigant is raised is when an instrument is passed through the working channel. In this

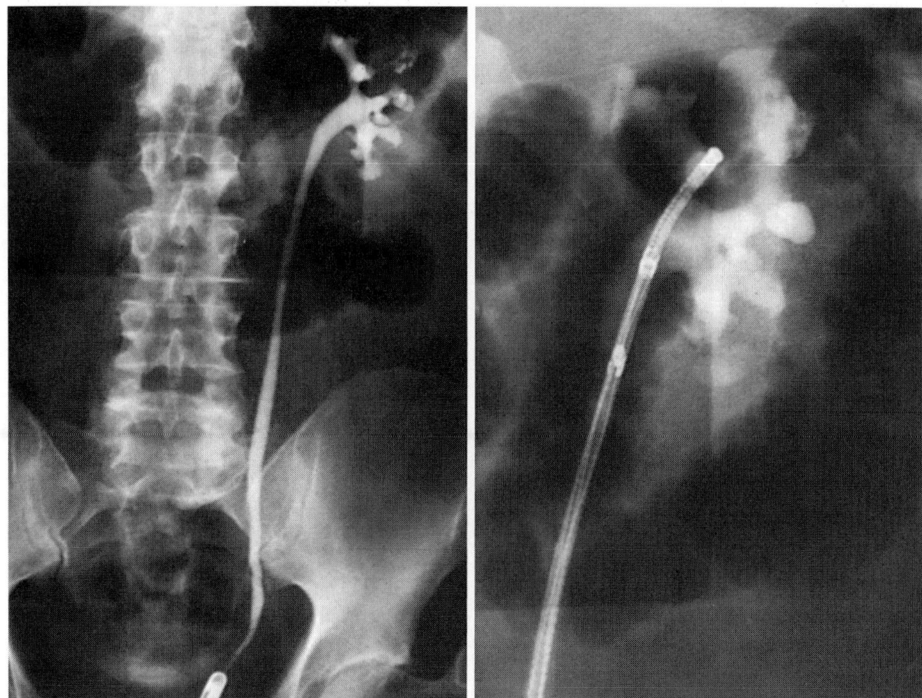

FIGURE 19.26. A retrograde ureterogram reveals poor filling of an upper-pole calyx. Flexible ureteroscopy revealed a papillary transitional cell carcinoma. The tumor was biopsied; however, because of its size and sessile nature, fulguration was not performed. The patient subsequently underwent a nephroureterectomy.

situation, the pressure on the irrigant may be increased to 150 mm Hg; as soon as the instrument is removed, the irrigant pressure should be returned to less than 50 mm Hg. Furthermore, throughout the procedure it is important not to introduce air into the collecting system. Not only will the presence of air make it more difficult to work because of the air-fluid interface and the reflection of light off of the air bubble, but also it may set up a situation in which an explosion can occur during electrocoagulation, resulting in extravasation and possible tumor spillage (9).

The goal of the treatment either is to resect or to coagulate the entire tumor. In the former circumstance, the resection is carried down flush with the urothelium. With the rigid ureteroscope this can be done with a small electrocautery loop. With the flexible ureteroscope, the cold-cup biopsy forceps is used to tediously resect the superficial portion of the tumor and biopsy the tumor's base, following which the base of the tumor is electrocoagulated or treated with the Nd:YAG laser (20 W); alternatively, the tumor can be vaporized and the base coagulated with the Ho:YAG laser. At the end of the procedure, a retrograde ureterogram is performed in order to rule out any extravasation. An indwelling ureteral stent and a urethral catheter are placed. The urethral catheter is removed on the next morning. The ureteral stent is removed in 3 to 5 days, unless a significant perforation has occurred, in which case the stent is left in place for approximately 4 to 6 weeks; in this case, a cystogram is performed before removing the urethral catheter to rule out ureteral extravasation.

The percutaneous approach is reserved for larger tumors (i.e., larger than 1 cm) (350,351). The method of resection appears to be continually evolving. Initially, a retrograde ureteral catheter usually is placed. This can be a 7-Fr, 11.5-mm balloon occlusion catheter; the balloon can be inflated in the renal pelvis and snugged down at the UPJ to preclude any tumor fragments from traveling into the ureter. The puncture into the collecting system is made such that the urologist both will have a straight approach to the tumor and yet enter the collecting system as far from the tumor as possible (Fig. 19.27). The tract is dilated to 30 Fr with a high-pressure balloon, and then a 30-Fr Amplatz working sheath is placed. The irrigant is kept at a pressure of less than 100 mm Hg. The tumor is resected piece by piece with a standard 24- or 26-Fr resectoscope. With each pass of the resectoscope loop, the tumor fragment is evacuated from the collecting system. The base of the tumor is biopsied with a cold-cup forceps and fulgurated using the Nd:YAG laser (at 20 to 30 W for 3-second exposures) or electrocautery (50 W) (125). The occlusion balloon catheter is then deflated and removed; an indwelling nephrostomy tube is positioned in the renal pelvis. Two days after the procedure, a nephrostogram is performed; if there is no extravasation, the nephrostomy tube is removed. Alternatively, the nephrostomy tube may be left in place for 9 to 12 weeks, during which

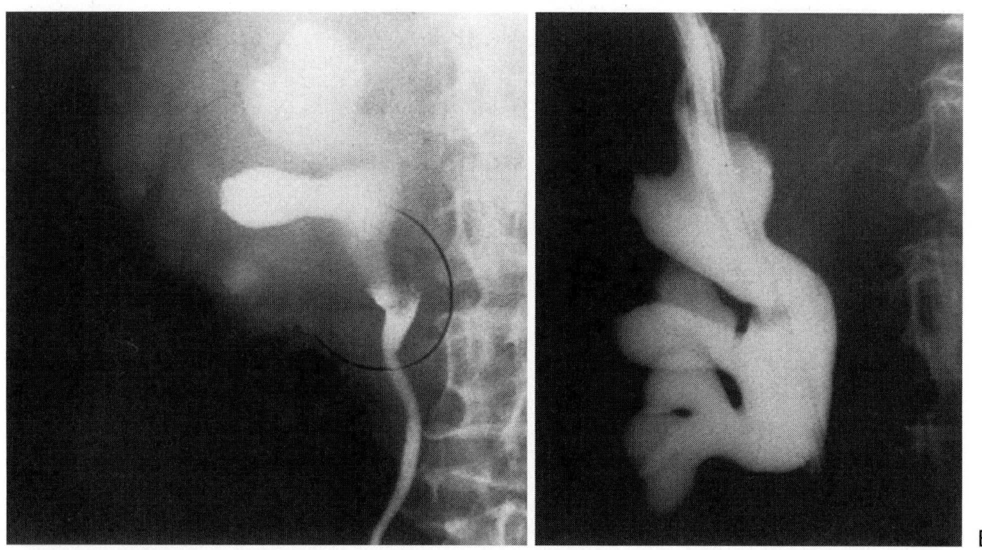

FIGURE 19.27. **A:** In a patient with a solitary kidney and hematuria, a retrograde ureterogram reveals a papillary filling defect at the level of the ureteropelvic junction. Subsequent ureteroscopy and biopsy showed the lesion to be a low-grade transitional cell cancer. **B:** A percutaneous nephrostomy was established via an upper-pole posterior calyx, thereby providing direct access to the tumor via a remote calyx. A standard resectoscope was then used to excise the tumor, and a nephrostomy tube was placed. (From Clayman RV, Kavousi LR. Endosurgical techniques for noncalculous disease. In: Walsh PC et al, eds. *Campbell's urology,* ed 6. Philadelphia: Saunders, 1992:2301, with permission.)

time instillation chemotherapy can be given on a weekly basis; similarly, by leaving the nephrostomy tube in place, second-look nephroscopy and tumor-base rebiopsy and fulguration can be accomplished at 6 or 12 weeks.

Results

The key question with regard to an endosurgical approach to TCCP is, To whom should this therapy be applied? Although there is consensus that for patients with low-grade, low-stage disease and with a solitary kidney, renal insufficiency, or high surgical risk that this minimally invasive approach is reasonable, there is significant concern about extending this approach to all patients with upper tract transitional cell cancer. In Table 19.10, series on the percutaneous treatment of TCCP are reviewed; the patients cited in these papers are also subdivided according to the grade or stage of their disease. What becomes clear is that even for low-grade or low-stage disease, the recurrence rate within the first 2 years after percutaneous resection is high: up to 33% (45,86,168,221,233,284). As such, multiple, subsequent endosurgical procedures can be expected. Also, among those patients with low-grade disease, approximately 75% underwent adjunctive therapy with iridium wires, instillation chemotherapy, or second-look procedures with further laser therapy to the tumor base. Despite all of this additional treatment, recurrences were still noted in one-third of patients. Also during the same 2- to 4-year follow-up period, 23% of patients required a nephroureterectomy (45,86,168,221,233,284).

The results of endosurgical therapy are only slightly better for patients with TCCP approached ureteroscopically; however, in most of these cases the tumors have been small (less than 1 cm) and usually low grade (G_1 to G_2) (Table 19.11). In 69 patients gleaned from various series with grade 1 tumors, there has been no report of local recurrence and no conversion to an open procedure at an average follow-up of 17 months; however, for 31 patients with grade 2 or 3 tumors, ureteroscopic resection was followed by local recurrence in up to half of the patients and conversion to an open procedure in 23% with an average follow-up of 32 months.

Although some authors have been able to identify a patient population in whom recurrence in the short term is low, this has not been the case in other series. Most series incorporate topical chemotherapy, following the initial percutaneous resection, as the management protocol for upper tract TCC. Jarrett and colleagues (168), using this regimen, noted that among their 11 patients with a solitary, stage 0/A, G_1 lesion, there were tumor recurrences in two patients during a greater than 4-year follow-up period; one was treated by endoscopic resection and one by nephroureterectomy due to large volume disease. Clark and colleagues (45) reported a 33% recurrence rate in their similar stage and grade patients with percutaneous management and topical BCG for upper tract TCC. Orihuela and Smith (279) noted several risk factors for recurrence: lack of use of postoperative BCG instillation, a sessile lesion, a tumor larger than 2 cm in diameter, positive preoperative cytology, positive random upper tract

TABLE 19.10. UPPER TRACT TCC: PERCUTANEOUS ENDOSURGICAL THERAPY

	No. of Patients												
	Tumor Grade				Stage								
Authors	G_1	G_2	G_3	CIS	O/A	B/C	Local Recurrence (%)	Bladder Recurrence (%)	Posttreatment Adjunctive Therapy (%)	Converted to Open (%)	Metastatic Disease (%)	Death from Cancer (%)	Average Follow-up (range) (mo)
Jarrett et al. (168)	11	12	13	—	31	5	33	Not specified	BCG × 6 wk	42	Not specified	17	56 (9–111)
Patel et al. (284)	11	11	1	1	25	0	23	31	^{192}Ir to tract	15	Not specified	7	45 (1–100)
Elliott et al. (86)	Not specified				5		25	—	0	43	Not specified	19	48 (20–117)
Martinez-Pineiro et al. (233)	Not specified				18		11	17	Thiotepa, mitomycin C, BCG, interferon	6	Not specified	14	31 (2–119)
Clark et al. (45)	6	8	4	0	18	0	33	Not specified	BCG × 6 wk	12	24	18	24 (2–76)
Lee et al. (221)	20	16	13	—	46	3	12	Not specified	0	20	12	24	36 (2–150)

TABLE 19.11. UPPER TRACT TCC: URETEROSCOPIC ENDOSURGICAL THERAPY

	No. of Patients												
	Tumor Grade				Stage		Local Recurrence (%)	Bladder Recurrence (%)	Posttreatment Adjunctive Therapy (%)	Converted to Open (%)	Metastatic Disease (%)	Death from Cancer (%)	Average Follow-up (range) (mo)
Authors	G_1	G_2	G_3	CIS	O/A	B/C							
Elliott et al. (86)	Not specified				16		38	—	0	43	Not specified	19	48 (20–117)
Martinez-Pineiro et al. (233)	Not specified				39		35	17	Thiotepa, mitomycin C, BCG, interferon	3	Not specified	14	31 (2–119)
Keeley et al. (185)	21	14	5				29	40	15 mitomycin C 7 BCG	17	0	0	30 (3–116)
Grasso et al. (122)	1	11	1	1	14	0	50	29	1 mitomycin and interferon 1 mitomycin	29	0	0	17 (6–31)

biopsies, and a prior history of transitional cell cancer of the bladder (TCCB).

Lee and colleagues (221) retrospectively reviewed 110 patients with localized TCC of the upper urinary tract, all of whom had 13-year follow-up. In this group, the results of open nephroureterectomy (60) and percutaneous resection (50) were compared. Of the disease-specific deaths, 65% (17 of 26) were in patients with grade 3 lesions, with a mean cancer survival period of 15.2 months after the initial procedure. Disease-specific survival rates after open and percutaneous approaches for grade 2 disease were 53.8 and 53.3 months, respectively.

Tumor grade remains the most important prognostic indicator in patients with renal TCC regardless of the surgical approach. Grade 3 tumors are more aggressive, presenting in an advanced stage, and recurrences are more often associated with metastasis. Nephroureterectomy is the management of choice in the surgical candidate. Percutaneous management of upper tract TCC is usually reserved for patients with a solitary kidney, bilateral disease, or chronic renal insufficiency. Percutaneous treatment of grade 1 or 2 renal TCCU in healthy individuals with a normal contralateral kidney mandates strict and lengthy follow-up.

Endourology for Transitional Cell Cancer of the Renal Pelvis: Adjunctive Measures

The efficacy of endosurgical therapy of TCCP has been obfuscated by the myriad treatment approaches, as previously described, and by variations in the use of instillation therapy and postresection adjunctive measures. Regarding instillation therapy, various agents have been instilled using a variety of schedules in an effort to prevent tumor recurrence. For example, de Kock and Breytenbach (69) performed local open excision of an upper tract transitional cell cancer and followed this treatment with six weekly and then ten monthly retrograde instillations of 60 mg of thiotepa in 150 mL of normal saline over 30 minutes; the ureter was not occluded. Over a 5-year follow-up period, there was no recurrence. In other series, Eastham and Huffman (83), Streem and Pontes (344), Inglis and Tolley (161), and Grossman and co-workers (125) used mitomycin C in the upper urinary tract with no adverse side effects. In these reports, one to five instillations of 20 to 40 mg of mitomycin C or two instillations of 5 mg of mitomycin C were given in the immediate postoperative period either through a nephrostomy tube or a 7-Fr, 90-cm single-J ureteral catheter. In the percutaneous method, Eastham and Huffman (83) reported giving the mitomycin C as a continuous drip infusion at 50 mL per hour (40 mg of mitomycin C in 1,000 mL of saline) for 20 hours. Pressure in the renal pelvis was maintained at 15 cm H_2O or less. In contrast, infusion by the ureteral catheter consists of slowly instilling 5 mg of mitomycin C in 20 mL of saline into the ureteral catheter; the ureteral and urethral catheters are then clamped for a 30-minute period, after which they are opened to drainage. This is done on postoperative days 1 and 2. It is essential with both methods that before instillation an antegrade nephrostogram via the nephrostomy tube or a retrograde nephrostogram via the ureteral catheter be performed; there should be no evidence of extravasation or intrarenal backflow before instillation of any chemotherapeutic agent.

The largest experience with instillation chemotherapy in the upper urinary tract is with BCG (141,366). In their series, Jarrett and colleagues (168) reported using BCG in 19 of 33 patients treated endoscopically. The BCG was administered as 50 mL through the nephrostomy tube in six weekly instillations. They were unable to demonstrate any significant difference in survival curves between the patients who received BCG and those not receiving this adjuvant therapy. Other investigators have used similar regimens with BCG following percutaneous resection of the tumor and have not conclusively demonstrated any benefit from this adjuvant therapy (45,233). Sharpe and associates (330) reported on 17 kidneys with positive selective upper tract cytology but negative radiographic studies. In these patients, a 6-week course of weekly BCG (Pasteur strain, 120 mg in 100 mL of normal saline) was given; the solution was instilled slowly over 1 hour via an external ureteral catheter. The height of the solution was kept 20 cm above the patient, who was placed in a supine position. The patients voided 1 hour after the therapy. Overall, 75% of the patients had normalization of their urinary cytology at an average follow-up of 3 years. Complications with this approach were predominantly of a minor nature (dysuria and transient hematuria). There was only one major complication: fever with BCG bacteremia. Similarly, Bellman and colleagues (26) reported only minor side effects from percutaneous transnephrostomy BCG therapy; in their series, BCG instillations did not have to be stopped because of any complications. Of interest, subsequent rebiopsy of the renal pelvis revealed asymptomatic granulomas in 25% of their patients; the presence of granuloma formation had no influence on the success of the therapy. Mukamel and colleagues (255) also have documented the lack of significant adverse reactions from BCG in the upper urinary tract among 13 patients with documented vesicoureteral reflux. As of yet, there have been no deaths from using BCG in the upper tract; however, meticulous attention to detail before and during BCG instillation is essential. Specifically, a preinstillation nephrostogram should reveal an intact collecting system, there should be no hematuria at the time of instillation, the urine must be sterile, and the instillation should always progress at a low inflow pressure (i.e., 20 cm H_2O) (36,297).

Other adjunctive treatment variations have been reported. For example, Nurse and co-workers (266), Nolan and associates (265), and Patel and colleagues (284) placed a radioactive iridium 192 wire in the nephrostomy tract for 3 to 8 days in order to deliver 4,000 to 4,500 cGy at 0.5 cm from the wire. With this regimen they experienced no seeding of the nephrostomy tract. Taking a different approach, Orihuela and Smith (279) followed the initial tumor resection with a second-look procedure and laser application to the base of the tumor. Presently, it is difficult at this stage to select a given regimen that produces reliable high-quality results. Only through further study and careful reporting of data will the optimal endosurgical approach to TCCP become clear. However, there is a suggestion that adjunctive instillation therapy, especially with BCG, and second-look biopsy or electroresection of the tumor base may reduce recurrence rates.

Endourology for Transitional Cell Cancer of the Renal Pelvis: Unsettled Issues

In addition to the aforementioned problems of the impact of technique on outcome, four other clinical issues directly affect the efficacy of an endosurgical approach to TCCP: accuracy of diagnosis, tumor implantation, recurrence, and surveillance. Unlike for TCCU, the accuracy in diagnosis of TCCP by ureteroscopic means is disconcertingly low. Huffman (150) and Huffman and colleagues (152) noted that undergrading or understaging occurred in 60% of the renal pelvic tumors approached ureteroscopically. This is a significant problem because the procedure itself is primarily of benefit only for low-stage, low-grade disease.

Tumor implantation caused by local seeding of the upper urinary tract or retroperitoneal extravasation remains an ongoing, albeit largely undocumented, concern. With regard to local seeding, Grasso and co-workers (123) have reported one case of ureteral and urethral seeding of a renal cell cancer after a flexible ureteroscopic procedure (9.8 Fr). However, there have been no published reports of ureteral transitional cell tumors occurring after endourologic treatment of a renal pelvic transitional cell tumor. Clayman has noted a case of extensive ureteral tumors developing after a combined percutaneous and flexible ureteroscopic procedure to treat a grade 2 noninvasive transitional cell tumor in the renal pelvis of a solitary kidney. The latter patient had no prior history of transitional cell cancer. He eventually required a ureterectomy and autotransplantation with a pyelovesicostomy; no metastatic disease developed. Whether this situation resulted from tumor dissemination or the multifocal nature of his transitional cell cancer remains unsettled. To date, there have been no other reports of extensive seeding of the ureter following ureteroscopy in patients with TCCP. A second area of concern is the potential for seeding of the retroperitoneum should ureteral perforation occur during ureteroscopy or from extravasation during placement of the percutaneous nephrostomy tract. Both fears have been realized, albeit in only one case each to date. Martinez-Pineiro and associates (233) noted local tumor recurrence in a patient with TCCP T_1, G_2 who underwent a ureteroscopic procedure followed by subsequent nephroureterectomy. During the ureteroscopic procedure, the ureter was perforated; extension of the tumor into the retroperitoneum was noted at the subsequent surgical procedure, and this patient went on to develop distant metastases and died of the cancer. In another case, Huang and colleagues (147) reported seeding of a nephrostomy tract 5 weeks after percutaneous transnephrostomy (36 Fr) biopsy of a grade 3 midureteral tumor. Although these represent only isolated case reports, the small number of patients undergoing these procedures, coupled with the lack of follow-up CT scan data and the relatively short follow-up period in all series, makes one cognizant that the retroperitoneal appearance of TCCP caused by extravasation during the procedure may be significantly higher than what has been reported to date.

Another area of potential problems centers around the possibility of pyelorenal backflow and the subsequent development of distant metastases. Lim and colleagues (223) noted in one patient that following ureteroscopy the nephroureterectomy specimen revealed submucosal migration of tumor cells into the renal venous and lymphatic spaces. However, these authors were using irrigation pressures as high as 200 mm Hg. Despite this disconcerting finding, no metastatic disease developed over the ensuing 6 months in their patient. Kulp and Bagley (208) noted no problems of tumor cell backflow in 13 patients; however, in all cases, only gravity irrigation or gentle hand irrigation was used. It would appear that if the irrigation pressure is kept below 100 mm Hg, this problem may not develop.

The next concern with regard to the endourologic management of upper tract transitional cell cancer is the problem of tumor recurrence or new tumor development in the ipsilateral intact upper urinary tract. Realizing that when a ureteral stump is left after nephrectomy for TCCP the recurrence rate in the ipsilateral ureter is 40%, one can hardly be surprised by the 20% to 75% recurrence rate reported at less than 2 years after percutaneous or ureteroscopic therapy for TCCP (205,346). This is really no different than the 23% recurrence rate in the upper tract after conservative open surgical therapy for grade 1 tumors or the 54% recurrence rate after similar conservative therapy for high-grade lesions (256,370).

Given the high rate of recurrent or newly developed tumors in the ipsilateral ureter and renal pelvis, postresection surveillance of the affected upper urinary tract is of major importance. Just as most urologists believe that cytology and cystography are inferior to cystoscopy for following patients with superficial bladder tumor, cytology and intravenous urography in large part may prove to be less reliable than ureteroscopy for following patients with TCCP. In the series reported by Grossman and colleagues (125), among patients with a *known* upper tract lesion, the cytology before the lesion was endoscopically removed was positive in only 8% of patients with a grade 1 lesion and 50% with a grade 2 lesion. Similarly, in Blute's experience among patients with a radiographically identifiable upper tract lesion, the combination of intravenous urography, retrograde ureterography, and cytology diagnosed only 55% of all renal pelvic tumors, whereas ureteroscopic evaluation correctly identified all renal pelvic tumors. As such, given the poor track record of nonendoscopic studies when a lesion is present, the use of these same modalities for surveillance appears to be ill advised; periodic ureteroscopy appears to be essential.

Problems with a ureteroscopic surveillance protocol arise if a patient is going to require intravenous sedation, a formal outpatient surgical visit, and an indwelling ureteral stent every time surveillance ureteroscopy is completed. If current recommendations for bladder tumor surveillance are applied to transitional cell tumors of the upper urinary tract, this would include at least six examinations during the first 2 years and annual ureteroscopy thereafter (108,322). This certainly is not as simple or as inexpensive as office cystoscopy. In an effort to reduce the cost and complexity of surveillance cystoscopy, Kerbl and Clayman (188) have reported deliberately unroofing the ureteral orifice and tunnel with an Orandi electrosurgical knife in two patients undergoing endourologic management of upper tract transitional cell cancers. In both patients, the resulting refluxing ureteral orifice was sufficiently patulous to permit flexible ureteroscopy without dilation or sedation in the office. To date, both patients have undergone routine surveillance, office-based ureteroscopy, for over 2 years. In one patient, a total of three diminutive upper tract recurrences have been noted and subsequently treated on an outpatient basis. In the other patient, there has been one upper tract recurrence also treated in a similar manner. Of note, these tumors were too small to be imaged on either retrograde ureterography or intravenous pyelography. However, the potential negative impact of a refluxing ureter in a patient with upper tract transitional cell cancer may be of concern because approximately one-third of these patients subsequently will develop bladder tumors. This may further compound the risk of recurrent or new tumor development on the previously affected upper urinary tract. Conflicting reports regarding the potential risk of reflux in a patient with TCCB already exist in the literature; although some authors have noted no risk of upper tract TCC development in patients with TCCB and vesicoureteral reflux, others have reported as high as a 20% incidence of upper tract tumors over a 2- to 9-year follow-up period (73,205,281).

Although one might argue that if ureteroscopy can be done safely in the office, the follow-up for TCCP should become identical to the follow-up for TCCB. The natural corollary to this reasoning is that the minimally invasive approach could then be used in all cases of low-grade, low-stage TCCP. However, the impetus for conservative, endoscopic bladder surgery is largely due to the fact that the bladder is a solitary organ, the removal of which is a major surgical undertaking associated with significant operative morbidity, lengthy hospitalization, and major changes in a patient's quality of life. For TCCP, a similar situation pertains only in the patient with a functionally or anatomically solitary kidney (319). Only in that circumstance does ablative surgery carry similar quality-of-life issues to removal of the bladder, specifically long-term dialysis and renal transplantation. Furthermore, the extension of minimally invasive therapy for TCCP to patients with two kidneys has a high price. For the dubious benefit of preserving the affected kidney, the middle-aged patient with at least a greater than 34-year life expectancy will have to undergo at least 34 separate surveillance ureteroscopic procedures in addition to the likelihood of requiring at least three additional minimally invasive procedures to treat recurrent, low-grade TCCP and a 10% to 20% likelihood of eventual nephroureterectomy because of recurrent but now invasive, extensive, high-grade, or overly extensive disease. Based on these considerations and the previously cited review of the literature, minimally invasive surgery for TCCP should be reserved only for patients with a solitary kidney, renal insufficiency, or high surgical risk; for the patient who has two kidneys and normal renal function, a nephroureterectomy remains the most expeditious, probably least expensive, and most definitive means of treatment. The possibilities that TCCP or TCCU will metachronously involve the contralateral kidney (1% to 2.5%) or that the patient with a now solitary kidney will develop renal insufficiency are not sufficient arguments to change current surgical practice for this entity in the patient with two otherwise normal kidneys (205).

Simple and Peripelvic Renal Cysts

Renal cystic disease spans the pathologic spectrum, including benign and malignant processes, acquired and inherited conditions, and infectious and noninfectious etiologies. Renal cysts may occur within the renal cortex, within the medulla, or within the peripelvic region; they may have a simple, nonloculated or a complex, septated configuration.

The most commonly occurring renal cysts are of a simple, acquired, tubular origin. Simple cysts are noted in approximately 50% of the adult population at autopsy; meanwhile, 20% to 40% of patients 50 to 80 years of age have simple renal cysts sufficiently large to be detected on CT of the kidneys (217). The prevalence of cysts appears to increase with patient age; over two-thirds of patients older than 80 years of age will have a cyst detectable by CT (217). Simple cysts are lined by detached immature tubular epithelium capable of transepithelial secretion. As such, cyst fluid contains sodium and chloride that are secreted into the cyst lumen possibly by an active transport mechanism; water osmotically follows the transfer of these ions. Fluid accumulation within the cyst also is determined by a host of pericystic regulatory factors: hormones (e.g., vasopressin, arginine), growth factors (e.g., epidermal growth factor), and other substances (e.g., prostaglandins E_1 and E_2) (120).

In this framework, the growth and, in some cases, the "malignant degeneration" of renal cysts become understandable outcomes.

In the differentiation of simple renal cysts from other, more concerning, renal masses, the diagnostic accuracy of renal US or CT is sufficiently high to preclude further invasive or costly radiographic studies. Often, this is the end of the evaluation; however, some urologists prefer to obtain a single follow-up study in 1 year to look for any changes in the size or overall appearance of the cyst in order to further corroborate its benign nature. In this regard, it is relatively rare for simple cysts to increase in size; Richter and colleagues (302) noted that only 6% of cysts increased in volume over a 1- to 10-year follow-up period. Instead, the number of cysts in a kidney is more likely to increase with time; in the study of Dalton and associates (64), approximately one-third of the patients developed additional cystic lesions during a follow-up period of 3.5 years.

Overall, simple renal cysts rarely become symptomatic. Symptoms, such as flank pain, occur when the cyst obstructs a portion of the collecting system or because of the sheer size of the cyst. Macroscopic hematuria and hypertension are extremely rare signs attributable to a renal cyst. By the same token, only in the symptomatic patient is treatment of an otherwise simple cyst indicated. Similar criteria also have been used to treat some patients with adult polycystic kidney disease either by percutaneous drainage or open surgical reduction (28). For other cystic masses, treatment is indicated only if the cyst is thought to be the result of a more serious malady, such as infection or malignancy.

Technique

There are two minimally invasive strategies for treating simple renal cysts: drainage with sclerosis or drainage with ablation. Drainage with sclerosis is performed under local anesthesia using ultrasonographic or CT guidance. First, a sheathed needle is directed into the cyst and the cavity is drained. The fluid is sent for chemical, cytologic, and bacterial evaluation. Next, the sheath of the needle is left in the cyst cavity and contrast is introduced. This enables the radiologist to carefully examine the contours of the cyst wall and determine whether the cyst communicates with the collecting system. If the cyst is smooth walled, is not peripelvic in location, and is excluded from the collecting system, a sclerosant can be instilled into the cyst cavity.

A variety of sclerosants are available (e.g., 95% ethanol, bismuth phosphate, fibrin glue, hypertonic glucose); however, ethanol is the most popular and, possibly, the most effective agent. In this technique, approximately 25% of the cyst fluid is replaced with alcohol. The alcohol is left in place for 20 minutes, during which time the patient is moved into a variety of positions to ensure bathing of the entire inner lining of the cyst. The alcohol is then drained from the cyst and the sheath is removed (21,280,290).

Drainage with ablation of a simple renal cyst or of a peripelvic renal cyst can be done in either an antegrade (percutaneous) or retrograde (ureteroscopic) manner. In the percutaneous technique, the cyst can be approached in one of three ways: transcystic, transparenchymal, or indirectly through the collecting system. In each situation, the procedure begins with passage of a retrograde ureteral catheter. This will enable the urologist to instill an indigo carmine–stained mixture of contrast material and saline into the collecting system, thereby making it easy to differentiate between entry into the collecting system (i.e., blue fluid) and entry into the cyst cavity (i.e., clear to yellow fluid).

In the percutaneous transcystic method, the cyst is punctured with a nephrostomy needle (Fig. 19.28, parts 1A to 1C). The needle is then directed across the cyst and into the renal pelvis; entry into the renal pelvis is confirmed by aspiration of blue fluid. A guidewire is passed down the ureter or coiled in the renal pelvis. The point of entry into the cyst is dilated, and a standard 24- to 26-Fr resectoscope equipped with a roller electrode is introduced. At this point, the inner lining of the cyst is electrocoagulated in all areas except where the cyst abuts the renal parenchyma or renal pelvis. Now, with the safety guidewire covered by a nonconductive angiographic catheter, the opening into the collecting system, if thin-walled, can be widened using a cold knife or electrosurgery. A transcystic nephrostomy tube is placed at the end of the procedure, such that its tip lies well within the renal pelvis.

In the percutaneous transparenchymal method, the cyst is entered by traversing the lateralmost portion of the renal parenchyma that overlies the cyst (Fig. 19.28, parts 2A,2B). Then a standard 24- to 26-Fr resectoscope is used to resect the outer, lateral cyst wall, thereby accomplishing a partial cyst decortication (148,291). The collecting system is never entered. If there is any bleeding at the end of the procedure, a catheter can be placed into the cyst cavity, thereby effectively tamponading the renal parenchyma.

In the percutaneous indirect method, a nephrostomy tract is placed in the kidney opposite the medial wall of the cyst (Fig. 19.28, parts 3A to 3C). A separate needle is passed percutaneously into the cyst cavity. By instilling an indigo carmine–stained mixture of contrast and sorbitol, the endoscopist is guided to the wall of the cyst that most closely abuts the collecting system and thus has a blue hue. With a resectoscope or a cold-knife urethrotome passed through the initial nephrostomy tract, the cyst wall is incised and the cyst is entered. Next, with use of a standard 24- to 26-Fr resectoscope equipped with a roller electrode, the far wall of the cyst is electrocoagulated. A nephrostomy tube is placed into the collecting system via the initial percutaneous puncture site, remote from the cyst cavity. This approach is of particular value when dealing with a peripelvic cyst (42,85, 156,199).

The ureteroscopic approach to cysts is limited to smaller cysts (i.e., less than 2 cm) that have a section of their wall

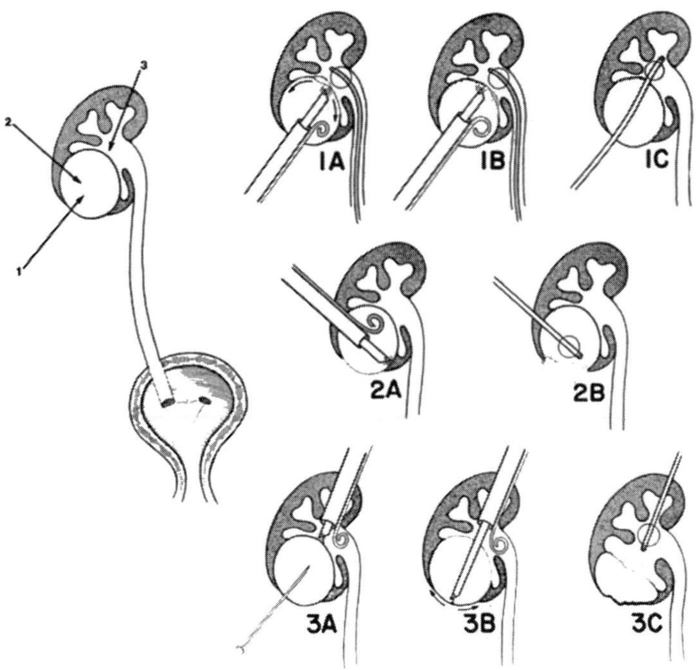

FIGURE 19.28. The three methods for percutaneously treating a renal cyst are depicted by the arrows: *1*, direct transcystic; *2*, direct transparenchymal; and *3*, indirect. **1A:** The cyst has been punctured directly and dilated; a 30-Fr Amplatz sheath has been passed, and through this a resectoscope has been introduced. The cyst wall abutting the collecting system is resected. Note that an occlusion balloon catheter has been passed up the ureter to assist in the recognition of the true collecting system. A safety guidewire catheter also has been placed in the cyst. **1B:** The remaining cyst wall is fulgurated with a roller electrode. **1C:** A transcystic nephrostomy tube is placed. **2A:** The parenchyma has been traversed in the process of entering the cyst. A 30-Fr Amplatz sheath is placed alongside a safety guidewire catheter. The outer wall of the cyst is resected, and other areas of the cyst wall are fulgurated. **2B:** A large-bore catheter is placed into the cystic cavity. The collecting system is not entered. **3A:** Via a remote calyx, the collecting system is entered and a 30-Fr Amplatz sheath is placed alongside a safety guidewire catheter. The presenting surface of the cyst is identified and resected. A needle has been placed into the cyst so that it can be readily drained and expanded, thereby aiding in its identification by the surgeon. Via the needle, normal saline stained with indigo carmine can be instilled into the cyst, thereby giving it a blue appearance and clearly delineating it from the normal collecting system. **3B:** The far wall of the cyst is fulgurated with a roller electrode. **3C:** A standard nephrostomy tube is placed in the collecting system.

bulging into a calyx or that share a common wall with the renal pelvis (i.e., peripelvic cyst) (182). If this approach is selected, it is still helpful to preplace a small percutaneous tube into the cyst cavity in order to fill the cyst with an indigo carmine–stained mixture of contrast and sorbitol. Then, via the rigid or flexible ureteroscope, a Ho:YAG laser or electrosurgical knife can be used to enter the cyst. Next, the inner surface of the cyst can be coagulated using either electrocautery or Nd:YAG laser energy (20 W).

In the rare event when a cyst has reformed despite ureteroscopic or percutaneous methods, a laparoscopic approach (i.e., drainage and cyst decortication) can be used.

Results

Drainage and sclerosis is the least invasive form of therapy for simple renal cysts. Short-term success rates for ethanol ablation are the highest of any sclerosant treatment at 97% to 100% (21,280). Cysts as large as 600 mL have been treated successfully with this method. Other sclerosants result in cyst disappearance in less than 50% of cases, especially when follow-up was extended beyond 2 years (144,290). Of note, the follow-up after ethanol ablation generally is under 1 year. Clearly, long-term follow-up studies on the durability of ethanol ablation are sorely needed.

The endoscopic treatment of renal cysts is indicated predominantly for peripelvic cysts or as salvage therapy for simple renal cysts when drainage and sclerotherapy fail. The percutaneous approach is still relatively rarely performed and hence the experience is small. For the percutaneous approach, the long-term success rate (i.e., complete cyst ablation) has been only 50% according to Plas and Hubner (291). In their series, with a median follow-up of 45.7 months, approximately 30% of the cysts recurred. The ureteroscopic approach has been reported only once (182). In one patient, the procedure was successful; however, the follow-up was less than 6 months.

Renal Abscess and Fungal Collections

A localized renal infection may occur either in the renal parenchyma (e.g., lobar nephronia, an infected renal cyst) or within the collecting system (e.g., pyocalyx caused by obstruction). The infections are due to *E. coli* in approximately one-third of cases; another one-third of patients are infected with either *Proteus mirabilis* or *Klebsiella pneumoniae* (174,307). Today, *Staphylococcus aureus* accounts for less than 10% of all renal abscesses (96). On rare occasion, a fungus is the underlying cause: *Candida albicans, Mucormycosis, Aspergillus,* or *Torulopsis glabrata* (169).

Presenting symptoms most commonly include fever, flank pain, or chills (60% to 90% of patients). Symptoms usually are present for up to 2 or more weeks before the diagnosis of a renal abscess is made. The most common associated illness is the presence of diabetes mellitus; these patients, as well as individuals with immunosuppressive disorders, are at greatest risk for developing life-threatening sequelae from an unrecognized renal abscess (96).

Today, the diagnosis of a renal abscess can be made more easily because of the advent of renal CT and US (Fig. 19.29). Fowler and Perkins (96) noted that among 61 consecutive patients with renal abscesses, CT or US provided a diagnostic accuracy of 96% and 92%, respectively.

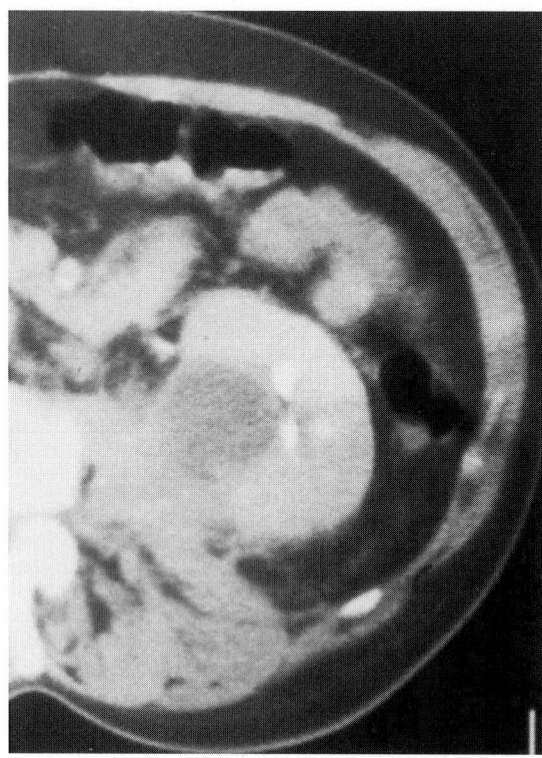

FIGURE 19.29. Computed tomography scan shows a cystic appearing lesion with debris. Puncture of the lesion confirmed the presence of a renal abscess. A drainage tube was subsequently placed inside the cavity as a therapeutic measure.

On CT scan a renal abscess classically has a cystic, albeit thick-walled, appearance; the CT density of the abscess is usually greater than that of a cyst (134). On the other hand, the ultrasonographic appearance of an abscess is that of an irregular mass with echo-producing intralesional debris and a poorly defined back wall (373).

Technique

Although antibiotic therapy alone has been reported to cure the rare patient with a renal abscess, this approach has not been widely adopted. The consensus is that renal abscesses should be aspirated and, in most cases, percutaneously drained as soon as they are diagnosed. This is most easily done under US or CT guidance. Following a confirmatory diagnosis by needle aspiration, a 7- or 8-Fr self-retaining (e.g., Cope locking loop) percutaneous drainage tube is placed within the abscess cavity. An infracostal percutaneous route is selected in order to avoid any possible pleural contamination.

If the problem is one of a fungal bezoar, a standard percutaneous technique may be undertaken after the patient has been given parenteral amphotericin B and achieved appropriate serum levels. The urine at this point should be sterile. Via two retrograde ureteral catheters, the renal pelvis is irrigated with amphotericin B (5 mg/100 mL) to decrease the chances of retroperitoneal contamination by the fungus. Next, via an infracostal percutaneous approach, the fungal bezoar is removed with grasping forceps or suctioned from the kidney using the ultrasonic lithotripsy probe. At the end of the procedure, a nephrostomy tube is placed; one of the ureteral catheters is also left in place. Postoperatively, once a nephrostogram shows no extravasation and no remaining fungal bezoars, the collecting system is irrigated through the ureteral catheter with amphotericin B (50 mg/L at 50 mL per hour) for 2 to 3 days (31,137,175,377).

Results

Over the past few years, a few clinicians have reported limited success with antibiotic therapy alone for treating a renal abscess. Chakroun and colleagues (39) noted that this therapy worked in 25% of their patients, whereas Gelabert and associates (104) had only a single success among 12 patients.

Overall, the consensus remains that a renal abscess is best treated by aspiration combined with ongoing percutaneous drainage. Only in Chakroun and co-workers' (39) series was aspiration alone a viable treatment option; in this series of 12 patients, only three patients eventually required percutaneous drainage. However, for Gelabert and colleagues (104), as well as Janetschek and associates (166) and other clinical investigators, percutaneous drainage was the most definitive and effective means for treating a renal abscess. In several series, this form of therapy was effective in 82% to 88% of patients; in Fowler and Perkin's (96) extensive report of 57 renal abscess patients treated with percutaneous drainage between 1972 and 1988, the success rate was even higher at 97% (60,96,111,134,166,167). However, percutaneous drainage of a renal abscess is not an innocuous procedure; approximately 10% of patients develop hemorrhage, recurrent abscess, or urosepsis after this procedure.

Failed percutaneous aspiration and drainage of a renal abscess is fortunately rare. Most failures are due to a loculated abscess or are associated with a fungal infection. The patient with a loculated abscess can at times be salvaged percutaneously by the placement of multiple percutaneous drainage tubes. For the patient with a fungal abscess, irrigation of the abscess cavity with amphotericin B (50 mg/L at 50 mL per hour) is sometimes helpful in resolving the problem (134). However, for the most part when initial percutaneous therapy fails, the next step is open surgery, with manual fragmentation of any loculations followed by placement of large drains or, if the kidney is functioning poorly, nephrectomy; this open approach may be necessary in up to 9% of cases.

Because of the advances in antibiotic and endourologic therapy, the mortality rate from renal abscess has fallen to 7% to 9%. Today, most fatalities from renal abscess result from a delay in diagnosis rather than therapeutic failure.

As with the previously described parenchymally based renal abscesses, the best mode of therapy for infection of an obstructed portion of the collecting system (i.e., pyonephrosis or a pyocalyx) is percutaneous drainage. In these cases, a percutaneous nephrostomy tube is placed into the obstructed area of the collecting system. This results in immediate relief of obstruction and drainage of the infection. When combined with appropriate antibiotic therapy, nephrostomy tube drainage is highly successful. In Janetschek and colleagues' (166) collected series of 21 cases, all patients with these conditions responded well to a percutaneous approach. However, two patients, despite percutaneous drainage, ultimately required a nephrectomy because of failure of the kidney to recover function (166).

Before the advent of endourologic techniques, urinary tract fungal bezoars usually were the harbinger of ureteral obstruction, urosepsis, and death; up to 80% of these patients succumbed. Today, however, successful therapy is achievable in the majority of these patients. A review of the endourologic literature reveals only a handful of cases of funguria with associated bezoar formation managed endourologically. In these cases, more than 80% of the patients have survived with an intact kidney following percutaneous drainage or extraction of the fungal mass (3,31,70, 76,137,162,163,175).

Post–renal transplantation

In the renal transplant population, the frequency of a urologic complication is closely associated with the type of ureteral reimplant performed at the time of renal transplantation. Most of these complications are secondary to ureteral obstruction; the remaining, less common complications are due to urinary tract fistula formation, ureteral necrosis, and urolithiasis.

With the traditional Leadbetter-Politano reimplantation, urinary tract complications occur in 5% to 11% of patients (355). However, with the more recent adaptation of routine primary ureteral stent placement at the time of the operation or an extravesical technique for performing a ureteroneocystostomy, the incidence of urologic complications has fallen to below 4% (355). However, up to two-thirds of these problems are still due to ureteral obstruction. The obstruction may be either of an intrinsic (i.e., ureteral stricture) or an extrinsic (i.e., perirenal fluid collection, such as lymphocele, urinoma, abscess, or hematoma) nature. The development of strictures usually occurs early in the postoperative course, but in some cases ureteral stricture formation may occur as late as 5 years postoperatively (178,195,355).

When faced with a rising creatinine in the renal transplant patient, the clinician must determine whether the apparent compromise in renal function is prerenal (i.e., arterial stenosis, renal vein thrombosis, or alteration in fluid status), renal (i.e., rejection), or postrenal (i.e., obstruction or fistula). To evaluate for a ureteric or perirenal postrenal problem, a renal US study or a CT scan is of particular benefit. Either study can reveal the presence of hydronephrosis or an extrinsic obstructive lesion and assess for intrarenal filling defects. With regard to perirenal lesions, the diagnostic accuracy of the CT is slightly better than sonography; in one review, sonography detected 73% of perirenal fluid collections, whereas CT was correct in 87% of the patients (sensitivity of 64% and specificity of 94%).

An advantage of renal US is that it can be performed with duplex Doppler scanning. As such, the renal vascular RI can be determined. When the RI exceeds 0.75, the chances of an obstructive process are high. However, a normal RI argues for a nonobstructive process, such as transplant rejection or a fistula. In a study of 35 renal transplant patients with pyelocaliectasis by Platt and associates (292), the RI was elevated (average of 0.81) in 13 patients with proven obstruction; there were two false-negative diagnoses, but in both patients the obstruction was associated with a fistula. The latter problem was probably responsible for the apparently normal RI. After placement of a percutaneous nephrostomy in the obstructed patients, the RI fell to 0.67.

When obstruction is suspected, the next step should be an antegrade nephrostogram (177). This is of both diagnostic and therapeutic value. The site of obstruction can be delineated clearly; the presence or absence of an associated ureteric fistula can be determined; if need be, a Whitaker pressure study can be performed; and a percutaneous nephrostomy can be left in place after the study is completed. The Whitaker test can be most helpful in distinguishing between an anatomic and a functional narrowing. In one study, up to 25% of ureteric strictures were functionally insignificant; in these four patients, the rise in creatinine was subsequently shown to be due to rejection (177).

The other two major areas of complications following transplantation in which endourology has had an impact are ureteral fistulae and perirenal collections. The most common site of a ureteral fistula is either at the site of the ureteral reimplantation or, more rarely, along the renal pelvis. Diagnosis of this condition can be made most clearly either during an antegrade nephrostogram or a retrograde ureterogram. In either case, a ureteral stent can then be placed to "put the ureter to rest." If an indwelling ureteral stent is placed retrograde, a urethral catheter also is indicated in order to preclude reflux and continued leakage at the fistula site. If the stent is inserted immediately after performing an antegrade nephrostogram, a percutaneous nephrostomy tube should be left in place to decompress the renal pelvis and prevent further passage of urine across the fistula.

Perirenal collections often produce symptoms of discomfort and a fullness in the lower abdomen; the usual sign is new-onset azotemia caused by ureteral obstruction. These collections may be due to one of four problems: urinoma, lymphocele, hematoma, or abscess. The CT scan is the most reliable method for diagnosing the presence of perirenal collection; at the same time the scan is done, the lesion can be drained and a self-retaining drainage tube can be placed. The obtained fluid can be sent for culture, cell blood count, and creatinine; these tests should effectively identify the nature of the collection.

Technique

The initial form of management for the majority of ureteral complications among renal transplant patients is placement of a percutaneous nephrostomy tube. Given the proximity of the transplanted kidney to the skin, the procedure can be accomplished rapidly and safely using either fluoroscopic or ultrasonographic imaging (336). The methods involved in dealing with ureteral strictures in the transplant kidney are the same as previously described for treatment of ureteral strictures in patients without a renal transplant. Likewise, the therapy for a ureteral fistula (i.e., placement of an indwelling ureteral stent) and for a perirenal collection (i.e., aspiration and drainage) do not differ from the techniques used to approach the same entities in patients with normal renal function and eutopic kidneys.

Results

Endourology has had a significant impact on the management of all types of ureteric and perirenal complications affecting the renal transplant patient. As previously noted, ureteric complications are usually due to either a ureteral stricture or a ureteral fistula. Ureteral strictures in the transplant patient have most commonly been treated with balloon dilation to 8 to 12 mm accompanied by ureteral stinting for 4 to 14 weeks with a 7- to 14-Fr ureteral stent. The success rate with this approach is 40% to 70% at an average follow-up of 2 years. Overall, strictures in the distal ureter or at the ureterovesical anastomotic site are more common than upper ureteral strictures and appear to respond better to endourologic management. In one study, the success rate with distal/ureterovesical junction (UVJ) ureteral strictures was 75%; however, only 16% of proximal ureteral strictures responded favorably to balloon dilation (93,172,177,192,283,333).

An alternative, albeit more invasive, approach to ureteric strictures is to endourologically incise the stricture. Conrad and colleagues (57) used a flexible wire-guided cold knife to endourologically treat 11 transplant patients with a ureteral stricture; all but two of the strictures were in the distal/UVJ portion of the ureter. An indwelling 14-Fr stent was placed for a period of 4 to 6 weeks. Success was achieved in 82% of patients with a mean follow-up of 28 months (2 to 61 months). Of interest, both UPJ obstructions and all six patients with very distal ureteral obstruction responded favorably to endoureterotomy; however, only two of four patients with middle or lower ureteral strictures had a favorable outcome. A similarly high rate of success has been reported by Youssef and associates (381a) using the Acucise device to cut the area of obstruction; a successful outcome was noted in five of six renal transplant patients. These data are similar to endoureterotomy data in the nontransplant patient population, among whom success rates for UPJ and distal ureteral obstruction are higher than for strictures lying in the lower or middle ureter that, after an endoureterotomy, have not been marsupialized into the renal pelvis or bladder, respectively. Overall, it would appear that an endourologic approach with balloon dilation or incision is a reasonable first step when dealing with posttransplant ureteral strictures, especially if the stricture involves the UPJ or UVJ area. Last, although endoureterotomy may be intrinsically more appealing to the urologic surgeon, at this point in time, given the small number of patients treated to date, there is no clear-cut difference in results between balloon dilation and endoureterotomy of distal strictures.

With regard to a ureteral fistula in the transplanted ureter, placement of an indwelling ureteral stent with either proximal (i.e., nephrostomy tube) or distal (i.e., urethral catheter) decompression is often effective. This is especially true if the leakage is associated with distal ureteral obstruction. However, ureteral fistulae are relatively rare, and experience with the endourologic management of this complication remains scant. In reviewing the available literature, the largest series of fistulae managed by stents was reported by Berger and co-workers (29); the procedure worked in only two of 12 patients. Subsequently, Hobarth and colleagues (143) and Irving and Kashi (164) independently reported an additional eight patients in whom either a ureteral stent or percutaneous nephrostomy was used to treat a ureteral fistula; a successful outcome was reported in five of the eight patients. One reason for the markedly improved results in the series of Irving and Kashi (164) is that these authors were careful to distinguish between a small ureteral fistula and total ureterovesical disruption as might occur with ureteral necrosis. In their series, patients with suspected ureteral necrosis were managed with direct surgical intervention. As such, endourologic methods were applied only to patients with small fistulae; among four patients with ureteral leakage unassociated with ureterovesical discontinuity, all were successfully managed endourologically.

Among perirenal collections, the most common type after renal transplantation is a lymphocele. In these cases, drainage may be followed by placement of a tube into the cavity; sclerotherapy with ethanol can be used if the lymphocele does not abut directly on the ureter or renal pelvis. Failing this, an open surgical procedure or, more recently, laparoscopic marsupialization can be performed. The latter has gained rapidly in popularity and today appears to be the treatment of choice should simple percutaneous drainage fail to resolve the problem (331). For other perirenal collections such as perirenal abscess, percutaneous drainage and appropriate antibiotic therapy is the first step. With regard to a nonexpanding hematoma, once the diagnosis is made, nothing further need be done unless the hematoma is causing extrinsic compression on the ureter. In this case, a ureteral stent can be placed until the hematoma resolves. Last, with regard to treating a perirenal urinoma, percutaneous drainage is the first step. Following this, the site of the fistula must be identified and appropriate endourologic or surgical therapy instituted (vide supra).

EXTRARENAL APPLICATIONS

Perirenal Abscess

Perirenal abscess can result from rupture of an acute renal abscess into the surrounding fatty tissue inside Gerota's fascia. Perirenal abscess formation usually arises as a complication of pyelonephritis, urolithiasis, penetrating trauma, and prior urologic procedures in the retroperitoneum or the collecting system. Perirenal abscess also may occur because of a secondary nonrenal etiology: enteric fistula, pancreatic abscess, and lumbar osteomyelitis. Hematogenous spread to the kidney from a cutaneous infection or intravenous drug usage also has been responsible for perirenal abscess formation. A significant number of patients with perirenal abscess will have diabetes mellitus or other coexisting debilitating conditions, such as underlying malignancy or immunosuppression.

The clinical course of a perirenal abscess is often insidious. The symptoms and signs are usually vague and nonspecific. Most commonly present is fever (58% to 83%), followed by flank or abdominal pain (20% to 70%), and a palpable mass (9% to 13%). Advanced cases may manifest with malaise, weight loss, and a draining sinus. Leukocytosis with a left shift is a routine finding. Urine cultures are usually positive; however, the bacteria isolated from the urine may not reflect the organisms isolated from the abscess in 19% of the cases. *E. coli* and *P. mirabilis* are the most common causative organisms; however, when the abscess results from hematogenous spread, *S. aureus* predominates (84,332).

Abdominal plain films may show scoliosis, loss of the psoas shadow and renal margin, urolithiasis, and gas within a perirenal mass. Intravenous pyelography can reveal thickening of Gerota's fascia, mottling of the perirenal fat, delayed renal function or nonfunction, focal or diffuse renal enlargement, presence of a mass effect, renal fixation, or hydronephrosis. Chest radiographs may be abnormal in up to 41% of cases; pleural effusion, lower-lobe consolidation, and elevation of the hemidiaphragm are the most common findings (87). Renal US characteristically will show round or oval hypoechoic lesions. However, abscesses containing large amounts of gas may be mistaken for bowel. Abscesses that contain a large amount of echogenic debris or with septations may have characteristics that are indistinguishable from a tumor (367). CT is the imaging modality of choice because it provides better definition of the extent of the abscess and its relationships to other structures than can be obtained with US. Typically, the mass has a soft tissue density (less than 20 HU) and may have a "rind sign" caused by vascular enhancement of the abscess wall after the administration of intravenous contrast (110). Rarely, scintigraphy with gallium- or indium-labeled white blood cells may be useful in determining the presence of an abscess when the diagnosis is uncertain.

Technique

Patients routinely are given broad-spectrum parenteral antibiotics before abscess drainage. The abscess is localized by US or CT. The abscess is then punctured with an 18-gauge, thin-walled needle. The puncture should be extraperitoneal and extrapleural (i.e., below the twelfth rib) to avoid seeding of the abscess contents into the peritoneal and thoracic cavities, respectively, which can result in peritonitis, pleural effusion, pyopneumothorax, and empyema. Contents of the abscess are aspirated and sent for Gram stain, culture, and sensitivities. A guidewire is advanced through the 18-gauge needle puncture and coiled in the abscess cavity. The tract is dilated with semirigid dilators under fluoroscopic or US guidance. A drainage catheter is then positioned and secured. The size of the drainage tube depends directly on the viscosity of the initial aspirate. Tube sizes generally range from 8 to 14 Fr, or occasionally, a vanSonnenberg sump catheter will be used for a very viscous collection. If the abscess is loculated, two or more catheters may be percutaneously placed to provide adequate drainage. Mean drainage times are between 5 and 20 days (213). Prolonged drainage should alert one to the possibility of an enteric or urinary tract fistula.

Saline irrigation of the catheters may be started after 48 hours to help clear debris from the cavity and prevent catheter occlusion. Sinograms may be obtained at the discretion of the urologist to monitor the size of the abscess cavity and to identify any fistulous tract. Once the drainage from the catheter has ceased, a sinogram is repeated. If the cavity is now small (i.e., not much larger than the drainage catheter), the catheter can be removed. Alternatively, if a substantial cavity persists, 95% ethanol can be used to attempt to sclerose the cavity. In this case, one must be certain that there is no communication between the abscess cavity and the collecting system or other viscera. Sclerosis is continued on a weekly basis for 3 to 6 weeks until the abscess cavity has completely collapsed around the drainage catheter, at which time the catheter can be removed.

Results

Perinephric abscess is a very serious problem that carries a high mortality rate, especially when prompt drainage and broad-spectrum antibiotics are delayed (Fig. 19.30). Even with timely percutaneous drainage, mortality rates are as high as 13%. Initial percutaneous drainage is the procedure of choice in the management of perirenal abscess and in select cases may be the only intervention necessary. Elyaderani and Moncman (87) reported that 2 of 6 peri-

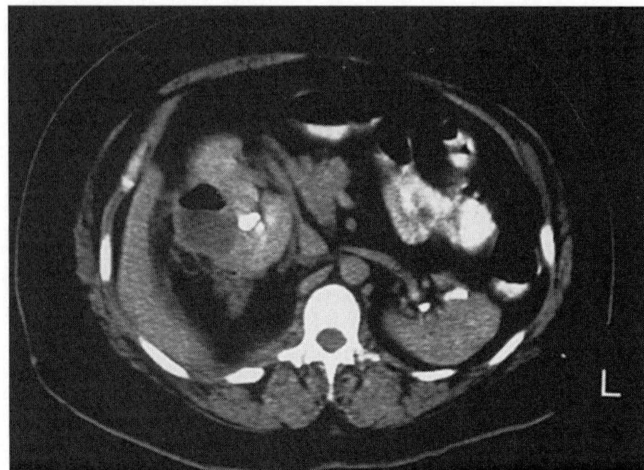

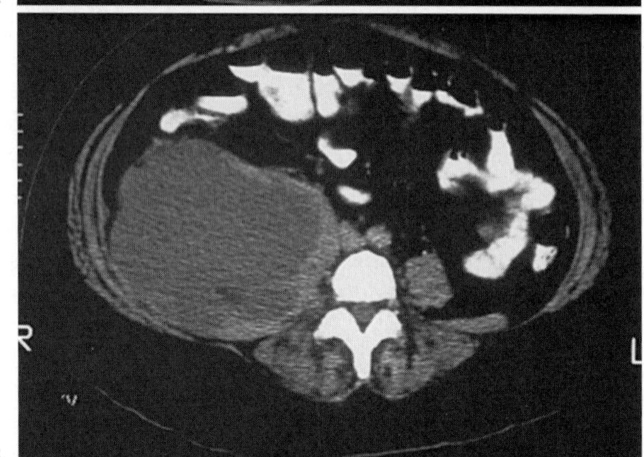

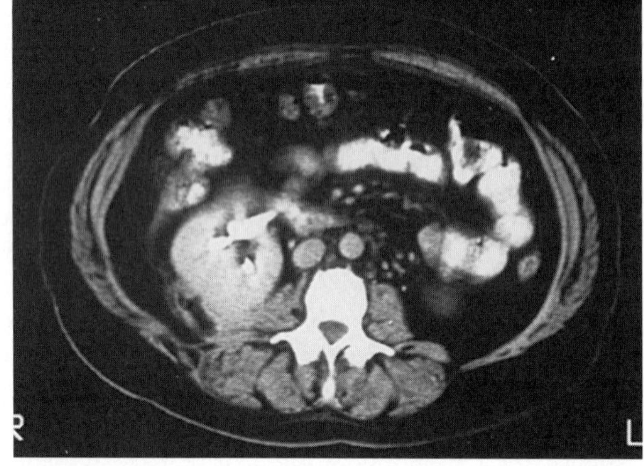

FIGURE 19.30. A: An obstructing upper-pole stone is present on this computed tomography scan. **B:** A large, retroperitoneal abscess caused by the obstruction and resulting infection. **C:** Three months after percutaneous stone removal and drainage of the abscess cavity, renal function has returned to normal and the abscess cavity has completely resolved.

renal abscesses treated with percutaneous drainage resolved completely without further intervention. Lang (213) reported that 9 of 10 perirenal abscesses resolved with percutaneous drainage. These data are in agreement with results reported independently by Haaga (134) and by Gerzof and Gale (110).

Urinoma

A perirenal urinoma results from renal or ureteral trauma, urologic surgical procedures, or upper tract obstruction with associated ureteral or renal extravasation (e.g., neoplasm, surgical ligation, calculus disease). Extravasation of urine into the perirenal space is usually due to a forniceal rupture. When the amount of urine extravasated exceeds the capacity for lymphatic clearance, a perirenal fluid collection develops. Inflammation and fibrosis at the site of leakage can lead to ureteral obstruction, progressive hydronephrosis, and ultimately loss of renal function (215).

Clinically, the symptoms and signs of a urinoma include vague abdominal or flank discomfort and sometimes a palpable mass. There may be several months' delay between the causative event and presentation and diagnosis of the urinoma. In cases of a left-sided collection, one must be certain that the fluid-filled mass does not represent a pancreatic pseudocyst.

Plain films of the abdomen may reveal a mass if the urinoma is large. Findings on intravenous urography may include decreased renal function or absence of renal function on the affected side, cephalad and lateral displacement of the kidney, or contrast in the urinoma on delayed images. CT is the optimal study to define the extent and the relationship of the urinoma to surrounding structures. The wall of the urinoma may be thickened and smooth; the density of the urinoma is between −10 and +30 HU. Homogeneous enhancement of the urinoma implies a functioning kidney and presence of a communication between the urinoma and the collecting system (215). A retrograde pyelogram or antegrade nephrostogram is useful in identifying the level of obstruction and the point of extravasation.

Technique

Under US or CT guidance, a percutaneous drain is placed in the most dependent aspect of the fluid collection. The aspirated fluid is sent for creatinine determination, blood cell count, culture and sensitivities, and when indicated, amylase. The creatinine content of a urinoma should be similar to the high creatinine content of the urine.

A 10-Fr biliary urinary drainage or locking Cope loop catheter is placed. In instances where there is no longer a communication with the collecting system and no ongoing obstruction, drainage usually ceases after 48 to 72 hours. In cases of prolonged drainage, placement of an indwelling ureteral stent and urethral catheter or a percutaneous nephrostomy generally provides diversion sufficient for spontaneous closure of the fistulous tract. There are rare instances in which there is persistent drainage despite renal and bladder catheter drainage. In these cases, the urinoma drainage tract can be dilated. An endoscope can be used to identify the point of communication with the renal collecting system (156). Biopsies may be taken of the cavity to rule out malignancy. If the point of communication is small and well away from the normal collecting system, the entire urinoma cavity and especially the base of the urinoma can be electrocoagulated with a roller electrode. If there is a larger communication, however, the urinoma cavity again can be electrocoagulated, following which a nephrostomy tube can be passed across the fistula and into the collecting system. The now dry cavity usually will collapse and seal around the shaft of the tube. In traumatic cases where there is devitalized tissue, an open surgical approach may be necessary for debridement and closure of the fistulous tract.

When the drainage has ceased, a sinogram is helpful to document collapse of the cavity. If there is still a large cavity, but drainage has stopped, and there is no demonstrable communication with the collecting system, ethanol sclerotherapy or repeat electrocoagulation can be used to facilitate collapse of the cavity.

Results

More than 90% of urinomas related to obstructive processes respond to drainage and correction of the underlying causes of obstruction. Ball and co-workers (18) found similar success in treating four pediatric patients with urinomas; all four patients responded well to percutaneous drainage of the urinoma. In urinomas resulting from trauma, success with percutaneous drainage is dependent on the viability of the tissue and the vascular supply near the fistulous tract. Cases in which there is a large amount of devitalized tissue, such as those associated with major trauma, may require open debridement and closure of the fistulous tract (248).

Lymphocele

For the urologist, a lymphocele occurs most commonly following pelvic lymphadenectomy, retroperitoneal lymph node dissection, or kidney transplantation. There is a 5% to 10% incidence of symptomatic lymphocele development following pelvic lymphadenectomy for malignancy (119). Khauli and colleagues (190) reported a 36% incidence of perirenal fluid collections following renal transplantation; among those patients, 7% had symptomatic lymphoceles that required intervention.

It is hypothesized that lymphoceles form when transected lymphatic channels are allowed to drain into a nonepithelialized space. Lymph fluid is devoid of platelets and has low concentrations of clotting factors; thus meticulous attention to ligation of the lymphatic vessels is necessary to prevent lymphocele formation. Perioperative heparin therapy, diuretic use, and high-dose corticosteroids also have been implicated as contributing factors to lymphocele formation (142,190).

The symptoms caused by a lymphocele result from compression of adjacent structures, lower-extremity edema, abdominal or pelvic mass, or bowel and bladder problems. In the transplant patient, the lymphocele may result in ureteral obstruction and a rise in serum creatinine. In the postpelvic lymph node dissection patient, the first sign of a pelvic lymphocele may be deep venous thrombosis and associated pulmonary embolus caused by partial obstruction of the external iliac vein by the lymphocele.

US is most commonly used to evaluate suspected pelvic fluid collections. In transplant patients, the US may reveal, in addition to the lymphocele, hydronephrosis or a mass effect on the bladder, colon, or iliac vessels. CT studies provide similar information.

Technique

The fluid collection is punctured under sonographic or CT guidance. The initial aspirate is sent for electrolytes, creatinine, cell count, and culture sensitivities. Additional studies that may be useful are determination of protein and cholesterol content along with cytologic analysis. The typical lymphocele fluid will have creatinine and electrolytes similar to serum, but the levels of cholesterol and protein are usually lower than serum values. Culture of the fluid should be sterile. Usually an 8- to 14-Fr drainage tube is left indwelling. When the drainage is less than 10 mL per 24 hours, the cavity is studied by contrast injection. If the cavity has collapsed around the drainage tube, the tube can be safely removed. If, despite 1 week of drainage, large amounts of fluid continue to be collected, sclerosis of the lymphocele may be attempted with 95% ethanol, povidone-iodine, tetracycline, or bleomycin (54,55,191,240). Sclerosis may be repeated, if necessary, at weekly intervals for several weeks. For patients with persistent or recurrent lymphoceles, laparoscopic intraperitonealization of the lymphocele is usually successful and has far less morbidity than an open approach (91,237,337).

Results

Small lymphoceles may not require treatment or may be managed by simple aspiration. Khauli and colleagues (190) reported an 86% spontaneous resolution rate in the management of asymptomatic posttransplant lymphoceles. For symptomatic lymphoceles, percutaneous drainage with or without sclerotherapy has a reported success rate of 69%; however, drainage may persist for up to 4 months following initial tube placement (55). For patients who fail percutaneous drainage and sclerosis and who have uninfected lymphoceles, the standard of care has been surgical exploration and intraperitoneal marsupialization with or without placement of a tag of omentum into the lymphocele cavity.

Laparoscopic intraperitonealization of the lymphocele has become popular (91,237,337). Fahlenkamp and associates (91) have reported the largest series to date with five patients all successfully treated by a laparoscopic peritoneal window procedure, although one patient required an additional percutaneous drainage of an undrained loculated portion of the lymphocele. The enthusiasm for this procedure must be tempered by the small series of patients and the potential complications of a laparoscopic procedure. One case of division of a transplant ureter during laparoscopic lymphocele drainage has been reported (334).

In some cases, the patient's anatomy precludes intraperitoneal marsupialization of the lymphocele. Lucas and colleagues (228) have reported the successful use of an internalized Tenckhoff catheter to drain posttransplant lymphoceles in three patients with a mean follow-up of 5.3 years. In a fourth patient, the Tenckhoff catheter became occluded. At reexploration the catheter was found to be encased in omentum. Three Tenckhoff catheters were placed in tandem, and the patient has done well during a 3-year follow-up period.

Another approach to the postpelvic lymph node dissection patient with an anatomically unfavorable (i.e., not amenable to a laparoscopic approach), unresponsive lymphocele is endoscopic fulguration. McDougall and Clayman (239) reported using this approach in a patient with a refractory lymphocele after a pelvic node dissection. With the patient under intravenous sedation, a short, rigid ureteroscope could be passed into the cavity and the base of the lymphocele could be electrocoagulated. The drainage tube was not replaced, and drainage rapidly ceased; it has not recurred.

CONCLUSIONS

With the passage of time, endourology has come to encompass a means of diagnosis and treatment for a whole host of maladies formerly approachable only by open surgery. In this regard, percutaneous and, more recently, ureteroscopic methods have prevailed, the latter being far less invasive than the former. The work that remains to be done is to further refine each of these techniques until its respective success rate routinely equals or exceeds the outcome of its open or laparoscopic surgical counterpart. To this end, the urologist and the bioengineer need to work hand in hand to develop and then critically test each new, less invasive treatment modality as it becomes available.

REFERENCES

1. Abdel-Hakim AM. Endopyelotomy for ureteropelvic junction obstruction: is long-term stenting mandatory? *J Endourol* 1987; 1:265.
2. Abdel-Razzak OM, Ehya H, Cubler-Goodman A, et al. Ureteroscopic biopsy in the upper urinary tract. *Urology* 1994; 44:451.
3. Abramowitz J, Fowler JE Jr, Falhuni K, et al. Percutaneous identification and removal of fungus ball from renal pelvis. *J Urol* 1986;135:1232.
4. Ahmad G, Segasothy M, Morad Z. Urinary erythrocyte morphology as a diagnostic aid in hematuria. *Singapore Med J* 1993;34:486.
5. Ahmadzadeh M. Use of a prototype 3-Fr needle electrode with flexible ureteroscopy of antegrade management of stenosed ureteroileal anastomosis. *Urol Int* 1992;49:215.
6. Aliabdi H, Reinberg Y, Gonzalez R. Percutaneous balloon dilation of ureteral strictures after failed surgical repair in children. *J Urol* 1990;144:486.
7. Amar AD, Das S. Upper urinary tract transitional cell carcinoma in patients with bladder carcinoma and associated vesicoureteral reflux. *J Urol* 1985;133:468.
8. Anderstrom C, Johansson SL, Pettersson S, et al. Carcinoma of the ureter: a clinicopathologic study of 49 cases. *J Urol* 1989; 142:280.
9. Andrews PE, Segura JW. Renal pelvic explosion during conservative management of upper tract urothelial cancer. *J Urol* 1991;146:407.
10. Badlani G, Eshghi M, Smith AD. Percutaneous surgery for ureteropelvic junction obstruction (endopyelotomy): technique and early results. *J Urol* 1986;135:26.
11. Bagley DH. Endoscopic ureteroureterostomy. *J Urol* 1990;143: 234A (abst 182).
12. Bagley DH. Intrarenal access with the flexible ureteropyeloscope: effects of active and passive tip deflection. *J Endourol* 1993;7:221.
13. Bagley DH, Allen J. Flexible ureteropyeloscopy in the diagnosis of benign essential hematuria. *J Urol* 1990;143:549.
14. Bagley DH, Huffman JL, Lyon ES. Flexible ureteropyeloscopy: diagnosis and treatment in the upper urinary tract. *J Urol* 1987;138:280.
15. Bagley DH, Liu J, Grasso M, et al. Endoluminal sonography in evaluation of the obstructed ureteropelvic junction. *J Endourol* 1994;8:287.
16. Bagley DH, Rivas D. Upper urinary tract filling defects: flexible ureteroscopic diagnosis. *J Urol* 1990;143:1196.
17. Bahnson RB. Silver nitrate irrigation for hematuria from sickle cell hemoglobinopathy. *J Urol* 1987;137:1194.
18. Ball WS, Towbin R, Strife JL, et al. Interventional genitourinary radiology in children: a review of 61 procedures. *AJR Am J Roentgenol* 1986;147:791.
19. Banner MP, Pollack HM. Dilatation of ureteral stenoses: techniques and experience in 44 patients. *AJR Am J Roentgenol* 1984;143:789.
20. Batata MA, Whitmore WF Jr, Hilaris BS, et al. Primary carcinoma of the ureter: a prognostic study. *Cancer* 1975;35:1626.
21. Bean WJ. Renal cysts: treatment with alcohol. *Radiology* 1981; 138:329.
22. Beckman CF, Roth RA. Secondary ureteropelvic junction stricture: percutaneous dilation. *Radiology* 1987;164:365.
23. Beckman CF, Roth RA, Bihrlie W III. Dilation of benign ureteral strictures. *Radiology* 1989;172:437.
24. Beckman CF, Roth RA, Bihrle W III. Retrograde balloon dilation for pelviureteric junction obstruction. *Br J Urol* 1993; 71:152.
25. Bellman GC, Brock WA, Smith AD. Endourologic management of obstructed hydrocalyx after blunt renal trauma. *Urology* 1994;43:546.
26. Bellman GC, Sweetser P, Smith AD. Complications of intracavitary bacillus Calmette-Guérin after percutaneous resection of upper tract transitional cell carcinoma. *J Urol* 1994;151:13.

27. Bennett JD, Brown TC, Kozak RI, et al. Transdiverticular percutaneous nephrostomy for caliceal diverticular stones. *J Endourol* 1992;6:55.
28. Bennett WM, Elzinga L, Golper TA, et al. Reduction of cyst volume for symptomatic management of autosomal dominant polycystic kidney disease. *J Urol* 1987;137:620.
29. Berger RE, Ansell JS, Tremann JA, et al. The use of self-retained ureteral stents in the management of urologic complications in renal transplant recipients. *J Urol* 1980;124:781.
30. Bloom NA, Vidone RA, Lytton B. Primary carcinoma of the ureter: a report of 102 new cases. *J Urol* 1970;103:590.
31. Blum JA. Acute monilial pyelohydronephrosis: report of a case successfully treated with amphotericin B continuous renal pelvis irrigation. *J Urol* 1966;96:614.

31a. Blute ML, Segura JW, Patterson DE, et al. Impact of endourology on diagnosis and management of upper urinary tract urothelial cancer. *J Urol* 1989;141(6):1298.

32. Bouchot O, Le Normand L, Couteau E, et al. The Whitaker test. Its reliability and place in the study of congenital malformative uropathies. *Ann Urol* 1989;23:58.
33. Brannen GE, Bush WH, Lewis GP. Endopyelotomy for primary repair of ureteropelvic junction obstruction. *J Urol* 1988; 139:29.
34. Bretland PM. The single compartment model applied to the large renal pelvis: a preliminary study. *Nucl Med Commun* 1992;13:106.
35. Brooks JD, Kavoussi LR, Preminger GM, et al. Comparison of open and endourologic approaches to the obstructed ureteropelvic junction. *J Urol* 1995;46:791.
36. Brosman SA, Lamm DL. The preparation, handling and use of intravesical bacillus Calmette-Guérin for the management of stage T_a, T_1 carcinoma *in situ* and transitional cell cancer. *J Urol* 1990;144:313.
37. Cassis AN, Brannen GE, Bush WH, et al. Endopyelotomy: review of results and complications. *J Urol* 1992;146:1492.
38. Chaiwatanarat T, Padhy AK, Bomanji JB, et al. Validation of renal output efficiency as an objective quantitative parameter in the evaluation of upper urinary tract obstruction. *J Nucl Med* 1993;34:845.
39. Chakroun M, Ladeb MF, Gharbi-Jemni H, et al. Non-surgical treatment of kidney abscesses. Apropos of 12 cases. *Ann Med Interne (Paris)* 1992;143:442.
40. Chandhoke PS, Clayman RV, Stone AM, et al. Endopyelotomy and endoureterotomy with the Acucise ureteral cutting balloon device: preliminary experience. *J Endourol* 1993;7:45.
41. Chang R, Marshall FF, Mitchell S. Percutaneous management of benign ureteral strictures and fistulas. *J Urol* 1987;137:1126.
42. Chehval MJ, Nepute JQ, Purcell MH. Nephroscopic obliteration of obstructing peripelvic renal cyst in conjunction with stone removal. *J Endourol* 1990;4:259.
43. Chow GK, Geisinger MA, Streem SB. Endopyelotomy outcome as a function of high versus dependent ureteral insertion. *Urology* 1999;54:999.
44. Chowdhury SD, Kenogbon J. Rigid ureteroscopic endopyelotomy without external drainage. *J Endourol* 1992;6:357.
45. Clark PE, Streem SB, Geisinger MA. 13-year experience with percutaneous management of upper tract transitional cell carcinoma. *J Urol* 1999;161:772.
46. Clark WR, Malik RS. Ureteropelvic junction obstruction: observations on the classic type in adults. *J Urol* 1987;138:276.
47. Clayman RV, Basler JW, Kavoussi L, et al. Ureteronephroscopic endopyelotomy. *J Urol* 1990;144:246.
48. Clayman RV, Castandea-Zuniga WR. Calyceal diverticulum. In: Clayman RV, Castandea-Zuniga WR, eds. *Techniques in endourology: a guide to the percutaneous removal of renal and ureteral calculi.* Dallas: Heritage Press, 1984.
49. Clayman RV, Denstedt JD. New technique: ureterorenoscopic urothelial endoureteroplasty: case report. *J Endourol* 1989; 3:425.
50. Clayman RV, Elbers J, Palmer JO, et al. Experimental extensive balloon dilatation of the distal ureter: immediate and long-term effects. *J Endourol* 1987;1:19.
51. Clayman RV, Lange PH, Fraley EE. Transitional cell cancer of the upper urinary tract. In: Javadpour N, ed. *Principles and management of urologic cancer,* ed 2. Baltimore: Williams & Wilkins, 1983.
52. Clayman RV, Stone AM, Chandhoke PS, et al. Endourological treatment of upper urinary tract obstruction with the Acucise catheter: an effective, less invasive approach. *J Urol* 1992;147: 471A.
53. Clayman RV, Surya V, Miller RP, et al. Pursuit of the renal mass: is ultrasound enough? *Am J Med* 1984;77:218.
54. Cohan RH, Saeed M, Schwab SJ, et al. Povidone-iodine sclerosis of pelvic lymphoceles: a prospective study. *Urol Radiol* 1988;10:203.
55. Cohan RH, Saeed M, Sussman SK, et al. Percutaneous drainage of pelvic lymphatic fluid collections in the renal transplant patients. *Invest Radiol* 1987;11:864.
56. Cohen TD, Gross MB, Preminger GM. Long-term follow-up of Acucise incision of ureteropelvic junction obstruction and ureteral strictures. *Urology* 1996;47:317.
57. Conrad S, Schneider AW, Tenschert W, et al. Endo-urological cold-knife incision for ureteral stenosis after renal transplantation. *J Urol* 1994;105:906.
58. Conway JJ. Well-tempered diuresis renography: its historical development, physiological and technical pitfalls, and standardized technique protocol. *Semin Nucl Med* 1992;22:74.
59. Cornud F, Mendelsberg M, Chretian Y, et al. Fluoroscopically guided percutaneous transrenal electroincision of ureterointestinal anastomotic strictures. *J Urol* 1992;147:578.
60. Cronan JJ, Armiag ES Jr, Dorfman GS. Percutaneous drainage of renal abscesses. *Am J Radiol* 1984;142:351.
61. Cubelli V, Smith AD. Transurethral ureteral surgery guided by fluoroscopy. *Endourology* 1987;2:8.
62. Cussenot O, Bassi S, Desgrandchamps F, et al. Outcomes of non–self-expandable metal prosthesis in strictured human ureter: suggestions for future developments. *J Endourol* 1993; 7:250.
63. Cuzin B, Abbar M, Dawahra M, et al. 100 percutaneous endopyelotomies. Technique, indications, results. *Prog Urol* 1992;2:409.
64. Dalton D, Neiman H, Grayhack JT. The natural history of simple renal cysts: a preliminary study. *J Urol* 1986;135:905.
65. Damico CF, Mebust WK, Valk WL, et al. Triamcinolone: adjuvant therapy for vesical neck contractures. *J Urol* 1973; 110:203.
66. Danuser H, Ackermann DK, Bohlen D, et al. Endopyelotomy for primary ureteropelvic junction obstruction: risk factors determine the success rate. *J Urol* 1998;159:56.
67. Davis DM. Intubated ureterotomy: a new operation for ureteral and ureteropelvic strictures. *Surg Gynecol Obstet* 1943;76:513.
68. Davis DM, Strong GH, Drake WM. Intubated ureterotomy: experimental work and clinical results. *J Urol* 1948;59:851.
69. de Kock MLS, Breytenbach IH. Local excision and topical thiotepa in the treatment of transitional cell carcinoma of the renal pelvis: a case report. *J Urol* 1986;136:461.
70. Dembner AG, Pfister RC. Fungal infection of the urinary tract: demonstration by antegrade pyelography and drainage by percutaneous nephrostomy. *AJR Am J Roentgenol* 1977;129:415.
71. Denovic M, Darzynkiewicz A, Kostryrka-Claps ML, et al. Flow cytometry of low stage bladder tumors. *Cancer* 1982;48:109.

72. Dervanian P, Castaigne D, Travagli JP, et al. Arterioureteral fistula after extended resection of pelvic tumors: report of three cases and review of the literature. *Ann Vasc Surg* 1992;6:362.
73. de Torres JA, Banus JM, Palou J, et al. Vesicorenal reflux and upper urinary tract transitional cell carcinoma after transurethral resection of recurrent superficial bladder carcinoma. *J Urol* 1987;138:49.
74. de Vries A. Clinical management of uric acid lithiasis. In: Roth RA, Finlayson B, eds. *Stones: clinical management of urolithiasis.* Baltimore: Williams & Wilkins, 1983.
75. Dierks SM, Clayman RV, Kavoussi LR, et al. Intraureteral surgery: appropriate cutting modality. *J Endourol* 1990;4:S114.
76. Doemeny JM, Banner MP, Shapiro MJ, et al. Percutaneous extraction of renal fungus ball. *Am J Radiol* 1988;150:1331.
77. Dourmashkin RL. Dilation of ureter with rubber bags in treatment of ureteral calculi: presentation of modified operating cystoscope; preliminary report. *J Urol* 1926;15:449.
78. Dourmashkin RL. Cystoscopic treatment of stones in the ureter. *J Urol* 1945;54:245.
79. Dowd PE, Mata JA, Arden C, et al. Ultrasound guided percutaneous renal biopsy using an automatic core biopsy system. *J Urol* 1991;146:1216.
80. Dowling RA, Corriere JN Jr, Sandler DM. Iatrogenic ureteral injury. *J Urol* 1986;135:912.
81. Doyle AJ, Gregory MC, Terreros DA. Percutaneous native renal biopsy: comparison of a 1.2 mm spring-driven system with a traditional 2 mm hand-driven system. *Am J Kidney Dis* 1994;23:498.
82. Dretler SP, Young RH. Stone granuloma: a cause of ureteral stricture. *J Urol* 1993;150:1800.
83. Eastham JA, Huffman JL. Technique of mitomycin C instillation in the treatment of upper urinary tract urothelial tumors. *J Urol* 1993;150(2 Pt 1):324.
84. Edelstein H, McCabe RE. Perinephric abscess. *Medicine* 1988; 67:118.
85. Eickenberg HU. Percutaneous surgery of renal cysts. *J Urol* 1985;133:200A.
86. Elliott DS, Blute ML, Patterson DE, et al. Long-term follow-up of endoscopically treated upper urinary tract transitional cell carcinoma. *Urology* 1996;47:819.
87. Elyaderani MK, Moncman J. Value of ultrasonography, fine-needle aspiration, and percutaneous drainage of perinephric abscess. *South Med J* 1985;78:685.
88. Eshghi M. Endoscopic incisions of the urinary tract. *AUA Update Series,* vol 8. Lessons 37 to 39, 1989.
89. Eshghi M, Tuong W, Fernandez R, et al. Percutaneous (endo) infundibulotomy. *J Endourol* 1987;1:107.
90. Faeber GJ, Richardson TD, Farah N et al. Retrograde treatment of ureteropelvic junction obstruction using the ureteral cutting balloon catheter. *J Urol* 1997;157:454.
91. Fahlenkamp D, Raatz D, Schonberger B, et al. Laparoscopic lymphocele drainage after renal transplantation. *J Urol* 1993; 150:316.
92. Farah RN, DiLoreta RR, Cerny JC. Transurethral resection combined with steroid injection in treatment of recurrent vesical neck contractures. *Urology* 1979;13:395.
93. Farah NB, Roddie M, Lord RHH, et al. Ureteric obstruction in renal transplants: the role of percutaneous balloon dilatation. *Nephrol Dial Transplant* 1991;6:977.
94. Figenshau RS, Clayman RV, Colberg JW, et al. Pediatric endopyelotomy: the Washington University experience. *J Urol* 1996;156:2025.
95. Figenshau RS, Clayman RV, Wick MR, et al. Acute histologic changes associated with endoureterotomy in the normal pig ureter. *J Endourol* 1991;5:357.
96. Fowler JE Jr, Perkins T. Presentation, diagnosis and treatment of renal abscesses: 1972–1988. *J Urol* 1994;151:847.
97. Fraley EE. Dismembered infundibulopyelostomy: improved technique for correcting vascular obstruction of the superior infundibulum. *J Urol* 1969;101:144.
98. Fuchs GJ, David RD. Flexible ureterorenoscopy, dilation of narrow caliceal neck, and ESWL. a new, minimally invasive approach to stones in caliceal diverticula. *J Endourol* 1989;3:255.
99. Gaboardi F, Bozzola A, Dotti E, et al. Conservative treatment of upper urinary tract tumors with Nd:YAG laser. *J Endourol* 1994;8:37.
100. Gallucci M, Alpi G. Antegrade transpelvic endopyelotomy in primary obstruction of the ureteropelvic junction. *J Endourol* 1996;10:127.
101. Garcia RL, Pontones J, Boronat F, et al. Extracorporeal shock-wave lithotripsy: an alternative treatment for lithiasis of caliceal diverticula. *Actas Urol Esp* 1992;16:467.
102. Gardiner RA, Weedon D, Sing J, et al. Replacement of ureteric segments by intubated neoureterotomies (modified Davis technique) using autologous bladder and omentum in dogs. *Br J Urol* 1984;56:354.
103. Gaylord GM, Johnsrude IS. Transrenal ureteral occlusion with Gianturco coils and gelatin sponge. *Radiology* 1989;172:1047.
104. Gelabert Mas A, Arango O, Bielsa O, et al. Percutaneous drainage of renal and perirenal abscesses. *Actas Urol Esp* 1992; 16:513.
105. Gelet A, Lopez JG, Cuzin B, et al. Endopyelotomy with the Acucise balloon device: preliminary results. XI Congress of the European Association of Urology, Berlin, abstract 59, p 31, July 13–16, 1994.
106. Gelet GS, Lopez JG, Cuzin B, et al. Long-term efficacy of percutaneous endopyelotomy. XI Congress of the European Association of Urology, Berlin, abstract 60, p 36, July 13–16, 1994.
107. Gelet A, Martin X, Dessouki T. Ureteropelvic invagination: reliable technique of endopyelotomy. *J Endourol* 1991;5:223.
107a. Gerber GS, Kim JC. Ureteroscopic endopyelotomy in the treatment of patients with ureteropelvic junction obstruction. *Urology* 55:198, 2000.
107b. Gerber GS, Alsikafi NF. Retrograde ureteroscopic incision for the treatment of nonureteroenteric ureteral strictures. *Tech Urol* 2000;6(1):12.
108. Gerber GS, Lyon ES. Endourological management of upper tract urothelial tumors. *J Urol* 1993;150:2.
109. Germinale F, Bottino P, Caviglia C, et al. Endourologic treatment of ureterointestinal strictures. *J Endourol* 1992;6:439.
110. Gerzof SG, Gale ME. Computed tomography and ultrasonography for diagnosis and treatment of renal and retroperitoneal abscesses. *Urol Clin North Am* 1982;9:185.
111. Gerzof SC, Johnson WC, Robbins AH, et al. Expanded criteria for percutaneous abscess drainage. *Arch Surg* 1985;120:227.
112. Gibbons RP, Bush WH Jr, Burnett LL. Needle tract seeding following aspiration of renal cell carcinoma. *J Urol* 1977; 118:865.
113. Gilbert R, Garra B, Gibbons MD. Renal duplex Doppler ultrasound: an adjunct in the evaluation of hydronephrosis in the child. *J Urol* 1993;150:1192.
114. Gittes RF. Management of transitional cell carcinoma of the upper tract: case for conservative local excision. *Urol Clin North Am* 1980;7:559.
115. Gittes RF, Varady S. Nephroscopy in chronic unilateral hematuria. *J Urol* 1981;126:297.
116. Glinz M, Ackermann D, Zingg EJ. The balloon-catheter Acucise: an important instrument for endoureterotomy. XI Congress of the European Association of Urology, Berlin, abstract 62, p 32, July 13–16, 1994.

117. Glinz M, Merz V, Ackermann D, Zingg EJ. Impact of the pelvicaliceal size on the success rate of endopyelotomy. XI Congress of the European Association of Urology, Berlin, abstract 63, p 33, July 13–16, 1994.
118. Gluckman GR, Stoller M, Irby P. Laparoscopic pyelocaliceal diverticula ablation. *J Endourol* 1993;7:315.
119. Goh M, Kantoff P, Kavoussi LR. Retroperitoneal lymphocele formation after selective laparoscopic retroperitoneal lymph node sampling. *J Urol* 1994;151:1626.
120. Grantham JJ. 1992 Homer Smith Award. Fluid secretion, cellular proliferation and the pathogenesis of renal epithelial cysts. *J Am Soc Nephrol* 1993;3:1841.
121. Grasso M, Bagley D. Small diameter, actively deflectable, flexible ureteroscopy. *J Urol* 1998;160:1648.
122. Grasso M, Fraiman M, Levine M. Ureteropyeloscopic diagnosis and treatment of upper urinary tract urothelial malignancies. *Urology* 1999;54:240.
123. Grasso M, McCue P, Bagley DH. Multiple urothelial recurrences of renal cell carcinoma after initial diagnostic flexible ureteroscopy. *J Urol* 1992;147:1358.
124. Greenberg R, Coleman JW, Quiguyan CC, et al. Bladder mucosal grafts: experimental use as a ureteral substitute and observation of certain physical properties. *J Urol* 1983;129:634.
125. Grossman HB, Schwartz SL, Konnak JW. Ureteroscopic treatment of urothelial carcinoma of the ureter and renal pelvis. *J Urol* 1992;148:275.
126. Gruntzig A. Transluminal dilatation of coronary artery stenosis [Letter]. *Lancet* 1978;1:263.
127. Guder WG, Hofmann W. Differentiation of proteinuria and haematuria by single protein analysis in urine. *Clin Biochem* 1993;26:277.
128. Guiliani L, Giberti C, Martovana G, et al. Results of radical cystectomy for primary bladder cancer: a retrospective study of more than two thousand cases. *Urology* 1985;26:243.
129. Gunther R, Klose K, Alken P. Transrenal ureteral occlusion with a detachable balloon. *Radiology* 1982;142:521.
130. Gunther R, Marberger M, Klose K. Transrenal ureteral embolization. *Diagn Radiol* 1979;132:317.
131. Gupta M, Smith AD. Crossing vessels at the ureteropelvic junction: do they influence endopyelotomy outcome? *J Urol* 1996;10:183.
132. Gupta M, Tuncay OL, Smith AD. Open surgical exploration after failed endopyelotomy: a 12 year perspective. *J Urol* 1997; 157:1613.
133. Guthman DA, Malek RS, Neves RJ, et al. Vesicoureteral reflux in the adult. V. Unilateral disease. *J Urol* 1991;146:21.
134. Haaga JR. Imaging intraabdominal abscesses and nonoperative drainage procedures. *World J Surg* 1990;14:204.
135. Hamm FC, Weinberg SR. Renal and ureteral surgery without intubation. *J Urol* 1955;73:475.
136. Hamm FC, Weinberg SR. Experimental studies of regeneration of the ureter without intubation. *J Urol* 1956;75:43.
137. Harrach LB, Burkholder GV, Goodwin WE. Renal candidiasis—a cause of anuria. *Br J Urol* 1970;42:258.
138. Heiken JP, Brink JA, Vannier MW. Spiral (helical) CT. *Radiology* 1993;189:647.
139. Hendren WH, Reda EF. Bladder mucosa graft for construction of male urethra. *J Pediatr Surg* 1986;21:189.
140. Heney NM, Nocks BH, Daly JJ, et al. Prognostic factors in carcinoma of the ureter. *J Urol* 1981;125:632.
141. Herr HW. Durable response of a carcinoma *in situ* of the renal pelvis to topical bacillus Calmette-Guérin. *J Urol* 1985; 134:531.
142. Heyman JH, Orron DE, Leiter E. Percutaneous management of postoperative lymphocele. *Urology* 1989;34:221.
143. Hobarth K, Hofbauer J, Marberger M. Interventional endourologic procedures after renal transplantation. *J Endourol* 1992;6:341.
144. Holmberg G, Hietala SO. Treatment of simple renal cysts by percutaneous puncture and instillation of bismuth phosphate. *Scand J Urol Nephrol* 1989;23:207.
145. Horgan JD, Maidenberg MJ, Smith AD. Endopyelotomy in the elderly. *J Urol* 1993;150:1107.
146. Hovnanian AP, Javadpour H, Gruhn JG. Reconstruction of the ureter by free autologous bladder mucosa graft. *J Urol* 1965;93:455.
147. Huang A, Low RK, White RD. Nephrostomy tract tumor seeding following percutaneous manipulation of a ureteral carcinoma. *J Urol* 1995;153:1041.
148. Hubner W, Pfab R, Porpaczy P et al. Renal cysts: percutaneous resection with standard urologic instruments. *J Endourol* 1990;4:61.
149. Huffman JL. Ureteroscopic management of transitional cell carcinoma of the upper urinary tract. *Urol Clin North Am* 1988;3:419.
150. Huffman JL. Endoscopic management of upper urinary tract urothelial cancer. *J Endourol* 1990;4:S141.
151. Huffman JL, Bagley DH, Lyon ES, et al. Endoscopic diagnosis and treatment of upper tract urothelial tumors. A preliminary report. *Cancer* 1985;55:1422.
152. Huffman JL, Morse MJ, Herr HW, et al. Ureteropyeloscopy: the diagnosis and therapeutic approach to upper tract urothelial tumors. *World J Urol* 1985;3:58.
153. Huffman JL, Morse MJ, Herr HW et al. Consideration for treatment of upper urinary tract tumors without topical therapy. *Urology* 1985;26:47.
154. Hulbert JC, Hernandez-Graulau JM, Hunter DW et al. Current concepts in the management of pyelocaliceal diverticula. *J Endourol* 1988;2:11.
155. Hulbert JC, Hunter D, Castaneda-Zuniga WR. Classification of and techniques for the reconstitution of acquired strictures in the region of the ureteropelvic junction. *J Urol* 1988;140:468.
156. Hulbert JC, Hunter D, Young AT, et al. Percutaneous intrarenal marsupialization of a perirenal cystic collection—endocystolysis. *J Urol* 1988;139:1039.
157. Hulbert JC, Lapointe S, Reddy PK, et al. Percutaneous endoscopic fulguration of a large volume caliceal diverticulum. *J Urol* 1987;138:116.
158. Hulbert JC, Reddy PK, Hunter DW, et al. Percutaneous techniques for the management of caliceal diverticula containing calculi. *J Urol* 1986;135:225.
159. Hwang T, Park Y. Endoscopic infundibulotomy in tuberculous renal infundibular stricture. *J Urol* 1994;151:852.
160. Inglis JA, Tolley DA. Ureteroscopic pyelolysis for pelviureteric junction obstruction. *Br J Urol* 1986;58:250.
161. Inglis JA, Tolley DA. Conservative management of transitional cell carcinoma of the renal pelvis. *J Endourol* 1988;2:27.
162. Irby PB, Stoller ML, McAninch JW. Fungal bezoars of the upper urinary tract. *J Urol* 1990;143:447.
163. Ireton RC, Krieger JN, Rudd TG, et al. Percutaneous endoscopic treatment of fungus ball obstruction in a renal allograft. *Transplantation* 1985;39:453.
164. Irving HC, Kashi SH. Complications of renal transplantation and the role of interventional radiology. *J Clin Ultrasound* 1992;20:545.
165. Janetschek G. Percutaneous intrarenal surgery for calyceal stones, infundibular stenosis, calyceal diverticula, and obstruction of the ureteropelvic junction. *J Urol* 1988;139:187A.
166. Janetschek G, Girstmair J, Semenitz E. Percutaneous drainage of computed infections of the upper urinary tract. *Wien Med Wochenschr* 1991;141:556.

167. Jaques P, Mauro M, Safrit H, et al. CT features of intraabdominal abscesses. *AJR Am J Roentgenol* 1986;146:1041.
168. Jarrett TW, Sweetser PM, Weiss GH, et al. Percutaneous management of transitional cell carcinoma of the renal collecting system: a 9-year experience. *J Urol* 1995;154:1629.
169. Jemni M, Jemni-Gharbi H, Zorgui A, et al. Renal and perirenal abscess and urinary tract obstruction caused by *Torulopsis glabrata* infection. *J Urol (Paris)* 1992;98:50.
170. Johnson DC, Oke EJ, Dunnick RN. Percutaneous balloon dilation of ureteral strictures. *AJR Am J Roentgenol* 1987; 148:181.
171. Jones JA, Lingeman JE, Steidle CP. The roles of extracorporeal shock wave lithotripsy and percutaneous nephrostolithotomy in the management of pyelocaliceal diverticula. *J Urol* 1991; 146:724.
172. Jones JW, Hunter DW, Matas AJ. Percutaneous treatment of ureteral strictures after renal transplantation. *Transplantation* 1991;55:1193.
173. Kadir S, White RI Jr, Engel R. Balloon dilatation of a ureteropelvic junction obstruction. *Radiology* 1982;143:263.
174. Kaneti J, Hertzanu Y. Renal abscess owing to *Salmonella* septicemia: percutaneous drainage. *J Urol* 1987;138:395.
175. Karlin GS, Rich M, Lee W, et al. Endourological management of upper-tract fungal infection. *J Endourol* 1987;1:49.
176. Karlin GS, Smith AD. Endopyelotomy. *Urol Clin North Am* 1988;15:433.
177. Kashi SH, Irving HC, Sadek SA. Does the Whitaker test add to antegrade pyelography in the investigation of collecting system dilatation in renal allografts? *Br J Radiol* 1993;66:877.
178. Kashi SH, Lodge JPA, Giles GR, et al. Ureteric complications of renal transplantation. *Br J Urol* 1992;70:139.
179. Kavoussi LR. Urothelial substitutes: ureter. *J Endourol* 1993; 17:419.
180. Kavoussi LR, Albala DM, Clayman RV. Outcome of secondary open surgical procedure in patients who failed primary endopyelotomy. *Br J Urol* 1993;72:157.
181. Kavoussi LR, Clayman RV, Basler J. Flexible actively deflectable fiberoptic ureteronephroscopy. *J Urol* 1989;142:949.
182. Kavoussi LR, Clayman RV, Mikkelsen DJ, et al. Ureteronephroscopic marsupialization of obstructing peripelvic renal cyst. *J Urol* 1991;146:411.
183. Kavoussi LR, Dierks S, Clayman R. Endoureterotomy: ureteronephroscopic treatment of ureteral strictures. *J Endourol* 1990; 4:S113.
184. Kavoussi LR, Meretyk S, Dierks SM, et al. Endopyelotomy for secondary ureteropelvic junction obstruction in children. *J Urol* 1991;145:345.
185. Keeley FX, Bibbo M, Bagley DH. Ureteroscopic treatment and surveillance of upper urinary tract transitional cell carcinoma. *J Urol* 1997;157:1560.
186. Keeley FX, Kulp DA, Bibbo M, et al. Diagnostic accuracy of ureteroscopic biopsy in upper tract transitional cell carcinoma. *J Urol* 1997;157:33.
187. Kerbl K, Chandhoke PS, Figenshau RS, et al. Effect of stent duration on ureteral healing following endoureterotomy in an animal model. *J Urol* 1993;150:1302.
188. Kerbl K, Clayman RV. Incision of the ureterovesical junction for endoscopic surveillance of transitional cell cancer of the upper urinary tract. *J Urol* 1993;150:1440.
189. Khan AM, Holman E, Pasztor I, et al. Endopyelotomy: experience with 320 cases. *J Endourol* 1997;11:243.
190. Khauli RB, Stoff JS, Lovewell T, et al. Post-transplant lymphoceles: a critical look into the risk factors, pathophysiology and management. *J Urol* 1993;150:22.
191. Khorram O, Stern JL. Bleomycin sclerotherapy of an intractable inguinal lymphocyst. *Gynecol Oncol* 1993;50:244.
192. Kim J, Banner MP, Ramchandani P, et al. Balloon dilation of ureteral strictures after renal transplantation. *Radiology* 1993; 186:717.
193. Kim SH, Yoon HK, Park JH, et al. Tuberculous stricture of the urinary tract: antegrade balloon dilation and ureteral stenting. *Abdom Imaging* 1993;18:186.
194. Kinn AC, Ohlsen H, Brehmer-Andersson E, et al. Therapeutic ureteral occlusion. *J Urol* 1986;135:29.
195. Kinnaert P, Hall M, Janssen F, et al. Ureteral stenosis after kidney transplantation: true incidence and long-term followup after surgical correction. *J Urol* 1985;133:17.
196. Kitamoto Y, Tomita M, Akamine M, et al. Differentiation of hematuria using a uniquely shaped red cell. *Nephron* 1993; 64:32.
197. Kletscher BA, Segura JW, LeRoy AJ, et al. Percutaneous antegrade endopyelotomy: review of 50 consecutive cases. *J Urol* 1995;153:701.
198. Koonings PP, Huffman JL, Schlaerth JB. Ureteroscopy: a new asset in the management of postoperative ureterovaginal fistulas. *Obstet Gynecol* 1992;80:548.
199. Korth K. Further indications for the percutaneous surgical technique on the kidney: percutaneous intrarenal marsupialization of renal cysts. In: Korth K, ed. *Percutaneous surgery of renal stones: techniques and tactics.* New York: Springer-Verlag, 1984.
200. Korth K, Kuenkel J. Unusual applications of ureteroscopy. *Urol Clin North Am* 1988;15:459.
201. Korth K, Kuenkel M, Karsch J. Percutaneous endopyelotomy and results: Korth technique. *J Endourol* 1996;10:121.
202. Kramolowsky EV, Clayman RV, Weyman PJ. Management of ureterointestinal anastomotic strictures: comparison of open surgical and endourological repair. *J Urol* 1988;139:1195.
203. Kramolowsky EV, Tucker RD, Nelson CMK. Management of benign ureteral strictures: open surgical repair or endoscopic dilation? *J Urol* 1989;141:285.
204. Krestin GP. Magnetic resonance imaging of the kidneys: current status. *Magn Reson Q* 1994;10:12.
205. Krogh J, Kvist E, Rye B. Transitional cell carcinoma of the upper urinary tract: prognostic variables and post-operative recurrences. *Br J Urol* 1991;67:32.
206. Krueger RP, Ash JM, Silver MM, et al. Primary hydronephrosis. Assessment of diuretic renography, pelvis perfusion pressure, operative findings, and renal and ureteral histology. *Urol Clin North Am* 1980;7:231.
207. Kuenkel M, Korth K. Endopyelotomy: results after long-term follow-up of 135 patients. *J Endourol* 1990;4:109.
208. Kulp DA, Bagley DH. Does flexible ureteropyeloscopy promote local recurrence of transitional cell carcinoma? *J Endourol* 1994;8:111.
209. Kumar R, Kapoor R, Mandhani A, et al. Optimum duration of splinting after endopyelotomy. *J Endourol* 1999;13:89.
210. Kumon H, Tsugawa M, Matumura Y, et al. Endoscopic diagnosis and treatment of chronic unilateral hematuria of uncertain etiology. *J Urol* 1990;143:554.
211. Lagha K, Martin X, Cuzin B, et al. Treatment of intradiverticular lithiasis by percutaneous methods. *Prog Urol* 1993;3:959.
212. Lang EK. Diagnosis and management of ureteral fistulas by percutaneous nephrostomy and antegrade stent catheter. *Radiology* 1981;138:311.
213. Lang EK. Renal, perirenal, and pararenal abscesses: percutaneous drainage. *Radiology* 1990;174:109.
214. Lang EK. Percutaneous infundibuloplasty: management of calyceal diverticula and infundibular stenosis. *Radiology* 1991; 181:871.

215. Lang EK, Glorioso LW II. Management of urinomas by percutaneous drainage procedures. *Radiol Clin North Am* 1986; 24:551.
216. Lang EK, Glorioso LW II. Antegrade transluminal dilation of benign ureteral strictures: long-term results. *AJR Am J Roentgenol* 1988;150:131.
217. Laucks SP Jr, McLachlan MSF. Aging and simple cysts of the kidney. *Br J Radiol* 1981;54:12.
218. Lagha K, Martin X, Cuzin B, et al. Treatment of intradiverticular lithiasis by percutaneous methods (19 caliceal diverticuli). *Prog Urol* 1993;3:959.
219. Leal JJ. A new procedure for biopsy of a solid renal mass: transurethral approach under fluoroscopic control. *J Urol* 1992; 148:98.
220. Lechevallier E, Eghazarian C, Ortega JC, et al. Retrograde Acucise endopyelotomy: long-term results. *J Endourol* 1999; 13:575.
221. Lee BR, Jabbour ME, Marshall FF, et al. 13-year survival comparison of percutaneous and open nephroureterectomy approaches for management of transitional cell carcinoma of renal collecting system: equivalent outcomes. *J Endourol* 1999; 13:289.
222. Levine SR, Emmett JL, Woolner LB. Cyst and tumor occurring in the same kidney (discussion). *Trans Am Assoc Genitourin Surg* 1963;55:126.
223. Lim DJ, Shattuck MC, Cook WA. Pyelovenous lymphatic migration of transitional cell carcinoma following ureterorenoscopy. *J Urol* 1993;149:109.
224. Lin DW, Bush WH, Mayo ME. Endourological treatment of ureteroenteric strictures: efficacy of Acucise endoureterotomy. *J Urol* 1999;162:696.
225. Lingeman JE, Siegel YI, Newman DM. Endopyelotomy for primary UPJ obstruction in the pediatric population. *J Urol* 1993;149:423A.
226. Lopez-Martinez RA, Singireddy S, Lang EK. The use of metallic stents to bypass ureteral strictures secondary to metastatic prostate cancer: experience with 8 patients. *J Urol* 1997;158:50.
227. Lossemore TM, Woodhouse CR, Shearer RJ. Role of ultrasound in the investigation of haematuria after normal intravenous urography and cystoscopy. *Eur Urol* 1991;19:6.
228. Lucas BA, Gill IS, Munch LC. Intraperitoneal drainage of recurrent lymphoceles using an internalized Tenkhoff catheter. *J Urol* 1994;151:970.
229. Lyon ES, Banno JJ, Schoenberg HW. Transurethral ureteroscopy in man using juvenile cystoscopy equipment. *J Urol* 1979;122:152.
230. Mahoney SA, Koletsky S, Persky L. Approximation and dilatation: the mode of healing of an intubated ureterostomy. *J Urol* 1962;88:197.
231. Maizels M, Firlit CF, Conway JJ, et al. Troubleshooting the diuretic renogram. *Urology* 1986;28:355.
232. Malden ES, Picus D, Clayman RV. Arteriovenous fistula complicating endopyelotomy. *J Urol* 1992;148:1520.
233. Martinez-Pineiro JA, Matres MJG, Martinez-Piniero L. Endourological treatment of upper tract urothelial carcinomas: analysis of a series of 59 tumors. *J Urol* 1996;156:377.
234. Mazeman E. Tumors of the upper urinary tract calyces, renal pelvis and ureter. *Eur Urol* 1976;2:120.
235. McCarthy CS, Sarker SD, Izquierdo G, et al. Pitfalls and limitations of diuretic renography. *Abdom Imaging* 1994;19:78.
236. Reference deleted in proofs.
237. McCullough CS, Soper NJ, Clayman RV, et al. Laparoscopic drainage of a posttransplant lymphocele. *Transplantation* 1991; 51:725.
238. McDonald JH, Calams JA. Experimental ureteral stricture: ureteral regrowth following ureterotomy with and without intubation. *J Urol* 1960;84:52.
239. McDougall EM, Clayman RV. Endoscopic management of persistent lymphocele following laparoscopic pelvic lymphadenectomy. *Urology* 1994;43:404.
240. McDowell GC, Babaian RJ, Johnson DE. Management of symptomatic lymphocele via percutaneous drainage and sclerotherapy with tetracycline. *Urology* 1991;37:237.
241. McMurtry JM, Clayman RV, Preminger GM. Endourologic diagnosis and treatment of essential hematuria. *J Endourol* 1987;1:145.
242. Melamed MR. Flow cytometry of the urinary bladder. *Urol Clin North Am* 1984;11:599.
243. Meretyk S, Albala DM, Clayman RV, et al. Endoureterotomy for treatment of ureteral strictures. *J Urol* 1992;147:1502.
244. Meretyk S, Clayman RV, Kavoussi LR, et al. Endourological treatment of ureteroenteric anastomotic strictures: long-term follow-up. *J Urol* 1991;145:723.
245. Meretyk I, Meretyk S, Clayman R. Endopyelotomy: comparison of ureteroscopic retrograde and antegrade percutaneous techniques. *J Urol* 1992;148:775.
246. Mikkelsen DJ, Kavoussi LR, Clayman RV, et al. Advances in flexible deflectable ureteronephroscopy (FDU): intrarenal surgery. *J Urol* 1989;141:192A.
247. Moon YT, Kerbl K, Gardner SM, et al. Evaluation of optimal stent size after endourologic incision of ureteral strictures. *J Urol* 1994;151:338A(abst 422).
248. Morano JU, Burkhalter JL. Percutaneous catheter drainage of post-traumatic urinoma. *J Urol* 1985;134:319.
249. Morris H. *Surgical diseases of the kidney and ureter.* London: Cassell, 1901.
250. Motola JA, Badlani GH, Smith AD. Endopyelotomy: long-term follow-up of 156 cases. *J Endourol* 1990;4:S139.
251. Motola JA, Badlani GH, Smith AD. Results of 212 consecutive endopyelotomies: an 8-year follow-up. *J Urol* 1993;149:453.
252. Motola JA, Fried R, Badlani GH, et al. Failed endopyelotomy: implications for future surgery on the ureteropelvic junction. *J Urol* 1993;150:821.
253. Muench PJ, Cates HB, Raney AM, et al. Endoscopic management of the obliterated ureteroileal anastomosis. *J Urol* 1987; 137:277.
254. Mukamel E, Nissenkorn I, Glanz I, et al. Upper tract tumors in patients with vesicoureteral reflux and recurrent bladder tumors. *Eur Urol* 1985;11:6.
255. Mukamel E, Vilkovsky E, Hadar H, et al. The effect of intravesical bacillus Calmette-Guérin therapy on the upper urinary tract. *J Urol* 1991;146:980.
256. Murphy DM, Zincke H, Furlow WL. Primary grade 1 transitional cell carcinoma of the renal pelvis and ureter. *J Urol* 1980;123:629.
257. Murphy LJT. The kidney. In: *The history of urology.* Springfield, Ill: Charles C. Thomas, 1972.
258. Nadler RB, Rao GS, Pearle MS, et al. Acucise endopyelotomy: assessment of long-term durability. *J Urol* 1996;156:1094.
259. Nakada SY, Elashry OM, Picus D, et al. Long-term outcome using flexible ureterorenoscopy in the diagnosis and management of lateralizing essential hematuria. *J Urol* 1997;157:776.
260. Nakada SY, Wolf JS, Brink JA, et al. Retrospective analysis of the effect of crossing vessels on successful retrograde endopyelotomy outcomes using spiral computerized tomography angiography. *J Urol* 1998;159:62.

261. Netto NR Jr, Ferreira U, Lemos GC, et al. Endourological management of ureteral strictures. *J Urol* 1990;144:631.
262. Newhouse JH, Pfister RC, Hendren WH, et al. Whitaker test after pyeloplasty: establishment of normal ureteral perfusion pressures. *Am J Radiol* 1981;137:223.
263. Nissenkorn I, Gdor Y. Nephrovesical subcutaneous stent: an alternative to permanent nephrostomy. *J Urol* 2000;163:528.
264. Nitze M. *Lehrbuch der Kystoscopie.* Wiesbaden, 1907:410.
265. Nolan RL, Nickel JC, Froud PJ. Percutaneous endourologic approach for transitional cell carcinoma of the renal pelvis. *Urol Radiol* 1988;9:217.
266. Nurse DE, Woodhouse CRJ, Kellett MJ, et al. Percutaneous removal of upper tract tumors. *World J Urol* 1989;7:131.
267. Oakley N, Raza A, Haq AU, et al. Endoburst: simple and safe is best. *J Endourol* 1998;12:423.
268. O'Brien WM, Maxted WC, Pahira JJ. Ureteral stricture: experience with 31 cases. *J Urol* 1988;140:737.
269. Oesterling JE, Fishman EK, Goldman SM, et al. The management of renal angiomyolipomas. *J Urol* 1986;135:1121.
270. Offringa M, Benbassat J. The value of urinary red cell shape in the diagnosis of glomerular and post-glomerular haematuria. *Postgrad Med J* 1992;68:648.
271. O'Flynn K, Hehir M, McKelvie G, et al. Endoballoon rupture and stenting for pelviureteric junction obstruction: technique and early results. *Br J Urol* 1989;64:572.
272. Older RA, Stoll HL, Omary RA, et al. Clinical value of renovascular resistive index measurement in the diagnosis of acute obstructive uropathy. *J Urol* 1997;157:2053.
273. Ono Y, Ohshima S, Kinukawa T, et al. Endopyeloureterotomy via a transpelvic extraureteral approach. *J Urol* 1992;147:352.
274. Oppenheimer R, Hinman F Jr. Ureteral regeneration: contracture vs. hyperplasia of smooth muscle. *J Urol* 1955;74:47.
275. Ordorica RC, Lindfors KK, Palmer JM. Diuretic Doppler sonography following successful repair of renal obstruction in children. *J Urol* 1993;150:774.
276. Osther PJ, Geersten U, Nielson HV. Ureteropelvic junction obstruction and ureteral strictures treated by simple high-pressure balloon dilation. *J Endourol* 1998;12:429.
277. O'Reilly PH. Diuresis renography 8 years later: an update. *J Urol* 1986;136:993.
278. O'Reilly PH, Lawson RS, Shields RA, et al. Idiopathic hydronephrosis—the diuresis renogram: a new non-invasive method of assessing equivocal pelvioureteral junction obstruction. *J Urol* 1979;121:153.
279. Orihuela E, Smith AD. Percutaneous treatment of transitional cell carcinoma of the upper urinary tract. *Urol Clin North Am* 1988;15:425.
280. Ozgun S, Cetin S, Ilken Y. Percutaneous renal cyst aspiration and treatment with alcohol. *Int Urol Nephrol* 1988;20:481.
281. Palou J, Farina LA, Villavicencio H, et al. Upper tract urothelial tumor after transurethral resection for bladder tumor. *Eur Urol* 1992;21:110.
282. Papadopoulos I, Wirth B, Bertermann H, et al. Diagnosis and treatment of urothelial tumors by ureteropyeloscopy. *J Endourol* 1990;4:55.
283. Pardalidis NP, Waltzer WC, Tellis VA, et al. Endourologic management of complications in renal allografts. *J Endourol* 1994;8:321.
284. Patel A, Soonawalla P, Shepherd SF et al. Long-term outcome after percutaneous treatment of transitional cell carcinoma of the renal pelvis. *J Urol* 1996;155:868.
285. Patterson DE, Segura JW, Benson RC Jr, et al. Endoscopic evaluation and treatment of patients with idiopathic gross hematuria. *J Urol* 1984;132:1199.
286. Pauer W, Lugmayr H. Metallic wall stents: a new therapy for extrinsic ureteral obstruction. *J Urol* 1992;148:281.
287. Payne SR, Coptcoat MJ, Kellet MJ, et al. Effective intubation for percutaneous pyelolysis. *Eur Urol* 1988;14:477.
288. Pearle MS, Moon YT, Endicott RC, et al. Comparison of retrograde endopyelotomy and endoballoon rupture (ENDOBRST) of the ureteropelvic junction in a porcine model. *J Urol* 1994;152:2232.
289. Perez-Castro EE, Martinez-Pineiro JA. Transurethral ureteroscopy: a current urologic procedure. *Arch Esp Urol* 1980;33:445.
290. Perugia G, Drudi FM, Carbone A, et al. Role of fibrin glue in percutaneous treatment of renal cysts. *J Endourol* 1991;5:225.
291. Plas EG, Hubner WA. Percutaneous resection of renal cysts: a long-term follow-up. *J Urol* 1993;149:703.
292. Platt JF, Ellis JH, Rubin JM. Renal transplant pyelocaliectasis: role of duplex Doppler US in evaluation. *Radiology* 1991; 179:435.
293. Preminger GM, Clayman RV, Nakada SY, et al. A multi-center clinical trial investigating the use of a fluoroscopically controlled cutting balloon catheter for the management of ureteral and ureteropelvic junction obstruction. *J Urol* 1997;157:1625.
294. Psihramis KE, Dretler SP. Extracorporeal shock wave lithotripsy of caliceal diverticula calculi. *J Urol* 1987;138:707.
295. Puppo P, Ricciotti G, Bottino P, et al. Exploration of the intrarenal collecting system using flexible fiberoscopy. *Arch Esp Urol* 1991;44:541.
296. Quillin SP, Brink JA, Heiken JP, et al. Helical (spiral) CT angiography for identification of crossing vessels at the ureteropelvic junction. *AJR Am J Roentgenol* 1996;166:1125.
297. Ramsey JC, Soloway MS. Instillation of bacillus Calmette-Guérin into the renal pelvis of a solitary kidney for the treatment of transitional cell carcinoma. *J Urol* 1990;143:1220.
298. Ramsey JWA, Miller RA, Kellet MJ, et al. Percutaneous pyelolysis: indications, complications, and results. *Br J Urol* 1984;56:586.
299. Ravi G, Motalib MA. Surgical correction of bilharzial ureteric stricture by Boari flap technique. *Br J Urol* 1993;71:535.
300. Reddy PK, Moore L, Hunter D, et al. Percutaneous ureteral fulguration: a non-surgical technique for ureteral occlusion. *J Urol* 1987;138:724.
300a. Renner C, Frede T, Seemann O, Rassweiler J. Laser endopyelotomy: minimally invasive therapy of ureteropelvic junction stenosis. *J Endourol* 1998;12(6):537.
301. Resnick MI. Radiolucent filling defects. In: Resnick MI, Caldamore AA, Spivnak JD, eds. *Decision making in urology.* St Louis: Mosby, 1985.
302. Richter S, Karbel G, Bechar R, et al. Should a benign renal cyst be treated? *Br J Urol* 1983;55:457.
303. Rodgers PM, Bates JA, Irving HC. Intrarenal Doppler ultrasound studies in normal and acutely obstructed kidneys. *Br J Radiol* 1992;65:207.
304. Rosen RJ, McLean GK, Freiman DB, et al. Obstructed ureteroileal conduits: antegrade catheter drainage. *AJR Am J Roentgenol* 1980;135:1201.
305. Rossleigh MA, Leighton DM, Farnsworth RH. Diuresis renography. The need for an additional view after gravity-assisted drainage. *Clin Nucl Med* 1993;18:210.
306. Ryan PC, Maher K, Hurley GD, et al. The Whitaker test: experimental analysis in a canine model of partial ureteric obstruction. *J Urol* 1989;141:387.
307. Sadi MU, Nardozza A Jr, Gionotti I. Percutaneous drainage of retroperitoneal abscesses. *J Endourol* 1988;2:293.
308. Sampaio FJB. Review: anatomic background for intrarenal endourologic surgery. *J Endourol* 1992;6:301.

309. Sampaio FJB, Favorito LA. Ureteropelvic junction stenosis: vascular anatomical background for endopyelotomy. *J Urol* 1993;150:1787.
310. Sarnacki CT, McCormack LJ, Kiser WS, et al. Urinary cytology and the clinical diagnosis of urinary tract malignancy: a clinicopathological study of 1400 patients. *J Urol* 1971; 106:761.
311. Sayer J, McCarthy MP, Schmidt JD. Identification and significance of dysmorphic versus isomorphic hematuria. *J Urol* 1990; 143:545.
312. Schenkman EM, Tarry WF. Comparison of percutaneous endopyelotomy with open pyeloplasty for pediatric ureteropelvic junction obstruction. *J Urol* 1998;159:1013.
313. Scardino PT, Scardino PL. Obstruction of the ureteropelvic junction. In: Bergman H, ed. *The ureter.* New York: Springer-Verlag, 1984.
314. Schmeller NT, Hofstetter AG. Laser treatment of ureteral tumors. *J Urol* 1989;141:840.
315. Schmeller N, Leitl F, Arnholdt H. Histology of ureter after unsuccessful endoscopic intubated incision. *J Urol* 1992; 147:450.
316. Schmidt JD, Hawtrey CE, Flocks RH, et al. Complications, results and problems of ileal diversion. *J Urol* 1973;109:210.
317. Schneider AW, Busch R, Otto V, et al. Endourological management of 41 stenosis in the upper urinary tract using the cold knife technique. *J Urol* 1989;141:208A.
318. Schneider AW, Conrad S, Busch R, et al. The cold-knife technique for endourological management of stenosis in the upper urinary tract. *J Urol* 1991;146:961.
319. Schoenberg MP, Van Arsdalen KN, Wein AJ. The management of transitional cell carcinoma in solitary renal units. *J Urol* 1991;146:700.
320. Schow DA, Vinson RK, Morrisseau PM. Percutaneous renal biopsy of the solitary kidney: a contraindication? *J Urol* 1992; 147:1235.
321. Scott R, Mohammed R, Gorham SD, et al. The evolution of a biodegradable membrane for use in urologic surgery: a summary of 109 *in vivo* experiments. *Br J Urol* 1988;62:26.
322. Seaman EK, Slawin KM, Benson MC. Treatment options for upper tract transitional-cell carcinoma. *Urol Clin North Am* 1993;20:349.
323. Segura J. Personal communication. 1994.
324. Selmy G, Hassouna M, Begin LR, et al. Effect of balloon dilation of ureter on upper tract dynamics and ureteral wall morphology. *J Endourol* 1993;7:211.
325. Semelka RC, Shoenut JP, Kroeker MA, et al. Renal lesions: controlled comparison between CT and 1.5-T MR imaging with nonenhanced and gadolinium-enhanced fat-suppressed spin-echo and breath-hold FLASH techniques. *Radiology* 1992; 182:425.
326. Shalhav AL, Giusti G, Elbahnasy AM, et al. Adult endopyelotomy: impact of etiology and antegrade versus retrograde approach on outcome. *J Urol* 1998;160:685.
327. Shalhav AL, Giusti G, Elbahnasy AM, et al. Endopyelotomy for high-insertion ureteropelvic junction obstruction. *J Endourol* 1998;12:127.
328. Shapira OM, Simon D, Rothstein H, et al. Unilateral ureteral obstruction secondary to rupture of liver echinococcal cyst. *J Urol* 1992;148:1888.
329. Shapiro MJ, Banner MP, Amendola MA, et al. Balloon catheter dilation of ureteroenteric strictures: long-term results. *Radiology* 1988;168:385.
330. Sharpe JR, Duffy G, Chin JL. Intrarenal bacillus Calmette-Guérin therapy for upper urinary tract carcinoma *in situ*. *J Urol* 1993;149:457.
331. Shaver TR, Swandson SJ III, Fernandez-Bueno C, et al. The optimal treatment of lymphoceles following renal transplantation. *Transpl Int* 1993;6:108.
332. Sheinfeld J, Erturk E, Spartara RF, et al. Perinephric abscess: current concepts. *J Urol* 1987;137:191.
333. Shokeir AA, El-Diasty AT, Ghoneim MA. Endourologic management of ureteric complications after live-donor kidney transplantation. *J Endourol* 1993;7:487.
334. Shokeir AA, Eraky I, El-Kappany H, et al. Accidental division of the transplanted ureter during laparoscopic drainage of lymphocele. *J Urol* 1994;151:1623.
335. Singal RK, Denstedt JD, Razvi HA, et al. Holmium:YAG laser endoureterotomy for treatment of ureteral stricture. *Urology* 1997;50:875.
336. Sjwierzewski SJ III, Konnak JUW, Ellis JH. Treatment of renal transplant ureteral complications by percutaneous techniques. *J Urol* 1993;149:986.
337. Slavis SA, Garner LD, Swift C, et al. Laparoscopic drainage of lymphocele after renal transplantation. *J Urol* 1992;148:96.
338. Smith AD. Management of iatrogenic ureteral strictures after urological procedures. *J Urol* 1988;140:1372.
339. Smith AD, Lange PH, Miller RP, et al. Percutaneous dilatation of ureteroileal strictures and insertion of Gibbons ureteral stents. *Urology* 1979;13:24.
340. Smith AD, Orihuela E, Crowley AR. Percutaneous management of renal pelvic tumors: a treatment option in selected cases. *J Urol* 1987;137:852.
341. Soloway MS, Masters S. Urothelial susceptibility to tumor cell implantation: influence of cauterization. *Cancer* 1980;46:1158.
342. Stefanini M, English HA, Taylor AE. Safe and effective, prolonged administration of epsilon aminocaproic acid in bleeding from the urinary tract. *J Urol* 1990;143:559.
343. Stephens FD. Ureterovascular hydronephrosis and the "aberrant" renal vessels. *J Urol* 1982;128:984.
344. Streem SB, Pontes EJ. Percutaneous management of upper tract transitional cell carcinoma. *J Urol* 1986;135:773.
345. Streem SB, Yost A. Treatment of caliceal diverticular calculi with extracorporeal shock wave lithotripsy: patient selection and extended follow-up. *J Urol* 1992;148:1043.
346. Strong DW, Pearse HD, Tank ES Jr, et al. The ureteral stump after nephroureterectomy. *J Urol* 1976;115:654.
347. Sutherland RS, Pfister RR, Koyle MA. Endopyelotomy associated ureteral necrosis: complete ureteral replacement using the Boari flap. *J Urol* 1992;148:1490.
348. Szewczyk W, Szkodny A, Noga A, et al. Endopyelotomy for ureteropelvic junction stenosis. *Int Urol Nephrol* 1992;24:105.
349. Talner LB. Obstructive uropathy. In: Pollack HM, ed. *Nuclear medicine techniques in clinical urology.* Philadelphia: Saunders, 1990.
350. Tasca A, Zattoni F. The case for a percutaneous approach to a transitional cell carcinoma of the renal pelvis. *J Urol* 1990; 143:902.
351. Tasca A, Zattoni F, Garbeglio A, et al. Endourologic treatment of transitional cell carcinoma of the upper urinary tract. *J Urol* 1992;6:253.
352. Tawfiek ER, Liu JB, Bagley DH. Ureteroscopic treatment of ureteropelvic junction obstruction. *J Urol* 1998;160:1643.
353. Tawfiek ER, Bagley DH. Ureteroscopic evaluation and treatment of chronic unilateral hematuria. *J Urol* 1998;160:700.
354. Terry JD, Rysavy JA, Frick MP. Intrarenal Doppler: characteristics of aging kidneys. *J Ultrasound Med* 1992;11:647.
355. Thiounn N, Benoit G, Osphal C, et al. Urological complications in renal transplantation. *Prog Urol* 1991;1:531.

356. Thomas R, Monga M, Klein EW. Ureteroscopic retrograde endopyelotomy for management of ureteropelvic junction obstruction. *J Endourol* 1996;10:141.
357. Timmons JW Jr, Malek RS, Hattery RR, et al. Caliceal diverticulum. *J Urol* 1975;114:6.
358. Tomita M, Kitamoto Y, Nakayama M, et al. A new morphological classification of urinary erythrocytes for differential diagnosis of glomerular hematuria. *Clin Nephrol* 1992;37:84.
359. Tosaka A, Ohya K, Yamada K, et al. Incidence and properties of renal masses and asymptomatic renal cell carcinoma detected by abdominal ultrasonography. *J Urol* 1990;144:1097.
360. Towbin RB, Wacksman J, Ball WS. Percutaneous pyeloplasty in children: experience in three patients. *Radiology* 1987; 163:381.
361. Upsdell SM, Testa HJ, Lawson RS. The F-15 diuresis renogram in suspected obstruction of the upper urinary tract. *Br J Urol* 1992;69:126.
362. Urban DA, Kerbl K, Clayman RV, et al. Endo-ureteroplasty with a free urothelial graft. *J Urol* 1994;152:910.
363. Van Baal JG, Smits NJ, Keeman JN, et al. The evolution of renal angiomyolipomas in patients with tuberous sclerosis. *J Urol* 1994;152:35.
364. Van Cangh PJ, Jorion JL, Wese FX, et al. Endoureteropyelotomy: percutaneous treatment of ureteropelvic junction obstruction. *J Urol* 1989;141:1317.
365. Van Cangh PJ, Wilmart JHF, Opsomer RJ, et al. Long-term results and late recurrence after endoureteropyelotomy: critical analysis of prognostic factors. *J Urol* 1994;151:934.
366. Van Helsdingen PJ, Rikken CHM. Treatment of urothelial carcinoma of the upper urinary tract following prostatocystectomy with mitomycin C instillation in the ileal loop. *J Urol* 1986;136:461.
367. Vehmas T, Paivansalo M, Taavitsainenn M, et al. Ultrasound in renal pyogenic infection: imaging and intervention. *Acta Radiol* 1988;29:675.
368. Vogeli AT, Mellin HE, Hopf B, et al. Ureteroscopy under local anaesthesia with and without intravenous analgesia. *Br J Urol* 1993;72:161.
369. von Schreeb T, Arner O, Skovsted G, et al. Renal adenocarcinoma: is there a risk of spreading tumor cells in diagnostic puncture? *Scand J Urol Nephrol* 1967;1:270.
370. Wallace DMA, Wallace DM, Whitfield HN, et al. The late results of conservative surgery for upper tract urothelial carcinomas. *Br J Urol* 1981;53:537.
371. Walther PJ, Robertson CN, Paulson DE. Lethal complications of standard self-retaining ureteral stents in patients with ileal conduit urinary diversions. *J Urol* 1985;133:851.
372. Webb EA, Smith BA Jr, Price WE. Plastic operations on the ureter without intubation. *J Urol* 1957;77:821.
372a. Webber RJS, Pandian SS, McClinton S, Hussey J. Retrograde balloon dilatation for pelviureteric junction obstruction: long-term follow-up. *J Endourol* 1997;11:239.
373. Weigert F, Schulz V, Kromer HD. Renal abscess: report of a case with sonographic, urographic, and CT evaluation. *Eur J Radiol* 1985;5:224.
374. Whitaker RH. An evaluation of 10 diagnostic pressure flow studies of the upper urinary tract. *J Urol* 1979;121:602.
375. Williams RD. Renal, perirenal, and ureteral neoplasms. In: Gillenwater JY, Grayhack JT, Howards SS, et al, eds. *Adult and pediatric urology,* ed 2. St Louis: Mosby, 1991.
376. Wills TE, Burns JR. Ureteroscopy: an outpatient procedure? *J Urol* 1994;151:1185.
377. Wise GJ. Amphotericin B in urological practice. *J Urol* 1990; 144:215.
378. Witherington R, Shelor WC. Treatment of postoperative ureteral stricture by catheter dilation: a forgotten procedure. *Urology* 1980;16:592.
379. Wolf JS, Elashry OM, Clayman RV. Long-term results of endoureterectomy for benign ureteral and ureteroenteric strictures. *J Urol* 1997;158:759.
380. Yoshida K, Nishimura T, Tsuboi N, et al. Clinical application of video image flexible ureteronephroscope for diagnosis of upper urinary tract disorders. *J Urol* 1991;146:809.
381. Young HH, McKay RW. Congenital valvular obstruction prostatic urethra. *Surg Gynecol Obstet* 1929;48:509.
381a. Youssef NI, Jindal R, Babayan RI, et al. The acucise catheter: a new endourological method for correcting transplant ureteric stenosis. *Transplantation* 1994;57(9):1398.
382. Yung BC, Sostre S, Gearhart JP. Normalized clearance-to-uptake slope ratio: a method to minimize false-positive diuretic renograms. *J Nucl Med* 1993;34:762.
383. Zincke H, Neves RJ. Feasibility of conservative surgery for transitional cell carcinoma of the upper urinary tract. *Urol Clin North Am* 1984;11:717.
384. Zungri E, Chechile G, Algaba F, et al. Treatment of transitional cell carcinoma of the ureter: is the controversy justified? *Eur Urol* 1990;17:276.

20

RENAL CYSTIC DISEASE

MARGUERITE C. LIPPERT

Renal cysts are abnormal dilations somewhere along the renal tubule between the glomerular capsule and the collecting system or are diverticulum-like structures possibly in continuity with the nephron. All renal cysts originate from microscopic renal tubules by proliferation of renal epithelial cells to form a diverticulum from the tubule wall and accumulation within the cyst of fluid from either glomerular filtrate or net transepithelial fluid secretion (144). Renal cysts may develop by heritable, developmental, or acquired processes. Renal cystic disease can involve both

M.C. Lippert: Department of Urology, University of Virginia Health Science Center, Charlottesville, VA 22908.

TABLE 20.1. CYSTIC DISEASE OF THE KIDNEY

Genetic

Autosomal-recessive (infantile) polycystic kidneys (ARPKD)

Autosomal-dominant (adult) polycystic kidneys (ADPKD)

Juvenile nephronophthisis–medullary cystic disease complex (NMCD):
- Juvenile nephronophthisis (autosomal recessive) (NPH)
- Medullary cystic disease (autosomal dominant) (ADMCKD)

Congenital nephrosis (autosomal recessive)

Cysts associated with multiple malformation syndromes

Nongenetic

Multicystic kidney (multicystic dysplasia) (MCDK)

Cystic nephroma (multilocular cyst)

Simple cysts

Medullary sponge kidneys (<5% inherited)

Acquired cystic kidney disease in chronic hemodialysis patients (ACKD)

Caliceal diverticulum (pyelogenic cyst)

Adapted from Glassberg K, et al. Renal dysgenesis and cystic disease of the kidney: a report of the Committee on Terminology, Nomenclature and Classification, Section on Urology, American Academy of Pediatrics. *J Urol* 1987;138:1085, with permission.

kidneys diffusely as autosomal-dominant polycystic kidney disease (ADPKD), one particular area of both kidneys as medullary sponge kidneys, or just one kidney or part of it as multicystic kidney. Alternatively, a cystic tumor can replace normal renal parenchyma as in multilocular cyst. Finally, simple cysts can occur alone or together anywhere in the kidney.

Classification of cysts for the purpose of simplifying concepts does not necessarily provide a practical, clinical framework for such diverse cystic diseases. Hence, although the classification of Osathanondh and Potter (290), based on microdissection studies, brought a basis for future research on the pathogenesis of renal cystic disease, the clinician was not aided in making a diagnosis from history, physical examination, and radiographic studies. Meaningful clinical classifications of renal cystic disease based on clinical and radiographic features, genetic investigation, and morphology, such as those of Bernstein (28) and Gardner and Evan (127), honestly portray the diversity of renal cystic diseases, but they do not lend themselves to a simple conceptual framework. Table 20.1 gives the 1987 classification from the Committee on Classification, Nomenclature, and Terminology of the American Academy of Pediatrics Section on Urology that offers broad genetic categories but still displays adequately the diversity of renal cystic diseases (137). The advent of ultrasonography (US), magnetic resonance imaging (MRI), and computed tomography (CT) have drastically improved the clinician's ability to diagnose and differentiate the various renal cystic diseases. There has been rapid recent progress in identification or chromosomal localization of responsible disease genes, giving insights into the pathophysiology of the genetic renal cystic diseases. The importance of a careful family history is emphasized by the classification of renal cystic diseases into genetic categories. Table 20.2 shows the known linkages of genetic renal cystic diseases.

AUTOSOMAL-DOMINANT POLYCYSTIC KIDNEY DISEASE

ADPKD is the most common form of cystic disease of the kidney and is caused by mutations in any one of at least three genes: PKD_1 on chromosome 16 (accounting for 85% of patients), PKD_2 on chromosome 4 (accounting for 15%), and the unmapped PKD_3 (probably accounting for rare families unlinked to the other two sites) (Table 20.3). It is the third most common cause of end-stage renal disease (ESRD), contributing 6% to 12% of patients receiving chronic renal dialysis. Fifty percent of patients typically develop chronic renal failure by age 60 (119). The highest incidence rate of ESRD from ADPKD is 1.5 per 100,000 population, occurring between the ages of 45 and 64 years (99). ADPKD occurs in about 1 in every 1,250 live births and is characterized by bilateral cystic disease in enlarged kidneys with a retained reniform shape. It is a systemic disease, and subsets of patients may develop

TABLE 20.2. GENETIC RENAL CYSTIC DISEASES—KNOWN LINKAGES

Disease	Inheritance	Chromosome
$ADPKD_1$	AD	16p31.1
$ADPKD_2$	AD	4q13-q23
ARPKD	AR	6p21
NPH_1	AR	2q12-q13
NPH_2	AR	9q23-q31
$ADMCKD_1$	AD	1q21
$ADMCKD_2$	AD	16q12
MKS_1	AR	17q21-q24
MKS_2	AR	11q13
VHL	AD	3p25.5
TSC_1	AD	9q34
TSC_2	AD	16p13.3

AD, autosomal dominant; ADMCKD, autosomal-dominant medullary cystic kidney disease; ADPKD, autosomal-dominant polycystic kidney disease; AR, autosomal recessive; ARPKD, autosomal-recessive polycystic kidney disease; MKS, Meckel's syndrome; NPH, nephronophthisis; TSC, tuberous sclerosis; VHL, von Hippel-Lindau disease.

TABLE 20.3. ADPKD—KNOWN LINKAGES

Disease	Inheritance	Chromosome	Gene	Mean Age Onset of ESRD (yr)	Gene Product
$ADPKD_1$	AD	16p31.1	PKD_1	54.3	Polycystin1
$ADPKD_2$	AD	4q13-q23	PKD_2	74	Polycystin2

AD, autosomal dominant; ADPKD, autosomal-dominant polycystic kidney disease.

extrarenal manifestations such as liver cysts or cerebral aneurysms.

Clinical Features

Typically, for the first 10 years of life, the kidneys are normal in function and anatomy. From age 10 to 30 years, US may show the presence of cysts, although the patient is asymptomatic. However, from 30 to 40 years, the patient may be diagnosed because of symptomatic presentation such as palpable kidneys, microscopic or gross hematuria, urinary tract infection (UTI), flank pain, or renal colic from passing clots. Although elevation of creatinine may begin between 40 and 50 years of age, dialysis or renal transplantation for ESRD does not typically become necessary until after age 50. Without dialysis or renal transplantation, the mean age of death for ADPKD is 50 years (81) and patients die of uremia (59%), heart failure, and cerebral hemorrhage. However, more recent studies suggest that many patients today are being diagnosed as having ADPKD without symptomatic presentation because of modern imaging and that these patients may remain without ESRD, death, or symptoms until their seventies (73,89).

Polycystic Liver Disease and Extrarenal Cysts

Liver cysts are the most common extrarenal manifestation in patients with both PKD_1 and PKD_2 mutations. Although about 50% of ADPKD patients have liver cysts (241), liver function remains normal except in rare cases of severe massive cystic disease compressing the biliary tree, leading to biliary obstruction and obstructive jaundice (102). Unlike renal cysts, in women, liver cysts are more numerous, occur earlier, and are more extensive in women (408). Multiparity and postmenopausal estrogen therapy increase the risk of massive hepatic cystic disease (109,353). Hepatic cyst development requires somatic inactivation of the normal allele coupled to a germline mutation just as in renal cysts (401). Polycystic liver disease has rarely occurred as a genetically distinct event with no association with ADPKD (190). Liver cysts rarely have been found in children with ADPKD, although they have been described in an 8-month-old ADPKD patient (272).

Although massive hepatic cystic disease usually does not impair hepatic function, a minority of patients complain of symptoms such as abdominal swelling, intermittent attacks of pain, shortness of breath, pain on stooping, dyspnea, early satiety, nausea, heartburn, and regurgitation (280,390). When the symptoms are disabling, initial treatment can include percutaneous drainage and sclerosis or laparoscopic fenestration, especially if there is one or a small number of dominant cysts (381). However, if there are many cysts, part of the liver is spared, allowing treatment with combined hepatic resection and fenestration (280). Occasionally, symptoms remain despite fenestration procedures, at which time orthotopic liver transplantation is considered (with or without kidney transplant depending on dialysis dependency) (204). Hepatic cyst infections, although rare, can be confused with renal cyst infections and are best treated with percutaneous drainage and antibiotics that concentrate in the biliary tree, such as trimethoprim-sulfamethoxazole (TMP-SMX) and fluoroquinolones (136).

In addition to liver cysts, ADPKD patients have developed cysts in the pancreas, lung, ovaries, esophagus, testes, bladder, thyroid, uterus, spleen, pineal gland, subarachnoid space, epididymis, seminal vesicles, and prostate. The estimated prevalence of pancreatic cysts is 98.5% in ADPKD patients older than 20 years of age (377). Complications of pancreatic cysts in ADPKD are rare, but chronic obstructive pancreatitis has been reported (254). Polycystin 1 has been found in epithelial cells of the pancreas.

Until the advent of US, seminal vesicle cysts were not described in ADPKD. However, when male ADPKD patients were screened with transrectal ultrasound (TRUS), 60% were found to have seminal vesicle cysts and 11% had prostate cysts (84). Hendry and associates (170) noted that although the TRUS appearances suggested seminal vesicle cysts in six male ADPKD patients, vasograms revealed dilation of the seminal vesicles from atonicity or failure to effectively contract with no evidence of seminal vesicle cysts (170). Ovarian cysts are not more prevalent in female ADPKD patients than in the general population (408).

Aneurysms and Hernias

Intracranial aneurysm (ICA) rupture is the most feared extrarenal complication of ADPKD. From 0% to 40% of ADPKD patients have asymptomatic, unruptured cranial aneurysms on autopsy, prospective angiographic imaging studies, and prospective noninvasive imaging studies (35,52,64,188,368,393). Currently, the prevalence of ICAs is approaching 10% in ADPKD patients, as opposed to 2% in the general population. Familial clustering of ICA in ADPKD patients does occur (212,406), with a prevalence of 16% in those families (408). ICAs have occurred in both PKD_1 and PKD_2 families.

The risk of rupture increases with the size of the aneurysm, with most aneurysms being less than 10 mm in size in ADPKD patients. Hence, the yearly risk of bleeding is low (0.5% to 2%) but the cumulative risk remains significant and depends on expected survival, which can be about 60 years in ADPKD patients (259). However, the average patient age when ICAs rupture in ADPKD is younger than in the general population and varies from 37 to 47 years of age (63). Although most acute neurologic events in ADPKD patients do not result from ruptured ICAs, these ruptured aneurysms can result in the potential sequelae of subarachnoid hemorrhage, with greater than 50% mortality and permanent disability; however, they are potentially preventable (63,259). Systematic screening of ADPKD patients with a positive ICA family history or previous aneurysmal rupture with MRI angiography beginning in the third decade of life is recommended (259). If angiography revealed an aneurysm, treatment with either microsurgical clipping or endovascular coiling should be recommended if the individual risk of rupture is higher than the risk of treatment. Such risk is dependent on the patient's age and health and the size and location of the ICA. In general, microsurgical clipping is still the treatment of choice, when feasible, because it is curative unless the patient is older, in which case endovascular coiling is a good alternative (259).

Cardiovascular abnormalities such as cardiac valve anomalies, dilation of the aortic root, dissections of the thoracic aorta, and coronary artery aneurysms have been reported to have an increased incidence in ADPKD patients (158,381). Routine echocardiography with Doppler analysis revealed 26% incidence of mitral valve prolapse, 31% incidence of mitral incompetence, 8% incidence of aortic incompetence, and 6% incidence of tricuspid prolapse in ADPKD patients (185). Symptoms of mitral prolapse (e.g., palpitations, nonexertional chest pain) are more common in ADPKD patients than in controls (119). PKD mutations may be responsible because polycystin 1 and polycystin 2 are strongly expressed in the medial myocytes of the elastic and large distributive arteries as well as in cardiac myocytes and valvular fibroblasts (149). Other nonrenal manifestations of ADPKD involve increased incidence of inguinal hernias, hiatal hernias, colonic diverticula, and cholangiocarcinoma. Polycystin 1 has been found in the epithelial cells of the intestine.

Pain

Pain is the most common presenting symptom of ADPKD, particularly in women (408). It antedates renal palpability and occurs in 59% of affected individuals (81). Pain usually occurs in the flank or lateral abdomen but may radiate to the epigastrium or suprapubic area. Acute pain can be secondary to cyst rupture or cyst hemorrhage. The more common dull pain increases as the disease progresses and cysts enlarge, and no etiology has been confirmed. Perhaps pain results from the stretching of the renal capsule, pressure on adjacent organs, or traction on the renal pedicle. Distinguishing this chronic dull pain from the pain of a simultaneous renal disease such as obstruction, hemorrhage, infection, or tumor is difficult but of great importance for the preservation of future renal function. These latter etiologies tend to cause pain of more recent onset. Abdominal pressure from massive hepatic cystic disease needs to be considered.

Hypertension

Mild to moderate hypertension antedates the onset of ESRD in about 60% of ADPKD patients. Before renal deterioration, ADPKD patients with hypertension have more renal cystic involvement than normotensive ADPKD patients (22). Cyst decompression can transiently lower blood pressure in hypertensive ADPKD patients until renal cystic volume increases again (103,115,384). Enlarging cysts could theoretically compress renal vessels, causing renal ischemia and thereby activating the renin-angiotensin-aldosterone system. Consequently, angiotensin-converting enzyme (ACE) inhibitors are widely prescribed as first-time agents for treating hypertensive patients with ADPKD. However, in hypertensive ADPKD patients with chronic renal insufficiency and massive cystic involvement, ACE inhibitor therapy can cause reversible renal failure (61). The mild to moderate hypertension in ADPKD responds well to drug treatment. Antihypertensive treatment may or may not retard the development of ESRD. Cardiovascular disease is the most common cause of death in ADPKD patients (408). Control of blood pressure is necessary to prevent accelerated hypertension and cardiovascular events. Mild to moderate hypertension in ADPKD patients may decrease on dialysis (326). PKD_1 patients have a fourfold increase in prevalence of hypertension compared with PKD_2 patients and have an earlier age of onset (34.8 versus 49.7 years) (376).

Hematuria; Flank Masses

Hematuria, gross or microscopic, is common, occurring in up to 64% of affected individuals (89). It is the presenting complaint in 35% (225). Hematuria can result from spontaneous or traumatic cyst rupture or concomitant calculi, infection, or neoplasm. An evaluation of hematuria in ADPKD patients should include all of these possibilities. Clots can cause renal colic and obstruction of the urinary tract. The most common inciting events precipitating hematuria in ADPKD patients are UTIs (42%), followed by sports or strenuous activity (20% in males and 11% in females) (225). Approximately 60% of ADPKD patients have palpable flank masses, of which one-third are bilateral and two-thirds are unilateral. However, it is a less common (15% of patients) finding at initial presentation.

ADPKD in Children

Less than 10% of cases of ADPKD present in the first decade of life (224). It is important to differentiate between children presenting at an early age with symptoms or complications leading to the diagnosis of ADPKD as opposed to those children of affected families in whom the diagnosis is made by family screening. Those identified in childhood by US family screening may have a benign early course (348), compared with those diagnosed *in utero* or by symptoms in the first few months of life, who have an estimated perinatal mortality of 43% with a 67% complication rate for the survivors by the age of 3 years (249). Children diagnosed as ADPKD *in utero* or in the first year of life have more severe renal cystic disease. In affected fetuses, oligohydramnios can occur earlier than in autosomal-recessive polycystic kidney disease (ARPKD) because the renal developmental abnormality occurs earlier in ADPKD than in ARPKD (154). Although most ADPKD infants survive, they have a more rapid decline in their renal function and more significant hypertension than their affected adult relatives. Of 24 children diagnosed with ADPKD prenatally or up to 1 year of life, 16 developed hypertension and required treatment at the mean age of 2.9 years; 3 of the 16 developed ESRD at the mean age of 2.8 years (249). Presenting symptoms in neonates include renomegaly in mild cases and respiratory distress or stillbirth in severe cases. Presenting symptoms after 1 year of age include renomegaly, hypertension, and hematuria.

Although simple renal cysts are common in adults, they are rare enough in children that any cyst on a renal US in a child at risk for ADPKD probably indicates the presence of ADPKD (121). When 106 children younger than 18 years of age who were at 50% risk of ADPKD were screened with US by these criteria as well as gene linkage analysis, 45% screened positive for ADPKD by both modalities. Fourteen children (13%) were positive for ADPKD by gene linkage analysis but had a normal initial US, although subsequent US examinations were positive for ADPKD during this analysis (121). The US false-negative rate was 25% using these criteria and highest in those children younger than 5 years of age. Since the development of present renal imaging techniques, the number of ADPKD cases discovered in childhood appears to be almost as high as that of ARPKD patients surviving the neonatal period (123).

Children with an early onset of severe ADPKD have a PKD_1 genotype and have an affected parent whose milder disease presented in adulthood. The increase in disease severity is limited to the kidney, which has a higher number of cysts and mostly glomerular cysts (289). Even though the child or fetus carries the same stable mutation as the affected parent, 45% of the subsequent gene carrier offspring have early-onset ADPKD, even with different partners (154). A modifying gene could be transmitted from the affected parent, which might alter the rate of somatic mutation at PKD_1 (289).

A less common cause of early onset of severe ADPKD occurs when both PKD_1 and TSC_2 [the more common gene causing tuberous sclerosis (TSC)] are both deleted, resulting in a phenotype with early-onset multiple renal cysts and/or early renal failure (50). This PKD_1–TSC_2 contiguous gene syndrome can occur because TSC_2 and PKD_1 are located a few nucleotides apart on chromosome 16. Patients may show findings of TSC [renal angiomyolipomas (AMLs), facial angiofibromas, and central nervous system (CNS) lesions resulting in mental retardation and/or seizures] before or after their early-onset severe renal cystic disease.

Morphology

On gross inspection, the ADPKD kidneys are huge because they are filled with hundreds of fluid-filled cysts (Fig. 20.1). Their surfaces are distorted by innumerable large cysts. However, unlike dysplastic kidneys, they retain their reniform shape. At autopsy, the mean combined kidney weight of clinically asymptomatic ADPKD patients was 512 g; of symptomatic patients, 930 g (165); and of ESRD ADPKD patients who came to renal dialysis, 2,600 g (23). The cut surface shows extensive parenchymal replacement of cortical and medullary cysts, which vary from a few millimeters to a few centimeters in diameter (Fig. 20.2). Cyst fluid varies from clear yellow to chocolate brown and from watery to gelatinous.

On microscopic study, islands of normal renal parenchyma are found, although most parenchyma has been replaced with cysts. The cysts are lined by a single layer of flattened cuboidal or columnar epithelium, but glomerular and tubular cysts may also be recognized. Cysts involve all elements of the nephron and collecting ducts. Estimates suggest that only 1% to 2% of the 2 million renal tubules develop cysts (147).

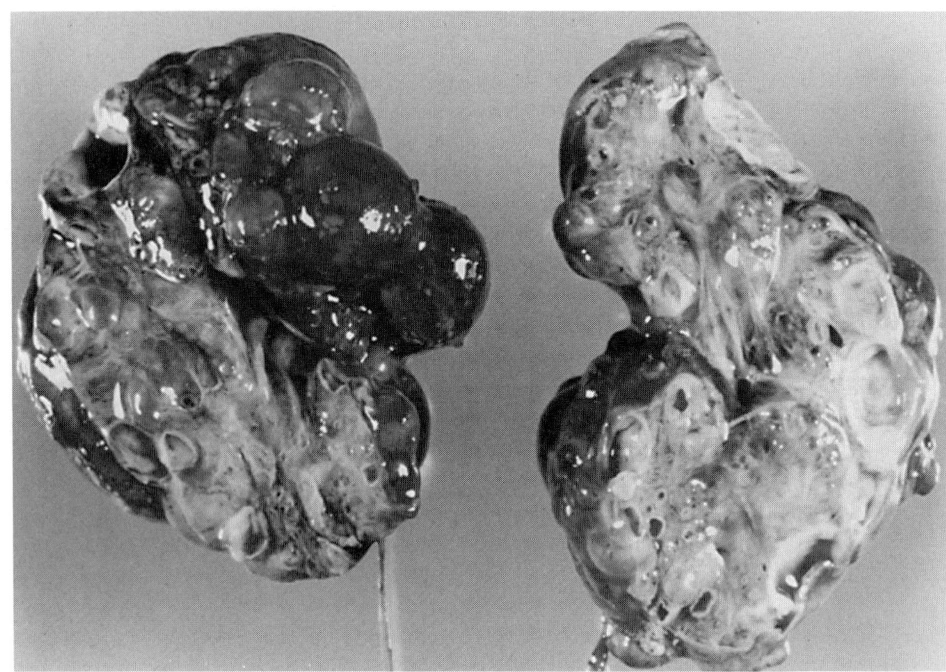

FIGURE 20.1. Autosomal-dominant polycystic kidney disease. Innumerable cysts distort the surfaces of these bilaterally enlarged kidneys. (Courtesy of Dr. S.E. Mills, Department of Pathology, University of Virginia Medical School, Charlottesville, VA.)

Pathogenesis

Fewer than 5% of the nephrons develop cysts in patients affected with ADPKD. Although every cell in the kidney harbors the dominant mutations in patients with ADPKD genotypes, a "second hit" mechanism must disable the wild-type allele before a solitary tubule cell begins to divide until a microcyst is formed. When cysts become 2 mm in diameter, 70% of them separate from the tubule of origin and fill with fluid exclusively by transepithelial secretion of sodium chloride (NaCl) and fluid under central control of cyclic adenosine monophosphate (cAMP) (145). Transepithelial fluid secretion and extracellular matrix remodeling are secondary factors (143).

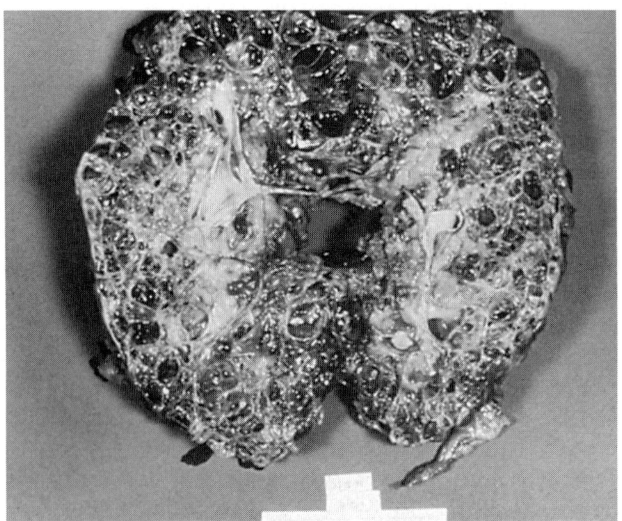

FIGURE 20.2. Autosomal-dominant polycystic kidney disease. Cut section reveals extensive parenchymal replacement by cortical and medullary cysts of varying sizes. (Courtesy of Dr. S.E. Mills, Department of Pathology, University of Virginia Medical School, Charlottesville, VA.)

Hence, the rate-limiting step in a two-step process of cyst formation is inactivation of the remaining normal allele as an acquired, or somatic, mutation in patients with a germline PKD_1 mutation (319) or with a germline PKD_2 mutation (226,307,378). Epithelial cells lining the renal and biliary ducts cysts appear to have "forgotten" how big the tubule is supposed to be and continue to proliferate. Kidneys from patients with ADPKD exhibit high levels of apoptosis (programmed cell death) as well as cellular proliferation (276), just as in embryonal renal development. Cysts may be viewed as survivors of programmed cell death, whereas the surrounding tubular epithelium may be unusually susceptible to the forces that cause apoptosis (145). Cyst enlargement seems insufficient to account for development of ESRD in ADPKD, but cysts may adversely affect adjacent renal parenchyma, resulting in cystic fibrosis through paracrine and endocrine factors (407) and hence renal failure.

Genetics and Diagnosis

The mutant gene in ADPKD, either PKD_1 or PKD_2, is expressed in an autosomal-dominant pattern, with a 50% chance of inheritance. However, within a given family, there is variable penetrance and variable ages of onset. As many as

25% of patients have no family history for ADPKD (165) because (a) affected relatives died of other causes before their disease was diagnosed, (b) affected living relatives may not be aware of their diagnosis, (c) nonpaternity, or (d) spontaneous new mutations. Spontaneous mutations occur in less than 10% of ADPKD patients (119). The mutation rate for ADPKD has been observed to be high and has been estimated to be 6.9×10^{-5} (92). By the age of 30, 70% penetrance has been estimated, and 99% has been estimated by the age of 55 (92). Humans homozygous for ADPKD have not been described (143).

In 1985, Reeders and colleagues established a linkage of a PKD locus to the α-globulin locus on the short arm of chromosome 16 using reverse genetics. Now christened PKD_1, this gene on chromosome 16p13.3 (15) has been mapped, fully sequenced, and characterized. Mutations on this long gene (52 kb) account for 85% of ADPKD patients who have the more severe form of ADPKD (191). PKD_1's protein product, polycystin 1, among the largest reported, is predicted to function as a membrane glycoprotein involved in cell–cell or cell–matrix interactions. Both the size of the gene and its complicated genomic structure with highly homologous loci elsewhere on chromosome 16 prevent direct mutation testing for the purpose of screening at-risk individuals. Linkage-based testing is feasible, but complicated by the existence of two distinct loci (227).

PKD_2, the mutated gene in the milder ADPKD phenotype, has been localized to chromosome 4q 13-23 (222,311) and characterized (273). Polycystin 2, the PKD_2 gene product, and polycystin 1 may be involved in a common signaling pathway that links extracellular adhesive events to alteration in ion transport, possibly regulating transmembrane Ca^{2+} fluxes (273,339,383).

Because 15% of ADPKD patients were found to have no linkage to PKD_1 (297,412), a search for PKD_2 began that was far more expeditious than the PKD_1 search because the PKD_2 gene has a far less complex genomic organization. Therefore gene-based diagnosis in PKD_2 is simpler than in PKD_1. However, because only 15% of ADPKD families have this form of the disease, it is less clinically useful in the absence of effective PKD_1 gene-based mutation detection. PKD_2 has a milder renal phenotype compared with PKD_1 as judged by age at onset of hypertension, ESRD, and cyst appearance (163,297,331,376). The existence of PKD_3, a third unmapped gene, would explain why some linkage studies do not link a few ADPKD families to either PKD_1 or PKD_2 (9,85); however, evidence is inconclusive (301).

Both forms of ADPKD are caused by a second hit mechanism that disables the wild-type allele. Within PKD_1 and PKD_2 families, phenotypic variability may be explained partially by gender and partially by random somatic events (i.e., the second hits) that inactivate the normal PKD_1 or PKD_2 allele. Because familial clustering of such ADPKD complications as intracranial saccular aneurysm occurs, attempts to find genetic heterogeneity to explain variability between families has been explored in addition to PKD_1 or PKD_2 mutations. Hateboer and associates (164) found differences only in the prevalence of hypertension and hernias between PKD_1 families secondary to the different PKD_1 mutations segregating to each family within their study.

Separate modifying genes may also affect the ADPKD phenotype by altering the chance of somatic mutation such as the ACE genotype. PKD_1 patients homozygous for the ACE deletion allele are at increased risk for developing ESRD before the age of 50 years; however, they do not have a greater prevalence of hypertension (310). Another example of a modifying gene may be mutant cystic fibrosis transmembrane conductance regulator protein (CFTR) because patients with ADPKD and cystic fibrosis (CF) had less severe polycystic kidney and liver disease (normal renal function, smaller renal volumes, absence of hypertension, and no liver cysts) as opposed to family members with only ADPKD (292).

Because of the technical demands and expense of both mutation detection and linkage analysis in ADPKD, identification of the genotype is not currently possible in most cases. There may be an exception in a subset of ADPKD families who reach ESRD late in life because this subset may be enriched for PKD_2 and gene-based diagnosis is simpler for PKD_2 (358). Gene-based diagnosis of PKD_1 is currently not practical because of complications engendered in detecting mutations in the reduplicated regions of the PKD_1 gene and because of the absence of recurrent mutations (358). Molecular genetic diagnosis of PKD_1 is best done by genetic linkage studies using intragenic and closely flanking polymorphic markers to overcome the problem of recombination.

Presently, the minimum requirement for the use of the test is the testing of two related clinically affected persons (120). Increasing the number of affected persons multiplies the degree of confidence in the recognition of the haplotype with which ADPKD is transmitted within each family. This requires large families, but in such a family, the predicated gene has a less than 5% error rate, which facilitates presymptomatic detection and prenatal diagnosis of ADPKD. When flanking markers for PKD_2 are used in conjunction with flanking markers for PKD_1, accuracy of diagnosis is improved. Individuals at risk for ADPKD who have less than two affected family members are dependent on US for diagnosis or potentially direct gene-based testing in PKD_2 families.

Although more accurate, molecular analysis of ADPKD is expensive and cannot be performed everywhere. US is the preferred method of diagnosis of ADPKD because it is highly sensitive, does not involve radiation or contrast material, and is widely available and inexpensive. The sensitivity of US for PKD_1 and PKD_2 patients older than 30 years of age is 100%. However, the sensitivity for PKD_1 patients younger than 31 years is 95.2%, and for PKD_2 patients younger than 31 years, it is only 66.6% (375). Therefore, for younger persons at risk in PKD_2 families, genetic testing is an option.

The early diagnosis of ADPKD facilitates improved genetic counseling and rational decision making about reproduction but will not necessarily lead to termination of an affected pregnancy. Linkage analysis can clarify gene status in potential living-related transplant donors. Many individuals at risk for ADPKD avoid presymptomatic diagnosis because of difficulty in getting life and medical insurance as well as future employment. A questionnaire-based study of ADPKD patients showed that 87% were concerned about the availability of health insurance, although 88% were covered. Fifty-seven percent of those with employer-based health insurance (83% of the total) had this availability determine their job choice (140).

Radiologic Findings and US Diagnosis

Contrast-enhanced CT scanning is the most sensitive diagnostic procedure for ADPKD. However, US has become the preferred diagnostic imaging method for children and adults because it is highly sensitive, does not involve radiation or contrast materials, and is widely available and inexpensive (Fig. 20.3). Renal US should pick up 95.2% of at-risk patients younger than 31 years of age in PKD_1 families and 66.6% in PKD_2 families (375). In those older than 30, US should pick up 100% of ADPKD because of the larger cyst size. The US diagnosis of $ADPKD_1$ depends on the patient's age. For patients aged younger than 30 years, two cysts, either bilateral or unilateral, must be present. Two cysts are necessary in each kidney for individuals aged 30 to 59 years, and at least four cysts are necessary in each kidney in individuals older than 60 years (322). A single cyst on US in an at-risk child is suggestive of ADPKD. Both US and CT are advantageous over intravenous pyelogram (IVP) because both allow a concomitant examination of the liver for cysts. IVP may reveal calyceal distortion on the pyelogram phase (mass effect), bilateral renal enlargement, and a Swiss-cheese appearance in the nephrogram phase (Fig. 20.4).

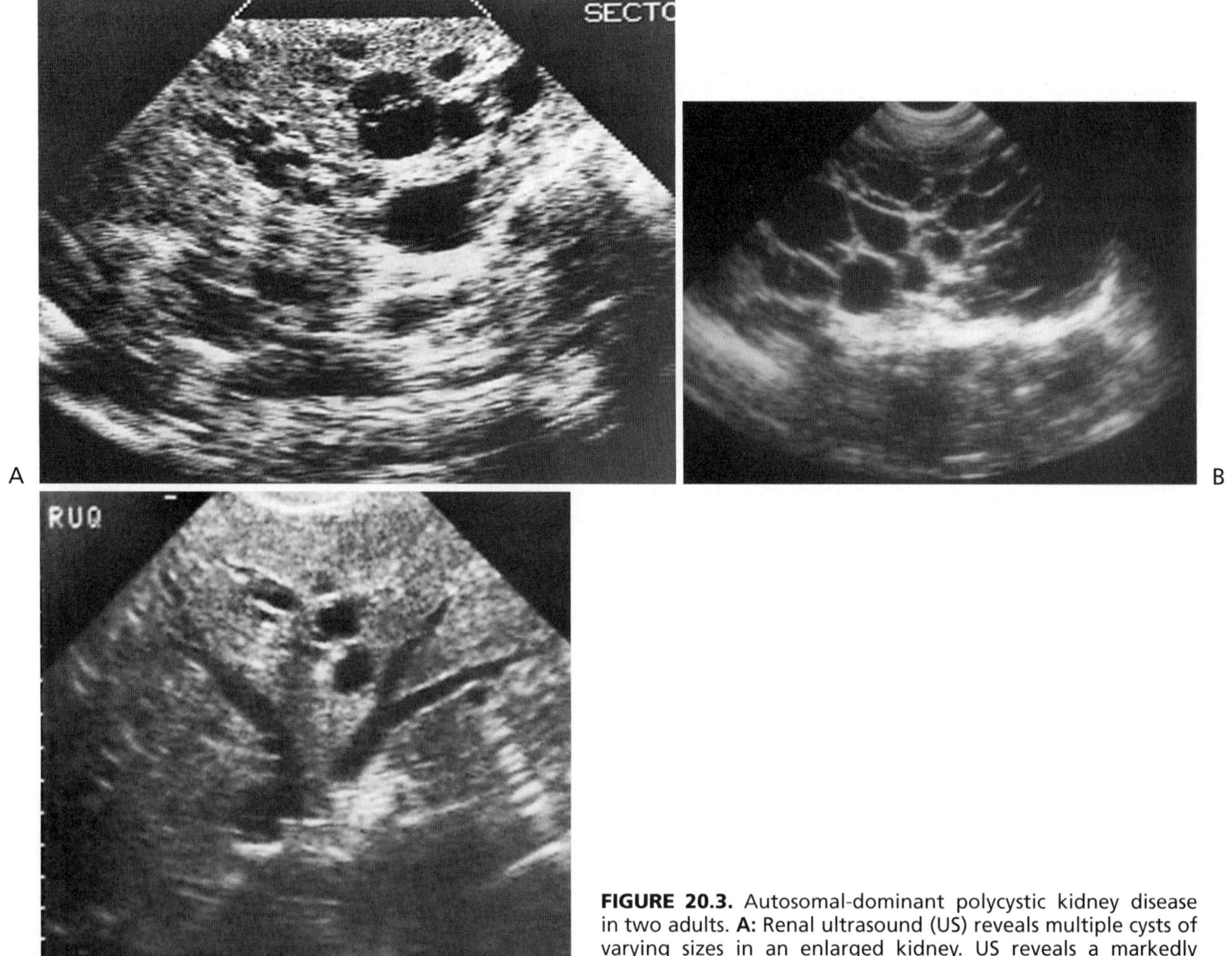

FIGURE 20.3. Autosomal-dominant polycystic kidney disease in two adults. **A:** Renal ultrasound (US) reveals multiple cysts of varying sizes in an enlarged kidney. US reveals a markedly enlarged kidney with numerous cysts of varying sizes **(B)** and two small cysts within the liver in a 37-year-old woman **(C).**

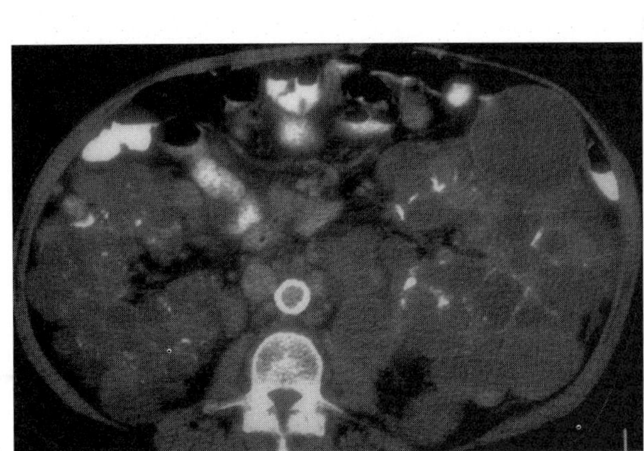
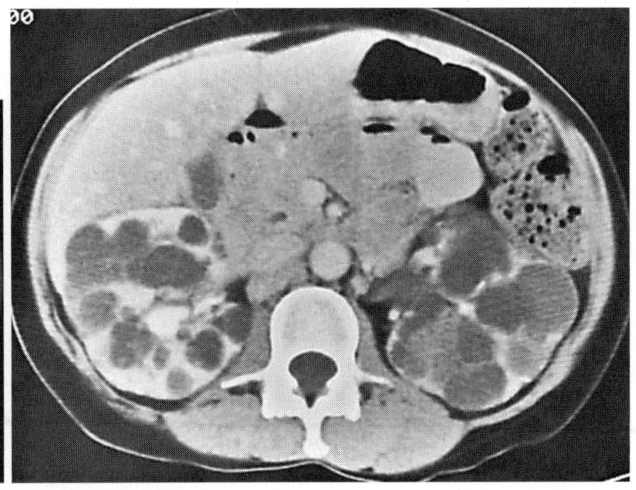

A B

FIGURE 20.4. Autosomal-dominant polycystic kidney disease in two adults. **A:** Unenhanced computed tomography (CT) scan revealing calcifications in walls of multiple cysts in enlarged kidneys. **B:** Enhanced CT scan in a 51-year-old woman reveals bilaterally markedly enlarged kidneys with multiple cysts of varying sizes, shapes, and attenuation values. There is some enhancing renal cortical tissue remaining, but excretion into the collecting system is identified only with difficulty.

Renal arteriography reveals stretching on vessels around avascular masses in large kidneys in the arterial phase and a mottled or Swiss-cheese appearance in the nephrogram phase (Fig. 20.5).

It is unfortunate that in a disease in which precise diagnosis of complications is crucial, the distorted anatomy of ADPKD kidneys often reduces the diagnostic accuracy of imaging procedures that are quite reliable in patients with normal kidneys (357). Contrast-enhanced CT scanning is the best technique for evaluating possible complications in ADPKD such as cyst or parenchymal infection, cyst hemorrhage, cyst calcifications, and renal calculi (242). Renal angiography can demonstrate renal cell carcinoma (RCC) in patients with ADPKD and can evaluate suspected renal hemorrhage and renovascular lesions. Both IVP and retrograde pyelography can localize the level of possible urinary tract obstruction in ADPKD. Retrograde pyelography should be avoided because of the high risk in ADPKD patients of introducing infection; however, it may be necessary when renal failure precludes satisfactory IVP and the level of obstruction needs to be localized. If intravenous contrast is contraindicated in an ADPKD patient, CT without contrast is the most useful test to rule out urinary tract obstruction (but not to find the level of obstruction) because US may not distinguish between parenchymal cysts and dilated calyces. Radiogallium scanning can help localize the cyst or parenchymal infection in ADPKD but false-positive and false-negative results may reduce the value of this test in individual patients. Indium-111 leukocyte scanning has potential to detect and localize infected cysts in patients with a polymorphonuclear leukocyte count greater than 2,000/mm^3 (49). MRI does not appear to offer advantages over CT, except perhaps to diagnose an acute renal hemorrhage.

Management

Therapy of ADPKD must be directed toward delaying and managing ESRD and toward managing the complications of ADPKD that occur before and after renal failure. Routine urologic diseases, such as urinary infections, calculi, and obstruction, can be very difficult problems in ADPKD patients and require special therapeutic consideration.

Renal Failure

Renal function is well preserved until late in ADPKD, at which time it decreases rapidly. Onset of renal failure is variable, but approximately 50% of ADPKD patients will have ESRD by 60 years of age (119). Time to development of ESRD in ADPKD patients is affected by genetic heterogeneity (PKD_1 versus PKD_2 mutations), random somatic events (second hits that inactivate PKD_1 or PKD_2 allele), and gender. A number of these factors predicting earlier ESRD in ADPKD patients can be identified early in ADPKD (206). For example, the median age of ESRD is 53 years for PKD_1 patients as opposed to 70 years in PKD_2 patients. Women had an additional 4 years until ESRD as compared with men (56 versus 52 years). Those patients diagnosed with ADPKD before age 30 developed ESRD at age 49 as compared with age 59 for those diagnosed after age 30. Hypertension does not appear to influence the rate of

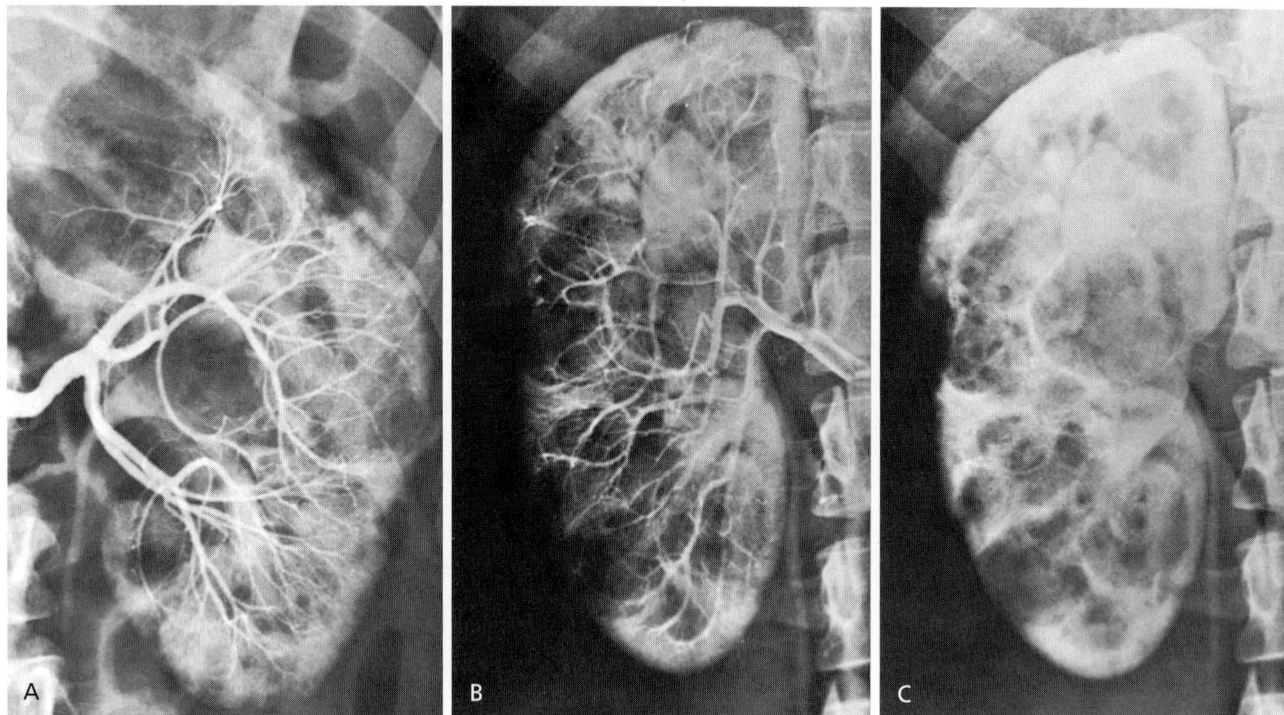

FIGURE 20.5. Autosomal-dominant polycystic kidney disease in two adults. **A:** The arterial phase of renal arteriography in a 23-year-old woman reveals stretching of the vessels around avascular masses in enlarged kidneys. **B:** The arterial phase of renal arteriography in a 30-year-old woman also reveals the intrarenal arterial branches to be stretched, elongated, and displaced by many cysts. **C:** The nephrogram phase of the same arteriogram reveals a mottled or Swiss-cheese appearance in both enlarged kidneys.

progression of renal failure in ADPKD, but the development of hypertension before age 35 reduced renal survival by 14 years compared with those developing hypertension after age 35. Earlier gross hematuria predicted earlier ESRD in ADPKD patients. Although female patients with ADPKD with three or more pregnancies had earlier onset of ESRD, Johnson and Gabow (206) also revealed that this effect was not significant independent of the patient's age at diagnosis and presence of hypertension.

The first sign of kidney failure in ADPKD is the inability to maximally concentrate urine. The renal concentrating defect in ADPKD can develop before glomerular filtration rate (GFR) decreases. There is loss of noncystic parenchyma replaced by fluid-filled cysts in a network of interstitial fibrosis, perhaps secondary to autocrine and paracrine factors (145). The noncystic nephrons compensate by increasing their function so that the GFRs are elevated very early in ADPKD; however, the compensatory mechanisms then fail, and other signs of renal failure follow.

General medical therapy for treatment of chronic renal failure includes low-sodium diets (326) and slowing of the development of osteodystrophy with aluminum hydroxide gel and treating metabolic acidosis. The Modification of Diet in Renal Disease (MDRD) Study revealed minimal benefit of a low-protein diet in ADPKD patients with moderate renal disease (GFR of 25 to 55 mL/min/1.73 m^2) but did suggest the benefit of protein restriction in advanced renal disease (GFR of 13 to 24 mL/min/1.73 m^2) (237).

Factors that predict a greater risk of renal failure include more severe proteinuria, UTIs in male patients, hepatic cystic disease in female patients, African-American race, and sickle cell trait in African-American patients (119). Management should include attempts to treat UTIs. Whether treatment of hypertension alters time of onset of ESRD in ADPKD patients is unknown, although control of blood pressure is necessary to prevent accelerated hypertension and cardiovascular events. Surgical cyst decompression does not slow progression of renal insufficiency in ADPKD (104).

Dialysis and Renal Transplantation

Fifty percent of ADPKD patients will eventually require dialysis or renal transplantation. Surprisingly, effective peritoneal dialysis has not been hindered by the large cystic renal and hepatic masses, hernias, or diverticulitis in ADPKD patients treated by continuous ambulatory peritoneal dialysis (157). When one takes into account ADPKD patients' older age at the time of dialysis, they do as well as other ESRD patients when receiving hemodialysis (18). When on hemodialysis, 5-year survival is 10% to 15% greater in ADPKD patients than in non-ADPKD patients, probably because of lower cardiac mortality in ADPKD patients

(313). Long-term renal dialysis also markedly reduces blood pressure in hypertensive ADPKD patients (326). While on hemodialysis, the prevalence of renal pain, gross hematuria, and renal infection is significantly greater in ADPKD patients, but these complications are rarely severe (313). ADPKD ESRD patients do as well as nondiabetic ESRD patients undergoing renal transplantation in that patient and graft survival are similar (18,113,160). Although Florijn and co-workers (116) found that ADPKD patients are at risk for cardiovascular disease after renal transplantation and Andreoni and colleagues found that ADPKD patients are at risk for gastrointestinal (GI) complications after renal transplantation, others have found no increased risk of coronary events or GI complications in ADPKD after renal transplantation (313). Cysts do not develop in the transplanted kidney in ADPKD patients any more than in other patients after renal transplantation (113). Despite superior results with living-related transplantation for non-ADPKD patients, this has been somewhat limited for ADPKD patients because the disease is familial. However, if an ADPKD patient has two clinically affected family members and if the ADPKD phenotype links with the PKD_1 or less common PKD_2 locus, living-related donors can be found at any age with use of linkage analysis. For the remaining ADPKD patients, living-related donors can be identified by negative radiographic findings when 30 years of age or older or at any age with direct gene-based mutation detection in PKD_2 families. Bilateral pretransplant nephrectomies are not routinely indicated in ADPKD because of high morbidity and mortality (116), but they are indicated in situations of recurrent pyelonephritis, hematuria requiring blood transfusions, and large renal size causing vena caval obstruction or precluding placement of renal allograft into the true pelvis (24).

Urinary Tract Infections

Symptomatic UTIs are common, with an overall incidence of 53% and recurrence rate of 61% in ADPKD patients. Complicated UTIs are less common but difficult to treat. The incidence of renal infection in PKD_2 was half that of PKD_1 (163). Of 23 female patients who had symptomatic UTIs, 12 (52%) had pyelonephritis, of whom 3 developed perinephric abscess (89). Up to 90% of UTIs in ADPKD occur in female patients (357). Urine culture may or may not be sterile, depending on the location of the infection. Sklar and associates (357) divide ADPKD renal infections into three types: (a) acute bacterial interstitial nephritis (infection of the noncystic parenchyma with an unobstructed collecting system), (b) pyonephrosis (infection of upper collecting system, which may be obstructed by stone, blood clot, or compressing cyst), and (c) pyocyst (infected cysts). Although a urine culture should be positive in acute bacterial interstitial nephritis, it may be negative in pyonephrosis and in pyocyst because of the confined infection. Distinguishing between these is helpful in choosing a treatment course. A poor response to antibiotics should suggest either pyocyst or an obstructed urinary tract (pyonephrosis). Infected cysts can be successfully treated with cyst-penetrating antibiotics (333). Failure of prolonged systemic antibiotics to treat infected cysts may make percutaneous puncture and drainage (62,295), laparoscopic decortication and drainage (168), open surgical drainage, or even nephrectomy necessary because of the attendant mortality of infected cysts. The retroperitoneal route of laparoscopic cyst decortication and drainage prevents intraperitoneal contamination and can be guided by laparoscopic US (168). The incidence of serious infections complicating ADPKD seems to be decreasing because the rates of infection (26%), nephrectomy (45%), and death (7%) in a 1983 study of ADPKD patients are higher than the respective rates of 16%, 12%, and 0% in a similar 1996 study (132). Radiologic diagnosis or localization of a pyocyst can be extremely difficult. CT or gallium scan may help localize the infection to a cyst, but ^{111}In leukocyte scanning may prove to be more sensitive in detecting and localizing infected cysts in ADPKD in renal failure (49). In some cases, the presence of debris or echogenic material on CT or US aid in the diagnosis (295). ADPKD patients with renal calculi are three times as likely to have UTIs than those without calculi and the infections are more complicated (242). Obstruction should be ruled out to eliminate pyonephrosis.

Few antibiotics penetrate the cysts, and of those available, fewer still are effective against Gram-negative organisms, which cause the vast majority of UTIs in ADPKD patients. Lipophobic antibiotics such as aminoglycosides, ampicillin, and cephalosporins penetrate cysts poorly but have a favorable activity against Gram-negative enteric organisms (26). Lipophilic antibiotics penetrate all cysts but have varying ranges of activity; examples of such antibiotics include (a) clindamycin or metronidazole for anaerobes; (b) vancomycin or erythromycin for staphylococci or streptococci (357); and (c) chloramphenicol (346), cefotaxime (26), TMP-SMX (105), ciprofloxacin (333), and norfloxacin for Gram-negative enteric organisms. Gibson and Watson (132) advocate initial therapy of complicated UTI in ADPKD patients with intravenous ampicillin and an aminoglycoside, realizing that failure to respond to these antibiotics would suggest a cyst infection because aminoglycosides do not penetrate cysts. Aminoglycosides should be withheld when renal function is compromised. Others recommend initial use of TMP-SMX and fluoroquinolones for infected renal cysts (408).

Urinary tract instrumentation (cystoscopy, retrograde pyelograms, and bladder catheterizations) should be avoided when possible in ADPKD patients because of the high association of infection and mortality despite sterile urine culture before instrumentation. Of 14 ADPKD patients who underwent urinary tract instrumentation, 6 (43%) developed symptomatic UTIs, of whom 3 had pyelonephritis that led to death in 2 despite parenteral antibiotic therapy (89). Most UTIs in ADPKD patients are believed to be ascending in origin and are more prevalent in women. With postmenopausal loss of estrogen protection, the vagina is colonized by Enterobacteriaceae instead of lactobacilli. Recurrent UTIs in postmenopausal women can be minimized by estrogen replacement therapy. Intravaginal estrogen cream may be helpful in postmenopausal ADPKD patients with recurrent UTIs if they do not have significant hepatic cystic disease.

Pain Management

Pain is reported in 61% of ADPKD patients (122) and must be evaluated to rule out obstruction, infection, neoplasms, and hemorrhage. If these causes are eliminated, chronic dull pain from ADPKD can be treated conservatively with analgesics such as acetaminophen. Nonsteroidal antiinflammatory drugs should be avoided because of their nephrotoxic potential. Pain clinics offer a multidisciplinary approach to help with this chronic pain. However, for those chronic pain ADPKD patients for whom such conservative methods have failed (usually a minority), cyst-decompression procedures are helpful. Percutaneous aspiration of three to five dominant superficial cysts under US guidance dramatically relieved pain in 11 narcotic-dependent ADPKD patients for 3 to 6 months (25). Percutaneous cyst aspiration accompanied by instillation with sclerosing agent results in a longer time period of cyst reduction than aspiration alone, but it also is likely to be limited to a lesser number of cysts decompressed as compared with open surgical drainage (384). Open surgical cyst decompression of 100 to 200 cysts per kidney in a 2- to 3-hour operation dramatically relieved pain in 80% of 26 narcotic-dependent ADPKD patients for 1 year and 62% for 2 years (104). Laparoscopic cyst decompression is limited to ADPKD patients with relatively few, but large, cysts because it provides inferior renal volume reduction compared with open surgical cyst decompression, although hospital stays and postoperative recovery are shorter (103). Cyst decortication and nephrectomy have been effectively performed laparoscopically for delayed recurrent pain after cyst aspiration and sclerosis, but only 1 to 62 cysts were decorticated at one sitting (101). Bilateral open transperitoneal cyst-reduction surgery for ADPKD allows drainage of 35 to greater than 1,000 cysts at one sitting with the option of simultaneous treatment of liver cysts by decortication or partial liver resection (115). Cyst-decompression procedures do not worsen or improve renal function in ADPKD patients long term (103).

Calculi

Flank pain in ADPKD can be secondary to obstruction of the urinary tract from clots, calculi, or cysts and is difficult to diagnose. Imaging studies must distinguish between obstructing calculi in the collecting system, renal parenchymal calcifications, and cyst wall calcifications. CT scanning with and without contrast best achieves these goals, and it can differentiate cysts from dilated calyces, which may not be possible on US (242). Levine and Grantham (242) found that CT scanning with and without contrast revealed 36% of ADPKD patients had renal calculi, whereas 25% had cyst calcifications. However, 20% of ADPKD patients were found to have nephrolithiasis when studied by review of IVPs and review of medical records, with nearly equal incidence in men and women (379). In this study, struvite was found in 10% of stones analyzed, although uric acid was found in 57% and calcium (phosphate, carbonate, and oxalate) in 77%; however, only 20% of the ADPKD stone patients had stones available for analysis. A common metabolic abnormality in ADPKD stone patients with normal renal function was hypocitricaciduria, whereas hyperuricemia was common in ADPKD stone patients taking diuretics or those with renal insufficiency (379). In all ADPKD patients (with or without calculi), hyperuricemia has been found in 71% (mean creatinine clearance of 69 mL per minute) and clinical gout in 24%, although the highest serum uric acid levels were found in ADPKD patients with the lowest GFR (268). Three times as many ADPKD patients with renal calculi have UTIs as those without renal calculi (242). There was no significant difference in the incidence of renal tract calculi between men and women or between PKD_1 and PKD_2 individuals (163). Obstructing ureteral and renal calculi have been successfully treated with extracorporeal shock wave lithotripsy (ESWL) (Fig. 20.6) in ADPKD. More than 82% of ESWL procedures were successful in ADPKD patients, but approximately half of them had residual fragments, which is higher than for patients without ADPKD (380). Retrograde procedures such as ureteroscopy with basket extraction, laser fragmentation, and ultrasonic fragmentation have been used successfully but can potentially cause ascending infections. Eighty percent of percutaneous procedures were successful in ADPKD patients (380). Alternatively, appropriate stone surgery can be done.

Obstruction, Hemorrhage, and Tumors

Obstruction of the urinary tract in ADPKD patients can also be caused by renal cyst compression, which can be treated by percutaneous, laparoscopic, or open surgical cyst decompression. Blood clots can also cause obstruction and can usually be managed conservatively. Bleeding in polycystic kidneys can usually be diagnosed by CT and treated with bed rest and observation. Cyst hemorrhage can be confined to the cystic space (causing acute pain), rupture into the collecting system (causing gross hematuria), and/or extend into the perinephric space. Intracyst hemorrhage has been treated successfully with desmopressin acetate and aprotinin administration (225). Severe hemorrhage can be treated by segmental renal artery embolization or percutaneous neph-

A

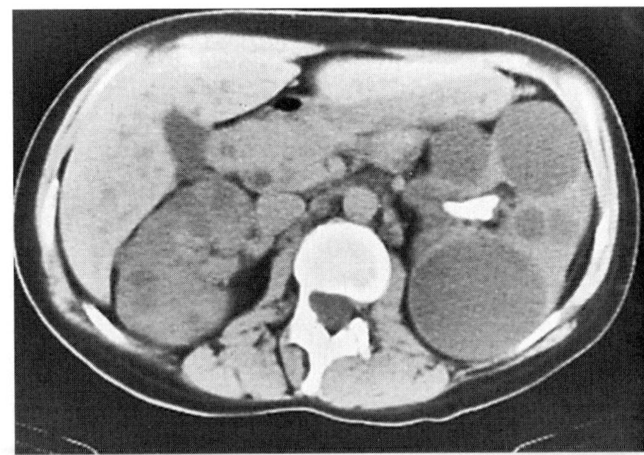

B

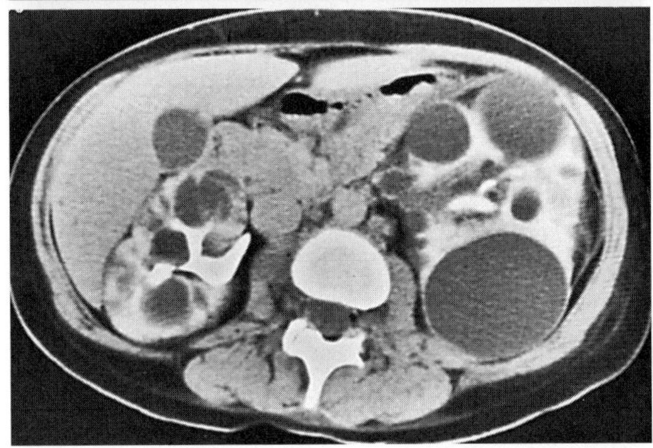

FIGURE 20.6. Autosomal-dominant polycystic kidney disease with left staghorn calculus treated by extracorporeal shock wave lithotripsy (ESWL) in a 31-year-old woman. **A:** Before ESWL, unenhanced computed tomography (CT) scan reveals a left staghorn calculus, bilaterally huge kidneys with multiple cysts of many sizes, and hepatic cysts. **B:** One day after ESWL, enhanced CT reveals no change in the renal cysts from ESWL. The residual gravel cannot be seen because of the contrast.

roscopic balloon occlusion of infundibuli to preserve some renal function in ADPKD patients. Alternatives to control hemorrhage include complete or partial nephrectomy.

RCC must be excluded in ADPKD patients with flank or abdominal pain, intrarenal hemorrhage, or hematuria. However, the risk of unilateral RCC in ADPKD patients is the same as the general population. However, ADPKD patients in renal failure who are receiving dialysis can develop acquired cystic kidney disease, which has a higher incidence of RCC. Both renal arteriography and MRI can help differentiate tumor from cyst (177) (Fig. 20.4).

AUTOSOMAL-RECESSIVE POLYCYSTIC KIDNEY DISEASE (INFANTILE TYPE)

ARPKD includes a spectrum of phenotypic appearances ranging from renal failure in infants to hepatic disease in older children. In addition, newborns with the severe common form of the disease can die of respiratory disorders within a few days after birth. Affected fetuses have bilaterally enlarged echogenic kidneys and oligohydramnios due to poor fetal urine output, usually after 20 weeks of gestation. These infants have the "Potter phenotype" (pulmonary hypoplasia, characteristic facies, and spine and limb deformities) because of their oligohydramnios. The incidence of ARPKD is about 1 in 20,000, with a heterozygosity frequency of 1 in 70 (417). ARPKD is characterized by bilateral cystic disease in enlarged kidneys with retained reniform shape. ARPKD is transmitted in an autosomal-recessive pattern only and is caused by a genetic defect on chromosome 6.

Clinical Features

The clinical picture of ARPKD covers a continuum of presentations of renal failure and hepatic disease developing at different ages and to different degrees. Newborns and infants suffer more from renal failure. Children presenting after infancy are more likely to have liver disease, although a continuum exists.

More than 75% of ARPKD patients present in the newborn period, at which time the child has massively enlarged kidneys (up to ten times normal size) (80,143), causing respiratory difficulties as a result of diaphragmatic elevation and pulmonary hypoplasia. Vaginal delivery may be impeded by the massive kidneys. Most deaths occur in the first month of life and are due to pulmonary atelectasis and respiratory failure from oligohydramnios (351). Survival of all but the most severely affected neonates is now the norm. Approximately 86% of children born with ARPKD are alive at 3 months and 79% at 12 months (214). Oliguria and Potter's facies may be present, but renal failure is not the cause of death. If the child survives the newborn period, he or she most likely will have eventual renal failure and systemic hypertension, which can be particularly severe in the first year of life (123). Seventy percent of ARPKD children require drug treatment for hypertension, which is insufficiently treated in 31.2% of these patients because of its severity (416). Blood pressure elevation is intermittent during the course of the disease. After the first month, growth failure and congestive heart failure are usually the major clinical problems (232). Some patients have secondary effects of chronic renal insufficiency such as anemia, growth failure, and renal osteodystrophy (416).

After the first year of life, the clinical presentation of ARPKD is more variable because of the spectrum of renal failure and hepatic disease. As children with ARPKD grow, the renal cystic dilation can regress as the kidneys become smaller (38). These children can have either slowly progressive renal insufficiency or simply a mild renal functional impairment such as a mild inability to concentrate urine. The percentage of patients with severe renal insufficiency increases with age from 11% at 2 years to 32% at 5 years, 36% at 10 years, 43% at 15 years, and 100% at 20 years (123). Zerres and others (418) showed a statistically significant sex difference in terms of more pronounced progress in girls. Girls with ARPKD had shorter survival probability (82% at 1 year) compared with boys (95% at 1 year) and more girls had impaired renal function, developed ESRD, and showed growth retardation (418). Systemic hypertension is common, but β-blockers and converting enzyme inhibitors are effective (123). UTIs occur in 30% to 43% of ARPKD patients but are more common in girls (43%) than in boys (20%) and occur earlier in girls (418).

However, with time, these older children with ARPKD can develop more severe hepatic involvement. The hepatic disease in ARPKD is called *congenital hepatic fibrosis* (CHF) because the liver has an increase in the number of portal bile ducts and fibrosis of the periportal spaces. Hepatic US can be used to confirm the presence of "biliary dysgenesis" in at least half of ARPKD patients (123). CHF presents clinically as portal hypertension, which can result in massive upper GI hemorrhage from ruptured esophageal varices. More commonly, the children with ARPKD develop splenomegaly as their initial or only sign of portal hypertension due to hepatic fibrosis (317). There is no hepatocellular disease. Caroli's disease (gross cystic dilation of the intrahepatic biliary tree) is often associated with ARPKD, and the two diseases may be overlapping syndromes (416). In this older age group (older than 6 years), CHF, not the renal cystic disease, may be responsible for death. However, the continuum of renal failure and hepatic disease in older children with ARPKD also includes children symptomatic from both kidney and liver disease (266). The clinical cause and

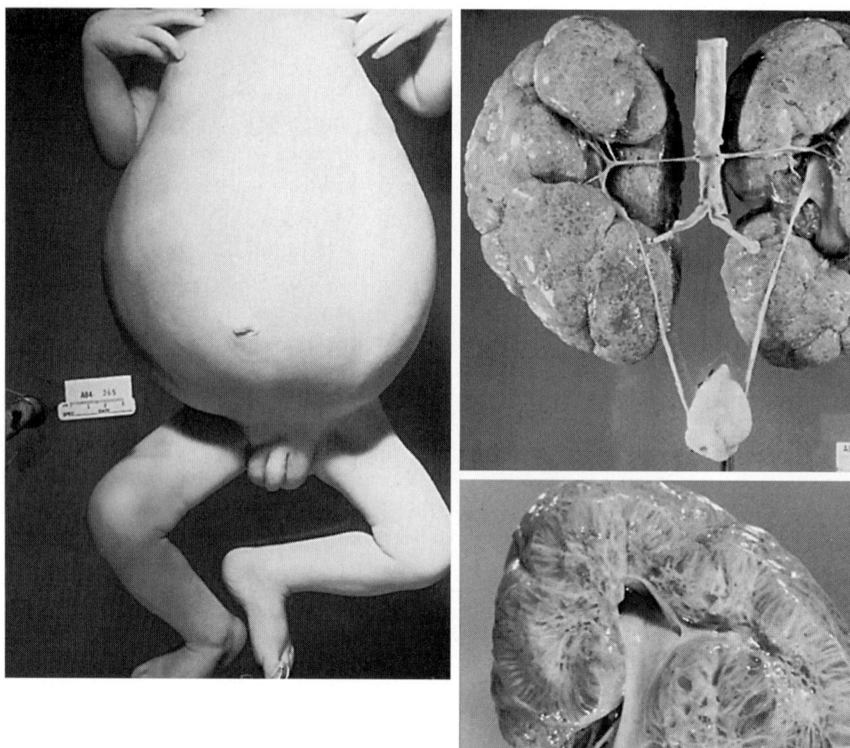

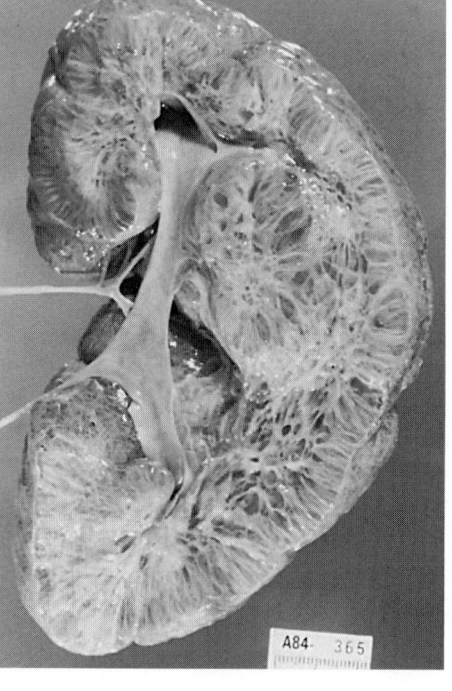

FIGURE 20.7. Autosomal-recessive polycystic kidney disease in a 7-month-old boy. **A:** Abdomen is markedly distended from the massively enlarged reniform kidneys **(B)**, which have minute cysts studding the kidney surface. **C:** Cut section reveals radial arrangement of tubular-shaped cysts. (Courtesy of Dr. S. Bova.)

pathologic expression of renal disease can be entirely dissimilar within the same family (125,173,215).

Morphology

The gross and microscopic characteristics of ARPKD kidneys vary with the age of the child at the time of presentation, but the disease is always bilateral. In newborns with the severe form of ARPKD, gross inspection reveals the kidneys to be adult size and reniform (Fig. 20.7). The kidney surface is smooth and studded with 1- to 2-mm cysts. The cut surface shows a striking radial arrangement of thin-walled channels extending from the pelvis to the cortex. Microscopically, these channels are dilated collecting tubules and ducts, which are the fusiform cysts of ARPKD. Interstitial edema is severe.

In children surviving the neonatal period, the kidneys become smaller, the collecting ducts become less dilated, and the remaining cysts are spherical as opposed to saccular (245). Also, variable degrees of corticotubular atrophy, basement membrane thickening, and interstitial fibrosis are present (173). These findings are also true for children who present with ARPKD after infancy. However, with time, these children are likely to develop CHF (317). Grossly, the liver in CHF is firm and enlarged with a granular surface. Microscopically, there are an excessive number of interlobular bile ducts. The liver is subdivided by bands of fibrous tissue in the periportal and interlobular spaces. Although portal hypertension is commonly attributed to a presinusoidal block because of the portal fibrosis or the portal vein abnormalities, a postsinusoidal block may be present in the same patients (31).

Pathogenesis and Genetics

The pathogenesis is unknown except that it is genetically transmitted as autosomal recessive. Heterozygotes are unaffected. Hence, a very careful family history covering at least three generations should be taken to exclude ADPKD. The ARPKD gene has been localized to chromosome region 6p21. The abnormal DNA results in the development of cysts in the renal collecting ducts, which expand to enormous size because of epithelial cell hyperplasia in the cyst walls and fluid accumulation within cyst cavities (143). Presenting newborns can have 80% of tubules involved, whereas patients presenting during adulthood have less renal involvement (10% of tubules) (351).

Because of the continuum of clinical presentation of ARPKD, four types were described by Blyth and Ockenden (40) with different ages of onset. Each type was to be transmitted as an autosomal-recessive allele and each type was to have occurred in all of the affected children of a family. However, further work has shown that not only do different clinical and pathologic courses occur within one family (125,173,215) but that ARPKD has a spectrum of phenotypic expressions and not just four genetically determined, rigidly defined subgroups (125,245). Deget and colleagues (87) revealed that intrafamilial variability of the clinical picture is small. Zerres and associates mapped the ARPKD gene locus to 6p21 codon in families with a mild ARPKD phenotype, and Guay-Woodford and associated (153) showed the severe perinatal form of ARPKD maps to the same chromosome. Together, these studies suggest there is a single ARPKD gene. Multiple allelism with only a few different alleles would account for the great variability of manifestations in different families and would also explain the relatively high intrafamilial concordance in manifestations (416).

Radiologic Findings

In infants with bilateral palpable abdominal masses, the initial study should be renal and abdominal US (Fig. 20.8). In newborns with the severe form of ARPKD, the kidneys are very large with diffusely increased parenchymal echogenicity. This increased echogenicity is caused by the sound beam bouncing off the innumerable dilated tubules. Some investigators have shown a more heterogeneous pattern with either "striped" or "pepper-and-salt" echoes (404), or a peripheral zone of normally echogenic cortex in some newborns (270). Occasionally, small cysts can be identified in the hyperechogenic medullary areas.

IVPs in infants with ARPKD may show only progressively dense nephrograms of these massive kidneys or may show the classic radial streaking of contrast in dilated collecting tubules. The collecting system is usually not seen, although contrast in the bladder may be seen on delayed films.

In the older child with ARPKD, the IVP pattern is less diagnostic because the kidneys are only somewhat enlarged and the renal pelvis and calyces are better visualized. The calyces may be blunted, or the pyramids may be opacified with a brushlike pattern. There may be an ectasia of the collecting tubules (215). US studies in the older child with ARPKD can demonstrate diffuse hyperechogenicity of the parenchyma or reveal a prominent rim of renal cortex with normal echogenicity surrounded by moderately echogenic medulla (270). Serial US studies in ARPKD patients surviving the neonatal period reveal that kidney size decreases (despite the child's linear growth) and echogenicity changed (38). Disseminated small cysts (less than 15 mm) are often visible and may be present from the neonatal period (123). US evaluation of the liver reveals increased echogenicity, dilated bile ducts, and no discrete cysts (173). CT of the kidneys in ARPKD can reveal accentuation of contrast material on the cortical layers and lacelike medullary cysts (211). CT without contrast commonly reveals bilateral renal calcifications in older ARPKD children with renal failure; however, these calcifications are not recognized on plain film (248). RARE-MR technique (rapid acquisition

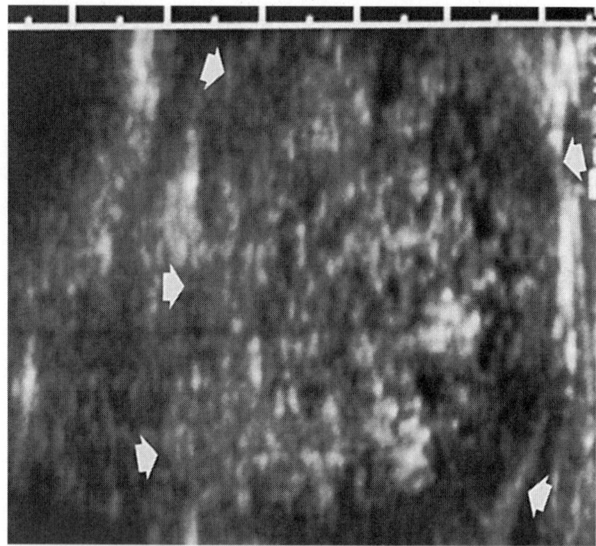

FIGURE 20.8. Autosomal-recessive polycystic kidney disease in newborn. Renal ultrasonography reveals marked renal enlargement with heterogenous pattern and myriad fine cysts. *Arrows* denote renal margin.

with relaxation enhancement) is a noninvasive imaging study that demonstrated the pathognomonic water-filled structures in all of eight ARPKD children evaluated (aged 3 months to 14 years) (219). Both magnetic resonance cholangiography (210) and hepatobiliary scintigraphy (400) have been used to diagnose Caroli's disease in ARPKD patients.

Diagnosis and Management

Families with a severely affected child carry a high risk that additional affected children will be severely affected as well, because intrafamilial variability of the clinical presentation is small (87). Because of the poor prognosis of the severe perinatal form of ARPKD, there is a strong demand for prenatal diagnosis. If a pathoanatomic examination of a previous affected child (liver biopsy or autopsy of fetus) is available, molecular linkage analysis is now feasible for prenatal diagnosis of subsequent pregnancies if DNA analysis of the parents and the one affected child has shown that markers linked to ARPKD are informative. Because direct mutation analysis in ARPKD is not available, correct clinical diagnosis of the first affected child is paramount for accurate prenatal diagnosis of subsequent pregnancies with molecular linkage analysis. The vast majority of families who meet these criteria were informative with the highly polymorphic markers of the ARPKD interval, with precise correlation between the genotype and the predicted phenotype (417). Mücher and co-workers (274) found that the large number of flanking polymorphic loci made genetic linkage-based prenatal diagnosis of ARPKD possible for more than 99% of the families that they analyzed.

In a prenatal differential diagnosis, ADPKD, Meckel's syndrome, and Bardet-Biedl syndrome should always be ruled out. Renal cystic changes can be seen in patients with CHF, which is also autosomal recessive. Adult ARPKD patients who present with mild renal failure can be diagnosed as ARPKD only if they have a negative family history and parents (older than 30 years of age) with normal renal US studies to exclude ADPKD. They can be diagnosed as having ARPKD if they have symptoms of portal hypertension or a liver biopsy revealing hepatic fibrosis (416).

The prenatal US picture of the enlarged kidneys and/or increased echogenicity is characteristic but not pathognomonic (415). Oligohydramnios occurs after 20 weeks of gestation in severe perinatal ARPKD. Related US measurements of kidney length may be the most useful parameter.

US (small renal cysts), liver biopsy (CHF), and family history (recessive inheritance) are usually sufficient to diagnose ARPKD (351). There is no known cure for ARPKD, but genetic counseling can inform parents that siblings of an affected child have a 25% chance of being affected and a 50% chance of being heterozygous carriers. Otherwise, treatment is supportive. Respiratory resuscitation and support may be necessary for newborns diagnosed with ARPKD. When the massively enlarged kidneys restrict diaphragmatic excursion, resulting in respiratory distress in addition to pulmonary hypoplasia, ARPKD newborns may require bilateral or unilateral nephrectomy. Unilateral nephrectomy may improve respiratory status and decrease feeding difficulties without inducing renal failure in ARPKD infants (20). Peritoneal dialysis can be instituted as they await renal transplantation (367). Older children may need antihypertensive medications for hypertension, digitalization for congestive heart failure, and alkali for metabolic acidosis to permit normal growth, as well as other supportive measures for treating renal failure in growing children. Chronic dialysis and renal transplantation may be necessary eventually, but liver involvement should be evaluated first. Jamil and co-authors (200) noted that liver disease did not progress rapidly after initiation of renal replacement therapy and did not subsequently present a clinical problem. Prophylactic portacaval shunting or combined liver–kidney transplantation was unnecessary. Portal hypertension may result from CHF in ARPKD and can be treated by portacaval shunting to treat esophageal varices. However, recurrent bleeding is controllable by sclerotherapy (200).

JUVENILE NEPHRONOPHTHISIS–RENAL MEDULLARY CYSTIC DISEASE COMPLEX

The juvenile nephronophthisis–medullary cystic disease complex (NMCD) consists of a group of hereditary diseases characterized by renal salt loss, renal cyst formation at the corticomedullary junction, and progressive renal failure. These diseases have different hereditary patterns and genetic heterogenicity but share similar clinical features and pathologic features. Both kidneys are small and reniform with small cysts at the corticomedullary junction. NMCD is uncommon, but it is the most common cause of renal failure in the adolescent.

Clinical Features and Genetics

Despite the genetic heterogeneity of NMCD, the pathologic and clinical features are similar except for the age of onset. The autosomal-recessive medullary cystic disease, juvenile nephronophthisis (NPH), affects mostly children and adolescents. The autosomal-dominant medullary cystic disease (ADMCKD) affects mostly adults. Finally, NMCD can rarely occur sporadically with no documented family history but consanguinity of parents should suggest the possibility of recessive inheritance.

NPH results in ESRD at about age 14 years and is the most common form of renal failure in adolescents (126). Because of severe salt wasting secondary to a severe defect in tubular function and the resultant inability to concentrate urine, children or adolescents present with polydipsia, polyuria, and secondary enuresis. Children can also present with growth retardation or skeletal deformity. The salt wasting occurs late in the disease and can be heralded by a decrease of already-present arterial hypertension. However, the polyuria and nocturia can be present for more than 10 years before ESRD occurs (54,60). Both sexes are affected equally. Urinary infections are not common.

Genetic heterogeneity exists within NPH (Table 20.4). Nephronophthisis type 1 (NPH_1, autosomal-recessive medullary cystic disease) has been mapped and localized to chromosome 2q12-13 (8). Within this region, the gene $NPHP_1$ was identified; this gene is deleted in more than 65% of patients with NPH_1 (175). NPH_1 is the most common type of NPH and NMCD. However, patients with the rare Senior-Løken syndrome (renal-retinal syndrome, autosomal-recessive medullary cystic disease, or NPH with retinitis pigmentosa) do not link to chromosome 2q12-13 (8). In addition, Gagnadoux and colleagues (124) described a group of infants who reached ESRD before 2 years of age with pathologic features similar to those of NPH. This disorder has been designated "infantile nephronophthisis" (NPH_2). Haider and associates (159) identified linkage of NPH_2 to chromosome 9q22-31 in a family with an autosomal-recessive mode of inheritance. Affected individuals developed hypertension, hyperkalemia, and rapid deterioration of renal function with ESRD by 3 years of age. There is emerging evidence that a third locus (NPH_3) exists for adolescence onset recessive nephronophthisis (176).

The autosomal-dominantly inherited disease, medullary cystic disease, is less common than juvenile nephronophthisis and results in ESRD at about 32 years of age (126). Many ADMCKD patients are hypertensive at an early stage of the disease, but some later develop hypotension due to excessive salt wasting. Polyuria and polydipsia are less intense in ADMCKD than in NPH. Some ADMCKD patients have gout and/or hyperuricemia (362). Christodoulou and associates (71) localized a gene ($ADMCKD_1$) for ADMCKD to chromosome 1q21 in two large Cypriot families. Affected family members also had hyperuricemia and gout, with a mean onset of ESRD at 62.6 years of age. Scolari and colleagues (347) described a second locus for medullary cystic disease, $ADMCKD_2$, on chromosome 16p12 in a large Italian family. Affected family members had hyperuricemia, gouty arthritis, and an average onset of ESRD at age 31.5 years. Diagnostic criteria for ADMCKD include (a) autosomal-dominant inheritance; (b) defective urine-concentration with polyuria, isosthenuria, and relatively normal urinalysis results; (c) normal or small-sized kidneys with occasional small medullary cysts; and (d) renal pathologic findings characterized by tubular-interstitial fibrosis (347). A third locus ($ADMCKD_3$) is possible (176).

Landing and colleagues (232) were correct that *medullary cyst disease* is not the name of a specific disease but is a useful term for a lesion that occurs in the later stages of several different genetically determined and other types of tubulointerstitial disease.

TABLE 20.4. NMCD COMPLEX—KNOWN LINKAGES

Disease	Inheritance	Chromosome	Mean Age Onset of ESRD
NPH_1	AR	2q12-q13	13 yr
NPH_2	AR	9q22-q31	7.8 mo
$ADMCKD_1$	AD	1q21	62.2 yr
$ADMCKD_2$	AD	16q12	31.5 yr

AD, autosomal dominant; ADMCKD, autosomal-dominant medullary cystic kidney disease; AR, autosomal recessive; ESRD, end-stage renal disease; NMCD, juvenile nephronophthisis–medullary cystic disease complex; NPH, nephronophthisis.

Morphology and Pathogenesis

On gross inspection, both kidneys in NMCD are contracted and pale with granular subcapsular surfaces. On cut section, there is poor demarcation between the medulla and the attenuated cortex. The cysts are actually diverticula of the distal convoluted tubules. When the cysts are macroscopic, they are typically located on cut section at the corticomedullary junction. They can range from microscopic to 1 cm in size. Cysts are usually present but occasionally are not especially early in the disease. Cysts are more common in ADMCKD than in NPH.

Microscopic examination reveals glomerular sclerosis, tubular atrophy, and interstitial fibrosis with chronic inflammation. The tubular basement membrane is markedly thickened. Without the presence of cysts, the pathologic findings resemble those of interstitial nephritis. Indeed, NMCD has been considered a primary interstitial nephritis by some (53). Therefore a renal biopsy can be misleading if the corticomedullary cysts are missed in the biopsy specimen. Such biopsy specimens have been diagnosed as chronic interstitial nephritis initially but were changed because a later examination of the entire kidney from a subsequent nephrectomy or autopsy may show the medullary cysts (53,318). Renal biopsies may also not reveal the cysts if the biopsies are done early in the disease.

The pathogenesis of NMCD is unknown, except that it can be genetically transmitted. The gene product of $NPHP_1$, nephrocystin, may play a role in the protein–protein interaction (e.g., in signal transduction at focal adhesions, the contact points between cells, extracellular matrix). A defect in cell–matrix interaction would help explain the tubular membrane disruption in NPH (176). Perhaps a tubular basement membrane defect causes the early occurrence of the decreased urine-concentrating ability. Both NPH and ADMCKD may be the results of defects in the same developmental or metabolic pathway. Potential similarities in mutated genes may result in similar phenotypes (71).

Radiologic Findings and Management

Radiographic findings vary with the stage of progression of NMCD. Occasionally, an IVP early in the disease may reveal characteristic patterns either as streaky contrast enhancement or ring-shaped retention of contrast material in the corticomedullary region (288). More commonly, an IVP reveals normal findings early in the disease but shows bilaterally small kidneys later in the disease, at which time high-dose nephrotomography could reveal renal cysts (332). However, an IVP is of little value very late in the disease when renal function is greatly reduced. US has been shown to reveal cysts in the corticomedullary zone ranging from 2 to 10 mm in size in both patients with early and late NMCD (288). US reveals disappearance of the corticomedullary differentiation at all but the early stages of NMCD as well as small kidneys and increased parenchymal echogenicity (128,332). Although US may not show cysts until later in the disease (39), thin-section CT may (106). US, CT, or both could complement renal biopsy to diagnosis NMCD if the cysts were missed on biopsy but revealed by US or CT.

Treatment of NMCD is directed toward general therapy for renal failure. If salt wasting is present, it can be treated with salt supplementation. Control of hypertension and a low-protein diet may prolong normal kidney function if patients are diagnosed early as a result of linkage data and available flanking markers (71). Dialysis and transplantation are successful. However, recognition of genetic variants is vital to avoid selecting a living donor for transplant who is personally at risk of developing the disease (13). Molecular genetic diagnosis of NPH_1 can be performed by demonstration of the presence of deletions or point mutations of the $NPHP_1$ gene (176). In addition, if glomerular cysts are found on renal biopsy, the patient should undergo liver biopsy before renal transplant to rule out hepatic disease. Hepatic disease has occasionally been associated with juvenile nephronophthisis, more commonly if glomerular cysts are found on renal biopsy. Because hepatic fibrosis can lead to portal hypertension, hepatic biopsy should be considered before renal transplant (33).

RENAL CYSTS ASSOCIATED WITH MULTIPLE MALFORMATION SYNDROMES

Renal cystic disease, macroscopic to microscopic, has been found in some hereditary disorders. Knowledge of these disorders is important for genetic counseling.

Chromosomal Disorders

Patients with trisomy 21 (Down syndrome), trisomy 18 (Edward's syndrome), trisomy 13 (Patau's syndrome), and trisomy C can develop microscopic cysts, usually of the glomerular spaces of the renal cortex.

Autosomal-recessive Syndromes

Renal cystic disease is commonly found in Meckel's syndrome (MKS) or Meckel-Gruber syndrome (occipital encephalocele, hepatic fibrosis, renal cystic dysplasia, and polydactyly) (176), in Jeune's syndrome (asphyxiating thoracic dystrophy—small chest and renal dysplasia), and in Zellweger's syndrome (cerebrohepatorenal syndrome—high forehead and hepatomegaly). The prognosis of MKS is guarded in cases with onset of renal insufficiency in the neonatal period. Two gene loci have been mapped for MKS (Table 20.2). MKS_1 is localized in 17q21-q24 (294) and MKS_2 is localized on 11q13 (334). Zellweger's syndrome is associated with renal microcysts and an almost complete lack of peroxisomes in renal tubular epithelial cells and defects in several peroxisomal enzymes (370). Renal cystic changes have been less commonly reported in a few other autosomal-recessive syndromes such as Goldston syndrome (cerebral malformations), Majewsky and Saldino-Noonan types of short rib polydactyly, lissencephaly (microcephaly, smoothness of the brain, and cystic renal dysplasia), and the Elijalde syndrome (acrocephalopolydactylous dysplasia—gigantism and renal dysplasia).

X-linked Dominant Syndrome

Renal cystic disease occurs later in life in the orofaciodigital syndrome, type I, and somewhat resembles ADPKD.

Autosomal-dominant Syndromes

Tuberous sclerosis (TSC) and von Hippel–Lindau disease (VHL) are most likely to require the attention of a urologist as opposed to the other multiple malformation syndromes. Hence, both autosomal-dominant syndromes are described in detail.

Von Hippel–Lindau Disease

VHL (cerebroretinal angiomatosis) is caused by a genetic defect in the short arm of chromosome 3 and results in renal cysts and clear-cell renal carcinomas as well as retinal angiomas; cerebellar, medullary, and spinal hemangioblastomas; pheochromocytomas; islet cell carcinomas, cystadenomas, and cysts of the pancreas; cystadenomas and cysts of the epididymis; and endolymphatic sac (inner ear) tumors (133,244,258). The disease is inherited as autosomal dominant with a high penetrance of more than 90% by age 65 (252). Most manifestations of VHL do not become apparent until after the patient has reached the end of his or her second decade. However, retinal angiomatosis often is the earliest manifestation and has been found in an asymptomatic patient as young as 9 years of age (239). Cerebellar hemangioblastomas were once the most common cause of death in VHL. As more patients survive the cerebellar lesions as a result of improved treatment methods, the incidence of renal cysts and renal tumors in patients has increased (304), such that RCC accounts for 50% of deaths in VHL and is the most common cause of death (216). In one study, CT of the abdomen and brain and indirect ophthalmoscopy were done as screening examinations on family members at risk. Of those who were diagnosed as having VHL, 35% had RCC and 76% had renal cysts (239). RCC was found only in those patients who had renal cysts (118,239). Unlike RCC in patients who do not have VHL, RCC in patients with VHL occurs in younger patients, has an equal sex distribution, and is usually bilateral and multicentric (304). These RCCs can invade locally and distantly metastasize (31).

The VHL gene maps to chromosome 3p25-26 (233). The VHL gene functions as a recessive tumor-suppressor gene, and inactivation of both alleles on the VHL gene is the critical event in the pathogenesis of VHL neoplasms (79). The allele from the affected parent has been inherited as mutated, and the wild-type allele from the nonaffected parent has been sporadically inactivated in the VHL neoplasms. If one or both alleles are unaffected, the VHL gene encodes proteins responsible for negative regulation of cell growth. Mutations of both alleles results in loss of functions of the encoded proteins with resultant uninhibited cell growth and malignant transformation. The VHL protein (pVHL) inhibits the stimulatory effects of Elongin on transcription by binding to the Elongin B and C subunits of this protein (279). Mutated pVHL cannot compete for binding to Elongins B and C and therefore regulation of transcriptional elongation is lost resulting in tumor growth. The VHL protein downregulates vascular endothelial growth factor (VEGF) (414). The mutated VHL gene upregulates VEGF so that clear-cell renal carcinomas, hemangioblastomas of the eye and CNS, and papillary cystadenoma of the epididymis secrete large amounts of VEGF, causing new blood vessels to infiltrate these tumors, which become hypervascular (236,279). Wild-type VHL is required for exit from the cell cycle, so RCC cells with mutant VHL continue to proliferate because they cannot exit the cell cycle (414). The VHL protein also is responsible for proper assembly of the extracellular fibronectin matrix and regulates expression of carbonic anhydrases 9 and 10 (414). Chromosome 3p allele loss was found in RCC, hemangioblastoma, pheochromocytoma, and pancreatic tumors, suggesting a common mechanism of tumorigenesis in all types of tumors in VHL disease (79).

Renal Lesions of VHL

The renal cysts of VHL are multiple and bilateral and are lined by variably hyperplastic epithelium. Benign renal cysts with clear-cell cytologic features were found only in kidneys of VHL patients (395). By extrapolating from microscopic evaluation, VHL kidneys have an estimated 1,100 cysts with clear-cell lining and 600 clear-cell solid neoplasms per kidney (395). The mean volume of these renal lesions was 0.46 mm^3. Hence, a constant morphology exists as the cysts grow. Clear-cell renal lesions in VHL patients ranging from cysts to microscopic RCC to macroscopic RCC show the loss of the VHL gene (247). Nodular hyperplasia within the cyst walls have been observed progressing to clear-cell carcinoma (28). DNA quantitative studies reveal that both the RCCs and the atypical cyst lining cells have the same DNA indices in VHL, suggesting that the atypical cyst lining cells evolve into RCC (189). However, serial CT renal imaging of VHL patients revealed that the majority of solid RCCs appeared to arise *de novo* and were not initially cystic (68). Conversion from cystic to solid lesions did occur in this serial CT renal imaging study but was not the predominant sequence of events in the development of RCC in VHL.

Loss of function of the VHL disease gene may be the initial event in the renal cellular transformation that results in the development of clear-cell cysts and tumors. It is unknown whether benign cysts with clear-cell lining progress to RCC or if benign cysts with clear-cell lining, atypical cysts, and renal clear-cell carcinomas represent different accumulations of genetic defects (315).

Genotype–phenotype Correlations

Differences in phenotypes in VHL patients can be secondary to either variable mutations in the single VHL gene or the effects of other modifying genes but not mutations in genes other than the VHL gene on chromosome 3p25-26. Therefore allelic heterogeneity and not locus heterogeneity can account for differences in VHL phenotypes. VHL can be caused by many different mutations in the VHL gene, with more than 162 different intragenic mutations described (279).

VHL germline mutations can be divided into those that produce truncated VHL proteins (type I) or those that produce intact VHL proteins with a change in a single amino acid (missense mutations) (type II) (65). Type I VHL patients may have retinal angiomas, spinal and cerebellar hemangioblastomas, pancreatic cysts, and kidney cancer. This is the most common form. Type II VHL patients may develop pheochromocytomas in addition to the tumors in type I (65,398). Type II families represent 7% to 20% of VHL families and rarely have renal and pancreatic cysts. Type II can be subdivided into certain VHL mutations with a low risk of clear-cell renal carcinomas and CNS lesions (type IIa) and high risks of clear-cell renal carcinomas and CNS lesions (type IIb). Type IIb is least common. No specific germline VHL mutation is associated with retinal angiomas or endolymphatic sinus tumors (414).

However, even related VHL family members with identical germline mutation can have variation in disease severity. Other genes may modify the effects of germline VHL mutations, such as the number of retinal angiomas in VHL patients (402). In addition, the greater the number of retinal angiomas, the greater the problem with RCC and hemangioblastoma later on.

Diagnosis, Screening, Surveillance, and Management

If the patient has a family history of VHL, the diagnosis is made if an individual has a single manifestation of the disorder as clear-cell renal carcinoma, retinal angioma, or pheochromocytoma (414). Also, multiple pancreatic cysts are uncommon in the general population and would be satisfactory for a VHL diagnosis in an at-risk individual, unlike renal and epididymal cysts (253). If there is no VHL family history, the diagnosis of VHL should be considered in an individual with two or more retinal or cerebellar hemangioblastomas; a single hemangioblastoma and a visceral tumor; familial or bilateral pheochromocytoma; familial, multicentric, or early-onset clear-cell renal carcinoma; or bilateral endolymphatic sac tumors (253). Recently, the frequency of VHL germline mutations in individuals with a single VHL manifestation without a VHL family history has been investigated with the following results: 1.6% of patients with sporadic renal carcinoma had a germline VHL manifestation, as did 2.5% to 5% of patients with an isolated retinal angioma (414). Germline VHL mutations are rare in isolated cases of pheochromocytoma but occur in 50% of patients with isolated familial pheochromocytoma or bilateral pheochromocytoma with no VHL family history (327). Some had been misdiagnosed as multiple endocrine neoplasia type 2.

Genetic linkage analysis with microsatellite flanking markers has been widely used in presymptomatic diagnosis in VHL families but is not possible for relatives of isolated cases or in families where necessary samples are not available (327). The cloning of the VHL tumor-suppressor gene has enabled direct mutation testing for VHL families. Once a patient is diagnosed as being affected, all at-risk relatives should be tested for the mutation because early detection of RCC and retinal hemangioblastoma significantly reduces morbidity and mortality. Prenatal diagnosis is possible. Annual physical and ophthalmologic examinations begin in infancy in individuals diagnosed with VHL. About 50% of VHL patients will have only one manifestation of the disease. Imaging of the abdominal organs and brain and spine should be added in teenagers and adults.

Radiographic evaluation of renal lesions in VHL is useful for screening family members and for following patients once they have been diagnosed as having VHL. IVP can reveal several mass lesions, but it cannot differentiate cysts from tumors. CT can reveal solid mass lesions and many reveal renal cysts, but it cannot differentiate between a small cyst and a small tumor, nor can it find a small tumor in the wall of the cyst. Thin-section (3 to 5 mm) contrast-enhanced CT is mandatory, and spiral geometry is desirable to decrease the chances a lesion is missed (69). US and, sometimes, angiography can fail to detect these small masses (239). US is critical to help determine whether a lesion is principally solid or cystic (69). CT scans can evaluate the adrenal glands for pheochromocytomas and the pancreas for islet cell carcinomas, cysts, and cystadenomas (186,244). Sequential CT studies are most sensitive in finding renal tumors before they become large enough to metastasize. However, a substantial proportion of renal lesions smaller than 1 cm were not detected by CT or US in VHL patients (201).

Annual studies are recommended once a diagnosis of VHL is made (216). MRI is especially useful in patients with renal failure in whom screening for RCC is still necessary (69). Contrast-enhanced MRI can be useful in determining whether a lesion is principally solid or cystic.

Annual CT renal imaging of VHL patients with renal lesions is recommended to determine the size and growth rate of the lesions and thus the appropriate management. Management can include continued observation, renal parenchymal sparing surgery, or nephrectomy. Bilateral nephrectomy can result in dialysis or renal transplantation. Walther and colleagues (397) noted no renal lesions 3 cm or smaller that metastasized in VHL patients. Renal parenchymal-sparing surgery was undertaken when the largest renal lesion reached 3 cm, at which time all visible tumors were resected from that kidney with use of intraoperative US to localize any additional tumors to be removed (397). Enucleation technique can be used because as many as 53 lesions have been removed from one kidney and lesions less than 3 cm have not been observed to penetrate this boundary, although they have invaded it (315). Because the remaining renal parenchyma in VHL patients has a high number of remaining microscopic lesions (395), these patients must be imaged annually with CT scans after renal parenchymal sparing surgery to detect when the largest residual renal lesion becomes radiographically evident and reaches 3 cm in size. At that time, nephrectomy or repeat parenchymal-sparing surgery can be considered. Excellent long-term survival is observed when partial nephrectomy is used to remove VHL renal lesions when technically possible regardless of lesion size (363). Despite a 51% local tumor recurrence in these VHL patients treated by partial nephrectomy when technically feasible, only 2 of 25 had concomitant metastatic disease and renal function was well preserved (363).

In VHL patients with renal lesions not amenable to renal parenchymal-sparing surgery or with local recurrence after such surgery, bilateral nephrectomy may eventually be necessary. Steinbach and others (363) noted that 23% of VHL patients eventually developed ESRD after treatment for localized RCC. Management options for ESRD in the VHL population includes dialysis or renal transplantation. Renal transplantation is attractive in these relatively young ESRD patients, but the risk of immunosuppression in VHL patients with multiple potential tumors must be considered. Goldfarb and associates (139) demonstrated no statistically significant difference in graft survival, patient survival, or renal function after renal transplantation in well-selected VHL patients compared with control patients without VHL. Of the 32 VHL patients, 3 died of metastatic RCC within 45 months of transplantation. For those VHL ESRD patients after bilateral nephrectomy for RCC with higher tumor stage (pT_3 and above) or large tumor burdens with a symptomatic presentation, waiting 2 years after nephrectomy to confirm that no metastatic disease develops before proceeding with renal transplantation seems reasonable. However, in VHL ESRD patients after bilateral nephrectomy for RCC that is low stage and was incidentally discovered, no waiting period may be necessary before renal transplantation.

Evaluation of living-related renal donors for VHL patients can now be performed with direct mutation testing to evaluate presymptomatic carriers of the VHL gene. A thorough evaluation is essential for all prospective living-related donors to VHL recipients.

Pheochromocytoma in VHL patients can be managed by either partial adrenalectomy or adrenalectomy (396).

Epididymal cystadenomas were found in 54% of VHL male patients screened by scrotal US (70). Two-thirds were bilateral. Their clinical course is benign, and scrotal US is useful for diagnosis (133). Surgical excision is necessary only if the lesions become symptomatic.

The care of VHL patients requires a multidisciplinary team and urologists need to be familiar with the nonurologic manifestations of VHL.

Tuberous Sclerosis

TSC is an autosomal-dominant disorder caused by a genetic defect on either chromosome 16 or 9; it results in the presence of hamartomas, which are benign tumors composed of cellular elements normally present in tissue. The CNS lesions of TSC include tubers (cortical dysplasia) in the cerebral cortex that can cause mental retardation, epilepsy, and autism. In addition, patients may have facial angiofibromas, renal AMLs, renal cysts, retinal hamartomas, ungual fibromas, bone tubers, and cardiac rhabdomyosarcomas. In patients with TSC, renal causes of death are second only to CNS causes (352).

Genetics

Although TSC is inherited as an autosomal-dominant trait with high penetrance, two-thirds of TSC patients have no family history of TSC and probably represent new mutations (sporadic cases from new mutations). Mutations in two different genes can result in the TSC phenotype, meaning that TSC exhibits locus heterogeneity. The TSC_1 gene is located at 16p13.3 and was cloned in 1993 (108). The TSC_2 gene is located at 9q34 and was cloned in 1997 (389). About 50% of TSC families link to TSC_1 and about 50% to TSC_2 (282,316). However, TSC_2 mutations are much more common in sporadic cases than TSC_1 mutations (12,229), so TSC_2 mutations are the more common genotypes. Most studies found no observable differences between TSC_1 and TSC_2 patients (229,282), although other studies found a higher incidence of mental retardation in TSC_2 patients than in TSC_1 patients (207) and a higher incidence of intellectual disability in TSC_2 sporadic cases than in TSC_1 sporadic cases (208). Complete clinical screening of the parents of supposedly sporadic cases reveals one of the parents to be a mosaic mutation carrier 10% of the time (391).

The TSC_2 gene encodes the protein tuberin, and the TSC_1 gene encodes the protein hamartin. Hamartin and tuberin directly interact, suggesting that they are components of a singular cellular pathway, which explains why TSC_1 and TSC_2 mutations have such similar phenotypes (389). Both TSC_1 and TSC_2 seem to act as tumor-suppressor genes because both germline mutations are inactivating and loss of allelic heterozygosity at 16p13 or 9q34 occurs in AMLs and rhabdomyomas in TSC patients (148,350). Loss of heterozygosity suggests that a TSC patient inherits (or spontaneously acquires through mutation) a deletion in one copy of the gene but develops lesions such as renal AMLs only when there is a somatic mutation in the other copy.

TSC_2, the more common gene causing TSC, and PKD_1, the gene causing 85% of ADPKD, are located a few nucleotides apart on chromosome 16 in a tail-to-tail orientation. Deletions involving both TSC_2 and PKD have been identified in a small subset of TSC patients with early-onset, multiple renal cysts and/or early renal failure (50). Thus the loss of TSC_2 and PKD_1 together describes a contiguous gene syndrome with a more severe infantile form of cystic disease than that found in TSC patients without loss of PKD_1 and a much earlier age of onset than normally found in ADPKD. Perhaps mutations of TSC_2 and PKD_1 have an additive or synergistic effect. The age of onset of renal failure in the TSC_2–PKD_1 contiguous gene syndrome sometimes varies significantly within the same family because of genetic mosaicism (338) (Fig. 20.9).

Renal Manifestations of Tuberous Sclerosis

Renal disease is the second most common cause of death in TSC patients after CNS causes (352). Common renal lesions are AMLs and renal cysts. Less common renal lesions are RCC and malignant epithelial AMLs. ESRD has been reported in 1% to 15% of TSC patients (67,74,345).

Renal Angiomyolipomas. AMLs are benign tumors consisting of variable proportions of fat-containing cells, smooth muscle cells, and arterial vessels whose thickened walls lack normal elastic tissue. AMLs have been detected in 49% (78) to 47% (364) of TSC patients but are a rare finding in the general population. Of TSC patients with AMLs, 91% had multiple lesions and 84% had bilateral AMLs, unlike the solitary AMLs in the general population (78). The incidence of AMLs increases with age in TSC patients (78), which supports the "two-hit" genetic process because the chance of somatic mutation of the second allele increases with age. AMLs in both TSC_1 and TSC_2 phenotypes have been observed to demonstrate loss of heterozygosity, which supports the idea that TSC_1 and TSC_2 act like tumor-suppressor genes (148,350). Other factors such as hormones modify the development of AMLs because pregnancy can accelerate AML growth and has been associated with rupture and hemorrhage of renal AML (96). In addition, AMLs in the general population are more common in women, AMLs in girls have a greater propensity for growth than in boys, and the larger renal AMLs occur after puberty (110). Henski and associates (171) found that 48% of renal AMLs in TSC patients (3 men and 18 women) had progesterone receptor immunoreactive smooth muscle cells but none contained estrogen receptor immunoreactive cells. Pulmonary lymphangiomyomatosis (LAM) is rare and is associated with TSC. It can have estrogen receptor and progesterone receptor immunoreactive smooth muscle cells (27). Female TSC patients with LAM can present with pneumothorax and hemothorax. The activity of the pulmonary lesions of LAM patients varies with physiologic hormonal changes and hormonal manipulation, so hormonal treatment can prolong survival and pulmonary disease (42).

The elastin-poor vascularity of AMLs makes them prone to hemorrhage into the retroperitoneum. Increasing AML size correlates with higher risk of retroperitoneal hemorrhage (91,385). AMLs are usually symptomatic if larger than 8 cm, but they tend to be asymptomatic if smaller than 4 cm (91). Rare instances of spread of AMLs to regional lymph nodes or into the inferior vena cava have been described, but no patient has had progression to widely disseminated disease (96). With regular screening of TSC patients, the incidence of AMLs may increase because routine US surveillance of affected children revealed 57% (mean age of 6.9 years) to have AMLs (110).

Renal Cysts. Renal cysts have been found in 32% (78) to 43% (278) of TSC patients. When children with TSC were routinely screened with renal US, 10% were found to have renal cysts at initial screening (mean age of 6.9 years), but 17% were found to at follow-up (mean age of 10.5 years) (110). Simple cysts may appear or disappear in children with TSC (110). Renal cysts and AMLs tend to occur in the same patients with cysts antedating the AMLs (278). Renal cysts are usually asymptomatic. Features of TSC may present after or before the renal cysts. Although rare, renal failure in TSC is more likely to occur in patients with renal cysts (287). Children presenting with early-onset multiple renal cysts and/or early-onset renal failure may have the TSC_2–PKD_1 contiguous gene syndrome (50). When 60 children with TSC were screened with renal US, polycystic kidneys as in ADPKD patients were seen in only 1 patient. The histopathologic studies of renal cysts distinguish between TSC and ADPKD because the renal cysts of TSC have eosinophilic cells in their hyperplastic epithelium (361).

Renal Malignancies. RCC has been described at a higher incidence in TSC patients than in the general population. TSC-associated RCC occurs at a younger age, is more likely to be bilateral, and is more likely to occur in women as opposed to sporadic RCC in the general population (31,399). Bjornsson and colleagues (36) described loss of heterozygosity in both TSC_1 and TSC_2 RCCs, indicating that increased risk is associated with both genotypes. Pea and associates (303) found alleged cases of TSC-associated RCC that were incorrectly diagnosed and concluded that RCC is less common in TSC than previously thought. Some cases called *TSC-associated RCC* were probably malignant epithelioid AMLs, and they suggested that all reported TSC-associated RCCs be reevaluated.

Renal Failure. ESRD has been reported in 1% to 15% of TSC patients (67,74,345). ESRD in TSC is more common in females than in males (80% versus 63.1%) (74,345). Reduction in the amount of functioning renal parenchyma secondary to nephrectomy, partial nephrectomy, and/or arterial embolization to remove malignancies or control hemorrhage, as well as replacement of renal parenchyma by AMLs and RCCs, was thought to be contributory in 32% to 40% of patients (74,345). Renal failure more commonly occurs in TSC patients with renal cysts (287). Although renal failure occurs earlier in TSC_2–PKD_1 contiguous gene syndrome, age of onset of ESRD is variable, even within the same family, and may not occur before the third decade because of genetic mosaicism (338). Clarke and associates (74) noted that on imaging, 4 of 10 TSC patients with ESRD had polycystic kidney disease.

Pathology

The pathologic findings vary with the degree of cystic involvement in TSC. Grossly, the kidneys can be enlarged, with cysts projecting throughout the renal cortex bilaterally. On cut section, multiple cysts (microscopic to 5 cm) are found throughout the cortex and medulla. Microscopically, renal cysts of TSC are easily differentiated from other renal cysts because of their hyperplastic epithelium of eosinophilic cells (361). Microdissection shows that cysts develop from all parts of the nephron.

Radiologic Findings

An IVP can reveal calyceal distortion and renal enlargement resulting from either the renal cysts of TSC or from the renal AMLs (76). US can differentiate the cysts from the hamartomas (Fig. 20.9). The AMLs appear sonographically as regions of increased echogenicity because of the presence of fat. In contrast, the cysts appear as anechoic lesions varying in size from 2 mm to 2 cm with thin uniform posterior walls and posterior enhancement (278). However, US cannot differentiate the renal cysts of TSC from those of ADPKD (unless multiple hepatic cysts are demonstrated, which would confirm the diagnosis of ADPKD). CT scanning can also demonstrate both the AMLs and the cysts of TSC. Demonstration of fat within the AML on CT makes the diagnosis of AML possible. In small AMLs (4 mm), detection of fat is difficult to achieve because of volume averaging, which makes CT confirmation of AMLs difficult. The detection of fat on US is far easier. Because all lesions seen on CT are detected by US, US is the preferred screening procedure for renal lesions of TSC (278). The renal angiographic manifestations of TSC consist of multiple AMLs, multiple renal artery aneurysms, renal cortical cysts, or some combination of these.

Management

A majority of TSC patients develop renal involvement, and a minority have significant morbidity. A baseline renal US in all TSC patients should be routine. Cooke and others (78) suggest serial renal US in TSC patients with no renal lesions and every 1 to 2 years in TSC patients with renal lesions. If there is any concern about a lesion, CT or MRI scan is appropriate. If extensive renal involvement is noted, renal function should be evaluated.

Any female TSC patient with AMLs should be monitored closely during pregnancy with renal US evaluations to allow for early diagnosis and intervention in renal hemorrhage. Female TSC patients should be cautioned about pregnancy and hormone replacement therapies. AMLs larger than 8 cm should be treated electively with arterial embolization or partial nephrectomy because most will cause complications if left untreated (91). AMLs smaller than 4 cm can be serially imaged because they are usually asymptomatic (91). AMLs between 4 and 8 cm have an unpredictable natural history because they are symptomatic 54% of the time (91). Modifying factors such as pregnancy potential should be taken into account, and patient counseling to recommend serial imaging versus elective renal sparing therapy is needed. TSC patients presenting with acute retroperitoneal hemorrhage from AML should be offered immediate arterial embolization to spare renal parenchyma (161).

MULTICYSTIC KIDNEY (MULTICYSTIC DYSPLASIA)

Multicystic kidney disease (MCDK) is the most common cause of an abdominal mass in the newborn. Although present at birth, a unilateral multicystic kidney can be clinically silent throughout adulthood. However, bilateral MCDK is fatal at birth because of insufficient renal function. The involved kidneys do not maintain a reniform shape but are replaced by clusters of cysts with fibrotic tissue. MCDK is a form of renal dysplasia and is rarely a genetically transmitted disorder (360).

Clinical Features

A multicystic kidney is present from birth but may be detected as early as 15 weeks *in utero* by prenatal US (365). Prenatal US has made *in utero* diagnosis the most common presentation of a multicystic kidney. The second most common presentation is in newborns as an asymptomatic abdominal mass that is mobile, irregular, and located in the flank and that may be transilluminated (394). Of those children diagnosed as having a MCDK, 90% were diagnosed before 1 year of age (365). A multicystic kidney is considered the most common or the second most common abdominal mass in the newborn, with congenital hydronephrosis as the alternative diagnosis (150). The widespread use of routine prenatal US has led to the observations that *in utero,* a multicystic kidney can involute and disappear. When the multicystic kidney disappears prenatally, the newborn is diagnosed as having unilateral renal agenesis, which may explain the cases of unilateral renal agenesis with an ipsilateral blind ending ureter (187). Postnatal follow-up US examinations in children with a unilateral multicystic kidney reveal that in the children followed 1 to 3 years, 47%

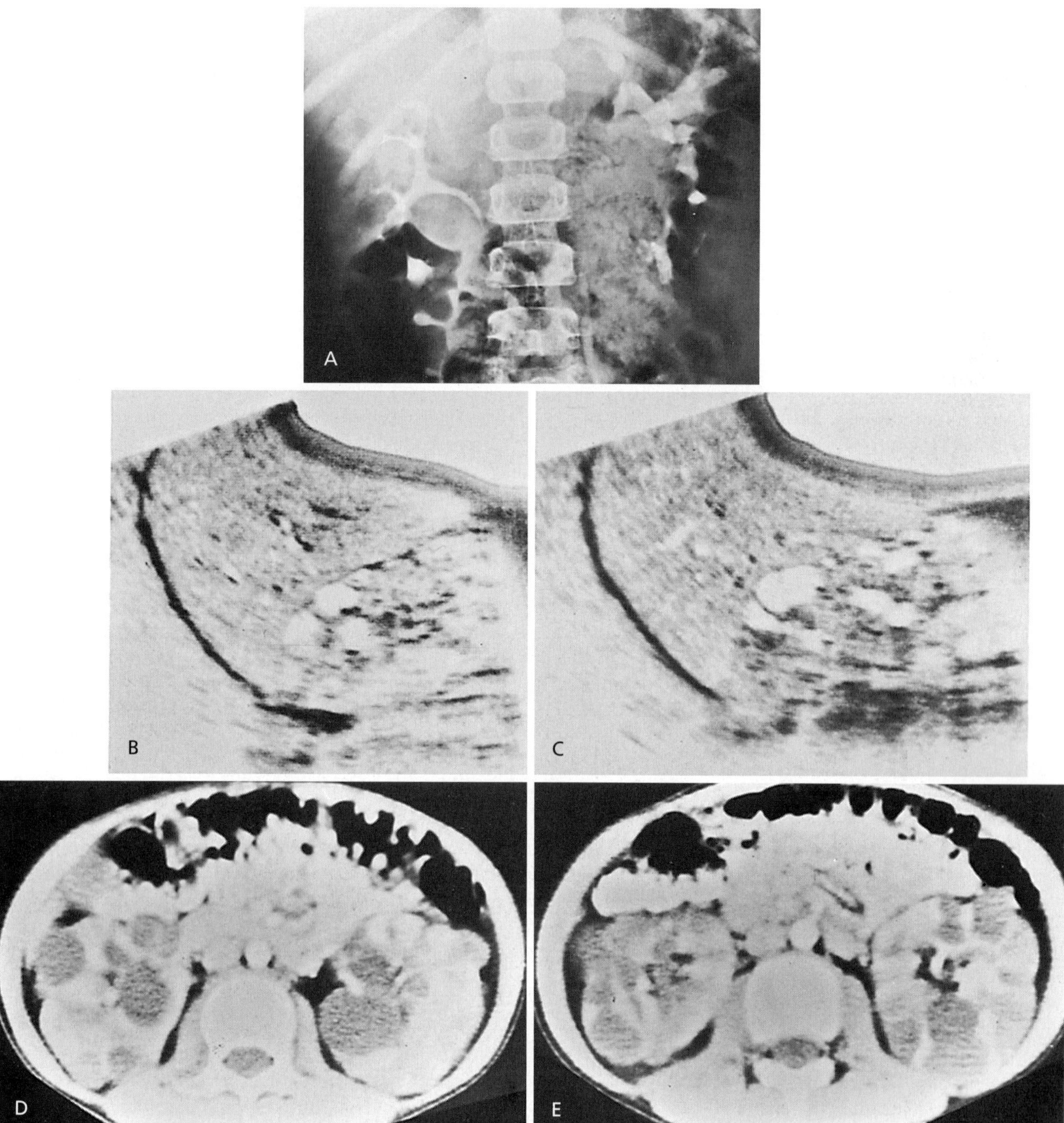

FIGURE 20.9. Tuberous sclerosis in a 10-year-old boy whose two brothers and mother were also affected. **A:** Intravenous pyelogram (IVP) reveals distortion of the collecting systems bilaterally. The splaying of the calyces could be secondary to either cysts or hamartomas. **B, C:** Renal ultrasonography reveals multiple cysts in both kidneys. **D, E:** Enhanced computed tomography reveals bilateral multiple renal cysts but no hamartomas. The presence of cysts can precede the presence of hamartomas. He had a seizure disorder, hypertension, and facial adenoma sebaceum. These radiologic findings in such a patient are typical for the TSC_2-PKD_1 contiguous gene syndrome.

of the kidneys decreased in size but were still detectable and 13% disappeared. In those children followed 3 to 5 years, 23% became undetectable on follow-up US (392). Over 4.5 years, White and associates (405) noted that 17% of MCDK kidneys involuted at a mean rate of 1.02 cm per year and 30% decreased in size at a mean rate of 0.38 cm per year, although they were still detectable. Twenty-six percent of MCDK kidneys grew at a rate of 1.16 cm per year over the 4.5 years. John and colleagues (205) noted that 48% of their MCDK patients had complete involution over 2.6 years, 32% had partial involution, and 4% (one child) had increase in size. Occasionally, a transient increase in size of a multicystic kidney would be followed by involution.

Contralateral compensatory hypertrophy has been noted in older MCDK patients regardless of whether or not the patient had a nephrectomy (151). When the length of the contralateral kidney is measured at birth in MCDK neonates, hypertrophy [defined as kidney length above 2 standard deviation scores (SDS)] was found in 24%, showing that hypertrophy starts *in utero* and continues throughout childhood (205). The other 76% of the MCDK neonates had renal lengths between mean and +2 SDS. All of the contralateral kidneys in MCDK children grew at a rate greater than normal (405). Length and volume of the contralateral kidney had the most remarkable increase during the first 6 months of life (205). The presence of abnormalities of the contralateral kidney did not affect the increased renal volume (205). Size increase, size decrease, or removal of the multicystic kidney did not alter the increased growth rate of the contralateral hypertrophy (405).

In older children and adults, a unilateral multicystic kidney can be found incidentally during radiographic study being done for unrelated reasons (230). A unilateral multicystic kidney can be entirely asymptomatic in these older patients or cause abdominal pain. Resultant imaging studies to evaluate the abdominal pain result in the diagnosis of MCDK (4,359).

Indications for Nephrectomy

Surgical exploration to confirm the diagnosis of a multicystic kidney is not necessary with the current use of renal US and radionuclide renal scans. Therefore indications for nephrectomy are controversial but include hypertension, infection, pain, increasing size, and malignancy. Renin-mediated hypertension in MCDK has been established. Of 441 cases reported to the multicystic kidney registry, no case has been documented with hypertension as a causative factor (392). Serial blood pressure measurements in MCDK patients followed for approximately 4 years revealed no cases of hypertension (205,405). Although hypertension is rare in MCDK, reported cases of hypertension in patients with MCDK who were treated by nephrectomy resulted in resolution of the hypertension in pediatric patients (7,107, 202) and not in adult patients (4).

Rudnik-Schöneborn and colleagues (336) found that 6 of their 204 MCDK pediatric patients required treatment with antihypertensive drugs for their hypertension. Two of the children had hypertension secondary to concomitant cardiovascular diseases, two children had spontaneous resolution of their hypertension after 6 months, one developed hypertension after nephrectomy, and one had no resolution of hypertension after nephrectomy.

Nephrectomy has rarely cured hypertension of long or unknown duration. Therefore, if patients with a MCKD are to be managed by surveillance, evaluation for hypertension must be rigorous (107) so that patients with hypertension and a multicystic kidney may benefit from a nephrectomy.

Infection involving a multicystic kidney is very rare (392) and is therefore not an indication for a prophylactic nephrectomy. UTIs may occur in patients with a multicystic kidney because of associated vesicoureteral reflux, which is more often contralateral than unilateral (114). Neither nephrectomy nor conservative management prevented the predisposition to UTI as a complication of MCDK (336). Although exceedingly rare, nephrectomy is appropriate therapy for an infected multicystic kidney (324). Pain is an indication for nephrectomy in a symptomatic patient, but this is uncommon. If the unusual circumstance of extraordinary growth of the multicystic kidney is noted over significant time or if the enlarging kidney is causing discomfort or feeding difficulty, nephrectomy is recommended (405).

Although nodular renal blastoma has been reported in multicystic kidneys (283), the development of malignancy in multicystic kidneys is so rare that prophylactic nephrectomy is unwarranted (21,392). There is a threefold to tenfold risk of Wilms' tumor compared with that in the general pediatric population (309). The mean age of presentation of MCDK children with Wilms' tumor is younger than the typical 3 to 4 years in the general pediatric population, with a mean age of 25 months (309). Screening renal US studies every 3 months up to 8 years of age is recommended to adequately screen MCDK patients for Wilms' tumor.

The Contralateral Kidney

Bilateral multicystic kidneys are less common than a unilateral multicystic kidney and are incompatible with life. Approximately 23% of fetuses with a multicystic kidney diagnosed by routine prenatal US screening were found to have bilateral disease, which is a higher incidence than that reported of births with a multicystic kidney (3,235). Bilateral disease can be associated with Potter's syndrome in which facial dysmorphia, pulmonary hypoplasia, and amnion nodosa all result from prolonged hydramnios, which results from low urinary output (47).

Males are more likely to be affected in unilateral MCDK than females at a ratio of 2.4 : 1, but females are twice as likely to have bilateral MCDK (235). Rarely, MCDK can involve only a portion of a kidney, such as in a kidney with a duplicated collecting system, when the segmental MCDK typically occurs in the upper pole with atresia of the upper moiety of proximal ureter and reflux into the ipsilateral functioning lower moiety (203). Although rarely reported, ipsilateral cystic dysplasia of the testis has been associated with MCDK (329). However, because cystic dysplasia of the testis is asymptomatic and boys with MCDK do not undergo routine scrotal US screening, this lesion may be more common than is currently believed.

The prognosis of patients with a unilateral multicystic kidney depends on the status of the contralateral urinary tract, irrespective of the removal of the multicystic kidney (88). Current imaging of patients with a multicystic kidney reveal that 39% have contralateral abnormalities (vesicoureteral reflux, 18%; ureteropelvic junction obstruction, 12%), 6% have bladder wall abnormalities, and 6% have ipsilateral reflux (11). If voiding cystourethrography is routinely performed as part of the initial evaluation on all infants with a multicystic kidney, 18% to 28% are found to have contralateral vesicoureteral reflux despite a normal renal US of the contralateral kidney in most cases (114,405). Vesicoureteral reflux grades I through IV were present, with 50% spontaneous resolution or downgrading to reflux grade I in 50% of patients over 2 to 4.5 years (336). Therefore careful study of the contralateral kidney is most important in evaluating a patient with a unilateral multicystic kidney and should include voiding cystourethrography because the prognosis is otherwise excellent.

Morphology

A multicystic kidney can appear grossly as a disorganized patternless mass of variably sized cysts. The calyces and pelvis are not recognizably present grossly, and the reniform shape may not be evident. Usually, part or all of the ureter is atretic. The vascular pedicle may be atretic (93). Microscopically, immature ducts, ductules, and glomeruli, along with cysts and islands of cartilage, reside within fibrous stroma or cellular mesenchyme. Mature glomeruli may be present, although rare. The cysts are lined by low cuboidal epithelium. Contrast injection into the cysts reveals communication between the cystic spaces via tubular structures (138,344).

Pathogenesis and Renal Dysplasia

A multicystic kidney is a category of renal dysplasia in which the kidney is totally affected and cystic. Serial US examinations have revealed a multicystic kidney to decrease to a small noncystic mass (dysplastic kidney) or even to complete disappearance (aplasia) (365). The appearance by US changes from a predominant cystic dysplasia to predominant dysplasia as first the cysts involute and then the kidney decreases in size. Hence, these forms of renal dysplasia can be considered as a heterogeneous continuum of totally or segmentally involved kidneys, which may be cystic, solid, or both.

The diagnosis of renal dysplasia is made from recognizing histologic criteria thought to represent the aborted remnants of the ureteral bud or its poorly induced progeny (371). Such histologic findings include primitive glomeruli, ductules, tubules, cartilage, and primitive ducts. However, all of these features except for the primitive ducts can also be found near renal scars or in renal inflammation. Hence, primitive ducts are the only noncontroversial histologic evidence of embryonic renal maldevelopment (112).

An association exists between renal dysplasia and urinary tract obstruction. Is the cause of the obstruction (e.g., a malfunctioning ureteral bud or its branch) also the cause of dysplasia in the associated kidney or segment (371)? Support is found in the association of unilateral renal dysplasia with unilateral ureteral obstruction, bilateral renal dysplasia with posterior urethral valves, and segmental renal dysplasia with segmental obstruction. Furthermore, although the severity of the renal dysplasia relates to the severity of obstruction, the severity of both could relate to the degree of malfunction of the ureteral bud.

A defect in the ability of the branching ureteric duct and the undifferentiated metanephric blastema to communicate appears to be the basic underlying principle for the formation of dysplasia (263). Cellular communication between the ureteric duct epithelium and the metanephric blastema cells involves cellular "cross-talk" using a network of ligands and receptors on both cell types. For example, hepatocyte growth factor is expressed predominantly in the metanephric blastema, while its receptor is localized in the ureteric bud epithelium, supporting the role of the ureteric duct as inducer of the metanephric mesenchyme (263). The multicystic dysplastic kidney likely begins with a normally determined stem cell population. Aberrant expression of genes involved in the cascade of renal differentiation could result in a renal malformation. A single gene mutation may alter the ability of the ureteric bud and metanephric blastema to communicate or to respond appropriately to their reciprocal signals (263). The final phenotypic expression of MCDK may be dependent on the dysregulation or altered expression of genes that have been affected by the primary gene defect.

The high incidence of contralateral renal defects associated with the isolated multicystic dysplastic kidney is more suggestive of a generalized defect in normal induction of kidney development than of an acquired unilateral insult (263). About 24% of MCDK fetuses diagnosed by prenatal US screening have bilateral disease (3,235), suggesting a common pathophysiologic mechanism. Numerous inherited syndromes with renal malformations, such as cystic dysplasia, have been described with known specific gene and protein defects. However, the variable penetrance of renal cystic dysplasia suggests that other genes may modify normal organogenesis (263). Associated nonrenal anomalies occur in up to 26% of unilateral MCDK patients and in 67% of instances of bilateral MCDK, suggesting an embryonic developmental field defect (235). Recent molecular techniques are expanding the understanding of the pathogenesis of MCDK.

Radiologic Findings

The frequency of the diagnosis of a multicystic kidney has increased because of the use of fetal US. A second-trimester US study is more likely to diagnose MCDK than late-trimester studies because the late-trimester studies may not identify the affected involuted kidney, thus altering the diagnosis to unilateral agenesis of unknown etiology (235). The accuracy of diagnosis in children has improved with the addition of radionuclide scanning to the point that the combination of US and renal scanning is so accurate that additional radiologic imaging is unnecessary. However, older patients may be diagnosed by other studies. A multicystic kidney appears as a nonfunctional mass on IVP. Contralateral compensatory hypertrophy occurs in 72% of children older than 2 years by US criteria (365). Because differentiation between a multicystic kidney and congenital hydronephrosis is necessary in evaluating an infant with a palpable abdominal mass, US features unique to a multicystic kidney have been described (366). The most useful criteria are (a) the presence of interfaces between cysts, (b) nonmedial location of the largest cyst, and (c) absence of an identifiable renal sinus (Fig. 20.10). Other confirmatory but not necessarily unique features on US are multiplicity of cysts that do not communicate and an absence of parenchymal tissue. Radionuclide scanning with Tc-99m DPTA reveals that 96% of multicystic kidneys demonstrate no uptake and that 4% have faint crescents of activity on delayed images (365). However, if Tc-99m DMSA is used as the tracer, 15% of MCDK kidneys show low-grade uptake, which correlates with the presence of mature cortical tissue found at nephrectomy (328). Renal angiography may show an absent or hypoplastic renal artery with no nephrogram (Fig. 20.11). Doppler US of the ipsilateral renal artery reveals marked abnormality of the waveform in a multicystic kidney (169). A retrograde urogram might reveal an atretic or absent ureter. CT is not commonly done on infants because of the requirement of prolonged periods of time without movement. However, when CT of a multicystic kidney in adults is performed, a small cystic kidney with or without calcifications can be revealed because the multicystic kidneys identified in adults tend to be smaller. Percutaneous injection of contrast material into cysts of multicystic kidneys in children has revealed communication between cysts (138,344).

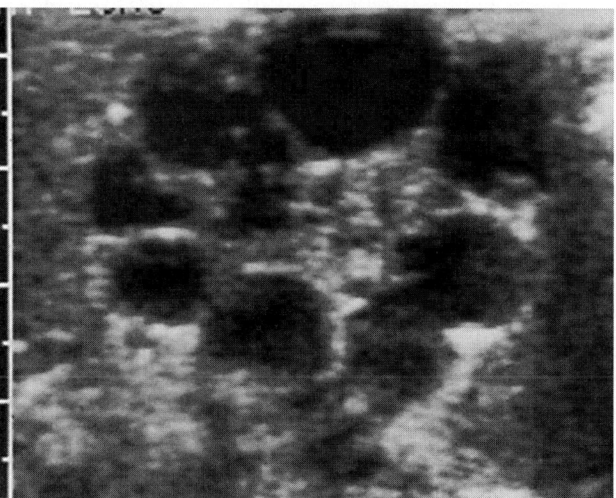

FIGURE 20.10. Multicystic kidney disease in female newborn. Renal ultrasonography at 1 week of age reveals multiple cysts in the right flank with septation between the cysts but no normal renal parenchyma. No communication was identified between the cysts, as would be present with hydronephrosis. The left kidney (not shown) was found to have ureteropelvic junction obstruction.

Management

In the past, multicystic kidneys were routinely removed for pathologic diagnosis. However, the characteristic appearance on US plus nonfunction on radionuclide scanning allow for an accurate diagnosis without nephrectomy. Prophylactic nephrectomy is probably not indicated for pain, infection, hypertension, or malignancy because of the rarity of these disorders. However, surveillance by US and blood pressure measurements of these patients must be maintained to discover the rare cases of hypertension and malignancy.

Serial renal US studies every 3 months until age 8 have been recommended to make a diagnosis of Wilms' tumor at an early stage because of its fast growth rate (309). Monthly abdominal examinations by the parents may be as effective at diagnosing Wilms' tumor, with renal US examinations at 6 months and every 1 to 2 years thereafter until the multicystic kidney has involuted and the contralateral kidney is deemed normal.

Voiding cystourethrography should be performed as part of the initial evaluation in infants with multicystic kidneys to diagnose vesicoureteral reflux because of the risk of scarring in a solitary functioning kidney. Prophylactic antibacterial therapy is necessary until the reflux resolves spontaneously (at about 20 months of age in most of these patients) (114). Evaluation of the contralateral kidney is essential. Nephrectomy for the rare patient with pain, hypertension, malignancy, infection, or respiratory embarrassment is appropriate although US-guided percutaneous cyst decompression has been reported to definitively treat respiratory embarrassment secondary to a multicystic kidney (181). Nephrectomy for the rare young patient with

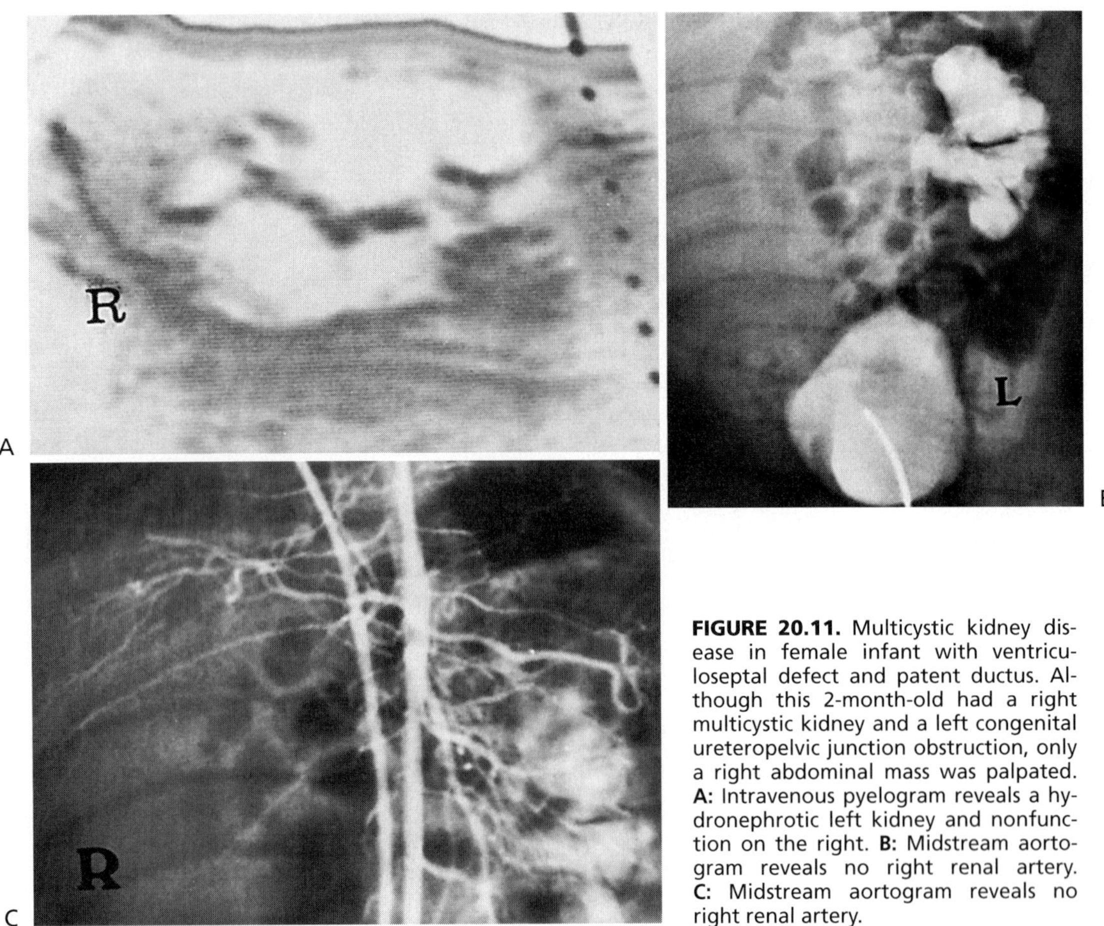

FIGURE 20.11. Multicystic kidney disease in female infant with ventriculoseptal defect and patent ductus. Although this 2-month-old had a right multicystic kidney and a left congenital ureteropelvic junction obstruction, only a right abdominal mass was palpated. **A:** Intravenous pyelogram reveals a hydronephrotic left kidney and nonfunction on the right. **B:** Midstream aortogram reveals no right renal artery. **C:** Midstream aortogram reveals no right renal artery.

extraordinary growth of a multicystic kidney may be appropriate (405).

CYSTIC NEPHROMA (MULTILOCULAR CYSTIC KIDNEY)

Cystic nephroma (CN) is a very rare benign cystic tumor of the kidney that is usually unilateral and compresses the adjacent normal renal tissue. Hence, although CN is listed as a cystic disease of the kidney, CN does not diffusely replace normal renal parenchyma bilaterally; instead, it compresses normal renal tissue unilaterally. CN is rare, with fewer than 200 cases reported (2). Children and adults are affected with equal frequency. The cysts are limited to the area of the kidney involved with the mass and vary in size from a few millimeters to 5 cm. The tumor is completely cystic, with no solid nodules.

Clinical Features

Although children and adults are affected equally with CN, 73% of cases occurring in children younger than 4 years of age are in boys; in contrast, 89% of cases in patients older than age 4 are in females (251). Children present with a nonpainful abdominal mass, whereas adults present with a symptom such as abdominal pain or hematuria. When hematuria does occur, it is usually associated with herniation of CN into the renal pelvis. CNs often replace substantial portions of the kidney and commonly herniate into the renal pelvis (251) or renal sinus (220). The cystic mass has been observed to grow slowly in some patients (3 years) and rapidly in others (2 months) according to sequential physical examination (251). These lesions primarily occur in whites, males before age 24 months, and females between 40 and 70 years of age (59).

Eble and Bonsib (96) consider CNs in children as a different entity than CNs in adults, despite similar radiographic features. Their review concludes that tumors in young children that have been classified as CN as well as those classified as cystic partially differentiated nephroblastoma (a rare cystic benign-behaving type of Wilms' tumor) represent a single entity. Both should be considered highly cystic Wilms' tumors with little or no capacity for invasion or metastasis, and both should be classified as cystic partially differentiated nephroblastoma. Both are currently treated the same regardless of whether elements of Wilms' tumor are found, so there is no need to distinguish between the two entities. Hence, Eble and Bonsib (96) conclude that the diagnosis of CN should no longer be applied to young children.

However, CN in adults has no connection to Wilms' tumor but is a benign cystic tumor that may rarely become malignant with secondary development of a sarcoma (96). Distinguishing CN from other extensively cystic renal neoplasms is not possible from preoperative imaging studies or fine-needle aspirates of these neoplasms (34,96). Intraoperative frozen-section analysis cannot always reliably distinguish CN from cystic RCC (34). Multilocular cystic lesions of the kidney are classified as Bosniak class 3 complicated cysts (17) in which imaging cannot distinguish malignancy from benign cystic lesions. Only 12% of RCCs are predominantly cystic, but these cystic RCCs have a slower growth rate, are identified at earlier stages and lower grades, are associated with a better prognosis and longer survival, and are even more likely to occur in males (96%) than conventional RCC (34). Fortunately, partial nephrectomy and radical nephrectomy are both effective treatments for both CN and cystic RCC because preoperative imaging and fine-needle aspirates cannot distinguish between the two entities and intraoperative frozen-section analysis could not identify malignancy in 3 of 8 cystic RCCs (although permanent sections could) (34).

Morphology and Pathogenesis

The pathologic criteria for establishing a diagnosis of CN were reformulated in 1956 by Boggs and Kimmelstiel (41). The criteria include (a) a multilocular mass, (b) no communication between cysts, (c) cysts lined by epithelium, (d) no communication between the cyst and pelvis, (e) remaining kidney essentially normal, and (f) no normal nephrons in the septa of the cysts. Joshi and Beckwith (209) further reformulated the criteria by specifying that the (a) tumor is composed entirely of cysts and their septa; (b) CN is a discrete well-demarcated mass; (c) septa are the sole solid component and conform to the outlines of the cyst without expansive nodules; (d) cysts are lined by flattened, cuboidal, or hobnail epithelium; and (e) septa contain fibrous tissue in which well-differentiated tubules may be present.

Grossly, the multilocular cystic mass is well circumscribed by a thick capsule and compresses normal adjacent renal tissue. Bilateral lesions are rare. Cut surface reveals multiple noncommunicating cysts, varying from a few millimeters to 5 cm in diameter. Microscopically, the cysts are lined by flattened or cuboidal epithelium. All cases of multilocular cystic kidneys have shown uniformly benign behavior. In adults, stromal septa have pronounced cellularity with a spindle cell pattern sometimes seen. Sarcoma was found in the septal stroma in 4 of 21 adults, with 3 of them developing metastasis containing the stromal element (251). These patients might have had multilocular sarcomas of the kidneys (59). The chemical content of the cyst fluid is similar to that of serum (1). The pathogenesis of CN is not known except that there is no familial tendency and that it behaves like a tumor in its growth and local recurrence. CN is not of developmental origin but is a cystic neoplastic lesion. The lack of normal renal tissue in its septa distinguishes CN from contiguous simple cysts and from congenital renal cystic disease with multiple cysts.

Radiologic Findings and Management

IVP of CN usually demonstrates an intrarenal mass in a normally functioning kidney. US can well visualize the multicystic nature of the tumor when the septa are seen to divide the mass into multiple loculi of regular distribution and similar size (129). CT reveals a cluster of cysts with thick walls and calcifications. However, when the cysts are small, it is more difficult for CT to confirm the cystic component of the mass (298). The septa on CT enhance with intravenous contrast medium (Fig. 20.12). MRI with gadolinium enhancement reveals enhancement of internal septa in all CN patients studied (220). Renal angiography usually reveals a hypovascular mass, sometimes with a tumor blush and neovascularity (2,251). Cytologic evaluation of cyst fluid is of limited value (2). In general, thickening of the septum to more than 1 mm, the presence of a solid component, calcification in the lesion, and neovascularity are potent signs of malignancy when imaging cystic renal tumors (82). However, US, dynamic CT, and dynamic MRI could not reliably distinguish between malignant and benign cystic tumors (178). Renal angiography was the most reliable imaging modality in distinguishing cystic RCC from benign cystic lesions by the presence or absence of tumor vessels (178), but neovascularization has been found in 20% of CNs (251).

Therefore surgical intervention is the only effective method to differentiate CN from a malignant lesion of the kidney. A preoperative diagnosis of CN versus cystic partially differentiated nephroblastoma is of little importance because chemotherapy and radiotherapy are not used to treat either, renal-sparing surgery can be appropriate for both if technically feasible, and the two can be considered the same entity in young children (96). Nephron-sparing surgery did not result in local recurrence with 3-year follow-up (59). Complete excision of childhood CN or cystic partially differentiated nephroblastoma is possible as conservative surgery, but special care must be taken to excise the cystic lesion that penetrates the renal pelvis (66). Because radiographic methods cannot rule out malignancy, a partial nephrectomy is adequate only after the surgeon has confirmed there is no malignancy in the surgical specimen pathologically, although histopathologic confirmation by frozen section can be wrong (34,337). Cystic RCC has such a favorable prognosis that conservative surgery is appropriate, as it is for CN if technically feasible (34). Treatment by nephrectomy is appropriate after assessment of the

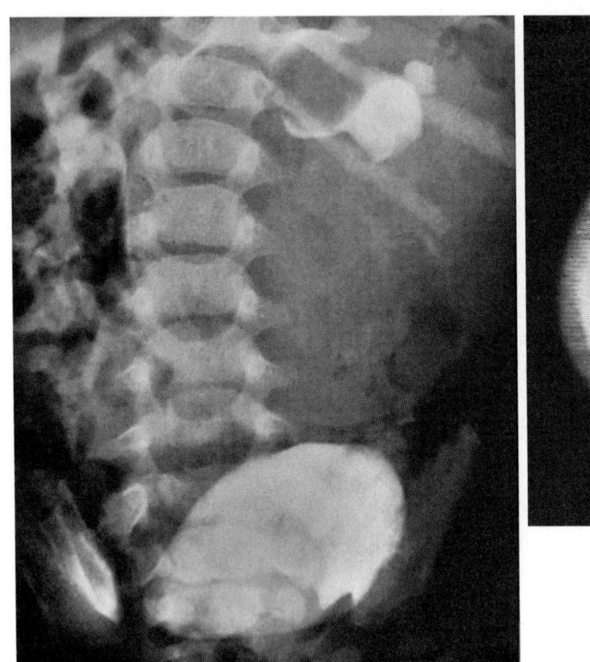

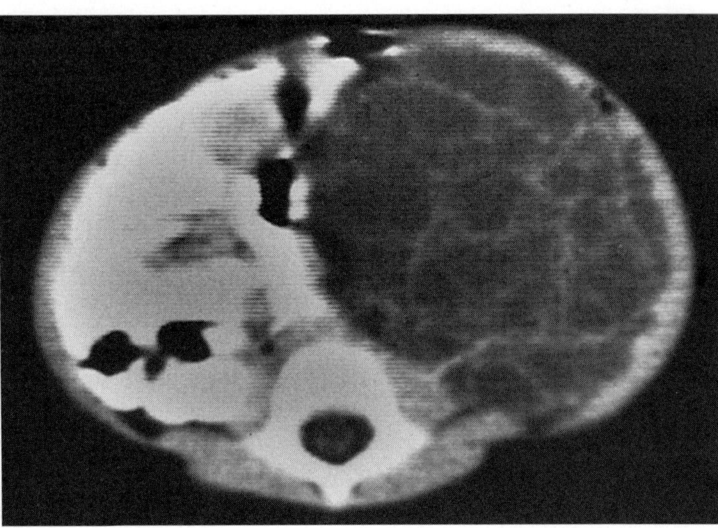

FIGURE 20.12. Cystic nephroma in a 4-year-old boy. **A:** KUB shows mass effect. **B:** Computed tomography scan with contrast reveals enhancing septa.

status of the contralateral kidney although bilateral cases are rare (66).

SIMPLE RENAL CYSTS AND COMPLEX RENAL CYSTS

Although simple cysts are an entity in their own right, concern regarding simple renal cysts is usually directed toward their differentiation from neoplastic renal masses because they are so frequently discovered as an incidental finding on radiographic studies. Indeed, 24% of routine abdominal CT scans in one study (234) and 20% in another (369) revealed unexpected simple renal cysts. Analyzing the data separately in both CT studies, 0% to 6% of patients younger than 40 years were found to have simple renal cysts, as opposed to 18% to 19% of patients 40 to 60 years of age and about 31% of patients older than 60. However, at autopsy, at least 50% of patients older than 50 years of age have grossly recognizable cysts of the renal parenchyma (223). Another autopsy study revealed a 39% overall incidence of renal cysts but a greater than 50% incidence in patients older than 50 (323). Forty-eight percent of patients had cysts less than 1 cm in diameter. These smaller cysts could have been missed by CT or US, which probably explains the discrepancy in frequency. By CT and US, the number of cysts per patient and the cyst diameter increased with the age of the patient (234,321). Such data suggest that simple renal cysts are acquired abnormalities, perhaps related to the aging process; however, the pathogenesis is unknown. They are not familial.

Renal Cysts in Children

Simple renal cysts are rare in children but may be detected at any age (373). A fetal simple renal cyst can rarely be identified by US in early pregnancy, but in the absence of associated anatomic or chromosome abnormalities, most fetal renal simple cysts will resolve during pregnancy without any sequelae (37). Before the routine use of IVP, US, and CT in children, the most common presentation of renal cysts in a child was that of an asymptomatic abdominal mass. However, in more recent series of pediatric patients, simple renal cysts were incidental findings on radiographic studies (19,141) with a reported frequency of 1 simple cyst for every 430 abdominal US studies performed (267).

Cyst Growth

Simple renal cysts are by definition unilocular, do not communicate with the collecting system, occur in a kidney that is otherwise normal, and have an epithelial lining that contains no renal elements. Grossly, cysts are tense and thin walled and vary in diameter from millimeters to 7 cm (Figs. 20.13 and 20.14). Microscopically, the cysts are lined with low cuboidal to attenuated flattened epithelium. Fluid of simple cysts has chemical features of an ultrafiltrate of plasma (223). A dynamic equilibrium exists between production and absorption of fluid in simple renal cysts such that the cyst fluid has levels of tritiated water that reach 73% of the serum level within 2 to 5 hours after an intravenous injection of tritiated water (199). Perhaps cyst growth is dependent on the ratio of fluid production to absorption. Serial US measurements of renal cysts reveal only 28% of cysts increased in size in a 2- to 3-year period. The size change was 1 to 2 cm, and 14% of the cysts decreased in size by 1 to 2 cm over 2 to 3 years (83). However, many US and CT studies reveal increasing prevalence of simple renal cysts with age (32,56,83,234,305) and increasing diameter of cysts with age (56,234,321).

Radiology and Classification

Radiographic methods to diagnose a simple renal cyst have improved tremendously over the last decade. Because IVP cannot differentiate between a solid renal mass and a cystic renal mass, both of which distort the pyelocaliceal system (Fig. 20.15), renal US should be the next study. If the US requirements for a simple renal cyst are completely met on a study, investigation of a simple cyst is complete (19). The US appearance of a simple renal cyst is an anechoic mass with sharply marginated smooth walls and posterior wall enhancement (Fig. 20.16). However, if sonographic criteria for a simple cyst are not met or if lesions contain calcium, septations, or irregular margins, a CT examination is necessary (44). US is preferable as an initial study because it costs less, is less invasive, delivers no radiation, and does not require the pediatric patient to remain motionless for an extended time. The CT criteria for diagnosis of a cyst are (a) sharp margination and demarcation from surrounding renal parenchyma, (b) smooth thin wall, (c) water density content that is homogeneous throughout, and (d) no enhancement after intravenous administration of contrast material (44).

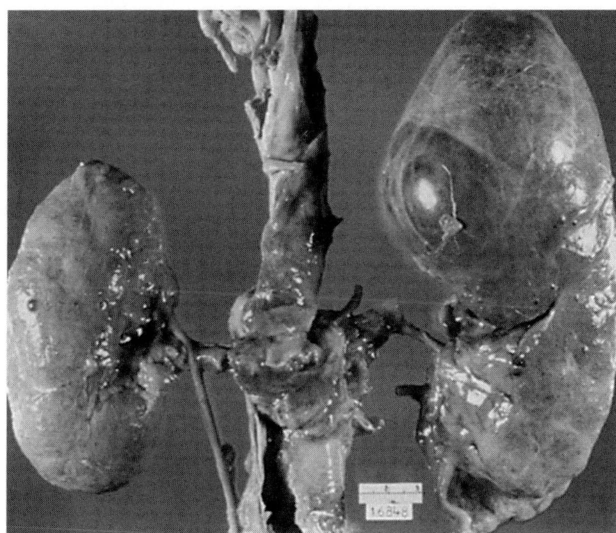

FIGURE 20.13. Simple cyst. A tense, thin-walled cyst is seen in the left upper pole. (Courtesy of Dr. S.E. Mills, Department of Pathology, University of Virginia Medical School, Charlottesville, VA.)

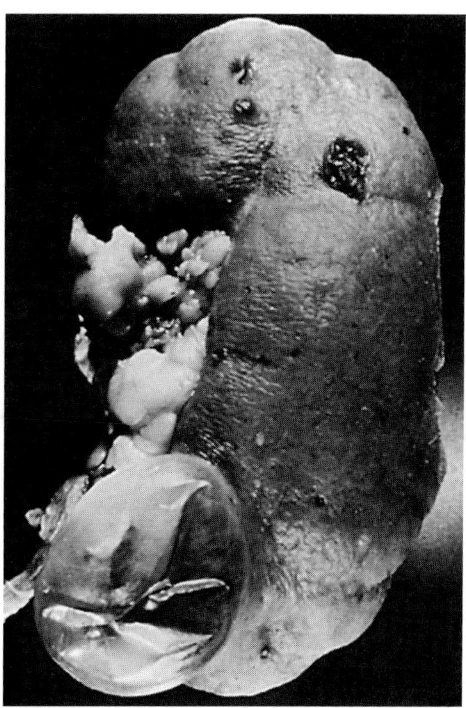

FIGURE 20.14. Simple cyst. A simple cyst is seen in the lower pole of this left kidney. Cyst was collapsed inadvertently at surgery. (Courtesy of Dr. S.E. Mills, Department of Pathology, University of Virginia Medical School, Charlottesville, VA.)

CT scanning to evaluate a renal cyst or mass found on another imaging modality should include non–contrast-enhanced scans through the lesion as well as contrast-enhanced scans and should include 5-mm-thick sections of the lesion while there is a high level of contrast media in the blood, unless the lesion is large enough that 10-mm-thick sections are adequate. Bosniak (44) has classified cystic lesions of the kidney into four categories based on a combination of CT and US imaging to help make clinical management decisions and to approximate the risk of malignancy. *Category I* lesions are benign simple cysts diagnosed definitively by CT or US. *Category II* lesions are benign but are minimally complicated because of worrisome radiologic findings in septated cysts, minimally calcified cysts, infected cysts, and high-density cysts. Such lesions do not require surgical exploration but may need to be followed. *Category III* lesions may be malignant and are more complicated cystic lesions because of thick or irregular calcifications or irregular thick septa with solid elements at the cyst wall attachments. Such lesions require confirmation by surgery in patients without poor operative risks. *Category IV* lesions

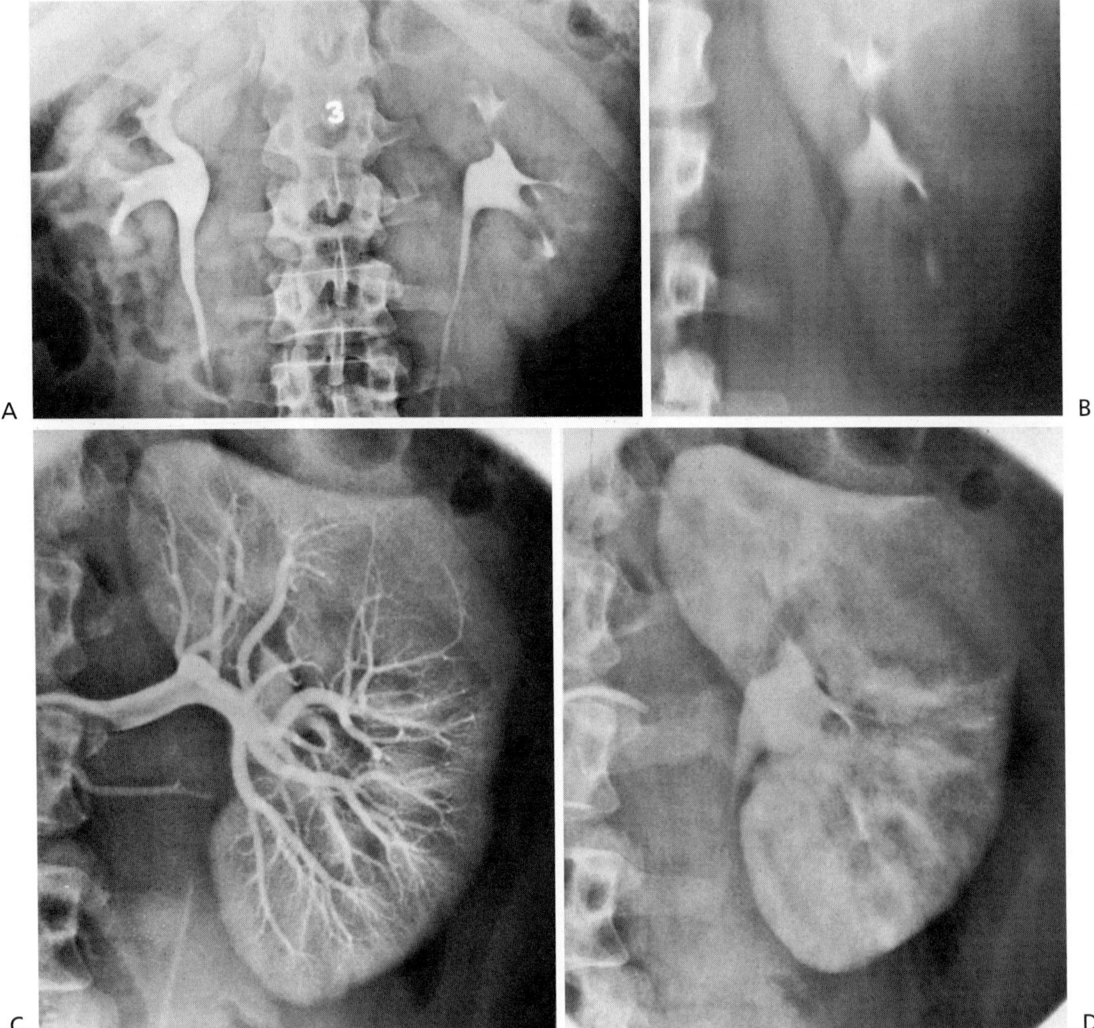

FIGURE 20.15. Simple cyst in a 36-year-old man. **A:** Intravenous pyelogram reveals bilaterally normal kidneys except for a spherical mass arising from the superolateral margin of the left kidney. **B:** Nephrotomography reveals the mass to be relatively lucent and to have smooth margins. **C, D:** Renal arteriography confirms the presence of a simple cyst by the draping of vessels around the mass, the lack of neovascularity, and its thin rim and "beaks" at its margin with the renal cortex.

are malignant cystic lesions and have irregular margins or solid vascular elements. They require surgical excision. Hyperdense renal cysts are in category II because they are assumed to be benign, usually contain old blood, are isodense or hypodense with surrounding renal parenchyma after intravenous contrast administration, and can be followed by serial CT (44) because cystic RCC can simulate a benign hyperdense cyst (162).

Sixteen pathologically proven cystic renal masses were retrospectively reviewed using the Bosniak classification by Aronson and colleagues (10). All category II lesions were benign, all category IV lesions were malignant, and of the seven category III lesions, three were benign and four were malignant. Similarly, 70 pathologically proven cystic renal masses were reviewed by Siegel and associates (354), with 0% Bosniak I malignant, 13% of Bosniak II malignant, 45% of Bosniak III malignant, and 90% of Bosniak IV malignant. However, Wilson and co-workers (409), in a similar retrospective review of pathologically proven cystic renal masses, found a high rate of malignancy in Bosniak categories II (80%), III (100%), and IV (100%). In addition, Cloix and associated (75), in a similar retrospective review of pathologically proven cystic renal masses, found a RCC that had been classified as a Bosniak I. However, the Bosniak classification requires devoted renal CT studies with 5-mm cuts. Cloix and colleagues (75) used 10-mm slices in their study, and not all patients had devoted renal CT scans. Only 9 of the 20 patients in Wilson and colleagues' study (409) had undergone dedicated thin-section renal CT examinations both before and after intravenous contrast administration. Siegel and associates (354) suggest that intraobserver variation in distinguishing Bosniak II and III lesions may explain the differences between these studies. Bosniak (45) amended his original classification system by adding class 2F for minimally complicated cysts that are "somewhat suspicious" and require follow-up with serial CT scans to establish stability instead of immediate surgical exploration. Despite any shortcomings of the Bosniak classification, it is the best system currently available to classify complex renal cysts.

Spiral CT scanning eliminates respiratory misregistration; therefore the walls of cystic lesions can be visualized with great precision and specificity in the diagnosis of simple renal cyst is increased. However, small lesions can be missed by spiral CT if scanning occurs too soon after contrast injection (46).

Renal angiography is less important in the diagnosis of a simple renal cyst but would show an avascular mass with renal cortex compressed at the margins. Both contrast-enhanced power Doppler sonography and delayed CT have shown promise in demonstrating tumor vascularity/enhancement in complex renal cysts (221,261). Percutaneous cyst puncture for cytology and injection of contrast is not now as commonly needed because of the high quality of US and CT available. Of course, the diagnosis of suspected infected cysts or abscesses is benefited by percutaneous aspirate, Gram stain, and culture. MRI can help differentiate between a simple cyst and a hemorrhagic cyst (Fig. 20.17). In addition, gadolinium-enhanced MRI scans and non–gadolinium-enhanced MRI scans can be used in patients unable to receive injections of contrast media for CT. Nonenhanced and gadolinium-enhanced T_1-weighted and T_2-weighted MRI has been evaluated to determine whether imaging features could distinguish between benign and malignant complex renal cysts (16). Although mural irregularity and intense mural enhancement strongly predicted malignancy in complex renal cysts, appearances of benign and malignant lesions overlap.

A

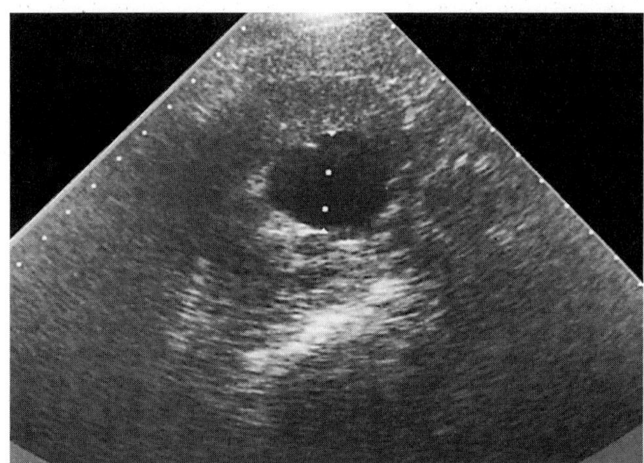

B

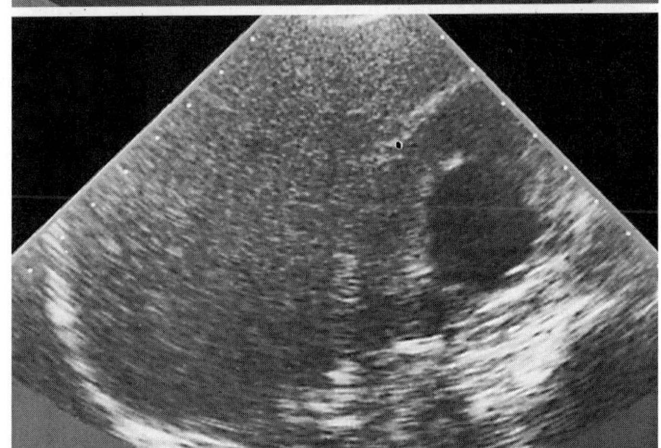

FIGURE 20.16. A, B: Simple cyst in 53-year-old woman. Renal ultrasonography reveals an anechoic renal mass with a smooth posterior wall and posterior wall enhancement.

Renal Sinus Cysts

Cysts in the renal sinus deserve mention. Parapelvic cysts are usually single, larger cysts in the renal sinus originating from adjacent parenchyma and are simple cysts. Peripelvic cysts are multiple, confluent, irregularly shaped cysts that appear to arise in the renal sinus itself and that may develop from lymphatic ectasia secondary to blockage of renal hilar lymphatics (6). Autopsy studies show a 1.3% to 1.5% incidence of sinus cysts in the older population. If a sinus cyst of any size happens to be appropriately located, symptoms such as hypertension, hematuria, and localized hydronephrosis can result if a renal sinus structure is compressed, such as a vascular structure or the collecting system (6). On US evaluation, peripelvic or renal sinus cysts may be mistaken for dilated calyces and pelvis. This potential for false diagnosis may be the only clinical relevance of this condition (300).

Management of Simple Cysts

Usually, simple cysts are asymptomatic coincidental findings on imaging studies and require no treatment. However, they occasionally can present as flank or abdominal pain, infection, hemorrhage, hypertension, and impairment of renal function. Case reports elucidate the rare presentation of simple cysts as hypertension in children (14,179) and in adults (330). Increased renin release from the affected kidney has been demonstrated as well as normalization of blood pressure after open surgical or percutaneous elimination of the cyst (14,330). In ADPKD, the cause of hypertension has been proposed to be activation of the renin-angiotensin-aldosterone system by cyst compression of adjacent renal vessels causing ischemia (62). A similar mechanism may account for the hypertension in the aforemen-

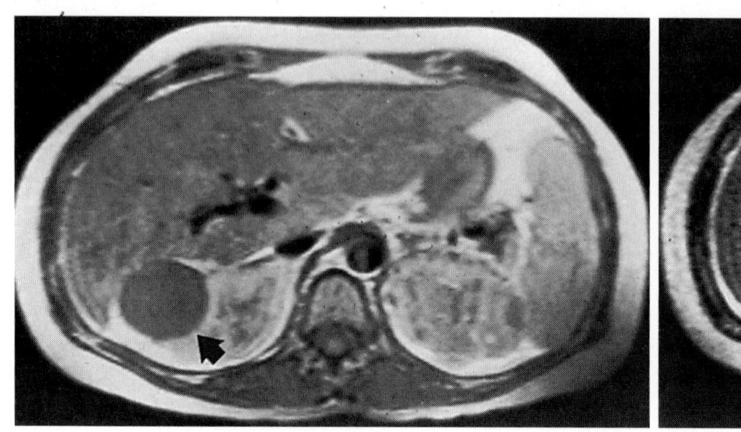

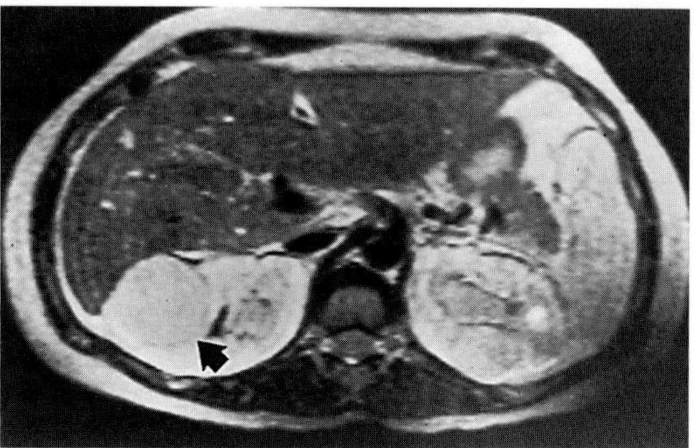

FIGURE 20.17. Simple cyst in a 44-year-old woman. **A:** Magnetic resonance imaging of a T_1-weighted image is characteristic of a simple right renal cyst *(arrow)* because of the distinct smooth margin and because of the low signal intensity (e.g., the cyst contents are very black). **B:** To confirm the diagnosis of a simple cyst, a T_2-weighted image demonstrates the cyst contents to have a high signal intensity (e.g., to be very white), which is consistent with water.

tioned case reports as well as hypertension in an aging population (305). More patients with simple renal cysts have hypertension (56). Not only are hypertension and simple renal cysts increasingly common with increasing age, but hypertension is significantly higher in individuals with cysts (305). Possibly, the association between simple renal cysts and higher arterial blood pressure arises from underlying renal disease causing both (306).

Approximately 6% of simple cysts hemorrhage, and although hemorrhagic cysts are extremely rare in children, they have been reported (325). Cyst hemorrhage can be spontaneous or secondary to trauma and may result in hematuria (296). Hyperdense renal cysts occasionally are incidentally found on CT imaging and are renal cysts containing old blood (44), suggesting minor cyst hemorrhage does not result in severe symptoms. Secondary cyst infections are rare but have been reported (131,256); these have been successfully treated with percutaneous drainage and systemic antibiotics (284). Acute urinary obstruction can cause extravasation of urine from the renal pelvis or calyces into a simple cyst (43). Except in rare cases when cysts cause calyceal or renal pelvic obstruction, simple renal cysts have no negative affect on renal function (184).

After the diagnosis of simple renal cyst has been made, no treatment is necessary except to treat symptoms such as abdominal or flank pain. Even though simple renal cysts are rare in the pediatric age group, once malignancy has been excluded appropriately by radiographic methods, no surgical exploration to confirm the diagnosis is necessary (141,320,355). Treatment of symptomatic renal cysts begins with percutaneous aspiration of the cyst to confirm that the symptom such as pain disappears. Cyst fluid can be analyzed cytologically as well as cultured to confirm diagnosis of simple cyst, but cyst fluid cytologic evaluation is not highly accurate. Twenty-four months after aspiration, cyst fluid will have reaccumulated, so there is no size difference between cysts that were aspirated and those that had no intervention (182). However, if the patient's symptom (pain) disappeared with aspiration and the cyst and symptom reoccurs, percutaneous aspiration should be repeated, followed by instillation of a sclerosing agent, such as urea cholohydrolactate, glucose, ethanol, phenol, tetracycline, bismuth phosphate, autologous blood, minocycline, Betadine (povidone-iodine), quinacrine, iophendylate, polidocanol, or ethanolamine (51,142,182,262,285,286,293, 386). Cyst and symptom recurrence are significantly lower after aspiration and instillation of a sclerosing agent than after aspiration alone (182,285); however, long-term cyst reduction occurs in only 50% of cases (183). Repeated injections of a sclerotherapeutic agent over a few days into an indwelling percutaneous drain into the cyst had a higher success rate, though. Three repeated ethanol injections over 2 days into an indwelling percutaneous drain resulted in complete disappearance of 97% of renal cysts at 3 months, with no recurrence during the mean 4-year follow-up (117). The drain was left to closed drainage between instillations.

Percutaneous resection of simple cysts is another treatment with the advantage of obtaining part of the cyst wall for pathologic analysis. Plas and Hubner (314) found that morbidity was minimal but that 50% of patients had residual or recurrent cyst tissue at 40 months, even though no patient had recurrence of their symptoms. Weichert-Jacobsen and others (403) described a modified percutaneous resection technique used only in patients with peripheral renal cysts and found no recurrence of cyst formation on US or symptoms at 19 months of follow-up. Laparoscopic excision of simple renal cysts has been reported through both abdominal and retroperitoneal approaches, with no evidence of recurrent cysts or symptoms in the initial series (155,275,281,335). Recurrence of a renal cyst but not symptoms has been reported after laparoscopic unroofing (217). A wide section of the cyst wall is obtained for pathologic review, as is the case for open surgical cyst excision. Open surgery does have the advantage of better control of bleeding.

Most symptomatic simple cysts can be effectively managed with percutaneous drainage and sclerosis. The repeat injections into an indwelling percutaneous drain have a high success rate. However, in those few simple cysts resistant to these techniques, the percutaneous resection is effective for peripheral simple renal cysts, as is laparoscopic decortication via either a transperitoneal or retroperitoneal approach or open surgical decortication.

Management of Peripelvic Cysts

Peripelvic cysts may lie between major hilar vessels and the renal pelvis. Sclerotherapy into peripelvic cysts is considered risky. Percutaneous sclerosis with multiple injections of povidone-iodine into an indwelling drain in four parapelvic cysts relieved symptoms in all patients with 7.2 months follow-up (312). Successful marsupialization of a peripelvic renal cyst using flexible ureteronephroscopy has been reported (218). Transperitoneal laparoscopic ablation of peripelvic cysts has been successful in alleviating pain but is technically challenging (180). Open surgical repair has succeeded after a failed retroperitoneal laparoscopic ablation of a peripelvic cyst (180).

Management of Complex Cysts

Bosniak category IV complex cysts can undergo partial or radical nephrectomy depending on the size and location of the complex cyst as well as the status of the contralateral kidney. Bosniak category III complex renal cysts can undergo open surgical exploration with preparedness to perform a partial nephrectomy (410). The cyst can be visualized directly while attempts are made to prevent tumor cell spillage, and the cyst fluid can be aspirated, and the external cyst wall and biopsies of the internal cyst wall can be sent for frozen analysis. Bosniak category IIF cysts can be followed by serial CT studies. Laparoscopic evaluation of 35 patients with Bosniak category II and III complex renal cysts revealed 5 patients (14%) with cystic RCC (341). At the time of laparoscopy, cyst fluid is aspirated and the cyst wall is excised and sent for pathologic evaluation, as are biopsies of the base of the cyst if suspicious. If the pathologist confirms malignancy, an immediate radical or partial nephrectomy can be performed (341).

MEDULLARY SPONGE KIDNEY

Medullary sponge kidney (MSK) is a relatively benign entity that is diagnosed by IVP. The diagnosis is usually made in adults who present for IVP for evaluation of calculi, hematuria, or infection. The male-to-female ratio is 2 : 1 (240). In MSK, the kidneys retain their reniform shape, and the incidence varies from 1 in 5,000 to 1 in 20,000 (228). Although described histologically to some extent in 1908 (100), it was the onset of IVP that made possible the description and classification of MSK as a disease by Cacchi and Ricci (55). Even today, IVP is the mainstay of diagnosis.

Clinical Features

MSK is most commonly diagnosed from 20 to 50 years of age, when patients have an IVP performed to evaluate their presenting symptom, which is either renal colic (50% to 60%), gross hematuria (10% to 18%), or UTI (20% to 33%) (228). Of those who have this radiographic diagnosis made, 60% will pass calculi at some time (228). However, an uncertain number are undiagnosed because they are asymptomatic. A small number of patients with MSK have been diagnosed when they were evaluated by IVP for other conditions, such as hypertensive screening, abdominal tumors, and so on. Hence, although 60% of patients diagnosed with MSK will pass calculi, it is uncertain what percentage of all patients with MSK will pass stones, have infections, and so forth. Nephrocalcinosis in MSK is clinically benign except that it leads to stone formation and passage of calculi. Of 70 kidneys examined in affected patients, 58 had intracavitary calculi ranging in number from one to infinity (100). Stone analysis reveals that calcium phosphate stones are the most common, with calcium oxalate stones making up most of the remainder.

In MSK, the medullary cysts are dilated collecting ducts in the pyramids and papillae. Urinary stagnation in these dilated or cystic tubules may be the cause of the calcifications found in these dilated ducts. Because metabolic disorders accounting for lithiasis are found less commonly in stone patients with MSK (60%) than in stone patients without MSK (93%), MSK may cause nephrolithiasis (134). Alternatively, perhaps the biochemical composition of the urine is altered in patients with MSK who have calculi (413). Defective urinary acidification might play an important role in the mechanism of hypercalcuria and hypocitraturia in MSK patients (291). From 40% to 90% of patients with nephrocalcinosis also have hypercalciuria (174). From 15% to 21% of patients with calcium stones were diagnosed as having MSK by IVP (299,413). Ginalski and colleagues (134) found MSK on 12% of IVPs in patients with nephrolithiasis and in 1% of IVPs of patients without nephrolithiasis and without a history of stones.

Progression of MSK, as evidenced by the size or location of the dilated collecting tubules on IVP, is uncommon (228). However, nephrocalcinosis in MSK is acquired (228). Sequential US studies on six children with MSK have revealed increasing echogenicity of the renal pyramids. This increasing echogenicity proved on CT to be calcifications, although the calcifications were too small to be seen on IVP (302). Three of these six children had hematuria, which was probably associated with their microlithiasis. Microlithiasis may be the cause of most of the hematuria seen in those MSK patients who have no demonstrable calcifications on IVP.

About 20% to 30% of patients with MSK have a UTI as their presenting symptom (228). UTI does not play a causal role in stone formation in most patients with MSK, most of whom have sterile urine (413); however, when present, infection has the potential of accelerating stone growth by alkalinizing the urine. Fortunately, infection in affected patients responds well to antibiotics, unlike in patients with ADPKD. In addition, patients affected with MSK have an incidence of hypertension similar to that found in the normal population. Occasionally, a mild urine-concentrating defect can be found in patients with MSK who otherwise have normal renal function.

Morphology, Pathogenesis, and Genetics

Grossly, the kidneys of MSK are of normal size or slightly larger and have kept their reniform shape. Cut surface reveals the larger of the dilated collecting duct cysts, which are present at the papillary tips of the renal pyramids (near the renal medulla). The smaller of the dilated collecting duct cysts may be visible only microscopically because they vary from 1 to 5 mm in diameter. Microscopically, the collecting ducts are lined by flattened epithelium, and the columns of Bertin are normal. As few as one or as many as all renal pyramids can have MSK and calcifications can be seen in the cysts clustered toward the papillary tips.

The pathogenesis of MSK is unknown, but it is probably congenital. Successive US studies in children with MSK show the progressive development of calcifications as the children grow as well as the presence of the disease in children (302). MSK has some basis for at least occasional genetic transmission because of documented family history in a few families (228) and its association with other congenital manifestations.

Radiologic Findings

The diagnosis of MSK is made by IVP (Fig. 20.18). The contrast medium stagnates in the dilated or cystic linear tubules in one or more renal papillae. These appear as linear radiations from the calyces and vary in shape from beads to strands. Whether a "pyramidal blush" is an early sign of MSK on IVP or is a normal finding is undecided. Calculi are located at papillary tips on a plain abdominal radiograph. US shows the medullary cysts only if they are large. However, in children, the renal medulla is better seen on US because there is less renal sinus fat and overlying muscle. As a result, hyperechoic areas of the pyramids are visualized and either represent ductal calcifications or dilated collecting ducts (302). On retrograde pyelography, the cysts or ectatic ducts either fail to fill with contrast or fill less prominently. The sensitivity of CT in the detection of MSK is markedly lower than that with IVP. However, CT is more sensitive than plain films and tomograms of IVP in the detection of the papillary calcifications of MSK (135).

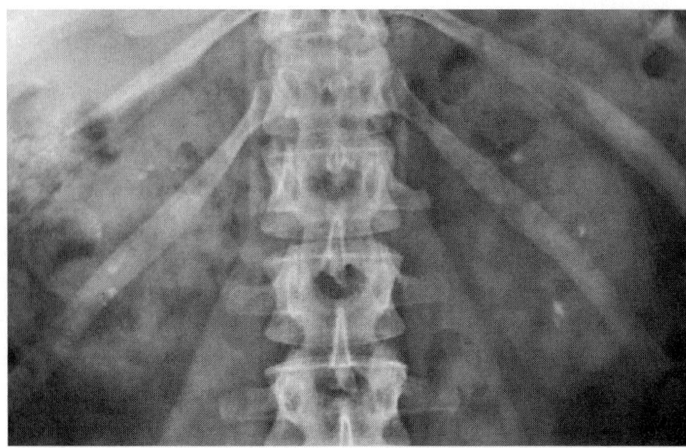
A

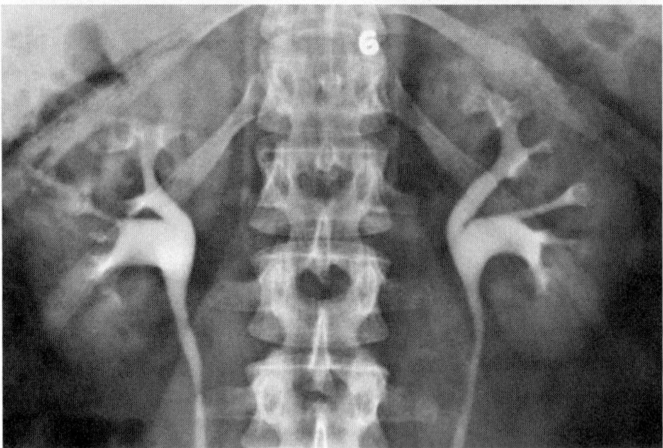

B

FIGURE 20.18. Medullary sponge kidney. **A:** A plain abdominal radiograph reveals bilateral nephrocalcinosis. The calculi are located at the papillary tips. **B:** An intravenous pyelogram in the same patient reveals linear radiations from the calyces. These radiations result from stagnation of contrast medium in the cystic or dilated collecting ducts.

Management

Some patients with MSK will have an asymptomatic course and require no medical intervention. Previously, 10% of the symptomatic patients had a poor prognosis because of recurrent renal calculi and infection (228), but with current therapies for infections and calculi, this number is probably lower. Infections in patients with MSK respond well to antibiotics. Prevention of stone formation can be attempted with increased fluid intake, thiazides, and inorganic phosphates (413). Urine alkalization may reduce the incidence of stone formation in these patients (90). Once calculi are formed, ESWL is effective in disintegrating symptomatic stones in the collecting system (90,277,387) but not in fragmenting the ductal (precaliceal) calcifications (90,387). Marked improvement in the frequency of renal colic and

UTIs was noted after ESWL, perhaps secondary to the reduction in stone mass and the reduced incidence of obstruction in the upper urinary tract (90). Transurethral extraction of ureteral calculi is appropriate with ureteroscopy as needed. Appropriate antibiotic prophylaxis during the perioperative period should be used because of the high risk of obstruction in these patients from passage of more calculi.

GLOMERULOCYSTIC KIDNEY DISEASE AND GLOMERULOCYSTIC KIDNEYS

Glomerulocystic kidney disease (GCKD) is a rare congenital bilateral cystic disease in which Bowman's space is dilated and thus appears as a glomerular cyst. The cysts contain some sort of glomerular tuft or tuft remnant. These multiple cysts are confined to the renal cortex in these reniform but very large kidneys. The tubular portion of the nephron is structurally normal. The lack of tubular involvement distinguishes GCKD from other cystic renal diseases in which proximal or distal tubule dilation leads to cyst formation in both the cortical and medullary regions (57).

Glomerulocystic kidneys occur in (a) GCKD, (b) heritable malformation syndromes, and (c) dysplastic kidneys (30). Glomerulocystic kidneys are a major component of heritable malformation syndromes such as ADPKD, TSC, orofaciodigital syndrome, brachymesomelia-renal syndrome, trisomy 13, short rib–polydactyly syndrome, Jeune syndrome, and familial juvenile nephronophthisis, and is a minor component in Zellweger's syndrome. Glomerular cysts can be a minor feature in dysplastic kidneys such as diffuse cystic dysplasia and renal-hepatic-pancreatic dysplasia (30). In contrast, GCKD comprises nonsyndromal heritable and sporadic forms of severely cystic kidneys in young children and to a lesser degree in adults.

GCKD has a broad range of clinical manifestations from death in early infancy to survival in adult life, with little handicap and with successful marriage and reproduction. Patients more commonly present in infancy or early childhood and have bilaterally palpable flank masses (265,349, 372). Renal function can deteriorate (265) or remain stable for an unknown amount of time (349). Glomerulocystic kidneys in young infants are a common expression of early onset ADPKD (32). Many of these newborns and young children have a family history of ADPKD, whereas others are sporadic. Because no differences are found between familial and sporadic cases, the sporadic cases are potentially new mutations of the same disease (30). Children with early onset of severe ADPKD have an affected parent whose milder disease presented in adulthood. The increase in disease severity is limited to the kidney that has a higher number of cysts and mostly glomerular cysts (289). Dedeoglu and co-workers (86) described an infant diagnosed with GCKD because of classic findings on his renal biopsy, normal renal US studies of his parents, and negative family history. Seven years later, his diagnosis was changed to ADPKD because a repeat renal US of his mother (30 years old) suggested ADPKD, pathologic examination of his kidneys after bilateral nephrectomies confirmed ADPKD, and gene linkage analysis was informative for the family for ADPKD. A positive family history can point the clinician in the right direction, which may be verified by linkage analysis. Glomerular cysts have also been identified in 40% of adult ADPKD kidneys examined for their presence (30).

Less commonly, GCKD is a cause of chronic renal insufficiency in older children (411). In rare instances, GCKD has been diagnosed in adults who can present with hypertension, flank pain, hematuria, mild chronic renal failure, and ESRD (57) or who can present as coincidental findings when patients undergo renal biopsies for another renal disease such as glomerulonephritis (58). Potentially, GCKD may be more common than realized because biopsies have not been performed on otherwise asymptomatic patients. GCKD in adults and older children may also be sporadic or familial. If familial, GCKD is dominant (269). Usually, patients progress to ESRD or stable chronic renal insufficiency (57). Poor prognosis may be related to extensive involvement with glomerular cysts at an early age. Survival beyond adolescence with only mild to moderate renal functional impairment and no associated congenital abnormalities appears to improve chances for maintaining adequate renal function (57). Another category of GCKD is hypoplastic GCKD, which is rare and dominant. Unlike other GCKD patients, these patients have small kidneys and abnormal pyelocaliceal anatomy. Amir and colleagues (5) suggest that GCKD may be acquired after hemolytic uremic syndrome.

GCKD kidneys are large and reniform, with cortical cysts that vary in diameter from a few millimeters to 7 cm (349). IVP demonstrates huge kidneys and can sometimes demonstrate calyceal distortion suggesting multiple renal cysts or masses (57). US demonstrates large kidneys and may show numerous small cysts, depending on cyst size (265). Therefore the kidneys appear strongly echogenic with cortical, subcortical, and subcapsular cysts (57). Selective renal arteriography can show intrarenal vessels stretched around numerous cortical cysts (349). A renal biopsy may be necessary to establish a diagnosis (57). MRI shows multiple cortical cysts and diffuse reduction of the intensity of the renal cortex with loss of the normal corticomedullary differentiation on T_1-weighted images (98).

Treatment is appropriate management of renal failure. Both dialysis and renal transplantation have been successful (265).

ACQUIRED CYSTIC KIDNEY DISEASE

Long-term maintenance dialysis therapy is now accepted therapy for patients with ESRD. However, dialysis has ushered in a new class of renal cystic disease called *acquired cystic kidney disease* (ACKD). ACKD was so named in 1977 by Dunnill and co-workers (95), who observed that 14 (47%) of 30 long-term dialysis patients had bilateral renal cystic disease at autopsy. None of these patients had renal cystic disease before beginning hemodialysis. Later studies revealed that hemodialysis patients and continuous ambulatory peritoneal dialysis (CAPD) patients have the same prevalence and severity of ACKD (196,343). Patients with longstanding renal insufficiency who have never been dialyzed also developed ACKD (48,72). In retrospect, ACKD was described in 1847 in patients with subacute glomerulonephritis causing such longstanding renal insufficiency (356). Because ACKD is asymptomatic in its early stages, ACKD can occur before ESRD is recognized. The uremic state promotes the development of ACKD, and dialysis extends the time that the cysts can develop. Serial CT scans of the kidneys of uremic patients suggest that cysts start to develop when serum creatinine is above 3 mg/dL (271). The incidence of ACKD in dialysis patients increases with the length of time the patient has received dialysis (241). Ishikawa and others (194) reported a 44% incidence of ACKD in patients who had undergone less than 3 years of hemodialysis, as opposed to an 80% incidence in patients who had more than 3 years. The reported prevalence rate of ACKD is increasing because of longer patient survival in dialysis therapies, higher rates of native kidney retention in transplant patients, and improved sensitivities of current imaging modalities (340). ACKD is bilateral, develops more quickly, and is more severe in men (77,198). The prevalence of ACKD in children undergoing CAPD and hemodialysis is just as high as that in adults (231,264).

Early on, ACKD patients are usually asymptomatic and are therefore not usually diagnosed unless screened radiologically as part of an evaluation for renal failure or transplantation. Alternatively, patients can present with severe intrarenal hemorrhage with or without gross hematuria. Among cases of ACKD with bleeding complications, only about 30% are related to tumor, whereas the rest are probably related to retroperitoneal hemorrhage due to rupture of a hemorrhagic cyst into the retroperitoneal space (130). Such hemorrhage can occur during anticoagulation therapy for hemodialysis, at which time patients may have such symptoms as sudden flank pain, hypotension, and decrease in hematocrit (192). Less commonly, ACKD patients may also develop a cyst infection, symptomatic distant metastases from RCC, matrix kidney stones (48), or increased erythropoietin production. The size increases of renal cysts over time in ACKD results in increased secretion of erythropoietin (97) and a rising hemoglobin (111).

Successful renal transplantation in dialysis patients can retard or lead to regression of established ACKD, as well as size reduction of the affected native kidneys (197,241), unless cyclosporine is used for immunosuppression (246). In cyclosporine-treated transplant patients, the prevalence of ACKD is essentially the same as that for hemodialysis patients. After a transplanted kidney undergoes chronic rejection, resulting in uremia, acquired renal cysts can develop in the grafted and native kidneys (195). The duration of uremia correlated with increased numbers of acquired renal cysts, just as prolongation of the dialysis period in ESRD increases not only the incidence of ACKD but also the number and size of acquired cysts.

Eighty-six percent of renal tumors in ACKD are asymptomatic and are found incidentally by imaging studies, although they can less commonly present with symptoms such as bleeding, pain, fever, hypercalcemia, or symptomatic metastatic disease. The prevalence of tumors increases with the duration of dialysis, just as kidney weight increases with duration. Increased kidney weight is secondary to increased cyst volume and epithelial proliferation, both of which can be considered premalignant. Cancer developed in 11% of tumors in ACKD kidneys weighing less than 150 g and 55.6% in ACKD kidneys weighing greater than 150 g. In addition, ACKD patients in the small kidney group did not have metastatic disease, whereas three patients in the large kidney group had metastatic disease (250). ACKD has an overall incidence of 43.6% of all dialysis patients surveyed. Renal tumors, usually multiple, are found in 7.1% of chronic dialysis patients but in 16.4% of the ACKD patients. Many of the tumors were small and were therefore considered adenomas, but 4.7% of the renal tumors had metastasized by the time of presentation (146). Considering only RCCs in ACKD, 20% are metastatic at presentation (260). In combined data from 13 studies, 4% of ACKD patients had RCC (defined as a tumor greater than 2 to 3 cm in diameter). However, this figure may be an underestimate because a pathologist will detect more tumors than a radiologist. The incidence of RCC in ACKD represents a fortyfold (in Japan) to fiftyfold (in the United States) increased risk of RCC compared with that of the general population (382).

RCC occurs at a younger age in ACKD than in the general population (45 versus 64 years) and has even higher male-to-female ratio in ACKD than the general population (6:1 versus 2:1). RCC is more common in African Americans than whites in the ACKD populations, but it is more common in whites than African Americans in the general population (260). In ACKD, RCC tends to be bilateral and multifocal, in contrast to solitary unilateral RCC in the general population.

Morphology, Pathogenesis, and Malignancy

Grossly, the renal cortex in ACKD is replaced by multiple, bilateral cysts; later, the medulla is involved to some extent. The kidneys are reniform and small initially as they decrease in size during the first 3 years of dialysis; however, they then increase in size secondary to acquired cyst development (260). Most cysts are 0.5 to 2.0 cm in diameter but can be 4 cm in diameter. Cyst fluid is clear to hemorrhagic.

Microscopically, few glomeruli remain. Microdissection studies reveal that the cysts mainly develop in proximal tubules that survive the sclerotic process leading to the end stage kidney (388). Most cysts are lined by low cuboidal or columnar epithelium. However, some cysts have atypical proliferations of columnar, multilayered living cells in papillary formation. Although epithelial proliferation in cystic kidneys does not invariably lead to the development of macroscopic tumors and malignancy, the relative infrequency with which adenocarcinomas are found in noncystic, compared with cystic, kidneys strongly suggests a causal relationship between epithelial hyperplasia and both cysts and tumors (31). The tumors found in ACKD can be categorized histologically into three groups: (a) papillary tumors that project into the cyst lumen without invading the cyst wall, (b) parenchymal tumors that reside adjacent to but not within the cyst, and (c) solid tumors that are sheets of less differentiated cells with either foamy or acidophilic cytoplasm. Central areas may have hemorrhage (94).

RCC in chronic dialysis patients has a papillary histologic pattern in 49% of cases, as opposed to 5% of the RCCs in the general population (193). Gains of chromosomes 7 and 17 and loss of Y have been observed in papillary RCCs in ACKD similar to sporadic papillary RCC, but the nonpapillary RCCs in ACKD patients did not show loss of chromosome 3p as in sporadic nonpapillary RCCs (152). Controversy exists over whether tumors less than 2 to 3 cm in size in ACKD patients should be called *adenomas* or *adenocarcinomas,* because there is no histologic difference and tumors greater than 3 cm had once to be less than 3 cm. Ishikawa and co-workers (193) suggest that all nonpapillary renal cell tumors in ACKD be diagnosed as RCCs and that the adenoma versus carcinoma question be limited to papillary renal tumors because of different genetic alterations and different natural histories. Specifically, a nonpapillary RCC can occur any time after starting dialysis, whereas papillary RCC and ACKD occur more frequently after long-term dialysis. Sant and Ucci (340) noted that renal neoplasms of 1.5 and 1.8 cm in native ACKD kidneys showed microscopic capsular invasion and suggested all renal adenomas be considered small adenocarcinomas with metastatic potential.

RCC can occur in the native kidneys in ACKD patients after successful renal transplantation (166,243,340). Renal transplantation reduces the frequency and severity of ACKD in ESRD patients but does not completely eliminate ACKD, even in all patients with good renal function, especially if the patient is treated with cyclosporine (246). Heinz-Peer and others (166) reported a 24.9% incidence of ACKD in native kidneys after successful renal transplantation and noted that 5% of the native kidneys with ACKD were found to have RCC. The genetic alterations in renal parenchymal cells undergoing epithelial proliferation during ACKD are important rate-limiting changes toward neoplastic growth. Therefore, although ACKD can be reversible in the native kidneys of individuals who have received functioning renal allografts, the final step in progression from cyst to adenoma to adenocarcinoma may not be reversible by correction of an uremic environment (144). The multistage process of oncogenesis may be beyond the bounds of physiologic control, so the malignant potential of ACKD may persist in renal transplant recipients, even after many years of normal function (166).

The pathogenesis of ACKD is unknown, but one theory involves the accumulation of biologically active substances such as cystogenic nephrotoxins that accumulate during hemodialysis, peritoneal dialysis, or chronic uremia. Such biologically active substances may cause kidneys to develop ACKD and renal tumors if these kidneys are exposed to the biologically active substance long enough. Support for this hypothesis lies in the fact that successful renal transplantation can result in regression of established ACKD. Because ACKD does occur in patients who have longstanding renal insufficiency before beginning dialysis, dialysate-leached chemicals are not believed to be the initiators of ACKD. Hence, this suggests that although hemodialysis and peritoneal dialysis prolong life, they are not complete kidney substitutes because they may allow some biologically active substance to accumulate (146).

Another theory suggests that the loss of functional renal mass such as a critical number of working nephrons increases production of renotropic factors that promote tubular cell hypertrophy and hyperplasia leading to cyst formation and, rarely, renal tumors (144,145). Hemodialysis and CAPD may fail to eliminate the substances that promote production of renotropic factors, although successful renal transplantation may retard or lead to the regression of ACKD. Increased expression of renotropic factors, epidermal growth factors, platelet-derived growth factor, and C-erb B-2 (a protooncogene) may be involved (172,260).

The hormonal theory offers another possibility for ACKD pathogenesis because ACKD occurs much earlier in male than in female patients. After 3 years of dialysis, ACKD incidence is 100% in males and 66% in females. Furthermore, after long-term dialysis, the severity of cystic transformation is far greater in male patients and the increase in renal volume in male ACKD patients is more than twofold that reported in female patients (77). However, the size of the kidney tends to plateau after 13 years of hemodialysis in male patients, whereas significant cystic changes developed in female patients receiving long-term (more than 18 years) hemodialysis (198). Perhaps the decreased androgen-to-estrogen ratio and the increased estrogen value could result in an estrogen receptor–mediated effect on tubular epithelial cell proliferation, which could be more pronounced in male tissues because they are less adapted to high estrogen values. In addition, androgen reduction (more severe in male patients) may upregulate epidermal growth factor (77).

Radiologic Findings, Screening, and Management

Because the incidence of ACKD increases with the length of time a patient has been receiving dialysis, asymptomatic dialysis patients should be screened after 3 years of dialysis treatment by either US or CT. A baseline predialysis renal US should be obtained for comparison purposes. If any US detects the presence of cysts, CT should be done to assess the presence of a renal tumor because ACKD patients are at increased risk for renal tumors. Unfortunately, it can be difficult for US to detect the small cysts of ACKD in these sonographically abnormal small kidneys of ESRD patients (146) (Fig. 20.19). Manns and others (257) were unable to identify 10% of the native kidneys in ACKD by US. Hence,

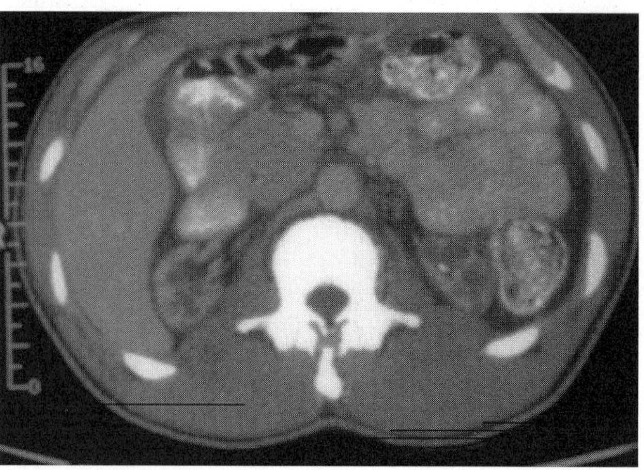

FIGURE 20.20. Acquired cystic kidney disease in a 46-year-old man on chronic dialysis who has had a left nephrectomy. Unenhanced computed tomography reveals a right small kidney with multiple cysts.

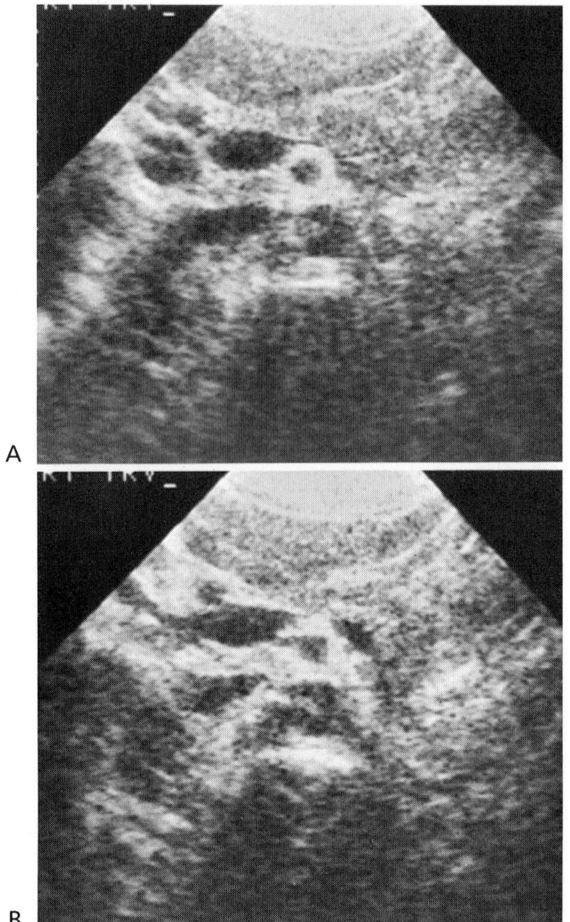

FIGURE 20.19. A, B: Acquired cystic kidney disease in a 52-year-old woman on chronic dialysis. Renal ultrasonography reveals small kidneys with increased cortical echoes as found in chronic renal disease. Multiple cysts are present and are of varying sizes.

if it were not for cost, contrast-enhanced CT would be preferable as a first test to diagnose ARCD as well as to diagnose tumor (Fig. 20.20). However, some authors have found US to be more accurate than CT to diagnose RCC in dialysis patients (374). If an ACKD patient becomes symptomatic with flank pain, hematuria, or any unexplained fever or systemic illness, appropriate imaging such as an enhanced CT scan is appropriate to evaluate for possible tumor, hemorrhage, or infected cyst. Annual CT screening of all long-term dialysis patients after 3 years would add $36 million to the Medicare budget, but data do not justify the expense (238). Screening ACKD patients on dialysis every 3 years by CT or US has been predicted to increase the 25-year life expectancy of a 20-year-old by 1.6 years but only increase the 5-year life expectancy of a 58-year-old by 4 to 5 days (342). More than half of the U.S. dialysis population would be unlikely to benefit from such screening because the median age of patients beginning dialysis is 62 years (342).

However, identification of subsets of ACKD patients most likely to benefit from annual screening is appropriate. For example, young patients with prolonged dialysis (255) and patients in good medical condition would benefit if annual renal imaging found localized RCC (238). In addition, subsets of ACKD patients with high-risk factors such as male gender (77) or large kidneys (250) would benefit. MRI is superior to US in depiction of simple and complex cysts of native kidneys in renal allograft recipients (167) but is not better than CT scanning even after gadolinium enhancement (382). The 1995 clinical practice guidelines of the American Society of Transplant Physicians for evaluation of renal transplant candidates do not recommend screening for ACKD and RCC because of the low frequency of cancer and reported regression of ACKD after transplantation (156). Gulanikar and associates (156) evaluated 206 consecutive adult patients for renal transplantation with a renal US and found 63 patients (30.6%) had ACKD and 8 (3.8%) had localized RCC (6 unilateral and 2 bilateral). Seven of the cancers were in the ACKD patients. Although US screening of the entire ESRD population for ACKD and tumors cannot be justified because of patient age and comorbidity limiting life expectancy, patients chosen for renal transplantation are younger and have less severe comorbidities. Given the expense and risk of renal transplantation, renal US screening for ACKD before renal transplantation is appropriate. Screening for tumors in native kidneys after transplantation with renal US may be justified in high-risk groups such as young men. Consideration should be given to scanning of native kidneys when a renal transplant patient undergoes US imaging of his or her graft (238).

In dialysis patients, renal tumors larger than 3 cm should undergo a radical nephrectomy unless the patient is a poor operative risk (382). Tumors less than 3 cm require radical nephrectomy if the patient is a transplantation candidate. Patients with tumors completely confined to the kidney can have a transplant immediately after the nephrectomy, but when tumors extend into the perinephric fat, a waiting period of 1 to 2 years is advised (308). Tumors less than 3 cm in the remaining ACKD patients require either radical nephrectomy or annual CT scans to access rate of growth to determine whether radical nephrectomy is appropriate. If a tumor is smaller than 3 cm and no rapid tumor growth is documented on serial imaging studies, but symptoms such as back pain or hematuria persist, nephrectomy is probably indicated because the tumor may be carcinoma and nephrectomy for intractable hematuria can reveal RCC that was not visualized preoperatively (130). Bilateral nephrectomy can be considered in ACKD-related RCC patients who are to undergo renal transplantation because posttransplant immunosuppression is a known risk factor for the development of renal neoplasms and because ACKD is a bilateral disease (382).

REFERENCES

1. Abt AB, Demers LM, Shochat SJ. Cystic nephroma: an ultrastructural biochemical study. *J Urol* 1979;122:539.
2. Alanen A, Nurmi M, Ekfors T. Multilocular renal lesions—a diagnostic challenge. *Clin Radiol* 1987;38:475.
3. Al-Khaldi N, et al. Outcome of antenatally detected cystic dysplastic kidney disease. *Arch Dis Child* 1994;70:520.
4. Ambrose SS, et al. Unilateral multicystic renal disease in adults. *J Urol* 1982;128:366.
5. Amir G, Rosenmann E, Drukker A. Acquired glomerulocystic kidney disease following haemolytic-uraemic syndrome. *Pediatr Nephrol* 1995;9:614.
6. Amis ES Jr, Cronan JJ. The renal sinus: an imaging review and proposed nomenclature for sinus cysts. *J Urol* 1988;139:1151.
7. Angermeier KW, Kay R, Levin H. Hypertension as a complication of multicystic dysplastic kidney. *Urology* 1992;39:55.
8. Antignac C, et al. A gene for familial juvenile nephronophthisis (recessive medullary cystic kidney disease) maps to chromosome 2p. *Nature Genet* 1993;3:342.
9. Ariza M, et al. A family with a milder form of adult dominant polycystic kidney disease not linked to the PKD_1 (16p) or PKD_2 (4q) genes. *J Med Genet* 1997;34:587.
10. Aronson S, et al. Cystic renal masses: usefulness of the Bosniak classification. *Urol Radiol* 1991;13:83.
11. Atiyeh B, Husmann D, Baum M. Controlled renal abnormalities in multicystic-dysplastic kidney disease. *J Pediatr* 1992; 121:65.
12. Au K-S, et al. Germ-line mutational analysis of the TSC2 gene in 90 tuberous-sclerosis patients. *Am J Hum Genet* 1998; 62:286.
13. Avasthi PS, Erickson DG, Gardner KD Jr. Hereditary renal-retinal dysplasia and the medullary cystic disease-n-nephronophthisis complex. *Ann Intern Med* 1976;84:157.
14. Babka JC, Cohen MS, Sode J. Solitary intrarenal cyst causing hypertension. *N Engl J Med* 1974;291:343.
15. Bachner L, Kaplan J. Molecular genetics and polycystic kidney diseases. *Adv Nephrol* 1989;18:3.
16. Balci NC, et al. Complex renal cysts: findings on MR imaging. *AJR Am J Roentgenol* 1999;172:1495.
17. Banner MP, et al. Multilocular renal cysts: radiologic pathologic correlation. *AJR Am J Roentgenol* 1981;136:239.
18. Barrett BJ, Parfrey PS. Autosomal dominant polycystic kidney disease and end stage renal disease. *Semin Dial* 1991;4:26.
19. Bartholomew TH, et al. The sonographic evaluation and management of simple renal cysts in children. *J Urol* 1980;123:732.
20. Bean SA, Bednarek FJ, Primack WA. Aggressive respiratory support and unilateral nephrectomy for infants with severe perinatal autosomal recessive polycystic kidney disease. *J Pediatr* 1995;127:311.
21. Beckwith JB. Should asymptomatic unilateral multicystic dysplastic kidneys be removed because of the future risk of neoplasia? *Pediatr Nephrol* 1992;6:511.
22. Bell PE, et al. Hypertension in autosomal dominant polycystic kidney disease. *Kidney Int* 1988;34:683.
23. Bennett AH, Stewart W, Lazarus JM. Bilateral nephrectomy in patients with polycystic renal disease. *Surg Gynecol Obstet* 1973; 137:819.
24. Bennett WM, Elzinga LW. Clinical management of autosomal dominant polycystic kidney disease. *Kidney Int* 1993;44[Suppl 42]:S74.
25. Bennett WM, et al. Reduction of cyst volume for symptomatic management of autosomal dominant polycystic kidney disease. *J Urol* 1987;137:620.
26. Bennett WM, et al. Cyst fluid antibiotic concentrations in autosomal-dominant polycystic disease. *Am J Kidney Dis* 1985; 6:400.
27. Berger U, et al. Pulmonary lymphangioleiomyomatosis and steroid receptors. *Am J Clin Pathol* 1990;93:609.
28. Bernstein J. A classification of renal cysts. In: Gardner KD Jr, ed. *Cystic diseases of the kidney.* New York: John Wiley & Sons, 1976:7.
29. Bernstein J. Congenital malformations of the kidney. In: Early LE, Gottschalk CW, eds. *Strauss Welt's diseases of the kidney,* 3rd ed. Boston: Little, Brown, 1979:1989.
30. Bernstein J. Glomerulocystic kidney disease—nosological considerations. *Pediatr Nephrol* 1993;7:464.
31. Bernstein J. Hepatic involvement in hereditary renal syndrome. *Birth Defects* 1987;23:115.
32. Bernstein J. Glomerular cysts in D-PKD. *Am J Med Genet* 1998;78:303.

33. Bernstein J, Landing BH. Glomerulocystic kidney disease. *Prog Clin Bio Res* 1989;305:27.
34. Bielsa O, et al. Cystic renal cell carcinoma: pathologic features, survival and implications for treatment. *Br J Urol* 1998;82:16.
35. Bigelow NH. The association of polycystic kidneys with intracranial aneurysms and other related disorders. *Am J Med Sci* 1953;225:485.
36. Bjornsson J, et al. Tuberous sclerosis-associated renal cell carcinoma: clinical, pathological and genetic features. *Am J Pathol* 1996;149:1201.
37. Blazer S, et al. Natural history of fetal simple renal cysts detected in early pregnancy. *J Urol* 1999;162:812.
38. Blickman JG, Bramson RT, Herrin JT. Autosomal recessive polycystic kidney disease: long term sonographic findings in patients surviving the neonatal period. *AJG* 1995;164:1247.
39. Blowey DL, et al. Ultrasound findings in juvenile nephronophthisis. *Pediatr Nephrol* 1996;10:22.
40. Blyth H, Ockenden BG. Polycystic disease of kidneys and children presenting in childhood. *J Med Genet* 1971;8:257.
41. Boggs LK, Kimmelstiel P. Benign multilocular cyst nephroma: report of two cases of so-called multilocular cyst of the kidney. *J Urol* 1956;76:530.
42. Bonetti F, Chiodera PL. Lymphangioleiomyomatosis and tuberous sclerosis: where is the border? *Eur Resp J* 1996;9:399.
43. Borge MA, Clark RL. Decompression of acute urinary tract obstruction by extravasation into a large simple cyst. *Urol Radiol* 1990;12:151.
44. Bosniak MA. The current radiological approach to renal cysts. *Radiology* 1986;158:1.
45. Bosniak MA. Difficulties in classifying cystic lesions of the kidney. *Urol Radiol* 1991;13:91.
46. Bosniak MA, Rofsky NM. Problems in the detection and characterization of small renal masses. *Radiology* 1996;198:638.
47. Bove KE. Pathology of selected abdominal masses in children. *Semin Roentgenol* 1988;23:147.
48. Branten AJW, Assmann KJM, Koene RAP. Matrix stones and acquired renal cysts in a non-dialyzed patient with chronic renal failure. *Nephrol Dial Transplant* 1995;10:123.
49. Bretan PN, Price DC, McClure RD. Localization of abscess in adult polycystic kidney by indium-111 leukocyte scan. *Urology* 1988;32:169.
50. Brook-Carter PT, et al. Deletion of the TSC2 and PKD1 genes associated with severe infantile polycystic kidney disease—a contiguous gene syndrome. *Nature Genet* 1994;8:328.
51. Brown B, Sharifi R, Lee M. Ethanolamine sclerotherapy of a renal cyst. *J Urol* 1995;153:385.
52. Brown RAP. Polycystic disease of the kidneys and intracranial aneurysms: The etiology and interrelationship of these conditions: review of recent literature and report of seven cases in which both conditions coexisted. *Glasgow Med J* 1951;32:333.
53. Brown RS, McClusky RT, Gang DL. Weekly clinicopathological exercises: case records of the Massachusetts General Hospital, case 48-n-1981. *N Engl J Med* 1981;305:1334.
54. Burke JR, et al. Juvenile nephronophthisis and medullary cystic disease—the same disease (report of a large family with medullary cystic disease associated with gout and epilepsy). *Clin Nephrol* 1982;18:1.
55. Cacchi R, Ricci V. Sopra una rara e forse ancora non descritta affezione cistica delle piramidi renali ("rene a spugna"). *Atti Soc Ital Urol* 1948;5:59.
56. Caglioti A, et al. Prevalence of symptoms in patients with renal cysts. *BMJ* 1993;306:430.
57. Carson RW, et al. Familial adult glomerulocystic kidney disease. *Am J Kidney Dis* 1987;9:154.
58. Carstens HB, Nassar RN. Glomerulocystic disease and lupus glomerulonephropathy. *Ultrastruct Pathol* 1994;18:137.
59. Castillo OA, Boyle ET, Kramer SA. Multiocular cysts of kidney. *Urology* 1994;37:156.
60. Chamberlin BC, Hagge WW, Strickler GB. Juvenile nephronophthisis and medullary cystic disease. *Mayo Clin Proc* 1997;52:485.
61. Chapman AB, Gabow PA, Schrier RW. Reversible renal failure associated with angiotensin-converting enzyme inhibitors in polycystic kidney disease. *Ann Intern Med* 1991;115:769.
62. Chapman AB, et al. The renin-angiotensin-aldosterone system and autosomal dominant polycystic kidney disease. *N Engl J Med* 1990;323:1091.
63. Chapman AB, Johnson AM, Gabow PA. Intracranial aneurysms in patients with autosomal dominant polycystic kidney disease: how to diagnose and who to screen. *Am J Kidney Dis* 1993;22:526.
64. Chapman AB, et al. Intracranial aneurysms in autosomal dominant polycystic kidney disease. *N Engl J Med* 1992;327:916.
65. Chen F, et al. Germline mutations in the von Hippel-Lindau disease tumor suppressor gene: correlations with phenotype. *Hum Mutations* 1995;5:66.
66. Cheng EY, et al. A rare case of bilateral multilocular renal cysts. *J Urol* 1997;157:1861.
67. Choyke PL. Inherited diseases of the kidney. *Radiol Clin North Am* 1996;34:925.
68. Choyke PL, et al. The natural history of renal lesions in von Hippel-Lindau disease: a serial CT study in 28 patients. *AJR Am J Roentgenol* 1992;159:1229.
69. Choyke PL, et al. von Hippel-Lindau disease: genetic, clinical and imaging features. *Radiology* 1995;194:629.
70. Choyke PL, et al. Epididymal cystadenomas in von Hippel-Lindau disease. *Urology* 1997;49:926.
71. Christodoulou K, et al. Chromosome 1 localization of a gene for autosomal dominant medullary cystic kidney disease (ADMCKD). *Hum Mole Genet* 1998;7:905.
72. Chung-Park M, Parveen T, Lam M. Acquired cystic disease of the kidneys and renal cell carcinoma in chronic renal insufficiency without dialysis treatment. *Nephron* 1989;53:157.
73. Churchill DN, et al. Prognosis of adult onset polycystic kidney disease re-evaluated. *Kidney Int* 1984;26:190.
74. Clarke A, et al. End-stage renal failure in adults with the tuberous sclerosis complex. *Nephrol Dial Transplant* 1999;14:988.
75. Cloix P, et al. Surgical management of complex renal cysts: a series of 32 cases. *J Urol* 1996;156:28.
76. Compton WR, et al. The abdominal angiographic spectrum of tuberous sclerosis. *AJR Am J Roentgenol* 1976;126:807.
77. Concolino G, et al. Acquired cystic kidney disease: the hormonal hypothesis. *Urology* 1993;41:170.
78. Cook JA, et al. A cross-sectional study renal involvement in tuberous sclerosis. *J Med Genet* 1996;33:480.
79. Crossey PA, et al. Molecular genetic investigations of the mechanism of tumourigenesis in von Hippel-Lindau disease: analysis of allele loss in VHL tumors. *Hum Genet* 1994;93:53.
80. Cussen LG, Stephens FD. Renal dysgenesis: a "urologic" classification. In: Stephens FD, ed. *Congenital malformations of the urinary tract.* New York: Praeger, 1983:463.
81. Dalgaard OZ. Bilateral polycystic disease of kidneys: a follow-up of 284 patients and their families. *Acta Med Scand (Suppl)* 1957;328:10.
82. Dalla-Palma L, Pozzi-Mucelli F, di Donna A. Cystic renal tumors: US and CT findings. *Urol Radiol* 1990;12:67.
83. Dalton D, Neiman H, Grayhack JT. The natural history of simple renal cysts: a preliminary study. *J Urol* 1986;136:905.

84. Danaci M, et al. The prevalence of seminal vesicle cysts in autosomal dominant polycystic kidney disease. *Nephrol Dial Transplant* 1998;13:2825.
85. Daoust MC, et al. Evidence for a third genetic locus for autosomal dominant polycystic kidney disease. *Genomics* 1995; 25:733.
86. Dedeoglu IO, et al. Spectrum of glomerulocystic kidneys: a case report and review of the literature. *Pediatr Pathol Lab Med* 1996;16;941.
87. Deget F, et al. Course of autosomal recessive polycystic kidney disease (ARPKD) in siblings: a clinical comparison of 20 sibships. *Clin Genet* 1995;47:248.
88. DeKlerk DP, Marshall FM, Jeffs RD. Multicystic dysplastic kidney. *J Urol* 1977;118:306.
89. Delaney VB, et al. Autosomal dominant polycystic kidney disease: Presentations, complications, and prognosis. *Am J Kidney Dis* 1985;5:104.
90. Deliveliotis C, et al. Management of lithiasis in medullary sponge kidneys. *Urol Int* 1996;57:198.
91. Dickinson M, et al. Renal angiomyolipoma: optimal treatment based on size and symptoms. *Clin Nephrol* 1998;49:281.
92. Dobin A, Kinberling WJ, Pettinger W, et al. Segregation analysis of autosomal dominant polycystic kidney disease. *Genet Epidemiol* 1993;10:189.
93. Donaldson JS, Shkolnik A. Pediatric renal masses. *Semin Roentgenol* 1988;23:194.
94. Dunnill MS. Acquired cystic disease. In: Grantham JJ, Gardner KD Jr, eds. *Problems in diagnosis and management of polycystic kidney disease.* Kansas City: PKR Foundation, 1985:211.
95. Dunnill MS, Millard PR, Oliver D. Acquired cystic disease of the kidneys. A hazard of long-term intermittent maintenance hemodialysis. *J Clin Pathol* 1977;30:868.
96. Eble JN, Bonsib SM. Extensively cystic renal neoplasms: cystic nephroma, cystic partially differentiated nephroblastoma, multilocular cystic renal cell carcinoma, and cystic hamartoma of the renal pelvis. *Semin Diagn Pathol* 1998;15:2.
97. Edmunds ME, et al. Plasma erythropoietin levels and acquired cystic disease of the kidney in patients receiving regular hemodialysis treatment. *Br J Hematol* 1991;78:275.
98. Egashira K, et al. MR imaging of adult glomerulocystic disease. A case report. *Acta Radiologica* 1991;32:251.
99. Eggers PW, Connerton R, McMullan M. The Medicare experience with end-stage renal disease: trends in incidence, prevalence, and survival. *Health Care Financing Rev* 1984;5:69.
100. Ekstrom T, et al. *Medullary sponge kidney.* Stockholm: Almqvist & Wiksel, 1959.
101. Elashry OM, et al. Laparoscopy for adult polycystic kidney disease: a promising alternative. *Am J Kidney Dis* 1996;27:224.
102. Elias TJ. Progressive hepatic failure secondary to adult polycystic kidney disease. *Aust NZ J Med* 1999;29:282.
103. Elzinga LW, Barry JM, Bennett WM. Surgical management of painful polycystic kidneys. *Am J Kidney Dis* 1993;22:532.
104. Elzinga LW, et al. Cyst decompression surgery for autosomal dominant polycystic kidney disease. *J Am Soc Nephrol* 1992;2: 1219.
105. Elzinga LW, et al. Trimethoprim-sulfamethoxazole in cyst fluid from autosomal dominant polycystic kidneys. *Kidney Int* 1987; 32:884.
106. Elzouki AY, et al. Thin-section computed tomography scans detect medullary cysts in patients believed to have juvenile nephronophthisis. *Am J Kidney Dis* 1996;27:216.
107. Emmert GK, King LR. The risk of hypertension is underestimated in the multicystic dysplastic kidney: a personal perspective. *Urology* 1994;44:404.
108. European Chromosome 16 Tuberous Sclerosis Consortium. Identification and characterization of the tuberous sclerosis gene on chromosome 16. *Cell* 1993;75:1305.
109. Everson GT. Hepatic cysts in autosomal dominant polycystic kidney disease. *Am J Kidney Dis* 1993;22:520.
110. Ewalt DH, et al. Renal lesion growth in children with tuberous sclerosis complex. *J Urol* 1998;160:141.
111. Fernandez A, et al. Anemia in dialysis: its relation to acquired cystic disease and serum levels of erythropoietin. *Am J Nephrol* 1991;11:12.
112. Filmer RB, Taxy JB, King LR. Renal dysplasia: Clinicopathological study. *Trans Am Assoc Genitourin Surg* 1974;66:18.
113. Fitzpatrick PM, et al. Long-term outcome of renal transplantation in autosomal dominant polycystic kidney disease. *Am J Kidney Dis* 1990;15:535.
114. Flack CE, Bellinger MF. The multicystic dysplastic kidney and contralateral vesicoureteral reflux: protection of the solitary kidney. *J Urol* 1993;150:1873.
115. Fleming TW, Barry JM. Bilateral open transperitoneal cyst reduction surgery for autosomal dominant polycystic kidney disease. *J Urol* 1998;159:44.
116. Florijn KW, et al. Long-term cardiovascular morbidity and mortality in autosomal dominant polycystic kidney disease patients after renal transplantation. *Transplantation* 1994;57:73.
117. Fontana D, et al. Treatment of simple renal cysts by percutaneous drainage with 3 repeated alcohol injections. *Urology* 1999; 53:904.
118. Frimodt-Moller PC, Nissen HM, Dyreborg U. Polycystic kidneys as the renal lesion in Lindau's disease. *J Urol* 1981; 125:868.
119. Gabow PA. Autosomal dominant polycystic kidney disease. *N Engl J Med* 1993;329:332.
120. Gabow PA, et al. Gene testing in autosomal dominant polycystic kidney disease: Results of National Kidney Foundation Workshop. *Am J Kidney Dis* 1989;13:85.
121. Gabow PA, et al. Utility of ultrasonography in the diagnosis of autosomal dominant polycystic kidney disease in children. *J Am Soc Nephrol* 1997;8:105.
122. Gabow PA, Ikle DW, Holmes JH. Polycystic kidney disease, prospective analysis of nonazotemic patients and family members. *Ann Intern Med* 1984;101:238.
123. Gagnadoux MF, et al. Cystic renal diseases in children. *Adv Nephrol* 1989;18:33.
124. Gagnadoux MF, et al. Infantile chronic tubulointerstitial nephritis with cortical myocysts: variant of nephronophthisis or new disease entity? *Pediatr Nephrol* 1989;3:50.
125. Gang DL, Herrin JT. Infantile polycystic disease of the liver and kidneys. *Clin Nephrol* 1986;25:28.
126. Gardner KD Jr. Juvenile nephronophthisis and renal medullary cystic disease. In: Gardner KD Jr, ed. *Cystic diseases of the kidney.* New York: John Wiley & Sons, 1976:173.
127. Gardner KD Jr, Evan AP. Cystic kidneys: an enigma evolves. *Am J Kidney Dis* 1984;3:403.
128. Garel LA, et al. Juvenile nephronophthisis: Sonographic appearance in children with severe uremia. *Radiology* 1984; 151:93.
129. Garrett A, Carty H, Pilling D. Multilocular cystic nephroma: report of three cases. *Clin Radiol* 1987;38:55.
130. Gehrig JJ, Gottheiner TJ, Swanson RS. Acquired cystic disease of the end-stage kidney. *Am J Med* 1985;79:609.
131. Gelet A, et al. Percutaneous treatment of benign renal cysts. European *Urology* 1990;18:248.
132. Gibson P, Watson ML. Cyst infection in polycystic kidney disease: a clinical challenge. *Nephrol Dial Transplant* 1998;13: 2455.

133. Gilcrease MZ, et al. Somatic von Hippel-Lindau mutation in clear cell papillary cystadenoma of the epididymis. *Hum Pathol* 1995;26:1341.
134. Ginalski JM, Portmann L, Jaeger P. Does medullary sponge kidney cause nephrolithiasis? *AJR Am J Roentgenol* 1990; 155:299.
135. Ginalski JM, et al. Medullary sponge kidney on axial computed tomography: comparison with excretory urography. *Eur J Radiol* 1991;12:104.
136. Gladziwa V, et al. Diagnosis and treatment of a solitary infected hepatic cyst in two patients with adult polycystic kidney disease. *Clin Nephrol* 1993;40:205.
137. Glassberg KI, et al. Renal dysgenesis and cystic disease of the kidney: A report of the Committee on Terminology, Nomenclature and Classification Section on Urology. *Am Acad Pediatr J Urol* 1987;138:1085.
138. Glassberg KI, Kassner EG. *Ex vivo* intracystic contrast studies of multicystic dysplastic kidneys. *J Urol* 1998;160:1204.
139. Goldfarb DA, et al. Results of renal transplantation in patients with renal cell carcinoma and von Hippel-Lindau disease. *Transplantation* 1997;64:1726.
140. Golin CO. Insurance for autosomal dominant polycystic kidney disease patients prior to end stage renal disease. *Am J Kidney Dis* 1996;27:220.
141. Gordon RL, et al. Simple serous cysts of the kidney in children. *Radiology* 1979;131:357.
142. Grabstald H. Catheterization of renal cyst for diagnostic and therapeutic purposes. *J Urol* 1954;71:28.
143. Grantham JJ. Polycystic kidney disease: hereditary and acquired. *Adv Intern Med* 1993;38:409.
144. Grantham JJ. Polycystic kidney disease: neoplasia in disguise. *Am J Kidney Dis* 1990;15:110.
145. Grantham JJ. Mechanisms of progression in autosomal dominant polycystic kidney disease. *Kidney Int* 1997;52:593.
146. Grantham JJ, Levine E. Acquired cystic disease: Replacing one kidney disease with another. *Kidney Int* 1985;28:99.
147. Grantham JJ, Geiser JL, Evan AP. Cyst formation and growth in autosomal dominant polycystic kidney disease. *Kidney Int* 1987;31:1145.
148. Green AJ, Smith M, Yates JRW. Loss of heterozygosity on chromosome 16p13.3 in hamartomas from tuberous sclerosis patients. *Nature Genet* 1994;6:193.
149. Griffin MD, et al. Vascular expression of polycystin. *J Am Soc Nephrol* 1997;8:616.
150. Griscom NT. The roentgenology of neonatal abdominal masses. *AJR Am J Roentgenol* 1965;93:447.
151. Griscom NT, Vawter GF, Fellers FX. Pelvoinfundibular atresia: the usual form of multicystic kidney: 44 unilateral and 2 bilateral cases. *Semin Roentgenol* 1975;10:125.
152. Gronwald J, et al. Chromosomal abnormalities in renal cell neoplasms associated with acquired renal cystic disease. A series studied by comparative genomic hybridization and fluorescence in situ hybridization. *J Pathol* 1999;187:308.
153. Guay-Woodford LM, et al. The severe perinatal form of autosomal recessive polycystic kidney disease maps to chromosome 6p21.1-p12: implications for genetic counseling. *Am J Hum Genet* 1995;56:1101.
154. Guay-Woodford LM, et al. Diffuse renal cystic disease in children: morphologic and genetic correlations. *Pediatr Nephrol* 1998;12:173.
155. Guazzoni G, et al. Laparoscopic unroofing of simple renal cysts. *Urology* 1994;43:154.
156. Gulanikar AC, et al. Prospective pretransplant ultrasound screening in 206 patients for acquired renal cysts and renal cell carcinoma. *Transplantation* 1998;66:1669.
157. Hadimeri H, et al. CAPD in patients with autosomal dominant polycystic kidney disease. *Peritoneal Dial Int* 1998;18:429.
158. Hadimeri H, Lamm C, Nyberg G. Coronary aneurysms in patients with autosomal dominant polycystic kidney disease. *J Am* Soc *Nephrol* 1998;9:837.
159. Haider NB, et al. A Bedouin kindred with infantile nephronophthisis demonstrates linkage to chromosome by homozygosity mapping. *Am J Hum Genet* 1998;63:1404.
160. Hamida MB, et al. Renal transplantation and autosomal dominant polycystic kidney disease: 20 year's experience. *Transplant Proc* 1993;25:2162.
161. Hamlin JA, et al. Renal angiomyolipomas: long term follow-up of embolization for acute hemorrhage. *Can Assoc Radiol J* 1997; 48:191.
162. Hartman DS, et al. Cystic renal cell carcinoma: CT findings simulating a benign hyperdense cyst. *AJR Am J Roentgenol* 1992;159:1235.
163. Hateboer N, et al. Comparison of phenotypes of polycystic kidney diseases types I and 2. European PKD_1-PKD_2 Study Group. *Lancet* 1999;353:103.
164. Hateboer N, et al. Familial phenotypic differences in PKD_1. *Kidney Int* 1999;56:34.
165. Hatfield PM, Pfister RC. Adult polycystic disease of the kidneys (Potter type 3). *JAMA* 1972;222:1527.
166. Heinz-Peer G, et al. Prevalence of acquired cystic kidney disease and tumors in native kidneys of renal transplant recipients: a prospective US study. *Radiology* 1995;195:667.
167. Heinz-Peer G, et al. Role of magnetic resonance imaging in renal transplant recipients with acquired cystic kidney disease. *Urology* 1998;51:534.
168. Hemal AK, et al. Retroperitoneoscopic management of infected cysts in adult polycystic kidney disease. *Urol Int* 1998;62:40.
169. Hendry PJ, Hendry GMA. Observations on the use of Doppler ultrasound in multicystic dysplastic kidney. *Pediatr Radiol* 1991;21:203.
170. Hendry WF, et al. Seminal megavesicles with adult polycystic kidney disease. *Hum Reprod* 1998;13:1567.
171. Henske EP, et al. Frequent progesterone receptor immunoreactivity in tuberous sclerosis-associated renal angiomyolipomas. *Mod Path* 1998;11:665.
172. Herrera GA. C-erb β-2 amplification in cystic renal disease. *Kidney Int* 1991;40:509.
173. Herrin JT. Phenotypic correlates of autosomal recessive (infantile) polycystic disease of kidney and liver: criteria for classification and genetic counseling. *Prog Clin Biol Res* 1989;305:45.
174. Higashihara E, Natahar K, Niijima T. Renal hypercalciuria and metabolic acidosis associated with medullary sponge kidney: effect of alkali therapy. *Urol Res* 1988;16:392.
175. Hildebrandt F, et al. A novel gene encoding an SH3 domain protein is mutated in nephronophthisis type 1. *Nature Genet* 1997;17:149.
176. Hildebrandt F, et al. Renal cystic disease. *Curr Opin Pediatr* 1999;11:141.
177. Hilpert PL, et al. MRI of hemorrhagic renal cysts in polycystic kidney disease. *AJR Am J Roentgenol* 1986;146:1167.
178. Hirai T, et al. Usefulness of color doppler flow imaging in differential diagnosis multilocular cystic lesions of the kidney. *J Ultrasound Med* 1995;14:771.
179. Hoard TD, O'Brien DP III: Simple renal cyst and high renin hypertension cured by cyst decompression. *J Urol* 1976; 115:326.
180. Hoenig DM, et al. Laparoscopic ablation of peripelvic renal cysts. *J Urol* 1997;158:1345.

181. Holloway WR, Weinstein SH. Percutaneous decompression: treatment for respiratory distress secondary to multicystic dysplastic kidney. *J Urol* 1990;144:113.
182. Holmberg G. Diagnostic aspects, functional significance and therapy of simple renal cysts. A clinical, radiologic, and experimental study. *Scand J Urol Nephrol Suppl* 1992;145:1.
183. Holmberg G, Hietala SO. Treatment of simple renal cysts by percutaneous puncture and instillation of bismuth-phosphate. *Scand J Urol Nephrol* 1989;23:207.
184. Holmberg G, et al. Significance of simple renal cysts and percutaneous cyst puncture on renal function. *Scand J Urol Nephrol* 1994;28:35.
185. Hossack KF, et al. Echocardiographic findings in autosomal dominant polycystic kidney disease. *N Engl J Med* 1988; 319:907.
186. Hough DM, et al. Pancreatic lesions in von Hippel-Lindau disease: prevalence, clinical significance, and CT findings. *AJR Am J Roentgenol* 1994;162:1091.
187. Hrair-George JM, Rushton, HG, Bulos D. Unilateral renal agenesis may result from *in utero* regression of multicystic renal dysplasia. *J Urol* 1993;150:793.
188. Huston III J, et al. Value of magnetic resonance angiography for the detection of intracranial aneurysms in autosomal dominant polycystic kidney disease. *J Am Soc Nephrol* 1993;3:1871.
189. Ibrahim RE, Weinberg DS, Weidner N. Atypical cysts and carcinomas of the kidneys in the phacomatoses. *Cancer* 1989; 63:148.
190. Iglesias DM, et al. Isolated polycystic liver disease not linked to polycystic kidney disease 1 and 2. *Dig Dis Sci* 1999;44:385.
191. International Polycystic Disease Consortium. Polycystic kidney disease: the complete structure of the PKD_1 gene and its protein. *Cell* 1995;81:289.
192. Ishikawa I. Uremic acquired cystic disease of the kidney. *Urology* 1985;26:101.
193. Ishikawa I, Kovacs G. High incidence of papillary renal cell tumors in patients on chronic hemodialysis. *Histopathology* 1993;22:135.
194. Ishikawa I, et al. Development of acquired cystic disease and adenocarcinoma of the kidney in glomerulonephritis chronic hemodialysis patients. *Clin Nephrol* 1980;14:1.
195. Ishikawa I, et al. Severity of acquired renal cysts in native kidneys and renal allograft with longstanding poor function. *Am J Kidney Dis* 1989;14:18.
196. Ishikawa I, Shikura N, Nagahara M, et al. Comparison of severity of acquired renal cysts between CAPD and hemodialysis. *Adv Peritoneal Dial* 1991;7:91.
197. Ishikawa I, et al. Regression of acquired cystic disease of the kidney after successful renal transplantation. *Am J Nephrol* 1983;3:310.
198. Ishikawa I, et al. Fifteen-year followup of acquired renal cystic disease—a gender difference. *Nephron* 1997;75:315.
199. Jacobsson L, et al. Fluid turnover in renal cysts. *Acta Med Scand* 1977;202:327.
200. Jamil B, et al. A study of long-term morbidity associated with autosomal recessive polycystic kidney disease. *Nephrol Dial Transplant* 1999;14:205.
201. Jamis-Dow CA, et al. Small (≤ 3 cm) renal masses: detection with CT versus US and pathologic correlation. *Radiology* 1996; 198:785.
202. Javadpour N, et al. Hypertension in a child caused by a multicystic kidney. *J Urol* 1970;104:918.
203. Jeon A, et al. A spectrum of segmental multicystic renal dysplasia. *Pediatr Radiol* 1999;9:309.
204. Jeyarajah DR, et al. Liver and kidney transplantation for polycystic disease. *Transplantation* 1998;66:529.
205. John U, et al. Kidney growth and renal function in unilateral multicystic dysplastic kidney disease. *Pediatr Nephrol* 1998; 12:567.
206. Johnson AM, Gabow PA. Identification of patients with autosomal dominant polycystic kidney disease at highest risk for end-stage renal disease. *J Am Soc Nephrol* 1997;8:1560.
207. Jones AC, et al. Molecular genetic and phenotypic analysis reveals differences between TSC_1 and TSC_2 associated familial and sporadic tuberous sclerosis. *Hum Mol Genet* 1997;6:2155.
208. Jones AC, et al. Comprehensive mutation analysis of TSC_1 and TSC_2 and phenotypic correlations in 150 families with tuberous sclerosis. *Am J Hum Genet* 1999;64:1305.
209. Joshi VV, Beckwith B. Multilocular cyst of the kidney (cystic nephroma) and cystic, partially differentiated nephroblastoma: terminology and criteria for diagnosis. *Cancer* 1989;64:466.
210. Jung G, et al. MR cholangiography in children with autosomal recessive polycystic kidney disease. *Pediatr Radiol* 1999;29:463.
211. Kaariainen H, et al. Polycystic kidney disease in children: Differential diagnosis between the dominantly and recessively inherited forms. *Prog Clin Biol Res* 1989;305:55.
212. Kaehny W, et al. Family clustering of intracranial aneurysms (ICA) in autosomal dominant polycystic kidney disease (ADPKD). *Kidney Int* 1987;31:204.
213. Kandt RS. Tuberous sclerosis: the next step. *J Child Neurol* 1993;8:107.
214. Kaplan BS, et al. Autosomal recessive polycystic kidney disease. *Pediatr Nephrol* 1989;3:43.
215. Kaplan BS, et al. Variable expression of autosomal recessive polycystic kidney disease and congenital hepatic fibrosis within a family. *Am J Med Genet* 1988;29:639.
216. Karsdorp N, Eldersen A, Wittebol-Post D. Von Hippel-Lindau disease: new strategies in early detection and treatment. *Am J Med* 1994;97:158.
217. Kattan SA. Immediate recurrence of simple renal cyst after laparoscopic unroofing. *Scand J Urol Nephrol* 1996;30:415.
218. Kavoussi LR, et al. Ureteronephroscopic marsupialization of obstructing peripelvic renal cyst. *J Urol* 1991;146:411.
219. Kern S, et al. RARE-MR-urography—a new diagnostic method in autosomal recessive polycystic kidney disease. *Acta Radiol* 1999;40:543.
220. Kettritz U, et al. Multilocular cystic nephroma: MR imaging appearance with current techniques, including gadolinium enhancement. *J MRI* 1996;1:145.
221. Kim AH, et al. Contrast-enhanced power doppler sonography for the differentiation of cystic renal lesions: preliminary study. *J Ultrasound Med* 1999;18:581.
222. Kimberling WJ, Kumar S, Gabow PA. Autosomal dominant polycystic kidney disease: localization of the second gene to chromosome 4q13-4q23. *Genomics* 1993;18:467.
223. Kissane JM. The morphology of renal cystic disease. In: Gardner KD Jr, ed. *Cystic diseases of the kidney.* New York: John Wiley & Sons, 1976:31.
224. Kissane JM, Smith MG. *Pathology of infancy and childhood,* 2nd ed. St. Louis: Mosby, 1975:587.
225. Klein AJP, Kozar RA, Kaplan LJ. Traumatic hematuria in patients with polycystic kidney disease. *Am Surg* 1999;65:464.
226. Koptides M, et al. Germinal and somatic mutations in the PKD_2 gene of renal cysts in autosomal dominant polycystic kidney disease. *Hum Mole Genet* 1999;8:509.
227. Korf BR. genetic testing for patients with renal disease: procedures, pitfalls, and ethical considerations. *Semin Nephrol* 1999; 19:319.
228. Kuiper JJ. Medullary sponge kidney. In: Gardner KD Jr, ed. *Cystic diseases of the kidney.* New York: John Wiley & Sons, 1976:151.

229. Kwiatkowska J, et al. Comprehensive mutational analysis of the TSC_1 gene: observations on frequency of mutations, associated features, and nonpenetrance. *Ann Hum Genet* 1998;62:277,
230. Kyaw MM, Koehler PR. Congenital multicystic kidney. In: Gardner KD Jr, ed. *Cystic diseases of the kidney.* New York: John Wiley & Sons, 1976:115.
231. Kyushu Pediatric Nephrology Study Group. Acquired cystic kidney disease in children undergoing continuous ambulatory peritoneal dialysis. *Am J Kidney Dis* 1999;34:242.
232. Landing BH, Gwinn JL, Lieberman E. Cystic diseases of the kidney in children. In: Gardner KD Jr, ed. *Cystic diseases of the kidney.* New York: John Wiley & Sons, 1976:187.
233. Latif F, et al. Identification of the von Hippel-Lindau disease tumor suppressor gene. *Science* 1993;260:1317.
234. Laucks SP, McLachlan SF. Aging and simple cysts of the kidney. *Br J Radiol* 1981;54:12.
235. Lazebnik N, et al. Insights into the pathogenesis and natural history of fetuses with multicystic dysplastic kidney disease. *Prenat Diag* 1999;19:418.
236. Leung SY, et al. Expression of vascular endothelial growth factor in von Hippel-Lindau syndrome-associated papillary cystadenoma of the epididymis. *Hum Pathol* 1998;29:132a.
237. Levey AS, et al. Dietary protein restriction and the progression of chronic renal disease: what have all of the results of the MDRD study shown? *J Am Soc Nephrol* 1999;10:2426.
238. Levine E. Renal cell carcinoma in uremic acquired renal cystic disease: incidence, detection and management. *Urol Radiol* 1992;13:203.
239. Levine E, et al. CT screening of the abdomen in von Hippel-Lindau disease. *AJR Am J Roentgenol* 1982;139:505.
240. Levine E, et al. Current concepts and controversies in imaging of renal cystic diseases. *Urol Clin North Am* 1979;24:523.
241. Levine E, Cook LT, Grantham JJ. Liver cysts in autosomal-dominant polycystic kidney disease: clinical and computed tomography. *AJR Am J Roentgenol* 1985;145:229.
242. Levine E, Grantham JJ. Calcified renal stones and cyst calcifications in autosomal dominant polycystic kidney disease: clinical and CT study in 84 patients. *AJR Am J Roentgenol* 1992; 159:77.
243. Levine LA, Gburak BM. Acquired renal cystic disease and renal adenocarcinoma following renal transplantation. *J Urol* 1994; 151:129.
244. Libutti SK, et al. Pancreatic neuroendocrine tumors associated with von Hippel-Lindau disease: diagnosis and management recommendations. *Surgery* 1998;124:1153.
245. Lieberman E, et al. Infantile polycystic disease of the kidneys and liver: clinical pathological and radiologic correlations and comparisons with congenital hepatic fibrosis. *Medicine (Balt)* 1971;50:277.
246. Lien YH, et al. Association of cyclosporin A with acquired cystic kidney disease of the native kidneys in renal transplant recipients. *Kidney Int* 1993;44:613.
247. Lubensky IA, et al. Allelic deletions of the VHL gene detected in multiple microscopic clear cell renal lesions in von Hippel-Lindau disease patients. *Am J Pathol* 1996;149:2089.
248. Lucaya J, et al. Renal calcifications in patients with autosomal recessive polycystic kidney disease: prevalence and cause. *AJR Am J Roentgenol* 1993;160:359.
249. MacDermot KD, et al. Prenatal diagnosis of autosomal dominant polycystic kidney disease (PKD_1) presenting *in utero* and prognosis for very early onset disease. *J Med Genet* 1998;35:13.
250. MacDougall ML, Welling LW, Wiegmann TB. Prediction of carcinoma in acquired cystic disease as a function of kidney weight. *J Am Soc Nephrol* 1990;1:828.
251. Madewell JE, et al. Multilocular cystic nephroma: a radiographic-pathologic correlation of 58 patients. *Radiology* 1983;146:309.
252. Maher ER, et al. Von Hippel-Lindau disease: a genetic study. *J Med Genet* 1991;28:443.
253. Maher ER, Kaelin WG. Von Hippel-Lindau disease. *Medicine* 1997;76:381.
254. Malka D, et al. Chronic obstructive pancreatitis due to a pancreatic cyst in a patient with autosomal dominant polycystic kidney disease. *Gut* 1998;42:131.
255. Mallofre C, et al. Acquired renal cystic disease in HD: a study of 82 nephrectomies in young patients. *Clin Nephrol* 1992; 37:297.
256. Manenti A, et al. Infection of a renal cyst, a rare complication of bronchopneumonia. *Acta Urologica Belgica* 1990;58:145.
257. Manns RA, et al. Acquired cystic disease of the kidney: ultrasound as the primary screening procedure. *Clin Radiol* 1990; 41:248.
258. Manski TJ, et al. Endolymphatic sac tumors. A source of morbid hearing loss in von Hippel-Lindau disease. *JAMA* 1997; 227:1461.
259. Mariani L, et al. Cerebral aneurysms in patients with autosomal dominant polycystic kidney disease—to screen, to clip, to coil? *Nephrol Dial Transplant* 1999;14:2319.
260. Marple JT, MacDougall M. Development of malignancy in the end stage renal disease patient. *Semin Nephrol* 1993; 13:306.
261. Mascari M and Bosniak MA. Delayed CT to evaluate renal masses incidentally discovered at contrast-enhanced CT: demonstration of vascularity with deenhancement. *Radiology* 1999; 213:674.
262. Mathe CP. Cystic disease of the kidney: diagnosis and treatment. *J Urol* 1949;61:319.
263. Matsell DG. Renal dysplasia: new approaches to an old problem. *Am J Kidney Dis* 1998;32:535-.
264. Mattoo TK, et al. Acquired renal cystic disease in children and young adults in maintenance dialysis. *Pediatr Nephrol* 1997;11:447.
265. McAlister WH, et al. Glomerulocystic kidney. *AJR Am J Roentgenol* 1979;133:536.
266. McClean RH, Gang DL, Herrin JT. Weekly clinicopathological exercises: Case records of the Massachusetts General Hospital, case 48-n-1978. *N Engl J Med* 1978;299:1294.
267. McHugh K, et al. Simple renal cysts in children: diagnosis and follow-up with US radiology. *Radiology* 1991;178:383.
268. Mejias E, et al. Hyperuricemia, gout, and autosomal dominant polycystic kidney disease. *Am J Med Sci* 1989;297:145.
269. Melnick SC, Brewer DB, Oldham JS. Cortical microcystic disease of the kidney with dominant inheritance: a previously undescribed syndrome. *J Clin Pathol* 1984;37:494.
270. Melson GL, et al. The spectrum of sonographic findings in infantile polycystic kidney disease with urographic and clinical correlations. *J Clin Ultrsound* 1985;13:113.
271. Mickisch O, et al. Multicystic transformation of kidneys in chronic renal failure. *Nephron* 1984;38:93.
272. Milutinovic J, Schabel SI, Ainsworth SK. Autosomal dominant polycystic kidney disease with liver and pancreatic involvement in early childhood. *Am J Kidney Dis* 1989;13:340.
273. Mochizuki T, et al. PKD_2, a gene for polycystic kidney disease that encodes an integral membrane protein. *Science* 1996;272: 1339.
274. Mücher G, et al. Fine mapping of the autosomal recessive polycystic kidney disease locus (PKD1) and the genes MUT, RDS, CSNK2B, and GSTA1 at 6p21-p12. *Genomics* 1998; 48:40.
275. Munch LC, Gill IS, McRoberts JW. Laparoscopic retroperitoneal renal cystectomy. *J Urol* 1994;151:135.
276. Murcia NS, Sweeney WE, Avner ED. New insights into the molecular pathophysiology of polycystic kidney disease. *Kidney Int* 1999;55:1187.

277. Nakada SY, Erturk E, Monaghan J. Role of extracorporeal shock wave lithotripsy in treatment of urolithiasis in patients with medullary sponge kidney. *Urology* 1993;41:331.
278. Narla LD, et al. The renal lesions of tuberous sclerosis (cysts and angiomyolipomas)—screening with sonography and computerized tomography. *Pediatr Radiol* 1988;18:205.
279. Neumann HPH, Zbar B. Renal cysts, renal cancer and von Hippel-Lindau disease. *Kidney Int* 1997;51:16.
280. Newman KD, et al. Treatment of highly symptomatic polycystic liver disease. *Ann Surg* 1990;212:30.
281. Nieh PT, Bihrle III W. Laparoscopic marsupialization of massive renal cyst. *J Urol* 1993;150:171.
282. Niida Y, et al. Analysis of both TSC_1 and TSC_2 for germline mutations in 126 unrelated patients with tuberous sclerosis. *Hum Mutat* 1999;14:412.
283. Noe HN, Marshall JH, Edwards OP. Nodular renal blastema in the multicystic kidney. *J Urol* 1989;142:468.
284. Ohkawa M, et al. Biochemical and pharmacodynamic studies of simple renal cyst fluids in relation to infection. *Nephron* 1991;59:80.
285. Ohkawa M, et al. Percutaneous injection sclerotherapy with minocycline hydrochloride for simple renal cysts. *Int Urol Nephrol* 1993;25:37.
286. Ohta S, Fujishiro Y, Fuse H. Polidocanal sclerotherapy for simple renal cysts. *Urol Int* 1997;58:145.
287. Okada RD, Platt MA, Fleishman J. Chronic renal failure in patients with tuberous sclerosis association with renal cysts. *Nephron* 1982;30:85.
288. Olsen A, Hojhus JH, Steffensen J. Renal medullary cystic disease: Findings at urography and ultrasonography. *Acta Radiol* 1988;5:527.
289. Ong AC. Cyst formation in ADPKD: new insights from natural and targeted mutants. *Nephrol Dial Transplant* 1999; 14:544.
290. Osathanondh V, Potter EL. Pathogenesis of polycystic kidneys: Historical survey. *Arch Pathol* 1964;77:459.
291. Osther PJ, et al. Urinary acidification and urinary excretion of calcium and citrate in women with bilateral medullary sponge kidney. *Urol Int* 1994;52:126.
292. O'Sullivan DA, et al. Cystic fibrosis and the phenotypic expression of autosomal dominant polycystic kidney disease. *Am J Kidney Dis* 1998;32:976.
293. Ozgur S, Cetin S, Ilker S. Percutaneous renal cyst aspiration and treatment with alcohol. *Int Urol Nephrol* 1988;20:481.
294. Paavola P, et al. The locus for Meckel syndrome with multiple congenital anomalies maps to chromosome 17q21-q24. *Nature Genet* 1995;11:213.
295. Palou J, et al. Percutaneous drainage by multiple and bilateral puncture of infected renal cysts in autosomal dominant polycystic kidney disease. *Nephrol Dial Transplant* 1998;13:1606.
296. Papanicolaou N, Pfister RC, Yoder IC. Spontaneous and traumatic rupture of renal cysts: diagnosis and outcome. *Radiology* 1986;160:99.
297. Parfrey PS, et al. The diagnosis and prognosis of autosomal dominant polycystic kidney disease. *N Engl J Med* 1990;323: 1085.
298. Parienty RA, et al. Computed tomography of multilocular cystic nephroma. *Radiology* 1981;140:135.
299. Parks JH, Coe FL, Strauss AL. Calcium nephrolithiasis and medullary sponge kidney in women. *N Engl J Med* 1982;306: 1088.
300. Patel U, Huntley L, Kellett MJ. Sonography features of renal obstruction mimicked by peripelvic cysts. *Clin Radiol* 1994; 49:481.
301. Paterson AD, Pei Y. Is there a third gene for autosomal dominant polycystic kidney disease? *Kidney Int* 1998;54: 1759.
302. Patriquin HB, O'Regan S. Medullary sponge kidney in childhood. *AJR Am J Roentgenol* 1985;145:315.
303. Pea M, et al. Apparent renal cell carcinomas in tuberous sclerosis are heterogeneous: the identification of malignant epithelioid angiomyolipoma. *Am J Surg Pathol* 1998;22:180.
304. Pearson JC, Weiss J, Tanagho EA. A plea for conservation of kidney in renal adenocarcinoma associated with von Hippel-Lindau disease. *J Urol* 1980;124:910.
305. Pedersen JF, Emamian SA, Nielsen MB. Simple renal cyst: relations to age and arterial blood pressure. *Br J Radiol* 1993; 66:581.
306. Pedersen JF, Emamian SA, Nielsen MB. Significant association between simple renal cysts and arterial blood pressure. *Br J Urol* 1997;79:688.
307. Pei Y, et al. Somatic PKD_2 mutations in individual kidney and liver cysts support a "two-hit" model of cystogenesis in type 2 autosomal dominant polycystic kidney disease. *J Am Soc Nephrol* 1999;10:1524.
308. Penn I. Renal transplant in patients with preexisting malignancies. *Transplant Proc* 1983;15:1079.
309. Perez LM, Naidu SI, Joseph DB. Outcome and rest analysis of operative versus nonoperative management of neonatal multicystic dysplastic kidneys. *J Urol* 1998;160:1207.
310. Perez-Oller L, et al. Influence of the ACE gene polymorphism in the progression of renal failure in autosomal dominant polycystic kidney disease. *Am J Kidney Dis* 1999;34:273.
311. Peters DJ, et al. Chromosome 4 localization of a second gene for autosomal dominant polycystic kidney disease. *Nature Genet* 1993;5:359.
312. Phelan M, Zajko A, Hrebinko RL. Preliminary results of percutaneous treatment of renal cysts with povidone-iodine sclerosis. *Urology* 1999;53:816.
313. Pirson Y, Christophe JL, Goffin E. Outcome of renal replacement therapy in autosomal dominant polycystic kidney disease. *Nephrol Dial Transplant* 1996;11:24.
314. Plas EG, Hubner WA. Percutaneous resection of renal cysts: a long-term follow-up. *J Urol* 1993;149:703.
315. Poston CD, et al. Characterization of the renal pathology of a familial form of renal cell carcinoma associated with von Hippel-Lindau disease: clinical and molecular genetic implications. *J Urol* 1995;153:22.
316. Povey S, et al. Two loci for tuberous sclerosis: one on 9q34 and on 16p13. *Ann Hum Genet* 1994;58:105.
317. Premkumar A, et al. The emergence of hepatic fibrosis and portal hypertension in infants and children with autosomal recessive polycystic kidney disease. *Pediatr Radiol* 1988; 18:123.
318. Proesmans W, Van Damme B, Macken J. Nephronophthisis and tapetoretinal degeneration associated with liver fibrosis. *Clin Nephrol* 1975;3:160.
319. Quian F, et al. The molecular basis of focal cyst formation in human autosomal dominant polycystic kidney disease type I. *Cell* 1996;87:979.
320. Ravden MI, et al. Evaluation of solitary simple renal cysts in children. *J Urol* 1980;124:904.
321. Ravine D, et al. An ultrasound renal cyst prevalence survey: specificity data for inherited renal cystic diseases. *Am J Kidney Dis* 1993;22:803.
322. Ravine D, et al. Evaluation of ultrasonographic diagnostic criteria for autosomal dominant polycystic kidney disease. *Lancet* 1994;343:824.
323. Reis M, et al. The small cystic and noncystic noninflammatory renal modules: a postmortem study. *J Urol* 1988;140:721.
324. Reitelman C, et al. Infected multicystic dysplastic kidney. *Urology* 1992;39:157.
325. Resnick MI. Hemorrhagic renal cyst. *Soc Pediatr Urol Newslett* 1989;Jan 15:8.

326. Reubi FC. Hypertension. In: Grantham JJ, Gardner KD Jr, eds. *Problems in management and diagnosis of polycystic kidney disease.* Kansas City: PKR Foundation, 1985:121.
327. Richards FM, et al. Molecular genetic analysis of von Hippel-Lindau disease. *J Intern Med* 1998;243:527.
328. Roach PJ. Renal dysplasia in infants: appearance on ^{99m}TcDMSA scintigraphy. *Pediatr Radiol* 1995;25:472.
329. Robson WLM, Thomason MA, Minette LJ. Cystic dysplasia of the testis associated with multicystic dysplasia of the kidney. *Urology* 1998;51:477.
330. Rockson SG, Stone RA, Gunnells JC. Solitary renal cyst with segmental ischemia and hypertension. *J Urol* 1974;112:550.
331. Roscoe JM, et al. Autosomal dominant polycystic kidney disease in Toronto. *Kidney Int* 1993;44:1101.
332. Rosenfield AT, et al. Gray scale ultrasonography in medullary cystic disease of the kidney and congenital hepatic fibrosis with tubular ectasia: new observations. *AJR Am J Roentgenol* 1977; 129:297.
333. Rossi SJ, et al. High dose ciprofloxacin in the treatment of a renal cyst infection. *Ann Pharmacother* 1993;27:38.
334. Roume J, et al. A gene for Meckel syndrome maps to chromosome 11q13. *Am J Hum Genet* 1997;34:1003.
335. Rubenstein SC, et al. Laparoscopic ablation of symptomatic renal cysts. *J Urol* 1993;150:1103.
336. Rudnik-Schöneborn S, et al. Clinical features of unilateral multicystic renal dysplasia in children. *Eur J Pediatr* 1998; 157:662.
337. Saathof PW, et al. Renal cell carcinoma in a multilocular renal cyst: a case report of a 27 year old female and review of literature. *Eur Urol* 1991;20:253.
338. Sampson JR, et al. Renal cystic disease in tuberous sclerosis: role of the polycystic kidney disease 1 gene. *Am J Hum Genet* 1997;61:843.
339. Sandford R, et al. Comparative analysis of the polycystic kidney disease I (PKD1) gene reveals an integral membrane glycoprotein with multiple evolutionary conserved domains. *Hum Mole Genet* 1997;6:1483.
340. Sant GR, Ucci AA. Acquired renal cystic disease and adenocarcinoma following renal transplantation—a current urological perspective. *Urol Int* 1998;60:108.
341. Santiago L, et al. Laparoscopic management of indeterminate renal cysts. *Urology* 1998;52:379.
342. Sarasin FP, et al. Screening for acquired cystic kidney disease: a decision analytic perspective. *Kidney Int* 1995;48:207.
343. Sasaki H, et al. Comparative study of cystic variations of the kidneys in haemodialysis and continuous ambulatory peritoneal dialysis patients. *Int Urol Nephrol* 1996;28:247.
344. Saxton HM, et al. Diagnostic puncture in renal cystic dysplasia (multicystic kidney). Evidence on the etiology of the cysts. *Br J Radiol* 1981;54:555.
345. Schillinger F, Montagnac R. Chronic renal failure and its treatment in tuberous sclerosis. *Nephrol Dial Transplant* 1996; 11:481.
346. Schwab SJ. Efficacy of chloramphenicol in refractory cyst infections in autosomal dominant polycystic kidney disease. *Am J Kidney Dis* 1985;5:258.
347. Scolari F, et al. Identification of a new locus for medullary cystic disease on chromosome 16p12. *Am J Hum Genet* 1999; 64:1655.
348. Sedman A, et al. Autosomal dominant polycystic kidney disease in childhood: a longitudinal study. *Kidney Int* 1987;31:1000.
349. Sellers B, Richie JP. Glomerulocystic kidney: proposed etiology and pathogenesis. *J Urol* 1978;119:678.
350. Sepp T, Yates JRW, Green AJ. Loss of heterozygosity in tuberous sclerosis hamartomas. *J Med Genet* 1996;33:962.
351. Shaikewitz ST, Chapman A. Autosomal recessive polycystic kidney disease: issues regarding the variability of clinical presentation. *J Am Soc Nephrol* 1993;3:1858.
352. Shepherd CW, et al. Causes of death in patients with tuberous sclerosis. *Mayo Clin Proc* 1991;66:792.
353. Shertha R, et al. Postmenopausal estrogen therapy selectively stimulates hepatic enlargement in women with autosomal dominant polycystic kidney disease. *Hepatology* 1997;26:1282.
354. Siegel CL, et al. CT of cystic renal masses: analysis of diagnostic performance and intraobserver variation. *AJR Am J Roentgenol* 1997;169:813.
355. Siegel MJ, McAlister WH. Simple cysts of the kidney in children. *J Urol* 1980;123:75.
356. Simon J. On subacute inflammation of the kidney. *Medico-Chir Trans* 1847;30:141.
357. Sklar AH, Caruana RJ, Lammers JE. Renal infections in autosomal dominant polycystic kidney disease. *Am J Kidney Dis* 1987;10:81.
358. Somlo S. The PKD_2 gene: structure, interactions, mutations, and inactivation. *Adv Nephrol* 1999;29:257.
359. Spence HM. Congenital unilateral multicystic kidney: an entity to be distinguished from polycystic kidney disease and other cystic disorders. *J Urol* 1955;74:693.
360. Srivastava T, Garola RE, Hellerstein S. Autosomal dominant inheritance of multicystic dysplastic kidney. *Pediatr Nephrol* 1999;13:481.
361. Stapleton FB, et al. The cystic renal lesion in tuberous sclerosis. *J Pediatr* 1980;97:574.
362. Stavrou C, et al. Medullary cystic kidney disease with hyperuricemia and gout in a large Cypriot family: no allelism with nephronophthisis type 1. *Am J Med Genet* 1998;77:149.
363. Steinbach F, et al. Treatment of renal cell carcinoma in von Hippel-Lindau disease. A multicenter study. *J Urol* 1995;153: 1812.
364. Stillwell TT, Gomez MR, Kelalis PP. Renal lesions in tuberous sclerosis. *J Urol* 1987;138:477.
365. Strife JL, et al. Multicystic dysplastic kidney in children: US follow-up. *Radiology* 1993;186:785.
366. Stuck KJ, Koff SA, Silber TM. Ultrasonic features of multicystic dysplastic kidney: expanded diagnostic criteria. *Radiology* 1982;143:217.
367. Sumfest JM, Burns MW, Mitchell MF. Aggressive surgical and medical management of autosomal recessive polycystic kidney disease. *Urology* 1993;42:309.
368. Suter W. Das kongenitale Aneurysma der basalen Gehirnarterien und Cystennieren. *Schweiz Med Wochenschr* 1949;79:471.
369. Tada S, et al. The incidence of simple renal cyst by computed tomography. *Clin Radiol* 1983;34:437.
370. Talwar D, Swaiman KF. Peroxisomal disorders: a review of a recently recognized group of clinical entities. *Clin Pediatr* 1987; 26:497.
371. Taxy JB. Renal dysplasia: a review. *Pathol Annu* 1985;20 (Pt 2):139.
372. Taxy JB, Filmer RB. Glomerulocystic kidney. *Arch Pathol Lab Med* 1976;100:186.
373. Teele RL, Share JC. The abdominal mass in the neonate. *Semin Roentgenol* 1988;23:175.
374. Terasawa Y, et al. Ultrasonic diagnosis of renal cell carcinoma in hemodialysis patients. *J Urol* 1994;152:846.
375. Torra R. Autosomal dominant polycystic kidney disease, type 2 (PKD2 disease). *Adv Nephrol* 1999;29:277.
376. Torra R, et al. Linkage, clinical features, and prognosis of autosomal dominant polycystic kidney disease types 1 and 2. *J Am Soc Nephrol* 1996;7:2142.

377. Torra R, et al. Pancreatic cysts in autosomal dominant polycystic kidney disease. *Clin Nephrol* 1997;47:19.
378. Torra R, et al. A loss-of-function model for cystogenesis in human autosomal dominant polycystic kidney disease type 2. *Am J Hum Genet* 1999;65:345.
379. Torres VE, et al. The association of nephrolithiasis and autosomal dominant polycystic kidney disease. *Am J Kidney Dis* 1988;11:318.
380. Torres VE, et al. Renal stone disease in autosomal dominant polycystic kidney disease. *Am J Kidney Dis* 1993;22:513.
381. Torres VE, et al. Extrarenal manifestations of autosomal dominant polycystic kidney disease. *Am J Kidney Dis* 1999; 34:xiv.
382. Truong LD, et al. Renal neoplasm in acquired cystic kidney disease. *Am J Kidney Dis* 1995;26:1.
383. Tsokias L, et al. Homo- and heterodimeric interactions between the gene products of PKD_1 and PKD_2. *Proc Natl Acad Sci USA* 1997;94:6965.
384. Uemasu J, et al. Effects of topical instillation of minocycline hydrochloride on cyst size and renal function in polycystic kidney disease. *Clin Nephrol* 1993;39:140.
385. van Baal JG, Smits NJ, Keeman JN. The evolution of renal angiomyolipomas in patients with tuberous sclerosis. *J Urol* 1994;152:35.
386. van der Ent CK, van Dalen A, Enterman JH. Antibiotic sclerotherapy for renal cysts. *Fortschr Rontgenstr* 1989;150:339.
387. Vandeursen H, Baert L. Prophylactic role of extracorporeal shock wave lithotripsy in the management of nephrocalcinosis. *Br J Urol* 1993;71:392.
388. Vandeursen H, et al. Acquired cystic disease of the kidney analyzed by microdissection. *J Urol* 1991;146:1168.
389. Van Slegtenhorst M, et al. Identification of the tuberous sclerosis gene TSC_1 on chromosome 9q34. *Science* 1997; 277:805.
390. Vauthey J-N, Maddern GJ, Blumgart LH. Adult polycystic disease of the liver. *Br J Surg* 1991;78:524.
391. Verhoef S, et al. High rate of mosaicism in tuberous sclerosis complex. *Am J Hum Genet* 1999;64:1632.
392. Wacksman J, Phipps L. Report of the multicystic kidney registry: preliminary findings. *J Urol* 1993;150:1870.
393. Wakabayashi T, et al. Polycystic kidney disease and intracranial aneurysms: early angiographic diagnosis and early operation for the unruptured aneurysm. *J Neurosurg* 1983;58:488.
394. Walker D, et al. Spectrum of multicystic dysplasia. *Urology* 1978;11:433.
395. Walther MC, et al. Prevalence of microscopic lesions in grossly normal renal parenchyma from patients with von Hippel-Lindau disease, sporadic renal cell carcinoma and no renal disease: clinical implications. *J Urol* 1995;154:2010.
396. Walther MC, et al. Management of hereditary pheochromocytoma in von Hippel-Lindau kindreds with partial adrenalectomy. *J Urol* 1999;161:395.
397. Walther MC, et al. Renal cancer in families with hereditary ren cancer: prospective size threshold for renal parenchyma sparing surgery. *J Urol* 1999;161:1475.
398. Walther MC, et al. Clinical and genetic characterization of pheochromocytoma in von Hippel-Lindau families: comparison with sporadic pheochromocytoma gives insight into natural history of pheochromocytoma. *J Urol* 1999;162:659.
399. Washecka R, Hanna M. Malignant renal tumors in tuberous sclerosis. *Urology* 1991;37:340.
400. Waters K, et al. Intrahepatic bile duct dilatation and cholestasis in autosomal recessive polycystic kidney disease demonstration with hepatobiliary scintigraphy. *Clin Nucl Med* 1995; 20:892.
401. Watnik TJ, et al. Somatic mutation in individual liver cysts supports a two-hit model of cystogenesis in autosomal dominant polycystic kidney disease. *Mole Cell* 1998;2:247.
402. Webster AR, et al. An analysis of phenotypic variation in the familial cancer syndrome von Hippel-Lindau disease: evidence for modifier effects. *Am J Hum Genet* 1998;63:1025.
403. Weichert-Jacobsen K, et al. Clinical experience with percutaneous renal cyst resection. *BJU Int* 1999;84:164.
404. Wernecke K, et al. Sonography of infantile polycystic kidney disease. *Urol Radiol* 1985;7:138.
405. White R, et al. Renal growth characteristics in children born with multicystic dysplastic kidneys. *Urology* 1998;52:874.
406. Wiebers DO, Torres VE. Screening for unruptured intracranial aneurysms in autosomal dominant polycystic kidney disease. *N Engl J Med* 1992;327:953.
407. Wilson PD, Du J, Norman JT. Autocrine, endocrine and paracrine regulation of growth abnormalities in autosomal dominant polycystic kidney disease. *Eur J Cell Biol* 1993; 61:131.
408. Wilson PD, Guay-Woodford L. Pathophysiology and clinical management of polycystic kidney disease in women. *Semin Nephrol* 1999;19:123.
409. Wilson TE, et al. Cystic renal masses: a reevaluation of the usefulness of the Bosniak classification system. *Acad Radiol* 1996;3:564.
410. Wolf JS. Evaluation and management of solid and cystic renal masses. *J Urol* 1998;159:1120.
411. Worthington JL, et al. Sonographically detectable cysts in polycystic kidney disease in newborn and young infants. *Pediatr Radiol* 1988;18:287.
412. Wright AF, Teague PW, Pound SE. A study of genetic linkage heterogeneity in 35 adult-onset polycystic kidney disease families. *Hum Genet* 1993;90:569.
413. Yendt ER. Medullary sponge kidney and nephrolithiasis. *N Engl J Med* 1982;306:1106.
414. Zbar B, et al. Third international meeting on von Hippel-Lindau disease. *Cancer Res* 1999;59:2251.
415. Zerres K, et al. Autosomal recessive polycystic kidney disease: Problems of prenatal diagnosis. *Prenat Diagn* 1988;8:215.
416. Zerres K, et al. Autosomal recessive polycystic kidney disease in 115 children: clinical presentation, course and influence of gender. *Acta Pediatr* 1996;85:437.
417. Zerres K, et al. Prenatal diagnosis of autosomal recessive polycystic kidney disease (ARPKD): molecular genetics, clinical experience, and fetal morphology. *Am J Med Genet* 1998; 76:137.
418. Zerres K, Rudnik-Schöneborn S, Mücher G. Autosomal recessive polycystic kidney disease: clinical features and genetics. *Adv Nephrol* 1996;25:147.

21

HYDRONEPHROSIS

JAY Y. GILLENWATER

Hydronephrosis is the distention of the renal calyces and pelvis with urine as a result of obstruction of the outflow of urine distal to the renal pelvis. Prolonged hydronephrosis results in renal parenchymal atrophy. Elevated renal pelvic pressures and decreased renal blood flow are postulated to be mechanisms of injury and cellular atrophy. Obstructive uropathy progressively impairs all renal functions except urinary dilution. The longer and more complete the obstruction, the more severe the pathophysiologic changes become.

Significant changes in experimental hydronephrosis have occurred in three areas in the last 4 years. There is a better understanding of which factors and vasoactive substances cause the decreased blood flow after 24 hours of complete unilateral ureteral obstruction (UUO). There is more information on causative factors leading to tubular loss and interstitial fibrogenesis. The differences between the pathophysiology of obstructive nephropathy in the newborn and adult have been further delineated, showing that in addition to tubular atrophy and interstitial fibrosis, obstruction in the maturing kidney impairs renal growth and development.

Recent research shows a complex series of pathophysiologic events after ureteral obstruction involving more than the anatomic, pathologic, and physiologic changes previously described. A variety of vasoactive compounds, growth factors, and cytokines are activated in response to ureteral obstruction. These factors include platelet-derived growth factor, transforming growth factor-β (TGF-β), epidermal growth factor, insulin-like growth factor, clusterin, nitric oxide, endothelin, atrial natriuretic peptide, and angiotensin II. There are also factors that cause leukocyte infiltration, such as osteopontin and arachidonic acid metabolites (eicosanoids).

Recent excellent reviews by Gulmi and colleagues (76), Chevalier (19), Ricardo and Diamond (169), and Klahr and Morrissey (113) define current knowledge of these vasoactive mediators. My interpretation of these data is that the etiology, pathophysiology, and consequence of UUO is significantly different in the newborn and the adult. Obstruction of the maturing kidney impairs renal growth and development in addition to causing tubular atrophy and interstitial fibrosis. The renin-angiotensin system (RAS) in the maturing kidney plays a greater role in normal develop-

J.Y. Gillenwater: Professor of Urology, University of Virginia Medical School, Charlottesville, VA 22908.

ment and pathophysiologic response than in the adult. In adult UUO, there is a better understanding of the development of fibrosis and the presence of various vasoactive compounds. There also appear to be species differences in responses to ureteral obstruction.

PATHOPHYSIOLOGY OF OBSTRUCTIVE UROPATHY

Historical Aspects of Hydronephrosis

Hinman first studied experimental hydronephrosis systematically (87,89,90). These studies showed that infection plus obstruction caused severe and rapid renal damage (87). Histologic changes were noted after 1 week of obstruction, with some histologic recovery after release of 60 days of obstruction in rats (87). Denervation of the kidney did not alter the course of hydronephrosis (94). Renal arterial or venous obstruction accentuated the damage in hydronephrosis (89,92,93). Release after 2 weeks of complete ureteral obstruction with contralateral nephrectomy resulted in the return of most function to the previously obstructed kidney. The same experiment with 3 weeks of complete obstruction resulted in only a 50% return of function. The animals could not survive release of obstruction lasting longer than 2 or 3 weeks if the opposite kidney was removed at the time of release of the ureteral obstruction. The animals could survive release after 30 to 60 days of unilateral hydronephrosis if the opposite normal kidney was damaged gradually after release of the ureteral obstruction.

Pathology

Urinary tract obstruction causes proximal dilation with anatomic changes in the proximal ureter, renal pelvis, and renal parenchyma. Initially, the proximal ureter and renal pelvis react with muscle hypertrophy and hyperplasia. Production of connective tissue consisting of collagen and elastic tissue occurs later and is thought to impair myogenic impulse transmission and cause disturbance of peristalsis (42,48,65,70,116). An increase in collagen, which acts as an inelastic collar preventing distention, has been found in the obstructing segments of the ureteropelvic junction and in megaureters (77,151,152). Studies of infants with ureteropelvic junction (UPJ) obstruction showed an increase in the inner longitudinal muscle bundles, in collagen between muscle bundles, and in elastin in the adventitia (191).

Hydronephrosis eventually causes tubular dilation with cellular atrophy and interstitial fibrosis. Within 7 days, atrophy is seen in the distal nephron. By 14 days, there is progressive dilation of the distal tubules and atrophy of the proximal tubular epithelial cells. At 28 days, there is loss of 50% of the medulla with marked atrophy of the proximal tubules and thinning of the cortex. Glomerular changes are not noted before 28 days of obstruction. There is no evidence of microscopic changes in the arteries to account for the substantially reduced blood flow observed in hydronephrosis. Venous drainage is impaired, causing some of the renal damage (2,46,91,97,164,180,182,193). Urinary tract obstruction causes proximal dilation, blunting of the renal papillae after 2 to 3 days, and gradual atrophy and thinning of the renal tissue. Microscopically, the renal tubules dilate with cellular atrophy beginning in the distal nephron. In longstanding hydronephrosis, the glomeruli become sclerotic. During obstruction, there is increased cellularity of the interstitium with leukocytes, fibroblasts, and macrophages, which may have vasoactive functions. No vascular obstruction is seen to account for the increased vascular resistance associated with chronic hydronephrosis.

Fluid Turnover in Hydronephrosis

Urine exits the renal pelvis in complete ureteral obstruction by extravasation, pyelolymphatic backflow, and pyelovenous backflow. Replacement glomerular filtration maintains the hydronephrosis. Thus there is an active turnover of urine in the hydronephrotic renal pelvis despite complete ureteral obstruction. Substances injected into the hydronephrotic renal pelvis have appeared in the systemic circulation, confirming the dynamic state of the hydronephrosis: strychnine (199), phenolsulfonphthalein (17), dye (138), and indigo carmine (96). Extravasation of urine first occurs through rupture of the fornix (10,96). Narath (146) and Olsson (155) studied urine backflow during ureteral obstruction. Initially, ureteral obstruction produces pyelocanalicular and pyelosinus backflow.

With acute obstruction and high pressures, as during retrogrades or with ureteral calculi, most of the fluid exits the renal pelvis by extravasation at the calyceal fornix. With low-pressure obstruction, much of the fluid exits into the lymphatic vessels. In chronic hydronephrosis, most of the fluid exits into the renal venous system.

Renal Counterbalance, Compensatory Renal Hypertrophy, and Renal Hypotrophy

The concepts of renal counterbalance, compensatory renal hypertrophy, and renal hypotrophy (disuse atrophy) were first introduced by Hinman in 1922 (88) and later summarized in 1926. The theory of renal counterbalance is based on the premise that there is a mechanism to monitor total renal function and that the function of each kidney can be modulated up or down as appropriate. Thus, if one kidney is removed or rendered nonfunctioning by obstruction, the opposite kidney would undergo compensatory hypertrophy. If additional renal tissue is added by release of unilateral obstruction or transplantation of additional kidneys, some mechanism would modulate total renal function downward by renal hypotrophy. Renal hypertrophy and hypotrophy involve changes in function. Some misunderstandings and controversy have resulted from efforts to comprehend renal counterbalance in terms of renal mass instead of function.

Studies have provided new information about compensatory renal hypertrophy. Two forms of renal growth have been postulated: obligatory growth thought to be under the stimulus of growth hormone and compensatory growth under an unknown humoral stimulus. Compensatory renal growth includes both hypertrophy and hyperplasia (161) and is not as great in older animals (84). After unilateral ureteral obstruction, there is a bilateral increase in renal mass the first week, followed by atrophy in the obstructed kidney and continued hypertrophy in the opposite unobstructed kidney. The increased mass in the obstructed kidney may be a local response to injury (229) or a response to the unknown humoral factor. In most models, the renotrophic factor is present in anephric animals. Renotrophic factor stimulates three forms of growth: embryonic growth, wound repair compensatory growth, and neoplastic growth (159). The renotrophic factor is thought to be humorally mediated and must be continually present to maintain compensatory growth (126). Similar renotrophic factors are present in urine and serum (80). During compensatory hypertrophy, glomeruli increase in size but not in number. Diabetes and pregnancy cause renal hypertrophy.

Chronic UUO in fetal sheep impairs growth of the obstructed kidney and stimulates compensatory growth in the contralateral kidney. The developing kidney is more susceptible to the effects of ipsilateral UUO. Adaptive growth of the contralateral kidney is also enhanced. Compensatory growth is reversible (187), whereas normal growth is not. Angiotensin acts as a growth factor in normal renal development and is not necessary in neonatal mouse. Insulin-like growth factor-1 plays a role in neonatal (but not adult) compensatory renal growth (143).

Renal hypotrophy (atrophy) is most easily understood in terms of function. When a hypertrophied kidney is experimentally transplanted into a recipient with a hypertrophied kidney, both kidneys return to their previous size (187,189). When two additional kidneys were transplanted into male rats with normal kidneys, there was no change in the size of either the two transplanted kidneys or the two normal kidneys. However, total renal blood flow and glomerular filtration showed no increase over normal conditions (170). Silber (187,189) found that after transplanting an additional kidney there was an increase in total renal mass and a 50% increase in total renal blood flow and glomerular filtration rate (GFR).

Studies in our laboratory showed that with release of unilateral complete obstruction, the obstructed kidney regains function over the next 4 months. Compensatory hypertrophy persists in the contralateral kidney during that time. Total renal function is not fully recovered to control values at 4 months. Studies in Chevalier's laboratory have confirmed the compensatory hypertrophy in the contralateral kidney in the neonate (19). These studies suggest both a humoral and a neural mechanism.

Return of Function After Complete Ureteral Obstruction

Recovery of renal function after release of complete ureteral obstruction varies with the species, total time of obstruction, presence or absence of infection, degree of pyelovenous and pyelolymphatic backflow, and whether the renal pelvis is intrarenal or extrarenal. In the dog with a normal contralateral kidney after release of 2 weeks of obstruction, the GFR can recover up to 46% of control function in 3 to 4 months. After release of 4 weeks of total ureteral obstruction, there was recovery of the GFR to 35% of control by 5 months. No return of function was noted with release after 6 weeks of total ureteral obstruction in the dog (201).

How long the human kidney can be completely obstructed and still regain function after release is not known for certain. Reports in the literature have been difficult to evaluate because the length and completeness of obstruction and the return of renal function are difficult to document adequately. With greater use of renal scanning and renal ultrasound and better awareness of possible ureteral obstruction after pelvic surgery, better documentation should be possible. The cases with the longest period of complete ureteral obstruction meeting the aforementioned criteria and showing some recovery of function are 56 and 69 days (74,120,166).

Prediction of Recovery Potential Before Release of the Obstruction

To make the right decision about nephrectomy or correcting an obstruction, the urologist needs to know whether the kidney will regain function after the obstruction is released. The two best means of assessing recoverability before surgery are the placement of temporary ureteral stents or nephrostomy tubes and the use of renal scans with sophisticated analysis. The simplest method is to place percutaneous nephrostomy tubes to relieve the obstruction and monitor creatinine clearances. If the previously obstructed kidney has not regained at least a 6 to 10 mL minute creatinine clearance by 2 to 3 months, I do not think it merits repair if the other kidney is normal.

Prediction of recoverability with the renal scans is more difficult and has not been successful in many studies. Evaluating cortical zones of interest by arbitrary mathematical analysis, however, has been successful: technetium (^{99}Tc) pentetic acid, diethylene triamine pentaacetic acid (DTPA) (121), ^{99m}Tc DMSA (dimercaptosuccinic acid) (132), and iodohippurate sodium labeled with iodine 131 (^{131}I hippuran) (66,108). That the different scanning agents measure various renal functions has not seemed to be as important as the method of quantitative analysis of the results. ^{131}I hippuran measures renal blood flow and correlates with the GFR. ^{99m}Tc DMSA accumulates in the cytoplasm of proximal tubular cells and is used to assess functioning cortical tissue. ^{99}Tc DTPA is eliminated by glomerular filtration and correlates with cortical renal blood flow. MacNeily and associates (125) believe it is important that measurement of the radioactivity be made between 1 and 3 minutes when the radioactivity is confined to renal blood vessels and functioning parenchyma. Before 1 minute, the radioactivity can be extrarenal; after 3 minutes, the accumulation of radioactivity in the renal pelvis can cause confusion.

Intrapelvic and Renal Tubular Pressures

Normal

Normal renal pelvic pressure is 6.5 mm Hg, which slightly exceeds the intraperitoneal, bladder, and ureteral pressures. Normal proximal tubular pressure is 14 mm Hg (134).

Unilateral Ureteral Obstruction

Ureteral and renal pelvic pressures after complete unilateral ureteral obstruction rise abruptly and then decrease within 24 hours to 50% of the peak values (202). Ureteral pressures continue to decline over the next 8 weeks to 15 mm Hg despite the continued completed obstruction (202). Thus static ureteral pressure measurements have never been helpful in determining the degree of ureteral obstruction.

The peak ureteral pressures with acute complete ureteral obstruction vary with hydration, osmotic diuresis, degree of ureteral contractions, and amount of reabsorption. The maximum pressure from filtration is the stop-flow pressure of 15 to 20 mm Hg [glomerular capillary pressure (60 mm Hg) minus capillary oncotic pressure (25 to 30 mm Hg) minus hydrostatic pressure in Bowman's capsule (15 mm Hg)]. The higher pressures measured during acute obstruction are a result of filtration pressure and active muscle contractions in the ureter and renal pelvis. Ureteral pressures of 50 to 70 mm Hg have been measured after acute ureteral obstruction in humans (5,97,130,134,144,153, 196). Ureteral pressure after obstruction can be further increased to 100 mm Hg by saline or mannitol diuresis (158,201).

Pressure transmitted back to the renal pelvis varies with the conditions of the obstruction. In acute unilateral obstruction in nondiuretic rats, the ureteral and proximal tubular pressure rises to 14 mm Hg, which is normal proximal tubule pressure (72,73). In diuretic rats, the maximum pressure in the ureter and proximal renal tubule rises to 40 mm Hg (72,73). Further elevation of ureteral pressure by injecting fluid to 80 mm Hg fails to transmit and does not raise proximal tubular pressure above 40 mm Hg, presumably because of compression of papillary foramina (72).

Within 24 hours, the elevated proximal tubular pressure is below normal as a result of afferent arteriole constriction (49,72). Another consequence of elevation of ureteral pressure is that the proximal and distal tubules become leaky to creatinine, mannitol, and sucrose. Studies have shown that the aqueous junctional complexes of membranes of adjacent cells are disrupted. The permeability is restored when tubular pressures return to normal (16,122).

When unilateral ureteral obstruction persists, ureteral pressure slowly declines to reach normal levels in 3 to 4 weeks (202). Michaelson (134) found an average decrease of intrapelvic pressures of 6.6 mm Hg after follow-up of six patients with partial obstruction for 8 weeks. Although ureteral and pelvic pressures decrease toward normal ranges with chronic obstruction, they must continue to be slightly elevated because something is sending signals maintaining the alterations seen in renal function during obstruction. Because relief of the obstruction promptly reverses the process, another possible explanation would be that the distention and increased tension are sending signals initiating the physiologic response.

Alterations of Renal Function During Unilateral Obstruction: Short-term Effects

Glomerular Filtration Rate

As previously described, within minutes of ureteral obstruction, the hydraulic pressure of the fluid proximal to the obstruction rises. As the proximal tubular pressure rises, the GFR falls. The decrease in the GFR is attributable to both the rise in tubular pressure and the decrease in the area of filtering membrane when the afferent arteriole constriction begins after 5 hours of obstruction. The GFRs in rats with complete obstruction were 52% at 4 hours, 23% at 12 hours, 4% at 24 hours, and 2% at 48 hours (79,162).

Renal Blood Flow

Ipsilateral renal blood flow and ureteral pressure have a triphasic relationship during the first 24 hours of acute unilateral ureteral obstruction (Fig. 21.1) (137). The initial transient (112-hour) response is an increase in renal blood flow and ureteral pressure, indicating a preglomerular vasodilation. Pretreatment with prostaglandin (PG) inhibitors prevents this vasodilation, indicating that PGE_2 and PGI_2, which dilate vessels and are produced in the kidneys, may be responsible (1,64,101,175). Nishikawa and associates (149) and Needleman and co-workers (147) measured increased production of the vasodilating prostaglandins during acute ureteral obstruction. The increase in renal blood flow caused by acute ureteral obstruction appears to be limited to cortical blood flow, with the inner cortex having the greatest

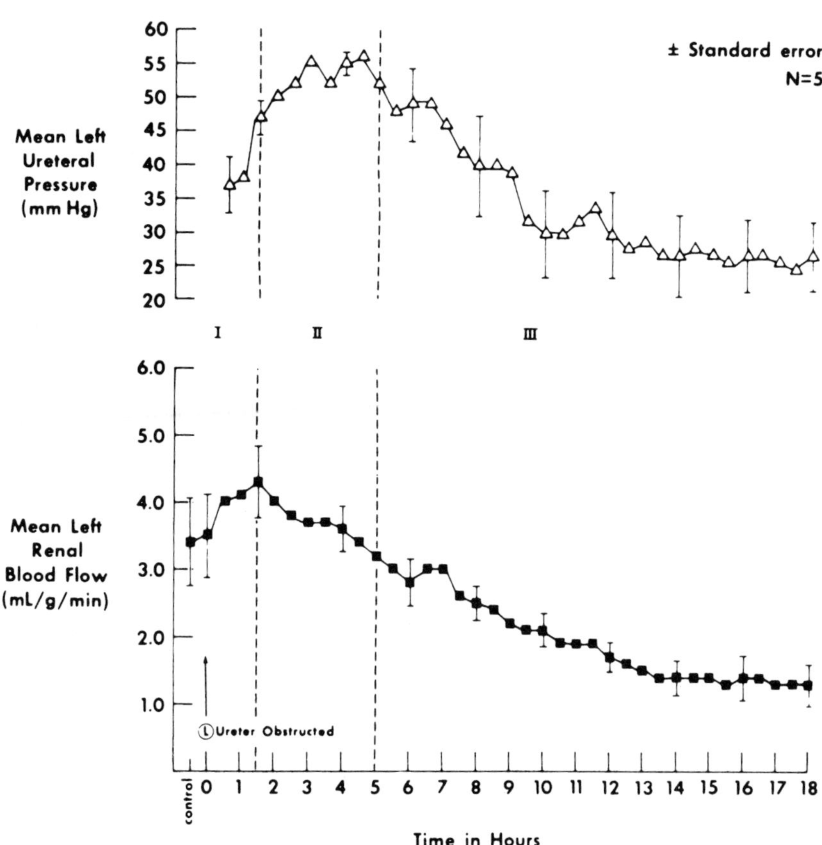

FIGURE 21.1. Triphasic relationship between ipsilateral renal blood flow and ureteral pressure during 18 hours of left complete ureteral obstruction in the dog. In phase I, both left renal blood flow and ureteral pressure increase. In phase II, left renal blood flow decreases, while ureteral pressure continues to increase. In phase III, left renal blood flow and ureteral pressure decline together. (From Vaughan ED Jr, Sorenson EJ, Gillenwater JY. The renal hemodynamic response to chronic unilateral complete ureteral occlusion. *Invest Urol* 1970;8:78, with permission.)

increase (190). The transient increase in renal blood flow is thought to be the result of a vasodilating prostaglandin release.

The second vascular phase, which consists of a decrease in renal blood flow with continuation of rising ureteral pressures, occurs 5 to 112 hours after the obstruction. The postulated mechanism is a rise in postglomerular vascular resistance.

During the third and chronic phase (5 to 18 hours), renal blood flow and ureteral pressure decrease. This fall in renal blood flow and ureteral pressure continues chronically (202). Preglomerular vasoconstriction causes the decrease in renal blood flow and lower ureteral pressure. Similar preglomerular vasoconstriction is seen in a single nephron with tubular obstruction (4).

Sheehan and associates (181) found reduced renal blood flow and thromboxane A_2 synthesis in dogs with partial ureteric obstruction. Increased renal blood flow to the nonobstructed side was associated with elevated PGE_2 formation. Elevated angiotensin I levels corresponded to maximal increases in prostaglandin synthesis.

Hemodynamic Changes in UUO

The role of vasodilator eicosanoids in phase I has been confirmed since the initial studies by Allen and associates (1), showing that pretreatment with indomethacin prevented the initial vasodilation seen with UUO. Studies have confirmed the role of vasodilator prostaglandin in causing the increased renal blood flow immediately after UUO (61,139).

The role of eicosanoids after phase III UUO is not as well established. Yarger and colleagues (227) showed a decrease in renal vasoconstriction in UUO after the administration of imidazole, a thromboxane A_2 synthesis inhibitor. Indomethacin, which decreases synthesis of both vasodilator and vasoconstrictor eicosanoids, did not increase renal blood flow.

The mechanism of the chronic preglomerular vasoconstriction in hydronephrosis has received the most experimental attention in the last 10 years. Unilateral ureteral obstruction results in decreased renal blood flow to the ipsilateral kidney and increased blood flow to the unobstructed contralateral kidney (56). The ipsilateral vasoconstriction is in part caused by thromboxanes, angiotensin, endothelin, and mesangial-cell contact (29,62,103,115, 118,139,140,185,227). Increased production of vasodilators as prostaglandins opposes the vasoconstriction in the ipsilateral kidney and, in part, causes the vasodilation of the contralateral kidney (101). Chronic UUO in the guinea pig increases angiotensin-dependent renal vasoconstriction independent of renal nerves (31). Vasodilation of the opposite kidney may be mediated by the renal nerves or contralateral renal renin suppressors (32,37). Thromboxanes have been shown to act as modulators of renal vascular resistance in UUO (78,227). Vasodilator prostaglandins appear to contribute to vasodilation of the intact opposite kidney (223).

Fern and co-workers (57) studied UUO mice with no to four functional copies of the angiotensin gene and found that angiotensin regulates at least 50% of the renal interstitial fibrotic response and that a functional renal-angiotensin system is not necessary for compensatory growth. UUO was also reported by Kinter and colleagues (112) to reduce renal antioxidant enzyme activities, including those seen with sodium depletion, thus contributing to the progression of renal injury in obstructive nephropathy.

Nitric oxide, an endothelial-derived relaxing factor (EDRF), is increased in the ipsilateral vasoconstricted rat kidney but not in the vasodilated contralateral kidney (33). Endogenous nitric oxide has a marked systemic and renal vasodilatory effect in the unobstructed normal rat (6,198, 205,209,228).

Haung (82) has pointed out that in normal renal physiology nitric oxide regulates local arteriolar tone, tubular sodium handling, and mesangial-cell proliferation and causes decreased synthesis and increased degradation of matrix protein. This suggests that nitric oxide may serve as an antifibrotic in the kidney. Administration of L-arginine before UUO resulted in nearly complete restoration of renal blood flow and GFR after release of obstruction and infusion of nitric oxide synthase (NOS) inhibitor before release of the obstruction resulted in complete loss of renal function in the affected kidney. Administration of L-arginine significantly decreased the infiltrating of macrophages into the interstitium of the obstructed kidney and improved GFR (82).

Glomeruli from the contralateral vasodilated kidney produce increased PGE_2 and 6-keto PGF_{1a} (223). The increased injury to the renal medulla in obstructive uropathy has been postulated to be due to reduced O_2 as a result of reduced nitric oxide formation (13,33).

Studies from Chevalier's laboratory at the University of Virginia have shown the following:

1. In neonatal obstruction, *in situ* localization of renin and mRNA was increased with ureteral obstruction (53). In contrast, adult rats with chronic unilateral ureteral obstruction of 24-hour and 4-week duration did not manifest an increase in the distribution of immunoreactive renin or renin mRNA in the obstructed kidneys (54).
2. In chronic unilateral ureteral obstruction in newborn rats studied by El-Dahr and co-workers (53), the renal sympathetic nerves modulated renin gene expression, which leads to increased renin distribution along afferent glomerular arterioles in both kidneys.
3. EDRF modulates basal arterial blood pressure, renal vascular resistance, GFR, and effective renal plasma flow in normal rats and in rats with unilateral release of bilateral ureteral obstruction of 24-hour duration (167).
4. Neonatal unilateral ureteral obstruction in newborn rats stimulates increased renin secretion in the obstructed kidney. The increased renin secretion is from recruitment of more renin-secreting renal cortical cells and is not blocked by chemical sympathectomy (150).

The pathophysiology of obstructive nephropathy in the newborn was recently reviewed by Chevalier (19) as summarized and partly quoted here. Obstruction to urinary flow results in a complex response by the developing kidney, manifested by impaired nephrogenesis, including delayed maturation of the renal vasculature, glomeruli, tubules, and interstitial cells. In the adult, UUO stimulates renal cell proliferation. These changes may result from a combination of factors, including loss of epithelial cell polarity, a reduction in the oncoprotein bcl-2 and epidermal growth factor (EGF), and increased expression of the fibrogenic cytokine TGF-β_1. UUO in the neonate causes impaired renal growth, renal tubular dilation, tubular atrophy, and interstitial fibrosis. Recent studies have focused less on the hemodynamic effects of obstruction and more on renal cellular response and the role of growth factors (18).

The developing kidney responds differently to chronic UUO than the adult kidney (18). The RAS plays a greater role in UUO in the neonate than in the adult kidney. In the neonate, there is enhanced activity of the entire RAS, which contributes to the very high renal vascular resistance during development, which normally gradually decreases. Chronic UUO in the neonatal rat results in a marked increase in renal renin gene expression, distributed along the length of the afferent arteriole and intratubular artery rather than being localized to the juxtaglomerular region. Angiotensin II is now recognized as a vasoconstrictor and an important growth factor that can stimulate proliferation or hypertrophy of renal tubular cells. Renal renin gene expression following UUO is ten times higher in the neonate than in the adult rat. Inhibition of angiotensin markedly reduces the progression of interstitial fibrosis and apoptosis (18). Compensatory renal growth in the neonate is primarily hyperplastic, whereas that in the adult is hypertrophic (47).

Activation of the RAS stimulates the expression of a variety of fibrogenic compounds, including TGF-β_1, platelet-derived growth factor, adhesion molecules, and α-smooth muscle actin. The functional consequences of obstructive nephropathy in early development are hyperfiltration by remaining nephrons, followed by a progressive decrease in the glomerular filtration rate that may only develop in later life.

Chronic UUO in the developing kidney slows renal maturation. There are similarities between the renal response to UUO and cystic kidney disease, possibly in part because of the constriction of the nephron in cystic kidneys. The progressive increase in renal expression of TGF-β_1

contributes to progressive interstitial fibrosis. In response to urinary tract obstruction, renal tubular cells lose their polarity. The EGF receptors normally located on the basal surface in the adult become localized to the apical surfaces (18).

In another laboratory, Gulbins and associates (75) found that in hydronephrotic rat kidneys physiologic control of basal vascular tone in larger preglomerular arterioles is modulated by an endothelium and EDRF. Efferent arteriolar tone is predominantly controlled by EDRF. Reyes and colleagues (167) state, "The role of some vasoconstrictors and vasodilators in altered renal hemodynamics occurring during ureteral obstruction [has] been studied. Angiotensin II (163), thromboxane A (113), and antidiuretic hormone (168) decrease GFR and ERPF. Prostaglandins and platelet-activating factor (PAF) tend to maintain GFR and ERPF. Inhibition of vasoconstrictors angiotensin II (163), thromboxane (113), and antidiuretic hormone (168) or giving platelet activating factor increases GFR and ERPF but not to normal levels indicating other nonactive factors are involved." Renal macrophages have been identified as the cellular source of prostanoids in hydronephrotic kidney (176).

The role of macrophages and reactive oxygen species in experimental hydronephrosis has recently been reviewed by Ricardo and Diamond (169). Reviewing the role of the infiltrating renal macrophage as a mediator of interstitial fibrosis after UUO, they postulate that "the mechanical disturbance of the proximal tubule resulting from complete ureteral ligation, elaborates a florid pro-inflammatory and pro-fibrogenic response. The initial injurious states results in the release of an array of chemoattractant signals by the tubular epithelium, including ICAM-1, osteopontin, and MCP-1, which lead to the facilitation and recruitment of macrophages into the renal interstitium. One of the many macrophage-derived products is TGF-beta, which promotes fibrogenesis by stimulating the synthesis of extracellular matrix proteins in parallel with the downregulation of matrix metalloproteins and the upregulation of matrix metalloprotein inhibitors" (169).

The role of growth factors, cytokines, and vasoactive compounds was recently reviewed by Klahr and Morrissey (113), who found that "renal interstitial inflammation and fibrosis occurs after ureteral obstruction. Fibrosis most likely develops as a consequence of an imbalance between extracellular matrix synthesis and deposition and the degradation and removal of matrix. Angiotensin II in turn upregulates other factors (TGF-β, tumor necrosis factor-α, nuclear factor-κB and several adhesion molecules and chemoattractants). Blockade of angiotensin II synthesis or inability of this peptide to bind to its receptor lessened the increased levels of mRNA for TGF-β and collagen-IV. Increased levels of angiotensin II have a major role in the development of tubulointerstitial fibrosis after ureteral obstruction" (113). The predominant physiologic alteration after 24 hours of ureteral obstruction is renal vasoconstriction. This may be due to an imbalance between vasoconstrictor and vasodilatory substances. Important vasoconstrictors include angiotensin II, thromboxane A_2, endothelin, and antidiuretic hormones. In bilateral ureteral obstruction, the leukotrienes have a vasoconstrictive effect. Vasodilators that may have a role include L-arginine (a precursor of nitric oxide), platelet-activating factor, and atrial natriuretic peptide. A decrease in these substances could cause vasoconstriction (113).

Recent studies in the research laboratory of Felsen and Vaughan have further explored the pathophysiology of UUO. The mouse kidney obstructed for 2 weeks expressed significantly more TGF-β, exhibited more tubular apoptosis and fibrosis, and had less inducible nitric oxide synthase (iNOS) expression and less total NOS activity than the contralateral unobstructed kidney. Treatment with the monoclonal antibody to TGF-β (ID11) significantly decreased tissue TGF-β concentration, tubular apoptosis, and fibrosis (136). Decreased nephrosis was accompanied by decreased p53 and increased bcl-2. Furthermore, iNOS expression in the obstructed kidney was restored by ID11 treatments, and tubular proliferation in both kidneys was significantly increased by ID11. These data suggest the possibility that ID11 can preserve the obstructed kidney in UUO.

The results using nitric oxide knockout mice demonstrate that nitric oxide appears to be protective against the apoptosis of UUO (135). Nitric oxide protects against the fibrosis of UUO (98). An *in vitro* study demonstrated that angiotensin II and mechanical stretch release NO and TGF-β from a renal tubule cell line and TGF-β is a negative regulator of NOS. In dogs, the nitric oxide system is activated during late UUO (177).

Experimental Studies of Postnatal Urinary Obstruction

Unilateral severe partial ureteral obstruction in the neonatal guinea pig results in renal growth arrest by 2 to 4 weeks (28). Three weeks after the obstruction in these animals, renal blood flow was decreased 50% and the GFR was decreased by 80%. The mechanism is thought to be ischemia caused by vasoconstriction from angiotensin II (29). Prostaglandins and thromboxane do not seem to mediate the vasoconstriction in this experimental model (26). The reduced GFR is thought to be the result of decreased renal blood flow, raised intratubular pressures, and reduced glomerular ultrafiltration coefficient. If the contralateral kidney is impaired or removed, there is less reduction of ipsilateral renal blood flow and some compensatory hypertrophy occurs in the partially obstructed neonatal kidney (21,28). The younger the age, the more compensatory hypertrophy of the contralateral unobstructed kidney is observed (195). Factors influencing the amount of injury from partial ureteral obstruction are age at the time of obstruction, severity of obstruction, and duration of obstruction. Brief (10-day) unilateral partial ureteral obstruction in the neonate results in permanent reduction of function in that kidney. If the obstruction is relieved at 5 days, there is less impairment of function than is seen after 10 days of obstruction (22,30).

Recovery of renal function in urinary obstruction is best achieved by early relief of obstruction. A few studies in experimental animals test whether some drugs further enhance recovery. Infusion of imidazole (a thromboxane inhibitor) or captopril (an angiotensin-converting enzyme inhibitor) significantly increased GFR and renal blood flow after release from 24 hours of complete ureteral obstruction in the adult rat (227). Long-term administration of captopril improved inulin clearance and renal mass after complete unilateral ureteral occlusion of 1- to 3-week duration in adult rats. Administration of indomethacin resulted in slight improvement of GFR but not of renal mass. McDougal (131) concluded from these studies that angiotensin II production and possibly thromboxane synthesis contribute to a loss of renal function after release of obstructive uropathy in adult rats.

Chevalier and Peach (29) found in the neonatal guinea pig that administration of enalapril during ureteral obstruction significantly lowered vascular resistance. After release of neonatal unilateral chronic partial ureteral obstruction, enalapril reciprocally altered angiotensin-mediated vascular tone of both kidneys. In those experiments in neonatal guinea pigs, enalapril (angiotensin-converting enzyme inhibitor) was administered after release from 5 to 10 days of unilateral partial ureteral obstruction. Vascular resistance was not reduced in the obstructed kidney to a greater extent than systemic vascular resistance. However, vascular resistance in the intact kidney was reduced after release of the obstruction in the opposite kidney. These studies suggest that the vascular tone of the intact kidney is increased after release of obstruction on the opposite side.

Tubular Function

In partial acute ureteral obstruction, urine volume decreases, osmolality increases, and urinary sodium concentration is reduced (86,194,219). These changes result from a slower rate of tubular flow caused by a decreased GFR and higher pressures. If the ureteral pressure is elevated to 70 mm Hg, there is a 50% reduction in maximum tubular clearance of glucose and *p*-aminohippuric acid (127). After complete acute ureteral obstruction, there is an additional decrease in the glomerular filtration rate and decreased sodium concentration in the distal tubule. After release of acute ureteral obstruction of 5 to 60 minutes at a pressure of 75 to 120 mm Hg, there is a temporary concentrating defect (58,106,110).

Summary

After acute ureteral obstruction ureteral and pelvic pressures rise as high as 50 to 70 mm Hg, depending on the diuretic state. This is a higher pressure than the 20 mm Hg net filtration pressure, indicating a component of muscle contraction. Renal blood flow and ureteral pressure relationships respond in a triphasic pattern to acute ureteral obstruction. The first phase (lasting 112 hours) is renal vasodilation from vasodilating prostaglandins associated with a rise in ureteral pressure. The second phase (5 to 112 hours) consists of a continued increase in ureteral pressure associated with a decrease in renal blood flow, indicating postglomerular vasoconstriction mediated in some unknown manner. The third and chronic phase exhibits both decreasing ureteral pressure and renal blood flow, as a result of preglomerular vasoconstriction mediated in part by thromboxanes and angiotensins. During acute complete ureteral obstruction, the GFR decreases and tubular function becomes impaired. With acute partial obstruction, tubular pressure rises and the GFR decreases with a resultant decrease in urine volume because of better reabsorption, increased osmolality, and lowered urine sodium concentration.

Long-term Effects of Partial Obstruction

Studies have been performed during chronic partial obstruction in patients and experimental animal models. Evaluation of renal function during the obstruction is important because there is a different environment after release of the obstruction. Studies by Suki and associates (194), Olesen and Madsen (154), Stecker and Gillenwater (192), and Wilson (213) show significant impairment in renal functions during mild degrees of obstruction. These studies during chronic unilateral partial ureteral obstruction show reductions in renal blood flow, GFR, concentrating ability, hydrogen excretion, and sodium reabsorption. Because tubular transit time is increased, sodium reabsorption must be impaired more than the filtration rate and tubule flow rate to account for the increased urinary sodium concentrations.

Most patient studies during partial obstruction have been with bilateral ureteral obstructions. All studies have shown impairment of urinary concentration (7,9,50,51,67,129, 142,200,217,218,230). Impairments of all phases of acidification (ammonia excretion, titratable acidity, and bicarbonate absorption) have been reported (7,9,51,67,129,217, 218,230).

Long-term Effects of Complete Obstruction

Ureteral and Tubular Pressures

Ureteral pressures peak 3 to 5 hours after complete unilateral ureteral obstruction and within 24 hours decrease to 50% of peak values. Ureteral pressures continue to decline over the next 6 to 8 weeks to approximately 15 mm Hg (202). Proximal tubular pressure may return to normal (4) or to 70% below normal (104,225). Numerous collapsed tubules are observed on the kidney surface (81,104). Glomerular capillary pressure is reduced (43).

Renal Blood Flow

Renal blood flow measured by flow probes during continued complete unilateral ureteral obstruction shows progressive decreases that are caused by afferent arteriole constriction. Measurement showed renal blood flow to be 70% of control at 24 hours, 50% at 72 hours, 30% by 6 days, 20% by 2 weeks, 18% at 4 and 6 weeks, and 12% at 8 weeks (137,202) (Fig. 21.2). Blood flow is decreased most in the outer cortex and inner medulla (186,190,226). The mechanism of the afferent arteriole vasoconstriction is discussed earlier in this chapter.

Glomerular Filtration Rate

Measurements of the GFR decrease progressively during complete ureteral obstruction in the dog, to 1.74 mL per minute at 1 week and 0.4 mL minute at 5 weeks of occlusion (145). The fluid exiting by pyelolymphatic, pyelovenous, and pyelotubular backflow is replaced by the continuing glomerular filtration. Immediately after ureteral obstruction is released, there is minimum urine flow. One week after release from 2 weeks of obstruction, the GFR was 15% of control; maximum recovery of the GFR after release from 2 weeks of obstruction was 46% of control (200). After release from 4 weeks of ureteral obstruction, the GFR was 3% and recovered to 35% of control at 5 months (201). No return of glomerular filtration was noted in dogs after 6 weeks of obstruction with a normal contralateral kidney.

Tubular Function

All tubular functions studied, with the exception of urinary dilution, are progressively impaired by complete ureteral obstruction. Perhaps urinary dilution is unimpaired because it is not a system that requires energy. Concentrating ability is severely impaired immediately after release. This tubular function is one of the first to be injured. Recovery of concentrating ability can be complete after release from 2 weeks of complete obstruction. After release from 4 weeks of obstruction, concentrating ability is permanently impaired.

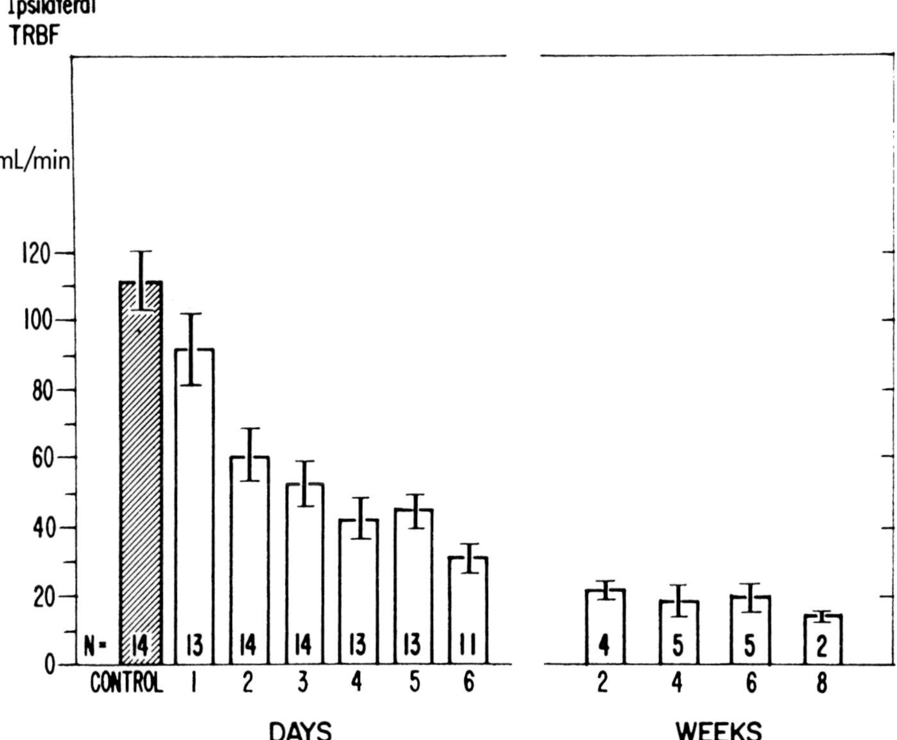

FIGURE 21.2. Changes in left renal blood flow with chronic total left ureteral occlusion in 14 dogs with chronic indwelling blood flow probes. TRBF, total renal blood flow. (From Moody TE, Vaughan ED Jr, Gillenwater JY. Relationship between renal blood flow and ureteral pressure during 18 hours of total unilateral occlusion. *Invest Urol* 1975;13:246, with permission.)

During short partial ureteral obstruction, urine osmolality is higher because of slow tubular transit times in the obstructed kidney. When the partial obstruction is released, urine osmolality falls (106).

Other tubular functions that have been shown to be impaired by chronic unilateral ureteral obstruction are maximum tubular excretory capacity of *p*-aminohippuric acid and glucose, potassium excretion, sodium reabsorption, and urinary acidification (8,36,109,201).

The main tubular effect is in concentrating ability. After release of up to 24 hours of obstruction, there is a normal flow rate of dilute urine with no sodium-losing tendency (214).

Contrasting Conditions During Ureteral Obstruction

Physiologic changes are different depending on whether the ureteral obstruction is unilateral or bilateral. With bilateral ureteral obstruction, the uremic state starts with retention of substances that are normally excreted, and one or more of these substances apparently affect renal hemodynamics and tubular function. Better understanding of clinical problems, such as postobstructive diuresis, has resulted from the study of this situation.

The surface tubules in rats look normal after 24 hours of bilateral ureteral obstruction, in contrast to the poorly perfused and filtering nephrons with collapsed tubules observed in unilateral ureteral obstruction. Proximal and distal tubular pressures are elevated in bilateral ureteral obstruction but are lower than normal in unilateral ureteral obstruction. Afferent arteriole pressure is increased in bilateral ureteral obstruction and decreased in unilateral ureteral obstruction. Glomerular capillary pressure increases to higher levels when both ureters are obstructed than when ureteral obstruction is unilateral. Renal blood flow is reduced to one-third of the control value after release of both bilateral and unilateral ureteral obstruction (24 hours). The single-nephron GFR is 40% of normal in bilateral ureteral obstruction. The reason for the decreased single-nephron GFR is the elevated tubular pressure because the glomerular capillary pressure is normal.

The explanation for the differences between the renal vascular responses in unilateral and bilateral ureteral obstruction is not known (44,81,105,133,197,206,213, 214,226).

Contrasting Studies After Release of Ureteral Obstruction

The contrast in the physiologic effects of chronic (24 hours or greater) unilateral and bilateral ureteral obstruction has provided a better understanding of postobstructive diuresis. The major difference is the significant natriuresis and diuresis occurring after release of bilateral ureteral obstruction. Through different mechanisms, renal blood flow and GFR are reduced to 33% of control in both unilateral and bilateral ureteral obstruction after release from 24 hours of obstruction. In unilateral ureteral obstruction, there is afferent arteriole constriction with abnormal distribution between the cortex and the medulla, with a shift of blood flow from the outer cortex to the inner cortex and medulla (104,105). In bilateral ureteral obstruction, there is efferent arteriole constriction and normal distribution of blood flow. The reduced GFR in unilateral ureteral obstruction is caused by the afferent arteriole constriction, and the reduced GFR in bilateral ureteral obstruction is the result of the increased proximal tubule pressure. After release of bilateral obstruction, the tubular pressure returns toward normal and the GFR remains low because of new afferent arteriole constriction (172,221). Wright (220) postulated that the new afferent arteriole constriction after release of bilateral ureteral obstruction is caused by the macula densa feedback mechanism responding to increased distal delivery of tubule fluid.

The role of nitric oxide is not the same in UUO and bilateral ureteral obstruction (BUO). Following release of BUO, renal nitric oxide synthase activity is decreased (167). Following UUO, NOS activity is increased, thereby counteracting the vasoconstrictor responses (33).

Urine flow is increased up to ten times that of control after release of bilateral ureteral obstruction, in contrast to the low rates of flow and solute excretion after release of unilateral ureteral obstruction. The excretion rates of potassium, phosphate, and urea are significantly increased. After release of bilateral ureteral obstruction, diuresis occurs despite the withholding of fluid and food during the period of obstruction. The diuresis persists for several days until sodium balance is restored. The concentrating defect persists several days longer than the salt loss. The impaired sodium reabsorption occurs in both the proximal and distal tubule (14,15,133). The mechanism of the postobstructive diuresis is not known, but cross-perfusion studies have shown a buildup of a natriuretic factor in the plasma of animals with bilateral ureteral obstruction (215). Wright and Howards (222) postulated that postobstructive diuresis results from two factors: (a) distention and damage to the collecting ducts by increased luminal pressure and (b) inhibition of proximal tubular sodium reabsorption by an unidentified factor that is normally excreted in the urine.

After release of 24 hours of unilateral ureteral obstruction, the previously obstructed kidney has a normal urine flow rate of dilute urine with no natriuresis. These conditions result from reduced renal blood flow and GFR, slightly impaired sodium reabsorption, and severely impaired concentrating ability.

Leahy and associates (117) studied renal injury and recovery in partial ureteric obstruction. Creatinine clearance after release of partial ureteric obstruction showed 8% of control with 60 days' obstruction, 31% of control with 28 days' obstruction, and normal function after 14 days' obstruction. Methyl-methacrylate extrusion casts of the renal microvasculature confirmed arteriolar constriction.

Clinical Postobstructive Diuresis

Patients rarely have a severe, life-threatening diuresis after release of urinary tract obstruction. Generally, diuresis occurs only if all nephron units were obstructed in a way similar to the animal studies described previously. Excellent reviews have been published by Goldsmith (68), Howards (100), Vaughan and Gillenwater (200), Wilson and Klahr (216), Klahr and Morrissey (113), Yarger (224), and Wright and Howards (222). A diuresis generally occurs after release of bilateral obstruction. The diuresis is physiologic, usually mild, and self-limiting. Patients with bilateral obstruction have a retention of sodium and water, and the diuresis is just restoring normal fluid and electrolyte balance (142).

The postulated mechanisms for the rare pathologically significant postobstructive diuresis are (a) impaired urine concentrating ability, (b) impaired sodium reabsorption, and (c) solute diuresis caused by retained urea or administered glucose. Transient peak urine flow rates of up to 69 mL per minute, with an average of 30 mL per minute, and cases of diabetes insipidus unresponsive to vasopressin have been reported (51,171).

In the clinical situation, a patient could develop major fluid and electrolyte problems if he or she had the rare pathologic sodium or water diuresis and it went unrecognized. Our plan of management after release of obstruction is to have the patient weighed and blood pressures recorded in the upright and supine positions and ask that the physician be notified if urine volume exceeds 200 mL per hour. The thirst mechanism will correct any abnormal water loss in the conscious and alert patient. Pathologic sodium loss with resultant contraction of extracellular fluid volumes can be recognized by orthostatic hypotension. Pathologic sodium loss can be replaced by 0.5N saline solution, initially at 50% of output to avoid perpetuating a possible salt and water overload. Pathologic diuresis from nephrogenic diabetes insipidus can be recognized from urine having a specific gravity value ranging from 1.000 to 1.004. Urine from patients with impaired sodium reabsorption should be isotonic.

Relationships of Hypertension and Hydronephrosis

There are two known mechanisms whereby hypertension can result from obstructive uropathy. During acute unilateral ureteral obstruction, renin-angiotensin-aldosterone secretion is increased, with an associated hypertension (208). Also, chronic partial or complete bilateral ureteral obstruction is associated with sodium, water, and urea retention, which produce a volume-related hypertension. In both types, the hypertension is corrected shortly after release of the obstruction. Vaughan and Sosa (203) have reviewed the subject extensively.

The incidence of hypertension with hydronephrosis is variable and not well documented. Most patients with bilateral chronic ureteral obstruction have a mild volume overload–related component to the hypertension, which is corrected by the postobstructive natriuresis and diuresis (200). In acute unilateral ureteral obstruction, patients had a 30% incidence of hypertension (178). In this same study, Schwartz (178) found the incidence of hypertension in patients to be 1.35% in chronic unilateral ureteral obstruction. Other studies have reported a 13% to 20% incidence of hypertension in chronic unilateral ureteral obstruction (12,207).

Thus most patients with chronic unilateral hydronephrosis are normotensive. Any hypertension is usually coincidental in most patients with chronic unilateral hydronephrosis. If significant, the kidney obstruction should be corrected to preserve renal function. In attempting to relate the hypertension and hydronephrosis, Vaughan and Sosa (203) point out that the patient's workup can be similar to renovascular hypertension if renin secretion is studied, contralateral renin suppression is shown, and a positive captopril test is obtained.

Fetal Hydronephrosis

Changing concepts in diagnosis and subsequent management of antenatal hydronephrosis were reviewed by Shokeir and Nijman (184). The increased use of ultrasonography for fetal–maternal screening has detected genitourinary abnormalities in 2 to 9 per 1,000 births, with a male-to-female ratio of 2:1. The major abnormality identified was hydronephrosis. A false-positive error rate of 9% to 22% is reported in the antenatal diagnosis of hydronephrosis. Explanations for the spontaneous resolution of antenatal hydronephrosis include the four- to six-times greater fetal urine flow rate than after delivery, fetal folds, and the increased compliance of the fetal ureter. The high fetal urine flow rate is attributed to differences in fetal renovascular resistances, GFR, and concentrating abilities. UPJ obstruction is the most common cause of antenatal hydronephrosis. Reflux is later diagnosed in 25% to 35% of cases.

The management of fetal hydronephrosis is controversial (184). Once hydronephrosis is diagnosed, ultrasound is repeated near term. If bilateral hydroureteronephrosis and a dilated bladder is diagnosed, ultrasound is recommended every 4 weeks. Other diagnostic tests available are amniocentesis, periumbilical blood sampling, chorionic villous sampling, and fetal urine sampling. None of these tests can accurately predict the degree of renal injury or predict the recoverability of renal function prenatally or postnatally. Prenatal intervention to relieve the obstruction has not been proven yet for routine use. Theoretically, the best opportunity would be in cases of urethral valves causing bladder outlet obstruction with progressive oligohydramnios. Shunting the urine from the obstructed bladder to the amniotic cavity should relieve the urinary obstruction and prevent the pulmonary hypoplasia associated with oligohydramnios. There are no large successful series showing the practicality of this procedure.

Screening for hydronephrosis shows a 2% incidence, with 21% of these having significant structural abnormalities requiring postnatal follow-up. Prenatal intervention for hydronephrosis gives similar outcomes as postnatal detection (39,60).

Congenital obstructive nephropathy is the principal cause of renal failure in infants and children. In the maturing kidney, urinary tract obstruction permanently impairs renal development (20).

Postnatal management of suspected hydronephrosis involves doing ultrasound several days after delivery. Unless serious abnormalities such as bilateral hydroureteronephrosis are detected, further ultrasounds are deferred until 1 month of life. Neonatal oliguria the first few days of life can mask hydronephrosis, which can be detected on the studies 4 weeks later. Diagnosis and management of the various conditions causing fetal urinary tract obstruction is dealt with in another chapter.

Glomerular Development

Chronic UUO interferes with both nephrogenesis and terminal maturation of glomeruli. Human fetuses with severe obstructive nephropathy have a reduced number of glomeruli (63). In experimental animals, relief of obstruction at 10 days does not increase the number of perfused glomeruli, but under certain conditions, GFR returns to normal, indicating that the remaining nephrons have hyperfiltration (23).

The effects of UUO on the developing tubule are profound, including suppression of proliferation, stimulation of apoptosis, and the maintenance of an immature phenotype by tubular epithelial cells. Expression of transforming growth factor-β_1 and clusterin are increased. Maturation of interstitial fibroblasts is delayed. Progression of tubular atrophy and interstitial cystitis results in part from continued activation of the RAS and oxygen radicals. Unlike in the adult, in the neonate, suppression of proliferation and stimulation of apoptosis are mediated at least in part through angiotensin II receptors (35).

Obstruction in the neonatal rat is attenuated by EGF (24). EGF stimulates renal tubule epithelial cell proliferation and maturation and reduces apoptosis in the neonatal rat kidney subjected to chronic UUO (25). During the critical period of nephrogenesis, impairment of the obstructed kidney and growth of the contralateral kidney are directly proportional to the duration of obstruction; thus earlier relief of obstruction may allow greater ultimate preservation of renal mass (34). However, after 5 days of obstruction in the neonatal rat, relief of obstruction does not reverse renal vascular, glomerular, tubular, and interstitial injury. Hyperfiltration and residual tubulointerstitial damage in the postobstructed kidney are likely to lead to deterioration of function in later life (27).

SURGICAL MANAGEMENT OF HYDRONEPHROSIS

All operative techniques for correction of ureteropelvic junction obstructions strive to achieve dependent drainage with an unobstructive anastomosis of the ureter to the renal pelvis. Attempts must be made to avoid parenchymal loss or ligation of any of the renal vessels. It must be remembered that any anastomosis heals by scar tissue, which will contract by about one-third of its original diameter as it matures. End-to-end or end-to-side anastomoses without spatulation of the ureter are doomed to failure.

Diagnostic Tests of Upper Urinary Tract Obstruction

Evaluation of the upper urinary tract is done (a) to determine whether it is dilated, (b) to determine whether the dilation represents a clinically significant obstruction, (c) to determine the effect of the obstruction on renal function, and (d) to determine the potential recoverability of function.

The tests used to diagnose upper urinary tract obstruction are ultrasonography, intravenous urography, diuretic renography, retrograde and antegrade pyelography, the Whitaker perfusion test, computed tomography (CT) scans (including helical CT scans), and magnetic resonance imaging with or without contrast agents. These tests have been recently reviewed by Shokeir (183).

Ultrasonography is often the first test used to screen for upper tract dilation. It is quick, noninvasive, accurate, readily available, and relatively inexpensive. The diuretic ultrasound has had limited usefulness to determine whether an obstruction is significant or not. Using Doppler ultrasound to determine the resistive index has been advocated by Platt and colleagues (160) to differentiate obstructive from nonobstructive dilation in adults. The resistive index is defined as peak systolic velocity minus lowest diastolic velocity divided by peak systolic velocity. A resistive index above 0.70 is used to differentiate obstruction from nonobstruction. In our hands, this test has not been very discriminatory.

Intravenous urography accurately depicts the anatomy of the calices, renal pelvis, and ureters but is not as accurate in quantitating the significance of any obstruction.

Diuretic renography was introduced by O'Reilly and associates in 1978 (157) and has since become an established method of diagnosing and evaluating upper urinary tract obstruction. In the diuretic renogram, an isotope is administered, and at a given time, a diuretic is administered intravenously. The ideal time activity curves under conditions of nonobstruction and obstruction are shown in Fig. 21.3. Adequate function is essential, and urethral catheters are necessary in most children. False-positive results from this test are seen in patients with poor renal function, in grossly dilated systems in which the rate of washout decreases even without obstruction, and when dehydration flattens the curves. False-negative results can occur in patients with a highly compliant (small volume, tight) renal pelvis, or when there is a forced diuresis. Accuracy is reported to be improved by deconvolutional analysis of the renogram with calculation of parenchymal transit time (212). The half-time of isotope drainage ($t_{1/2}$) after a diuretic is commonly used for evaluation. Kidneys with a $t_{1/2}$ of less than 10 minutes are considered unobstructed, and kidneys with a $t_{1/2}$ of greater than 20 minutes are considered obstructed. Those in between are equivocal. In my opinion, the accuracy of this technique is highly variable, depending on the institution where it is performed.

Connolly and associates (38) reviewed the variability of diuresis renography interpretation resulting from the different methods used for determining postdiuretic renal pelvic clearance half-times. They found a 27.8% variation between the four methods of $t_{1/2}$ determinations, emphasizing the individual variations of studies in different institutions.

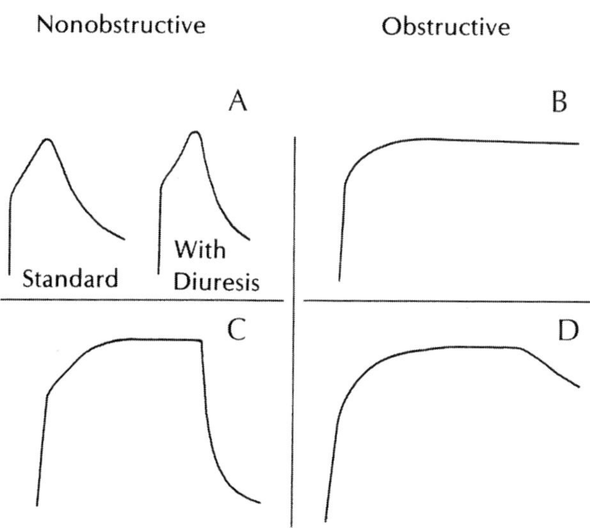

FIGURE 21.3. Typical diagrammatic diuresis renograms. *D* is where diuretics were administered; *A* is nonobstructive; *B* is obstructed with no washout; *C* is nonobstructive after diuresis; *D* is obstructive with no washout after diuresis. (Modified from Lupton EW, Richards D, Testa HJ, et al. A comparison of diuresis renography, the Whitaker test, and renal pelvic morphology in idiopathic hydronephrosis. *Br J Urol* 1985;57:119, with permission.)

Retrograde pyelography is rarely used except to define the anatomy better in certain situations. Rapid emptying of the contrast indicates no obstruction. If a percutaneous nephrostomy tube is inserted, antegrade pyelography should be done to help define whether the system is obstructed and the site of the obstruction.

The technique and interpretation of the Whitaker test (210) requires the collecting system to be filled completely before beginning the test. Other sources of error are urine leaks when there are high urine outputs and not using a urethral catheter. Koff and colleagues (114) classified the pressure-flow patterns as simple or complex. This procedure, properly done, will help define obstruction in equivocal cases such as massively dilated systems with poor function. The obvious disadvantage is the invasiveness of placing a nephrostomy tube.

The unenhanced helical CT has become the test of choice to diagnose acute urinary tract obstruction from kidney stones and can give valuable information in other conditions with dilated upper urinary tracts.

Accuracy of the Various Tests

The available literature regarding the accuracy of these tests to determine whether an upper urinary tract dilation represents a significant obstruction was reviewed by Lupton and associates (124) and O'Reilly (156). In general, there is good correlation of the tests when there is clear-cut severe obstruction or clear-cut nonobstruction. On the equivocal cases, however, there is much disagreement.

Two studies (40,124) showed excellent correlation between diuresis renography and mean transit time through the renal parenchyma. Studies comparing diuresis renography with perfusion pressure flow studies have reported variable results, with reported correlations of 86% (179), 84% (83), 67% (124), 53% (211), and 54% (69).

Studies comparing diuresis renography with renal pelvic morphology report an 87.5% correlation between the two tests (55,71,123). Israel (102) reported a 100% correlation between diuresis renography and synchronous intrapelvic pressure measurements.

Equivocal washout studies present clinical problems. If the kidney has good function and the patient is well hydrated, O'Reilly (156) thinks an equivocal response indicates partial obstruction. When renal function is impaired, it is difficult to distinguish whether an equivocal response is caused by obstruction or by the renal impairment itself. By O'Reilly's analysis (156), 15 of 188 patients (8%) had obstruction on the diuresis renograms but normal perfusion-pressure studies. O'Reilly stated that two cases had intermittent obstruction and the other 13 had gross hydronephrosis, poor renal function, or both. Of the 188 cases, 48 (25%), including 32 previously reported by Hay and colleagues (83), had normal diuresis renograms but abnormal perfusion-pressure studies.

A possible explanation put forward by O'Reilly for the discrepancies is that the systems tolerated lower flow rates but not the 10 mL per minute used in the perfusion-pressure studies.

The intrarenal resistive index is a physiologic parameter that indirectly reflects the degree of resistance in the intrarenal vasculature. In a review of the literature, Rawashdek and associates (165) concluded that the intrarenal resistive index measurements are still in a developmental phase and that this technique has yet to be recognized as a dependable parameter to determine whether a dilated renal pelvis represents significant obstruction.

Indications for Surgery

The major indications for surgical repair of hydronephrosis are relief of pain or relief of significant obstruction that will destroy renal function. Intermittent hydronephrosis classically occurs during a marked diuresis and is best demonstrated by radiologic studies during the symptomatic episodes (148). Determination of whether a mild partial obstruction is significant is more difficult. The best studies are the intravenous urogram to demonstrate calyceal clubbing and dilation, diuretic renograms, Whitaker renal perfusion studies, retrograde pyelograms with washout studies, or longitudinal follow-up urograms showing progressive dilation of the renal pelvis and calyces. When an individual case is first seen with mild to moderate dilation of the renal pelvis, it is not always possible to forecast its natural history.

Ryan and associates (172) have reported that *in situ* double-J stents impair upper urinary tract motility and experimental calculus transit time and may delay passage of ureteric calculi.

Forty-one kidneys in infants and newborns were studied with diuretic renography, showing partial obstruction or dilation with obstruction that washed out with diuretics. Twelve-month follow-up showed deterioration to significant obstruction in 20%. The deterioration was more likely to occur in the markedly hydronephrotic units (99). Bilateral hydronephrosis detected antenatally was followed for up to 7 years in 26 children. Operations were never performed on 34 kidneys, and operations were performed on 18 kidneys. There was no consistent difference in final filtration rates of the two groups (107).

I have seen patients whose previous radiologic studies showed a mild hydronephrosis, presenting with significant hydronephrosis that had progressed over periods of 1 to 10 years. Thus ureteropelvic junction obstruction is progressive in some patients.

A 17-year follow-up of 36 adults with UPJ obstruction managed without surgery showed little change in function or worsening of hydronephrosis. Forty-seven patients who had pyeloplasty (and presumably more hydronephrosis) showed split function of the obstructed kidney from 40.8% to 47.1% of total function after pyeloplasty, but total GFR did not improve (111).

Lennon and associates (119) studied *in vitro* the pharmacologic options for the treatment of acute ureteric colic. Morphine was confirmed to have a spasmogenic effect on ureteric activity, which was unaffected by naloxone. Both indomethacin and diclofenac produced an abrupt inhibition of ureteral contraction, which, because of spasmolytic effects, may be indicated as therapy for the acutely obstructed ureter.

Selection of Operative Procedures

All of the operative techniques provide a dependent and progressive funneling of the ureteropelvic junction. The two basic techniques are the use of some type of pelvic flap (41,59,173) and the dismembered pyeloplasty (3,59). Recently, balloon dilations have become popular, and they were 80% successful in 40 cases (128). Endopyelotomies have been successful as well (86%) (141). The most commonly used surgical procedure is the dismembered pyeloplasty. All the operations work, and one should not be dogmatic in declaring that one or another of the operations is best.

Meticulous care and delicate handling of the renal pelvis and ureter are essential for the success of the pyeloplasty. Small, sharp scissors and fine vascular forceps are essential to prevent crush damage of the tissues. Tissues that are frequently lifted or held should have sutures placed for traction, or skin hooks should be used. Tissue must be approximated with fine sutures (I prefer chromic catgut 4-0 or 5-0 wedged on an atraumatic needle). Knots should be placed on the outside. I prefer to use interrupted sutures beginning at the apex to avoid a "dog-ear" in this location.

I agree with Blandy (11) that too much time has been wasted arguing over whether to use stents or nephrostomies. Any urologist should know how to use both. Stents should be used if the anastomosis appears likely to kink or is obstructed by edema during the first few days. Nephrostomies are needed if renal function is unclear or if there is a high likelihood of leakage or obstruction. I generally favor using both stents and nephrostomies. In bilateral hydronephrosis, if one side is infected, that side should be repaired first. In uninfected hydronephrosis, if one side has poorer function, that side should be repaired first.

Ureteral strictures in association with ureteropelvic junction obstruction are uncommon in my experience. Ureteral strictures can be corrected during the pyeloplasty. The Davis intubated ureterotomy (45) or end-to-end anastomosis can be used.

Foley Y-plasty

The Foley Y-plasty (59) was designed for the correction of an obstructive, congenital high insertion of the ureter into the renal pelvis (Fig. 21.4). The pelvis and ureter must be dissected free. Careful planning of the pelvic incisions is essential. The anterior and posterior pelvic incisions and the ureteral incision should be approximately the same length. I have found it helpful to mark the end of each planned incision with a 4-0 silk suture. The anterior pelvic incision is started at the ureteropelvic junction and extended laterally and downward toward the hilum of the kidney. The posterior incision is then similarly made, completing the V portion of the Y incision. The ureteral incision is then made down the lateral margin (the side facing the renal pelvis). The sharp tip of the pelvic flap is rounded off. Before closure, the nephrostomy tube and stent are placed, if they are being used. Interrupted 4-0 or 5-0 chromic catgut is used for closure, starting at the tip to avoid leaving a dog-ear in the renal pelvis. I drain the area with two drains. All tubes and drains are brought out the posterior part of the wound, because it has less sensation than the anterior portion. The Foley Y-type ureteropelvioplasty can be combined with a Davis intubated ureterotomy (45) when the ureteral structure is longer than can be corrected with the Foley Y-plasty alone (Fig. 21.5). Use of stents is essential in the Davis intubated ureterotomy to provide scaffolding for new growth. I usually place several sutures loosely from the edges across the catheter to ensure that the sides lie flat and do not curl up. Davis states that the healing by secondary intention requires 6 weeks. When exposing the

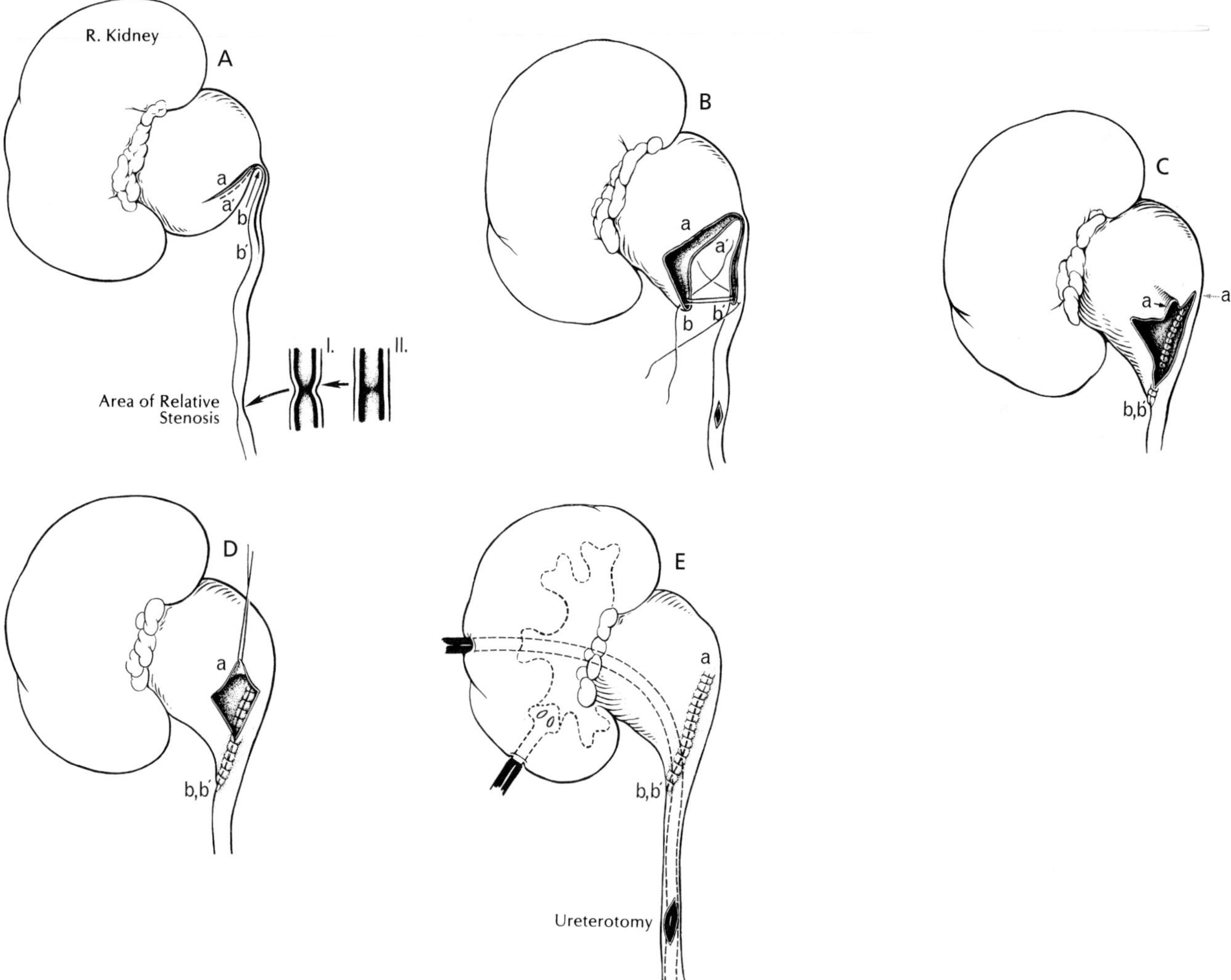

FIGURE 21.4. Classic Foley Y-plasty. **A:** Anterior and posterior pelvic incisions should be the same length as the ureteral incision. **B:** The tip of the flap and the lower end of the ureterotomy should be approximated first. **C, D:** The closure is started at *(b,b′)* and extended upward to *(a,a′)*. A dog-ear may form at point *a*. *I* and *II* illustrate the infrequent relative narrowing of the ureter, which is occasionally seen lower in the ureter. **E:** If there is a narrow segment, it can be treated by a ureterotomy or dilation. (Modified from Smart WR. Surgical correction of hydronephrosis. In: Harrison JH et al, eds. *Campbell's urology,* ed 4. Philadelphia: Saunders, 1979, with permission.)

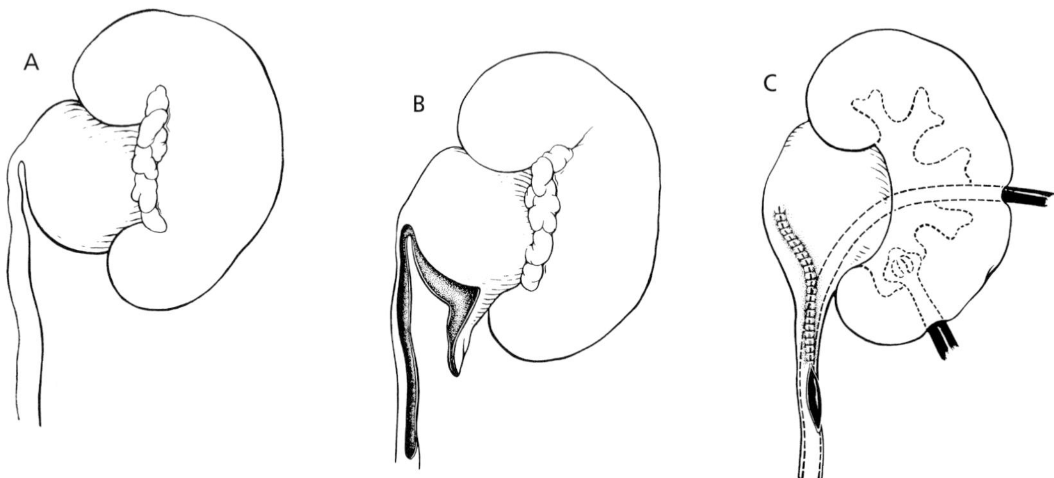

FIGURE 21.5. The classic Foley Y-plasty for high ureteral insertion with a long obstructing ureteral defect. **A:** The high insertion of the ureter into the renal pelvis. **B:** The long ureterotomy and funneling flap in the renal pelvis. **C:** The closure of the renal pelvis with the lower portion of the ureteral incision left open as a Davis intubated ureterotomy.

ureter, there should be minimum dissection to preserve the blood supply. Careful nontraumatic handling of the tissues is essential.

Dismembered Ureteropyelostomy

The operation first described by Foley in 1937 (59) and Anderson and Hynes in 1949 (3) is the most commonly used pyeloplasty and works well in most situations. The operation consists of suturing a spatulated ureter to a generous V-shaped pelvic flap. The pelvic flap is essential to provide the funneling. The kidney and ureter are dissected free, noting carefully whether there are any lower pole vessels. It is important to know how long the narrow upper ureteral segment is to plan the pelvic flap. If needed, additional length can be gained by mobilizing the kidney. Preoperative evaluation should have provided information about the length of the narrowed ureteral segment. If additional information is needed, one can open the renal pelvis and pass down a calibrating ureteral catheter or bougie à boule.

Before opening the pelvis, I plan and map out the incision, the pelvic flap, and any excess renal pelvis I am going to remove, placing marking sutures or using a marking pen. I always mark the lateral edge of the ureter where I plan to do the spatulation to prevent rotation and cutting the ureter in the incorrect place. Proper orientation is essential. It is easy to misplace the anastomosis and cause rotations or angulation if one does not pay attention, stay oriented, and properly mark the tissues. A nice aspect of this operation is that it can be used with either an intrarenal oran extrarenal pelvis. There are several ways one can fashion the renal pelvic flap (Figs. 21.6 to 21.9) (11).

Ureterocalyceal Anastomosis

The ureterocalyceal anastomosis can be used when there seems to be no other option for anastomosing the kidney. This anastomosis is most useful when the renal pelvis cannot be dissected out or used. The procedure is more difficult and will have a higher failure rate than other procedures. The two different methods are removing a button of renal parenchyma over the lower calyx (Fig. 21.10) or opening the lower calyx by incising down to the calyx in the medial portion of the lower pole of the kidney (Fig. 21.11).

In ureterocalyceal anastomosis, one usually is not able to adequately dissect out the renal pelvis because of scar tissue. Usually, there is a longer narrowed segment of ureter. The ureter is cut back to normal tissue and spatulated on the lateral border. If the renal pelvis can be entered, I pass a sound down to the lower calyx and cut out an adequate button of renal parenchyma, marking the mucosal edges of the calyx for later anastomosis. If the renal pelvis cannot be entered, a guillotine type of procedure will provide access to the lower calyx.

The other type of procedure that can be used in some circumstances is the ureterocalicostomy. This procedure was devised to correct a narrow infundibulum. The renal pelvis is opened and a right-angle clamp is passed into the lower calyx. Before making the cut it is advisable to place a bulldog clamp around the renal artery, because bleeding from large veins can be tremendous. The parenchyma is cut, including the mucosa of the lower calyx. The ureter is cut on

Text continued on page 899

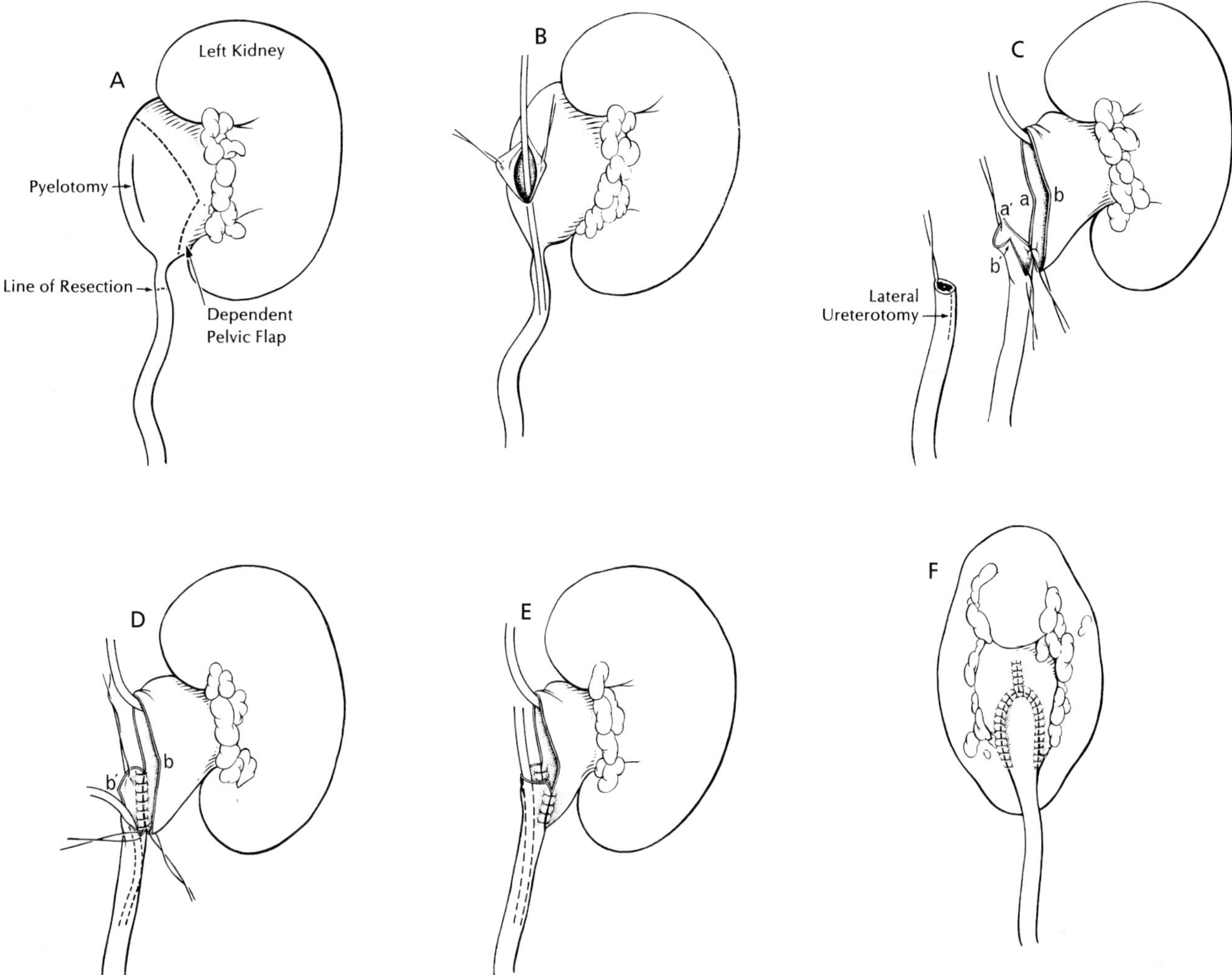

FIGURE 21.6. Dismembered Foley Y-plasty operation. The obstructing segment is excised and a dependent funneling of the pelvis is achieved. **A:** The pyelotomy and ureterotomy incisions are planned and marked. **B:** The pyelotomy incision is started. **C:** The lateral ureterotomy is done and ureteral stent passed after excising the ureteral segment. **D:** Suturing with 3-0 or 4-0 absorbable sutures is started on the posterior surface at the apex. **E:** Traction sutures are used to approximate the edges. It is important not to crush the tissue with heavy forceps. The tip of the flap is sewn to the ureterotomy. It is important to start at the apex. **F:** The funnel is completed, and any redundant pelvis can be resected. The pelvis is reconstituted. (Modified from Smart WR. Surgical correction of hydronephrosis. In: Harrison JH et al, eds. *Campbell's urology,* ed 4. Philadelphia: Saunders, 1979, with permission.)

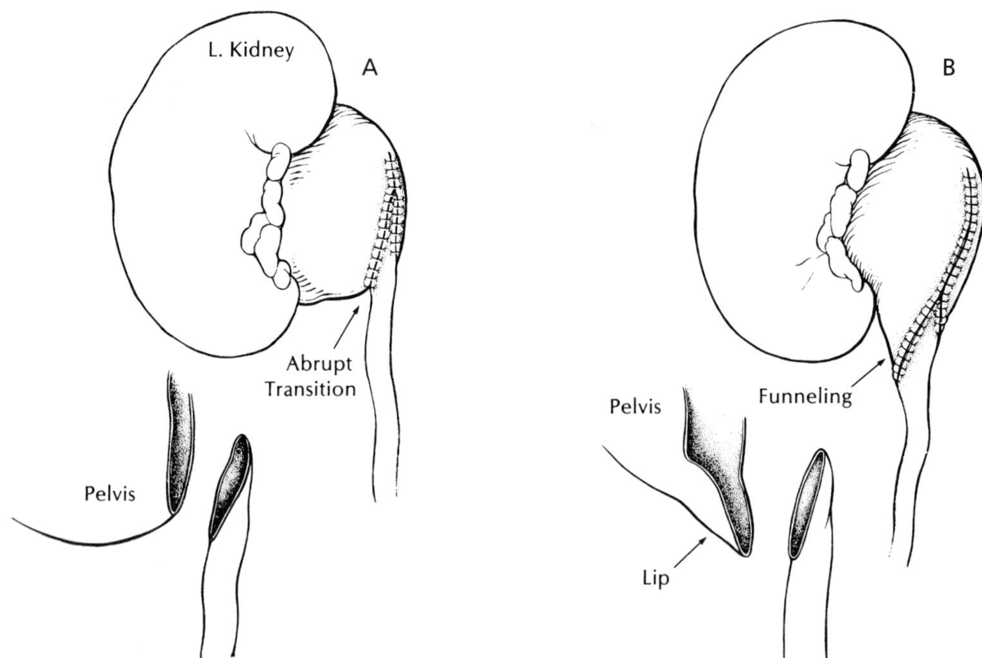

FIGURE 21.7. The value and importance of creating a funnel **(B)** in the pelvis as opposed to creating an abrupt transition between the pelvis and the ureter **(A).** Proper funneling gives dependent drainage with a nice transition between the pelvis and ureter. (Modified from Smart WR. Surgical correction of hydronephrosis. In: Harrison JH et al, eds. *Campbell's urology,* ed 4. Philadelphia: Saunders, 1979, with permission.)

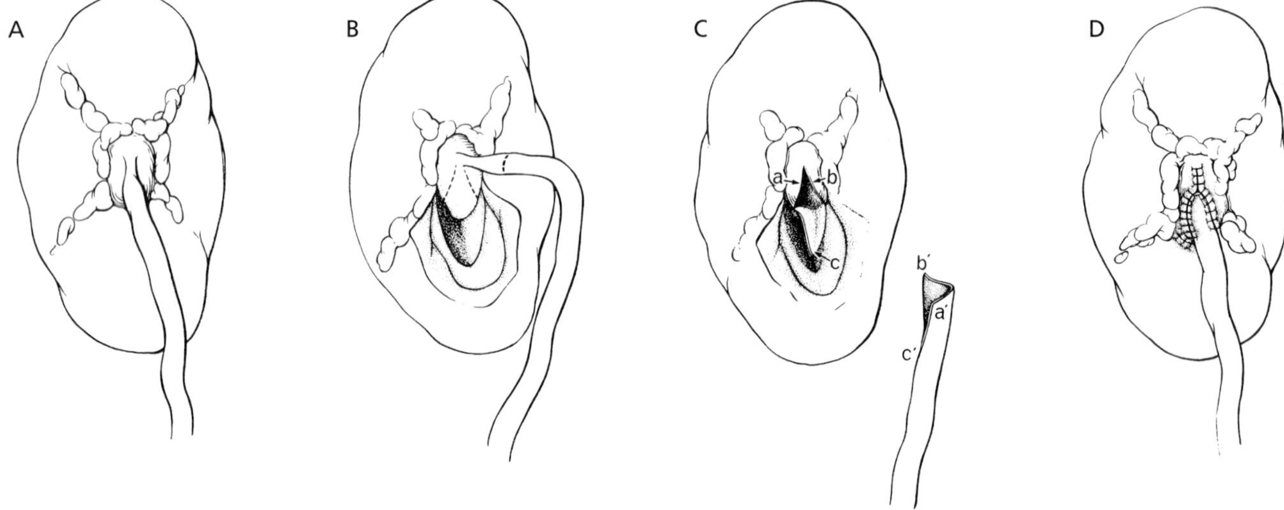

FIGURE 21.8. Difficult high-insertion repair. The Foley Y-plasty can be adapted to patients with a small extrarenal pelvis. **A:** The area of narrowing in the upper ureter with small extrarenal pelvis. **B:** Resection of renal parenchyma to expose the large intrarenal pelvis. **C:** The ureter is cut distal to the obstruction and spatulated. The pelvis flap is also formed after resection of the stenotic segment. Approximate *a-a′, b-b′,* and *c-c′.* **D:** The anastomosis is completed with a funneled and dependent pelvis. (Modified from Smart WR. Surgical correction of hydronephrosis. In: Harrison JH et al, eds. *Campbell's urology,* ed 4. Philadelphia: Saunders, 1979, with permission.)

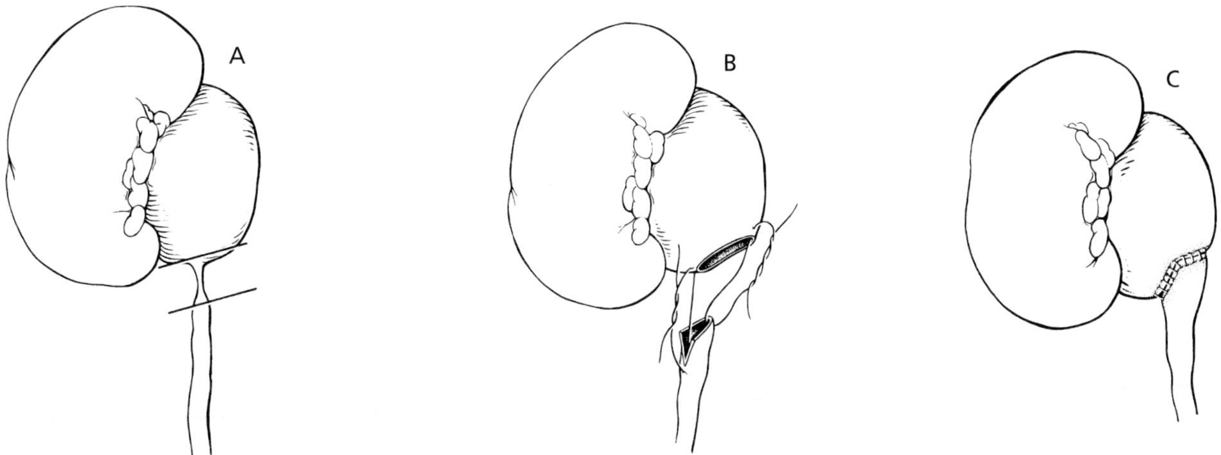

FIGURE 21.9. Simple pyeloplasties in children have been successful. The narrow segment **(A)** is excised, leaving the pelvis tunneled, and the ureter is spatulated **(B).** Closure is with 3-0 or 4-0 absorbable sutures **(C).** (Modified from Zincke H et al. Ureteropelvic obstruction in children. *Surg Gynecol Obstet* 1974;139:873, with permission.)

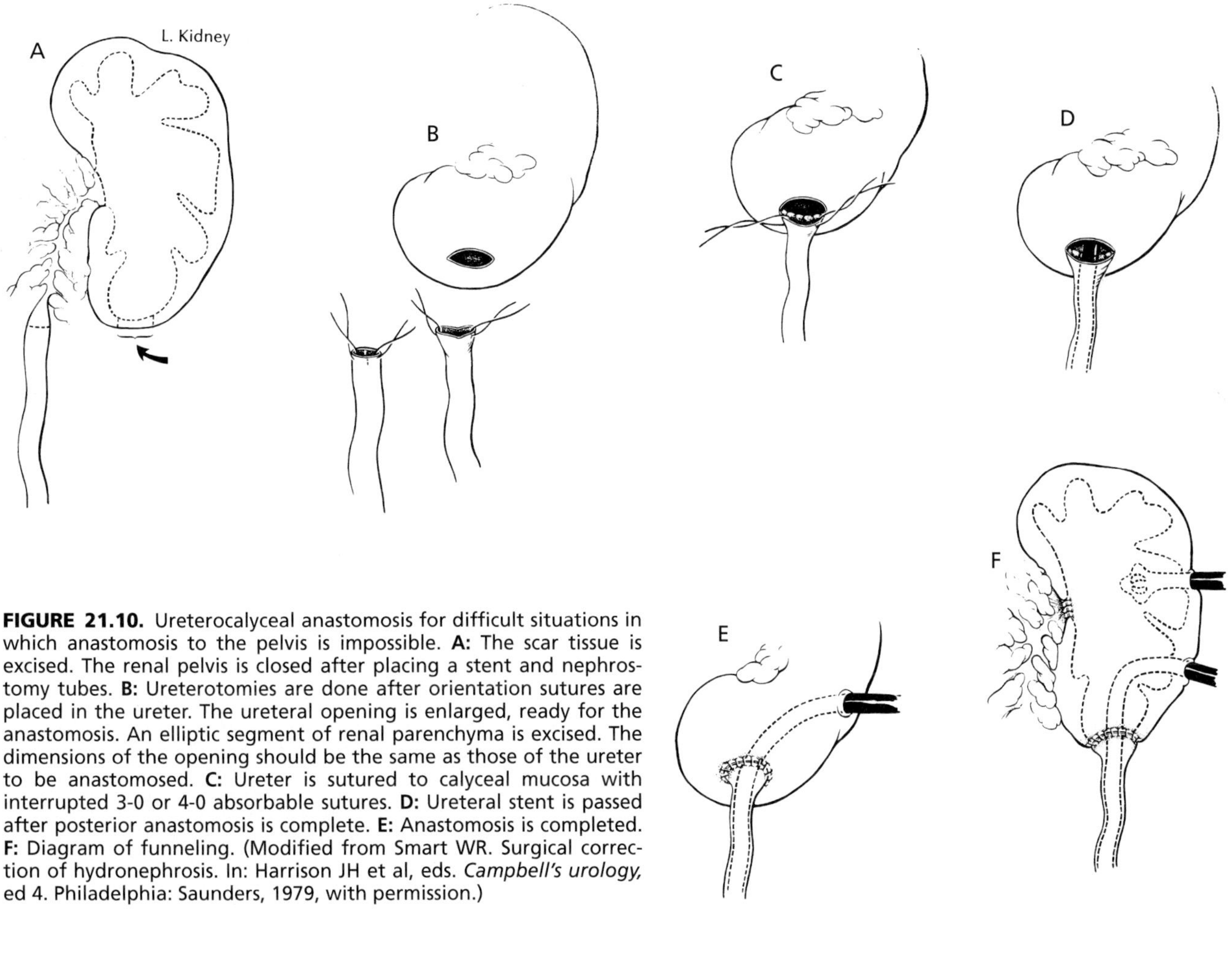

FIGURE 21.10. Ureterocalyceal anastomosis for difficult situations in which anastomosis to the pelvis is impossible. **A:** The scar tissue is excised. The renal pelvis is closed after placing a stent and nephrostomy tubes. **B:** Ureterotomies are done after orientation sutures are placed in the ureter. The ureteral opening is enlarged, ready for the anastomosis. An elliptic segment of renal parenchyma is excised. The dimensions of the opening should be the same as those of the ureter to be anastomosed. **C:** Ureter is sutured to calyceal mucosa with interrupted 3-0 or 4-0 absorbable sutures. **D:** Ureteral stent is passed after posterior anastomosis is complete. **E:** Anastomosis is completed. **F:** Diagram of funneling. (Modified from Smart WR. Surgical correction of hydronephrosis. In: Harrison JH et al, eds. *Campbell's urology,* ed 4. Philadelphia: Saunders, 1979, with permission.)

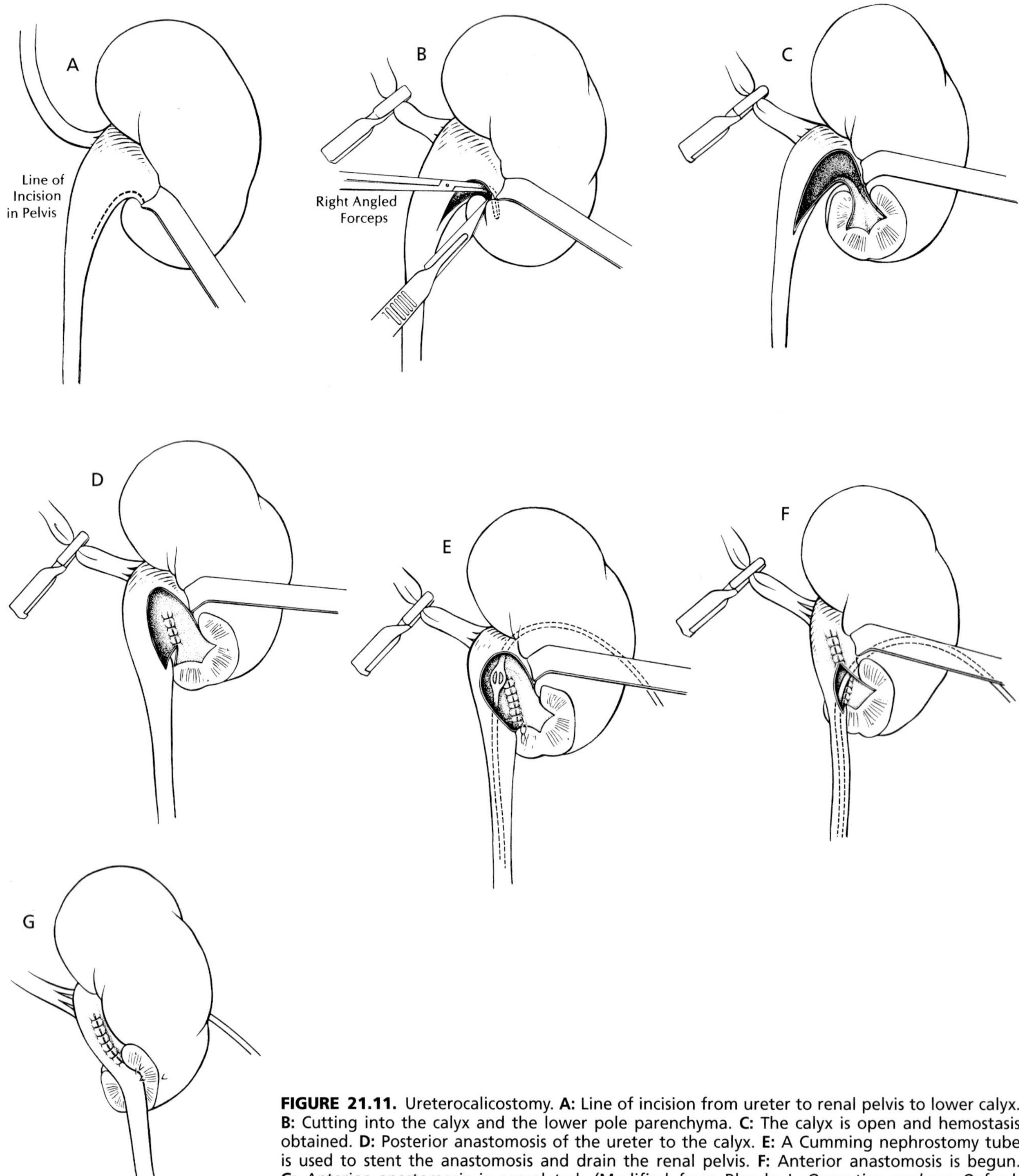

FIGURE 21.11. Ureterocalicostomy. **A:** Line of incision from ureter to renal pelvis to lower calyx. **B:** Cutting into the calyx and the lower pole parenchyma. **C:** The calyx is open and hemostasis obtained. **D:** Posterior anastomosis of the ureter to the calyx. **E:** A Cumming nephrostomy tube is used to stent the anastomosis and drain the renal pelvis. **F:** Anterior anastomosis is begun. **G:** Anterior anastomosis is completed. (Modified from Blandy J. *Operative urology.* Oxford: Blackwell Scientific, 1978, with permission.)

its lateral border and sutured with 3-0 or 4-0 chromic sutures to the calyceal mucosa. The sutures should be interrupted at the apex. Nephrostomy tubes and stents should always be used, because these operations have a higher risk of failure.

Extrinsic Vascular Obstruction

The Hellstrom vascular relocation procedure (85) is a simple technique for correcting renal outlet obstruction from a crossing vessel (Fig. 21.12). This procedure should be used solely when there is extrinsic obstruction only. One has to be careful that there is no intrinsic obstruction. I have operated on at least six hydronephrotic kidneys with intrinsic obstruction that previously had been thought to have only extrinsic obstruction. Intrinsic obstruction cannot be ruled out by passing a catheter through the area in question. Some of the obstructions are caused by impaired function, not intrinsic or extrinsic scarring. If there is any doubt about an area of intrinsic obstruction, I think it should be corrected at the time of surgery. In the Hellstrom procedure, the anterior herniation of the renal pelvis is placed behind the vessels, and the vessel is fixed to the renal pelvis to relieve the extrinsic obstruction.

Hydronephrosis in a Horseshoe Kidney

Hydronephrosis can occur in horseshoe kidneys. The obstruction is usually ureteropelvic junction obstruction and is not from pressure where the ureter crosses the kidney. The isthmus is usually medial to the obstruction and is not causing the obstruction. The problem with routine cutting of the isthmus is that one can injure major renal vessels or enter the collecting system. In my experience, most pyeloplasties can be accomplished without having to divide the isthmus. If the isthmus is thin, it should be divided with lateral placement of the lower poles.

The pyeloplasty can be done like any other pyeloplasty. The dismembered pyeloplasty is usually the preferred procedure. To expose the horseshoe kidney, one needs to make a midline or paramedian incision. The bowel is mobilized medially. The kidney usually lies in the region of the bifurcation of the aorta. Renal vessels come from the aorta and iliac arteries.

Hydronephrosis from Retrocaval Ureter

The retrocaval ureter is a congenital anomaly in which the right ureter passes behind the vena cava, causing obstruction (Fig. 21.13). The abnormality is caused by persistence of the posterior cardinal vein as the major portion of the infrarenal inferior vena cava. The kidney is approached through a flank or an abdominal incision. The renal pelvis is dissected down to where the ureter passes under the vena cava. The ureter can be cut here. The normal ureter is located as it crosses anterior to the vena cava and is cut. One then spatulates the distal ureter segments and does an anastomosis with a U-shaped flap of the renal pelvis.

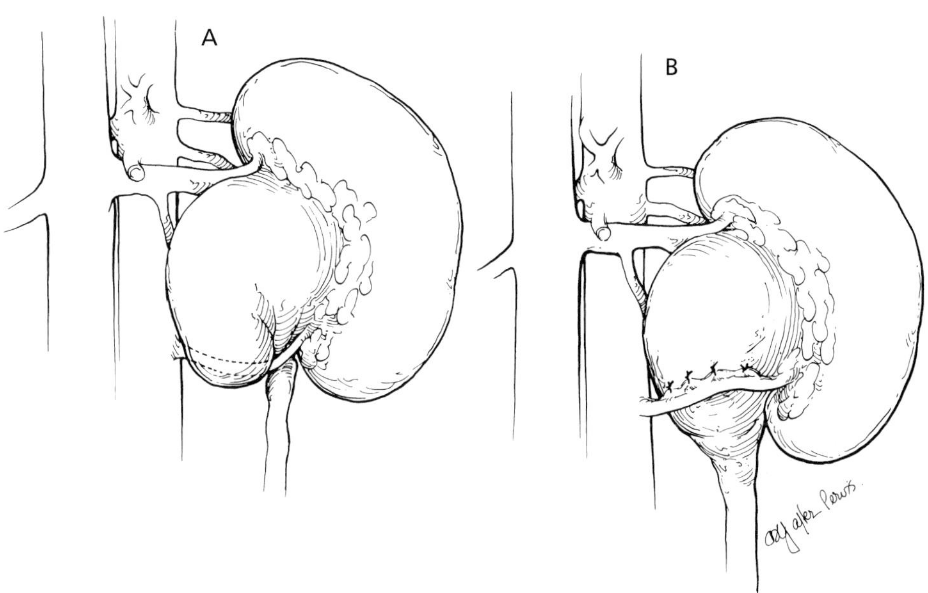

FIGURE 21.12. Hellstrom technique. The obstructing vessel is moved to a nonobstructing position. An intrinsic defect should be carefully ruled out by perfusion studies on the operating table. **A:** Anterior herniation of the renal pelvis over an obstructing renal vessel. **B:** Fixation of the renal vessels in a nonobstructing position. (Modified from Smart WR. Surgical correction of hydronephrosis. In: Harrison JH et al, eds. *Campbell's urology,* ed 4. Philadelphia: Saunders, 1979, with permission.)

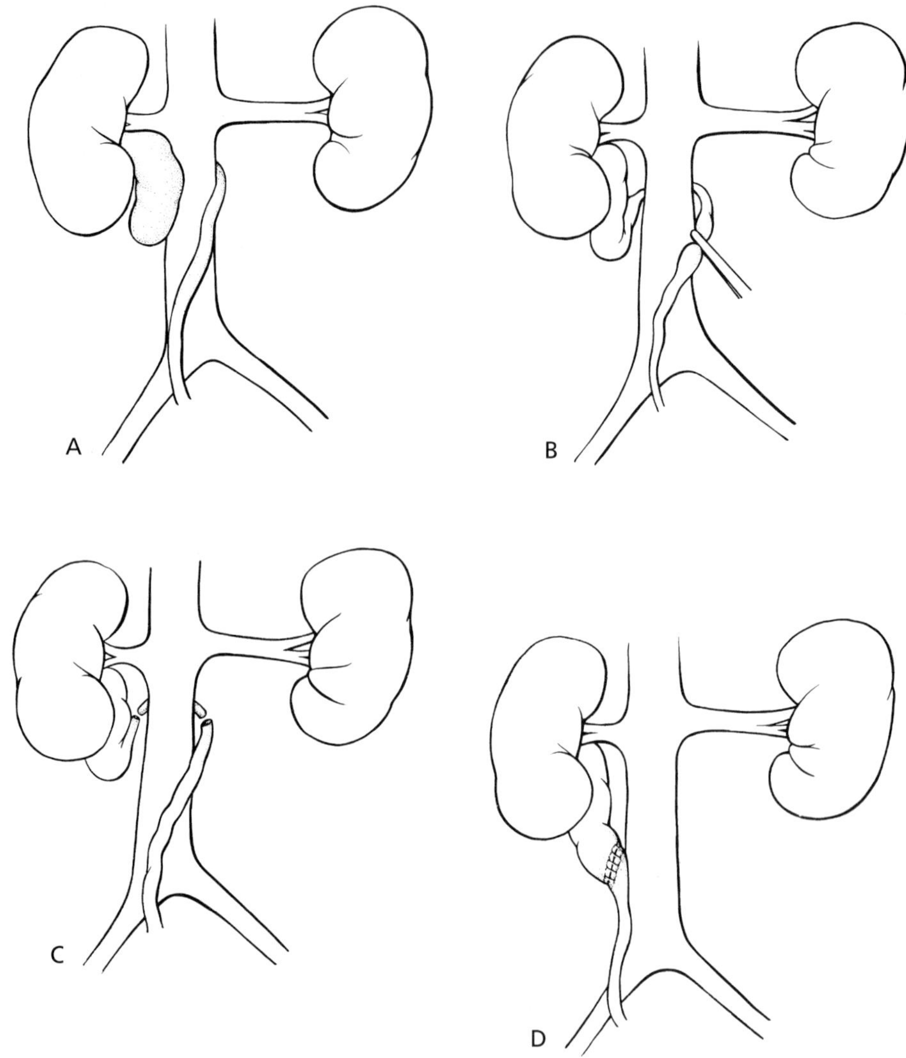

FIGURE 21.13. **A:** Retrocaval ureter. **B:** The renal pelvis is dissected down to where the ureter passes under the vena cava. **C:** The ureter can be cut here; the normal ureter is located as it crosses anteriorly to the vena cava, and is cut. **D:** The distal ureter segment is then spatulated, and an anastomosis with a U-shaped flap of the renal pelvis is performed.

REFERENCES

1. Allen JT, Vaughan ED Jr, Gillenwater JY. The effect of indomethacin on renal blood flow and ureteral pressure in unilateral obstruction in awake dogs. *Invest Urol* 1978;15:324.
2. Altschul R, Fedor S. Vascular changes in hydronephrosis. *Am Heart J* 153;46:291.
3. Anderson JC, Hynes W. Retrocaval ureter; case diagnosed preoperatively and treated successfully by plastic operation. *Br J Urol* 1949;21:209.
4. Arendshorst WJ, Finn WF, Gottschalk CW. Nephron stop-flow pressure response to obstruction for 24 hours in the rat kidney. *J Clin Invest* 1974;53:1497.
5. Backlund L, Nordgren L. Pressure variations in the upper urinary tract and kidney at total ureteric occlusion. *Acta Soc Med Ups* 1966;71:285.
6. Baylis C, Harton P, Engels K. Endothelial-derived relaxing factor controls renal hemodynamics in the normal rat kidney. *J Am Soc Nephrol* 1991;1:875.
7. Berlyne GM. Distal tubular function in chronic hydronephrosis. *Q J Med* 1961;30:339.
8. Berlyne GM, Macken A. On the mechanism of renal inability to produce a concentrated urine in chronic hydronephrosis. *Clin Sci* 1962;22:315.
9. Better OS, Arieff AI, Massry SG, et al. Studies on renal function after relief of complete unilateral ureteral obstruction of three months' duration in man. *Am J Med* 1973;54:234.
10. Bird CE, Moise TS. Pyelovenous backflow. *JAMA* 1926; 86:661.
11. Blandy J. *Operative urology.* Oxford: Blackwell Scientific, 1978:55.
12. Brasch WF, Walters W, Hammer HJ. Hypertension and the surgical kidney. *JAMA* 1940;115:1837.

13. Brezis M, Heyman SN, Dinour D, et al. Role of nitric oxide in renal medullary oxygenation. Studies in isolated and intact rat kidneys. *J Clin Invest* 1991;88:390.
14. Buerkert J, Alexander E, Purkerson ML, et al. On the site of decreased fluid reabsorption after release of ureteral obstruction in the rat. *J Lab Clin Med* 1976;87:397.
15. Buerkert J, Head M, Klahr S. Effects of acute bilateral ureteral obstruction on deep nephron and terminal collecting duct function in the young rat. *J Clin Invest* 1977;59:1055.
16. Bulger RE, Lorentz WB Jr, Colindres RE, et al. Morphologic changes in rat renal proximal tubules and their tight junctions with increased intraluminal pressure. *Lab Invest* 1974;30:136.
17. Burns JE, Schwartz EO. Absorption from the renal pelvis in hydronephrosis due to permanent and complete occlusion of the ureter. *J Urol* 1918;2:445.
18. Chevalier RL. Nephrological aspects of urinary tract obstruction. *Curr Opin Urol* 1997;7:320.
19. Chevalier RL. Pathophysiology of obstructive uropathy in the newborn. *Semin Nephrol* 1998;18:585.
20. Chevalier RL. Molecular and cellular pathophysiology of obstructive nephrology. *Pediatr Nephrol* 1999;13:612.
21. Chevalier RL, Gomez RA, Jones CE. Impaired hemodynamic recovery following release of chronic partial ureteric obstruction: effect of age. *Pediatr Res* 1987;21:473(abst).
22. Chevalier RL, Gomez RA, Jones CE. Release of neonatal unilateral chronic partial ureteral obstruction reciprocally alters angiotensin-media vascular tone of both kidneys. *Pediatr Res* 1987;21:473(abst).
23. Chevalier RL, Gomez RA, Jones CA. Developmental determinants of recovery after relief of partial ureteral obstruction. *Kidney Int* 1988;33:775.
24. Chevalier RL, Goyal S, Wolstenholme JT, et al. Obstructive nephropathy in the neonate is attenuated by epidermal growth factor. *Kidney Int* 1998;54:38.
25. Chevalier RL, Goyal S, Thornhill BA. EGF improves recovery following relief of unilateral ureteral obstruction in the neonatal rat. *J Urol* 1999;162:1532.
26. Chevalier RL, Jones CE. Contribution of endogenous vasoactive compounds to renal vascular resistance in neonatal chronic partial ureteral obstruction. *J Urol* 1986;136:532.
27. Chevalier RL, Kim A, Thornhill BA, et al. Recovery following relief of unilateral ureteral obstruction in the neonatal rat. *Kidney Int* 1999;55:793.
28. Chevalier RL, Kaiser DL. Chronic partial ureteral obstruction in the neonatal guinea pig: influence of uninephrectomy on growth and hemodynamics. *Pediatr Res* 1984;18:1266.
29. Chevalier RL, Peach MJ. Hemodynamic effects of enalapril on neonatal chronic partial ureteral obstruction. *Kidney Int* 1985; 28:891.
30. Chevalier RL, Sturgill BC, Jones CE, et al. Morphologic correlates of renal growth arrest in neonatal partial ureteral obstruction. *Pediatr Res* 1987;21:338.
31. Chevalier RL, Thornhill BA. Ureteral obstruction in the neonatal guinea pig: interaction of sympathetic nerves and angiotensin. *Pediatr Nephrol* 1995;9:441.
32. Chevalier RL, Thornhill BA. Ureteral obstruction in the neonatal rat: renal nerves modulate hemodynamic effects. *Pediatr Nephrol* 1995;9:447.
33. Chevalier RL, Thornhill BA, Gomez RA. EDRF modulates renal hemodynamics during unilateral ureteral obstruction in the rat. *Kidney Int* 1992;42:400.
34. Chevalier RL, Thornhill BA, Wolstenholme JT, et al. Unilateral ureteral obstruction in early development alters renal growth: dependence on the duration of obstruction. *J Urol* 1999;161:309.
35. Chevalier RL, Thornhill BA, Wolstenholme JT. The renal cellular response to ureteral obstruction: role of maturation and angiotensin II. *Am J Physiol* 1999;277:F41.
36. Chisholm GD. Bilateral renal clearance studies in experimental obstructive uropathy. *Proc R Soc Med* 1964;57:571.
37. Chung KH, Chevalier RL. Arrested development of the neonatal kidney following chronic ureteral obstruction. *J Urol* 1996; 155:1139.
38. Connolly LP, Zurakowski D, Peters CA, et al. Variability of diuresis renography interpretation due to method of post-diuretic renal pelvis clearancer half-time determination. *J Urol* 2000;164:467.
39. Coplen DE, Hare JY, Zderic SA, et al. Ten-year experience with prenatal intervention for hydronephrosis. *J Urol* 1996; 156:1142.
40. Cosgriff DF, Berry JM. A comparative assessment of deconvolution and diuresis renography in equivocal upper urinary tract obstruction. *Nucl Med Commun* 1982;53:377.
41. Culp OS, DeWeerd JH. Pelvic flap operation for certain types of ureteropelvic obstruction: preliminary report. *Mayo Clin Proc* 1951;26:483.
42. Cussen LJ, Tymms A. Hyperplasia of ureteral muscle in response to acute obstruction of the ureter. *Invest Urol* 1972; 9:504.
43. Dal Canton A, Corradi A, Stanziale R, et al. Effects of 24-hour unilateral ureteral obstruction on glomerular hemodynamics in rat kidney. *Kidney Int* 1979;15:457.
44. Dal Canton A, Corradi A, Stanziale R, et al. Glomerular hemodynamics before and after release of 24-hour bilateral ureteral obstruction. *Kidney Int* 1980;17:491.
45. Davis DM. Intubated ureterotomy; new operation for ureteral and ureteropelvic stricture. *Surg Gynecol Obstet* 1943;76:513.
46. Deming CL. The effects of intrarenal hydronephrosis on the components of the renal cortex. *J Urol* 1951;65:478.
47. Dicker SE, Shirley PG. Compensatory renal growth after unilateral nephrectomy in the newborn rat. *J Physiol* 1973; 228:193.
48. Djurhuus JC, Nerstrom B, Gyrd-Hansen N, et al. Experimental hydronephrosis. *Acta Chir Scand* 1976;472:17.
49. Dominguez R, Adams RB. Renal function during and after acute hydronephrosis in the dog. *Lab Invest* 1958;7:292.
50. Dorhout-Mees EJ. Reversible water losing state, caused by incomplete ureteric obstruction. *Acta Med Scand* 1960; 168:193.
51. Earley LE. Extreme polyuria in obstructive nephropathy: report of a case of "water-losing nephritis" in an infant with a discussion of polyuria. *N Engl J Med* 1956;255:600.
52. El-Dahr SS, Gomez RA, Gray MS, et al. *In situ* localization of renin and its mRNA in neonatal ureteral obstruction. *Am J Physiol* 1990;258:F854.
53. El-Dahr SS, Gomez RA, Gray MS, et al. Renal nerves modulate renin gene expression in the developing rat kidney with ureteral obstruction. *J Clin Invest* 1991;87:800.
54. El-Dahr SS, Gomez RA, Khare G, et al. Expression of renin and its mRNA in the adult rat kidney with chronic ureteral obstruction. *Am J Kid Dis* 1990;15:575.
55. English PJ, Testa HJ, Gosling JA, et al. Idiopathic hydronephrosis in childhood—a comparison between diuresis renography and upper urinary tract morphology. *Br J Urol* 1982; 54:603.
56. Felsch W, Lou MH, Vaughan ED Jr. Effect of ureteral obstruction on renal hemodynamics. *Semin Urol* 1991;5:160.
57. Fern R, Yesko CM, Thornhill BA, et al. Reduced angiotensin expression attenuates renal interstitial fibrosis in obstructive nephropathy in mice. *J Clin Invest* 1999;103:39.

58. Finkle AL, Karg SJ, Smith DR. Parameters of renal functional capacity in reversible hydroureteronephrosis in dogs: II. Effects of one hour of ureteral obstruction upon urinary volume, osmolality, TcH_2O, C_{PAH}, RBF_{kr} and pUO_2. *Invest Urol* 1968; 6:26.
59. Foley FEB. New plastic operation for strictures at ureteropelvic junction; report of 20 operations. *J Urol* 1937;38:643.
60. Freedman AL, Bukowski TP, Smith CA, et al. Fetal therapy for obstructive uropathy: specific outcomes diagnosis. *J Urol* 1996; 156:720.
61. Frokiaer J. Obstructive nephropathy in the pig: aspects of renal hemodynamics and hormonal changes during acute unilateral ureteral obstruction. *APMIS* 1998;106[Suppl 82]:7.
62. Frokiaer J, Pederson EB, Knudsen L, et al. The impact of total unilateral ureteral obstruction on intrarenal angiotensin II production in the polycalyceal pig kidney. *Scand J Urol Nephrol* 1992;26:289.
63. Gasser B, Mauss Y, Ghnassia JP, et al. A quantitative study of normal nephrogenesis in the human fetus: its implication in the natural history of kidney changes due to low obstructive uropathies. *Fetal Diagn Ther* 1993;8:371.
64. Gaudio KM, Siegel NJ, Hayslett J, et al. Renal perfusion and intratubular pressure during ureteral occlusion in the rat. *Am J Physiol* 1980;238:F205.
65. Gee WE, Kiviat MD. Ureteral response to partial obstruction: smooth muscle hyperplasia and connective tissue proliferation. *Invest Urol* 1975;12:309.
66. Gillenwater JY, Teates D, Marion DN. Prediction of recoverability in hydronephrosis with ^{131}I hippuran renograms. Presented at annual meeting, American Urological Association, New York, May 13-17, 1979.
67. Gillenwater JY, Westervelt FB Jr, Vaughan ED, et al. Renal function after release of chronic unilateral hydronephrosis in man. *Kidney Int* 1975;7:179.
68. Goldsmith C. Postobstructive diuresis. *Kidney* 1968;2:1.
69. Gonzalez R, Chiou RK. Diagnosis of upper urinary tract obstruction in children: comparison of diuresis renography and perfusion-pressure flow studies. *J Urol* 1985;133:646.
70. Gosling JA, Dixon JS. Species variation in the location of upper urinary tract pacemaker cells. *Invest Urol* 1974;11:418.
71. Gosling JA, Dixon JS. Functional obstruction of the ureter and renal pelvis: a histological and electron microscopic study. *Br J Urol* 1978;50:145.
72. Gottschalk CW, Mylle M. Micropuncture study of pressures in proximal tubules and peritubular capillaries of the rat kidney and their relation to ureteral and renal venous pressures. *Am J Physiol* 1956;185:430.
73. Gottschalk CW, Mylle M. Micropuncture study of pressures in proximal and distal tubules and peritubular capillaries of the rat kidney during osmotic diuresis. *Am J Physiol* 1957;189:323.
74. Graham JB. Recovery of kidney after ureteral obstruction. *JAMA* 1962;181:993.
75. Gulbins E, Hoffend J, Zou AP, et al. Endothelin and endothelium-derived relaxing factor control of basal renovascular tone in hydronephrotic rat kidneys. *J Physiol* 1993;469:571.
76. Gulmi FA, Felsen D, Vaughan ED Jr. Pathophysiology of urinary tract obstruction. In: Walsh PC et al, eds. *Campbell's urology*, ed 7. Philadelphia: Saunders, 1998.
77. Hanna MK, Jetts RD, Sturgess JM, et al. Ureteral structure and ultrastructure: II. Congenital ureteropelvic junction obstruction and primary obstructive megaureter. *J Urol* 1976;116:725.
78. Harris KPG, Schreiner GF, Klahr S. Effect of leukocyte depletion on the function of the reobstructed kidney in the rat. *Kidney Int* 1989;36:210.
79. Harris RH, Gill JM. Changes in glomerular filtration rate during complete ureteral obstruction in rats. *Kidney Int* 1981; 19:603.
80. Harris RH, Hise MK, Best CF. Renotrophic factors in urine. *Kidney Int* 1983;23:616.
81. Harris RH, Yarger WE. Renal function after release of unilateral ureteral obstruction in rats. *Am J Physiol* 1974;227:806.
82. Haung A. The role of nitric oxide in obstructive nephropathy. *J Urol* 2000;163:1276.
83. Hay AW, Norman WJ, Price ML, et al. A comparison between diuresis renography and the Whitaker test in 64 kidneys. *Br J Urol* 1984;56:561.
84. Hayslett JP. Effect of age on compensatory renal growth. *Kidney Int* 1983;23:599.
85. Hellstrom J, Giertz G, Lindblom K. Pathogenesis and treatment of hydronephrosis. In: *VIII Congreso de la Sociedad Internacional de Urologia*. Paris: Libraire Gaston Doin, 1949.
86. Hermann W. Sitzungsberichte d. k. Akad, der Wissensch. zu Wein. *Math-Naturwiss* 1859;36:349. Cited in Cushny AR. *The secretion of the urine*. London: Longmans, Green, 1917.
87. Hinman F. Experimental hydronephrosis: repair following ureterocystoneostomy in white rats with complete ureteral obstruction. *J Urol* 1919;3:147.
88. Hinman F. Renal counterbalance: an experimental and clinical study with reference to significance of disuse atrophy. *Trans Am Soc Genitourin Surg* 1922;15:241.
89. Hinman F. Renal counterbalance. *Arch Surg* 1926;12:1105.
90. Hinman F. Pathogenesis of hydronephrosis. *Surg Gynecol Obstet* 1934;58:356.
91. Hinman F. Hydronephrosis: I. The structural change. II. The functional change. III. Hydronephrosis and hypertension. *Surgery* 1945;17:816.
92. Hinman F, Hepler AB. Experimental hydronephrosis: the effect of changes in blood pressure and in blood flow on its rate of development: I. Splanchnotomy: increased intrarenal blood pressure and flow; diuresis. *Arch Surg* 1925;11:578.
93. Hinman F, Hepler AB. Experimental hydronephrosis: The effect of changes in blood pressure and in blood flow on its rate of development: II. Partial obstruction of the renal artery: diminished blood flow, diminished intrarenal pressure and oliguria. *Arch Surg* 1925;11:649.
94. Hinman F, Hepler AB. Experimental hydronephrosis: the effect of changes in blood pressure and in blood flow on its rate of development, and the significance of the venous collateral system: III. Partial obstruction of the renal vein without and with ligation of all collateral veins. *Arch Surg* 1925;11:917.
95. Hinman F, Hepler AB. Experimental hydronephrosis: the effect of ligature of one branch of the renal artery on its rate of development: IV. Simultaneous ligation of the posterior branch of the renal artery and the ureter on the same side. *Arch Surg* 1926;12:830.
96. Hinman F, Lee-Brown RK. Pyelovenous outflow, its relation to pelvic reabsorption, to hydronephrosis and to accidents of pyelography. *JAMA* 1924;82:607.
97. Hinman F, Morison DM. An experimental study of the circulatory changes in hydronephrosis. *J Urol* 1924;21:435.
98. Hochberg DA, Chen J, Vaughan ED Jr, et al. Interstitial fibrosis is exacerbated in unilateral ureteral obstruction (UUO) in mice lacking the gene for inducible nitric oxide synthase. *J Urol* 1998;159:68.
99. Homsy YL, Saad F, Laberge I, et al. Transitional hydronephrosis of the newborn and infant. *J Urol* 1990;144:578.
100. Howards SS. Postobstructive diuresis: a misunderstood phenomenon. *J Urol* 1973;110:537.

101. Ichikawa I, Brenner BM. Role of local intrarenal vasoconstrictor-vasodilator interactions in mild partial ureteral obstruction. *Am J Physiol* 1979;236:F131.
102. Israel AR. Validation of the diuretic renogram with simultaneous intrapelvic pressure monitoring. Presentation to the 77th Annual Meeting of the American Urological Society, Kansas City, 1982.
103. Ito S, Johnson CS, Carretero OA. Modulation of angiotensin II–induced vasoconstriction by endothelium-derived relaxing factor in the isolated microperfused rabbit afferent arteriole. *J Clin Invest* 1991;87:1656.
104. Jaenike JR. The renal response to ureteral obstruction: a model for the study of factors which influence glomerular filtration pressure. *J Lab Clin Med* 1970;76:373.
105. Jaenike JR. The renal functional defect of postobstructive nephropathy: the effects of bilateral ureteral obstruction in the rat. *J Clin Invest* 1972;51:2999.
106. Jaenike JR, Bray GA. Effects of acute transitory urinary obstruction in the dog. *Am J Physiol* 1960;199:1219.
107. Josephson S, Dhillon HK, Ransley PG. Post-natal management of antenatally detected, bilateral hydronephrosis. *Urol Int* 1993; 51:79.
108. Kalika V, Bard RH, Iloreta A, et al. Prediction of renal functional recovery after relief of upper urinary tract obstruction. *J Urol* 1981;126:301.
109. Kerr WS Jr: Effect of complete ureteral obstruction for one week on kidney function. *J Appl Physiol* 1954;6:762.
110. Kessler RH. Acute effects of brief ureteral stasis on urinary and renal papillary chloride concentration. *Am J Physiol* 1960;199: 1215.
111. Kinn AC. Ureteropelvic junction obstruction: long-term followup of adults with and without surgical treatment. *J Urol* 2000;164:652.
112. Kinter M, Wolstenholme JT, Thornhill BA, et al. Unilateral ureteral obstruction impairs renal antioxidant enzyme activation during sodium depletion. *Kidney Int* 1999;55:1327.
113. Klahr S, Morrissey JJ. The role of growth factors, cytokines and nasoactive compounds in obstructive nephropathy. *Semin Nephrol* 1998;18:622.
114. Koff SA, Hayden LJ, Cirulli C, et al. Pathophysiology of ureteropelvic junction obstruction: experimental and clinical observations. *J Urol* 1986;136:333.
115. Kuhl PG, Schonig G, Schweer H, et al. Increased renal biosynthesis of prostaglandin E_2 and thromboxane B_2 in human congenital obstructive uropathy. *Pediatr Res* 1990;27:103.
116. Ladefoged O, Djurhuus JC. Morphology of the upper urinary tract in experimental hydronephrosis in pigs. *Acta Chir Scand* 1976;472:29.
117. Leahy AL, Ryan PC, McEntee GM, et al. Renal injury and recovery in partial ureteric obstruction. *J Urol* 1989;142:199.
118. Lefkowith JB, Okegawa T, DeSchryver-Keekemeti K, et al. Macrophage-dependent arachidonate metabolism in hydronephrosis. *Kidney Int* 1984;26:10.
119. Lennon GM, Bourke J, Ryan PC, et al. Pharmacological options for the treatment of acute ureteric colic. *Br J Urol* 1993; 71:401.
120. Lewis HY, Pierce JM. Return of function after relief of complete ureteral obstruction of 69 days' duration. *J Urol* 1962; 88:377.
121. Lome LG, Pinsky S, Levy L. Dynamic renal scan in the nonvisualizing kidney. *J Urol* 1979;121:148.
122. Lorentz WB Jr, Lassiter WE, Gottschalk CW. Renal tubular permeability during increased intrarenal pressure. *J Clin Invest* 1972;51:484.
123. Lupton EW, O'Reilly PH, Testa HJ, et al. Diuresis renography and morphology in urinary tract obstruction. *Br J Urol* 1981; 51:449.
124. Lupton EW, Richards D, Testa HJ, et al. A comparison of diuresis renography, the Whitaker test and renal pelvic morphology in idiopathic hydronephrosis. *Br J Urol* 1985;57:119.
125. MacNeily AE, Maizels M, Kaplan WE, et al. Does early pyeloplasty really avert loss of renal function? A retrospective review. *J Urol* 1993;150:769.
126. Malt RA. Humoral factors in regulation of compensatory renal hypertrophy. *Kidney Int* 1983;23:611.
127. Malvin RL, Kutchai H, Ostermann F. Decreased nephron population resulting from increased ureteral pressure. *Am J Physiol* 1964;207:835.
128. McClinton S, Steyn JH, Hussey JK. Retrograde balloon dilation for pelviureteric junction obstruction. *Br J Urol* 1993; 71:152.
129. McCrory WW, Shibuya M, Leumann E, et al. Studies of renal function in children with chronic hydronephrosis. *Pediatr Clin North Am* 1971;18:445.
130. McDonald JR, Mann FC, Priestly JT. The maximum intrapelvic pressure (secretory) of the kidney of the dog. *J Urol* 1937; 37:326.
131. McDougal WS. Pharmacologic preservation of renal mass and function in obstructive uropathy. *J Urol* 1982;128:418.
132. McDougal WS, Flanigan RC. Renal functional recovery of the hydronephrotic kidney predicted before relief of the obstruction. *Invest Urol* 1981;18:440.
133. McDougal WS, Wright FS. Defect in proximal and distal sodium transport in postobstructive diuresis. *Kidney Int* 1972; 2:304.
134. Michaelson G. Percutaneous puncture of the renal pelvis, intrapelvic pressure, and the concentrating capacity of the kidney in hydronephrosis. *Acta Med Scand (Suppl)* 1974;559:1.
135. Miyajima A, Chen J, Kirman I, et al. Interaction of nitric oxide and transforming growth factor-β1 induced by angiotensin II and mechanical stretch in rat reveal tubular epithelial cells. *J Urol* 2000;164:1729.
136. Miyajima A, Chen J, Stern J, et al. Antibody to transforming growth factor-beta prevents renal tubular apoptosis in unilateral ureteral obstruction. *J Urol* 2000;163:84.
137. Moody TE, Vaughan ED Jr, Gillenwater JY. Relationship between renal blood flow and ureteral pressure during 18 hours of total unilateral occlusion. *Invest Urol* 1975;13:246.
138. Morison DM. Routes of absorption in hydronephrosis: experimentation with dyes in the totally obstructed ureter. *Br J Urol* 1929;1:30.
139. Morrison AR, Nishikawa K, Needleman P. Unmasking of thromboxane A_2 synthesis by ureteral obstruction in the rabbit kidney. *Nature* 1977;267:259.
140. Morrison AR, Nishikawa K, Needleman P. Thromboxane A_2 biosynthesis in the ureter-obstructed isolated perfused kidney of the rabbit. *J Pharmacol Exp Ther* 1978;205:1.
141. Motola JA, Badlani GH, Smith AD. Results of 212 consecutive endopyelotomies: an 8-year follow up. *J Urol* 1993;149:453.
142. Muldowney FP, Duffy GJ, Kelly DG, et al. Sodium diuresis after relief of obstructive uropathy. *N Engl J Med* 1966;274: 1294.
143. Mulroney SE, Haramadi A, Roberts CT Jr, et al. Renal IGF-1 mRNA levels are enhanced following unilateral nephrectomy in immature but not adult rats. *Endocrinology* 1989;128:2660.
144. Murphy GP, Scott WW. The renal hemodynamic response to acute and chronic ureteral occlusions. *J Urol* 1966;95:636.
145. Naber KG, Madsen PO. Renal function in chronic hydronephrosis with and without infection and the role of lymphatics: an experimental study in dogs. *Urol Res* 1974;2:1.

146. Narath PA. The hydromechanics of the calix renalis. *J Urol* 1940;43:145.
147. Needleman P, Bronson SD, Wyche A, et al. Cardiac and renal prostaglandin I_2 biosynthesis and biological effects in isolated perfused rabbit tissues. *J Clin Invest* 1978;61:839.
148. Nesbit RM. Diagnosis of intermittent hydronephrosis: importance of pyelography during episodes of pain. *J Urol* 1956; 67:787.
149. Nishikawa K, Morrison A, Needleman P. Exaggerated prostaglandin biosynthesis and its influence on renal resistance in the isolated hydronephrotic rabbit kidney. *J Clin Invest* 1977;59: 1143.
150. Norwood VF, Carey RM, Geary KM, et al. Neonatal ureteral obstruction stimulates recruitment of renin-secreting renal cortical cells. *Kidney Int* 1994;45:1333.
151. Notfrey RG. The structural basis for normal and abnormal ureteral motility. *Ann R Coll Surg Engl* 1971;49:250.
152. Notfrey RG. Electron microscopy of the primary obstructive megaureter. *Br J Urol* 1972;44:229.
153. Obniski. *Centralbl Physiol* 1907;21:548. Cited in Cushny A. *The secretion of the urine.* London: Longmans, Green, 1917.
154. Olesen S, Madsen PO. Renal function during experimental hydronephrosis: function during partial obstruction following contralateral nephrectomy in the dog. *J Urol* 1968;99:692.
155. Olsson O. Studies on back-flow in excretion urography. *Acta Radiol (Suppl)* 1948;29:70.
156. O'Reilly PH. Diuresis renography eight years later: a critical update. *J Urol* 1986;136:993.
157. O'Reilly PH, Testa HJ, Lawson RS, et al. Diuresis renography in equivocal urinary tract obstruction. *Br J Urol* 1978;50:76.
158. Papadopoulou ZL, Slotkoff LM, Eisner GM, et al. Glomerular filtration during stop-flow. *Proc Soc Exp Biol Med* 1969;130: 1206.
159. Patt LM, Houck JC. Role of polypeptide growth factors in normal and abnormal growth. *Kidney Int* 1983;23:603.
160. Platt JF, Rubin JM, Ellis HM, et al. Duplex Doppler US of the kidney: differentiation of obstructive from nonobstructive dilatation. *Radiology* 1989;17:515.
161. Preuss HG. Compensatory renal growth symposium—an introduction. *Kidney Int* 1983;23:571.
162. Provoost AP, Molenaar JC. Renal function during and after a temporary complete unilateral ureter obstruction in rats. *Invest Urol* 1981;18:242.
163. Purkerson ML, Klahr S. Prior inhibition of vasoconstrictors normalizes GFR in postobstructed kidneys. *Kidney Int* 1989;35: 1306.
164. Rao NR, Heptinstall RH. Experimental hydronephrosis: a microangiographic study. *Invest Urol* 1968;6:183.
165. Rawashdek YF, Djurhuss JC, Mortensen J, et al. The intrarenal resistive index as a pathophysiological marker in obstructive uropathy. *J Urol* 2001 *(in press).*
166. Reisman DD, Kamholz JH, Kantor HI. Early deligation of the ureter. *J Urol* 1957;78:363.
167. Reyes AA, Martin D, Settle S, et al. EDRF role in renal function and blood pressure of normal rats and rats with obstructive uropathy. *Kidney Int* 1992;41:403.
168. Reyes AA, Robertson G, Klahr S. Role of antidiuretic hormone in obstructive nephropathy. *Proc Soc Exp Biol Med* 1991; 197:49.
169. Ricardo SD, Diamond JR. The role of macrophages and reactive oxygen species in experimental hydronephrosis. *Semin Nephrol* 1998;18:612.
170. Rist M, Lee S, Gittes RF. Glomerular filtration rate and effective renal plasma flow in four-kidney rats. *Surg Forum* 1975; 26:577.
171. Roussak NJ, Oleesky S. Water-losing nephritis, a syndrome simulating diabetes insipidus. *O J Med* 1954;23:147.
172. Ryan PC, Lennon GM, McLean PA, et al. The effects of acute and chronic JJ stent placements on upper urinary tract motility and calculus transit. *Br J Urol* 1994;74:434.
173. Scardino PL, Prince CL. Vertical flap ureteropelvioplasty: preliminary report. *South Med J* 1953;46:325.
174. Schnermann J, Wright FS, Davis JM, et al. Regulation of superficial nephron filtration rate by tubulo-glomerular feedback. *Pflugers Arch* 1970;318:147.
175. Schramm LP, Carlson DE. Inhibition of renal vasoconstriction by elevated ureteral pressure. *Am J Physiol* 1975;228:1126.
176. Schreiner GF, Harris KPG, Purkerson ML, et al. Immunological aspects of acute ureteral obstruction: immune cell infiltrate in the kidney. *Kidney Int* 1988;34:487.
177. Schulsinger DA, Marion DN, Kim FY, et al. The nitric oxide system is activated during late unilateral ureteral obstruction. *J Urol* 1997;157:209.
178. Schwartz DT. Unilateral upper urinary tract obstruction and arterial hypertension. *N Y State J Med* 1969;69:668.
179. Senac MU Jr, Miller JH, Stanley P. Evaluation of obstructive uropathy in children; radionuclide renography versus the Whitaker test. *Am J Radiol* 1985;1:11.
180. Sheehan HL, Davis JC. Experimental hydronephrosis. *Arch Pathol* 1959;68:185.
181. Sheehan SJ, Moran KT, Dowsett DJ, et al. Renal haemodynamics and prostaglandin synthesis in partial unilateral ureteric obstruction. *Urol Res* 1994;22:279.
182. Shimamura T, Kissane JM, Gyorki F. Experimental hydronephrosis: nephron dissection and electron microscopy of the kidney following obstruction of the ureter and in recovery from obstruction. *Lab Invest* 1966;15:629.
183. Shokeir AA. The diagnosis of upper urinary tract obstruction. *BJU Int* 1999;83:893.
184. Shokeir AA, Nijman RJM. The changing concepts in diagnosis and subsequent management of antenatal hydronephrosis. *BJU Int* 2000;85:987.
185. Shultz PJ, Schorer AE, Rau L. Effects of endothelium-derived relaxing factor and nitric oxide on rat mesangial cells. *Am J Physiol* 1990;258:F162.
186. Siegel NJ, Feldman RA, Lytton B, et al. Renal cortical blood flow distribution in obstructive nephropathy. *Circ Res* 1977; 40:379.
187. Silber S. Compensatory and obligatory renal growth in babies and adults. *Aust N Z J Surg* 1974;44:421.
188. Silber S. Growth of baby kidneys transplanted into adults. *Surg Forum* 1975;26:579.
189. Silber S, Malvin RL. Compensatory and obligatory renal growth in rats. *Am J Physiol* 1974;226:114.
190. Solez K, Pouchak S, Buono RA, et al. Inner medullary plasma flow in the kidney with ureteral obstruction. *Am J Physiol* 1976;231:1315.
191. Starr NT, Maizels M, Chou P, et al. Microanatomy and morphometry of the hydronephrotic "obstructed" renal pelvis in asymptomatic infants. *J Urol* 1992;148:519.
192. Stecker JR, Gillenwater JY. Experimental partial ureteral obstruction: I. Alteration in renal function. *Invest Urol* 1971; 8:377.
193. Strong KC. Plastic studies in abnormal renal architecture: the parenchymal alterations in experimental hydronephrosis. *Arch Pathol* 1940;29:77.
194. Suki W, Eknoyan G, Rector FC Jr, et al. Patterns of nephron perfusion in acute and chronic hydronephrosis. *J Clin Invest* 1966;45:122.

195. Taki M, Goldsmith DI, Spitzer A. Impact of age on effects of ureteral obstruction on renal function. *Kidney Int* 1983;24:602.
196. Taylor MJ, Ullmann E. Glomerular filtration after obstruction of the ureter. *J Physiol* 1961;157:38.
197. Thirakomen K, Kozlov N, Arruda J, et al. Renal hydrogen ion secretion following the release of unilateral ureteral obstruction. *Am J Physiol* 1976;231:1233.
198. Tolins JP, Palmer RMJ, Moneda S, et al. Role of endothelium-derived relaxing factor in regulation of renal hemodynamic responses. *Am J Physiol* 1990;258:H655.
199. Tuffier M. Étude clinique et experimentale sur l'hydronephrose. *Ann Mal Org Genitourin* 1894;12:14. Cited in Cushny A. *The secretion of the urine.* London: Longmans, Green, 1917.
200. Vaughan ED Jr, Gillenwater JY. Diagnosis, characterization and management of postobstructive diuresis. *J Urol* 1973; 109:286.
201. Vaughan ED Jr, Shenasky JH II, Gillenwater JY. Mechanism of acute hemodynamic response to ureteral occlusion. *Invest Urol* 1971;9:109.
202. Vaughan ED Jr, Sorenson EJ, Gillenwater JY. The renal hemodynamic response to chronic unilateral complete ureteral occlusion. *Invest Urol* 1970;8:78.
203. Vaughan ED Jr, Sosa RE. Hypertension and hydronephrosis. In: Brenner BM, Laragh JH, eds. *Hypertension: pathophysiology, diagnosis and management.* New York: Raven Press, 1990.
204. Vaughan ED Jr, Sweet RE, Gillenwater JY. Unilateral ureteral occlusion: pattern of nephron repair and compensatory response. *J Urol* 1973;109:979.
205. Walder CE, Thienermann C, Vane JR. The involvement of endothelium-derived relaxing factor in the regulation of renal cortical blood flow in the rat. *Br J Pharmacol* 1991;102:967.
206. Walls J, Buerkert JE, Purkerson JL, et al. Nature of the acidifying defect after relief of ureteral obstruction. *Kidney Int* 1975; 7:304.
207. Wanner C, Luscher TF, Schollmeyer P, et al. Unilateral hydronephrosis and hypertension: cause or coincidence? *Nephron* 1987;45:236.
208. Weidmann P, Beretta-Piccoli C, Hirsch D, et al. Curable hypertension with unilateral hydronephrosis: studies on the role of circulating renin. *Ann Intern Med* 1977;87:437.
209. Welch WJ, Wilcox CS, Aisaka K, et al. Nitric oxide synthesis from L-arginine modulates renal vascular resistance in isolated perfused and intact rat kidneys. *J Cardiovasc Pharmacol* 1991; 17:S165.
210. Whitaker RH. Methods of assessing obstruction in dilated ureters. *Br J Urol* 1973;45:15.
211. Whitaker RH, Buxton-Thomas MS. A comparison of pressure-flow studies and renography in equivocal upper urinary tract obstruction. *J Urol* 1984;131:446.
212. Whitfield HN, Britton KE, Hendry WF, et al. The distinction between obstructive nephropathy and uropathy by radionuclide transit times. *Br J Urol* 1978;50:433.
213. Wilson DR. Micropuncture study of chronic obstructive nephropathy before and after release of obstruction. *Kidney Int* 1972;2:119.
214. Wilson DR. The influence of volume expansion on renal function after relief of chronic unilateral ureteral obstruction. *Kidney Int* 1974;5:402.
215. Wilson DR, Honrath U. Cross-circulation study of natriuretic factors in postobstructive diuresis. *J Clin Invest* 1976;57:380.
216. Wilson DR, Klahr S. Urinary tract obstruction. In: Schrier RW, Gottschalk CW, eds. *Diseases of the kidney.* Boston: Little, Brown, 1993.
217. Winberg J. Renal function in congenital bladder neck obstruction. *Acta Chir Scand* 1958;116:332.
218. Winberg J. Renal function in water-losing syndrome due to lower urinary tract obstruction before and after treatment. *Acta Pediatr* 1959;48:149.
219. Winton FR. Influence of increase of ureteral pressure on the isolated mammalian kidney. *J Physiol* 1931;71:381.
220. Wright FS. Intrarenal regulation of glomerular filtration rate. *N Engl J Med* 1974;291:135.
221. Wright FS, Briggs JP. Feedback regulation of glomerular filtration rate. *Am J Physiol* 1977;233:F1.
222. Wright FH, Howards SS. Obstructive injury. In: Brenner BM, Rector FC, eds. *The kidney.* Philadelphia: Saunders, 1979.
223. Yanagisawa H, Morrissey J, Morrison AR, et al. Eicosanoid production by isolated glomeruli of rats with unilateral ureteral obstruction. *Kidney Int* 1990;37:1528.
224. Yarger WE. Urinary tract obstruction. In: Brenner BM, Rector FC: *The kidney.* Philadelphia: WB Saunders, 1991.
225. Yarger WE, Aynedjian HS, Bank N. A micropuncture study of postobstructive diuresis in the rat. *J Clin Invest* 1972;51:625.
226. Yarger WE, Griffith LD. Intrarenal hemodynamics following chronic unilateral obstruction in the dog. *Am J Physiol* 1974; 227:806.
227. Yarger WE, Schocken DD, Harris RH. Obstructive uropathy in the rat: possible roles for the renin-angiotensin system, prostaglandins, and thromboxanes in postobstructive renal function. *J Clin Invest* 1980;65:400.
228. Zatz R, DeNucci G, Michelazzo SM, et al. Effects of acute nitric oxide inhibition on rat glomerular microcirculation. *Am J Physiol* 1991;261:F360.
229. Zelman SJ, Zenser TV, Davis BB. Renal growth in response to unilateral ureteral obstruction. *Kidney Int* 1983;23:594.
230. Zetterstrom R, Ericsson NO, Winberg J. Separate renal function studies in predominantly unilateral hydronephrosis. *Acta Paediatr* 1958;47:540.

22

RENAL TRANSPLANTATION

STUART M. FLECHNER
ANDREW C. NOVICK

continued

S.M. Flechner and A.C. Novick: Cleveland Clinic Foundation, Cleveland, OH 44195.

Recent years have witnessed an explosive growth in the number of patients experiencing end-stage renal disease (ESRD), as well as the number of centers providing therapeutic modalities such as hemodialysis, peritoneal dialysis, and renal transplantation. Data from the United States Renal Data System (303) reveals an annual growth in the prevalent population of ESRD patients of more than 10% (Fig. 22.1), with many treated by center hemodialysis. Currently, more than 220,000 patients with ESRD require treatment. There is an age-dependent increase in the incidence of new patients with ESRD (Fig. 22.2). The mean age is 61 years, and more than half are older than 65 years. The continued aging of the U.S. population will undoubtedly ensure continued growth of the ESRD population.

Although there has been continued improvement in patient survival for both dialysis and transplantation (Fig. 22.3), the mortality rate of the ESRD population continues to be approximately 20% per year. Patients with ESRD enjoy only 20% to 25% of the life expectancy of the general population (8.8 years versus 31.8 years, respectively, at ages 45 to 49). Cardiovascular events are the most common cause of death in patients with ESRD. As Fig. 22.4 indicates, death rates for dialysis patients increase dramatically for each cause among patients older than 65 years of age.

The annual cost for the ESRD population in 1997 was more than $15 billion (Fig. 22.5). This is more than $43,000 per patient, with approximately 75% of this cost being absorbed by the federal Medicare program and additional amounts paid by state medicaid programs and private sources. These figures significantly underestimate the true expense because costs related to lost time from work and other expenses are not reflected.

As a result of economic considerations, quality of life, and outcomes, renal transplantation has emerged as the preferred treatment modality for most patients with ESRD (67). However, the number of transplants performed has not kept pace with the ESRD population growth (Table 22.1), and more than 42,000 patients are now awaiting transplantation (9). As apparent from Table 22.1, the number of kidney transplants has increased over 10 years by one-third from about 8,600 to 12,000 per year. However, this has been inadequate to meet the rising number of waiting patients, which has increased more than 250% during the same period. Although there have been slight increases in the number of cadaveric organ donors, this has been attributed to an increased use of older donors (older than age 60) and those with extended criteria of organ quality (e.g., ischemia, hypertension). There has been a doubling in the number of live donor transplants in the last decade, as improved immunosuppression has permitted the use of more distant relatives and even unrelated (spouses) individuals (Fig. 22.6). Experimental work on the use of animal xenografts as a source of donor organs remains many years away from being a clinical reality (13,224), but it continues to represent the best hope to resolve the worldwide organ donor shortage problem. The severe shortage of available donor organs has had more marked implications in extrarenal (e.g., heart, liver) transplants as numerous patients awaiting transplantation die each year, and significant concerns have arisen with respect to assurance that available organs will be allocated to needy recipients in a fair and equitable manner. Federal legislation created the National Organ Procurement and Transplant Network, and the United Network for Organ Sharing (UNOS) was awarded the federal contract to develop policies for equitable organ distribution.

IMMUNOBIOLOGY OF TRANSPLANTATION

Advances in molecular biology have aided our understanding of the immunobiology of organ transplantation and rejection. A *locus* is the location of a gene on a chromosome. *Alleles* are alternative forms of a gene at a given locus on homologous chromosomes. The *major histocompatibility complex* (MHC) is a series of cell surface antigens encoded by closely linked genes. A *haplotype* is the sum of genetic material or unit of inheritance contributed by each parent. Each individual inherits a distinct haplotype from each parent. The *phenotype* is the total histocompatibility antigens expressed by an individual without distinguishing which antigens are maternally or paternally derived. The *genotype* is the total of histocompatibility antigens expressed

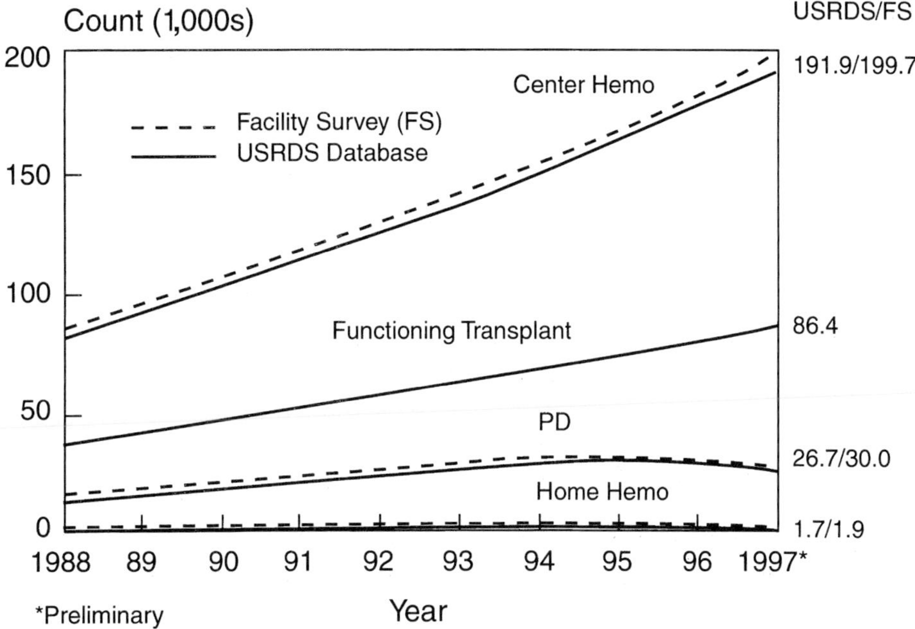

FIGURE 22.1. Point prevalence counts of patients with end-stage renal disease alive on December 31, by treatment modality and year, 1988–1997. Medicare patients only. PD, peritoneal dialysis. (From United States Renal Data System 1999 Annual Data Report. III. Treatment modalities for ESRD patients [Review]. *Am J Kidney Dis* 1999;34[2 Suppl 1]:S53, with permission.)

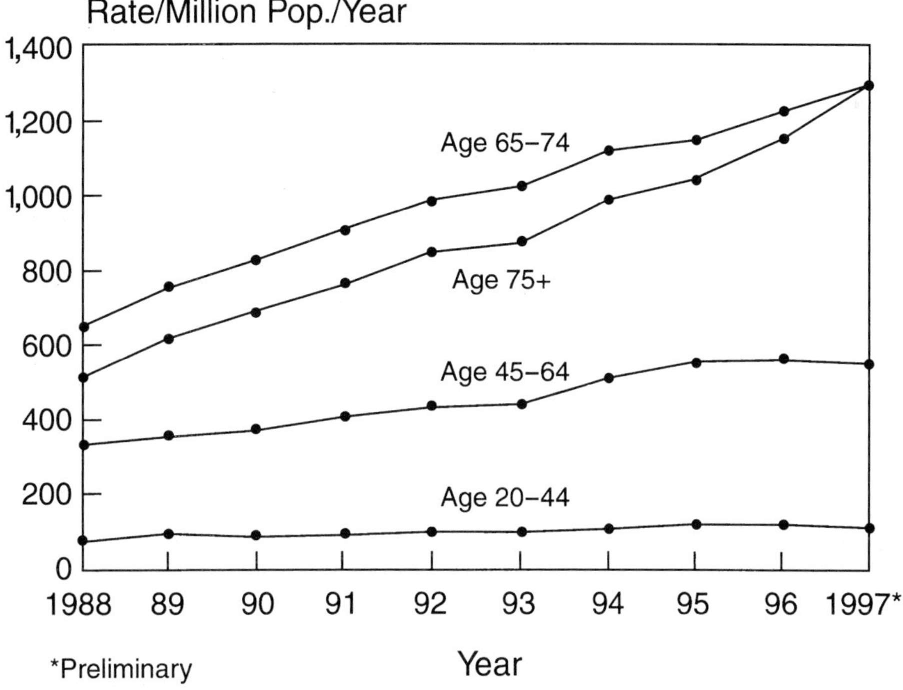

FIGURE 22.2. Incidence rates of treated end-stage renal disease per million population, by age group, 1988–1997. Medicare patients only. (From United States Renal Data System 1999 Annual Data Report. II. Incidence and prevalance of ESRD. *Am J Kidney Dis* 1999;34[2 Suppl 1]:S45, with permission.)

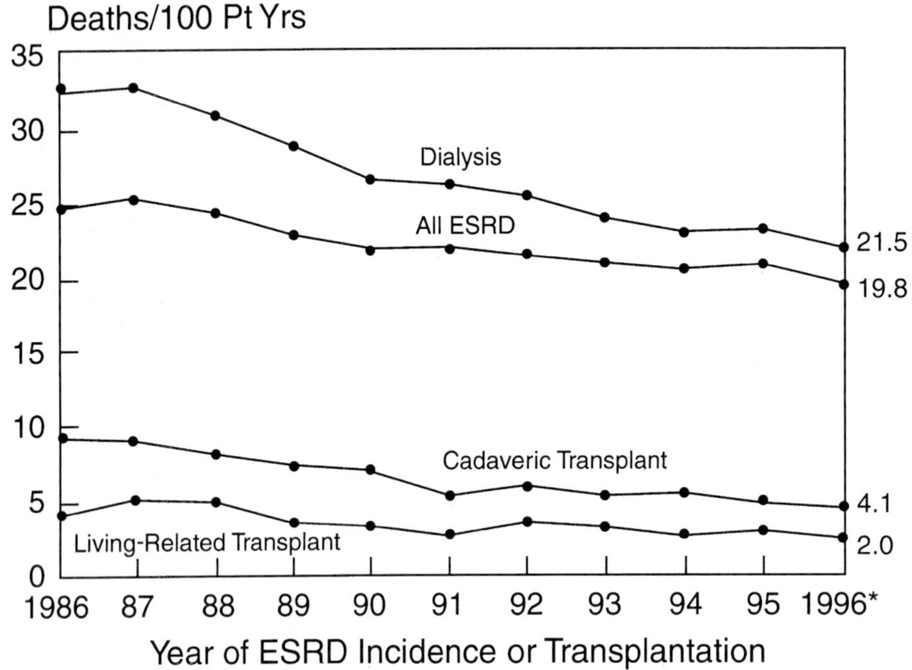

FIGURE 22.3. Death rates based on estimates from proportional hazards regression models by modality and year of end-stage renal disease *(ESRD)* incidence or of first transplantation. For each category, death rates are adjusted by age, race, sex, and diabetes to the average patient in a corresponding standard population. [From USRDS 1999 annual data report. *Am J Kidney Dis* 1999;34(2 Suppl 1):S77, with permission.]

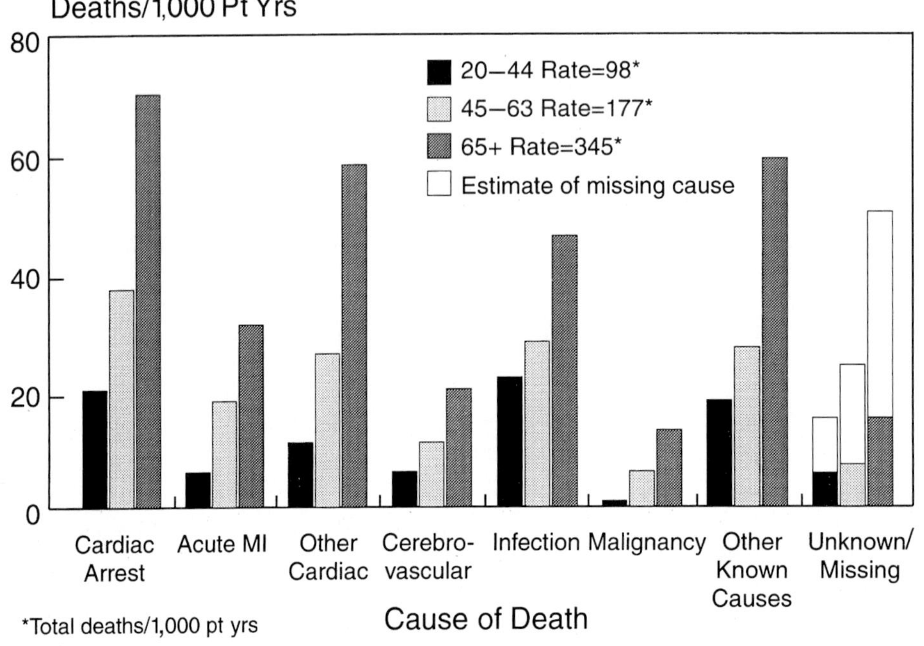

FIGURE 22.4. Cause-specific death rates for all dialysis patients by age, 1995–1997. The categories are collapsed from a death notification form. Patients younger than 20 years of age are excluded. MI, myocardial infarction. [From USRDS 1999 annual data report. *Am J Kidney Dis* 1999;34(2 Suppl 1):S88, with permission.]

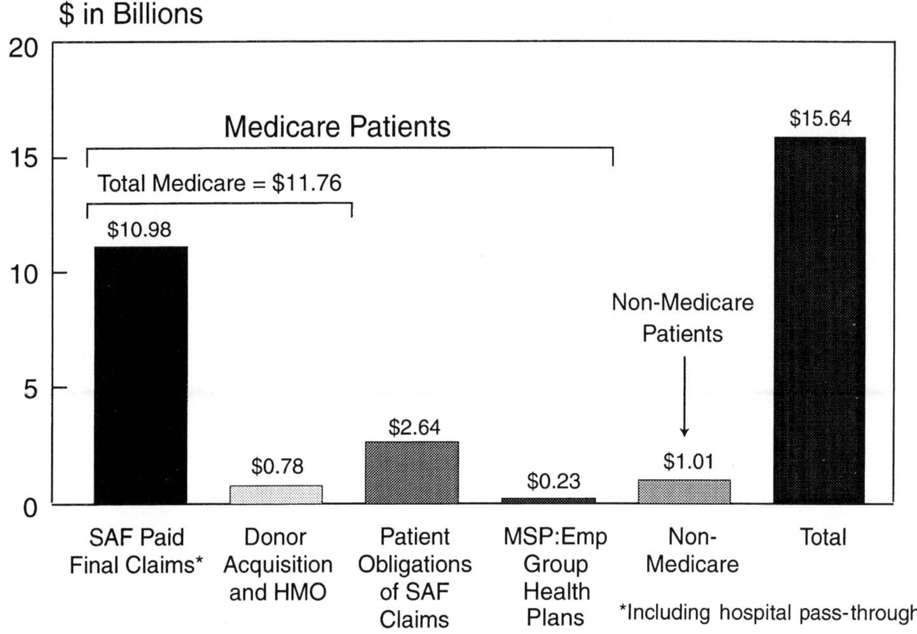

FIGURE 22.5. Estimated total direct monetary cost of treating end-stage renal disease in the United States, 1997. Separate estimates of cost are reported according to eligibility for Medicare insurance. HMO, health maintenance organization; SAF, Standard Analysis Files. [From USRDS 1999 annual data report. *Am J Kidney Dis* 1999;34(2 Suppl 1):S128, with permission.]

by an individual, designating the maternal and paternal contributions.

Many of the basic observations on transplant rejection were made through research into the mechanisms of tumor resistance. Following is a brief historical review of some of the investigators who have advanced our current knowledge of transplant immunobiology. In 1902, Carrel and Guthrie, during the development of vascular suture techniques, performed canine kidney autotransplants (same individual), allotransplants (members of same species), and xenotransplants (between species) (40). They observed that the autografts survived indefinitely, whereas the allografts and xenografts were rejected. Landsteiner (148) described the ABO blood group antigens. Haldane (103) theorized that transplanted tissues were rejected due to differences in alloantigens that were similar to differences in blood group antigens. Little and Tyzzer (156) noted that tumors survived when transplanted between mice of the same strain, but rejected when transplanted to other strains. Gorer (96), noting these observations, correlated these findings with the existence of an allelic blood group antigen that was able to be serologically detected. This important observation demonstrated that tumor rejection is not dependent on tumor-specific antigens, but on antigens present in normal tissues.

Snell (259) confirmed that it was the histocompatibility loci, and their encoded antigens, that account for both tumor and skin graft rejection. He reasoned that the distribution of these "transplantation antigens" followed a Mendelian pattern. Medawar (176) demonstrated that the rejection response was primarily a reaction rather than humorally mediated hypersensitivity. He performed full-thickness rabbit skin grafts and a few weeks later regrafts using the same

TABLE 22.1. NUMBERS OF RENAL TRANSPLANTS, CADAVERIC DONORS, AND WAITING PATIENTS, 1989–1998

	1989	1990	1991	1992	1993	1994	1995	1996	1997	1998
Cadaveric transplants	6,753	7,323	7,281	7,203	7,509	7,638	7,691	7,722	7,769	8,011
Live donor transplants	1,903	2,094	2,393	2,236	2,850	3,006	3,354	3,596	3,844	4,151
Total transplants	8,656	9,417	9,674	9,439	10,359	10,644	11,045	11,318	11,613	12,162
Cadaveric donors	3,810	4,306	4,268	4,276	4,606	4,798	5,001	5,037	5,081	5,341
Patients waiting	16,294	17,883	19,352	22,376	24,937	27,498	31,149	34,646	38,270	42,392

From 1999 annual report of the U.S. Scientific Registry of Transplant Recipients and the Organ Procurement and Transplantation Network transplant data 1989–1998. Richmond, VA: UNOS; and Bethesda, MD: Division of Organ Transplantation, Bureau of Health Resources, U.S. Department of Health and Human Services.

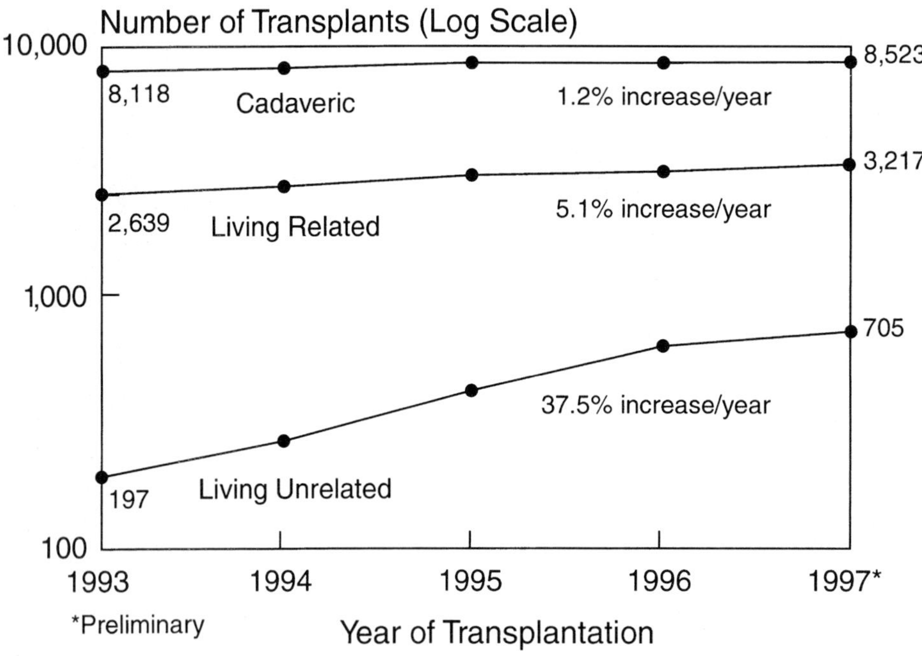

FIGURE 22.6. Total number of renal transplants by donor source and year (1993–1997) shown on log scale. Largest increase in living unrelated category. [From USRDS 1999 annual data report. *Am J Kidney Dis* 1999;34(2 Suppl 1):S96, with permission.]

donors into the same recipients, and demonstrated the phenomenon of accelerated rejection. Billingham and associates (22), expanding on the observations of Medawar, demonstrated the phenomenon of second set or accelerated rejection in recipients sensitized by prior exposure to the donor alloantigen (i.e., the more rapid rejection of a second graft from the same donor from which a first graft had been rejected).

Through the work of these and many other investigators, the field of clinical organ transplantation has evolved. However, the success of clinical renal transplantation currently rests on the use of drugs to achieve nonspecific immune suppression to prevent allograft rejection. The ultimate goal of organ transplantation is to induce the development of *donor-specific tolerance* (defined as the state of immune unresponsiveness to the donor MHC antigens, but the host maintains the ability to respond to other foreign antigens). Several hypotheses exist regarding mechanisms of tolerance induction, which has been observed primarily in animal models, but also anecdotally seen in transplant recipients who were taken off immunosuppressive medications for medical reasons or occasionally in noncompliant patients who stopped taking their medications. These include *clonal deletion*—elimination of immunoreactive T cells; *clonal anergy*—prevention of activation and proliferation of donor antigen–specific T cells; *suppression*—inducing other cells or mechanisms to prevent the triggering of a donor-specific immune response; and *chimerism*—persistence of a small number of hematopoietic cells of donor origin in the recipient (10). Although presently not a clinical reality, tolerance induction remains the goal of transplant research worldwide.

THE HUMAN MAJOR HISTOCOMPATIBILITY COMPLEX

The immune response of a patient when exposed to the "foreign" tissue of an organ transplant continues to represent the major barrier to success in spite of the many advances that have been made in immunosuppression. The human major histocompatibility complex is the primary target of immune-reactive cells that make up the rejection process. The MHC describes a region of genes that encode proteins that are responsible for the rejection of tissues between different species or between members of the same species. More important, these cell surface proteins serve as identity markers on cells interacting with T lymphocytes carrying out specific immune functions. The cell surface MHC markers are called human leukocyte antigens (HLAs) because they were first identified on white blood cells.

The HLA gene complex is found on the short arm of chromosome 6 (Fig. 22.7). Two classes of antigens, class I (HLA-A, HLA-B, and HLA-C) and class II (HLA-DR, HLA-DQ, and HLA-DP), can be differentiated by their molecular structure and their tissue distribution. The class I HLAs consist of a 44-kDa, transmembrane glycoprotein α-chain that is noncovalently associated with β_2-microglobulin on the cell surface. These molecules are found in varying densities on essentially all cells in the body.

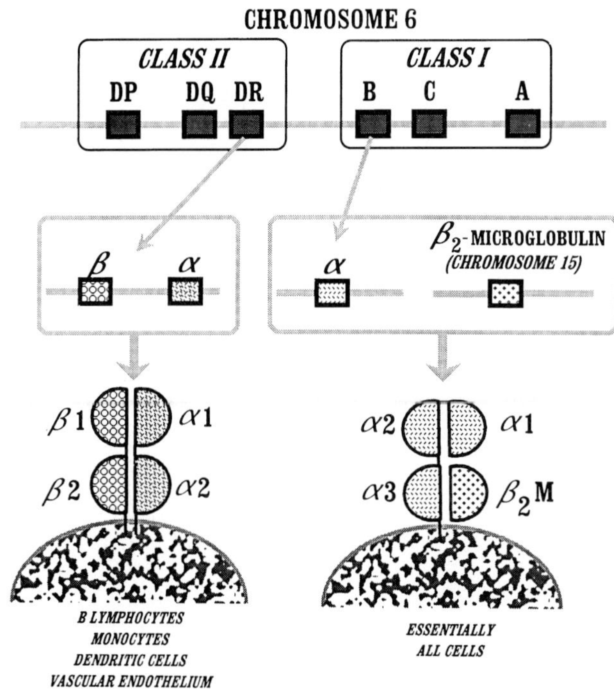

FIGURE 22.7. A simplified illustration of HLA genes and molecules.

HLA class II molecules are made up of two transmembrane glycoproteins, an α-chain of approximately 34 kDa and a β-chain that is slightly smaller (28 kDa). Their tissue distribution is much more restricted than that seen with class I. The B lymphocytes, which express both class I and class II, are commonly used to identify class II antigens in the laboratory. The involvement of HLA class II in transplant rejection results from the presence of these molecules on the surface of vascular endothelial cells of the graft, as well as on "passenger leukocytes" that are present in the organ.

The MHC genes are codominantly expressed, meaning that each individual expresses the HLAs that are inherited from either parent. What makes this system unique is the degree of polymorphism that is found, resulting in a great many alleles or variants of these antigens that have been identified in the population. Table 22.2 illustrates the HLA-A, HLA-B, HLA-C, HLA-DR, and HLA-DQ antigens that can be identified using standard lymphocytotoxicity methodologies. Using polymerase chain reaction (PCR)–based DNA-level testing, it is becoming abundantly clear that the degree of polymorphism is much greater than was previously thought. In 1994, the numbers of alleles that had been identified at the DNA level included 50 at

TABLE 22.2. LISTING OF RECOGNIZED HUMAN LEUKOCYTE ANTIGEN SPECIFICITIES*

HLA-A	HLA-B		HLA-C	HLA-DR	HLA-DQ
A1	B5	B51 (5)	Cw1	DR1	DQ1
A2	B7	B5102	Cw2	DR103	DQ2
A203	B703	B5103	Cw3	DR2	DQ3
A210	B8	B52 (5)	Cw4	DR3	DQ4
A3	B12	B53	Cw5	DR4	DQ5 (1)
A9	B13	B54 (22)	Cw6	DR5	DQ6 (1)
A10	B14	B55 (22)	Cw7	DR6	DQ7 (3)
A11	B15	B56 (22)	Cw8	DR7	DQ8 (3)
A19	B16	B57 (17)	Cw9 (w3)	DR8	DQ9 (3)
A23 (9)	B17	B58 (17)	Cw10 (w3)	DR9	
A24 (9)	B18	B59		DR10	
A2403	B21	B60 (40)		DR11 (5)	
A25 (10)	B22	B61 (40)		DR12 (5)	
A26 (10)	B27	B62 (15)		DR13 (6)	
A28	B35	B63 (15)		DR14 (6)	
A29 (19)	B37	B64 (14)		DR1403	
A30 (19)	B38 (16)	B65 (14)		DR 1404	
A31 (19)	B39 (16)	B67		DR15 (2)	
A32 (19)	B3901	B70		DR16 (2)	
A33 (19)	B3902	B71 (70)		DR17 (3)	
A34 (10)	B40	B72 (70)		DR18 (3)	
A36	B4005	B73			
A43	B41	B75 (15)		DR51	
A66 (10)	B42	B76 (15)		DR52	
A68 (28)	B44 (12)	B77 (15)		DR53	
A69 (28)	B45 (12)	B7801			
A74 (19)	B46	NM5			
	B47				
	B48	Bw4			
	B49 (21)	Bw6			
	B50 (21)				

*Revised Jan. 14, 1993.
Adapted from *Histocompatibility laboratory manual.* The Cleveland Clinic Foundation.

HLA-A, 97 at HLA-B, 34 at HLA-C, 106 at HLA-DR, 26 at HLA-DQ, and 59 at HLA-SP (24). All of the class I polymorphism is found in the α-chain, β_2-microglobulin being invariant, and the number of class II alleles given are for the β-chains, which are much more polymorphic than the class II α-chains.

One other system that plays a major role in histocompatibility is the ABO blood group antigens. Incompatibility at ABO can result in hyperacute rejection of a transplanted organ. The same general rules that apply for transfusion are relevant for transplantation (i.e., type O is the universal donor, type AB is the universal recipient, and so on), and confirmation of ABO compatibility should always be performed before transplantation of an organ.

HISTOCOMPATIBILITY TESTING FOR TRANSPLANTATION

Three areas of histocompatibility testing are relevant for organ transplantation: (a) the typing of patient and donor to determine the degree of *match;* (b) assessment of the level of *sensitization* to HLAs in patients who have been exposed to foreign antigens via pregnancies, transfusions, or transplant; and (c) *crossmatching,* in which the serum of the patient is examined for the presence of preformed antidonor antibodies that would be potentially harmful to the graft. By examining all of these factors, it is possible to assess the degree of risk for rejection in a particular donor–recipient combination.

The mainstay of histocompatibility testing is the complement-mediated, lymphocytotoxicity assay (285). This technique involves the incubation of lymphocytes with antibodies that react with HLAs, addition of a source of complement that results in lysis of the cells if antibody is bound to their surface, and the scoring of cell death using a vital stain. T lymphocytes, which express HLA-A, HLA-B, and HLA-C, are used only for class I typing, and B lymphocytes, which express class II, are used to identify HLA-DR, HLA-DQ, and HLA-DP. The sources of HLA reagents include allosera obtained from sensitized individuals as a result of pregnancy, transfusion, or transplant rejection, and in some cases monoclonal antibodies specific for HLA. Because individuals are seldom exposed to a single mismatched HLA, a considerable amount of screening of sera is required to obtain reagents appropriate for HLA typing. HLA typing at the DNA level is a rapidly developing technology that holds much promise (204). Here it is the nucleotide sequences of the DNA that are identified, rather than the epitopes found on the HLA molecules that recognized using antibodies. Once the DNA sequence of an HLA molecule is determined, it is relatively simple to produce reagents that can identify the polymorphic sequences. This general approach has almost unlimited potential for the identification of the many HLA alleles.

Individuals inherit one set, a haplotype, of HLAs from each of their parents. Therefore matching for HLA involves two antigens each at three HLA loci. Most data regarding HLA matching have included antigens at the HLA-A, HLA-B (class I), and HLA-DR (class II) loci, including anywhere from zero to six antigens matched. However, for solid organ transplantation, the concern is to avoid mismatched antigens that the patient would recognize as foreign. Therefore assessing the number of mismatches is the more appropriate method for determining compatibility at HLA in solid organ transplantation. Sometimes fewer than six antigens are identified, which may result from an individual who inherits the same antigen at a particular locus from each parent (homozygous).

Presensitization to HLAs is the major obstacle faced by many kidney transplant candidates. The same events that provide potential sources of HLA reagents in some individuals, such as pregnancy, transfusion, and transplant rejection, may sensitize a potential transplant candidate. To assess the degree of presensitization, a patient's serum is tested against a panel of lymphocytes from individuals of known HLA type, using essentially the same lymphocytotoxicity assay used for HLA typing. A value is obtained, the percent panel reactive antibody (PRA), that represents the percentage of the population that the patient's serum would be expected to react against. Many laboratories take this a step further, identifying HLA specificities of the antibodies, as well as identifying HLAs that the patient does not have antibodies against and therefore would be "acceptable" mismatches for the patient. In general, sera are obtained and screened on a monthly basis for patients waiting for a kidney transplant. The PRA may vary from month to month, necessitating frequent antibody screening to provide current information should a donor become available. Patients not previously exposed to HLAs may be screened at longer intervals, assuming that it is possible to document changes in their status (e.g., transfusion).

Perhaps the most important activity of the histocompatibility laboratory is performing the crossmatch test. It has been known for years that the presence of antidonor antibodies, particularly IgG, anti–T cell (class I) reactions, is associated with a significant risk of hyperacute rejection (209). The class of antigen recognized by the antibodies (class I or II) by using T and B cells as targets can be determined, as can the class of antibody (IgG or IgM) using a variety of permutations of the lymphocytotoxicity technique. Not all types of antibody reactions are associated with a high degree of risk of rejection, so characterization of the reaction can assist in determining compatibility between patient and donor. Sometimes reactions may also be due to an autoantibody, which can be removed by absorption with "self" lymphocytes.

Standard crossmatching techniques have made hyperacute rejection a rare occurrence. However, the observation that a number of transplants resulted in grafts that never functioned and that this was more likely to occur in presensitized recipients has led to the development of more sensitive crossmatching techniques. Two approaches use antibody reagents that bind to human IgG to enhance the sensitivity. In the antiglobulin crossmatch, a second anti-IgG antibody is used, allowing the detection of weak reactions and those involving noncomplement-binding IgG using lymphocytotoxicity. The flow cytometry crossmatch uses a fluorescent-labeled anti-IgG reagent, and the binding of the patient's antibodies, not the donor lymphocytes, is measured using a flow cytometer. Both the antiglobulin approach (137) and the flow cytometry technique (51) can be used to identify patients who are at high risk of graft loss, and these techniques are especially effective in cases involving retransplants.

Using the information provided by the degree of mismatch, the PRA information and the crossmatch allow an assessment of the degree of compatibility between patient and donor. In general, an extremely well-matched graft, such as an O-A, B, DR antigen mismatch, can be expected to do well. An antibody specificity against a donor antigen found in a recent serum is of more concern than one from months or years before the transplant, particularly if there is crossmatch activity (115). In terms of crossmatch reactivity, IgG is of more concern than IgM, T cell (class I) more than B cell (class II), and recent serum more than historical (114); reactions involving autoreactive antibodies, which are often IgM, do not appear to be deleterious. Essentially all transplants involve some degree of risk of rejection, but using the histocompatibility results can help avoid recipient–donor combinations at the greatest risk.

MECHANISMS OF IMMUNOLOGIC RESPONSE—ANTIGEN RECOGNITION; CELLULAR AND HUMORAL RESPONSE

The purpose of the immune system is to protect the host by identifying and eradicating potentially harmful invaders and foreign substances. The cells and molecules responsible for immunity constitute the immune system, and their collective and coordinated response to the introduction of foreign substances is called the immune response. The immune response can be divided into nonspecific-innate immunity and specific-adaptive immunity. The nonspecific arm includes cells such as neutrophils and macrophages, which can phagocytose pathogens, and inflammatory molecules such as complement, which can directly kill cells. The specific arm of the immune system by contrast is able to selectively identify foreign molecules and respond and adapt to only those foreign cells. Furthermore, the specific arm exhibits memory, such that reexposure prompts a more rapid and vigorous response. It is the specific arm of the immune system that is most important in transplant rejection (296).

Adaptive immunity can be further divided into humoral (antibody) and cellular components. The humoral response derives from B cells that recognize foreign antigens via antibody receptors on the B-cell surface. When activated, the B cell matures into a plasma cell, which secretes a large quantity of its specific antibody. When a pathogen is coated by these specific antibodies, cell death can occur by complement activation or phagocytosis by other cells that recognize and bind to the "tail" of the antibody (opsonization). In organ transplantation, the presence of "preformed" antibodies in the recipient that are specific for the donor organ results in the rapid destruction of the organ (hyperacute rejection). These antibodies bind immediately to the vascular endothelium of the graft and trigger complement-dependent cytotoxicity, eventually leading to complete vascular thrombosis.

The T lymphocyte is the central component of the cellular arm of the immune response (298). T cells recognize protein antigen through their T-cell receptor only after an antigen has been processed into peptide fragments and presented on carrier MHC molecules by antigen-presenting cells (APCs). Intracellular antigens are usually presented to T cells by class I MHC molecules. Extracellular antigens, however, must first be phagocytosed by a specialized APC such as a macrophage or dendritic cell, which presents peptides bound to class II MHC molecules. The result is that the T cell must recognize both MHC and peptide in a particular arrangement for antigen-specific activation to take place (Fig. 22.8). The types of responses are also controlled by the specificity of the MHC antigens on the APCs themselves. Those T cells bearing CD8 that are programmed to

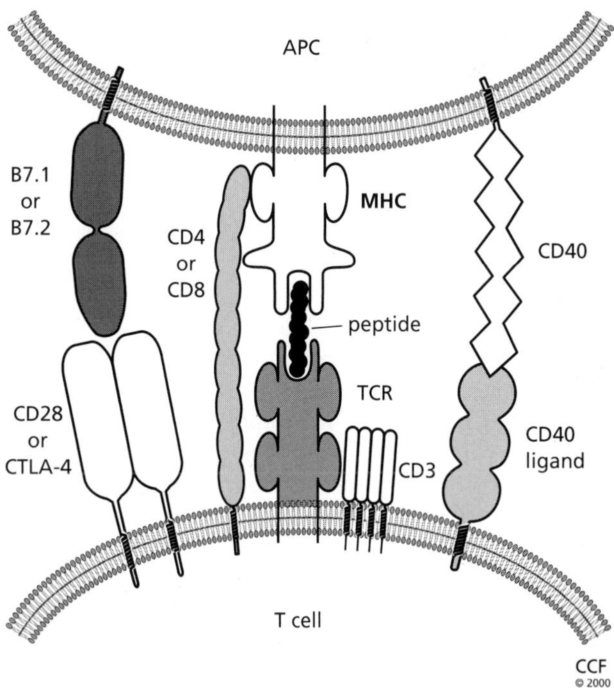

FIGURE 22.8. Presentation of foreign peptide antigen to host T cell. Signal 1 delivered as peptide is processed and presented in MHC groove of APC to T-cell receptor. Signal 2 is delivered by APC costimulatory molecule B7 or CD40 to T-cell ligand CD28 or CD40 L, respectively. T cell CD4 or CD8 molecule stabilizes the interaction.

be cytotoxic require APCs to present antigen in context of MHC class I molecules; those T cells bearing CD4 that are programmed to become helper T cells require antigen to be presented in context of MHC class II molecules (178).

The overall scheme of allograft rejection can be divided into five stages:

1. Antigen recognition
2. T-cell activation—requires two signals
3. Signal transduction and cytokine release
4. Cellular differentiation and proliferation
5. Target cell destruction

Graft alloantigens provide a unique potential for host T-cell activation because they themselves serve both as immunogens and as components of the activation mechanism. When a kidney is transplanted into a recipient, it brings with it an array of tissue-bound class I and II MHC molecules, as well as antigen-presenting cells. These APCs are included in the group of donor-derived white cells referred to as *passenger leukocytes,* which can be adherent to blood vessels or within the interstitial tissues. The activation of recipient T cells requires two distinct signals. Signal 1 requires the presentation of the peptide–MHC complex on an APC to the T-cell receptor of a resting T cell. Signal 2 is a costimulatory signal that is transmitted by surface glycoproteins on the APC, which interact with their ligand on the T-cell surface. The most important costimulatory signals are the B7 or CD40 molecules on an APC binding to their T-cell surface ligands CD28 (or CTLA-4) or CD40 ligand (CD154), respectively. The triggering of the T-cell receptor by signal 1 alone leads to anergy or nonresponsiveness. An APC that provides both signals 1 and 2 leads to activation of protein kinase C and other signal transduction pathways in the T cell. The resting T cell then progresses through the cell cycle from the "G_0" phase to clonal proliferation.

The immune response is provided two distinct pathways for allorecognition (99). A *direct presentation* pathway is provided by *donor APCs,* which present peptide–MHC complexes to recipient T cells. The foreign MHC molecules presented to the recipient can be a myriad of alloantigens, including the allogenic MHC molecule itself plus the many different peptides derived from endogenous proteins. Direct presentation is thought to be responsible for early acute rejection episodes. The recipient can also engage alloantigens through the *indirect presentation* pathway dependent on *recipient APCs.* Indirect presentation requires the uptake and processing of donor MHC molecules (to form peptide fragments) by recipient APCs, which present peptide–MHC complexes to the recipient T-cell receptor. Peripheral recipient APCs migrate to the graft to pick up soluble donor MHC molecules for processing. The actual site of indirect pathway T-cell activation occurs in recipient lymph nodes and is thus "self" MHC restricted. The indirect route becomes more important with time as donor APCs (required for direct recognition) diminish by senescence. The indirect pathway is thought to be more important for the development of chronic allograft rejection.

Once the recipient immune system is activated, the allograft can be attacked by several mechanisms. Recipient CD8 T cells that recognize foreign MHC class I molecules can directly damage donor cells by drilling holes in their cell membranes with a class of molecules called perforins (133). Some cytokines released by CD4 T cells can damage the allograft directly, such as tumor necrosis factor-α. Natural killer (NK) cells, which are not MHC specific but which are attracted during the immune response by opsonins, can also cause direct cell damage. Antibodies produced by B cells can fix complement, attract platelets, and destroy the organ through vascular rejection.

MODIFICATION OF THE IMMUNE RESPONSE—PREVENTION OF REJECTION

Blood Transfusion Effect

For more than 30 years, the effect of blood transfusions in renal transplantation has been investigated and debated. As clinical transplantation has developed, the policies and practices regarding the avoidance or use of blood transfusions has changed dramatically on several occasions. Before 1973, transfusions were avoided in dialysis patients awaiting transplantation because of concern that they would develop deleterious antibodies (sensitization), which would have an adverse impact on success (16). Opelz and colleagues (205) described improved results in a large number of recipients who had received transfusions compared with those who had not been transfused. Subsequently, numerous reports revealed a 10% to 20% improvement in graft survival in transfused patients and a near-uniform policy of all patients receiving at least two to five transfusions before transplantation was adopted. However, over the ensuing years, refinements in HLA typing and crossmatching, as well as the development of new immunosuppressive medications, especially cyclosporine, appeared to diminish the transfusion effect. As Fig. 22.9 indicates, no discernible difference has been seen between transfused and nontransfused recipients of first cadaver transplants since 1988 (286).

Similar results have been reported relative to the use of transfusions in recipients of living-related renal transplants. Salvatierra and colleagues (243) demonstrated that donor-specific (blood from the intended donor) transfusion greatly improved results in recipients of 1-haplotype–matched kidneys. This benefit was substantiated as donor-specific transfusion (DST) protocols became commonplace. Again, however, the transfusion benefits appeared to wane with the introduction of newer immunosuppressive medications (77). The major disadvantages of transfusions include the possible transmission of viral diseases and sensitization of the patient to disparate HLA phenotypes. In addition, the

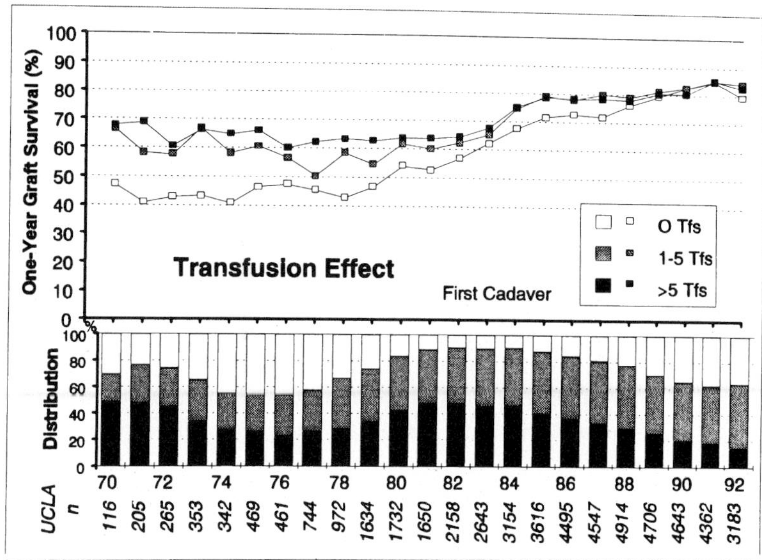

FIGURE 22.9. Effect of blood transfusions in recipients of first cadaver transplants by year, 1970–1992, demonstrating no benefit since 1988. (From Terasaki PI, Yuge J, Cecka DW, et al. Thirty year trends in clinical kidney transplantation. In: Terasaki PI, Cecka JM, eds. *Clinical transplants, 1993.* Los Angeles: UCLA Tissue Typing Laboratory, 1994, with permission.)

availability of synthetic erythropoietin (66) has led to a substantial reduction in the number of centers currently using pretransplant transfusions.

Immunosuppressive Agents

As the molecular events in the alloantigen processing pathways have become more apparent, so has the nonspecificity of long-standing immunosuppressive therapy whose toxicities have derived from the broad impact on the body's immune system ("overimmunosuppression"). Although the ideal immunosuppressant that selectively targets only specific steps in allograft rejection while sparing all other immunologic components is not yet available, numerous promising agents are being investigated. The chemical structures of agents in current clinical use, as well as newer ones being studied, are depicted in Figs. 22.10 through 22.12. Their proposed mechanism of action, available results, and toxicities are reviewed next; several more comprehensive reports are available (106,279,293,296).

Chemical Immunosuppression

Corticosteroids

Since the initial observations more than 35 years ago that corticosteroids could prevent and treat renal allograft rejection (120), they have become the cornerstone of immunosuppressive therapy. Corticosteroids have numerous effects on the immune system (294), and their effect on T lymphocytes appears greater than that on B lymphocytes. Sequestration of lymphocytes in lymph nodes and the bone marrow results in the often observed lymphopenia. Glucocorticoids become bound to intercellular receptors, and conformational changes in the steroid–receptor complex allow for genetic interference with cytokine production. The primary immunosuppressive affect of corticosteroids is inhibition of production and monocyte release of interleukin (IL)-1with subsequent inhibition of IL-2 and interferon-γ, thus interfering with lymphocyte activation and production of effector cells.

Systemic toxicities of corticosteroids, including cushingoid features, hypercholesterolemia, hyperlipidemia, hyperglycemia, weight gain, aseptic necrosis of bone and osteoporosis, poor wound healing, growth retardation, psychiatric disturbances, and increased susceptibility to infection, are

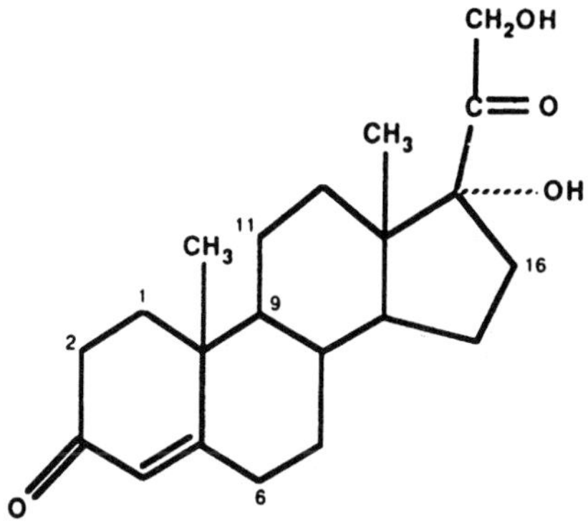

	$C_1 - C_2$	C_6	C_9	C_{11}	C_{16}
METHYLPREDNISOLONE	DOUBLE BOND	···CH_3	–H	◀OH	–H
PREDNISOLONE	DOUBLE BOND	–H	–H	◀OH	–H
PREDNISONE	DOUBLE BOND	–H	–H	=O	–H

FIGURE 22.10. Chemical structure of corticosteroids. (From Thomson AW, Woo J, Cooper M. Mode of action of immunosuppressive drugs with particular reference to the molecular basis of macrolide-induced immunosuppression. In: Thomson AW, ed. *The molecular biology of immunosuppression.* New York: Wiley, 1992:161, with permission.)

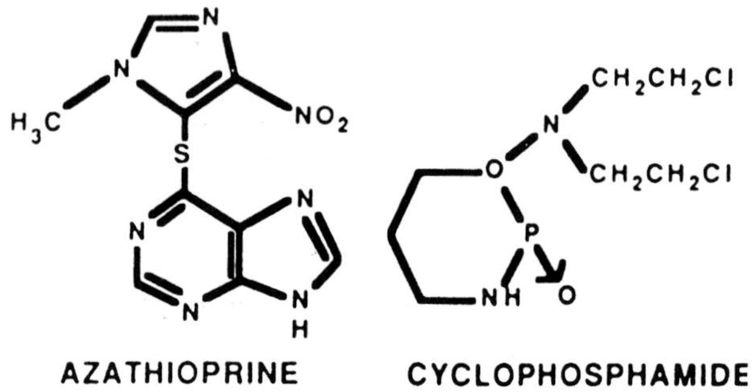

AZATHIOPRINE CYCLOPHOSPHAMIDE

FIGURE 22.11. Chemical structure of azathioprine and cyclophosphamide. (From Thomson AW, Woo J, Cooper M. Mode of action of immunosuppressive drugs with particular reference to the molecular basis of macrolide-induced immunosuppression. In: Thomson AW, ed. *The molecular biology of immunosuppression.* New York: Wiley, 1992:157, with permission.)

known to all clinicians and have resulted in intense efforts to reduce steroid dosage. Alternate-day steroid dosing appears beneficial for growth in children (283), but complete steroid withdrawal appears more problematic. There have been several trials attempting to withdraw steroids form stable transplant patients (2,245). The benefits include lower blood pressure, improved lipid profiles, and diminished physical side effects attributed to steroids. However, early graft stability is often followed by acute rejection in about one-third of the patients. If attempted, withdrawal should be entertained in well-matched recipients, 1 year or more after transplant, with no prior episodes of rejection. Living-related recipients who demonstrate *in vitro* hyporesponsiveness to the donor can usually be safely withdrawn (77).

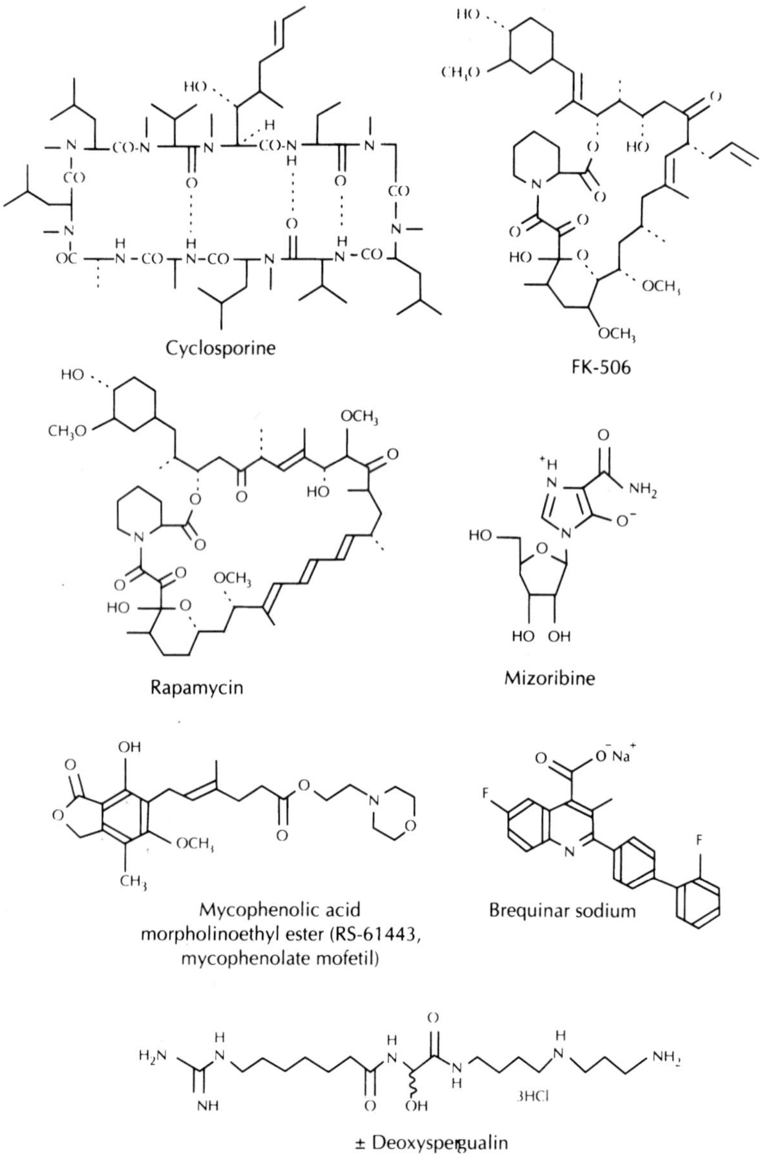

Cyclosporine

FK-506

Rapamycin

Mizoribine

Mycophenolic acid morpholinoethyl ester (RS-61443, mycophenolate mofetil)

Brequinar sodium

± Deoxyspergualin

FIGURE 22.12. Names and chemical structures of cyclosporine and newer xenobiotic immunosuppressive agents. (From Lewis RM. Developments and issues in immunosuppressive therapy. *Curr Opin Urol* 1994;4:100, with permission.)

Antiproliferative Drugs

Azathioprine

Initial efforts with immunosuppression in renal transplant recipients occurred using 6-mercaptopurine and its imidazole derivative azathioprine (185). Azathioprine is metabolized *in vivo* to 6-mercaptopurine, and the antimetabolites block DNA synthesis by inhibiting purine synthesis and metabolism via competitive enzyme inhibition. Early proliferation, especially in rapidly dividing cells (lymphoblast), is inhibited, although there is no effect against activated lymphocytes (effector phase). As such, azathioprine is most effective if given immediately after antigen presentation to prevent rejection and is ineffective in treating ongoing rejection.

Adverse effects of azathioprine include myelosuppression with leukopenia and thrombocytopenia, alopecia, hepatotoxicity, cholestatic jaundice, and increased risk of infection and neoplasia. Toxicity from azathioprine will usually respond to dose reduction, although occasionally drug substitution is required. When compared directly with another antiproliferative agent, mycophenolate mofetil, azathioprine is not as potent in rejection prophylaxis. Therefore its use has been diminishing rapidly over the past few years.

Cyclophosphamide

Cyclophosphamide has historically been used in place of azathioprine, although it is much less commonly used today. It is an alkylating agent that is biotransformed by the hepatic microsomal oxidase system to active alkylating metabolites. It inhibits DNA replication and, like azathioprine, affects rapidly dividing cells and is most effective immediately after antigen presentation. Xenotransplants have renewed interest in cyclophosphamide's ability to block B-cell proliferation (268). Cyclophosphamide has a narrower therapeutic-to-toxic ratio than azathioprine, and adverse effects include myelosuppression with leukopenia, fertility disorders, and hemorrhagic cystitis.

Mycophenolate Mofetil

Mycophenolate mofetil (MMF), developed specifically as an immunosuppressant, is a semisynthetic morpholinoethyl ester derivative of the fungal antibiotic mycophenolic acid (5). It is a noncompetitive inhibitor of the enzyme inosine monophosphate dehydrogenase, resulting in the inhibition of purine biosynthesis. MMF has markedly increased oral bioavailability compared with the parent compound mycophenolic acid, and it inhibits the proliferation of activated T and B cells and blocks antibody formation (225). It is thought to be more specific for lymphocytes, which rely primarily on *de novo* purine synthetic pathways. In experimental models, MMF prolongs the survival of skin, kidney, heart, and pancreatic islet allografts, as well as reversing ongoing rejection (183). Its role would seem to be as a substitute for azathioprine due to a decreased incidence of significant myelosuppression or hepatotoxicity. MMF is well tolerated at dosages up to 2,000 to 3,000 mg/day, with dose-related gastrointestinal (GI) disorders being its major toxicity. Initial multicenter trials comparing MMF with azathioprine in addition to cyclosporine and steroid maintenance therapy demonstrated a marked decrease in acute rejection episodes during the first year, from approximately 50% to 35% (107,262). However, patient and graft survival were not statistically different. Nevertheless, the diminished acute rejection rates translate into less clinical morbidity, and this agent has replaced azathioprine in many centers. *In vitro* MMF is a more potent inhibitor to B-cell responses than azathioprine, and it is hoped that this may have a beneficial effect on the development or severity of chronic rejection. Longer follow-up will be needed to confirm this hypothesis.

Antilymphocyte Drugs

Cyclosporine

One of the most significant advances in clinical transplantation was the isolation of cyclosporine from *Tolypocladium inflatum Gams,* a soil fungus, and the demonstration by Borel and colleagues (25) of its immunosuppressive properties, which were lymphocyte specific. Cyclosporine is a cyclic peptide that is soluble only in lipids or organic solvents. Detailed accounts of cyclosporine's proposed mechanisms of action, pharmacokinetics, results, and toxicities have been summarized (129).

Significant insight into mechanism of action was gained with the identification of immunophilins (cytosolic binding proteins). Cyclosporine binds to its specific immunophilin, cyclophilin, resulting in conformational changes and subsequent binding of calcineurin (105). Ultimately, the inhibition of calcineurin prevents the downstream gene transcription of IL-2 and other cytokines required for T-cell activation and proliferation (279). Thus cyclosporine is the prototype of a class of drugs now referred to as calcineurin inhibitors. Cyclosporine's actions are directed primarily toward T helper (CD4+) cells with less effect on other T-lymphocyte subsets, and although the blockade occurs early in the lymphocyte activation pathway, it is slightly later than corticosteroid activity, thus allowing for synergistic therapy.

Initial clinical results with cyclosporine revealed significantly improved 1-year allograft survival in cadaveric recipients compared with conventional therapy with prednisone and azathioprine (37), and this improved 1-year allograft survival has withstood the test of time. Improved results led to enthusiasm to investigate cyclosporine monotherapy without steroids, although problems similar to those discussed previously for steroid withdrawal, including increased rejection and graft loss, have been experienced (282). Therefore the agent is most commonly administered in combination with steroids and an antiproliferative agent.

Despite the marked improvements seen and broad experience gained with cyclosporine, difficulties with its use continue to be encountered. Diminished bioavailability, especially in the immediate posttransplant period, and variable patient pharmacokinetic profiles have resulted in numerous dosing strategies (129), with both 12- and 24-hour schedules widely used. Cyclosporine is metabolized by the hepatic P-450 cytochrome system, and drugs that inhibit or stimulate this enzyme system can significantly affect cyclosporine blood levels, thus making it imperative for clinicians to be informed of drug changes and their interactions (147). Primarily related to the cost of cyclosporine, drugs with more pronounced inhibition of the P-450 system, including diltiazem and ketoconazole, have been used to increase cyclosporine blood levels, thus reducing the required dosage (89). The introduction of an oral encapsulated cyclosporine has improved patient compliance (56), and a new oral cyclosporine microemulsion appears promising in addressing these concerns. Neoral is a microemulsion formulation that has been demonstrated to have more consistent absorption (increased bioavailability) and diminished pharmacokinetic variability (256).

However, the most distressing component of cyclosporine has been its toxicity, especially acute and chronic nephrotoxicity. Acute cyclosporine nephrotoxicity is mediated by pronounced vascular and, to a lesser degree, tubular alterations (239) and is manifested by oligoanuria and azotemia, clinically indistinguishable from acute rejection, and severe acute tubular necrosis in the immediate post–cadaveric transplant setting (81). Associated hyperkalemia, hyperuricemia, hypertension, hypomagnesemia, and renal tubular acidosis can also occur. A dose-dependent reduction in renal blood flow and glomerular filtration rate occur in acute cyclosporine nephrotoxicity, and although data are somewhat confusing, it appears to be mediated through an imbalance of the prostaglandin-thromboxane system rather than the renin-angiotensin system (48,141). Unfortunately, the findings of cyclosporine-induced decreased levels of vasodilating prostaglandins and elevated levels of the potent vasoconstrictor thromboxane A_2 have not resulted in the identification of specific agents effective in ameliorating cyclosporine nephrotoxicity. A number of prostaglandin analogues have been evaluated, and although some have resulted in improvement in renal function, this has not been universal. A large, multicenter, prospective, randomized, double-blind study failed to demonstrate any difference in cyclosporine toxicity in patients receiving placebo or Enisoprost (1). Similar conflicting results have been reported with the use of thromboxane synthetase inhibitors (239), and further studies will be needed to assess the potential benefit of these agents.

A number of theoretic and observed properties render calcium channel blockers ideal candidates for the treatment of cyclosporine nephrotoxicity. In addition to reducing the dosage requirement, they are effective in treating the associated hypertension. The cyclosporine-induced renal mesangial cell uptake of Ca^{2+} and resultant enhanced contractility and vasoconstriction may well be blocked by calcium antagonists, which also reverse afferent arteriolar vasoconstriction. In addition to reducing cyclosporine nephrotoxicity, verapamil administration has been associated with fewer rejection episodes, possibly related to direct immunosuppressive actions (58).

Chronic nephropathy with progressive renal deterioration was encountered in early experiences with higher doses of cyclosporine. Fortunately, fears related to high rates of graft loss have not been realized, and stable renal function has been demonstrated with long-term cyclosporine use (153). Similarly, higher incidences of lymphoproliferative disorders, including non-Hodgkin's lymphomas, appear related to excessive dosages (212). Other adverse effects of cyclosporine include hepatotoxicity, hyperglycemia, hyperlipidemia, hirsutism, gingival hyperplasia, myalgias, arthralgias, and neurotoxicity (131). Dosage reduction will often mitigate against these effects, although it must be done carefully to avoid increased risk of rejection. Cessation of cyclosporine therapy, like steroid withdrawal, has been accompanied by increased rejection and even late graft loss (244).

Tacrolimus

Tacrolimus is a fungal macrolide antibiotic isolated from *Streptomyces tsukubaensis* with very similar effects on T-cell function as cyclosporine, and it is also classified as a calcineurin inhibitor. Like cyclosporine, it binds to a cytosolic receptor protein (FKBP, a distinctly separate immunophilin class), which leads to the inhibition of a transcription activator, necessary for lymphokine (e.g., IL-2) gene expression. These events result in the inhibition of T-cell activation and proliferation (292). *In vitro,* tacrolimus is 10 to 100 times more potent than cyclosporine on a per weight basis, permitting diminished dosing. In multicenter trials, tacrolimus was found to be comparable in immunosuppressive efficacy to cyclosporine in kidney transplantation (172,222). However, the agent has a similar toxicity profile to cyclosporine. In particular, it may be just as nephrotoxic and requires careful dosage adjustments. Interestingly, histopathologic findings similar to those ascribed to cyclosporine toxicity have been seen in biopsies of tacrolimus-treated patients (231). Tacrolimus may permit a lower maintenance dosage of steroids, but it has been associated with an increased incidence of posttransplant diabetes (125). Trials of tacrolimus to reverse chronic rejection in patients initially given other agents were not successful, although (surprisingly, given the mechanism of action) it has been effective in "rescuing" ongoing rejection refractory to steroids and antilymphocytic therapy (128).

Rapamycin (Sirolimus)

Rapamycin is a macrolide antibiotic derived from *Streptomyces hygroscopicus* with potent immunosuppressive activity. It has similar molecular structure to the calcineurin inhibitors (Fig. 22.12) and binds to the same cytosolic receptor protein (FKBP) as tacrolimus. However, its mode of action appears to be distinct from the other agents (254). Although it is a potent inhibitor of lymphocyte responses to cytokines such as IL-2, IL-4, and IL-6, it has no direct effect on the synthesis of these lymphokines. The rapamycin–FKBP complex appears to block a distinct p70 kinase called mTOR (molecular target of rapamycin). The inhibition of mTOR blocks IL-2 signal transduction pathways that prevent cell-cycle progression from G_1 to S phase in T cells. In experimental animals, rapamycin prolonged the survival of skin, heart, kidney, pancreas, and small bowel allografts. It also produced synergism with cyclosporine, which suggests an initial approach to its clinical use (although it appears antagonistic with tacrolimus). In initial clinical trials, rapamycin did not cause nephrotoxicity, unlike cyclosporine and tacrolimus. It is not hepatotoxic, nor does it induce hyperglycemia. However, it can induce thrombocytopenia and causes significant hyperlipidemia in approximately 20% of patients (27). Significant increases in cholesterol and triglycerides usually require the use of both dietary control and statin drugs. Rapamycin was first used in combination with cyclosporine and steroids in doses of 2 and 5 mg, and it was compared with cyclosporine, steroids, and azathioprine in the pivotal multicenter trials. With 2 years of follow-up, there was no significant difference in patient or graft survival between the groups. However, the incidence of acute rejection at 6 months was less, 23% versus 43%, in the patients given sirolimus (130). This exciting new agent may offer effective immunosuppression without nephrotoxicity, and it is currently being evaluated in combination with other agents.

Antilymphocyte Antibodies

Polyclonal Antibodies

Polyclonal antibodies directed against human lymphoid cells were initially used in renal transplant recipients more than 30 years ago (269). Antibodies are produced by injecting (immunizing) animals such as horses, goats, sheep, or rabbits with cells from human lymphoid tissue. Immune sera from several animals is usually pooled and the gamma globulin fractions extracted. Desired antibodies are recovered, and unwanted antibodies are removed. Minnesota antilymphoblast globulin (MALG) and antithymocyte globulin (ATGAM, Upjohn Co.), both equine derived, have been most widely used in clinical transplantation, although the former is no longer available. Recently, a rabbit-derived antithymocyte antibody (thymoglobulin, Sangstat) has been introduced.

Once injected, the antibodies bind to lymphocytes, resulting in a rapid lymphopenia. Although the exact mechanism is not known, it is probably related to complement-mediated cell lysis with clearance by the reticuloendothelial system, or the antibody may mask T-cell surface antigens, thus blocking the cell's function. A prolonged immunosuppressive effect may be the result of suppressor cell inhibition of proliferation. Polyclonal antibodies have been used primarily in cadaveric renal transplantation for the prevention and treatment of rejection. In a meta analysis including thousands of patients who received antilymphocyte induction therapy, there appeared to be both short-term advantages and long-term improvements in graft survival (280). In randomized trials, the rabbit product thymoglobulin was shown to be more effective than the equine product ATGAM in reversing acute rejection (88% versus 76%) and for rejection prophylaxis during induction therapy (30).

Because of their strong immunosuppressive effects, polyclonal antibodies are limited to short courses and other immunosuppressive agents are significantly reduced during polyclonal antibody administration. Adverse effects include fever, chills, and arthralgias related to the injection of foreign proteins and possibly the release of cytokines. These effects can be minimized by pretreatment with corticosteroids and antihistamines. There is a significant "batch-to-batch" variability, and pretreatment is required before each administration. More serious adverse effects include increased susceptibility to infections (especially viral), serum sickness, and anaphylaxis.

Monoclonal Antibodies

The introduction of hybridoma technology has opened the door for the development of more highly specific antibodies directed against single elements at the molecular level (144). Mice are generally used for the production of monoclonal antibodies after immunization with human lymphocytes. Antibody-producing B cells are recovered from the spleen and fused with an immortal murine myeloma cell line. The resulting hybrid cells (hybridomas) are isolated and grown in culture. The desired clones are then chosen for the specific antibody production. Numerous monoclonal antibodies are currently being investigated for possible use in transplantation (250). These antibodies, like polyclonal antibodies, exert their effects through a variety of mechanisms. In addition to complement-mediated lysis, blockade and inactivation of cell surface molecules, and opsonization with phagocytosis, these antibodies can induce cytotoxicity and modulation of cell surface molecules on target tissues.

OKT3 (Orthoclone)

OKT3 was the first commercially available monoclonal antibody used in transplantation. It is a murine (mouse) antibody directed against the CD3 antigen complex, a component of the T-cell receptor, which exists on the surface of all T cells. The CD3 molecule plays an important role in signal transduction and subsequent T-cell proliferation and activation. After a standard 5-mg dose, OKT3 inhibits the CD3 complex with resultant lymphocyte inactivation and results in depletion of CD3-positive T cells from the circulation via opsonization. After a few days, lymphocytes reappear but are modulated with the CD3 complex internalized or shed from the cell surface. OKT3, like polyclonal antibodies, has been used to delay the initiation of cyclosporine and for prophylaxis and treatment of rejection episodes (181).

Adverse effects of OKT3 include a first-dose response that simulates a severe flulike syndrome, consisting of fever, chills, nausea, vomiting, diarrhea, myalgias, headache, general malaise, and in severe cases, aseptic meningitis and pulmonary edema. These symptoms are caused by initial activation of resting T cells by OKT3, which is a xenoantibody, and the release of cytokines such as tumor necrosis factor and interferon-γ (43). Many of these symptoms can be diminished by pretreatment with corticosteroids (219). The use of OKT3 for induction therapy has been shown to diminish early acute rejection episodes and improve long-term graft survival (111,193). A recent randomized trial using a low-dose (2.5-mg) regimen for induction, with mycophenolate mofetil and timed doses of corticosteroid pretreatment, demonstrated that a 16% rate of acute rejection and diminished side effects could be achieved (84).

Anti–Interleukin-2 Receptor Antibodies

Another selective site for monoclonal antibody targeting of the immune response is the IL-2 receptor or Tac (CD25), present on the surface of activated immune-competent T cells. Previous studies in animals demonstrated the utility of CD25 blockade for immunosuppression using murine-derived monoclonal antibodies. However, the rapid translation of this model to the clinic has come about due to the development of humanized and chimeric forms of anti–IL-2R antibody through the use of recombinant DNA technology. Both a chimeric anti-CD25 (basiliximab) and a humanized anti-CD25 (daclizumab) bind to different epitopes on the α-chain of the T-cell IL-2 receptor, preventing further signal transduction and T-cell proliferation. The chimeric form is genetically engineered to combine human heavy and light chain constant regions with murine heavy and light chain variable regimens, which contain the antibody binding sequences. The humanized form uses multiple amino acid substitutions of human for mouse sequences to produce a more "humanlike" IgG antibody. The net effect is to produce a hybrid IgG that retains the specific anti-CD25 binding characteristics with a less xenogenic backbone. In clinical trials, each agent was shown to produce excellent antirejection prophylaxis with a diminished side effect profile (309). We have recently compared basiliximab to OKT3 for induction therapy and found comparable rates of acute rejection, 16% versus 12%, p = NS, and less cytokine release with basiliximab (82). These newer drugs appear easier to use than previous anti–T cell agents, and they are becoming the preferred agents for induction therapy presuming these results will be durable over several years.

Costimulatory Blockade

As previously mentioned in the section on immune activation, a new and exciting area of investigation is the role of costimulation in immune responsiveness. Blocking the costimulatory signal 2 prevents T-cell activation from occurring. Future clinical trials are anticipated to test the efficacy and safety of this approach. Agents such as the fusion protein CTLA-4 Ig, which blocks the B7–CD28 interaction, and anti-CD154, which interrupts CD40–CD40 ligand interaction, may provide a new avenue for control of allograft rejection.

Additional Agents Under Investigation

15-Deoxyspergualin

15-Deoxyspergualin is an antitumor antibiotic extracted from *Bacillus laterosporus* that has shown immunosuppressive activity in animal models. Its mechanism of action has not been elucidated, although it appears to decrease cytotoxic T-lymphocyte proliferation and inhibit antibody production by preventing lymphocyte maturation. It also may downregulate the expression of class II antigens on immune-competent cells. In experimental animals, 15-deoxyspergualin prolonged survival and reversed rejection in skin, pancreatic islet, heart, liver, and kidney allografts (234). The drug has been used clinically in Japan as part of induction therapy in living related and cadaveric renal transplantation. Although a number of reports appeared promising, in one study the drug was not as potent as steroids in reversing acute rejection, and its precise role is currently under consideration. Side effects were significant, including leukopenia and thrombocytopenia (199).

Mizoribine

Mizoribine is an imidazole antibiotic that has been available for clinical use in Japan. Like azathioprine, it inhibits purine biosynthesis and abrogates both cell-mediated humoral immune responses. Although it may posses less immunosuppressive potency than other agents, it apparently does not cause significant myelosuppression or hepatotoxicity. In clinical trials of mismatched living related renal transplants, mizoribine was used in combination with cyclosporine and prednisone. When compared with other patients treated with cyclosporine, azathioprine, and prednisone, there was no difference in outcome (301). Data among recipients of cadaveric kidneys are not yet available. GI toxicity was reported to be related to the blood levels of the drug, which must be adjusted in patients with diminished renal function (101). It is recommended that the agent not be given to significantly oligoanuric patients, which may limit its use in cadaveric transplantation.

RECIPIENT SELECTION AND PREPARATION

The increasing demand for transplantation is a natural trend that parallels the improved results enjoyed by current recipients compared with previous generations of transplanted patients (42,68). Diminished morbidity, coupled with improved graft survival, have encouraged more and more patients to seek the transplant option. At the same time, improved results have expanded the pool of potential recipients for which transplantation can be safely performed. Absolute criteria that in the past would render a patient too old, too young, too small, too debilitated, too atherosclerotic, or diabetic have been liberalized or even eliminated by most transplant centers. The primary indication for transplantation today is the patient-driven desire to return to preillness levels of activity, well-being, self-image, employment status, and sexual performance. Although a functioning renal allograft is not a cure for renal failure, renal transplantation provides the best opportunity to achieve these goals (45,68,78). However, the proper evaluation of every potential recipient and donor is of critical importance to ensure the best clinical outcome and the best use of a limited resource.

The option of renal transplantation should be entertained by any patient with permanent renal failure, even though not every patient would be medically suitable or desire a surgical form of therapy. In addition, the unique risks and responsibilities required of an individual receiving chronic immunosuppression would not be appropriate for all patients. Nevertheless, a complete discussion of treatment options can be useful to permit patients the opportunity to participate in treatment planning.

The timing of renal transplantation may also have a significant impact on outcome. Some renal physicians advocate a mandatory period of dialysis before transplantation so that patients can "get used to" their diagnosis of ESRD. In some circumstances, this may be psychologically beneficial, especially when renal function has been waxing and waning or when the etiology of renal failure is unknown. Clearly, transplantation should not be performed as an emergency, and patients who first present in florid uremia may require acute dialysis and stabilization. However, for those with slowly progressing renal failure, many highly motivated individuals have requested that the transplant be performed before the need for chronic dialysis (86,179). These patients see elective or preemptive transplantation as less disruptive to their lives, and they can avoid or delay the additional surgery required to create vascular access. Such an approach in carefully screened and selected patients can be done successfully, especially when a living donor is available. Therefore the patient with ESRD has several options to consider in the choice and timing of renal replacement therapy (Fig. 22.13).

The ever-increasing worldwide shortage of donor organs necessitates a strategy of donor allocation that provides for the best possible outcome among a given ESRD population. The altruism of donor families, which is the engine that drives organ donation, depends on the doctrine that needy recipients will have equitable access to organs and that recipient selection will be based on sound medical criteria. Therefore the option of renal transplantation should not be entertained when the risks of the surgical procedure and attendant lifelong use of immunosuppressive drugs outweigh the benefits of a functioning kidney. Each individual must be carefully evaluated for any coexisting medical or psychosocial problem that would lead to a poor outcome if left uncorrected (300).

Primary Renal Diseases

The diagnoses listed in Table 22.3 represent the most commonly encountered causes of ESRD. This large spectrum includes both congenital and acquired renal disease, those isolated to the kidney, as well as systemic diseases with renal complications. With few exceptions, patients with any of these primary diagnoses have been successfully transplanted with either a cadaveric or living-related

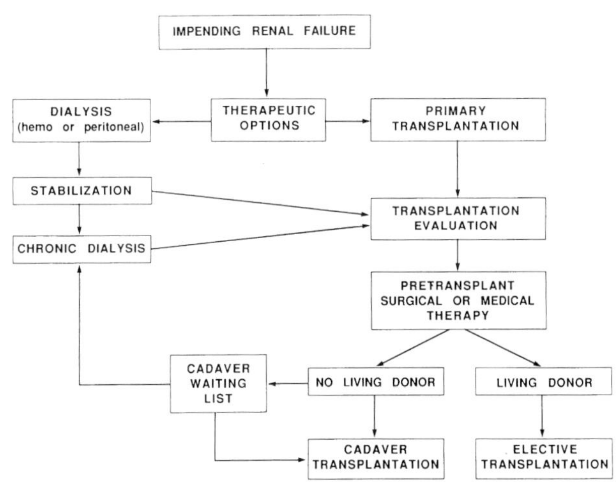

FIGURE 22.13. Patient options with end-stage renal disease.

TABLE 22.3. MOST COMMON FORMS OF CHRONIC RENAL FAILURE LEADING TO RENAL TRANSPLANTATION

Glomerular disease	Neurogenic bladder
Membranoproliferative glomerulonephritis	Congenital (meningomyelocele)
Rapidly progressive glomerulonephritis	Acquired
Anti–glomerular basement membrane disease	Hereditary diseases
Membranous nephropathy	Polycystic kidney disease
IgA nephropathy (Berger's)	Medullary cystic disease
Focal segmental glomerulosclerosis	Alport's syndrome
Diabetic nephropathy	Nephrolithiases
Arteriolar nephrosclerosis	Infection stones
Essential hypertension	Hyperoxaluria
Malignant hypertension	Cystinuria
Bilateral renovascular disease	Systemic diseases
Interstitial disease	Lupus erythematosus
Chronic pyelonephritis	Hemolytic uremic syndrome
Analgesic nephropathy	Amyloidosis
Toxic nephropathy	Scleroderma
Congenital disorders	Polyarteritis nodosa
Renal agenesis	Henoch-Schönlein purpura
Renal dysplasia	Infections
Posterior urethral valves	Tuberculosis
Vesicoureteral reflux	Schistosomiasis
Prune-belly syndrome	Surgical nephrectomy
Ureteropelvic junction obstruction	Trauma
	Renal malignancy

kidney. According to data among U.S. residents reported to the Health Care Financing Administration at the end of 1991, more than 58% of the individuals receiving dialysis were older than age 50 and 46% were female (302). In addition, nearly 30% of the transplants done that year were in individuals older than age 44 and nearly 40% were female (302).

There has also been a shift in the most commonly encountered renal failure diagnoses among those patients eventually receiving a kidney transplant. Although all forms of glomerulonephritis are still the most common etiology (26%), diabetes is now the second most commonly encountered diagnosis (21%), followed by hypertension (14%), cystic disease of the kidney (8%), other causes (8%), urologic disorders (previously obstructive uropathy) (6%), cause unknown (7%), and missing information (9%). It is not unusual for patients to seek medical attention after they are in far advanced stages of chronic renal failure and have small, shrunken kidneys. At such a late stage, it is often impossible to determine the true cause of renal failure with a biopsy, hence the unknown etiology category. Interestingly, more than 11,000 new patients entering dialysis for the first time each year enter into this category.

As might be predicted, patients with primary glomerular diseases may develop recurrent disease in the transplanted kidney. Recurrence rates as high as 50% have been reported on posttransplant biopsies in some patients with anti–glomerular basement membrane (anti-GBM) disease, IgA nephropathy, focal sclerosis, and membranoproliferative glomerulonephritis (11,21,98,171,175). It has been postulated that the continuous use of immunosuppressive drugs after transplant may significantly slow the progression of recurrent disease. This may be true because the actual rate of graft loss from recurrent disease is quite small (218). *De novo* glomerular disease, such as membranous nephropathy, has also been reported (253,272). Although the fear of recurrence should not alter the decision to proceed with transplantation, the timing of the transplant should be considered carefully. Patients with a very rapid and aggressive course to renal failure, such as those with focal segmental sclerosis, rapidly progressive glomerulonephritis, or high titers of anti-GBM antibody, should probably wait 6 to 12 months on dialysis until the disease is quiescent.

Insulin-dependent diabetic patients make up a steadily increasing percentage of the ESRD population (302). Although not a cure for diabetes, patients with uremic diabetes often experience dramatic improvement in exercise tolerance, mobility, and well-being after renal transplantation. Much of this improvement is due to a reversal of uremic neuropathy, which often compounds the peripheral neuropathy of diabetes (200). Diabetic patients with severely compromised vision often experience a similar degree of rehabilitation as sighted patients and should not be excluded from transplantation (102). Unfortunately, progressive vasculopathy continues after transplant, which leads to a higher rate of myocardial infarction, stroke, and amputation than in the nondiabetic transplant population (151). For this reason, it is important to screen diabetic patients for correctable coronary artery, carotid, and peripheral vascular lesions before transplantation. The improving results with simultaneous pancreas–kidney transplantation may provide an additional opportunity for selected patients to slow the progression of diabetic vasculopathy (135,190).

Arteriolar nephrosclerosis, often associated with malignant hypertension, is another common cause of renal failure, especially in young African American males. Although some patients have a dramatic improvement in blood pressure control with the onset of dialysis, others may require nephrectomy to prevent cardiovascular and cerebrovascular accidents. It should be noted that control of blood pressure with medication may significantly improve renal function in previously untreated patients as well (164). Such patients should not be transplanted until irreversible renal failure has been established. The successful transplantation of patients with metabolic, hereditary, and systemic diseases can usually be accomplished. However, patients should be advised that recurrences have been reported. An especially troubling group are those patients with primary oxalosis. Oxalate deposition and stone formation in the new transplant kidney has been observed frequently, with nonimmune graft loss as a result of recurrent disease (242). For this reason, there has been increasing enthusiasm for the simultaneous transplant of both a liver and a kidney to correct the metabolic abnormality. The transplantation of patients with a previous history of self-destructive behavior leading to renal failure, such as those with analgesic abuse nephropathy, intravenous drug abuse nephropathy, and similar behaviors, must be carefully screened and evaluated. A period of observation with required compliance to the medical regimen and random drug screens may be appropriate in certain situations. It may be helpful to seek the input of various family, community, social service, and religious support services (91,316).

Age

Chronologic age has often been a barrier to transplantation, with arbitrary cutoffs established for upper and lower age ranges in many centers. In the past, the ideal candidate may have been between 15 and 45 years of age, but improved transplant practice and delivery of immunosuppression has permitted the transplantation of small children less than 10 kg in weight and older patients in their sixties and seventies. The physiologic age of the patient is a more significant determinant of outcome (122,162). Older candidates should be aggressively screened for active cardiovascular disease. Posttransplant myocardial infarction, stroke, and peripheral vascular disease remain the most common causes of morbidity and mortality in these patients, whether they are transplanted or remain on dialysis (117). Therefore careful history and physical examination and the liberal use of noninvasive and invasive (angiography) studies, when indicated, best determine suitability for transplantation (62). The older-age patient with atherosclerotic disease should have realistic goals regarding rehabilitation and physical activity. Those patients with severe, noncorrectable atherosclerotic disease and little expectation for physical rehabilitation are probably best served by chronic dialysis, regardless of their chronologic age. On the other hand, patients with identifiable atherosclerotic lesions should have them repaired by surgery or angioplasty before transplant (61).

Small children less than 20 kg in weight have been considered high-risk recipients because of the technical difficulties associated with surgery and dialysis in this group (180). In addition, many small babies with progressive uremia are severely malnourished and have somatic and neurologic growth retardation. Refinements in pediatric anesthesia, intensive care practice, and surgical technique have substantially improved transplant outcome, and size alone should no longer be considered a contraindication (49,174,188). Although some have advocated the transplantation of small infants on an urgent basis, such practice is rarely, if ever, indicated. Small uremic children can be safely stabilized with peritoneal dialysis (72). During this time, they can be nutritionally repleted. The use of small nasogastric tubes for enteral hyperalimentation during continuous peritoneal dialysis has been a major advance. Because many such children have willing parental donors, the once high-risk endeavor of transplanting small children can now proceed in an orderly, elective fashion.

Urologic Evaluation

The purpose of the urinary tract evaluation is to uncover any functional or anatomic abnormalities that would predispose the recipient to posttransplant complications. An initial history should address the onset of renal failure and its presentation, in an attempt to identify such problems as recurrent urinary tract infection, pyelonephritis, stone disease, gross hematuria, and the presence of irritative or obstructive voiding symptoms or incontinence. Routine evaluation should include a urinalysis, urine culture, 24-hour urine collection for volume, creatinine clearance, protein excretion, and a voiding cystourethrogram. Some studies may be limited in patients with oligoanuria, and others may be required only for those with specific complaints. Patients with hematuria, filling defects, incontinence, significant prostatism, or a history of previous lower urinary tract pathology should undergo cystoscopy. Retrograde pyelograms may be required in certain patients. Selected urodynamic studies may be used for those with incontinence or suggestion of a neurogenic bladder. It should be noted that virtually all ESRD patients with a defunctionalized bladder (less than 200 mL per day urine output) demonstrate high voiding pressures, uninhibited contractions, and low flow rates. These findings invariably resolve when normal voided volumes are restored after transplantation. Men older than age 50 should have a prostate-specific antigen (PSA) blood test to screen for occult prostate cancer (41). Posttransplant prostate cancer was detected in 5.8% of men after kidney transplant in a previously unscreened recipient population (163). This suggests that the disease will become more prevalent in men as older-age patients are referred for transplant.

The increase in the number of men older than age 55 who elect the option of transplantation includes many with symptoms of prostatism. Those who produce more than 1 L per day of urine should undergo standard evaluation, and if significantly obstructed, undergo transurethral (electroresection or laser-assisted) prostatectomy. However, patients who produce small urine volumes are difficult to evaluate and have a propensity to develop bladder neck contractures and strictures after a resection (23). Such patients should await definitive management until urine volumes return to normal after transplantation. The role of pharmacotherapy for prostatic obstruction is currently evolving. Patients who develop posttransplant retention can be successfully managed by intermittent clean catheterization until definitive therapy is instituted. Patients with urethral stricture disease should be treated by direct-vision internal urethrotomy. More complete reconstructions should be completely healed before transplant. If stricture patients produce small urine volumes, daily self-catheterization of the urethra may be required to prevent recurrent stricture disease.

The adequacy of the bladder to both store and empty can usually be elicited by history and voiding cystourethrogram, although an occasional patient may need a more detailed urodynamic assessment. If unresolved, bladder filling, emptying, and continence can be reliably tested before transplant by the placement of a small percutaneous suprapubic tube and graduated saline irrigation (143). Patients with large flaccid bladders (some diabetics) that empty poorly can be managed after transplant using intermittent catheterization if their continence mechanism is intact (76). Most small defunctionalized bladders (even those less than 50 mL) will dilate nicely after transplantation, even when anuria has been present for many years (255). However, a few patients may have contracted noncompliant and fibrosed bladders most often secondary to tuberculosis, radiation, schistosomiasis, or severe interstitial cystitis. The bladders in such patients, as well as those with total incontinence or high-pressure neurogenic bladders, are not suitable for transplantation and will require the use of intestinal segments (191,291).

If the patient has a noncompliant, high-pressure, small-capacity bladder with an intact continence mechanism, bladder augmentation with a segment of large or small bowel can be performed. If no satisfactory urethral continence mechanism remains, an abdominal reservoir with a continent stoma (a Kock pouch or variation thereof) may be considered. For many, the standard ileal loop conduit may be the procedure of choice (110). The implantation of an artificial urinary sphincter for incontinent patients can be safely performed in selected patients (201). Reconstructive bowel surgery should be performed at least 4 to 6 weeks before transplantation to permit complete healing.

PRELIMINARY SURGERY

The use of continuous chemical immunosuppression after transplant increases the risk of complications for elective or emergency surgical procedures. For example, wound healing is impaired, sutured anastomoses have a greater tendency to leak, and wound hematomas are more frequently encountered. Otherwise, minor postoperative complications such as pulmonary problems or urinary tract infections may become more difficult to resolve in the immunosuppressed patient. For this reason, it is preferable to perform any necessary elective surgery before transplantation. This includes more common procedures such as hernia repair, hemorrhoids, cosmetic surgery, skin biopsies, extensive dental work, and orthopedic procedures. The following major surgical procedures may also be required to prepare a recipient for transplantation and should be completed and healed before the introduction of continuous immunosuppression.

Nephrectomy

Routine bilateral native nephrectomies are no longer considered a prerequisite for transplantation. The intended indication, removal of the stimulus that triggered immune-mediated renal injury, has been superseded by improved immunosuppression. Another common indication, hypertension, has been made more manageable by the introduction of new classes of antihypertensive agents such as α- and β-adrenergic blockers, vasodilators, calcium channel blockers, and converting enzyme inhibitors. For dialysis-dependent patients, the retention of native kidneys has distinct advantages. They contribute to red cell production and calcium homeostasis and provide an additional source of fluid and potassium loss. A number of specific indications remain for pretransplant nephrectomy, which is required in approximately 10% to 15% of patients. These indications include recurrent bacterial pyelonephritis, infected renal cysts, active stone passage, high-grade vesicoureteral reflux with residual urine, hypertension refractory to oral agents, renal tumors, and patients with severe proteinuria causing malnutrition and edema. On occasion, patients may have massive polycystic kidneys that cause abdominal symptoms, gross hematuria, or cyst infection, or become so large that they preclude placement of the graft in the iliac fossa, and must be removed. In patients with reflux, tuberculosis, hydronephrosis, or other ureteral pathology, a nephroureterectomy may be required.

Splenectomy

Surgical removal of the spleen for the purpose of augmenting immunosuppression was once thought to be an integral component of pretransplant preparation, especially for those recipients undergoing retransplantation. Earlier reports of improved graft survival were no doubt the result of a greater tolerance for azathioprine in splenectomized patients (90). Leukopenia, which often limited the use of antiproliferative agents such as azathioprine in patients with intact spleens, is now less common in cyclosporine-treated patients. In addition, splenectomized patients are known to have a greater long-term risk of sepsis, which has further diminished the enthusiasm for this procedure (3). The rare patient may benefit from splenectomy if pancytopenia secondary to massive hypersplenism is present. More recently, recipients of ABO-mismatched kidneys have been salvaged by the combination of splenectomy, plasmapheresis, and antilymphocyte preparations (4). The spleen is apparently an essential site for the production of anti-ABO isohemagglutinins.

Parathyroidectomy

Most ESRD patients suffer from secondary hyperparathyroidism, which can be managed with oral phosphorus binders and is readily reversible with a kidney transplant. However, a few develop tertiary hyperparathyroidism often accompanied by peptic ulcer disease, metastatic calcification, pancreatitis, itching, and severe bone mineral reabsorption. Many of these patients have serum calcium levels at the upper limit of normal, but radioimmunoassay parathormone levels are elevated 10 to 100 times. These patients should undergo subtotal parathyroidectomy before transplantation.

GASTROINTESTINAL DISEASE

Transplant recipients with active peptic ulcer disease are at high risk for bleeding or perforation in the early posttransplant period when doses of corticosteroids are highest (277). Therefore patients with active disease, recurrent ulcers, and a history of significant bleeding requiring transfusion should have an acid-reducing procedure before transplant. The selective vagotomy has become the preferred procedure. It is prudent to document complete healing by endoscopy before the introduction of immunosuppression.

The mortality rate associated with acute cholecystitis in transplant recipients has been reported to be up to 30%. Therefore patients with active gallbladder disease, as well as those with asymptomatic cholelithiasis, should undergo cholecystectomy before transplant (157). Laparoscopic techniques have revolutionized the management of this disease, permitting a more rapid recovery time (8). The laparoscopic approach has also been used successfully in ESRD patients who are treated with peritoneal dialysis.

The presence of colon diverticula in patients older than age 45 is of concern. Those patients with a well-documented history of diverticulitis should have a prophylactic colectomy (usually on the left side) if they are to be immunosuppressed. The mortality rate of posttransplant colon perforation has been reported to be as high as 50% (46,202). Patients with scattered diverticula and no history of bowel symptoms need to be appraised of the possibility of perforation and its consequences. Although prophylactic colectomy in these patients seems hard to justify, the decision to proceed with transplantation should not be taken lightly. If possible, these patients should have the renal allograft placed on the right side.

GENERAL MEDICAL EVALUATION

It is imperative that each potential recipient undergo a complete evaluation before transplantation by the team responsible for the patient's surgery and immunosuppression (Table 22.4). The majority of this evaluation can be done as an outpatient; in a few specific instances, some tests may require hospitalization to complete. The main purpose of this evaluation is to uncover any preexisting medical or psychosocial conditions that could lead to increased posttransplant morbidity or mortality. Any such condition, if identified, should be corrected before transplant surgery and the administration of immunosuppressive therapy. The absolute list of studies performed may vary from center to center based on different practice philosophies and the distribution of various groups of ESRD patients (230). Whatever the circumstance, it is incumbent on all transplant practitioners to ensure that patients are thoroughly prepared and can therefore maximize their opportunity for a successful outcome (121).

History

The initial history should address the onset of renal failure and its presentation. Hypertension, proteinuria, edema, fever, or weight gain may have resolved or may remain active. The cause of the disease and any available biopsy material should be reviewed. Associated problems, such as recurrent urinary tract infections, pyelonephritis, stone disease, or gross hematuria, should be explored. If a patient still produces urine, voiding patterns should be ascertained in an effort to diagnose bladder outlet obstruction. Symptoms related to vascular disease should be elicited, specifically looking for coronary or carotid artery disease and peripheral vascular disease. A careful GI history is important to uncover gallbladder, pancreatic, liver, or peptic ulcer disease symptoms. The family history may uncover a pattern of cancer, bleeding disorders, or inherited renal disease. Previous use of immunosuppressive drugs and any complications should be noted. The quantity and time of administration of blood products should be recorded.

Physical Examination

The initial physical examination may reflect patient compliance with dialysis and with medical therapy. Fluid overload and edema may represent intentional noncompliance. The eyes may reveal lipid abnormalities or cataracts, and the fundi can demonstrate the degree of diabetic retinopathy or arterial pathology. The cardiac examination may reveal new murmurs that have an infectious origin. All major blood vessels from the carotids to the dorsal pedis should be palpated. Diminished pulses or bruits should be evaluated further. Sources of occult infection such as otitis, dental abscesses, genital or perirectal abscesses, and the lower extremities of diabetics should be carefully inspected. The presence of lymphadenopathy in the inguinal, cervical, and axillary regions should be identified. A pelvic examination in females should include a Papanicolaou smear if not

TABLE 22.4. PRETRANSPLANT EVALUATION FOR POTENTIAL RECIPIENTS

General studies
- History and physical examination
- Pelvic examination, Pap smear
- Stool for occult blood
- Chest radiograph, electrocardiogram

Blood chemistry
- Electrolytes, blood urea nitrogen, creatinine, Ca, PO_4, alkaline phosphatase, parathyroid hormone
- Bilirubin, ALT/AST, LDH
- Amylase, uric acid
- Cholesterol, triglycerides

Hematologic studies
- Complete blood count and differential
- Platelets, prothrombin time, partial thromboplastin time
- Direct Coombs' test
- Cold agglutinins

Serology
- Cytomegalovirus, Epstein-Barr virus, herpes simplex virus, Venereal Disease Research Laboratory test
- Human immunodeficiency virus
- Hepatitis A, B, C

Urologic studies
- Urinalysis
- 24-Hour urine for creatinine clearance, protein
- Voiding cystourethrogram

Radiologic studies
- Ultrasonography of kidneys, liver
- Radiograph of mandible, sinuses

Cultures
- Urine, blood, nasal

Selected studies
- Pulmonary function tests
- Arterial blood gases
- Mammogram (age older than 40)
- Barium enema/colonoscopy (age older than 50)
- Upper GI endoscopy
- Cystoscopy
- Urodynamic studies
- Abdominal computed tomography
- Vascular Doppler studies
- Stress thallium/coronary angiography
- Echocardiogram

Immunologic studies
- Serum immunoglobulins
- Serum complement
- T-cell subsets
- Panel mix lymphocyte culture (MLC)
- Spontaneous blastogenesis
- Skin testing, purified protein derivative, mumps, *Candida*, histoplasmosis

Tissue typing
- ABO and Rh
- HLA-A, HLA-B, HLA-DR
- Anti-HLA cytotoxic antibody screen
- Donor-specific MLC

GI, gastrointestinal; LDH, lactate dehydrogenase.

previously done, and the rectal examination should screen for occult blood.

Laboratory Tests

Blood chemistry and serology studies are important to uncover any abnormalities or exposure to infectious agents that could complicate the transplant procedure or subsequent immunosuppressive therapy. The goal should be to normalize metabolic balance and nutrition for each potential recipient. All potential recipients should be tested for antibody to the HIV virus using confidentiality procedures and Western blot confirmation as appropriate (136). Prior or current exposure to cytomegalovirus (CMV), Epstein-Barr virus, herpes simplex virus, and hepatitis A, B, or C virus should be ascertained. Patients with positive blood or urine cultures should be treated after the source of the infection is identified. Cultures should be repeated after treatment to ensure complete response. Patients with an autoimmune etiology for kidney failure such as those with systemic lupus erythematosus, anti-GBM disease, or rapidly progressive glomerulonephritis should be screened for low complement levels, high titers of anti-GBM antibody, or circulating immune complexes. If any are present, these patients should wait 6 to 12 months on dialysis before proceeding with transplantation, to diminish the risks of recurrent disease.

Radiographic Studies

In addition to a chest radiograph, the native kidneys should be examined by ultrasound to rule out stones, tumors, acquired cystic disease, hydronephrosis, and so on. Ultrasound of the gallbladder and pancreas is necessary to screen for stones or pancreatic disease. Patients with a history of peptic ulcer disease or current symptoms should have an upper GI series or endoscopy. Patients older than 50 who may harbor diverticula or polyps or those with occult blood in the stool should have a barium enema or colonoscopy. Plain films of the sinuses, mandible, and teeth can uncover small microabscesses.

Selected Studies

Patients with extensive smoking history are instructed to stop before transplantation. Such patients, as well as those with a history of frequent pulmonary infections, should have pulmonary function tests and blood gases. Reversible bronchospasm should be corrected medically if identified. Coronary artery disease is a significant cause of morbidity and mortality after transplant, especially in older-age patients and diabetics (75,151). Patients older than 50 with any cardiac symptoms should initially be screened with a treadmill or exercise-induced stress thallium scan (7). However, these tests are often inconclusive in diabetics and patients who fail to produce a maximal-effort heart rate (116,168). Therefore, in sedentary patients and diabetic patients, a screening coronary angiogram is strongly recommended (158,165). Potential recipients with critical coronary artery lesions should have them repaired either by angioplasty or bypass surgery before transplantation (166). Doppler studies are useful to screen for carotid and peripheral vascular lesions, especially in symptomatic patients or those with audible bruits.

LIVE DONOR EVALUATION AND PROCUREMENT

Donor Evaluation

Healthy, willing, and highly motivated living relatives of the recipient such as siblings, parents, and children make up approximately 20% of the kidneys transplanted. More distant relatives such as aunts, uncles, grandparents, or cousins may also be suitable donors in certain circumstances. A second source of live donor kidneys comes from non–biologically related individuals. A healthy spouse is the most likely representative of this group, but unusually motivated "friends" of the recipient have been used in highly selective circumstances. The use of a living-related donor (LRD) in human renal transplantation has created a unique ethical dilemma for those involved with the daily care of transplant patients. In no other area in medicine is an otherwise healthy individual asked to subject himself or herself to the potential morbidity or mortality of major surgery for no apparent physical benefit. There are two basic reasons why LRD transplants are done, and each presents a variable degree of significance for a given donor recipient pair. First, LRD kidneys work better and last longer (42). This fact has been continuously observed using virtually all combinations of nonspecific chemical immunosuppression during the past 30 years. Second, there is a global shortage of cadaver kidneys (67,266). Therefore LRD transplantation will expedite the process for some recipients and may permit transplantation to be done in some patients who have been unable to secure a crossmatch-negative cadaver kidney while waiting for an extended period. These benefits, solely to the recipient, must be balanced against the potential short- and long-term harm to the donor. If more than one donor is available to a particular recipient, donors are selected based on their degree of histocompatibility, assuming that medical and psychosocial parameters are equal. Table 22.5 lists, in descending order, the degree of tissue similarity among potential donors and suggests the order of preference for a specific recipient.

Despite compelling arguments for the use of living donors, such procedures should not be done if significant morbidity or mortality were to be experienced by the donor. The concept of self-sacrifice and organ donation has been extensively examined by the medical, ethical, and legal professions. Postdonation analyses have consistently found that the donor experience was an overwhelmingly positive one, although sometimes tempered by recipient outcome (126,249). Clearly, renal donation is not an innocuous procedure; all donors experience some degree of anxiety, physical pain, and disruption of their employment schedule, schooling, and home life. In addition, a degree of pressure and coercion can be present among family members that is not readily apparent to health care professionals. For this reason, each donor must be given the opportunity to give his or her independent, informed consent to this decision. We have found that it is very important to counsel the spouse of the potential donor and to permit his or her input into the process as well. It is also helpful to allow the potential donor to determine the pace of the evaluation. Some may truly be undecided and may require more time to evaluate their commitment or desire to opt out of the process. These complex social interactions make it difficult to consider minors younger than age 18 as potential donors in all but the most unusual circumstances.

What then is the potential risk to the renal donor? Although the number of donor deaths worldwide is quite low, they have occurred. It has been reported that the 5-year life expectancy of a unilaterally nephrectomized 35-year-old healthy male donor is 99.1%, as compared with 99.3% for a matched control with two kidneys (177). Another estimate is that the mortality rate for donor nephrectomy is less than 0.1% (150). The long-term risk by actuarial methods has been calculated to equal that of commuting in a car 16 miles each working day. Fortunately, major postoperative complications such as life-threatening cardiopulmonary events or infections are rare, but minor complications such as atelectasis and urinary tract infections are reported to occur in 10% to 20% of cases (314). A flurry of concern has been generated from the findings of Brenner and colleagues (31) that rats who underwent renal ablation were subject to

TABLE 22.5. DONOR SELECTION BY IMMUNOLOGIC SIMILARITY

Monozygotic twins
HLA-identical siblings
Haploidentical siblings, parents, children, relatives
Less than haploidentical siblings, parents, children, relatives
Distant relatives
Unrelated living donors (e.g., spouse)
Cadaveric donors

hyperfiltration in the remnant kidney. This process led to glomerular sclerosis and deterioration of renal function, which was related to protein intake and time. However, several studies of renal donors with more than 20 years of follow-up failed to identify this problem in humans (238,308). Progressive renal deterioration is not observed, and the incidence of hypertension was consistent with that of the population at large. Some uninephrectomized donors did have an increased urinary protein excretion, but the implications of this are presently unknown. In an interesting comparative report, adult kidney donors followed for more than 20 years were compared with their siblings who did not donate for other than medical reasons (187). Both groups had similar renal function at the time of kidney donation. There was no significant difference in serum creatinine, creatinine clearance, blood urine nitrogen, blood pressure, or proteinuria between the kidney donors or their siblings with two kidneys. Proper informed consent and risk appraisal should continue to be the cornerstone of live donor evaluation.

The use of kidneys from living unrelated individuals, primarily a spouse, has increased in recent years. The enthusiasm for using living unrelated donors comes from three general observations. First, the continued increase in the number of waiting potential recipients and a stagnant supply of suitable cadaver organs continues to drive efforts to expand the organ donor pool (152,266). Second, the bond between two individuals, such as husband and wife, is arguably as firm as that between blood relations. The same satisfaction in helping a loved one that is attributed to living-related donation can be conveyed by spousal donation. Third, as the results of transplantation continue to improve, the expectations for success with living unrelated donors has never been better. In fact, 1-year patient and graft survival in excess of 90% has been reported using living unrelated donors (287,318). The elimination of warm ischemic injury and preservation injury to the live donor kidney, similar to that enjoyed with the LRD kidney, improves transplant outcome. One underlying concern and criticism of living unrelated transplantation relates to the possibility of commercialization and coercion of the donor. Precisely these considerations have made the sale and trafficking of human organs and tissues illegal in the United States (public law 98-507) and have been decried by virtually every transplantation organization (39,52). The decision to use living unrelated donors is not a trivial one and should be carefully individualized by any transplant unit considering this approach (317).

The purpose of the donor evaluation is to uncover any preexisting renal disease or predilection for renal disease in the potential donor. In addition, patients are screened for risk factors that would preclude major surgery and general anesthesia. Certain conditions may be identified that will not only lead to exclusion of the donor, but may require medical or surgical therapy for the donor's benefit. Therefore, before evaluation, every potential donor must be informed as to the nature of these studies and how the information will be used. It is important to maintain a strict doctor/patient relationship with donors and to accede to their requests for confidentiality. Table 22.6 lists the most commonly encountered problems that lead to exclusion of a potential donor.

TABLE 22.6. EXCLUSION CRITERIA FOR LIVING DONORS

Age younger than 18 and older than 65 years
Hypertension, >140/90 mm Hg, long-standing use of medications
Diabetes, abnormal GTT, HbA_{1c}, islet cell antibody
Proteinuria, >250 mg per 244 hr
Stones
GFR <80 mL/min
Significant renal abnormalities, horseshoe, fused ectopia, etc., resulting in a solitary normal kidney
Obesity >30% ideal body weight
Psychosocial problems

GFR, glomerular filtration rate; GTT, glucose tolerance test.

History and Physical Examination

Potential donors should be adults (age 18 or older) who are competent to give their own informed consent for renal donation. It is unusual that potential donors older than 65 would be suitable candidates (12). Donors should not have unexplained fevers, urinary tract infections, pyelonephritis, hematuria, or stone disease. Any history of urologic surgery should be documented. In general, donors with hypertension, diabetes, cerebrovascular disease, or systemic illnesses involving the kidneys are excluded. Daily medications, nonprescription drug use, and allergies should be noted. The sexual history of the donor is recorded. Donors should be reassured that donation will not alter present sexual performance (34).

Laboratory Tests

Screening chemistry and hematologic studies should be consistent with a normal physiologic state. Abnormalities such as elevated liver transaminases or prolonged coagulation profiles should be further evaluated. Serologic studies and cultures are necessary to identify present or past exposure to transmissible diseases. Donors with a previously unknown history of exposure to venereal disease should be completely treated before consideration for renal donation. Potential donors who are infected with hepatitis B or C virus or HIV should not donate organs or tissues (64,240). However, some have advocated the use of hepatitis C–positive donor organs in recipients with prior hepatitis C infection. Donors with previous exposure to CMV may place recipients at increased risk for primary CMV disease, which will require appropriate prophylaxis.

Renal function studies are essential and should be performed in triplicate. Although no absolute criteria have been established, renal donors should have a creatinine clearance in excess of 80 mL per minute. It is not uncommon to find donors with a serum creatinine less than the laboratory-suggested 1.5 mg/dL who have a creatinine clearance under 80 mL per minute. Such donors, often thin, middle-aged women, may require an inulin clearance or radionuclide determination of the glomerular filtration rate for confirmation. The 24-hour urinary protein excretion should be less than 250 mg in adults. Patients with crystalluria on urine analysis require metabolic stone evaluation.

Radiographic Studies

The final piece to the donor evaluation confirms the anatomic integrity of the donor kidneys. An excretory urogram is performed initially to document two functioning renal units of generally normal size, shape, and position. Abnormalities, such as a solitary kidney, severe atrophy or scarring, stones, obstruction, horseshoe kidney, or tumors would exclude renal donation. If the urogram is normal, an angiogram is done to identify the abdominal aorta; determine number, position, and patency of renal vessels; and further delineate the renal parenchyma. This can be done by either standard catheter angiography or the somewhat less invasive digital subtraction techniques (79,265). Spiral computed tomography (CT) imaging is currently under evaluation as a noninvasive method to identify renal vascular and parenchymal anatomy.

DONOR NEPHRECTOMY TECHNIQUE

If one kidney has a minor abnormality on radiographic studies, such as a renal scar, a single small simple cyst, or an abnormal calyx, it is considered prudent to remove that renal unit, leaving the donor with the more anatomically normal one. If both renal units are normal, the left kidney is preferred by most transplant surgeons because the left renal vein is longer, making recipient transplantation easier to perform. Multiple renal arteries exist in approximately 20% of potential donors, and removal of the kidney with a single renal artery is preferred. If a kidney with two renal arteries is necessary for transplantation, *ex vivo* bench surgery techniques can be used to facilitate transplantation in the recipient. However, the use of kidneys with more than two renal arteries of substantial size is generally not recommended. Kidneys with duplicated collecting systems have been used successfully for live donor transplantation, if care is taken to remove the ureters in a common sheath with the blood supply protected.

The surgical technique for live donor nephrectomy should in principle use the minimum surgical insult required to remove an anatomically intact and physiologically maintained kidney for transplantation. An extraperitoneal and extrapleural flank incision is suitable in most cases. The nephrectomy can be done in most cases without removing a rib. A Turner-Warwick supracostal twelfth rib incision is preferred (299). A transperitoneal nephrectomy may occasionally be used if multiple renal vessels are involved. However, this incision has been associated with an increased rate of morbidity, such as bowel obstruction and splenic injury.

During the last few years, several centers have begun to remove donor kidneys using laparoscopic methods. The left kidney is usually removed by placement of intraperitoneal ports, and a second counterincision is made for the surgeon to place a hand in the abdomen to remove the intact kidney. Those who perform the procedure state that it causes less pain and provides for a more rapid recovery (87). The kidneys removed by laparoscopy are anatomically and physiologically inferior to those removed by open nephrectomy, but appear to function normally after a short period (85). The procedure requires a dedicated team of skilled laparoscopists so as to avoid technical complications such as ureteral necrosis (192). Randomized comparative trials are lacking to compare the open and the laparoscopic approach, but the procedure is becoming more popular, especially in centers that have invested in laparoscopic equipment.

The goal of donor nephrectomy is to remove the kidney without sustaining any ischemic injury. A well-preserved kidney, when transplanted into the recipient, should function promptly and avoid posttransplant dialysis requirements.

Four things can be done by the transplant surgeon to minimize the ischemic damage to the live donor kidney. First, ischemic injury can be minimized by decreasing the energy-requiring oxidative metabolism of the kidney. Glomerular filtration is passive, driven by cardiac output, but the tubular reabsorption of the kidney requires energy expenditure, primarily by the mitochondria. Flooding the kidney with salt and water diminishes tubular reabsorption. This is done with intensive preoperative hydration of the donor, usually 150 to 200 mL per hour of intravenous fluid, which will result in a urine specific gravity less than 10.010. During the surgical procedure, diuresis can also be maintained with use of a hyperosmolar agent such as mannitol.

Second, renal ischemia can be minimized by avoiding vasospasm of the renal circulation. This is most often caused by traction on the kidney during the surgical dissection. If the kidney becomes soft or dusky in color during dissection, it is best to stop and allow the spasm to break. The application of local vasodilator drugs such as papaverine or lidocaine may be useful. Dissection can commence when the kidney becomes full and pink in color. The same problem can occur if the renal artery is surrounded with a vessel loop that is secured by a weighted metal clamp.

Third, warm ischemic injury to the kidney can be minimized by cooling the kidney after it is removed from the donor. Iced saline or perfusate at 40°C will retard mitochondrial oxidative metabolism.

Fourth, the kidney when removed is subject to cellular swelling due to the paralysis of the oxygen-dependent Na^+-K^+-ATPase pump. By perfusing the *ex vivo* kidney with a hyperosmolar solution that mimics the intracellular ionic concentrations of sodium and potassium, cellular swelling can be minimized.

It is also important during surgical nephrectomy to remove the kidney when it is in an active state of diuresis. Therefore the previously mentioned techniques to avoid spasm should be used when the kidney is removed.

The integrity of the blood supply to the ureter is essential to avoid ureteral necrosis and fistula formation in the recipient. This is done by removing a wide area of periureteral tissue with the specimen. It is generally satisfactory to transect the ureter at the pelvic brim, which will provide adequate length for transplantation.

A small rent in the peritoneum should be oversewn with absorbable suture. After the kidney is removed, the incision should be filled with water or saline and the lungs inflated to check for a rent in the pleura. A small tear can usually be oversewn around a 16-Fr Red Robinson catheter. The wound can then be closed in layers around the catheter. When closure is complete, the lungs should be expanded by the anesthesiologist, and the air in the chest can be evacuated by placing the end of the catheter under a water seal. Air bubbles will cease when the lung is fully expanded. If there is a very large hole in the pleura or the pneumothorax is not diagnosed until the patient is in the recovery room, a chest tube will have to be placed temporarily for expansion of the lung. A Foley catheter, which is placed during the induction of anesthesia, can be removed on the first postoperative day as the patient is encouraged to ambulate. We have found that the use of a patient-controlled analgesic delivery system is useful for some patients to control pain. The use of an epidural catheter for postoperative pain control and the use of intravenous ketorolac for up to 48 hours are also helpful, and decrease narcotic use (which predisposes to ileus). Donors should remain on nothing-by-mouth status for 1 to 2 days to avoid an ileus. They can generally be discharged 2 to 3 days after surgery and can return to full activity in about 3 to 4 weeks.

CADAVER DONOR EVALUATION AND PROCUREMENT

Most renal transplant recipients will not have a willing family donor, and therefore they must rely on an organ from a cadaver. A well-functioning cadaveric kidney will provide the same opportunity for rehabilitation from ESRD as a live donor organ. However, a number of complicating factors in cadaveric transplantation arise from the fact that organ availability is both a limited and random event, which makes the surgical procedure nonelective in nature. Cadaver kidneys are preferably transplanted within 24 hours of recovery, but they can produce acceptable results after up to 48 to 60 hours of preservation. During this period, a previously evaluated and waiting recipient is identified and prepared for surgery. This may include dialysis or metabolic adjustments for the recipient, as well as transport of the recipient or the kidney across the country. As mandated by UNOS with some local variance, the kidney is usually placed by using a weighted system encompassing ABO blood type, tissue type, length of wait, and possibly other medical or local criteria (304).

Donor Evaluation and Maintenance

Potential renal donors generally come from individuals who have suffered irreversible head trauma, cerebrovascular accident, or anoxic brain injury (57). They should preferably be between 5 and 60 years of age. There should be no history of systemic diseases that involve the kidneys, such as nephrolithiasis, hypertension (longstanding with drug therapy), diabetes mellitus, or autoimmune disease. Patients with a history of malignant tumors other than localized brain or nonmelanoma skin cancer should not be used as organ donors. There should be no history of transmissible infectious disease or active untreated infection. A history of longstanding use of analgesics may indicate chronic renal injury. It is best not to consider individuals with high-risk behavior for HIV disease such as documented intravenous drug users, active homosexuals, hemophiliacs requiring blood transfusions, or those with known infected sexual partners (64,241). One of the great uncertainties associated with cadaver renal transplantation relates directly to the adequacy of the medical history of the cadaver donor. Many posttransplant recipient problems can be minimized or even avoided by an accurate donor history. This can be a special problem when the mortal injury occurs far from the patient's home. It is always important to obtain a medical history from someone who has had close recent contact with the individual, not merely a relative or friend.

Organs for transplantation cannot be removed until the surviving family gives specific permission for this act and brain death has been declared. The act of donation is therefore completely dependent on the good will and altruism of the public at large. The use of a signed donor card on the back of a driver's license is not sufficient consent and has been of marginal value in increasing the donor supply. Interestingly, one of the greatest impediments to identifying donors and obtaining family consent has been delayed referral or nonreferral to local organ procurement agencies by hospital personnel. It is hoped that increased local and national education policies, as well as "required request" legislation, will expand the pool of potential donors through greater public awareness (221).

Donor Management

The process of organ procurement can begin only when an individual has been declared brain dead and family consent has been obtained. In most states, the diagnosis of brain death requires strict medical criteria to be met, and a signed declaration must be made by two physicians, neither of whom can be a member of the transplant team. Brain death remains a clinical diagnosis (Table 22.7), but it can be supported by other objective tests (208). To be declared brain dead the patient should be comatose, be unable to breathe without mechanical assistance, and have absent cranial nerve function and reflexes. The absence of perfusion of the brain on an isotopic cerebral blood flow scan is a useful confirmatory test due to its ease of performance and reliability (252). The absence of flow is not compatible with the return of brain function. It is important to make this diagnosis after ruling out hypothermia, drug intoxication, metabolic encephalopathy, and shock as confounding diagnoses.

Once declared brain dead, the donor should be kept in a state as close to normal homeostasis as possible. Appropriate ventilatory support is required, and normothermia should be maintained. Maintenance of pulmonary care, nasogastric suction to prevent aspiration, lubrication and protection of the eyes, removal of all intravascular catheters placed without sterile technique, monitoring of vital organ function with a central venous and arterial pressure catheter, and a Foley catheter are usually required. Blood transfusion is not routinely necessary, except in cases of ongoing hemorrhage. Often, donors are volume contracted and dehydrated (the appropriate management for brain injury) and must be resuscitated with fluids. Ringer's lactate is usually sufficient. Deterioration of brain function and loss of central neurohumoral regulatory control may result in severe systemic hypertension (Cushing's reflex) due to elevated circulating catecholamines and sympathetic activity. β-Blockers can be useful to protect the myocardium when this occurs. In some donors, brain herniation may result in bradycardia, hypotension, and diminished organ perfusion. Adequate systolic blood pressure, usually more than 100 mm Hg, is recommended. The use of vasopressors such as dopamine, which maintains renal blood flow, can be helpful. Urine output in adults should be maintained at more than 1 mL/kg per hour. Frequently, donors may develop massive urine output (more than 500 mL per hour) as a result of central diabetes insipidus, due to low levels of circulating antidiuretic hormone from the destroyed hypothalamic-pituitary axis. The resulting excessive free water loss can lead to hypokalemia, hypernatremia, hypocalcemia, and hypophosphatemia. This condition can be treated with exogenous vasopressin, which can be delivered intranasally.

TABLE 22.7. DIAGNOSIS OF BRAIN DEATH

I. Clinical criteria
  a. Unresponsiveness to external stimuli (pain, sound, light, noxious, ice water calorics)
  b. Absence of spontaneous breathing
  c. No cranial nerve function
  d. Above findings present with body temperature >90°F
  e. Absence of CNS-depressant drugs

II. Clinical criteria can be supported by
  a. Isoelectric electroencephalogram
  b. Lack of cerebral perfusion by angiogram or radiographic flow scan
  c. Absence of evoked potentials

CNS, central nervous system.

The serum creatinine in the cadaver donor should be less than 2.0 mg/dL. A rising creatinine may be due to prolonged hypotension, which may cause irreversible renal ischemia. A rising serum creatinine, coupled with a markedly diminished urine output of less than 30 mL per hour before removal of the kidneys, is associated with permanent renal injury. The maintenance of the donor before surgical nephrectomy is one of the most important factors that contribute to immediate graft function after revascularization and the diminished need for posttransplant dialysis (160). Older donor kidneys, older than age 60, are especially susceptible to adverse prerecovery donor function, and every effort should be made to normalize physiologic parameters in these patients.

Donor Procurement Technique

The goals of cadaver kidney removal are to recover two anatomically intact kidneys with good physiologic function. The kidneys are removed en bloc with the midportion of the aorta and vena cava so as to preserve the origins of the renal blood vessels. Currently, most organ donors have an extra renal organ removed at the same time. If multiple organs are to be removed, the preferred sequence is the heart or lungs first, liver or pancreas second, and then the kidneys. It is important to keep the donor hemodynamically stable as long as possible during organ recovery. Most cadaver donors are given a large dose of corticosteroids to deplete circulating donor lymphocytes. Intravenous mannitol in doses of up to 1 g/kg is useful to ensure diuresis and provide some ischemic protection. A large dose of systemic heparin (10,000 to 20,000 units) is given just before organ removal. Some have advocated the use of α-blockers, calcium channel blockers, or dopamine to diminish renal vasospasm secondary to surgical manipulation.

In multiple organ recoveries, the procedure begins with a long incision from the sternum to the pubis. In kidney-only procurement, this may be modified with a xiphoid-to-pubis incision that may be widened with a cruciate extension. The right colon and duodenum are mobilized, exposing the great vessels. The aortic bifurcation is isolated and a cannula is placed for cooling. A similar cannula is placed near the bifurcation of the vena cava. The suprarenal aorta is mobilized above the celiac trunk, as well as the suprarenal vena cava. If liver or pancreas procurement is to be done, this is more easily accomplished after the abdominal organs are removed. The ureters are divided deep in the pelvis with a generous amount of periureteral tissue intact. Once the superior mesenteric and celiac arteries are ligated, the kidneys can be flushed with ice-cold preservation fluid and circulatory arrest can ensue. Iced slush can be placed around the kidneys for additional surface cooling. At this point, wide excision of the kidneys with Gerota's fascia and the great vessels can be done, with care being given to avoid any dissection in the hilum of the kidney or posterior to the great vessels without direct visualization.

The entire en bloc specimen with aorta vena cava in both kidneys is then removed from the patient and placed in a pan of ice-cold perfusate for further dissection on a back table (Fig. 22.14). A large amount of Gerota's fat and fascia should be removed, confirming the complete flushing of all renal segments. This is rarely a problem if the return perfusate from the vena cava is clear while the organs are *in situ.* The kidneys should always be separated first by dividing the aorta on its posterior surface and then anteriorly, to leave a generous cuff of right or left aortic wall with the renal arterial circulation. This will include multiple renal arteries if present. The left renal vein can be divided flush with the vena cava and the left kidney removed separately. The right renal vein should always be kept intact with the vena cava to permit renal venous extension procedures if required in the recipient.

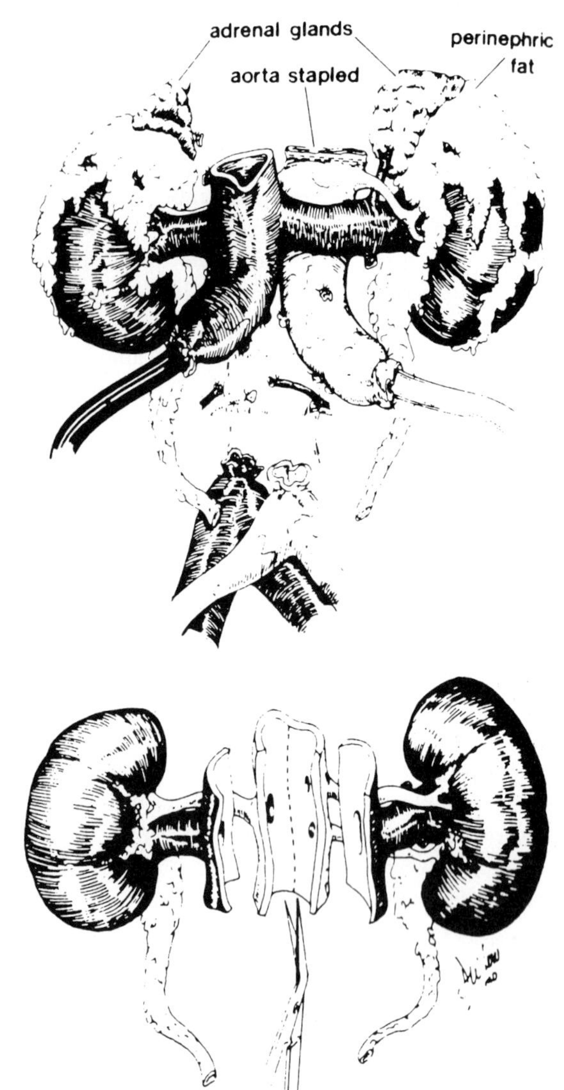

FIGURE 22.14. Technique for cadaver kidney removal. Specimen should include midaorta and vena cava with attached renal vessels. Once removed, the great vessels should be divided on their posterior surface to identify the number and location of the renal vessels. (From Barker CF, et al. Renal transplantation. In: Sabiston DC, ed. *Textbook of surgery.* Philadelphia: Saunders, 1986, with permission.)

Organ Preservation

The clinical practice of a cadaver renal transplantation requires the ability to store and preserve the kidney *ex vivo* for hours or even days. Because the acquisition of a renal donor is random, may occur at any hour, and must permit the transport of the organ over great distances, organ preservation techniques must be relatively simple, mobile, and inexpensive. In most circumstances, the process of tissue typing, crossmatching, and identification and preparation of a recipient takes at least 10 to 12 hours. In larger UNOS regions, and factoring in mandatory sharing of phenotypically identical donor–recipient pairs, this process may take up to 48 hours. In unusual circumstances, up to 60 hours of *ex vivo* time has been required. The goal of organ preservation is to provide an organ that will be protected from ischemic hypoxic damage and will function promptly in the host when revascularized.

Diminished blood flow and oxygen delivery to an organ results in ischemic injury (73). In kidney transplantation, there are two clinicopathologic consequences of ischemic injury. The first, due to a milder degree of ischemia, is acute tubular necrosis (ATN), which is reversible and results in delay of graft function after transplant. Pathologically, ATN results in sloughing and regeneration of the renal tubular epithelium with intact basement membranes. Blood flow is maintained, although glomerular filtration rate is minimal. The kidney may produce a filtrate (nonoliguric ATN) but does not remove waste products. The second form of ischemic injury is more severe and irreversible, termed *cortical necrosis.* Pathologically, necrosis of the entire renal cortex is found. Such kidneys never function (primary nonfunction), have poor blood flow characteristics, and ultimately fibrose. These pathologic findings are similar to the renal injuries suffered by patients who experience massive cardiogenic or hemorrhagic shock.

Kidneys can suffer ischemic injury at several points during organ recovery and preservation (18). *In situ* ischemia can occur in the cadaver donor during the terminal phases of brain death and organ retrieval. Hypotension is the proximate cause. Warm ischemia occurs from the time of circulatory arrest until the kidney is cooled and flushed. A human kidney can tolerate up to 20 to 30 minutes of warm ischemia, although current methods of organ procurement attempt to keep this time to zero. Beyond this time, irreversible injury ensues. Cold ischemic time refers to the period of *ex vivo* cold storage before reestablishment of the renal circulation in the recipient. A variable period of ambiothermic (room temperature) ischemia can occur during the surgical time required for anastomosis of the kidney blood vessels, although this can also be minimized by surface cooling with iced slush.

On a cellular level, ischemic injury renders the tissues hypoxic and retards oxidative, energy-requiring metabolic functions, often found in the mitochondria. One such function is the formation of high-energy phosphonucleotides such as adenosine triphosphate (ATP), required for the plasma membrane–situated Na-K and Ca pumps. Hypoxic cells lose the intermediate purine substrates required for ATP formation through degradation by xanthine oxidase. Loss of these pump functions leads to cellular swelling due to the influx of sodium and water into the cell and efflux of potassium across strong diffusion gradients. In addition, anaerobic glycolysis predominates, which produces lactic acid and hydrogen ions with resultant cellular acidosis. Acidosis is responsible for activation of lysosomal enzymes that lead to mitochondrial and cell membrane lysis. Another destructive process is the formation of superoxide anions during ischemia. These so-called oxygen free radicals can cause tissue injury during reperfusion of the kidney if they have accumulated.

Therefore solutions for organ preservation have been developed that attempt to counteract the metabolic consequences of hypoxia and anaerobic metabolism (Table 22.8). An essential ingredient in organ preservation is hypothermia. Rapid cooling at the onset of organ removal is done with iced saline slush. Perfusion and storage of the kidney at 4° to 10°C will minimize ischemic injury. Hypothermia reduces oxygen demand, slows metabolism, conserves energy in the form of adenine nucleotides, and retards catabolic enzyme activity. In addition, the ideal preservation solution would prevent acidosis, provide substrate for regenerating high-energy phosphate compounds (ATP), prevent reperfusion injury due to oxygen free radicals, and minimize cellular swelling.

TABLE 22.8. MAJOR COMPONENTS OF KIDNEY PRESERVATION SOLUTIONS

Collins Solution	UW Solution
Potassium chloride	Hydroxethyl starch
Potassium phosphate	Lactobionate
Glucose	Potassium phosphate
Sodium bicarbonate	Magnesium sulfate
Magnesium sulfate	Raffinose, glutathione
Osmolality 360 mOsm/L	Allopurinol, adenosine, insulin
	Osmolality 320 mOsm/L

The most commonly used preservation solution for kidneys was first developed by Collins more than 20 years ago. Its essential constituents mimic the intracellular rather than the extracellular fluid compartment with high K and low Na concentrations. It is made hyperosmolar with sugars to diminish the intracellular uptake of water, which causes cellular swelling. Similar preservation solutions have been made using either mannitol or sucrose as the primary osmotic agent. Each can produce adequate cold storage for up to 48 hours.

However, the advent of extrarenal organ transplantation in the 1980s required further refinements. The liver, which can metabolize glucose under preservation conditions more efficiently than the kidney, was not well maintained by the Collins solution. Therefore researchers at the University of Wisconsin (UW) developed a perfusate more suitable for the liver and pancreas, which may also provide better preservation for the kidney (226). The UW solution uses lactobionate in place of glucose as an impermeable anion to prevent cellular swelling. Raffinose and hydroxymethyl starch provide additional osmotic and colloid support for the extracellular space. The absence of glucose diminishes anaerobic glycolysis and subsequent acidosis, and adenosine provides substrate for regenerating ATP during reperfusion. Allopurinol may help reduce the formation of oxygen free radicals. The use of UW solution may extend renal preservation up to 72 hours (264).

Once cooled and perfused through the renal artery, kidneys are generally kept in a container filled with the perfusate on ice. A container with each kidney is then transported to the transplant center. This technique (so-called simple cold storage) is used by the majority of transplant centers worldwide. Some have advocated the use of machine pulsatile perfusion to preserve kidneys, which may provide for lower rates of delayed graft function with extended preservation times. The machine pulsatile perfusion method can allow the determination of perfusion pressures, resistance to flow, pH, and metabolic products, which some have suggested correlate with renal viability. Although it is more cumbersome and expensive, the machine preservation technique may be most helpful for kidneys preserved beyond 48 hours.

RENAL TRANSPLANT OPERATION

Renal transplant recipients are particularly susceptible to poor healing and infection because of the complications of uremia and the altered host responses induced by immunosuppressive therapy. These considerations demand meticulous attention to detail in performing transplantation surgery, with careful handling of tissues and strict adherence to basic operative principles of asepsis and hemostasis.

In most cases, the renal allograft is implanted into one or the other iliac fossa (197). In determining which iliac fossa to use for transplantation, one should consider both the anteroposterior relationships of the renal vessels and the anticipated method of arterial anastomosis. When end-to-side arterial anastomosis to the hypogastric artery seems likely, as in performing single-artery transplantation in young patients, it is customary to place the right kidney in the left iliac fossa, and vice versa. When end-to-end arterial anastomosis to the external or common iliac artery is expected, as in older patients or when using a Carrel aortic patch with multiple donor arteries, the right kidney will lie more comfortably in the right iliac fossa and the left kidney in the left iliac fossa. These are only relative considerations, and with proper positioning of the graft and renal vessels, either kidney may be inserted into either iliac fossa. A relative advantage of using the right iliac fossa is that the right iliac vein has a more horizontal course than the left and is more accessible for the venous anastomosis. This may assume clinical significance when transplanting a kidney with an unusually short renal vein.

In patients with a history of lower extremity thrombophlebitis, silent thrombosis of the iliac veins may have occurred and transplantation should be performed preferentially into the opposite iliac fossa. If ipsilateral transplantation is being considered, preoperative venography should be done to verify iliac venous patency. In patients with a prior failed renal transplant, the second graft is always placed in the unoperated contralateral iliac fossa.

When the recipient is anesthetized, a 20-Fr urethral catheter is inserted in the bladder. A urine specimen is sent for culture, or if the patient is anuric, the bladder is irrigated with saline and this fluid is cultured. The bladder is filled by gravity with 100 to 200 mL of 1% neomycin sulfate solution, and the catheter is clamped and connected to a closed drainage system. Shaving of the operative site is done in the operating room, and the skin is prepared with an iodine solution for 10 minutes. Before commencing the operation, a single intravenous bolus of broad-spectrum antibiotics is given.

A lower-quadrant transverse semilunar skin incision is made, extending from the midline to just above the anterior superior iliac spine (Fig. 22.15). Throughout the operation, care is taken to achieve absolute hemostasis and to minimize blood loss. The external oblique, internal oblique, and transversus abdominis muscles are divided in line with the incision. The inferior epigastric vessels are identified lateral to the rectus muscle and are then secured and divided. The rectus muscle is either retracted medially or, if exposure of the bladder is not adequate, divided at its tendinous insertion into the symphysis pubis. The round ligament in the female is ligated and divided. The spermatic cord in the male is mobilized and retracted medially to obviate postoperative hydrocele formation, which commonly occurs following high cord ligation.

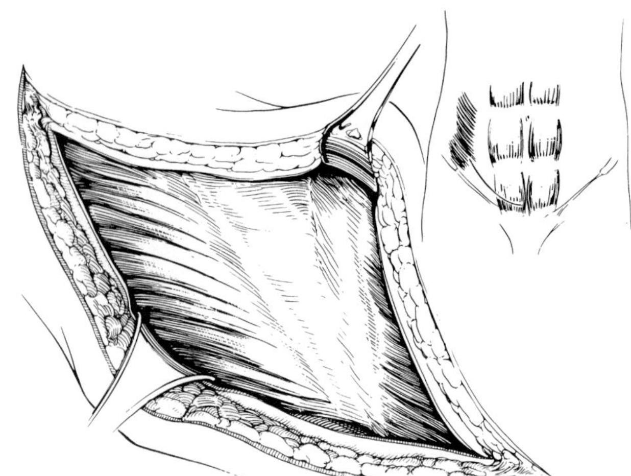

FIGURE 22.15. Lower quadrant transverse semilunar incision is used to perform renal transplantation. (From Novick AC, Streem SB, Pontes JE, et al, eds. *Stewart's operative urology.* Baltimore: Williams & Wilkins, 1989, with permission.)

Extraperitoneal exposure of the iliac fossa is obtained by reflecting the peritoneum superiorly to the common iliac artery and medially to the bladder. A self-retaining ring retractor is then inserted to maintain exposure of the operative field (Fig. 22.16). The lateral blade of the retractor is doubly padded to avoid injury to the lateral femoral cutaneous nerve. The superior retractor blade is positioned to avoid compression of the common iliac artery, which may interfere with allograft perfusion following revascularization.

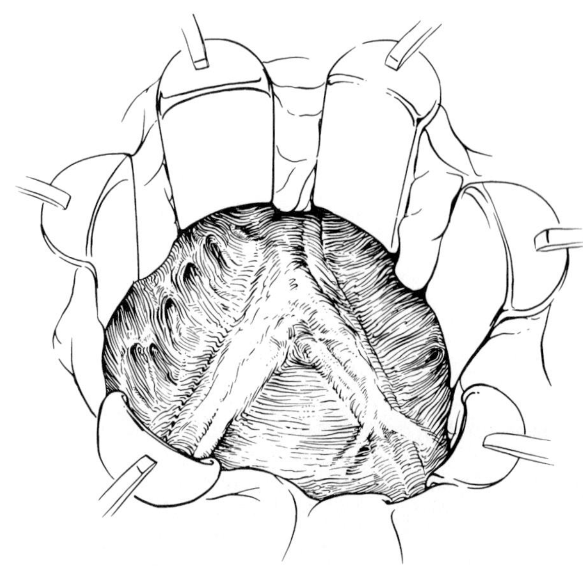

FIGURE 22.16. Extraperitoneal exposure of the iliac fossa is maintained with a self-retaining retractor. (From Novick AC, Streem SB, Pontes JE, et al, eds. *Stewart's operative urology.* Baltimore: Williams & Wilkins, 1989, with permission.)

The external iliac vein is mobilized from the internal iliac origin to the femoral junction. To avoid postoperative lymphatic complications, all overlying lymphatic tissue is ligated and divided. If the donor kidney has a short renal vein, the internal iliac vein is divided to allow elevation of the external iliac vein and thereby facilitate the venous anastomosis. End-to-end anastomosis of the renal artery to the hypogastric artery is preferred, and the latter vessel is then mobilized from its origin to the major anterior and posterior branches. Again, all overlying lymphatic vessels are ligated and divided. In such cases, it is unnecessary to mobilize the common and external iliac arteries (Fig. 22.17).

Vascular clamps are placed proximally and distally on the external iliac vein. A venotomy is performed by excising a narrow longitudinal ellipse from the anterolateral aspect of the vein. The hypogastric artery is temporarily occluded proximally, the major branches are ligated distally, and the artery is divided proximal to the ligatures. If mild atherosclerosis of the hypogastric artery is present, endarterectomy is performed to render this vessel suitable for anastomosis to the renal artery. Heparin solution is instilled into the lumen of the hypogastric artery and external iliac vein.

The kidney is then brought into the operative field and the artery and vein are examined. Any residual tissue surrounding the origin of these vessels is removed and, if the renal vein appears short, this is mobilized from the renal sinus to obtain greater length. The kidney is lowered into the incision and end-to-side anastomosis of the renal vein to the external iliac vein is performed with a continuous 5-0 vascular suture. End-to-end anastomosis of the renal artery to the hypogastric artery is performed with interrupted 6-0 sutures after aligning these vessels carefully to avoid angulation or kinking. After the arterial anastomosis is completed, all vascular clamps are removed and circulation to the kidney is restored (Fig. 22.18).

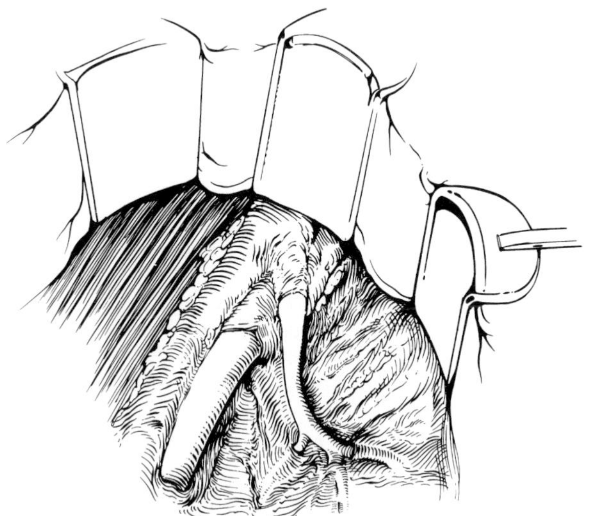

FIGURE 22.17. The external iliac vein and hypogastric artery are mobilized. (From Novick AC, Streem SB, Pontes JE, et al, eds. *Stewart's operative urology.* Baltimore: Williams & Wilkins, 1989, with permission.)

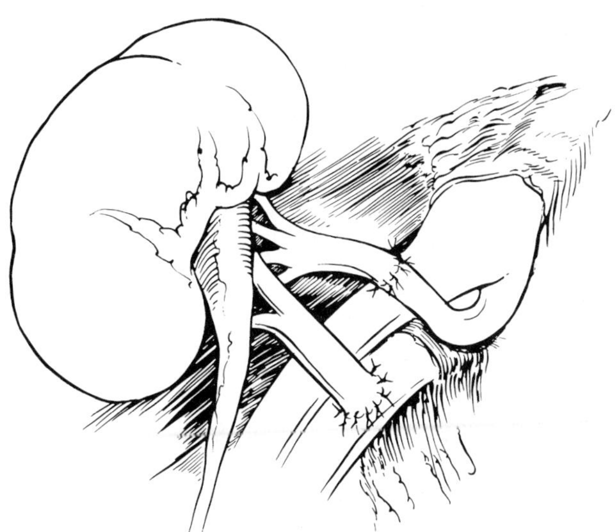

FIGURE 22.18. The renal vein is anastomosed end-to-side to the external iliac vein; the renal artery is anastomosed end-to-end to the hypogastric artery. (From Novick AC, Streem SB, Pontes JE, et al, eds. *Stewart's operative urology.* Baltimore: Williams & Wilkins, 1989, with permission.)

The indications for end-to-side arterial anastomosis to the common or external iliac artery are extensive atherosclerosis of the hypogastric artery, significant discrepancy in size between the renal and hypogastric arteries, or multiple donor renal arteries encompassed by a Carrel aortic patch. In such cases, the external iliac artery and a contiguous segment of the common iliac artery are mobilized. Vascular clamps are placed across the common iliac, hypogastric, and external iliac arteries, and an arteriotomy in the recipient vessel is performed. In general, our preference is to perform end-to-side arterial anastomosis to the common iliac artery because of its larger caliber. This may not be possible when renal arterial length is insufficient or when there is significant atherosclerosis of the common iliac artery. In such cases, arterial anastomosis is to the external iliac artery, which lies in closer proximity to the renal hilus and is less often diseased than the common iliac artery. An interrupted-suture technique with 6-0 sutures is used unless anastomosis of a Carrel aortic patch is performed, in which case a continuous 5-0 suture is used (Fig. 22.19).

After completion of the vascular anastomosis, urinary tract reconstruction is achieved by ureteroneocystostomy. This method is preferred over ureteroureterostomy or ureteropyelostomy because of a lower incidence of postoperative urinary fistulae. In performing ureteroneocystostomy, one should use the shortest length of ureter that will reach the bladder without tension because the allograft ureter receives its blood supply exclusively from branches of the renal artery. Since 1983, we have preferentially used the extravesical ureteroneocystostomy technique originally described by Lich (Fig. 22.20).

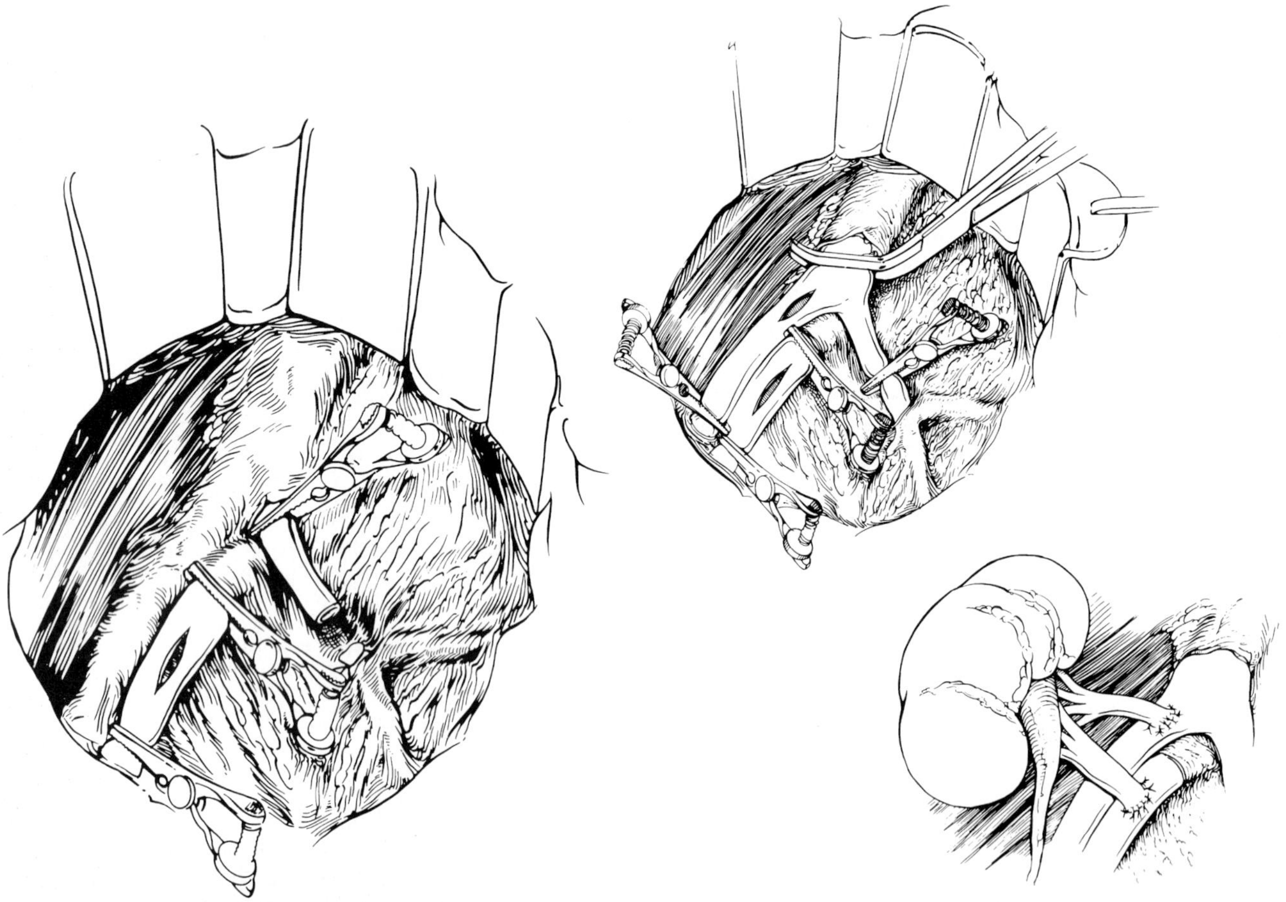

FIGURE 22.19. The renal vein is anastomosed end-to-side to the external iliac vein, and the renal artery is anastomosed end-to-side to the common iliac artery. (From Novick AC, Streem SB, Pontes JE, et al, eds. *Stewart's operative urology.* Baltimore: Williams & Wilkins, 1989, with permission.)

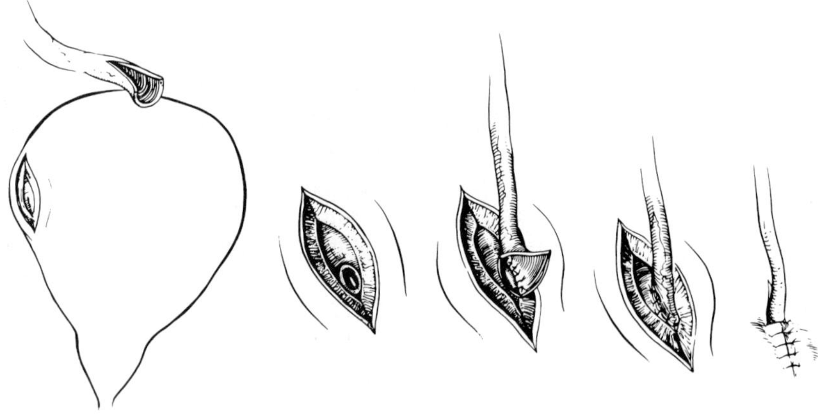

FIGURE 22.20. Extravesical ureteroneocystostomy technique. (From Novick AC, Streem SB, Pontes JE, et al, eds. *Stewart's operative urology.* Baltimore: Williams & Wilkins, 1989, with permission.)

A 3-cm incision is made on the posterolateral aspect of the bladder. The perivesical fat, adventitia, and muscle of the bladder wall are incised to expose the mucosa over the entire length of the incision. The edges of the bladder muscle are undermined by pushing the mucosa away from the muscle. The distal end of the allograft ureter is spatulated for a short distance. A small opening is made in the bladder mucosa at the distal end of the incision, and mucosa-to-mucosa anastomosis is done between the ureter and the bladder, using interrupted or continuous 4-0 chromic sutures. At the distal aspect of the suture line, one or two bites are inserted through the entire bladder wall to anchor the ureter and prevent it from pulling out of the tunnel. The bladder muscle then is reapproximated loosely over the ureter with interrupted 3-0 chromic sutures.

As an alternative to this method, a transvesical ureteroneocystostomy technique may be used. The bladder is opened through an anterior cystotomy and a stab incision is made in the posterolateral bladder wall. The donor ureter is brought through the stab incision, and a 2- to 3-cm submucosal tunnel, directed toward the bladder neck, is fashioned. The ureter is then brought through the tunnel, taking care to avoid torsion on its longitudinal axis. The ureter is spatulated and anastomosed to the bladder with interrupted 4-0 or 5-0 chromic sutures. The sutures fixing the distal aspect of the ureter to the bladder are inserted deeply into the muscularis, while the remaining sutures are placed only through the bladder mucosa. The mucosa overlying the stab incision is closed with a continuous 5-0 chromic suture. The cystostomy incision is closed in three separate layers, with the second and third layers slightly overlapping the immediately underlying layer, to ensure a watertight repair.

The transvesical ureteroneocystostomy technique is preferred for transplantation of kidneys with a double ureter. The two ureters are left in their common adventitial sheath and are brought through the posterior bladder wall and submucosal tunnel together, as with a single ureter. Both ureteral ends are spatulated, the medial ends are sutured together, and the lateral and distal aspects are anastomosed to the bladder as with a single ureter (Fig. 22.21).

After all anastomoses have been completed and adequate hemostasis has been achieved, the wound is irrigated with 2,000 mL of normal saline solution. This is an important local measure both in debriding the wound of small nonviable pieces of tissue and in minimizing the influence of inadvertent intraoperative contamination. The transplant incision is always closed without drainage in two separate musculofascial layers. The subcutaneous layer and the skin are also closed separately, and a pressure dressing is then used to cover the wound.

In the early postoperative period, fluid and electrolyte balance is maintained by monitoring central venous pressure, blood pressure, pulse rate, urinary output, and body weight. When oligoanuria is present despite normovolemia, 12.5 g of mannitol and 40 mg of furosemide are given intravenously. The amount of furosemide may be doubled to a maximum dose of 160 mg. Some cadaver allograft recipients remain oliguric following these measures due to vasomotor nephropathy. This diagnosis can be established only after excluding hyperacute rejection or technical problems by examining the incision for drainage, ensuring a patent urethral catheter, and obtaining an ultrasound study and an isotope renal scan. In contrast, living related allograft recipients often experience a profound postoperative osmotic diuresis, which necessitates vigorous fluid and electrolyte replacement.

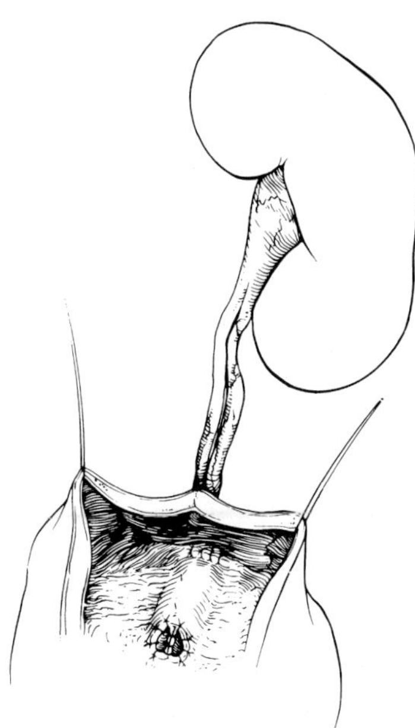

FIGURE 22.21. Transvesical ureteroneocystostomy technique for donor kidney with double ureter. (From Novick AC, Streem SB, Pontes JE, et al, eds. *Stewart's operative urology.* Baltimore: Williams & Wilkins, 1989, with permission.)

Within the first 24 hours postoperatively, a technetium renal scan is routinely done to verify the patency of the transplanted renal artery. If uptake of isotope by the allograft is lacking or questionable, renal arteriography should be performed to evaluate the possibility of arterial thrombosis or hyperacute rejection. The initial surgical dressing is removed 24 hours postoperatively and is changed daily thereafter, using strict sterile technique. Systemic antibiotic therapy is administered only to patients with documented infection. A urethral catheter is left indwelling for 3 to 7 days, and the sutures from the transplant wound are removed 10 days postoperatively.

MULTIPLE RENAL VESSELS

Multiple renal arteries occur unilaterally and bilaterally in 23% and 10% of the population, respectively. Important

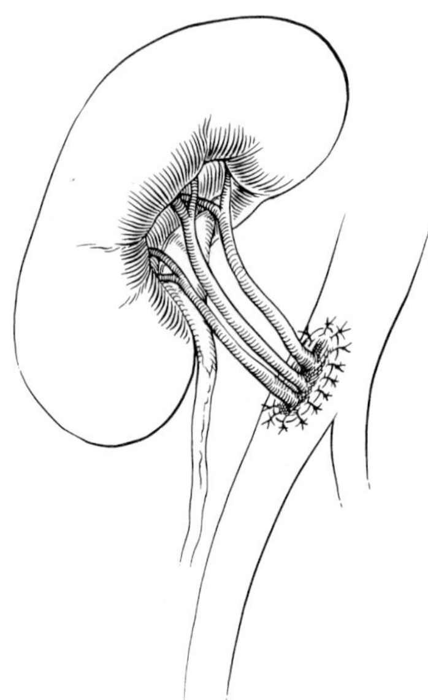

FIGURE 22.22. End-to-side anastomosis of the Carrel aortic patch with multiple renal arteries to the common iliac artery. (From Novick AC, Streem SB, Pontes JE, et al, eds. *Stewart's operative urology.* Baltimore: Williams & Wilkins, 1989, with permission.)

prerequisites to successful transplantation of kidneys with multiple arteries are proper techniques of organ procurement, thorough arteriographic evaluation of potential living donors, and selection of an appropriate method of arterial revascularization. When such kidneys are transplanted, failure to recognize and preserve an accessory renal artery may eventuate in ureteral necrosis, graft rupture, segmental renal infarction, postoperative hypertension, or calyceal fistula formation. A variety of techniques are available for performing multiple artery renal transplantation (195).

Anastomosis of a Carrel aortic patch encompassing all renal arteries to the recipient common or external iliac artery is the preferred method for arterial anastomosis of cadaver kidneys with multiple arteries (Fig. 22.22). This requires that cadaver donor nephrectomy be performed en bloc with the aorta and vena cava. Use of such an aortic patch is not possible when kidneys are harvested separately, when polar vessels are injured inadvertently during removal, when there is significant atherosclerosis of the perirenal aorta, or when the renal arteries are widely separated on the aorta. Likewise, in live donor renal transplantation, a cuff of aorta should never be taken because of the increased risk to the donor.

When two adjacent renal arteries of comparable size are present, our preferred method is extracorporeal side-to-side anastomosis of the two vessels to create a common ostium (Fig. 22.23). This is done just before implantation, with the kidney cooled in ice saline solution. Continuous 6-0 or 7-0 vascular sutures are used for the repair, with optimal magnification provided by 3.5× loupes. Revascularization in the recipient involves only a single arterial anastomosis, preferably end-to-end to the hypogastric artery, with no increase in the warm renal ischemia time. This method is technically simple and, hemodynamically, yields less resistance to flow than do separate vascular anastomoses because of the greater cross-sectional area of the coapted vessels.

When two renal arteries of disparate caliber are present, our preferred technique is end-to-side reimplantation of the smaller artery into the larger one (Fig. 22.24). A short linear arteriotomy is made in the side of the larger artery, without removing any of the vessel wall, to obviate narrowing of the arterial lumen. The smaller artery is spatulated, and end-to-side anastomosis to the larger vessel is done with interrupted 7-0 vascular sutures, using microvascular instruments and 3.5× loupes for magnification. A small catheter or probe may be placed through the suture line during its construction to prevent accidental entrapment of the back wall. The completed anastomosis is tested for patency and integrity by gentle perfusion of the main renal artery. The transplant operation is then done as with a single renal artery. The advantages of this method are that it is technically simple, it involves anastomosis of vessels that are similar in thickness, only one arterial anastomosis is required in the recipient, and warm renal ischemia time is not prolonged. This technique can also be used for transplant kidneys supplied by more than two renal arteries of varying caliber.

Another method for transplanting kidneys with multiple renal arteries involves fashioning these into a single artery before implantation with a branched graft of autogenous hypogastric artery (Fig. 22.25). If atherosclerosis is present in the hypogastric artery, this can be removed after its procurement using the eversion endarterectomy technique.

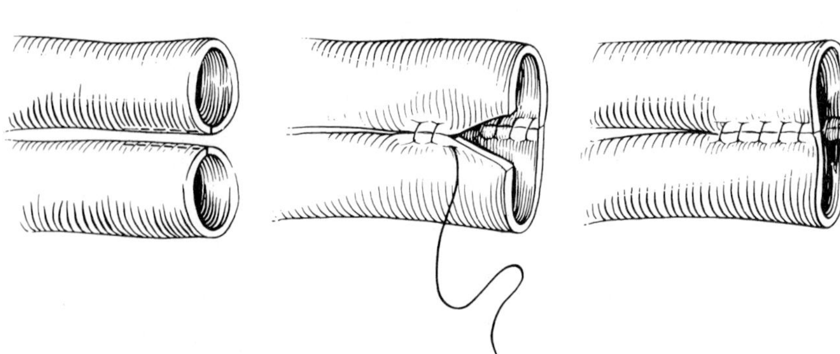

FIGURE 22.23. Side-to-side conjoined anastomosis for two renal arteries of equal caliber. (From Novick AC, Streem SB, Pontes JE, et al, eds. *Stewart's operative urology.* Baltimore: Williams & Wilkins, 1989, with permission.)

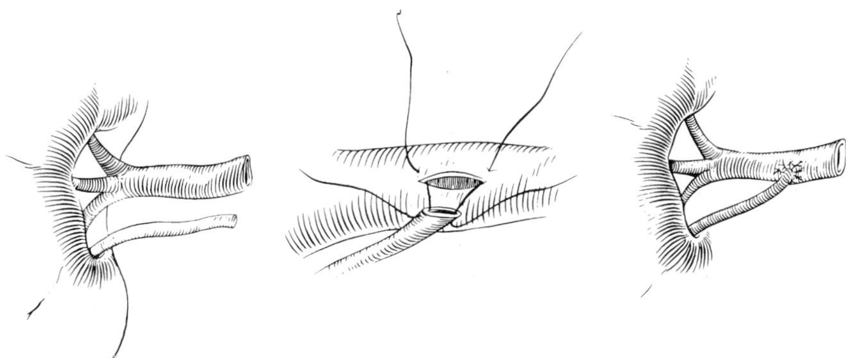

FIGURE 22.24. End-to-side reimplantation of small renal artery into larger one. (From Novick AC, Streem SB, Pontes JE, et al, eds. *Stewart's operative urology.* Baltimore: Williams & Wilkins, 1989, with permission.)

Donor arterial repair is done extracorporeally under surface hypothermia with end-to-end anastomosis of the graft branches of the distal renal arteries. The kidney is then transplanted as with a single renal artery, with no added warm ischemia time. This technique is particularly useful to transplant kidneys with more than two renal arteries or when insufficient arterial length is present to permit use of the previous two methods described. Should extensive calcification of the hypogastric artery render it unsuitable as a reconstructive graft, a branched saphenous vein graft can be used alternatively in the same fashion.

Additional techniques for performing multiple artery transplantation include arterial anastomoses to the branches of the hypogastric artery, separate arterial anastomoses to the external or common iliac arteries, separate arterial anastomoses to the hypogastric and external iliac arteries, and polar artery anastomosis to the inferior epigastric artery. These techniques all require performance of multiple arterial anastomoses *in situ* that result in a prolonged warm ischemia time. Therefore, when a Carrel aortic patch is not available, we prefer extracorporeal arterial reconstruction using one of the three methods described previously. These latter techniques have proven to be readily applicable, either individually or in combination, to most anatomic variants presented by kidneys with multiple arteries.

Multiple renal veins are less common than multiple arteries and more frequently involve the right kidney. Small renal veins can be ligated without risk. When double renal veins of equal size are present, both of these must be preserved to avoid increased intrarenal venous pressure after revascularization. The optimal method involves implanting these together with a cuff of vena cava obtained at the time of nephrectomy. When this is not available, extracorporeal venous reconstruction is performed as described for multiple arteries with either a conjoined or an end-to-side anastomosis of the two veins.

TRANSPLANTATION IN CHILDREN

There are special surgical considerations when renal transplantation is performed in young pediatric patients. In children weighing less than 20 kg, the iliac fossa is too small to accommodate a kidney from an adult donor. In this event, the graft must be inserted in a more cephalad location.

A midline transperitoneal incision is made, and the cecum and ascending colon are reflected medially to expose the aorta, the vena cava, and the common iliac vessels. The graft is placed retrocecally with end-to-side anastomosis of the renal vein either to the vena cava or to the right common

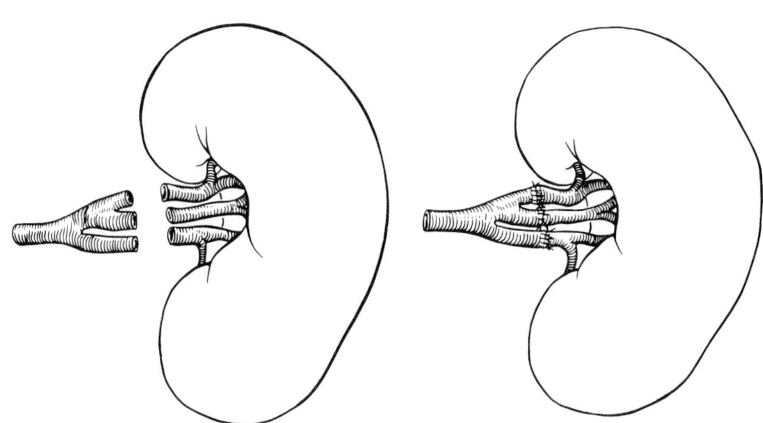

FIGURE 22.25. Use of branched autologous vascular graft to reconstruct multiple renal arteries. (From Novick AC, Streem SB, Pontes JE, et al, eds. *Stewart's operative urology.* Baltimore: Williams & Wilkins, 1989, with permission.)

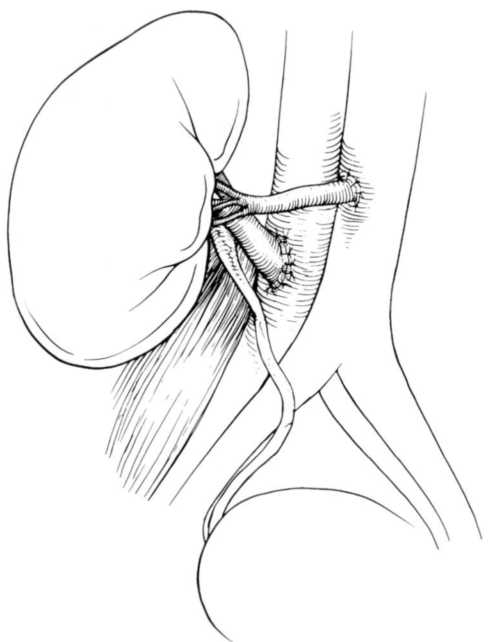

FIGURE 22.26. Technique of retrocecal renal transplantation for placement of adult donor kidney into small child. (From Novick AC, Streem SB, Pontes JE, et al, eds. *Stewart's operative urology.* Baltimore: Williams & Wilkins, 1989, with permission.)

iliac vein. The renal artery is anastomosed end-to-side to either the aorta or the right common iliac artery (Fig. 22.26). Immediately after revascularization of the allograft, 300 mL of albumin is administered as an intravenous bolus to replenish the suddenly depleted intravascular volume and to ensure adequate renal perfusion. The ureter generally reaches the bladder easily, remaining retroperitoneal throughout its course, and a ureteroneocystostomy is performed. An alternative surgical approach for performing transplantation in children involves the use of extraperitoneal incision extending from the tip of the twelfth rib to the symphysis pubis. This method is particularly helpful in children who have been managed with peritoneal dialysis. Very small children, weighing less than 8 kg, require transplantation of a pediatric cadaver graft.

TRANSPLANTATION WITH URINARY DIVERSION

In some patients, the bladder may be unsuitable for transplantation due either to severe neurogenic disease or to postinflammatory contracture. In such cases, renal transplantation must be performed in conjunction with supravesical urinary diversion. The most common technique involves the creation of an intestinal (generally ileal) conduit with a lower quadrant stoma at a separate operation before transplantation; 4 to 6 weeks later, the transplant operation is performed (161).

The preferred method for performing transplantation into an ileal conduit is to place the allograft retrocecally, as in pediatric transplantation, with anastomosis of the renal vessels either to the aorta and vena cava or to the common iliac vessels. This allows gravity-dependent urinary drainage and a more direct ureteroenteric anastomosis than when transplantation into the iliac fossa is done (Fig. 22.27).

In some patients with ESRD, diversion with cutaneous ureterostomy has been performed previously and a well-functioning stoma is present. In such cases, the stoma and a short contiguous segment of distal ureter can be preserved at the time of bilateral nephrectomy. Transplantation is then performed with anastomosis of the allograft ureter to the retained native ureter just below the abdominal wall, thus obviating the need for an intestinal segment (Fig. 22.28). Using this method, satisfactory urinary drainage is achieved through the normal peristaltic ability of the allograft ureter, and the retained dilated ureter functions solely as a short conduit and stoma (161).

RENAL ALLOGRAFT REJECTION

Preventive Immunosuppressive Protocols

Immunosuppressive protocols using the agents discussed previously can be divided into two phases: induction and maintenance. *Induction* describes initial high-dose immunosuppression designed to prevent a primary immune response during the first 7 to 10 days of engraftment. Numerous factors (e.g., patient selection, organ quality) can influence immunosuppressive decisions, and transplant physician experience and judgment are key determinants of

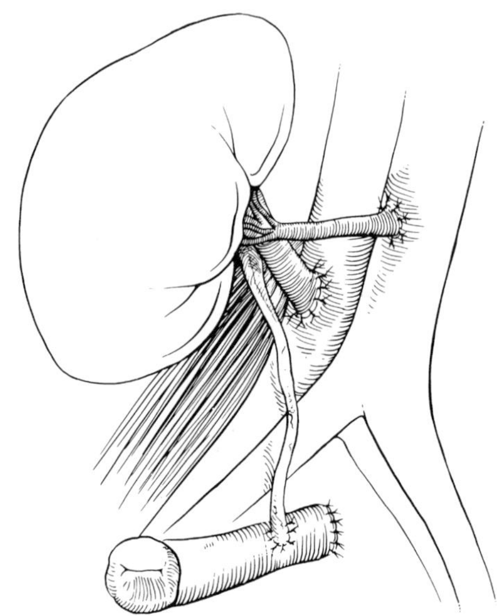

FIGURE 22.27. Technique of renal transplantation into an intestinal conduit. (From Novick AC, Streem SB, Pontes JE, et al, eds. *Stewart's operative urology.* Baltimore: Williams & Wilkins, 1989, with permission.)

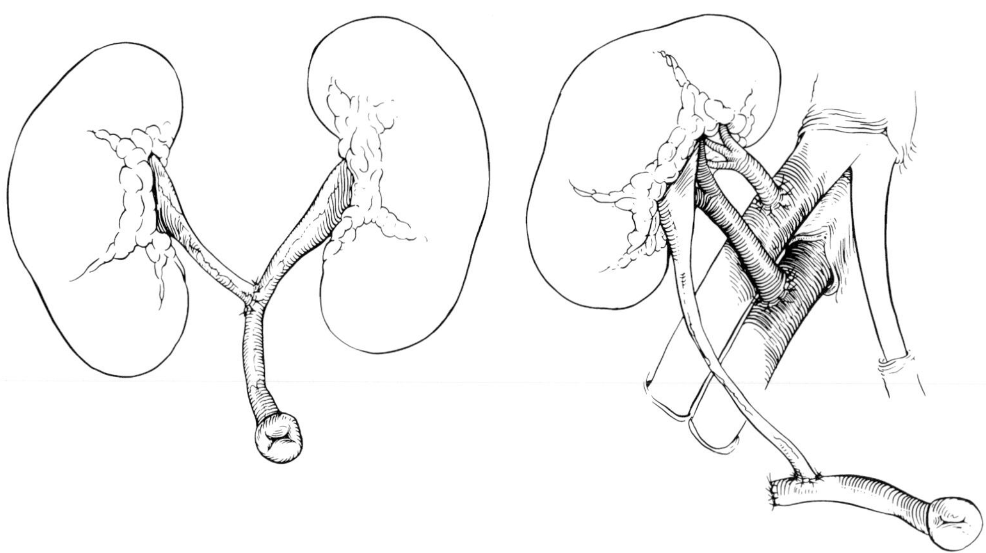

FIGURE 22.28. Technique of renal transplantation using existing cutaneous ureterostomy stoma. (From Novick AC, Streem SB, Pontes JE, et al, eds. *Stewart's operative urology.* Baltimore: Williams & Wilkins, 1989, with permission.)

patient management. Currently, induction therapy involves either polyclonal or monoclonal antilymphocyte agents. As previously mentioned, these agents are often used as sequential therapy with a delay in the institution of a calcineurin inhibitor drug until the kidney has sufficiently recovered from ischemic preservation injury. In general, if preservation times are short, under 12 to 18 hours, calcineurin agents can be introduced earlier without an increased risk of delayed graft function. However, when preservation times are 24 hours or longer, delayed graft function rates of 30% or more can occur, and the duration will be prolonged by the immediate introduction of calcineurin inhibitor drugs. Another consideration in induction therapy is the choice between polyclonal and monoclonal agents. Most studies have found these two classes of agents to be equally effective with respect to rejection prevention and allograft survival. The polyclonal agents are usually administered for 7 to 14 days and require central venous access due to the high protein load and vein sclerosis that occurs. The monoclonal agents can be given peripherally and are more suitable for early hospital discharge. The newer anti–IL-2 receptor blocking agents have longer half-lives and can be given only on days 0 and 4 with prolonged immunosuppression present for several weeks.

Maintenance therapy describes the lowest doses of immunosuppressive drugs necessary to prevent rejection. Unfortunately, this is often arrived at by trial and error and results in much interpatient variability. The principles of drug interactions and synergism that have been developed from multidrug protocols for cancer chemotherapy also apply to rejection prophylaxis. Multiple drugs with different mechanisms of action can be used together to permit lower dosages and less toxicity than would be obtained from higher dosages of single agents. Most centers have arrived at triple-drug maintenance regimens consisting of a calcineurin inhibitor drug (cyclosporine or tacrolimus), an antiproliferative agent (mycophenolate mofetil or azathioprine), and corticosteroids. Rapamycin is being evaluated either in combination with a calcineurin drug or as a replacement.

The following is a description of current immunosuppressive protocols used at The Cleveland Clinic Foundation and a brief review of their rationale.

Live Donor Recipients

HLA-identical siblings receive corticosteroids and cyclosporine. Cyclosporine is begun at 6 to 8 kg per day in divided doses approximately 36 hours before transplantation and subsequently adjusted to maintain trough blood levels at about 200 ng/mL. One gram of intravenous methylprednisolone is given perioperatively, and prednisone is begun at 2 mg/kg per day in divided doses from postoperative day 1. Prednisone is tapered to 30 mg per day by day 8, to 25 mg at 1 month, and lowered by 2.5 mg per month to 7.5 mg per day. Steroids are sometimes tapered off by 1 year.

Mismatched live donor recipients (1-haplotype, 0-haplotype, and live unrelated) recipients are managed with cyclosporine-based triple-drug therapy. Again, cyclosporine is begun 36 hours before transplantation at 6 to 8 mg/kg per day and adjusted by trough blood level monitoring. Steroids are given in doses similar to those described for HLA-ID recipients. Mycophenolate mofetil is begun on day 1 at 1 g twice daily and left at this dose unless specific toxicity necessitates dosage reduction. We have recently experienced a fall in acute rejection rates to single digits in mismatched live donor recipients with the addition of basiliximab (82). The IL-2 receptor blocking antibody has now been incorporated into our protocol.

Cadaveric Recipients

Our initial concerns of cyclosporine's potentiation of ischemic injury in kidneys with prolonged preservation times were confirmed by a randomized study in which kidneys from a single donor were transplanted separately into one of two groups, the first receiving initial cyclosporine therapy while the second received sequential therapy with a delay in initiation of cyclosporine (194). Patients receiving cyclosporine had an increased incidence of delayed graft function and primary nonfunction, resulting in a diminished overall allograft survival. This was further substantiated in an experimental model in which cyclosporine was administered to rats subjected to varying times of renal ischemia (132). A protocol using sequential, quadruple therapy (MALG plus prednisone, azathioprine, and cyclosporine) was instituted at that time. Subsequent to the availability of OKT3, we initiated a randomized, prospective comparison of OKT3 versus ALG in patients with acute renal failure following cadaveric renal transplantation (270). The results revealed no difference in patient or allograft survival or rejection rates, although there was a slight increase in side effects in the OKT3 group. We subsequently demonstrated that OKT3 side effects could be diminished using lower doses and steroid pretreatment (84).

Currently, cadaveric recipients receive steroids and mycophenolate mofetil in a manner similar to that for live donor recipients. Basiliximab is given at 20 mg on days 0 and 4. The T-cell activation marker CD25 is obtained to confirm efficacy. Cyclosporine is begun after return of adequate renal function (serum creatinine 4.0 mg/dL or lower) at approximately 6 mg/kg per day and adjusted to keep trough levels at 200 to 250 ng/mL the first month. In cases of prolonged ATN, cyclosporine is delayed until day 8 to 10 and advanced more slowly.

DIAGNOSIS OF REJECTION

The prompt diagnosis of rejection as the cause of allograft dysfunction is imperative to minimize irreversible damage to the kidney. Depending on the time from transplantation and the preceding level of renal function, the diagnosis can be obscure. The more classic findings of fever; a swollen, painful kidney; and diminished urine output are often absent in patients receiving cyclosporine. Differential diagnoses include ATN, nephrotoxicity, urinary obstruction or fistula, and vascular complications. A renal ultrasound (see Surgical Complications) will assist in assessing the latter causes. The findings resulting in the diagnosis of rejection are those related to renal nuclear scanning and a renal allograft biopsy.

Renal Scan

The value of sequential renal scans in the evaluation of renal transplant recipients has long been established (71). Technetium 99m diethylenetriamine pentacetic acid (^{99m}Tc DTPA) (173) and iodine-labeled orthoiodohippurate (I-OIH) (319) have been the most widely used radiopharmaceuticals. However, we now use technetium 99m mercaptoacetyl-triglycine (^{99m}Tc MAG3) to image renal transplant recipients (38,198). MAG3 is a primarily tubular-excreted compound; it shares equivalent physiologic properties with OIH that, in combination with its availability as a technetium-labeled agent, make it a preferable alternative as the radionuclide pharmaceutical. Images obtained with MAG3 are distinctly superior to those previously seen with DTPA and OIH.

Representative MAG3 scans for various clinical scenarios are depicted in Figs. 22.29 through 22.36. Figure 22.29 is that of the allograft of a living-related recipient immediately after transplant and demonstrates excellent perfusion and function. There is prompt uptake of the radiopharmaceutical with early peak accumulation and a rapid excretion and clearance from the allograft. Episodes of renal function deterioration will be demonstrated in the scan, primarily manifested as a delay in uptake with the failure to reach peak accumulation (the allograft continues to accumulate throughout the duration of the study) and diminished excretion and clearance. Figure 22.30 demonstrates an immediate posttransplant cadaveric recipient with acute tubular necrosis. Figure 22.31 reveals significant improvement in the scan 1 week later as the acute tubular necrosis has resolved. Failure of the scan to demonstrate improvement in this setting or a sudden deterioration in the appearance in the scan would implicate other causes of renal failure. Figure 22.32 is a 24-hour posttransplant scan in a living-related recipient with excellent function. One month after transplant, the patient experienced an acute rise in his serum creatinine with associated deterioration of the scan (Fig. 22.33). A percutaneous renal biopsy revealed acute cellular rejection. He underwent antirejection therapy with improvement in renal function (Fig. 22.34). Figure 22.35 is that of an immediate posttransplant living-related recipient; Fig. 22.36 was obtained approximately 4 days later associated with a rise in the patient's serum creatinine. The patient was noted to have elevated cyclosporine levels, and his dosage was reduced with improvement in his renal function.

Percutaneous Renal Allograft Biopsy

Although clinical and radiographic clues can arouse suspicion, the certainty of rejection requires histopathologic examination of allograft tissue. A percutaneous needle

Text continued on page 949

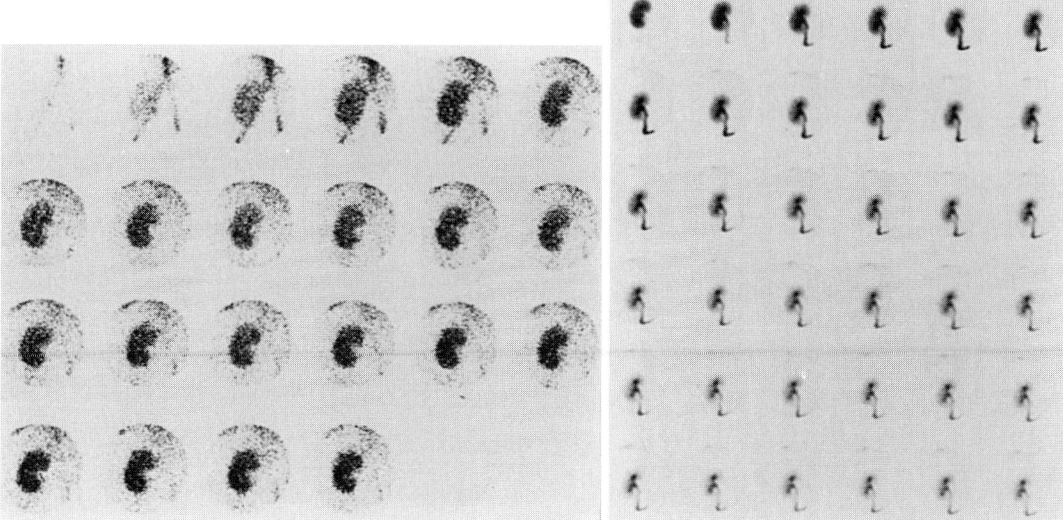

FIGURE 22.29. Renal scan in living related recipient 1 day postoperatively demonstrating excellent perfusion and function with rapid uptake and time to peak accumulation and prompt excretion and clearance.

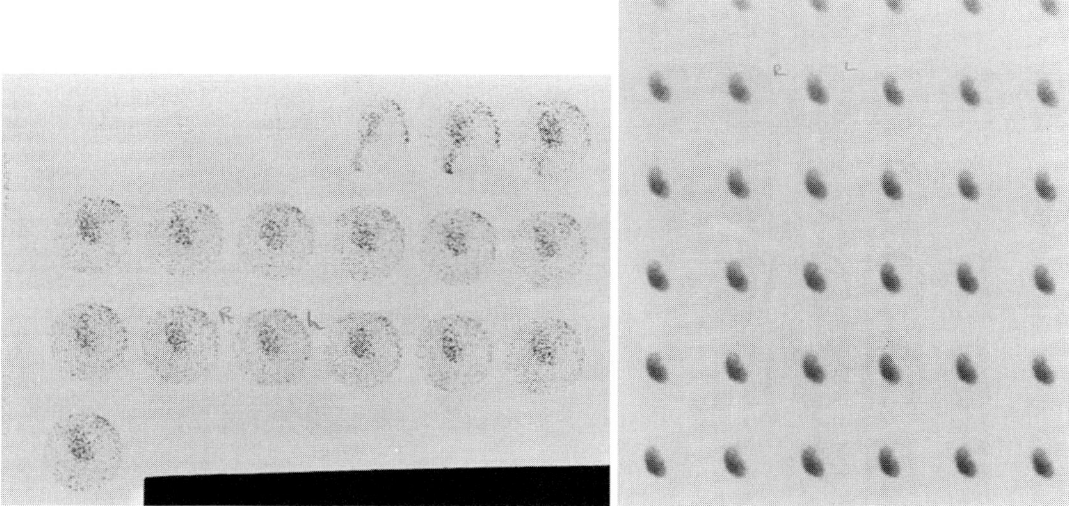

FIGURE 22.30. Baseline renal scan in cadaveric recipient with acute tubular necrosis illustrating a delay in uptake with persistent accumulation throughout the study and diminished excretion and clearance.

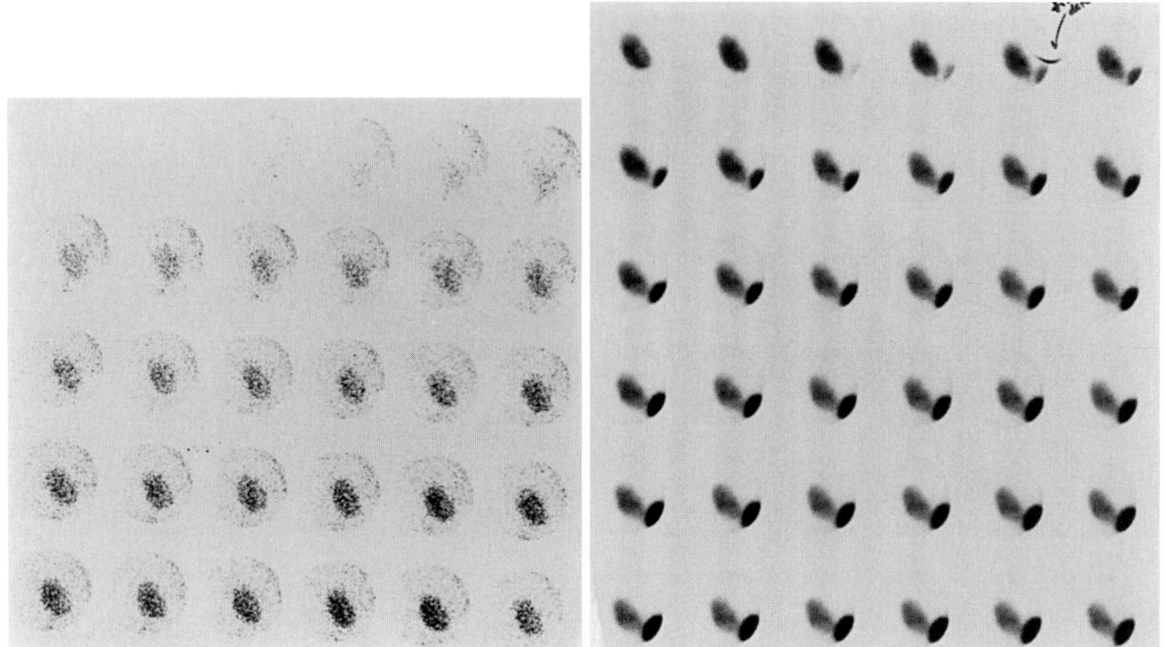

FIGURE 22.31. Renal scan in the same patient as Fig. 22.30, 1 week later, revealing improvement with resolution of acute tubular necrosis.

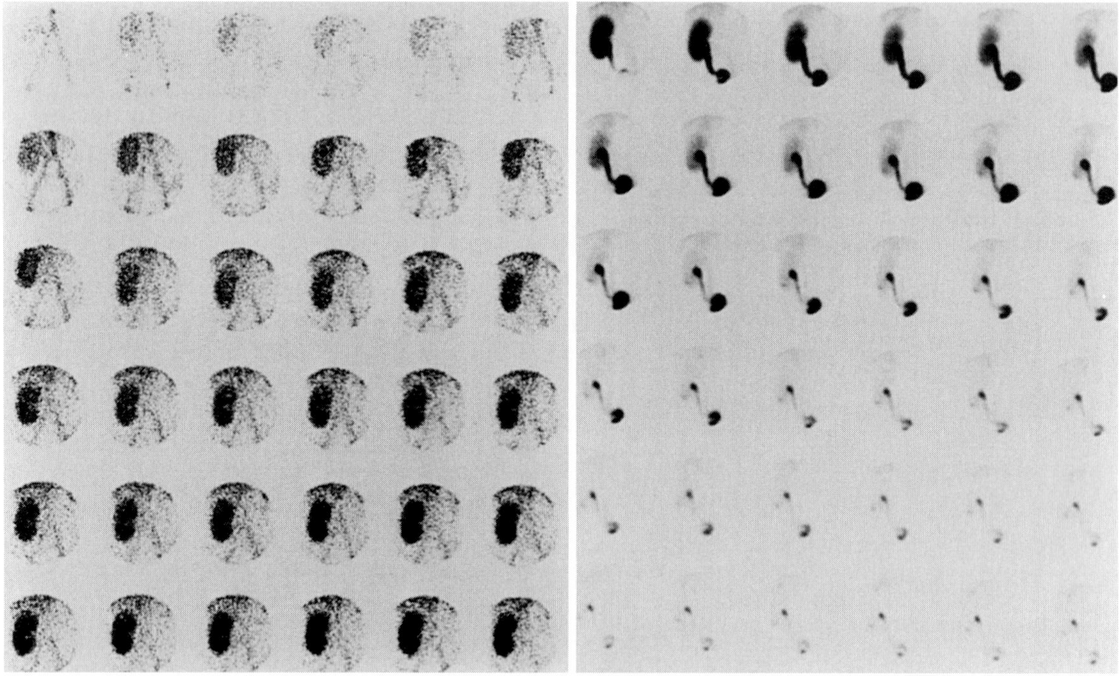

FIGURE 22.32. Baseline scan in living-related recipient with good perfusion and function.

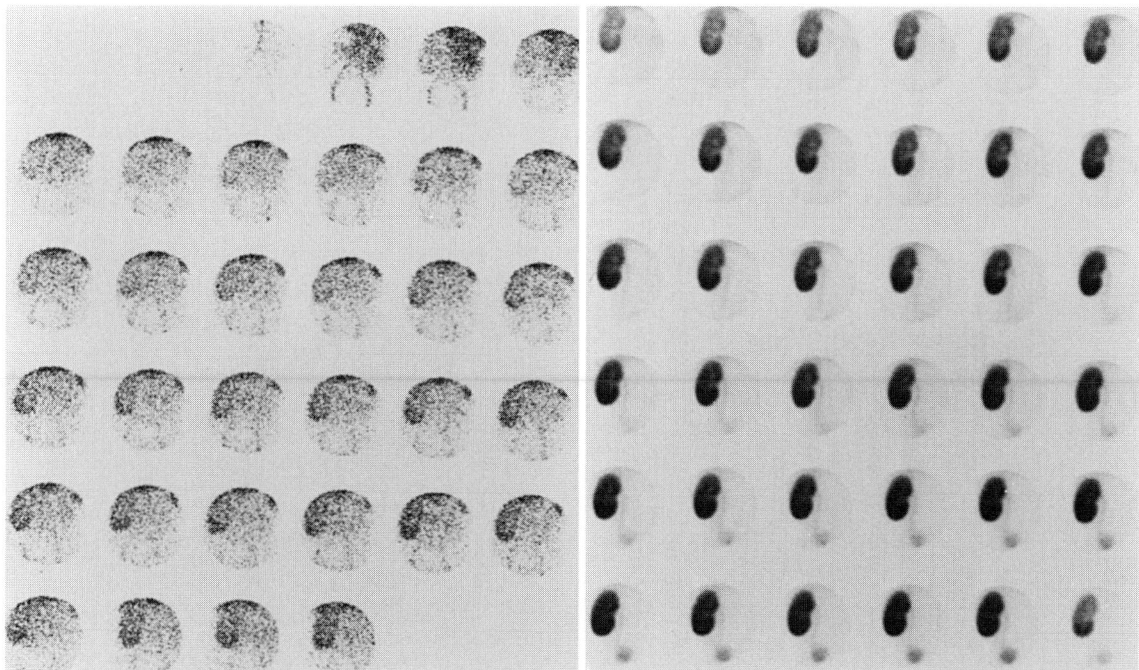

FIGURE 22.33. Scan in same patient as Fig. 22.32, 1 month later, with biopsy-proven rejection illustrating diminished perfusion and function.

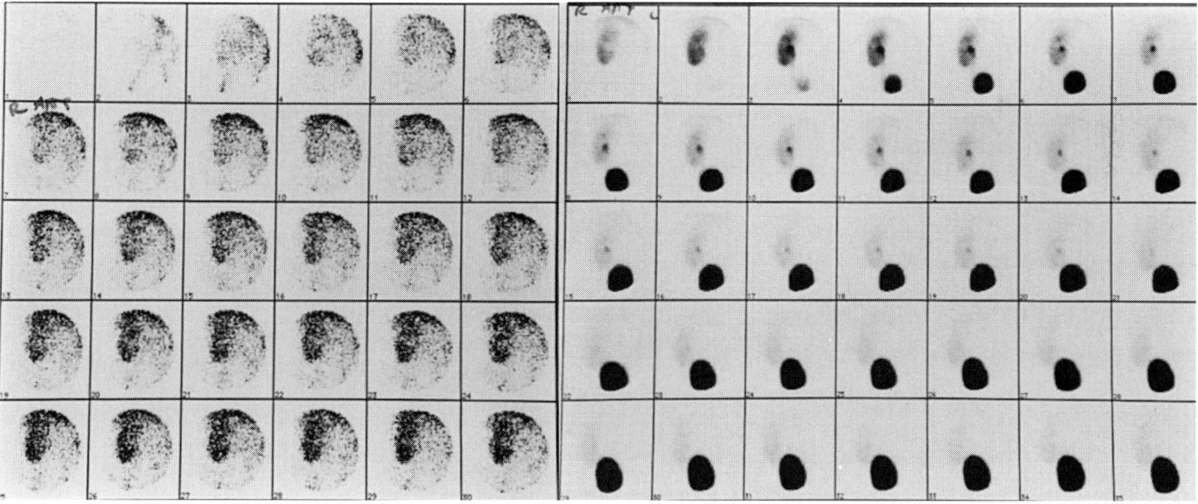

FIGURE 22.34. Scan in same patient as Fig. 22.32 following antirejection therapy with improvement in renal function.

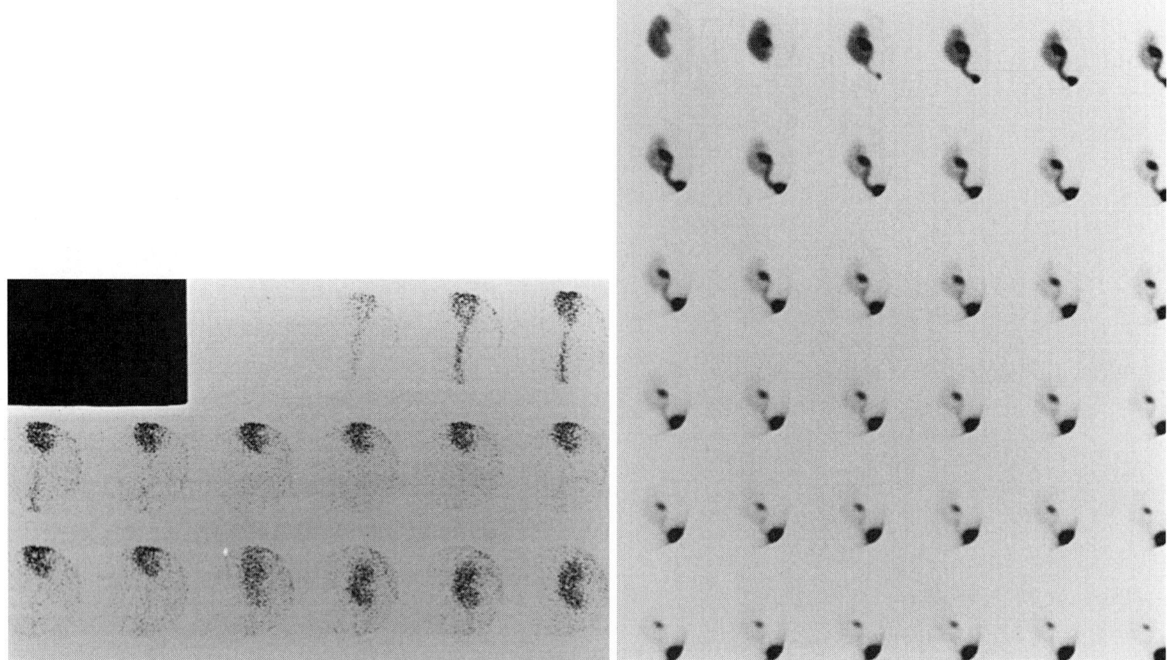

FIGURE 22.35. Baseline scan in living-related recipient, demonstrating good perfusion and function.

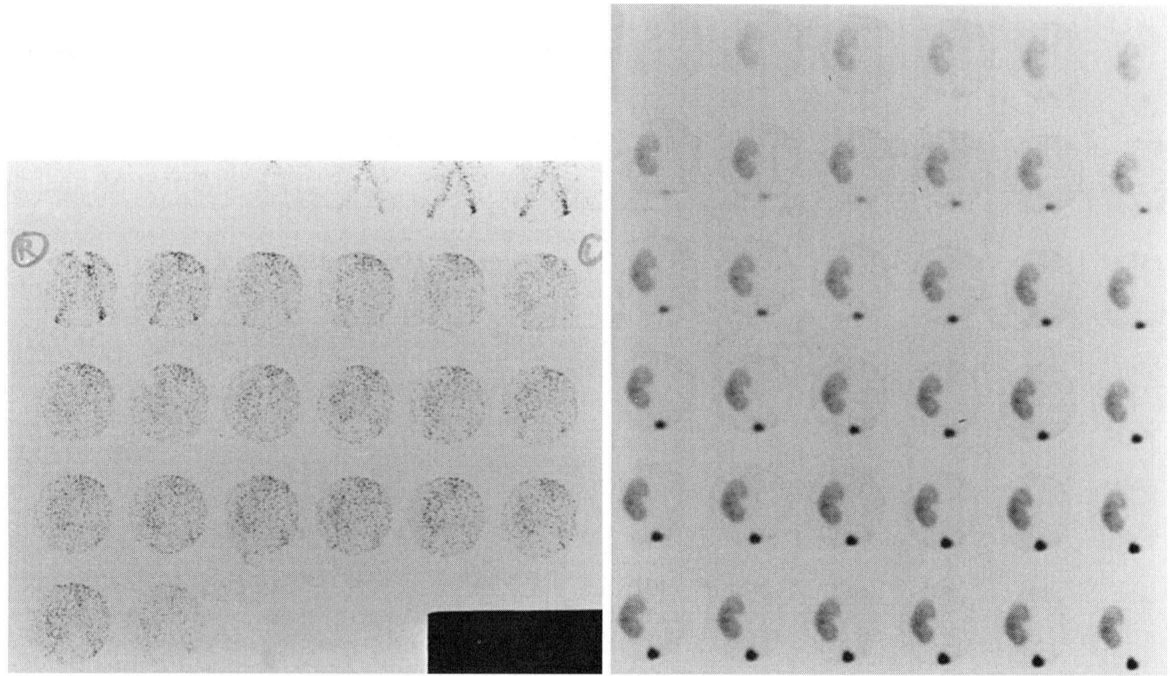

FIGURE 22.36. Scan in same patient as Fig. 22.35, approximately 4 days later, with elevated creatinine and cyclosporine levels.

TABLE 22.9. THE BANFF SCHEMA SIMPLIFIED

Biopsy Findings	Banff Classification	Possible Clinical Approach
Normal, minor changes, or infiltrates *without* tubular invasion	Normal or "other" (nonspecific changes)	No treatment, or treat other entity
Mild lymphocytic invasion of tubules (tubulitis)	Borderline changes	No treatment, or treat other entity
Widespread interstitial infiltrate with moderate invasion of tubules	Mild acute rejection (grade I)	Treat for rejection if there are clinical signs
Widespread interstitial infiltrate with severe invasion of tubules and/or mild or moderate intimal arteritis	Moderate acute rejection (grade II)	Treat for rejection, consider ALG or OKT3 if refractory to steroids
Severe intimal arteritis and/or "transmural" arteritis, fibrinoid change, and medical smooth muscle cell necrosis often with patchy infarction and interstitial hemorrhage	Severe acute rejection (grade III)	Treat for rejection unless clinical course suggests rejection cannot be reversed, in which case consider abandoning the graft
Hyaline arteriolar thickening (new onset, not present in implantation biopsy), and/or extensive isometric vacuolization of tubules, smooth muscle degeneration, thrombotic microangiopathy	"Other," cyclosporine toxicity	Reduce cyclosporine therapy
Tubular cell loss and necrosis, regenerative changes	"Other," acute tubular necrosis	Await recovery
Interstitial fibrosis, tubular atrophy (new-onset arterial fibrous intimal thickening suggests chronic rejection)	Chronic transplant nephropathy	Temporize

From Solez K, Axelson RA, Banner B, et al. International standardization of nomenclature and criteria for the histologic diagnosis of renal allograft rejection: the Banff working classification of kidney transplant pathology. *Kidney Int* 1993;44:411, with permission.

biopsy of the kidney is often easily performed; including in the outpatient clinic, especially under ultrasound guidance. We currently perform approximately 80% of biopsies in this setting. Although the potential for significant complications, including bleeding, exists, a core biopsy can be performed safely with a high likelihood of providing needed information (140). A proposed standardized classification (Banff schema) was developed based on the premise that some findings (including tubulitis and intimal arteritis) are specific for rejection, whereas others (e.g., a cellular infiltrate) are nonspecific (Table 22.9) (261). A more recent update of the schema focused on so-called borderline cases of interstitial inflammation and severe vascular rejection (228).

TREATMENT OF REJECTION

Pulse Corticosteroids

As they have been for more than three decades, increased (pulse) doses of corticosteroids are the initial antirejection therapy in most programs. There are few data to support any given dose (0.5 g versus 1 g per day) or a particular route of administration (intravenous versus high-dose oral) (59). Currently, rejection episodes at our center are initially treated with 0.5 g of methylprednisolone (Solu-Medrol) per day for 3 days (271). If the rejection has not been reversed after 3 days of corticosteroid therapy or if more ominous findings are present in the biopsy (e.g., severe vasculitis), more aggressive therapy is initiated with antilymphocyte agents. Corticosteroids are administered before a biopsy is performed, and all patients undergo a biopsy before receiving antilymphocyte preparations to ensure that rejection is the cause of allograft dysfunction, as opposed to other etiologies such as acute tubular necrosis or cyclosporine nephrotoxicity.

Antilymphocyte Preparations

Both polyclonal (MALG) (274) and monoclonal (OKT3) (206) antilymphocyte preparations are extremely effective in reversing rejection when compared with corticosteroids. Although reported as primary therapy by some centers (289), we have generally reserved the use of these agents for steroid-resistant rejection episodes because of the toxicities mentioned previously. Both agents have been extremely effective with reversal rates of 70% to 90% for steroid-resistant rejection (193), although there is a slightly higher rate of re-rejection following treatment. Interestingly, approximately 50% of these rejection episodes occurring after treatment with antilymphocyte preparations for steroid-resistant rejection will respond to a course of steroids. Before re-treating with OKT3, the patient must be checked for the presence of antibodies to OKT3.

Although direct comparative studies are few, results with ALG and OKT3 for steroid-resistant rejection appear to be similar. A prospective, randomized, although small, study found slightly improved results in patients treated with OKT3 for steroid-resistant rejection compared with those receiving ALG (113). MALG is given at dosages of 15 to 20 mg/kg per day for 10 to 14 days, and OKT3 is given at a dosage of 5 mg per day for 7 to 14 days.

Plasmapheresis

Although OKT3 has been shown to be of benefit in some patients with "vascular" rejection (251), there currently exists no universally effective treatment for antibody-mediated rejection. As plasmapheresis had been shown to be successful in treating various immunologically mediated renal diseases (211), attempts were directed at using it for humoral rejection. Initial anecdotal reports indicated that plasmapheresis would be efficacious in treating antibody-mediated rejection; however, more in-depth reviews (59,211) of available data including controlled studies have failed to confirm its role in this setting. More sensitive posttransplant monitoring, such as flow cytometry cross-matches (50), may allow for antibody production detection before organ damage and thus potentially enhance the effectiveness of plasmapheresis. Additional applications of plasmapheresis have included the removal of anti–blood group antibodies in patients undergoing ABO-incompatible transplants (297). Backman and colleagues (14) reported on the use of plasmapheresis to remove anti-HLA antibodies from highly sensitized patients, thus allowing 14 of 17 patients to undergo transplantation who otherwise would have remained on dialysis. However, numerous logistical problems (e.g., waiting time before a cadaver kidney becomes available, necessity for availability of plasmapheresis at any time) have limited this potential application of plasmapheresis.

MEDICAL COMPLICATIONS

Medical complications experienced by renal transplant recipients are manifestations of underlying systemic diseases (e.g., diabetes), medication-specific adverse effects, or the result of acquired immunodeficiency. Complications encompass essentially all organ systems, and virtually every recipient will require therapeutic intervention for management of medical diseases. These complications can occur at any time in the posttransplant course (early or late), and thus lifelong surveillance of the transplant recipient is necessary.

Infection

Broad-spectrum antimicrobials and prophylactic protocols aimed at more serious infectious agents (including viral) have diminished but not eradicated the significant morbidity and mortality rates suffered by immunocompromised renal transplant hosts. More than half of renal transplant recipients will experience at least a single episode of infection in the first year after transplant (240), and septicemia is second only to cardiovascular events as the leading cause of death in the posttransplant setting (302). Immunosuppressed patients are at risk not only for the usual bacterial infections experienced by the immunocompetent host, but opportunistic infections as well. Pulmonary infections have been the leading contributor to the morbidity and mortality rates seen in renal transplant recipients, and causative agents include bacterial *(Pseudomonas, Mycobacteria, Listeria monocytogenes, Legionella,* and *Nocardia asteroides),* viral (CMV, herpesvirus), and fungal *(Candida, Pneumocystis carinii, Aspergillus,* and *Cryptococcus)* (240). Significant morbidity is associated with a delay in the accurate diagnosis, which is often not possible based on sputum specimens and may require transtracheal or transbronchial aspiration or biopsy or even percutaneous or open lung biopsy. Improvements in immunosuppressive strategies (especially decreased corticosteroids) have been associated with a reduction in the incidence of and death from pneumonia in renal transplant recipients (182), which are approximately 10% and 2%, respectively, in the cyclosporine era (112). Morbidity from *Pneumocystis carinii* pneumonia, which occurs in 5% to 10% of transplant recipients, has been virtually eliminated with trimethoprim-sulfamethoxazole prophylaxis (169), which also protects against *Nocardia asteroides* and *Listeria monocytogenes.*

Urinary tract infections are by far the most common bacterial infection occurring in the renal transplant recipient, with an incidence of 35% to 79% in the nonprophylaxed patient. Approximately 60% of episodes of Gram-negative sepsis in renal transplant patients originate from the urinary system (240). The morbidity of urinary tract infections is closely linked to the timing from transplantation, with those infections in the first few months more often being associated with pyelonephritis, bacteremia, and frequent relapses, compared with those infections occurring more than 6 months after transplant, which are usually more benign. Risk factors for urinary tract infection include indwelling Foley catheters, lower urinary tract anatomic abnormalities, stones, ureteral stents, and neurogenic bladder. In addition to the described pulmonary benefit, trimethoprim-sulfamethoxazole significantly reduces the incidence of urinary tract infection and resultant bacteremia in this patient population (88). We currently administer one single-strength trimethoprim-sulfamethoxazole tablet daily in the posttransplant period. In patients with an allergy to sulpha drugs, low-dose quinoline (norfloxacin or ciprofloxacin) may be substituted, although this results in a loss of the pulmonary prophylaxis.

Chronic liver disease occurs in 10% to 15% of renal transplant recipients and is the cause of death in 8% to 28% of survivors greater than 10 years after transplant (28). Viral hepatitis is the major cause of morbidity. Much has been learned with regard to hepatitis B virus (HBV) in this setting, and numerous questions regarding hepatitis C virus (HCV) have emerged as major considerations. The presence of a specific, sensitive, and rapid screening test for hepatitis B surface antigen (HBsAg) has rendered the transmission of hepatitis B by transplantation (with the associated risk of fulminant hepatitis), as well as the transplantation of chronically infected individuals destined to do poorly, relatively uncommon (240). A study of several thousand cadaveric organ donors revealed a prevalence of HCV by antibody testing to be approximately 5% compared with approximately 1% for healthy blood donors (215). The prevalence of virus as detected by polymerase chain reaction (PCR) was 2.4%, suggesting that half of the donors would not have transmitted virus. However, PCR is not currently available as a screening tool. A separate study from the New England Organ Bank identified 29 recipients of organs from 13 HCV antibody donors (216,217). One hundred percent of the recipients had detectable virus by PCR, although only 62% seroconverted. Forty-eight percent of the recipients developed hepatitis, including 12 with chronic liver disease and 1 with subfulminant hepatic failure. The development of chronic liver disease in posttransplant HCV disease appears more indolent than that of HBV. Rao and Andersen (232) reported a higher incidence of chronic progressive hepatitis, chronic active hepatitis, cirrhosis, and death from hepatic failure in patients 10 years after renal transplant with chronic hepatitis B compared to those with non-HBV chronic liver disease, thought to represent HCV. Until the risks are better defined, it appears that a policy of avoiding the use of HCV antibody–positive donors is appropriate, whereas the presence of HCV in a potential recipient does not represent an absolute contraindication to transplantation.

CMV is the most frequently encountered infection in renal transplant recipients, and risk factors include the serologic status of donor and recipient, as well as the immunosuppressive regimen used (240). CMV infection is reported to occur in 20% to 70% of renal transplant recipients. CMV infection occurs via one of three mechanisms. Primary infection results from the transmission of virus form a seropositive donor to a seronegative recipient; reactivation occurs when a seropositive recipient experiences reactivation of latent virus; and superinfection is a result of the transmission of a different strain (serotype) from a seropositive donor to a seropositive recipient. The term *CMV infection* is used to describe the growth of CMV in the blood or urine of the recipient. Symptomatic CMV disease describes viral growth accompanied by clinical symptoms. The most common is a clinical syndrome of fever and leukopenia. However, tissue-invasive disease involving the lungs, liver, GI tract, bone marrow, or central nervous system can occur. Approximately 60% of recipients at risk for primary infection will develop symptomatic CMV disease.

The nucleoside analogues acyclovir and ganciclovir have been used to treat CMV infection. High-dose acyclovir (800 mg four to five times a day) (15) and CMV hyperimmune globulin (260) have been used to diminish the incidence or severity of primary disease. They appear to be somewhat less effective when donors are seropositive or when antilymphocyte preparations, especially OKT3, are used. Intravenous ganciclovir at doses of 5 mg/kg twice a day for 2 to 3 weeks has proven effective in the treatment of CMV infection, as well as for preemptive therapy in patients receiving antilymphocyte preparations (210).

An oral preparation of ganciclovir has been introduced for CMV prophylaxis, although it has significantly decreased bioavailability compared with the intravenous blood levels achieved. We performed a randomized trial of oral ganciclovir versus oral acyclovir for CMV prophylaxis in renal transplant recipients considered at high risk due to induction with OKT3 (83). Only 2% of ganciclovir-treated patients compared with 36% of acyclovir-treated patients developed CMV infection. Most acyclovir failures occurred when donors were seropositive for CMV. We now administer oral ganciclovir for 90 days for all recipients of CMV-seropositive donors.

Malignancy

Renal transplant patients experience an increased susceptibility to malignancy, and the Cincinnati Tumor Registry reports a higher incidence of lymphomas, lip cancer, Kaposi's sarcoma, carcinomas of the kidney, carcinomas of the vulva and perineum, and hepatobiliary tumors as compared with the general population (214). Skin cancers are the most common and occur with similar frequency in both groups, although squamous cell predominates in the transplant patients and basal cell is more common in the general population. Lymphomas account for 20% of all cancers in transplant patients, compared with 5% of all cancers in the general population. Posttransplant lymphoproliferative disorders (PTLDs) represent a serious threat to the transplant patient. PTLDs differ from the lymphomas in the general population in that the overwhelming majority (94%) are non-Hodgkin's lymphomas and arise predominantly (86%) from B lymphocytes. Extranodal involvement is more common in PTLDs (70%); approximately 25% involve the central nervous system and 20% involve the allograft itself. Although initial reports suggested a higher incidence of PTLDs in OKT3-treated patients, it is probably a result of overall overimmunosuppression rather than a single immunosuppressive agent (214) and appears to be related to the induction of B-cell proliferation by Epstein-Barr virus (EBV) infection in the immunosuppressed patient. These relationships were demonstrated dramatically in a small series of patients in which a 12.5% incidence of PTLD was noted in patients receiving MALG induction followed by OKT3 for rejection (47). In the same study, patients at risk for primary EBV infection had a 23.1% of incidence of

PTLD compared with 0.7% for EBV-seropositive patients. Polyclonal B-cell PTLD appears to be more responsive to therapeutic measures including reduction of immunosuppression (189) than monoclonal B-cell PTLD, which appears to have a more malignant course (possibly representing progression in the continuum of the disease). The role of ganciclovir in the treatment of PTLDs is unknown at present.

Hypertension

In the cyclosporine era, 60% to 70% of patients experience hypertension following transplantation, compared with 40% to 50% before the introduction of cyclosporine, with a significant impact on patient and allograft survival (53,74). Not only has cyclosporine altered the prevalence of hypertension in the posttransplant patient, but it has also changed the mechanism and nature, and thus the treatment, of hypertension in this setting (53,74). Although the causes of posttransplant hypertension are numerous, before the introduction of cyclosporine renin-mediated causes appeared to be primarily responsible, often related to native kidney contributions or chronic rejection in the allograft. Currently, direct effects from cyclosporine predominate as the etiology of hypertension in most patients. Discussed previously (see section on cyclosporine), calcium channel blockers have emerged as the antihypertensive treatment of choice in these patients, assuming that corticosteroids and cyclosporine have been reduced to as low a dose as possible without risking rejection. Angiotensin-converting enzyme (ACE) inhibitors should be used with extreme caution because they can induce renal insufficiency, even in the absence of renal artery stenosis, as well as exacerbate existing hyperkalemia. However, the observation that posttransplant patients treated with ACE inhibitors were experiencing unexplained anemia has lead to a therapeutic benefit (310). Approximately 10% to 15% of posttransplant patients experience erythrocytosis, and through mechanisms poorly understood (although possibly related to alterations in erythropoietin production), judicious use of ACE inhibitors has been proven effective in lowering the hematocrit without creating the adverse effects mentioned previously, thus obviating the need for frequent phlebotomies, which had been the mainstay of previous treatment for posttransplant erythrocytosis (92). Provided rejection, recurrent disease, and renal artery stenosis in the allograft have been excluded, patients whose hypertension does not respond to medical therapy should be considered candidates for bilateral native nephrectomies (54).

Hyperlipidemia

Hyperlipidemia occurs in 50% to 80% of renal transplant recipients and, like hypertension, is the result of multifactorial causes, occurs with at least the same if not greater frequency since the introduction of cyclosporine, and serves as a potential risk factor for significant cardiovascular-related patient morbidity and death (119,167). Posttransplant hyperlipidemia appears to be more closely related to corticosteroid dose than cyclosporine dose (307), although unfortunately a reduction or withdrawal of steroids does not ameliorate the hyperlipidemia, and a concomitant reduction in high-density lipoprotein cholesterol with total cholesterol raises considerable doubt with regard to the cardiovascular benefit (119). Dietary management, exercise, and optimization of steroid and cyclosporine dosing constitute primary therapy for posttransplant hyperlipidemia. Persistent hyperlipidemia despite these measures requires drug intervention, and 3-hydroxy-3-methylglutaryl coenzyme A (HMG-CoA) reductase inhibitors have become the preferred treatment in this setting. Although adverse effects, especially rhabdomyolysis, have been observed with higher doses of HMG-CoA, especially with higher cyclosporine doses, the cautious use of lower doses and proper monitoring of liver function test and creatinine phosphokinase levels appears to be safe and effective (44).

Hyperparathyroidism

Posttransplant hypercalcemic hyperparathyroidism occurs in approximately 30% of patients despite the normalization of urinary phosphate excretion and renal synthesis of calcitriol, defects seen in uremic hyperparathyroidism (127). Patients with a longer duration of dialysis and larger hyperplastic parathyroid glands appear to be at greater risk because glandular involution after transplant is size and time dependent. However, most patients who have spontaneous resolution and parathyroidectomy, necessary in approximately 6% to 10%, should be reserved for patients experiencing significant complications such as marked or symptomatic hypercalcemia and progressive bone disease, especially osteonecrosis (55). Transient hypocalcemia can be seen following parathyroidectomy, although long-term calcium supplementation is usually not required.

SURGICAL COMPLICATIONS

Surgical problems following renal transplantation are predominantly related to either vascular or urologic complications. Improvements in surgical technique and meticulous attention to both the donor and recipient operations has led to a significant decrease in the surgical complication rate. Equally important in minimizing the morbidity associated with renal transplantation are anticipation of surgical complications and their prompt treatment when they occur (196). Surgical complications continue to occur in 10% of transplant recipients but, fortunately, are rarely the cause for allograft loss today.

Hemorrhage

Acute postoperative hemorrhage can result from disruption of a vascular suture line. Additional causes include inadequate preparation of the graft bed, an undetected or poorly ligated branch of the hypogastric artery, inappropriately ligated epigastric vessels, an unrecognized vessel in the renal pelvis, abnormal coagulation mechanisms of the recipients, and spontaneous graft rupture. The incidence of postoperative hemorrhage is increased when hemodialysis is required in the immediate postoperative period. The diagnosis of postoperative hemorrhage is usually evident on clinical grounds. The patient complains of excruciating pain around the kidney, in the back and flank. Hypovolemic shock can develop rapidly. Perinephric hematoma formation can cause functional allograft impairment by compression of the renal parenchyma, renal vessels, or ureter. Emergency exploration is usually necessary. If vascular repair or reconstruction cannot be accomplished within a reasonable time, allograft nephrectomy is indicated. Evacuation of the hematoma is important to prevent bacterial infection.

Late hemorrhage, arising months or years after transplantation, is rare but can occur as a result of rupture of a pseudoaneurysm at the anastomotic site. Hemorrhage as a result of percutaneous needle allograft biopsy has also been reported (313). The use of smaller-gauge automated needle biopsy under real-time ultrasound guidance should decrease this complication (65). Rupture of a mycotic aneurysm is another disastrous event that is fortunately rare (145). It is usually the result of a deep wound infection with secondary involvement of the vascular suture line. Transplant nephrectomy with ligation of the iliac artery and drainage of the area is the most expeditious and effective procedure (97). Salvage of the ipsilateral limb is possible with an extraanatomic revascularization procedure such as a femoral-femoral or axillofemoral bypass.

Renal Artery Thrombosis

Arterial thrombosis is a rare (less than 1%) complication that may occur as a result of hyperacute rejection, postoperative hypotension, faulty technical performance of the anastomosis, trauma to the intima of the donor artery during harvesting or perfusion, severe atherosclerosis in the recipient vessels, or wide disparity in the calibers of the donor and recipient vessels. Cyclosporine toxicity has been implicated in some cases of renal artery thrombosis on the basis of a hypocoagulable state (237). If the transplant recipient is anuric postoperatively and there is no uptake of isotope with a technetium renal scan, renal arteriography should be performed immediately. In most cases, the kidney is beyond salvage by the time the diagnosis is made, and transplant nephrectomy is the treatment of choice.

Renal Vein Thrombosis

Renal vein thrombosis is a rare (less than 1%) complication. It may result from a technical error in performing the venous anastomosis, ipsilateral femoroiliac thrombosis, external compression of the iliac or renal vein by perinephric fluid collection, or compression of the left common iliac vein between the right common iliac or aorta and the sacral promontory (silent iliac compression syndrome) (263). Additional causes in pediatric recipients include extrinsic compression in the iliac fossa (26) and kidneys from young donors less than 5 years old (109). An increased incidence of venous thromboembolism has also been noted in the cyclosporine era (306).

Venous thrombosis should be suspected when a transplant recipient has oliguria, graft enlargement, heavy proteinuria, and ipsilateral lower extremity edema. Renal flow scan shows delayed uptake with little or no excretion of the isotope. Renal venography is diagnostic and is useful in delineating the extent of the thrombus. Graft survival with renal vein thrombosis occurring within 1 month of transplantation has been poor. Early diagnosis and prompt thrombectomy occasionally have resulted in graft salvage, but more commonly, prolonged venous stasis will lead to a nonviable graft when surgical exploration is undertaken and nephrectomy is then performed. Renal vein thrombosis occurring more than 1 month after transplantation is best treated with systemic anticoagulation because, by that time, established collateral venous channels are adequate to prevent graft loss.

Renal Artery Stenosis

Hypertension following renal allotransplantation is common and may be secondary to rejection, ischemic allograft damage, retained native kidneys, steroid therapy, cyclosporine therapy, recurrence of primary renal disease in the allograft, or renal artery stenosis. Renal artery stenosis has been reported in 1% to 12% of transplant recipients and can occur at the site of anastomosis, in the donor renal artery, or in the recipient hypogastric artery (207). The causes include faulty suture technique, damage to the donor arterial intima during perfusion, intimal damage from rejection, improper apposition of the donor and recipient vessels with torsion, excessive length of the renal artery leading to angulation, or atherosclerosis in the recipient artery. An increased incidence of renal artery stenosis has been observed following transplantation of small pediatric cadaver donor kidney.

Renal arteriography is indicated whenever an allograft recipient has severe hypertension or unexplained deterioration in renal function (104). Renal vein renin measurements and captopril renography are of limited diagnostic value in this setting. Revascularization of the allograft is indicated when arterial stenosis is considered the cause

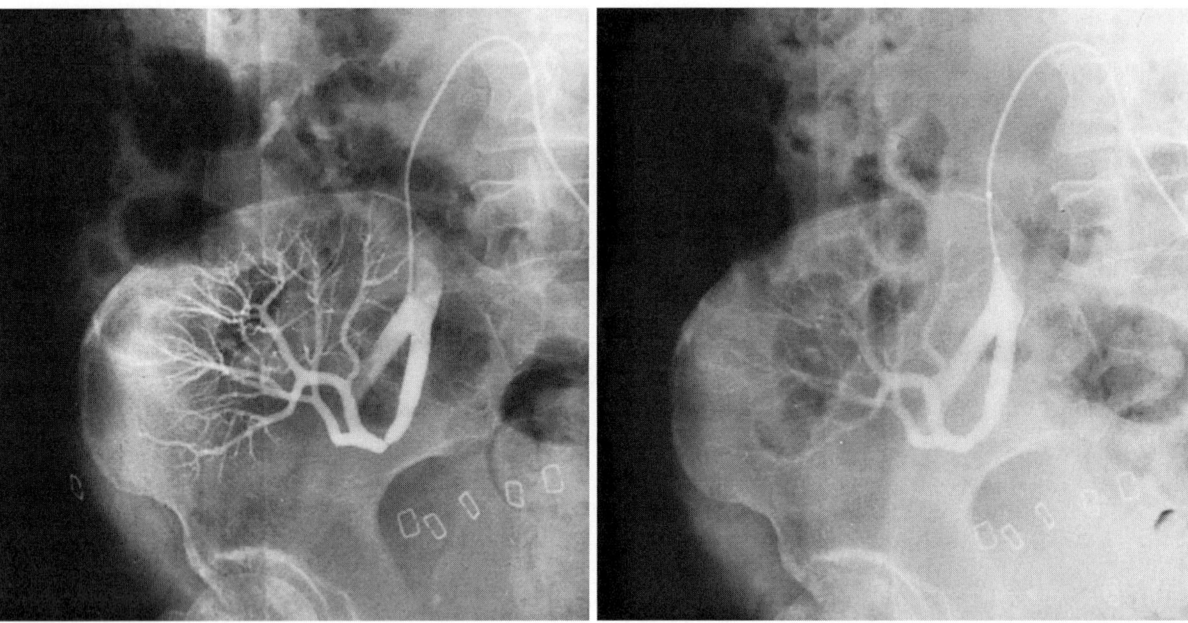

FIGURE 22.37. A: Transplant arteriogram demonstrates significant stenosis at the site of anastomosis of the recipient hypogastric artery to the donor artery. **B:** Following percutaneous transluminal angioplasty, a repeat transplant arteriogram shows complete resolution of the arterial stenosis.

of intractable hypertension or renal dysfunction. Percutaneous transluminal angioplasty has yielded satisfactory results in these patients and is an appropriate initial option (100,233) (Fig. 22.37). Secondary surgical revascularization is indicated if angioplasty cannot be done or is unsuccessful.

A variety of techniques have been described for performing secondary arterial revascularization of a renal allograft. These include segmental arterial resection with end-to-end anastomosis, saphenous vein bypass for the proximal common iliac artery or aorta, direct reimplantation into the common or external iliac artery, patch angioplasty, or anastomosis to the hypogastric artery if this vessel is available. These are technically complex operations due to the frequent presence of dense scar tissue around the allograft; the renal vein and ureter are also often adherent to the renal artery. The results of surgical revascularization in these patients are generally satisfactory but less so than those obtained with primary revascularization of the native or transplant kidney (Table 22.10) (60,63,146,296). These operations should be performed through a transabdominal incision, which facilitates identification of the transplant renal artery. We have found that a saphenous vein bypass graft from the common iliac artery or aorta to the distal disease-free transplant renal artery is a relatively straightforward, versatile, and effective technique (Fig. 22.38). Occasionally, with a long renal artery and a short focal area of stenosis, segmental resection with reanastomosis is a satisfactory option.

Renal Artery Pseudoaneurysm

Renal arterial pseudoaneurysm formation is a potentially devastating complication of renal transplantation that occurs in less than 1% of patients (94,145,235,236). Pseudoaneurysms may result from infection, injury to the renal artery during procurement or preservation, ischemic damage from excessive stripping of the artery and its vasa vasorum, faulty suture technique, or external traumatic injury. These mechanisms produce disruption of the arterial wall, usually at the site of arterial anastomosis, leading to the development of a communicating sac lined by fibrous and adventitial tissue.

The natural history of transplant renal artery pseudoaneurysm is not known, although it is clear that rupture can

TABLE 22.10. RESULTS OF SURGICAL REVASCULARIZATION FOR TRANSPLANT RENAL ARTERY STENOSIS

	No. of Patients	No. of Successful
Dickerman, 1980[63]	16	12
Rijksen, 1982	25	18
Tilney, 1984[296]	21	14
Benoit, 1987	40	32
Lacombe, 1988[146]	63	51
DeMeyer, 1989[60]	16	15
Total	181	142 (78%)

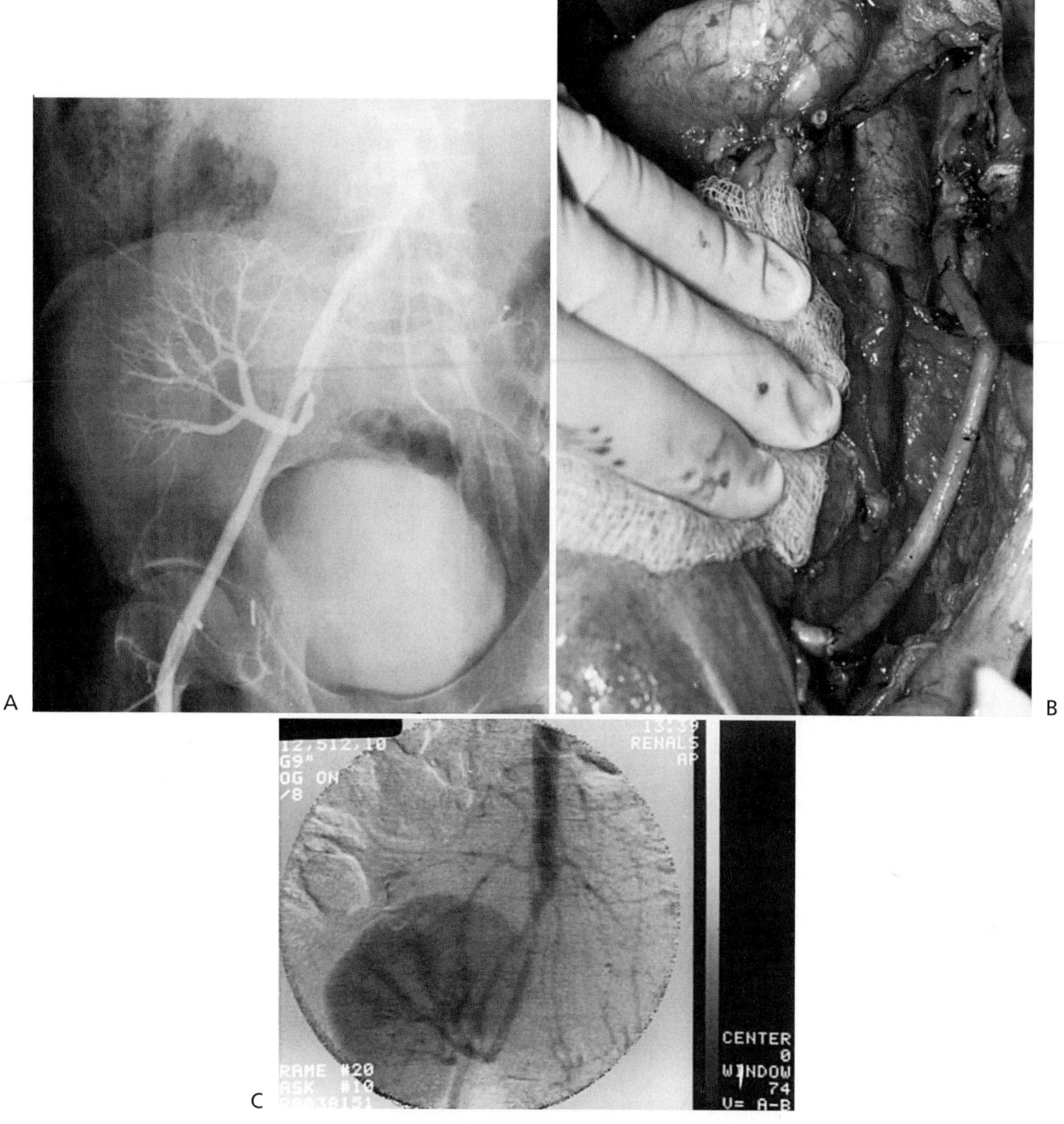

FIGURE 22.38. A: Pelvic arteriogram shows severe stenosis of proximal artery to right renal allograft. **B:** Operative photograph of completed aortorenal saphenous vein bypass. **C:** Postoperative intravenous digital subtraction angiogram shows patent bypass to renal allograft.

occur even if the aneurysm is not affected. Hypertension and deterioration of renal function also can result from pseudoaneurysm formation, usually through extrinsic compression of the renal vessels with consequent diminished allograft perfusion. Transplant nephrectomy generally has been performed to prevent rupture (94,145,235), while *in situ* reconstruction and allograft salvage have only rarely been described (236).

We recently treated a transplant recipient with stable graft function and a 6.5-cm renal artery pseudoaneurysm causing severe hypertension and sciatic pain. Excision of the pseudoaneurysm and reconstruction were indicated to prevent rupture, reduce hypertension, and maintain stable allograft function. At surgery, extensive fibrosis was observed around the pseudoaneurysm, which enveloped the external iliac artery and renal vessels. The renal allograft together with the pseudoaneurysm and a segment of the external iliac artery were removed en bloc, and the allograft was quickly flushed with cold Collins solution. The excised segment of external iliac artery was replaced with an interposition synthetic graft. Extracorporeal renal vascular reconstruction was performed, and the repaired graft was autotransplanted into the contralateral iliac fossa (Fig. 22.39). This approach allowed allograft revascularization to be done in a previously unoperated area using healthy recipient vessels. Extracorporeal reconstruction and autotransplantation of a renal allograft has not previously been reported but can be an effective salvage technique for selected patients with complex vascular lesions involving the transplant kidney (35).

Allograft Rupture

Spontaneous allograft rupture is an uncommon complication that usually occurs within the first month after transplantation (196). Graft rupture is most often seen in transplant recipients undergoing an acute rejection episode. Although this complication was formerly observed in 1% to 10% of patients, it is now only rarely encountered (less than 1%) because patients on cyclosporine maintenance therapy do not generally experience severe graft enlargement during acute rejection. Trauma, ureteral obstruction, and recent open renal biopsy are additional predisposing factors for graft rupture. Routine capsulotomy at the time of transplantation does not obviate postoperative graft rupture. The clinical picture includes sudden pain and swelling of the graft, a palpable flank mass, oliguria, and vascular collapse.

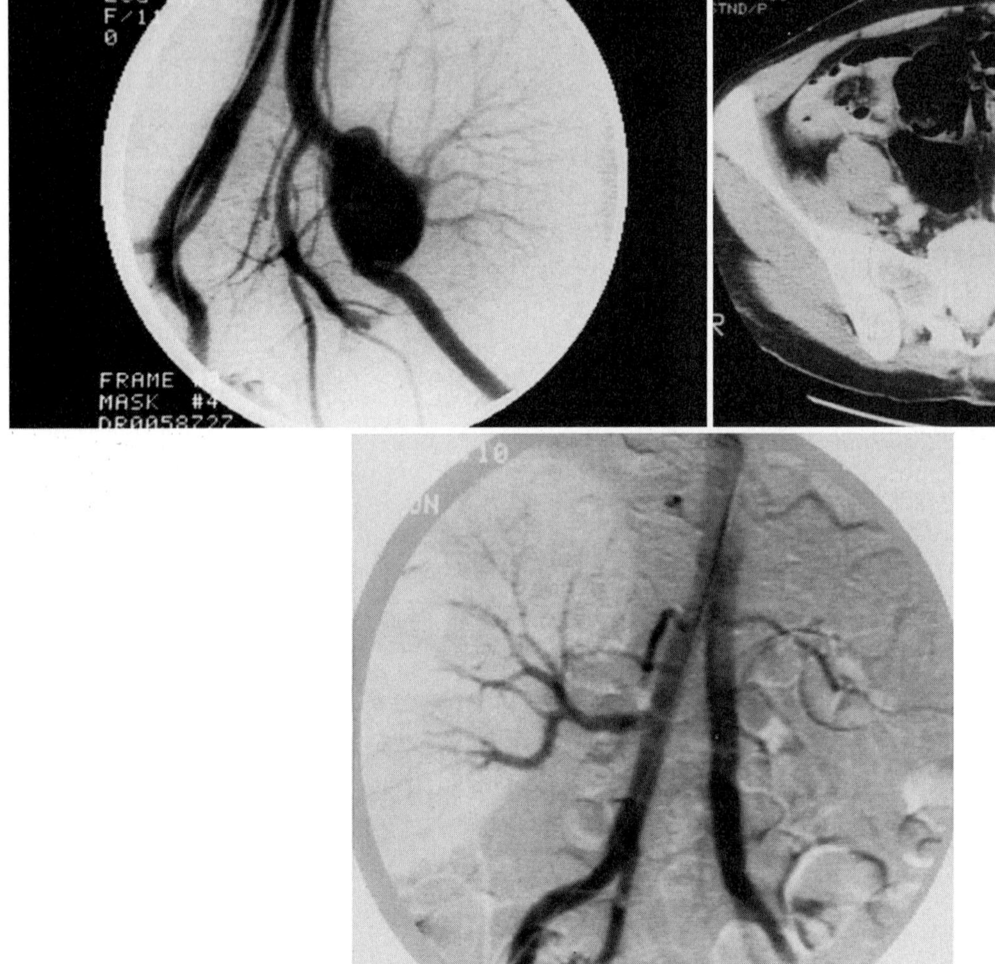

FIGURE 22.39. A: Arteriogram reveals large pseudoaneurysm arising near arterial anastomosis between renal artery and left external iliac artery. Intrarenal vasculature can be seen lateral to pseudoaneurysm. **B:** Pelvic computed tomography scan shows large renal artery pseudoaneurysm extending posteriorly in left iliac fossa. **C:** Following extracorporeal revascularization and autotransplantation, arteriogram shows patent anastomosis of reconstructed renal artery to right common iliac artery. (From Campbell SC, Gill I, Novick AC. Delayed allograft autotransplantation after excision of a large symptomatic renal artery pseudoaneurysm. *J Urol* 1993;149:361, with permission.)

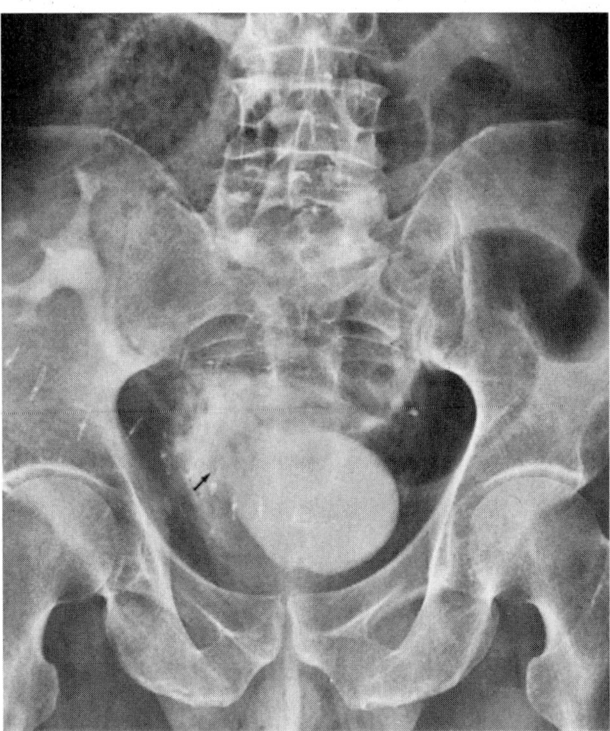

FIGURE 22.40. Intravenous pyelogram shows extravasation of contrast material from a distal ureteral fistula. (From Novick AC, Straffon RA, eds. *Vascular problems in urologic surgery.* Philadelphia: WB Saunders, 1982, with permission.)

If the graft is functionally salvageable and it is technically feasible, the laceration should be repaired. If the graft has been irreversibly damaged by rejection or if multiple areas of rupture preclude a satisfactory repair, nephrectomy provides the optimum treatment.

Ureteral Fistula

Ureteral fistulae most often manifest early in the posttransplant course and may be heralded by pain or swelling over the allograft. Unilateral leg edema may also be present; occasionally, fluid will egress from the wound. A definitive diagnosis can be made by determination of electrolyte, urea, and creatinine concentrations in any fluid collected from the incision or from fluid aspirated percutaneously. This will help differentiate urine from serum or lymph. Diagnostic radiographic studies include intravenous pyelography (Fig. 22.40), ultrasound, and CT (33,220). When renal function is adequate, intravenous contrast can be given during CT scanning to differentiate urine from other fluid collections. A plain film can be taken immediately after the CT to obtain anatomic information equivalent to that with intravenous urography. As is the case for patients with transplant ureteral obstruction, however, the level of function at the time the urinary extravasation is diagnosed may not be adequate to allow administration of intravenous contrast. Retrograde studies can be difficult and have often been replaced by routine percutaneous nephrostomy placement and antegrade pyelography. In this setting, the percutaneous nephrostomy allows early proximal diversion and access for subsequent follow-up studies. It also allows precise delineation of the level of extravasation to plan further management.

Ureteral fistulae almost always result from compromise of ureteral vascularity, the result of which is ureteral necrosis and sloughing. As such, the distal ureter is most commonly involved, although the necrosis can involve the entire ureter. Less often, the ureteral fistula is a result of a local technical factor associated with the ureteroneocystostomy that then results in a distal ureteral leak. In any case, standard intervention for a ureteral fistula is immediate open operative intervention (196,248). For fistulae limited to the distal ureter or ureteroneocystostomy itself, a repeat ureteral reimplant can be performed and a stent temporarily left indwelling. If viability of the more proximal transplant ureter is in question, repeat ureteroneocystostomy is not appropriate. In these cases, the ureter is resected back as far as necessary to ensure that it has an adequate blood supply. Options for reconstruction then include ureteroureterostomy with anastomosis of the native ureter to the proximal transplant ureter or, when the entire allograft ureter is nonviable, a ureteropyelostomy (Fig. 22.41). In all cases, an internal stent is left indwelling for these secondary reconstructive procedures (20). If associated infection is also a factor, externalized drains should be placed near the anastomosis, and in some cases, nephrostomy drainage should be implemented (95).

Percutaneous nephrostomy drainage has gained a role for adjunctive and at times definitive management of ureteral fistulae (154,275). When a ureteral fistula is diagnosed, institution of percutaneous nephrostomy drainage allows early proximal diversion and access for radiographic studies that allow precise delineation of the site of extravasation. Such antegrade studies are especially important when compromised renal function does not allow administration of intravenous contrast for urography or CT. When a percutaneous nephrostomy has been placed for diagnostic purposes, it can be left indwelling during the postreconstructive period to allow proximal urinary diversion and access for postoperative radiographic evaluation.

In some cases, percutaneous techniques can be used to obviate entirely the need for secondary operative reconstruction. Successful endourologic management of ureteral fistulae is a likely result only in select patients in whom antegrade studies suggest extravasation limited to the distal ureter and in whom contrast enters the bladder during antegrade pyelography. Proximal extravasation or failure of contrast to enter the bladder suggests extensive ureteral loss, and in such cases, percutaneous treatment will rarely prove definitive. When percutaneous management is selected, the optimal approach involves placement of a guidewire, and subsequently a stent, across the site of extravasation into the bladder. Ultimately, the patient should be left with an

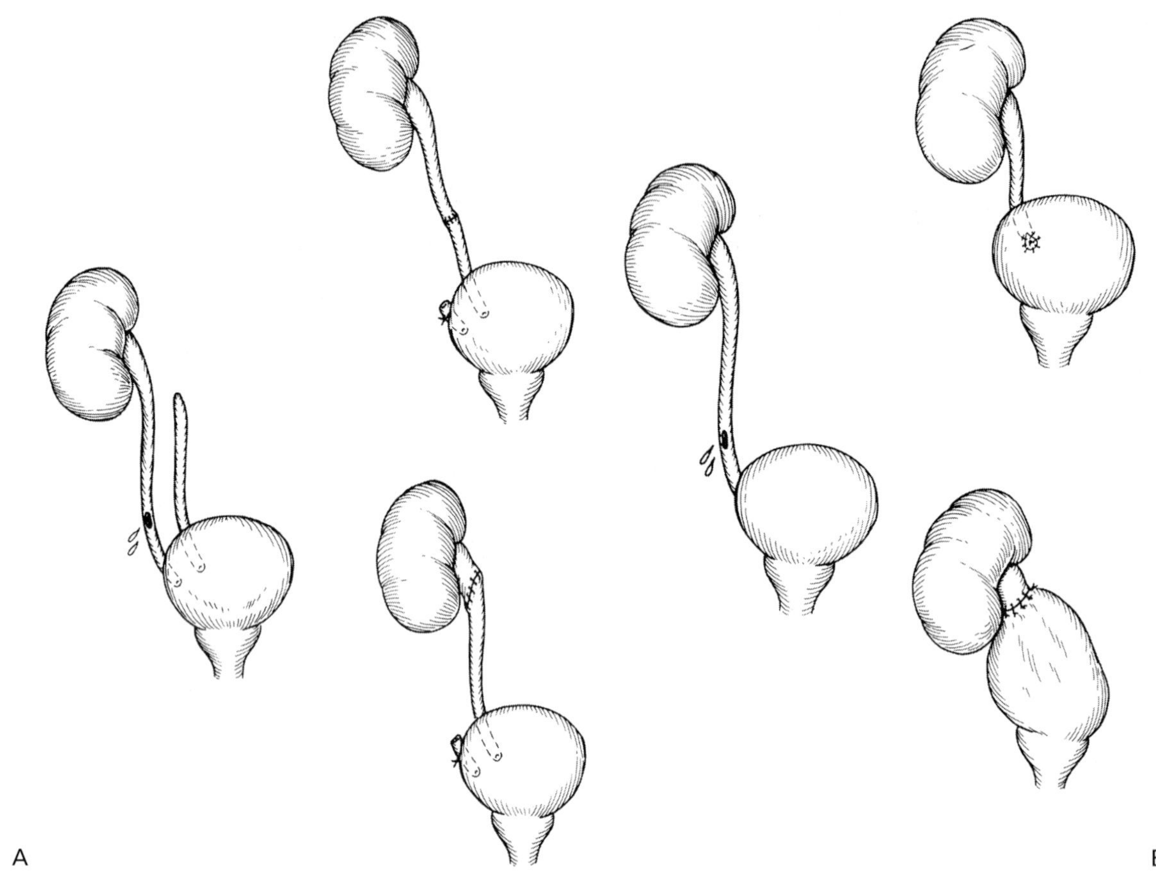

FIGURE 22.41. A: When ipsilateral native ureter is available, ureteral fistula can be repaired with ureteroneocystostomy *(top)* or ureteropyelostomy *(bottom).* **B:** When ipsilateral native ureter is absent, ureteral fistula can be repaired with ureteroneocystostomy *(top)* or pyelovesicostomy *(bottom).* (From Novick AC, Straffon RA, eds. *Vascular problems in urologic surgery.* Philadelphia: WB Saunders, 1982, with permission.)

internal stent and a nephrostomy tube for drainage or an internal-external stent for external drainage. Percutaneous management can be continued as long as the patient remains stable clinically and serial radiographic studies show the fistula to be resolving. Separate percutaneous drainage of a urinoma should be performed if it is infected, particularly large, or in any way symptomatic.

Although percutaneous techniques can provide long-term definitive management for some transplant ureteral fistulae, success rates will be limited. As such, we believe the primary roles of percutaneous techniques in this setting are for diagnosis and as therapeutic adjuncts before definitive operative reconstruction. In our experience, definitive percutaneous management of transplant ureteral fistulae has had a success rate of only 36%, even in highly selected patients (36).

Calyceal Fistula

Calyceal fistula is now a rare complication of renal transplantation that is essentially always the result of segmental renal infarction. Contemporary vascular techniques for management of multiple renal arteries have relegated this to a rare cause of urinary fistula. Standard intervention historically involved open exploration with debridement and drainage, along with primary closure of the involved collecting system. Unfortunately, such management was associated with unacceptably high rates of graft loss and mortality. Improved results were subsequently reported with operative placement of nephrostomy tubes and institution of external drainage. More recently, calyceal fistulae have been shown to resolve with external drainage alone. The contemporary management of this uncommon complication should consist of institution of percutaneous catheter drainage at the site of extravasation. If there is any degree of urinary obstruction associated with the fistula, percutaneous nephrostomy drainage or internal stenting should also be instituted. With adequate percutaneous drainage, calyceal fistulae should resolve without the need for open operative intervention.

Bladder Fistula

The incidence of bladder fistulae has decreased with the increasingly infrequent use of an extravesical, rather than a transvesical, ureteroneocystostomy to restore urinary continuity at the time of transplantation (93,295). The diagnosis of a bladder fistula is relatively easy to establish with a cystogram, which generally reveals extravasation of contrast. If a catheter had not been indwelling at the time the extravasation became evident, a cautious trial of standard catheter bladder drainage alone can be instituted, although separate percutaneous drainage of a urinoma may be indicated as described earlier. Failure of this management to result in resolution should prompt open exploration with debridement and repair.

A bladder fistula diagnosed in the presence of an extravesical ureteroneocystostomy is generally diagnostic of leakage at the ureteroneocystostomy itself. In such cases, catheter drainage alone will rarely be successful. However, if the extravasation is limited to the distal ureter as defined by intravenous or antegrade pyelography, a trial of percutaneous management can be instituted as described for ureteral fistulae. A failure of or contraindication to percutaneous management necessitates prompt open operative intervention as for ureteral fistulae.

Ureteral Obstruction

Ureteral obstruction is generally a late complication of renal transplantation. The contemporary incidence has decreased to less than 5% to 10% of renal allograft recipients, but this complication still accounts for up to one-third of all significant urologic complications (139). The diagnosis is usually made during evaluation of azotemia in an otherwise asymptomatic patient, at which time standard radiographic study with ultrasonography will identify hydronephrosis. If renal

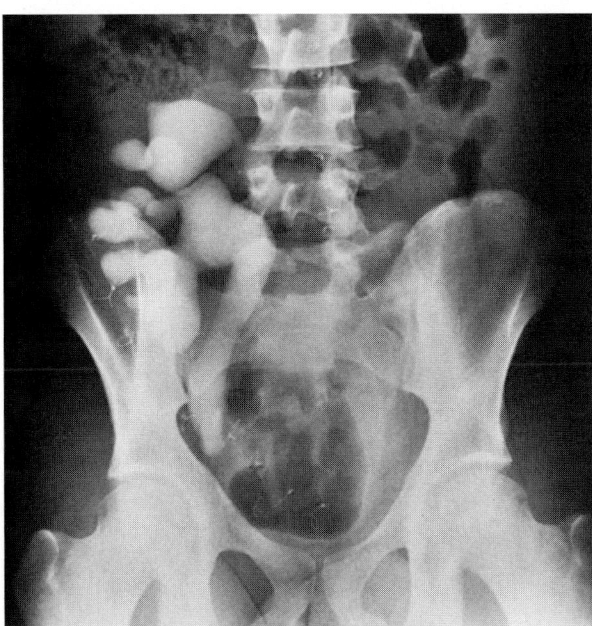

FIGURE 22.42. Intravenous pyelogram demonstrates hydronephrosis from distal ureteral obstruction. (From Novick AC, Straffon RA, eds. *Vascular problems in urologic surgery.* Philadelphia: WB Saunders, 1982, with permission.)

function is adequate, intravenous urography may allow delineation of the site of obstruction (Fig. 22.42). Retrograde pyelography may be attempted to define the site of obstruction, although difficulty in cannulation of the neoureteral orifice has generally led to abandonment of this study in favor of percutaneous nephrostomy placement with antegrade pyelography. In some cases, the functional significance of a mildly dilated collecting system may be unclear. In these cases, the effect on renal function of prolonged percutaneous drainage can provide a definitive answer. Further evaluation with antegrade pressure/perfusion studies may also be of benefit in select cases. Definitive operative reconstruction of transplant ureter obstruction is dependent on the etiology and site of obstruction. The most common problem is distal obstruction that involves the ureteroneocystostomy. Although technical factors at the time of transplantation may have played a role, ureteral ischemia should be considered. This is especially true when longer segments of the ureter appear to be involved. Less common causes of ureteral obstruction include extrinsic compression by hematoma, lymphocele or abscess, ureteral kinking, or less commonly, previously unrecognized intrinsic ureteropelvic junction obstruction. Rarely, intermittent obstruction can result from placement of the ureteral anastomosis in the mobile anterior dome of the bladder.

If the obstruction is limited to the very distal ureter, a repeat ureteroneocystostomy can be performed (196). In these cases, intraoperative placement of a soft, self-retaining internal stent that is left indwelling for 4 to 6 weeks should be considered. For extensive ureteral involvement, a nearly universally applicable reconstructive technique uses the native ureter for a ureteropyelostomy to the transplant renal pelvis (247). This avoids the need for extensive dissection of the transplant ureter and at the same time obviates the need to use a transplant ureter that may be of marginal quality. When the native ureter is used, the proximal native ureter can generally be ligated and the native kidney left *in situ* (159). However, in the presence of infection, native nephrectomy should be performed. An alternative to nephrectomy is anastomosis of the native ureter in a side-to-side fashion to the transplant renal pelvis (142). This precludes the possibility of a late complication associated with simple ligation of that ureter. Again, an internal stent is left indwelling during the early postoperative period. If a percutaneous nephrostomy had been placed before definitive repair, this also can be left indwelling during the initial postoperative period to provide temporary urinary diversion and access for postreconstructive radiographic studies.

When the native ureter is not available or is otherwise inappropriate for use in reconstruction, a variety of salvage reconstructive procedures may be used. These include vesicopyelostomy during which the bladder is anastomosed directly to the renal pelvis, with or without a bladder flap (229). An alternative to vesicopyelostomy for complicated reconstruction is an ileal interposition. In rare cases in which the transplant renal pelvis cannot be accessed either because of peripelvic fibrosis or an intrarenal anatomy, consideration can be given to native ureterocalicostomy or vesicocalicostomy (123,312).

In recent years, transplant ureteral obstruction has been managed entirely with an endourologic approach by combining percutaneous nephrostomy drainage with transluminal ureteral dilation or endoscopic incisional ureterotomy. Those patients best suited for an endourologic approach are those with short, discrete strictures limited to the distal ureter or ureterovesical anastomosis itself (276). Midureteral narrowing suggests extrinsic compression, and long areas of stricture suggest extensive fibrosis, in which case endourologic management is unlikely to prove definitive. Similarly, ureteropelvic junction obstruction in transplanted kidneys generally results from unrecognized intrinsic ureteropelvic junction obstruction in the donor organ or from kinking at the time of transplantation. In either case, simple ureteral dilation is again unlikely to be successful. As an endourologic alternative, percutaneous endopyelotomy may have a definitive role. Reports of endourologic management of transplant ureteral stenosis have become available in larger numbers of patients, and these results suggest a 45% to 70% success rate, even after extended periods of follow-up (19,276).

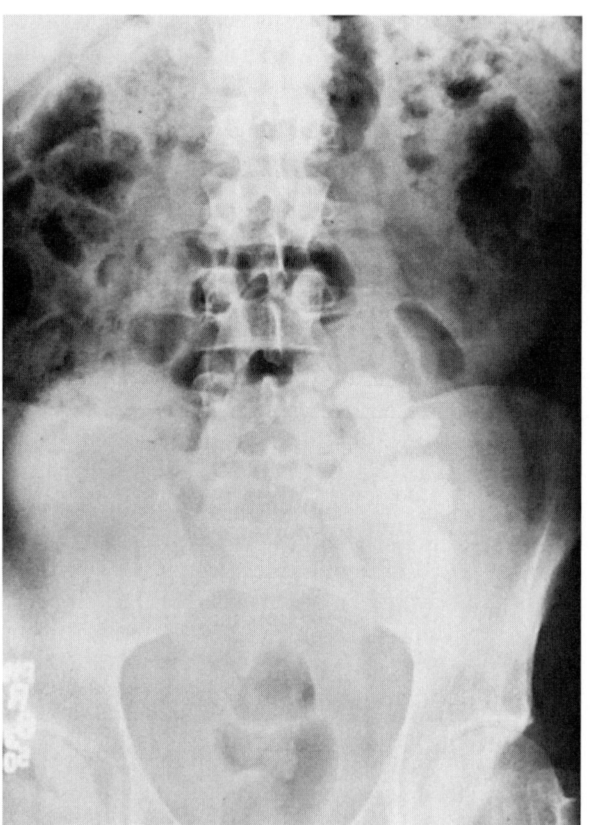

FIGURE 22.43. Intravenous pyelogram demonstrates hydronephrosis and bladder displacement from a large pelvic lymphocele. (From Novick AC, Straffon RA, eds. *Vascular problems in urologic surgery.* Philadelphia: WB Saunders, 1982, with permission.)

Lymphocele

A *lymphocele* is a collection of lymph around the allograft. Lymphoceles may be unilocular or multilocular or encapsulated, ranging in size from a small, insignificant collection to a large obstructing mass containing more than 1,000 mL of fluid. A lymphocele is caused by lymphatic leakage from the allograft bed or the allograft itself. Care in ligation of perirenal lymphatics during donor nephrectomy and recipient lymphatics during preparation of the iliac fossa is essential in preventing this complication. Normally, severed lymphatics close within 48 hours and regenerate within 7 to 10 days. However, in transplant recipients, several factors can predispose to prolonged lymphatic leakage. These factors include rejection, open transplant biopsy, and the use of various medications such as steroids, diuretics, and anticoagulants. Retransplantation has also been implicated in the development of lymphoceles (273).

The most common initial signs and symptoms of a lymphocele are urinary frequency, suprapubic pressure, a ballottable mass adjacent to the allograft, and edema of the ipsilateral thigh and genitalia. Findings suggestive of rejection, such as hypertension, oliguria, decreased renal function, and proteinuria, may also be present. With a significant lymphocele, intravenous pyelography usually shows hydronephrosis or displacement of the bladder, with no extravasation of contrast material (Fig. 22.43). Cystography will confirm extrinsic bladder compression and the absence of extravasation. Currently, ultrasonography and CT scanning are the diagnostic methods of choice for establishing the presence, location, and extent of perinephric fluid collections. If a urinary fistula is suspected, a CT scan with contrast should be performed. Needle aspiration and determination of the creatinine and urea content of the fluid can also distinguish urinoma from lymphocele.

Small, loculated, low-density perinephric fluid collections are relatively common following transplantation. If the patient is clinically asymptomatic with no radiographic evidence of obstructive uropathy or urinary extravasation, no treatment is necessary.

When a significant lymphocele is present, a drainage procedure is indicated. Percutaneous aspiration of the lymphocele with injection of a sclerosing agent may be performed but has a variable success rate (288,315). Definitive therapy is provided by internal marsupialization of the lymphocele into the peritoneal cavity (134,320). This was formerly accomplished through a surgical abdominal incision, but laparoscopic internal lymphocele drainage can now be performed with excellent results (69,138,184,311).

Hydrocele

The incidence of ipsilateral hydrocele formation after renal transplantation has been reported to be as high as 68% when the spermatic cord is transacted at the time of transplantation (213). Therefore this practice has largely been abandoned. Transection of the spermatic cord results in interference with lymphatic drainage of the testicle and leads to accumulation of hydrocele fluid. In addition, the testicle is rendered ischemic due to interruption of the main blood supply, making its viability totally dependent on collateral circulation. Hydrocelectomy in these patients is fraught with the potential complications of testicular loss and abscess formation (213). Aspiration of a hydrocele with tetracycline sclerotherapy is an alternative and effective treatment modality (246). Fortunately, the majority of hydroceles after renal transplantation are asymptomatic, and only a few require treatment. Symptoms are usually related to discomfort, pain, interference with sexual activity, or embarrassment related to size. The diagnosis is usually evident on physical examination and by transillumination. Ultrasound may be used to document the size and pattern of the hydrocele, to assess the testicle, and as an adjunct to aspiration and sclerotherapy.

RESULTS OF RENAL TRANSPLANTATION

More sensitive histocompatibility crossmatching techniques, which have virtually eliminated hyperacute rejection episodes; careful patient selection with appropriate preoperative evaluation, reducing immediate postoperative complications; refinements in surgical techniques, minimizing technical losses; development of newer immunosuppressive drugs and strategies, lowering the incidence of early rejection; and enhanced therapy against infections, especially antiviral agents, have all contributed to an improvement in the success of renal transplantation in the past few years. One-year patient survival now exceeds 95% for all transplant groups, and 1-year allograft survival exceeds 85% for cadaveric and 95% for one-haplotype and HLA-identical recipients, respectively (Fig. 22.44). As depicted in Fig. 22.45, this enhanced 1-year survival has resulted in a slowly increasing graft survival half-life for cadaveric as well as living donor recipients (42).

During the 1990s, there was a slow but persistent improvement in long-term renal allograft survival. This is best analyzed by comparing the survival half-lives of kidneys. The introduction of cyclosporine in the early 1980s resulted in improved 1-year survivals of up to 80%, but little improvement in cadaveric half-life of more than 7 to 8 years. However, further incremental advances in immunosuppression and patient management have now produced a significant prolongation in survival half-life of 21.6 years for live donor and 13.8 years for cadaveric donor recipients (108). It has been suggested that these findings may be a direct result of the decreased rates of acute rejection during the first posttransplant year, because these early rejection episodes have been shown to be a major cause of chronic rejection and late graft loss (6,70,80,124).

The influence of HLA matching on graft survival is obvious between live donor and cadaveric recipients (42). As illustrated in Fig. 22.46, 5-year survival rates are 87%, 75%, and 60% with corresponding half-lives of 24.8 years, 13.9 years, and 9 years for HLA-identical, one-haplotype, and cadaver recipients, respectively. However, the exact benefit of HLA matching within subgroups, especially cadav-

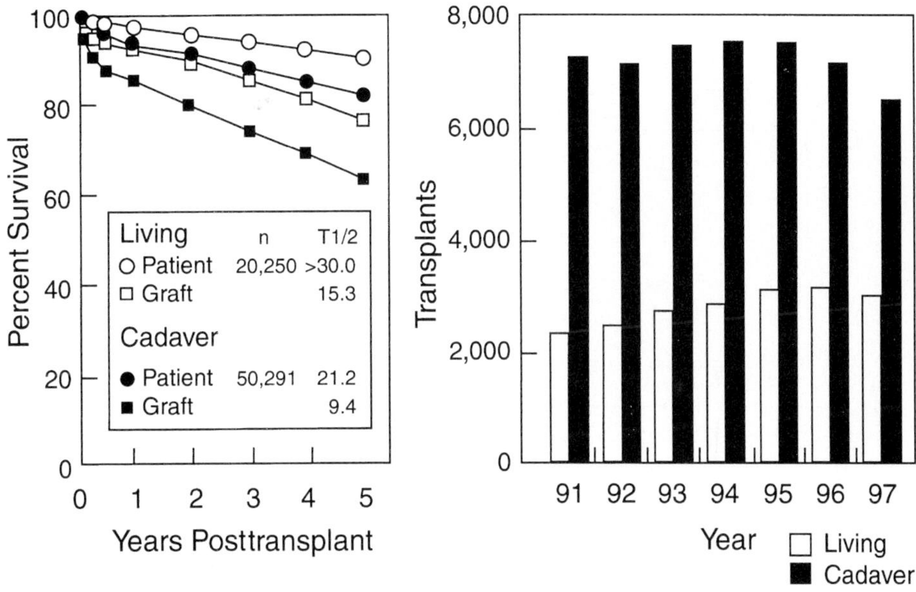

FIGURE 22.44. Patient and allograft survival by year based on donor relationship. (From Cecka JM. The UNOS scientific renal transplant registry. In: Terasaki PI, Cecka JM, eds. *Clinical transplants, 1998.* Los Angeles: UCLA Tissue Typing Laboratory, 1998:2, with permission.)

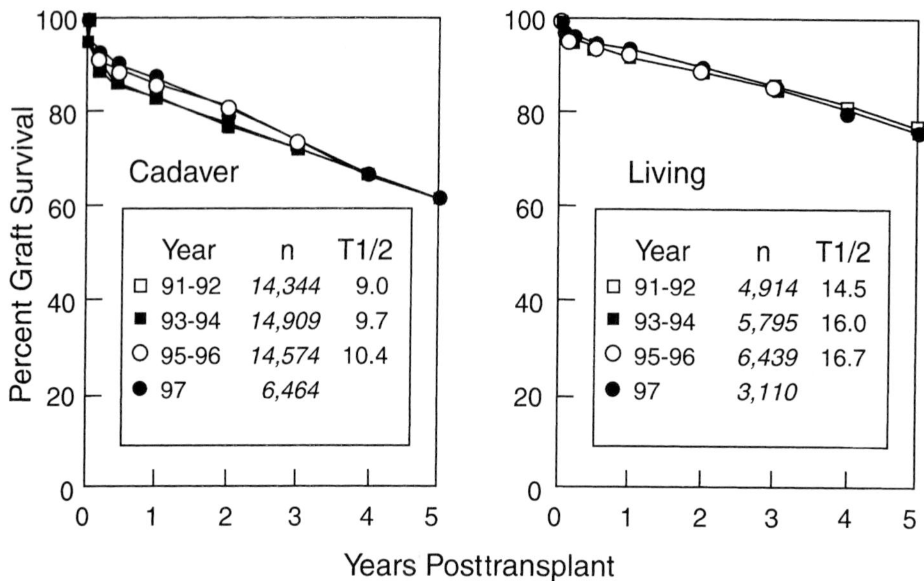

FIGURE 22.45. Allograft survival rates by year for major subgroups. (From Cecka JM. The UNOS scientific renal transplant registry. In: Terasaki PI, Cecka JM, eds. *Clinical transplants, 1998.* Los Angeles: UCLA Tissue Typing Laboratory, 1998:2, with permission.)

eric recipients, is not so obvious. The data demonstrate 5-year graft survival of 70% for six-antigen matched kidneys versus 58% for zero-antigen matched cadaver kidneys (Fig. 22.46). More impressively, six-antigen matched kidneys exhibited a half-life of 12.7 years compared with 8.0 years for kidneys with one or more mismatched antigens. It would appear reasonable to continue policies aimed at ensuring that best matched transplants are maximized (281). Unfortunately, incremental benefits (e.g., three-antigen versus four-antigen) are not as impressive (203). One reason for this latter observation is that prolonged cold ischemia times and shipping of kidneys have a detrimental effect on graft survival. Prolonged cold ischemia times increase the incidence of delayed graft function after

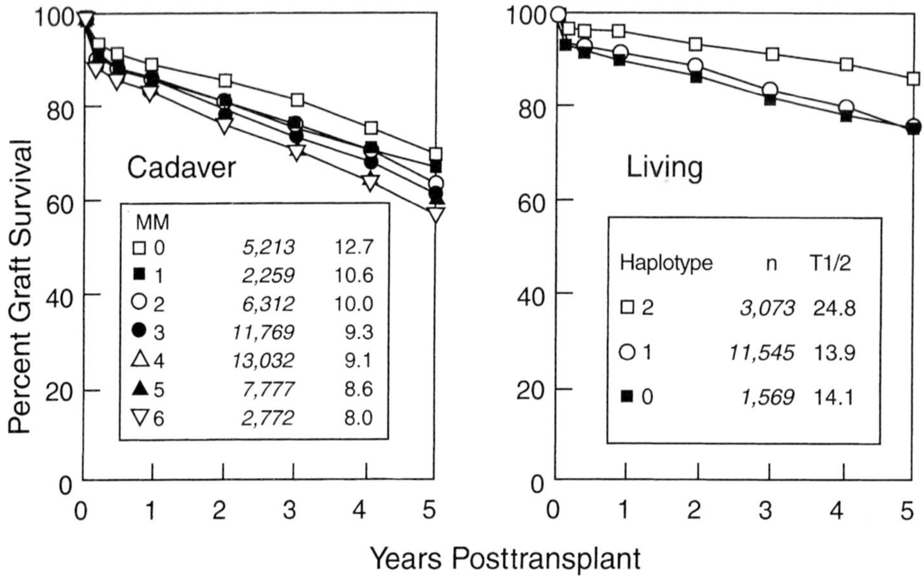

FIGURE 22.46. Rate of cadaveric and live donor graft loss at 5 years based on HLA matching. Data from more than 65,000 transplants, 1991–1997. Cadaveric transplants ranged from zero to six mismatched HLA antigens. (From Cecka JM. The UNOS scientific renal transplant registry. In: Terasaki PI, Cecka JM, eds. *Clinical transplants, 1998.* Los Angeles: UCLA Tissue Typing Laboratory, 1998:10, with permission.)

transplant (Fig. 22.47). This is especially true for older-age cadaver kidneys. Delayed graft function in turn may negate any small advantage from fewer degrees of HLA matching.

The most commonly cited cause of allograft failure after the first year is chronic rejection. Unfortunately, chronic rejection is largely an ill-defined, poorly understood process that results in unrelenting, progressive renal damage (80,118,124,170). The diagnosis of chronic rejection is usually based on histopathology, which includes among other findings interstitial fibrosis, tubular atrophy, arteriolar intimal thickening with narrowing of the lumen, and glomerulosclerosis (261). No specific treatment exists for chronic rejection other than preventing precipitating events and treating potential exacerbating factors (e.g., hypertension). A number of studies have implicated acute rejection as a risk factor for chronic rejection and subsequent allograft loss (6,70,80). Ferguson (70) reported a half-life of 16.9 years in patients experiencing no rejection versus 3.9 years in recipients experiencing more than one rejection episode. However, it is clear that not all patients experiencing acute rejection are destined to develop chronic rejection and allograft loss. In reviewing 53 patients at our institute who had functioning grafts surviving more than 20 years, Braun and colleagues (29) reported that 58% had experienced acute rejection episodes. Nevertheless, the recent increase in survival half-lives appears to be enjoyed by patients who experienced no acute rejection episodes during the first year (Fig. 22.48). Although predicting who develops chronic rejection after an acute rejection episode may not be possible, the data suggest that preventing an acute rejection episode is the most effective way to achieve long-term graft success.

Death with a functioning allograft has emerged as a major cause of long-term graft loss, especially in older recipients and diabetics. Matas and colleagues (171) have indicated that survival rates calculated counting death with a functioning graft as a cause of allograft loss are dramatically different from those calculated censoring patients who die with a functioning graft, and they have suggested that results should be reported both ways. In their series, nondiabetic living donor non–HLA-identical recipients greater than age 50 had a half-life of 9 years when death with function was considered graft loss, compared with a half-life of 62 years when data with function were censored. Other centers have reported similar results and have even demonstrated better survival in older recipients than young ones (suggesting less immunologic graft loss) when death with a functioning graft was censored (223,290). As more high-risk patients, especially diabetic and older patients, are transplanted and survive the early posttransplant period, death with a functioning graft is likely to become the predominant cause of graft loss in centers where it has not already done so.

Delayed graft function also adversely affects long-term survival, although the primary effect may be earlier (42,186,257). Although donor and organ preservation factors clearly affect the quality of initial function of the kidney

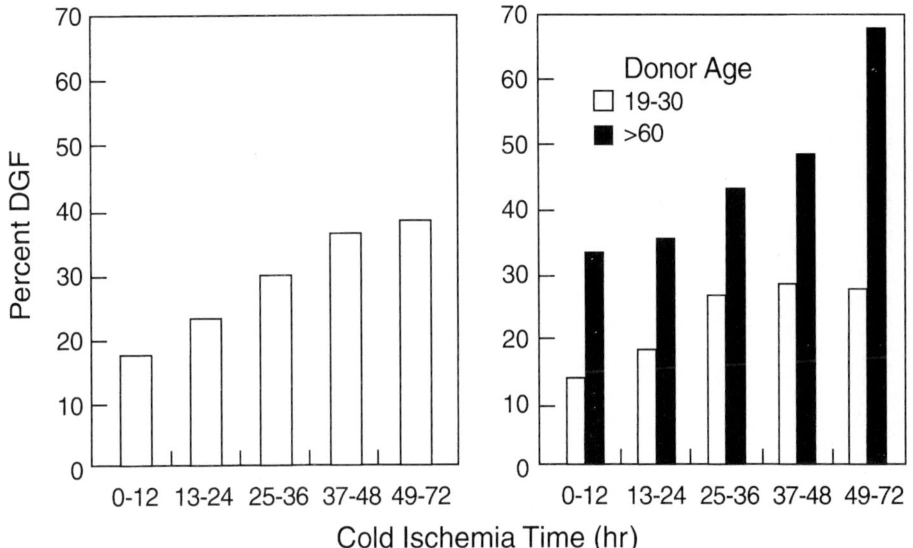

FIGURE 22.47. The effect of cold ischemia time on incidence of delayed graft function. Kidneys older than age 60 were especially susceptible, demonstrating twice the rate of delayed graft function at each 12-hour interval compared with kidneys age 19 to 30. (From Cecka JM. The UNOS scientific renal transplant registry. In: Terasaki PI, Cecka JM, eds. *Clinical transplants, 1998.* Los Angeles: UCLA Tissue Typing Laboratory, 1998:8, with permission.)

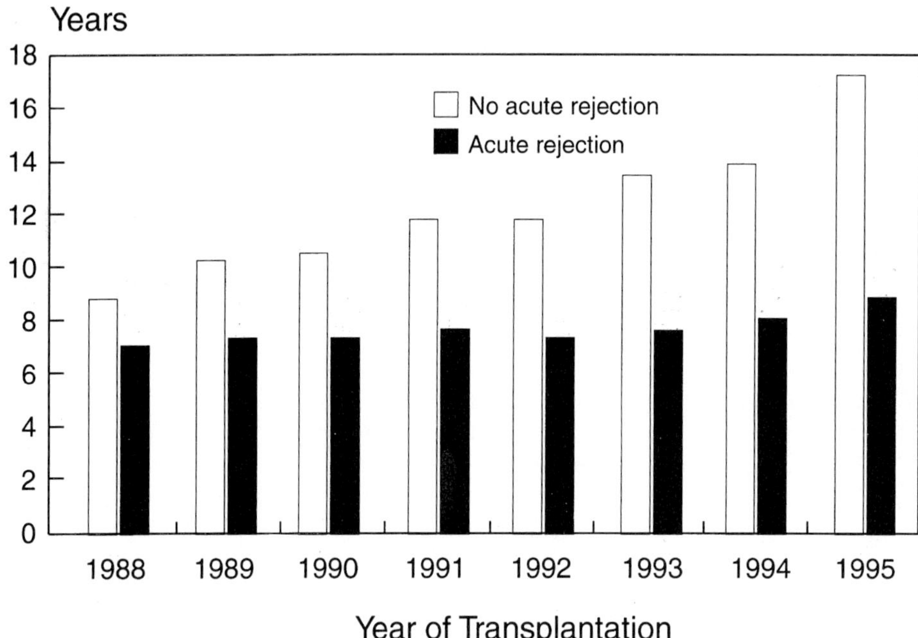

FIGURE 22.48. Projected half-life of grafts from cadaveric donors according to the presence or absence of clinical acute rejection during the first year after transplantation. (From Hariharan S, Johnson CP, Bresnahan BA, et al. Improved graft survival after renal transplantation in the United States 1988–1996. *N Engl J Med* 2000;342:605.)

following transplantation, evidence exists suggesting that immunologic factors contribute as well. Animal models have demonstrated increased MHC antigen expression related to ischemia (258). In addition, brain death itself may cause an upregulation of cell surface immunoreactive products and release of cytokines that promote both ischemic renal injury and immunologic injury (227). Other nonimmunologic causes may be responsible for long-term graft loss as well. Brenner and colleagues (31), noting diminished results with pediatric donors, female donors, and transplants into larger recipients, suggest that "one size may not fit all" and recommend matching of kidneys based on nephron dosing as well as HLA matching. Terasaki and colleagues (284) observed that elevated serum creatinines at the time of discharge from the hospital following transplantation correlated with decreased graft survival. They suggested that the hyperfiltration hypothesis (32) could explain diminished results seen in transplants using kidneys from infant and older donors, using kidneys from female donors to male recipients, occurring in obese patients, or following early acute rejection episodes.

As stated earlier, the ultimate goal for long-term success in renal transplantation is the induction of donor-specific tolerance in the recipient. Although this is not clinically achievable at present, recent observations have generated hope of its accomplishment in the near future. Using DNA typing and other technologies, Starzl and colleagues (267) have demonstrated the peripheral migration of donor cells (chimerism) in patients with long-term allograft survival who exhibit donor-specific nonreactivity following renal transplantation. Although a direct cause and effect of microchimerism and donor-specific hyporesponsiveness has not been demonstrated, it has allowed for investigation of immunosuppressive strategies. The infusion of donor allogeneic bone marrow into a recipient who has undergone myeloablation can lead to tolerance of allografts from the same donor (278). This involves the creation of a new immune system that becomes "educated" to recognize the alloantigens as "self." However, because of toxicity, the use of myeloablation has been limited to animals. A clinical trial using donor bone marrow and concomitant T-cell depletion with polyclonal antibodies has been encouraging, but has not resulted in tolerance (17). More recently, tolerance induction has been demonstrated in animals by blocking costimulatory signals to T cells. Costimulation is required for T-cell activation and to prevent T-cell anergy. Tolerance can be induced in animal models using blockade of the CD28–B7 interaction with a soluble recombinant fusion protein called CTLA-4Ig (155). In addition, blockade of CD154 (ligand of CD40) by monoclonal antibodies can tolerize murine skin and cardiac allografts (149). Clinical trials of costimulatory blockade are anticipated. Future improvement in results of renal transplantation will depend on utilization of knowledge of molecular events to develop more highly specific immunosuppressive agents—or, preferably, induce donor-specific tolerance, obviating the need for immunosuppressive agents altogether.

REFERENCES

1. Adams M, the Enisoprost Renal Transplant Study Group. Enisoprost in renal transplantation. *Transplantation* 1992;53:338.
2. Ahsan N, Hricik D, Matas A, et al. Prednisone withdrawal in kidney transplant recipients on cyclosporine and mycophenolate mofetil. *Transplantation* 1999;68:1865.
3. Alexander JW, First M, Majeski J, et al. The late adverse effect of splenectomy on patient survival following cadaver renal transplantation. *Transplantation* 1984;37:467.
4. Alexandre EP, Squifflet JP, DeBruyere M, et al. Splenectomy as a prerequisite for successful ABO incompatible renal transplantation. *Transplant Proc* 1985;17:138.
5. Allison AC, Eugui EM. Mycophenolate mofetil, a rationally designed immunosuppressive drug. *Clin Transplantation* 1993; 7:96.
6. Almond PS, Matas A, Gillingham K, et al. Risk factors for chronic rejection in renal allograft recipients. *Transplantation* 1993;55:752.
7. American College of Physicians Health and Public Policy Committee: Efficacy of exercise thallium-201 scintigraphy in the diagnosis and prognosis of coronary artery disease. *Ann Intern Med* 1990;113:703.
8. An analysis of 1518 laparoscopic cholecystectomies. The Southern Surgeons Club. *N Engl J Med* 1991;324:1073.
9. *1999 annual report of the US Scientific Registry for Transplant Recipients and the Organ Procurement and Transplantation Network—transplant data: 1989-1998.* Richmond, Va: Transplantation Network–UNOS; and Bethesda, Md: Division of Organ Transplantation, Bureau of Health Resources Development, Health Resources and Services Administration, US Department of Health and Human Services.
10. Aradhye S, Turka L. Will tolerance become a clinical reality? *Am J Med Sci* 1997;313:310.
11. Artero M, Biava C, Amend W, et al. Recurrent focal glomerulosclerosis. Natural history and response to therapy. *Am J Med* 1992;92:375.
12. Askari A, Novick A, Braun W, et al. The older living related donor. Prognosis for the donor and recipient. *J Urol* 1980; 129:779.
13. Auchincloss H, Sachs DH. Xenogenic transplantation. *Annu Rev Immunol* 1998;16:433.
14. Backman U, Fellstrom B, Frodin L, et al. Successful transplantation in highly sensitized patients. *Transplant Proc* 1989; 21:762.
15. Balfour HH, Chace BA, Stapleton JT, et al. A randomized placebo-controlled trial of oral acyclovir for the prevention of cytomegalovirus disease in recipients of renal allografts. *N Engl J Med* 1989;320:1381.
16. Banowsky LHW, Braun WE, Magnusson MO, et al. Current status of adult renal transplantation at the Cleveland Clinic Foundation. *J Urol* 1974;111:578.
17. Barber WH. Donor-specific transfusions in renal transplantation. *Clin Transplantation* 1994;8:204.
18. Belzer FO, Southard JH. Principles of solid organ preservation by cold storage. *Transplantation* 1988;44:673.
19. Benoit G, Alexander L, Moukarzel M, et al. Percutaneous antegrade dilations of ureteral strictures in kidney transplants. *J Urol* 1993;150:37.
20. Berger RE, Ansell TS, Treemann JA, et al. The use of self-retained ureteral stents in the management of urologic complications in renal transplant recipients. *J Urol* 1980;124:781.
21. Berger J, Yaneva H, Nabarva B, et al. Recurrence of mesangial deposition of IgA after renal transplantation. *Kidney Int* 1975; 7:232.
22. Billingham RE, Brent L, Medawar PB. The antigenic stimulus in transplantation immunity. *Nature* 1956;178:514.
23. Bissada NK. Incidence of vesical neck contracture complicating prostatic resection in hemodialysis patients. *J Urol* 1977; 117:192.
24. Bodmer JG, Marsh SGE, Albert, ED, et al. Nomenclature for factors of the HLA system. *Tissue Antigens* 1994;44:1.
25. Borel JF, Feurer C, Gubler HU, et al. Biological effects of cyclosporine A. A new antilymphocytic agent. *Agents Actions* 1976;6:468.
26. Borowicz MR, Hanevold CD, Cfer JB, et al. Extrinsic compression in the iliac fossa can cause renal vein occlusion in pediatric kidney recipients but graft loss can be prevented. *Transplant Proc* 1994;26:119.
27. Brattstrom C, Wilczek H, Tyden G, et al. Hyperlipidemia in renal transplant recipients treated with sirolimus (rapamycin). *Transplantation* 1998;65:1272.
28. Braun WE. Nephrology forum: long-term complications of renal transplantation. *Kidney Int* 1990;37:1363.
29. Braun WE, Popowniak KL, Gifford RW, et al. 20 year renal allograft successes do not confirm current dicta that acute rejection and delayed function portend chronic rejection and allograft failure. *Proc Am Soc Transplant Physicians* 1994;13: 87(abst).
30. Brenner BM, Cohen RA, Milford EL. In renal transplantation, one size may not fit all. *J Am Soc Nephrol* 1992;3:162.
31. Brenner B, Meger TL, Hostetter T. Dietary protein intake and the progressive nature of kidney disease. *N Engl J Med* 1982; 307:652.
32. Brennan DC, Flavin K, Lowell JA, et al. A randomized double-blinded comparison of thymoglobulin vs. ATGAM for induction therapy in adult renal transplant recipients. *Transplantation* 1999;67:1011.
33. Bretan PN Jr, Hodge E, Streem SB, et al. Diagnosis of renal transplant urinary fistulas. *Transplant Proc* 1989;21:1962.
34. Buszta C, Steinmuller DR, Schreiber M, et al. Pregnancy after donor nephrectomy. *Transplantation* 1985;40:651.
35. Campbell SC, Gill I, Novick AC. Delayed allograft autotransplantation after excision of a large symptomatic renal artery pseudoaneurysm. *J Urol* 1993;149:361.
36. Campbell SC, Streem SB, Zelch M, et al. Percutaneous management of transplant ureteral fistulas: patient selection and long-term results. *J Urol* 1993;150:1115.
37. Canadian Multicentre Transplant Study Group. A randomized clinical trial of cyclosporine in cadaveric renal transplantation. *N Engl J Med* 1983;309:809.
38. Carmody E, Greene A, Brennan P, et al. Sequential Tc mercaptoacetyl-triglycine (MAG3) renography as an evaluator of early renal transplant function. *Clin Transplantation* 1993;7:245.
39. Carpenter C, Ettenger R, Strom T. "Free market" approach to organ donation. *N Engl J Med* 1984;310:395.
40. Carrell A, Guthrie CC. Functions of a transplanted kidney. *Science* 1905;22:473.
41. Catalona WI, Smith DS, Ratliff T, et al. Measurement of prostate specific antigen in serum as screening test for prostate cancer. *N Engl J Med* 1991;324:1156.
42. Cecka JM, Terasaki PI. The UNOS scientific renal transplant registry. In: Terasaki PI, Cecka JM, eds. *Clinical transplants.* Los Angeles: UCLA Tissue Typing Laboratory, 1998.
43. Chatenoud L, Ferran C, Reuter A, et al. Systemic reaction to the anti–T cell monoclonal antibody OKT3 in relation to serum levels of tumor necrosis factor and interferon-gamma. *N Engl J Med* 1989;320:1420.

44. Cheung AK, De Vault GA Jr, Gregory MC. A prospective study on treatment of hypercholesterolemia with lovastatin in renal transplant recipients receiving cyclosporine. *J Am Soc Nephrol* 1993;3:1884.
45. Christiansen AJ, Holman JM, Turner CW. Quality of life in ESRD. Influence of renal transplantation. *Clin Transplantation* 1989;3:46.
46. Church IM, Fazio V, Braun WE, et al. Perforation of the colon in renal homograft recipients. *Ann Surg* 1986;203:69.
47. Cockfield SM, Preiksaitis JK, Jewel LD, et al. Posttransplant lymphoproliferative disorder in renal allograft recipients. Clinical experience and risk factor analysis in a single center. *Transplantation* 1993;56:8896.
48. Coffman T, Carr D, Yarger W, et al. Evidence that renal prostaglandin and thromboxane production is stimulated in chronic cyclosporine nephrotoxicity. *Transplantation* 1987; 43:282.
49. Conley SB, Flechner SM, Rose G, et al. The use of cyclosporine in pediatric renal transplant recipients. *J Pediatr* 1985;106:45.
50. Cook DJ, Klingman LL, Koo AP, et al. Quantitative flow cytometry crossmatching (QFXM) for precise measurement of donor-specific alloreactivity. *Transplant Proc* 1994;26:2866.
51. Cook DJ, Terasaki PI, Iwaki Y, et al. An approach to reducing early kidney transplant failure by flow cytometry crossmatching. *Clin Transplants* 1987;1:253.
52. Council of the Transplantation Society. Commercialization in transplantation. The problems and some guidelines for practice. *Lancet* 1985;2:715.
53. Curtis JJ. Hypertension following kidney transplantation. *Am J Kidney Dis* 1994;23:471.
54. Curtis JJ, Luke RG, Diethelm AG, et al. Benefits of removal of native kidneys in hypertension after renal transplantation. *Lancet* 1985;2:739.
55. D'Alessandro AM et al. Tertiary hyperparathyroidism after renal transplantation: operative indications. *Surgery* 1989;106: 1049.
56. Dandavino R, Boucher A, Gagne M, et al. A pharmacoeconomic intrapatient comparison of Sandimmune capsules and Sandimmune oral solution in the kidney transplant recipient. *Transplant Proc* 1991;23:985.
57. Darby JM, Stein K, Grenuik A, et al. Approach to management of the heartbeating "brain dead" organ donor. *JAMA* 1989; 261:2222.
58. Dawidson I, Rooth P, Fry W, et al. Prevention of acute cyclosporine-induced renal blood flow inhibition and improved immunosuppression with verapamil. *Transplantation* 1989; 48:575.
59. Delmonico FL, Tolkoff-Rubin N. Treatment of acute rejection. In: Milford EL, ed. *Renal transplantation: contemporary issues in nephrology.* New York: Churchill Livingstone, 1989.
60. DeMeyer M, Pirson Y, Dautrebande J, et al. Treatment of renal graft artery stenosis. *Transplantation* 1989;47:784.
61. DeMeyer M, Wyns W, Dion R, et al. Myocardial revascularization in patients on renal replacement therapy. *Clin Nephrol* 1991;36:147.
62. Derfler K, Kletler K, Balcke P, et al. Predictive value of thallium-201 dipyridamole myocardial stress scintigraphy in chronic hemodialysis patients and transplant recipients. *Clin Nephrol* 1990;36:192.
63. Dickerman RM, Peters PC, Hull AR, et al. Surgical correction of post-transplant renovascular hypertension. *Ann Surg* 1980; 192:639.
64. Erice A, Phame FS, Heussner RC, et al. HIV infection in organ transplant recipients. *Rev Infect Dis* 1991;13:537.
65. Erturk E, Rubens DJ, Panner BJ, et al. Automated core biopsy of renal allografts using ultrasonic guidance. *Transplantation* 1991,5:1311.
66. Eschbach J, Egrie JC, Downing MR, et al. Correction of anemia of ESRD with recombinant human erythropoietin. *N Engl J Med* 1987;316:73.
67. Evans RW. Need, demand, and supply in kidney transplantation: a review of the data, an examination of the issues, and projections through the year 2000. *Semin Nephrol* 1992; 12:234.
68. Evans RW. The benefits of transplantation. Survival and quality of life. In: Evans RW, Manninen DL, Dong F, eds. *The national cooperative transplantation study.* Seattle: Battelle Research Center, 1991.
69. Fahlenkamp D, Raatz D, Schonberger B, et al. Laparoscopic lymphocele drainage after renal transplantation. *J Urol* 1993; 150:316.
70. Ferguson R. Acute rejection episodes—best predictor of long-term primary cadaveric renal transplant survival. *Clin Transplantation* 1994;8:328.
71. Figueroa JE, Rodriguez-Antunez A, Nakamoto S, et al. The scintigram after renal transplantation in man. *N Engl J Med* 1965;273:1406.
72. Fine R. Peritoneal dialysis in children. *J Pediatr* 1982;100:1.
73. Finn WF. Prevention of ischemic injury in renal transplantation. *Kidney Int* 1990;37:171.
74. First MR, Neylan JF, Rocher LL, et al. Hypertension after renal transplantation. *J Am Soc Nephrol* 1994;4:S30.
75. Fischel RJ, Payne WD, Gillingham KJ, et al. Long term outlook for renal transplant recipients with one year function. *Transplantation* 1992;51:118.
76. Flechner SM, Conley SB, Brewer E, et al. Intermittent clean catheterization. An alternative to diversion in continent transplant recipients. *J Urol* 1983;130:878.
77. Flechner SM, Kerman RH, Van Buren CT, et al. The use of cyclosporine in living-related renal transplantation. Donor-specific hyporesponsiveness and steroid withdrawal. *Transplantation* 1984;38:685.
78. Flechner SM, Novick AC, Braun WE, et al. Functional capacity and rehabilitation of recipients with a functioning renal allograft 10 years or more. *Transplantation* 1983;35:572.
79. Flechner SM, Sandler CM, Houston GK, et al. 100 living related kidney donor evaluations using digital subtraction angiography. *Transplantation* 1985;40:675.
80. Flechner SM, Modlin CS, Serrano DP, et al. Determinants of chronic renal allograft rejection in cyclosporine treated recipients. *Transplantation* 1996;62:1235.
81. Flechner SM, Van Buren C, Kerman R, et al. The nephrotoxicity of cyclosporine in renal transplant recipients. *Transplant Proc* 1983;2689.
82. Flechner SM, Goldfarb DA, Fairchild R, et al. A randomized prospective trial of OKT3 vs. Basiliximab for induction therapy in renal transplantation. *Transplantation* 2000;69:S1.
83. Flechner SM, Avery RK, Fisher R, et al. A randomized prospective controlled trial of oral acyclovir vs. oral ganciclovir for CMV prophylaxis in high risk kidney transplant recipients. *Transplantation* 1998;66:1682.
84. Flechner SM, Goldfarb A, Fairchild R, et al. A randomized prospective trial of low dose OKT3 induction therapy to prevent rejection and minimize side effects in recipients of kidney transplantation. *Transplantation* 2000;69:2374.
85. Flechner SM. Laparoscopic live donor nephrectomy: a critical review of the initial experience. *Transplantation Reviews* 2000; 14:96.

86. Flom LS, Riesman EM, Donovan JM, et al. Favorable experience with preemptive renal transplantation in children. *Pediatr Nephrol* 1992;6:258.
87. Flowers JL, Jacobs SC, Cho E, et al. Comparison of open and laparoscopic live donor nephrectomy. *Am Surg* 1997;226:483.
88. Fox BC, Sollinger HW, Belzer FO, et al. A prospective, randomized, double-blind study of trimethoprim-sulfamethoxazole for prophylaxis of infection in renal transplantation: Clinical efficacy, absorption of trimethoprim-sulfamethoxazole, effects on microflora and the cost benefit of prophylaxis. *Am J Med* 1990;89:255.
89. Frey FJ. Pharmacokinetic determinations of cyclosporine and prednisone in renal transplant patients. *Kidney Int* 1991;39:1034.
90. Fryd D, Sutherland D, Simmons R, et al. Results of a prospective randomized study on the effect of splenectomy vs. no splenectomy in renal transplantation. *Transplant Proc* 1981;13:48.
91. Garcia LL, Agueru AE, Cavalli J, et al. Kidney transplantation: absolute and relative psychological contraindications. *Transplant Proc* 1991;23:1344.
92. Gaston RS, Julian BA, and Curtis JJ. Posttransplant erythrocytosis: an enigma revisited. In-depth review. *Am J Kidney Dis* 1994;24:1.
93. Gibbons WS, Barry JM, Hefty TR. Complications following unstented parallel incision extravesical ureteroneocystostomy in 1,000 kidney transplants. *J Urol* 1992;148:38.
94. Goldman MH, Tilney NL, Vineyard GC, et al. A twenty year survey of arterial complication of renal transplantation. *Surg Gynecol Obstet* 1975;141:758.
95. Goldstein I, Choi SI, Olsson CA. Nephrostomy drainage for renal transplant complications. *J Urol* 1981;126:159.
96. Gorer PA. The genetic and antigenic basis of tumor transplantation. *J Pathol Bacteriol* 1937;44:691.
97. Gorey TF, Bulkey GB, Spees EK, et al. Iliac artery ligation: the relative paucity of ischemic sequelae in renal transplant patients. *Ann Surg* 1979;190:753.
98. Goss JA, Cole BR, Jendrisak MD, et al. Renal transplantation for systemic lupus erythematosus and recurrent lupus nephritis. *Transplantation* 1991;52:805.
99. Gould DS, Auchincloss H. Direct and indirect recognition: the role of MHC antigens in graft rejection. *Immunology Today* 1999;20:77.
100. Greenstein SM, Verstanig A, McLean GK, et al. Percutaneous transluminal angioplasty: the procedure of choice in the hypertensive renal allograft recipient with renal artery stenosis. *Transplantation* 1987;43:29.
101. Gregory CR, Gourley IM, Cain GR, et al. Mizoribine serum levels associated with enterotoxicity in the dog. *Transplantation* 1991;51: 877.
102. Haber W, Hoffken B, Freiling U, et al. Professional, training for the blind diabetic with nephropathy. *Diabetic Nephropathy* 1985;4:88.
103. Haldane JBS. The genetics of cancer. *Nature* 1933;132:265.
104. Halloran P. Immunosuppressive agents in clinical trials in transplantation. *Am J Med Sci* 1997;313:282.
105. Halloran P, Mathew T, Tomlanovich S, et al. Mycophenolate mofetil in renal allograft recipients: a pooled efficacy analysis of three double-blind clinical studies in the prevention of rejection. *Transplantation* 1997;63:39.
106. Hamway S et al. Impaired renal allograft function: a comparative study with angiography and histopathology. *J Urol* 1979;122:292.
107. Handschumacher RE, Harding MW, Rice J, et al. Cyclophilin: a specific cytosolic binding protein for cyclosporine A. *Science* 1984;226:544.
108. Hariharan S, Johnson CP, Bresnahan BA, et al. Improved graft survival after renal transplantation in the United States 1988–1996. *N Engl J Med* 2000;342:605.
109. Harmon WE, Stablein D, Alexander SR, et al. Graft thrombosis in pediatric renal transplant recipients: a report of the American Pediatric Renal Transplant Cooperative Study. *Transplantation* 1991;51:406.
110. Hatch DA, Belitsky P, Barry JM, et al. Fate of renal allografts transplanted in patients with urinary diversion. *Transplantation* 1993;56:838.
111. Henry ML, Elkhammas M, Bumgardner G, et al. A prospective randomized trial of Neoral and CellCept with and without OKT3 induction. *Proc ASTS* 1998;24.
112. Hesse UJ, Fryd DS, Chatterjee SN, et al. Pulmonary infections: the Minnesota randomized prospective trial of cyclosporine versus azathioprine-antilymphocyte globulin for immunosuppression in renal allograft recipients. *Arch Surg* 1986;121:1056.
113. Hesse UJ, Wienand P, Baldamus C, et al. Preliminary results of a prospectively randomized trial of ALG vs OKT3 for steroid-resistant rejection after renal transplantation in the early post-operative period. *Transplant Proc* 1990;22:2273.
114. Hodge E, Novick A, Lewis R, et al. Results of transplantation with remote-positive proximate-negative T cell antiglobulin crossmatches. *Transplant Proc* 1987;19:789.
115. Holley JL, Fenton RA, Arthur RS. Thallium stress testing does not predict cardiovascular risk in diabetic patients with ESRD undergoing cadaver renal transplantation. *Am J Med* 1991;90:563.
116. Hobart MG, Modlin CS, Kapoor A, et al. Transplantation of pediatric en bloc kidneys into adult recipients. *Transplantation* 1998;66:1689.
117. Horina JH, Holzer H, Reisinger EC, et al. Elderly patients and chronic hemodialysis. *Lancet* 1992;339:183.
118. Hostetter TH. Chronic transplant rejection. *Kidney Int* 1994;46:266.
119. Hricik DE. Posttransplant hyperlipidemia: the treatment dilemma. *Am J Kidney Dis* 1994;23:766.
120. Hume DM, Magee JH, Kauffman HM Jr. Renal homotransplantation in man in modified recipients. *Ann Surg* 1963;158:608.
121. Hunt J. Pretransplant evaluation and outcome. *Semin Nephrol* 1992;12:227.
122. Hutchinson TA, Thomas DC, MacFibbon B. Predicting survival in adults with ESRD. An age equivalency index. *Ann Intern Med* 1982;96:417.
123. Jarowenko MV, Flechner SM. Recipient ureterocalicostomy in a renal allograft. *J Urol* 1985;133:844.
124. Jindal RM, Hariharan S. Chronic rejection in kidney transplants: an in depth review. *Nephron* 1999;83:13.
125. Johnson C, Ahsan N, Gonwa T, et al. Randomized trial of tacrolimus in combination with azathioprine or mycophenolate vs. cyclosporine with mycophenolate after cadaveric kidney transplantation. *Transplantation* 2000;69:834.
126. Johnson EM, Anderson K, Jacobs C, et al. Long term followup of living kidney donors. *Transplantation* 1999;67:717.
127. Jordan ML. Immunosuppressive therapy and results of renal transplantation. *Curr Opin Urol* 1993;3:126.
128. Julian BA, Quarles LD, Niemann KM. Musculoskeletal complications after renal transplantation: pathogenesis and treatment. *Am J Kidney Dis* 1992;19:99.
129. Kahan BD, ed. *Cyclosporine.* Orlando: Grune & Stratton, 1988.

130. Kahan BD for US and Global Multicenter Sirolimus Trial Group. Two year follow up of the pivotal multicenter trials of sirolimus. *Transplantation* 2000;69:5361.
131. Kahan BD, Flechner SM, Lorber M, et al. Complications of cyclosporine therapy. *World J Surg* 1986;10:348.
132. Kanazi G, Stowe N, Steinmuller D, et al. Effect of cyclosporine upon the function of ischemically damaged kidneys in the rat. *Transplantation* 1986;41:782.
133. Kataoka K, Naomoto Y, Shiozaki S, et al. Infiltration of perforin-positive mononuclear cells into the rejected kidney allograft. *Transplantation* 1992;53:240.
134. Kay R, Fuchs E, Barry JM. Management of postoperative pelvic lymphoceles. *Urology* 1980;15:345.
135. Kennedy WR, Navarro X, Goetz F, et al. The effects of pancreas transplantation on diabetic neuropathy. *N Engl J Med* 1990;322:1031.
136. Kerman R, Flechner SM, Van Buren C, et al. Investigation of HIV serology in a renal transplant population. *Transplantation* 1987;43:241.
137. Kerman RH, Van Buren CT, Lewis RM, et al. Improved graft survival for flow cytometry and antihuman globulin crossmatch-negative retransplant recipients. *Transplantation* 1990;49:52.
138. Khauli RB, Mojerthal AC, Caushaj PE. Treatment of lymphocele and lymphatic fistula following renal transplantation by laparoscopic peritoneal window. *J Urol* 1992;147:1353.
139. Kinnaert P, Hall M, Janssen F, et al. Ureteral stenosis after kidney transplantation: true incidence and long term follow-up after surgical correction. *J Urol* 1985;133:17.
140. Kiss D, Landmann J, Mihatsch M, et al. Risks and benefits of graft biopsy in renal transplantation under cyclosporine A. *Clin Nephrol* 1992;38:132.
141. Klassen DK, Solez K, Burdick JF. Effects of cyclosporine on human renal allograft renin and prostaglandin production. *Transplantation* 1989;47:1072.
142. Kockelbergh RC, Millar RJ, Walker RG, et al. Pyeloureterostomy in the management of renal allograft ureteral complications: an alternative technique. *J Urol* 1993;149:366.
143. Kogan S, Levitt S. Bladder evaluation in patients before undiversion in previously diverted urinary tracts. *J Urol* 1977; 118:443.
144. Kohler G, Milstein C. Continuous cultures of fused cells secreting antibody of predefined specificity. *Nature* 1975;256:495.
145. Kyriakides GK, Simmons R, Najarian JS. Mycotic aneurysms in transplant patients. *Arch Surg* 1976;111:472.
146. Lacombe M. Renal artery stenosis after renal transplantation. *Ann Vasc Surg* 1988;2:155.
147. Lake KD. Cyclosporine drug interactions: a review. *Card Surg* 1988;2:617.
148. Landsteiner K. Uber agglutination serscheinungen normalen menschliachen blutes vivien. *Klin Wochenschr* 1901;14:1132.
149. Larsen CP, Elwood ET, Alexander DZ, et al. Long term acceptance of skin and cardiac allografts after blocking CD40 and CD28 pathways. *Nature* 1996;381:434.
150. Leary F, DeWeerd J. Living donor nephrectomy. *J Urol* 1973; 109:947.
151. Lemmers MJ, Barry JM. Major role for arterial disease in morbidity and mortality after kidney transplantation in diabetes. *Diabetes Care* 1991;14:295.
152. Levery A, Hou S, Bash H. Sounding board: kidney transplantation from unrelated living donors. *N Engl J Med* 1986;314:914.
153. Lewis R, Podbielski J, Sprayberry S, et al. Stability of renal allograft glomerular filtration rate associated with long-term use of cyclosporine A. *Transplantation* 1993;55:1014.
154. Lieberman RP, Glass NR, Crummy AB, et al. Nonoperative percutaneous management of urinary fistulas and strictures in renal transplantation. *Surg Gynecol Obstet* 1982;155:667.
155. Lin H, Bolling SF, Linsley P, et al. Long term acceptance of MHC mismatched cardiac allografts induced by CTLA-4Ig plus donor specific transfusion. *J Exp Med* 1993;178:1801.
156. Little CC. In: Snell GD, ed. *The biology of the laboratory mouse.* New York: Dover, 1941.
157. Lorber M, Van Buren CT, Flechner SM, et al. Hepatobiliary complications of cyclosporine therapy in 466 renal transplant recipients. *Transplantation* 1987;43:35.
158. Lorber MI, Van Buren CT, Flechner SM, et al. Pretransplant coronary artery angiography for diabetic renal transplant recipients. *Transplant Proc* 1987;19:1539.
159. Lord RHH, Pepera T, Williams G. Ureteroureterostomy and pyeloureterostomy without native nephrectomy in renal transplantation. *Br J Urol* 1991;67:349.
160. Lucas BA, Vaughn WK, Spees EK, et al. Identification of donor factors predisposing to high discard rates of cadaveric kidneys and increased graft loss within one year post transplant. Transplantation 1987;43:253.
161. Malavaud B, Hoff M, Miedouge M, et al. PSA based screening for prostate cancer after renal transplantation. *Transplantation* 2000;69:2461.
162. Macgregor P et al. Renal transplantation in end-stage renal disease patients with existing urinary diversion. *J Urol* 1986; 135:686.
163. Mayer AD, Dmetrewski J, Squifflet J, et al. Multicenter randomized trial comparing tacrolimus and cyclosporine in the prevention of renal allograft rejection. *Transplantation* 1999; 64:436.
164. Mailloux LV, Bellucci AG, Wilkes BM, et al. Mortality in dialysis patients: analysis of the causes of death. *Am J Kidney Dis* 1991;18:326.
165. Mamdani B. Recovery of prolonged renal failure in patients with accelerated hypertension. *N Engl J Med* 1974;291:1343.
166. Manske C, Thomas W, Wang Y. Screening diabetic transplant candidates for coronary artery disease: identification of a low risk subgroup. *Kidney Int* 1993;44:617.
167. Manske C, Wang Y, Wilson RF, et al. Coronary revascularization in insulin dependent diabetics with chronic renal failure. *Lancet* 1992;340:998.
168. Markell MS, Armenti V, Danovitch G, et al. Hyperlipidemia and glucose intolerance in the post-renal transplant recipient. *J Am Soc Nephrol* 1994;4:S37.
169. Marwick TH, Steinmuller DR, Underwood DA, et al. Ineffectiveness of dipyridamole thallium imaging as a screening technique for coronary artery disease in patients with ESRD. *Transplantation* 1989;49:100.
170. Masur H. Prevention and treatment of *Pneumocystis* pneumonia. *N Engl J Med* 1992;327:1853.
171. Matas AJ, Gillingham KJ, Sutherland DE. Half-life and risk factors for kidney transplant outcome: importance of death with function. *Transplantation* 1993;55:757.
172. Matthew TH. Recurrence of disease following renal transplantation. *Am J Kidney Dis* 1988;12:85.
173. McConnell JD, Sagalowsky AI, Lewis SE, et al. Prospective evaluation of renal allograft dysfunction with technetium diethylenetriaminepentaacetic acid renal scans. *J Urol* 1984;131:875.
174. McEnery PT, Stablein DM, Arbus G, et al. Renal transplantation in children. Report of the North American Pediatric Renal Transplant Cooperative Study. *N Engl J Med* 1992;326:1727.
175. McLean RH, Geiger H, Burke B, et al. Recurrence of membranoproliferative GN following kidney transplantation. *Am J Med* 1976;60:60.

176. Medawar PB. The behavior and fate of skin autografts and skin homografts in rabbits. *J Anat* 1944;78:176.
177. Micelli MC, Parnes J. The role of CD4 and CD8 in T cell activation and differentiation. *Adv Immunol* 1993;53:59.
178. Merrill JP. Moral problems of artificial and transplanted organs. *Ann Intern Med* 1964;61:355.
179. Migliori RJ, Simmons R, Payne WD, et al. Renal transplantation done safely without prior chronic dialysis therapy. *Transplantation* 1987;43:51.
180. Moel DI, Butt K. Renal transplantation in children less than two years of age. *J Pediatr* 1981;99:535.
181. Monaco AP. Clinical aspects of monoclonal antibody therapy in kidney transplantation. *Transplant Sci* 1992;2:9.
182. Moore FD Jr, Kohler TR, Strom TB, et al. The declining mortality of pneumonia in renal transplant recipients. *Infect Surg* 1983;2:13.
183. Morris RE, Wang J, Blum JR, et al. Immunosuppressive effects of the morpholinoethyl ester of mycophenolic acid (RS-61443) in rat and non-human primate recipients of heart allografts. *Transplant Proc* 1991;23:19.
184. Mulgaonkar S, Jakobs MG, Viscuso R, et al. Laparoscopic internal drainage of lymphocele in renal transplants. *Am J Kidney Dis* 1992;19:490.
185. Murray JE, Merrill JP, Harrison JH, et al. Prolonged survival of human-kidney homografts by immunosuppressive drug therapy. *N Engl J Med* 1963;268:1315.
186. Naimark DMJ, Cole E. Determinants of long-term renal allograft survival. *Transplant Rev* 1994;8:93.
187. Najarian JS, Chavers B, McHugh L, et al. Twenty years or more of follow up of living kidney donors. *Lancet* 1992; 340:807.
188. Najarian JS, Frey DJ, Matas AJ, et al. Renal transplantation in infants. *Ann Surg* 1990;212:353.
189. Nalesnik MA, Makowka L, Starzl TE. The diagnosis and treatment of posttransplant lymphoproliferative disorders. *Curr Probl Surg* 1988;25:367.
190. Nathan DM, Fogel H, Xiorman D, et al. Long term metabolic and quality of life results with pancreatic renal transplantation. *Transplantation* 1991;52:85.
191. Nogueria JM, Cangro C, Fink JC, et al. A comparison of recipient outcome with laparoscopic vs. open live donor nephrectomy. *Transplantation* 1999;67:722.
192. Nguyen DH, Reinberg Y, Gonzalez R, et al. Outcome of renal transplantation after urinary diversion and enterocytoplasty. *J Urol* 1990;144:1349.
193. Norman DJ, Barry JM, Bennett WM, et al. The use of OKT3 in cadaveric renal transplantation for rejection that is unresponsive to conventional anti-rejection therapy. *Am J Kidney Dis* 1988;11:90.
194. Novick AC, Ho Hsieh H, Steinmuller D, et al. Detrimental effect of cyclosporine on initial function of cadaver renal allografts following extended preservation: results of a randomized prospective study. *Transplantation* 1986;42:154.
195. Novick AC, Magnusson M, Braun WE. Multiple-artery renal transplantation: emphasis on extracorporeal methods of donor arterial reconstruction. *J Urol* 1979;122:731.
196. Novick AC. Surgery of renal transplantation and complications. In: Novick AC, Straffon RA, eds. *Vascular problems in urologic surgery.* Philadelphia: Saunders, 1982.
197. Novick AC. Technique of renal transplantation. In: Novick AC, Streem SB, Pontes JE, eds. *Stewart's operative urology.* Baltimore: Williams & Wilkins, 1989.
198. Oei HY, Surachno S, Wilminek JM, et al. Measurement of ^{99m}Tc-MAG3 uptake in renal transplant population. *Contrib Nephrol* 1990;79:113.
199. Ohlman S, Ganndeahl G, Tyden G, et al. Treatment of renal transplant rejection with 15 deoxyspergualin: a dose-finding study in man. *Transplant Proc* 1992;24:318.
200. Okiye S, Engen D, Sterioff S, et al. Primary and secondary renal transplantation in diabetes. *JAMA* 1983;249:492.
201. O'Malley KJ, Kickey D, Kapoor A, et al. Artificial urinary sphincter insertion into renal transplant recipients. *Urology* 1999;54:923.
202. O'Malley KJ, Flechner SM, Kapoor A, et al. Acute colonic pseudo-obstruction (Ogilvie's syndrome) early post renal transplantation. *Am J Surg* 1999;177:492.
203. Opelz G. Correlation of HLA matching with kidney graft survival in patients with or without cyclosporine treatment. *Transplantation* 1985;40:240.
204. Opelz G, Mytilineous J, Scherer S, et al. Survival of DNA HLA-DR typed and matched cadaver kidney transplants. *Lancet* 1991;338:461.
205. Opelz G et al. Effect of blood transfusions on subsequent kidney transplants. *Transplant Proc* 1973;5:253.
206. Ortho Multicenter Transplant Study Group. A randomized trial of OKT3 monoclonal antibody for acute rejection of cadaveric renal transplants. *N Engl J Med* 1985;313:337.
207. Palleschi J, Novick AC, Braun WE, et al. Vascular complications of renal transplantation. *Urology* 1980;16:61.
208. Pallis C. Brainstem death. The evolution of a concept. In: Morris PJ, ed. *Kidney transplantation: principles and practice.* London, UK: Grune & Stratton, 1984.
209. Patel R, Terasaki PI. Significance of the positive crossmatch test in kidney transplantation. *N Engl J Med* 1969;280:735.
210. Patel R, Snydman D, Rubin R, et al. CMV prophylaxis in solid organ transplant recipients. *Transplantation* 1996;61:1279.
211. Patten E. Therapeutic plasmapheresis and plasma exchange. *Crit Rev Clin Lab Sci* 1986;23:147.
212. Penn I. Cancers following cyclosporine therapy. *Transplantation* 1987;43:32.
213. Penn I, Mackie G, Halgrimson CG, et al. Testicular complications following renal transplantation. *Ann Surg* 1972;176:697.
214. Penn I. Occurrence of cancers in immunosuppressed organ transplant recipients. In: Teraski PI, ed. *Clinical transplants 1990.* Los Angeles: UCLA Tissue Typing Laboratory, 1991.
215. Pereira BJG, Kirkman RL, Bryan CF, et al. National collaborative study of anti-HCV in cadaver donors: reduced organ wastage using a second generation anti-HCV test. *J Am Soc Nephrol* 1992;3:875(abst).
216. Pereira BJG, Milford EL, Kirkman RL, et al. Prevalence of HCV RNA in hepatitis C antibody positive cadaver organ donors and their recipients. *N Engl J Med* 1992;273:910.
217. Pereira BJG, Milford EL, Kirkman RL, et al. Transmission of hepatitis C virus by organ transplantation. *N Engl J Med* 1991;325:454.
218. Perez R, Matas AJ, Gillingham KJ, et al. Lessons learned and future hopes: three thousand renal transplants at the University of Minnesota. In: Terasaki PI, ed. *Clinical transplants 1990.* Los Angeles: UCLA Tissue Typing Laboratory, 1991.
219. Pescovitz M, Milgram M, Leapman S, et al. Corticosteroid inhibition of the OKT3 induced febrile and nephrotoxic responses during treatment of renal allograft rejection. *Transplantation* 1998;57:529.
220. Petronis J, Kittur DS. The use of technetium DTPA for detecting post-transplantation urinary extravasation. *Transplantation* 1988;46:910.
221. Phillips MG, ed. *Organ procurement, preservation, and distribution in transplantation.* Richmond, Va: UNOS, 1991.
222. Pirsch J, Miller J, Deirhoi M, et al. A comparison of tacrolimus and cyclosporine for immunosuppression after cadaveric renal transplantation. *Transplantation* 1997;68:977.

223. Pirsch JD, D'Alessandro AM, Sollinger HW, et al. The effect of donor age, recipient age and HLA-match on immunologic graft survival in cadaver renal transplant recipients. *Transplantation* 1992;53:55.
224. Platt JL, Bach FH. The barrier to xenotransplantation. *Transplantation* 1991;52:937.
225. Platz K, Sollinger H, Gullet D, et al. RS-61443, a new potent immunosuppressive agent. *Transplantation* 1990;51:27.
226. Ploeg R. Kidney preservation with the UW and Euro-Collins solutions. *Transplantation* 1990;49:281.
227. Pratscke J, Kusaka M, Wilhem M, et al. Brain death and its influence on donor organ quality and outcome after transplantation. *Transplantation* 1999;67:343.
228. Racusen L, Solez K, Colvin R, et al. The Banff 1997 working classification of renal allograft pathology. *Kidney Int* 1997; 55:713.
229. Rajfer J, Koyle MA, Ehrlich RM, et al. Pyelovesicostomy as a form of urinary reconstruction in renal transplantation. *J Urol* 1986;136:372.
230. Ramos EL, Kasiske BL, Alexander SR, et al. The evaluation of candidates for renal transplantation. Current practice of U.S. transplant centers. *Transplantation* 1994;57:490.
231. Randhawa PS, Shapiro R, Jordan MI, et al. The histopathological changes associated with allograft rejection and drug toxicity in renal transplant recipients maintained on FK506. Clinical significance and comparison with cyclosporine. *Am J Surg Pathol* 1993;17:60.
232. Rao KV, Andersen RC. Long-term results and complications in renal transplant recipients. Observations in the second decade. *Transplantation* 1988;45:45.
233. Raynaud A, Bedrossian J, Remy P, et al. Percutaneous transluminal angioplasty of renal transplant arterial stenoses. *AJR Am J Roentgenol* 1986;146:853.
234. Reichensparner H. Does 15 deoxyspergualin induce graft nonreactivity after cardiac and renal transplantation in primates? *Transplantation* 1990;50:181.
235. Renigers SA, Spigos DG. Pseudoaneurysm of the arterial anastomosis in a renal transplant. *AJR Am J Roentgenol* 1978; 131:525.
236. Richardson AJ, Liddington M, Jaskowski A, et al. Pregnancy in a renal transplant recipient complicated by rupture of a transplant renal artery aneurysm. *Br J Surg* 1990;77:228.
237. Rigotti JP, Flechner SM, VanBuren CT, et al. Increased incidence of renal allograft thrombosis under cyclosporine immunosuppression. *Int Surg* 1986;71:38.
238. Robitaille P, Lortie L, Mongean J, et al. Long term follow up of patients who underwent unilateral nephrectomy in childhood. *Lancet* 1985;1:1297.
239. Rossi SJ, Schroeder TJ, Hariharan S, et al. Prevention and management of the adverse effects associated with immunosuppressive therapy. *Drug Safety* 1993;9(2):104.
240. Rubin RH. Infectious disease complications of renal transplantation. *Kidney Int* 1993;44:221.
241. Rubin RH, Jenkins RL, Shaw BW, et al. The acquired immunodeficiency syndrome and transplantation. *Transplantation* 1987;44:1.
242. Saborio P, Scheinman JI. Transplantation for primary oxaluria in the United States. *Kidney Int* 1999;56:1094.
243. Salvatierra O, Vincenti F, Amend W, et al. Deliberate donor-specific blood transfusion prior to living related renal transplantation. A new approach. *Ann Surg* 1980;192:543.
244. Sanders CE, Curtis JJ, Julian BA, et al. Tapering or continuing of cyclosporine for financial reasons: a single center experience. *Am J Kidney Dis* 1993;21:9.
245. Sandrini S, Maiorca R, Scolari F, et al. Prospective randomized trial of azathioprine addition to cyclosporine vs. cyclosporine monotherapy at steroid withdrawal. *Transplantation* 2000;69: 1861.
246. Sankari BR, Boullier JA, Garvin PJ, et al. Sclerotherapy with tetracycline for hydroceles in renal transplant patients. *J Urol* 1992;148:1188.
247. Schiff M Jr, Lytton B. Secondary ureteropyelostomy in renal transplant recipients. *J Urol* 1981;126:723.
248. Schiff M Jr, McGuire EJ, Weiss RM, et al. Management of urinary fistulas after renal transplantation. *J Urol* 1976; 115:251.
249. Schover LR, Streem SB, Boparai N, et al. The psychosocial impact of donating a kidney: long term follow up from a urology based center. *J Urol* 1997;157:1596.
250. Schroeder T, First MR. Monoclonal antibodies in organ transplantation. *Am J Kidney Dis* 1994;23:138.
251. Schroeder T, Weiss MA, Smith RD, et al. The efficacy of OKT3 in vascular rejection. *Transplantation* 1991;51:312.
252. Schwartz J, Baxter J, Bull D. Radionuclide cerebral imaging confirming brain death. *JAMA* 1983;249:246.
253. Schwartz A, Krause PH, Offerman G, et al. Recurrent and *de novo* renal disease after kidney transplantation. *Am J Kidney Dis* 1991;17:524.
254. Sehgal S. Rapamune: mechanism of action immunosuppressive effect results from blockade of signal transduction and cell cycle progression. *Clin Biochem* 1998;311:335.
255. Serrano DP, Flechner SM, Modlin CS, et al. Transplantation into the long term defunctionalized bladder. *J Urol* 1996; 156:885.
256. Shah MB, Martin JE, Schroeder T, et al. The evaluation of the safety and tolerability of two formulations of cyclosporine: Sandimmune and Neoral. *Transplantation* 1999;67:1411.
257. Shoskes DA, Cecka JM. Deleterious effects of delayed graft function in renal transplant recipients independent of acute rejection. *Transplantation* 1998;66:1697.
258. Shoskes DA, Parfrey NA, Hallorhan PF. Increased major histocompatibility complex antigen expression in acute tubular necrosis in mouse kidney. *Transplantation* 1990;49:201.
259. Snell GD. Methods for the study of histocompatibility genes. *Journal of Genetics* 1948;49:87.
260. Snydman DR, Werner BG, Heinze-Lacey B, et al. Use of cytomegalovirus immune globulin to prevent cytomegalovirus disease in renal transplant recipients. *N Engl J Med* 1987;317: 1049.
261. Solez K, Axelson RA, Banner B, et al. International standardization of nomenclature and criteria for the histologic diagnosis of renal allograft rejection: the Banff working classification of kidney transplant pathology. *Kidney Int* 1993;44:411.
262. Sollinger HW for the US Renal Transplant Mycophenolate Mofetil Study Group. Mycophenolate for the prevention of acute rejection in cadaveric renal allograft recipients. *Transplantation* 1995;60: 225.
263. Sorenson BL, Hold T, Nissen HM. Silent iliac compression syndrome as a cause of renal vein thrombosis after transplantation. *Scand J Urol Nephrol* 1972;15:75.
264. Southard JH, Van Gulik TM, Ametani MS, et al. Important components of the UW solution. *Transplantation* 1990;49:251.
265. Spencer W, Streem S, Geisinger MA, et al. Outcome of angiographic evaluation of living renal donors. *J Urol* 1988;140: 1364.
266. Spital A. The shortage of organs for transplantation: where do we go from here? *N Engl J Med* 1991;325:1243.
267. Starzl TE, Demetris AJ, Trucco M, et al. Chimerism and donor-specific nonreactivity 27 to 29 years after kidney allotransplantation. *Transplantation* 1993;55:1272.

268. Starzl TE, Fung J, Tzakis A, et al. Baboon-to-human liver transplantation. *Lancet* 1993;341:65.
269. Starzl TE, Marchioro TL, Porter KA, et al. The use of heterologous antilymphoid agents in canine renal and liver homotransplantation and in human renal homotransplantation. *Surg Gynecol Obstet* 1967;124:301.
270. Steinmuller DR, Hayes JM, Novick AC, et al. Comparison of OKT3 with ALG for prophylaxis for patients with acute renal failure after cadaveric renal transplantation. *Transplantation* 1991;52:67.
271. Steinmuller RD, Hodge E, Boshkos C, et al. Prophylaxis and treatment of post renal transplant rejection. *Cleve Clin J Med* 1991;58:125.
272. Steinmuller DR, Stilmont M, Idelson B, et al. *De novo* development of membranous nephropathy in cadaveric renal allografts. *Clin Nephrol* 1978;9:210.
273. Streem SB, Novick AC, Braun WE, et al. Low dose maintenance prednisone and antilymphocyte globulin for the treatment of acute rejection. *Transplantation* 1983;35:420.
274. Streem SB, Novick AC, Steinmuller DR, et al. Percutaneous techniques for the management of urological renal transplant complications. *J Urol* 1986;135:456.
275. Streem SB, Novick AC, Steinmuller DR, et al. Long-term efficacy of ureteral dilation for transplant ureteral stenosis. *J Urol* 1988;140:32.
276. Stephanian E, Matas AJ, Gores P, et al. Retransplantation as a risk factor in lymphocele formation. *Transplantation* 1992; 53:676.
277. Stuart FP, Reckard C, Schulak J, et al. Gastroduodenal complications in kidney transplant recipients. *Ann Surg* 1981; 194:339.
278. Sykes M, Sachs DH. Bone marrow transplantation as a means of inducing tolerance. *Semin Immunol* 1990;2:401.
279. Suranyi MG, Halloran PF, Hall BM. Recent developments in renal transplantation. *Curr Nephrol* 1994;17:385.
280. Szczech LA, Berlin JA, Aradhye S, et al. Effect of antilymphocyte induction therapy on renal allograft survival: a meta analysis. *J Am Soc Nephrol* 1997;8:1771.
281. Takemoto S, Terasaki PI, Cecka JM, et al. Survival of nationally shared HLA-matched kidney transplants from cadaveric donors. *N Engl J Med* 1992;327:834.
282. Tarantino A, Aroldi A, Stucci L, et al. A randomized prospective trial comparing cyclosporine monotherapy with triple drug therapy in renal transplantation. *Transplantation* 1991;52:53.
283. Tejani A, Butt KMH, Rajpoot D, et al. Strategies for optimizing growth in children with kidney transplants. *Transplantation* 1989;47:229.
284. Terasaki PI, Koyama H, Cecka TM, et al. The hyperfiltration hypothesis in human renal transplantation. *Transplantation* 1994;57:1450.
285. Terasaki PI, Mandell M, Van de Water J, et al. Human blood lymphocyte cytotoxicity reactions with allogenic antisera. *Ann N Y Acad Sci* 1964;120:322.
286. Terasaki PI, Yuge J, Cecka JM, et al. Thirty year trends in clinical kidney transplantation. In: Terasaki PI, Cecka JM, eds. *Clinical transplants, 1993.* Los Angeles: UCLA Tissue Typing Laboratory, 1994.
287. Terasaki PI, Cecka JM, Gjertson DW, et al. High survival rates of kidney transplants from spousal and other living unrelated donors. *N Engl J Med* 1995;333:333.
288. Teruel JL, Martin Escobar E, Quereda C, et al. A simple and safe method for management of lymphocele after renal transplantation. *J Urol* 1983;130:1058.
289. Tesi RJ, Elkhammas EA, Henry ML, et al. OKT3 for primary therapy of the first rejection episode in kidney transplants. *Transplantation* 1993;55:1023.
290. Tesi RJ, Elkhammas EA, Davies EA, et al. Renal transplantation in older people. *Lancet* 1994;343:461.
291. Thomalla JV, Mitchell M, Leapman S, et al. Renal transplantation into the reconstructed bladder. *J Urol* 1989;141:265.
292. Thompson A. FK506—profile of an important new immunosuppressant. *Transplant Rev* 1990;4:1.
293. Thomson AW, Starzl TE. New immunosuppressive drugs: mechanistic insights and potential therapeutic advances. *Immunol Rev* 1993;17:71.
294. Thomson AW, Woo J, Cooper M. Mode of action of immunosuppressive drugs with particular reference to the molecular basis of macrolide-induced immunosuppression. In: Thomson AW, ed. *The molecular biology of immunosuppression.* New York: Wiley, 1992.
295. Thrasher JB, Temple DR, Spees EK. Extravesical versus Leadbetter-Politano ureteroneocystostomy: a comparison of urological complications in 320 renal transplants. *J Urol* 1990; 144:1105.
296. Tilney NL, Rocha A, Strom TB, et al. Renal artery stenosis in transplant patients. *Ann Surg* 1984;199:454.
297. Toma H. ABO-incompatible renal transplantation. *Urol Clin North Am* 1994;21:299.
298. Tilney NL, Strom TB, Paul L, eds. *Transplantation biology: cellular and molecular aspects.* Philadelphia: Lippincott Raven, 1997.
299. Turner-Warwick R. The supracostal approach to the renal area. *Br J Urol* 1965;37:671.
300. Ubel PA, Arnold RM, Caplan A. Rationing failure. The ethical lessons of the retransplantation of scarce vital organs. *JAMA* 1993;270:2469.
301. Uchida H, Mita K, Bekku Y, et al. Advantages of triple therapy with mizoribine, cyclosporine and prednisone over other types of triple or double therapy. *J Toxicol Sci* 1991;16:181.
302. United States Renal Data System. *USRDS 1993 annual data report.* Bethesda, MD: National Institutes of Health, National Institute of Diabetes and Digestive and Kidney Diseases, 1993.
303. United States Renal Data System. Annual data report. *Am J Kidney Dis* 1999;34[Suppl 1]:2.
304. UNOS update. Richmond, VA: United Network for Organ Sharing. 1989;5:9.
305. UNOS update. Richmond, VA: United Network for Organ Sharing. 1994;10:4.
306. Vanrenterghem Y, Roel SL, Lerut T, et al. Thromboembolic complications and haemostatic changes in cyclosporine treated cadaveric kidney allograft recipients. *Lancet* 1985;1:999.
307. Vathsala A, Weinberg RB, Schoenberg L, et al. Lipid abnormalities in cyclosporine-prednisone-treated renal transplant recipients. *Transplantation* 1989;48:37.
308. Vincenti F, Amend W, Kaysen G, et al. Long term renal function in kidney donors. *Transplantation* 1984;36:626.
309. Vincenti F, Kirkman R, Light S, et al. Interleukin-2 receptor blockade with daclizumab to prevent acute rejection in renal transplantation. *N Engl J Med* 1998;336:161.
310. Vlahakos DV, Canzanello VJ, Madaio MP, et al. Enalapril-associated anemia in renal transplant recipients treated for hypertension. *Am J Kidney Dis* 1991;17:199.
311. Voeller G, Butts A, Vera S. Kidney transplant lymphocele: treatment with laparoscopic drainage and omental patching. *J Laparoendosc Surg* 1992;19:490.
312. Von Son WJ, Hooykaas AP, Sloof MJH, et al. Vesicocalicostomy as ultimate solution for recurrent urologic complications after cadaveric renal transplantation in a patient with poor bladder function. *J Urol* 1986;136:889.

313. Waltzer WC, Miller F, Arnold A, et al. Value of percutaneous core needle biopsy in the differential diagnosis of renal transplant dysfunction. *J Urol* 1987;137:1117.
314. Weiland D, Sutherland D, Chavers B, et al. Information on 628 living related kidney donors at a single institution with long term follow up on 472 cases. *Transplant Proc* 1984;16:5.
315. Williams G, Howard N. Management of lymphatic leakage after renal transplantation. *Transplantation* 1981;31:134.
316. Wolcott D, Norquist G. Psychiatric aspects of kidney transplantation. In: Danovitch G, ed. *Handbook of kidney transplantation.* Boston: Little, Brown, 1992.
317. World Health Organization. Guiding principles on human organ transplantation. *Lancet* 1991;337:1470.
318. Wyner L, Novick AC, Streem S, et al. Improved success of living unrelated renal transplantation with cyclosporine. *J Urol* 1993;149:706.
319. Zaki SK, Bretan PN, Go RT, et al. A simple and accurate grading system for orthoiodohippurate renal scans in the assessment of posttransplant renal function. *J Urol* 1990;143:1099.
320. Zinke H, Woods JE, Leary FJ, et al. Experience with lymphoceles after renal transplantation. *Surgery* 1975;77:444.

Adult and Pediatric Urology, 4/e, edited by Jay Y. Gillenwater, John T. Grayhack, Stuart S. Howards, and Michael E. Mitchell.
Lippincott Williams & Wilkins, Philadelphia © 2002

23

RENOVASCULAR HYPERTENSION AND ISCHEMIC NEPHROPATHY

E. DARRACOTT VAUGHAN, JR.
R. ERNEST SOSA

Sixty million Americans have high blood pressure. Hypertension secondary to renovascular disease is a leading cause of secondary hypertension in adults. The incidence of renovascular hypertension (RVH) is not known. It has been estimated that 3% to 5% of all hypertensive patients have RVH (44). An improved understanding of the renin-angiotensin-aldosterone system has permitted researchers to establish more sensitive and specific diagnostic screening tests for RVH. Advances in pharmacology, renal revascularization, and interventional radiology have steadily improved the efficacy and safety of treatment for patients diagnosed to have renovascular hypertension (127). The challenge for the physician is to accurately diagnose RVH and to select a treatment strategy suitable for his or her patient.

The importance of diagnosing RVH is multifold. First, sustained hypertension is a leading risk factor for premature illness and death. Poorly controlled or uncontrolled pressure elevation leads to small-vessel disease and end-organ damage, principally affecting the heart, kidneys, and central nervous system (59). Moreover, renin-dependent hypertension results in more severe vascular damage and hence in a higher incidence of myocardial infarctions and strokes at a younger age than is found in patients with normal or low renin hypertension, who are generally older (10). Second, RVH is difficult to manage medically (49). Even if adequate blood pressure control is maintained by pharmacologic means, progression of arterial disease is not prevented (103,135) and renal ischemia may actually worsen when the pressure is lowered to clinically desirable levels (1). Third, RVH is potentially curable by renal revascularization (21) or

E.D. Vaughan, Jr., and R.E. Sosa: Department of Urology, Weill-Cornell Medical Center; Department of Urology, New York-Presbyterian Hospital, New York, NY 10021.

angioplasty, and renal function can be stabilized or enhanced by renal revascularization (134). Fourth, renal arterial disease can lead to ischemic nephropathy, renal failure, if not diagnosed and treated (79).

This chapter presents the current understanding of the natural history and pathophysiology of RVH. A strategy for a cost-effective and reliable diagnostic evaluation of RVH is described. Established and new options for treatment are discussed and compared.

DEFINITIONS

Hypertension

It is estimated that 60 million individuals in the United States have hypertension. At what blood pressure is a person said to be hypertensive? It is difficult to define a precise cutoff that marks the upper limit of acceptable blood pressure, but it is generally acknowledged that the higher the blood pressure, the worse the resultant risk of morbidity and mortality (89). As a working definition, the 1984 Joint National Committee on Detection, Evaluation and Treatment of High Blood Pressure recommended that a sustained blood pressure of 140/90 mm Hg be considered the cutoff point between normal blood pressure and mild hypertension for all patients older than 18 years of age. Children with a sustained increase in arterial pressure greater than or equal to the 90th percentile for age are considered hypertensive. Whatever the patient's age, an elevation in blood pressure should be documented on at least three separate occasions, when measured with an appropriate-sized blood pressure cuff, to justify the diagnosis of hypertension. It is not unusual to find that a patient who is hypertensive at an initial evaluation remains normotensive at subsequent measurements (12).

Renovascular Disease

Renal disease has been recognized in association with hypertension since the early nineteenth century (8). In 1898, Tigerstedt and Bergmann (121) demonstrated that a water-soluble extract that they called renin, derived from the renal cortex of a healthy rabbit, could produce a marked and sustained hypertension when injected intravenously into a second rabbit. Interest in the relationship between renal disease and hypertension did not flourish, however, until the classic experiments by Goldblatt and associates (37) in the dog demonstrated that reversible elevation in the systemic arterial pressure could be produced by clamping the main renal artery of one of two healthy kidneys. The blood pressure returned to normal on removal of the kidney or the clamp.

The development and widespread use of arteriography in the 1950s focused attention on renal arterial disease in hypertensive patients and led to advances in renovascular surgery (34). It quickly became apparent, however, that lesions of the renal artery could be demonstrated angiographically in normotensive patients. Moreover, the results of the national cooperative study on renovascular surgery for treatment of hypertension revealed a sobering 34% failure rate in hypertensive patients subjected to renal revascularization (33). It became clear that angiographic documentation of renal artery disease in a hypertensive patient was not sufficient to justify surgical correction of the arterial lesion.

Greater insight into the pathophysiology of renal artery disease was gained by experiments in vessel hemodynamics. It was determined that the internal diameter of an artery must be reduced by greater than 70% for a significant decrease in blood flow to occur (66) and that a pressure gradient greater than 40 mm Hg across a stenosis in the renal artery was necessary to produce a significant decrease in the renal plasma flow, glomerular filtration rate (GFR), urinary sodium excretion, and urine flow rate (106).

The discovery of angiotensin (7,85) and the determination of its sequence (108) led to the eventual development of accurate radioimmunoassays to quantify the activity of the renin-angiotensin system. Researchers established that a significant decrease in blood flow to a kidney results in the activation of the renin-angiotensin-aldosterone cascade, establishing a hypertensive state. Correction of the stenosis or removal of the ischemic kidney eliminates the hyperreninemic state, allowing the blood pressure to return to normal levels.

Accordingly, *renovascular hypertension* can be defined as a sustained blood pressure elevation secondary to a physiologically significant renal artery stenosis that is correctable by repair of the lesion or by removal of the kidney. From a clinical point of view, however, it is imperative to be able to diagnose RVH prospectively. The availability of pharmacologic agents that block different steps in the renin-angiotensin-aldosterone cascade, such as converting enzyme inhibitors (CEIs) and technical advances in interventional radiology, have contributed to our understanding of the pathophysiology of RVH. On the basis of this knowledge, sensitive and specific tests that prospectively identify patients with RVH are in current clinical use.

PATHOLOGY AND NATURAL HISTORY OF RENAL ARTERY DISEASE

Atherosclerosis and fibromuscular disease of the renal artery account for most cases of RVH. Two-thirds of patients with RVH have atheromatous lesions of the renal artery. Atherosclerotic plaques typically are located in the proximal 2 cm of the main renal artery, but they also may involve the distal artery and its branches. The earliest morphologic change is vascular smooth muscle hypertrophy and hyperplasia. Angiotensin II is an important growth factor in vascular smooth muscle cells (101). The chronic administration of angiotensin-converting enzyme inhibitors will reverse many changes of vascular hypertrophy in experimental animal models and will improve vascular compliance in the hypertensive patient. Following the onset of vascular smooth muscle hypertrophy and hyperplasia, lipid deposition occurs, with necrosis, inflammation, and formation of atherosclerotic intimal plaques that protrude into the lumen. Blood pressure elevation appears to aggravate the severity of atheromatous lesions. Calcification, surface erosion with thrombus formation, or dissection of the vessel wall may ensue (96).

Atheromatous renal arterial disease predominantly afflicts men in older age groups. The disease is often diffuse, affecting the aorta and its major branches, as well as the coronary and cerebral arteries. The renal arteries are involved bilaterally in up to 40% of cases. In the national cooperative study on RVH, patients with bilateral disease had the lowest cure rate and the highest morbidity (33). A review by Schreiber and colleagues (103) of 85 patients with atheromatous renovascular disease treated medically and followed up for a mean of 52 months revealed that the disease was progressive in over 44% of patients, with progression to complete occlusion of the renal artery in 16% of renal units. Reducing the blood pressure alone has not been shown to reduce the risk of atherosclerotic complications of hypertension. Bilateral progression has been found in 20% to 30% of patients (100).

Fibromuscular diseases of the renal artery are responsible for one-third of cases of RVH. Four pathologically different types of renal artery dysplasia have been described (114). Intimal fibroplasia accounts for approximately 10% of the fibromuscular diseases. This disorder primarily involves the intima by the circumferential accumulation of collagen, compromising the arterial lumen. The disease is progressive, and dissecting hematomas may form. Children and young male adults are principally afflicted. Vessels other than the renals may be involved. Angiographically, a smooth focal stenosis is typically seen at the midrenal artery or its branches. Dissection may alter the appearance of the stenosis and of the vessel. Because of the progressive nature of this disease, prompt repair of the lesion is advised.

Fibromuscular hyperplasia is the rarest of the fibrous dysplasias. It is characterized by hyperplasia of the smooth muscle and fibrous tissue, producing a concentric thickening of the renal artery wall. This disease afflicts children and young adults and is progressive.

Medial fibroplasia accounts for 75% to 80% of the fibromuscular dysplasias. On angiogram the diseased artery has the appearance of a string of beads. This angiographic pattern is caused by a series of collagenous rings alternating with aneurysmal dilations, involving the media of the main renal artery, often extending into its branches. Women in their thirties or forties are usually afflicted. This lesion does not dissect, and complete occlusion has not been reported. Schreiber and co-workers (103) followed up a group of 75 patients with this disease for a mean of 65 months and noted that progression of the lesions occurred in 33% of patients regardless of their age. Correction of the lesion by angioplasty is the treatment of choice.

In perimedial fibroplasia, a collar of dense collagen envelops the renal artery just beneath the adventitia. The lesions are tightly stenotic, and therefore extensive collateral vessels are commonly identified on angiography. Young women, 15 to 30 years of age, are most commonly afflicted. The lesion may be progressive, and repair is recommended.

PHYSIOLOGY OF THE RENIN-ANGIOTENSIN SYSTEM

The renin-angiotensin-aldosterone system plays an important role in the regulation of blood pressure and sodium-volume homeostasis. The renin-angiotensin system (RAS) is involved in the maintenance of a constant arterial blood pressure despite extremes of sodium intake. A decrease in sodium intake increases the formation and secretion of angiotensin II by mechanisms that are discussed later in this chapter. Angiotensin II enhances aldosterone biosynthesis by the glomerulosa cells of the adrenal cortex and increases sodium reabsorption at the proximal tubule. In states of increased sodium intake, the activity of the RAS is depressed, and excess sodium is excreted to maintain balance.

The RAS also protects the organism from the potential catastrophic effects of rapid-onset hypotension by responding to a sudden pressure decrease with an immediate increase in renin release. As discussed later, renin initiates a cascade of enzymatic reactions, resulting in the formation of angiotensin II. Angiotensin II is a potent vasopressor that helps restore the systemic blood pressure. It is particularly effective in constricting the precapillary and postcapillary resistance vessels. In addition, in the peripheral nerves angiotensin II potentiates the effects of norepinephrine at the noradrenergic neuroeffector junctions by increasing norepinephrine release, decreasing norepinephrine uptake, and increasing vascular sensitivity to norepinephrine. In summary, RAS buffers a decrease in blood pressure by direct constriction of resistant vessels, by interaction with the noradrenergic receptors in the vascular smooth muscles.

Renin is a proteolytic enzyme formed in modified smooth muscle cells known as the *juxtaglomerular cells* of the afferent arteriole. The juxtaglomerular cells are in intimate proximity of the macula densa of the distal tubule. Together, these microstructures are known as the juxtaglomerular apparatus. Renin is primarily released in response to (a) low renal perfusion pressure in the afferent arteriole (baroreceptor mechanism), resulting from either renal artery stenosis or a decrease in the mean systemic arterial pressure (this response is independent of renal innervation or of the GFR); (b) a low chloride (or sodium) concentration in the filtrate reaching the distal convoluted tubule (macula densa

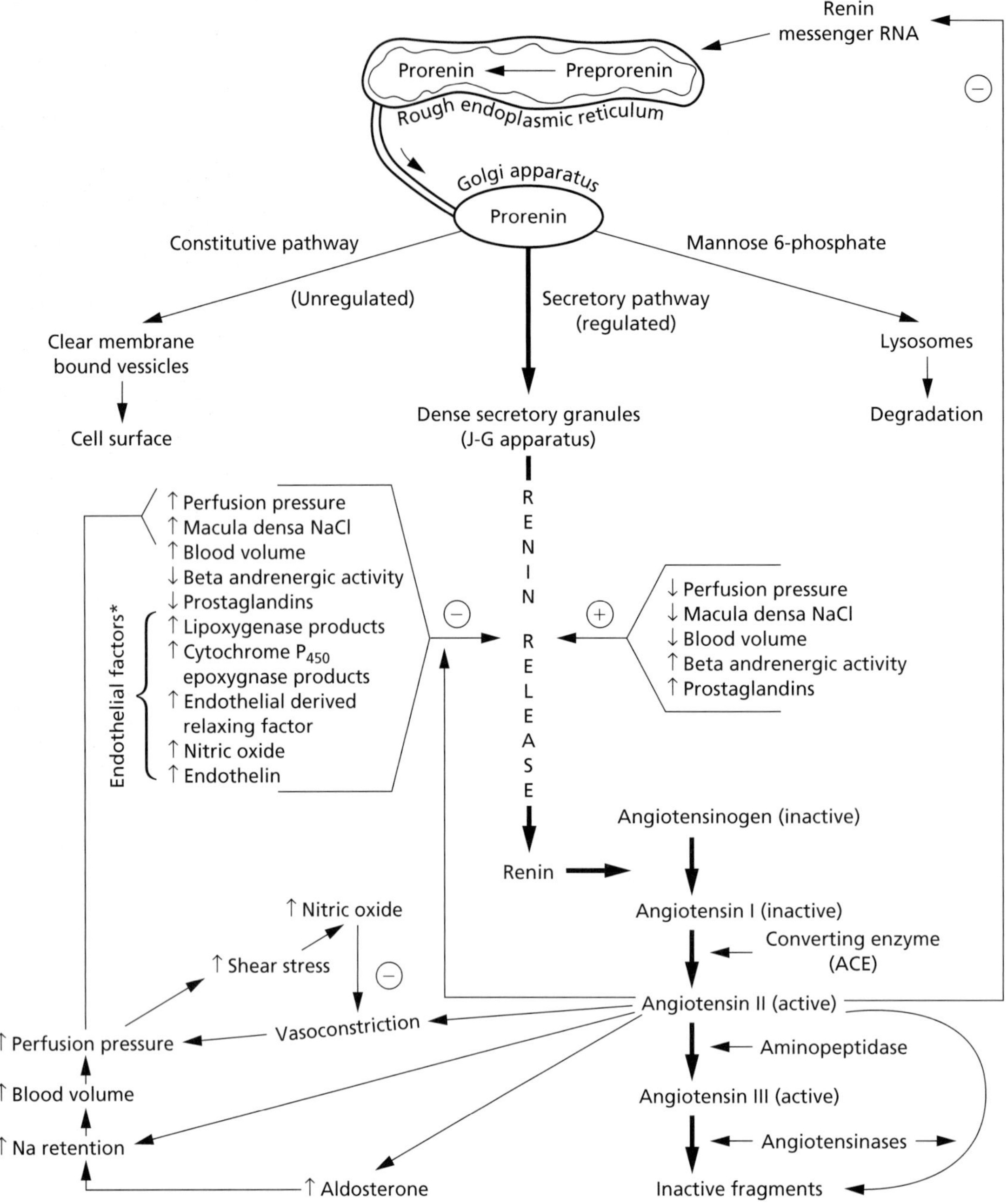

FIGURE 23.1. Renin-angiotensin-aldosterone system. (Modified from Felsen D, Vaughan ED Jr. In: Rajfer J, ed. *Urologic endocrinology.* Philadelphia: Saunders, 1986:112, with permission.)

mechanism); and (c) adrenergic stimulation of the β_1-adrenergic receptors in the juxtaglomerular cells. In the intact animal, decreases in mean arterial pressure and central blood volume activate baroreceptor and volume reflexes, eliciting adrenergic efferent signals that stimulate renin release (Fig. 23.1).

The enzymatic action of renin splits angiotensin I off the α_2-globulin angiotensinogen. Angiotensin I generally is considered an inactive molecule. Angiotensin-converting enzyme then cleaves a dipeptide off angiotensin I to produce angiotensin II.

Angiotensin II has a wide range of biologic activities. It is the protagonist through which the RAS regulates blood pressure and fluid-volume homeostasis. It is believed that angiotensin II plays an important role in renal autoregulation at low renal perfusion pressures. Normal dogs with an intact RAS subjected to graded decreases in mean renal perfusion pressure are able to maintain normal GFR. However, if the activity of the RAS is blocked by high salt intake or by CEIs, a decrease of mean renal perfusion pressure to the same levels is associated with a decrease in GFR (41). At low renal perfusion pressures, angiotensin II produces a selective efferent arteriolar vasoconstrictor to increase the glomerular capillary hydrostatic pressure and thus maintain GFR. Clinically, it has been shown that use of CEIs in patients with bilateral renal artery stenosis or stenosis of a renal artery to a solitary kidney is associated with azotemia that reverses when the drug is suspended. However, lowering of the pressure to the same level with antihypertensives that do not interfere with the RAS does not appear to compromise renal function (1,95,97). Use of CEIs in patients with unilateral renal artery stenosis also has been shown to decrease the GFR and renal blood flow of the ipsilateral kidney but not of the contralateral normal kidney (131).

PATHOPHYSIOLOGY OF RENOVASCULAR HYPERTENSION

Our current understanding of the pathophysiology of RVH has been derived to a large extent from work in experimental models of hypertension. Goldblatt and associates (37) first demonstrated that clamping one renal artery in a normal dog produced hypertension that was correctable by removing the clamp or the ischemic kidney. Currently, two models of RVH have been identified and characterized. The two kidney–one clip model is prepared by clipping the renal artery to one of the two kidneys. The ischemic kidney is designated by the ipsilateral kidney, and the untouched kidney is the contralateral kidney. In the one kidney–one clip model, the renal artery to the one kidney is clipped, and the contralateral kidney is removed. The degree of hypertension is similar for these two hypertensive models, but the mechanisms of hypertension differ in some respects.

The decrease in perfusion pressure and blood flow to the ipsilateral kidney in the two kidney–one clip model is associated with a decrease in the ipsilateral GFR, filtered sodium load, and urine sodium excretion (113). An increase in the reabsorption of water and electrolytes is dictated by glomerular-tubular balance in the ipsilateral kidney, increasing the urinary concentration of nonreabsorbable solutes and hence of urine osmolality. The decrease in mean renal perfusion pressure stimulates the baroreceptor mechanism and the decrease in the filtered load sodium (or chloride) activates the macula densa mechanism to increase renin secretion from the ischemic kidney.

The increase in the plasma renin activity invokes an angiotensin II–induced increase in mean systemic arterial blood pressure. The contralateral GFR does not change significantly, but a pressure-induced natriuresis and diuresis can be observed (112). Contralateral renin secretion is totally suppressed as the baroreceptor and macula densa mechanisms are turned off by the described physiologic changes. Tubular absorption of electrolytes and water is less marked than in the ipsilateral kidney because GFR is maintained. The contralateral urine osmolality is accordingly lower than that of the ipsilateral kidney.

The increase in arterial blood pressure in the one kidney–one clip model of hypertension is initially maintained by the vasoconstrictive properties of angiotensin II. If the renal artery clip is maintained for several weeks in the dog or rat, plasma renin activity is noted to return to normal or below normal levels. In this "chronic phase" of RVH, the degree of pressure elevation is equal to that observed in the acute phase, but salt and volume retention primarily account for the hypertension. The short-term administration of RAS blockers does not have a significant depressor effect. Sodium deprivation at this point increases the plasma renin activity and reestablishes sensitivity to the depressor effects of RAS blockers (35).

There is also evidence that other mechanisms are active. These include decreased nerve traffic (57) and increased production of nitric oxide. Nitric oxide inhibitors exacerbate hypertension in experimental renovascular models (76). In addition, there is evidence for a role of prostaglandin endoperoxides because the $T_xA_2/PC\text{-}H_2$ receptor antagonist (ifetroban) also lowers blood pressure in both the acute and chronic phase of the two kidney–one clip model (132).

PHARMACOLOGIC PROBES FOR THE RENIN-ANGIOTENSIN SYSTEM

Insight into the physiology of the RAS has been gained from the development of pharmacologic compounds that inhibit the release of the renin, block the conversion of angiotensin II, or are specific angiotensin II receptor analogs (Fig. 23.1).

The first drug that specifically blocked the action of angiotensin II was saralasin. Saralasin is an angiotensin II analog with affinity for the angiotensin II receptor, but with partial agonist activity (86). Administration of saralasin to two kidney–one clip hypertensive models or to patients with RVH produces a depressor response. However, saralasin lost favor as a screening agent for RVH because of its agonist activity, which produces an increase in blood pressure and hence an underestimation of the contribution of angiotensin II to the maintenance of hypertension.

CEIs prevent the conversion of angiotensin I to angiotensin II. Naturally occurring CEIs initially were found in snake venom (3). Captopril, an orally active synthetic CEI with a rapid onset of action, currently is used in a screening role for renin-dependent hypertension (see Single-dose Captopril Test) and to treat RVH in select cases.

More recently, a number of oral drugs have been developed that block the action of angiotensin II at the receptor level. Losartan is the prototype. At present, the angiotensin II subtype AT_1 receptor appears to be the primary angiotensin receptor in the kidney and vasculature (38).

CLINICAL EVALUATION OF RENOVASCULAR HYPERTENSION

It is now clear that the angiographic finding of a stenosed renal artery in a hypertensive patient is insufficient evidence on which to diagnose RVH. In this regard, hypertensive patients with a renal artery stenosis may not improve after renal revascularization (33). Moreover, radiologic (28) and autopsy (46) series have shown that normotensive patients can have severely diseased renal arteries. Patients with atherosclerotic disease elsewhere have a 20% to 50% chance of having renal arterial disease (129,136).

Until recently, means by which to reliably identify patients with a physiologically significant renal artery stenosis have eluded the clinician. There are no pathognomonic clinical characteristics that reliably lead to the diagnosis (107), but certain clinical features should arouse suspicion that RVH may be present (Table 23.1).

Taking these clinical findings altogether, Mann and Pickering (67) have defined patients who are at low, moderate, or high risk for renovascular hypertension (Table 23.2). Patients at moderate or high risk warrant further study (90).

The lack of reliable clinical clues stimulated further study in laboratory animals in pursuit of understanding the physiologic profiles that characterize laboratory models of Goldblatt's hypertension. These endeavors have resulted in the delineation of a variety of approaches to screen for patients with RVH.

The emergence of methods to reliably assay the activity of the RAS and the development of pharmacologic probes that block specific steps in the renin-angiotensin cascade have led to the use of renin determinations to diagnose RVH. Goldblatt's initial animal work led to the assumption that the underlying derangement in RVH is excess renin secretion resulting in angiotensin II formation. The hypertensive animal model most analogous to human RVH is the two kidney–one clip Goldblatt preparation. In this model, the hypertension initially is depending on the increased renin secretion from the clipped kidney. The administration

TABLE 23.1. CLINICAL CLUES SUGGESTIVE OF RENOVASCULAR HYPERTENSION (RVH)

Clues	Comment
Historical	
Hypertension in the absence of any family history of hypertensive disease	Suspect if family history negative; however, about ⅓ of patients with RVH have a positive family history.
Age of onset of hypertension <25 or >45 yr	The average age of onset for essential hypertension is 31 ± 10 (SD) yr. Children and young adults usually have fibromuscular disease; adults >45 yr are more likely to have atherosclerotic narrowing of arteries.
Abrupt onset of moderate to severe hypertension	Essential hypertension usually begins with a "labile" phase before mild hypertension becomes established; usually has a more telescoped natural history, often first appearing as moderate hypertension of recent onset.
Development of severe or malignant hypertension	RVH often becomes moderately severe and is prone to produce acceleration- or malignant-phase hypertension; both forms of hypertension involve markedly increased renin release.
Headaches	Essential hypertension is usually asymptomatic. There seem to be more headaches with RVH, possibly related to its severity or to high levels of angiotensin II, a potent cerebrovascular vasconstrictor.
Cigarette smoking	In a survey (78a), 74% of patients with fibromuscular renal artery stenosis were smokers; 88% of those with atherosclerotic disease smoked.
White race	RVH is uncommon in the African American population.
Resistance to or escape from blood pressure control with standard diuretic therapy or antiadrenergic	Probably the most typical feature of RVH is that it responds poorly to diuretics and often only transiently to antiadrenergic drugs.
Excellent antihypertensive response to CEIs such as captopril	CEIs block the RAS most effectively and are therefore highly specific agents.
Examination and routine laboratory results	
Retinopathy	Hemorrhages, exudates, or papilledema indicate acceleration or malignant phase.
Abdominal or flank bruit	A helpful clue, but commonly present in elderly individuals, and occasionally it is present in younger patients who have no apparent vascular stenosis.
Carotid bruits or other evidence of large-vessel disease	Commonly the vascular disease is not limited to the renal bed.
Hypokalemia—in the untreated state or in response to a thiazide diuretic	Increased aldosterone stimulation by the RAS tends to reduce the serum potassium level. In untreated essential hypertension this does not occur. Thiazide diuretics accentuate this phenomenon in RVH.

CEIs, converting enzyme inhibitors; RAS, renin-angiotensin system.
From Vaughan ED Jr, Case CB, Pickering TG, et al. Clinical evaluation of renovascular hypertension and therapeutic decisions, *Urol Clin North Am* 1984;11:393, with permission.

of CEIs or competitive angiotensin II analogs (9) can prevent or reverse the hypertension. This early phase of two kidney–one clip hypertension exhibits four characteristics: increased secretion of renin from the clipped kidney, absence of renin secretion from the opposite kidney, decreased renal blood flow to the clipped kidney, and elevated pressure secondary to angiotensin II–induced vasoconstriction. The identification of these characteristics permitted the development of a rational approach to the use of plasma renin activity determinations and angiotensin blockade in the diagnosis of RVH (90,127) (Fig. 23.2).

TABLE 23.2. TESTING FOR RENOVASCULAR HYPERTENSION: CLINICAL INDEX OF SUSPICION AS A GUIDE TO SELECTING PATIENTS FOR WORKUP

Index of Clinical Suspicion
Low (should not be tested)
▪ Borderline, mild, or moderate hypertension in the absence of clinical clues
Moderate (noninvasive tests recommended)
▪ Severe hypertension (diastolic blood pressure >120 mm Hg)
▪ Hypertension refractory to standard therapy
▪ Abrupt onset of sustained moderate to severe hypertension at age <20 or >50 yr
▪ Hypertension with a suggestive abdominal bruit (long, high-pitched, and localized to the region of the renal artery)
▪ Moderate hypertension (diastolic blood pressure >105 mm Hg) in a smoker, a patient with evidence of occlusive vascular disease (cerebrovascular, coronary, peripheral vascular), or a patient with unexplained but stable elevation of serum creatinine
▪ Normalization of blood pressure by an angiotensin-converting enzyme inhibitor in a patient with moderate or severe hypertension (particularly in a smoker or patient with recent onset of hypertension)

Modified from reference 90.

Until recently, the combined analysis of the peripheral renin level and determination of differential renal vein renin levels was the standard methodology for identifying potentially curable patients with renovascular hypertension (127). Less invasive tests that give both anatomic and physiologic evidence for curable renovascular hypertension are currently being explored. These tests include captopril renography, color Doppler sonography, spiral computed tomography (CT) angiography, and magnetic resonance angiography (MRA) (52,88).

However, before discussing these tests, it is important to review the use of renin determinations to understand the pathophysiology of renovascular hypertension.

PERIPHERAL PLASMA RENIN ACTIVITY

Peripheral ambulatory plasma renin activity samples are collected in a standardized setting that requires that the patient be salt replete and off all antihypertensive medicines that influence plasma renin activity for at least 2 weeks. In addition, the plasma renin activity is sampled after 4 hours of ambulation and is indexed against a 24-hour urine sodium determination.

The rationale for emphasizing the peripheral plasma renin activity determination is that it is an index of renin secretion (105). In a study of hypertensive patients who had

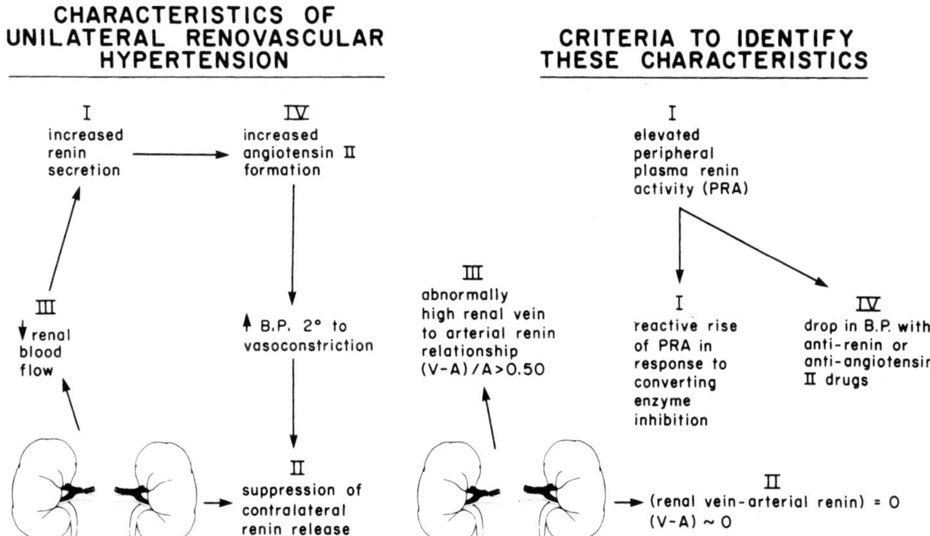

FIGURE 23.2. Characteristics of the early phase of two kidney–one clip Goldblatt's hypertension in the rat *(left)* and the criteria derived from the animal model that identify the patient with correctable renal hypertension. (From Vaughan ED Jr, Case DB, Pickering TG, et al. Clinical evaluation of renovascular hypertension and therapeutic decisions. *Urol Clin North Am* 1984;11:393, with permission.)

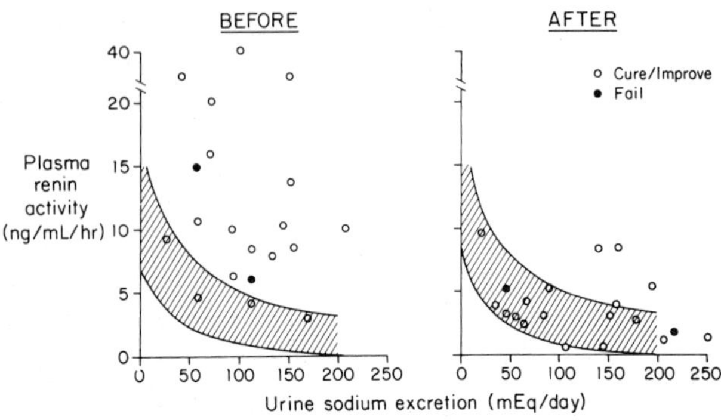

FIGURE 23.3. Effect of angioplasty on peripheral plasma renin activity indexed against 24-hour sodium excretion. *Left panel:* Before angioplasty. *Right panel:* 6 months after angioplasty. *Hatched area* shows normal range. (From Pickering TG, Sos TA, Vaughan ED Jr, et al. Predictive value and changes of renin secretion in hypertensive patients with unilateral renovascular disease undergoing successful renal angioplasty. *Am J Med* 1984;76:394, with permission.)

successful angioplasty, the peripheral plasma renin activity was elevated in 80% before angioplasty (93). The plasma renin activity always decreased and usually returned to normal after successful angioplasty (Fig. 23.3).

The 20% false-negative rate places definitive limitations on the use of peripheral plasma renin activity as a screening test for RVH. In addition, many patients with proved RVH have severe, life-threatening hypertension that precludes cessation of antihypertensive medications before blood sampling. Performance of plasma renin activity determinations while the patient is taking medication invalidates the accuracy of the test and eliminates the quantification of peripheral plasma renin activity as a practical screening tool. A third factor is the finding that 16% of patients with essential hypertension also have high plasma renin activity when indexed against a 24-hour urine sodium determination (10). Thus the positive predictive value is poor.

Enhanced Accuracy of Peripheral Plasma Renin Activity by Stimulation with Angiotensin-blocking Agents

The first angiotensin-blocking agent used for testing in human hypertension was saralasin. The initial results demonstrated that the compound, as predicted, lowered blood pressure in high-renin forms of hypertension (9).

A second approach to the use of angiotensin blockade to expose RVH came from experience after the development of CEIs that block angiotensin II formation. One of the peptides, teprotide, was shown to block the vasopressor effect of angiotensin II, and it was possible to demonstrate a close direct correlation between the pretreatment level of plasma renin activity and the magnitude of the depressor response (17).

The success of teprotide was a potent stimulus to the development of the orally active CEI captopril. Captopril has the potential for use as a diagnostic probe, like teprotide, because it has a rapid onset of action (within 10 to 15 minutes), reaching a peak effect by 90 minutes (16) (Fig. 23.4).

During the early studies of the effect of these agents on blood pressure in hypertensive patients, it was noted that

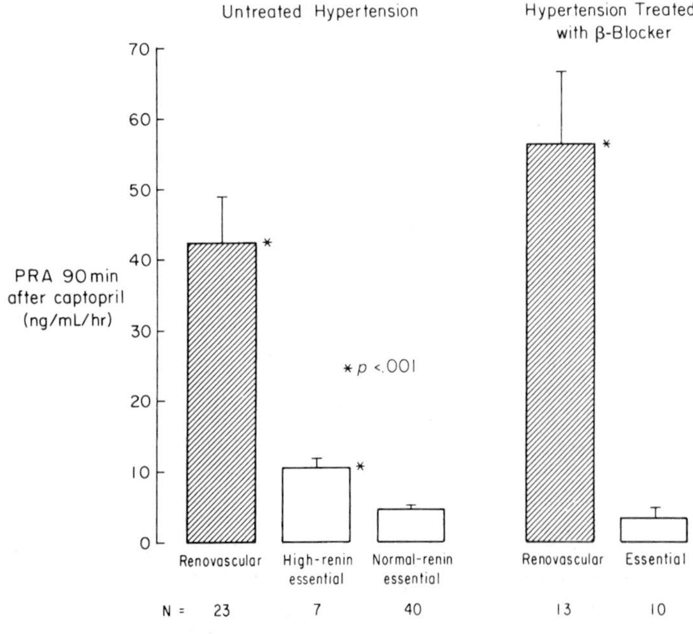

FIGURE 23.4. Levels of plasma renin activity in renovascular hypertension (RVH) and essential hypertension 90 minutes after a single dose of captopril. A marked reactive hyperreninemia was found in the group with RVH whether or not they were already receiving β-blocker therapy. (From Case DB, Atlas SA, Laragh JH. Physiologic effects and blockade. In: Laragh JH, Buhler FR, Seldin DW, eds. *Frontiers in hypertension research.* New York: Springer-Verlag, 1982, with permission.)

angiotensin blockade resulted in a marked rise in plasma renin activity in selected patients. Accordingly, the induction of marked rises in plasma activity appeared to be a more specific test for RVH than the induction of depressor responses.

Single-dose Captopril Test

The captopril test is a reliable screening test well suited for outpatient use. Diuretics and preferably all other antihypertensive medications are discontinued at least 2 weeks before testing. Patients are advised not to restrict their salt intake. Twenty to thirty minutes before testing, the patient is seated comfortably in a quiet room, during which time an intravenous catheter is placed for blood sampling, and baseline blood pressure is taken for a baseline plasma renin activity determination before the oral administration of 25 mg of captopril. Blood pressure measurements are then taken every 15 minutes for 1 hour. Venous blood sampling is repeated at 30 and 60 minutes after captopril administration. A depressor renin activity level (92) is seen in patients with renin-dependent hypertension (diastolic pressure decrease of 15% or more). However, the change in blood pressure has low specificity, because patients with essential hypertension also may have a depressor response.

Formation of angiotensin II is greatly decreased by captopril. The resulting decrease in systemic blood pressure in patients with renin-dependent hypertension further decreases the blood flow to the ischemic kidney. The lower perfusion pressure produces a decrease in the glomerular capillary hydrostatic pressure, diminishing the GFR. In addition, the efferent arteriole, which undergoes angiotensin II–induced vasoconstriction at low perfusion pressures to maintain glomerular filtration, relaxes as angiotensin II formation is blocked, thus decreasing the ipsilateral GFR further. The macula densa and baroreceptor mechanisms are activated, and more renin is released from the ischemic kidney. In renin-dependent hypertension, but not in essential hypertension, inhibition of the converting enzyme is associated with a rise in plasma renin activity to 12 ng/mL per hour or greater, an increment in plasma renin activity of 10 ng/mL per hour or more above baseline levels, and a percent increase in plasma renin activity of 170% or more (or 400% if the baseline plasma renin activity was less than 3 ng/mL per hour). If these three criteria are present in a patient with normal renal function off diuretics, RVH can be distinguished from essential hypertension with a specificity of 100% and a sensitivity of 95% (75). Prior sodium depletion by diuretics or by dietary restraint increases plasma renin activity and abolishes the specificity of this test. Patients in treatment with β-adrenergic blockers remain responsive to captopril as described previously unless their baseline plasma renin activity is less than 2.5, in which case the test may be unreliable (Table 23.3).

TABLE 23.3. SINGLE-DOSE CAPTOPRIL TEST

Drugs
- Discontinue all antihypertensive medicines for at least 2 wk, if possible; otherwise, maintain β-blocker but avoid diuretics, CEIs, and nonsteroidal antinflammatory drugs for at least 1 wk, ideally 2 wk.

Diet
- A diet with normal or high sodium content is necessary. Too low a sodium intake will produce false-positive results. If there is a question about diet, a 24-hr urine collection for sodium will closely reflect the intake.

Procedure
- The patient is seated comfortably for 20–30 min before testing and maintained in this position for the duration of the test.
- Blood pressure is measured at 20, 25, and 30 min (obtain three stable baseline measurements), then blood is sampled for plasma renin activity (in a lavender top Vacutainor kept at room temperature).
- A 25-mg captopril tablet is crushed (to ensure that it dissolves) and 30 mL of water added to prepare a suspension. The patient is instructed to drink the suspension, wash the contents out twice, and drink those also.
- Blood pressure and plasma renin activity are remeasured after 30 and 60 min.

CEIs, converting enzyme inhibitors.
From Vaughan ED Jr, Case DB, Pickering TG, et al. Clinical evaluation of renovascular hypertension and therapeutic decisions. *Urol Clin North Am* 1984;11:393, with permission.

In summary, the single-dose captopril test appears to accurately separate patients with RVH from those with essential hypertension. In addition, a 24-hour urine collection is not necessary, and the patient can remain on β-blockade.

Captopril Renogram Insert

The captopril renogram is performed in a similar fashion as the single-dose captopril test. A crushed tablet of 25 mg of captopril is given 1 hour before the procedure. Numerous isotopes have been used (Table 23.3), with ^{99m}Tc mercaptoacetylglycylglycyl-glycine (MAG3) being most commonly used today. Interpretation depends on the isotope chosen and the parameter calculated. Commonly used parameters are (a) split renal function percent uptake left to right; (b) maximum activity (A_{max}); (c) single-kidney GFR or renal blood flow, depending on which isotope is used; (d) time to peak activity (T_{max}); (e) the transit time; and (f) residual cortical activity indicating slow isotopic washout. Often, the renogram curves are graded. If the test is positive, imaging studies are necessary because there can be positive tests in patients with parenchymal disease (78). Table 23.4 lists the recent literature concerning the captopril scan, including predictive value (88). False-negative scans can occur in azotemic patients with segmental branch disease. Taken altogether, along with color Doppler sonography, the captopril renogram is gaining popularity as the initial test to identify RVH.

Contralateral Suppression of Renin Secretion and an Elevated Renal Vein-to-Arterial Renin Relationship: Use of Differential Renal Vein Renin Determinations

The emergence of the captopril renogram coupled with noninvasive imaging of the renal arteries has relegated renal vein renin determinations to a supportive role in difficult cases. However, the understanding of renal vein renin secretion enhances our understanding of RVH.

In view of limitations of the traditional renal vein ratio analysis, a method for analysis of renal values has been devised and is based on the characteristics of experimental two kidney–one clip Goldblatt's hypertension (Table 23.5) (Fig. 23.2).

Hypersecretion of renin, as determined by the renin-sodium index or captopril stimulation, serves as the primary criterion for the diagnosis of RVH. A second criterion is the demonstration of the absence of renin secretion from the contralateral (or noninvolved) kidney. Suppression of renin secretion from this kidney can be determined by subtracting the arterial plasma renin activity (A) from the renal venous renin activity (V). Because the inferior vena caval (IVC) renin and aortic renin are the same, the IVC renin value can be substituted for A in this equation (105). Hence, patients with curable RVH exhibit an absence of renin secretion from the opposite kidney; that is, $V - A = 0$, also called *contralateral suppression of renin* (115,123). Contralateral suppression of renin indicates that the noninvolved kidney is responding in an appropriate, "normal" fashion to the elevated blood pressure, increased circulatory angiotensin II levels, or increased sodium chloride at the macula densa by shutting off renin secretion. This phenomenon is at times present not only in patients with unilateral renal arterial lesions but also in patients with bilateral disease demonstrated by arteriograms who have a dominant lesion on one side (91).

A third criterion is based on studies of renal vein and arterial vein relationships in patients with essential hypertension. The mean renal venous renin level has been determined to be about 25% higher than arterial plasma renin activity (105). Hence, a total renin increment (both kidneys) of approximately 50% is necessary to maintain a given peripheral renin level: $(V - A)/A = 50\%$. However, a reduction in renal blood flow also influences the renal venous renin level. In this setting, the renal venous renin

TABLE 23.4. ANGIOTENSIN-CONVERTING ENZYME INHIBITOR RENOGRAPHY WITH DIFFERENT TRACERS IN DIAGNOSING RENAL ARTERY STENOSIS

Reference	RAS	EH	Sensitivity	Specificity (%)	Positive Predictive Value	Negative Predictive Value
DTPA						
Pedersen, et al. (1989)	14	10	93	100	100	91
Dondi, et al. (1990)	52	80	92	96	97	95
Chen, et al. (1990)	23	27	91	93	91	93
Mann, et al. (1991)	35	20	51	100	100	54
Setaro, et al. (1991)	58	55	91	87	88	91
Svetkey, et al. (1991)	31	109	74	44	27	86
Pedersen, et al. (1992)	26	16	76	94	94	96
Dey, et al. (1993)	45	43	89	84	85	88
Mittal, et al. (1996)	45	41	82	90	90	82
IOH						
Mann, et al. (1991)	35	20	43	90	88	47
Erbsloh-Moller, et al. (1991)	28	22	96	95	95	96
Svetkey, et al. (1991)	31	109	71	41	26	83
MAG_3						
Nitzsche, et al. (1991)	18	50	94	88	74	98
Roccatello and Picciotto (1997)						
Standard evaluation	29	20	79	70	79	76
Expected renogram	29	20	79	95	96	76
DTPA or IOH						
Geyskes, et al. (1987)	15	19	80	100	100	86
Fommei, et al. (1991)	208	157	63	84	85	63
Roccatello, et al. (1992)	35	32	92	94	94	91

DTPA, ^{99m}Tc-diethylenetriaminopentaacetate; EH, essential hypertension; IOH, ^{133}I or ^{125}I-ortoiodohippurate; MAG_3, ^{99m}Tc-mercaptoacetylgycylglycylglycine; RAS, renal artery stenosis.
Modified from Pedersen EB: New tools in diagnosing renal artery stenosis. *Kidney Int* 2000;57:2657.

TABLE 23.5. RENIN VALUES FOR PREDICTING CURABILITY OF RENOVASCULAR HYPERTENSION

Collection of samples (moderate sodium intake ± 100 mEq/day)	
Ambulatory peripheral renin and 24-hr urine sodium excretion under steady state conditions (i.e., not on day of arteriography)	
Collection of blood for PRA before and after converting enzyme blockade	
Collection of supine:	
Renal vein renin from suspect kidney (V1) and inferior vena caval renin (A1)	
Renal vein from contralateral kidney (V2) and inferior vena caval renin (A2)	
Enhancement of renin secretion by converting enzyme blockade if initial renin sampling is inconclusive	
Criteria for predicting cure	
High PRA in relation to UNaV	Measurement of hypersecretion of renin
Contralateral kidney: (V2 – A2) = 0	An indicator of absent renin secretion from the contralateral kidney
Suspect kidney: (V1 – A1)/A1 = 0.50	Measurement of reduced renal blood flow
$\frac{(V-A)}{A} + \frac{(V-A)}{A} = 0.50$ in patients with high PRA means	
Incorrect sampling	
Segmental disease	Repeat with segmental sampling

PRA, plasma renin activity.
From Vaughan ED Jr, Sosa TA, Sniderman KW, et al. Renal vein renin secretory patterns before and after transluminal angioplasty in patients with renovascular hypertension: verification of analytic criteria. In: Laragh JH, ed. *Frontiers in hypertension research.* New York: Springar-Verlag, 1981, with permission.

concentration is misleadingly high, shifting the renal vein–to–arterial renin relationships upward. Thus the elevation of the increment above approximately 50% becomes an index of the severity of the reduction in blood flow consequent to the obstructing vascular lesion (Fig. 23.5). The combination of these criteria found in a group of patients managed by renal revascularization is shown in Fig. 23.6 (124).

An additional aid to renal vein sampling is the utilization of segmental renal venous sampling (102), especially in cases in which sampling of blood from the major renal vein fails to demonstrate a combined renin increment of 50% from both kidneys, suggesting either a technical error or segmental disease. This approach may be particularly helpful in children with segmental parenchymal disease (87).

The patterns of renal vein renin activity in bilateral RVH are less consistent than in unilateral disease (92).

Validation of the Four Criteria

In addition to a favorable clinical response to renal angioplasty, we also have had the unique opportunity to study the effect of restoration of blood flow on renal vein renin concentration and renin excretion (92,126). To accomplish this goal we have monitored the immediate effect of successful angioplasty on renal renin secretion. Thirty minutes after angioplasty, a marked reduction was noted in the renal vein renin from the previously stenotic side (Fig. 23.7). The residual ipsilateral increment of renal vein renin was approximately 50% above the peripheral level, whereas contralateral renin suppression persisted. This 50% increment has been predicted previously to occur in the setting of unilateral renin secretion and normal renal blood flow (105).

The finding that the renal renin secretory characteristics of RVH reverse after successful angioplasty with correction of the hypertension is strong support that they truly reflect the abnormal secretory behavior of renin in curable RVH.

Color Doppler Sonography

Renal sonography has rapidly evolved from a technique that gave only anatomic information to a functional test. The advances include the use of a Doppler probe (116), the color

ESSENTIAL HYPERTENSION

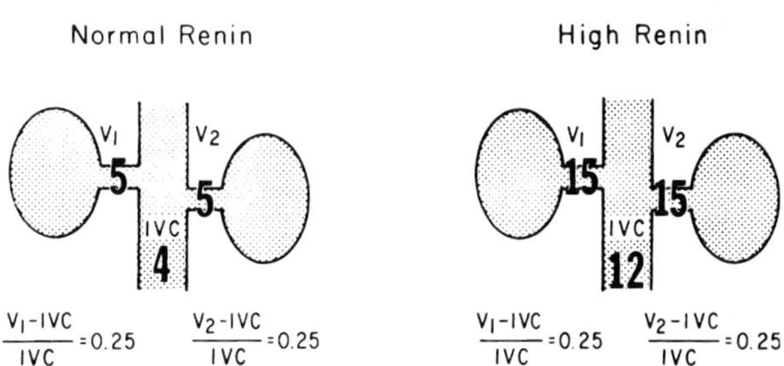

RENOVASCULAR HYPERTENSION

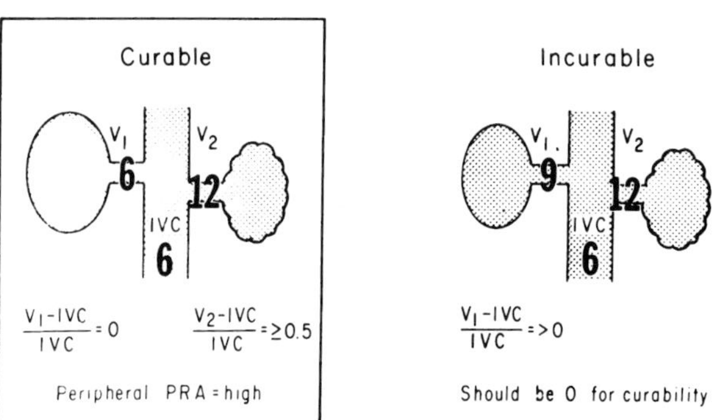

FIGURE 23.5. Renal vein renin diagnostic pattern. In essential hypertension *(top)* at all levels of renin secretion the renin level of each renal vein is approximately 25% greater than either the peripheral arterial or venous levels. In the setting of unilateral renin secretion (curable RVH) the active kidney is solely responsible for maintaining the peripheral renin levels. Hence, the increment is 50% (0.5) and becomes progressively greater as renal blood flow is reduced. Unequal bilateral renin secretion *(bottom right)* indicates bilateral disease and decreases the chance of cure after corrective unilateral surgery. (From Laragh JH, Sealey JE. Renin sodium profiling: why, how and when in clinical practice. *Cardiovasc Med* 1977;2:1503, with permission.)

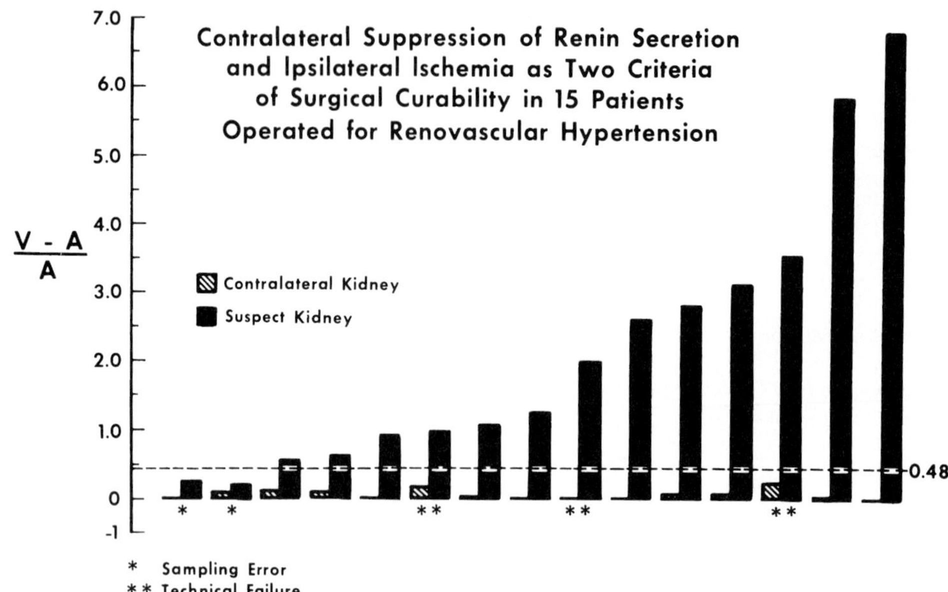

FIGURE 23.6. Of 15 patients with renovascular hypertension, 13 exhibited (V – A)/A in excess of 48% from the suspect kidney and a suppressed value from the contralateral kidney. V is renal venous plasma renin activity; A is arterial or infrarenal inferior vena cava plasma renin activity. Asterisks (**) denote the three patients who had values suggesting surgical curability yet had residual or recurrent hypertension resulting from technical failure. (From Vaughan ED Jr, Carey RM, Ayers CR, et al. A physiologic definition of blood pressure response to renal revascularization in patients with renovascular hypertension. *Kidney Int* 1979;15:S83, with permission.)

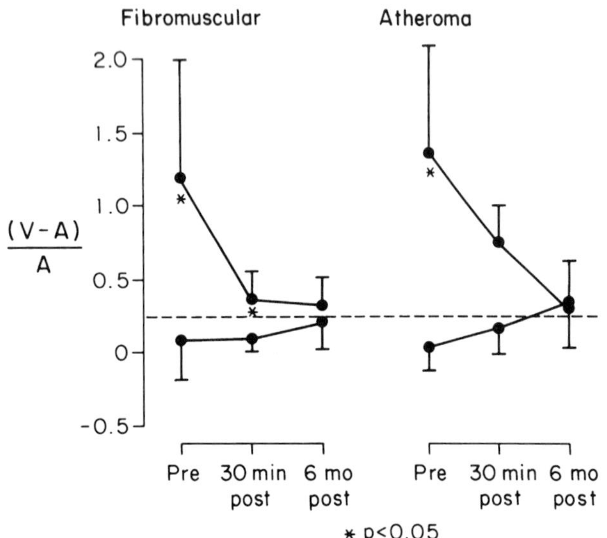

FIGURE 23.7. Effect of angioplasty on renal vein renins. Samples were taken immediately before angioplasty, 30 minutes after, and 6 months later. The higher values were for the ischemic kidney, the lower for the contralateral kidney. Asterisks (*) indicate significant difference between the two kidneys, and the *dotted line* is the normal level of (V – A)/A (0.24). (From Pickering TG, Sos TA, Vaughan ED Jr, et al. Predictive value and changes of renin secretion in hypertensive patients with unilateral renovascular disease undergoing successful renal angioplasty. *Am J Med* 1984;76:398, with permission.)

technique, the use of contrast (74), and the captopril Doppler sonogram (128). Similar to the captopril renogram, several indexes have been used: peak systolic velocity, renal aortic ratio, end-systolic index, acceleration time, and acceleration index. The overall results as compiled by Pedersen (88) are shown in Table 23.6.

The major difficulties have been in the development of competent personnel with experience. Moreover, obesity and intestinal gas are limitations. Other variables include whether attention is placed on intrarenal vessels, which cannot always be localized (99), or directly on the main renal artery (73). Regardless of differences in technique, the test is gaining wider usage (52). Again, a positive test requires anatomic confirmation.

Imaging Studies

Following a positive screening test, the traditional approach has been renal angiography followed immediately by angioplasty if possible. In a patient in whom there is a high index of clinical suspicion, angiography is still preferred (Fig. 23.8) (90).

Recently, two newer, less invasive techniques are being used to diagnose renal artery stenosis.

Spiral Computed Tomography Angiography

The development of spiral CT has permitted data acquisition during a single breath hold. The scanning time is

TABLE 23.6. COLOR DOPPLER SONOGRAPHY IN DIAGNOSING RENAL ARTERY STENOSIS

	Patients N		Arteries N						
Reference	EH or Controls	RAS	Controls	Stenotic Arteries	Degree of Stenosis	Sensitivity	Specificity (%)	Positive Predictive Value	Negative Predictive Value
Postma, et al. (1992)	46	24		29	50	63	86	83	68
Stavros, et al. (1992)	30	26		32	60	95	97	92	98
Kliewer, et al. (1993)	23	23		28	80	66	67		
Schwerk, et al. (1994)	53	19		19	50	82	92		
Olin, et al. (1995)			63	124	60	98	98	99	97
Spies, et al. (1995)			153	42	50	93	92	77	98
Krumme, et al. (1996)	47	88		107	50	89	92	92	88
Miralles, et al. (1996)	34	44	98	58	60	87[c]/76[d]	91[c]/92[d]	86[c]/86[d]	92[c]/87[d]
Missouris, et al. (1996)			24	16	60	85[e]/94[f]	79[e]/88[f]		
Postma, et al. (1996)	52[d]	19			50	47	97		
Nazzal, et al. (1997)			70	73	50	89[b]/63[g]	92[b]/98[g]	85[b]/91[g]	94[b]/87[g]
Riehl, et al. (1997)	161	53		59	70	93	96	93	98

[a]Technical failure in 15 of 61 patients.
[b]Test parameter was acceleration index.
[c]Test parameter was peak systolic velocity in the renal artery.
[d]Technical failures in 5 of 57 patients.
[e]Without ultrasound contrast enhancement.
[f]With ultrasound enhancement.
[g]Test parameter was acceleration time.
[h]Test parameter was renal/aortic ratio.
EH, essential hypertension; RAS, renal artery stenosis.
From Pederson EB. New tools in diagnosing renal artery stenosis. *Kidney Int* 2000;57:2657.

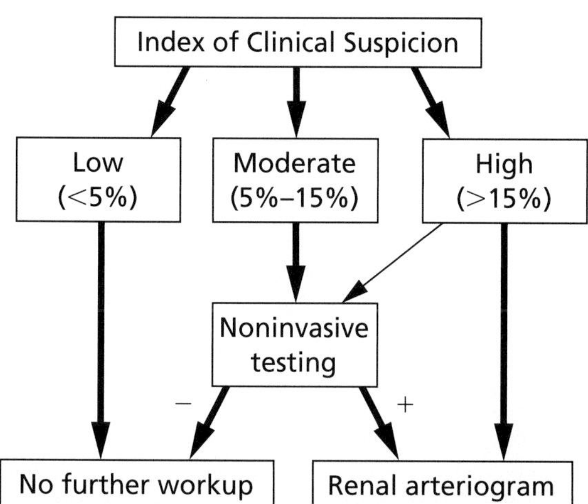

FIGURE 23.8. Suggested workup of a patient suspected of having renovascular disease. (From Pickering TG, Blumenfield JD. Renovascular hypertension and ischemic nephropathy. In: Brenner BM, ed. *The kidney.* Philadelphia: WB Saunders, 2000:2007.)

approximately 35 seconds, the examination time is approximately 20 minutes, and the data analysis takes approximately 30 minutes. The results are impressive (Fig. 23.9). This technique is now being used routinely to evaluate renal donors (94). The reported sensitivity ranges from 88% to 98% and the specificity ranges from 82% to 98%, giving a positive predictive value greater than 85% (88). The one caveat is that a relatively high volume (150 mL) of contrast is given peripherally; thus there is a risk of nephrotoxicity. In addition, the accuracy appears to be decreased in azotemic patients.

Magnetic Resonance Angiography

The two MRA techniques used are time-of-flight and phase-contrast sequences. MRA avoids the problem of renal toxicity but is limited to visualization of the main renal artery and the larger branches (39) (Fig. 23.10). The use of gadolinium may enhance the sensitivity of the technique (109). The technique is most useful in patients with atherosclerotic

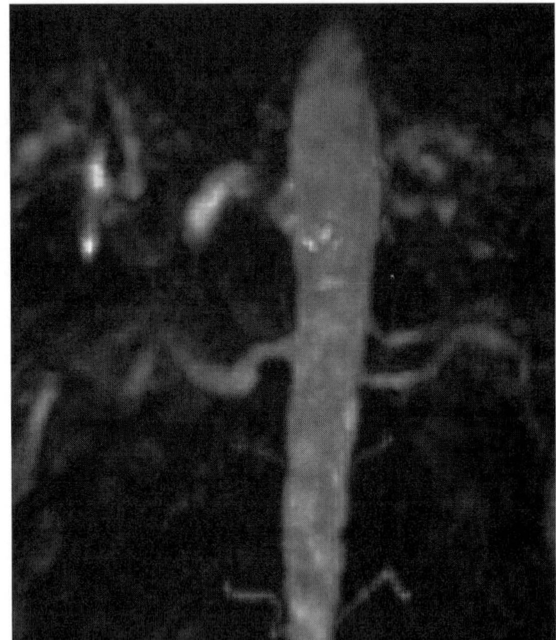

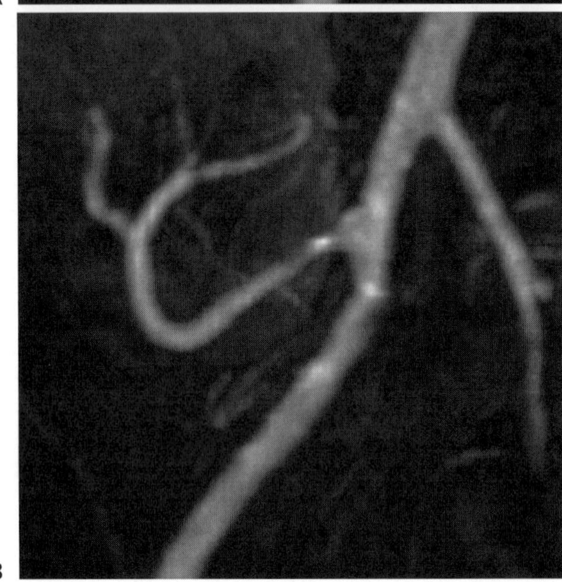

FIGURE 23.9. Spiral computed tomography scans showing bilateral renal artery stenosis **(A)** and stenosis of a transplant renal artery **(B)**.

disease where the lesion is in the proximal renal artery, particularly if the patient has impaired renal function.

Identifying the Potentially Curable Patient

The approach of Pickering and Blumenfeld (90) already alluded to (Fig. 23.8) seems rational. Thus the low-risk patient, in whom screening tests have low predictive value, is initially treated without evaluation. In contrast, for high-risk patients (Table 23.2), angiography is the initial study. Patients at moderate risk begin their evaluation with either a captopril renogram or a color duplex Doppler scan. If the test is negative, no additional studies are done. If the initial test is positive, anatomic localizing tests are necessary.

Ischemic Nephropathy

The other entity associated with renal artery stenosis is ischemic nephropathy. Thus renal artery stenosis is an important cause of chronic renal insufficiency due to a reduction in GFR (50,79,100).

Hypertension is now the most common cause of end-stage renal disease (ESRD) in patients older than 65 years of age (56). The subset of these patients with renal artery stenosis is unclear. However, in one study, 83 of 687 dialysis patients (12%) were found to have renal artery disease (65). Novick and colleagues (82) established the following criteria

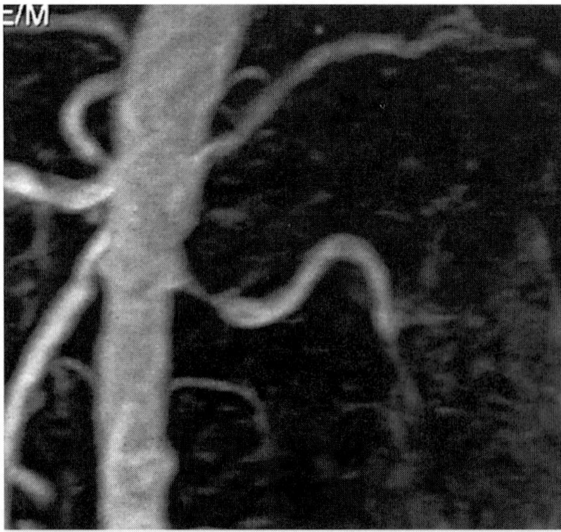

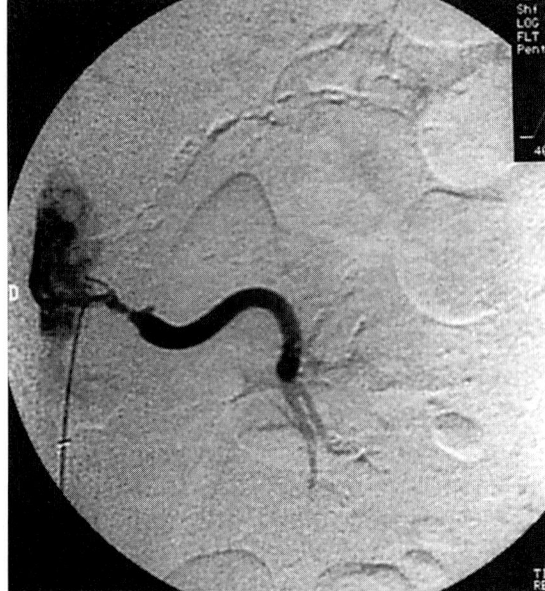

FIGURE 23.10. Three-dimensional, gadolinium-enhanced magnetic resonance angiography showing a thrombosis of the left renal artery and severe stenosis of the left renal artery. [From Grenier N, Trilland M. 2000;86(Suppl):84.]

for screening for atherosclerotic renal artery disease: (a) evidence of generalized atherosclerosis, (b) a unilateral small kidney, and (c) mild to moderate azotemia (serum creatinine greater than 1.5 mg/dL). If the patient was found to have a high-grade stenosis (greater than 75%) bilaterally or in a solitary kidney, intervention was recommended (82).

Preservation of renal function has been demonstrated after renal revascularization (4) or angioplasty (13,104). However, randomized trials, now in progress, are necessary to prove that intervention is more successful than medical management in forestalling ESRD.

In addition, the evaluation previously described using peripheral and renal vein renin determinations are often inaccurate in azotemic patients. Thus color Doppler or MRA studies are necessary to exclude ischemic nephropathy as the cause of azotemia.

TREATMENT OF RENOVASCULAR HYPERTENSION

The therapeutic options for the treatment of RVH include percutaneous transluminal angioplasty, renal artery stent placement, surgical revascularization, autotransplantation, pharmacologic interference of the RAS, and removal of the ischemic kidney.

Renal Artery Angioplasty for Renovascular Hypertension

Percutaneous transluminal angioplasty was first introduced by Dotter and Judkins in 1964 for the treatment of peripheral vascular stenoses. The introduction of flexible, double-lumen balloon catheters by Gruntzig and Hopff (40) permitted the development of percutaneous transluminal angioplasty of renal artery stenoses. The fibromuscular dysplasias and unilateral, nonostial, nonoccluded atherosclerotic renal artery stenoses are the most suitable lesions for treatment with percutaneous transluminal renal angioplasty (PTRA). The ability to avoid a general anesthetic and the relatively low morbidity of this procedure have allowed renal revascularization in patients who might have been deemed unsuitable for surgery secondary to concurrent present diseases. However, PTRA does have inherent limitations and is not suitable for dilation of ostial lesions or arterial occlusions. Therefore careful patient selection is necessary. In addition, percutaneous transluminal angioplasty is not universally available because it can be performed only by well-trained and skilled interventional radiologists with a vascular surgical team backup.

Technical success is defined as complete if the residual stenosis is 50% or less and as partial if the residual stenosis is 50% to 70% (110). The criteria to determine blood pressure are those of the national cooperative study on RVH (33). A decrease in the diastolic blood pressure to less than 90 mm Hg in the absence of antihypertensive medication is considered a cure, and a decrease in diastolic blood pressure of 15% or greater with or without antihypertensive medication is considered an improvement. A decrement in diastolic blood pressure of less than 15% is considered a failure.

Renal artery angioplasty is technically successful in approximately 80% of patients with atherosclerotic renal disease. However, the cure rate is only about 30%, with 50% improved, probably due to generalized disease. Nonostial, nonoccluded unilateral lesions were noted to be most amenable to angioplasty. Ostial lesions, total renal artery occlusions, and bilateral lesions, which often tend to be ostial and occluded, did not respond satisfactorily to angioplasty. The technical success rate in these patients as a group was 12% (110). Ostial lesions result from aortic plaques that impinge on the renal artery orifice. Inflation of the balloon catheter displaces the plaque, with recoil and assumption of the original position, occurring at deflation of the balloon. Martin and colleagues (70) reported a 25% blood pressure benefit with no cures for a group of 20 patients with ostial lesions. The development of renal artery stents now allows ostial lesions to be treated successfully with percutaneous angiographic techniques. In patients with bilateral RVH, the cure rate was a disappointing 5% and the improvement rate 41% in contrast to a 25% cure and a 47% improvement rate for patients with unilateral disease.

Renal artery angioplasty has been more successful in the treatment of the fibromuscular dysplasias. In approximately 90% of patients, the stenosed arteries are dilated successfully. Of this subgroup, 88% enjoyed a blood pressure benefit as a result of the treatment (38% cured and 50% improved). Restenosis after dilation occurred in fewer than 5% of cases in a review of long-term follow-up (117).

Complications of PTRA are reported in 10% of cases and include trauma to the access vessels (femoral or axillary) with hemorrhage. Renal artery damage by dissection, aneurysm formation, perforation, and balloon malfunction or rupture has been reported (19,31,117). Cholesterol embolization of the kidney with resulting loss in renal function or of the lower extremities resulting in distal vascular compromise have been reported. Complications of angioplasty resulting in the loss of renal unit have been infrequent, and associated deaths have been rare.

Renal Artery Stents

Patients whose renal artery strictures cannot be adequately dilated by angioplasty or whose arteries restenose following an initially successful dilation have limited therapeutic alternatives. However, an exciting alternative treatment currently is being used for these patients. A stainless steel balloon-expandable stent may be placed across a stricture to reestablish the renal artery lumen. The stents (Fig. 23.11) are 1 to 3 cm in length and may be expanded to a diameter of 4 to 9 mm (medium stents) or 8 to 12 mm (large stents).

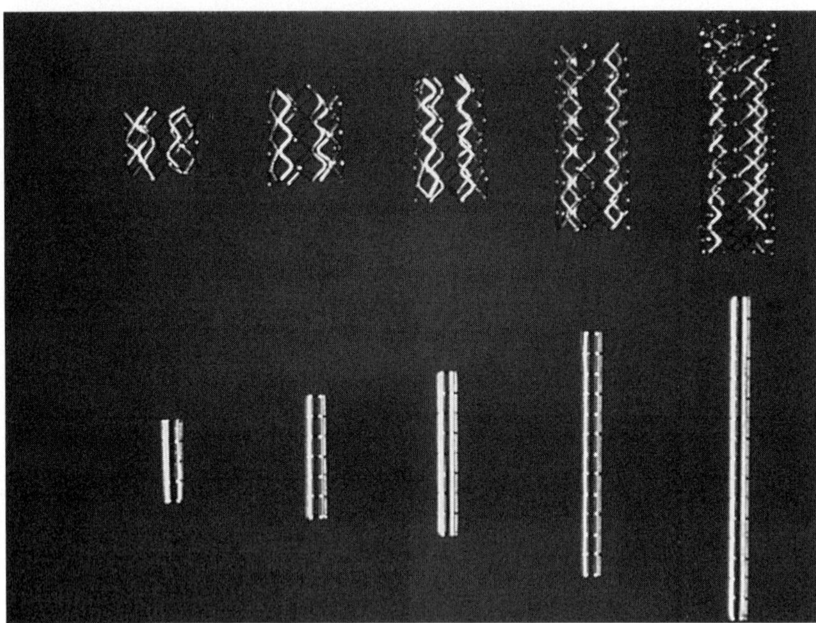

FIGURE 23.11. Palmaz stents for treatment of renal artery stenosis. Stents of various lengths are seen in the *lower row*. The *upper row* shows the stents after balloon expansion.

The renal artery stents are placed by angiographic techniques. Percutaneous transluminal angioplasty precedes introduction of a renal artery stent. If adequate dilation is not established, a stent is positioned across the renal artery stricture and is balloon expanded to reestablish the lumen. The Department of Radiology at the New York Hospital–Cornell Medical Center placed 24 stents to treat 23 renal artery stenoses in 21 patients between May 1989 and December 1993 (122). One patient was treated for a transplant renal artery stenosis. The remaining 20 patients had ostial, atherosclerotic renal artery lesions, which are generally refractory to percutaneous angioplasty. Eight stents (33%) were placed immediately following an inadequate percutaneous renal artery angioplasty. Sixteen stents (66%) were placed following a restenosis.

The percent stenosis for this group of patients was angiographically determined to be 86.3% ± 9.8%. Immediately after stent placement, the percent stenosis decreased to 1.67% ± 8.1%. At a mean angiographic follow-up of 7.6 months (range of 3 to 12 months), the percent stenosis was found to be 44% ± 23% ($p < .0001$ when compared with the prestent angiogram). Restenosis appeared to be due to endothelial ingrowth into the stent and not to stent compression or kinking. In 11 patients, the hypertension was cured (3 patients) or improved (8 patients). Although individual patients enjoyed improvement in renal function (7 of 11 patients with a creatinine greater than 1.5 mg/dL improved), the change in renal function for this small group as a whole was not statistically significant. Of 21 patients, 15 (71%) benefited from this procedure by an improvement in renal function, an improvement in blood pressure control, or both.

In looking at these preliminary results, it must be borne in mind that patients with recurrence of ostial renal artery lesions have a high failure rate when managed by angioplasty alone. Surgical revascularization is associated with much greater morbidity and mortality rates than angioplasty. Medical management can be complicated by progressive loss of renal function despite good blood pressure control. Table 23.7 reviews renal function after angioplasty (90).

Case I

A 73-year-old woman, following a right nephrectomy many years before, had a 30-year history of hypertension. She was found to have a significant ostial lesion that could not be dilated by percutaneous transluminal angioplasty (Fig. 23.12). She underwent renal stent placement (Fig. 23.13). Seven months after stent placement, her renal artery remains patent and her creatinine and blood pressure are improved and stable (Fig. 23.14).

Case II

A 53-year-old white woman with a long history of hypertension has bilateral atherosclerotic ostial lesions. Percutaneous transluminal angioplasty on two lesions failed to correct her stenoses. The patient had diabetes mellitus, hypertension, and gradients of 100 mm Hg across each stenosis (Fig. 23.15). Renal artery stents were placed bilaterally (Fig. 23.16), with disappearance of the gradients and improvement in her blood pressure control.

Surgical Treatment for Renovascular Hypertension

The first surgical treatment described for RVH was nephrectomy (61). During the 1940s and 1950s, small kid-

TABLE 23.7. RENAL FUNCTION AFTER RENAL ANGIOPLASTY

		Outcome			
Reference	**Patients**	**Improved**	**Stable**	**Worse**	**Death**
Luft, et al. 1983 (64)	12	3 (25)	5 (42)	4 (43)	0 (0)
Pickering, et al., 1986 (93)	55	26 (47)	19 (35)	10 (18)	NA
Bell, et al., 1987 (5)	20	7 (35)	10 (50)	3 (15)	0 (0)
O'Donovan, et al., 1992 (84)	17	9 (53)	2 (12)	6 (35)	5 (29)
Martin, et al., 1992 (69)	79	34 (43)	45 (57)[b]		1 (1)
Canzanello, et al., 1989 (11)	69	36 (52)[c]		33 (48)	
Dorros, et al., 1998 (26)	163				3 (2)
	124 unilateral	41 (33)	41 (33)	42 (34)	
	39 bilateral	15 (38)	16 (42)	8 (21)	
Total	**415**	**171 (41)**	**138 (33)**	**106 (26)**	**9 (2)**

[a]Indicates renal artery stent placement during angioplasty.
[b]Indicates sum of stable and worse.
[c]Indicates improved and stable.
( ), percent of patients from each study; NA, data not available.

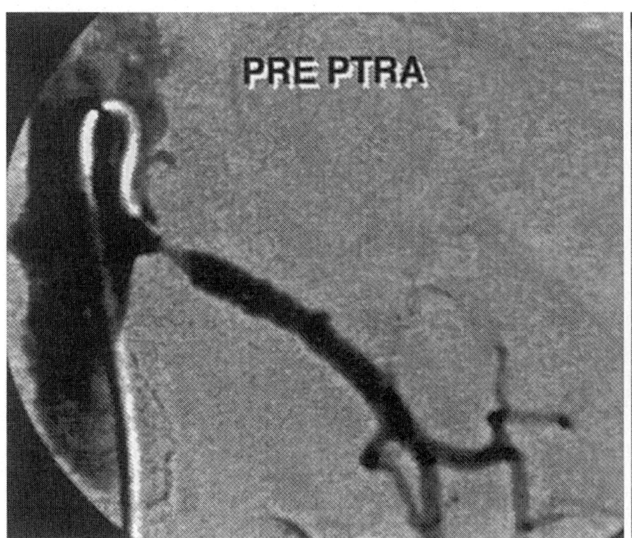

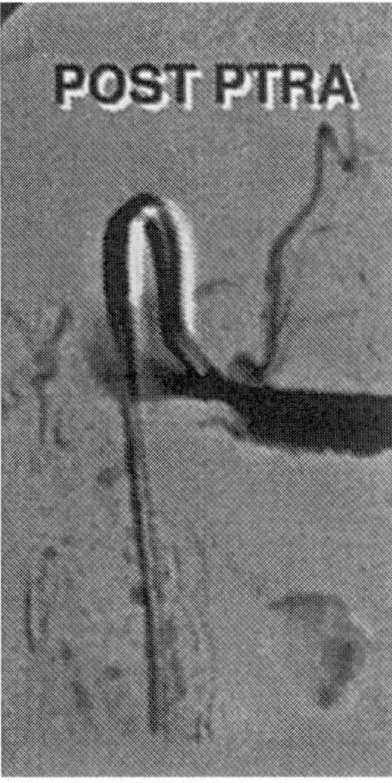

FIGURE 23.12. An ostial, left renal artery lesion is angiographically defined before percutaneous transluminal renal angioplasty **(PTRA).** After dilation, the lumen is larger. The renal artery stent can be positioned on an angioplasty balloon across the stenosis and expanded.

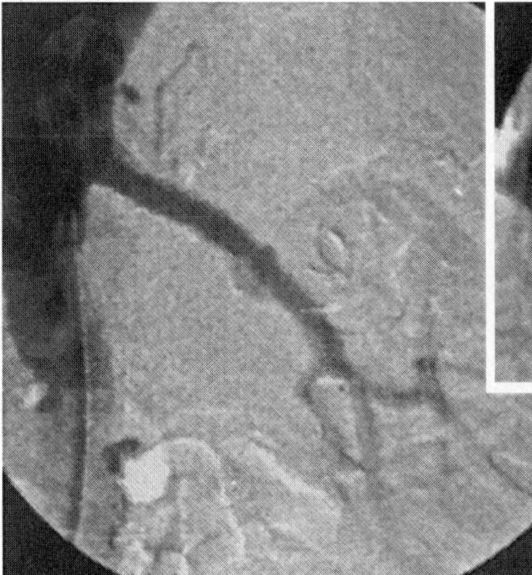

FIGURE 23.13. Poststent. A wide-caliber ostium and renal artery can be seen after the stent is expanded. The cone-down view on the inset allows the expanded stent to be recognized across the ostium and proximal renal artery.

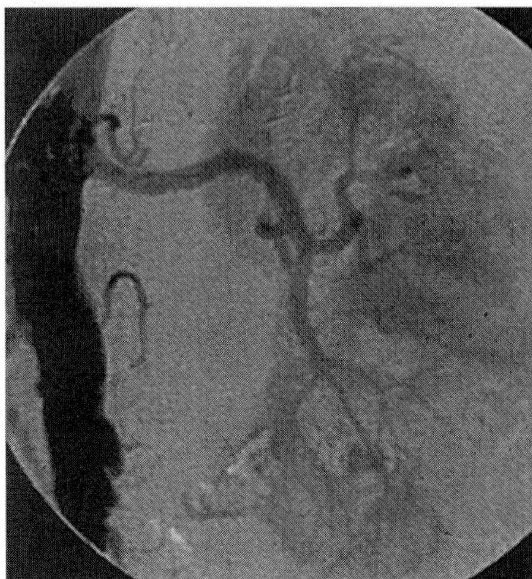

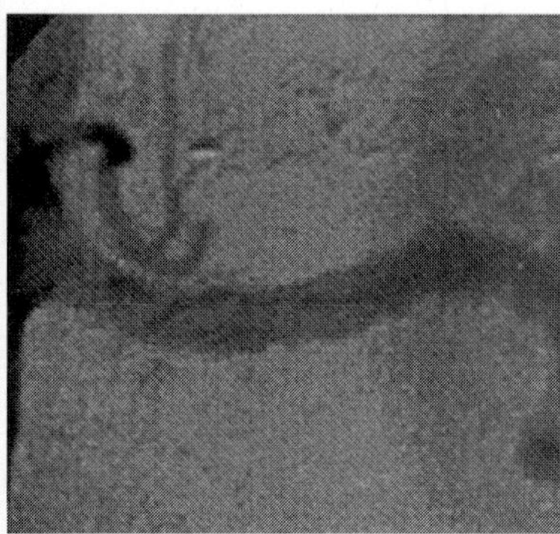

FIGURE 23.14. At a 7-month angiographic follow-up, the left renal artery and ostium remain open.

neys were removed from hypertensive patients with the idea of controlling the blood pressure. In 1956, a careful review of the effects of nephrectomy on the treatment of hypertension revealed a dismal 19% success rate. However, it was appreciated that patients with unilateral renovascular disease fared somewhat better than patients with unilateral renal parenchymal disease (120). This observation plus the development and widespread use of angiography in the 1950s redirected the focus of surgical treatment of renovascular disease to revascularization of ischemic kidneys. Freeman and colleagues (34) pioneered revascularization of ischemic kidneys by performing aortic and bilateral renal artery thromboendarterectomy to treat hypertension. Aortorenal bypass quickly became the preferred method of renal revascularization, and angiography was relied on as the definitive test to predict blood pressure response to surgical correction.

The national cooperative study on RVH (33) reviewed the efficacy of surgically correcting renal artery lesions to cure hypertension. Despite a 51% cure rate, the results revealed a disappointing 34% failure rate and an unacceptable operative mortality rate approaching 10%. The patients at highest risk for operative morbidity and mortality were those with concurrent coronary or cerebrovascular disease or with bilateral renovascular disease often associated with azotemia.

In the past decade, the results of surgical renal vascularization have improved as a result of better patient selection, which can be attributed to a better understanding of the natural history of renal artery disease, to a better under-

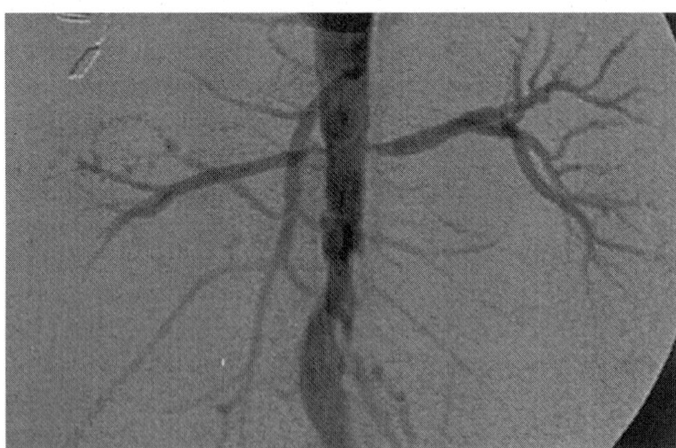

FIGURE 23.15. The angiogram of a 53-year-old white female with IDDM, hypertension, and an abdominal bruit reveals bilateral atherosclerotic ostial lesions. The gradient measured across each stenosis was 100 mm Hg (see Case II).

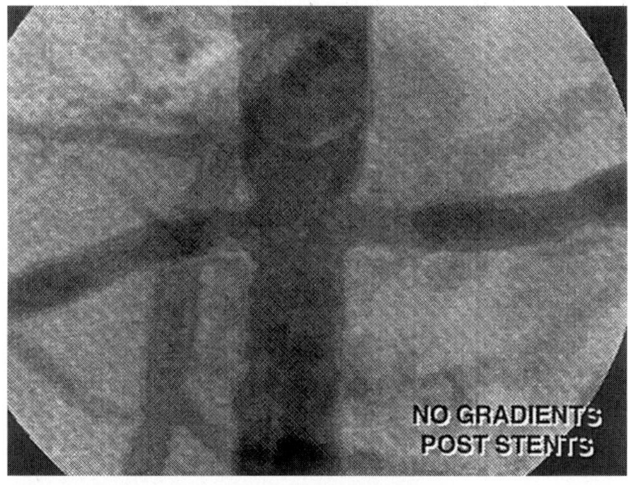

FIGURE 23.16. An angiogram performed immediately following bilateral renal stent placement reveals wide-open lumina. There was no pressure gradient across the ostia.

TABLE 23.8. RENAL FUNCTION AFTER SURGICAL REVASCULARIZATION

		Outcome			
Reference	Patients	Improved	Stable	Worse	Death
Luft, et al., 1983 (64)	12	8 (67)	2 (17)	2 (17)	2 (17)
Jamieson, et al., 1984 (51)	23	15 (65)	0 (0)	8 (35)	4 (17)
Novick, et al., 1987 (83)	153	93 (61)	50 (33)	140 (6)	5 (3)
Hallett, et al., 1987 (42)	91	20 (22)	48 (53)	23 (25)	6 (7.1)
Hansen, et al., 1989 (43)	25	12 (48)	11 (44)	2 (8)	2 (8)
Dean, et al., 1991 (24)	53	31 (59)	15 (28)	7 (13)	5 (9)
Messina, et al., 1992 (71)	17	12 (71)	2 (12)	3 (18)	1 (6)
Bredenberg, et al., 1992 (6)	40	22 (55)	10 (25)	8 (20)	NA
Libertino and Beckmann, 1994 (62)	91	45 (46)	31 (32)	15 (16)	6 (7)
Fergany, et al., 1994 (30)	18	4 (22)	13 (72)	1 (6)	0 (0)
Total	**523**	**262 (50)**	**182 (35)**	**79 (15)**	**31 (6)**

( ), percent of patients.

standing of the physiology and pathophysiology of the renin-angiotensin-aldosterone system, and to the development of pharmacologic probes that serve as highly reliable screening tests. There is growing recognition that patients with decreased renal function, even those with total occlusion of a renal artery, may recover renal function and enjoy a blood pressure benefit after renal revascularization (63). In the latter group, angiography demonstrates a delayed nephrogram because of a rich network of collateral vessels that preserve renal morphology and function. In patients with a preoperative serum creatinine level of less than 3 mg/dL, postoperative renal function was stable and improved in 89%. Conversely, renal revascularization in patients with a baseline serum creatinine level of greater than 4 mg/dL was not worthwhile because advanced underlying renal parenchymal disease prevented improvement in renal function. Table 23.8 reviews renal function after surgical revascularization (90).

The previously unacceptable operative morbidity and mortality rates associated with renal revascularization have improved substantially by careful patient selection and preparation. It has been recognized that concurrent coronary and cerebrovascular disease and bilateral renovascular disease with azotemia greatly increase the risk of operative intervention (81). Accordingly, cardiac and cerebral revascularization are performed, when appropriate, before renal revascularization. Using this protocol, operative morbidity and mortality rates have been greatly reduced. Novick and colleagues (81) achieved a 91% blood pressure benefit in 100 consecutive renal revascularizations for atherosclerotic RVH. Bilateral revascularization is not routinely performed. Instead, the more severely affected kidney is revascularized first. Contralateral repair is reserved for patients with persistent hypertension in whom repeat renal vein renins lateralize to the unoperated side.

Aortorenal bypass with an autogenous vascular graft is the surgical treatment of choice for renal revascularization. The saphenous vein is employed most commonly. Patients with branch renal artery stenosis can be treated with multiple branch grafts employing microsurgical techniques *in vivo* or with *ex vivo* bench surgery (82). Branch intraparenchymal stenoses also may be amenable to intraoperative dilation with rigid dilators (Fig. 23.17) or angiographic-type balloon catheters introduced through the main renal artery. Most patients with bilateral disease require repair of only one side (82,118). If a bilateral repair is planned, it is performed most safely as a staged procedure.

In patients with severe aortoiliac disease, it is possible to revascularize the kidneys without performing a complete aortic replacement. Libertino and colleagues (63) developed and described hepatorenal and splenorenal bypass opera-

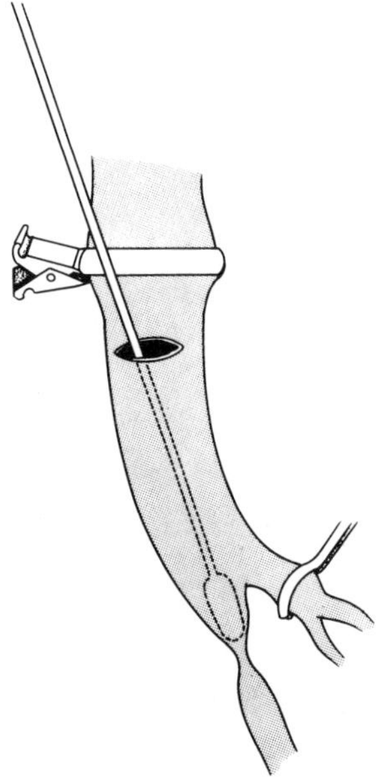

FIGURE 23.17. Intraoperative dilation of a stenosed renal artery branch with a rigid dilator.

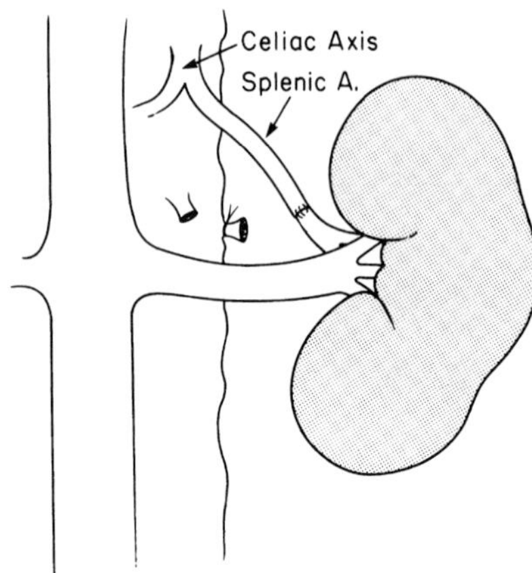

FIGURE 23.18. End-to-end splenorenal bypass to the left kidney.

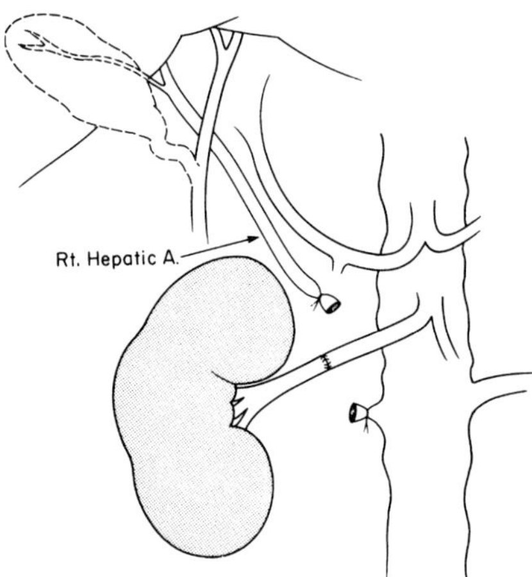

FIGURE 23.20. End-to-end hepatorenal bypass from the right hepatic artery to the right renal artery. An adjunctive cholecystectomy is necessary, because the gallbladder loses its nutrient artery.

tions to revascularize the right and left kidneys, respectively (18). The splenorenal bypass requires patent celiac and splenic arteries. A single end-to-end vascular anastomosis is fashioned (Fig. 23.18). The spleen is preserved and nourished by collateral short gastric arteries.

The hepatic artery is ideal for bypass to the right kidney because this vessel rarely is involved by atherosclerotic disease. The most common method of hepatorenal bypass is interposition of a saphenous vein graft, end-to-side to the common hepatic artery, just beyond the gastroduodenal artery (Fig. 23.19). If the right hepatic artery is used, the gallbladder becomes ischemic, and an adjunctive cholecystectomy is necessary (Fig. 23.20). An end-to-end gastroduodenal-renal anastomosis with saphenous vein interposition also is feasible (Fig. 23.21), although the gastroduodenal artery is difficult to mobilize. Results of follow-up studies of 1 to 8 years (mean of 4 years) after hepatorenal bypass are encouraging (18). The operation was successful in 33 of 36 patients (92%). There was no evidence of permanent hepatic impairment, graft stenosis, or late complications within this period of follow-up.

Renal autotransplantation and iliorenal bypass with a long saphenous vein graft are useful alternative techniques for renal revascularization in patients with severe aortic atherosclerosis and absence of severe iliac disease (Figs. 23.22 and 23.23). However, the atherosclerotic process may progress to involve the iliac vessels and compromise the blood flow of the revascularized kidney. Accordingly, Novick and colleagues (82) recommend that renal autotransplantation be considered only when a splenorenal or hepatorenal bypass cannot be performed. Early results after renal revascularization are favorable. However, data on the durability of vascular anastomoses and the long-term blood pressure benefit are more limited. Dean (22) reviewed

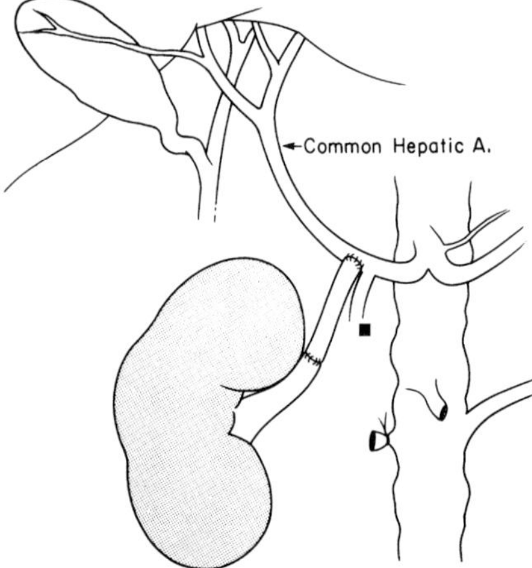

FIGURE 23.19. End-to-side hepatorenal bypass, from the common hepatic artery to the right renal artery with a saphenous vein graft interposition.

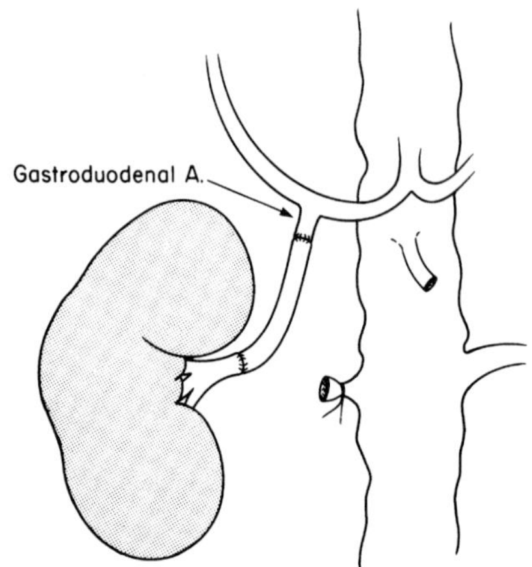

FIGURE 23.21. End-to-end gastroduodenal-renal artery anastomosis with a saphenous vein interposition.

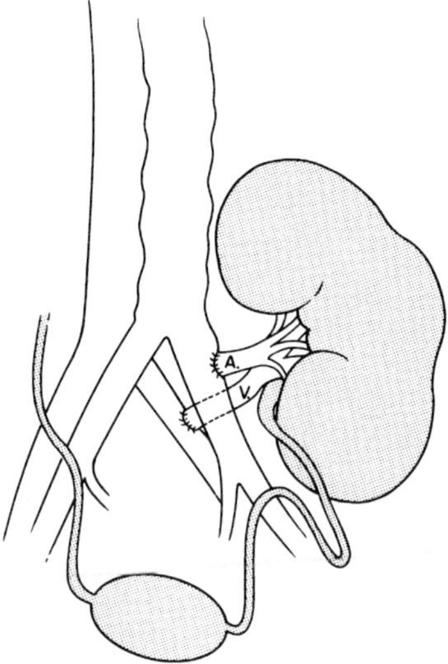

FIGURE 23.22. Renal revascularization by autotransplantation leaving the ureter intact.

the 20-year experience at Vanderbilt University with aortorenal bypass. He found that blood pressure was cured or improved in 95% of patients with fibromuscular renal artery disease and in 78% of patients operated on for atheromatous renal artery disease. The beneficial effect of operative treatment was maintained in this group over a follow-up period of up to 23 years. Dean (22) noted that the fate of a bypass graft is determined by several factors. These include the graft material, its length, and the flow through the conduit, as well as the surgical prevision of the anastomosis. A short graft length and high flow rate are favorable for

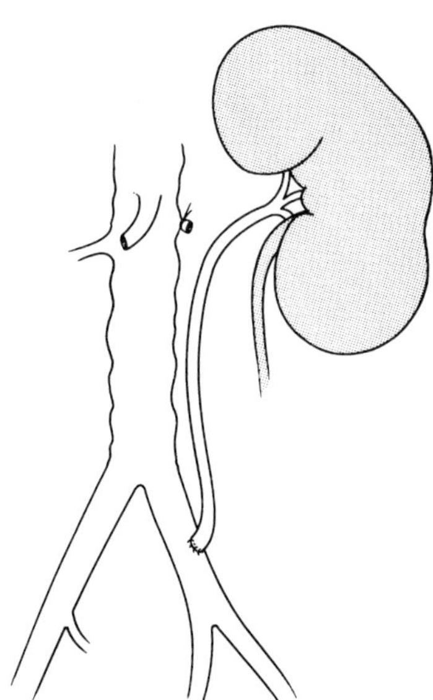

FIGURE 23.23. Renal revascularization by ileorenal bypass by means of a long saphenous vein graft.

long-term patency. An autogenous artery would seem the ideal graft to use.

Wylie (133) used the hypogastric artery for renal revascularization. He reported 98% patency and no late degenerative changes at a 5-year follow-up. The hypogastric autograft has particular appeal in the pediatric patient, because the graft enlarges with age in proportion to the increased demand for flow. However, the iliac arteries are not immune from the fibromuscular and atherosclerotic diseases involving the renal arteries and may succumb to these same disease processes or may already be involved at the time that renal revascularization is planned.

Venous autografts are structurally weaker than arterial autografts and represent an increased risk for aneurysmal degeneration. The saphenous vein has been used frequently in aortorenal revascularization. There is a 3% to 7% degeneration in follow-up of at least 1 year (22,27). Dacron was previously employed as a synthetic graft, but recently, polytetrafluoroethylene (Gore-Tex) grafts are preferred because of greater ease in suturing. Synthetic grafts also have the advantage of being available in a variety of sizes. However, they are subject to anastomotic aneurysmal degeneration and stenosis.

The results of surgical revascularization from the experience at the Cleveland Clinic are shown in Table 23.9 (80). The surgical techniques used in this series are shown in Table 23.10. The postoperative renal function was improved or stabilized in 89% of the patients with atherosclerotic renovascular disease who underwent renal revascularization.

Darling and co-workers (21) recently published a large series that emphasizes the success of renal artery reconstruction in a series of 568 complex cases. The cases were selected because of extensive disease in the angioplasty era. For example, 406 patients had a coexisting abdominal aortic aneurysm, 125 had aortoiliac occlusive disease, and in only 156 (23%) was renal revascularization the primary procedure. Remarkably, the death rate was only 5.5% and the occlusion rate was only 2.8% (21). Moreover, the long-term (5 years) patency rate was 95%. In patients who underwent reconstruction for symptomatic lesions, 26% improved, 68% stabilized, and 6% worsened.

Medical Management of Renovascular Hypertension

Medical management of RVH has been unsatisfactory in the past. Hunt and colleagues (49) followed up 214 patients with RVH for 7 to 14 years. One hundred patients were selected for surgical therapy after failing to respond to 3 months of medical therapy. Patients treated medically had a higher mortality rate (40% versus 16%) and overall less effective control of their blood pressure than their surgically treated counterparts. Dean and colleagues (23) medically treated 41 patients with RVH. They found that the arterial

TABLE 23.9. RESULTS OF SURGICAL REVASCULARIZATION OF RENOVASCULAR HYPERTENSION AT THE CLEVELAND CLINIC

	No. of Patients	Postoperative Blood Pressure			Follow-up (mo)
		Cured (%)	Improved (%)	Failed (%)	
Atherosclerosis	180	55 (31)	110 (61)	15 (6)	6–117
Fibrous dysplasia	104	66 (63)	31 (30)	7 (7)	10–115

From Novick AO. Surgical management of renovascular hypertension. In: Kaplan NM, Brenner BM, Laregh JH, eds. *The kidney in hypertension.* New York: Raven Press, 1987, with permission.

stenosis progressed in 41% of patients and that progression to complete occlusion occurred in 12%. In all fairness to the medical management of RVH, it must be pointed out that the drugs used in these studies were far less specific to control a hyperactive RAS than the β-adrenergic blockers and CEIs available today. These newer drugs have been more effective in controlling blood pressure in patients with fibromuscular dysplasia than in those with atherosclerotic renovascular disease. Patients in the latter group tend to be older, have more target organ damage, and require more drugs for blood pressure control than the younger patients with fibromuscular disease.

Despite the greater specificity of these drugs for the RAS, their safety and efficacy in the treatment of RVH remain in doubt. Many reports have documented the onset of reversible decrease in renal function associated with use of CEIs in patients with bilateral renal artery stenosis or stenosis of the renal artery to a solitary kidney (54). The decrement in renal function does not appear to be caused entirely by the depressor effect of these drugs, because lowering the blood pressure to the same degree with a drug that does not interfere with the RAS does not usually lead to a comparable decrease in renal function. Micropuncture studies suggest that at low perfusion pressures the glomerular capillary hydrostatic pressure is increased by an angiotensin II–dependent constriction of the efferent arteriole (41). Inhibition of angiotensin II formation in the setting of a decreased perfusion pressure lowers glomerular filtration. Discontinuation of the CEI restores renal function to baseline.

TABLE 23.10. SURGICAL REVASCULARIZATION TECHNIQUE FOR RENAL ARTERY DISEASE AT THE CLEVELAND CLINIC

	Atherosclerosis (n = 254)	Fibrous Dysplasia or Aneurysm (n = 126)
Aortorenal bypass	138	82
Splenorenal bypass	42	4
Hepatorenal bypass	29	0
Iliorenal bypass	19	0
Autotransplantation	8	1
Aortic replacement	11	0
Ex vivo repair and autotransplantation	0	37
Other	7	2

From Novick AO. Surgical management of renovascular hypertension. In: Kaplan NM, Brenner BM, Laregh JH, eds. *The kidney in hypertension.* New York: Raven Press, 1987.

Unfortunately, the drug-induced decrease in renal function is not limited to patients with bilateral renal artery disease. Experimental administration of CEIs in two kidney–one clip animals reveals that the ischemic kidney has a severe decline in GFR, whereas the contralateral kidney remains unaffected (130). Clinically, Wenting and colleagues (131) demonstrated, with the use of nuclear renal scans, significant impairment of renal function in the ischemic kidney of patients with unilateral renal artery stenosis treated with captopril.

Textor and colleagues (118) argued against medical management for RVH beyond the use of CEIs, possibly to implicate a wide range of antihypertensive medications. In eight patients with bilateral renal artery disease in which both renal arteries had luminal stenoses of 75% or greater, decreasing the blood pressure from a baseline of approximately 200/100 to 140/85 mm Hg by graded increases in intravenous nitroprusside produced significant decreases in total renal plasma flow and GFR. Nitroprusside is known to increase renin secretion, and therefore interference with the autoregulatory actions of angiotensin II cannot be implicated. It appears that renal units whose blood flow is already compromised cannot tolerate reduction in blood pressure to clinically relevant levels.

Four of those eight patients underwent unilateral renal revascularization of the more ischemic kidney. Although renal function per se was not significantly improved by surgery, repeated challenge with graded nitroprusside infusions, attaining the same lower levels of blood pressure, did not lower renal plasma flow or GFR. This observation strongly suggests that revascularization may protect the kidneys from loss of renal function when the blood pressure is lowered to clinically desirable levels by antihypertensive medicines (118).

Finally, it must be borne in mind that RVH is a vascular disease whose manifestations can include loss of renal function and renin-dependent hypertension. Pharmacologic treatment of the hypertension does not address the cause of the problem. However, despite the superior results generally achieved by the revascularization of a renal artery stenosis, there is a role for medical management in the treatment of RVH. Medical management must be employed in patients who have not benefited from angioplasty or surgical revascularization, in patients who are not candidates for intervention because of the presence of other serious diseases, and in those who have refused intervention. Whatever the case, all patients with RVH who are treated pharmacologically must be evaluated carefully and routinely for changes in renal function and size (25).

REFERENCES

1. Arzilli S, Giovannetti R, Meola M, et al. ACE-inhibition vs. surgical treatment in the outcome of ischemic kidneys of renovascular patients: a one-year follow-up. *High Blood Pressure* 1992;1:47.
2. Ayers CR, Harris RH, Lefer LG. Control of renin release in experimental hypertension. *Circ Res* 1969;24/25[Suppl 1]:103.
3. Bakhle YS. Conversion of angiotensin I to angiotensin II by cell-free extracts of dog lung. *Nature* 1968;220:919.
4. Bedoya L, Ziegelbaum M, Didt DG, et al. The effect of baseline renal function on the outcome following renal revascularization. *Cleve Clin J Med* 1989;56:415.
5. Bell GM, Reid J, Buist TAS. Percutaneous transluminal angioplasty improves blood pressure and renal function in renovascular hypertension. *Q J Med* 1987;63:393.
6. Bredenberg CE, Sampson LN, Ray FS, et al. Changing patterns in surgery for chronic renal artery occlusive diseases. *J Vasc Surg* 1992;15:1018.
7. Braun-Menendez E, Fasciolo JC, Leloir LR, et al. The substance causing renal hypertension. *J Physiol* 1940;98:283.
8. Bright R. Causes and observations, illustrative of renal disease accompanied with the secretion of albuminous urine. *Surg Hosp Rep* 1836;1:338.
9. Brunner HR, Gavras H, Laragh JH, et al. Angiotensin II blockade in man by SAR^1-Ala^8-angiotensin II for understanding and treatment of high blood pressure. *Lancet* 1973; 2:1045.
10. Brunner HR, Laragh JH, Baer L, et al. Essential hypertension: renin and aldosterone, heart attack, and stroke. *N Engl J Med* 1972;286:441.
11. Canzanello VJ, Millan VG, Spiegel JE, et al. Percutaneous transluminal renal angioplasty in management of atherosclerotic renovascular hypertension: results in 100 patients. *Hypertension* 1989;13:163.
12. Carey RM, Reid RA, Ayers CR, et al. The Charlottesville blood pressure surgery; value of repeat blood pressure measurement to define the prevalence of labile and sustained hypertension. *JAMA* 1976;236:847.
13. Casarella WJ. Non-coronary angioplasty. *Curr Probl Cardiol* 1986;11:3.
14. Case DB, Atlas SA, Laragh JH. Reactive hyperreninemia to angiotensin blockade identified renovascular hypertension. *Clin Sci* 1979;57[Suppl]:313.
15. Case DB, Atlas, SA, Larach JH. Physiologic effects and blockade. In: Laragh JH, Bjhler FR, Seldin DW, eds. *Frontiers in hypertension research.* New York: Springer-Verlag, 1982.
16. Case DB, Atlas, SA, Larach JH, et al. Clinical experience with blockade of the renin-angiotensin-aldosterone system by an oral converting enzyme inhibitor (AQ 14225, captopril) in hypertensive patients. *Prog Cardiovasc Dis* 1978;21:195.
17. Case DB, Wallace JM, Keim HJ, et al. Estimating renin participation in hypertension: superiority of converting enzyme inhibitor over saralasin. *Am J Med* 1976;61:790.
18. Chibaro EA, Libertino JA, Novick AC. Use of hepatic circulation for renal revascularization. *Ann Surg* 1984;199:406.
19. Cohn DJ, Sos TA, Saddekni A, et al. Transluminal angioplasty for atherosclerotic renal artery stenosis. *Semin Intervent Radiol* 1984;1:279.
20. Colapinto RF, Stronell RD, Harries-Jones PE, et al. Percutaneous translumination dilatation of the renal artery; follow-up studies on renovascular hypertension. *AJR Am J Roentgenol* 1982;139:727.
21. Darling CR, Krenbreck PD, Chang BD, et al. Outcome of renal artery reconstruction analysis of 687 procedures. *Ann Surg* 1999;230:524.
22. Dean RH: Renovascular hypertension: an overview. In: Rutherford RB, ed. *Vascular surgery.* Philadelphia: Saunders, 1984.
23. Dean RH, Keiffer RW, Smith BM, et al. Renovascular hypertension: anatomic and functional changes during drug therapy. *Arch Surg* 1981;116:1408.
24. Dean RH, Tribble RW, Hansen KJ, et al. Evolution of renal insufficiency in ischemic nephropathy. *Ann Surg* 1991; 213:446.
25. Devoy MA, Tomson CR, Edmunds ME, et al. Deterioration in renal function associated with CEI therapy is not always reversible. *J Int Med* 1992;232:493.
26. Dorros G, Laff M, Mathiak L, et al. Four-year follow-up of Palmz-Schatz stent revascularization as treatment for atherosclerotic renal artery stenosis. *Circulation* 1998;98:642.
27. Ernst CB, Stanley JC, Marshall FF, et al. Renal revascularization for atherosclerotic renovascular hypertension: prognostic implications of focal renal arterial versus overt generalized arteriosclerosis. *Surgery* 1973;73:859.
28. Eyler WR, Clark MD, Garman JE, et al. Angiography of the renal areas including a comparative study of renal arterial stenosis in patients with and without hypertension. *Radiology* 1962;78:879.
29. Felson D, Vaughan ED Jr. Endocrine function of the renal parenchyma. In: Rajfer J, ed. *Urologic endocrinology.* Philadelphia: Saunders, 1986.
30. Fergany A, Novick AC, Goldfarb DA. Management of atherosclerotic renal artery disease in younger patients. *J Urol* 1994; 151:10.
31. Fletchner SM. Percutaneous transluminal dilatation: a realistic appraisal in patients with stenosing lesions of the renal artery. *Urol Clin North Am* 1984;11:515.
32. Fommei E, Ghione S, Palla F, et al. Renal scintigraphic captopril test in the diagnosis of renovascular hypertension. *Hypertension* 1987;10:212.
33. Foster JH, Maxwell MH, Franklin SS, et al. Renovascular occlusive disease: results of operative treatment. *JAMA* 1975; 231:1043.
34. Freeman NE, Leeds FM, Elliott W. Thromboendarterectomy for hypertension due to renal artery occlusion. *JAMA* 1954; 156:1077.
35. Gavras H, Brunner HR, Vaughan ED Jr, et al. Angiotensin-sodium interaction in blood pressure maintenance of renal hypertensive and normotensive rats. *Science* 1973;180:1369.

36. Geyskes GG, Oei HP, Puylaert CBAJ, et al. Unilateral renal failure after captopril in patients with renovascular hypertension. In: Glorioso N et al, eds. *Renovascular hypertension.* New York: Raven Press, 1987.
37. Goldblatt H, Lynch J, Hanzal RF, et al. Studies on experimental hypertension. I. The production of persistent elevation of systolic blood pressure by means of renal ischemia. *J Exp Med* 1934;59:347.
38. Goodfriend T, Elliott ME, Katt KJ. Angiotensin receptors and their antagonist. *N Engl J Med* 1996;334:1649.
39. Grist TM. Magnetic resonance angiography of renal artery stenosis. *Am J Kidney Dis* 1994;24:700.
40. Gruntzig A, Hopff H. Perkutane Rekanalization chronischer arterieller Verschluse mit einem neuen Dilatationskatheter: Modifikation der Dotter-Technick. *Deutsch Medication Wochenschr* 1974;99:2502.
41. Hall JE, Coleman TG, Guyton AC, et al. Control of glomerular filtration rate by circulating angiotensin II. *Am J Physiol* 1981;241:R190.
42. Hallett JWJ, Fowl R, O'Brien PC, et al. Renovascular operations in patients with chronic renal insufficiency: do the benefits justify the risks? *J Vasc Surg* 1987;257:498.
43. Hansen KJ, Dietsheim JA, Metropol SH, et al. Management of renovascular hypertension in the elderly population [Comments]. *J Vasc Surg* 1989;10:266.
44. Herrera AH, Davidson RA. Renovascular disease in older adults. *Clin Geriatr Med* 1998;14:237.
45. Holland GA, Dougherty L, Carpenter JP, et al. Breath-hold ultrafast three-dimensional gadolinium-enhanced MR angiography of the aorta and the renal and other visceral abdominal arteries. *AJR Am J Roentgenol* 1996;166:971.
46. Holley KE, Hunt JC, Brown AL, et al. Renal artery stenosis: a clinical-pathologic study in normotensive patients. *Am J Med* 1964;37:14.
47. Horn ML, Conklin VM, Keenan RE, et al. Angiotensin II profiling with saralasin: summary of the Eaton Collaborative Study. *Kidney Int* 1979;9[Suppl]:S115.
48. Howard JE, Berthrong N, Gould D, et al. Hypertension resulting from unilateral renovascular disease and its relief by nephrectomy. *Johns Hopkins Med J* 1954;94:51.
49. Hunt JC, Sheps SC, Harrison EG, et al. Renal and renovascular hypertension: a reasoned approach to diagnosis and management. *Arch Intern Med* 1974;133:988.
50. Jacobson HR. Ischemic renal disease: an overlooked terminal entity. *Kidney Int* 1988;34:729.
51. Jamieson GG, Clarkson AR, Woodroffe AJ, et al. Reconstructive renal vascular surgery for chronic renal failure. *Br J Surg* 1984;71:338.
52. Johansson M, Jensen G, Aruell M, et al. Evaluation of duplex ultrasound and captopril renography for detection of renovascular hypertension. *Kidney Int* 2000;58:774.
53. Johnson JA, Davis JO, Witty RT. Effects of catecholamines and renal nerve stimulation on renin release in the non-filtering kidney. *Circ Res* 1971;29:646.
54. Johnson RJ, Alpers CE, Yoshimura A, et al. Renal injury from all mediated hypertension. *Hypertension* 1992;19:464.
55. Kaplan-Pavlobcic S, Koselji M, Obrez I, et al. Percutaneous transluminous angioplasty: follow-up studies in renovascular hypertension. *Przegl Lek* 1985;43:342.
56. Klag MJ, Whelton PK, Randall BL, et al. Blood pressure and end-stage renal disease in men. *N Engl J Med* 1996;334:13.
57. Kooner JS, Peart WS, Mathias CJ. The sympathetic nervous system in hypertension due to unilateral renal artery stenosis in man. *Clin Auton Res* 1991;1:195.
58. Kuhlman S, Mandalim R, Raovr K, et al. Percutaneous transluminal dilatation of renal artery stenosis. *Am J Med* 1985; 79:792.
59. Laragh JH. Basic principles for the office evaluation and treatment of high blood pressure: part I. *Cardiol Rev Rep* 1981;2: 1318.
60. Laragh JH, Sealey JE. Renin sodium profiling: why, how and when in clinical practice. *Cardiovasc Med* 1977;2:1503.
61. Leadbetter WF, Burkland CF. Hypertension in unilateral renal disease. *J Urol* 1938;39:611.
62. Libertino JA, Beckmann CF. Surgery and percutaneous angioplasty in the management of renovascular hypertension. *Urol Clin North Am* 1994;21:235.
63. Libertino JA, Zinman L, Breslin DJ, et al. Renal artery revascularization: restoration of renal function. *JAMA* 1980;244:1340.
64. Luft FC, Grim CE, Weinberger MH. Intervention in patients with renovascular hypertension and renal insufficiency. *J Urol* 1983;130:654.
65. Mailloux LU, Napolitano B, Belluci AG, et al. Renovascular disease causing end-stage renal disease, incidence, clinical correlates, and outcomes: a 20-year clinical experience. *Am J Kidney Dis* 1994;24:622.
66. Mann FC, Herrick JF, Essex HE, et al. The effect on the blood flow of decreasing lumen of a blood vessel. *Surgery* 1938:4:249.
67. Mann SJ, Pickering TG. Detection of renovascular hypertension: state of the art: review 1992. *Ann Intern Med* 1992; 117:845.
68. Martin EC, Maltern RF, Baer L, et al. Renal angioplasty for hypertension: predictive factors for long-term success. *AJR Am J Roentgenol* 1981;137:921.
69. Martin LG, Cork RD, Kaufman SL. Long-term results of angioplasty in 110 patients with renal artery stenosis. *J Vasc Interv Radiol* 1992;3:619.
70. Martin LG, Price RB, Casarella WJ, et al. Percutaneous angioplasty in clinical management of renovascular hypertension: initial and long-term results. *Radiology* 1985;155:629.
71. Messina LM, Zelenock GB, Yao KA, et al. Renal revascularization for recurrent pulmonary edema in patients with poorly controlled hypertension and renal insufficiency; a distinct subgroup of patients with arteriosclerotic renal artery occlusive disease. *J Vasc Surg* 1992;15:73.
72. Miller G, Ford KK, Barun SD, et al. Percutaneous transluminal angioplasty vs surgery for renovascular hypertension. *AJR Am J Roentgenol* 1985;144:447.
73. Miralles M, Cairols M, Cotillas J, et al. Value of Doppler parameters in the diagnosis of renal artery stenosis. *J Vasc Surg* 1996;23:428.
74. Missouris CG, Allan GM, Balan FG, et al. Non-invasive screening for renal artery stenosis with ultrasound contrast enhancement. *J Hypertens* 1996;14:519.
75. Muller FB, Sealey JE, Case DB, et al. The captopril test for identifying renovascular disease in hypertensive patients. *Am J Med* 1986;80:633.
76. Nakamoto H, Ferrario CM, Fuller SB, et al. Angiotensin (1-7) and nitric oxide interaction in renovascular hypertension. *Hypertension* 1995;25:796.
77. Nally JV. Use of captopril renography for the diagnosis of renovascular hypertension. *World J Urol* 1989;7:72.
78. Nally JV, Chen C, Fine E, et al. Diagnostic criteria of renovascular hypertension with captopril renography. *Am J Hypertens* 1991;4:749S.

78a. Nicholson JP, Teichman SL, Alderman MH, et al. Cigarette smoking and renovascular hypertension. *Lancet* 1983;2:765.

79. Nobert CF, Libertino JA. Ischemic nephropathy. *Curr Opin Urol* 1998;8:129.
80. Novick AC. Surgical management of renovascular hypertension. In: Kaplan MN, Brenner BM, Laragh JH, eds. *The kidney in hypertension.* New York: Raven Press, 1987.
81. Novick AC, Straffon RA, Stewart BH, et al. Diminished operative morbidity and mortality in renal revascularization. *JAMA* 1981;256:749.
82. Novick AC, Textor SC, Brodie B, et al. Renovascularization to preserve renal function in patients with atherosclerotic renovascular disease. *Urol Clin North Am* 1984;11:477.
83. Novick AC, Ziegelbaum M, Vidt DG, et al. Trends in surgical revascularization for renal artery disease. Ten years experience. *JAMA* 1987;257:498.
84. O'Donovan RM, Gutierrez OH, Izzo JLJ. Preservation of renal function by percutaneous renal angioplasty in high-risk elderly patients; short term outcome. *Nephron* 1992;60:187.
85. Page IH, Helmer OM. A crystalline pressor substance (angiotonin) resulting from the reaction between renin and renin activatory. *J Exp Med* 1940;71:29.
86. Pals DT, Masucci FDS, Denning GS Jr, et al. Role of the pressor action and angiotensin II in experimental hypertension. *Circ Res* 1971;29:673.
87. Parrott TS, Woodward JR, Trulock TS, et al. Segmental renal vein renins and partial nephrectomy for hypertension. *J Urol* 1984;131:736.
88. Pedersen EB. New tools in diagnosing renal artery stenosis. *Kidney Int* 2000;57:2657.
89. Pickering G. Hypertension definitions, natural histories and consequences. In: Laragh JH, ed. *Hypertension manual.* New York: Yorke Medical Books, 1973.
90. Pickering TG, Blumenfeld JD. Renovascular hypertension and ischemic nephropathy. In: Brenner BM, ed. *The kidney.* Philadelphia: WB Saunders, 2000:2007.
91. Pickering TG, Case DB, Sos TA, et al. Unilateral suppression of renin secretion in patients with bilateral renal artery stenosis. *Clin Res* 1983.
92. Pickering TG, Sos TA, James GD, et al. Comparison of renal vein renin activity in hypertensive patients with stenosis of one or both renal arteries. *J Hypertens* 1985;3:1.
93. Pickering TG, Sos TA, Saddekni S, et al. Renal angioplasty in patients with azotemia and renovascular hypertension. *J Hypertens* 1986;4[Suppl 5]:S667.
94. Posniak MA, Lee FT Jr. Computed tomographic angiography in the preoperative evaluation of potential renal transplant donors. *Curr Opin Urol* 1999;9:165.
95. Postma CT, Hoefnagels WH, Barentsz JO, et al. Occlusion of unilateral stenosed renal arteries—relation to medical treatment. *J Hum Hypertens* 1989;3:185.
96. Ratliff NB. Renal vascular disease: pathology of large blood vessel disease. *Am J Kidney Dis* 1985;5:893.
97. Ribstein J, Mourad G, Mimran A. Contrasting acute effects of captopril and nifedipine on renal function and renovascular hypertension. *Am J Hypertens* 1988;1:239.
98. Richardson D, Stella A, Geonetti G, et al. Mechanisms of renal release of renin by electrical stimulation of the brainstem in the cat. *Circ Res* 1974;34:425.
99. Riehl J, Schmitt H, Bongaitz D, et al. Renal artery stenosis: evaluation with colour duplex ultrasonography. *Nephrol Dial Transplant* 1997;12:1608.
100. Rimmer JM, Gennari FJ. Atherosclerotic renovascular disease and progressive renal failure. *Ann Intern Med* 1993;118:712.
101. Rosendorff C. Reversal of structural changes in hypertensive arteries: a major prospect for the future. *Afr Med J* 1991; [Suppl]:4.
102. Schambelan MJ, Glickman M, Stockigt JR, et al. The selective renal vein renin sampling in hypertensive patients with segmental renal lesions. *N Engl J Med* 1974;29:1153.
103. Schreiber MJ, Pohl MA, Novick AC. The natural history of atherosclerotic and fibrous renal artery disease. *Urol Clin North Am* 1984;11:383.
104. Schwarten DE. Percutaneous transluminal renal artery angioplasty. In: Kaplan NM, Brenner BM, Laragh JH, eds. *The kidney and hypertension.* New York: Raven Press, 1987.
105. Sealey JE, Buhler FR, Laragh JH, et al. The physiology of renin secretion in essential hypertension: estimation of renin secretion rate and renal plasma flow from peripheral and renal vein renin levels. *Am J Med* 1973;55:391.
106. Selkurt EE. The effect of pulse pressure and mean arterial pressure modification of renal hemodynamics and electrolyte and water excretion. *Circulation* 1951;4:541.
107. Simon N, Franklin SS, Bleifer KH, et al. Clinical characteristics of renovascular hypertension. *JAMA* 1972;220:1209.
108. Skeggs LT Jr, Lentz KE, Kahn JR, et al. Amino acid sequence of hypertension II. *J Exp Med* 1956;104:193.
109. Snidow JJ, Johnson MS, Harris DJ, et al. Three-dimensional gadolinium-enhanced MR angiography for aortoiliac in-flow assessment plus renal artery screening in a single breath hold. *Radiology* 1996;198:725.
110. Sos TA, Pickering TG, Phil D, et al. Percutaneous transluminal renal angioplasty in renovascular hypertension due to atheroma or fibromuscular dysplasia. *N Engl J Med* 1983;309:274.
111. Sosa RE. Effects of converting enzyme inhibition on renal function in chronic 2-kidney, 1-clip hypertensive dogs. *J Urol* 1987;137:209(abst 424).
112. Sosa RE, Vaughan ED Jr. Evaluation of surgically curable hypertension. *Am Urol Assoc Update* 1983;2:Lesson 31.
113. Stamey TA, Nudelman IJ, Good TH, et al. Functional characteristics of renovascular hypertension. *Medicine* 1961;40:347.
114. Stewart BH. Renovascular hypertension: surgical treatment. *Monogr Urol* 1981;5:3.
115. Stockigt JR, Noakes CA, Collins RD, et al. Renal-vein renin in various forms of renal hypertension. *Lancet* 1972;1:1194.
116. Strandness DE Jr. Duplex imaging for the detection of renal artery stenosis. *Am J Kidney Dis* 1994;24:674.
117. Tegtmeyer CJ, Tegtmeyer VL, Kellum CD, et al. Percutaneous transluminal angioplasty: the treatment of choice for vascular lesions caused by fibromuscular dysplasia. *Semin Intervent Radiol* 1984;1:289.
118. Textor SC, Tarazi RC, Novick AC, et al. Regulation of renal hemodynamics and glomerular filtration in patients with renovascular hypertension during converting enzyme inhibition with captopril. *Am J Med* 1984;76:29.
119. Thibonnier M, Joseph A, Sassano P, et al. Improved diagnosis of unilateral renal artery lesions after captopril administration. *JAMA* 1984;251:56.
120. Thompson JE, Smithwick RH. Human hypertension due to unilateral renal disease, with special reference to renal artery lesions. *Angiology* 1957;3:493.
121. Tigerstedt R, Bergmann TG. Niere und kreislauf. *Skand Arch Physiol* 1898;8:233.
122. Trost D, Sos TS. Renal stents. Personal communication.
123. Vaughan ED Jr, Buhler FR, Laragh JH, et al. Renovascular hypertension; renin measurements to indicate hypersecretion and contralateral suppression, estimate renal plasma flow and score for surgical curability. *Am J Med* 1973;55:402.
124. Vaughan ED Jr, Carey RM, Ayers CR, et al. A physiologic definition of blood pressure response to renal revascularization in patients with renovascular hypertension. *Kidney Int* 1979;15:S83.

125. Vaughan ED Jr, Case DB, Pickering TG, et al. Clinical evaluation of renovascular hypertension and therapeutic decisions. *Urol Clin North Am* 1984;11:393.
126. Vaughan ED Jr, Sos TA, Sniderman KW, et al. Renal vein renin secretory patterns before and after transluminal angioplasty in patients with renovascular hypertension: verification of analytic criteria. In: Laragh JH, ed. *Frontiers in hypertension research.* New York: Springer-Verlag, 1981.
127. Vaughan ED Jr, Sosa RE. Clinovascular hypertension and other renovascular diseases. In: Walsh PC et al, eds. *Campbell's urology,* ed 7. Philadelphia: Saunders, 1998.
128. Veglio F, Frascisco M, Melchio R, et al. Assessment of renal resistance indexed after captopril tests by Doppler in essential and renovascular hypertension. *Kidney Int* 1995;48:1611.
129. Wachtell K, Ibsen H, Olsen MH, et al. Prevalence of renal artery stenosis in patients with peripheral vascular disease and hypertension. *J Hum Hypertens* 1996;10:83.
130. Wallace ECH, Morton JM. Chronic captopril infusion in two-kidney, one-clip rats with normal plasma renin concentration. *J Hypertens* 1984;2:285.
131. Wenting GJ, Tan-tjong HL, Derkx FHM, et al. Split renal function after captopril in unilateral renal artery stenosis. *BMJ* 1984;288:886.
132. Wilcox CS, Cardozo J, Welch WJ. A21 and $TtxA_2$/PGH_2 receptors maintain hypertension throughout 2K,1C Goldblatt hypertension in the rat. *Am J Physiol* 1996;271:R891.
133. Wylie EJ. Endarterectomy and autogenous arterial grafts in the surgical treatment of stenosing lesions of the renal artery. *Urol Clin North Am* 1975;2:351.
134. Ying CY, Tifft CP, Gavras H, et al. Renal revascularization in the azotemic hypertensive patient resistant to therapy. *N Engl J Med* 1984;311:1070.
135. Zierler RE, Bergelin RO, Davidson RC, et al. A prospective study of disease progression in patients with atherosclerotic renal artery stenosis. *Am J Hypertens* 1996;9:1055.
136. Zierler RE, Berglin RO, Polissar NL, et al. Carotid and lower extremity arterial disease in patients with renal artery atherosclerosis. *Arch Intern Med* 1998;158:761.

Adult and Pediatric Urology, 4/e, edited by Jay Y. Gillenwater, John T. Grayhack, Stuart S. Howards, and Michael E. Mitchell.
Lippincott Williams & Wilkins, Philadelphia © 2002

24

THE URETER

ROBERT M. WEISS

The function of the upper urinary tract is to transport urine from the minor calyces toward the bladder and to protect the renal parenchyma and cranial portions of the urinary tract from distally generated backflow and back-pressure. Peristaltic activity begins with the origin of the electrical activity at pacemaker sites situated in the proximal portion of the renal collecting system (20,34,66,106,211,231, 242). The electrical activity is transmitted distally from cell to cell and gives rise to the ureteral contraction wave, which propels the bolus of urine distally. Efficient collection and propulsion of urine is dependent on the passive and active properties of the ureter and on the ability of the ureter to coapt its walls completely (240). Urine passes into the bladder via the ureterovesical junction (UVJ), which under normal conditions permits antegrade transport of urine from the ureter into the bladder and prevents retrograde passage of urine from the bladder into the ureter.

ANATOMY

Gross Anatomy

The ureter is a 25- to 30-cm-long tube extending from the renal pelvis to the bladder. The three narrowest areas of the ureter are (a) at the ureteropelvic junction (UPJ), (b) at the site where the ureter crosses the iliac vessels, and (c) at the intramural portion of the distal ureter. It is at these sites that calculi most frequently become impacted.

As the ureter descends in a medial direction from the kidney, it lies on the psoas muscle in close apposition to the peritoneum, to which it is attached. In its abdominal course, both ureters are crossed anteriorly by the gonadal vessels, and they in turn cross anterior to the genitofemoral nerve (Fig 24.1A). On the right side, the descending portion of the duodenum usually lies in front of the ureter, and more distally the right ureter is crossed anteriorly by the right colic and ileocolic vessels in the root of the mesentery (Fig. 24.1B). The appendix may overlie the right ureter. On the left side, the ureter is crossed anteriorly by the left colic vessels, and as it passes over the pelvic brim, it passes behind the sigmoid colon.

As the ureters descend into the true pelvis, they pass over the terminal portion of the common or the first portion of the external iliac arteries (Fig. 24.1C). At this point, the two ureters are approximately 5 cm apart. After crossing into the pelvis, the ureters first diverge laterally and then converge medially toward the trigone. In the male, the pelvic ureter passes anterior to the internal iliac (hypogastric) artery and then just before it enters the bladder it is crossed anteriorly by the vas deferens (Fig. 24.1D). In the female, the pelvic ureter passes anterior to the internal iliac (hypogastric) artery, below the root of the broad ligament of the uterus,

R.M. Weiss: Section of Urology, Department of Surgery, Yale University School of Medicine, Yale–New Haven Hospital, New Haven, CT 06520.

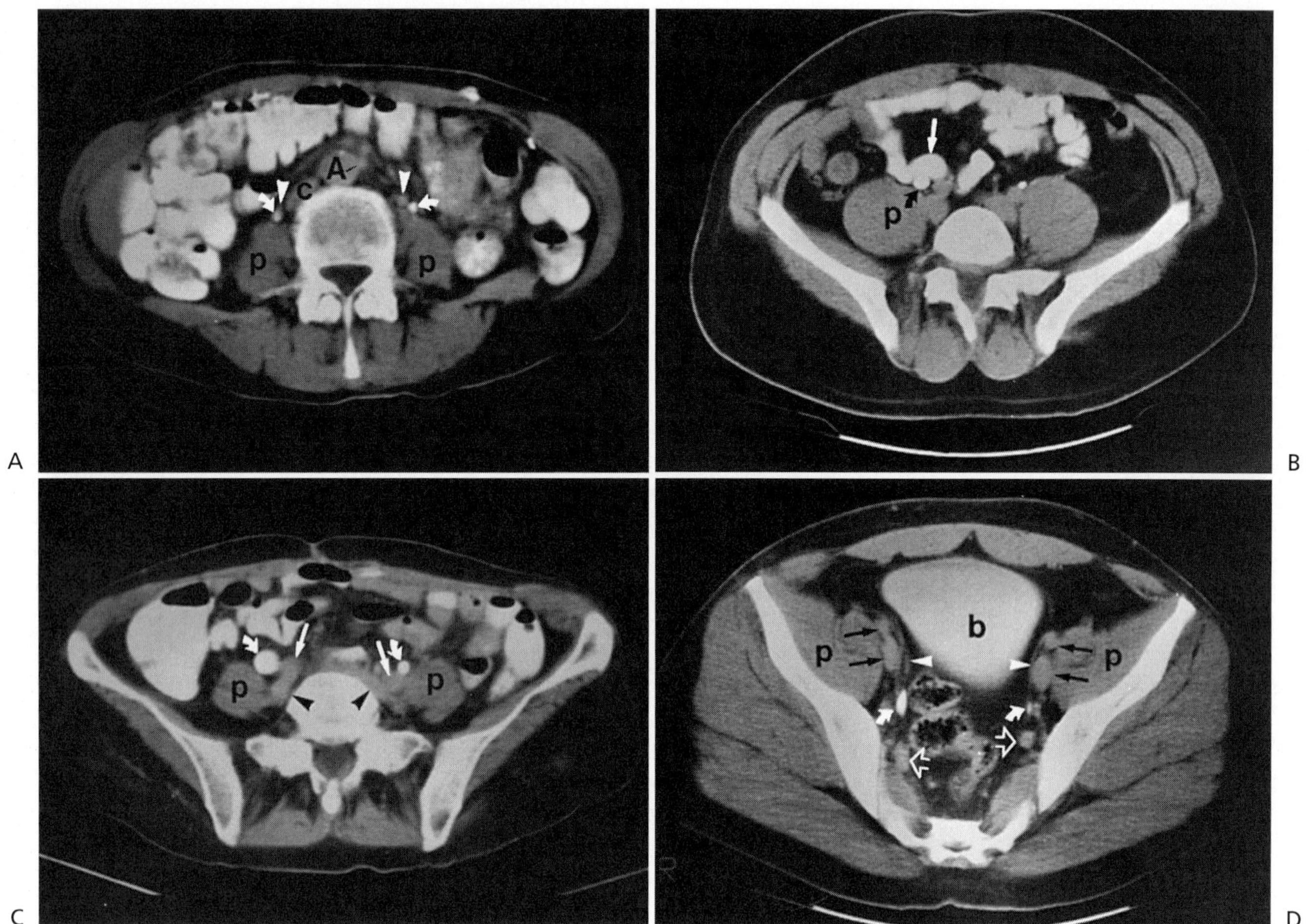

FIGURE 24.1. Computed tomography scans. **A:** Transverse section showing ureters *(curved arrows)* lying on top of psoas muscle *(p)*. The gonadal vessels *(arrowheads)* are located anterior and medial to the ureter. A, aorta; C, vena cava. **B:** Close relationship between right ureter *(curved arrow)* and bowel *(straight arrow)*. Right ureter is dilated. p, psoas muscle. **C:** Ureters *(curved arrows)* passing over common iliac arteries *(straight arrow)* and veins *(arrowheads)*. Ureters are dilated. p, psoas muscle. **D:** Ureters *(curved arrows)* are crossed anteromedially by vasa deferentia *(arrowheads)*. *Straight arrows* show external iliac arteries and veins; *open arrows* show hypogastric vessels. p, iliopsoas muscle; b, bladder.

and then runs along the lateral aspect of the cervix, passing under the uterine artery. The ureter is crossed by the obliterated umbilical vessels in both males and females.

Blood Supply

The ureter is supplied by a variable number of segmental arteries that arise from the aorta and from a variety of its branches or subbranches, including the renal, gonadal, adrenal, common iliac, internal iliac, external iliac, superior vesical, inferior vesical, vesiculodeferential, uterine, obturator, gluteal, vaginal, and middle hemorrhoidal arteries (39). As these segmental vessels reach the ureter, they divide into ascending and descending branches that run in the adventitial layer of the ureter. The descending branches of proximally located segmental arteries anastomose with the ascending branches of more distally located segmental vessels, thus forming long, longitudinally running vascular channels. These anastomosing arteries may give off secondary branches that form arterial plexuses in the adventitial layer of the ureter. Tributaries from the adventitial plexus pierce the muscular coat and form delicate plexuses in the submucosal layer.

Lymphatic Supply

Ureteral lymph vessels begin in communicating submucosal, intramuscular, and adventitial plexuses (239). Lymphatics from the proximal ureter may join lymphatics of the kidney, which follow the course of the renal vein to end in the lateral aortic nodes, or they may drain directly into the lateral aortic nodes near the origin of the gonadal arteries.

Lymphatics from the midureter drain into the lumbar nodes along the aorta and inferior vena cava, and lymphatics from the lower ureter terminate in the common, external, and internal iliac glands.

Nerve Supply

In a syncytial-type smooth muscle such as the ureter, there is a diffuse release of transmitter from nerve bundles, with the subsequent spread of excitation from one muscle cell to another (25). The lack of discrete neuromuscular junctions in such a system accounts for the difficulty in anatomically demonstrating the presence of ureteral innervation.

The nerves to the ureter arise from the celiac, aorticorenal, and mesenteric ganglia and also from the aortic, superior hypogastric, and inferior hypogastric plexuses. The sympathetic fibers arise from T-11 to L-1. The parasympathetic fibers to the upper ureter are derived from the vagus, and those to the lower ureter are from S-2 to S-4. In humans, the lower ureter receives a denser innervation than the upper ureter (49).

The ureter also is supplied by capsaicin-sensitive primary afferent nerve fibers that contain the tachykinins, substance P (SP), neurokinin A (NKA), neuropeptide K (NPK), and calcitonin gene–related peptide (CGRP) (45,88,130,189). The afferent innervation is densest proximally and decreases caudally (136).

Cross-sectional Anatomy

Histologically, the ureter is composed of three layers:

1. An inner mucosal layer, consisting of urothelium and its supporting lamina propria
2. A muscular layer
3. An outer adventitial layer

The inner lining of the ureter, or urothelium, is composed of transitional cell epithelium. In the contracted state, the urothelium assumes a stellate appearance, with the lumen of the ureter being completely occluded. Beneath the urothelium and separating it from the muscular coat is the lamina propria, which contains both elastic and collagenous fibers.

In humans, typical spindle-shaped smooth muscle cells, grouped together in compact bundles and rich in nonspecific cholinesterase, originate in the distal part of each minor calyx (43). These cells, which compose the outer muscle layer of the calyces and renal pelvis, are continuous with the muscular coat of the ureter.

There have been a variety of descriptions of the arrangement of the fibers in the muscular coat of the ureter. A classic description is that the muscular coat consists of an inner and outer longitudinal layer separated by a circular layer (37). Satani (179) noted that the musculature of the upper ureter ran haphazardly in all directions, whereas that of the lower ureter consisted of inner longitudinal and outer circular fibers. Murnaghan (149) described the muscle bundles as a long spiral that begins proximally as longitudinal strands in the outer region of the musculature, forms a middle circular layer as the spiral turn is made, and terminates in a distal longitudinal inner layer. Tanagho (204) emphasized that ureteral muscle bundles assume a helical or spiral configuration. More recently, Gosling and Dixon (67) noted that individual muscle bundles do not spiral around the ureter but rather form a complex meshwork of interweaving and interconnecting smooth muscle bundles without distinct longitudinal and circular layers. A scanning electron microscopic study of the guinea pig ureter showed a primarily circular arrangement in the upper ureter with a few outer longitudinal and obliquely oriented fibers, a highly irregular orientation of interlacing muscle bundles in the midureter, and predominantly longitudinally oriented muscle bundles with an underlying circular muscle coat in the lower ureter (201). The adventitia of the ureter is composed of areolar and fibroelastic connective tissue, which contains the blood vessels, lymphatics, and nerve fibers that subdivide, ramify, and enter the ureter proper.

Cellular Anatomy

The primary functional anatomic unit of the ureter is the smooth muscle cell, whose main function is to contract. The cell is extremely small, approximately 250 to 400 μm long and 5 to 7 μm in diameter, which permits a significant proportion of the calcium (Ca^{2+}) involved in the contractile process to enter the cell from extracellular sources at the time of excitation. The nucleus of the cell is ellipsoid and contains a darkly staining body, the nucleolus, and the genetic material of the cell. Surrounding the nucleus is the cytoplasm or sarcoplasm, which contains the structures involved in cell function. In the cytoplasm, frequently in close approximation to the nucleus, are *mitochondria,* which perform many of the nutritive functions of the cell (Fig. 24.2). Also within the cytoplasm are lattice-shaped structures called *endoplasmic* or *sarcoplasmic reticulum.* These structures serve as a site for internal storage of calcium, which plays an important role in the contraction of the smooth muscle cell.

Dispersed in the sarcoplasm are the contractile proteins, actin and myosin, which interact—depending on the local Ca^{2+} concentration—to result in contraction or relaxation. The actin is dispersed through the sarcoplasm in hexagonal clumps and is interspersed with the less numerous clumps of the more deeply staining myosin. Attachment plaques are dark bands along the cell surface that serve as attachment devices for the actin. Any process that leads to an increase in Ca^{2+} concentration in the region of the contractile proteins results in contraction, and, conversely, any process that leads to a decrease in Ca^{2+} concentration in the region of the contractile proteins results in relaxation.

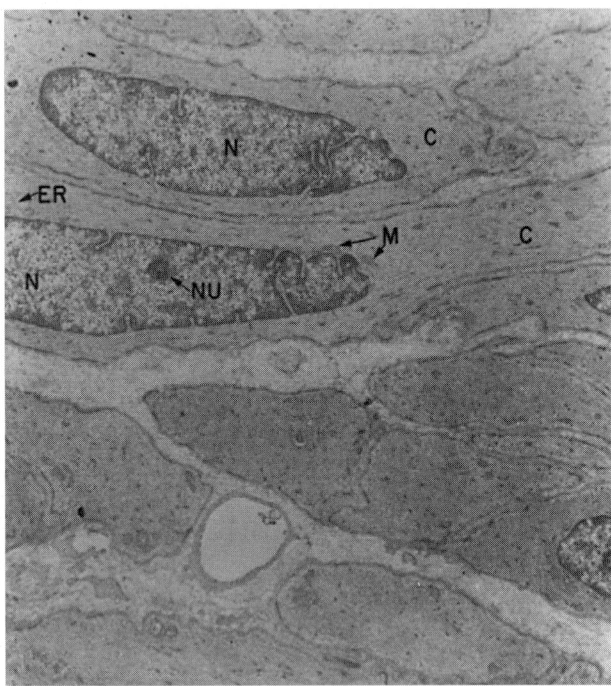

FIGURE 24.2. Electron micrograph of human ureter. C, cytoplasm (sarcoplasm); ER, endoplasmic (sarcoplasmic) reticulum; M, mitochondria; N, nucleus; NU, nucleolus. (Modified from Weiss RM. Ureteral function. *Urology* 1978;12:114, with permission.)

Along the periphery of the cell are numerous cavitary structures, some of which open to the outside of the cell, referred to as *caveolae.* These structures may serve a role in the nutritive functions of the cell or in the transport of ions across the cell membrane. Surrounding the cell is a doubled layer cell membrane. The *inner plasma* membrane surrounds the entire cell, whereas the *outer basement membrane* is absent at areas of close cell-to-cell contact, referred to as *intermediate junctions* (Fig. 24.3).

PHYSIOLOGY

Electrical Activity

The electrical properties of excitable tissues depend on the distribution of ions on the inside and outside of the cell membrane and on the relative permeability of the cell membrane to these ions (81). When a ureteral muscle cell is in a nonexcited or resting state, the electrical potential difference across the cell membrane, or transmembrane potential, is referred to as the resting membrane potential (RMP). The RMP is primarily determined by the distribution of potassium ions (K^+) across the cell membrane and by the preferential permeability of the resting membrane to potassium (76,222). In the resting state, the tendency for the positively charged K^+ ions to diffuse from the inside of the cell, where they are more concentrated, to the outside of the cell, where they are less concentrated, creates an electrical gradient in which the inside of the cell membrane is more negative than the outside. The electrical gradient that is formed tends to oppose the further movement of K^+ ions outward across the cell membrane along its concentration gradient. Thus an equilibrium is reached with a greater concentration of K^+ on the inside of the membrane and with the inside of the cell membrane being negatively charged with respect to the outside of the cell membrane.

The RMP in smooth muscle is lower than that which would be expected if the resting cell membrane were exclusively permeable to potassium. The RMP in the ureter is in the range of -33 to -70 mV (99,222). In the resting state, the sodium concentration on the outside of the cell membrane is greater than that on the inside. If the resting membrane were somewhat permeable to Na^+, both the concentration and electrical gradient would support an inward movement of Na^+ across the cell membrane, with a resultant decrease in the electronegativity of the inner surface of the cell membrane. Such a process could be a factor in the maintenance of a low RMP in smooth muscle. The RMP also may be maintained in part by an active mechanism capable of extruding Na^+ from within the cell against a concentration and an electrochemical gradient, and also by the relative permeability and distribution of chloride (Cl) ions across the cell membrane (105).

The transmembrane potential of an inactive or resting ureteral cell remains stable until it is excited by an external stimulus, whether electrical, mechanical (stretch), or chemi-

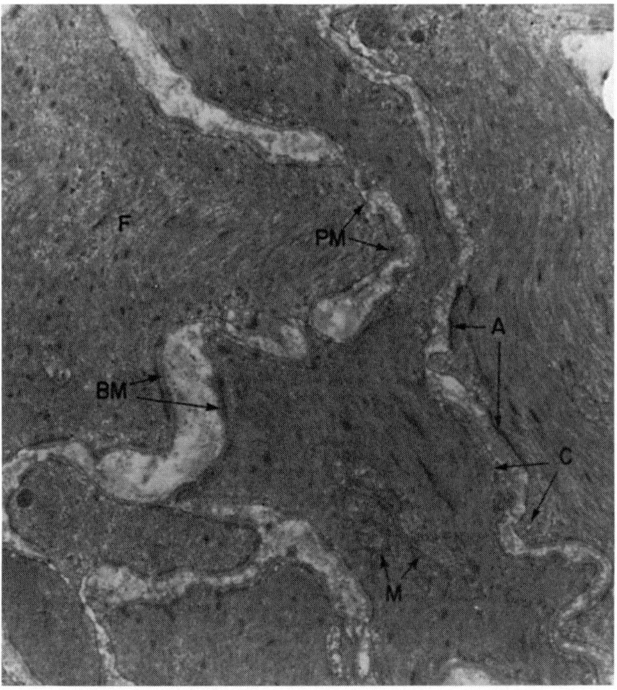

FIGURE 24.3. Electron micrograph of human ureter. A, attachment plaques; BM, basement membrane; C, caveolae; F, actin and myosin filaments; M, mitochondria; PM, plasma membrane. (From Weiss RM. Ureteral function. *Urology* 1978; 12:114, with permission.)

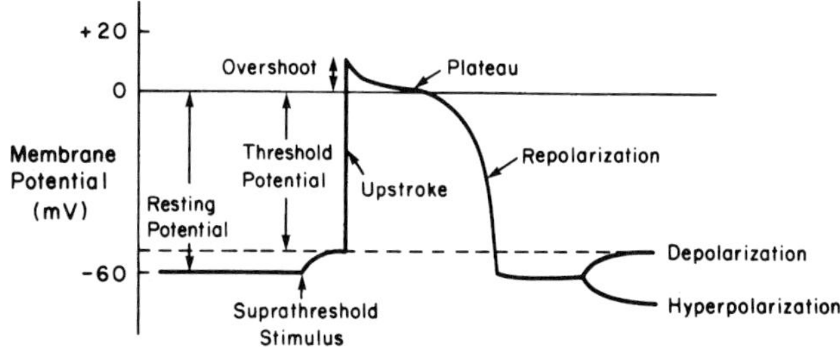

FIGURE 24.4. Schematic diagram of ureteral action potential.

cal, or by conduction of electrical activity from an already excited adjacent cell. When a ureteral cell is stimulated, depolarization occurs, with the inside of the cell membrane becoming less negative than it was before stimulation. If a sufficient area of the cell membrane is depolarized rapidly enough to reach a critical level of transmembrane potential, referred to as the *threshold potential,* a regenerative depolarization, or action potential, is initiated (Fig. 24.4). The action potential has the capacity to act as the stimulus for excitation of adjacent quiescent cells, and through a complicated chain of events gives rise to the ureteral contraction.

When the ureteral smooth muscle cell is excited, its membrane loses its preferential permeability to K^+ and becomes more permeable to Na^+ and Ca^{2+} ions, which move inward across the cell membrane and give rise to the upstroke of the action potential (21,100,188,218,219). As the positively charged Na^+ and Ca^{2+} ions move inward across the cell membrane, the inside of the membrane becomes less negative with respect to the outside and may even become positive with respect to the outside at the peak of the action potential, a state referred to as *overshoot.* The rate of rise of the upstroke of the ureteral action potential is relatively slow, 1.2 ± 0.06 V per second in the cat (99), and accounts in part for the slow conduction velocity in the ureter.

After reaching the peak of its action potential, the ureter maintains its potential for a period of time (plateau of the action potential) before the transmembrane potential returns to its resting level (repolarization). The plateau phase appears to depend on the persistence of a high inward Na^+ conductance, and the repolarization phase appears at least in part to be due to an outward movement of K^+ across the cell membrane (21,103,104,188). The duration of the action potential in the cat ranges from 259 to 405 milliseconds (98).

In summary, the transmembrane potential of the resting ureteral cell (RMP) is approximately −33 to −70 mV and is primarily determined by the distribution of K^+ ions across the cell membrane and by the relative selective permeability of the resting cell membrane to K^+. When excited by a suprathreshold stimulus, the membrane becomes less permeable to K^+ ions and more permeable to Na^+ and Ca^{2+} ions, which move inward across the cell membrane and provide the ionic mechanism for the development of the upstroke of the action potential. Calcium also plays a prominent role in the contractile mechanism. After reaching the peak of its action potential, the membrane maintains a depolarized state (plateau of the action potential) for a time before the membrane potential of the activated cell returns to its resting level, repolarization. The plateau appears to be related to a persisting inward Na^+ current, and repolarization of the membrane probably is related to a decrease in the membrane permeability to Na^+ and Ca^{2+} and a renewed increase in permeability to K^+.

Pacemaker Potentials and Pacemaker Activity

Cells that develop electrical activity spontaneously are referred to as *pacemaker cells.* Pacemaker cells differ from nonpacemaker cells in that their resting transmembrane potential tends to be lower (less negative) than nonpacemaker cells (108) and does not remain constant but rather undergoes a slow spontaneous depolarization. If the spontaneously changing membrane potential reaches the threshold potential, the upstroke of an action potential occurs.

Dixon and Gosling (42,43,65,66,68) provided morphologic evidence of specialized pacemaker tissues in the proximal portion of the urinary collecting system. In humans, Dixon and Gosling (43) identified atypical smooth muscle cells in the region of attachment of each minor calyx to the renal parenchyma that are devoid of nonspecific cholinesterase. These distinctive cells, loosely arranged and separated from one another by connective tissue, form a thin sheet of muscle that covers each minor calyceal fornix. The atypical cells run across the renal parenchyma that lies between the renal attachments of the minor calcyes and thus serve as a connector between the minor calyces. Atypical cells are arranged longitudinally as an inner layer of the muscle coat of the minor and major calyces and of the renal pelvis. They appear to be closely applied to and to interconnect with typical muscle cells in these structures, but they do not extend beyond the UPJ into the ureter. The atypical cells may act as pacemaker cells or as a preferential conduction pathway. Lang and colleagues (107) described fibroblast-like cells in the proximal portion of the guinea pig renal pelvis that resemble the interstitial cells of Cajal that act as pacemaker cells in the intestine.

In the multicalyceal kidney, Morita and associates (146,147), using extracellular electrodes, recorded low voltage potentials, which appear to be pacemaker potentials, from the junction of the minor calyces and the major calyx. They noted that the contraction rhythm varied in each calyx. Calyceal contractions, with resultant coaptation of the walls of the calyces, facilitate outflow of urine from the papillae and protect the renal parenchyma from pressure increases transmitted from the renal pelvis. At normal urine flow rates in the multicalyceal kidney, pacemaker contractions of the calyces occur at a rate of approximately six per minute. At normal rates of flow, the contraction waves are frequently blocked in the renal pelvis or at the UPJ (146). With increasing flow, there is a cessation of this block, and a 1:1 relationship is observed between pacemaker and ureteral contractions (33). In other words, at high flows, ureteral contractions occur at the same frequency as that of the calyces, whereas at low flows, calyceal contraction frequencies are greater than those of the ureter.

Under normal conditions, electrical activity arises proximally and is conducted distally from one muscle cell to another across the intermediate junctions (113,212). These close cellular contacts are similar to nexuses, which have been shown in other smooth muscles to be low-resistance pathways for cell-to-cell conduction (8). Although the primary pacemaker for ureteral peristalsis is located in the proximal portion of the collecting system, latent pacemakers are present in all regions of the ureter (90,140). Action potentials arising at these sites can propagate proximally and distally. Under normal conditions, these latent pacemaker regions are dominated by activity arising at the primary pacemaker sites. When the latent pacemaker sites are freed of their domination by the primary pacemaker, they in turn may act as a pacemaker.

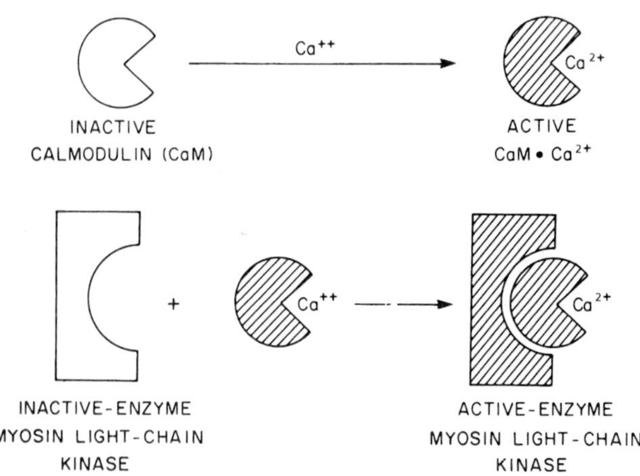

FIGURE 24.5. Schematic representation of contractile process in smooth muscle. Calmodulin is activated by Ca^{2+}. The activated calcium–calmodulin complex activates the enzyme myosin light-chain kinase. (Modified from Weiss RM. Physiology and pharmacology of the renal pelvis and ureter. In: Walsh PC, et al, eds. *Campbell's urology,* ed 5. Philadelphia: Saunders, 1986, with permission.)

Contractile Activity

The contractile event is dependent on the concentration of free sarcoplasmic Ca^{2+} in the region of the contractile proteins actin and myosin. Any process that results in an increase in Ca^{2+} in the region of the contractile proteins favors the development of a contraction; any process that results in a decrease in Ca^{2+} in the region of the contractile proteins favors relaxation.

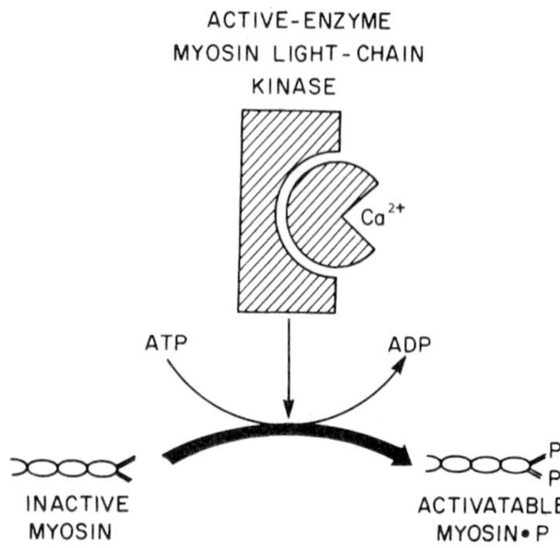

FIGURE 24.6. Schematic representation of contractile process in smooth muscle. The activated enzyme, myosin light-chain kinase, catalyzes the phosphorylation of myosin. Myosin must be phosphorylated for actin to activate myosin ATPase. (Modified from Weiss RM. Physiology and pharmacology of the renal pelvis and ureter. In: Walsh PC, et al, eds. *Campbell's urology,* ed 5. Philadelphia: Saunders, 1986, with permission.)

Contractile Proteins

In smooth muscle, the most widely accepted theory suggests that phosphorylation of myosin is involved in the contractile process. With excitation, there is a transient increase in the sarcoplasmic Ca^{2+} concentration from a steady state concentration of 10^{-8} M to 10^{-7} M to a concentration of 10^{-6} M or higher. At this higher concentration, Ca^{2+} forms an active complex with the calcium-binding protein calmodulin (223) (Fig. 24.5). Calmodulin without Ca^{2+} is inactive. The calcium–calmodulin complex activates a calmodulin-dependent enzyme, myosin light-chain kinase, which in turn catalyzes the phosphorylation of the 20,000-Da light chain of myosin (Fig. 24.6). Phosphorylation of the myosin light chain is a prerequisite for activation by actin of myosin Mg^{2+}-adenosine triphosphatase (ATPase) activity, with resultant hydrolysis or adenosine triphosphate (ATP) and the development of smooth muscle tension or shortening (Fig. 24.7).

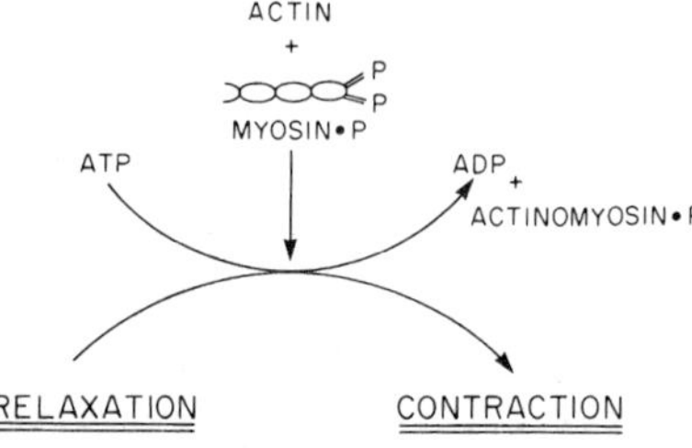

FIGURE 24.7. Schematic representation of contractile process in smooth muscle. Actin activates ATPase activity of phosphorylated myosin with the resultant development of contraction. (Modified from Weiss RM. Physiology and pharmacology of the renal pelvis and ureter. In: Walsh PC, et al, eds. *Campbell's urology,* ed 5. Philadelphia: Saunders, 1986, with permission.)

When the Ca^{2+} concentration in the region of the contractile proteins is low, myosin light-chain kinase is not activated, because calmodulin requires Ca^{2+} to activate the enzyme. This prevents activation of the contractile appara-

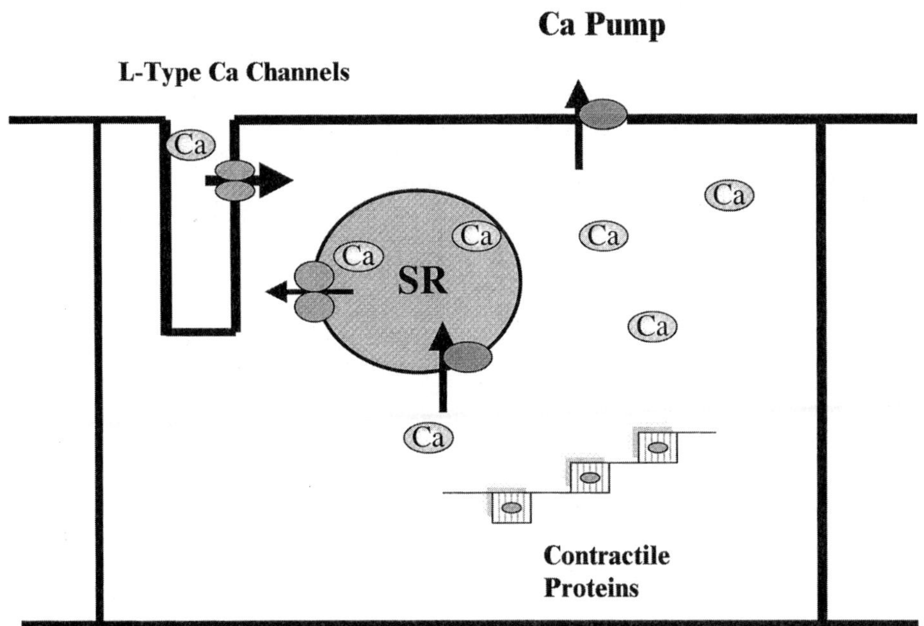

FIGURE 24.8. Schematic representation of calcium *(Ca)* movements involved in ureteral contraction. Ca involved in contractile process may be derived from extracellular sources or from tightly bound intracellular storage sites. SR, sarcoplasmic reticulum.

tus, because the myosin light chain cannot be phosphorylated, a process that must precede tension development. Furthermore, a phosphatase dephosphorylates the myosin light chain, preventing actin activation of myosin ATPase activity, and relaxation results.

The calcium involved in the ureteral contraction is derived from two main sources (Fig. 24.8). Because smooth muscle cells have a small diameter, the inward movement of extracellular Ca^{2+} into the cell through L-type calcium channels during the upstroke of the action potential provides a significant source of sarcoplasmic calcium (79,125). Calcium release from a more tightly bound storage site, that is, the endoplasmic (sarcoplasmic) reticulum, is another possible source of sarcoplasmic calcium (218), although pharmacologic evidence suggests that Ca^{2+} release from the sarcoplasmic reticulum does not play a significant role in ureteral contractions, at least in the guinea pig (122,124, 125). Relaxation results from a decrease in the concentration of free sarcoplasmic Ca^{2+} in the region of the contractile proteins. The decrease in sarcoplasmic Ca^{2+} can result from uptake of Ca^{2+} into intracellular storage sites (124, 125) or from extrusion of Ca^{2+} from the cell (24).

Role of Nervous System in Ureteral Function

The ureter is a syncytial type of smooth muscle without discrete neuromuscular junctions. Because peristalsis may persist after transplantation (155) or denervation (234), and because normal antegrade peristalsis persists after reversal of a segment of ureter *in situ* (142), it is apparent that ureteral peristalsis can occur without innervation. Further evidence indicating that an intact innervation is not required for ureteral peristalsis is that neither pacemaker activity nor the propagation of ureteral peristalsis is affected by the neural poison tetrodotoxin (61,185). It is, however, also apparent that the nervous system plays at least a modulating role in ureteral peristalsis. Autonomic drugs may affect the rate of urine transport through the ureter by modulating not only peristaltic frequency but also bolus volume (148). There is strong evidence to support the presence of excitatory α-adrenergic and inhibitory β-adrenergic receptors in the ureter (139,171,225). Support for the presence of excitatory α-adrenergic and inhibitory β-adrenergic receptor mechanisms in the ureter includes the demonstration of adenylyl cyclase activity in the ureter (230,236), the demonstration of α- and β-adrenergic receptors in the ureter using receptor binding techniques (110,111), and the finding that the application of a given intraluminal pressure results in a greater degree of ureteral deformation in rabbits depleted of catecholamines by the administration of reserpine than results from the application of the same pressure load to a ureter of a normal non–reserpine-treated animal (226). Furthermore, electrical stimulation with high-intensity, high-frequency, short-duration pulses has been shown to release catecholamines, presumably from neural tissue intrinsic within the wall of the ureter (225) and renal calyx (116), and catecholamine-containing nerve fibers and cells have been demonstrated in the ureter (163).

Available data suggest that cholinergic (parasympathetic) agonists potentiate ureteral and renal pelvic contractility by directly stimulating cholinergic receptors (128,164,220) or by indirectly causing the release of catecholamines (171). The ureter contains acetylcholinesterase-positive nerve fibers and cells, with the intravesical ureter being the most densely innervated (164), and cholinergic (muscarinic) receptors have been demonstrated in the ureter (110,111). DelTacca's demonstration (41) of acetylcholine release from isolated guinea pig, rabbit, and human ureters during field stimulation, and the inhibition of this release by the neural poison tetrodotoxin, provides further evidence for a role of the parasympathetic nervous system in the control of ureteral activity.

Anatomic support for a role of the nervous system in the modulation of peristalsis is provided by the demonstration of adventitial nerves in the human ureter (152,153) and the immunohistochemical demonstration of nerves and nerve cells beneath the muscularis and adventitia in the human and pig ureter (93).

Release of the tachykinins SP, NKA, and NPK from capsaicin-sensitive sensory nerves of the ureter has an excitatory effect on ureteral peristalsis, whereas release of CGRP from these nerves has an inhibitory effect on ureteral peristalsis (87). The excitatory effect of the tachykinins involves excitation of NK2 receptors in guinea pig and human ureters (158). The inhibitory effect of CGRP is associated with an increase in cyclic adenosine monophosphate (cAMP) (177). Maggi and associates (132) noted that the excitatory effects of tachykinins are more prominent in the renal pelvis than in the ureter and that the inhibitory effects of CGRP are more prominent in the ureter than in the renal pelvis. Histochemical studies have shown that the tachykinins and CGRP colocalize in the same nerves in the guinea pig and human ureter (88). Peptidergic neurons containing neuropeptide Y (NPY) and vasoactive intestinal polypeptide (VIP) also are present in the rat, cat, guinea pig, and human ureters (3,5,49,162). NPY potentiates the contractile responses to norepinephrine (162). VIP decreases ureteral peristaltic frequency and amplitude (109).

Nitric oxide (NO) and NO donors cause an increase in cyclic guanosine monophosphate (cGMP), with resultant relaxation of the renal pelvis and ureter (91,92). Nerves displaying immunoreactivity for nitric oxide synthase (NOS) or nicotinamide-adenine-dinucleotide phosphate (NADPH) diaphorase are present in the human ureter (60,91,193). There is some evidence that NO may be a transmitter in the ureter and renal pelvis, but there may be species and anatomic differences. NOS inhibitors have been shown to block nonadrenergic, noncholinergic (NANC) nerve-mediated relaxations of pig intravesical ureter (77), but they do not influence the spontaneous motility of isolated guinea pig renal pelvis or guinea pig and sheep ureter (57,127).

Physiology of the Ureteropelvic Junction

Griffiths and Notschaele (70) described the dynamics of urine transport within the ureter. As the renal pelvis fills, there is a rise in renal pelvic pressure, and urine is ultimately extruded into the upper ureter, which is initially in a collapsed state. After transporting the urine into the upper ureter, renal pelvic pressure declines to its baseline value, and the cycle of pelvic filling, increase in pressure, and launching of urine into the ureter occurs again. The closed UPJ may be protective to the kidney in dissipating backpressure from the ureter, because ureteral contractile pressures are higher than renal pelvic pressures.

The mechanism for urine launching into the upper ureter is not completely understood, and abnormalities in a rather complicated regulatory mechanism may cause the hydronephrosis associated with functional UPJ obstructions in which urine transport is impaired, even though large-caliber catheters can be passed readily through the UPJ. Whereas in the normal system, peristalsis is controlled by pacemaker cells that generate high-frequency action potentials in the proximal pelvicalyceal region, in the chronically dilated system, the frequency gradient in the renal pelvis is lost. This can be associated with latent pacemakers initiating dystropic orthograde peristaltic activity or retrograde contractions. Obstruction alters the hierarchic organization of the multiple coupled pacemakers that normally coordinate peristaltic activity (31). Such disruption causes uncoordinated pelvic contractions that may result in hypertrophy of the renal pelvic smooth muscle and impaired transport of urine into the ureter. Whether these functional changes are secondary to or the cause of the dilation is not certain.

Murnaghan (150) related the functional abnormality at the UPJ to an alteration in the configuration of the muscle bundles, and Foote and associates (54) observed a decrease in musculature at the UPJ in patients with a UPJ obstruction. Hanna (73) noted in severe UPJ obstruction abnormalities in the musculature of the renal pelvis and disruption of intercellular relationships at the UPJ itself. Gosling and Dixon (64) also observed histologic abnormalities in the dilated renal pelvis. In some instances, there may be areas of actual narrowing or valvelike processes at the UPJ. Furthermore, a vessel or adhesive band crossing the UPJ may potentiate the degree of dilation in any of the forms of UPJ obstruction.

Propulsion of Urinary Bolus

Following extrusion into the ureter, the urine forms a bolus owing to a ureteral contraction ring that completely coapts the ureteral walls (70). The contraction ring at the rear end of the bolus progresses distally at a constant velocity, while the velocity of the leading edge of the bolus varies along the ureter (46). Therefore the width and length of the bolus is not uniform as it moves from the renal pelvis to the bladder. The bolus of urine that is pushed distally in front of the contraction ring lies almost entirely in a passive, noncontracting part of the ureter (224). Contraction waves normally occur two to six times per minute in the normal human ureter (47) and are conducted at a velocity of

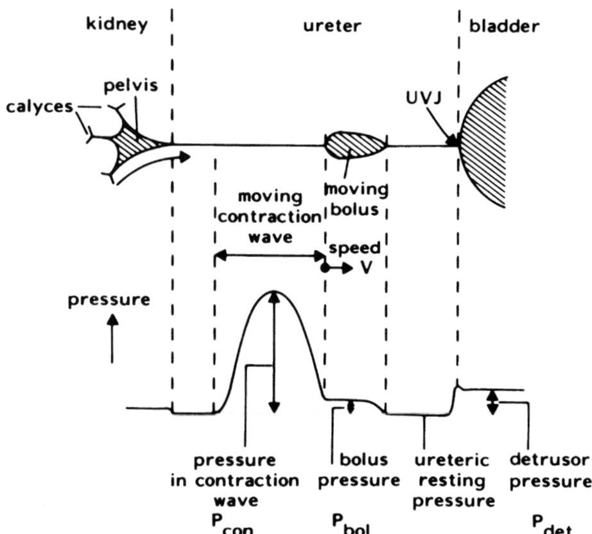

FIGURE 24.9. Schematic representation of a single bolus in the ureter moving from the renal pelvis to the bladder. Corresponding distribution of pressure within the urinary tract is shown *(lower tracing).* UVJ, ureterovesical junction; V, speed of bolus movement. (From Griffiths DJ, Notschaele C. The mechanics of urine transport in the upper urinary tract. I. The dynamics of the isolated bolus. *Neurol Urodynam* 1983;2:155, with permission.)

approximately 2 to 5 cm per second (26). Baseline (resting) ureteral pressure is approximately 0 to 5 cm H_2O, and contractile pressures may range from 20 to 60 cm H_2O (47). The major component of the recorded pressure is derived from the contraction wave, with only a small component derived from the bolus pressure. The urine bolus is forced into the bladder by the advancing contraction wave, which dissipates at the UVJ (Fig. 24.9). When functioning properly, the UVJ ensures one-way transport of urine.

As with any tubular structure, the ureter can transport a set maximum amount of fluid per unit time. Under normal flows, in which bolus formation occurs, the amount of urine transported per unit time is significantly less than the maximum transport capacity of the ureter. At high flows, the ureteral walls do not coapt, and fluid is transported in a continuous column rather than in a series of boluses.

Changes in the dimensions of the ureter that occur in pathologic states may in themselves account for inefficient urine transport, even if the contractile force of the individual fibers remains unchanged (11,70,227). The Laplace equation expresses the relationship between the variables that affect intraluminal pressure:

$$\text{Pressure} = \frac{\text{Stress} \times \text{Wall Thickness}}{\text{Radius}}$$

An increase in ureteral diameter in itself can cause a decrease in intraluminal pressure and result in inefficient urine transport.

The Laplace relationship also may provide a rationale for ureteral tapering of the dilated ureter. With ureteral tapering, muscle thickness and the ability of the ureter to contract remain unchanged. The decrease in radius occurring with ureteral tapering may in itself account for higher intraluminal pressure, with resultant improved urine transport. The tapered ureter can coapt its walls more readily and generate a higher intraluminal pressure, even though the material itself has not been changed (227). Diagrammatically, with ureteral tapering, force or the number of blocks remains unchanged, but intraluminal pressure increases as the load is supported over a smaller area; thus pressure or the height of the pile of blocks increases (Fig. 24.10).

Effect of Diuresis on Ureteral Function

The upper urinary tract alters its characteristics according to the amount of urine to be transported. Smooth muscle function is affected by the amount of stretch and the rate with which the stretch is applied. The initial response of the ureter to an increase in urine flow is an increase in the frequency of peristalsis. At relatively low flow rates, small increases in flow result in large increases in peristaltic frequency. At higher flow rates, relatively large increases in flow result in only small increases in peristaltic frequency. With increasing urine flow, peristaltic frequency increases to a maximum, and further increases in urine transport occur by means of increases in bolus volume (32). As the volume of the bolus increases, the leading edge of the bolus approximates the contraction ring of the preceding bolus. The pressure in the bolus increases because of increased resistance at the leading edge of the bolus, where it touches the preceding contraction wave. At very high flows, the pressure within the bolus exceeds the contraction pressure in the ring, and the contraction pressure is no longer sufficient to coapt the ureteral wall. The boluses then coalesce, and the ureter becomes filled with a column of fluid and dilates. At high flows, urine is transported through an open tube by columnar flow rather than by a series of boluses.

Physiology of the Ureterovesical Junction

Griffiths (71) analyzed the factors involved in urine transport across the UVJ. Under normal conditions and at normal flow rates, the contraction wave that occludes the ureteral lumen propagates distally with the urine bolus in front of it. When the bolus reaches the UVJ, the pressure within the bolus must exceed intravesical pressure for the bolus of urine to pass across the UVJ into the bladder. For the contraction wave to coapt the ureter walls and move the urine bolus distally, the pressure generated by the contraction wave must exceed the pressure within the urinary bolus. The UVJ does not relax (228).

Blok and co-workers (14) demonstrated fast and slow pressure waves at the UVJ. The fast pressure waves originate from intrinsic ureteral contractions, are related to retraction of the distal ureter within its sheaths, and are accompanied by bolus ejection of fluid into the bladder. This telescoping,

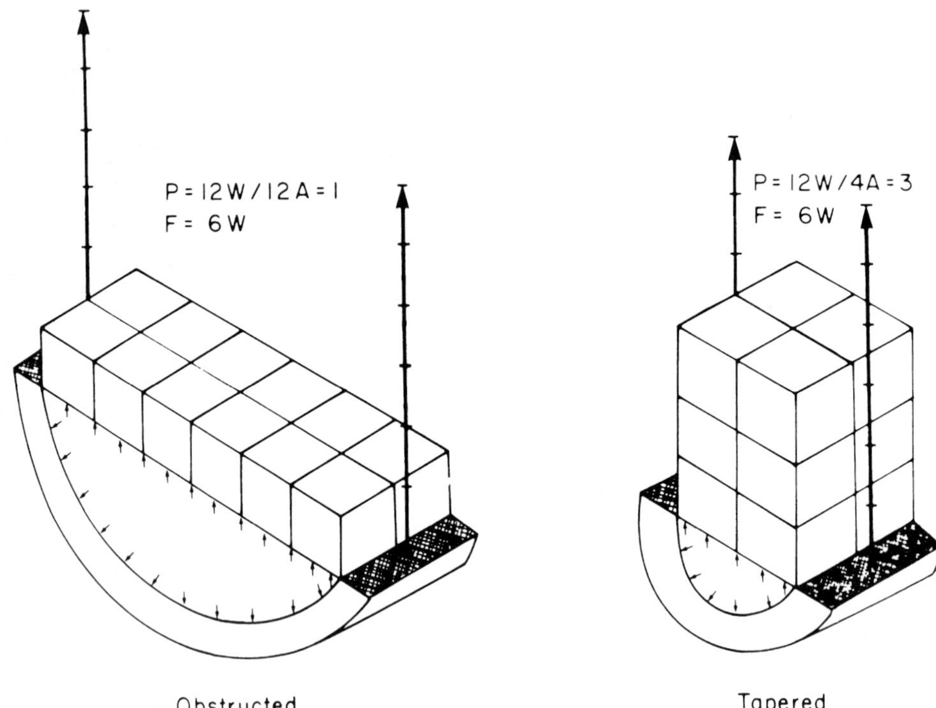

FIGURE 24.10. Diagrammatic representation of changes that occur with tapering of the obstructed ureter. A, area over which force is distributed; F, force developed by each half of ureter; P, pressure; W, blocks or weights representing load proportional to force. (From Weiss RM, Biancani P. A rationale for ureteral tapering. *Urology* 1982;20:482, with permission.)

dynamic event decreases the UVJ resistance to flow and thus facilitates urine passage into the bladder. The slow pressure waves originate from the surrounding detrusor muscles and represent the influence of detrusor activity on flow through the UVJ. Coolsaet and associates (36) demonstrated that resistance to flow through the UVJ is due to (a) stretch of the bladder base and UVJ, (b) intravesical pressure transmitted to the submucosal ureteral segment, (c) activity of the detrusor muscle surrounding the UVJ, and (d) dynamics of the ureteral segment composing the UVJ.

The relationship between upper urinary tract function and resistance to outflow at the UVJ is of major clinical importance. The pressure within the bladder during the storage phase is of paramount importance in determining the efficacy of urine transport across the UVJ. This is the pressure that the ureter must work against for the greatest period of time. During filling of the normal bladder, sympathetic impulses and the viscoelastic properties of bladder wall inhibit the magnitude of the intravesical pressure rise. With filling, the normal bladder maintains a relatively low intravesical pressure (138). The low intravesical pressure facilitates urine transport across the UVJ and prevents ureteral dilation.

Renal function and the functional integrity of the upper urinary tract are at risk in individuals with noncompliant or hyperactive bladders. In the noncompliant fibrotic bladder and in some forms of neurogenic vesical dysfunction, the bladder is autonomous, and relatively small increases in bladder volume result in large increases in intravesical pressure with impairment of ureteral emptying. Regular emptying of these bladders may not be sufficient to protect the upper tracts, and intravesical pressure may need to be lowered by reduction in detrusor tonus. Furthermore, outflow resistance at the UVJ may be high in the overdistended bladder even at low intravesical pressures. This results from stretch of the UVJ and decreased retractability of the submucosal ureteral segment. Intravesical volume thus should be kept at reasonable levels, which may require intermittent catheterization. Increased resistance to bolus outflow across the UVJ can occur when there is obstruction at the UVJ, when intravesical pressure or volume is excessive, or when flow rates are so high as to exceed the transport capacity of the UVJ. Under such conditions, in which the bolus of urine cannot freely pass into the bladder, the pressure within the bolus, propelled by the ureteral contraction ring, increases and may exceed the pressure within the contraction ring. Under these conditions, the contraction wave will be unable to coapt the ureteral wall and intraureter reflux will occur. This impaired bolus transport will cause secondary widening of the ureter and weaker ureteral contractions, with only a fraction of the bolus volume passing distally. Griffiths (71) presented theoretic evidence to show that a similar situation of impaired bolus transport across the UVJ would be expected if the ureter was wide or weakly contracting, even if the UVJ was perfectly normal. Under these conditions, a similar breakdown of bolus discharge into the bladder can occur in the wide or weakly contracting ureter at high flow rates, even if the UVJ is normal.

There is some evidence that gravity may assist urine transport and that the erect position, by enhancing hydrostatic loading of the UVJ, may facilitate urine transport across the UVJ, especially in individuals with wide upper tracts (181). From a clinical viewpoint, some workers have suggested that bed rest may be deleterious to renal function in the patient with urinary retention and dilated upper urinary tracts (58).

Relationship Between Vesicoureteral Reflux and Ureteral Function

The intravesical ureter is approximately 1.5 cm long and takes an oblique course through the bladder wall. It is composed of an intramural segment, which is surrounded by detrusor muscle, and a submucosal segment, which lies directly under the bladder urothelium (203). The relationship between the length and diameter of the intravesical segment of ureter appears to be a factor in the prevention of vesicoureteral reflux (156). Trigonal function also may be a factor in the prevention of vesicoureteral reflux (202). Furthermore, the development of vesicoureteral reflux in individuals with bladder outlet obstruction and neurogenic vesical dysfunction provides evidence that increased intravesical pressures also may be a factor in certain instances of reflux.

Although an abnormality of the UVJ is the primary etiologic factor in most cases of reflux, there is evidence to suggest that decreased ureteral peristaltic activity may be a contributory factor (96,141,228). Support for this contention may be derived from the findings that a normal ureter may not reflux, even when reimplanted into a bladder without a submucosal tunnel (40), and that a defunctionalized refluxing ureter may cease to reflux when a proximal diversion is taken down and urine flow through the ureter is reinstated (206,233). Furthermore, the success rate of antireflux procedures is less with poorly functioning dilated ureters, and, although this may be related to technical factors, decreased peristaltic activity may be a reason for failure in many instances.

Studies in normal and mildly refluxing systems have shown that there is a high-pressure zone in the distal ureter with a resultant pressure gradient across the UVJ (228). With bladder filling, the resultant UVJ–bladder pressure gradient increases in nonrefluxing systems, whereas it decreases and may disappear in refluxing systems (228) (Fig. 24.11). This decrease in the pressure gradient in refluxing systems may be related to lateralization of the ureteral orifice and shortening of the intravesical tunnel and may correspond to the time when reflux occurs.

Effect of Infection on Ureteral Function

Infection within the upper urinary tract may impair urine transport. Bacteria and endotoxins have been shown to inhibit ureteral activity (95,165,205), and pyelonephritis in the monkey has been associated with decreased peristaltic activity (168). Furthermore, Rose and Gillenwater (170) have shown that infection can potentiate the deleterious effects of obstruction on ureteral function.

In humans, irregular peristaltic contractions, often with a decreased amplitude, have been recorded with infection. In more severe cases, absence of activity has been noted (173). Furthermore, ureteral dilation may occur with retroperitoneal inflammatory processes secondary to appendicitis, regional enteritis, ulcerative colitis, or peritonitis (134). Infection also may reduce the compliance of the intravesical ureter and permit reflux to occur in situations in which the UVJ is intrinsically of marginal competence (35).

Effect of Calculi on Ureteral Function

Factors that can affect the spontaneous passage of calculi include the size and shape of the stone (213); areas of narrowing within the ureteral lumen; ureteral peristalsis; the hydrostatic pressure of the column of urine proximal to the calculus (190); and edema, inflammation, and spasm of the ureter at the site of the stone (82).

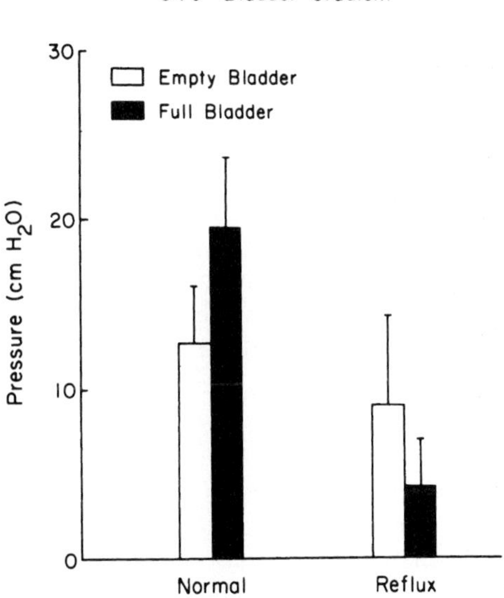

FIGURE 24.11. Pressure gradient across the ureterovesical junction *(UVJ)* in normal and mildly refluxing (grades II and III) systems. (From Weiss RM, Biancani P. Characteristics of normal and refluxing ureterovesical junctions. *J Urol* 1983;129:858, with permission.)

Two factors that appear to be most useful in facilitating stone passage are an increase in hydrostatic pressure proximal to a calculus and relaxation of the ureter in the vicinity of the stone. In support of the theory that increased hydrostatic pressure facilitates stone passage, it has been shown in the rabbit and dog ureter that artificial concentrations with holes move more slowly than those without holes (190). Furthermore, ureteral ligation proximal to a concretion has been shown to decrease hydrostatic pressure, with resultant inhibition of stone passage (190). Theoretically, high fluid intake will increase hydrostatic pressure proximal to a stone and thus may aid in its passage; however, the elevated hydrostatic pressure, if prolonged, is potentially deleterious to the kidney.

With respect to the potential facilitative effect of ureteral relaxation on stone passage, Peters and Eckstein (161) showed that the spasmolytic agents phentolamine, an α-adrenergic antagonist, and orciprenaline, a β-adrenergic agonist, dilated the canine ureter at the level of an artificial concretion and thus permitted increased fluid flow beyond a partially obstructive concretion. It appears that resistance to urine flow in this experimental model was caused in part by the artificial concretion and in part by local spasm and that the resistance could be decreased by spasmolytic drugs, such as phentolamine and orciprenaline. Although it has not been determined whether this spasmolytic effect would aid in stone passage, the same principle has been used to float upper ureteral stones proximally into the renal pelvis as a prelude to percutaneous nephrostolithotomy. Obstruction of the ureter with a balloon catheter leads to dilation of the ureter, with the impacted stone then being able to migrate proximally (9). Furthermore, placement of a nephrostomy tube proximal to a steinstrasse appears to facilitate passage of the stones. This may result from decreasing peristaltic activity that acts as a spasmodic factor in the region of the stone.

Although these data can be interpreted to imply that ureteral relaxation in the region of a concretion would aid in stone passage, a controlled study currently is not available. Such a study with an agent known to have strong relaxant effects on the ureter, such as theophylline (69,230), would be of value, but the interpretation of the data obtained might be difficult because of the marked variability of spontaneous stone passage in the clinical setting.

Ureterolithotomy

With the advent of ureteroscopy, percutaneous nephrostolithotomy, and extracorporeal shock wave lithotripsy (ESWL), open ureterolithotomy has become a less frequently used procedure. However, it may still be the preferred technique for the removal of large midureteral stones that are impacted at the level of the iliac vessels. For upper ureteral calculi, a standard flank incision below or through the bed of the twelfth rib has been the standard approach, although a posterior lumbotomy has a role in the management of larger, well-impacted calculi. During the procedure, avoidance of stone migration, especially proximally, should be ensured by control of the ureter above and below the calculus with vessel loops or Babcock forceps. A longitudinal incision in the ureter is made directly over the stone, and the stone is extracted. A small catheter is passed proximally into the renal pelvis for irrigation and to ensure that the system is unobstructed. Although distal passage of the catheter into the bladder can be used to assess distal obstruction, it can cause edema at the UVJ, with prolongation of flank drainage postoperatively. For this reason, the use of distal catheter passage can be individualized depending on the clinical situation.

Some authors favor a loose closure of the ureter with only one or two fine sutures, and others seek a watertight closure with either interrupted or continuous fine sutures. Both methods work. Our preference is multiple interrupted 5-0 chromic adventitial sutures, which avoid excessive prolonged leakage yet provide a means for urine egress, if necessary. One or two Penrose drains brought to the exterior through a stab wound provide for drainage.

The technical details for removal of midureteral stones are essentially the same as for upper ureteral calculi. The approach can either be via a subcostal flank incision or via an anterior extraperitoneal approach, using a horizontal incision beginning below the tip of the twelfth rib and extending anteriorly, with the patient in the supine position with a roll of towels beneath the shoulder and buttock. This approach, classically employed for sympathectomy, can involve muscle splitting, or the muscle layers can be divided.

Lower ureteral calculi can be approached through a modified Gibson's incision as used for renal transplantation or through a vertical suprapubic incision with retraction of the bladder toward the contralateral side. At times, with a periureteral inflammatory reaction or scarring from previous surgery, the ureter and stone may be difficult to identify. Identification of the ureter proximally, where it crosses the bifurcation of the common iliac artery, may facilitate its localization, and opening the peritoneum with visualization of the ureter through the posterior parietal peritoneum can be helpful. Identification and division of the obliterated umbilical vessels also can aid in localizing the ureter and facilitating removal of the calculus. The technique for stone removal is similar to that employed for higher stones, and early control of the ureter proximal to the calculus with a vessel loop is imperative.

For calculi in the most distal portions of the ureter, such as in the intramural portion of the UVJ, a transvesical approach can be used. If the stone can be palpated with the bladder open, an incision is made in the vesical mucosa directly over the calculus. If the stone is somewhat more proximal, proximal ureteral control with a vessel loop is obtained extravesically, and the incision in the ureter can be extended proximally from within the bladder. If there is concern about distal ureteral damage in cases in which there is significant periureteral inflammation, a ureteroneocystostomy using a short submucosal tunnel may be required and would be preferable to the development of a ureteral obstruction necessitating a secondary procedure. In women, a transvaginal approach can be used for distal ureteral calculi.

Effect of Pregnancy on Ureteral Function

Hydroureteronephrosis of pregnancy begins in the second trimester of gestation and subsides within the first month after parturition. It is more severe on the right than on the left side, and ureteral dilation does not occur below the pelvic brim. Roberts (169) presented a strong argument in favor of obstruction as the primary etiologic factor in the development of hydroureteronephrosis of pregnancy. Others have suggested a hormonal mechanism for the ureteral dilation of pregnancy (216). As emphasized by Roberts (169):

1. Elevated baseline (resting) ureteral pressures consistent with obstruction have been recorded above the pelvic brim in pregnant women, which decrease when positional changes permit the uterus to fall away from the ureters (176).
2. Normal ureteral contractile pressures have been recorded in pregnant women, suggesting that hormonally induced ureteral atony is not the prime factor in ureteral dilation of pregnancy.
3. Women whose ureters do not cross the pelvic brim, that is, those with pelvic kidneys or ileal conduits, do not develop ureteral dilation of pregnancy.
4. Hydronephrosis of pregnancy usually does not occur in quadripeds whose uterus hangs away from the ureters (210).
5. Elevated ureteral pressures in the pregnant monkey return to normal when the uterus is elevated from the ureters at laparotomy or when the fetus and placenta are removed from the uterus.

Studies of the effects of hormones of pregnancy on ureteral function have been conflicting. Although several studies have shown an inhibitory effect of progesterone on ureteral function (89,102) this has not been a universal finding (159,182). Progesterone has been noted to increase the degree of ureteral dilation during pregnancy and to retard the rate of disappearance of hydroureter in postpartum women (119). Furthermore, hydronephrosis has been reported in women taking oral contraceptives (72,137). Others, however, failed to induce changes in ureteral activity in women by the administration of estrogen, progesterone, or a mixture of these drugs (29,135). Thus, although obstruction appears to be the primary factor in the development of hydronephrosis of pregnancy, it is possible that a combination of hormonal and obstructive factors is involved (52).

Effect of Age on Ureteral Function

Aging affects the structure and function of the ureter. In a human autopsy study of subjects ranging in age from 12 weeks of gestation to 12 years of age, Cussen (38) noted a progressive increase in the population of smooth muscle cells and a small increase in the overall size of the individual smooth muscle cells with age. This is accompanied by an irregular increase in the number of elastic fibers. A progressive increase in ureteral cross-sectional muscle area is also observed in the ureter of the guinea pig between 3 weeks and 3 years of age, accompanied by an increase in developed force (85) (Fig. 24.12). The increase in force developed between 3 weeks and 3 months of age seems to be attributable to an increase in contractility, because there is an associated increase in active stress, or force per unit area of muscle. The increase in force developed between 3 months and 3 years of age can be explained by an increase in muscle mass alone, because there is no change in active stress between these two age groups (Fig. 24.13). Although changes in the force–length relationships of guinea pig ureter occur with age, the force–velocity relationships do not change with age (12).

The response of the ureter to pathologic insults depends not only on the magnitude and duration of the pathologic insult but also on the age of the individual affected. The neonatal rabbit ureter undergoes greater degrees of deformation in response to an applied intraluminal pressure than does the adult rabbit ureter (1). This decrease in compliance with age also is noted clinically, where more marked degrees

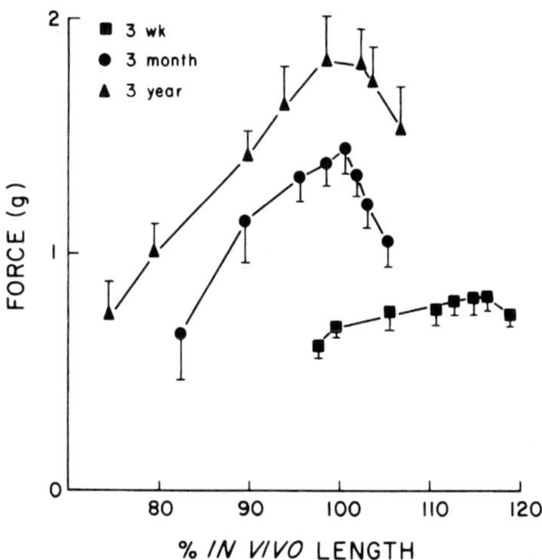

FIGURE 24.12. Active force–length curves of isolated guinea pig ureteral segments as a function of age. Developed force increases with age. Data are shown as mean ± SEM. (Modified from Hong KW, Biancani P, Weiss RM. Effect of age on contractility of guinea pig ureter. *J Urol* 1980;17:459, with permission.)

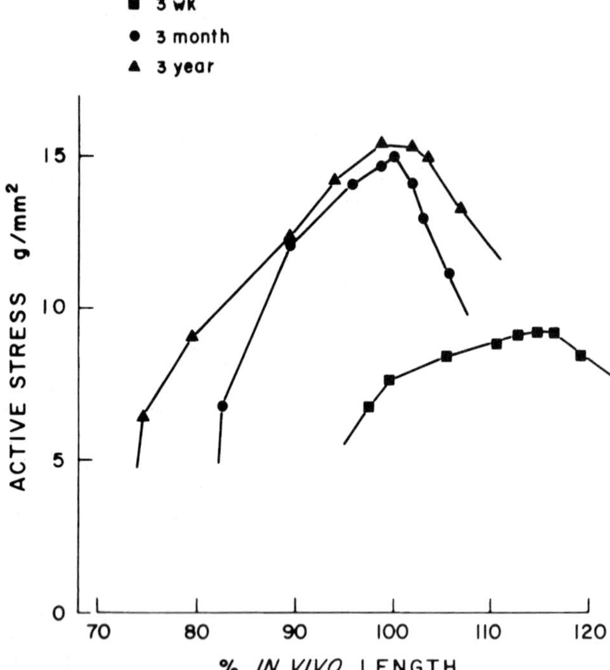

FIGURE 24.13. Active stress (force/unit area) – length curves of isolated guinea pig ureteral segments as a function of age. Stress increases between the 3-week and 3-month age groups and then remains constant with further aging. (Modified from Hong KW, Biancani P, Weiss RM. Effect of age on contractility of guinea pig ureter. *J Urol* 1980;17:459, with permission.)

of ureteral dilation occur in the neonate and young child in response to obstruction than in the adult. Experimental data suggest that aging has effects on the mechanical and biochemical properties of the ureter (1,85,236), and these changes may affect the response of the ureter to pathologic insult.

URETERAL PHARMACOLOGY

The ureter is affected by both the parasympathetic (cholinergic) and sympathetic (adrenergic) branches of the autonomic nervous system.

Parasympathetic (Cholinergic) System

Acetylcholine (ACh), the prototype cholinergic agonist, serves as the neurotransmitter at (a) neuromuscular junctions of somatic motor nerves (nicotinic sites), (b) preganglionic parasympathetic and sympathetic neuroeffector junctions (nicotinic sites), and (c) postganglionic parasympathetic neuroeffector sites, such as smooth muscle cells (muscarinic sites). ACh, synthesized in the nerve terminals from acetyl coenzyme A (CoA) and choline by the enzyme choline acetyltransferase, is released into the synaptic cleft and interacts with postganglionic receptor sites to elicit a functional response. ACh subsequently is hydrolyzed (degraded) by the enzyme acetylcholinesterase (AChE). The muscarinic effects of cholinergic agonists can be blocked by the parasympatholytic agent atropine. The effects of nicotinic agonists can be blocked by nondepolarizing ganglionic blocking agents or by high concentrations of the nicotinic agonist itself, which may cause ganglionic blockade by desensitization of receptor sites after an initial period of ganglionic stimulation.

ACh and other cholinergic agonists, such as methacholine, carbamylcholine (carbachol), and bethanechol (Urecholine), have in general been observed to have an excitatory effect on ureteral function, that is, they increase the frequency and force of contractions (171,220). The excitatory responses to carbachol and ACh appear to be more marked in ureters from younger than from older guinea pigs (232).

Anticholinesterases (anti-ChEs) prevent hydrolysis of ACh by cholinesterases and thus potentiate the actions of ACh. The effects of anti-ChEs, such as physostigmine and neostigmine, parallel the excitatory effects of ACh and other parasympathomimetics on the ureter (121). Although atropine, a competitive antagonist of the muscarinic effects of ACh, has been shown to inhibit the excitatory effects of parasympathomimetic agents (121,220) and physostigmine (121) on a variety of ureteral and calyceal preparations, the majority of studies have shown that atropine itself has little direct effect on ureteral activity in many species, including humans (94,167). Even when atropine has been observed to inhibit ureteral activity, its effects are frequently minimal and inconsistent (172), providing little rationale for its use in the treatment of ureteral colic.

Sympathetic (Adrenergic) System

Most investigators have noted that α-adrenergic agonists, such as norepinephrine and phenylephrine, stimulate ureteral activity (74,139,171,220,225). Norepinephrine, the chemical mediator responsible for adrenergic transmission, is synthesized in the neuron from tyrosine. Once released from the nerve terminal, some of the norepinephrine combines with postsynaptic receptors on the effector organs, such as smooth muscle, leading to a physiologic response. There are both α_1- and α_2-postsynaptic receptors in smooth muscle, and stimulation of either results in a contractile response. Presynaptic α_2-adrenergic receptors in the neuron inhibit the release of norepinephrine from the nerve terminal, and thus excitation of these receptors is inhibitory to smooth muscle function (Fig. 24.14). Reuptake or neuronal uptake of norepinephrine into the neuron limits the amount of time that norepinephrine is in contact with the innervated tissue and thus regulates the magnitude and duration of the catecholamine-induced response. Agents such as cocaine and imipramine (Tofranil), which inhibit neuronal uptake, potentiate the physiologic response to norepinephrine. The enzymes monoamine oxidase (MAO) and catechol-*O*-methyltransferase (COMT) provide degradation pathways for norepinephrine.

β-Adrenergic agonists, such as isoproterenol, inhibit ureteral activity (139,171,220,225). The relaxant effects of isoproterenol are greater in ureters from young than from old guinea pigs (232,235). It appears that the β-adrenoceptor subtype involved in the relaxation response is species specific (209). Tyramine, whose adrenergic agonist effects are primarily due to the release of norepinephrine from adrenergic terminals, has a stimulatory effect on the upper urinary tract (53,115).

The α-adrenergic antagonists phentolamine and phenoxybenzamine (Dibenzyline) have been shown to inhibit the stimulatory effects of norepinephrine and other α-adrenergic agonists in a variety of ureteral preparations (53,74,115,139,171,220,225). The β-adrenergic antagonist propranolol has been shown to block the inhibitory effects of β-adrenergic agonists, such as isoproterenol, in a variety of ureteral preparations. A prototype α_1-adrenergic antagonist is prazosin, and a prototype α_2-adrenergic antagonist is yohimbine.

Second Messengers

Adrenergic and cholinergic agonists regulate physiologic processes via their interaction with a variety of specific membrane-bound receptors (6,56), and the responses to these agonists are mediated via "second messengers," such as cAMP, cGMP, Ca^{2+}, inositol 1,4,5-trisphosphate (IP_3), and diacylglycerol (DG).

cAMP mediates the relaxing effects of β-adrenergic agonists in a variety of smooth muscles including the ureter (230,235,236). The β-adrenergic agonist, such as isoproterenol, combines with a receptor on the outer surface of the cell membrane (Fig. 24.15). The β-adrenergic agonist itself does not enter the cell. The agonist–receptor complex in turn activates the enzyme adenylyl cyclase on the inner surface of the cell membrane with the conversion of ATP to cAMP. A stimulatory guanine nucleotide-regulatory protein (G protein), G_s, acts as a functional communication between the hormone-occupied receptor and the catalytic or active unit of the adenylyl cyclase. Age-dependent changes in the ability of isoproterenol to activate adenylyl cyclase play a role in the effect of age on isoproterenol-induced ureteral relaxation (236). cAMP acts as a second or "internal" messenger for the response elicited by the β-adrenergic agonist. cAMP, through activation of a protein kinase and subsequent phosphorylation of proteins, has been suggested to lead to the uptake of Ca^{2+} into intracellular storage sites, such as the endoplasmic reticulum, with a resultant decrease in free sarcoplasmic Ca^{2+} and the development of relaxation (7).

cAMP levels may be increased by increasing its synthesis or by decreasing its degradation. Synthesis of cAMP involves activation of the enzyme adenylyl cyclase, and degradation of cAMP involves activation of the enzyme phosphodiesterase. Two agents that relax ureteral smooth muscle increase cAMP levels: isoproterenol, by increasing synthesis, and theophylline, by decreasing degradation (28,196,229, 230). Further support for a role of cAMP in relaxation of smooth muscles can be derived from the finding that

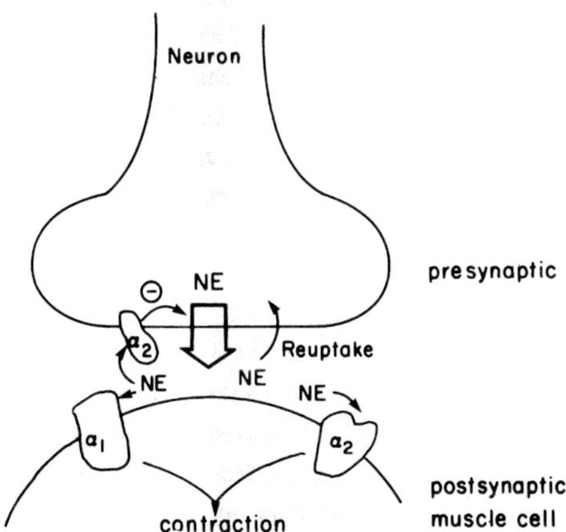

FIGURE 24.14. Diagrammatic representation of the role of presynaptic and postsynaptic α-adrenergic receptors. Norepinephrine *(NE)* released from nerve terminals may combine with postsynaptic α_1- and α_2-adrenergic receptors on smooth muscle to cause contraction. Norepinephrine combining with presynaptic α_2-adrenergic receptors on the nerve terminal prevents further release of NE from the neuron.

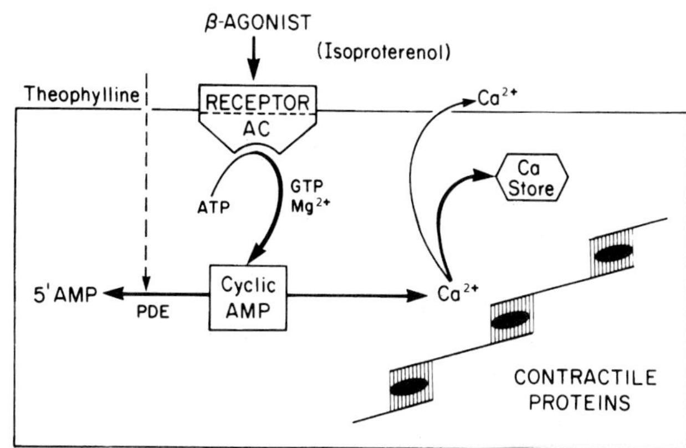

FIGURE 24.15. Diagrammatic representation of the role of cyclic adenosine monophosphate (cAMP) in β-adrenergic agonist–induced relaxation of smooth muscle. Agonist combines with receptor on the outer surface of the cell membrane. The receptor–agonist complex, in turn, activates the enzyme adenylyl cyclase on the inner surface of the cell membrane, which in the presence of Mg^{2+} and guanosine triphosphate (GTP) results in the conversion of adenosine triphosphate (ATP) to cAMP. cAMP is postulated to cause an increased uptake of Ca^{2+} into intracellular storage sites with a resultant decrease in Ca^{2+} in the region of the contractile proteins, resulting in relaxation. cAMP also may act directly on the contractile proteins to inhibit the contractile process. The enzyme phosphodiesterase *(PDE)* degrades cAMP to 5'AMP. Theophylline is a PDE inhibitor and thus also can increase cAMP with resultant smooth muscle relaxation.

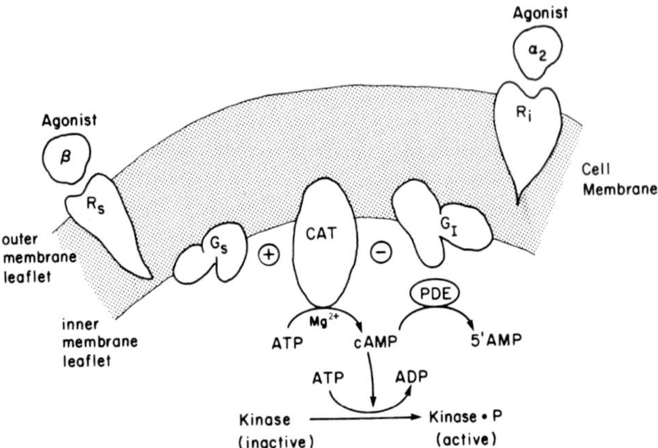

FIGURE 24.16. Diagrammatic representation of the relationship between the functional response to β- and α_2-adrenergic agonists and the cyclic nucleotide system. β-Adrenergic agonists activate the enzyme adenylyl cyclase and increase cyclic adenosine monophosphate *(cAMP)* production by working through a stimulatory receptor, R_S, and a stimulatory G protein, G_S. α_2-Adrenergic agonists inhibit adenylyl cyclase activity by working through an inhibitory receptor, R_i, and an inhibitory G-protein, G_I. The enzyme phosphodiesterase *(PDE)* degrades cAMP to 5′AMP. CAT, catalytic subunit of adenylyl cyclase.

dibutyryl cAMP, which more readily diffuses into the intact cell and is more resistant to breakdown by phosphodiesterase than cAMP, can relax smooth muscle (235).

Some of the actions of the α_2-adrenergic and muscarinic cholinergic agonists appear to involve the inhibition of adenylyl cyclase via stimulation of an inhibitory G protein, G_i (Fig. 24.16) (114). Other actions of muscarinic cholinergic agonists and some actions of α_1-adrenergic agonists and a number of hormones or neurotransmitters, whose actions are associated with an increase in intracellular Ca^{2+}, are related to changes in inositol lipid metabolism. Interaction of these agents with a receptor leads to the hydrolysis of polyphosphatidylinositol 4,5-biphosphate (PIP_2) by a phosphodiesterase (phospholipase C) with the formation of IP_3 and DG (10) (Fig. 24.17). IP_3 is involved in Ca^{2+} mobilization from intracellular stores, such as the endoplasmic reticulum (198). IP_3 initiates the flow of information in the calmodulin branch of the calcium messenger system and is thought to be responsible either for brief contractile responses or for the initial phase of sustained responses (157). DG binds to protein kinase C (PKC), causes its translocation to the cell membrane, and, by reducing the Ca^{2+} requirements for PKC activation, allows the enzyme to become more active. The physiologic response to DG depends on protein phosphorylation (151). The PKC branch of the calcium messenger system is thought to be responsible for the sustained phase of the contractile response (157) and is responsive to hormonally induced changes in intracellular calcium. DG, by activating phospholipase A, serves as a source of arachidonic acid (AA), the substrate for prostaglandin synthesis (133). Arachidonic acid may be involved in the stimulation of guanylyl cyclase with the formation of cGMP (10). This would explain the calcium-dependent increase in cGMP associated with the smooth muscle contractions induced by the cholinergic agonist, carbachol, and the α_1-adrenergic agonist, norepinephrine. These increases in cGMP follow the onset of the contractile event. cGMP itself appears to be inhibitory to smooth muscle function. 8-Bromo cGMP relaxes the ureter and other smooth muscles, and sodium nitroprusside–induced smooth muscle relaxation is associated with an increase in cGMP (27,184).

Studies indicate that NO is a mediator of smooth muscle relaxation (23). NOS converts L-arginine to NO and citrulline (Fig. 24.18). The NO, in turn, activates an enzyme, guanylyl cyclase, that converts guanosine triphosphate (GTP) to cGMP, which results in smooth muscle relaxation. Nitric oxide also may cause smooth muscle relaxation by opening potassium channels (16,78).

There are multiple isoforms of NOS. Neuronal NOS (nNOS) is Ca^{2+} and NADPH dependent (22). Neuronal excitation activates this enzyme, and the NO produced may result in smooth muscle relaxation. Endothelial NOS (eNOS) is also Ca^{2+} and NADPH dependent (186). Inducible NOS (iNOS) is NADPH dependent but Ca^{2+} independent and has been identified in ureteral (194) and other

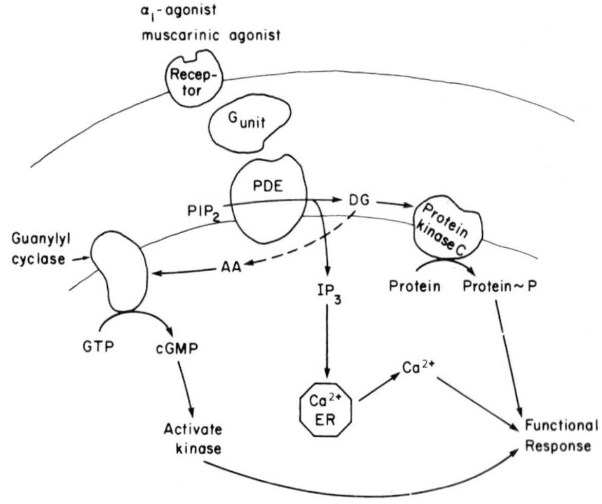

FIGURE 24.17. Diagrammatic representation of the role of inositol lipid metabolism in smooth muscle function. Agonists, such as α_1-adrenergic agonists and some muscarinic agonists, interact with a receptor, with the resultant hydrolysis of polyphosphatidylinositol 4,5 biphosphate (PIP_2), by a phosphodiesterase (phospholipase C) with the formation of 1,4,5-trisphosphate (IP_3), and diacylglycerol (DG). The functional response resulting from IP_3 is related to Ca^{2+} mobilization. DG activates protein kinase C, with the resultant functional response being dependent on protein phosphorylation. There is some evidence that DG may cause an increase in cyclic guanosine monophosphate (cGMP), which may explain the increase in cGMP observed in association with the contractile response to some autonomic agonists. AA, arachidonic acid; ER, endoplasmic reticulum; GTP, guanosine triphosphate.

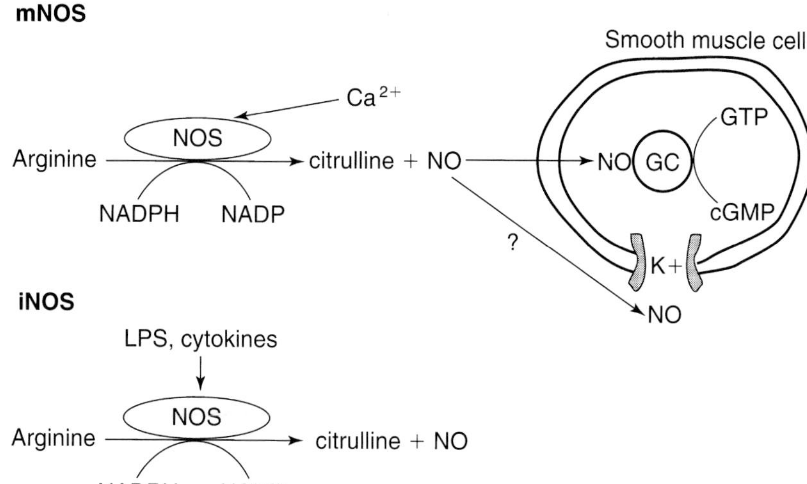

FIGURE 24.18. Schematic representation of nitric oxide synthase (mNOS, iNOS). GC, guanylyl cyclase; K^+, calcium-dependent potassium channel; LPS, lipopolysaccharide.

smooth muscles, and NOS-immunoreactive nerve fibers have been demonstrated in human ureter (195,197). NOS has been reported to colocalize with VIP, NPY, and tyrosine hydroxylase in nerves supplying the human ureter, including the intravesical segment (48,91,193).

Studies of isolated human ureteral segments suggest that the NO pathway may be involved in human ureteral relaxation (197). The NO donor 3-morpholinosyndonimine (SIN-1) can relax human ureteral segments, an action inhibited by the guanylyl cyclase inhibitor, methylene blue. The L-arginine–NO–cGMP pathway also may play a role in the function of the ureterovesical junction (91). NO donors inhibited agonist-induced contractions of isolated pig and human intravesical ureteral segments, and this inhibition was associated with an increase in cGMP levels.

Other Pharmacologic Agents

There are numerous reports of the excitatory effects of morphine and meperidine (Demerol) on the ureter, although these findings have not been universal (94,172). Both morphine and meperidine may have ureteral spasmogenic effects that theoretically would detract from their value in the management of ureteral colic. The efficacy of these agents in treating ureteral colic depends on their central nervous system actions, which decrease the perception of pain.

The primary prostaglandins (PGs), PGE_1, PGE_2, and $PGF_{2\alpha}$, are synthesized from the fatty acid, arachidonic acid. Two cyclooxygenase (COX) isoforms, COX-1 and COX-2, are the key regulatory enzymes in the biosynthesis of PGs from arachidonic acid (217). Indomethacin and aspirin can inhibit PG synthesis, and relatively specific COX-1 and COX-2 inhibitors have been developed. The functional response to PGs varies with the specific smooth muscle. In the ureter, PGE_1 activates adenylyl cyclase activity (236), increases cAMP levels (221), and inhibits activity. In contrast, $PGF_{2\alpha}$ is excitatory (19,30). Prostacyclin (PGI_2), a prostanoid, is synthesized in the urothelium of the ureter (2).

Indomethacin has been employed in the management of ureteral colic (83). COX inhibitors such as indomethacin inhibit pyeloureteral motility (30,177,208,242). The pain relief resulting from indomethacin, however, probably is due to inhibition of the prostaglandin-mediated vasodilation that occurs subsequent to obstruction (4,191). This prostaglandin-mediated vasodilation aids in preserving renal function, and thus, although indomethacin may provide pain relief, it is potentially deleterious to renal function (160). Endothelins (ETs) are potent vasoconstrictor peptides that exist in three isoforms (i.e., ET-1, ET-2, and ET-3). Endothelins have been shown to initiate contractions in isolated guinea pig and porcine ureters (50,129). There are two major endothelin receptor subtypes, ET_A and ET_B, with the ET_A receptor subtype being the predominant subtype in the ureter (112).

Histamine and the H_1-receptor agonist 2-(2-pyridyl) ethylamine cause contraction of the ureter, an effect that is antagonized by the H_1-receptor antagonist dimethindene. The H_2-receptor antagonist cimetidine does not affect the contractile response to histamine. These data show that the excitatory effects of histamine are mediated by the H_1-receptor subtype (44). Histamine and the H_2-receptor agonist impromidine relax precontracted ureteral segments, actions that are antagonized by cimetidine. These data are consistent with H_2-receptors mediating ureteral relaxant effects (44). 5-Hydroxytryptamine induces concentration-dependent contractions of isolated human ureteral segments (59).

Because Ca^{2+} is necessary for the development of the action potential and contraction of the ureter, agents that block the movement of Ca^{2+} into the cell would be expected to depress ureteral function. Calcium channel blockers, such as verapamil, diltiazem, and nifedipine, have been shown to inhibit ureteral activity (62,80,84,125,174,175,218), and calcium antagonist receptors are present in the ureter (241). L-type voltage-dependent calcium channels mediate K^+-induced contractions in the guinea pig ureter (127). This is supported by the finding that the L-type calcium agonist Bay K 8644 potentiates K^+-induced contractions.

Potassium channel openers, such as pinacidil, cromakalim, and BRL 38227, hyperpolarize smooth muscle membranes and decrease spontaneous activity of the smooth muscle (55). BRL 38227 and cromakalim have been shown to inhibit ureteral activity (101,126). The effects of cromakalim are inhibited by glibenclamide (126).

In the clinical situation, the ureter's relatively sparse blood supply limits the distribution of drug to the ureter. In addition, many drugs that have theoretic potential use in the management of ureteral pathology have untoward side effects when used in the necessary concentrations. Although many drugs can affect ureteral function, their current clinical usefulness is limited.

URETERAL REPLACEMENT

Many clinical conditions have provided an impetus for the use of ureteral substitutes. Indications for ureteral replacement include recurrent calculi, ureteral trauma, hydronephrosis, ureterovaginal fistulae, ureteral obstruction, inflammatory disease, ureteral tumors, retroperitoneal fibrosis, and a variety of undiversions. Methods for ureteral replacement can be classified as synthetic prostheses, free grafts, and pedicle grafts. The use of free grafts and prosthetics has primarily been experimental, with most of the success being found with pedicle grafts.

A variety of synthetic materials have been used as ureteral substitutes, including Vitallium (117), tantalum (118), polyvinylchloride (215), silicone (183), Teflon (214), Dacron (13), polyethylene tubing (75), and silicone rubber (15). These materials have not gained general acceptance because of the occurrence of salt deposits and the lack of peristalsis, resulting in a functional obstruction. Studies continue toward finding a suitable biocompatible synthetic material. A tube of collagen sponge has been tried in an effort to capitalize on the regenerative growth potential of the ureter (200). The collagen sponge acts as a biodegradable scaffold for the regenerative activity of the ureter.

Free grafts have included bladder mucosa (86), peritoneum (51), vessels (187), stomach (145), and fetal umbilical vessels (97). Disruption and the lack of peristalsis have interfered with the clinical use of these materials.

In clinical practice, ureteral replacement has in general involved the use of pedicle grafts. Bladder flaps (Boari flaps), with or without hitching the bladder to the psoas muscle, have been a highly effective means of replacing the lower ureter (154). Flaps of the renal capsule have been used to enlarge the UPJ (207). Although pedicle flaps of the fallopian tube and appendix have been tried, they have not provided the required peristaltic function, and hydronephrosis has resulted (143,180).

Ileum has been the most widely used pedicle graft and the most successful (18,63,192). Proponents of the use of the ileum for replacement of the entire ureter have cautioned against its use in individuals with a serum creatinine level of 2 mg/dL or greater because of the ensuant electrolyte abnormalities (17). Middleton (144) suggested that the absorptive surface of the ileal ureter could be minimized by tapering the segment. This procedure also could aid in the construction of an antirefluxing ileovesical anastomosis. When using the ileum to replace the ureter, the ileum should be used in an isoperistaltic manner, and there should be no evidence of distal obstruction. Immediately following the procedure, there may be considerable mucus in the urine, but this tends to clear with time. Normal saline or acetylcysteine (Mucomyst) may aid in preventing mucous clogging of the urinary tract. Colon also has been used as a ureteral substitute, but less widely (199).

Lytton and Schiff (120) used a short, isolated segment of ileum to replace a segment of ureter, with the distal anastomosis of the ileum being to the ureter. This interposition, rather than replacement, gives one the opportunity to take advantage of a normal, nonrefluxing UVJ and diminishes the risk of electrolyte disturbances, especially in the patient with mild renal insufficiency. The ileal segment is tapered on its distal antimesenteric surface and, if possible, placed retroperitoneally by passing it through a window in the mesentery. The long-term results with this procedure have been excellent.

REFERENCES

1. Akimoto M, Biancani P, Weiss RM. Comparative pressure-length diameter relationship of neonatal and adult rabbit ureters. *Invest Urol* 1977;14:297.
2. Ali M, Angelo-Khattar M, Thulesius L, et al. Urothelial synthesis of prostanoids in the ovine ureter. *Urol Res* 1998; 26:171.
3. Allen JM, Rodrigo J, Kerle DJ, et al. Neuropeptide Y (NPY)–containing nerves in mammalian ureter. *Urology* 1990;35:81.
4. Allen JT, Vaughan ED Jr, Gillenwater JY. The effect of indomethacin on renal blood flow and ureteral pressure in unilateral obstruction in awake dogs. *Invest Urol* 1978;15:324.
5. Alm P, Alumets R, Håkanson R, et al. Origin and distribution of VIP (vasoactive intestinal polypeptide) nerves in the genitourinary tract. *Cell Tissue Res* 1980;205:337.
6. Alquist RP. Study of adrenotropic receptors. *Am J Physiol* 1948;153:586.
7. Andersson R, Nilsson K. Cyclic AMP and calcium in relaxation in intestinal smooth muscle. *Nature* 1972;238:119.
8. Barr L, Berger W, Dewey MM. Electrical transmission at the nexus between smooth muscle cells. *J Gen Physiol* 1968; 51:347.
9. Beckmann CF, Roth RA. Use of retrograde occlusion balloon catheters in percutaneous removal of renal calculi. *Urology* 1985;25:277.

10. Berridge MJ. Inositol trisphosphate and diacylglycerol as second messengers. *Biochem J* 1984;220:345.
11. Biancani P, Hausman M, Weiss RM. Effect of obstruction on ureteral circumferential force-length relations. *Am J Physiol* 1982;243:F204.
12. Biancani P, Onyski JH, Zabinski MP, et al. Force velocity relationships of the guinea pig ureter. *J Urol* 1984;131:988.
13. Block NL, Stover E, Politano VA. A prosthetic ureter in the dog. *Trans Am Soc Artif Intern Organs* 1977;23:367.
14. Blok C, van Venrooij GEPM, Coolsaet BLRA. Dynamics of the ureterovesical junction: a qualitative analysis of the ureterovesical pressure profile in the pig. *J Urol* 1985;134:818.
15. Blum J, Skemp C, Reisner M. Silicone rubber ureteral prosthesis. *J Urol* 1963;90:276.
16. Bolotina VM, Najibi S, Palacino J, et al. Nitric oxide directly activates calcium-dependent potassium channels in vascular smooth muscle. *Nature* 1994;368:850.
17. Boxer RJ, Fritzsche P, Skinner DG, et al. Replacement of the ureter by small intestine: clinical application and results of the ileal ureter in 89 patients. *J Urol* 1979;121:728.
18. Boxer RJ, Johnson SF, Ehrlich RM. Ureteral substitution. *Urology* 1978;12:269.
19. Boyarsky S, Labay P. Ureteral motility. *Annu Rev Med* 1969; 20:383.
20. Bozler E. The activity of the pacemaker previous to the discharge of a muscular impulse. *Am J Physiol* 1942;136:543.
21. Brading AF, Burdyga THV, Scripnyuk ZD. The effects of papaverine on the electrical and mechanical activity of the guinea-pig ureter. *J Physiol (Lond)* 1983;334:79.
22. Bredt DS, Snyder SH. Isolation of nitric oxide synthase, a calmodulin requiring enzyme. *Proc Natl Acad Sci USA* 1990; 87:682.
23. Bult H, Boeckxstaens GE, Pelckmans PA, et al. Nitric oxide as an inhibitory NANC neurotransmitter. *Nature* 1990;345:346.
24. Burdyga THV, Magura IS. Effects of temperature and Na^+ on the relaxation of phasic and tonic tension of guinea-pig ureter muscle. *Gen Physiol Biophys* 1988;7:3.
25. Burnstock G. Structure of smooth muscle and its innervation. In: Bulbring E, Brading AF, Jones AW, et al, eds. *Smooth muscle.* Baltimore: Williams & Wilkins, 1970.
26. Butcher HR Jr, Sleator W Jr. A study of the electrical activity of intact and partially mobilized human ureters. *J Urol* 1955; 73:970.
27. Cho YH, Biancani P, Weiss RM. Adenyl and guanyl nucleotide induced relaxation of ureteral smooth muscle. *Fed Proc* 1984; 43:353.
28. Cho YH, Wheeler MA, Weiss RM. Ontogeny of phosphodiesterase and of calmodulin levels in guinea pig ureter. *J Urol* 1988;139:1095.
29. Clayton JD, Roberts JA. Radionuclide postpartum evaluation of the urinary tract during anovular therapy. *Surg Gynecol Obstet* 1973;137:215.
30. Cole RS, Fry CH, Shuttleworth KED. The action of the prostaglandins on isolated human ureteric smooth muscle. *Br J Urol* 1988;61:19.
31. Constantinou CE, Djurhuus JC. Pyeloureteral dynamics in the intact and chronically-obstructed multicalyceal kidney. *Am J Physiol* 1981;241:R389.
32. Constantinou CE, Grenato JJ Jr, Govan DE. Dynamics of the upper urinary tract: accommodation in the rate and stroke volume of ureteral peristalsis as a response to transient alteration in urine flow rate. *Urol Int* 1974;29:249.
33. Constantinou CE, Yamaguchi O. Multiple-coupled pacemaker system in renal pelvis of the unicalyceal kidney. *Am J Physiol* 1981;241:R412.
34. Constantinou CE. Renal pelvic pacemaker control of ureteral peristaltic rate. *Am J Physiol* 1974;226:1413.
35. Cook WA, King LR. Vesicoureteral reflux. In: Harrison JH, Gittes RF, Perlmutter AD, et al, eds. *Campbell's urology.* Philadelphia: Saunders, 1979.
36. Coolsaet BLRA, van Venrooij GEPM, et al. Detrusor pressure versus wall stress in relation to ureterovesical resistance. *Neurourol Urodynam* 1982;1:105.
37. Copenhaver WM, Johnson DD, eds. *Bailey's textbook of histology,* ed 14. Baltimore: Williams & Wilkins, 1958.
38. Cussen LJ. The structure of the normal human ureter in infancy and childhood: a quantitative study of the muscular and elastic tissue. *Invest Urol* 1967;5:179.
39. Daniel O, Shackman R. The blood supply of the human ureter in relation to ureterocolic anastomoses. *Br J Urol* 1952; 24:334.
40. Debruyne FMJ, Wijdeveld PGAB, Koene RAP, et al. Ureteroneo-cystomy in renal transplantation: is an antireflux mechanism mandatory? *Br J Urol* 1978;50:378.
41. DelTacca M. Acetylcholine content of and release from isolated pelviureteral tract. *Naunyn Schmiedebergs Arch Pharmacol* 1978; 302:293.
42. Dixon JS, Gosling JA. The fine structure of pacemaker cells in the pig renal calices. *Anat Rec* 1973;175:139.
43. Dixon JS, Gosling JA. The musculature of the human renal calices, pelvis and upper ureter. *J Anat* 1982;135:129.
44. Dodel RC, Hafner D, Borchard U. Characterization of histamine receptors in the ureter of the dog. *Eur J Pharmacol* 1996;318:395.
45. Dray A, Hankins MW, Yeats JC. Desensitization and capsaicin-induced release of substance P–like immunoreactivity from guinea-pig ureter *in vitro. Neuroscience* 1989;31:479.
46. Durbin G, Gerlach R, Eichhorn G, et al. The time distance diagram: a new method to analyze ureteral peristalsis by cineradiography. *J Urol* 1980;18:207.
47. Edmond P, Ross JA, Kirkland IS. Human ureteral peristalsis. *J Urol* 1970;104:670.
48. Edyvane KA, Smet PJ, Trussell DC, et al. Patterns of neuronal colocalization of tyrosine hydroxylase, neuropeptide Y, vasoactive intestinal polypeptide, calcitonin gene–related peptide and substance P in human ureter. *J Auton Nerv Sys* 1994;48:241.
49. Edyvane KA, Trussell DC, Jonavicius J, et al. Presence and regional variation in peptide-containing nerves in the human ureter. *J Auton Nerv Sys* 1992;39:127.
50. Eguchi S, Kozuka M, Hirose S, et al. Unique contractile action of endothelins on porcine isolated ureter and characterization of the endothelin-binding sites. *Biomed Res* 1991;12:35.
51. Eposti PL. Regeneration of smooth muscle fibers of the ureter following plastic surgery with free flaps of the parietal peritoneum. *Minerva Chir* 1956;11:1208.
52. Fainstat T. Ureteral dilatation in pregnancy: a review. *Obstet Gynecol Surv* 1963;18:845.
53. Finberg JPM, Peart WS. Function of smooth muscle of the rat renal pelvis—response of the isolated pelvis muscle to the angiotensin and some other substances. *Br J Pharmacol* 1970; 39:373.
54. Foote JW, Blennerhassett JB, Wiglesworth FW, et al. Observations on the ureteropelvic junction. *J Urol* 1970;104:252.
55. Foster CD, Fujii K, Kingdon J, et al. The effect of cromakalim on the smooth muscle of the guinea-pig urinary bladder. *Br J Pharmacol* 1989;97:281.
56. Furchgott RF. Receptor mechanisms. *Annu Rev Pharmacol Toxicol* 1964;4:21.
57. Garcia-Pascual A, Costa G, Labadia A, et al. Characterization of nitric oxide synthase activity in sheep urinary tract: functional implications. *Br J Pharmacol* 1996;118:905.
58. George NJR, O'Reilly PH Jr, Barnard RJ, et al. Practical management of patients with dilated upper tracts and chronic retention of urine. *Br J Urol* 1984;56:9.

59. Gidener S, Gumustekin M, Kirkali Z. Pharmacological analysis of 5-hydroxytryptamine effects on human isolated ureter. *Pharmacol Res* 1999;39:487.
60. Goessl C, Grozdanovic Z, Knispel HH, et al. Nitroxergic innervation of the human ureterovesical junction. *Urol Res* 1995;23:189.
61. Golenhofen K, Hannapel J. Normal spontaneous activity of the pyeloureteral system in the guinea pig. *Pflügers Arch* 1973; 341:257.
62. Golenhofen K, Lammel E. Selective suppression of some components of spontaneous activity in various types of smooth muscle by iproveratril (verapamil). *Pflügers Arch* 1973;331:233.
63. Goodwin WE, Winter CC, Turner RD. Replacement of the ureter by small intestine: clinical application and results of the ileal ureter. *J Urol* 1959;81:406.
64. Gosling JA, Dixon JS. Functional obstruction of the ureter and renal pelvis: a histological and electron microscopic study. *Br J Urol* 1978;50:145.
65. Gosling JA, Dixon JS. Morphologic evidence that the renal calyx and pelvis control ureteric activity in the rabbit. *Am J Anat* 1971;130:393.
66. Gosling JA, Dixon JS. Species variation in the location of upper urinary tract pacemaker cells. *Invest Urol* 1974;11:418.
67. Gosling JA, Dixon JS. Upper urinary tract: structure. In: Whitfield HN, Hendry WF, eds. *Textbook of genito-urinary surgery.* Edinburgh: Churchill Livingstone, 1985.
68. Gosling JA. Atypical muscle cells in the wall of the renal calix and pelvis with a note on their possible significance. *Experientia* 1970;26:769.
69. Green DF, Glickman MG, Weiss RM. Preliminary results with aminophylline as smooth muscle relaxant in percutaneous renal surgery. *J Endourol* 1987;1:243.
70. Griffiths DJ, Notschaele C. The mechanics of urine transport in the upper urinary tract. I. The dynamics of the isolated bolus. *Neurourol Urodynam* 1983;2:155.
71. Griffiths DJ. The mechanics of urine transport in the upper urinary tract. II. The discharge of the bolus into the bladder and dynamics at high rates of flow. *Neurourol Urodynam* 1983; 2:167.
72. Guyer PB, Delaney D. Urinary tract dilatation and oral contraceptives. *BMJ* 1970;4:588.
73. Hanna MK. Some observations on congenital ureteropelvic junction obstruction. *Urology* 1978;12:151.
74. Hannappel J, Golenhofen K. The effect of catecholamines on ureteral peristalsis in different species (dog, guinea pig and rat). *Pflügers Arch* 1974;55:350.
75. Hardin CA. Experimental repair of ureters by polyethylene tubing and ureteral and vessel grafts. *Arch Surg* 1957;68:57.
76. Hendrickx H, Vereecken RL, Casteels R. The influence of potassium on the electrical and mechanical activity of the guinea pig ureter. *Urol Res* 1975;3:155.
77. Hernandez M, Prieto D, Orensanz LM, et al. Nitric oxide is involved in the NANC inhibitory neurotransmission of the pig intravesical ureter. *Neurosci Lett* 1995;186:33.
78. Hernandez M, Prieto D, Orensanz LM, et al. Involvement of a glibenclamide sensitive mechanism in the nitrergic neurotransmission of the guinea pig intravesical ureter. *Br J Pharmacol* 1997;120:609.
79. Hertle L, Nawrath H. Stimulation of voltage-dependent contractions by calcium channel activator Bay K 8644 in the human upper urinary tract *in vitro. J Urol* 1989;141:1014.
80. Hertle L, Nawrath H. Calcium channel blockade in smooth muscle of the upper urinary tract. *J Urol* 1984;132:1265.
81. Hodgkin AL. Ionic movements and electrical activity in giant nerve fibers. *Proc R Soc Lond (Biol)* 1958;148:1.
82. Holmlund D, Hassler O. A method of studying the ureteral reaction to artificial concrements. *Acta Chir Scand* 1965; 130:335.
83. Holmlund D, Sjoden JG. Treatment of ureteral colic with intravenous indomethacin. *J Urol* 1978;120:676.
84. Hong KW, Biancani P, Weiss RM. "On" and "off" responses of guinea pig ureter. *Am J Physiol* 1985;248:C165.
85. Hong KW, Biancani P, Weiss RM. Effect of age on contractility of guinea pig ureter. *Invest Urol* 1980;17:459.
86. Hovanian AP, Kingsley IA. Reconstruction of the ureter by free autologous bladder mucosa graft. *J Urol* 1966;96:167.
87. Hua XY, Lundberg JM. Dual capsaicin effects on ureteric motility: low dose inhibition mediated by calcitonin gene–related peptide and high dose stimulation by tachykinins? *Acta Physiol Scand* 1986;128:453.
88. Hua XY, Theodorsson-Norheim E, Lundberg JM, et al. Co-localization of tachykinins and calcitonin gene–related peptide in capsaicin-sensitive afferents in relation to motility effects on the human ureter *in vitro. Neuroscience* 1987;23:693.
89. Hundley JM Jr, Diehl WK, Diggs ES. Hormonal influences upon the ureter. *Am J Obstet Gynecol* 1942;44:858.
90. Imaizumi Y, Muraki K, Takeda M. Ionic currents in single smooth muscle cells from the ureter of the guinea pig. *J Physiol (Lond)* 1989;411:131.
91. Iselin CE, Alm P, Schaad NC, et al. Localization of nitric oxide synthase and hemoxygenase, and functional effects of nitric oxide and carbon monoxide in the pig and human intravesical ureter. *Neurourol Urodyn* 1997;16:209.
92. Iselin CE, Alm P, Schaad NC, et al. Nitric oxide inhibits contraction of isolated pig ureteral smooth muscle. *J Urol* 1996;155:763.
93. Karahan ST, Krammer HJ, Kühnel W. Immunohistochemical demonstration of nerves and nerve cells in human and porcine ureters. *Ann Anat* 1993;175:259.
94. Kiil F. *The function of the ureter and renal pelvis.* Philadelphia: Saunders, 1957.
95. King WW, Cox CE. Bacterial inhibition of ureteral smooth muscle contractility. I. The effect of common urinary pathogens and endotoxin in an *in vitro* system. *J Urol* 1972;108:700.
96. Kirkland IS, Ross JA, Edmond P, et al. Urethral function in vesicoureteral reflux. *Br J Urol* 1971;43:289.
97. Klippel KF, Hohenfellner R. Umbilical vein as ureteral replacement. *Invest Urol* 1979;16:447.
98. Kobayashi M, Irisawa H. Effect of sodium deficiency on the action potential of the smooth muscle of ureter. *Am J Physiol* 1964;206:205.
99. Kobayashi M. Effect of calcium on electrical activity in smooth muscle cells of cat ureter. *Am J Physiol* 1969;216:1279.
100. Kobayashi M. Effects of Na and Ca on the generation and conduction of excitation in the ureter. *Am J Physiol* 1965; 208:715.
101. Kotani H, Ginkawa M, Sakai T. A simple method for measurement of ureteric peristaltic function *in vivo* and the effect of drugs acting on ion channels applied from the ureter lumen in anesthetized rats. *Jpn J Pharmacol* 1993;62:331.
102. Kumar D. *In vitro* inhibitory effect of progesterone on extrauterine smooth muscle. *Am J Obstet Gynecol* 1962;84:1300.
103. Kuriyama H, Osa T, Toida N. Membrane properties of the smooth muscle of guinea-pig ureter. *J Physiol (Lond)* 1967; 191:225.
104. Kuriyama H, Tomita T. The action potential in the smooth muscle of the guinea pig Taenia coli and ureter studied by the double sucrose-gap methods. *J Gen Physiol* 1970;55:147.
105. Kuriyama H. The influence of potassium, sodium and chloride on the membrane potential of the smooth muscle of Taenia coli. *J Physiol (Lond)* 1963;166:15.

106. Lammers WJEP, Ahmad HR, Arafat K. Spatial and temporal variations in pacemaking and conduction in the isolated renal pelvis. *Am J Physiol* 1996;270:F567.
107. Lang RJ, Exintaris B, Teele ME, et al. Electrical basis of peristalsis in the mammalian upper urinary tract. *Clin Exp Pharmacol Physiol* 1998;25:310.
108. Lang RJ, Zhang Y. The effect of K channel blockers on the spontaneous electrical and contractile activity in the proximal renal pelvis of the guinea pig. *J Urol* 1996;155:332.
109. Larsen JJ, Otteson B, Fahrenkrug J, et al. Vasoactive intestinal polypeptide (VIP) in the male genitourinary tract. *Invest Urol* 1981;19:211.
110. Latifpour J, Kondo S, O'Hollaren B, et al. Autonomic receptors in urinary tract: sex and age differences. *J Pharmacol Exp Ther* 1990;253:661.
111. Latifpour J, Morita T, O'Hollaren B, et al. Characterization of autonomic receptors in neonatal urinary tract smooth muscle. *Dev Pharmacol Ther* 1989;13:1.
112. Latifpour, J, Fukimoto Y, Weiss RM. Regional differences in the density and subtype specificity of endothelin receptors in rabbit urinary tract. *Naunyn Schmiedberg's Arch Pharmacol* 1995;352:459.
113. Libertino JA, Weiss RM. Ultrastructure of human ureter. *J Urol* 1972;108:71.
114. Londos C, Cooper DMF, Rodbell M. Receptor-mediated stimulation and inhibition of adenylate cyclases: the fat cell as a model system. *Adv Cyclic Nucleotide Res* 1981;14:163.
115. Longrigg N. Autonomic innervation of the renal calyx. *Br J Urol* 1974;46:357.
116. Longrigg N. Minor calices as primary pacemaker sites for ureteral activity in man. *Lancet* 1975;1:253.
117. Lord JW Jr, Eckel JH. The use of Vitallium tubes in the urinary tract of the dog. *J Urol* 1942;48:412.
118. Lubash S. Experience with tantalum tubes in the reimplantation of the ureters into the sigmoid in dogs and humans. *J Urol* 1947;57:1010.
119. Lubin S, Drexler LS, Bilotta WA. Post-partum pyeloureteral changes following hormone administration. *Surg Gynecol Obstet* 1941;73:391.
120. Lytton B, Schiff M. Interposition of an ileal segment for repair of ureteral injuries. *J Urol* 1981;125:739.
121. Macht DI. On the pharmacology of the ureter. II. Actions of drugs affecting the sacral autonomics. *J Pharmacol Exp Ther* 1916;8:261.
122. Maggi CA, Giuliani S, Santicioli P, et al. Role of intracellular calcium in the K channel opener action of CGRP in the guinea-pig ureter. *Br J Pharmacol* 1996;118:1493.
123. Maggi CA, Giuliani S, Santicioli P. CGRP inhibition of electromechanical coupling in the guinea pig isolated renal pelvis. *Naunyn Schmiedebergs Arch Pharmacol* 1995;352:529.
124. Maggi CA, Giuliani S, Santicioli P. Effect of the Ca^{2+}-ATPase inhibitor, cyclopiazonic acid, on electromechanical coupling in the guinea-pig ureter. *Br J Pharmacol* 1995;114:127.
125. Maggi CA, Giuliani S, Santicioli P. Effect of Bay K 8644 and ryanodine on the refractory period, action potential and mechanical response of the guinea pig ureter to electrical stimulation. *Naunyn Schmiedebergs Arch Pharmacol* 1994;349:510.
126. Maggi CA, Giuliani S, Santicioli P. Effect of cromakalim and glibenclamide on spontaneous and evoked motility of the guinea pig isolated renal pelvis and ureter. *Br J Pharmacol* 1994;111:687.
127. Maggi CA, Giuliani S. A pharmacological analysis of calcium channels involved in phasic and tonic responses of the guinea-pig ureter to high potassium. *J Auton Pharmacol* 1995;15:55.
128. Maggi CA, Giuliani S. Nonadrenergic noncholinergic excitatory innervation of the guinea-pig renal pelvis. Involvement of capsaicin-sensitive primary afferent neurons. *J Urol* 1992;141:1394.
129. Maggi CA, Santicioli P, del Bianco E, et al. Local motor responses to bradykinin and bacterial chemotactic peptide formyl-methionyl-leucyl-phenylalanine (FMLP) in the guinea-pig isolated renal pelvis and ureter. *J Urol* 1992;148:1944.
130. Maggi CA, Santicioli P, Giuliani S, et al. The motor effect of the capsaicin-sensitive inhibitory innervation of the rat ureter. *Eur J Pharmacol* 1986;126:333.
131. Maggi CA, Santicioli P, Giuliani S. Role of cyclic AMP and protein kinase A in K channel activation by CGRP in the guinea-pig ureter. *J Auton Pharmacol* 1995;15:403.
132. Maggi CA, Theodorsson E, Santicioli P, et al. Tachykinins and calcitonin gene–related peptides as co-transmitters in local motor responses produced by sensory nerve activation in the guinea pig isolated renal pelvis. *Neuroscience* 1992;46:549.
133. Mahadevappa VG, Holub BJ. Degradation of different molecular species of phosphatidylinositol in thrombin-stimulated human platelets. *J Biol Chem* 1983;258:5337.
134. Makker SP, Tucker AS, Izant RJ Jr, et al. Nonobstructive hydronephrosis and hydroureter associated with peritonitis. *N Engl J Med* 1972;287:535.
135. Marchant DJ. Effects of pregnancy and progestational agents on the urinary tract. *Am J Obstet Gynecol* 1972;112:487.
136. Marfurt CF, Echtenkamp SF. Sensory innervation of the rat kidney and ureter as revealed by the antegrade transport of wheat germ agglutinin–horseradish peroxidase (WGA-HRP) from dorsal root ganglia. *J Comp Neurol* 1991;311:389.
137. Marshall S, Lyon RP, Minker D. Ureteral dilatation following use of oral contraceptives. *JAMA* 1966;198:206.
138. McGuire EJ. Physiology of the lower urinary tract. *Am J Kidney Dis* 1983;2:402.
139. McLeod DG, Reynolds DG, Swan KG. Adrenergic mechanisms in the canine ureter. *Am J Physiol* 1973;224:1054.
140. Meini S, Santicioli P, Maggi CA. Propagation of impulses in the gunea-pig ureter and its blockade by calcitonin gene–related peptide (CGRP). *Naunyn Schmiedebergs Arch Pharmacol* 1995; 351:79.
141. Melick WF, Brodeur AE, Herbig F, et al. Use of a ureteral pacemaker in the treatment of ureteral reflux. *J Urol* 1966; 95:184.
142. Melick WF, Naryka JJ, Schmidt JH. Experimental studies of ureteral peristaltic patterns in the pig. II. Myogenic activity of the pig ureter. *J Urol* 1961;86:46.
143. Melnikoff AE. Sur le replacement de l'uretere par une anse isolee de l'intestin grele. *Rev Clin J Urol* 1912;1:601.
144. Middleton AW Jr. Tapered ileum as ureter substitute in severe renal damage. *Urology* 1977;9:509.
145. Morelle VR. Replacement of the ureter by a segment of the stomach in pigs and dogs. *Arch Chir Neerl* 1963;15:293.
146. Morita T, Ishizuka G, Tsuchida S. Initiation and propagation of stimulus from the renal pelvic pacemaker in pig kidney. *Invest Urol* 1981;19:157.
147. Morita T, Kondo S, Suzuki T, et al. Effect of calyceal resection on pelviureteral peristalsis in isolated pig kidney. *J Urol* 1986; 135:151.
148. Morita T, Wada I, Saekai H, et al. Ureteral urine transport: changes in bolus volume, peristaltic frequency, intraluminal pressure and volume of flow resulting from autonomic drugs. *J Urol* 1987;137:132.
149. Murnaghan GF. Mechanisms of congenital hydronephrosis with reference to factors influencing surgical treatment. *Ann R Coll Surg Engl* 1958;23:25.

150. Murnaghan GF. The dynamics of the renal pelvis and ureter with reference to congenital hydronephrosis. *Br J Urol* 1958; 30:321.
151. Nishizuka Y. The role of protein kinase C in cell surface signal transduction and tumor production. *Nature* 1984;308:693.
152. Notley RG. Electron microscopy of the lower ureter in man. *Br J Urol* 1970;42:439.
153. Notley RG. Electron microscopy of the upper ureter and pelviureteric junction. *Br J Urol* 1968;40:37.
154. Ockerblad NF. Reimplantation of the ureter into the bladder by a flap method. *J Urol* 1947;57:845.
155. O'Conor VJ Jr, Dawson-Edwards P. Role of the ureter in renal transplantation. I. Studies of denervated ureter with particular reference to ureteroureteral anastomoses. *J Urol* 1969;82:566.
156. Paquin AJ Jr. Ureterovesical anastomosis: the description and evaluation of a technique. *J Urol* 1959;82:573.
157. Park S, Rasmussen H. Activation of tracheal smooth muscle contraction: synergism between Ca^{++} and activators of protein kinase C. *Proc Natl Acad Sci USA* 1985;82:8835.
158. Patacchini R, Santicioli P, Zagorodnyuk V, et al. Excitatory motor and electrical effects produced by tachykinins in the human and guinea-pig isolated ureter and guinea-pig renal pelvis. *Br J Pharmacol* 1998;125:987.
159. Payne FL, Hodes PJ. The effect of the female hormones and of pregnancy upon the ureters of lower animals as demonstrated by intravenous uropathy. *Am J Obstet Gynecol* 1939;37:1024.
160. Perlmutter A, Miller L, Trimble LA, et al. Toradol and NSAID used for renal colic decreases renal perfusion and ureteral pressure in a canine model of unilateral ureteral obstruction. *J Urol* 1993;149:926.
161. Peters HJ, Eckstein W. Possible pharmacological means of treating renal colic. *Urol Res* 1975;3:55.
162. Prieto D, Hernandez M, Rivera L, et al. Distribution and functional effects of neuropeptide Y on equine ureteral smoth muscle and resistance arteries. *Regul Peptides* 1997;69:155.
163. Prieto D, Hernández M, Rivera L, et al. Catecholaminergic innervation of the equine ureter. *Res Vet Sci* 1992;54:312.
164. Prieto D, Simonsen U, Martin J, et al. Histochemical and functional evidence for a cholinergic innervation of the equine ureter. *J Auton Nerve Sys* 1994;47:159.
165. Primbs K. Untersuchungen über die Einwirkung von Bakterientoxinen auf der überlebenden Meerschweinchenureter. *Z Urol Chir* 1913;1:600.
166. Raz S, Ziegler M, Caine M. Hormonal influence on the adrenergic receptor of the ureter. *Br J Urol* 1972;44:405.
167. Reid RE, Herman R, Teng C. Attempts at altering ureteral activity in the unanesthetized, conditioned dog with commonly employed drugs. *Invest Urol* 1976;12:74.
168. Roberts JA. Experimental pyelonephritis in the monkey. III. Pathophysiology of ureteral malfunction induced by bacteria. *Invest Urol* 1975;13:117.
169. Roberts JA. Hydronephrosis of pregnancy. *Urology* 1976;8:1.
170. Rose JG, Gillenwater JY. Pathophysiology of ureteral obstruction. *Am J Physiol* 1973;225:830.
171. Rose JG, Gillenwater JY. The effect of adrenergic and cholinergic agents and their blockers upon ureteral activity. *Invest Urol* 1974;11:439.
172. Ross JA, Edmond P, Griffiths JM. The action of drugs on the intact human ureter. *Br J Urol* 1967;39:26.
173. Ross JA, Edmond P, Kirkland IS. *Behaviour of the human ureter in health and disease.* Edinburgh: Churchill Livingstone, 1972.
174. Sakanashi M, Kato T, Miyamoto Y, et al. Comparative effects of diltiazem and glycerol trinitrate on isolated ureter and coronary artery of the dog. *Pharmacology* 1986;32:11.
175. Sakanashi N, Kato T, Miyamoto Y, et al. Comparison of the effects of nifedipine in ureter and coronary artery isolated from the dog. *Drug Res* 1985;35:584.
176. Sala NL, Rubi RA. Ureteral function in pregnant women. II. Ureteral contractility during normal pregnancy. *Am J Obstet Gynecol* 1967;99:228.
177. Santicioli P, Carganico G, Meini S, et al. Modulation by stereoselective inhibition of cyclooxygenase of electromechanical coupling in the guinea-pig isolated renal pelvis. *Br J Pharmacol* 1995;114:1149.
178. Santicioli P, Morbidelli L, Parenti A, et al. Calcitonin gene–related peptide selectively increases cAMP levels in the guinea-pig ureter. *Eur J Pharmacol* 1995;289:17.
179. Satani Y. Histological study of the ureter. *J Urol* 1919;3:247.
180. Schein CJ, Sanders AR, Hurwitt ES. Experimental reconstruction of the ureters. *Arch Surg* 1956;73:47.
181. Schick E, Tanagho E. The effect of gravity on ureteral peristalsis. *J Urol* 1973;109:187.
182. Schneider DH, Eichner E, Gordon MB. An attempt at production of hydronephrosis of pregnancy, artificially induced. *Am J Obstet Gynecol* 1953;65:660.
183. Schreiber B, Homann W, Mlynek M, et al. Ureteral replacement with a new prosthesis. *Trans Am Soc Artif Intern Organs* 1979;25:61.
184. Schultz K, Bohme E, Volker AWK, et al. Relaxation of hormonally-stimulated smooth muscular tissues by the 8-bromo derivative of cyclic GMP. *Naunyn Schmiedebergs Arch Pharmacol* 1979;306:1.
185. Seki N, Suzuki H. Electrical properties of smooth muscle cell membrane in renal pelvis of rabbits. *Am J Physiol* 1990;259: F888.
186. Sessa W. The nitric oxide synthase family of proteins. *J Vasc Res* 1994;31:131.
187. Sewell WH. Failure of freeze-dried homologous arteries used as arterial grafts. *J Urol* 1955;74:600.
188. Shuba MF. The effect of sodium-free and potassium-free solutions, ionic current inhibitors and ouabain on electrophysiological properties of smooth muscle of guinea-pig ureter. *J Physiol (Lond)* 1977;264:837.
189. Sikri KL, Hoyes AD, Barber P, et al. Substance P–like immunoreactivity in the intramural nerve plexus of the guinea pig ureter: a light and electron microscopical study. *J Anat* 1981; 133:425.
190. Sivula A, Lehtonen T. Spontaneous passage of artificial concretions applied in the rabbit ureter. *Scand J Urol Nephrol* 1967; 1:259.
191. Sjoden JG, Wahlberg J, Persson AEG. The effect of indomethacin on glomerular capillary pressure and pelvic pressure during ureteral obstruction. *J Urol* 1982;127:1017.
192. Skinner DG, Goodwin WE. Indications for the use of intestinal segments in management of nephrocalcinosis. *J Urol* 1975; 113:436.
193. Smet PJ, Edyvane KA, Jonavicius J, et al. Colocalization of nitric oxide synthase with vasoactive intestinal peptide, neuropeptide Y and tyrosine hydroxylase in nerves supplying human ureter. *J Urol* 1994;152:1292.
194. Smith SD, Wheeler MA, Nishimoto T, et al. The differential expression of nitric oxide synthase in guinea pig urinary tract. *J Urol* 1993;149:248A.
195. Stief CG, Taher A, Meyer M, et al. A possible role of nitric oxide (NO) in the relaxation of renal pelvis and ureter. *J Urol* 1993;149:492A.
196. Stief CG, Taher A, Truss M, et al. Phosphodiesterase isoenzymes in human ureteral smooth muscle: identification, characterization, and functional effects of various phosphodiesterase inhibitors *in vitro.* *Urol Int* 1995;55:183.

197. Stief CG, Uckert S, Truss MC, et al. A possible role for nitric oxide in the regulation of human ureteral smooth muscle tone *in vitro*. *Urol Res* 1996;24:333.
198. Streb H, Irvine RF, Berridge MJ, et al. Release of Ca^{++} from a non-mitochondrial store in pancreatic acinar cell by inositol, 1,4,5-triphosphate. *Nature* 1983;306:67.
199. Struthers NW, Scott R. Reconstruction of the upper ureter with colon. *J Urol* 1974;112:179.
200. Tachibana M, Nagamatsu GR, Addonizio JC. Ureteral replacement using collagen sponge tube grafts. *J Urol* 1985; 133:866.
201. Tachibana S, Takeuchi M, Uehara Y. The architecture of the musculature of the guinea-pig ureter as examined by scanning electron microscopy. *J Urol* 1985;134:582.
202. Tanagho EA, Hutch JA, Meyers FH, et al. Primary vesicoureteral reflux: experimental studies of its etiology. *J Urol* 1965;93:165.
203. Tanagho EA, Meyers FH, Smith DE. The trigone: anatomical and physiological considerations: 1. In relation to the ureterovesical junction. *J Urol* 1968;100:623.
204. Tanagho EA. Ureteral embryology, developmental anatomy, and myology. In: Boyarsky S, Gottschalk GW, Tanagho EA, et al, eds. *Urodynamics: hydrodynamics of the ureter and renal pelvis.* New York: Academic Press, 1971.
205. Teague N, Boyarsky S. The effect of coliform bacilli upon ureteral peristalsis. *Invest Urol* 1968;5:423.
206. Teele RL, Lebowitz RL, Colodny AH. Reflux into the unused ureter. *J Urol* 1976;115:310.
207. Thompson IM, Kovacsi L, Portersfield J. Reconstruction of the ureteropelvic junction with pedicle grafts and renal capsule. *J Urol* 1963;89:573.
208. Thulesius O, Angelo-Khattar M, Ali M. The effect of prostaglandin synthesis inhibition on motility of the sheep ureter. *Acta Physiol Scand* 1987;131:51.
209. Tomiyama Y, Hayakawa K, Shinagawa K, et al. Beta-adrenoceptor subtypes in the ureteral smooth muscle of rats, rabbits and dogs. *Eur J Pharmacol* 1998;352:269.
210. Traut HF, Kuder A. Inflammation of the upper urinary tract complicating the reproductive period of woman: collective review. *Int Abst Surg* 1938;67:568.
211. Tsuchida S, Yamaguchi O. A constant electrical activity of the renal pelvis correlated to ureteral peristalsis. *Tohoku J Exp Med* 1977;121:133.
212. Uehara Y, Burnstock G. Demonstration of "gap junctions" between smooth muscle cells. *J Cell Biol* 1970;44:215.
213. Ueno A, Kawamura T, Ogawa A, et al. Relation of spontaneous passage of ureteral calculi to size. *Urology* 1977;10:544.
214. Ulm AH, Krauss L. Total unilateral Teflon ureteral substitutes in the dog. *J Urol* 1960;83:575.
215. Ulm AH, Lo MC. Total bilateral polyvinyl ureteral substitutes in the dog. *Surgery* 1959;45:313.
216. van Wagenen G, Jenkins RH. An experimental examination of factors causing ureteral dilatation of pregnancy. *J Urol* 1939;42: 1010.
217. Vane JR. Cyclooxygenase 1 and 2. *Annu Rev Pharmacol Toxicol* 1998;38:97.
218. Vereecken RL, Hendrickx H, Casteels R. The influence of calcium on the electrical and mechanical activity of the guinea pig ureter. *Urol Res* 1975;3:149.
219. Vereecken RL, Hendrickx H, Casteels R. The influence of sodium on the electrical and mechanical activity of the guinea pig ureter. *Urol Res* 1975;3:159.
220. Vereecken RL. *Dynamical aspects of urine transport in the ureter.* Louvain, Belgium: Acco, 1973.
221. Vermue NA, Den Hertog A. The actions of prostaglandins on ureter smooth muscle of guinea pig. *Eur J Pharmacol* 1987; 142:163.
222. Washizu Y. Grouped discharge in ureter muscle. *Comp Biochem Physiol* 1966;19:713.
223. Watterson DM, Harrelson WG Jr, Keller PM, et al. Structural similarity between the Ca^{++}-dependent regulatory proteins of 3′:5′-cyclic nucleotide phosphodiesterase and actomyosin ATPase. *J Biol Chem* 1976;251:4501.
224. Weinberg SL. Ureteral functions. I. Simultaneous monitoring of ureteral peristalsis. *Invest Urol* 1974;12:103.
225. Weiss RM, Bassett AL, Hoffman BF. Adrenergic innervation of the ureter. *Invest Urol* 1978;16:123.
226. Weiss RM, Biancani P, Zabinski MP. Adrenergic control of the ureteral tonus. *Invest Urol* 1974;12:30.
227. Weiss RM, Biancani P. A rationale for ureteral tapering. *Urology* 1982;20:482.
228. Weiss RM, Biancani P. Characteristics of normal and refluxing ureterovesical junctions. *J Urol* 1983;129:858.
229. Weiss RM, Hardman JG, Wells JN. Resistance of a separated form of canine ureteral phosphodiesterase activity to inhibition by xanthines and papaverine. *Biochem Pharmacol* 1981;30: 2371.
230. Weiss RM, Vulliemoz Y, Verosky M, et al. Adenylate cyclase and phosphodiesterase in rabbit ureter. *Invest Urol* 1977;15:15.
231. Weiss RM, Wagner ML, Hoffman GF. Localization of pacemaker for peristalsis in the intact canine ureter. *J Urol* 1967; 5:42.
232. Weiss RM, Wheeler MA, Biancani P. Age related changes in the response of ureteral smooth muscle to autonomic agonists. *Fed Proc* 1985;44:506.
233. Weiss RM. Clinical implications of ureteral physiology. *J Urol* 1979;121:401.
234. Wharton LR. The innervation of the ureter, with respect to denervation. *J Urol* 1932;28:639.
235. Wheeler MA, Cho YH, Hong KW, et al. Age dependent alterations in β-adrenergic receptor function in guinea pig ureter. In: Sperelakis N, Wood J, eds. *Frontiers in smooth muscle research,* vol 327. New York: Alan R. Liss, 1990.
236. Wheeler MA, Housman A, Cho YH, et al. Age dependence of adenylate cyclase activity in guinea pig ureter homogenate. *J Pharmacol Exp Ther* 1986;239:99.
237. Whitaker RH. Methods of assessing obstruction in dilated ureters. *Br J Urol* 1973;45:15.
238. Whitaker RH. The Whitaker test. *Urol Clin North Am* 1979; 6:529.
239. Williams PL, Warwick R, eds. *Gray's anatomy.* Philadelphia: Saunders, 1980.
240. Woodburne RT, Lapides J. The ureteral lumen during peristalsis. *Am J Anat* 1972;133:255.
241. Yoshida M, Latifpour J, Weiss RM. Age-related changes in calcium antagonist receptors in rabbit ureter. *Dev Pharm Ther* 1992;
18:100.
242. Zhang Y, Lang RJ. Effects of intrinsic prostaglandins on the spontaneous contractile and electrical activity of the proximal renal pelvis of the guinea pig. *Br J Pharmacol* 1994;113:431.

INDEX

C

D

E

F

G

H

I

J

K

L

M

O

P

Q

R

T

U

V